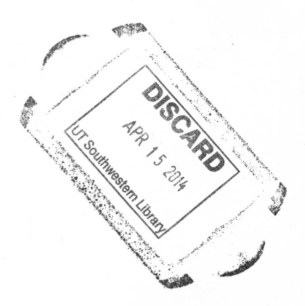

Scientific Foundations
of
Otolaryngology

Edited by

RONALD HINCHCLIFFE

B.Sc., M.D., Ph.D., M.R.C.P. (Edin.), D.L.O.

Reader in Neuro-otology, Institute of Laryngology and Otology,
University of London; Honorary Consultant in Neuro-otology, Royal National
Throat, Nose and Ear Hospital, London; Examiner
in Audiology to the Universities of Manchester
and Southampton

and

DONALD HARRISON

M.D., M.S., F.R.C.S., D.L.O.

Professor of Laryngology and Otology, Institute
of Laryngology and Otology, University of London;
Civilian Consultant to the Navy in Otolaryngology

A WILLIAM HEINEMANN MEDICAL BOOKS PUBLICATION

DISTRIBUTED BY

YEAR BOOK MEDICAL PUBLISHERS, INC.

35 EAST WACKER DRIVE

CHICAGO

1976

First published 1976

Distributed in Continental North, South and Central America,
Hawaii, Puerto Rico and The Philippines by
Year Book Medical Publishers Inc.

ISBN 0–8151–4425–3

by arrangement with William Heinemann Medical Books Ltd.

Library of Congress Catalog Card Number 76–17666

Printed in Great Britain

THIS BOOK
IS DEDICATED
BY THE
CONTRIBUTORS
AND THE EDITORS
TO
THEIR
MENTORS

IA—24 pp.

CONTENTS

CONTRIBUTORS   xiii

FOREWORD   xvii
    J. ANGELL-JAMES, CBE, MD, FRCP, FRCS

PREFACE   xix
    R. HINCHCLIFFE and D. F. N. HARRISON

ACKNOWLEDGEMENTS   xxi

SECTION I
QUANTITATIVE METHODS

1. MEASUREMENT   2
    R. HINCHCLIFFE

2. STATISTICS   9
    R. HINCHCLIFFE

3. COMPUTERS   31
    A. R. D. THORNTON

SECTION II
PHYSICS

4. BASIC ELECTRICITY   15
    R. I. DAMPER

5. ELECTRONICS   69
    R. I. DAMPER

6. ACOUSTICS   87
    F. J. FAHY

7. ELECTROACOUSTICS   101
    W. TEMPEST

8. PHYSICS OF HEAT   111
    D. D. LINDSAY

SECTION III
GENETICS

9. GENETICAL BASIS FOR OTOLARYNGOLOGICAL DISORDERS   121
    G. R. FRASER

SECTION IV
ENVIRONMENTAL SCIENCES

10. EPIDEMIOLOGY   133
    R. HINCHCLIFFE

11. HEARING CONSERVATION AND NOISE REDUCTION   151
    A. M. MARTIN

CONTENTS

SECTION V

EAR-STRUCTURE

12. ORGANOGENESIS OF EAR 173
    T. van de Water and R. Ruben

13. COMPARATIVE ANATOMY OF EAR 184
    Ade Pye and R. Hinchcliffe

14. ULTRASTRUCTURE OF EAR 202
    I. Friedmann

15. APPLIED MORPHOLOGY OF EAR 211
    D. Garfield Davies

SECTION VI

EAR-FUNCTION

16. MECHANICS OF THE AUDITORY APPARATUS 237
    J. Tonndorf and S. M. Khanna

17. AUDITORY TUBAL FUNCTION 252
    H. J. Holmquist

18. INTRATYMPANIC MUSCLES 257
    S. D. Anderson

19. ACOUSTIC IMPEDANCE 281
    D. N. Brooks

20. LABYRINTHINE FLUIDS 290
    S. K. Bosher

21. COCHLEAR ELECTROPHYSIOLOGY 303
    J. M. Aran and M. Portmann

22. AUDITORY NERVOUS SYSTEM 312
    W. D. Keidel and S. Kallert

23. APPLICATION OF AUDITORY ELECTRONEUROPHYSIOLOGICAL TESTS 334
    H. A. Beagley

24. PSYCHOACOUSTICS 344
    S. D. G. Stephens

25. APPLICATION OF PSYCHOACOUSTICS TO CENTRAL AUDITORY DYSFUNCTION 352
    S. D. G. Stephens

26. VESTIBULAR SYSTEM—EXPERIMENTAL PATHOPHYSIOLOGY 361
    M. Igarashi

27. VESTIBULAR PHYSIOLOGY 371
    T. D. M. Roberts

28. NEURO-OTOLOGY 383
    R. Hinchcliffe

SECTION VII

OROFACIAL STRUCTURES

29. EMBRYOLOGY OF FACIAL STRUCTURES   421
      L. BERNSTEIN

30. FACIAL NERVE   429
      J. GROVES

31. SALIVARY APPARATUS   460
      H. DIAMANT

32. TASTE   468
      R. I. HENKIN

33. PALATE   484
      B. FRITZELL

SECTION VIII

NOSE

34. OLFACTION   495
      E. DOUEK

35. NOSE—FILTRATION ASPECTS   502
      A. C. HILDING

36. NOSE—AIR CONDITIONING FUNCTION   513
      POUL STOKSTED and MUNIR KHAN

37. NASAL FUNCTION—ACOUSTIC ASPECTS   523
      J. KYTTÄ

SECTION IX

THROAT

38. DEVELOPMENTAL ANATOMY OF LARYNX   529
      M. HAST

39. COMPARATIVE ANATOMY OF LARYNX   536
      SUSAN DENNY

40. LARYNX—NEUROLOGY   546
      B. D. WYKE and J. A. KIRCHNER

41. LARYNX—MEASUREMENT OF FUNCTION   574
      H. VON LEDEN

42. DEGLUTITION   591
      W. LUND

SECTION X

VOICE, SPEECH AND LANGUAGE

43. VOICE AND SPEECH   599
      D. B. FRY

44. LANGUAGE AND SPECIFIC LANGUAGE DISORDERS IN CHILDREN   609
      M. RODDA

SECTION XI
OTOLARYNGOLOGICAL BIOLOGY AND PATHOLOGY

45. VIROLOGY   625
    K. E. K. ROWSON

46. BACTERIOLOGY   638
    T. A. L. REES

47. MYCOLOGY   645
    MYRA MCKELVIE

48. PARASITOLOGY   661
    F. E. G. COX

49. PATHOLOGY OF NOSE AND THROAT   667
    L. MICHAELS

SECTION XII
MATERIA OTOLARYNGOLOGICA

50. GENERAL ASPECTS   703
    R. HINCHCLIFFE

51. CYTOTOXIC DRUGS   725
    I. BURN

52. RADIOTHERAPY   733
    J. M. HENK and J. F. FOWLER

53. BLOOD TRANSFUSION   749
    J. BOXALL

54. SURGICAL IMPLANTS   762
    PETER MCKELVIE

55. TRACHEOSTOMY TUBES   766
    R. PRACY

56. AUDIOMETERS   772
    M. C. MARTIN

57. AUDIOMETRY   788
    J. J. KNIGHT

58. CONDITIONS FOR HEARING TESTS   800
    L. FISCH

59. AUDITORY PROSTHESES   805
    M. C. MARTIN

60. SELECTION OF HEARING AIDS   824
    A. MARKIDES

61. ELECTROACOUSTIC REHABILITATION EQUIPMENT OTHER THAN HEARING AIDS   830
    ELIZABETH KNOX

62. AUDITORY REHABILITATION   839
    R. J. BENCH and K. P. MURPHY

SECTION XIII

TOXICOLOGY

63. OTOTOXIC DRUGS   849
    J. C. BALLANTYNE

64. RHINOTOXIC DRUGS   862
    L. CAPEL

SECTION XIV

RECONSTRUCTIVE SURGERY

65. EAR   865
    B. H. COLMAN

66. NOSE   882
    T. R. BULL

67. LARYNX   894
    J. H. OGURA and G. J. SPECTOR

68. TRACHEA   919
    B. W. PEARSON

SECTION XV

FINALE

69. ETHICAL AND LEGAL CONTROL OVER ACQUISITION AND APPLICATION OF
    OTOLARYNGOLOGICAL KNOWLEDGE   935
    DOREEN HINCHCLIFFE and R. HINCHCLIFFE

APPENDICES

1. NUMBER SYSTEMS   947

2. SYSTEME INTERNATIONAL   947

3. CONVERSION TABLES   949

4. DECLARATION OF HELSINKI   949

5. ETHICAL CANONS (CIOMS)   950

6. SHORT MULTILINGUAL DICTIONARY   951

INDEX   956

LIST OF CONTRIBUTORS

STEWART ANDERSON MSc
Research Assistant, Institute of Laryngology and Otology, University of London.

J. M. ARAN Ing.
Laboratoire d'Audiologie Expérimentale, Clinique Universitaire d'O.R.L. et Centre Régional d'Audio-Phonologie, Université de Bordeaux, France.

J. A. ARROYO MD
Head of Diagnostic Department, Institute of Communication Disorders, Mexico City, Mexico.

JOHN BALLANTYNE FRCS
Consultant ENT Surgeon, Royal Free Hospital, London.

H. A. BEAGLEY FRCS, DLO
Consultant Otologist, Royal National Throat, Nose and Ear Hospital, London.

R. J. BENCH PhD
Principal Scientific Officer, Audiology Research Unit, Royal Berkshire Hospital, Reading, U.K.

LESLIE BERNSTEIN MD, DDS
Professor and Chairman, Department of Otorhinolaryngology, School of Medicine, University of California, Davis, California, U.S.A.

KEITH BOSHER PhD, FRCS
Reader in Otology, Ferens Institute, Middlesex Hospital Medical School, London.

JOHN BOXALL FIMLT
Chief Technician, Department of Pathology and Bacteriology, Institute of Laryngology and Otology, University of London.

D. N. BROOKS MSc
Director, Manchester Audiology Clinic, Manchester, U.K.

T. R. BULL MB, FRCS
Consultant Surgeon, Royal National Throat, Nose and Ear Hospital and Metropolitan Ear, Nose and Throat Hospital; Lecturer, Institute of Laryngology and Otology, University of London.

IAN BURN FRCS
Consultant Surgeon, Charing Cross Hospital, London.

L. H. CAPEL MD, FRCP
Physician, The London Chest Hospital and the Royal National Throat, Nose and Ear Hospital, London.

YVES CAZALS
Laboratoire d'Audiologie Expérimentale, Clinique Universitaire d'O.R.L. et Centre Régional d'Audio-Phonologie – Université de Bordeaux, France.

B. H. COLMAN MA, BSc, ChM, FRCS (Ed)
Consultant Surgeon, Department of Otolaryngology, The Radcliffe Infirmary, Oxford.

F. E. G. COX PhD, DSc
Professor of Zoology, King's College, University of London.

ROBERT DAMPER MSc, MIEE, MInstP
Research Assistant, Institute of Laryngology and Otology and Department of Electrical Engineering, Imperial College, University of London.

D. GARFIELD DAVIES FRCS
Consultant Otolaryngologist, Middlesex Hospital and Ferens Institute, Middlesex Hospital Medical School; Consultant Surgeon the Royal National Throat, Nose and Ear Hospital, London; Lecturer, Institute of Laryngology and Otology, University of London.

SUSAN P. DENNY BSc
Research Assistant, Institute of Laryngology and Otology, University of London.

H. DIAMANT MD
Professor and Head, University ENT Clinic, Umeå, Sweden.

ELLIS DOUEK FRCS
Consultant Otologist, Guy's Hospital, London.

F. J. FAHY PhD
Institute of Sound and Vibration Research, University of Southampton, U.K.

L. FISCH MD, DLO
Consultant in Audiology, The Hospital for Sick Children, London; Director, Hearing Clinics, Tottenham and Heston; Senior Lecturer and Research Fellow, Institute of Laryngology and Otology, University of London.

J. F. FOWLER PhD, FInstP
Director, Cancer Research Campaign's Research Unit on Radiobiology, Mount Vernon Hospital, Northwood, Middlesex, U.K.

G. R. FRASER MD, PhD, FRCP(C)
Professor of Medical Genetics, Memorial University of Newfoundland, St. John's, Newfoundland, Canada.

I. FRIEDMANN MD, DSc, FRCPath
Emeritus Professor of Pathology, University of London; Hon. Consultant Pathologist, Clinical Research Centre, Northwick Park Hospital, Harrow, Middlesex, U.K.

BJÖRN FRITZELL MD
Department of Phoniatrics, Huddinge University Hospital, Karolinska Institute, Stockholm, Sweden.

D. B. FRY PhD
Professor of Experimental Phonetics, University of London.

JOHN GROVES MB, FRCS
Consultant Ear, Nose and Throat Surgeon, Royal Free Hospital, London.

D. F. N. HARRISON MD, MS, FRCS, DLO
Professor of Laryngology and Otology, Institute of Laryngology and Otology, University of London.

MALCOLM H. HAST PhD
Professor and Director of Research, Department of Otolaryngology and Maxillofacial Surgery, Northwestern University Medical School, Chicago, Ill., U.S.A.

J. M. HENK FFR
Consultant Radiotherapist, Velindre Hospital, Cardiff, U.K.

ROBERT I. HENKIN MD
Chief, Section on Neuroendocrinology, National Heart and Lung Institute, National Institutes of Health, Bethesda, Maryland, U.S.A.

A. C. HILDING MD, PhD
Research Laboratory, St. Luke's Hospital, Duluth, Minnesota, U.S.A.

RONALD HINCHCLIFFE BSc, MD, PhD, MRCP(Ed), DLO
Reader in Neuro-otology, Institute of Laryngology and Otology, University of London; Honorary Consultant in Neuro-otology, Royal National Throat, Nose and Ear Hospital, London; Examiner in Audiology to the Universities of Manchester and Southampton.

DOREEN HINCHCLIFFE LLB, PhD, Barrister-at-Law
Institute of Advanced Legal Studies, University of London.

H. J. HOLMQUIST MD
Chief of Otolaryngology, Central Hospital, Karlstad, Sweden.

MAKOTO IGARASHI MD
Professor and Director of Research, Department of Otolaryngology, Baylor College of Medicine, Houston, Texas, U.S.A.

S. KALLERT MD
I. Physiologisches Institut der Universität Erlangen-Nürnberg, West Germany.

W. D. KEIDEL MD
Professor and Director, 1. Physiologisches Institut der Universität Erlangen-Nürnberg, West Germany.

MUNIR A. KHAN MD
University Hospital, Odense, Denmark.

SHYAM M. KHANNA PhD
Fowler Memorial Laboratory, College of Physicians and Surgeons, Columbia University, New York, U.S.A.

JOHN A. KIRCHNER MD
Professor and Head, Department of Otolaryngology, Yale University, New Haven, U.S.A.

J. J. KNIGHT PhD, FInstP
Physicist, Institute of Laryngology and Otology, University of London; Examiner in Audiology to the University of Salford, U.K.

ELIZABETH C. KNOX BSc
Scientific Officer, Technical Department (Scotland), Royal National Institute for the Deaf, Glasgow, U.K.

JYRKI KYTTÄ MD, PhM
Turun Yliopistollinen Keskussairaala, Turku, Finland.

HANS VON LEDEN MD
Institute of Laryngology and Voice Disorders, Los Angeles, California, U.S.A.

D. D. LINDSAY MA, AFRAeS, FInstP
Lecturer, Department of Medical Physics, University of Aberdeen, U.K.

WILLIAM LUND MS, FRCS
Consultant Surgeon, Department of Otolaryngology, Radcliffe Infirmary, Oxford, U.K.

MYRA McKELVIE MB, MRCP
Consultant Dermatologist, Wexham Park Hospital,

Mt. Vernon Hospital and Canadian Red Cross Memorial Hospital, U.K.

PETER McKELVIE MD, ChM, FRCS, DLO
Consultant Surgeon, The London Hospital, and the Royal National Throat, Nose and Ear Hospital, London; Consultant Otolaryngologist, Royal Postgraduate Medical School and Hammersmith Hospital, London.

ANDREAS MARKIDES PhD, MEd, DipAud
Institute of Sound and Vibration Research, University of Southampton, U.K.

A. M. MARTIN BSc, MSc, PhD, MInstP
Hearing Conservation Unit, Institute of Sound and Vibration Research, University of Southampton, U.K.

M. C. MARTIN BSc
Head of Scientific and Technical Department, Royal National Institute for the Deaf, London.

FRANCA MERLUZZI MD
Institute of Occupational Medicine, University of Milan, Italy.

LESLIE MICHAELS MD, FRCPath, FRCP(C)
Professor and Director, Department of Pathology and Bacteriology, Institute of Laryngology and Otology, University of London.

K. P. MURPHY PhD
Audiology Research Unit, Royal Berkshire Hospital, Reading, U.K.

JOSEPH H. OGURA MD, FACS
Lindburg Professor and Head, Department of Otolaryngology, Washington University School of Medicine, St. Louis, U.S.A.

BRUCE W. PEARSON MD, FRCS(C)
Department of Otorhinolaryngology, Mayo Clinic, Rochester, Minnesota, U.S.A.

M. PORTMANN MD
Clinique Universitaire d'O.R.L. et Centre Régional d'Audio-Phonologie - Université de Bordeux, France.

ROBERT PRACY FRCS
Consultant Ear, Nose and Throat Surgeon, Royal National Throat, Nose and Ear Hospital and Hospital for Sick Children, London.

ADE PYE PhD
Research Zoologist, Institute of Laryngology and Otology, University of London.

T. A. L. REES BSc, PhD
Lecturer in Microbiology, Department of Pathology and Bacteriology, Institute of Laryngology and Otology, University of London.

T. D. M. ROBERTS PhD
Reader, Institute of Physiology, University of Glasgow, U.K.

MICHAEL RODDA BSc, PhD, ABPsS
Statistics and Research Division, Department of Health and Social Security, London.

K. E. K. ROWSON MA, MD, MRCPath
Senior Lecturer in Virology, Dept. of Pathology and Bacteriology, Institute of Laryngology and Otology, University of London.

R. J. RUBEN MD
  Professor and Chairman, Department of Otorhino-
  laryngology, Albert Einstein College of Medicine,
  Yeshiva University, New York, U.S.A.

ALEXANDER SOKOLOVSKI MD, PhD
  Professor of Otolaryngology, University of Giessen,
  West Germany.

GERSHON J. SPECTOR MD, FACS
  Associate Professor, Department of Otolaryngology,
  Washington University School of Medicine, St. Louis,
  U.S.A.

S. D. G. STEPHENS BSc, MB, MPhil
  Consultant in Audiological Medicine, Royal National
  Throat, Nose and Ear Hospital, London.

PAUL STOKSTED MD
  University Hospital, Odense, Denmark.

WILLIAM TEMPEST PhD
  Reader in Electrical Engineering, University of Salford,
  U.K.

A. R. D. THORNTON PhD
  Institute of Sound and Vibration Research, University
  of Southampton, U.K.

JUERGEN TONNDORF MD PhD
  Research Professor, Fowler Memorial Laboratory,
  Department of Otolaryngology, College of Physicians
  and Surgeons, Columbia University, New York,
  U.S.A.

THOMAS VAN DE WATER MS
  Department of Otorhinolaryngology, Albert Einstein
  College of Medicine, Yeshiva University, New York,
  U.S.A.

B. D. WYKE MD, BS
  Senior Lecturer, Royal College of Surgeons of England,
  London.

FOREWORD

For those who desire to practise, teach or engage in research as well as those who are in training in the wide field or otolaryngology and all its allied sciences, an authoritative source of information on the previous fundamental scientific work is invaluable. This book has been compiled to fill such a need. The two editors with international reputations in their particular fields have drawn upon the expert assistance of leaders in many of the profound and challenging subjects that are encompassed in the specialty. The available and published works are too vast to be covered in every detail but selected references will guide the reader in further study. Many chapters are rightly contributed by practising otolaryngologists but inevitably some subjects have called for an author in the field of pure science. The inclusion of some historical notes will be appreciated and the use of the *Système International d'Unités* (*International System of Units*) is in keeping with the latest practice.

In a work of composite authorship some subjects are inevitably dealt with in greater depth than others, but in general a very good balance will be found. The labour of compiling this volume will be more than justified in the saving of countless hours by individuals in many departments where workers are engaged in this field. With many new papers being published every day supplements or new additions will inevitably be called for but this volume will stand as a reference covering a long and productive epoch.

J. Angell-James

PREFACE

There is little doubt that at the beginning of this century, otorhinolaryngology was amongst the Cinderellas of the surgical specialties. However, dramatic changes have occurred and as we enter the fourth quarter of the twentieth century we find this specialty encompassing a range of sophisticated surgical and scientific techniques undreamt of by the practitioners of yesteryear.

The scientific basis of this specialty is now widespread and it is the modest ambition of this book to portray this in as representative a manner as is feasible. Although the title refers to "Scientific Foundations", it is conceded that much that is discussed will be in respect not of science but of technology, and not of foundations but of superstructure. However, the two are interrelated and the whole we hope fulfils the ambitions of the publishers and the needs of our readers. It is hoped that this book will be of use to those who are about to embark upon a career in one or other of the many facets of otorhinolaryngology, providing them with both factual information and stimulating thought.

The book is not designed however, with a view to preparing candidates for any particular attainment examination.

We are fully conscious of the role that has been played by editors and publishers in the development of terminologies and the need to persuade all concerned to adopt international agreed systems. The editors, therefore, placed some of their few constraints upon contributors in this respect, i.e. that they should use the International System of Units, proposed or recommended International Non-Proprietary names for drugs, which are issued by W.H.O. (as given in Marler's Pharmacological and Chemical Synonyms), current English language versions (as given in the 35th edition of Gray's Anatomy) of anatomical terms that are listed in the latest Nomina Anatomica, and Snell's terminology for transplants. Unfortunately, some of the illustrations are reproductions of previously published figures; they may therefore, not have been labelled using this current international terminology.

The editors are indebted to the contributors not only for providing their individual chapters, but also for their constructive criticisms, advice and encouragement. The secretarial services of Miss Susan Damps and of Miss E.M. Foster and her staff of Tape Typing (London) were invaluable, particularly in the final preparation of the manuscripts. We would also wish to acknowledge the editorial assistance of George Buchanan, F.R.C.S., Anthony Cheesman, F.R.C.S., and Robert Damper, M.Sc., M.I.E.E. Finally, and most important, the editors are most indebted to Mr. Christopher Jarvis of Heinemann Medical Books Ltd., for his patience and understanding of the difficulties of translating manuscripts to printed page.

April, 1975   R. Hinchcliffe
                                                       D. F. N. Harrison

ACKNOWLEDGEMENTS

The Editors and Contributors wish to thank the following authors, or organizations, and their publishers, for permission to reproduce particular illustrations or other material:

The late Professor Barry Anson and Professor James Donaldson for Figures 2, 5, 6 and 10 in Chapter 30 (from their book *Surgical Anatomy of the Temporal Bone*, published by Saunders); Professors John Bordley and Pal Kapur for Figure 8 in Chapter 10 (from their paper on "The Histopathological Changes in the Temporal Bone resulting from Acute Smallpox and Chickenpox Infection", in *Laryngoscope*, 1972); Dr. A. R. de C. Deacock, Royal National Throat Nose and Ear Hospital, for data used in Chapter 2; Sir Richard Doll of Oxford University for Fig. 13 in Chapter 10; Down Bros. and Mayer and Phelps for illustrations of tracheostomy tubes in Chapter 55; Doctors A. Eberstein and J. Goodgold of New York University for Figure 12 in Chapter 30 (from their book *Electrodiagnosis of Neuromuscular Disorders*, published by Williams and Wilkins); Professor Hans Engström, Uppsala University for Figure 2 in Chapter 63; Doctors U. C. G. Engzell and A. W. Jones for Figs. 8 to 11 in Chapter 47 (from their paper on "Rhinosporidiosis in Uganda" in the *Journal of Laryngology and Otology*, 1973); Dr. Alfio Ferlito, University of Padua, for Fig. 12 in Chapter 47 (from his paper on "Primary Aspergillosis of the Larynx" in the *Journal of Laryngology and Otology*, 1974); Professor Ugo Fisch for Fig. 3 in Chapter 30 (from his chapter in *Disorders of the Skull Base Region*, edited by C. A. Hamberger and J. Wersäll and published by Almqvist and Wiksell); Professors J. E. Hawkins Jr., and L-G. Johnsson, University of Michigan, for Figs. 4, 5 and 6 in Chapter 63 (from their articles on experimental ototoxicity in *Laryngoscope*, 1972); Professors O. P. and R. M. Gupta, Benares Hindu University for Fig. 4 in Chapter 47 (from their article on histoplasmosis in *Laryngoscope*, 1970); Hearing Conservation Limited, London, for Fig. 2 in Chapter 56; The Institute of Physics for permission to reproduce their summary of the International System of Units (SI) in Appendix 2; Professor Frank Martinson, University of Ibadan, for Figures 5, 6 and 7 in Chapter 47; Dr. Jacob Meiry, Massachusetts Institute of Technology, and Professors Melvill Jones, McGill University, and Lawrence Stark, University of California, for Figs. 4, 3 and 2 in Chapter 28 (from their illustrations in *The Control of Eye Movements* edited by Paul Bach-y-Rita and Carter Collins and published by Academic Press who hold the copyright); Doctors M. M. Merzenich and R. A. Schindler for Fig. 1 in Chapter 54 (from their paper on "Chronic Intracochlear Electrode Implantation" in *Annals of Otology, Rhinology and Laryngology*, 1974); Mullard Limited, London, for Fig. 20 in Chapter 59; Dr. Suchitra Prasansuk, Mahidol University, for unpublished data used in Chapter 2; Dr. Bruce Proctor for Fig. 3 in Chapter 15 (from his paper on "Surgical Anatomy of the Posterior Tympanum" published in the *Annals of Otology, Rhinology and Laryngology*, 1969); Professor David Pye, University of London, for Fig. 1 in Chapter 13; Joselen Ransome F.R.C.S. for Fig. 7 in Chapter 63 (from her article on hexadimethrine toxicity in the *Journal of Laryngology and Otology*, 1966); Professor Harold Schuknecht, Harvard University, for Figs. 22 and 23 in Chapter 15 (from his book *Pathology of the Ear* published by

Harvard University Press) and Figs. 7 to 10 in Chapter 65 (from his book *Stapedectomy* published by Little, Brown and Co.); Navnit Shah F.R.C.S. for Fig. 3 in Chapter 2 (from his paper on "Secretory Otitis Media" in the *Journal of Laryngology and Otology*, 1971); Albert Shalom F.R.C.S. for data used in Chapters 2 and 53; P. M. Shenoi F.R.C.S. for Figure 8 in Chapter 63 (from his paper on the "Ototoxicity of absorbable Gelatin Sponge" in the *Proceedings of the Royal Society of Medicine*, 1973); Gordon Smyth F.R.C.S. for Fig. 4 in Chapter 30 (from his paper on "The Facial Nerve in Acoustic Tumor Surgery" in the *Archives of Otolaryngology*, 1973); and Professor H. Stupp, University of Düsseldorf, for Figures 9 and 10 in Chapter 63 (from his article on ototoxicity in *Audiology*, 1973); Doctors A. White and P. L. Verma for Fig. 8 in Chapter 30 (from their paper on the "Spatial Arrangement of Facial Nerve Fibres" in the *Journal of Laryngology and Otology*, 1973).

SECTION I

QUANTITATIVE METHODS

PAGE

1. MEASUREMENT   2

2. STATISTICS   9

3. COMPUTERS   31

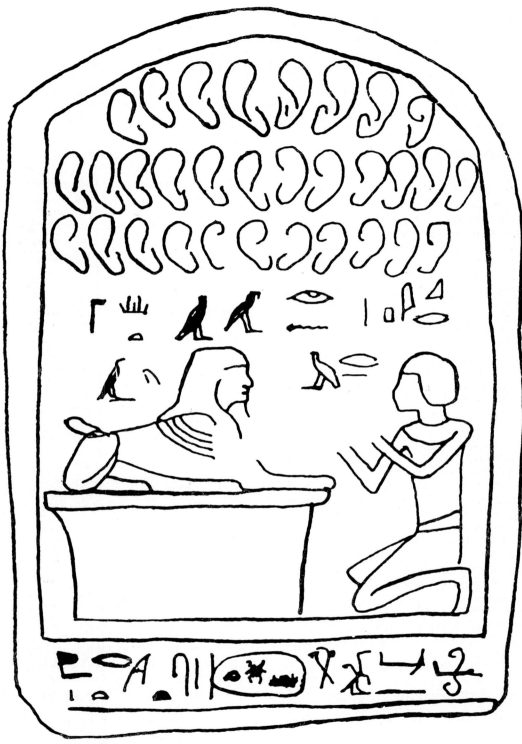

Fig. 1. Tablet excavated from Temple of Amenhotep II. (After Hassan, 1949.)

1. MEASUREMENT
(Numbers, scales, units, functions)

R. HINCHCLIFFE

INTRODUCTION

As Stevens (1951) pointed out, *measurement*, in its broadest sense, is the assignment of numerals to objects or events according to certain rules. And the fact that numerals can be assigned under different rules leads to different kinds of *scales* and different kinds of measurements. The system whereby these rules are applied constitutes *mathematics*. Thus mathematics is not a science in itself but a system of logic. The stature of a science is commonly measured by the degree to which it makes use of mathematics. Conversely, it has been asserted that if something cannot be measured, one cannot know anything about it. This, however, may not be so serious a statement as it would first appear. In the simplest state of affairs, an object or event may be present or absent. Such occurrences or non-occurrences may be represented by 1 or 0 (*binary* system), and can actually be subjected to a sophisticated mathematical analysis (Boolean algebra—devised by George Boole in 1874 for a mathematical analysis of logic). With this in mind, one can then more readily accept Lord Kelvin's dictum that "whatever exists, exists in some quantity, and can therefore be measured". Measurement has a great historical background. It was an integral part of the science of the ancient Egyptian civilization. Figure 1 shows a tablet recovered from the Temple of Amenhotep II (1448–1420 B.C.), which is adjacent to the Sphinx. The tablet is dedicated by the scribe Mer to "Hor-em-Akhet, the Great God who hears". It is of note that not only were ears and hearing prominent in the ancient Egyptian mythology but quantification was also apparent. Nevertheless, even today we persist in using descriptive terms where quantification is possible. Simpson (1963) has shown, for example, that the descriptive terms "practically always", "frequently", "as often as not", "occasionally" and "almost never" correspond to actual frequency values of 91 per cent, 74 per cent, 50 per cent, 23 per cent and 3 per cent respectively.

NUMBERS AND NUMBER SYSTEMS

A number is a symbol (digit), or combination of symbols (digits), designating "how many". Most systems of numeration are based on a repetitive procedure that makes it possible to show larger numbers by combining symbols for smaller numbers. Some preliterate peoples are, however, only able to count "one", "two", "many, many, many". The Roman numeration system (I, II, III, IV . . .) was based upon the cardinal principle (*principle of corres-pondence*) and was able to denote magnitudes only. A numeration system capable of being used as a basis for an arithmetic required a knowledge of the *principle of position*, which was already known to the Babylonian civilization, whose later records also contained a symbol for zero. It was, however, left to the Indian mathematicians of the 5th and later centuries A.D. to develop an arithmetic based upon this principle of position and using a symbol, first a dot, then a circle, to denote "nothing".

The *base* (*radix*) of a *number system* is equal to the number of available discrete characters (coefficients). Thus, in the decimal system, there are ten discrete characters, 0 to 9 inclusive, in any column. Therefore the base of this system is 10. The binary system possesses only two characters (0 and 1), the octal, 8 (0 to 7 inclusive), and the hexadecimal, 16 (0, 1, 2, 3, 4, 5, 6, 7, 8, 9, A, B, C, D, E and F). Strictly speaking, whenever a number is given, a subscript should be employed to indicate the number system which is being used. This subscript corresponds to the base of that particular number system. Thus a number expressed as 10110_2 in the binary system will correspond to 22_{10} in the decimal system. (In general usage, where the decimal system is employed, and when computers are not involved, we would just write "22" for this number.) The use of the subscript "2" would indicate that the number "10110" that we have given is not ten thousand one hundred and ten. Usually, confusions do not arise between binary and decimal notations but they might between decimal, octal and hexadecimal notations. Thus "17" writen in hexadecimal notation would be the same as "23" in decimal notation. Consequently, the first number should be written "17_{16}". Any base is of course possible. The choice of the base 10 is, of course, an anatomical accident and provides further evidence for the anthropomorphic basis of even our mathematics. A number system with a base of 60 was employed by the Babylonians and this still persists in our measures of time (seconds and minutes). Although in the seventeenth century, the mathematician Leibniz dwelt at length on the binary system, the application of this number system, together with the octal and hexadecimal, was dependent upon recent developments in computer science. Thus the simplest (binary) number system is used not only by some preliterate peoples, but also by the twentieth century digital computer (see page 34). This is because two numerals can be represented by an electrical switch that is "open" for one number and "closed" for the other. A digit in the binary system is frequently referred to as a *bit* (contraction of "binary digit"). Since digital computers work on the binary system, a simple method must be available for converting from decimal to binary and vice versa. Just as each position in a decimal number corresponds to a power of ten, so this position in a binary number corresponds to a power of two. Thus the binary number 10111 can be expressed as a series of powers of two, i.e.

$$10111_2 = (1 \times 2)^4 + (0 \times 2)^3 + (1 \times 2)^2 + (1 \times 2)^1 + (1 \times 2)^0 \quad (1.1)$$
$$= 16 + 0 + 4 + 2 + 1$$
$$= 23_{10} \quad (1.2)$$

(note that any value raised to the power zero is unity). The octal number system came into existence because of the difficulty of dealing with long strings of binary 0's and 1's and converting them into decimals. Conversion is awkward because of the absence of a simple relationship between powers of two (binary system) and powers of ten (decimal system). The octal system is a shorthand method of writing a group of three binary digits as a single octal digit. Reference to Appendix 1 (p. 947) shows that the binary number 101 corresponds to the octal number 5. Consequently, the binary number 101 111 011 corresponds to the octal number 573. Octal numbers can be converted to decimal numbers by multiplying each digit by the position coefficient and adding the resulting products. Thus

$$573_8 = (3 \times 8^0) + (7 \times 8^1) + (5 \times 8^2) = 3 + 56 + 320 = 379_{10} \quad (1.3)$$

The converse operation of converting a decimal number to an octal or a binary one is performed by successive divisions of the quotient by the radix. The remainders give the number in the new number system. Thus conversion of 379_{10} to an octal number gives successive quotients of 47 and 5 with remainders of 3, 7 and 5 (equivalent to $3 \times 8^0 + 7 \times 8^1 + 5 \times 8^2$).

The hexadecimal notation is in use since there are sixteen possible combinations of the four binary digits which are required to represent the ten decimal characters (although values of 7 and less can be expressed by a 3 bit code, the values 8 and 9 in the decimal system require that the binary digits be increased to four). The hexadecimal code ensures that none of the six unused combinations in a four-bit-code are wasted.

CLASSIFICATION OF NUMBERS

Whole numbers are known as *integers*. A *fraction* is a ratio of integers. Signed (positive or negative) integers or fractions constitute *rational* numbers, i.e. these can all be obtained by rational operations. Rational operations involve addition, subtraction, multiplication, division and evolution (or exponentiation, i.e. raising to a power). A number not of this type is termed *irrational*, e.g. $\sqrt{2}$. If written in decimal form, the latter number is 1·4142135 . . ., i.e. the digits continue endlessly but no sequence will repeat. By contrast, if a rational number is converted into decimal form, its digits either terminate or repeat. Irrational numbers which cannot be obtained as a result of algebraic

operation, such as extraction of a root, are termed *transcendental*. Examples of the latter class of numbers include π, the ratio of the circumference of a circle to its diameter, and e the base of natural (Napierian) logarithms.

SCALES

When numerals are assigned to events or objects according to some rule, a *scale* results. Table 1 shows Stevens'

TABLE 1

SCALES OF MEASUREMENT
(After Stevens, 1951)

Scale	Basic Empirical Operations	Permissible Statistics	Examples
Nominal	Determination of equality	Number of cases Mode Contingency correlation	Assignment of type to Békésy audiograms or to tympanoplasties
Ordinal	Determination of greater or less	Median Percentiles Order correlation	Grading of malignancy of cancers
Interval	Determination of equality of intervals	Mean Standard deviation Product-moment correlation	Temperature (Fahrenheit and Celsius); calendar time; position
Ratio	Determination of equality of ratios	Geometric mean Coefficient of variation Logarithms, decibels	Numerosity; length; mass, absolute (thermodynamic) temperature (kelvin); density; resistance; loudness (sones); pitch (mels)

(1946; 1951) hierarchical classification of scales of measurement. The scales of measurement found in otolaryngology occur in all four groups. These scales range in sophistication from the numerical designation of types of Békésy audiograms or of tympanoplastic operations to the numerical designation of the subjective magnitude of sound intensity (loudness) or of sound frequency (pitch). The decibel scale, which is a logarithmic ratio scale, is mentioned on several occasions later in this book.

Some scales of measurement used in otolaryngology are composite scales which include multi-dimensional or mixed scales. Thus the TNM classification of neoplasms, first proposed by Denoix (UICC, 1968; 1973) is, on first appearances, a composite of three ordinal scales (Tumour; Nodes, lymph, regional; Metastases, distant) which are expressed as an alphanumeric code of the type TaNbMc, where a, b and c refer to measures (expressed as integers) which indicate the hierarchical severity or progression on each scale. Thus for a malignancy of the nasal part of pharynx which extends beyond this region, involves bone and is associated with fixed regional lymph nodes and distant metastases, a, b and c would have values 4, 3 and 1 respectively. Thus such a tumour would be designated as T4N3M1. However, inspection of Table 2 shows that both

TABLE 2

VALUES OF INDICES IN TNM CLASSIFICATION

(After UICC, 1968; 1973)

Index	T		N	M
0	No evidence of primary		Regional lymph nodes not palpable	No evidence of distant metastases
1	Localized; small; movable	V A	Movable homolateral nodes	Distant metastases present
2	Larger	R I	Movable contralateral or bilateral nodes	—
3	Extending beyond region	A B	Fixed nodes	—
(4)	Bone involvement	L E	—	—

the range for, and the meaning to be attached to, a given value of "a" is variable, being dependent on the tumour site. Moreover, M actually represents a binary character, so that leaves us only with N as a possibly truly ordinal scale. However, this property is jeopardized in those cases where the clinician is permitted to subdivide N1 and N2 (into e.g. N1a and N1b) according to whether or not he judges the palpable node to contain growth. Although the modifications and extensions suggested by Sakai and Masaki (1971) are an improvement, it is nevertheless not surprising that the TMN classification presents a metrologist's or taxonomist's nightmare. Harrison (1970) has indicated that, although the system is both effective and accurate in some sites, in the laryngeal part of pharynx, for example, this is not so. Moreover, Lederman (1970) points out that the UICC (Union Internationale Contre le Cancer) makes no recommendation as to how the various TNM categories should be grouped so as to provide a small practical number of clinical stages. The American Joint Committee for Cancer Staging (1962) recommends four clinical stages and suggests a way in which the TNM categories could be grouped, placing emphasis on the presence of lymph node metastases as being the decisive factor in prognosis. However, as Lederman points out, one other factor requires consideration, in regard to the larynx at least. This is the fixation of the affected part. The 4-digit code advocated by the American Cancer Society (1968) to designate the morphology of neoplasms presents an even greater metrologist's nightmare. The first three digits refer to the type of tumour and thus constitute a nominal scale. However, the fourth digit basically refers to an ordinal scale of malignancy. It is this composite nature of codings of

neoplasms which severely restricts their value. This is notwithstanding the additional flaw in these ordinal scalings of malignancy of using a number at one end of the scale to designate an undetermined degree of malignancy. Thus the fourth digit code of the American Cancer Society's malignancy grading, which has values ranging from 3 to 8, uses the value 3 to designate "differentiation not determined or stated". It would have been better to use a central value or the symbol * ("not known" or "not knowable") as used by taxonomists. Indeed, a more rigorous study of the requirements and possibilities of cancer classification and grading should enable one to produce a single composite measure of malignancy magnitude. In other words, the goal of the oncological metrologist should be to produce a composite quantitative measure analogous to Burns and Robinson's (1970) noise immission level (NIL) or to Robinson's (1969) noise pollution level. The NIL is defined as the A-weighted (see Chapter 11) noise immission (an index of the total noise energy incident on the ear over a specified period of time) expressed in decibels relative to a specified datum. Burns and Robinson showed that the NIL is quantitatively related to the degree of noise-induced hearing loss in industry. The noise pollution level (L_{NP}) is a single index which expresses the nuisance value of successive noises, e.g. aircraft or motor vehicle. It is based upon two terms, one representing the equivalent continuous noise level on the energy basis, the other representing the augmentation of annoyance when fluctuations of noise level occur. Audiology may appear to be a far cry from oncology, the two perhaps representing each end of the spectrum of otolaryngological specialities, but, as Politzer, the father of otology, is reported to have said "Everything is related to everything".

UNITS

Two equal quantities may be represented by different numbers if they are measured in different units. For example, 1 mile = 1,760 yards = 1,609 metres. Consequently there have been attempts at both national and international levels to standardize units, and some of these standards are legally enforceable. Because of the need for an international language in which to communicate the measurements of commerce and of science, the CIPM (Comité International des Poids et Mesures) formulated the Système International d'Unités (SI) in 1960. The CGPM (Conférence Général des Poids et Mesures) has met at three to four yearly intervals since then and produced further resolutions and recommendations to improve this system of units. An English translation of the French "Système International d'Unités", which was published by the International Bureau of Weights and Measures (BIPM—Bureau International des Poids et Mesures), became available from Her Majesty's Stationery Office in 1973 (National Physical Laboratory, 1973). The present set of units are shown in Appendix 2 (page 947). In 1967, the Conference of the Joint Committee on Metrication of the Royal Society and the Council of Engineering Institutions strongly recommended that "SI units" be increasingly used in University and College teachings in the U.K. Now, at the international level, the Council of

European Communities has issued directives that the SI system should replace all other systems of units in national legislation. In this context, public health legislation was explicitly mentioned.

This international system is both metric and decimal and its advantages, as Peach (1969) points out, are:

(1) There are at present only seven base units which are precisely defined.

(2) All other units may be derived from these seven base units, i.e. the system is *coherent*.

(3) The unit of energy in all forms is a joule (newton-metre), i.e. the system is *consistent*.

(4) The same set of multiples and sub-multiples are applied to all units. These multiples and sub-multiples are powers of 10.

(5) The unit of force—the newton—is independent of the earth's gravity. The introduction of the earth's gravitational acceleration "g" is often unnecessary. (An approximation to "g" is 10 m.s^{-2}, which assists in calculations.)

(6) Electrical units are consistent from both electro-magnetic and electrostatic viewpoints.

Nevertheless, the system still has room for improvement. For example, not only is the base unit of mass (the kilogram) still not defined in terms of natural processes but its name already contains a multiplying prefix (kilo).

Other points to note in this International System are:

(1) In accordance with Resolution 7 of the 9th CGPM (1948) lower case is used for *symbols* of units unless the symbol is derived from a proper name, in which instance, an initial capital letter is used. These symbols are not followed by a full stop (period).

(2) Unit symbols do not change in the plural.

(3) Irrespective of whether a unit's name is derived from a proper name or not, it is always written in small case.

(4) According to Recommendations R31 and R100 of Technical Committee ISO/TC 12 of ISO (International Organisation for Standardisation), a solidus (/) must not be repeated on the same line unless ambiguity is avoided by parentheses. In complicated cases, negative powers or parentheses should be used. For example, it is preferable to write m.kg.s^{-3}.A^{-1} (and not m.kg/s^3/A.), for expressing electrical field strength.

(5) Amongst units deprecated by the system are the "calorie" and the "micron".

(6) The 12th CGPM (1964) recommended that the name *litre* should not be employed to give the results of high accuracy volume measurements.

(7) The word *"weight"* should be avoided since it is ambiguous, sometimes meaning "mass", and at other times "mechanical force".

(8) The only SI unit for temperature is the kelvin (symbol K), the unit of thermodynamic temperature. The 13th CGPM (1967) decided that the kelvin should always be used to express an interval or a difference of temperature, as well as a magnitude of temperature. This Conference also agreed that the unit "degree

Celsius" (symbol °C) is equal to the unit "kelvin". The 1964 General Conference had adopted the name "degree Celsius" to denote the degree of temperature instead of "degree centigrade".

(9) Considering the advice of IUPAP (International Union of Pure and Applied Physics), IUPAC (International Union of Pure and Applied Chemistry) and ISO (International Organisation for Standardisation) on the need to define a unit of amount of substance, the 14th CGPM (1971) decided on the *mole* (symbol "mol"). This is defined as the amount of substance of a system which contains as many elementary entities as there are atoms in 0·012 kg of carbon 12. As Owen and his colleagues (1970) point out, a number of benefits accrue from the use of the mole:

(a) It brings terminology in physiology and medicine more into line with that in chemistry and physics.

(b) It goes a long way toward providing a uniform system of physiological concentration units. Although enzyme concentrations cannot usually be expressed in terms of moles, the expression of plasma enzyme activities in IUs (micromoles of substrate converted per unit time per litre of plasma) at least brings enzyme concentrations into line with those of simple substances.

(c) It avoids ambiguities arising in the use of the "equivalent" or of its sub-unit, the "milliequivalent". For example, it resolves the problem of concentration units for polyvalent ions such as phosphate whose degrees of protonation and, therefore, effective equivalent weight, depends on the pH.

(d) It allows ready appreciation of the *osmolal* significance of plasma components and a ready calculation of the *osmolality* (property resulting from the lowering of solvent activity due to the presence of a solute), of a fluid of a known composition.

(e) Therapeutic doses expressed in moles would avoid confusion when pharmacologically active substances may be supplied in several different forms. For example, the molecular weights of histamine and of histamine diphosphate are 111 and 307 respectively. Thus a dose prescribed in micrograms would differ by a factor of 3. However, prescribing a dose in millimoles would specify a given amount of histamine regardless of the salt used.

The Commission on Quantities and Units in Clinical Chemistry (CQUCC), formed jointly by IUPAC (International Union of Pure and Applied Chemistry) and IFCC (International Federation of Clinical Chemistry) have broadly endorsed the SI system (especially the mole as a unit) and recommended its adoption for reporting biochemical measurements. However, CQUCC wish to see the litre retained for the present as a unit of volume but it envisaged that, within a number of years, it may well be decided to rescind the litre and express volumes in terms of cubic metres. CQUCC also proposed the systematic use of factors which are powers of 10 with exponents that are whole multiples of three. In other words, the use of hecto-, deca-, deci and centi- would be discouraged. This proposal has been criticized by van Assendelft and his colleagues (1973) as being too restrictive. Such a proposal, if accepted, would, for example, exclude length being expressed in centimetres. These authors also endorse the plea of Owen and his colleagues to retain the concept of pH (negative logarithm of the hydrogen ion activity) and not replace it by expressing hydrogen ion activity as substance concentration.

The implications for medicine in general and for otolaryngology in particular of adopting the Système International are perhaps not yet widely appreciated. A haemoglobin concentration previously expressed as 14·8 g/100 ml now becomes 9·2 mmol.l^{-1}, a blood pressure of 135/90 mm Hg becomes 18/12 kPa (kilopascals), and a middle ear pressure of -150 mm H_2O becomes $-1·5$ kPa. Moreover, when using SI units, an obese patient, instead of being given an 850 kilocalorie diet, should be given a 3 560 kJ one (note SI convention of dividing up numbers in groups of three but inserting neither dots nor commas in the spaces between groups).

Units Outside the International System

The 1969 CIPM recognized that there were a number of units which were outside the system, but were accepted as being "in use with the International System". Into this category come the minute, the hour and the day. In addition to these units, there are units which are not mentioned by the Système International. We have already cited pH.

A *decibel* (dB) is one tenth of a *bel*, which is the logarithm of the ratio of two particular sound intensities. Since the acoustician measures sound pressure and not sound intensity, and pressure is proportional to the square root of intensity, the decibel scale is also derived from the ratio of the square of two sound pressures. This is the same as saying that the number of decibels is equal to 20 times the logarithm of two pressure ratios. Thus one decibel corresponds to a 12 per cent increase in sound pressure. Unless stated otherwise, the reference pressure is taken to be 20 μPa (micropascals). This was formerly expressed as 0·000 02 newtons per square metre (and, before that, 0·000 2 dynes per square centimetre). In this case, the particular sound level should be expressed in terms of dB SPL (sound pressure level). In audiology, the acoustic reactance presented to a source of sound by the external and middle ear is usually expressed in terms of the equivalent volume of air instead of in coherent units. However, Lilly (1972) points out that an ear with a given acoustic reactance may, when expressed in terms of an equivalent volume of air, be within the normal range in Miami but within the "otosclerotic" range in Santa Fe. This is because "the equivalent volume" values depend on the altitude of the location where the measurements have been done.

FUNCTIONS

A *function* is defined as the expression in mathematical symbols of the relationship between variables. Thus if x and y represent real numbers, then y is a function of x if y is uniquely determined by the value of x. For example, the equation

$$y = 6x \qquad (1.4)$$

states that y is a function of x because, for every real number substituted for x, there can be only one real number for the value of y. Thus if $x = 1$, $y = 6$; if $x = 4$, $y = 24$; if $x = -2·5$, $y = -15$. An equation of the form:

$$y = ax + b \qquad (1.5)$$

defines a *linear function* and is thus termed a linear equation. The word "linear" is derived from the fact that the graph of such a function is a straight line. However, as perhaps might be expected, many functions encountered in otolaryngology are non-linear. Of particular importance are logarithmic, exponential, power and Gompertzian functions.

A *logarithmic function* is defined by the expression

$$y = \log_b x \qquad (1.6)$$

where $b =$ the base of the logarithms.

The logarithm of the number x to a given base, b, is the power y to which the base must be raised to equal the number, i.e.

$$x = b^y \qquad (1.7)$$

The value of the base may be any positive number except 1. If the base is 10, the logarithms are termed *common* or *Briggsian*, after an English professor of geometry who originated these in the seventeenth century. If the base is e (2·71828), the logarithms are termed *natural* or *Napierian*, after the Scot who originated these in the seventeenth century also. The natural logarithm of a number x may be referred to as $\log_e x$ or $\ln x$.

A logarithmic equation of the general type

$$y = c(\log_b x) + k \qquad (1.8)$$

gives a straight line graph when y is plotted against $\log_b x$. Both c and k are constants, c being the slope and k the intercept (point where the graph crosses the y axis).

An obvious example of the use of common logarithms in otolaryngology is the decibel scale where the number of decibels is given by 20 times the logarithm of the ratio of two sound pressures,

i.e. $$L = 20 \log_{10} \frac{P_2}{P_1} \qquad (1.9)$$

where L is the sound level in dB of a particular sound (having a pressure P_2 pascals) relative to another sound having a pressure of P_1 pascals.

An example of natural logarithms is in the Nernst equation which is referred to in Chapter 20. This relates the size of the resting (transmembrane) potential across biological cell membranes to the ratio of the concentrations of permeable ions. Thus, for sodium and potassium, the potential difference

$$(E_i - E_0) = \frac{RT}{F} \ln \frac{[K^+]_0}{[K^+]_i} = \frac{RT}{F} \ln \frac{[Na^+]_0}{[Na^+]_i} \qquad (1.10)$$

where

R = gas constant

T = absolute temperature

F = Faraday's constant

$[K^+]_0$ = concentration of potassium in compartment (o)

$[K^+]_i$ = concentration of potassium in compartment (i)

$[Na^+]_0$ = concentration of sodium in compartment (o)

$[Na^+]_i$ = concentration of sodium in compartment (i).

The *exponential function* is the inverse of a logarithmic function, so that

$$y = b^x \qquad (1.11)$$

where b is commonly e (base of natural logarithms) so that

$$y = e^x \qquad (1.12)$$

or, in general form,

$$y = ce^{kx} \qquad (1.13)$$

where c and k are constants.

The attenuation of X-rays is governed by an exponential law such that

$$I = I_0 e^{-\mu x} \qquad (1.14)$$

where I = intensity of X-ray beam after passage through a homogeneous medium

I_0 = initial intensity of X-ray beam

x = thickness of material

μ = linear attenuation coefficient (this is characteristic of the attenuating material and the radiation energy concerned)

As pointed out in Chapter 51, malignant tumour growth rate is essentially exponential with time. Emanuel' and Evseenko (1970) provide extensive data to support Breur's (1966) thesis. Their kinetic law of tumour growth is expressed

$$\Phi = \Phi_0 e^{\phi t} \qquad (1.15)$$

where Φ = volume or diameter of tumour at time t

Φ_0 = volume or diameter of tumour at time t_0

and ϕ = self-acceleration factor.

Dose-response curves of several anti-tumour agents may also be exponential (Berenbaum, 1969) and so described by the expression:

$$F = e^{-cD} \qquad (1.16)$$

where F = surviving fraction of cell population

D = dose of anti-tumour agent

c = a constant.

A special type of exponential function is the *logistic* function. These functions are of the type:

$$\text{logistic } (x) = \frac{e^x}{1 + e^x} \qquad (1.17)$$

which it is more convenient to express for typographical reasons as

$$\text{logistic } (x) = \{\exp (x)\}/[1 + \{\exp (x)\}] \qquad (1.18)$$

Scheiblechner (1974) has used this function to relate measured hearing levels to noise exposure.

A logistic equation has also been used by Sacher and Trucco (1966) to describe the behaviour of steady-state populations which is useful in discussing the kinetics of cancer treatment. This equation is expressed

$$F_t = F/\{F + (1 - F) \exp -(kt)\} \qquad (1.19)$$

where F_t = fractional size of population at time t after depletion (or increase) to a fraction F of its original size

and k = recovery constant

The *power function* is defined by the equation

$$y = kx^n \qquad (1.20)$$

where k = a constant

therefore

$$\log y = n \log x + \log k \qquad (1.21)$$

Thus when $\log y$ is plotted against $\log x$, a straight line is obtained with a slope n and intercept $\log k$.

The magnitude of sensation, including loudness and both subjective smell and subjective taste intensities, was, for over a hundred years, considered to be a logarithmic function of the magnitude of the physical (or chemical) stimulus (Weber–Fechner Law). In a series of investigations over the past quarter of a century, Stevens and his colleagues have shown that such a function does not fit the experimental data (Stevens, 1962). The psychophysical law is now accepted as an example of a power function,

i.e.

$$\psi = k\phi^\beta \qquad (1.22)$$

where ψ = subjective magnitude of stimulus

ϕ = physical magnitude of stimulus

The value for the exponent β depends on the particular sensory continuum concerned. Thus, for loudness, it has a value of 0·6, for the intensity of coffee odour, 0·55, for the taste intensity of both salt and sucrose, 1·3. Near threshold, as Scharf and Stevens (1961) have shown in respect of loudness in particular, the psychophysical law should be modified to fit the experimental data as follows:

$$\psi = k(\phi - \phi_0)^\beta \qquad (1.23)$$

where ϕ_0 = threshold intensity of stimulus.

The psychophysical law undoubtedly has a physiological basis. In experimental animals, the electrophysiological response for the first auditory neurone has been shown to be related, in the form of a power function, to the physical magnitude of the sound stimulus. The rate of neural discharges from the vestibular ganglion is a power function of the angular acceleration to which an animal is subjected (Correia and Landolt, 1973). Ottoson's (1956) data show that the amplitude of the electro-olfactogram is a power function of the physical intensity of the odorous substance.

Nordling (1953) has shown that the death rate from cancer rises with the sixth power of the age. He therefore suggested that carcinogenesis might depend on a series of mutations in affected cells and that the clinical manifestations were dependent on the cumulative effects of this series of mutations. In 1969, Ashley reported that mean annual death rates for, for example, gastric carcinoma, showed a straight line graph when plotted as a function of age on double logarithmic graph paper. In other words, the death rate is a power function of the age. This supports the 1954 hypothesis of Armitage and Doll for a multiple "hit" theory of carcinogenesis. As Ashley points out, the steps in a multi-stage carcinogenesis are often equated with somatic mutations, changes in the genetic material of the cell, the first of which may be inherited in nature. The depressing implication of all this is that it makes the possibility of there being a single cause for cancer, inasmuch as there is for other disorders, remote. This in turn points to the need for us to look to epidemiology to identify environmental carcinogenic factors.

The *Gompertz function* is defined by the equation

$$Y = Vg^{h^x} \qquad (1.24)$$

where both g and h are constants and V is a limiting value of Y. Here the data give a straight line if one plots the logarithm of the difference between the logarithms of Y and of V against x. The slope of this line is the logarithm of h and the intercept is the logarithm of the logarithm of g. As mentioned in Chapter 3, a Gompertz function can be fitted to noise-induced temporary threshold shift due to short duration impulse sound.

In Chapter 51, it is mentioned that, although over the greater part of its life, a tumour may exhibit exponential growth, there is a decay in growth as it becomes larger. A Gompertz function is then found to give a better fit to the data. Indeed, biological growth in general is best represented by a Gompertz function (Laird, 1966, 1967; Laird *et al.*, 1965). Using knowledge of these functions and available data, Berenbaum (1969) has presented equations for determining the relationship between the dose and the interval between doses for therapeutic regimens to eliminate populations growing either exponentially or according to the Gompertz growth equation and to conserve at a steady-state level populations normally maintained in a steady state by homoeostasis. Regimens may therefore be chosen that selectively damage one cell population while allowing another in the same individual to survive. The model suggests that, in some circumstances, the fates of two cell populations in the same individual may be reversed by manipulating the therapeutic regimen.

Of course, since most conditions are multifactorial, a particular measure will frequently be found to be a function of more than one variable. Yet, at the same time, some variables are not, contrary to expectations, related to the measure in question. For example, we may consider the data presented by Sellars (1969) on the closure of tympanic membrane (*pars tensa*) perforations by trichloroacetic acid cautery. For a series of perforations, which were neither total nor associated with cholesteatoma, Sellars recorded the age of the patient, the chronicity of the lesion, the site and size of the perforation and the number of treatments required. Inspection of the published data indicated that chronicity and perforation site were not important factors. The principal factor appeared to be the patient's age, with the size of the perforation as a secondary factor. Thus one might postulate that the number of treatments required for these central perforations by this technique was, say, a power function of the patient's age and, say, a logistic function of the perforation size, e.g.

$$N = 0 \cdot 4 \left(\frac{e^x}{1 + e^x} \right) A^{0 \cdot 8} \qquad (1.25)$$

where N = number of weekly treatments required,

x = size of perforation in mm,

and A = patient's age in years.

The logistic function would be required to account for a negligible difference in the number of treatments required by a subtotal and a 2·5 mm diameter perforation, yet with the suggestion of a small difference in the number of treatments between a 2·5 mm and a 1·5 mm perforation. This mathematical model could be tested by a more extensive study. The experimental design for such a study and the subsequent analysis of the data, together with curve fitting, is a matter for statistics. This is the subject of the next chapter.

REFERENCES

American Cancer Society (1968), *Manual of Tumor Nomenclature and Coding*. American Cancer Society Inc.

Armitage, P. and Doll, R. (1954), "The Age Distribution of Cancer and a Multi-stage Theory of Carcinogenesis," *Brit. J. Cancer*, **8**, 1.

Ashley, D. J. B. (1969), "The Two 'Hit' and Multiple 'Hit' Theories of Carcinogenesis," *Brit. J. Cancer*, **23**, 313.

Assendelft, O. W. van, Mook, G. A. and Zijlstra, W. G. (1973), "International System of Units (SI) in Physiology," *Pflügers Arch.*, **339**, 265.

Berenbaum, M. C. (1969), "Dose, Response Curves for Agents that Impair Cell Reproductive Integrity," *Brit. J. Cancer*, **23**, 426, 434.

Breur, K. (1966), "Growth Rate and Radiosensitivity of Human Tumours." *Europ. J. Cancer*, **2**, 157.

Burns, W. and Robinson, D. W. (1970), *Hearing and Noise in Industry*. London: HMSO.

Correia, M. J. and Landolt, J. P. (1973), "Spontaneous and Driven Responses from Primary Neurons of the Anterior Semicircular Canal of the Pigeon," *Adv. oto-rhino-laryng.*, **19**, 134.

Emanuel', N. M. and Evseenko, L. S. (1970), "Kolichestvennye osnovy klinicheskoĭ onkologii," *Izdatel'stvo* "*Meditsina*". Moscow.

Harrison, D. F. N. (1970), "Pathology of Hypopharyngeal Cancer in Relation to Surgical Management," *J. Laryng.*, **84**, 349.

Hassan, S. (1949), *The Sphinx*. Cairo: Government Press.

Laird, A. K. (1966), "Postnatal Growth of Birds and Mammals," *Growth*, **30**, 349.

Laird, A. K. (1967), "Evolution of the Human Growth Curve," *Growth*, **31**, 345.

Laird, A. K., Tyler, S. A. and Barton, A. D. (1965), "Dynamics of Normal Growth," *Growth*, **29**, 233.

Lederman, M. (1970), "Radiotherapy of Cancer of Larynx," *J. Laryng.*, **84**, 867.

Lilly, D. J. (1972), "Ch. 23" in *Handbook of Clincial Audiology* (J. Katz, Ed.). Baltimore: Williams and Wilkins.

National Physical Laboratory (1973), *SI: The International System of Units*. London: HMSO.

Nordling, C. O. (1953), "A New Theory on the Cancer-inducing Mechanism," *Brit. J. Cancer*, **7**, 68.

Ottoson, D. (1956), "Analysis of the Electrical Activity of the Olfactory Epithelium," *Acta physiol. scand.* Suppl. 122.

Owen, J. A., Edwards, R. G. and Coller, B. A. W. (1970), *The Mole in Biology and Medicine*. Edinburgh and London: Livingstone.

Peach, J. (1969), *Kempe's Metrication Handbook*. London: Morgan Grampian.

Robinson, D. W. (1969), *The Concept of Noise Pollution Level*. NPL Aero Report Ac38. Teddington, Mx.: National Physical Laboratory.

Sacher, G. A. and Trucco, E. (1966), "Theory of Radiation Injury and Recovery in Self-Renewing Cell Populations," *Radiation Res.*, **29**, 236.

Sakai, S. and Masaki, N. (1971), "Proposal for a TNM Classification and its Extended Application for Maliganant Tumours of the Head and Neck Regions," *Acto oto-laryng.* (Stockh.), **72**, 370.

Scharf, B. and Stevens, J. C. (1961), "The Form of the Loudness Function Near Threshold," *Proc. III Int. Congr. Acoustics*, Vol. 1. Amsterdam: Elsevier.

Scheiblechner, H. (1974), "The Validity of the 'Energy Principle' for Noise-induced Hearing Loss," *Audiology*, **13**, 93.

Sellars, S. L. (1969), "The Closure of Tympanic Membrane Perforations by Cautery—A Reappraisal," *J. Laryng.*, **83**, 487.

Simpson, R. H. (1963), "Stability in Meanings for quantitative Terms: A Comparison Over 20 Years," *Q. J. Speech*, **49**, 146.

Stevens, S. S. (1946), "On the Theory of Scales of Measurement," *Science*, **103**, 677.

Stevens, S. S. (1951), "Mathematics, Measurement and Psychophysics," Chapter 1 in *Handbook of Experimental Psychology* (S. S. Stevens, Ed.). New York: Wiley.

Stevens, S. S. (1962), "In Pursuit of the Sensory Law." Second Public Klopsteg Lecture. Northwestern University, Evanston, Ill., U.S.A.

UICC (1968), *TNM Classification of Malignant Tumours*. Geneva: Union International Contre le Cancer.

UICC (1973), *Supplement to TNM Classification of Malignant Tumours*. Geneva: Union International Contre le Cancer.

2. STATISTICS

R. HINCHCLIFFE

The word "statistics" has, unfortunately, three meanings. First, it may refer to quantitative data affected to a marked extent by a multiplicity of causes. Secondly, it may refer to a set (usually a pair or a triad) of numbers which specifies a large body of data. Thirdly, it may be used to describe that branch of mathematical knowledge which is able to draw rigorous conclusions from variable material, the conclusions being framed in terms of *probability*. Probability refers to the likelihood that some event will occur or that some proposition is true. It is expressed on a scale of 0–1 where "0" denotes a complete impossibility and "1" a complete certainty that something will happen or is true. Events that have a "50–50" chance, i.e. even chance, of happening, e.g. a coin coming down heads after tossing it, would have a probability of 0·5, usually written as $p = 0·5$. Similarly, an event which has a 1 in 20 chance of happening would be written as $p = 0·05$ and a 1 in 100 chance as $p = 0·01$.

Applications of the statistical method can be classified into three categories, which are not distinct but merge into one another, i.e. *Descriptive Statistics, Analytical* (or *Inferential*) *Statistics* and *Predictive Statistics*.

Descriptive Statistics refers to the condensation of a large body of data into a few numbers (statistics) which present the relevant information. Analytical Statistics deals with methods that enable conclusions to be drawn from a mass of data. The application of statistics for predictive purposes requires an intimate knowledge of the particular situation for which the prediction is made.

DESCRIPTIVE STATISTICS

Whereas a *constant* is a quantity which always has the same value (e.g. π, the ratio of a circle's circumference to its diameter, which equals approximately 3·1416), a *variable* is a quantity which, as its name implies, does not take a fixed value. Thus the term variable may, for example, refer to the sex of a person or his hearing level measured by bone conduction at 500 Hz. Although variables are frequently used as synonymous with *measures*, Stevens (1951) sought to distinguish between a measure and an *indicant*. An indicant is a correlate bearing an unknown relationship to an underlying phenomenon. Thus, for example, the most comfortable loudness level shows an inverse correlation with phonophobia and therefore might be regarded as an indicant of the latter. Once the actual relationship has been established, e.g. that of a frequency scale in hertz to the pitch scale in mels, then the indicant of pitch (the frequency scale) becomes known as a *calibrated indicant*. The more mature a science, the more it makes use of calibrated indicants.

The term *variate* is sometimes used as synonymous with variable but, strictly speaking, the term should only be used when referring to a quantity with which a specific probability distribution is associated, e.g. the height of individuals or their hearing levels.

Numerical taxonomy (Sokal and Sneath, 1963), which is a special branch of statistics dealing with quantitative methods for classification purposes, refers to measures and indicants as *attributes* or *characters*. Moreover, it subdivides characters into quantitative, qualitative or binary characters. *Quantitative characters* are those which are measurable on ordinal, interval or ratio scales (*see* Chapter 1). Qualitative characters are measurable on nominal scales and the binary character is one which can assume one of two states only, e.g. present or absent; positive or negative.

Presentation of Data

In addition to presenting statistical data in the form of tables, they may be presented visually in forms dependent on whether we are dealing with:

(1) the proportionate breakdown of a given total value,
(2) a time series,
(3) the relationship between two variates, or
(4) a frequency distribution.

The *proportionate breakdown* of a given total value, e.g. the different findings at operation during revision stapedectomy, can be conveniently represented in a *pie chart* (Fig. 1).

A *time series*, e.g. the number of tympanoplasties performed each year, may be represented pictorially by pictograms, by graphs or by bar charts. A *pictogram* involves the use of pictures to represent data. The same picture, always of the same size, is shown repeatedly. The quantity represented is indicated by the number of pictures shown. A picture would represent one or several units of the quantity being measured and fractions of the picture would indicate appropriate fractions of the unit. Thus, in our example, the drawing of an eardrum could represent

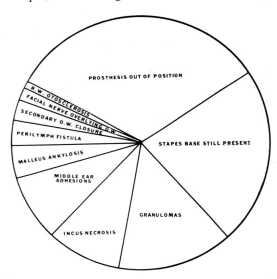

Fig. 1. Pie-chart showing proportionate breakdown of findings at operation during revision stapedectomy. (After Feldman and Schuknecht, 1970.)

20 tympanoplasties and a quarter of an eardrum drawing five tympanoplasties. However, a time series is perhaps best represented by a *graph*, i.e. a continuous line joining the data points. It is frequently convenient to smooth out a time series, e.g. the monthly incidence of acute otitis media, by performing a moving (running) average on the data. Several examples of this are shown in Chapter 10. Figure 2 shows the effects of applying a moving average to the monthly incidence data of Bell's palsy in Alexandria. The effect here is to exclude the irregular monthly fluctuations and make a seasonal fluctuation more clearly discernible. A moving average treatment of data is performed by summing

the first n observations and dividing by n. This gives a trend value for the middle period of the n observations, i.e. for the period corresponding to the $\left(\dfrac{n+1}{2}\right)$th observation. The calculation of the next moving average is then done for the next period by taking the next n observations after

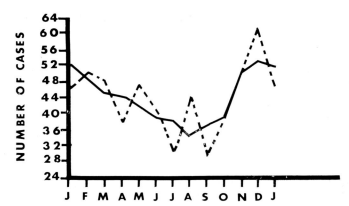

Fig. 2. Monthly incidence of Bell's palsy. The interrupted line represents actual values; the continuous line shows a three-monthly moving average. (After El-Ebiary, 1971.)

excluding the first observation in the series. In looking for seasonal fluctuations in monthly incidence data, the author has found it convenient to give n a value of 3. This is the same as saying that the "smoothed" value for a given month is obtained by taking the value for that particular month, together with the values for each month on either side and then calculating the average for these three values. A *bar chart* uses vertical bars, which are separated from one another. The height of a given bar is directly related to the variable which it represents.

The relationship between two *variates* is best presented visually in the form of a graph, where the horizontal (x) axis or abscissa represents the independent variable and the vertical (y) axis or ordinate represents the dependent variable. The two axes together are known as the co-ordinates. Points corresponding to each pair of values (x_i, y_i) for the two variates, are plotted on the graph. The purpose is to see from inspection whether or not there appears to be any relationship between the two variates. If there does appear to be a relationship, the first question is "Is the curve which could be fitted to the data a straight line or, at any rate, not significantly different from a straight line?" Statistical tests can be applied to ascertain whether or not a straight line is the curve of best fit to the data and, if so, the *method of least squares* (*see* later) can be applied to specify precisely the equation of this line of best fit. Strictly speaking, if, in such a visual presentation of the data, the points are not joined, or otherwise fitted, by a line (or family of curves or lines), then the figure is known as a *scattergraph* (Fig. 3) or scatter diagram. Use of different symbols for paired values (x_i, y_i) or of different lines (a family of curves) enables a third variable (z) to be included. Thus a point then indicates three quantities (x_i, y_i, z_i). Needless to say, the variable z must, in such a case, be restricted to representing discrete steps. In these cases where a third variable is represented, this variable is sometimes referred to as a *parameter*. This is in accord with at least one dictionary definition of the term which defines it as "a quantity which is constant in a particular case considered, but which varies in different cases", i.e. a parameter is both a constant and a variable! This is readily understandable in a given case since a given curve of the family of curves would have an equation in which a particular value of z would appear as a constant in that equation. However, z would have a different value in the other equations relating

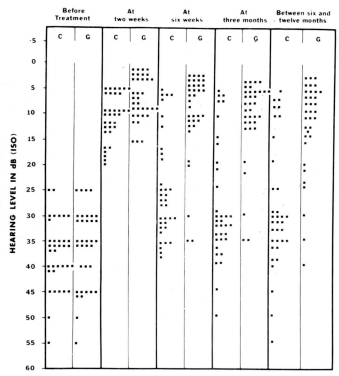

FIG. 3. Scatter diagram showing distribution of hearing levels in control ears (C) and in ears with grommets (G) at two weeks, six weeks, three months and between six and twelve months post-operatively. Indicated hearing levels are the average for those at frequencies of 500, 1000 and 2000 Hz. (After Shah, 1971.)

to each of the other curves in that family. Nevertheless, perhaps in view of the misgivings about the use of the word "parameter" which were expressed in a leading article in the *British Medical Journal* in 1966, the use of the term should be restricted to variables which partly or wholly characterize a probability distribution (Armitage, 1973). Incidentally, Hogben suggested the word *metameter* to designate a measurement, or transformation of such measurement, that is used in evaluating biological tests (Bacharach *et al.*, 1942).

A *frequency distribution* can be illustrated visually by a *histogram*. The values of the variable are represented on the horizontal scale and the frequency, i.e. a relative or absolute number of observations, on the vertical scale. Where discrete, ungrouped variables are concerned, as in a *binomial* or a *Poisson* distribution, a *line histogram* should be used. Where continuously variable, but grouped, measures are concerned, as in a *Gaussian* distribution, a *rectangular*

histogram should be used. (These three different types of probability distributions are discussed later). If instead of the steps shown on a rectangular histogram, it is desired to represent the data by a single curve, the mid-points of the tops of the rectangles are joined by straight lines. This produces the *frequency polygon*. A smoothed frequency polygon is known as a *frequency curve*. A *cumulative frequency curve* or *ogive* is the name given to the curve obtained when the cumulative frequencies of a distribution are graphed. In the case of a Gaussian distribution, the ogive is sigmoid (*see* Fig. 18) when plotted on a linear scale. Thus the normal articulation function of the speech audiogram resembles an ogive. Indeed, Alusi and his colleagues (1974) have presented evidence that the form of the normal speech audiometric curve with word lists in any language is that of a cumulative frequency distribution.

Binomial Distribution

The binomial distribution is applicable to cases where one knows both the number of times an event did occur and the number of times it did not. With one toss of a coin, the probability of it coming down heads and not tails is 0·5 (denoted by $p = 0·5$), and the probability of it coming down tails and not heads is also 0·5 (denoted by $q = 0·5$). The probability of either happening is unity ($p + q$). For two tosses of a coin, the possibilities are two heads and no tails (probability $= p^2$), one head and one tail (probability $= 2pq$) and no heads but two tails (probability $= q^2$),

i.e.
$$p^2 + 2pq + q^2 = 1 \qquad (2.1)$$

This expression is of course the expansion of

$$(p + q)^2 \qquad (2.2)$$

Thus n tosses of the coin would give possible combinations and probabilities determined by the expansion of $(p + q)^n$. As Armitage (1973) points out, a particular example of this binomial distribution is the sex distribution in families of 4. The possible composition of such families are: 4 girls; one boy and 3 girls; 2 of each sex; 3 boys and one girl; or, all boys. These five composition types have probabilities of

$$p^4 + 4p^3q + 6p^2q^2 + 4pq^3 + q^4 \qquad (2.3)$$

i.e. the expansion of

$$(p + q)^4 \qquad (2.4)$$

where p = probability of boy at birth in general population and q = probability of girl at birth in general population. If values of 0·51 and 0·49 are assigned to p and q respectively, then the probabilities come out at 0·0576 (all girls), 0·24 (one boy, 3 girls), 0·3747 (2 boys, 2 girls), 0·26 (one girl, 3 boys) and 0·0677 (all boys). The numerical coefficients, termed the binomial coefficients, in the above equations, i.e. 1, 4, 6, 4 and 1, can be determined from a table known as Pascal's Triangle, after the French mathematician who devised it. This binomial coefficient is often indicated as $\binom{n}{k}$, which is a shorthand way of saying the number of combinations of n things taken k at a time.

Poisson Distribution

There are a number of conditions in which, as for the binomial distribution, the number of times an event did occur is known, but, unlike the binomial distribution, the number of times it did not occur is not known. For these conditions, the Poisson distribution is applicable. This is named after another French mathematician, Poisson (1781–1840) who showed that a particular distribution can describe the occurrence of isolated events in a continuum. If the expected or average number of occurrences of an event is z, then the probability of observing the occurrences of 0, 1, 2, 3, etc., events is given by the successive terms of the expansion:

$$e^{-z}, ze^{-z}, \frac{z^2}{2!} \cdot e^{-z}, \frac{z^3}{3!} \cdot e^{-z} \dots \frac{z^n}{n!} \cdot e^{-z} \quad (2.5)$$

Note that "2!" means *factorial* 2. A factorial number is the product of an integer number and all lower integers, excluding zero. (But factorial zero is taken as unity.) For example, "3!" means $3 \times 2 \times 1$. Characteristically, the Poisson distribution has a single parameter, z, which represents both the mean and the variance (*see* later). In 1957, Bateman reported the number of times he had had to perform myringotomy (equivalent to the occurrence of an event) in 54 ears affected by secretory otitis media. The actual data are tabulated in Table 1 and shown also in Fig. 4 (line histogram). Thus 54 ears required a total of 70 myringotomies, which gives an average (z) number of

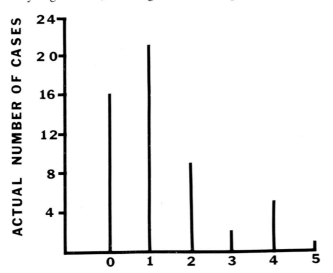

Fig. 4. Line histogram showing distribution of cases (ears) which required the stated number of myringotomies (horizontal axis) in treatment of secretory otitis media. (After Bateman, 1957.)

myringotomies per ear of 1·3. If a Poisson distribution applies to these circumstances, the probabilities of requiring 0, 1, 2, 3, 4 and 5 myringotomies are given by the successive terms:

$$e^{-1\cdot3}, 1\cdot3e^{-1\cdot3}, \frac{(1\cdot3)^2 e^{-1\cdot3}}{2!}, \frac{(1\cdot3)^4 e^{-1\cdot3}}{3!},$$

$$\frac{(1\cdot3)^4 e^{-1\cdot3}}{4!} \text{ and } \frac{(1\cdot3)^5 e^{-1\cdot3}}{5!} \quad (2.6)$$

i.e. 0·27, 0·35, 0·23, 0·1, 0·03 and 0·008 respectively. Since there were a total of 54 ears, the expected number of ears requiring 0, 1, 2, 3, 4 and 5 myringotomies is $54 \times 0\cdot27$, $54 \times 0\cdot35$, $54 \times 0\cdot23$, $54 \times 0\cdot1$, $54 \times 0\cdot03$ and $54 \times 0\cdot008$ respectively, i.e. 15, 19, 12, 5, 2 and 0 (to the nearest whole numbers) (Table 3 and Fig. 5). Thus the number of

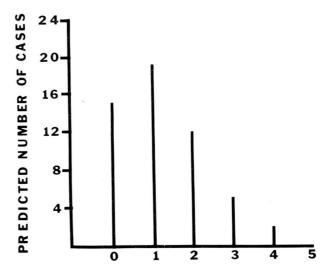

Fig. 5. Line histogram of distribution of predicted number of cases (ears) which would require myringotomy on the assumption that the distribution shown in Fig. 4 is a Poisson one.

myringotomies which Bateman found were required to treat secretory otitis media agrees fairly well with a Poisson distribution.

TABLE 1

ACTUAL AND THEORETICAL (BASED ON POISSON DISTRIBUTION) NUMBER OF EARS REQUIRING STATED NUMBER OF MYRINGOTOMIES IN A SERIES OF CHILDREN WITH SECRETORY OTITIS MEDIA

(After Bateman, 1957)

No. of Myringotomies	No. of Ears Requiring Stated No. of Myringotomies	
	Actual	Theoretical
0	16	15
1	21	19
2	9	12
3	2	5
4	5	2
5	1	0

The goodness of fit of data to a Poisson distribution can be tested either visually or numerically. Plotting the data on Poisson probability paper gives a vertical straight line if the data is so distributed. The usual statistical test is "Student"* (1907) Poisson heterogeneity test. For class

* The pseudonym of W. S. Gossett.

values of less than 5, Fisher's exact test should be used (*see later*).

Gaussian Distribution

In contrast to the binomial and Poisson distributions, which both relate to a discrete variable, the Gaussian distribution relates to a continuous probability distribution. In other words, the Gaussian (or *normal*) distribution relates to quantities whose magnitude is continuously variable, e.g. height or hearing level. This particular distribution is frequently attributed to Gauss (1777–1855), the German mathematician. The distribution was, however, independently discovered by both de Moivre (an Englishman of French origin) and by Laplace (the French mathematician) in 1733.

Figure 6 shows a rectangular histogram relating to the distribution of air conduction hearing levels at 500 Hz for ears in a random sample of the general population which gave a Rinne positive response but which showed scarring or perforation of the tympanic membrane. The histogram is unimodal, i.e. has only one peak, and is roughly symmetrical. This is the pattern of a Gaussian distribution.

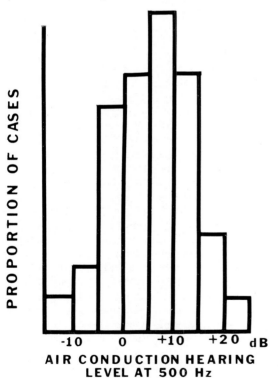

FIG. 6. Rectangular histogram showing actual air conduction hearing levels at 500 Hz for ears in a random sample of the general population which gave a Rinne positive response but showed scarring or perforation of the tympanic membrane. (After Hinchcliffe and Littler, 1961.)

Figure 7 shows not only the Gaussian distribution curve which has been fitted to this particular histogram but also a Gaussian curve fitted to another histogram for similar, but Rinne negative, ears in the same random sample population. Each curve is bell shaped and is characterized by two measures only, i.e. the mean ($\bar{x}$) and the standard deviation (σ). These are sometimes referred to as parameters of *central tendency* and of *dispersion* respectively. (A parameter of central tendency refers to one or other of the

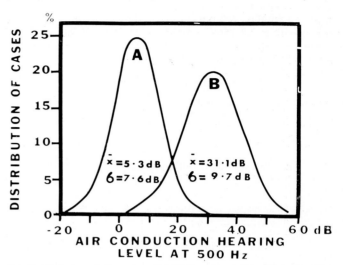

FIG. 7. Bell-shaped Gaussian distribution curve (A) which has been fitted to the data shown in Fig. 6. In addition, there is a second Gaussian curve (B) which has been fitted to similar data in the same random sample of a general population but which refers to ears giving a Rinne negative response. (After Hinchcliffe and Littler, 1961.)

"average" values. Dispersion refers to the spread of values.) These two measures uniquely describe a Gaussian curve. Not only do the two curves shown in Fig. 7 have different means, i.e. averages (5·3 and 31·1 dB), but also different standard deviations (7·6 and 9·7 dB). The greater standard deviation in the case of "B" serves to make that curve squatter. Populations which have different standard deviations are said to be *heteroscedastic*; those which have the same standard deviation are *homoscedastic*.

There are a number of measures of dispersion (i.e scatter or variation) of data, viz. the *range*, the *interquartile distance*, the *mean deviation*, the *variance* and the *standard deviation*. The range, i.e. the difference between the maximum and minimum values of a measurement, has three disadvantages. First, it is based on two only of the original observations. Secondly, it will depend on the number of observations. Thirdly, calculations based on extremes are undependable. The interquartile distance avoids the disadvantages inherent in using extreme values. It is the distance between the lower quartile (Q_1), i.e. the value below which one-quarter of the ordered observations fall, and the upper quartile (Q_3), i.e. the value above which one-quarter of the ordered observations fall. It is better, however, to use all the deviations from the mean, i.e. ($x_i - \bar{x}$), where the subscript for the first x tells us that we are dealing with an array of numbers, and the bar over the second x identifies it as the mean. Since the mean of the deviations will always be zero, one must ignore the sign in counting these deviations, i.e. the mean deviation is

$$\frac{\sum_{i=1}^{n} |x_i - \bar{x}|}{n} \quad \text{or, more simply,} \quad \frac{\sum |x_i - \bar{x}|}{n} \quad (2.7)$$

where the vertical lines indicate that the sign of the value between them is ignored and the Greek capital letter sigma means "the sum of". Division by the total number of observations (n) gives the mean deviation. Unfortunately, this parameter is difficult to handle mathematically. A more easily handled parameter is the *variance*. This is the mean value of the squared deviations. The *standard deviation* is the square root of the variance and is frequently denoted by the small Greek letter sigma, σ.

$$\sigma = \sqrt{[\{\sum(x_i - \bar{x})^2\}/(n - 1)]} \qquad (2.8)$$

Since
$$\sum(x_i - \bar{x})^2 = \sum x^2 - (\sum x)^2/n \qquad (2.9)$$

Equation (2.8) can be expressed as

$$\sigma = \sqrt{[\{\sum x^2 - (\sum x)^2/n\}/(n - 1)]} \qquad (2.10)$$

This equation will be found more useful in actual calculations. Note that, instead of "n" as denominator, we have $(n - 1)$. This is a consequence of statistical methods of inference where the collection of observations being analysed is considered to be a sample drawn from a much larger group (*population*) of measurements. A better estimate of the population variance is obtained by using the devisor $(n - 1)$ instead of n. For normally distributed (i.e. Gaussian) measurements, two-thirds of measurements lie within plus or minus one standard deviation of the mean, 95 per cent within two standard deviations and less than 1 per cent more than three standard deviations away from the mean. The equation for a Gaussian curve is

$$y_i = \frac{1}{\sigma\sqrt{(2\pi)}} \cdot e^{-\frac{(x_i - \bar{x})^2}{2\sigma^2}} \qquad (2.11)$$

where y_i = height of curve at point x_i along scale of x, i.e. the probability associated with that particular value x_i of the variate x.

σ = standard deviation of x

π = ratio of circumference of a circle to its diameter (approx. 3·1416)

and e = base of natural (Napierian) logarithms (approx. 2·7183).

Since the equation for a normal curve involves the value "e", the equation is a particular case of an *exponential function*. For typographical reasons, the expression "exp" should be used for the exponential function when the argument (in this case, $(x_i - \bar{x})^2/2\sigma^2$) is larger than a single compact group of symbols. Thus the Gaussian curve equation may be written:

$$y_i = [1/\{\sigma\sqrt{(2\pi)}\}] \exp -\{(x_i - \bar{x})^2/(2\sigma^2)\} \qquad (2.12)$$

In practice, it will be found more convenient to have a Gaussian distribution expression which is applicable to histograms, where values of the variate are grouped. In this case

$$n_i = [(Nd_i)/\{\sigma\sqrt{(2\pi)}\}] \exp -\{(x_i - \bar{x})^2/(2\sigma^2)\} \qquad (2.13)$$

where n_i = number of expected observations in the particular histogram rectangle, i.e. cell group or class interval, which is centred on x_i, the mean value of class interval of width d_i.

N = total observations made.

The Gaussian distribution is of the utmost importance in statistics as a prerequisite to the application of statistical tests, since many powerful tests depend on the assumption that the variates concerned are normally distributed. It is therefore mandatory that a set of measurements be examined to see whether or not they conform to a Gaussian distribution. If they do not, then the next step would be to see how a transformation of the measurements could be made to obtain a Gaussian distribution.

Five procedures can be adopted to see how well a Gaussian curve fits the data:

(1) Visual inspection,
(2) Plotting on *arithmetical probability paper*,
(3) Calculating a *coefficient* of *kurtosis*,
(4) Applying a χ^2 (chi-squared) test (*see* later), and
(5) Tukey's "*hanging rootogram*" (Healy, 1968).
(6) Calculating a *coefficient of skewness*.

It has already been mentioned that a histogram showing the frequency distribution of a variate should be unimodal, symmetrical and of a particular bell-shped configuration. Few variates have other than unimodal distributions. An exception is, for example, the threshold of taste for phenylthiourea (phenylthiocarbamide), which is bimodally distributed. Thus this particular taste threshold cannot be normally distributed. The many unimodal distributions found in medicine in general, and in otolaryngology in particular, may not be symmetrical. They are said to be *skewed*. Skewness and the question of whether or not they can be transformed to a Gaussian distribution will be discussed later. If the frequency distribution of the data appears to be unimodally and symmetrically distributed, then it should be plotted on arithmetical probability paper (Fig. 8). Here the cumulative percentage distribution is plotted on a graph paper that is so constructed that the characteristic sigmoid curve of the ogive (cumulative frequency distribution) is straightened out to a straight line curve. As a corollary, data which are plotted on this type of graph paper and do not conform to a straight line are not normally distributed. Figure 8 shows that a straight line can be fitted to the cumulative percentage distribution of our example of air conduction hearing levels at 500 Hz.

Kurtosis describes the peakedness of a distribution. If the distribution is narrow humped, it is said to be *leptokurtic*, if broad humped, *platykurtic*. Kurtosis represents a departure from a normal distribution and should not be confused with the slenderness or otherwise of normal (Gaussian) distributions. This latter feature is expressed as Pearson's *coefficient of variation* (the ratio of the standard deviation to the mean expressed as a percentage). The degree of kurtosis is measured by the fourth moment (the first moment about the origin is the mean itself, the second moment about the mean is the variance and the third moment is used in measuring the degree of skewness) divided by the fourth power of the standard deviation, i.e.

the coefficient of kurtosis $c = \{\sum(x_i - \bar{x})^4\}/n\sigma^4$ (2.14)

This coefficient has a value of 3 for a Gaussian distribution. Values in excess of 3 indicate a leptokurtic, and less than 3 a platykurtic, distribution.

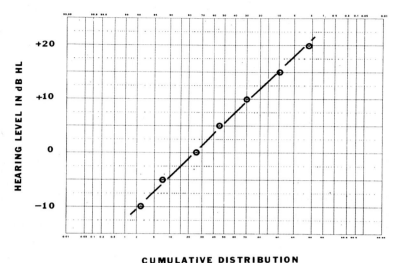

FIG. 8. Cumulative percentage distribution of data shown in histogram form in Fig. 6 which is here plotted on arithmetical probability paper. Note that the plotted points conform to a straight line.

The χ^2 test is mentioned later. In Tukey's "hanging rootogram", the frequencies are plotted on a square root scale with the observed frequencies "hanging down" from the expected values. About 95 per cent of the discrepancies between observed and expected values should lie within the range -1 to $+1$, which are represented by two parallel lines above and below the horizontal axis.

Skewness, i.e. asymmetry, of a distribution can be measured by tests based on the knowledge that only with a completely symmetrical distribution will the mean, median and mode coincide (the mean is the "average", the median is the middle observation when the values for the variate are arranged in decreasing order, and the mode is the value of the variate where the frequency distribution reaches a peak). These measures are

(1) Pearson's coefficient of skewness

$$k = (\bar{x} - m)/\sigma \qquad (2.15)$$

where $\bar{x}$ = arithmetic mean

m = mode

and σ = standard deviation

(2) Modified Pearson coefficient

$$k = \{3(\bar{x} - w)\}/\sigma \qquad (2.16)$$

where w = median,

(3) Bowley's coefficient of skewness

$$k = \{2(Q_3 + Q_1 - 2Q_2)\}/(Q_3 - Q_1) \qquad (2.17)$$

where Q_1 = first quartile

Q_2 = second quartile, i.e. median (w of equation 2.16)

Q_3 = third quartile

(4) Third moment about the mean divided by the cube of the standard deviation to convert it to a relative form, i.e.

$$k = \{\sum(x_i - \bar{x})^3\}/n\sigma^3 \qquad (2.18)$$

For symmetrical distributions, the above coefficients will be zero; for a distribution skewed to the right, i.e. where the mean, median and a longer tail are to the right of the mode, the coefficient will be positive, for one skewed to the left, it will be negative. (This terminology of the direction of skew is, of course, the converse of what one might expect.) However, visual inspection of a histogram will usually indicate where a distribution is significantly skewed. Thus Fig. 9 shows a histogram of middle ear compliances

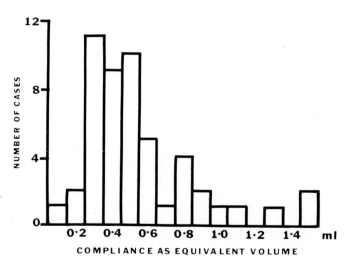

FIG. 9. Rectangular histogram of middle ear compliances (measured as equivalent volume) of a population of young Thai adults. The volumes along the horizontal axis indicate the lower boundaries of the data groups (categories) which are denoted by the appropriate rectangles. The size of each of these classes is 0·1 ml. Note the skewing (termed "skewed to the right"). (After Prasansuk, 1974.)

(measured as equivalent volume) of a population of young Thai adults. The histogram is clearly positively skewed. In such cases, the first thing to do is to take a logarithmic transform of the variate (in this case, equivalent volume in ml). A Gaussian curve of best fit is then calculated and the best theoretical histogram for such a logarithmic transformed variate is shown in Fig. 10 (the variate has

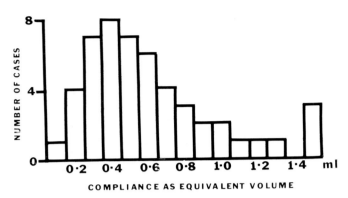

FIG. 10. Rectangular histogram corresponding to best-fit Gaussian distribution of the logarithmically transformed variate (equivalent volume) of data shown in Fig. 9. (The variate has been converted back to the linear measurement for comparison with Fig. 9.)

been converted back to the linear measurement in ml for purposes of comparison with the original data). A broadly-similar skewed histogram has been produced. However, other transformations of the variate are possible in order to convert skewed distributions into symmetrical ones. It is in the selection of the particular transformation that knowledge of the particular branch of science involved is so

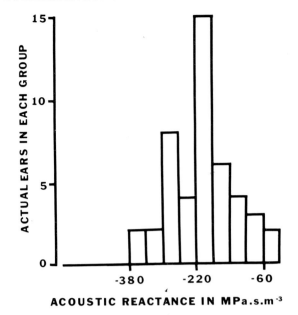

FIG. 12. Histogram of transformed measures of data shown in Fig. 9. Note that the transformation from equivalent volume to MPa.s.m^{-3} is associated with eradication of the skewness.

show a basically normal (Gaussian) distribution. A histogram (Fig. 12) shows an essentially symmetrical curve, for such transformed measures, in contrast to the skewed curve (Fig. 9) for the untransformed measures in

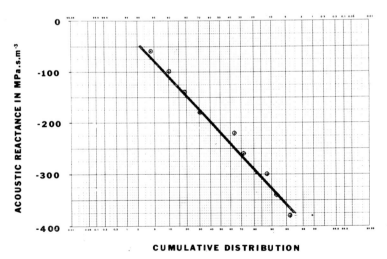

FIG. 11. Cumulative percentage distribution of data shown in Fig. 9 which is here expressed in terms of acoustic reactance in MPa.s.m^{-3} (a reciprocal function of equivalent volume).

valuable. The equivalent volume which is used as a measure of the acoustic compliance of the middle ear is in fact inversely related to the acoustic reactance of the middle ear. Thus we should look at the frequency distribution of these measures after converting to MPa.s.m^{-3}. Figure 11 shows such transformed measures plotted on arithmetical probability paper. The data conform reasonably well to a straight line, indicating that such transformed measures

millilitres. The best fit (to a Gaussian distribution) of this data is shown in histogram form in Fig. 13 and, when the best fit Gaussian distribution is transformed back to measures as equivalent volumes we have the histogram shown in Fig. 14. Visual comparison of this histogram and that of Fig. 10 (derived from a logarithmic transform) with the histogram from the original data (Fig. 9) indicates that the histogram of Fig. 14 is a better representation.

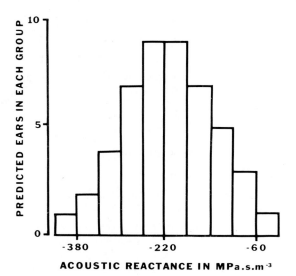

FIG. 13. Histogram of best-fit Gaussian distribution of data shown in Fig. 12.

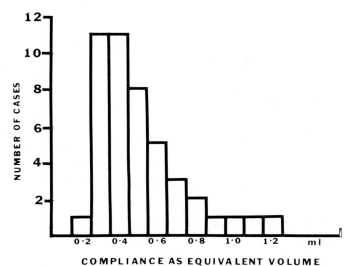

FIG. 14. Histogram showing distribution of predicted number of cases based on the assumption that the measures shown in Fig. 9 are normally distributed when expressed in terms of acoustic reactance, but with conversion of values derived from the best-fit Gaussian distribution in SI acoustic impedance units back to equivalent volume. Note that the frequency distribution in this figure shows a greater similarity to that in Fig. 9 than does that of Fig. 10.

ANALYTICAL STATISTICS

The principal value of analytical statistics in otolarnygology is to assess the value of diagnostic tests and to compare different methods of treatment. In the future, one may hope to see in otolaryngology an extension from general medicine of disease diagnosis using Bayesian, or other, statistics.

Assessment of Tests

A valuable diagnostic test is one that, *inter alia*, is valid, reliable and sensitive. *Validity* of a test refers to the ability of the test to measure that which it sets out to measure. The validity of a new test is usually determined by seeing how well it correlates with other tests which are used to measure a particular function. Thus validity is sometimes considered to be synonymous with accuracy and to be a measure of the closeness with which a measured value agrees with the "true" value (Bahn, 1972). *Reliability* means the degree of reproducibility of the test, i.e. the test-retest reliability. It can thus be measured by the degree of correlation of the measures obtained from the first and second (or subsequent) applications of a test. *Sensitivity* is discussed in Chapter 10.

Depending upon the scales of measurement involved, the degree of relationship between two variables can be expressed quantitatively as

(1) *Contingency correlations* (for measurements on nominal scales)
(2) *Order correlations* (for measurements on ordinal scales)
(3) *Product-moment correlations* (for measurements on interval scales).

Two contingency correlation coefficients for two dichotomous variables, i.e. *A, not A, B* and *not B*, and due to Yule are (i) *coefficient of association* and (ii) *coefficient of colligation*.

The coefficient of association is given by

$$Q = (ad - bc)/(ad + bc) \qquad (2.19)$$

where $a = A \text{ and } B$

$b = B \text{ and } not\ A$

$c = A \text{ and } not\ B$

$d = not\ A \text{ and } not\ B$

TABLE 2

A 2 × 2 CONTINGENCY (FOURFOLD) TABLE

	A	*not A*
B	a	b
not B	c	d

as shown in Table 2, for which the standard error is given by

$$\varepsilon = \{(1 - Q^2)/2\} \Big/ \sqrt{\left(\frac{1}{a} + \frac{1}{b} + \frac{1}{c} + \frac{1}{d}\right)} \qquad (2.20)$$

The coefficient of colligation is given by

$$Y = \{1 - \sqrt{(bc/ad)}\}/\{1 + \sqrt{(bc/ad)}\} \qquad (2.21)$$

and for this the standard error is given by

$$\varepsilon = \{(1 - Y^2)/4\} \sqrt{\Big/\left(\frac{1}{a} + \frac{1}{b} + \frac{1}{c} + \frac{1}{d}\right)} \qquad (2.22)$$

An example of the application of these coefficients of association and colligation is shown in Table 3, where the data refer to the results of the Weber and Rinne tests on a random sample population.

The coefficient of association in this example is given by

$$Q = \{(9 \times 684) - (25 \times 4)\}/ \quad (2.23)$$
$$\{(9 \times 684) + (25 \times 4)\}$$

i.e. $Q = \underline{0.97}$ (2.24)

TABLE 3

A 2 × 2 CONTINGENCY TABLE IN RESPECT OF TUNING FORK RESPONSES OF A RANDOM SAMPLE OF A RURAL POPULATION
(After Hinchcliffe and Littler, 1961)

Lateralization to Suspect Ear	Rinne Response		
	True Negative	Otherwise	Total
Yes	9	25	34
No	4	684	688
TOTAL	13	709	722

with a standard error of 0·02. This means that the true value of the coefficient of association lies between two standard errors of the calculated value, i.e. in the range 0·93 and 1·01. The latter value is, however, impossible since the coefficient cannot exceed the value of unity. Thus one should say that the true value of the coefficient of association lies between 0·93 and 1·0. The coefficient of colligation based upon the same example is given by

$$Y = [1 - \sqrt{\{(25 \times 4)/(9 \times 684)\}}]/ \quad$$
$$[1 + \sqrt{\{(25 \times 4)/(9 \times 684)\}}] \quad (2.25)$$

i.e. $Y = \underline{0.77}$ (2.26)

with a standard error given by

$$\varepsilon = [\{1 - 0.77)^2\}/4] \sqrt{\left(\frac{1}{9} + \frac{1}{25} + \frac{1}{4} + \frac{1}{684}\right)} = 0.06 \ (2.27)$$

Thus we see that when we compare the Weber and Rinne test results with one another, the measure of correlation with one statistical test is 0·97, with a standard error of 0·02; with another test, 0·77, with a standard error of 0·06.

In view of the difference in values obtained by these two coefficients it is important that the particular coefficients used should be specified.

For variables on ordinal scales, a number of measures of correlation are available. *Spearman's rank order*, or *rank-difference, correlation coefficient*, ρ (rho), is given by

$$\rho = 1 - [6\sum d^2/\{n(n^2 - 1)\}] \quad (2.28)$$

where d = difference between the rankings of the same item in each series,

and n = number of items ranked.

Where ties occur, i.e. equal rankings are given, a correction factor must be introduced. This gives a tie-corrected correlation coefficient, $\rho_{corr.}$, where

$$\rho_{corr} = \{n(n^2 - 1) - 6\sum d^2 - 6(t' + u')\}/$$
$$\sqrt{[\{n(n^2 - 1) - 12t'\}}$$
$$\{n(n^2 - 1) - 12u'\}] \quad (2.29)$$

where t' and u' are tie-corrections for the first and second variables respectively, and where

$$t' = \sum[\{t^2(t - 1)\}/12] \quad (2.30)$$

and $u' = \sum[\{u^2(u - 1)\}/12] \quad (2.31)$

Where $n \geqslant 10$, the significance of ρ is given by

$$t = \rho\sqrt{\{(n - 2)/(1 - \rho^2)\}} \quad (2.32)$$

where t = Student's t (*see* later) and is distributed with $(n - 2)$ degrees of freedom.

Rank order coefficients can also be used to compare two variables where one is on an ordinal scale and the other is on an interval or ratio scale. For example, a study was recently made of blood loss during stapedectomy under conventional anaesthesia (Deacock, 1971). Blood in the suction line was washed through into a trap and a sample of these washings compared colorimetrically with a known dilution of the patient's blood. The operation was also timed so that measures of both the total blood loss and the rate of blood loss were available. The surgeon assessed the bleeding according to whether it was "excellent", "very good", "good", "average", "poorish", "poor" or "bad"

TABLE 4

MEASURED BLOOD LOSSES (TOTAL AND RATES) IN A SERIES OF STAPEDECTOMY OPERATIONS UNDER CONVENTIONAL ANAESTHESIA TOGETHER WITH THE SURGEON'S ASSESSMENT OF THE BLOOD LOSS
(After Deacock, 1971)

Surgeon's Assessment	Measured Blood Loss	
	Total	Rate
Excellent	0·46 ml	8·4 μl. min^{-1}
Very good	0·28	6·5
Very good	0·45	7·6
Very good	0·30	10·0
Very good	0·35	15·9
Good	0·67	19·7
Good	0·70	21·2
Good	0·32	22·9
Good	0·58	29·0
Average	0·92	40·0
Average	1·82	55·2
Poorish	0·88	38·3
Poor	1·16	40·0
Poor	2·00	40·8
Poor	1·05	42·0
Poor	0·93	44·3
Poor	1·60	47·1
Poor	1·46	56·2
Bad	1·88	64·8

(Table 4). These qualitative judgements can be considered to represent the rank order of subjective magnitude of blood loss and the measured blood losses can themselves be transformed from actual measures to rank order losses, as in Table 5. Calculation of Spearman's rank order

TABLE 5
TABULATION OF DATA SHOWN IN TABLE 4 IN TERMS OF RANK ORDERS

Rank Orders			Differences		Differences²	
A (Surgeon's Assessment)	B (Total Blood Loss)	C (Rate of Blood Loss)	(A–B)	(A–C)	(A–B)²	(A–C)²
1	6	3	−5·0	−2·0	25	4
3·5	1	1	2·5	2·5	6·25	6·25
3·5	5	2	−1·5	1·5	2·25	2·25
3·5	2	4	1·5	−0·5	2·25	0·25
3·5	4	5	−0·5	−1·5	0·25	2·25
7·5	8	6	−0·5	1·5	0·25	2·25
7·5	9	7	−1·5	0·5	2·25	0·25
7·5	3	8	4·5	−0·5	20·25	0·25
7·5	7	9	0·5	−1·5	0·25	2·25
10·5	11	11·5	−0·5	−1·0	0·25	1
10·5	17	17	−6·5	−6·5	42·25	42·25
12	10	10	2·0	2·0	4·00	4
15·5	14	11·5	1·5	4·0	2·25	16
15·5	19	13	−3·5	2·5	12·25	6·25
15·5	13	14	2·5	1·5	6·25	2·25
15·5	12	15	3·5	0·5	12·25	0·25
15·5	16	16	−0·5	−0·5	0·25	0·25
15·5	15	18	0·5	−2·5	0·25	6·25
19	18	19	1·0	0·0	1	0

correlation coefficient for the surgeon's assessment and the total blood loss gives a value of 0·88 (tie-corrected, 0·87) and for the assessment and the rate of blood loss of 0·91 (with or without tie-correction). A similar study by the same author, but for stapedectomies done under neuroleptanaesthesia, gave results as shown in Tables 6 and 7.

TABLE 6
MEASURED BLOOD LOSSES (TOTALS AND RATES) IN STAPEDECTOMY OPERATIONS UNDER NEUROLEPT-ANAESTHESIA, TOGETHER WITH THE SURGEON'S ASSESSMENT OF THE BLOOD LOSS
(After Deacock, 1971)

Surgeon's Assessment	Measured Blood Loss	
	Total	Rate
Very good	0·34 ml	7·9 μl. min^{-1}
Very good	0·86	14·6
Very good	1·53	21·9
Good	0·73	20·3
Good	0·45	28·1
Good	1·14	30·8
Average	0·95	31·7
Average	0·88	44·0
Fair	2·00	40·0
Fair	1·21	46·5
Poor	1·16	50·4
Bad	3·20	123·0

TABLE 7
TABULATION OF DATA GIVEN IN TABLE 6 IN TERMS OF RANK ORDERS

Rank Orders			Differences		Differences²	
A (Surgeon's Assessment)	B (Total Blood Loss)	C (Rate of Blood Loss)	(A–B)	(A–C)	(A–B)²	(A–C)²
2	1	1	1	1	1	1
2	4	2	−2	0	4	0
2	10	4	−8	−2	64	4
5	3	3	2	2	4	4
5	2	5	3	0	9	0
5	7	6	−2	−1	4	1
7·5	6	7	1·5	0·5	2·25	0·25
7·5	5	9	2·5	−1·5	6·25	2·25
9·5	11	8	−1·5	1·5	2·25	2·25
9·5	9	10	0·5	−0·5	0·25	0·25
11	8	11	3	0	9	0
12	12	12	0	0	0	0
SUM			0	0	106	15

Here, the descriptive terms used by the surgeons were: "Very good", "good", "average", "fair', "poor" and "bad". Spearman's rank order correlation coefficient calculated for the judgements versus the total blood loss and for the judgements versus the rate of blood loss were 0·63 and 0·95 respectively. It would thus appear from this study that a surgeon can assess the rate of blood loss with considerable accuracy. There appears to be a better correlation with rate of blood loss than with total blood loss, at least for these micro-surgical procedures. These results provide an example of the ability of human beings to judge relative frequencies and proportions very accurately (Peterson and Beach, 1967).

Other indices for comparing two sets of measures on ordinal scales are a rank correlation coefficient based upon Kendall's statistic, the Mann–Whitney U test and Wilcoxon's matched-pairs signed ranks test. Salomon (1974) uses Friedman's (1937) rank order test to analyse responses to ERA (electric response audiometry). These tests just mentioned are known as *distribution-free* (i.e. non-parametric) methods since they do not depend upon assumptions that the variate concerned has a particular, e.g. Gaussian, distribution.

Pearson's product-moment correlation coefficient (r) is used to express the degree of relationship between two sets of measures which are measurable on interval or ratio scales. The coefficient provides a measure of the degree of *linear* relationship between the two variates. This coefficient also has a value ranging from −1 to +1. Measures which are completely correlated would have values of +1 or −1, depending on whether the slope of the linear regression is positive or negative. Measures which are completely uncorrelated would have a coefficient of zero. The data for two variates should therefore first be plotted on graph paper to ascertain whether or not any relationship

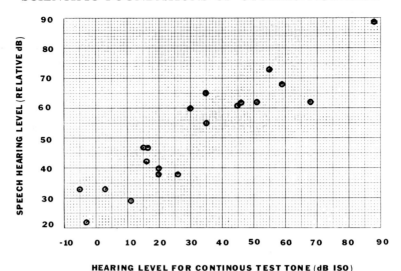

FIG. 15. Scattergraph showing relationship of speech hearing level to the hearing
level for a continuous test tone of 2000 Hz.

appears to exist and to ascertain whether or not this relationship is a linear one. Figure 15 shows such a plot for data on hearing levels for speech material and for continuous, automatically recorded (with a Békésy audiometer) pure tones, which data are also given in Table 8. A basically

TABLE 8

TABULATION OF SPEECH HEARING LEVELS TOGETHER
WITH CORRESPONDING HEARING LEVELS AT 2000 Hz
FOR BOTH CONTINUOUS AND PULSED TEST TONES FOR
A SERIES OF 20 EARS

Speech Hearing Level (in relative decibels) (y_i)	Hearing Level at 2000 Hz (From Békésy Audiogram)	
	Continuous Test Tone (x_i)	Pulsed Test Tone (w_i)
40	20	−10
55	35	33
73	55	55
62	46	35
38	26	25
60	30	30
65	35	33
33	−5	−5
38	20	20
47	15	14
42	16	26
89	88	88
22	−3	−3
29	11	0
33	3	0
62	51	51
68	59	59
47	15	15
61	45	35
62	68	68
1026	630	569

linear relationship appears to hold. (Let us forget for the moment that the decibel scale is a logarithmic scale and use the values as though they were on linear scales for the purposes of our argument.) Pearson's correlation coefficient is equal to the *covariance* of the two variates (x and y, say) divided by the square root of the product of the variances of these two variates,

i.e. $r_{x.y} = (1/n)\{\sum(x_i - \bar{x})(y_i - \bar{y})\}/(\sigma_x . \sigma_y)$ (2.33)

For purposes of facilitating the calculation, this equation can be more conveniently expressed as:

$$r_{x.y} = (n\sum xy - \sum x \sum y)/\sqrt{[\{n\sum x^2 - (\sum x)^2\}}$$
$$\{n\sum y^2 - (\sum y)^2\}]   (2.34)$$

If we consider the two variates, y and x of Table 8, to calculate $r_{x.y}$, we obtain

$$r_{x.y} = (146\ 640)/\sqrt{[\{229\ 340\}}$$
$$\{110\ 324\}] = 0.92   (2.35)$$

Similarly, a correlation coefficient ($r_{w.y}$) calculated for the speech hearing levels (y) and the automatically recorded thresholds using a pulsed test tone (w) gives

$$r_{w.y} = (152\ 926)/\sqrt{[\{261\ 419\}}$$
$$\{110\ 324\}] = 0.90   (2.36)$$

These two values of r show a very high correlation between the measured speech hearing levels and the pure tone hearing levels at 2000 Hz, whether a continuous test tone or a pulsed test tone is used.

Another index, the *coefficient of determination*, provides a measure of association between two variates since it is the ratio of the explained variation to the total variation. This coefficient is the square of Pearson's product–moment correlation coefficient. Thus where, as in our example, $r = 0.92$, then the coefficient of determination is 0.85; where $r = 0.90$, the coefficient of determination is 0.81. This is the same as saying that, in the first case, 85 per cent of the variance in y (speech hearing level) is attributable to the regression of y on x (hearing level for a continuous 2000 Hz test tone); in the second case, 81 per cent of the variance in y is attributable to regression of y on w (hearing level for a pulsed 2000 Hz test tone). In general, it will also be seen that only when $r > 0.7$ will 50 per cent or more of the variance of y be due to the regression of y on x.

Having calculated a correlation coefficient between two variables, we may then wish to determine an equation, termed a *regression equation*, which will enable us to obtain the best prediction of the value of one variate knowing the value of the other variate. However, estimating x from y is not just the reverse of estimating y from x. This is because an estimation of y from x using the regression equation minimizes the sum of the squares (*see Method of Least Squares* later) of the discrepancies in y; an estimation of x from y minimizes the sum of the squares of the discrepancies in x. Thus the regression equation for y on x is

$$(y_i - \bar{y}) = r(\sigma_y/\sigma_x)(x_i - \bar{x}) \qquad (2.37)$$

And for x on y,

$$(x_i - \bar{x}) = r(\sigma_x/\sigma_y)(y_i - \bar{y}) \qquad (2.38)$$

Thus, in our example above, we can predict the speech hearing level (y_i) from the 2000 Hz continuous test tone threshold (x_i) as

$$(y_i - 51) = 0.92(17/24.6)(x_i - 31.5) \qquad (2.39)$$

(Equation (2.10) gives the method for calculating the standard deviations),

i.e. $$y_i = 0.64x_i + 31 \qquad (2.40)$$

Similarly, $(x_i - 31.5) = 0.92(24.6/17)(y_i - 51) \qquad (2.41)$

so that $$x_i = 1.33y_i - 36 \qquad (2.42)$$

Note that equation (2.42) is not the corollary of equation (2.40). If we calculate y_i as a function of x_i from equation (2.42), we obtain

$$y_i = (x_i + 36)/1.33 = 0.75x_i + 27 \qquad (2.43)$$

The degree of uncertainty of regression estimates is assessed by an index known as the *standard error of estimate*. According to whether we are predicting y or x, it is given by

$$S_y = \sigma_y\sqrt{(1 - r^2)} \qquad (2.44)$$

and $$S_x = \sigma_x\sqrt{(1 - r^2)} \qquad (2.45)$$

Thus, for our example,

$$S_y = 17\sqrt{\{1 - (0.92)^2\}} = 6.7 \text{ dB} \qquad (2.46)$$

and $$S_x = 24.6\sqrt{\{1 - (0.92)^2\}} = 9.6 \text{ dB} \qquad (2.47)$$

In about 95 per cent of cases, the actual value will lie within plus or minus two standard errors of the value predicted for the regression equation.

As Oldham (1968) points out, the regression equation is not necessarily the description of a mathematical law connecting two functions. Regression is concerned simply with the behaviour of the average value of a particular variable, the dependent variable, as other quantities are set at different values. The existence of a regression curve may not answer any questions but instead direct attention to questions to be answered. Let us therefore take a fresh look at the regression equation (2.40) in our example. The variates, x and y, are both measured on a logarithmic (decibel) scale, where the values are given by

$$x = 20 \log_{10} (p_x/p_{x_0}) \qquad (2.48)$$

and $$y = 20 \log_{10} (p_y/p_{y_0}) \qquad (2.49)$$

where p_x = sound pressure of 2000 Hz tone at threshold of hearing in pascals.

p_{x_0} = reference sound pressure for the decibel scale used in indicating 2000 Hz tone magnitude in pascals.

p_y = sound pressure of speech material corresponding to 50 per cent intelligibility in pascals.

and p_{y_0} = reference sound pressure for the decibel scale used in indicating speech level in pascals.

If equations (2.48) and (2.49) are substituted in equation (2.40) we obtain

$$20 \log_{10} (p_y/p_{y_0}) = 0.64\{20 \log_{10} (p_x/p_{x_0})\} + 31 \quad (2.50)$$

i.e. $$p_y = (p_x)^{0.64}\{(35.48\, p_{y_0})/(p_{x_0})^{0.64}\} \qquad (2.51)$$

The value of the term within the brackets { }, which is essentially a scaling factor, will depend upon the values of p_{x_0} and of p_{y_0}, i.e. upon the calibration of the two audiometers. Each of these constants could well have values of the order of 50 μPa (equivalent to 8 dB SPL). If this were so, the term in brackets would have a value of unity and equation (2.51) would become

$$p_y = (p_x)^{0.64} \qquad (2.52)$$

Expressed in words this would be "the sound pressure corresponding to the threshold of speech intelligibility is a power function of the sound pressure corresponding to the threshold for a 2000 Hz tone". (Power functions are discussed in Chapter 1.) The fact that there is not a one-to-one ratio may merely reflect that, in the sample studied, the hearing threshold of 2000 Hz deteriorated at a greater rate than the other (lower) frequencies involved in speech perception. (Highly likely since this is what happens in presbyacusis and many other sensorineural hearing losses.)

Another example where a power function might provide a more logical equation relating to variates is in connection with estimates of pre-operative blood loss. We have previously mentioned the study where the subjective magnitude of blood loss at operation was assessed on a category scale. Another study at the same centre required the surgeon to give a subjective estimate of the blood loss in millilitres (Shalom, 1964). The data are reproduced in Table 9 and graphed in Fig. 16. Inspection of the graph shows not only a good correspondence of the surgeon's estimate with the actual measurement of blood loss but also a suggestion that there is a linear relationship. It would therefore seem appropriate to calculate Pearson's product-moment correlation coefficient. Analysis of the data by the methods already described gives a value for this coefficient in this example of 0.83. This indicates a very good correlation. Consultation of Fisher and Yates' (1963) Tables shows that, for the size of the sample studied, this correlation coefficient is significant at the $p < 0.001$ level. The coefficient of determination $(r_{xy})^2$, is 0.69. In

regression equation calculated as described previously gives the expression

$$y_i = x_i + 292 \qquad (2.53)$$

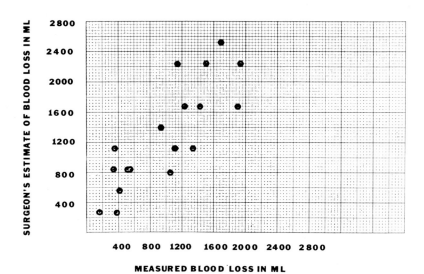

Fig. 16. Scattergraph showing relationship of subjective estimates of blood loss as a function of measured blood loss. (After Shalom, 1965.)

TABLE 9

TABULATION OF BOTH MEASURED AND SUBJECTIVELY ESTIMATED VOLUMES OF BLOOD LOSS IN A SERIES OF MAJOR FACE AND NECK OPERATIONS

(After Shalom, 1964)

Measured Blood Loss in millilitres (x)	Surgeon's Subjective Estimate of Loss in millilitres (y)
518	840
349	840
1124	1120
947	1400
1514	2240
1932	1680
1435	1680
530	840
1060	840
1687	2520
1345	1120
382	250
1930	2240
1245	1680
174	280
1150	2240
417	560
363	1120

This would imply that the average surgeon in that study overestimated the blood loss by about 300 ml. We should, however, question the meaningfulness of this regression equation when we note that it implies that, for zero blood loss, the surgeon would give an estimated value of 292 ml. Moreover, according to Stevens' (1962) psychophysical law, subjective magnitudes are known to be a power function of physical magnitudes. It might therefore be rewarding if we were to replot the data on double logarithmic co-ordinates, where a straight line plot would indicate that the variates were related by a power function. What in effect is the same as plotting the logarithms of the values for the two variates on ordinary (arithmetic) graph paper is to use double logarithmic graph paper. This has been done and is shown in Fig. 17. A straight line plot for this graph seems just as plausible as one for that of Fig. 16. The *method of least squares* can be used to obtain the best fit straight line to the data. With this method, the data are considered to fit a straight line, i.e. of the general formula

$$y = ax + b \qquad (2.54)$$

where the gradient (a) is given by the expression

$$a = \{\textstyle\sum xy - (\sum x \sum y/N)\}/\{\sum x^2 - (\sum x)^2/N\} \qquad (2.55)$$

and the intercept (b) by the expression

$$b = (\textstyle\sum x \sum xy - \sum y \sum x^2)/\{(\sum x)^2 - N(\sum x^2)\} \qquad (2.56)$$

Equation (2.54) then becomes

$$y = 0.783x + 0.7588 \qquad (2.57)$$

other words, this linear regression model explains 69 per cent of the total variation in the surgeon's estimates. A

However, since x and y refer to the logarithmic transforms of our variates, the expression is actually

$$\log y' = 0.783 \log x + 0.7588 \qquad (2.58)$$

where y' = predicted estimate of blood loss in ml, and

x = actual measured blood loss in ml.

This is equivalent to the power function

$$y' = 5.74x^{0.783} \qquad (2.59)$$

If we accept that the power function best describes the relationship between the two variates in this example, then

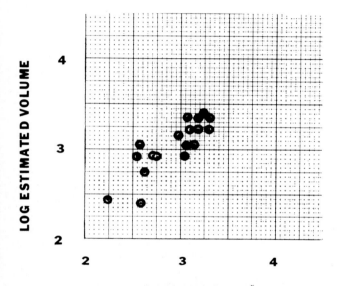

LOG ESTIMATED VOLUME

LOG MEASURED VOLUME

FIG. 17. A scattergraph showing the inter-relationship of logarithmic transforms of the variates given in Fig. 16.

neither this example nor the previous one (speech hearing levels regressing on 2000 Hz threshold measurements) are linear regression models. Therefore, non-linear correlation coefficients are more appropriate. As Yeomans (1968) points out, in contrast to the approach described for linear regression models, correlation coefficients for non-linear models can be calculated only after the regression coefficients have been evaluated. Since the correlation coefficient is equal to the square root of the *coefficient of determination*, this must first be evaluated. The coefficient of determination is given by

$$r^2 = \frac{\text{explained variation}}{\text{total variation}} = \frac{\sum_i (y_i' - \bar{y})^2}{\sum_i (y_i - \bar{y})^2} \qquad (2.60)$$

where y_i' = predicted value of y at x_i

y_i = measured value of y at x_i

and $\bar{y}$ = mean value of y.

The value for the denominator is more conveniently expressed as in equation (2.9). For this example, the coefficient of determination is found to be 0.72 and the coefficient of non-linear correlation $\sqrt{0.72}$, i.e. 0.85. These are higher values than those derived from the linear

regression model. With this power function model, the explained variation accounts for 72 per cent of the total variation in the regression estimates. It is interesting to consider what might be the theoretical value of the exponent (0.783) in equation (2.59). If we consider that a surgeon's estimate is governed by Stevens (1962) psychophysical power law, then what sensory continua are involved? Since the surgeon's estimate in operations of the type included in this study is based primarily on the extent of bloodstained drapes and other materials, it would appear that the visual subjective magnitude of area should be involved. Stevens and Guirao (1963) reported the exponent for this particular sensory continuum to be 0.7. This exponent compares favourably with the exponent determined from Shalom's study.

If linearization of the relationship of two variables is not possible, then an attempt should be made to fit a *polynomial* equation of second degree or more (the ordinary linear regression equation constitutes a first degree polynomial). The general polynomial model is of the type

$$y = \alpha + \beta_1 x + \beta_2 x^2 + \ldots + \beta_n x^n \qquad (2.61)$$

The highest power of x, denoted here by n, is referred to as the degree of the polynomial. A polynomial of the second degree (parabola) gives the quadratic equation:

$$y = \alpha + \beta_1 x + \beta_2 x^2 \qquad (2.62)$$

of the third degree ($n = 3$), the cubic equation:

$$y = \alpha + \beta_1 x + \beta_2 x^2 + \beta_3 x^3 \qquad (2.63)$$

and of the fourth degree ($n = 4$), the quadratic equation:

$$y = \alpha + \beta_1 x + \beta_2 x^2 + \beta_3 x^3 + \beta_4 x^4 \qquad (2.64)$$

Curves fitted to polynomial equations exhibit a number of *points of inflection* (bends). The actual number is one less than the degree of the polynomial.

As an example, Fig. 18 shows a speech audiogram obtained from an individual with a sensorineural hearing loss. The audiogram exhibits not only a loss in gain compared to the normal, but also a discrimination loss (failure to reach 100 per cent word recognition score) and a "roll off" (*see* Chapter 11). Although it was mentioned earlier that a normal speech audiogram can be fitted by an ogive as on the left of Fig. 18, this is not the case for abnormal speech audiograms of the type shown on the right of the same figure. The curve in that figure shows two points of *inflection* so that, in attempting to fit a polynomial equation, we should first explore the possibility of using a third-degree polynomial, i.e. the type shown in equation (2.63). To find the value of the coefficients α, β_1, β_2 and β_3 in that equation, four *normal equations*, derived from the procedure for minimizing the sum of squares, must be solved:

$$\sum y = \alpha n + \beta_1 \sum x + \beta_2 \sum x^2 + \beta_3 \sum x^3 \qquad (2.65)$$

$$\sum xy = \alpha \sum x + \beta_2 \sum x^2 + \beta_2 \sum x^3 + \beta_3 \sum x^4 \qquad (2.66)$$

$$\sum x^2 y = \alpha \sum x^2 + \beta_1 \sum x^3 + \beta_2 \sum x^4 + \beta_3 \sum x^5 \qquad (2.67)$$

$$\sum x^3 y = \alpha \sum x^3 + \beta_1 \sum x^4 + \beta_2 \sum x^5 + \beta_3 \sum x^6 \qquad (2.68)$$

It should be noted that it is not possible to produce single formula for the coefficients, so that the four equations must be solved simultaneously. The data which are visually presented in Fig. 18 are tabulated in Table 10. When the above four equations are solved using the data in Table 10, the coefficients are found to have the following values: 120 (α), $-7\cdot7$ (β_1), $0\cdot135$ (β_2) and $-6\cdot464 \times 10^{-4}$ (β_3).

derived by first calculating the coefficient of determination and taking the square root of this value, as described previously. For this model, the value of the numerator in equation (2.60) is given by

$$\sum(y' - y)^2 = (\alpha\sum y + \beta_1\sum xy + \beta_2\sum x^2 y \\ + \beta_3\sum x^3 y) - \{(\sum y)^2/n\} \quad (2.70)$$

SPEECH AUDIOGRAM.

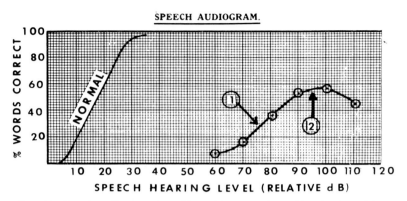

FIG. 18. Speech audiogram of a subject with a sensorineural hearing loss. Note the two points of inflection (labelled 1 and 2) on this curve.

Thus a third-degree polynomial fitted to the speech audiogram of Fig. 18 has the form

$$y = 120 - 7\cdot7x + 0\cdot135x^2 - 6\cdot464 \times 10^{-4}x^3 \quad (2.69)$$

where y = per cent words correctly repeated
and x = speech material sound level in relative dB.

TABLE 10

ACTUAL AND PREDICTED (FROM BEST-FIT THIRD DEGREE POLYNOMIAL EQUATION) SPEECH AUDIOMETRIC SCORES FOR A SUBJECT WITH A SENSORINEURAL HEARING LOSS

Speech Hearing Level (in relative decibels) (x)	% Correct Word Recognition	
	Actual (y)	Predicted (y')
60	8	4
70	16	21
80	36	37
90	52	49
100	56	54
110	44	46

This is not to suggest that that either the normal or the abnormal speech audiogram is best treated as a cubic regression curve. A more sophisticated statistical treatment of speech audiometric data by Lyregaard (1973) has shown that the distributions of scores is of a generalized binomial type, although the simple binomial distribution offers a good approximation.

Since equation (2.69) represents a non-linear regression model, a coefficient of non-linear correlation must be

When these equations are solved, the coefficient of determination is found to have a value of 0·97. In other words, 97 per cent of the total variation in the recorded speech intelligibility scores for our sample subject can be attributed to the regression of this score on the speech hearing level according to a third-degree polynomial equation. Since the coefficient of determination is the square of the correlation coefficient, the *coefficient of curvilinear correlation* in this sample is $\sqrt{0\cdot97} = 0\cdot98$. As with all coefficients of non-linear correlation, this value, it should be noted, has no sign since the regression line slope is positive at one point, and negative at another.

Curvilinear regressions, other than those represented by polynomials, also exist. A *periodic regression*, in which regression equations have a sinusoidal form, is illustrated in Chapter 10 (Figs 4–6).

When a number of measurements are made of a function, or an object, it is frequently assumed, quite plausibly, that (a) a number of tests may be measuring the same thing, or basic factor, and (b) some or all of these measures may be influenced by more than one basic factor. This concept underlies *Factor Analysis*. This is a statistical procedure, initially adapted and developed by psychologists, whereby the performance of subjects on a large number of tests could be examined for the presence or absence of common factors. There are a number of different methods of factor analysis (Kendall, 1957; Seal, 1964). One, termed the *maximum likelihood* solution, is statistically the most respectable. Computer programmes are available for this and a number of other methods of factor analysis. Indeed, were assistance from computers not available, these analyses would be much less frequently performed. The required calculations are otherwise too tedious. Unfortunately, no acceptable statistical criteria yet exist for determining the number of factors necessary to account for the observed correlations. One method of multivariate analysis, *Principal Component Analysis* (Hotelling, 1933) produces as many components as there are tests. This method has previously been used for the statistical analysis of caloric test measures (Hinchcliffe, 1967a).

Disease Diagnosis

Assessment of the validity and reliability of the various diagnostic tests by the statistical methods that we have just outlined, together with epidemiological data on the frequency of particular disorders in relevant populations, should be a prerequisite to the diagnosis of disease using statistical procedures. *Inter alia*, these studies will enable us to define the frequency of *characters* (diagnostic test results, including elementary measures such as age and sex) in individual diseases. From this data base, *Bayes' theorem of conditional probability* may be applied to produce probabilities for different diagnoses (Ledley and Lusted, 1959). Bayesian statistics (Lindley, 1965; Phillips, 1973) takes its name from its originator, Thomas Bayes (1702–61), an English clergyman. The operation of Bayesian statistics is best explained by an example. An otolaryngologist may entertain the hypothesis: "This patient is suffering from disease X". By regarding this patient as a random member of a large group of patients presenting themselves at his clinic, he may be able to associate this hypothesis with a certain probability, i.e. the long-term proportion of patients afflicted with disease X. This probability is termed the *prior probability*, since it can be ascertained from retrospective observations. The otolaryngologist now makes certain observations or measurements. He then again considers the probability of the hypothesis "this patient is suffering from disease X". This reassessed probability is termed the *posterior probability* since it refers to the situation after new observations have been made. Bayes' theorem always takes the same basic form, i.e. prior probabilities are converted to posterior probabilities by multiplication in proportion to *likelihoods* (probabilities of a particular outcome on different hypotheses). Bayesian statistics are frequently used in what is termed *computer-assisted diagnosis*. This technique has, for example, been used in the diagnosis of thyroid disorders with a 96 per cent accuracy (Fitzgerald and Williams, 1964). Boyle and his associates (1966) used both a Bayesian model and a *relative likelihood model* for their studies of computer-assisted diagnosis of thyroid disorders. The relative likelihood model was superior in that it did not fail to diagnose thyroid carcinoma when this was otherwise apparent clinically. However, the Bayesian model missed three out of 19 carcinoma cases which were clinically obvious. A computer programme in Arkansas (Oddie *et al.*, 1971) uses knowledge about the statistical features of thyroid function tests in that area. Shifts in the average values and changes with the precision of individual tests which may result from changes in laboratory methods, environmental iodine levels or the dietary habits of the community can be constantly monitored and the diagnostic criteria appropriately adjusted. As Baron and Fraser (1965) pointed out, if the initial classification and weighting of characters (measurements including symptoms and signs) is based upon a sufficiently wide experience, so that its validity is accepted,

this technique will make fewer mistakes than the non-specialist physician (and perhaps even the specialist!) In this respect, it has been said that such a computer programme acts as a "super-consultant": it will always arrive at the probability of every possible programmed diagnosis for any complex of characters that are supplied to it for analysis. By this means, a disease could be accurately diagnosed by the otolaryngolosist even though he had never previously encountered the disease. Of course, the method cannot identify a disease for which a model has not yet been set up. It is also assumed that, for a valid diagnosis, a valid classification of the group of disorders to which the disorder in question belongs has been established. Too often this is not the case. The classification of disease (nosology), especially in otolaryngology, is a neglected study. The techniques of *numerical taxonomy* (better termed *taxonometry*, since the classification of numbers is not under consideration) have already been successfully applied to the classification of diseases. Taxonometry (Sokal and Sneath, 1963) depends on making as many different measurements as possible on a large group of objects (patients for example) and then expressing the relationship between any two objects, or patients, as an index, the *similarity coefficient*. This coefficient varies in value between zero (no relationship) and one (identical). A matrix of coefficients is thus obtained. A *cluster analysis* then groups together patients who are most similar. The clusters are distributed in multi-dimensional space and those clusters which are sufficiently isolated can be regarded as disease entities. A taxonometric study of the idiopathic vertiginous disorders, including Ménière's disorder, by the author failed to reveal other than a single cluster of disorders (Hinchcliffe, 1967b). This would indicate that many disorders that are considered by some as distinct from Ménière's disorder are actually *formes frustes* or variants of that disorder. A study of the anatomical features of the middle ear of members of the Heteromyidae, a family of rodents containing the pocket- "mice" and "rats", included a taxonometric analysis (Hinchcliffe and Pye, 1969). The results were able to support one of a number of competing suggested classifications for the members of this family.

The *efficacy* of diagnostic tests may be assessed by a statistical technique known as *discriminant analysis*. Hollingsworth (1959) sought the best group of tests for diagnosing suspected cases of primary carcinoma of the bronchus and lung. He found that 14 measures obtained from symptoms, clinical signs and cytological and radiological examination could provide an 85 per cent effective diagnosis.

Assessing Methods of Treatment

The assessment of potential methods of treatment hinges statistically on making *tests of significance*. An observed result is said to be *statistically significant* at the chosen level of probability. As stated previously, probability (p) is expressed on a scale of 0–1. A level of $p < 0.05$, i.e. a 1 in 20 chance of happening, is the level usually accepted in medicine for some difference being considered to be significant. Miller (1966) has suggested that we use the terms "decisive" and "conclusive" for the levels $p < 0.01$ and $p < 0.001$ respectively. The exact procedure in making a test of significance will depend on the nature of the relevant data. Nevertheless, in the experimental assessment of therapeutic procedures, a particular sequence of events, as Smart (1970) points out, is followed. First, a hypothesis, termed the *null hypothesis*, which is appropriate to the problem, is set out. An appropriate null hypothesis in a clinical trial of a new treatment might be that the proportion of patients improved by the new treatment is not different from the proportion improved by another treatment, or that the average value of some clinically relevant measurement, e.g. hearing level, in the group receiving the new treatment is not different from the corresponding value in the group receiving the other treatment. Secondly, the null hypothesis must be translated into appropriate quantitative terms in an experiment designed to test it. Thirdly, the experiment must be executed correctly. Finally, one must calculate, if the null hypothesis is true, the probability of the observed result having arisen by random sampling variation.

The *design of experiments* is a major branch of statistics. Indeed some have considered it a subject in its own right and defined it as the science of obtaining unambiguous results of the highest possible accuracy from experiments on variable material. It is possible to plan elaborate experiments in which several factors can be taken into account statistically at the same time (Cochran and Cox, 1957; Cox, 1958). The main principles of experimental design for therapeutic trials are:

(1) Comparison.
(2) Replication.
(3) Randomization.
(4) Objectivity.

The comparative basis of "controlled" clinical trials is fundamental; indeed they should be termed *comparative therapeutic trials*. This is merely an extension of Sir Henry Dale's dictum that all measurement is essentially comparative. The drug or procedure with which a new remedy is compared may be an already accepted drug or an established procedure. In the case of drugs, one may use an inert preparation (*placebo*) which appears to be physically identical to the naked eye with the active preparation. There are individuals who, for psychological reasons, are *placebo responders*. Any treatment must normally be applied to more than one patient. This provides greater accuracy than can be obtained from a single observation, since the experimental errors tend to cancel out. Moreover, replication provides a measure of the experimental error derived from the variability between replicates. The decision as to which patient should receive, or should not receive, treatment should include a random element. This randomization is directed towards the elimination of bias. The latter should be confirmed by showing that the two samples (treated and untreated) are matched, so far as possible, in every way, particularly as regards their age and sex stratification. In certain experiments, one may have to consider *order* and/or *sequence* effects. Order effects refer to the influence on the results of the order (i.e. first-,

second-, third- . . .) in which a test was given. Sequence effects refer to the influence of the type of preceding or succeeding stimuli. The *Latin Square* design caters for order effects only. It has the same number of columns and rows as the number of tests or treatments studied. It is thus a square array of n letters each repeated n times and disposed so that each letter occurs just once in every row and column. Thus if we wish to measure responses to the conventional bithermal (dual temperature) caloric test on a given population we could use a Latin Square design as shown in Table 11.

TABLE 11

LATIN SQUARE DESIGN OF AN INVESTIGATION USING CALORIC TEST RESPONSES WHERE THE EXPERIMENT HAS BEEN DESIGNED TO ANNUL POSSIBLE ORDER EFFECTS

44°R	44°L	30°R	30°L
30°L	44°R	44°L	30°R
30°R	30°L	44°R	44°L
44°L	30°R	30°L	44°R

With chronic or episodic disorders, one is able to obtain serial observations on a patient. It is therefore possible to measure how a single patient responds to different treatments. Such experiments constitute *cross-over* trials and help eliminate inter-subject variation.

The previous paragraphs have described procedures to ensure that the results of therapeutic trials are not biased by factors operating at the beginning of the trial. In an attempt to eradicate bias in the assessment of responses to treatment, a *double-blind* trial should be used if possible. It is termed "double-blind" in the sense that neither the doctor nor the patient knows which treatment is being given. Clearly, such trials are difficult, if not impossible, where physical methods of treatment, including surgery, are being used. Nevertheless, it is only by this procedure that objectivity can be achieved. In experiments using animals, "dummy" operations can be used, as was done by Sokolovski (1973) in investigating the effect of stapedial tenotomy on noise-induced hearing loss in cats.

The particular statistics to be used in analysing data from therapeutic trials will depend on the type of data. If we are dealing with proportions, then χ^2 (chi-squared) tests are appropriate, if with continuous distributions, then tests for *difference between means* or *analysis of variance* would be appropriate.

Cody and Taylor's (1973) analysis of the long-term results of tympanoplasty was based mainly on χ^2 tests. They showed that there was no statistically significant difference, on the one hand, between different methods of repair, and, on the other hand, different (active or inactive disease) ears grafted. The χ^2 test which was first described by Pearson, enables one to assess the probability of the difference between, for example, observed and expected values having arisen by chance. As Moroney points out, the χ^2 distribution is one of the most versatile in statistical theory. Its value is given by the expression

$$\chi^2 = \sum\{(O - E)^2/E\} \tag{2.71}$$

where O = observed frequency

and E = expected frequency, i.e. frequency expected on the basis of the model to be tested.

Dividing by the expected value simply brings the squared difference into proportion. If the observed and expected frequencies are equal, then χ^2 will be zero. The greater the difference between observed and expected values, the greater must be the value of χ^2. Consequently, the greater the value of χ^2, the lower the probability of the finding being due to chance. Graphs and tables for values of χ^2 have been constructed (Fisher and Yates, 1963) and inspection of these indicates whether or not the discrepancy could be due to chance. However, before entering a χ^2 table one must first determine the number of *degrees of freedom* (*df*). The concept of degrees is, as Oldham points out, central to the theory of exact tests of significance. The number of degrees of freedom is defined as the number of independent contributions to a theoretical sampling distributon (e.g. χ^2, *t* and *f* distributions). A particular application of the χ^2 test is in assessing *goodness of fit* of experimental distributions to theoretical ones—binomial, Poisson or Gaussian. In calculating the degrees of freedom in these cases, one must bear in mind that the number of *df* is equivalent to the number of categories less the number of sample characteristics needed to obtain the expected frequencies. Thus for both binomial and Poisson distributions, the *df* is two less than the number of categories since two sample characteristics (mean and sample size) are required from the sample. With Gaussian distributions, the *df* is three less than the number of categories or class groups since three sample characteristics (mean, standard deviation and sample size) are required from the sample. In general, the χ^2 test should not be used if any expected frequency is less than unity or if more than 20 per cent of the expected frequencies are less than 5. This difference may be circumvented by pooling adjacent categories. As an example, let us look at the observed frequencies for the distribution of middle ear compliance (measured in MPa.s.m^{-3}) (Fig. 12) and comparing them with the expected frequencies shown in Fig. 13. To obviate small expected frequencies, the first two categories (shown as rectangles in the histogram) are pooled, as are the eighth and subsequent categories, giving a total of 7 categories. χ^2 is calculated and found to be 7·656. The number of degrees of freedom is 4 ($df = 7 - 3 = 4$) and the decision criterion for a 5 per cent significance level is found from Fisher and Yates' tables to be 9·488. Since $\chi^2_{calc.}$ is less than $\chi^2_{0.05}$, one must accept that the sample population shown in Fig. 12 could have been drawn from a population having the same

distribution as in Fig. 13, a Gaussian distribution. Table 12 shows an application of the χ^2 test to the goodness of fit of a Poisson distribution. This is in respect of the data in Table 1 (in view of the small numbers involved, the last three

TABLE 12

χ^2 TEST APPLIED TO TEST GOODNESS OF FIT OF POISSON DISTRIBUTION TO NUMBER OF EARS REQUIRING MYRINGOTOMY

Category	O	E	$(O{-}E)$	$(O{-}E)^2$	$\dfrac{O{-}E^2}{E}$
0	16	15	0	1	0·0667
1	21	19	2	4	0·2105
2	9	12	−3	9	0·7500
3⎫ 4⎬ 5⎭	8	7	1	1	0·1429
				$\chi(calc.) =$	1·1701

categories were collapsed into one for this analysis). In this case, $\chi^2_{calc.} = 1·17 < \chi^2_{0.05} = 5·991$ ($df = 4 - 2 = 2$). So one must accept that the sample population could have been drawn from a population with a Poisson distribution.

The simplest, but yet a special, case of the χ^2 test is when it relates to a dichotomous (division into two classes only) variable. In this case, results can be shown in a *fourfold* or 2×2 contingency table as in Table 2. In this case, χ^2 is given by

$$\chi^2 = \{N(ad - bc)^2\}/$$
$$\{(a + c)(b + d)(c + d)(a + b)\} \tag{2.72}$$

where N = total sample size.

However, since this presentation is binomial in essence and the χ^2 distribution is a continuous one, a correction is required. This correction (Yates') consists in decreasing by a half those values in the table which exceed expectation, and increasing by a half those values which are less than the expected value. An example of an application of the χ^2 test to a fourfold table is in connection with a clinical trial of thonzylamine in the treatment of the common cold (Smart, 1970). The results are shown in Table 13. The value of χ^2 *without* Yates' correction is

$$\chi^2 = [1156\{(278 \times 334) - (301 \times 243)\}^2]/$$
$$\{(278 + 243)(401 + 334)(243 + 334)$$
$$(278 + 301)\} = \underline{4·063} \tag{2.73}$$

The value of χ^2 *with* Yates' correction is

$$\chi^2 = [1156\{(277·5 \times 333·5) - (301·5 \times 243·5)\}^2]/$$
$$\{(277·5 + 243·5)(301·5 + 333·5)$$
$$(243·5 + 333·5)(277·5 + 301·5)\}$$
$$= \underline{3·828} \tag{2.74}$$

The value of χ^2 in equation (2.73) would be significant at the $p < 0.05$ level but that in equation (2.74) is not.

With small frequencies, even with this continuity correction, as Armitage (1973) points out, there is doubt about the adequacy of the χ^2 approximation. In such cases, i.e. when

TABLE 13

A 2×2 CONTINGENCY (FOURFOLD) TABLE TO SHOW THE RESPONSE OF THE COMMON COLD TO THON-ZYLAMINE AND TO A COMPARISON PREPARATION

(After Smart, 1970)

Drug	Improved or Cured	
	Yes	No
Thonzylamine	278	301
Comparison	243	334

the smallest number in any square of the fourfold table is less than 5, the Fisher–Irwin–Yates exact 2×2 *probability test* should be applied. In this case

$$p = \{(a + b)!(c + d)!(a + c)!(b + d)!\}/$$
$$(n!\, a!\, b!\, c!\, d!) \qquad (2.75)$$

A survey may present data on the proportion of individuals with a particular disorder in a single sample of a population. It is then desirable to estimate what the true proportion of such individuals is likely to be in the general population. Since proportions are also considered to have distributions, termed *sampling distributions*, which are normally distributed, this estimate involves a determination of the standard deviation of this distribution. The term *standard error* is used to describe this standard deviation. We have already met it before in connection with estimates from regression equations. It is thus the standard deviation of a frequency distribution which represents how some quantity calculated from limited data might vary under the chance effects of sampling. It is therefore a hypothetical quantity measuring uncertainty about the accuracy of an estimate. This value is conventionally written after the value for an estimate but preceded by the symbol "$\pm$". The standard error of a proportion, $\varepsilon_{\text{prop}}$, is given by

$$\varepsilon_{\text{prop}} = \pm\sqrt{(pq/n)} \qquad (2.76)$$

where p = proportion of conditions in population from which the sample was drawn

$\quad q = (1 - p)$

and $\quad n$ = sample size.

For sample sizes greater than 50, it is considered that the sample proportion can be used for the population proportion in equation (2.76). Thus, if we found that, in a sample of 400 people, 191 were women, then the proportion of women in that sample would be 0·4775, and

$$\varepsilon_{\text{prop}} = \pm\sqrt{[\{0\cdot4775(1 - 0\cdot4775)\}/n]} = \pm0\cdot025 \quad (2.77)$$

Thus the 95 per cent confidence level is the sample proportion $\pm1\cdot96(\varepsilon_{\text{prop}})$, i.e. $0\cdot4775 \pm 0\cdot049$. Thus the true proportion of women in the population from which the sample was drawn would be between 43 and 53 per cent. In other words, the data do not support any sex difference in this case. For smaller samples and samples with smaller proportions, Limits of Expectation Tables, as given by Fisher and Yates (1963), should be consulted.

The concept of standard error can also be used in dealing with continuously distributed variables. Thus the standard error of the estimate of a mean is given by

$$\varepsilon = \pm\sigma/\sqrt{n} \qquad (2.78)$$

where σ = standard deviation of sample
and $\quad n$ = sample size

Thus the 95 per cent confidence limits of the mean are

$$\bar{x} \pm 1\cdot96\,\sigma/\sqrt{n} \qquad (2.79)$$

i.e. there is a 95 per cent probability that the true mean of the population from which the sample was drawn lies between the limits given by equation (2.79). Thus, in our sample of blood losses during major face and neck operations (Table 9), the mean loss was 1 006 ml, the standard deviation 573 ml, and the sample size 18. Thus the 95 per cent confidence limits of the mean are $\pm(1\cdot96 \times 573)/\sqrt{18}$, i.e. ±265 ml. In other words, we would expect that the average blood loss in major face and neck operations would be somewhere in the range 0·74–1·27 l. The size of this uncertainty is attributable not only to the relatively small size of the sample but also to the variation, the effect of which is enhanced by the platykurtic nature of the distribution.

For *comparing the means* of two samples of size greater than about 50, the standard error of the difference in the means is given by

$$\varepsilon = \pm\sqrt{\{(\sigma_1^2/n_1) + (\sigma_2^2/n_2)\}} \qquad (2.80)$$

The factor "1·96" for multiplying the ratio of the standard deviation to the square root of a sample in order to obtain the 95 per cent confidence limits is strictly applicable only to samples of infinite size. For a sample size of 60, a value of 2 would be appropriate and for samples less than 60 in size, a value greater than 2 would be appropriate. The various values for this factor, termed *Student's t*, are given in Fisher and Yates' Statistical Tables. The actual value depends upon the level of confidence required and upon the degrees of freedom (in this context, one less than the sample size). Thus, if we consider our data on total blood loss during stapedectomy (Tables 4 and 6) and compare the mean values for the two methods of anaesthesia, we obtain

$$t = (\bar{x}_1 - \bar{x}_2)/\sqrt{\{(s^2/n_1) + (s^2/n_2)\}} \qquad (2.81)$$

where s is a combined estimate of the standard deviation. Its value is given by

$$s^2 = \{\sum(x_i - \bar{x}_1)^2 + \sum(x_j - \bar{x}_2)^2\}/$$
$$(n_1 + n_2 - 2) \qquad (2.82)$$

Thus for our example,

$$s^2 = (5 \cdot 8605 + 6 \cdot 5577)/(20 + 12 - 2) =$$
$$0 \cdot 4139 \quad (2.83)$$

and

$$t = (0 \cdot 938 - 1 \cdot 204)/\sqrt{\{(0 \cdot 4139/20) + (0 \cdot 4139/12)\}} = -1 \cdot 132 \quad (2.84)$$

The negative sign merely indicates the direction of the difference between the means. Whether or not this value of t is significant can be determined by consulting Fisher and Yates' tables for the distribution of t. For 30 df (i.e. $20 + 12 - 2$), t must reach $2 \cdot 042$ to be significant at the 95 per cent level. Thus this difference between the two samples is not significant.

the number of subjects in the study was determined either before the start of the trial or at least by some circumstances independent of the results themselves. As Armitage (1954) points out, there are strong ethical reasons both in prophylactic and in therapeutic trials that the results be subject to continuous analysis as they become available. In this way, it may thus be possible to discontinue a trial as soon as it can safely be concluded that one treatment is more effective than another. Such trials, known as *sequential trials*, are based upon Wald's (1947) method of *sequential analysis*. They have been used for the comparison of diamorphine and pholcodine as cough suppressants (Snell and Armitage, 1957), and for the comparison of calcium chloride and epinephrine as bronchial dilators (Kilpatrick and Oldham, 1954) and for studying the effect

TABLE 14

FORMAT FOR SETTING OUT RESULTS OF ANALYSIS OF VARIANCE

(Note that $\bar{\bar{y}}$ is the overall mean for all the samples; n is the number of values in each sample; $\bar{y}$ represents the mean for a given sample; y refers to individual values, which is subscripted, e.g. y_2, if a particular sample is denoted; $(k - 1)$ refers to the number of degrees of freedom associated with the between sample sum of squares; $(N - k)$ refers to the degree of freedom associated with the scatter of the sample mean about the overall mean; k refers to the number of samples and N to the total number of observations in all the samples combined. Since the mean of each sample represents n values, its squared deviation is multiplied by n to bring it into line with other sources of variation which are to be regarded as within samples.)

Source of Variation	Sum of Squares	df	V		F
Between samples	$\Sigma n(\bar{y} - \bar{\bar{y}})^2$	$k - 1$	$\{\Sigma n(\bar{y} - \bar{\bar{y}})^2\}/(k - 1)$	(B)	B/E
Within samples	$\Sigma(y_1 - \bar{y}_1)^2 + \ldots + \Sigma(y_n - \bar{y}_n)^2$	$N - k$	$\dfrac{\{\Sigma(y_1 - \bar{y}_1)^2 + \ldots \Sigma(y_n - \bar{y}_n)^2\}}{(N - k)}$	(E)	
Total	$\Sigma(y - \bar{\bar{y}})^2$	$N - 1$			

Although Student's t test is a useful method for comparing two samples, it cannot be used for more than two samples. For this purpose, Fisher's *Analysis of Variance* is used. As its name implies, this test depends on a comparison of the variance between samples with the variance within samples. The results for an analysis of variance are usually set out as in Table 14. If the variance "between samples" is large compared with the variance "within samples", then it is unlikely that the samples have been drawn from the same population. The variance ratio test, as analysis of variance is sometimes referred to, is also referred to as Snedecor's F test, since Snedecor computed tables for the variance ratio distribution and named the ratio F in honour of Fisher. To make a test of significance, one needs to know this variance ratio and the numbers of degrees of freedom associated with the two sums of squares, i.e. $(k - 1)$ and $(N - k)$, where k is the number of samples and N is the total number of observations. Consequently, the distribution of F is three-dimensional. Thus the appropriate tables give values of F which would be exceeded in random sampling with various probabilities for various pairs of df.

The statistical methods that have been described so far for testing the significance of observed differences between groups, normally applied at the end of a trial, assume that

of auditory tubal irradiation with strontium 90 implants in children with middle ear disease (Siedentop and Eggert, 1973) (the irradiation was ineffective). Although the planning of a sequential experimental design involves more work than does a conventional comparative trial, once calculated, a sequential channel may be used for any number of problems requiring decisions within the same statistical limits (Trehub and Scherer, 1958).

CONCLUSIONS

This chapter has provided an all too brief account of how statistics might be applied to otolaryngological data. Such statistical treatment might serve merely to present results in a succinct form or to make deductions regarding the truth or otherwise of some hypothesis. The latter might be in respect of the validity or reliability of a particular measure or test or it might be in respect of the efficacy of some drug or therapeutic procedure. However, in an attempt to ensure that an experiment or investigation is as flawless as possible, it is most important that the experimental design be discussed with a statistician *before* the study is undertaken.

If a comparative prophylactic or therapeutic trial is envisaged on man or other animals, consideration will have to be given as to whether it should involve a fixed number of patients or it should proceed sequentially. The choice between the two is to some extent related to the statistical philosophy adopted, i.e. *frequentist, Bayesian* or *likelihoodist*. These three viewpoints are discussed by Plackett (1966). However, as Gehan and Schneiderman (1973) point out, differences between viewpoints have not led to markedly different ways of conducting prophylactic or therapeutic trials. According to the frequentist philosophy, in a comparative trial, the size of the sample to be studied is determined by:

    (a) The level of significance required.

    (b) The value of the desired power of the test (the chance that a particular trial will declare a given real difference in response as statistically significant).

    (c) The difference between treatment success rates that it is important to detect.

Cochran and Cox (1957) give tables which indicate the requisite number of subjects that would meet these criteria. For example, a standard method of treatment may be known to give a 40 per cent response rate and it is desired to conduct a clinical trial to determine whether a new treatment results in a better response rate. If it is desired to detect with a 90 per cent probability a 10 per cent improvement in that response rate, which results are significant at the $p = 0.05$ level, then 420 subjects would be required. However, if the new drug is twice as effective as the standard drug, it would be detected with the same probability and at the same level of significance with only 24 subjects.

As a final note, attention should be drawn to a point that has been emphasized by Békésy (1960) and others: It is virtually impossible to prove the negative of a hypothesis.

For our conclusions to this chapter we can perhaps do no better than quote Moroney from his introductory chapter: "A statistical analysis, properly conducted, is a delicate dissection of uncertainties, a surgery of suppositions. The surgeon must guard carefully against false incisions with his scalpel. Very often he has to sew up the patient as inoperable."

REFERENCES

Alusi, H. A., Hinchcliffe, R., Ingham, B., Knight, J. J. and North, C. (1974), "Arabic Speech Audiometry," *Audiology*, **13**, 212.

Armitage, P. (1954), "Sequential Tests in Prophylactic and Therapeutic Trials," *Quart. J. Med.*, **23**, 255.

Armitage, P. (1973), *Statistical Methods in Medical Research.* Oxford: Blackwell.

Bacharach, A. L., Coates, Marie E. and Middleton, T. R. (1942), "A Biological Test for Vitamin P Activity," *Biochem. J.*, **36**, 407.

Bahn, Anita K. (1972), *Basic Medical Statistics.* New York: Grune and Stratton.

Baron, D. N. and Fraser, Patricia M. (1965), "Digital Computer in Classification and Diagnosis of Diseases," *Lancet*, **ii**, 1066.

Bateman, G. H. (1957), "Secretory Otitis Media," *J. Laryng.*, **71**, 261.

Békésy, G. von (1960), *Experiments in Hearing.* New York: McGraw-Hill.

Boyle, J. A., Greig, W. R., Franklin, D. A., Harden, R. McG., Buchanan, W. W. and McGirr, E. M. (1966), "Construction of a Model for Computer-assisted Diagnosis. Application to the Problem of Non-toxic Goitre," *Quart. J. Med.*, **35**, 565.

Cochran, W. G. and Cox, G. M. (1957), *Experimental Designs.* New York: Wiley.

Cody, D. T. R. and Taylor, W. F. (1973), "Tympanoplasty: Long-term Results," *Ann. Otol.*, **82**, 538.

Cox, D. R. (1958), *Planning of Experiments.* New York: Wiley.

Deacock, A. R. de C. (1971), "Aspects of Anaesthesia for Middle-ear Surgery and Blood Loss during Stapedectomy," *Proc. roy. Soc. Med.*, **64**, 1226.

El-Ebiary, H. M. (1971), "Facial Paralysis: A Clinical Study of 580 Cases," *Rheum. phys. Med.*, **11**, 100.

Feldman, B. A. and Schuknecht, H. F. (1970), "Experiences with Revision Stapedectomy Procedures," *Laryngoscope*, **80**, 1281.

Fisher, R. A. and Yates, F. (1963), *Statistical Tables for Biological, Agricultural and Medical Research.* Edinburgh: Oliver and Boyd.

Fitzgerald, L. T. and Williams, C. M. (1964), "Medical Program for Computer Diagnosis of Thyroid Disease," *Radiology*, **82**, 334.

Friedman, M. (1937), "The Use of Ranks to Avoid the Assumption of Normality Implicit in the Analysis of Variance," *J. Amer. statist. Ass.*, **32**, 675.

Gehan, E. A. and Schneiderman, M. A. (1973), "Ch. VIII," in *Cancer Medicine* (J. F. Holland and E. Frei, Eds.). Philadelphia: Lea and Febiger.

Healy, M. J. R. (1968), "The Disciplining of Medical Data," *Brit. med. Bull.*, **24**, 210.

Hill, A. B. (1967), *Principles of Medical Statistics.* London: Lancet.

Hinchcliffe, R. (1967a), "Validity of Measures of Caloric Test Response," *Acta oto-laryng. (Stockh.)*, **63**, 69.

Hinchcliffe, R. (1967b), "An Attempt to Classify the Primary Vertigos," *J. Laryng.*, **81**, 849.

Hinchcliffe, R. and Littler, T. S. (1961), "The Detection and Measurement of Conductive Deafness," *J. Laryng.*, **75**, 201.

Hinchcliffe, R. and Pye, Ade (1969), "Variations in the Middle Ear of the Mammalia," *J. Zool. (Lond.)*, **157**, 277.

Hollingsworth, T. H. (1959), "Using an Electronic Computer in a Problem of Medical Diagnosis," *J. roy. statist. Soc.*, Series A., **122**, 221.

Hotelling, H. (1933), "Analysis of a Complex of Statistical Variables into Principal Components," *J. educ. Psychol.*, **24**, 417.

Kendall, M. G. (1957), *A Course in Multivariate Analysis.* London: Griffin.

Kilpatrick, G. S. and Oldham, P. D. (1954), "Calcium Chloride and Adrenaline as Bronchodilators, Compared by Sequential Analysis," *Brit. med. J.*, **2**, 1388.

Leading Article (1966), "Pause at the Parameter," *Brit. med. J.*, **1**, 1063.

Ledley, R. S. and Lusted, L. B. (1959), "Reason Foundations of Medical Diagnosis," *Science*, **130**, 9.

Lindley, D. V. (1965), *Introduction to Probability and Statistics from a Bayesian Viewpoint.* Cambridge: Cambridge University Press.

Lyregaard, P. E. (1973), "On the Statistics of Speech Audiometry Data," NPL Acoustics Report Ac 63. National Physical Laboratory, U.K.

Miller, D. A. (1966), " 'Significant' and 'Highly Significant'," *Nature (Lond.)*, **210**, 1190.

Moroney, M. J. (1953), *Facts from Figures.* London: Penguin Books.

Oddie, T. H. (1971), "Computer Diagnosis from Tests of Thyroid Function," *J. clin. Endocr.*, **32**, 167.

Oldham, P. D. (1968), *Measurement in Medicine: The Interpretation of Numerical Data.* London: English Universities Press.

Peterson, C. and Beach, L. R. (1967), "Man as an Intuitive Statistician," *Psychol. Bull.*, **68**, 29.

Phillips, L. D. (1973), *Bayesian Statistics for Social Scientists.* London: Nelson.

Plackett, R. L. (1966), "Current Trends in Statistical Inference," *J. roy. statist. Soc.*, Series A., **129**, 2.

Prasansuk, S. (1974). Submitted for publication.

Salomon, G. (1974), "Electric Response Audiometry (ERA) Based on Rank Correlation," *Audiology*, **13**, 181.

Seal, H. L. (1964), *Multivariate Statistical Analysis for Biologists.* London: Methuen.

Shah, N. (1971), "Use of grommets in 'glue' ears," *J. Laryng.*, **81**, 283.

Shalom, A. S. (1964), "Blood Loss in Ear, Nose and Throat Operations," *J. Laryng.*, **78**, 734.

Siedentop, K. H. and Eggert, R. A. (1973), "Eustachian Tube Irradiation with Strontium 90 in Children," *Arch. Otolaryng.*, **98**, 302.

Smart, J. V. (1970), *Elements of Medical Statistics*. London: Staples.

Snell, E. S. and Armitage, P. (1957), "Clinical Comparison of Diamorphine and Pholcodine as Cough Suppressants by a New Method of Sequential Analysis," *Lancet*, **i**, 860.

Sokal, R. R. and Sneath, P. H. A. (1963), *Principles of Numerical Taxonomy*. San Francisco and London: Freeman.

Sokolovski, A. (1973), "The Protective Action of the Stapedius Muscle in Noise-induced Hearing Loss in Cats," *Arch. klin. exp. Ohr.-, Nas.-u. Kehlk. Heilk.*, **203**, 289.

Stevens, S. S. (1951), "Mathematics, Measurement and Psychophysics," in *Handbook of Experimental Psychology*, Chap. 1 (S. S. Stevens, Ed.). New York: Wiley.

Stevens, S. S. (1962), *In Pursuit of the Sensory Law*, Second Public Klopsteg Lecture. Evanston, Ill.: Northeastern University.

Stevens, S. S. and Guirao, Miguelina (1963), "Subjective Scaling of Length and Area and the Matching of Length to Loudness and Brightness," *J. exp. Psychol.*, **66**, 177.

"Student" (1907), "On the Error of Counting with a Haemocytometer," *Biometrika*, **5**, 351.

Trehub, A. and Scherer, I. W. (1958), "The Clinical Application of Sequential Analysis," *J. clin. Psychol.*, **14**, 86.

Wald, A. (1947), *Sequential Analysis*. New York: Wiley.

Yeomans, K. A. (1968), *Statistics for the Social Scientists*. Harmondsworth: Penguin Books.

3. COMPUTERS

A. R. D. THORNTON

"But the age of chivalry is gone. That of sophisters, economists and calculators, has succeeded; and the glory of Europe is extinguished forever."
(Edmund Burke, *Reflections on the Revolution in France*, 1792)

THE COMPUTER

The computer is a tool at the third stage of development. Man has used tools to aid him in his work for thousands of years; and a hand tool, such as a screwdriver, represents the first stage of development. Here the tool is designed for a specific function, but, in order to carry out this function, a human must supply the power required by muscular effort, and he must provide control of the action. The second stage may be exemplified by a tool such as an electric drill. Here, as far as the drilling is concerned, the human muscle is replaced by an electric motor, and the human operator is required only to provide control. The third stage machine is automatic; it has automatic control of an operation or a sequence of operations. The machine has the capability of deciding which operations to perform according to rules which form a basic part of the machine structure. Simple examples of this stage are refrigerators and central heating systems which are controlled by thermostats. More complex examples include auto-change record players, automatic weaving looms and, of course, computers.

Computers can perform simple functions with great reliability and at a high speed, and are used, basically, as an aid to calculation and decision making. Historically, many calculating devices have been invented, which form a part of the development of the modern computer.

Two rulers can be used to perform addition and subtraction, and the calculation of $2 + 3 = 5$ is illustrated in Fig. 1. The introduction of logarithms by Napier and Briggs did much to simplify computation as the manipulations of multiplication and division were reduced to those of addition and subtraction. Figure 2 shows the calculation of $2 \times 3 = 6$ using two rulers with logarithmic scales. This principal forms the basis of the slide rule, which is one example of an analogue machine. These machines represent the magnitude of numbers by some physical quantity such as length or voltage; and, while slide rules are widely used for the solution of simple problems, the analogue computer uses electronic circuit elements to provide the arithmetical functions used in the solution of more complex problems. The main use of

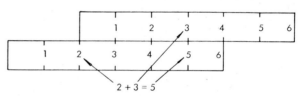

FIG. 1. Calculation of $2 + 3 = 5$, using two rulers.

analogue computers lies in the domain of simulation, or providing an electrical analogy, of dynamical systems such as muscular activity, heart action, respiration and similar continuous functions. The accuracy of the results depends upon the accuracy of the functional elements. An ordinary

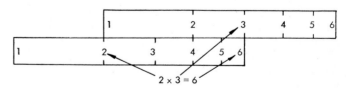

FIG. 2. Calculation of $2 \times 3 = 6$, using two rulers with logarithmic scales.

slide rule can produce results which are correct to within one per cent. However, the accuracy of an arithmetical process is limited only by the number of figures or digits that are used; and it is digital machines which are most commonly applied to computational problems.

The earliest digital calculating machine was the abacus which, initially, comprised pebbles placed in grooves made in the sand; each groove representing units, tens, hundreds, etc. Later the device was constructed in a frame, the pebbles being replaced by beads strung on wires. The abacus was not greatly used in Western Europe, but is still in use in some Eastern countries, where, in the hands of a skilled operator, remarkable speeds of calculation can be achieved. In 1946, the American Army arranged a competition, involving arithmetic operations, between one Private Wood, who used a desk calculator, and a Japanese clerk, who used an abacus. Kiyoshi Matsuzaki, the Japanese clerk, was the clear winner.

In 1642, Blaise Pascal, at the age of 19, designed and built a mechanical calculator which could carry out addition and subtraction. John Napier, in about 1690, produced his "multiplying bones". These were small bones, which could be carried in the pocket, inscribed with multiplication tables. Each bone bore the table for a particular digit, and allowed the user to effect a multiplication by adding certain numbers. That such basic aids were required at that time reflects the scarcity of individuals who had a working knowledge of even simple arithmetic calculations. In 1662, Pepys, who was later to become President of the Royal Society and who was, for that era, a well educated man, was appointed to the contracts branch of the Admiralty. In order to carry out the tasks required by this post, he had to arrange for special tuition so that he could learn his multiplication tables. In contrast, Leibnitz, in 1694, was able to improve on Pascal's calculator by inventing a machine which carried out multiplication by repeated addition. It was not a successful commercial proposition, and mechanical calculators were not commercially exploited until the 1880's, and even then received no extensive use until the 1920's.

Charles Babbage was born in 1792, and has been called the father of modern computation. He was the first person to visualize an automatic computer, and he outlined the fundamental principles of today's digital computers.

The French Government had instigated a project for the computation of mathematical tables. The project employed three or four mathematicians who decided upon the method of calculation, about seven people who reduced this method to a series of operations involving only addition and subtraction and about eighty "human computers" who actually carried out these operations.

In 1812, Babbage designed his Difference Engine which was intended to replace the eighty "human computers" in the calculation of mathematical tables. He constructed a small working model which he demonstrated in 1822, but a complete machine was never finished. In 1833 he conceived the idea of the Analytical Engine, which would be able to perform any type of calculation. The functions and specifications of this machine are essentially the same as those of present day computers. Although Babbage devoted the rest of his life, and much of his fortune, to an attempt to perfect the Analytical Engine, a working model was never built. However, sufficient detail remains to estimate the approximate timings involved which are about 1 s for an addition and 1 min for a multiplication.

It was not until 1944 that the first automatic digital computer was built. This was an electromechanical device, and was followed in 1946 by the first electronic digital computer (ENIAC). ENIAC was built at the Moore School of Electrical Engineering in the University of Pennsylvania, and represented a major advance in the computer field. The increased speed of electronic operations is reflected in the times for addition (0·2 ms) and for multiplication (28 ms).

By this time computer development was being carried out at many centres, and, as the basic electronic circuit elements became more robust and capable of operating at higher frequencies, so digital computers became more reliable and faster in operation. A modern computer might well require only 1 μs for an addition and 3 μs for a multiplication. Together with this hardware development came corresponding progress in the software, the sets of instructions comprising programs and subroutines, which define the actions of the computer.

TERMINOLOGY AND OPERATION

A digital computer is a machine capable of performing operations on numbers represented in digital form. The unit which performs these operations is called the central processor, and, in order to provide the data and to obtain the results, it is connected to input and to output devices. These enable us to communicate with the computer, and use various means to translate the data from the digital format used by the central processor to a format which is more readily understandable. As they are external to the processor, they are known as peripheral units.

The most common peripheral unit is the teleprinter or teletype,* which is an electrical or electronic typewriter used to type in commands or data to the processor, and, under the control of the processor, to type out information. Many teletypes include a paper tape reader and punch in addition to the keyboard. It is a slow device which operates at rates of about 10 characters per second.

Paper tape has been used as an input/output medium since the start of digital computers. 5-track paper tape devices were already part of the telegraph system, and these were adapted for computer use. The coding of information onto 5-track tape soon brought problems because there is not sufficient coding capacity for the full range of symbols and characters required.

Nowadays, 8-track tape is more commonly used, which takes 7 tracks for data and 1 track for a parity bit. This allows a set of 2^7 or 128 characters or symbols to be coded as combinations of holes punched across the 1 in. wide paper tape. There are 10 characters to the inch punched along the paper tape, which makes it a compact and cheap medium. In addition to the electromechanical teletype reader and punch there are high speed punches operating at up to 300 characters per second, and photoelectric readers operating at up to 2000 characters per second.

One of the disadvantages of paper tape is that if a single character has been typed incorrectly then the whole tape may need to be repunched. This difficulty is overcome with

---

* Teletype is a registered trademark of the Teletype Corporation of the U.S.A.

cards, where a set of data is punched onto many rectangular cards, each usually containing 80 columns. A character is represented by a combination of holes punched in a column. Cards are prepared on a special punch which has a keyboard and arrangements for feeding and collecting cards from the punch face. The peripheral unit at the computer, the card reader, is an input device only. It comprises a card hopper which takes a stack of punched cards, and a card track which passes cards individually to

third type, which is becoming more widely used, has a single, moving writing head which strikes the ribbon with a set of rods to form a dot matrix. This is a cheaper but much slower system.

Often the data to be fed to the computer will not be in the form of numbers, but will be represented by an analogue voltage. Electrical activity from the brain (EEG) or muscle (EMG) as well as the outputs from various transducers will produce a voltage signal. In order to obtain numbers for

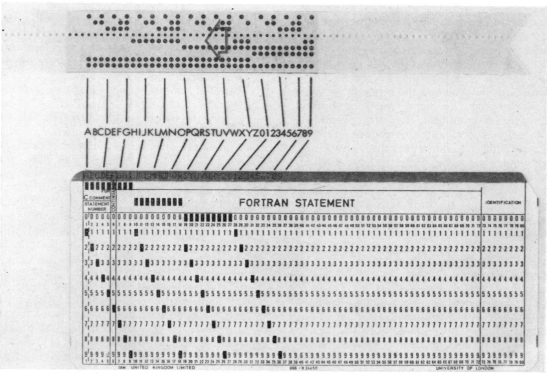

FIG. 3. Coding of paper tape and punched card.

the reading head. As with paper tape systems, the reading head may be electromechanical, but, more often, it is a photo-electric reader which permits rates of about 1000 cards per minute, or a maximum of about 1300 characters per second. Figure 3 illustrates the punched card and paper tape formats.

Alphanumeric data, that is, both alphabetical characters and numbers, can be output by the teletype at low speeds; but a device called a line printer will produce typed output at rates from 300 to 2000 lines per minute, or a maximum rate of about 5300 characters per second. There are two main types of line printer: chain printers, where a chain of type characters moves continuously across the width of the paper, and barrel printers, where a series of wheels, one at each print position across the paper, revolve to bring the type characters past the papers. Both work on the same principle. In order to print a character at a certain position across the paper, an electrical signal is sent to a hammer at that position, at a time when the appropriate type character is facing the paper. The hammer strikes the paper and an ink ribbon against the typeface to print the character. A

the central processor the voltage signal is sampled by an analogue-to-digital converter and the numerical value of the sample is passed to the processor. Nyquist, in 1924, showed that all the information in an analogue signal could be contained in a set of samples of that signal, provided that the time between samples did not exceed a value which is determined by the highest frequency component of the signal. Thus, provided that an adequate sampling rate has been set, a series of values can be obtained from an analogue-to-digital converter which allows a digital computer to acquire analogue, electrical signals.

In a similar manner digital-to-analogue converters can provide voltage outputs which may be used to control other devices or to drive a visual display unit or cathode-ray tube. These are screens on which waveforms, diagrams and text may be displayed. Some systems provide photographic or photocopying devices to obtain a hard copy of the screen display, but the majority of textual output is handled by a teletype or line printer, and graphical output is dealt with by an incremental plotter. Such a plotter is controlled by the computer and has a pen which can be raised, lowered and moved left and right through a small, fixed distance. Similarly, the plotter paper can be moved up and down, enabling any type of waveform or symbol to be drawn.

The central processor unit (CPU) is the nerve centre of the computer. It co-ordinates and controls the operation of the peripheral units and performs logical and arithmetical operations on the data according to the program* instructions. These operations are carried out with electronic and electrical devices which have two stable states, that is: switches can be on or off, lamps can be illuminated or not, transistors and diodes can perform as switches and be "open" or "closed". Thus it is much more convenient for the electronic logical and arithmetical units which are available, to use an arithmetic which is based on two states rather than the normal arithmetic system which has ten states. So, both the data and the program instructions within the computer are represented as binary numbers instead of decimal numbers. The various number systems are distinguished in Chapter 1. Binary numbers rapidly become very lengthy, and, whilst this is no problem to the computer hardware, it becomes awkward for the programmers to handle and to remember large binary numbers. By noting that $2^3 = 8$, binary numbers may be arranged in groups of three binary digits and each group can be represented by a single digit of a base eight number system. Unless one actually has to work with these numbers, it would appear that adding an octal system (base eight) to the decimal (base ten) and binary (base two) systems is an unnecessary complication, but in practice it is really most useful.

In order to distinguish between the systems, in cases where there is the possibility of confusion, the base of the number system being used follows the number as a suffix; e.g. 12_8. Translation between the various systems represents no problem, and the decimal, octal and binary representations of some commonly encountered values are given in Appendix I (page 947).

The binary numbers are stored, manipulated and controlled by three separate hardware sections of the CPU, the memory unit, the arithmetic unit and the control unit.

The internal memory provides the storage within the processor. Small ferrite rings, or cores, can store a binary digit, or bit, as each ring can be magnetized in either a clockwise direction (which could represent the 0 condition) or in an anticlockwise direction (the 1 condition). The magnetic state of each ferrite ring can be set and can be detected by wires which pass through the centre. Thus a bit may be "written" into the core storage or "read" from the core storage. To represent any number greater than 1, several bits must be used. The exact number of bits used vary from one computer to another but 12, 18, 24 and 36 bits are commonly found. Such a collection of bits is called a word, and this is the basic unit of the processor memory and arithmetic operations. The range of values that can be stored in a word will depend upon the word length, a 12 bit word can store 4095 ($2^{12} - 1$) values, an 18 bit word can store 262143 ($2^{18} - 1$) values and so on.

* Program is used to distinguish between a computer program and a programme of events.

If the accuracy or range of a single word is not adequate, values can be represented by two words, called double precision operation, or a different system using two or more words, to give floating point representation can be utilized. The location of a word within the core memory is called the address, and the function of the circuitry which connects to the memory is to read or write the value of a word at a given address.

The arithmetic unit contains one or more special word stores called registers in which the arithmetic operations of addition, subtraction, multiplication and division can be performed. The basic register for addition and subtraction is called the accumulator, and, in general, a number fed in from a peripheral unit will enter into the accumulator directly, and will then be passed from the accumulator to the memory.

Similarly, if two numbers, stored in the core memory, are to be added together and the sum stored back in the memory, then the accumulator will first be cleared, the first number extracted from memory and added to the accumulator, the second number added in the same way and, finally, the value in the accumulator will be stored in the memory.

The third section of the processor, the control unit, provides the facilities needed for the operations. It has several special registers to enable it to locate addresses in the memory, identify which instruction is to be obeyed and to transfer data from the memory and the arithmetic unit. In fact, modern computer design uses this third section only as the CPU and treats the memory and arithmetic units as peripherals. This allows parallel operations in which more than one instruction can be dealt with at a time, giving a significant increase in the speed of operation.

In order for the processor to deal with data, the data values must be in the core store. However, such store is expensive and several cheaper forms of storage, called backing storage, are used to supplement the internal memory. Backing storage is provided by peripheral devices such as magnetic tape or disc, and, in order to deal with numbers stored on these devices, the appropriate sections of the data are read into core memory, processed, and, if necessary, written out to the storage device before the next section of data is dealt with. Programs, as well as data, are usually kept on the backing store and each program is read into core as required.

Digital magnetic tape systems are similar to a conventional tape recorder with the exceptions that the tape is generally wider, multi-track recordings are made and pulses, representing bits, are recorded together with timing marks and an addressing system. Disc stores comprise a number of flat circular steel plates coated with magnetic material. These are rotated at high speed past read and write heads which access the data.

Some peripheral units, such as disc and magnetic tape, will often contain their own sub-processors which allow them to access the memory directly without the data having to pass through the accumulator and without having to involve the main processor. Direct memory access devices can transfer data whilst the main processor is performing other functions, and this feature enables computation to proceed much more quickly, and exemplifies the modern trend towards parallel operation mentioned earlier.

Figure 4 shows a block diagram of a straightforward computer system. In practice, computer systems differ greatly, dependent upon the particular type of work involved. Even in the medical field, they range from small, on-line computers which are "dedicated" to a particular job, to large, central, multi-user systems. It is possible for several users to run different programs on the same computer by time-sharing. This is based on the fact that

clear the main arithmetic register, that is, set the accumulator to zero. Codes 2000_8 and 3000_8 could mean "add" and "store" respectively; so that a program to add together two numbers, which are in locations 100_8 and 120_8 in the memory, and to store the sum in location 300_8, could be coded as:

```
1000   (Clear the accumulator)
2100   (Add the contents of location 100₈)
2120   (Add the contents of location 120₈)
3300   (Store the sum in location 300₈)
```

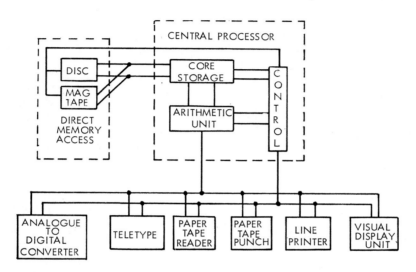

PERIPHERAL UNITS

FIG. 4. Block diagram of a computer system.

the central processor will take approximately a millionth of a second to perform a simple instruction, whereas data coming in, from a teletype will take a minimum time of about 100 ms, or a factor of 100 000 times longer, to input a character. This huge disparity between the working rates of the central processor and its peripherals make it desirable that the processor, instead of waiting for the next input from a terminal, should service other terminals or continue with other programs in the intervening 100 ms period. Even the time required by the peripheral units is fast compared to human working rates, and so, as far as the user is concerned, the various terminals are run simultaneously.

PROGRAM LANGUAGES

In order to solve a particular problem, or to carry out a certain function, the computer has to implement a series of instructions which is called a program. The user must first supply the program, and there are many different ways which he can use to write the instructions.

The most direct method is to use the binary coding which is used in the computer memory, or, for the sake of brevity, to use the equivalent octal numbers in writing the program and to change these to binary as they are fed into the memory. For example, the code 1000_8 could mean

Whilst this is the most straightforward method as far as the computer is concerned, it is not an easy task for the programmer. An easier system is to write the program in a *symbolic* language, or an *assembly code*, in which mnemonics will correspond to the binary arithmetic instructions, and labels or tags will correspond to memory locations. Taking the coding examples defined above, the mnemonics CLR (Clear accumulator), ADD (Add to accumulator) and STO (Store the accumulator) would correspond to the values 1000_8, 2000_8 and 3000_8 respectively. Similarly, the programmer would define labels for locations where data are stored, and a program to add the two numbers stored in locations A and B, and store the sum at location C would be written as:

```
CLR
ADD A
ADD B
STO C
```

Somewhere else in the program the locations would be entered:

```
A, 3
B, 2
C, 0
```

After the program has been executed the contents of location C would be equal to 5.

In order to translate this symbolic language into binary code, a special program called an *assembler* is used. The assembler will read the mnemonic symbol, look it up in a table from which it will obtain the binary code, replace the labels by memory address values, and thus generate the binary program.

There are a large number of operations which are common to many programs, such as reading numbers from the teletype, typing numbers on a line printer, etc. The sequence of instructions which control these operations could be written as a subroutine, a section of program which can be entered from any location in the main program and which will return to the following location. A program to read a number from the teletype and to store it in location A could be written as:

JMP READTTY   (Jump to teletype read sub-
                     routine)
STO A   (Subroutine will return here with
                     the number in the accumulator.
                     The number is then stored in
                     location A)

With simple assemblers the symbolic code for these subroutines will be on the back-up storage device and the programmer will have to add the code to his program before assembly. More advanced assemblers can have the binary of the subroutine stored, and, at assembly time, will automatically add any subroutine required from the subroutine library.

The next stage of simplification for the programmer is to use a *problem-orientated* language. In such languages there is a syntax which governs command statements in a standardized form of English, and mathematical statements. A program to read two numbers from the teletype and to print out the sum could be written as:

READ A   (Read first number and store in A)
READ B   (Read second number and store in B)
C = A + B   (Set location C equal to the sum)
WRITE C   (Print out the sum)

Whilst the task has become easier for the programmer, the computer has the difficult task of translating this language to a binary code. This is achieved by another special program called a *compiler*, which has to generate one or more words of symbolic code for each statement, and to create calls to the correct subroutines.

For example, the mathematical statement:

$$C = A + B,$$

is compiled to:

CLR
ADD A
ADD B
STO C,

and the command statement READ A, is compiled to:

JMP READTTY
STO A.

Once this stage has been reached, the compiler automatically hands over control to an assembler which produces the binary code and adds the required subroutines from the library. In practice the compiler and assembler are usually combined into one program.

ALGOL (Algorithmic Language) and FORTRAN (Formula Translation) are examples of problem orientated high level languages for scientific and mathematical use, in which the source program statements comprise algebraic formulae and standardized, but understandable English. COBOL (Common Business Orientated Language) is another high level language developed for commercial use.

An alternative form of high level languages is provided by *interpreters*, which have all the mathematical and peripheral handling subroutines in the memory plus specialized subroutines which translate from the high level language to binary code as the program is being executed. As far as the operator is concerned, there is no compilation nor assembly, he merely writes a statement in a high level language which can be executed immediately. For example, in the interpretive language FOCAL* (Formula Calculator) the operator could enter on the teletype the statement:

$$TYPE \ (3 + 6)/2$$

and the computer would immediately respond by typing the answer: 4·500. Alternatively, an ordered series of statements forming a program can be written by prefacing each line with a number. Again, the program to read two numbers and type their sum would be:

1.1 ASK N1, N2
1.2 SET A = N1 + N2
1.3 TYPE "SUM=", A

and the program could be executed immediately.

Each of these languages has advantages and disadvantages which are summarized below.

Symbolic language (assembly code) allows the programmer the maximum flexibility as he is not committed to fixed subroutines, and has control of every peripheral device in the system. In any particular situation the most efficient coding can be achieved, and, in situations where the program has to operate at the highest possible speed, machine code is often the only coding method that can be used. The disadvantages include the large number of instruction mnemonics that the programmer has to use, and the large number of instructions required; it could take several hundred instructions to read a non-integer decimal number from the teletype.

High level languages (using compilers) greatly simplify the task of the programmer, particularly for complex calculations. The language is only moderately difficult to learn and bears some resemblance to English. However, the final binary program, in

---

* FOCAL is a registered trade mark of Digital Equipment Corporation, Maynard, Massachusetts, U.S.A.

general, is not optimally coded and so the programs, when executed, are slower in operation than machine code. The programmer is dependent upon the library subroutines, and not all peripheral devices may be handled thereby decreasing the flexibility of the system. If an error is made in the source program, the programmer will have to correct the source program, and then carry out the compilation and assembly procedures again.

High level languages (interpreters) simplify the task of the programmer even more. Not only are direct statements accepted as well as program lines, but, generally the language is easier to learn and closer to English. If a mistake is made in the source program it can be corrected and the program re-run immediately. The disadvantages are that such languages produce programs that run more slowly than the compiled languages, and, because all the subroutines are loaded into the memory, instead of just those subroutines required by the particular program, there is less room in the memory for program and data storage.

PROBLEM SOLVING

It has been shown how a computer can carry out arithmetical functions, either directly for addition and subtraction, or by using subroutines for more complex functions such as sine, cosine and logarithm. In a similar manner, it is capable of logical decisions such as whether a variable is less than, equal to or greater than some value. Finally the computer can transfer data, either within the memory or to and from peripheral devices. Thus, any problem which the computer can solve must be definable in terms of arithmetical, logical and transfer operations.

Given a problem to be solved the following stages have to be carried out in order to arrive at a computer program.

(i) A mathematical or logical model of the problem must be derived and the equations formulated.

(ii) If necessary, a numerical method of solving the equations which is suitable for a digital computer must be selected.

(iii) A graphical representation of the logical sequence of operations involved in the computation is required. This is the *flow diagram*, and it will show how the problem can be solved by operations which are possible on the computer.

(iv) Based on the flow diagram, the operations must be defined in a language suitable for the computer.

The flow diagram, or flow chart, uses different symbols to represent terminal points in the program (such as the beginning and the end), decision points, and arithmetic functions or processes. Although standards have been produced for these symbols there is a great deal of work published in non-standard formats, and the reader should be prepared for changes in format. Here, the following symbols will be used:

⬭ Terminal point

▭ Processing (data transfer and arithmetic)

◇ Decision point

○ Continuation (for a diagram comprising several sections)

A simple program to read in three numbers and to type out their sum would have the flow diagram shown in Fig. 5. This comprises an *initialization* section in which the

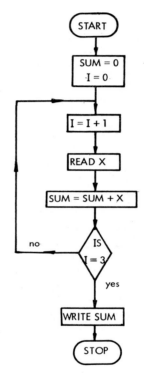

FIG. 5. Flow diagram of a program to add three numbers.

values of SUM and of the counter, I, are set to zero. This is followed by a *loop* in which the value of I is *incremented* or increased by 1, a number X is read, and the SUM set equal to its old value plus the value of X. A decision point completes the loop; if I is not equal to 3 then more input is required and the program goes back to ask for another input value. If $I = 3$, all the numbers have been read and the program will type out the sum and halt.

If the three numbers were 3, 7 and 9, the following table gives the values of the variables at different stages of the program.

Figure 6 shows how an everyday action would be itemized in a flow diagram.

A more practical example of flow diagrams results from the following problem. Suppose that audiometric thresholds at 1000 Hz have been measured for a large number of patients who are suffering from a particular disorder.

In order to describe the data mathematically, the mean and the variance of the sample are required.

GETTING UP IN THE MORNING

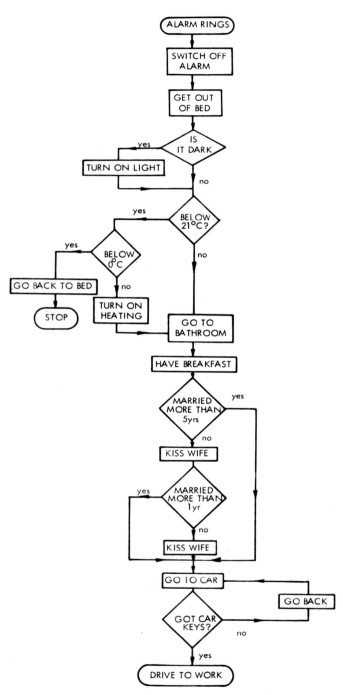

FIG. 6. Flow diagram example.

The first step in the procedure is easily completed as the model of the problem is already in mathematical terms, and the standard statistical equations are:

$$\text{mean,} \qquad \bar{x} = \frac{1}{n} \sum_{i=1}^{n} x_i,$$

$$\text{and variance,} \qquad S^2 = \frac{1}{(n-1)} \sum_{i=1}^{n} (x_i - \bar{x})^2$$

One numerical method for the computation is that suggested by the equations themselves. First read in the

TABLE I

STATES OF THE VARIABLES OF FIG. 5

State	I	X	SUM
Initialized	0	–	0
1st Pass of loop	1	3	3
2nd Pass of loop	2	7	10
3rd Pass of loop	3	9	19

data, store them and calculate the sum, from this obtain the mean and compute the sum of the squares of each datum minus the mean $\left(\sum_{i=1}^{n} (x_i - \bar{x})^2 \right)$. Finally, divide this by $(n-1)$ to obtain the variance, and write out the values. The corresponding flow diagram is shown in Fig. 7, and, whilst this program will work satisfactorily, it requires that the data be stored as an array $X(1)$, $X(2) \ldots X(N)$, and it involves N passes around two loops. A much better numerical method as far as computation is concerned can be derived by noting that

$$\sum_{i=1}^{n} (x_i - \bar{x})^2 = \sum_{i=1}^{n} x_i^2 + \sum_{i=1}^{n} \bar{x}^2 - 2\bar{x} \sum_{i=1}^{n} x_i \qquad (3.1)$$

$$= \sum_{i=1}^{n} x_i^2 + n \left(\frac{\sum_{i=1}^{n} x_i}{n} \right)^2 - \frac{2}{n} \sum_{i=1}^{n} x_i \sum_{i=1}^{n} x_i \qquad (3.2)$$

$$= \sum_{i=1}^{n} x_i^2 - (\sum_{i=1}^{n} x_i)^2/n \qquad (3.3)$$

Thus, the variance may be computed directly from the values of the sum and the sum of squares of the data. The new method involves calculating the sum and the sum of squares for each datum as it is acquired. The flow diagram is shown in Fig. 8, and requires only one loop and does not need to store the original data.

In general this is a good numerical method, but it is not without its drawbacks. Sometimes, calculation of the variance from the formula

$$\frac{1}{(n-1)} \left(\sum_{i=1}^{n} x_i^2 - \frac{1}{n} \left\{ \sum_{i=1}^{n} x_i \right\} \right)^2$$

can involve calculating a very small difference between two very large numbers, and unless the computer has sufficient accuracy, gross errors can result. For example, the three numbers 5001, 5002, and 5003 have a mean of 5002 and a

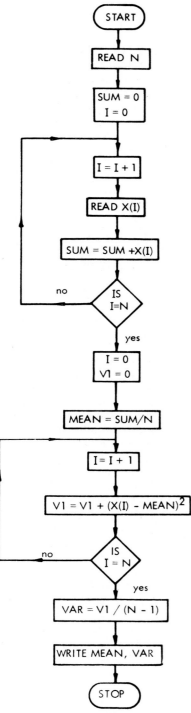

FIG. 7. Flow diagram for the calculation of mean and variance (1).

In order to arrive at the correct answer the computer must have an accuracy of better than 1 part in 38 million. This problem can be overcome by calculating the running mean and variance as each number is read, thus avoiding the use of very large values given by sums of squares.

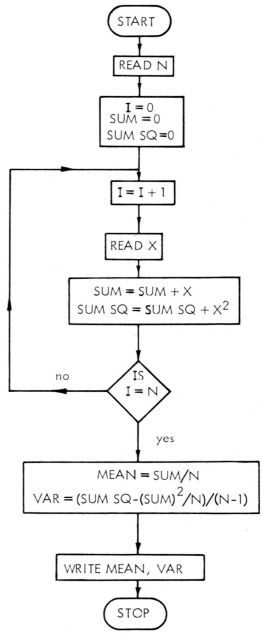

FIG. 8. Flow diagram for the calculation of mean and variance (2).

variance of 1. To compute this by the method discussed above involves the subtraction:

$$75\,060\,014\,-$$
$$75\,060\,012$$
$$=\qquad 2$$

Normally, the detail of the *algorithm*, or the procedure used in the solution of a problem, need not concern the user. However, the user should be aware of what steps are involved in obtaining a computer-based result to a problem, and should realize that only those problems which can be expressed in terms of arithmetic functions and logical decisions, albeit in some cases in a highly complex manner, are capable of solution.

ON-LINE APPLICATIONS

On-line applications of computer programs describe the situation in which the patient is effectively treated as a peripheral device, which supplies information of some sort, or as a link between peripheral devices to provide interaction with different parts of the computer system. Computer-controlled automatic audiometry (Wood, 1971) is an example of the patient providing a link between peripheral units.

Many of the on-line measurements in medicine are electrophysiological. Electrocardiography and electro-encephalography are accepted techniques. In the otological field, the measurement of the electrical potentials produced by the cochlea and the neural activity of the auditory system, are becoming increasingly important. These potentials differ from those recorded in ECG's and EEG's in two fundamental aspects.

Firstly, they are not spontaneous potentials; they have to be evoked by an acoustical stimulus. Secondly, the magnitude of the evoked potentials is much less than that of other electrical activity which is recorded at the same site. The background activity comprises ongoing EEG, myogenic potentials and electrical noise, and, as it is larger than the auditory potentials, will completely obscure any direct recording. Although direct measurement is impossible, several computer techniques are available for extracting these low amplitude responses from the background noise; the most common of which is *Time Domain Averaging*.

It has been pointed out that, provided a suitable sampling rate had been chosen, an analogue voltage could be recorded, and stored in the computer memory, by digital sampling. Thus, the electrical activity from the recording electrode can be passed to the core storage. Time domain averaging involves obtaining the average, or the sum, of a series of digital samples of the record waveform, and is applied as follows:

The parameters of the acoustic stimulus are fixed, and the computer starts to sample the signal from the electrode. A fixed time later the acoustical stimulus is presented and at a still later moment the sampling is stopped. The digital sample values are stored in the computer memory and form a record of the first sweep. The whole procedure is repeated, and the values of the second sweep are added to those of the first, building a record of the sum of all the sweeps. After, say 100 sweeps, the process is stopped. As the response always occurs at a fixed time after the stimulus, a point on the response waveform will always be referred to the same memory address, which will now contain a value equal to 100 times the value of the point in the original response. Thus the summed sweeps contain a record of the response at 100 times its original magnitude. The background noise is not *time-locked* to the stimulus but is comprised of processes which are independent of the occurrence of an acoustical signal. Therefore, at any

point in the sweep the value of the noise will sometimes be positive, sometimes negative, and will tend to cancel. This means that, whereas the final record contains the response waveform at 100 times its original magnitude, the final value of the noise process will not be anywhere near 100 times its original value. Thus the signal-to-noise ratio has been improved by averaging, and the averaging procedure can be continued until the response waveform can be clearly defined. A more exact description of the signal-to-noise ratio improvement with averaging is given in the appendix to this chapter.

Figure 9 shows the results of averaging for an *auditory evoked response* (*see* Chapters 22 and 23) recorded at the vertex.

In 1961, Goldstein reported on the use of averaging in measuring acoustical evoked responses, and Davis (1965) described an evoked potential, recorded from the vertex, whose largest positive peak had a latency of about 160 ms. The potential has a peak-to-peak amplitude of the order of 20 μV at high levels of stimulation, and its use in estimating auditory thresholds has been reported by Rapin (1964), by Davis (1965) and by Barnet (1965). Whilst close agreement can be obtained between audiometric and evoked response thresholds, there is considerable variability in the latter.

The technique of estimating threshold in this way has become widely applied and is known as Electric Response Audiometry (ERA). Hyde (1973) has carried out fundamental researches in this field and has described the parameters required for clinical testing. The properties of the response vary considerably with the psychological state of the patient and with the use of anaesthesia.

The computer's task in obtaining a response is straightforward. The signal is comprised of low frequencies (in the range 0–20 Hz) and digital sampling need only be at a low rate. In general some 40 sweeps are required to elicit a clear response which must then be written to a graph plotter to obtain a permanent record.

The *cochlear potentials* (*see* Chapters 21 and 23) evoked by acoustical click stimuli were first extensively recorded in man by Ruben *et al.* (1960). In 1967 Portman and his associates recorded these potentials using a technique in which a needle electrode is passed through the eardrum and across the middle ear to rest on the bony promontory between the stapes base (footplate) and the niche of the fenestra cochleae (round window). Aran *et al.* (1971) reported how the technique is applied to clinical patients and Aran and Negrevergne (1973) showed the difference in response functions obtained from different types of disorders. These peripheral responses appear to be unaffected by sedation or anaesthesia.

The role of the computer in obtaining these responses is similar to its use in the evoked vertex response recordings, but there are some additional requirements which make the task more complex.

The peak-to-peak amplitude of the response is of the order of 6 μV at high levels of stimulation and hence some 200–300 sweeps are required to elicit a clear response. The latency varies between about 1 and 4 ms depending upon the intensity, and the response is only about 1 ms in

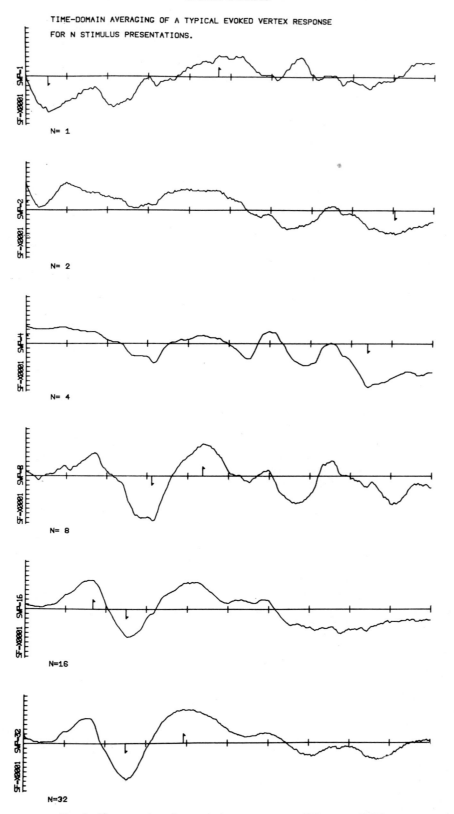

Fig. 9. The averaging of an evoked vertex response. (Thornton, 1973.)

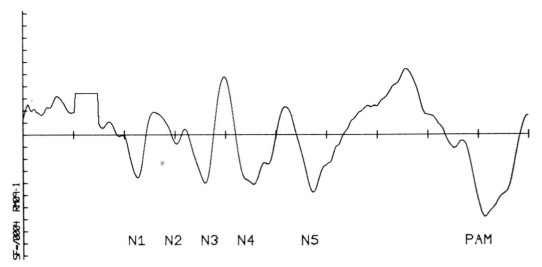

FIG. 10. Vestibulo-cochlear nerve, brainstem nuclei and post-auricular myogenic responses recorded in a normal subject. (Thornton, 1973.)

duration. Thus the sampling rate must be very much higher and the computer has to operate at higher speeds.

The cochlear potentials comprise not only the action potentials (AP) of the vestibulocochlear nerve, but also the cochlear microphonic (CM), a voltage response which follows approximately the pressure wave of the signal. The AP is always a negative going wave irrespective of the stimulus polarity. Thus, if the click stimuli are alternately positive and negative the CM will be alternately positive and negative and will cancel in the average. If, in addition to this basic averaging, each alternate sweep record is inverted and averaged in a separate section of the computer memory, the AP will itself be alternating and will cancel in this average. Thus the computer can extract both the CM and AP from the noise, and isolate the CM and AP responses in different averages.

Sohmer and Feinmesser (1967) and Thornton (1972), using surface electrodes with the active electrode sited at the earlobe or on the mastoid respectively, have reported the measurement of not only the cochlear microphonic and vestibulocochlear nerve response, but also responses from the auditory brainstem nuclei. Animal studies by Lev and Sohmer (1971) which used simultaneous recordings taken from both intracranial and surface electrodes led them to ascribe the sources of the five neural responses as:

N1: Vestibulocochlear,
N2: Cochlear nucleus,
N3: Superior olivary complex,
N4 ⎫
N5 ⎭ : Inferior colliculus.

These responses have latencies ranging from 1 to 7 ms, and, in addition, an auditory specific *myogenic response* can be recorded at about 12 ms latency from the post-auricular muscles. Figure 10 shows the set of neural and myogenic responses recorded from a normal subject. The post-auricular muscle responses can be used to estimate

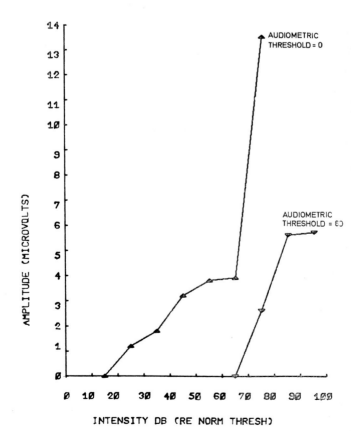

FIG. 11. Comparison between audiometric thresholds and those estimated from post-auricular muscle responses. (Thornton, 1973.)

threshold. Figure 11 shows a comparison between the levels at which the myogenic response disappears; and the audiometric thresholds recorded from a patient with a unilateral loss. The neural responses are much smaller in magnitude than those recorded with the trans-tympanic technique and, consequently, are not as good a threshold indicator. However, this measurement of brainstem function provides an aid in the diagnosis of retro-cochlear and neurological disorders, and research into the normal limits of the responses and the results obtained with selected pathologies is being carried out. (Lieberman et al., 1973; Rutt et al., 1973.)

This technique involves all the computational problems associated with the trans-tympanic technique, and, because the largest neural responses are only of about $0.5 \mu V$ magnitude, some 2000–3000 sweeps are required. This represents the worst signal-to-noise ratio of all the measurements, and, in some cases, the averaged data are stored on tape or disc for further computer analysis.

Plattig (1970) has applied time domain averaging to the study of the evoked vertex potentials obtained in response to taste stimuli. The stimuli were combinations of electrical pulses applied to the tongue, and the taste sensations they produced had been evaluated by subjective experiments. He found a clear correlation between the stimulus-response functions obtained by electrophysiological recording and those obtained from psychophysical studies.

Finally, a good example of the use of a computer to *control, run and analyse* an experiment is provided by studies of auditory/visual reaction times and visual perception times. This experiment forms part of a series of tests of central auditory function (Stephens and Thornton, 1972), and is based on the rationale that, in a unilateral lesion of the auditory cortex, the reaction times to auditory stimuli presented to the contralateral ear are prolonged; and in bilateral lesions the auditory reaction times show an increase from the normal value, whereas visual reaction times should be normal. Work is in progress to define more accurately these normal limits and to investigate the effect in more detail by utilizing the concept of auditory/visual simultaneity (Sanford, 1971).

The first part is achieved in the following manner. A programmable clock in the computer is set to measure time intervals in increments of 0.1 ms. The experimenter presses a teletype key to start the test and, after a random time interval, the computer switches on the clock and either a visual or auditory stimulus. The patient presses a button which stops the clock, the time interval is computed and stored on digital magnetic tape for later analysis.

The second part of the test is similar to the first, but requires two actions from the patient. In addition to supplying an auditory stimulus and measuring the reaction time, the computer displays a clock face on the screen which utilizes a moving dot instead of clock hands. The position of the dot, when the stimulus is presented, is recorded and when the patient presses the response button the dot is removed from the display. The patient is asked to define the dot position when the stimulus was given and his answer is entered on the teletype. In this case, both the

auditory reaction time and the visual perception time are stored on the tape.

At the end of the experiment the data are recalled from the tape and analysed.

GENERAL APPLICATIONS

A great deal of computation is carried out without a patient connected directly into the system, and many computer analyses are common to a number of fields of measurement and of research. Here these applications are divided into three main areas; analyses, modelling and records.

(a) Analyses

These comprise numerical and statistical analyses of data from patients, data manipulation and plotting. In common with any discipline involving measurement, basic statistical analysis is performed by the computer.

Data manipulation can be exemplified by reference to the electrocochleographic studies described earlier. The averaged responses, which have been stored on digital magnetic tape, can be affected by the following:

(i) A positive shift due to electrode contact potentials, drift in the equipment, etc.
(ii) Contamination in the pre-stimulatory region by electrical artifacts from the stimulus generator.
(iii) Residual noise which remains after the averaging process and tends to obscure the response.

Figure 12 shows how these factors may be dealt with on the computer. 12(A) shows the basic average. In 12(B) the data have been set to zero mean, and, in 12(C), the electrical artifact has been removed and the data digitally smoothed. Finally, in 12(D) the position of the acoustical stimulus has been marked and the data expanded to a more convenient scale.

Such a sequence of operations requires the operator to depress a few teletype keys, one for each function, and takes only one or two seconds.

In addition to obtaining a clear record and a graphical output, the numerical values of amplitude and latency for each peak are required. Again, this can be arranged as a semi-automatic function of the computer program. The operator has control of two cursors which he places before the first peak of interest and after the last. The program will then type out the latency, amplitude and peak to peak amplitude for all turning points in the waveform which lie between the two cursors.

If the individual sweeps are stored on disc or on magnetic tape, then several possibilites exist whereby the average may be improved. Individual sweeps may be scanned for large artifacts which, if present, will exclude that sweep from the average. Alternatively, a preliminary average may be produced from all sweeps, the mean and variance calculated, and then individual sweeps may be rejected on a statistical criterion. Access to the individual records provides the opportunity for much more detailed statistical analyses to be implemented and for studies of the basic

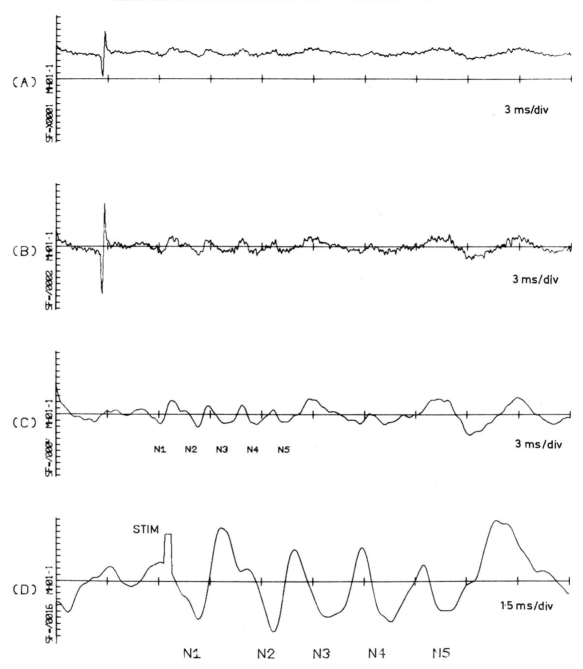

FIG. 12. Illustration of data manipulation techniques using an electrocochleographic response. (Thornton, 1973.)

characteristics of the response to be carried out. Hyde (1973) has studied the non-stationary properties of the evoked vertex response, and Fig. 13 shows an example of the growth function for the P_{180} peak (the peak of the positive wave at 180 ms latency). Here the sum of the values of a point, corresponding to P_{180} in the final average, is plotted against the number of sweeps. It can be seen that, at 35 sweeps the peak is negative, at 49 sweeps, it is zero, and finally, at 100 sweeps it is positive. Studies such as these outline the underlying properties of these responses, and stress the importance of using a technique that will

minimize possible errors in interpretation when applying these methods to clinical practice.

These lead on to the next stage of computer evaluation of biological signals which involves the automatic detection, recognition or classification of the signals.

The automatic detection of auditory evoked responses can be dealt with in many ways. Cross-correlation of a high level response with records obtained from lower level signals is one example of template-matching techniques which has been used (Friedman, 1968) as have statistical methods which evaluate the probability of obtaining the measured waveform if there was only random noise in the original signal.

The use of matched digital filters to evaluate evoked responses has been reported (Donchin, 1968). In this technique the computer synthesizes an "optimum" filter to match the data from a particular patient or experimental series. This technique has been used in conjunction with Wald's sequence test by Ott *et al.* (1973) to provide an automatic response detection system.

investigation of the motion of the basilar membrane under the effects of capillary forces from the cochlear fluids. Fant (1972) has used modelling techniques and compared the theoretical predictions with experimental findings (Fujimura and Lindquist, 1971) in his studies of the *vocal tract*. The main purpose here was to extend the theoretical basis for calculating the damping of vocal tract resonance modes.

Statistical models are often used, or at least implied, in

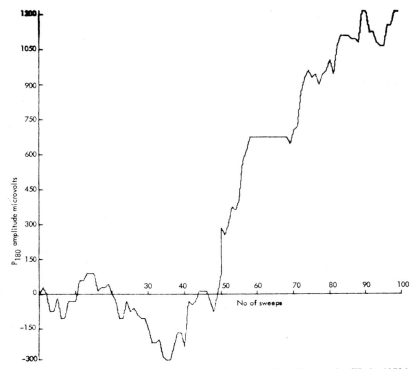

FIG. 13. Example of non-stationarity: the growth function for a P_{180} peak. (Hyde, 1973.)

Classification of the types of response can be obtained by extracting certain features of the response and comparing these using multidimensional vector techniques (Feldman, 1971). Such techniques have also been applied to automatic *speech recognition* by Green and Ainsworth (1973), who described a system for the recognition of continuous speech; and by Crichton and Fallside (1973) for both computer analysis and synthesis of speech.

Sayers and Hinchcliffe (1974) are using functions of weighted regression line approximations to the slow phase of nystagmus to examine and quantify electronystag-mographic records taken from patients with vestibular disorders.

(b) Modelling

The computer greatly facilitates the use of mathematical models of physiological mechanisms. Such modelling may involve a representation of the functional properties of the mechanism, or may be a non-functional statistical computation or curve-fitting procedure.

Computer models have been widely used to display *basilar membrane* movement (Crane, 1972) and in the study of cochlear mechanics. Clifton (1972) carried out an

almost any process of analysis. A simple example of multidimensional regression analysis can illustrate the approach. A control experiment, with normally hearing subjects, was carried out to measure both the pure tone audiometric thresholds at 500, 1 000 and 2 000 Hz and the speech intelligibility threshold for each subject. This was to provide normative data on the relationship between speech and audiometric thresholds. It was expected that the speech threshold would equal some constant plus weighted values of the three audiometric thresholds. Explicitly, the statistical model is:

$$S_i = \beta_0 + \beta_1 f_{1i} + \beta_2 f_{2i} + \beta_3 f_{3i} + e_i, \qquad (3.4)$$

where S_i = speech intelligibility threshold,

$$\left.\begin{matrix} f_{1i} \\ f_{2i} \\ f_{3i} \end{matrix}\right\} = \text{audiometric thresholds}$$

$$\left.\begin{matrix} \beta_0 \\ \beta_1 \\ \beta_2 \\ \beta_3 \end{matrix}\right\} \text{ are constants,}$$

and e_i is a random error term.

A regression analysis gave the following values (Thornton, 1973):

$$S_i = 4\cdot4 + 0\cdot29f_1 - 0\cdot23f_2 - 0\cdot04f_3$$

This provides an example of why such modelling should be explicit so that the computed results may be interpreted correctly. Here the interpretation of the results is that, given a subject's audiometric thresholds, the best prediction available to estimate his speech threshold is given by substituting the values in the equation shown above. The equation must *not* be interpreted as a functional relationship, in which case the interpretation would be that, as the

cases. Firstly, where the measurements have been taken for x values of equal interval; secondly, where the x values are of equal ratio. Fortunately, these conditions are merely a reflection of the normal experimental procedure and do not form an experimental constraint. Thus, it is possible to solve the equation and to determine V, g and h from three values of x and Y. Figure 14 shows a comparison between experimental data from Carter and Kryter (1962) and the Gompertz function calculated from three equal ratio values. These and other results show that it is reasonable to use Gompertz functions to predict the maximum TTS likely to result from various noise patterns.

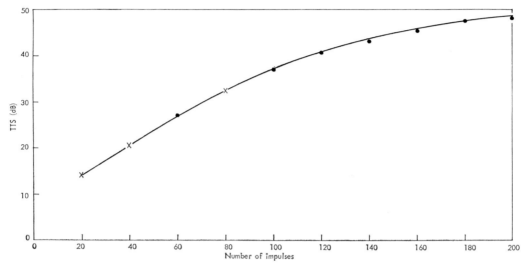

FIG. 14. Comparison of experimental TTS data (·) with a Gompertz function calculated from three experimental points (x). (Carter and Kryter, 1962.)

coefficient of f_2 is negative, then the greater the hearing loss at 1000 Hz the better will be the speech intelligibility. Such is clearly not the case.

Regression analysis basically represents *curve-fitting* according to some statistical criterion designed to minimize errors. Other types of curve-fitting can be carried out which use particular solutions of the equation to define the curve. Temporary threshold shift (TTS) data are used to estimate the amount of permanent damage to the hearing system by measuring the TTS_2 (TTS 2 min after exposure to the noise in question). Walker (1970) studied this TTS_2 measure for short duration impulse sounds. His findings were similar to those of Carter and Kryter (1962) who had proposed a mathematical relationship to fit the measured curves. This relationship gives a family of curves, known as Gompertz functions, and takes the form

$$Y = Vg^{h^x} \tag{3.5}$$

where Y is the TTS_2 for a given number of impulses, X; V is the maximum value of TTS_2 that would be reached for a particular noise pattern, and g and h are constants. From the experimental results, various values of x are known and the corresponding values of Y have been measured. It is possible to obtain a simple analytical solution for the Gompertz function in two particular

The advantage of this technique is that it allows the maximum level of TTS to be predicted from TTS values which are relatively small.

(c) Records

Some examples of the storage and retrieval of electrophysiological data recorded from patients have been given earlier. Full patient records involve material of much wider applicability than is pertinent here. Unfortunately, in the current computer-based systems, very little specific otolaryngological data are included. However, as such systems develop and cover more details of clinical tests, it is to be expected that such data will be included, and so a brief outline of patient record facilities is included here.

Generally, such a facility is based upon a central computer with a large backing store, which is accessed by many remote terminals at different locations. Teletypes and visual display units form the majority of the terminals, but, in more complex systems, digital interfaces with laboratory equipment may well be added.

This allows the automatic handling of patient admission, transfer, discharge and charging (IBM(a)) and provides fast access to information concerning the current status of a patient and his comparative condition over the last week, plus full details of laboratory analyses (IBM(b)). Hospital administration and internal communication are therefore greatly improved. However, as Abrams *et al.* (1968) point out, full details of a patient's condition may involve not only a single hospital department, but also physiotherapists, general practitioners and dentists, as well as research workers. Each group will have some kind of patient record facility, much of which will be duplicated. Moreover, as general practice consultations account for about 55 per cent of all patient contacts in the U.K., there is obviously a requirement for an integrated health record system. Systems have been detailed (Bowden, 1967) which could provide an integrated system for all the medical and para-medical services concerned with patients.

A further refinement is the development of techniques that will facilitate the classification of patients into different diagnostic, therapeutic and prognostic groups. The number of variables involved could mean that the computational power needed and the time required to print all the possible combinations would be prohibitive. However, Hall, Hallen and Selander (1971) using linear discriminatory techniques have reported a method which allows the analysis of a large number of variables without the need for a great deal of computer time.

There is no doubt that, as specialization increases, and the number of people concerned with the treatment of a patient grows, there will be an increasing requirement for fast-access, accurate and legible records.

CONCLUSIONS

It is clear that computers are becoming increasingly involved in many areas of everday life, and have an important role to play in otolaryngological as well as other medical fields. This means that the otolaryngologist should be aware not only of the advantages but also of the limitations of computers. He should have some knowledge of the kind of problems which are amenable to computer evaluation and should have a basic understanding of their function. There may well come a time when he will be called upon to decide whether or not to accept standardized reports, and be prepared to define his work in terms of logical decisions, if he is to benefit from computer technology.

The modern computer, by now a very distant relation to Babbage's analytical engine, has had far-reaching effects on almost all branches of measurement and research. Whilst the examples given here represent only a small fraction of the total application, it is hoped that the position of the computer in the field of otolaryngology has been placed in perspective.

APPENDIX

Time Domain Averaging

It is convenient to consider the signal, $s(t)$, which is taken from the recording electrode, as comprised of two separate components; $r(t)$, the response and $n(t)$, the background noise. Thus,

$$s(t) = r(t) + n(t) \tag{3.6}$$

and, at a point in the sweep we can write

$$s = r + n, \tag{3.7}$$

where r is the value of a point on the response waveform and is constant, and n is the same point on the noise process which, it is assumed, is a process which is normally distributed with mean $= 0$, and variance $= \sigma^2$. That is,

$$n \sim N(0, \sigma^2). \tag{3.8}$$

Now, the signal-to-noise ratio can be defined as

$$(S/N) = \text{rms (response)}/\text{rms (noise)}, \tag{3.9}$$

where rms indicates the root mean square value.

Initially, the signal-to-noise ratio

$$(S_i/N_i) = \text{rms } (r)/\text{rms } (n), \tag{3.10}$$

which

$$= (r/\sigma), \tag{3.11}$$

as r is a constant, and n has mean $= 0$, and variance $= \sigma^2$. If we average the signal over m sweeps, we have

$$\frac{1}{m} \sum_{i=1}^{m} S_i = \frac{1}{m} \sum_{i=1}^{m} r_i + \frac{1}{m} \sum_{i=1}^{m} n_i. \tag{3.12}$$

Now,

$$\frac{1}{m} \sum_{i=1}^{m} r_i = \bar{r} = r \tag{3.13}$$

(where $\bar{r}$ indicates the mean value of r, which is equal to r as r is a constant), and,

$$\frac{1}{m} \sum_{i=1}^{m} n_i = \bar{n}, \tag{3.14}$$

which is normally distributed with mean $= 0$ and variance $= \sigma^2/m$, or,

$$\frac{1}{m} \sum_{i=1}^{m} n_i = \bar{n} \sim N(0, \sigma^2/m). \tag{3.15}$$

Thus, the output signal-to-noise ratio from the averaged record

$$(S_0/N_0) = \text{rms } (\bar{r})/\text{rms } (\bar{n}), \tag{3.16}$$

which

$$= r/(\sigma\sqrt{m}). \tag{3.17}$$

Thus,

$$(S_0/N_0) = r/(\sigma/\sqrt{m}) = \sqrt{m}.(r/\sigma), \tag{3.18}$$

which, from (6), gives,

$$(S_0/N_0) = \sqrt{m}. (S_i/N_i). \tag{3.19}$$

Therefore, the signal-to-noise ratio has been improved by a factor equal to the square root of the number of sweeps used to obtain the average.

REFERENCES

Abrams, M. E., Bowden, K. F., Chamberlain, J. and MacCullum, I. R. (1968), *J. Roy. Coll. Gen. Practit.*, **16**, 415.

Aran, J-M. and Negrevergne, M. (1973), *Audiology*, **12**, 488.

Aran, J-M., Pelerin, J., Lenoir, J., Portmann, Cl. and Darrouzet, J. (1971), *Revue Lar.*, suppl., 602.

Barnet, A. B. (1965), *Acta Otolaryng.*, suppl. 206, 143.

Bowden, K. F. (1967). Personal communication.

Carter, N. L. and Kryter, K. D. (1962), *Rep. no.* 949 (Bolt, Beranek and Newman, Eds.).

Clifton, R. J. (1972), *I.S.V.R. Memo No.* 466. University of Southampton.

Crane, H. D. (1972), *J. Aud. Res.*, **12** (1), 36.

Crichton, R. G. and Fallside, F. (1973), Proc. B.S.A. Meeting, April 1973: Session B: Paper 73SHB7.

Davis, H. (1965), *Acta Otolaryng.*, **59**, 179.

Donchin, E. (1968), *Average Evoked Potentials* (Donchin and Lindsley, Eds.), p. 199. NASA SP-191.

Fant, G. (1972), STL-QPSR 2–3/(72) (KTH, Stockholm): 28.

Feldman, J. F. (1971), *Computers in the Neurophysiology Laboratory*, Vol 1, p. 63. D.E.C. Mass. U.S.A.

Friedman, D. (1968), *Detection of Signals by Template Matching*. The Johns Hopkins Press.

Fujimura, O. and Lindquist, J. (1971), *J. acoust. Soc. Amer.*, **49**, 541.

Goldstein, M. H. (1961), *Electroenceph. clin. Neurophysiol*, suppl. 20.

Green, P. D. and Ainsworth, W. A. (1973), Proc. B.S.A. Meeting, April 1973: Session C: Paper 73SHC4.

Hall, P., Hallen, B. and Selander, H. (1971), *Meth. Inform. Med.*, **10** (2), 96.

Hyde, M. L. (1973), Ph. D. Thesis, University of Southampton, England.

I.B.M. (a) Application Brief: GKZO-0630-0.

I.B.M. (b) Application Brief: GKZO-0637-0.

Lieberman, A., Sohmer, H. and Szabo, G. (1973), *Arch. Ohr.-Nas.-, u. Kehlk Heilk.*, **201**, 79.

Nyquist, H. (1924), *Bell Syst. tech. J.*, **3** (2), 324.

Ott, N., Meder, H. G. and Schmitt, H. G. (1973), I.B.M. Publication 73, 10.001.

Plattig, K. H. (1970), *Gustation and Olfaction*, p. 73 (G. Ohloff and A. F. Thomas, Eds.). London and New York: Academic Press.

Portman, M., Le Bert, G. and Aran, J.-M. (1967), *Rev. Laryng.*, *Paris*, **88**, 157.

Rapin, I. (1964), *Ann. N.Y. Acad. Sci.*, **112**, 182.

Ruben, R. J., Broadley, J. E., Nager, G. T., Secula, J., Knickerbocker, G. G. and Fisch, U. (1960), *Ann. Otol.*, **69**, 459.

Rutt, N. S., Stephens, S. D. G. and Thornton, A. R. D. (1973), *J. Physiol.*, **232**, 109.

Sanford, A. J. (1971), *Quart. J. exp. Psychol.*, **23**, 296.

Sayers, B. McA. and Hinchcliffe, R. (1974). Personal communication.

Sohmer, H. and Feinmesser, M. (1967), *Ann. Otol.*, **76**, 427.

Stephens, S. D. G. and Thornton, A. R. D. (1972), Annual Report of the Institute of Sound and Vibration Research: Sec. 5B.1 (iii).

Thornton, A. R. D. (1972), *E.R.A. J.*, **22**, 4.

Thornton, A. R. D. (1973). Unpublished data.

Walker, J. G. (1970), *Ann. Occup. Hyg.*, **13**, 51.

Wood, T. J. (1971), *J. Aud. Res.*, **11**, 325.

SECTION II

PHYSICS

		PAGE
4. BASIC ELECTRICITY		51
5. ELECTRONICS		69
6. ACOUSTICS		87
7. ELECTROACOUSTICS		101
8. PHYSICS OF HEAT		111

4. BASIC ELECTRICITY

R. I. DAMPER

INTRODUCTION

This chapter is intended to introduce the basic concepts and terminology necessary for an understanding of the "Electronics" chapter which follows. It is aimed at the reader with little formal knowledge of mathematics beyond differentiation and integration. Topics such as the vector and complex number notations are introduced, but are explained either in the text or in appendices.

The reader who has had little contact with electrical theory or electronics may be forgiven for wondering what its relevance to otolaryngology might be. In fact, it is considerable; and can be divided into four broad categories. The first of these concerns the measurement of physical parameters. In both clinical practice and research applications, electrical methods of measurement are extremely common. Examples of such techniques include the measurement of laryngeal function by electroglottography (electrolaryngology) and the recording of the cochlear microphonic potential, as in the technique of electrocochleography, at present coming into clinical prominence.

The second area of importance involves equipment for otolaryngology. This embraces topics such as the design of hearing aids, and the production of devices for audiological investigation (e.g. tone generators for audiometry, or noise generators to be used for masking purposes). A further area where electrical science plays a prominent role is that of modelling of certain physiological systems. Møller's model of the middle ear (1961) and Flanagan's electrical model of basilar membrane displacement (1962) are examples in point. Many other such examples will be found throughout the rest of the book. The facility with which diverse physical systems can be modelled by electrical means is but one by-product of the recent huge advances in this branch of science.

Finally, a number of techniques have been evolved for the treatment and analysis of electrical systems, which can also be applied to other situations. Some of these situations are of interest in otolaryngology. Examples include the many statistical methods developed in the telephone and communication industries which can be used in the study of speech and hearing. After reading the following two chapters, it is hoped that the medically-orientated worker will be better able to appreciate the material appearing in the literature, much of it written by engineers and technologists, on topics such as these.

In attempting to present a readable yet useful account of basic electricity, many simplifications have had to be made. Accordingly, the subject matter is neither exhaustive nor rigorous. Interested readers will, however, find many suggestions for further study in the bibliography at the end of the chapter.

SI units have, of course, been used throughout. The definitions of common electrical units have been collected together in an appendix, in order to avoid confusion in the main text.

CHARGE AND THE ELECTRIC FIELD

The concept of charge is of major importance in understanding both electric current and the structure of matter. The forces existing between charges in a vacuum were investigated by Coulomb (1788). He found that the force was inversely proportional to the square of the distance between charges and proportional to the magnitudes of the charges. Hence for two charges at a fixed distance:

$$F \propto \frac{q_1 q_2}{r^2}$$

F—force exerted by charges on each other (units: newton)
q_1, q_2—respective magnitude of charges involved (units: coulomb)
r—distance between charges (units: metre).

Introducing a constant of proportionality:

$$F = \frac{k q_1 q_2}{r^2}$$

In the International System of units (SI), now universally adopted for scientific and technological work (*see* Chapter 1), the constant of proportionality is given by:

$$k = \frac{1}{4\pi\varepsilon_0}$$

ε_0—permittivity of free space, equal to $8\cdot85 \times 10^{-12}$ $C^2.N^{-1}.m^{-1}$

So that:

$$F = \frac{q_1 q_2}{4\pi\varepsilon_0 r^2} \tag{4.1}$$

The reader may wonder why such a complicated constant is chosen. In fact, the use of this constant to relate force and charge has a very considerable simplifying effect on the unitary system. This arises from the SI definition of electric current in terms of the force between moving charge elements.*

* *See* Appendix I for definitions of electrical units in the SI system.

Following Coulomb's work, there was considerable argument over the agency by which a charge at some point could exert a force upon other charges placed in its vicinity. Such arguments can be circumvented by introducing the extremely useful concept of an *electric field*, E, relating the force, F, experienced by a charge, q, by the equation:

$$\mathbf{F} = q\mathbf{E}* \qquad (4.2)$$

We shall return frequently to the topic of the electric field

POTENTIAL, POTENTIAL DIFFERENCE AND ELECTROMOTIVE FORCE

Since a charge in an electric field experiences a force, work must be done to move charge from one point in the field to some other point. The work done in moving unit positive charge between points an infinitely small distance, ds, apart against this force is called the *potential difference* between those points. Denoting potential difference by dV, we have:

$$\mathrm{d}V = \text{work done per unit charge}$$
$$= \frac{\text{externally applied force} \times \text{distance}}{\text{charge}}$$
$$= \frac{\mathbf{F}_e \cdot \mathbf{ds}}{q}†$$

But by (4.2)

$$\mathbf{F} = q\mathbf{E}$$

So that the external force required to overcome this is:

$$\mathbf{F}_e = -q\mathbf{E}$$
$$\therefore \mathrm{d}V = -\mathbf{E} \cdot \mathbf{ds}$$

Hence

$$V = -\int \mathbf{E} \cdot \mathbf{ds} \qquad (4.3)$$

and (in scalar notation):

$$\mathrm{E} = \frac{-\mathrm{d}V}{\mathrm{d}s}$$

Because of this equality, electric field is often referred to as potential gradient. Although only the difference of potential between points has any fundamental significance, it is occasionally convenient to choose the reference point for zero potential at infinity. The *absolute potential* at a point then becomes the work necessary to bring a unit positive charge from infinity to the specified point. The units of potential are joules per coulomb or, more commonly, volts.

An "electrostatic" potential difference, as described above, cannot be used to cause charge to move around a closed circuit. This is because the work done in moving charge from a point, A, to another point, B, is exactly equal and opposite to the work done in moving the same charge from B to A. Hence the net work around a closed path is

zero. Useful engineering applications of electricity demand that work be performed by current moving around just such a closed circuit. This means that the potential difference available to move charge must also be a source of energy. Such a source is said to be characterized by its *electromotive force*, usually abbreviated emf. Emf, like electrostatic potential difference, has units of volts and, for this reason, the two are often confused. The distinction between them is that only an emf can provide energy to cause current in a closed circuit, although engineers use the term *voltage* for both emf and potential difference.

ELECTRICAL PROPERTIES OF MATTER

As is well known, all matter is composed of *atoms*. An understanding of electrical phenomena on the macroscopic scale demands an appreciation of the microscopic details of the structure of matter. This is so because the integrity, both of the atoms themselves and of ensembles of atoms forming materials, rests upon the attraction or repulsion of unlike or like charges respectively.

In every atom there is a positively charged nucleus around which are grouped negatively charged *electrons*. The charge on each electron is minute, being $1·602 \times 10^{-19}$ coulombs. Since electrons are indivisible, this is the smallest quantity of electric charge that can exist as a separate entity. Such amounts, that cannot be further divided, are termed *quanta* in the terminology of modern physics.

The electrons can be thought of as arranged in shells or orbits surrounding the nucleus. The maximum number of electrons which can be accommodated in each orbit, are found from simple, well known rules.* Normally, the orbits associated with the lowest energies (those closest to the nucleus) are filled in preference to all others. The electrons in the outermost shell, furthest from the nucleus, are termed *valence* electrons and are important in bonding between atoms to form materials.

The nucleus generally contains both *protons* and *neutrons*. These elementary particles have approximately the same mass, but are each some 1 835 times heavier than the electron, which has a mass of $9·108 \times 10^{-31}$ kg. Therefore the number of protons and neutrons in the nucleus can be taken as determining the mass of the atom, the much lighter electron making little contribution.

The proton has positive charge equal in magnitude to that of the electron, whereas the neutron is so named because it is electrically neutral. It follows that the normal (electrically neutral) atom must have the same number of electrons and protons. This number, equal to the quanta of nuclear charge, is called the *atomic number*.

The force of attraction between the oppositely charged electrons and nuclei is one of the most important forces acting to maintain the integrity of the atom. If large enough external forces are applied to the electrons bound to atoms, particularly the valence electrons furthest from the nucleus, they may be removed, or dissociated. It is the sustained motion of free electrons such as these under the influence of an applied electric field which constitutes *electric current*

---

* The reader should note that this is a vector equation. The significance of vectors and vector equations is outlined in Appendix II.

† *See* Appendix II for an explanation of the vector dot product.

* The nth shell can accommodate a maximum of $2n^2$ electrons.

in most materials. The atom which remains, after removal of one or more of its electrons, has net positive charge and is termed an *ion*. In some cases the flow of electric charge associated with ions actually constitutes the electric current. This is particularly important in biological situations. For instance, the currents which flow across the nerve cell membrane when an action potential is propagated are due to the movement of simple ionic species.

In some elements the atoms have a tendency to associate with available electrons rather than lose them, and so gain a net negative charge. One way that atoms of different species can combine to form solids is for one species to lose an electron from its atoms to produce positive ions. These electrons then associate with atoms of another species, yielding negative ions. The so-called ionic compound is then held together by the force of attraction between the oppositely charged ions. Solids formed in this way are generally very poor conductors of electricity since there are few free electrons in the material to carry the current. The ionic compounds include sodium chloride and potassium iodide. Materials such as these, which do not easily allow the passage of current, are termed *insulators* or dielectrics.

Many other bonding mechanisms exist, one of which is peculiar to metals. This group of elements is characterized by the possession of a small number of valence electrons relative to the number of valency *orbitals* (that is, the number of electrons that could be accommodated in a full shell). This leads to a situation where the atoms of the material aggregate, when forming a solid, so that valence electrons occupy as many as possible of the valency orbitals. These electrons are thus not localized between atoms but are free to move throughout the body of the material. Such free electrons are often called *conduction* electrons and are distinct from bound valence electrons. When an external electric field is applied they are able to move along the resulting potential gradient, giving rise to an electric current. Materials that possess this property are termed *conductors*, and the metals form the most important class of conductors. Copper, for instance, has approximately 10^{29} free electrons per cubic metre of material.

The final bonding scheme of interest to us here is the so-called covalent bond. In this case mutual sharing of one or more valence electrons between atoms occurs. Attractive forces between the shared electron and the nuclei provide cohesion in the material. In the covalent compounds it is possible to liberate some of the bound charges and so allow current to flow. These bound charges can be freed by thermal vibrations, by the application of large external electric fields or even by incident radiation such as light. Materials that are normally poor conductors, but can be made to conduct relatively well by elevating their temperature (so that conduction electrons are produced by thermal vibration), are termed *semiconductors*, and are of paramount importance in modern electronics. It is from semiconductors that transistors, as well as many other very useful devices, are made. Silicon and germanium are two important examples of this class of materials.

The value of semiconductors lies in the fact that their conductivity can be altered within quite wide ranges by the introduction of carefully chosen impurities, or *dopants*.

Material without such impurities is called intrinsic, whereas semiconductor that has been doped is termed extrinsic. We expect that extrinsic conductivity is much higher than intrinsic conductivity as explained below. Another most important fact is that the mode of conduction in the extrinsic material depends upon the properties of the doping material. This is a difficult topic to discuss in elementary terms; a realistic description requiring the use of quantum mechanics. However, we shall simply describe those salient points necessary for an understanding of the electronic devices treated in the next chapter.

As previously stated, conduction electrons can be produced in a semiconductor by thermal vibration of the constituent atoms, so that conductivity rises with temperature over a certain range. These *excited* electrons are then free to take part in conduction processes. Such an electron can be considered to leave behind it a conceptual "vacancy" or *hole*, when moving from its normal state to an excited state. Conduction can, in fact, occur via holes, just as it does via electrons. When this happens, the vacant site (holes) may become occupied by electrons under the influence of an applied field in such a way that the hole effectively appears to move through the material (corresponding to a flow of current). This differs from conduction by electrons in that the electrons occupying the holes are not excited (they have a lower energy than the excited, conduction electrons), nor are they free to move any appreciable distance under the action of an applied field.

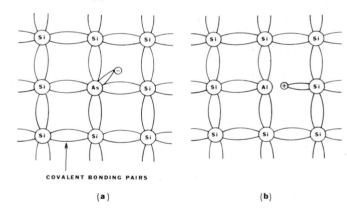

FIG. 1. (a) Pentavalent dopant (e.g. arsenic, phosphorus) in silicon crystal lattice. (b) Trivalent dopant (e.g. indium, aluminium) in silicon lattice.

We are now ready to consider the outcome of introducing two different types of impurity atom into the material. Silicon, widely used for the production of semiconductor devices, has four electrons in its outer or valence shell. If impurities such as phosphorus or arsenic, which have five valence electrons, are used for doping purposes then one more electron will exist in the vicinity of the impurity atom than is necessary for bonding purposes. This is shown diagrammatically in Fig. 1a. This extra electron is held much less tightly to the parent nucleus than the electrons which participate in bonding, and so requires only a small energy absorption in order to free it to take part in conduction processes. Pentavalent species can therefore be used to raise the conductivity of semiconductors by donating electrons, which can participate in the carrying of electric current. Hence such dopants are called *donors*. Material into which such atoms have been introduced is called *n-type* (or negative type) material.

In similar manner, if a trivalent species, such as indium or aluminium, is used as a dopant, there will be insufficient electrons in the vicinity of the impurity atom to satisfy the bonding requirements. This is shown in Fig. 1b. In other words, holes will be introduced into the material which can participate in conduction processes by combining with nearby electrons. Dopants of this type are therefore referred to as *acceptors*, whereas the doped material is called *p-type* (or positive type). The junction formed between *p*- and *n*-type materials has important electrical properties which form the basis of the principle of operation of modern semiconductor devices, such as the transistor, to be discussed in the next chapter.

THE MAGNETIC FIELD

The electric field is a useful concept when dealing with charges at rest. However, the situation is greatly complicated when moving charges are considered. A discussion of effects due to charges in motion is facilitated by the introduction of the *magnetic field*.

Ampere (1820) described the force existing between two parallel current-carrying wires in a vacuum. He found that, for currents in the same direction, the force was one of attraction; whereas when one of the currents was reversed, the force became one of repulsion. The forces were found to vary with the magnitude of the currents and also their directions (i.e. relative positions of the conductors), emphasizing the vector nature of the phenomenon. This, then, is an example of force associated with moving charges. The force per unit length between parallel wires in vacuum is found to be given by the following proportionality:

$$F \propto \frac{I_1 I_2}{a}$$

F—force in newtons per metre
I_1, I_2—respective currents in the two conductors in amperes
a—distance between conductors in metres.

The constant of proportionality for this equation in the International System is written $\mu_0/2\pi$ so that:

$$F = \frac{\mu_0 I_1 I_2}{2\pi a} \qquad (4.4)$$

μ_0 has the value $4\pi \times 10^{-7}$ N.C^{-2} . s^2 and is called the *permeability of free space*. The value of this constant is chosen so as to introduce numerical consistency between electrical, magnetic and mechanical phenomena. In fact, equation (4.4) is used to define the unit of current, the ampere (*see* Appendix I). If there is some material (other than vacuum) between the wires then F is increased by a factor μ_r, the *relative permeability* of the material.

We now introduce the magnetic field concept. The characteristic of this field is that a charge, q, moving through it with a velocity, v, experiences a force, F. Denoting the magnetic field by B, the force is given by:

$$F = qvB$$

In the vector notation:

$$\mathbf{F} = q\mathbf{v} \times \mathbf{B}* \qquad (4.5)$$

Equation (4.5) is often called the Lorentz equation, in honour of the Dutch physicist, H. A. Lorentz.

The magnetic field, **B**, has units of tesla, abbreviated T (previously weber per square metre).

A charge, q, moving with velocity, **v**, for a distance, **l**, gives rise to a current, I, so that an alternative form of (4.5) is:

$$\mathbf{F} = I\mathbf{l} \times \mathbf{B}$$

relating force, current and magnetic field.

It follows that current in a conductor produces a magnetic field. The magnetic field, **B**, is often characterized by the so-called *magnetic flux*, ϕ, passing through an area, A. **B** is then referred to as the magnetic flux density and is given by:

$$B = \frac{d\phi}{dA} \qquad (4.6)$$

ϕ has units of webers; hence the one-time use of webers per square metre for the units of **B** before the tesla was adopted.

CURRENT IN CONDUCTORS; OHM'S LAW

We have seen above that electric current is the manifestation of a flow of charge. Current, i, can then be defined as the rate of change of charge, q, at a point, so that:

$$i = \frac{dq}{dt} \qquad (4.7)$$

$$\text{charge } (q) = \begin{array}{c} \text{number of electrons} \\ \text{in material } (N') \end{array} \times \begin{array}{c} \text{charge on each} \\ \text{electron } (e) \end{array}$$

i.e. $\qquad q = N'e$

Consider a block of material, area A, length x; with N electrons per cubic metre (Fig. 2):

$$N' = N \times \text{volume}$$
$$= NAx$$

The current through area A is therefore given by:

$$i = \frac{d}{dt}(NAxe)$$

$$= NAe . \frac{dx}{dt}$$

$$\therefore i = NAev \qquad (4.8)$$

v—mean velocity of the ensemble of charge carrying particles (electrons).

* *See* Appendix II for explanation of vector cross product.

Hence current is seen to be proportional to the mean velocity in equation (4.8). This mean velocity, in conductors,

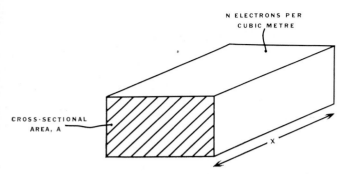

N ELECTRONS PER CUBIC METRE

CROSS-SECTIONAL AREA, A

x

FIG. 2. Block of conducting material, illustrating outline proof of Ohm's law.

is influenced solely by the externally applied field, under conditions of constant temperature, etc., so that:

$$\mathbf{v} \propto \text{electric field, } \mathbf{E} \qquad (4.9)$$

Introducing a constant of proportionality, μ:

$$\mathbf{v} = \mu\mathbf{E}$$

μ, the mean velocity per unit electric field, is termed the *mobility* of the charge carriers.

For a length, l, of conducting material with a potential difference (or voltage), V, between its ends, the electric field is uniform and is given in scalar notation by equation (4.3) as:

$$\mathbf{E} = \frac{V}{l}$$

$$\therefore \text{velocity, } v = \frac{\mu V}{l}$$

and substitution in (4.8) gives:

$$i = NAe \frac{\mu V}{l} \qquad (4.10)$$

so that $\qquad\qquad i \propto V$

This is the fundamentally important relation for conducting materials that was discovered experimentally by G. S. Ohm (1827). He designated the constant of proportionality between voltage, V, and current, I, as *resistance*, R, so that Ohm's law in its familiar form is:

$$V = IR \qquad (4.11)$$

When voltage, V, is expressed in volts and current, I, in amperes, then the resistance, R, has units of ohms (symbol Ω).

Ohm's law can then be stated as follows:

For a length of conducting material of constant cross-sectional area, at constant temperature and pressure, the potential difference between the ends of the conductor is directly proportional to the current flowing at any point.

Comparing equations (4.10) and (4.11) gives:

$$R = \frac{l}{NAe\mu}$$

or

$$R \propto \frac{l}{A}$$

This indicates that resistance varies directly with the length of the conductor and inversely with cross-sectional area. Introducing a constant of proportionality, ρ, gives:

$$R = \frac{\rho l}{A} \qquad (4.12)$$

ρ is termed the *resistivity* of the material (units: ohm-metre).

The resistivity, ρ, is by definition the inverse of the conductivity, σ.

Hence:

$$\text{conductivity, } \sigma = Ne\mu \qquad (4.13)$$

Equation (4.13) tells us that the more free electrons a material possesses, and the higher their mobility, the better will that material conduct electric current.

APPLICATION OF OHM'S LAW TO ELECTRIC CIRCUITS; KIRCHHOFF'S LAWS

The great practical importance of Ohm's law lies in the fact that, as well as describing the voltage–current relation in lengths of conductor (possessing the inherent property of resistance) it can also be applied to electric circuits composed of assemblies of elements.

These elements are of three basic types: resistors, capacitors and inductors. Capacitors and inductors will be dealt with in a later section but something will be said here concerning resistors.

Resistors, as circuit elements, are simply fabricated from coils of conductive material. Consider the case of a number of resistors of resistance R_1, R_2, R_3, etc., connected in series (Fig. 3a). Applying Ohm's law (4.11) to each resistor we have for the potential difference across each:

$$V_1 = IR_1$$
$$V_2 = IR_2$$
$$V_3 = IR_3$$

etc.

Now applying Ohm's law to the complete circuit:

$$V = IR'$$

R'—total resistance.

But $\quad V = V_1 + V_2 + V_3 + \ldots$ (*see below*)
$$\therefore V = I(R_1 + R_2 + R_3 + \ldots)$$

So total resistance is given by:

$$R' = R_1 + R_2 + R_3 + \ldots$$

For n resistors in series:

$$R' = \sum_{i=1}^{n} R_i \qquad (4.14)$$

In the case of resistors connected in parallel, the voltage across each is the same (Fig. 3b). Hence:

$$V = I_1 R_1 = I_2 R_2$$

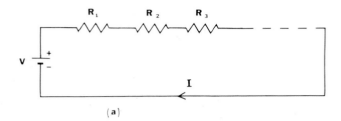

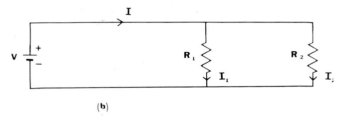

FIG. 3. (a) Resistors in series. (b) Resistors in parallel.

Again applying Ohm's law to the complete circuit:

$$V = IR'$$

But
$$I = I_1 + I_2 \quad (\textit{see below})$$

$$\therefore \quad V = (I_1 + I_2)R'$$

or
$$I_1 R_1 = (I_1 + I_2)R'$$

since
$$I_1 R_1 = I_2 R_2$$
$$I_2 = I_1(R_1/R_2)$$

$$\therefore \quad I_1 R_1 = (I_1 + I_1(R_1/R_2))R'$$

$$R' = \frac{R_1}{1 + R_1/R_2}$$

Total resistance is therefore given by:

$$R' = \frac{R_1 R_2}{R_1 + R_2}$$

Generalizing to the case of n resistors in parallel:

$$1/R' = \sum_{i=1}^{n} (1/R_i) \qquad (4.15)$$

In some circuit arrangements the simple rules of resistors in series and parallel cannot easily be employed. In these cases two rules, formulated by Kirchhoff (1845), can be used with advantage:

(i) The sum of voltage sources (emf's) in a closed circuit is equal to the sum of the voltages dropped across the elements of the circuit. For a resistive circuit:

$$V = \sum IR \qquad (4.16)$$

This rule is a simple consequence of the principle of conservation of energy.

(ii) The sum of currents flowing into or out of a circuit junction is zero, i.e.

$$\sum_i I_i = 0 \qquad (4.17)$$

This equality is a result of the fact that charge cannot accumulate at a point in a circuit. That is, the principle of conservation of charge cannot be violated.

The use of these rules is illustrated using the circuit of Fig. 4. The object is to find the currents in each limb of the circuit, given the values of the resistors and the emf's. Closed paths or loops (A, B, C) are constructed such that each limb is included at least once. Next (4.17) is used to label currents in each limb as shown.

Equation (4.16) is now applied, remembering that according to convention, positive current flows from points of positive to points of negative potential.

Loop A: $V_1 = I_1 R_1 + (I_1 + I_3)R_2$
Loop B: $V_2 = -I_1 R_1 + I_2 R_3$
Loop C: $-V_2 = (I_2 - I_3)R_4 - (I_1 + I_3)R_2$

These three simultaneous equations are then solved for I_1, I_2 and I_3 in terms of the known voltage sources and resistances.

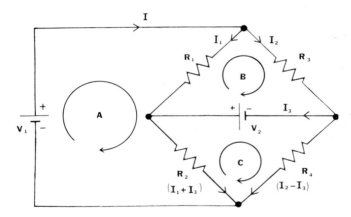

FIG. 4. Circuit illustrating use of Kirchhoff's rules.

Before we leave the subject of Ohm's law for the present, two comments are appropriate. Firstly, the law describes a *linear* relation between voltage and current and therefore cannot strictly be used to solve non-linear circuits; that is, a circuit containing elements or devices in which voltages and currents are not proportional. Proportionality between voltage and current is a consequence of mean charge carrier velocity being directly related to electric field, as in (4.9). Many materials and devices do not meet this basic requirement. As we shall see in the next chapter, transistors are, in fact, non-linear devices. However, Ohm's law can often be applied, as many devices are effectively linear over an appreciable range of voltage and current. Care must be taken in such cases that the limits of linearity are not exceeded.

Secondly, the reason for the use of electrical circuits as analogues for diverse physical situations can now be partly appreciated. Ohm's law is in fact only one form of a quite universal linear thermodynamic relation relating generalized "forces" and "flows". Here, the force driving the flow of charge, or current, is potential difference. In, say, a hydraulic system the driving force is pressure, producing flow of fluid material. Hence, hydraulic systems, such as the blood circulation, can in many respects be represented conceptually by an appropriate electric circuit; by exploiting the dualities between pressure and voltage, and flow and current.

DIRECT AND ALTERNATING CURRENTS

For the simple case of a source of voltage connected across a purely resistive conductor or circuit element, Ohm's law, equation (4.11), tells us that the current, because it is directly proportional to the voltage, follows the same time variation as the voltage. Formally:

$$V(t) = R \cdot I(t)$$

where V and I are now functions of time
Two cases are of major importance. These are:

(i) The situation where voltage is time invariant (or constant). The resulting current, which is not a function of time, is called *direct current* or dc.
(ii) Voltage varies sinusoidally. That is, its variation is described by the equation:

$$V(t) = A \cdot \sin(\omega t) \qquad (4.18)$$

In this case the resulting current is termed *alternating current*, abbreviated ac. For the purposes of illustration, such a sinusoidal function can be considered as being generated by a vector, magnitude A, rotating counterclockwise about its origin at an angular velocity of ω radians per second. This is illustrated in Fig. 5.

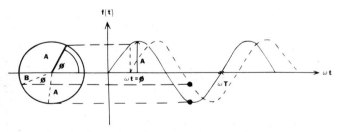

FIG. 5. Generation of sine waves by a rotating vector.

The resulting function, $f(t)$, varies cyclically and has amplitude, A, as shown by the full line in the illustration. Let us denote the first zero-crossing point of the ωt axis, excluding the origin, by ωT. This point corresponds to a complete rotation of the generating vector, that is through an angle of 2π radians. Hence the angle ϕ shown in the diagram is now given by:

$$\phi = 2\pi$$

and $\therefore$
$$\omega T = 2\pi$$

hence
$$\omega = \frac{2\pi}{T} \qquad (4.19)$$

The time, T, between zero-crossings of the sinusoidal function is termed the *period*. T, therefore, gives the time taken to generate a complete *cycle*. A very useful way of describing an alternating quantity, either voltage or current, is with reference to the number of cycles occurring in unit time. This quantity is called the *frequency* of the waveform, and is simply determined from the inverse of the period. Hence:

$$\text{frequency}, f = \frac{1}{T}$$

Frequency has units of hertz (Hz); previously cycles per second.

Substituting in (4.19)
$$\omega = 2\pi f \qquad (4.20)$$

so that the sinusoidal function in (4.18) becomes:

$$f(t) = A \sin 2\pi f t \qquad (4.21)$$

Suppose that in Fig. 5, instead of having a single generating vector, **A**, we also had another vector, **B**, of the same amplitude and rotating at the same angular frequency as **A**, but displaced by the angle, ϕ, as shown. In this case, two sinusoidal functions are generated; the only difference between them being that the waveform due to **B** (shown dotted) is displaced in time relative to the waveform generated by **A**. The two functions are said to exhibit a *phase difference*. The waveform depicted by the dotted line is said to "lag" that depicted by the full line, by the phase angle ϕ. In this case the relation (4.21) describing the dotted waveform becomes:

$$f(t) = A \sin(2\pi f t - \phi) \qquad (4.22)$$

If in (4.22) the phase angle ϕ is positive then $f(t)$ is said to "lead" the reference waveform.

If $\phi = +90°$ (or $\pi/2$ radians):
$$f(t) = A \sin(2\pi f t + \pi/2)$$
$$= A \cos 2\pi f t$$

and the waveform is described by a cosine function.

There are, of course, many other more complicated forms of voltage or current variation with time (other than constant or sinusoidal relations), such as rectangular pulses or "sawtooth" waves. This in no way detracts from the importance of sinusoidal variations in electric circuits, since for complex variations, analysis can be performed in terms of superimposed sine and cosine functions. Thus, if the behaviour of a linear circuit for sinusoidal applied voltages is known, the behaviour for all complex waveforms of interest can be found. This is a consequence of the very important Fourier theorem (1807), which states that any time-varying function fulfilling certain basic conditions, can be described as a sum of sine and cosine functions at various frequencies. These conditions are satisfied in all cases of practical importance.

HEATING EFFECT OF A CURRENT: POWER

When a potential difference causes current to flow in a conductor, the mobile electrons gain energy and are accelerated. However, this acceleration does not continue indefinitely because the electrons eventually collide with the fixed ionic lattice of the material. A process something like this has already been implicity assumed in our earlier discussion of mean velocity. In these collisions energy is imparted to the ions causing thermal vibrations, and so raising the temperature of the material. It is this loss of energy by collision that is manifested as the resistance of the conductor.

The work done, dW, in moving charge, dq, against this resistance is given by:

$$dW = Vdq$$

where V is the potential difference across the resistance.

The rate at which work is done, defined as *power*, is then:

$$P = \frac{dW}{dt} = V\frac{dq}{dt}$$

$$\therefore P = VI \qquad (4.23)$$

The units of power are watts (joules per second).

By Ohm's law, $V = IR$, (4.23) can also be written as:

$$P = VI = I^2R = \frac{V^2}{R} \qquad (4.24)$$

The last two expressions are only applicable if Ohm's law holds.

The work necessary to maintain the flow of current can be obtained in various ways. The simplest expedient is to convert chemical energy to electrical energy, as in the electrolytic cell or battery. Commercially, electrical energy is often produced at the expense of mechanical energy, essentially by rotating a conductor in a magnetic field. The principle which is utilized, that of electromagnetic induction, will be dealt with further when induced emf's are discussed.

A complication arises when we wish to measure power in ac circuits, since in this case the voltages and currents do not have unique, steady values. The expedient adopted to overcome this difficulty is to define *effective values* in the following manner. The effective values of current and voltage in an ac circuit are the corresponding dc values that would develop the same power. Consider an alternating current, i, passing through a resistance, R, for a time, t. Then:

$$\text{power dissipated} = I_{\text{eff}}^2 Rt$$

$$I_{\text{eff}} - \text{effective current.}$$

The instantaneous rate of power dissipation is i^2R, so that:

$$\text{power dissipated in time } t' = \int_0^t i^2R \, dt$$

Hence

$$I_{\text{eff}}^2 Rt' = \int_0^{t'} i^2R \, dt$$

But i is an alternating current:

$$\therefore i = I_0 \sin \omega t$$

$$I_{\text{eff}}^2 Rt' = \int_0^{t'} I_0^2 R \sin^2 \omega t \, dt$$

$$I_{\text{eff}}^2 = \frac{I_0^2}{t'} \int_0^{t'} \sin^2 \omega t \, dt$$

But $\sin^2 x = \frac{1}{2}(1 - \cos 2x)$:

$$\therefore I_{\text{eff}}^2 = \frac{I_0^2}{2t'} \int_0^{t'} (1 - \cos 2\omega t) \, dt$$

Integrating over an integer number of half-cycles ($\omega t' = n\pi$):

$$I_{\text{eff}}^2 = \frac{I_0^2}{2}$$

Taking square roots:

$$I_{\text{eff}} = \frac{I_0}{\sqrt{2}} \qquad (4.25)$$

Similarly for the effective voltage:

$$V_{\text{eff}} = \frac{V_0}{\sqrt{2}}$$

Because of the method of obtaining these effective values, they are generally referred to as *root-mean-square* (rms) values and are of considerable importance in expressing ac power. If Ohm's law holds:

$$\text{ac power} = V_{\text{rms}} I_{\text{rms}} = \frac{I_{\text{rms}}^2}{V_{\text{rms}}} = \frac{V_{\text{rms}}}{R}$$

Note that:

$$V_{\text{rms}} I_{\text{rms}} = \frac{V_0}{\sqrt{2}} \cdot \frac{I_0}{\sqrt{2}} = \frac{V_0 I_0}{2}$$

so that the ac power is half the product of the peak voltages and currents.

Occasionally it is convenient to express power in ratio form, relative to some standard power. In order to render the measure arithmetically tractable, the ratio is generally expressed on a logarithmic scale. Thus:

$$\text{relative power level of } P_2 = \log_{10} \frac{P_2}{P_1}$$

P_1—reference power level.

The unit of relative power in this scheme is the bel, symbol B, named after Alexander Bell. It has become common practice to quote relative power levels in decibels (dB), so that:

$$\text{relative power level (dB)} = 10 \log_{10} \frac{P_2}{P_1} \qquad (4.26)$$

The reader will no doubt be familiar with the method of expressing sound pressure levels (SPL) in dB. The electrical analogue to pressure is, of course, voltage; and the electrical engineer also finds it convenient to express the relation between two voltage levels in decibels. Since power

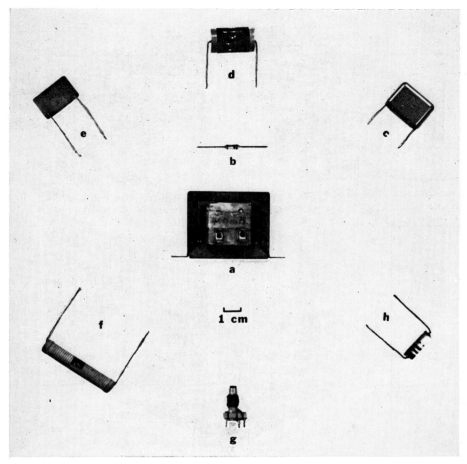

FIG. 6. Some commonly used resistors, capacitors and inductors: (a) 400 mH inductor, (b) carbon resistor (¼ W power dissipation), (c) capacitor with polycarbonate dielectric, (d) capacitor with paper dielectric, (e) silvered mica capacitor, (f) wire-wound resistor, (g) variable miniature inductor, (h) carbon resistor (1 W power dissipation).

is proportional to the square of voltage (equation (4.24)) we have:

$$\text{relative voltage level (dB)} = 20 \log_{10} \frac{V_2}{V_1}$$

The reference voltage, V_1, may be chosen variously as the input voltage to a circuit, or the peak voltage, or any other convenient value.

If power, P_2, is twice the reference power, P_1, (4.26) becomes:

$$\text{relative power level} = 10 \log_{10} 2 \text{ dB}$$
$$= 3{\cdot}01 \text{ dB}$$

So the half-power situation corresponds approximately to a 3 dB difference. This half-power point is extensively used in characterizing the performance of amplifiers and filters (see later).

CAPACITANCE AND INDUCTANCE

We have already seen how the movement of charge (i.e. current) through a conductor under the influence of an electric field leads to the concept of resistance. However, in many practical electric circuits, elements are used whose action depends upon them either actually storing charge, or upon effects due to charge moving through a changing magnetic field. The former elements are called *capacitors*, whereas the latter elements are known as *inductors*. Both capacitors and inductors are extremely important in electrical circuits. These will now be dealt with in turn. Figure 6 illustrates some commercially available resistors, inductors and capacitors in everyday use.

A capacitor is a device for storing charge. The *capacitance*, C, of a capacitor is defined as the charge stored per unit potential, i.e.

$$C = Q/V \qquad (4.27)$$

The unit of capacitance is the farad, named in honour of Michael Faraday.

The larger the capacitance, the greater is the amount of charge that must be added in order to raise the potential by 1 V.

In order to exhibit capacitance (i.e. to store charge) a conductor must be *isolated* so that stored charge cannot easily leak off; that is, it must be separated from closed circuit contact with other conducting bodies by an insulator.

The usual geometrical configuration employed is that of two conducting sheets separated by a dielectric. This is the so-called parallel-plate capacitor, illustrated schematically in Fig. 7.

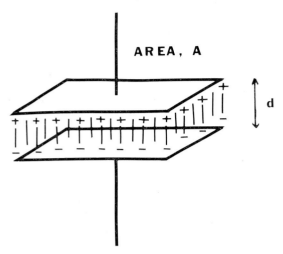

FIG. 7. The parallel-plate capacitor.

The calculation of the capacitance of the parallel-plate capacitor is a little involved, but is given in outline below.

Firstly, we generalize Coulomb's law (equation (4.1)) for the case of the force on a test charge, q, in the region of a number of other charges, q_i, in a vacuum:

$$F = \frac{1}{4\pi\varepsilon_0} \int \frac{q\,\mathrm{d}q_i}{r^2}$$

So the electric field is given, by equation (4.2), as:

$$E = \frac{F}{q} = \frac{1}{4\pi\varepsilon_0} \int \frac{\mathrm{d}q_i}{r^2}$$

For the case of the electric field at a point close to a plane distribution of charge (as with the parallel plate capacitor), E can be found from the above equation by integrating the contributions $\mathrm{d}q_i$ over the total surface to give:

$$E = \frac{Q}{2\varepsilon_0 A}$$

Q—total charge.
A—area over which this charge is uniformly distributed.

For *two* parallel plates:

$$E = Q/\varepsilon_0 A$$

From equation (4.3):

$$V = -\int_0^d \mathbf{E} \cdot \mathbf{ds}$$

$$\therefore\ V = \frac{Qd}{\varepsilon_0 A}$$

And $C = Q/V$

Hence $C = \dfrac{\varepsilon_0 A}{d}$ (4.28)

The above discussion holds only when the insulating material is free space (i.e. vacuum). It is found that (Faraday, 1838) if a dielectric (insulating) material is introduced between the plates, the capacitance is increased by a factor which is constant for any specific material. This factor is termed the *relative permittivity*, ε_r (previously called dielectric constant). Denoting the capacitance with a vacuum between the plates as C_v and the capacitance of the same capacitor with a dielectric material between the plates as C_d, we have:

$$\varepsilon_r = \frac{C_d}{C_v}$$

It follows from (4.28) that, for the capacitor with dielectric between the plates:

$$C_d = \frac{\varepsilon_0 \varepsilon_r A}{d}   (4.29)$$

Free space has a relative permittivity of 1 (by definition); air has the value 1·0006 (and so is usually taken as equivalent to free space); mica, often used in commercially produced capacitors, has a value of about 5; and water has the value 80.

Note the analogy between relative permittivity and relative permeability.

Just like resistors, capacitors are often connected in circuits in series or parallel combinations. Figure 8a shows

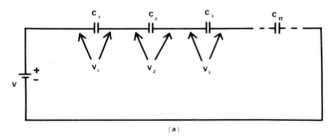

(a)

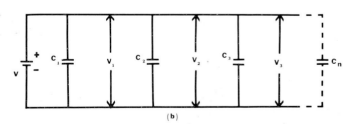

(b)

FIG. 8. (a) Capacitors in series. (b) Capacitors in parallel.

a series arrangement. The charge stored on one plate of a capacitor must, by the principle of charge conservation, be equal and opposite to the charge on the other plate. Since one plate of capacitor C_1 is connected directly to one plate of C_2 it follows that the charge, Q, on each capacitor will be equal. That is:

$$Q = Q_1 = Q_2 = Q_3 = \ldots = Q_n$$

The total voltage will therefore be given by:

$$V = V_1 + V_2 + V_3 + \ldots$$

But by (4.27):

$$V = Q/C$$

$$\therefore \quad Q/C_{\text{total}} = Q_1/C_1 + Q_2/C_2 + Q_3/C_3 + \cdots$$

Cancelling through by Q ($= Q_1 = Q_2$, etc.):

$$\frac{1}{C_{\text{total}}} = \frac{1}{C_1} + \frac{1}{C_2} + \frac{1}{C_3} + \cdots$$

For n capacitors:

$$\frac{1}{C_{\text{total}}} = \sum_{i=1}^{n} \frac{1}{C_i} \qquad (4.30)$$

So the equation for the series combination of capacitors is of the same form as that for the parallel combination of resistors, equation (4.15).

Similarly for n capacitors in parallel (Fig. 8b), using the relations:

(i) $V = V_1 = V_2 = V_3$, etc., and

(ii) $Q = Q_1 + Q_2 + Q_3 + \cdots$

We find:

$$C_{\text{total}} = \sum_{i=1}^{n} C_i \qquad (4.31)$$

We now turn to the matter of inductance. Consider a length, l, of conductor moving through a magnetic field in a direction, x, perpendicular to both the field and the conductor length. That is to say, vectors $\mathbf{B}$, $\mathbf{l}$ and $\mathbf{x}$ are mutually perpendicular. By equation (4.5) the force experienced by a test charge, q, will be:

$$\mathbf{F} = q\mathbf{v} \times \mathbf{B}$$

where

$$\mathbf{v} = \frac{d}{dt} \cdot \mathbf{x}$$

The force on this charge will (if the charge is free to move, as in the case of the conductor) produce charge separation, and hence a potential difference across the ends of the conductor. If, however, instead of a single length of material, we had a closed loop of dimensions $l \times b$ (where $\mathbf{l}$ is still the direction perpendicular to both motion and field), current would flow around the circuit. That is, the motion of a conducting coil through a magnetic field produces an emf. The magnitude of this emf can be determined from (4.5) as follows:

suppose the loop moves from point 1, at which:

$$t = t_1$$
$$x = x_1$$
$$B = B_1$$
$$F = F_1$$

to point 2 where:

$$t = t_2$$
$$x = x_2$$
$$B = B_2$$
$$F = F_2$$

Then the work done, W, by the magnetic forces in carrying charge, q, around the loop is:

$$W = \mathbf{F} \cdot \mathbf{dl}$$
$$= (F_2 - F_1)l$$
$$= qv \mid B_2 - B_1 \mid l$$

The sign of the right hand side will be positive if $\mathbf{F}$, $\mathbf{v}$ and $\mathbf{B}$ form a right hand set and negative if they form a left hand set, as a consequence of the definition of the vector cross product (*see* Appendix II). Here for convenience we take the negative sign, and assume that the corresponding work will be positive (*see* discussion of Lenz's principle below). Hence:

$$W = -q \left(\frac{x_2}{t_2} - \frac{x_1}{t_2} \right) \mid B_2 - B_1 \mid l$$

Substituting for B from (6) in terms of flux density:

$$W = -q \frac{\Delta x}{\Delta t} \left[\frac{\phi_2}{A} - \frac{\phi_1}{A} \right] l$$
$$= -q \frac{\Delta \phi}{\Delta t} \cdot \frac{l\Delta x}{A}$$

But $\qquad A = l\Delta x$

$$\therefore \qquad W = -q \frac{\Delta \phi}{\Delta t}$$

In the limit, as Δt tends to zero:

$$\frac{W}{q} = -\frac{d\phi}{dt}$$

The induced emf, ε, is simply the work done per unit charge, so that:

$$\varepsilon = -\frac{d\phi}{dt} \qquad (4.32)$$

The induced emf is seen to be equal in magnitude to the rate of change of flux.

Although we have obtained this result for the case of a conductor moving through a magnetic field, Faraday (1832) showed experimentally that the same result holds for conductors where the magnetic field itself is changing rather than the position of the conductor. It is also of interest to note that the relation holds even when there is no conductor present. Equation (4.32) is often called Faraday's law of electromagnetic induction.

Lenz (1834) showed that the direction of the induced emf is always in such a sense as to oppose the flux change that produced it. This is one simple consequence of the principle of conservation of energy, generally called *Lenz's law*, and justifies the assumption made above regarding the sign of the work term.

For N turns of coil moving in a magnetic field, (4.32) becomes:

$$\varepsilon = -N \frac{d\phi}{dt} \qquad (4.33)$$

The principle formulated in this equation is the basis of the production of electricity by commercial generators, in which a coil with a large number of turns is rotated in a magnetic field.

One way in which flux can change in a coil, is for there to be a change of current in a closely adjacent coil. This arises from the fact, previously noted, that current through a conductor produces a magnetic field.

Passive circuit devices that make use of this phenomenon are called *inductors*. The emf induced in the turns of a coil can either be produced as a result of flux change in a physically separate, but close, coil; or in other turns of the same coil. In the former case we talk of *mutual inductance*, whereas in the latter case we talk of *self inductance*.

Self inductance is conventionally given the symbol, L; whereas M denotes mutual inductance.

If the current in a coil, subscript 1, changes at a rate di_1/dt, then the self inductance is defined via the equation:

$$\varepsilon_1 = -L_1 \frac{d}{dt} i_1 \qquad (4.34)$$

where ε_1 is the emf induced in the coil.

If the same current change in coil 1 induces an emf ε_2 in a coil, subscript 2, close by, the mutual inductance between the two is defined via the equation:

$$\varepsilon_2 = -M_{12} \frac{d}{dt} i_1 \qquad (4.35)$$

Since $M_{12} = M_{21}$ for the same two coils it follows that:

$$\varepsilon_1 = -M_{12} \frac{d}{dt} i_2$$

Mutual inductance is the principle behind the operation of the *transformer*.

The unit of inductance (both self and mutual) is the henry. From (4.34) and (4.35) it can be seen that the henry is equivalent to one volt-second per ampere ($V.s.A^{-1}$).

The rules for evaluating the total inductance of series/parallel combinations of inductors depend upon whether or not there is any flux linkage (i.e. mutual inductance) between them. For three non-interacting self inductances in series (Fig. 9a) we have:

$$-L \frac{di}{dt} = -L_1 \frac{di}{dt} - L_2 \frac{di}{dt} - L_3 \frac{di}{dt}$$

So that the total inductance is given by:

$$L = L_1 + L_2 + L_3$$

In general, for n inductors in series:

$$L = \sum_{i=1}^{n} L_i \qquad (4.36)$$

Similarly for n non-interacting inductors in parallel:

$$1/L = \sum_{i=1}^{n} 1/L_i \qquad (4.37)$$

Note that the equations are of exactly the same form as those for resistor combinations.

Figure 9b shows two inductors with a mutual inductance, M, between them. Adding induced emf's to find the total gives:

$$\varepsilon = \varepsilon_1 + \varepsilon_2 + \varepsilon_{12} + \varepsilon_{21} \qquad (4.38)$$

ε_{12} = emf induced in coil 1 by coil 2
ε_{21} = emf induced in coil 2 by coil 1.

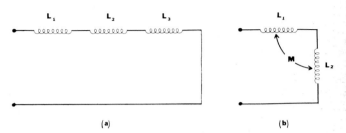

FIG. 9. (a) Inductors in series. It is assumed that there is no mutual inductance between them. (b) Two inductors in series; with mutual inductance M between them.

Since mutual inductance is a property of the pair of coils and the same current flows through each:

$$\varepsilon_{21} = \varepsilon_{12}$$

The mutual inductance terms, ε_{12} and ε_{21}, might either add to the total flux or give flux in a direction opposite to that of the self induction. Hence:

$$\varepsilon_{12} = \varepsilon_{21} = \pm M \frac{di}{dt}$$

Therefore (4.38) becomes:

$$\varepsilon = -L \frac{di}{dt} = -L_1 \frac{di}{dt} - L_2 \frac{di}{dt} \pm 2M \frac{di}{dt}$$

$$\therefore L = L_1 + L_2 \pm 2M \qquad (4.39)$$

The evaluation of the total inductance of parallel combinations of inductors with flux linkage is relatively more complex than the series case, and will not be dealt with here.

Since inductors are, in practice, fabricated from coils of conducting wire, they must possess some resistance. Also there will be some capacitance between adjacent turns of coil, which are separated by insulating material, In general, any circuit element will possess some finite resistance, capacitance and inductance, whatever its intended nature. Thus charge will leak off a capacitor through its inherent resistance, and a resistor will have some capacitance and inductance. Occasionally these effects cannot be ignored. This applies particularly at high frequencies.

REACTANCE, IMPEDANCE AND COMPLEX NOTATION

Consider a capacitor, C, connected to an alternating emf, v (Fig. 10a). The current through the capacitor is found by differentiating equation (4.27) to give:

$$i = C \frac{dv}{dt}$$

Since v is an alternating voltage, from equation (4.18):

$$v = V_0 \sin \omega t$$

$$\therefore i = C \frac{d}{dt} \cdot V_0 \sin \omega t$$

$$i = CV_0 \cos \omega t \qquad (4.40)$$

The voltage, v, and current, i, are shown plotted on the same axes in Fig. 10b. From this illustration it is apparent

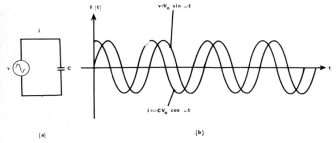

FIG. 10. (a) Capacitor connected to source of alternating emf. (b) Current and voltage variations with time for a capacitor.

that the current through a capacitor leads the voltage by a phase angle of $\pi/2$ radians (90°). This result is also obtainable from equation (4.40) and the trigonometrical relation:

$$\cos \omega t = \sin (\omega t + \pi/2)$$

so that $\qquad i = CV_0 \sin (\omega t + \pi/2)$

The amplitude of the current, I_0 is given by (4.40) when $\cos \omega t$ takes its maximum value of 1:

$$I_0 = \omega C V_0$$

$$\therefore V_0 = \frac{I_0}{\omega C} \qquad (4.41)$$

It is instructive to compare this equation with that describing Ohm's law for a simple resistance, equation (4.11). We see that the two equations are of the same form, except that resistance, R, is replaced by a term $(1/\omega C)$. This quantity, analogous to resistance in current–voltage relationships, is called *capacitative reactance* (units: ohms); often given the symbol X_c. Hence, for the circuit of Fig. 10a:

$$V_0 = I_0 X_c$$

In similar manner, we now consider the case of an inductor in series with an alternating voltage source (Fig. 11a). By Kirchhoff's first law, equation (4.16):

$$v + \varepsilon_L = 0$$

where $\qquad \varepsilon_L = -L \frac{di}{dt}$ (from equation (4.34))

$$\therefore v = L \frac{di}{dt}$$

$$\frac{di}{dt} = \frac{1}{L} \cdot v$$

Since we have an alternating voltage:

$$v = V_0 \sin \omega t$$

$$\frac{di}{dt} = \frac{V_0}{L} \sin \omega t$$

$$i = \frac{V_0}{L} \int \sin \omega t \, dt$$

$$i = -\frac{V_0}{\omega L} \cos \omega t \qquad (4.42)$$

From Fig. 11b it can be seen that the current through the inductor lags the voltage across it by a phase angle

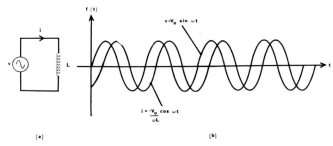

FIG. 11. (a) Inductor connected to a source of alternating emf. (b) Current and voltage variations with time for an inductor.

of $\pi/2$ rad. Again this can also be demonstrated by writing the trigonometrical relationship:

$$-\cos \omega t = \sin (\omega t - \pi/2)$$

so that: $\qquad i = \frac{V_0}{\omega L} \cdot \sin (\omega t - \pi/2)$

The amplitude of the current, I_0, is given by:

$$I_0 = \frac{V_0}{\omega L}$$

$$\therefore V_0 = \omega L I_0 \qquad (4.43)$$

Comparing this equation to the general form of Ohm's law, as before, we see that resistance is replaced by a term, ωL, known as *inductive reactance*, X_L; units: ohms. Equation (4.43) then becomes:

$$V_0 = I_0 X_L$$

Figure 12a illustrates a circuit consisting of an inductor, capacitor and resistor in series with an alternating voltage source, V_0. We now wish to solve the circuit in terms of voltages and current. One way that this can be done is to utilize the ideas of vector addition and subtraction (*see* Appendix II). We have already seen how an alternating quantity can be represented as a rotating vector. However, strictly speaking, vectors have attributes of magnitude and direction. Electrical quantities possess the characteristic of phase, rather than direction. That is to say, it is the phase relationships between currents and voltages that are of importance. For this reason these quantities are generally referred to as *phasors*, but the rules of vector addition and subtraction still apply. Now:

$$\mathbf{V}_0 = \mathbf{V}_R + \mathbf{V}_L + \mathbf{V}_C \qquad (4.44)$$

where the magnitudes are given by:

$$V_R = IR$$
$$V_L = I\omega L$$
$$V_C = I/\omega C$$

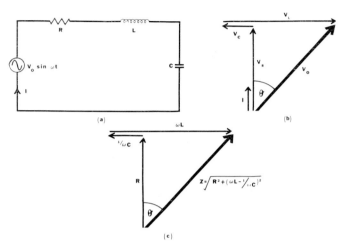

FIG. 12. (a) Series RLC circuit. (b) Voltage phasor (vector) diagram for RLC circuit. (c) Reactance—resistance phasor diagram for RLC circuit; produced from (b) by division of all moduli by I.

We can now draw a phasor diagram for these three voltages, using the results that:

(i) $\mathbf{V}_C$ lags $\mathbf{I}$ by a phase angle of 90°
(ii) $\mathbf{V}_L$ leads $\mathbf{I}$ by 90°
(iii) $\mathbf{V}_R$ is in phase with $\mathbf{I}$.

This phasor diagram is shown in Fig. 12b.

It should be noted that when voltage and current across a circuit element are out of phase, the power dissipated is no longer given by the product of V and I. In fact, it is given by the scalar product of the phasors $\mathbf{V}$ and $\mathbf{I}$ (Appendix II):

$$P = VI \cos \delta$$

where δ is the phase angle.

When $\delta = \pm 90°$, as in the case of capacitors and inductors, we have the important result that the power dissipated by a reactive element is zero.

The resultant voltage, $\mathbf{V}_0$, can also be depicted on Fig. 12b and is shown from equation (4.44) to be identical to the source voltage. In other words, counter-clockwise rotation of $\mathbf{V}_0$ produces a voltage (*see* p. 57) which corresponds exactly to that produced by counter-clockwise rotation of the combination of vectors, $\mathbf{V}_C$, $\mathbf{V}_L$ and $\mathbf{V}_R$.

Instead of proceeding in this way, we could scale the vectors by dividing by the magnitude of $\mathbf{I}$. The situation when this is done is depicted in Fig. 12c. The phasor diagram is of exactly the same form as Fig. 12b, except that $\mathbf{V}_R$ is replaced by $\mathbf{R}$, $\mathbf{V}_L$ is replaced by $\omega\mathbf{L}$ and $\mathbf{V}_C$ is replaced

by $\mathbf{C}'/\omega$ (where $C' = 1/C$). In this case the resultant, labelled Z, can be found from the theorem of Pythagoras:

$$Z = \sqrt{R^2 + (\omega L - 1/\omega C)^2} \qquad (4.45)$$

Putting total reactance,

$$X = X_L - X_C$$
$$= \omega L - 1/\omega C$$

yields $Z = \sqrt{R^2 + X^2}$

It follows from the fact that Fig. 12c is a scaled-down version of Fig. 12b that:

$$Z = V_0/I_0 \qquad (4.46)$$

and so has units of ohms. The quantity, Z, is termed the *impedance* of the ac circuit and is formally similar to resistance in a dc circuit. Equation (4.45) holds for the series *RLC* circuit; for the parallel arrangement (in analogous way to combining resistors in parallel) we have:

$$\frac{1}{Z} = \sqrt{\frac{1}{R^2} + \left(\frac{1}{X_L} - \frac{1}{X_C}\right)^2}$$

For a given set of values of R, L and C, the impedance, Z, given by equation (4.45):

$$Z = \sqrt{R^2 + (\omega L - 1/\omega C)^2}$$

varies with frequency. In particular, when:

$$\omega_0 L = 1/\omega_0 C$$

i.e. $$\omega_0 = \frac{1}{\sqrt{LC}}$$

the impedance has a minimum value and is purely resistive. For this condition the current is maximal. ω_0 is called the *resonant frequency* of the circuit. Resonance occurs when the voltages across the inductance and capacitance are equal and opposite, so that the phase angle between current and applied voltage is zero. If the circuit resistance is very small, the current at resonance may be very large and, hence, the potential difference across each of the inductor and the capacitor may be very large (although the total voltage will be zero).

Resonance has tremendous significance, not just in electronics, but in many other fields. For instance, in acoustics, resonance occurs in enclosures, where the resonant frequency depends basically upon the enclosure dimensions. This is of great importance in the production of speech, where nasal and other (pharyngeal and oral) cavities are used to produce resonances at particular frequencies.

The parallel *RLC* circuit also displays resonant behaviour; except that impedance is at a maximum, and current is therefore minimal, at an angular frequency given by $1/\sqrt{LC}$.

Referring back to the equations for V_L and V_C it is seen that the appearance of the scalar term, ω, multiplying the current in the inductive case indicates a phase lead of 90° with respect to the voltage, whereas the term $(1/\omega)$ indicates that the current leads voltage by 90° in the capacitative case. Consider now a vector **A** as depicted in Fig. 13a. If **A** is multiplied by (−1) the outcome of this is to effectively rotate **A** through π radians (180°) as shown. In other words, multiplication by the *operator* (−1) rotates the vector **A** through 180°. Now, if we can find an operator which rotates a vector through 90°, it can be used to describe the situation occurring with inductive and capacitative circuit elements. Two multiplications by this operator, which we shall call j, correspond to 180° rotation. Hence:

$$j^2 = -1$$

and
$$j = \sqrt{-1} \qquad (4.47)$$

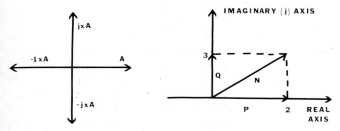

FIG. 13. (a) Multiplication of a vector, **A**, by powers of the complex operator, j. (b) Representation of a complex number in analogous manner to a vector.

So multiplication by j produces a counter-clockwise rotation through 90°, whereas division by j produces a clockwise rotation by a similar amount, since:

$$\frac{1}{j} = \frac{j}{j^2} = -j$$

and
$$-j = (j^2)j = j^3$$

and three successive shifts by 90° counter-clockwise are equivalent to a clockwise rotation by 90°.

The so-called complex operator, j, has no arithmetic significance whatsoever, since the square root of a negative number cannot be assigned a value. Therefore, quantities involving j as a multiplier are referred to as being *imaginary*. A *complex number* is one possessing both arithmetically valid (or *real*) parts, and imaginary parts: e.g.

$$N = 2 + j3$$

N can, however, be plotted in the *complex plane* as shown in Fig. 13b, using the knowledge that multiplication by j rotates the real number 3 through 90° onto a vertical, or imaginary axis. This representation is analogous to the representation of the vector, **N**, resulting from addition of vectors **P** and **Q**, shown in the figure, having magnitudes of 2 and 3 respectively.

In vector notation:

$$\mathbf{N} = \mathbf{P} + \mathbf{Q}$$

In complex notation:

$$N = 2 + j3$$
$$= P + jQ$$

By Pythagoras' theorem, the magnitude of *N* is given as:

$$N = \sqrt{P^2 + Q^2}$$

Hence complex notation can be considered as a compact way of describing vectors.*

Returning to equations (4.43) and (4.41), these can be rewritten as:

$$V_L = (j\omega L)\, I_L$$

and
$$V_C = \frac{1}{j\omega C}\, I_C$$

where the j's multiplying the angular velocity terms, ω, now indicate the phase relations between voltage and current for these reactive elements. Hence:

$$X_L = j\omega L$$

$$X_C = \frac{1}{j\omega C}$$

$$= \frac{j}{j^2\omega C} \qquad \left(\begin{array}{l}\text{multiplying numerator and}\\ \text{denominator by j}\end{array}\right)$$

$$\therefore \; X_C = -j/\omega C$$

In a series combination of inductance and capacitance:

total reactance, $\quad X = j\omega L - j/\omega C$

$$= j\left(\omega L - \frac{1}{\omega C}\right)$$

The complex expression for the impedance, *Z*, for a series *RLC* circuit will now be:

$$Z = R + jX$$

$$= R + j\left(\omega L - \frac{1}{\omega C}\right)$$

This equation can be seen to describe the situation shown in the vector diagram of Fig. 12c. We know from the example above that the magnitude of a complex number can be found by squaring the real and imaginary parts, adding them and taking the square root. Hence:

$$Z = \sqrt{R^2 + \left(\omega L - \frac{1}{\omega C}\right)^2}$$

which is the same result as equation (4.45), obtained without the necessity to draw vector diagrams. The phase angle, θ, can also be found from the trigonometrical relation:

$$\tan\theta = \frac{\text{imaginary part}}{\text{real part}}$$

In this case:

$$\tan\theta = \frac{\omega L - 1/\omega C}{R}$$

<hr/>

* This analogy should not, however, be taken too literally. For instance, one can divide an expression by a complex number, but division by a vector is not defined.

GENERAL PRINCIPLES OF ELECTRICAL MEASUREMENT

The effects due to the passage of a current, some of which have been outlined in the earlier parts of the chapter, give a convenient means of making electrical measurements. For instance, the heating effect of a current, given by equation (4.24) as I^2Rt (when the current flows for a time, t) can be utilized. One instrument, the hot-wire ammeter, uses the linear expansion of a conducting wire with increasing temperature, to move a pointer or needle across a graduated scale. The deflection of this needle is therefore proportional to the square of the current passing through the test wire.

The most useful effect, however, as far as the measurement of electric current is concerned is the magnetic effect. In the *moving coil meter* the current to be measured flows through a coil, to which is attached a pointer (Fig. 14). The coil is mounted on bearings and is free to rotate in a radial magnetic field. This field is produced by a suitably shaped permanent magnet, as shown in the figure. The extent of any rotation of the coil is indicated by the pointer on a scale. From the Lorentz equation, written as:

$$\mathbf{F} = I\mathbf{l} \times \mathbf{B}$$

it is seen that current-carrying conductors in a magnetic field experience a force, as described previously. The magnitude of this force is proportional to the current flowing. In an N turn coil, the total force is N times that given by the equation above.

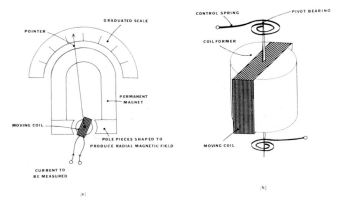

FIG. 14. The moving coil meter; (a) component parts and (b) details of the moving coil assembly. The current to be measured is often passed through the coil via the control spring and pivot.

The principle of operation of this meter can therefore be simply described as follows. The current to be measured is passed through the moving coil element, and experiences a force. By convention, when the current is flowing from the positive to the negative terminal of the meter, this force gives rise to a deflection of the pointer in a positive direction. This deflection is opposed by *control springs*, which have the purpose of damping down the meter's movement, so that a steady state deflection is quickly obtained. The position of the pointer, in the steady state, is thus proportional to the current to be measured which can be read off a suitably calibrated scale.

Although this is a device for the measurement of current, the voltage between the meter terminals can be found from Ohm's law, if the coil resistance is accurately known. The range of measurement, of either current or voltage, is determined by the current through the coil which will produce full-scale deflection (fsd). The fsd current, and hence the range of the meter, can be changed by incorporating high-quality resistors of predetermined value either in series or parallel with the meter coil. Series resistors used in this way are termed *multipliers*, whereas the parallel resistors are called *shunts*. Multipliers are added to increase the ranges of voltage measurement, and shunts to increase the ranges of current measurement.

The moving coil meter, as described above, is obviously only of value for the measurement of dc quantities. An alternating current applied to the coil will produce oscillations of the pointer and a steady state reading will not be possible. However, by rectifying (*see* next chapter) the alternating current or voltage, rms readings are possible.

Considerable care must be taken in the reliance placed on measures of current and voltage taken with meters such as these. To take the reading literally implies that connection of the meter in the circuit has not significantly affected the pre-existing voltages and currents. This will only be the case if:

    (i) when measuring voltages the resistance of the meter coil is much greater than the circuit resistance between the meter terminals.

    (ii) when measuring currents the meter coil resistance is much less than the circuit resistance through which the current flows.

If these conditions are not met, corrections have to be made to the reading obtained. This is done by estimating the change in the voltage or current caused by the introduction of the meter coil resistance into the circuit. With a typical instrument, using the dc voltage scale, the resistance introduced will be of the order of $2 \text{ k}\Omega \cdot \text{V}^{-1}$, whereas on the dc current ranges the voltage drop across the terminals will be about $\frac{1}{2}$ V for fsd. Performance on ac ranges is somewhat inferior to this.

Instead of using the force on current carrying conductors in a magnetic field to produce a measurable deflection, it is possible to utilize the deflection of electrons travelling perpendicular to an electric field (equation (4.2)) for measurement purposes. This is the principle of the *cathode ray oscilloscope* (CRO), shown diagrammatically in Fig. 15a. Here electrons are produced at the cathode by thermionic emission (*see* next chapter) and are accelerated by a high positive potential, in the direction of a phosphor-coated screen. When the electrons strike this screen a bright spot is seen. Intermediate between the electron source and the screen are arranged two sets of mutually perpendicular parallel plates, commonly called the x- and y-plates of the CRO. A potential difference applied to the x-plates will produce a deflection along the horizontal (or x) axis of the screen. On the other hand, potential differences between the y plates will produce deflections along the vertical (or y) axis of the screen. In one common application of this instrument, a sawtooth waveform is applied to the x-plates (Fig. 15b).

This produces a spot pattern which moves slowly across the screen from one side to the other and then moves back in the opposite direction in a very short time (the "fly-back" time) such that there appears to an observer to be a continuous movement of the spot. If a voltage waveform is now applied to the y-plates, the time course of the waveform will be traced out on the oscilloscope screen. By calibrating deflection in the y-direction, amplitude measures can be obtained. Similarly, a knowledge of the rise time of the slow component of the sawtooth waveform (that is, a known *time base*) makes frequency and period measures possible. The CRO is extremely useful both for ac and dc measurements, and for the examination of complex waveforms. Many of these instruments have dual-trace facilities (i.e. two sets of y-plates) allowing relative phases to be found.

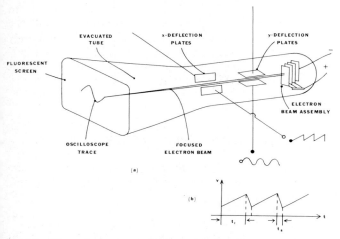

FIG. 15. The cathode ray oscilloscope (CRO). (a) Component parts of CRO. (b) Saw-tooth (time-base) waveform as applied to the x-plates of the oscilloscope. t_t—time for electron beam to trace out the waveform in the forward direction. t_B—"fly-back" time.

The CRO is an unusual measuring instrument in that it is effectively inertia-less. Therefore no damping system (like the control springs of the moving coil meter) is required; and steady state measures are obtained very quickly.

In the measurement of bioelectric potentials contact has to be established between the biological medium and the measuring equipment. In most cases this is done by attaching suitable electrodes. The properties of these electrodes influence to a large extent the measures obtained. Therefore, it is a matter of some importance for the user to be aware of the electrical characteristics of the electrodes used. A very good account of electrode properties and types for auditory research has been given by Dallos (1973). In addition, Cooper *et al.* (1968) have discussed many commonly used electrodes, principally those used for surface recording.

Most electrophysiological potentials are rather small, and so some amplification of these potentials is generally necessary. The next chapter will deal with this important topic. (Note, however, that the cathode ray oscilloscope described above incorporates x- and y-deflection amplifiers.)

It should be emphasized that only the most elementary

considerations have been discussed above in the context of voltage and current measurement. For a discussion of many other important and relevant topics, such as bridge methods, the reader is referred to the book by Baldwin; details of which appear below.

APPENDIX I

A Glossary of Electrical Quantities; Definitions and SI Units

Current: 1 *ampere* is that current which, flowing through two infinitely long parallel conductors in vacuum separated by 1 metre, gives rise to a force of 2×10^{-7} newtons (per metre length) between the conductors. The ampere is a base unit of the International System (SI).

Charge: 1 *coulomb* of charge is that quantity of electricity which corresponds to a current of 1 ampere when moving past a fixed point in a time of 1 second.

Electrical potential: the potential of a point is 1 *volt* when the work required to move 1 coulomb of charge from infinity to the specified point is 1 joule.

Potential difference: the potential difference between two points is 1 *volt* when the work required to move 1 coulomb of charge from one of the points to the other is 1 joule.

Resistance: 1 *ohm* is that resistance through which a current of one ampere flows when the potential difference across the resistance is 1 volt.

Frequency: the frequency of a sinusoidal quantity is 1 *hertz* when the time between successive maxima is 1 second.

Capacitance: the capacitance of a body is 1 *farad* when the charge stored by the body for a potential difference of 1 volt is 1 coulomb.

Inductance: an inductance of 1 *henry* gives rise to an induced emf of 1 volt when current charges through the inductance at the rate of 1 ampere per second.

Magnetic flux: a flux of 1 *weber* gives rise to an emf of 1 volt across the ends of a conductor moving perpendicularly through the region in which this flux exists in a time of 1 second.

APPENDIX II

Vectors

A *vector* can be defined as a quantity, possessing magnitude, which acts in a specified direction, e.g. force, velocity, magnetic field. It is therefore distinct from scalar quantities which possess magnitude only, e.g. mass, speed, potential.

A very compact way of specifying vectors is in terms of *cartesian coordinates*. In this system three mutually perpendicular *basis vectors* of unit magnitude are specified; usually denoted $\mathbf{x}$, $\mathbf{y}$ and $\mathbf{z}$. Components of the vector in question, say $\mathbf{V}$, in the $\mathbf{x}$, $\mathbf{y}$ and $\mathbf{z}$ directions can then be found by taking scalar products:

$$V_x = Vx \cos \alpha$$
$$V_y = Vy \cos \beta$$
$$V_z = Vz \cos \gamma$$

where α, β and γ are the angles between $\mathbf{V}$ and the x, y and z axes respectively.

The vector **V** can now be written as:

$$\mathbf{V} = V_x\mathbf{x} + V_y\mathbf{y} + V_z\mathbf{z}$$

or more compactly as:

$$\mathbf{V} = (V_x, V_y, V_z)$$

As well as the *rectangular* cartesian coordinates described above, polar coordinates may be similarly used to advantage in certain situations.

Two vectors, **a** and **b**, are said to be equal if their moduli (i.e. magnitudes) are equal and they act in parallel directions *in the same sense*. Formally:

$$\mathbf{a} = \mathbf{b}$$

The magnitudes of **a** and **b** are written $|\mathbf{a}|$ and $|\mathbf{b}|$ (or simply a and b) respectively.

If the moduli are not equal, that is, a is λ times larger than b, then we write:

$$\mathbf{a} = \lambda\mathbf{b} \qquad (4.\text{I})$$

Equation (4.I) defines the operations of scalar multiplication.

If **a** and **b** have equal magnitudes but act in parallel directions in opposite senses then:

$$\mathbf{a} = -\mathbf{b}$$

Vector addition and subtraction are defined according to the so-called vector triangle rule. Figure 16 shows the addition of vectors **p** and **q** to produce a vector, **r**:

$$\mathbf{r} = \mathbf{p} + \mathbf{q}$$

Vector **r** is termed the *resultant* of **p** and **q**.
By the theorem of Pythagoras:

$$r = \sqrt{p^2 + q^2} \qquad (4.\text{II})$$

Subtraction of **q** from **p**, say, is understood to mean addition of **p** to a negative vector **q**. Here the magnitude

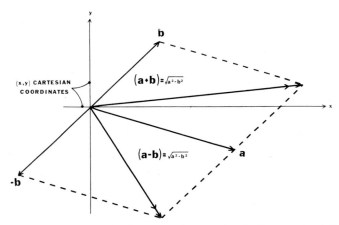

FIG. 16. Addition and subtraction of vectors by the "vector triangle" method.

will be given by equation (4.I), but the direction will differ from that of **r** above, as shown in Fig. 16.

Division by a vector is not defined.

Multiplication by vector quantities is of two types:

(i) scalar (or dot) product.

The scalar product of two vectors, **a** and **b** is defined as:

$$\mathbf{a} \cdot \mathbf{b} = ab \cos \theta$$

where θ is the angle between **a** and **b**.
Note that the resulting product, **a** . **b**, is a scalar.

(ii) vector (or cross) product.

This is defined as:

$$\mathbf{a} \times \mathbf{b} = ab \sin \theta\hat{\boldsymbol{\epsilon}}$$

θ is the angle between **a** and **b**.
$\hat{\boldsymbol{\epsilon}}$ is a vector of unit modulus, perpendicular to the plane defined by **a** and **b** in such a direction that **a**, **b** and $\hat{\boldsymbol{\epsilon}}$ form a *right-handed set*. By this is meant that, in moving from vector **a** to **b**, through the angle θ, rotation around the direction of $\hat{\boldsymbol{\epsilon}}$ is in a clockwise sense. This terminology derives from the use of the so-called right-hand and left-hand rules to work out the directions of motion of conductors in electric generators and motors respectively.

SUGGESTIONS FOR FURTHER READING

Archenhold, W. F. (1971), *Electromagnetism and Electrostatics Using SI Units*, 2nd Edition. Edinburgh: Oliver and Boyd.
Baldwin, C. T. (1973), *Fundamentals of Electrical Measurements*, 2nd Edition. London: Harrap.
Brookes, A. M. P. (1963), *Basic Electrical Circuits*. Oxford: Pergamon.
Cotton, H. (1973), *Basic Electrotechnology*. London: Macmillan.
Duffin, W. J. (1973), *Electricity and Magnetism*, 2nd Edition. London: McGraw-Hill.
Lancaster, G. (1974), *Dc and Ac Circuits*. Oxford: Clarendon Press.
Perkins, G. D. (1971), *Principles of Electrical Science*. London: English Universities Press.
Morley, A. and Hughes, E. (1972), *Principles of Electricity in SI Units*, 3rd Edition. London: Longman.

REFERENCES

Ampère, A. M. (1820), *Ann. Chim. et Phys.*, **15**, 59.
Cooper, R., Osselton, J. W. and Shaw, J. C. (1969), *EEG Technology*. London: Butterworths.
Coulomb, C. A. (1788), *Mem. Acad. Roy. Soc.*, 1785 volume: 569.
Dallos, P. (1973), *The Auditory Periphery: Biophysics and Physiology*. New York: Academic Press.
Faraday, M. (1832), *Phil. Trans. Roy. Soc. Lond.*, **122**, 125.
Faraday, M. (1838), *Phil. Trans. Roy. Soc. Lond.*, **128**, 268.
Flanagan, J. L. (1962), *Bell. Syst. Tech. J.*, **41**, 959.
Fourier, J. B. J. (1807) Unpublished.*
Kirchhoff, G. R. (1845), *Pogg. Annal.*,†**64**, 497.
Lenz, H. F. E. (1834), *Pogg. Annal.*, **31**, 483.
Møller, A. R. (1961), *J. Acoust. Soc. Am.*, **33**, 168.
Ohm, G. S. (1827), *Die galvanische Kette mathematisch bearbietet*. Berlin: T. H. Riemann.

* This paper, read before the Institut de France in December 1807, is the subject of a book by I. Grattan-Guiness: *Joseph Fourier, 1768–1830*. M.I.T. Press (1972).
† *Poggendorf's Annalen der Physik*.

5. ELECTRONICS

R. I. DAMPER

INTRODUCTION

In recent years striking advances have been made in the field of applied electronics. The most important of these have been concerned with aspects such as:

(1) The reduction of size of electronic devices, with a concomitant reduction of power requirements and increased convenience.

(2) Improved reliability both of devices and electronic assemblies.

(3) Greater diversity of device types and characteristics; and of techniques in electronic science.

Important developments in this context have been the invention of the transistor, the introduction of printed circuits and, more recently, the advent of *microelectronics* whereby whole circuits are fabricated on a small "chip" of suitable semiconducting material, such as silicon.

This has led to the situation where electronics now plays a very important role in almost all of the applied sciences, including many branches of medicine. The general scheme of applications of electronics to otolaryngology has been outlined in the early part of the previous chapter. Here, however, attention is focused upon some further properties of passive* circuits, active devices and their many uses; and recent innovations in microelectronics.

PASSIVE R, L AND C NETWORKS

Referring back to equations (4.27) and 4.7) in the previous chapter, for charge, Q, stored by capacitance, C, we have:

$$Q = CV$$

and current,

$$i = dQ/dt$$

Hence,

$$i = C \frac{dV}{dt}$$

The current through a capacitor is therefore proportional to the rate of change of voltage across it. This equation bears some similarity to (4.34) in the previous chapter, relating current and induced emf in an inductance:

$$\varepsilon = -L \frac{di}{dt}$$

In fact, these two equations tell us something of great importance about the circuit behaviour of capacitors and inductors, namely that:

(i) The current flowing through an inductor cannot change abruptly.

(ii) The voltage across a capacitor cannot change abruptly.

* Passive circuit elements are those not needing a source of energy for their action, e.g. resistors, capacitors, inductors. Active devices (transistors, triode valves, etc.) require an energy source before they can operate.

If this were not so, the changes would produce emf's and currents (respectively) which would be infinite, since they are proportional to the derivatives of the changes with respect to time. This is, of course, physically impossible. It should be borne in mind, however, that the resulting emf's and currents can themselves change abruptly provided that their magnitudes are finite.

Figure 1a shows a resistor and capacitor in series with a dc source and an open switch. If the switch is closed

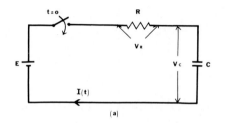

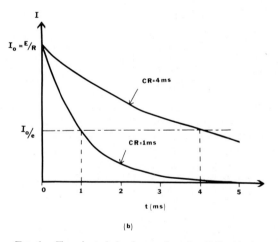

FIG. 1. Transient behaviour of series RC circuit. (a) Circuit diagram; (b) current versus time for step input voltage, for two different values of time constant, CR.

at time $t = 0$, this amounts to applying a step input (i.e. voltage *transient*) to the RC network. Applying Kirchhoff's first rule gives:

$$E = V_R + V_C$$

$$= IR + Q/C$$

or

$$R \frac{dQ}{dt} + Q/C = E$$

Solving this simple differential equation for Q (assuming no charge is stored initially on the capacitor) yields:

$$Q = EC(1 - \exp(-t/CR))$$

That is, the charge, Q, stored on the capacitor reaches its final value, EC, exponentially. The current can be found by differentiation of the above equation.

$$I = \frac{dQ}{dt} = EC \frac{d}{dt} \{1 - \exp(-t/CR)\}$$

$$\therefore \quad I = \frac{E}{R} \exp(-t/CR) \qquad (5.1)$$

Figure 1b shows current plotted against time for two different values of the term CR. Several points of interest should be mentioned. Firstly, the initial current (I_0) is given simply by the ratio of E to R. Secondly, the value of CR is seen to determine the rate at which current falls off exponentially. This can be simply demonstrated by differentiating (5.1) with respect to time and substituting $t = 0$ to give the initial rate of decrease as:

$$\left(\frac{dI}{dt}\right)_{t=0} = -\frac{1}{CR} \cdot \frac{E}{R}$$

$$= -\frac{I_0}{CR}$$

For this reason CR is referred to as the *time constant* of the circuit, and is a parameter of some significance as will be shown below. Note that CR has units of time.

Finally, it should be noted that when $t = CR$, the current is given by:

$$I = \frac{E}{R} \exp(-1)$$

$$\therefore \quad I = I_0/e$$

Hence the time constant of a series RC circuit can be defined as the time taken for the current to fall to $1/e$ (approximately 37 per cent) of its initial value, when a voltage-step transient is applied.

The same considerations apply for the series RL circuit of Fig. 2a. Here application of Kirchhoff's first rule gives:

$$E = V_R + V_L \qquad \text{(where } V_L = -\varepsilon\text{)}$$

$$= IR + L\frac{dI}{dt}$$

Solution of this differential equation yields the result:

$$I = \frac{E}{R}(1 - \exp(-Rt/L)) \qquad (5.2)$$

In this case, the time constant for the circuit is L/R, which again has units of seconds. The time constant is defined here as the time taken for the current to reach $(1 - 1/e)$ of its final value; given by E/R (Fig. 2b).

The practical importance of time constants is very considerable. Suppose an electrophysiological signal, such as an EEG potential, is to be recorded. Generally in EEG work one is much more interested in the variations of potential than their absolute value. For this reason, a *coupling capacitor*, together with a resistance to earth, is often inserted in the path between electrode and EEG recording machine to block the slowly varying potentials. In other

words, the fact that the voltage across a capacitor cannot change abruptly (and hence fast variations are transmitted) is utilized in order to remove dc and low frequency components from the signal. Because of this, such an RC network is referred to as a *high-pass filter* since only high frequency components can pass. The time constant of the coupling network determines the lowest frequency component which is transmitted without significant attenuation

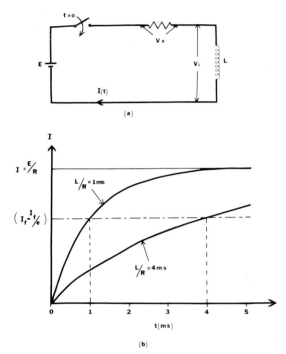

FIG. 2. Transient behaviour of series RL circuit. (a) Circuit diagram; (b) current versus time for step input voltage, for two different values of time constant, L/R.

—the so-called *cut-off frequency* of the filter. This is discussed further below.

Figure 3a shows a graph relating coupling time constant to the frequency at which a given percentage loss in sensitivity is suffered. Figure 3b shows the effect of different time constant values for the simple high-pass RC network on responses both to a square wave voltage function and a 1·5 Hz sinusoidal voltage. In particular, the phase displacement of the sine wave should be noted. It is an inherent property of an electrical network exhibiting attenuation which is a function of frequency, that a phase shift is introduced between input and output which also varies with frequency. In some applications this can be a considerable nuisance (e.g. in signal processing operations) but occasionally use can be made of this property. An example of such a case is the RC phase-shift network employed in some simple oscillators (*see later*).

If a network allows slowly varying potentials to pass unattenuated, but rejects high frequency components, it is called a *low-pass filter*.

Figure 4a shows four simple passive filter networks; two of which are high-pass and two low-pass. In each case

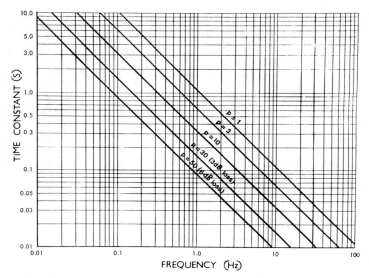

FIG. 3(a). Graph showing the relation between frequency and time constant for a number of values of percentage loss, p, of sensitivity.

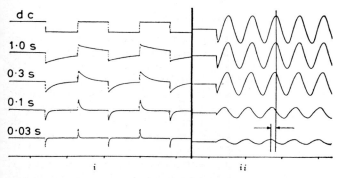

FIG. 3(b). (i) Effect of different time constant values on the response to a step function (square wave) signal. (ii) Corresponding effect on a 1·5 Hz sine wave signal. Note the time (phase) displacements. (Reproduced from Cooper, Osselton and Shaw (1969) by kind permission of the authors and publishers.)

the expression for output voltage in terms of the input voltage is given. The complex ratio of output to input voltages (i.e. in terms of jω) is generally called the *transfer function* of the network, T (jω) i.e.:

$$\frac{V_{\text{out}}}{V_{\text{in}}} = T(\text{j}\omega) \tag{5.3}$$

Figure 4b shows amplitude and phase variations with angular frequency, ω, for these simple circuits. The cut-off frequency mentioned above is defined, for both high- and low-pass filters, as that frequency at which a sinusoidal input voltage is attenuated by 3 dB. For this reason, the cut-off frequency is often referred to as the *3 dB point*, as indicated in the previous chapter. At the 3 dB point:

$$20 \log_{10} \left| \frac{V_{\text{out}}}{V_{\text{in}}} \right| = -3$$

From equation (5.3):

$$20 \log_{10} | T(\text{j}\omega_c) | = -3$$

where ω_c is the angular cut-off frequency.

$$\therefore \quad | T(\text{j}\omega_c) | = \frac{1}{\sqrt{2}}$$

For the low-pass RC filter, circuit (ii) of Fig. 4a:

$$| T(\text{j}\omega_c) | = \left| \frac{1}{1 + \text{j}\omega_c CR} \right| = \frac{1}{\sqrt{2}}$$

$$\therefore \quad | 1 + \text{j}\omega_c CR | = \sqrt{2}$$

$$(1 + \omega_c^2 C^2 R^2)^{\frac{1}{2}} = \sqrt{2}$$

and

$$\omega_c = \frac{1}{CR} \tag{5.4}$$

Hence the angular cut-off frequency is inversely related to the time constant of the circuit.

Similarly, for the high-pass RL filter we have:

$$\left| \frac{\text{j}\omega_c (L/R)}{1 + \text{j}\omega_c (L/R)} \right| = \frac{1}{\sqrt{2}}$$

and $\therefore$

$$\left| \frac{1 + \text{j}\omega_c (L/R)}{\text{j}\omega_c (L/R)} \right| = \sqrt{2}$$

Multiplying top and bottom by $-\text{j}\omega_c (L/R)$:*

$$\left| \frac{-\text{j}\omega_c (L/R) + \omega_c^2 (L/R)^2}{\omega_c^2 (L/R)^2} \right| = \sqrt{2}$$

$$| 1 - \text{j}\omega_c^{-1} (L/R)^{-1} | = \sqrt{2}$$

$$(1 + \omega_c^{-2} (L/R)^{-2})^{\frac{1}{2}} = \sqrt{2}$$

$$1 + \frac{1}{\omega_c^2 (L/R)^2} = 2$$

* It is a standard technique for rationalizing complex numbers (i.e. to reduce a ratio to a single term) to multiply top and bottom of the expression by the complex conjugate of the denominator. The complex conjugate is simply found by changing the sign of the imaginary term.

and
$$\omega_c = \frac{1}{(L/R)} \qquad (5.5)$$

In general, for these simple R, L and C filters, the cut-off frequency is related to the inverse of the time constant, as evidenced by equations (5.4) and (5.5).

The properties of a filter network are conveniently described by the variations of the modulus and phase of $T(j\omega)$ with frequency. These two variations are termed the gain response and phase response; $A(\omega)$ and $\phi(\omega)$ respectively. Plots of $A(\omega)$ and $\phi(\omega)$ versus ω are very useful in practical terms, and are known as *Bode plots* after H. W. Bode (1945), who did a large amount of work on filter circuits. Figure 4b shows Bode plots for the networks of Fig. 4a.

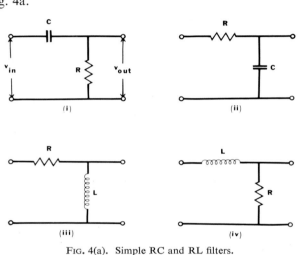

FIG. 4(a). Simple RC and RL filters.

(i) high-pass RC filter
$$V_{out} = \frac{j\omega CR}{1 + j\omega CR} \cdot V_{in}$$

(ii) low-pass RC filter
$$V_{out} = \frac{V_{in}}{1 + j\omega CR}$$

(iii) high-pass RL filter
$$V_{out} = \frac{j\omega(L/R)}{1 + j\omega(L/R)} \cdot V_{in}$$

(iv) low-pass RL filter
$$V_{out} = \frac{V_{in}}{1 + j\omega(L/R)}$$

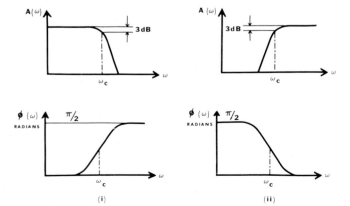

FIG. 4(b). Amplitude and phase responses, $A(\omega)$ and $\phi(\omega)$, for (i) simple low-pass filter and (ii) simple high-pass filter.

Connecting together a number of such high-pass filters (with comparable 3 dB points) has the effect of increasing the fall-off of $A(\omega)$ in the attenuation band; similarly for the low-pass filter. Cascading together a high- and low-pass filter produces a network which will only allow frequency components within a certain range to pass without attenuation. This is called a *band-pass filter*. The *bandwidth* of the network is defined as the difference in frequency between the 3 dB points of the high-pass and low-pass sections respectively.

The high-pass network is sometimes referred to as a *differentiator*, since its effect is to perform the mathematical operation of differentiation upon the input voltage function. By a similar argument, the low-pass network is often spoken of as an *integrator*.

Although such simple filters as these are frequently used in recording electrophysiological signals (and for several other applications) one gets much better performance from more complex designs or from active filters (*see later*). In particular, the use of inductors should be avoided where possible because of their bulk and cost.

PHYSICAL ELECTRONICS: VACUUM TUBES

In the vacuum tube device, or *valve*, free electrons are produced by a process called *thermionic emission*. A metal element or electrode, the *cathode*, is heated to such a temperature that the electrons acquire sufficient thermal energy to escape from the surface. They then produce the so-called *space charge* in the region of the cathode. The material of the cathode is usually coated with an oxide layer which lowers the temperature at which thermionic emission can occur.

If another element (with a low working temperature) is incorporated in the device, and held at a positive potential with respect to the cathode, an electric field exists between the two electrodes. This additional element is termed the *anode*; and an electron flux results from cathode to anode. In other words, current flows from positive to negative electrodes. This two-electrode device is termed a *diode*. The valve is evacuated so that gas molecules do not retard or scatter the electron flux by inter-particle collisions.

The magnitude of the anode to cathode current in this device is limited by the rate at which electrons can be emitted from the cathode. When the current is so limited it is no longer a function of anode-cathode potential difference, V_a, and the device is said to be *saturated*. Within a wide range, the saturation current can be increased by increasing the cathode temperature. Below the minimum saturation voltage, the current is said to be *space charge limited* (since it then depends upon the rate at which electrons enter and leave the space charge) and can be shown to be proportional to $V_a^{3/2}$ (Child, 1911; Langmuir, 1913). The vacuum tube device does not, therefore, obey Ohm's law; it is non-linear. Figure 5a depicts typical current-voltage curves, or *characteristic curves*, for the vacuum diode at various cathode temperatures.

If the anode is made negative with respect to the cathode, electrons produced by thermionic emission do not experience a force in the direction of the anode because the electric field is in the wrong sense. Therefore, current only flows when V_a is positive. Advantage is often taken of this ability to pass a current in one direction only. That is, the diode is used as a *rectifier*, to produce direct current from alternating current. Figure 5b shows a simple circuit for half-wave retification. The output waveform can be made to resemble more closely a constant dc voltage by the process

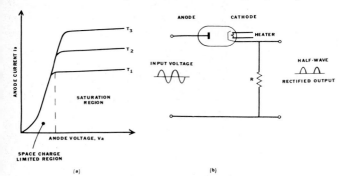

FIG. 5. The vacuum diode. (a) Typical current-voltage characteristic. T_1, T_2, T_3 denote cathode temperatures where $T_3 > T_2 > T_1$. (b) Simple circuit for half-wave rectification.

of "smoothing". This is usually done by passing the rectified voltage through a simple RC low-pass filter (Waidelich, 1941).

The diode may also be used as a peak-limiter or "clipper", ensuring that the potential at a point in a circuit never exceeds a predetermined value.

Current flow in the diode (from anode to cathode) depends, in the space charge limited region, upon the potential gradient. This can be modified by the inclusion of a third element, or *grid*, intermediate between the other two electrodes. This grid consists of an open network of wire, which allows the passage of most of the electrons. Such a device is called a *triode* (de Forest, 1906). Figure 6 illustrates the construction of the triode.

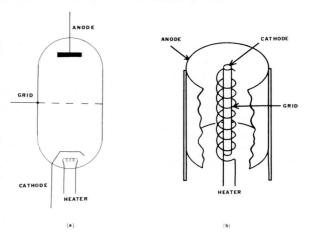

FIG. 6. The triode valve. (a) Schematic representation and (b) details of construction.

If a negative potential is applied to the grid it will tend to repel electrons back to the cathode. If this negative potential is made large enough, no electrons will leave the space charge cloud and the valve is said to be "cut off".

It is the effect that the grid potential has on current flow that accounts for the amplifying properties of the triode. Because the control grid is physically much closer to the cathode than is the anode, it has a much more profound effect on current flow than does anode voltage. That is to say, a small change in grid voltage produces a relatively large change in anode current. So a small alternating potential applied to the grid will produce a large amplitude alternating current in the anode circuit. Further, there is practically no current flow into the grid because of its open mesh geometry. Hence, sensitive control of anode current can be achieved for minimal power expenditure. This is a desirable property for any amplifier.

Figure 7a shows typical curves of anode current, I_a, versus grid voltage, V_g, for constant values of anode

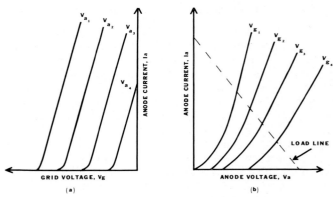

FIG. 7. Triode valve characteristics. (a) Transfer characteristic and (b) anode characteristic with a load line shown. In (a) $V_{a_1} > V_{a_2} > V_{a_3} > V_{a_4}$; in (b) $V_{g_1} > V_{g_2} > V_{g_3} > V_{g_4}$.

voltage, V_a. This plot is known as the *transfer characteristic*. The slope of this graph in its linear region is termed the *mutual conductance* of the valve, g_m. Hence:

$$g_m = \frac{\Delta I_a}{\Delta V_g}\bigg]_{\text{constant } V_a} \qquad (5.6)$$

As implied above, this slope will be large for an amplifying device.

Figure 7b shows another very useful curve, the anode characteristic, where anode current is plotted versus anode voltage for constant grid voltage. This curve will be of the same form as that obtaining for the diode. In this case, the slope of the linear region represents the conductance of the valve. This is the reciprocal of the *anode slope resistance*, r_a:

$$\frac{1}{r_a} = \frac{\Delta I_a}{\Delta V_a}\bigg]_{V_g} \qquad (5.7)$$

The voltage *amplification factor* of the valve, μ, is given simply by the change in anode voltage for a change in grid potential at constant anode current. That is:

$$\mu = \frac{\Delta V_a}{\Delta V_g}\bigg]_{I_a}$$

$$= \frac{\Delta V_a}{\Delta I_a} \cdot \frac{\Delta I_a}{\Delta V_g}$$

$$\therefore \ \mu = r_a g_m \qquad (5.8)$$

Hence, the amplification factor is simply found from the anode and transfer characteristics. μ may be as large as 200–300.

Many valves have been produced in which extra electrodes are incorporated for special applications (e.g. tetrode and pentode). These will not be dealt with further.

Although the development of valve amplifiers, which are briefly discussed in a later section, was a topic of great importance in the earlier days of electronics, in the past 20 years semiconductor devices have all but made valves obsolete. These new devices require a far smaller power supply for their operation and are more reliable, robust and physically smaller. We shall now consider the principle of operation of these most important devices.

PHYSICAL ELECTRONICS: SEMICONDUCTOR DEVICES

In order to achieve current flow from anode to cathode in the linear region of the thermionic valve characteristic, there must be a large potential difference (perhaps 150–250 V) between the two electrodes. This necessity to provide a high voltage supply has severe drawbacks in respect of the convenience, size, reliability and safety of electronic equipment incorporating vacuum tube devices. By contrast, semiconductor devices require very low powers and low working temperatures for their operation. Whereas valve power supplies are generally derived from mains electricity, small batteries can be used to power semiconductor circuitry.

The basic physics of materials, including semiconductors, has been outlined in the previous chapter ("Basic Electricity"); and the distinction between p- and n-type impurity semiconductors has been made. We now consider the very important properties of the junction between two such materials; the pn junction. The n-type material, although electrically neutral, possesses high-energy conduction electrons, whereas the p-type material has holes in valence states. These mobile charge carriers, due to the impurities introduced by dopant species during manufacture, are termed *majority carriers*. By contrast, carriers of opposite sign, due to the intrinsic conductivity of the semiconductor, are called *minority carriers*. In order to understand the conditions existing at the pn junction it is convenient to suppose that the p- and n-materials are initially separate, but are subsequently joined together in such a way that there is crystal lattice continuity at the interface (Fig. 8). We now consider the events leading up to the establishment of a dynamic equilibrium at the junction.

Majority carriers (electrons) from the n-type region tend to diffuse into the p-type region where the mobile electron density is very much less. Also, the majority carriers (holes) in the p-type region diffuse in the opposite direction along the concentration gradient. The effect of these two processes is to make the n-type region electrically positive, and the p-type region negative. Hence, a potential barrier builds up across the junction which tends to oppose the further diffusion of majority carriers. However, it assists the movement of the oppositely charged minority carriers.

Equilibrium is reached when the current due to majority carriers (limited by the potential barrier) is equal to that due to minority carriers; yielding a net zero current across the junction.

Three comments are appropriate regarding the description above. Firstly, we have seen that current flow can be due to the existence of a concentration gradient of charge carriers. This is distinct from the situation (encountered in the previous chapter) where current flow is due to charge moving along a potential gradient, or electrical field. In

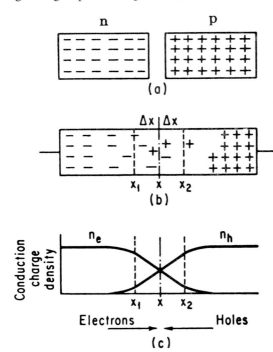

FIG. 8. A pn junction: (a) electron and hole distribution before joining; (b) same after joining, showing depletion region and (c) variation of charge density magnitude. (Reproduced from Ryder (1964) by kind permission of the publishers.)

the former case, we talk of *diffusion current*, whereas in the latter case we talk of *drift current*. Secondly, in the equilibrium situation, diffusion currents are limited to a narrow region between x_1 and x_2, as shown in Figs. 8b, c. This region, some 1 μm thick, is called the *depletion layer* or barrier layer. Finally, in practical terms, pn junction devices are not produced by joining together p- and n-type regions as above. In fact, the two different dopants are introduced during manufacture into different, adjacent areas of the same single crystal of semiconductor material.

Having briefly examined the equilibrium condition at the junction, we now discuss the effect of applying a potential difference. Suppose a battery is connected with its positive pole contacting the n-type region, and its negative pole contacting the p-type region (Fig. 9a). In this case, mobile electrons will be drawn towards the positive pole of the battery in the n-type region; and mobile holes will similarly move away from the junction region in the p-type material. Hence, the potential barrier at the interface will increase, severely limiting the diffusion of majority carriers, although there will be a very small current due to minority carriers. The *pn* junction is said to be *reverse biased*. On increasing the battery voltage, the reverse current will increase until all the minority carriers in the junction region are involved. The current then becomes almost independent of voltage; that is, it is equal to the *reverse saturation current*, I_0, shown in Fig. 9c.

If the battery connections are now reversed, the potential barrier at the junction is reduced, so allowing a considerable current due to majority carriers to flow (Figs. 9b, c). The junction is now said to be biased in the *forward direction*. Hence, we see that the *pn* junction device possesses a property of the thermionic diode, in that it exhibits a low resistance to current flow in one direction and a high resistance when biased in the other direction. For this

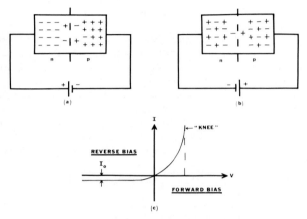

FIG. 9. (a) Reverse-biased *pn* junction, (b) forward-biased *pn* junction, (c) characteristic curve for semiconductor diode, showing reverse saturation and "knee" voltage.

reason, the *pn* junction device described above is called the *semiconductor diode*; and is extensively used for purposes of rectification.

Originally semiconductor diodes were manufactured almost exclusively using germanium (Ge) as the basic material. However, silicon (Si) has a lower intrinsic conductivity than germanium and so there are fewer minority carriers under the same conditions. Thus, the reverse saturation current for a silicon diode is much less than for a germanium diode. Further, the "knee" of the characteristic curve shown in Fig. 9c (that is the forward bias at which resistance markedly decreases) occurs at a much higher voltage (about 0·7 V) in Si diodes, compared with about 0·3 V for Ge diodes. These two desirable properties mean that, these days, silicon is generally the material of choice for semiconductor devices.

We have seen that the triode is derived from the diode valve by the addition of a control grid. In a similar way, the transistor differs from the semiconductor diode in that it possesses three distinct, differently doped regions; rather than two (Bardeen and Brattain, 1948). Here we consider the *npn* junction transistor (Shockley *et al.*, 1951), which consists of a thin *p*-type region between two *n*-type regions, although *pnp* transistors are also available. Devices of this construction are called *bipolar transistors*. The three

sections of the device (Fig. 10a) are termed the *emitter*, *base* and *collector*. Ohmic (non-rectifying) contacts are made to the three regions.

The transistor can be conveniently considered as two *pn* junctions. With the bias arrangement of Fig. 10a, one

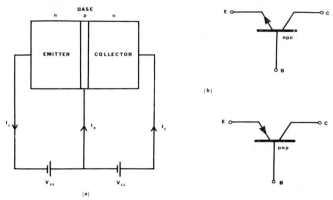

FIG. 10. (a) *npn* transistor showing bias arrangement in common base connection. (b) Circuit symbols for *npn* and *pnp* transistors. The arrow at the emitter indicates the normal direction of current flow.

of these (the emitter-base junction) is forward biased, whereas the other (the base-collector junction) is reverse biased. Hence, there is a large flow of majority carriers (electrons) across the emitter-base junction, producing the emitter current, I_E. Some of these electrons will recombine with holes in the base to produce base current, I_B. However, if the base is made very thin during manufacture (perhaps of the order 10–20 μm) many electrons will have sufficient energy to reach the base-collector junction. Thereafter, current flow is aided by the positive battery potential connected to the collector. Hence, in this device, current flow, I_E, in the low resistance* emitter-base circuit is transferred to current flow, I_C, in the high resistance (reverse biased) base-collector circuit. In fact, the name "transistor" is a contraction of the term *transfer resistor*. It is this property which enables the transistor to be used as an amplifier.

Since the transistor is a three-terminal device, one terminal must be common to both input and output in circuit applications. This common terminal determines the name of the connection. That is, the circuit of Fig. 10a is called the common base connection; common emitter and common collector connections are also used. Table 1 summarizes the salient features of these three configurations.

Applying Kirchhoff's second rule to the common base circuit of Fig. 10a:

$$I_E = I_B + I_C \qquad (5.9)$$

The base current is due to recombination of electrons and holes. Since only about 2 per cent of mobile charge carriers fail to reach the collector from the emitter, we have:

$$I_E \simeq I_C$$

and
$$\frac{\Delta I_C}{\Delta I_E} \simeq 0·98$$

* Strictly "low impedance" because of the capacitance of the junction.

TABLE 1

PROPERTIES OF THE THREE TRANSISTOR CIRCUIT CONFIGURATIONS

Feature	Common Base	Common Emitter	Common Collector
Current gain	< 1 (0.95–0.98)	≫ 1 (50–200)	≫ 1 (50–200)
Voltage gain	≫ 1 (~ 1,000)	≫ 1 (~ 1,000)	< 1
Power gain	medium (~ 900)	high (~ 15,000)	low
Input impedance	low (35Ω)	fairly low (1 kΩ)	high (1 MΩ)
Output impedance	high (1 MΩ)	fairly low (50 kΩ)	low (300 Ω)
Uses	used where low input impedance and/or high frequency operation is required	multistage amplifiers where high gains are required	buffer stages

The ratio of collector current to emitter current for constant collector voltage defines the *current gain*, α, of the transistor in the common base configuration:

$$\alpha = \frac{\Delta I_C}{\Delta I_E}\bigg]_{V_C \text{ const}} \qquad (5.10)$$

Note that the current gain is always less than unity, but that power gain is still a feature of the device. This occurs because of the wide ratio between the low input resistance into which charges are injected and the high output resistance at which they are extracted.

Here we have ignored the effect of minority carriers. In fact, the collector current has two components; one due emitter current and the other due to minority carriers. This latter component, I_{CO}, is dependent upon temperature and can, if large enough, severely limit performance or even damage the device. It is called *leakage current*. So:

$$\text{total collector current} = I_E + I_{CO}$$

In the common base mode, the base is analogous with the cathode of the triode valve. Similarly, the collector is analogous with the anode, whereas the emitter performs the control function of the grid. Because of the essential symmetry of the device, the transistor could conceivably be operated "back-to-front", i.e. with collector and emitter interchanged. However, this may produce lower current gains because, at manufacture, the collector is often made physically larger than the emitter. This is done in order to enhance the charge-collecting function of the collector.

In the common emitter configuration, the base performs the analogous control function to the triode grid. The current gain, β, in the common emitter configuration, will then be defined in similar manner to equation (5.10) as:

$$\beta = \frac{\Delta I_C}{\Delta I_B}\bigg]_{V_C \text{ const.}}$$

The base current, however, results largely from recombination losses of only a few percent; so that β may reach values as high as 200.

From equations (5.9) and (5.10):

$$\Delta I_C = \alpha \, \Delta I_E$$

and

$$\Delta I_B = \Delta I_E - \Delta I_C$$
$$= \Delta I_E (1 - \alpha)$$

$$\therefore \quad \beta = \frac{\Delta I_C}{\Delta I_E (1 - \alpha)} = \frac{\alpha}{1 - \alpha} \qquad (5.11)$$

For a typical value of α of 0.98:

$$\beta = \frac{0.98}{0.02}$$
$$\simeq 50$$

Because of its much higher current gain, and consequently larger power gain, the common emitter configuration is favoured for general applications such as multistage amplifiers (*see next section*).

Just as with the triode, characteristic curves are found to be very useful in describing transistor operation, and in designing circuits with specific devices. Figure 11 shows a few typical characteristics; and the non-linearity of the transistor can be clearly seen from these. Note, however,

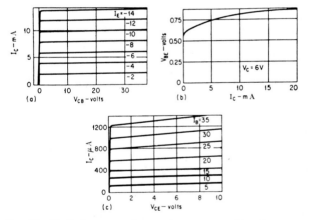

FIG. 11. Typical common-base and common-emitter characteristics. In (a) values of I_E are given in milliamperes; in (c) values of I_B are in microamperes. (Reproduced from Ryder (1964) by kind permission of the publishers.)

that there exists a large region in which the device is effectively linear. In such regions, linear analysis may be employed; and a number of linear equivalent circuits for the transistor exist, details of which will be found in most of the books detailed in the bibliography. These greatly simplify detailed design and analysis.

Referring to Figs. 11a and 11c it can be seen that the transistor can be considered either to be "on" or "off". That is to say, collector current, I_C, is close either to zero or some constant value depending upon emitter or base current. In this way, the transistor can be considered as a two-state (binary) device, or switch. Such a binary device is the basic unit of the digital computer. Lack of space precludes discussion of the important topic of digital electronics here, but the interested reader is referred to the book by Harris *et al.*, mentioned in the bibliography.

Recently, another type of three terminal semiconducting device has been increasingly used. This device, the field effect transistor (FET), operates on a somewhat different principle to the bipolar transistor (Shockley, 1952). The basis of the operation of this device is that the resistance (strictly impedance) to current flow between two terminals, the *source* and *drain*, is modulated by the potential at the third terminal, the *gate*. In this sense, the field effect transistor is much more similar to the triode valve than is the biploar transistor. Common source, common drain and common gate connections are possible.

There are basically two types of field effect transistor:
(1) The junction FET.
(2) The insulated gate FET (IGFET)—some of which are often called metal-oxide-semiconductor transistors (MOST's) because of their construction.

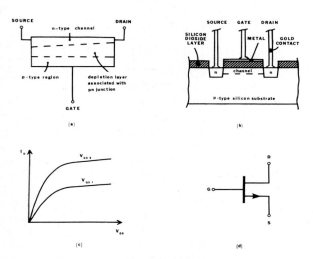

FIG. 12. (a) *n*-channel junction FET, (b) *n*-channel MOST, (c) typical drain characteristics of FET for two different gate potentials, $V_{GS_2} > V_{GS_1}$, (d) circuit symbol for *n*-channel FET. The direction of the arrow will be reversed in the case of the *p*-channel device.

Figure 12 shows schematic drawings for these two devices, along with the drain current I_D, versus drain-source voltage, V_{DS}, characteristic for constant values of gate-source bias, V_{GS}.

In the *n*-channel junction FET (Fig. 12a) there is a depletion layer (containing no free charge carriers) forming one boundary of the conducting channel. A bias voltage applied to the gate will affect the width of this depletion layer, and hence will modulate source-to-drain current. Because of its resistance, there is a voltage drop along the length of the channel, so that bias effectively increases from source to drain, as indicated in the figure.

In the MOST or IGFET (Fig. 12b) the gate is insulated from the channel by a layer of silicon dioxide (*see later*). The channel may either be present initially (a doped impurity region) or it may be induced electrostatically by a field between the gate and the substrate. As in the

junction FET, the gate potential modulates the channel impedance, thus giving a means of controlling current flow.

AC AND DC AMPLIFIERS

In the foregoing discussion we have seen how triode valves and transistors possess the ability to amplify signals. Figure 13 shows a typical amplifier circuit using a triode

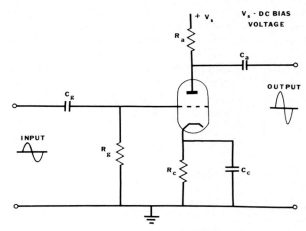

FIG. 13. Typical triode amplifier circuit.

valve. The capacitor, C_g, is incorporated to block dc potentials. Its value is chosen such that the reactance $1/\omega C_g$ is small compared with the grid resistance, R_g. Hence, most of the signal voltage will appear at the grid. Note that this condition will only be satisfied for large ω; so that the inclusion of this capacitor affects the low frequency response of the amplifier. The cathode resistance, R_c, and the anode (or load) resistance, R_a, are chosen so that the valve is biased correctly. That is, in the absence of an input signal (the *quiescent* condition) the dc potentials and voltages that obtain are in the central part of the linear region of the characteristic.

This can be illustrated by applying Kirchhoff's first rule to the dc path via R_a and R_c:

$$V_B = I_a R_a + V_a + I_a R_c$$

$$\therefore \quad I_a = \frac{V_B}{(R_a + R_c)} - \frac{V_a}{(R_a + R_c)} \qquad (5.12)$$

Hence, there is a linear relation between I_a and V_a in the dc condition. The straight line given by equation (5.12) can be drawn in on the anode characteristic. This has been done in Fig. 7b, which appears earlier. This line is called the *load line*, and intercepts the I_a and V_a axes at $I_a = V_B/(R_a + R_c)$ and $V_a = V_B$ respectively. The intersection of the load line with the anode characteristic gives the quiescent point for a particular grid bias.

The quiescent point is arranged to be at the centre of the linear region to ensure that maximum current and voltage excursions can take place without the range of linearity being exceeded. If the device operates in the non-linear region of its characteristic, distortion of the output waveform will occur. Many other bias arrangements are possible.

The capacitor, C_c, across the cathode resistance is included to maintain the cathode voltage approximately constant, even though there are rapid variations of anode current due to the input signal. To achieve this the time constant R_cC_c should be large compared with the period of the signal frequency. In other words, the reactance $1/\omega C_c$ should be much smaller than R_c; so that C_c affects the low frequency response of the amplifier, as does C_g.

As explained earlier, a small variation of the signal voltage applied to the grid leads to a relatively large change in anode current, causing the potential difference across the anode resistance, R_a, to change. This potential difference is taken as the amplifier output. The overall gain of the amplifier will, by definition, be given as:

$$\text{gain} = \left| \frac{\Delta V_{\text{out}}}{\Delta V_{\text{in}}} \right| \simeq \frac{\Delta V_{\text{out}}}{\Delta V_g}$$

$$\Delta V_{\text{out}} = \Delta I_a \cdot R_a$$

But

$$\Delta I_a = \frac{\Delta V_a}{R_a + r_a + R_c}$$

where r_a is the anode slope resistance of the vacuum tube device.

$$\therefore \quad \Delta V_{\text{out}} = \frac{\Delta V_a \cdot R_a}{R_a + r_a + R_c}$$

and

$$\text{gain} = \frac{\Delta V_{\text{out}}}{\Delta V_g} = \frac{\Delta V_a}{\Delta V_g} \cdot \frac{R_a}{R_a + r_a + R_c}$$

$$\therefore \quad \text{gain} = \frac{\mu R_a}{R_a + r_a + R_c} \tag{5.13}$$

From equation (5.13) we see that μ represents the theoretically maximum gain (for $R_a \gg r_a + R_c$). However, it is not possible to keep increasing the gain by progressively increasing R_a. This is so because, for large R_a, the anode voltage will approach zero as all the bias voltage is dropped across R_a. Note also that the inclusion of the resistor R_c (used to obtain suitable bias conditions) has the effect of reducing the gain. This important effect, which is called *negative feedback*, is further discussed below.

The considerations outlined above are very similar when an FET is used in place of the triode valve. Bipolar transistors are also very commonly used but the design parameters are rather different. Valves are, in fact, very rarely used these days for simple amplifiers. For this reason, we will consider FET or bipolar transistor circuits only from this point onwards.

If a single stage of voltage amplification is inadequate, as is often the case, then further stages must be added; so that each stage amplifies the output of the previous one. The overall gain, A_T, will be given by the products of the individual stage gains:

$$A_T = \prod_i A_i \tag{5.14}$$

In coupling the stages together it is important that the quiescent conditions of each of the individual devices do not adversely affect each other. In this case the stages are effectively isolated and can be designed separately. If ac signals only are to be amplified the problem is easily solved. A capacitor can be used to couple the output of one stage to the input of the next. Figure 14 shows a two-stage amplifier, using *n*-channel FET's and an RC coupling arrangement. The resistance, R, at the gate of the second transistor is necessary to give a resistive path between gate and source of that transistor. This prevents a build-up of charge at the gate. The time constant of the RC combination determines the lowest frequency which can be amplified.

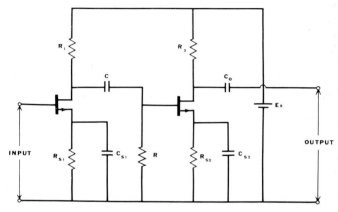

FIG. 14. Two stage RC coupled FET amplifier.

A considerable problem arises if slowly varying signals, or signals having some average value with respect to zero potential, are to be amplified. In this case it is not possible to use reactive elements, such as capacitors and inductors, to give the circuit signal characteristics which are different from bias characteristics. It is impossible in such circuits to distinguish between thermal effects, changes in device characteristics or bias conditions ("drift") and signals of interest. This objection holds also for the case of the single stage amplifier. Emitter or source resistors (analogous to R_c in Fig. 13) must not be bypassed by capacitors.

If only the lowest frequencies are of interest, it is possible to "chop" the dc signal, by periodically connecting the signal input to earth, thus producing an ac version of the waveform which can be demodulated after the various stages of amplification. With this system (*chopper amplifier*) it is obviously not possible to amplify frequency components greater than half the chopping frequency, so high frequency performance is limited. This problem can be partly overcome by using a high quality wideband dc amplifier in parallel with a chopper amplifier. The output of the latter amplifier is used to modify the overall output, thus correcting the drift in the wideband amplifier. This arrangement is known as *chopper stabilization*.

If the signals of interest are very small (so that drift is appreciable in comparison) and the required gain and bandwidth are large, careful design is essential. Here the use of semiconductor devices has important advantages over valve designs. In particular, the much lower supply voltages and absence of heater circuits gives much lower drift. Also, transistors are much less noisy (*see below*) than valves at low frequencies; and the low supply voltages simplify interstage coupling.

Figure 15 shows an extremely important dc amplifier design, using two bipolar transistors in common emitter configuration. This type of amplifier uses balanced operation at the input (and succeeding stages) to eliminate drift. The design is therefore called a *balanced amplifier* (or differential amplifier). The circuit is arranged so that, for instance, temperature-dependent signals (such as collector leakage current) tend to cancel. It can be seen that, by symmetry, similar signals at both inputs ($v_{in\,1} = v_{in\,2}$) will produce similar signals at the two collectors. Hence, the total output, v_{out}, will be zero. This phenomenon is termed *common-mode rejection* (or *in-phase rejection*) since in-phase signals cancel. It is only the out-of-phase component (that is, the difference of the two signals) that is amplified, hence the name "differential" amplifier.

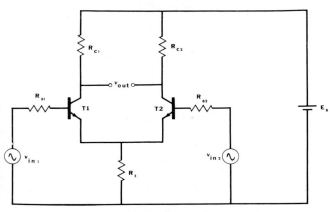

FIG. 15. The differential amplifier.

It is apparent that, for good common-mode rejection, any change in the base-emitter voltage of one transistor (caused by thermal effects, say) must be exactly balanced by an equal change in the other transistor. To achieve this, the transistors are generally selected to have the same characteristics and to respond to equivalent temperature changes in the same way. Sometimes they are sealed in the same canister so that environmental temperatures are comparable. This is the reason for the term "balanced" in connection with this amplifier.

The *common-mode rejection ratio* is defined as the output for out-of-phase inputs (say $v_{in\,1} = v_{in\,1}$; and $v_{in\,2} = 0$) divided by the output for in-phase inputs ($v_{in\,1} = v_{in\,2}$). This ratio may be several thousand for a good design using modern transistors.

In order to take advantage of the common-mode rejection of this amplifier it is necessary to derive a differential input. That is, the signal to be amplified must be applied not only to the base of transistor T1 but must also appear, although equal and opposite, at the base of T2. This is relatively easily achieved; and the amplifier is then said to have a *push-pull* input.

One very important consequence of the common-mode rejection property of differential amplifiers is the minimization of effects due to interference from mains supplies; so often a problem in electrophysiological recording. 50 Hz (or 60 Hz in the U.S.A.) mains contamination in

the output is minimal, since it appears in-phase at both amplifier inputs.

FEEDBACK: FOLLOWER CIRCUITS AND OSCILLATORS

From the previous section, it is apparent that the requirements for a good (precision) amplifier can be stated as follows:

(i) The output voltage should be proportional to the input voltage, but (usually) much greater in amplitude, under all working conditions.

(ii) The attachment of the amplifier to the signal source must not significantly alter the signal waveform.

(iii) The attachment of a load (such as a recording device) to the amplifier output must not adversely alter the output voltage waveform.

All of these requirements can be achieved to a greater or lesser degree by the use of feedback, as we will show below.

Condition (i) above requires that the gain of the amplifier is a constant, and is therefore independent of frequency, over the whole frequency range of interest. So, if (for instance) neural spikes are to be amplified undistorted, the bandwidth of the amplifier used must, in theory, be infinite. Further, the voltage amplifications should be independent of variations both in supply voltages and in the characteristics of the devices used (which should be linear), due perhaps to temperature changes or ageing effects.

Another requirement is that the amplifier does not generate extraneous signals, or *noise*, internally. The noise produced can be found by looking at the amplifier output under operating conditions, but in the absence of an input. This noise is usually due to random thermal motions of free charges in circuit elements or electronic devices. The energy of such noise is uniformly distributed over the whole of the frequency spectrum. In fact, it is possible to show (Johnson, 1928; Nyquist, 1928) that the noise voltage, E_n, generated within a certain bandwidth, Δf hertz, in a resistance, R ohms, is given by:

$$E_n = \sqrt{4kTR\,\Delta f}$$

k — Boltzmann's constant (1.38×10^{-23} J.K^{-1})

T — Absolute temperature (K)

The noise source can therefore be considered as a voltage generator, E_n, in series with a noiseless resistor, R.

Noise in transistors, although also due to random thermal effects, differs from noise in resistors in that the power per unit bandwith varies inversely with frequency. Thus, it is maximal at low frequencies. The extent of noise depends upon choice of quiescent point, and is usually reduced by lowering collector supply voltage (in the common-emitter mode).

Condition (ii) above, namely that the amplifier should not adversely affect the signal source, requires that no current flows into the input terminal. In other words, the *input impedance* of the amplifier (the impedance between the input terminals) must be very large; at least in comparison with the source impedance. Similarly, (iii) requires that the input impedance of the recording device be large with respect to the output impedance of the amplifier. For this reason, the output impedance should be as low as possible.

The problem of obtaining a high enough input impedance is particularly relevant when recording from high impedance sources, such as glass micro-electrodes. It is the inherently high input impedances of FET's (gate may be virtually isolated from rest of device) that is so attractive in applications such as this.

The expedient of feeding back the output voltage, or a certain fraction of it, to the input can improve gain stability, reduce noise and distortion, increase input impedance and decrease output impedance (Black, 1934).

Figure 16 shows an amplifier, gain A, considered as a *four-terminal network* (i.e. with discrete input and output connections, and with none of the detailed circuitry shown). Another four-terminal network is used to feed a proportion, β, of the output voltage back in series with the input. This arrangement is called *voltage feedback* to distinguish it from the case where a proportion of the output current is fed-back. From the diagram:

$$v_0 = Av_{\text{in}}$$

and

$$v_{\text{in}} = v_{\text{s}} + \beta v_0$$

$$\therefore \quad v_0 = Av_{\text{s}} + A\beta v_0 \qquad (5.15)$$

$$v_0 (1 - A\beta) = Av_{\text{s}}$$

The gain with feedback, A_{f}, is, by definition, given as:

$$A_{\text{f}} = \frac{v_0}{v_{\text{s}}}$$

$$\therefore \quad A_{\text{f}} = \frac{A}{1 - A\beta} \qquad (5.16)$$

A_{f} is generally called the *closed-loop gain*; and $A\beta$ is termed the *open-loop gain*, since it corresponds to the gain of amplifier and feedback network when the feedback loop is disconnected. *Positive feedback* occurs when the term $A\beta$ is positive; and the effective gain is increased from A to A_{f}. *Negative feedback* occurs when the term $A\beta$ is negative; and the effective gain is decreased. Negative $A\beta$ implies that the feedback network phase-shifts the output by π rad (180°), if we assume that the amplifier without feedback introduces no phase shift. If the amplifier does in fact introduce a shift, the requirement for negative feedback remains that the fed-back voltage should be in antiphase with the input.

Suppose that the amplifier were a two-stage amplifier with stage gains A_1 and A_2 respectively, i.e.:

$$A = A_1 A_2 \quad \text{(from equation (5.14))}$$

Further suppose that, as a result of some noisy component, a noise voltage, N, appears at the input of the second stage. The output with feedback is then found by adding an additional term $A_2 N$ to equation (5.15):

$$v_0 = Av_{\text{s}} + A\beta v_0 + A_2 N$$

$$\therefore \quad v_0 (1 - A\beta) = Av_{\text{s}} + A_2 N$$

$$= A \left\{ v_{\text{s}} + \frac{N}{A_1} \right\}$$

$$v_0 = \frac{A}{1 - A\beta} \left\{ v_{\text{s}} + \frac{N}{A_1} \right\}$$

Since with negative feedback $| 1 - A\beta | > 1$, the noise voltage is reduced due to feedback, together with the output, Av_{s}. However, the noise is further reduced with respect to the output by a factor A_1 (the gain preceding the noise source). The use of feedback therefore decreases the effect of internally generated noise in the amplifier.

Gain stability can be examined by differentiating equation (5.16):

$$dA_{\text{f}} = \frac{(1 - A\beta)\, dA + A\beta\, dA}{(1 - A\beta)^2}$$

$$= \frac{dA}{1 - A\beta} + \frac{A\beta}{(1 - A\beta)^2} \cdot dA$$

Dividing through by A_{f}:

$$\frac{dA_{\text{f}}}{A_{\text{f}}} = \frac{1}{1 - A\beta} \cdot \frac{dA}{A_{\text{f}}} + \frac{A\beta}{(1 - A\beta)^2} \cdot \frac{dA}{A_{\text{f}}}$$

Substituting from equation (5.16):

$$\frac{dA_{\text{f}}}{A_{\text{f}}} = \frac{dA}{A} + \frac{\beta}{1 - A\beta} \cdot dA$$

$$= \frac{dA}{A} \left\{ 1 + \frac{A\beta}{1 - A\beta} \right\}$$

$$\frac{dA_{\text{f}}}{A_{\text{f}}} = \frac{1}{1 - A\beta} \cdot \frac{dA}{A}$$

Hence, the fractional change in gain with feedback, $dA_{\text{f}}/A_{\text{f}}$, is $(1 - A\beta)$ times less then the corresponding change, dA/A, without negative feedback. The gain can therefore be stabilized quite effectively by the use of negative feedback.

Referring again to Fig. 16, the input impedance with feedback is Z_{in}' and the output impedance with feedback is Z_0'. As before:

$$v_{\text{in}} = v_{\text{s}} + \beta v_0$$

and

$$v_0 = Av_{\text{in}}$$

$$\therefore \quad v_{\text{in}} = \frac{v_{\text{s}}}{1 - A\beta} \qquad (5.17$$

The input current with feedback is:

$$i_{\text{f}} = \frac{v_{\text{s}}}{Z_{\text{in}}'} = \frac{v_{\text{in}}}{Z_{\text{in}}}$$

where Z_{in} is the input impedance without feedback.

$$\therefore \quad Z_{\text{in}}' = \frac{v_{\text{s}}}{v_{\text{in}}} \cdot Z_{\text{in}}$$

$$Z_{\text{in}}' = (1 - A\beta)Z_{\text{in}} \quad \text{(from equation (5.17))}$$

So the input impedance is increased by a factor $1 - A\beta$ (greater than unity for negative feedback).

Similarly, it can be shown that the output impedance with feedback, $Z_o{}'$, is less than it would otherwise be (Z_o) by the factor $(1 - A\beta)$ when employing voltage feedback.

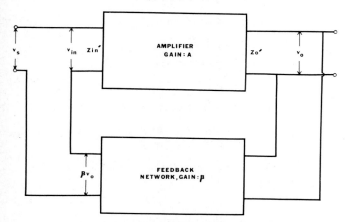

FIG. 16. Schematic diagram for voltage feedback arrangement.

Below, we shall see that, if *current feedback* is applied (i.e. a proportion of the output current is fed-back to the input), the output impedance is increased over and above that without feedback.

Figure 17 shows a most important negative voltage-feedback circuit; the *source follower*. This is the FET analogue of the well-known *cathode follower* (Richter, 1943), long used in physiological applications for its high input impedance.

The circuit in the illustration is drawn to depict small changes only. In other words, for the sake of simplicity, no attempt has been made to represent bias circuitry.

For a feedback amplifier:

$$v_s = v_{in} - \beta v_o$$

From the diagram, Fig. 17a:

$$\beta v_o = - v_o$$

$$\therefore \quad \beta = -1$$

Hence the feedback is negative and:

$$v_s = v_{in} + v_o$$
$$= v_{in} + A v_{in}$$
$$= (1 + A) v_{in}$$

Comparing Figs. 17a and b:

$$v_g = v_{in}$$

and

$$v_o = v_d$$

$$\therefore \quad v_s = (1 + A) v_g$$

and

$$v_d = R_s i_d$$

The mutual conductance, or *transconductance*, of an FET, g_m, is defined in analogous manner to that for the vacuum tube (equation (5.6)).

i.e.

$$g_m = \frac{\Delta I_D}{\Delta V_G} = \frac{i_d}{v_g} \quad *$$

$$\therefore \quad i_d = g_m v_g$$

and

$$v_d = g_m R_s v_g$$

Now, the gain without feedback is given by:

$$A = \frac{v_o}{v_{in}}$$

$$= \frac{v_d}{v_g}$$

$$A = g_m R_s \qquad (5.18)$$

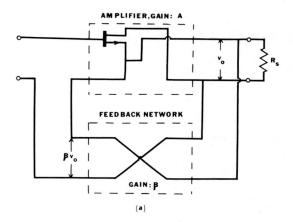

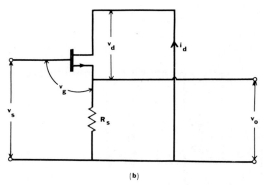

FIG. 17. The source follower as a voltage feedback amplifier. Circuits drawn for small changes only: (a) showing explicitly how the output voltage is fed back to the input in antiphase and (b) conventional circuit representation.

The closed loop gain is:

$$A_f = \frac{v_o}{v_s}$$

$$= \frac{A}{1 + A} \text{ (since } \beta = -1)$$

Typically, g_m may be 5 millisiemens (5 mS—1 siemen is equal to 1 reciprocal ohm) and the source resistance may

---

* This notation, using lower case letters for small changes or alternating quantities, is extremely useful and has been used earlier in the chapter.

be about 20 kΩ. Hence, from equation (5.18) the gain without feedback will be about 100.

$$A = g_\mathrm{m}R_\mathrm{s} \gg 1$$

and
$$A_\mathrm{f} \simeq \frac{A}{A}$$
$$= 1$$

So the output of the source follower is approximately independent of g_m (i.e. of device parameters) and virtually "follows" the input without phase-reversal; hence the name of the circuit.

The input impedance is increased by a factor $(1 + g_\mathrm{m}R_\mathrm{s})$, whereas the output impedance is reduced by a similar fraction, when feedback is applied. Follower circuits are therefore extensively used as the first stage of an amplifier, when recording from a high impedance source.

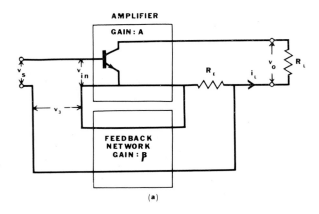

(a)

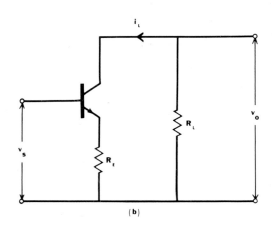

(b)

FIG. 18. (a) Common emitter amplifier employing current feedback. (b) Conventional circuit representation.

The bipolar transistor equivalent of the source follower is the emitter follower. The emitter follower is a common-collector circuit (*see* Table 1). Figure 18 depicts a bipolar transistor circuit employing current feedback, via the emitter resistor, R_E. We now obtain an expression for the output impedance with feedback, Z_o', for this amplifier.

The important theorem of Thévenin (1883) states that the output impedance of a network is given by the output

voltage obtaining when the output terminals are open-circuited, divided by the current that flows when the terminals are short-circuited.

i.e.
$$Z_\mathrm{o}' = \frac{\text{open-circuit voltage}}{\text{short-circuit current}} = \frac{v_\mathrm{oc}}{i_\mathrm{sc}}$$

$$v_\mathrm{oc} = Av_\mathrm{in}$$

and
$$v_\mathrm{in} = v_\mathrm{s} + R_\mathrm{E}i_\mathrm{L}$$

When the output is open-circuited, $i_\mathrm{L} = 0$.

$$\therefore \quad v_\mathrm{oc} = Av_\mathrm{s} \qquad (5.19)$$

By Ohm's law, the short-circuit current will be:

$$i_\mathrm{sc} = \frac{Av_\mathrm{in}}{Z_\mathrm{o} + R_\mathrm{E}} \qquad (5.20)$$

where Z_o is the output impedance without feedback. As before:

$$v_\mathrm{in} = v_\mathrm{s} + \beta R_\mathrm{E}i_\mathrm{L}$$

When the output is short-circuited, $i_\mathrm{L} = i_\mathrm{sc}$.

$$\therefore \quad v_\mathrm{in} = v_\mathrm{s} + \beta R_\mathrm{E}i_\mathrm{sc}$$

Substituting in equation (5.20):

$$i_\mathrm{sc} = \frac{A(v_\mathrm{s} + \beta R_\mathrm{E}i_\mathrm{sc})}{Z_\mathrm{o} + R_\mathrm{E}}$$

$$\therefore \quad i_\mathrm{sc}(Z_\mathrm{o} + R_\mathrm{E} - A\beta R_\mathrm{E}) = Av_\mathrm{s}$$

$$i_\mathrm{sc} = \frac{Av_\mathrm{s}}{Z_\mathrm{o} + R_\mathrm{E}(1 - A\beta)}$$

From (5.19):

$$i_\mathrm{sc} = \frac{v_\mathrm{oc}}{Z_\mathrm{o} + R_\mathrm{E}(1 - A\beta)}$$

$$Z_\mathrm{o}' = \frac{v_\mathrm{oc}}{i_\mathrm{sc}} = Z_\mathrm{o} + R_\mathrm{E}(1 - A\beta)$$

For the circuit of Fig. 18b, $\beta = -1$, and the output impedance with current feedback is increased by a factor $R_\mathrm{E}(1 + A)$. This is essentially the only difference between current and voltage feedback.

We now consider an application of positive feedback. By equation (5.16):

$$\frac{v_\mathrm{out}}{v_\mathrm{in}} = \frac{A}{1 - A\beta}$$

If the open loop gain, $A\beta$, is purely real and equal to 1 then the overall gain with feedback (the closed loop gain) becomes infinite. Theoretically, this means that it is possible to obtain an output from an amplifier without applying a signal, simply by feeding any output voltage that does appear back to the input without phase-shift. Such a feedback amplifier arrangement is called an *oscillator*. The reader may be familiar with the problem of oscillation caused by positive feedback in hearing aids when used with poorly fitting ear moulds.

Initially, the output will be due to internally generated (wideband) noise but as this is fed back regeneratively, the output amplitude will grow until it is limited only by the gain characteristic of the system or by external circuitry. The frequency of the output will be that for which:

$$A\beta = 1 + j0$$

So, if the amplifier introduces a phase-shift of π rad (180°) as, for example, a single stage transistor amplifier might do, the feedback network must introduce a further 180° phase-shift at the required frequency for oscillation. The network shown in Fig. 19a employing identical resistors and capacitors can be used for this purpose.

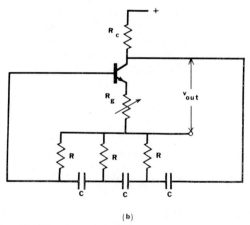

(a)

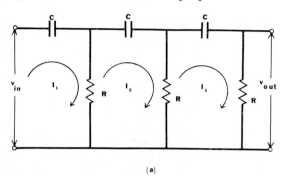

(b)

FIG. 19. The phase shift (RC) oscillator. (a) RC feedback network, (b) oscillator circuit.

Applying Kirchhoff's rules to this circuit:

$$v_{in} = -jX_c i_1 + R(i_1 - i_2)$$
$$0 = -jX_c i_2 + R(i_2 - i_3) + R(i_2 - i_1)$$
$$0 = -jX_c i_3 + R i_3 + R(i_3 - i_2)$$

These three equations can be solved for i_3 to yield:

$$i_3 = \frac{R^2 v_{in}}{(R^3 - 5X_c^2 R) + j(X_c^3 - 6X_c R^2)}$$

Now: $v_{out} = i_3 R$

so $\beta = \frac{R^3}{(R^3 - 5X_c^2 R) + j(X_c^3 - 6X_c R^2)}$

and the condition for oscillation in the circuit of Fig. 19b is that β, equal to $\frac{v_{out}}{v_{in}}$, is real with a modulus of -1.

Hence, all imaginary terms must vanish.

$$\therefore \quad X_c^3 = 6X_c R^2$$
$$X_c^2 = 6R^2$$
$$\frac{1}{\omega_0^2 C^2} = 6R^2$$
$$\omega_0 = \frac{1}{\sqrt{6}RC} \qquad (5.21)$$

Equation (5.21) gives the frequency of oscillation. At this frequency:

$$\beta = \frac{R^3}{R^3 - 5X_c^2 R}$$
$$= \frac{R^3}{R^3 - 5R(6R^2)}$$
$$\beta = -\frac{1}{29}$$

So, for the open loop gain to equal $1 + j0$ the amplifier gain, A, should be equal to -29.

A variety of passive feedback networks are used for the design of oscillators, some of which introduce zero phase-shift. These are used, for example, when the amplifier has two stages giving an overall phase change of zero. Resonant circuits, for instance, are used in the RL family of oscillators. Factors which should be considered in oscillator design include frequency stability and the spectral content (the distribution of energy with frequency) of the output. Ideally, the output should be a pure sine wave; but if its amplitude is limited only by saturation-type non-linearities it will be contaminated with harmonics.

Having seen that the open loop gain, $A\beta$, is generally frequency-dependent, a difficulty in the design of negative feedback amplifiers becomes apparent. An amplifier designed to utilize negative feedback within a particular frequency range may well, outside that range, have the feedback voltage in phase with the signal; giving positive feedback and perhaps causing oscillation. In this case the amplifier would have to be redesigned.

Finally, it should be pointed out that feedback is a very important concept, not only in electronic circuits, but in many of the applied sciences also. These include physiology and medicine. The function of a system incorporating negative feedback is, as we have seen in the case of electronic amplifiers, to produce an output which faithfully reproduces the system input. If the system input can be considered to represent some constant reference value, then we have a *control system* which acts as a *regulator*. That is, it acts to maintain an effectively constant output, equal to the reference input. Such regulatory systems abound in physiology, where they are termed *homeostatic* control mechanisms. Some examples of parameters controlled within tolerable limits by this means are blood sugar concentrations and the rates of some enzyme reactions.

If, however, the system input is variable, the negative feedback control system produces an output which follows the input variations. Such a system is termed a *servo-mechanism*. An example of a biological servomechanism is the visual-tracking mechanism, where the output can be considered to be the angular position of the lens. The system acts to keep the subject of interest centred broadly on the fovea (the most visually acute region of the retina).

Positive feedback systems have received less attention in this field, but epidemics and psychiatric disorders are occasionally viewed in this light (Milsum, 1968).

THE OPERATIONAL AMPLIFIER

Circuit design and manufacturing techniques have lately advanced to the stage where it is possible to produce amplifiers having almost all of the attributes mentioned above (e.g. very high gain, very high input impedance, ultra-wide bandwidth, etc.). The *operational amplifier* is an ultra-high gain, phase-reversing amplifier (usually having a differential input) which, for the purposes of circuit design and analysis, is considered to have the following properties:

(i) The gain is effectively infinite in magnitude (practical value $\simeq 10^4$ or 10^5), real and negative.
(ii) The input impedance is infinite, so that input current is zero.
(iii) The output impedance is zero.
(iv) The bandwidth is infinite.
(v) Any feedback network can be employed without affecting the stability of the amplifier.

Figure 20a shows an operational amplifier, gain $- A$, with an impedance Z_1, between the signal source and the positive input, and feedback via an impedance, Z_2.

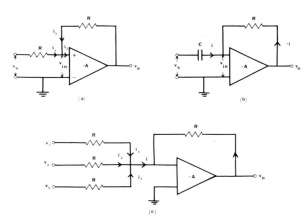

FIG. 20. The operational amplifier: (a) connection in feedback circuit, (b) the operational amplifier differentiator, (c) the summing amplifier.

By Kirchhoff's second rule:

$$i_1 - i_2 + i_3 = 0$$

But, for the operational amplifier, the input current, i_2, is assumed zero:

$$\therefore \quad i_1 = - i_3 \qquad (5.22)$$

Now:

$$v_o = - Av_{in}$$

$$\therefore \quad v_{in} = - \frac{v_o}{A}$$

Since A is considered infinite, $v_{in} \simeq 0$.

But

$$v_s - v_{in} = Z_1 i_1$$

$$\therefore \quad v_s \simeq Z_1 i_1 \qquad (5.23)$$

and

$$v_o - v_{in} = Z_2 i_3$$

$$\therefore \quad v_o \simeq Z_2 i_3$$

Substituting from (5.22)

$$v_o = - Z_2 i_1 \qquad (5.24)$$

Dividing (5.23) into (5.24) gives the overall gain with feedback, A_f, as:

$$A_f = \frac{v_o}{v_s} = - \frac{Z_2}{Z_1} \qquad (5.25)$$

This important equation for the closed loop gain implies that the operational amplifier can be used to obtain a wide variety of desired transfer functions, simply by choosing appropriate combinations of resistor and capacitor for Z_1 and Z_2. (Note that inductors need not be used as the effect of an inductance in the feedback loop can be simulated by placing a capacitor in the input lead.) By this means feedback amplifiers having applications such as active filters, analogue computer elements (summers, differentiators and integrators) and sample-and-hold amplifiers can be designed. To illustrate this, reference is made to Figs. 20b, c.

In Fig. 20b, equation (5.23) becomes:

$$v_s = X_c i$$

The current through the capacitor is given by:

$$i = C \frac{dv_s}{dt}$$

By equations (5.22) and (5.24):

$$v_o = - Ri$$

$$v_o = - CR \frac{d}{dt} v_s \qquad (5.26)$$

This circuit, therefore, behaves as a differentiator: the output voltage is the time-derivative of the input voltage. Note, however, from our previous comments that the mathematical operation of differentiation corresponds to the signal operation of high-pass filtering. It is easy to show that interchanging R and C in this circuit produces an integrator (or low-pass filter) by interchanging v_o and v_s in equation (5.26) above.

Consider now the circuit of Figure 20c:

$$v_o = - iR'$$

and

$$i = i_1 + i_2 + i_3$$

$$= \frac{V_1}{R} + \frac{V_2}{R} + \frac{V_3}{R}$$

$$\therefore \quad v_{\mathrm{o}} = -\frac{R'}{R}\,(V_1 + V_2 + V_3) \qquad (5.27)$$

Hence, the output of the amplifier is proportional to the sum of the input voltages. This circuit arrangement is therefore called a *summing amplifier* and is much used in analogue computers, together with differentiators and integrators, for finding solutions to differential equations.

The reader is referred to any of the operational amplifier handbooks produced by the major manufacturers for further information on these versatile and most useful devices.

MICROELECTRICS

As we have seen, transistors can be fabricated by diffusing dopant material into a block of semiconductor, or *substrate*. This diffusion process must be carried out at high temperatures. Silicon is the material of choice for the substrate because it is cheap and abundant (in fact, it is the second commonest element, after oxygen), has good electrical properties, as described earlier, and possesses an oxide (SiO$_2$) of high relative permittivity, $\varepsilon_{\mathrm{r}} \simeq 13$, which can therefore be used for insulation purposes. Silicon dioxide layers can be "grown" on the substrate material and, when so produced, are found to be mechanically highly compatible with the silicon. This arises because they have similar crystal lattice structures and comparable coefficients of thermal expansion, so that the Si/SiO$_2$ interface is effectively homogeneous.

Because of these properties, the *silicon planar process* for the production of bipolar transistors, has become important over the last 10 years. The term "planar" in this context implies that all the necessary processing of the silicon chip is carried out on one surface only. This represented a significant advance compared to earlier methods where both lateral surfaces of the substrate had to be processed.

Figure 21 illustrates schematically the important stages in the planar manufacturing method. The starting point for the process is a single crystal of silicon, uniformly doped *n*-type. An oxide layer is then grown on top of this by passing oxygen at 1300–1600 K (about 1000–1300°C) over the surface. Subsequently the oxide is coated with a photo-resistive material. This is selectively exposed to ultra-violet (uv) radiation through an appropriately shaped mask. Following the exposure, those regions of the coated surface which have been subject to ultra-violet irradiation are resistant to removal with a suitable developing fluid. The photo-resist on the masked surfaces, however, is easily removed by application of the developer, to expose the oxide layer beneath. The remaining photo-resist is cured by heat treatment at about 400 K. Hydrofluoric acid (HF) is then used to etch the exposed silicon dioxide. The cured photo-resist protects the remaining, underlying oxide from the action of the acid.

The *p*-type base diffusion is now effected by treatment with gaseous boron bromide (BBr$_3$) at 1200–1500 K. The oxide layer acts as a barrier to diffusion. When the base diffusion is completed, any cured photo-resist is removed with hot sulphuric acid (H$_2$SO$_4$). The basic steps

of the process are then repeated using the mask appropriate for the emitter diffusion, and phosphorus oxychloride (POCl$_3$) vapour at stage (f) to produce an *n*-type region. All that remains is for metal contacts to be made to the base, emitter and collector, and for the device to be hermetically sealed.

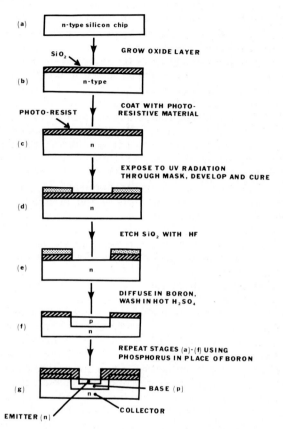

FIG. 21. Transistor production by the silicon planar method. Metallized connections and device sealing and packaging remain to be effected.

Early developments in silicon planar technology quickly led to the situation where it was possible to produce several active devices on a single chip of semiconductor. At this stage, however, difficulty was experienced in fabricating passive devices (resistors, capacitors and inductors) by the planar process. The advent of methods of producing resistors and capacitors by evaporating films of suitable material onto inert ceramic chips meant that whole circuits could be produced by fabricating active devices on silicon substrates, passive devices on ceramic chips and interconnecting them. Circuits produced in this way were termed *integrated circuits* (IC's) and were said to be of the *hybrid* type. *Monolithic* IC's also became available, where the passive devices were fabricated directly upon the silicon substrate.

These integrated circuits revolutionized electronic practice by making fairly complex circuit functions available cheaply in extremely small packages, perhaps only two or three times larger than previously available single transistors. It is often convenient to distinguish between

IC packages intended for digital applications and *linear* IC's, such as operational amplifiers.

Examination of Fig. 10b suggests that FET's could also be produced using the techniques above. In fact, a considerable part of the present prominence of MOS FET's is the facility with which they can be fabricated; requiring, as they do, fewer masking and diffusion operations.

Recently progress has been made in the use of the bulk resistivity of silicon, suitably doped, to produce resistors in microelectronic circuits. For a time the capacitance of the *pn* junction (arising from the fact that there is charge separation to either side of the depletion layer) was used for capacitor fabrication. However, it is now considered better to use the dielectric properties of silicon dioxide for this purpose. Great difficulty is still experienced with integrated circuit inductors. The principal problem here is to find a high permeability material having the desired physical properties for ease of manufacture and reliability.

A few years ago, it was realized that a limit to the exploitation of the then current IC technology was set by the packaging and interconnection of the modules. Much attention was therefore focused upon producing greater and greater numbers of devices upon single chips of silicon. Fairly obviously, this aim can be achieved either by increasing the packing density of the devices or increasing the size of the silicon chip. Progress has recently been made in both of these areas. The chief difficulty with increasing the size of the substrate is the increased probability of a serious crystallographic defect in either semiconductor or oxide rendering a module unusable. This has been overcome to an extent by employing the technique of *discretionary wiring*, whereby only the patent devices are connected after manufacture. Problems in increasing the packing density occur because of diffusion interactions and the necessity for the devices to be electrically isolated from one another. At present, it is possible to fabricate complex circuitry or repetitive arrays (large numbers of similar circuits) upon a single piece of substrate. This technology is generally referred to as either *medium scale integration* (MSI) or *large scale integration* (LSI), depending upon the number of devices incorporated. The dividing line between MSI and LSI is not really well defined. However, whereas MSI structures may be linear or digital, the repetitive nature of logical (digital) functions means that only they have been realised using LSI.

In producing large or medium scale integration systems for particular applications, a choice must be made between bipolar and MOS active devices. Generally bipolar transistors can be made to give much faster switching times in digital circuits, but MOST's also have inherent advantages. These include very high input impedance, good thermal stability and greater ease of manufacture. Currently, two production schemes are of importance. The first of these, employing bipolar transistors, achieves high packing densities and fewer manufacturing steps by an ingenious method of device isolation. In this scheme, part of the collector diffusion itself is used for isolation purposes. This is known as *collector diffusion isolation* (CDI)*.

The second technique exploits the advantages of com-

* CDI is a trademark of Ferranti Ltd.

plementary symmetry in MOS MSI or LSI systems. Complementary symmetry can be defined as the use of two complementary transistors (i.e. *npn* and *pnp* bipolar in devices, or *p*-channel and *n*-channel FET's) in a circuit in place of a single device. MOS integrated circuits produced in this way are known as COSMOS circuits. A number of advantages may be obtained by employing complementary symmetry (*see* for instance the chapter on complementary circuits in Hemingway's book). In COSMOS digital circuits, faster switching times and lower power consumptions are perhaps the most important of these.

It is felt that, within the next few years, further exploitations of techniques such as COSMOS and CDI LSI may well lead to complex electronic assemblies becoming small enough and cheap enough to play a major role in the practice of medicine.

CONCLUDING REMARKS

The material presented above is necessarily somewhat inhomogeneous and simplified. An attempt has been made to give an appreciation not only of the basic science of electronics, but also of the areas where recent technological innovation may bring advances. Several topics which the author would like to have briefly covered have been omitted in order to keep the account a reasonable length. One such topic which perhaps deserves mention here is the matter of signal recovery techniques. These techniques aim to improve the detection or intelligibility of signals, to which is added a significant amount of noise. Two such techniques are the use of the phase-sensitive detector and signal averaging.

The mode of operation of the phase-sensitive detector has been simply described by Abernethy (1973) and the interested reader is referred to this work. Signal averaging, and some of its applications to otolaryngology, are described in the chapters by Thornton, by Aran and Portmann and by Beagley.

A selection of books covering some of the topics of this chapter in a little more detail are given in the bibliography below.

REFERENCES

Abernethy, J. D. W. (1973), *Phys. Bull.*, **24**, 591.
Bardeen, J. and Brattain, W. H. (1948), *Phys. Rev.*, **74**, 230.
Black, H. S. (1934), *Elec. Eng.*, **53**, 114.
Bode, H. W. (1945), *Network Analysis and Feedback Amplifier Design*. Princeton, New Jersey: Van Nostrand-Rheinhold.
Child, C. D. (1911), *Phys. Rev.* (1st series), **32**, 492.
Cooper, R., Osselton, J. W. and Shaw, J. C. (1969), *EEG Technology*. London: Butterworths.
de Forest, L. (1906), *Amer. Inst. Elec. Eng. Proc.*, **24**, 719.
Johnson, J. B. (1928), *Phys. Rev.*, **32**, 97.
Langmuir, I. (1913), *Phys. Rev.*, **2**, 450.
Milsum, J. H. (Ed.) (1968), *Positive Feedback*. Oxford: Pergamon.
Nyquist, H. (1928), *Phys. Rev.*, **32**, 110.
Richter, W. (1943), *Electronics*, **16**, 112.
Ryder, J. D. (1964), *Electronic Engineering Principles*. Englewood Cliffs, New Jersey: Prentice-Hall.
Shockley, W., Sparks, M. and Teal, G. K. (1951), *Phys. Rev.*, **83**, 151.
Shockley, W. (1952), *Proc. IRE*, **40**, 1365.
Thévenin, L. (1883), *Annales Télégraph*, **10**, 222.
Waidelich, D. L. (1941), *Trans. A.I.E.E.*, **60**, 1161.

SUGGESTIONS FOR FURTHER READING

Clayton, J. B. (1974), *Operational Amplifiers*, 2nd edition. London: Butterworths.

Close, K. J. and Yarwood, J. (1971), *An Introduction to Semiconductors*. London: Heinemann.

Faulkner, E. A. (1966), *Principles of Linear Circuits*. London: Chapman and Hall.

Harris, J. N., Gray, P. E. and Searle, C. L. (1966), *Digital Transistor Circuits*. New York: Wiley.

Hemingway, T. K. (1970), *Electronic Designers' Handbook*, 2nd edition. London: Business Books.

Hibberd, R. G. (1972), *Integrated Circuit Pocket Book*. London: Newnes-Butterworths.

Pridham, G. J. (1973), *Solid-State Circuits*. Oxford: Pergamon.

Smith, R. J. (1971), *Circuits, Devices and Systems*, 2nd edition. New York: Wiley.

Yanof, H. M. (1972), *Biomedical Electronics*, 2nd edition. Philadelphia: F. A. Davis.

6. ACOUSTICS

F. J. FAHY

PHYSICAL NATURE OF SOUND

Inertia and Elasticity

Sound is both a physical phenomenon and a subjective sensation. The present chapter is intended to introduce the reader to the physical nature and behaviour of sound. Perhaps the most remarkable feature of sound is its ability to travel over great distances and through many different types of material. For example, sound which originates in a water cistern in the loft can travel to the farthest reaches of a house, via the water in the pipes, via the solid material of the pipes and of the structure of the house, eventually to reach the ear via the air in a room; it is literally all pervading.

We may ask what properties these various materials have in common which allow them each to carry sound. The answer is that they are those properties which are essential to most mechanical vibration processes, namely inertia (mass) and elasticity (stiffness); the former may be loosely defined as the resistance to acceleration and the latter as the resistance to deformation. The type of deformation associated with sound in fluids, i.e. gases and liquids, is generally different from those associated with sound in solids because fluids cannot resist shearing deformations (like cards in a pack sliding over each other) whereas solids, by definition, can.

Before discussing the nature of sound further it might be helpful to consider these properties of inertia and elasticity in more detail. We shall, at this stage, take a macroscopic view of matter; that is to say we shall consider materials to be continuous, rather than deal with the microscopic world of atoms and molecules. We each have subjective experience of the fact that it takes a force to change the direction or speed of a moving body; this is a manifestation of the possession of inertia by matter. Just as a large material body possesses inertia, so does every small portion, or element, of that body. Just as it takes a force to alter the direction or speed of motion of a large body, so it takes a force to alter the motion of each small element. Consequently the motion of each element within a material is controlled by the forces imposed upon it by surrounding elements, and also in some cases by external influences such as gravitational or electromagnetic force fields. We shall not be concerned with such external forces in the present discussion.

The phenomenon of elasticity concerns the relationship between the relative displacements of elements and the forces they impose upon each other as a result of these displacements. As has already been stated, fluids and solids behave somewhat differently in this respect. Some concrete examples may help to clarify the picture. Consider first the behaviour of a gas, specifically air, in respect of various types of deformation. If we take a bicycle pump, put a finger over the connector attachment hole, push the handle in slowly until considerable resistance is felt, and then release the handle, it will move back some distance. We infer from this observation that the response of the mass of air in the pump to an imposed change of volume is the generation of internal forces between elements which act so as to resist the imposed deformation; then forces act equally in all directions. The elements adjacent to the piston apply force to the piston so as to move it and increase the volume, and thereby reduce the internal forces. We characterize the magnitude of these internal forces by the force that the fluid exerts on *unit area* of any solid surface in contact with it, such as the walls of the pump; this quantity we call *pressure*. We term the ratio of mass of the gas to its volume, *density*. Hence we observe that an increase in density leads to an increase in pressure, and that this process is at least partly reversible; this is an example of the property of elasticity as exhibited by a gas. An attempt to gently pull out the handle, and then release it, will demonstrate the reduction in pressure due to a decrease in density. Strictly speaking the change in gas pressure corresponding to a given change in density will depend upon the rate of the compression-expansion process. This need not concern us here, although it is interesting to note that Newton theoretically calculated the speed of propagation of sound disturbance through the air incorrectly because he used the wrong pressure-density relationship.

The stiffness of air may also be nicely demonstrated by holding a thin sheet of plywood of about 0·1 metre square above, and parallel to, a table top. If the sheet is tapped with the knuckles and brought slowly down towards the table, the pitch of the sound will increase because the air adds its own stiffness to that of the sheet.

Another form of deformation of a gas is also possible. It is a well established fact that when a flat surface of a solid object is moved through the air in a direction tangential to that surface, the air immediately next to the surface does not move relative to that surface, but moves with it; this is the boundary layer phenomenon. Consider what happens if we send a playing card sliding fast along a shiny table top. It often lifts slightly off the surface and sits on a thin layer of air. Eventually it slows down and falls back on the table—it shows no tendency to return to the sender. In this case the air is deformed in shear because it moves with the card at the top of the layer and stays still at the table surface. The effect of the internal forces developed by this type of deformation is to retard the card, not in a reversible manner, but only so as to convert its mechanical energy into heat. This is an example of the effect of the phenomenon of viscosity. It is a physical property of gases and liquids which is not essential to the existence of sound; on the contrary, it is partly responsible for the diminution of sound as it travels over long distances.

Liquids exhibit the properties of elasticity and viscosity in much the same manner as gases, but the magnitude of the internal pressure forces developed by a given *fractional* change of density are about 20 000 times larger; we say that gases are more compressible than liquids. Solids, on the other hand, can resist shear deformation in an elastic manner, as can be observed by attempting to slide a soft block of rubber along a table while at the same time pressing down on it, and then releasing the force. They are also elastically compressible in the manner of liquids and solids, although the presence of the free surfaces of solid bodies influences their behaviour to a great extent. Homogenous solids are generally even less compressible than liquids, although the presence of pores, as for instance in cork, can greatly increase their compressibility, as can the presence of gas bubbles in liquids.

Air possesses the property of inertia because it has mass. The force that the wind exerts on a body in its path is mainly due to change of speed imposed on the air by the presence of the body. Since sound involves motion of air particles about an equilibrium position it is clear that forces act on each particle: these are the pressure forces which arise from deformation of the surrounding elements of air.

We are now in a position to consider the role that elasticity and inertia play in the phenomenon of sound. We shall initially consider sound in air. Sound is often considered as a vibration of the air, which implies an oscillatory motion about some mean equilibrium condition. Although many common continuous sounds do involve vibrations of the air, it is misleading to think of an element of air as a kind of pendulum which oscillates to and fro for a long time following a disturbance from equilibrium. Consider, for example, what happens when a balloon bursts. The quiescent air around the balloon is at a static pressure of about 10^5 pascals (newtons per square metre—oddly enough 1 newton is about the weight of a medium sized apple). This pressure is caused by the weight of the atmospheric air above the surface acting like the force on the piston in the pump and compressing the air at the surface

to a density where the resulting pressure forces are sufficient to support the surmounting column of air. Air which has been compressed in the balloon by the action of inflation and the elastic stretching forces of the rubber, and which is hence at a higher pressure than the surrounding air, is no longer constrained by the rubber and therefore accelerates into the immediately surrounding air in all directions. This surrounding air cannot be displaced instantly because it has inertia, and the volume previously available for it now has to contain an additional mass of air. The density increases, and the pressure increases, which creates an imbalance of internal elastic forces between the immediately surrounding "layer" and the air outside it, which results in a further outward motion, increase in density, and so on. This process would seem to give rise to a mass exodus of air away from the original position of the balloon; we have, however neglected the role of inertia and the fact that pressure acts equally in all directions. The very increase in pressure that the initial release of air creates immediately around the balloon, due to its ingress, acts not only on the surrounding air but on the released air itself so as to retard its outward motion. It does not stop moving immediately because it has inertia and takes time to come to rest; however, it eventually does so and then returns to a state of equilibrium with the surrounding air. This reversal of motion occurs in all the surrounding layers of air following the passage of the disturbance (that is to say, the passing of the pulse of pressure higher than the static pressure to regions of air further and further removed from the origin.) It is clear that an element of air does not act like a pendulum, or mass-spring system, because it does not continue to oscillate once the disturbance has passed.

A study of disturbances travelling along a weak coil spring (such as a "Slinky" toy) is of great help in visualizing the type of motion described above which is known as wave motion (Fig. 1). However, there is an important

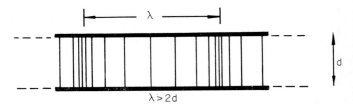

Fig. 1. Plane waves in a duct: the density of the lines denotes degree of compression of the air. λ is the wavelength.

difference between the motion of a spring and that arising from the burst balloon. The disturbance carried by the spring is constrained to move in one direction only; this is known as one-dimensional, or plane, wave motion. The nature of fluid pressure is to act equally in all directions so that the bang of the balloon spreads out in all directions. Only in special cases do sound waves in gases travel in one direction only; the most commonly met example is sound in a pipe or duct of relatively small cross-section.

Speed of Sound

The magnitude of the rise in pressure by even such an unpleasantly loud noise as a balloon burst is very small compared with the static pressure of the air. The range of magnitude of normally-experienced pressure disturbances, of which the extremes may be represented, for example, by those perceptible as sound on a very quiet night in the country, and those produced by the balloon extends from about one thousand millionth (10^{-9}), to about one thousandth (10^{-3}) of the atmosphere static pressure respectively—very small disturbances indeed! Such small disturbances travel through the air at a speed which is independent of their magnitude, so that disturbance patterns (waveforms) are faithfully reproduced at a distance from their origin. Figure 2 illustrates this point. This

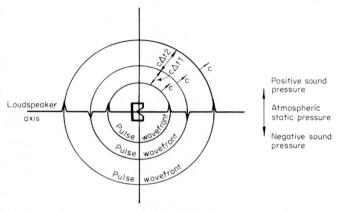

FIG. 2. Pulse wavefronts emitted from a loudspeaker to which positive and negative steady voltages are applied: the time interval between the first and second reversals is Δt_1 seconds, and between second and third reversals is Δt_2 seconds.

speed c is determined by ratio of the air stiffness to air density or, what is equivalent, simply by the temperature of the air. A quite accurate formula for air is $c = 20 \cdot 25 \sqrt{T}$ metres per second, where c is the speed of sound and T is the thermodynamic temperature in Kelvins, K (K = ^{0}C + 273). At sea level and room temperature c is about 340 m. s^{-1}. The speed of sound in homogeneous liquids is considerably higher than that in gases because, although they are more dense, they are proportionately even less compressible. For example the speed of sound in water, or in animal tissue which is largely composed of water, is about 1500 m. s^{-1}. In bone, which is inhomogeneous, the speed is about 570 m. s^{-1}.

The speed of sound in solids depends upon the mode of deformation since solids can deform elastically in many different ways. Compressional deformations of the type associated with sound in fluids propagate at 4000–5000 m.s^{-1}. Other forms of deformation such as those associated with bending vibrations in bars and plates, propogate at speeds which are dependent upon the rate of change of deformation; these are known as dispersive waves. The dispersive character of bending waves leads to a complex interaction behaviour between sound in fluids and solids. An important result of this behaviour is that the transmission of sound from air through such structures as partitions is extremely efficient at certain frequencies; the phenomenon is known as *coincidence*.

Frequency

Many sources of sound are continuous in time, unlike the balloon burst. Such a source could be constructed from a loudspeaker mounted in one side of a small closed box. If a battery is applied to the terminals the loudspeaker cone moves out (or in) once and remains in a displaced position. A single pulse wavefront of positive sound pressure higher than static (or lower than static) moves outwards in all directions from the loudspeaker, rather as it does from the balloon. If the battery leads are repeatedly reversed a series of pulses of alternately positive and negative sound pressure will propagate away from the loudspeaker at the speed of sound as shown in Fig. 2. As explained later, the magnitude of the pulse will vary along a wavefront with angle from the loudspeaker axis. If, instead of a series of discrete changes of voltage, the voltage is varied smoothly from positive to negative, and vice versa, the pressure variations will also be smooth, and the sound will lose its explosive character.

At this stage we must introduce a concept which is fundamental to the analysis and synthesis of time-dependent quantities such as the small variations of pressure about the mean static pressure that we perceive as sound: the concept is that of *frequency*. Here we will use the term frequency in its strictly scientific sense as distinct from the common usage to describe the rate of repetition of discrete events such as frequency of a bus service. The scientific concept of frequency is specifically associated with the concept of sinusoidal, or simple harmonic, variation of a quantity. This form of variation is readily explained in terms of motion of a point in a circle at constant speed. For instance, if we observe a stone being whirled round in a horizontal circle on the end of a string from a fairly distant vantage point on a level with the plane of the motion, we will observe a sinusoidal variation of position with time (Fig. 3); we call this *simple harmonic motion*. It is the type of vibrational motion that simple mechanical systems undergo after displacement from equilibrium. The rate of repetition of such a type of variation is termed the frequency; the time for one complete cycle is called the period. The unit of frequency is the hertz (previously—cycles per second); frequency in Hz is the inverse of period in seconds. Frequency is also measured in radians per second; this relates to the circular motion shown in Fig. 3, 2π radians corresponding to once round the circle. Hence, frequency in radians per second equals 2π times frequency in hertz (Hz). The symbol for frequency in hertz is normally f, and that for frequency in radians per second is normally ω. The maximum observed excursion of the aforementioned stone from the centre point of the motion is termed the *amplitude* of the variation, which we may symbolize by a. Hence displacement in simple harmonic motion is described by the expression $a \sin(\omega t)$ or $a \sin (2\pi f t)$.

A discussion of why this type of variation should be fundamental to the analysis of time-dependent oscillatory motion is beyond the scope of this chapter. However, the sinusoidal form of variation of sound pressure with time is of special significance in the realm of musical acoustics because it is only certain combinations of sounds having such a simple form which sound harmonious to the ear. It is therefore natural to study the behaviour of simple harmonic sound disturbances, because small amplitude sound has a speed of propagation which is not only independent of amplitude, but is also independent of frequency, so that the "mix" of sinusoidal components in a complex sound remains the same as the sound propagates freely

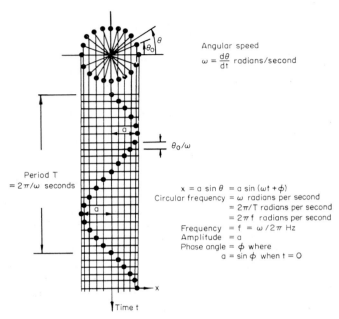

Angular speed

$$\omega = \frac{d\theta}{dt} \text{ radians/second}$$

Period T
$= 2\pi/\omega$ seconds

θ_0/ω

$x = a \sin \theta = a \sin (\omega t + \phi)$
Circular frequency $= \omega$ radians per second
$\qquad\qquad\qquad = 2\pi/T$ radians per second
$\qquad\qquad\qquad = 2\pi f$ radians per second
Frequency $= f = \omega/2\pi$ Hz
Amplitude $= a$
Phase angle $= \phi$ where
$\qquad\qquad a = \sin \phi$ when $t = 0$

Time t

FIG. 3. Relationship between circular motion at constant speed and simple harmonic motion.

through the air. Dissipatory forces may cause the higher frequency components to diminish more rapidly than the lower frequency components in propagation over large distances so that the character of the sound varies slowly with distance from the source. This means that the form of variation in time of the pressure at a point in space is identical to the form of variation in pressure in space along the direction of propagation although the magnitude of the variation will normally diminish with distance from the source, (Fig. 4). It is perhaps unfortunate that many elementary textbooks on acoustics introduce simple harmonic motion and frequency without clearly explaining that, although it is most uncommon to encounter pure, single frequency, simple harmonic sound (or vibration) outside the laboratory, the Fourier theorem allows us to synthesize sound fields of any time dependence—even a balloon burst—from a combination of the elementary motions which the books describe.

Other good reasons for the study of simple harmonic (or pure tone) sound, having one frequency only, are as follows:

(a) The sensitivity of the ear is a function of frequency of sound; it is also a function of amplitude as will be described in the book.

(b) The assumption of simple harmonic time dependence greatly simplifies mathematical analysis of sound fields.

(c) Sound waves of low frequency interact very differently from low frequency sound waves with material obstacles.

(d) The performance of most noise control systems is frequency sensitive.

(e) Certain mechanical and acoustic systems respond very strongly to disturbances of certain frequencies (resonance frequencies).

One must distinguish between subjectively assigned frequency, termed *pitch*, and the mathematically defined frequency components of a sound, such as a note of a woodwind instrument, or even a short burst of sound produced by a laboratory oscillator which is designed to generate sinusoidally varying voltage outputs. In the former case, the sound consists of a fundamental frequency, which usually produces the subjective impression of pitch, together with a series of harmonics of the fundamental frequency which partly account for the tone or timbre of the instrumental sound. The harmonics are sound components having frequencies which are integer multiples (1, 2, 3, 4, etc.) of the fundamental frequency. In the latter case, a pitch will be assigned to the tone burst even if only one complete cycle of oscillation is heard, whereas Fourier analysis of this sound will indicate components of many frequencies to be present in varying degree, with a major contribution at the frequency set on the oscillator dial. We should not normally assign a pitch to a balloon burst because no oscillation occurs; however, Fourier analysis indicates that such a disturbance can be synthesized from an infinite number of equal strength frequency components covering a frequency range of (0–infinity) Hz. We are therefore not suprised that no definite sensation of pitch occurs.

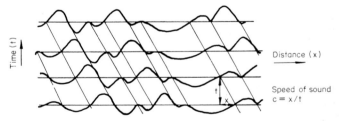

Time (t)

Distance (x)

Speed of sound
$c = x/t$

FIG. 4. Sound waves normally propagate in an unchanging form.

Referring back to Fig. 2, which illustrates a train of pulses radiated by a loudspeaker which has a regularly reversed steady voltage difference applied across the coil, we may expect that a sensation of pitch will be produced by a sufficiently rapid rate of reversal of polarity. This is indeed the case, the pitch corresponding to a frequency of half the reversal rate.

Wavelength

Having clarified what we mean by frequency in respect of variation of sound pressure in time, we may now introduce a measure of the variation of sound pressure in space, or more specifically, variation in the direction of propagation. We have seen that the non-dispersive nature of speed (speed of propagation independent of frequency) creates identical spatial and temporal forms of variation of sound pressure in a freely propagating wave. Hence a simple harmonic time dependence is associated with a simple harmonic space dependence—a sine wave in space. A measure of the "space-frequency" can be derived in a manner similar to that for time frequency. The period of time between successive maximum positive or negative deviations of pressure from the static value is called the period, T, in seconds, and the inverse, $1/T$, is called the frequency, f, in Hz. The distance between successive maximum deviations in space is clearly equal to the period, T, times the distance travelled in one second, i.e. the speed of propagation of sound, c. We call this distance the *wavelength* and represent it by the symbol λ; it is measured in metres and it is clearly related to the frequency and the speed of sound by the following formulae:

$$\lambda = cT$$
$$\text{or } \lambda(1/T) = c$$
$$\text{or } \lambda f = c \qquad (6.1)$$

Equation (6.1) should be committed to memory, together with the most commonly used value of the speed of sound, which is $c = 340$ m. s^{-1} at 288K (15°C), a typical atmospheric temperature at sea level.

It has been stated above that frequency is of significance partly because the sensitivity of hearing varies with frequency. Similarly, wavelength is of significance for the purely physical behaviour of sound when it encounters solid obstacles, as we shall see in the sections on enclosures and on scattering and diffraction. As a rough guide we may assume that short, high frequency sound waves behave like rays of light in respect of reflection from surfaces, transmission through apertures, and the production of shadows by solid objects (Fig. 5). Long wavelength (low frequency) sound waves do not behave at all like rays; if

Interference

Interference is a phenomenon which is a characteristic feature of wave behaviour. It is associated with the principle of superposition in linear systems; this means that small variations about a mean static value, such as sound pressures, which arise from different sources, can be simply added together at any one time and place to give the total variation at that time and place. This may seem self-evident until we consider a non-linear system such as a washing line. The first wet garment to be suspended causes a significant droop in the line at the point of suspension. The addition of further garments of equal weight at the same point will cause progressively smaller and smaller droops, because the system is non-linear, i.e., the relationship between suspended weight and droop, if plotted on a graph would not show a straight line relationship. This is not so with normally-encountered levels of sound, although non-linear effects are common in physiological mechanisms, as for instance, the hearing mechanism. Increases in subjective response to equal incremental increases of sound pressure get progressively smaller as the total sound pressure rises. The system is said to *saturate*.

Intereference can lead to two commonly observed phenomena. One is that of "beats" whereby two simple harmonic components of sound with slightly differing frequencies are generated, usually by different sources. Beating may often be observed when one's car slowly passes a lorry on a hill and the engine or gear box noises contain such components. The level of the source varies slowly in an oscillatory fashion. What is happening is that the total sound pressure at the ear of the observer is made up of contributions from both the simple harmonic, or pure tone, waves. Because one wave has a slightly higher frequency than the other it goes through reversals of sound pressure at a slightly greater rate than the other wave. Hence, at one instant the total pressure, which equals the

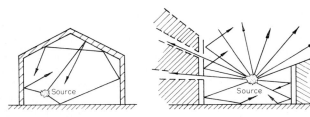

FIG. 5. Ray concept for enclosures, apertures and barriers.

they did you would not, for example, be able to talk to your neighbour who is out of sight over a high garden wall! In addition, long wavelength sound does not pass easily or at all through small apertures in partitions, or passing into, or out of, openings in small pipes. We see therefore that sound wavelength is a very important parameter of which we must be aware when considering the physical behaviour of sound. Of course, if a complex sound can be synthesized from many frequency components, so the complex wave can be synthesized from many different wavelength components, the long and the short components behaving rather differently.

sum of the component pressures, is equal to the addition of two maximum positive pressures (a loud part of the beat cycle). After some time the total pressure will equal the sum of one positive contribution and one negative contribution (a quiet part of the cycle). The frequency of occurrence of maximum (or minimum) total sound pressures is equal to the difference between the frequencies of the individual harmonic components. Figure 6 illustrates the phenomenon. Beats are normally only distinctly observed if the difference is less than about 5 Hz.

A second result of interference between sound waves is the generation of standing wave patterns in space. Only simple harmonic components of *equal* frequency can generate such a pattern of pressure variation which does not travel in the manner we have previously discussed, but stays apparently fixed in space while varying sinusoidally in time. The most commonly observed example of such interference is created by reflection of a pure tone sound wave from a large flat surface, such as a wall. Of course, the reflected wave has a frequency equal to the incident wave and they interfere. From the practical point of view one of the most important manifestations of interference by reflection is the establishment in rooms excited by a single frequency source of sound of very large variations of sound pressure amplitudes from place to place.

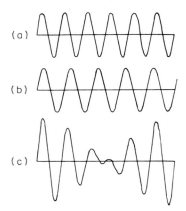

Fig. 6. Interference in time of two sound sources with slightly different frequencies, resulting in beats.

In addition to these two examples, the phenomenon of interference is the cause of directivity of sources of sound. For example, a loudspeaker radiates the low frequency components of sound more or less uniformly around it, whereas it tends to concentrate the higher frequency components directly forward in preference to the side and the rear; so, too, does a human mouth. This is the result of interference between the sound waves radiated from the different areas of the radiator together with the effect of the geometry of the mounting in which the source is located, e.g. baffle, head, etc. The directional characteristics of human speech are of considerable importance in determining the intelligibility of speech, because the high frequency components, which are radiated more directionally, carry most of the information content; the lower frequencies simply determine the loudness.

Diffraction and Scattering

The rather forbidding title of this section refers to the distortion of an otherwise freely spreading sound wave by the presence of solid obstacles. This has been the subject of study and analysis over many years by mathematical physicists—we need not get so involved in the technical details. Suffice to say that components of sound having wavelengths considerably smaller than a typical dimension of the object (e.g. width of a human head, height of a barrier, diameter of a tree trunk) are reflected from the object as though it were a mirror reflecting light, with the

resulting formation of fairly sharp shadows (quiet zones) behind the obstacles. Similarly, waves will pass through an aperture in an obstacle like rays of light, if the diameter of the hole is much larger than an acoustic wavelength. On the other hand, components of sound having wavelengths long compared to an obstacle will tend to bend round it and pass on almost unhindered, i.e. no distinct shadow zone is formed. Also, there is considerable reflection of low frequency sound from apertures of diameter substantially smaller than a wavelength, e.g. the opening of the outer ear, the outlet of a car exhaust pipe. A given physical barrier to sound is therefore likely to be far more efficient at high frequencies than at low frequencies.

The diffraction of sound by the human head is at least partly responsible for the directional faculty of the hearing mechanism. At low frequencies (< 300 Hz) the sound waves are barely distorted and it is considered that the directional sense is associated with the time interval between the hearing of substantially the same pressure variations by each ear. At high frequencies the head creates a substantial shadow and an ear which is shaded from the source senses lower sound pressure amplitudes than the unshaded ear. This seems to be an excellent example of accommodation of the organism to the physical behaviour of the environment in such a way as to obtain more comprehensive information about its surroundings.

Sound in Enclosures

So far we have concentrated on the behaviour of freely spreading sound in the open air. Enclosure of a source of sound produces multiple reflection of the sound waves from the enclosure surfaces. The nature of the resulting fields depend greatly upon the dimensions of the enclosure in relation to the wavelength of the sound. We therefore consider small, medium sized and large enclosures separately: it must be clearly understood that the classification of a given enclosure depends upon wavelength of the sound component considered.

At very low frequencies, when the dimensions are very small in terms of λ, wave effects are not apparent and the air undergoes uniform compression and expansion. This can lead, in the case of an enclosure penetrated by an opening, to a *resonance* (preferred frequency of vibration having attendant high sound pressures) on which the mass of air in the opening "bounces" on the enclosed air, which acts as a spring. This system is known as a Helmholtz resonator and accounts for the boom commonly experienced in cars with an open window.

At frequencies for which λ is rather similar to the enclosure dimensions, wave interference effects cause the air in the enclosure to vibrate strongly at preferred (resonance) frequencies and less strongly at intermediate frequencies. Vibration at the resonance frequencies is associated with large variations of sound pressure over the volume of the enclosure. Typical pressure patterns and resonance frequencies are shown in Fig. 7. Similar interference effects at low frequencies can cause covers (hoods) placed close to vibrating machine surfaces to be less effective than their weight per unit area would normally suggest, and throw the burden of noise control onto the stiffness performance of the enclosure. Resonance effects in boiler enclosures can, in some circumstances, influence combustion source noise.

At frequencies for which λ is less than the enclosure dimensions, the ray concept of sound can be used, as with single obstacles (Fig. 5). Sound from an enclosed source will suffer multiple reflections from the enclosure walls to form a *reverberant field* in which the sound pressures are rather uniform, except for pure tone sources, in which

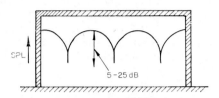

Fig. 7. SPL distribution in a simple standing wave in an enclosure.

case there are always large variations, even at high frequencies. Because the waves returning to the source position have travelled a considerable distance and have been partially absorbed by the walls, they are weaker than the sound as it leaves the source. Consequently a region remains around the source in which the sound field is unaffected by wall reflection. This is termed the *direct field* (Fig. 8). The general effect of reverberation is to raise the sound pressures in the reverberant field above that in the absence of enclosure and to cause sound waves to travel in many directions inside the enclosure. If the

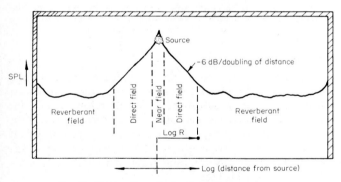

Fig. 8. Field regions for a source in an enclosure.

field is sufficiently omni-directional it is referred to as a *diffuse field*.

Ducts form a special class of enclosure in which, normally, only one of the three dimensions are large compared with an acoustic wavelength. The duct wall reflections cause the wave field in ducts to take the form of one-dimensional *plane waves* below frequencies for which the duct width is less than $\lambda/2$. These waves travel parallel to the duct walls (Fig. 1). They do not traverse regions of a duct in which the cross-sectional area changes sharply. Indeed they are strongly reflected at such sections. This behaviour forms the basis for such noise control devices as automobile mufflers. However, in general, plane waves are not substantially reflected at bends in constant section

ducts, and these cannot be relied upon to give significant reductions in sound energy passing along a duct.

Sound Energy

Sound is a form of mechanical energy. As such it cannot be destroyed but only converted into another form. Hence it is appropriate to describe the generation process by rate of energy production, or the *sound power* generated by the source. This quantity is of fundamental importance to noise calculation and control procedures. Also of great importance is the rate at which energy passes through unit area of space. This is a measure of energy concentration and is known as *intensity*. It is not easy to measure the intensity of sound waves, but fortunately there are a number of conditions which can be approximately satisfied in practice under which the sound intensity is simply related to the time averaged value of the squared acoustic pressure (*mean square pressure*) which can be measured with a *sound level meter* (*see* later). Figure 9 illustrates the formation of the mean square pressure, conventionally written as $\bar{p}^2$.

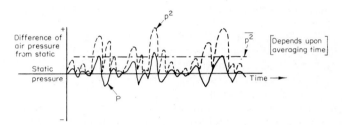

Fig. 9. Mean square pressure.

The conditions are as follows:

(a) A *plane*, uni-directional travelling wave, as illustrated in Fig. 1.

Plane waves are not commonly encountered except in ducts carrying low frequency sound. They do not, however, usually travel in one direction only along the duct because they suffer reflection at any discontinuities or bends. Consequent interference effects between the waves travelling in the two directions form *standing waves*, in which the intensity, or rate of flow of energy per unit cross-section of the duct, is not simply related to $\bar{p}^2$.

(b) A spherically, or hemispherically, spreading wave field, many wavelengths from a complex source, in which the relationship between intensity and $\bar{p}^2$ is the same as in a plane wave.

(c) A field in a large reflective enclosure, which is many wavelengths in size. Large industrial rooms can produce approximately diffuse field conditions provided that they do not have low ceilings by comparison with their width and do not have the form of a corridor. Ideally, only under any one of the above circumstances can intensity, and, hence source power, be measured with a microphone. In practice, less ideal conditions have to be lived with, in which case use of the above intensity $\bar{p}^2$ relationship incurs some error.

The sound energy generated by a source spreads out over a larger and larger area as the wave travels away from the source. Hence the concentration of energy, or the intensity normally reduces with distance from a source. This fact can be used to advantage in noise control design, where the sensitive areas are kept as far as possible from the noisiest source. When the sound field is spherical, as from a simple source in free space, the intensity, is given by $W/4\pi R^2$, where W is the power of the source and R is the radius of observation. Hence $\bar{p}^2$ varies as $1/R^2$; the well known inverse square law. If such a source is located near a large plane surface such as the ground, the field is *hemi-spherical* but $\bar{p}^2$ varies in the same way with R^2.

As previously described when a source is large and complex the wave field is only spherical at large distances from the source. Hence the inverse square law is not applicable near to such sources, in the so-called *near-field*, but only in the *far field*, many wavelengths from the source. The extent of the near field depends upon the acoustic wavelength and the dimensions of the source; it may in practice be taken to extend to a distance of two times the major source dimensions or four times the centre-of-source height above any reflecting plane; whichever is the larger.

The fact that sound is a form of energy and cannot be destroyed means that redirection of sound by barriers and partitions is normally only a partial noise control solution. Special structures called *absorbers*, which are capable of turning sound into heat with high efficiency, must also be employed. Normal constructional materials such as brick, timber, steel and asbestos are not efficient absorbers of sound and must normally be supplemented by special absorbing materials.

SOUND SOURCES

Sound sources are so diverse that it is difficult to generalize about them. However, some degree of classification may be arrived at on the basis of the following source characteristics: acoustic efficiency, frequency characteristics, directionality.

Acoustic Efficiency

The *acoustic efficiency* is the ratio of acoustic power generated by a source to that mechanical, chemical or electrical power which is supplied to the noise-producing device. It normally lies between 10 per cent (siren, loud-speaker) and 0·001 per cent (gas jets).

Many noise sources consist of vibrating surfaces, such as machinery casings, pipework and general steel work. The efficiency of radiation can be thought of as the acoustic power generated per unit area of surface, per unit of vibratory motion. In general the radiation efficiency of a vibrating surface increases as the surface dimensions are increased in relation to a wavelength, and also as the stiffness of the surface increases. This is why sounding boards are necessary for string instruments; the strongly vibrating strings are extremely inefficient radiators. Similar behaviour occurs with pipe and valve systems wherein the turbulent flow uses the structure as a sounding board. It will be realized that strongly vibrating mechanical and fluid systems must be isolated from potential sounding boards. A common example of this problem is the attachment of system inlet and outlet pipes to enclosure walls.

Frequency Characteristics

Some sources, such as siren compressors, electric motors and gear boxes, emit noise at a number of discrete frequencies (*tones*), others, such as flow control valves and fin-coolers, emit sound over a continuous range of frequencies (*broad band*). The frequency distribution of acoustic energy is described by a *frequency spectrum*. Some characteristic ranges of machinery noise frequencies are shown in Fig. 10. Standard spectral representations of sound are described in more detail in Chapter 11.

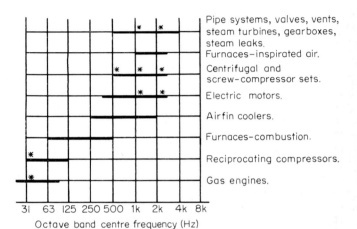

Pipe systems, valves, vents, steam turbines, gearboxes, steam leaks.
Furnaces—inspirated air.
Centrifugal and screw-compressor sets.
Electric motors.
Airfin coolers.
Furnaces—combustion.
Reciprocating compressors.
Gas engines.

31 63 125 250 500 1k 2k 4k 8k
Octave band centre frequency (Hz)

FIG. 10. Petroleum processing equipment which is likely to contribute significantly to community noise. An asterisk denotes areas where throb or pure-tone characteristics are likely to be important.

Directionality

As previously described, few complex sources radiate sound energy with equal intensity in all directions. However, in general, sources radiate more uniformly at low frequencies when they are small in relation to an acoustic wavelength, then at high frequencies, when they are large compared with an acoustic wavelength. Listening to a normal loud-speaker driven at low and high frequencies will soon convince anyone of this fact.

WAVES IN PANELS, WALLS AND PARTITIONS: SOUND TRANSMISSION

Single leaf homogeneous panels, walls and partitions constructed of solid materials are widely used to control noise. It is therefore important to gain at least a qualitative understanding of the nature of the interaction of sound waves with such structures. The term "wall" will be used to include all such structures.

Sound which is incident upon a plane wall causes transverse vibratory motion of the wall (bending) by virtue of the fluctuating pressures imposed upon the wall surface (Fig. 11). First consider the wall as a limp structure, having no resistance to distortion (*stiffness*), but simply having a certain *mass per unit area* (m). Newton's law of motion states that the acceleration (a) of the wall will be inversely proportional to m for a given surface sound pressure (P_1). Also, the sound pressure (P_2) produced by the wall motion is proportional to the surface velocity (v) of the wall. For

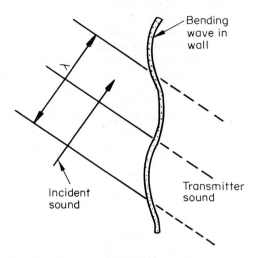

FIG. 11. Sound wave incident on plane wall.

a sound of a given frequency (f) the velocity is equal to (acceleration/$2\pi \times$ frequency). Hence:

$$P_2 \propto v = a/2\pi f = [(P_1/m)/(2\pi f)]. \qquad (6.2)$$

Thus $P_2/P_1 \propto 1/mf$.

The ratio of transmitted pressure to incident pressure is seen to be inversely proportional to the product of the mass per unit area of the wall and the frequency of the incident sound. The effectiveness of the limp wall as a barrier (*sound insulation*) *increases* with its *surface mass* and with the frequency of the sound, and the sound transmission is said to be mass controlled. This is the basis of the *Mass Law* which we shall meet again later.

In reality, walls have a resistance to bending which depends upon their thickness, and on the elastic modulus of the wall material. The combined effect of mass and stiffness is to allow the propagation of transverse motion in the form of *bending waves* to occur, rather as the mass and elasticity of air allow sound waves to occur. The natural speed of bending waves in a wall is not independent of frequency, as it is for sound waves in air, but depends upon the square root of the frequency. For a given wall, therefore the speed of sound and of bending waves can be equal (*see* Fig. 12). This frequency is known as the *coincidence* (or *critical*) *frequency* (f_c) and it depends upon wall thickness (h), wall material density (ρ) and wall material elastic modulus (E), thus:

$$f_c = \left(\frac{c_0^2}{1 \cdot 8h}\right)\left(\sqrt{\frac{\rho}{E}}\right) \qquad (6.3)$$

where c_0 is the speed of sound in air. It will be seen that f_c increases with the wall density and decreases with wall thickness and elastic modulus. Critical frequencies for common materials are given in Table 1.

At frequencies near to f_c sound transmission is rather

TABLE 1

CRITICAL FREQUENCIES OF SOME COMMON MATERIALS

Material	Critical Frequency × Surface Density (Hz × kg. m⁻²)
Lead	600 000
Fibre board	134 000
Steel	97 700
Reinforced concrete	44 000
Brick	42 000
Glass	38 000
Asbestos cement	33 600
Aluminium	32 200
Hardboard	30 600
Plasterboard	29 200
Plywood	13 200
Flaxboard	13 200

easy, and the insulation is correspondingly poor. The insulation in the *coincidence region* is largely controlled by the *damping* of the walls, whereas damping has a negligble effect at frequencies below f_c. At frequencies above the coincidence region sound insulation increases rapidly with frequency. Ideally, a single wall to be used as part of a room-type enclosure should be heavy and have a low

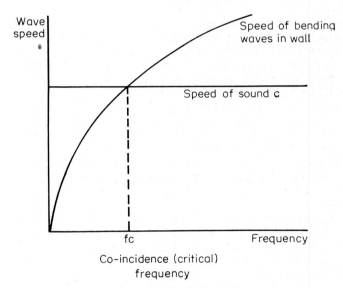

FIG. 12. Illustration of coincidence frequency.

bending stiffness. In contrast, as mentioned previously, close fitting hoods for *low frequency* (< 200 Hz) noise reduction depend largely upon stiffness for their effect.

Lightweight double walls, having an air gap separating the walls, can give sound insulations higher than that which combined masses of the walls would give according to the mass law. Lightweight double walls of plasterboard, timber and glass can suffer from a special type of resonance at the lower audio frequencies if the air gap is not sufficiently large, as it is not in thermal double glazing. The effect is illustrated in Fig. 13. The incorporation of acoustic absorbent material, such as a 30 mm thick fibreglass or mineral wool blanket, is normally necessary to eliminate such effects and to improve the overall insulation. There is little benefit to be gained from using heavy double masonry walls, instead of the equivalent weight single wall, for all except very special noise control problems.

It is interesting to note that masonry walls do not, in general, follow the mass law because they have low co-incidence frequencies in the 150–300 Hz range.

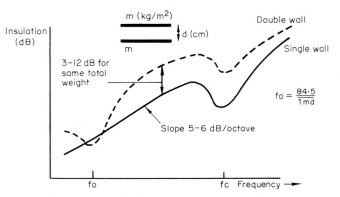

FIG. 13. Generalized insulation performance curves of single and double wall of the same total weight.

SOUND ABSORPTION

In most cases of practical interest, sound energy is absorbed by being converted into heat via dissipative viscous fluid—or visco-elastic solid—forces. The efficiency of absorption is measured in terms of the absorption coefficient which is defined as the fraction of energy incident upon the surface of an absorbing material, or structure, which is converted into heat, and thereby not reflected. Porous materials, such as fibreglass, mineral wool and porous plastic foam must be sufficiently open to allow the sound wave to enter the air-containing channels, and yet closed sufficiently to present a considerable resistance to wave motion in these channels. A good "rule of thumb" test of the potential absorbing capacity of a material is to try to blow through it. A good material will allow the air to pass, but not without a fair amount of effort on the part of the lungs. This property is measured in terms of flow resistance. For porous material attached directly to a rigid surface (wall) there is an optimum flow resistance for each particular material thickness. In general porous layers on rigid backing surfaces are not very efficient below the frequency at which the sound wavelength is greater than ten times the distance from the wall to the outside of the layer. Their general behaviour is illustrated in Fig. 14. In some absorbers, such as gypsum ceiling tiles, the effective flow resistance is reduced and the effective thickness is increased by perforation or slotting of the surface.

Porous layers (Fig. 14a) may be covered with perforated sheets for protection and containment. The effect is to reduce the frequency of maximum absorption, and to substantially reduce high frequency absorption as seen in Fig. 14b. In practice this effect is only significant for perforations of open area of less than 30 per cent. It must be

realized that the absorption coefficient (energy absorbed/ energy incident) of a porous material is highly dependent upon the angle at which sound is incident upon it. The absorption coefficient normally quoted is the random incidence (diffuse field) absorption coefficient. One should not, therefore, expect to obtain this performance in a duct in which most of the sound energy travels parallel to the material surface (grazing incidence).

Porous layers are in general not much good at absorbing low frequency sound (< 500 Hz) unless large air backing spaces (> 15 cm) can be provided. Special purpose low frequency absorbers are illustrated in Fig. 14d, e. The most practical type is the panel absorber, which can be readily made with layers of roofing felt, or plywood panels, mounted on frames over a backing space. The absorption curve is peaked about a frequency given by:

$$f = \frac{60}{\sqrt{md}} \qquad (6.4)$$

where m is the cover mass in kg. m^{-2} and d is the depth of the backing space in m. Such absorbers may be used to reduce low frequency, pure tone sound levels in boiler houses. The use of the Helmholtz resonator is not recommended because it is too tricky to predict its performance.

Absorption coefficients of some common constructional materials are given in Table 2.

TABLE 2

ABSORPTION COEFFICIENTS OF SOME COMMON CONSTRUCTIONAL MATERIALS

Material	Frequency (Hz)						
	63	125	200	500	1000	2000	4000
Brickwork	0·05	0·05	0·04	0·02	0·05	0·05	
Concrete	0·05	0·02	0·02	0·04	0·05	0·05	
4 mm glass sheet		0·3		0·1		0·05	
6 mm glass sheet		0·1		0·04		0·02	
Plaster on solid backing	0·05	0·03	0·03	0·02	0·03	0·04	0·05
Wood boards on joists	0·1	0·15	0·2	0·1	0·1	0·1	0·1
Wood block floor	0·05	0·02	0·04	0·05	0·05	0·1	0·05
Asbestos sheet	0·15	0·10	0·06	0·05	0·04	0·02	0·02

QUANTATIVE MEASURES OF SOUND

Sound Pressure Level

The variation of pressure about the static value is the most useful, and easily measurable, quantity associated with acoustic disturbances in gases and liquids; it is termed the *sound pressure*. In air, the static value is the atmospheric pressure which normally undergoes only very

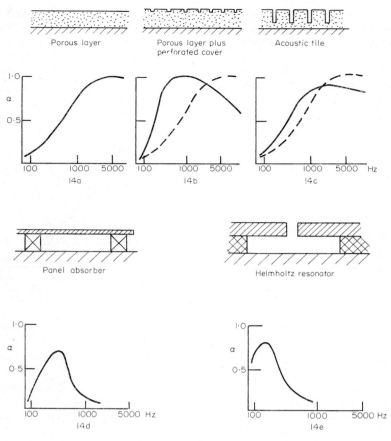

FIG. 14. Wall absorbers.

slow changes, as indicated by a wall barometer. Most sounds consist of alternate increases of pressure above (positive sound pressure), and decreases of pressure below (negative sound pressure), the static value at each point in the field (Fig. 9). The variations may take a very complex form in time and, as has previously been stated, are rarely of the simple harmonic, or sinusoidal form, that some textbooks would have us believe. It is not normally necessary to have a detailed description of the "time-history" of a sound—a measure of the relative contributions of the various harmonic components is generally of greater use, particularly in relationship to the matters of subjective assessment and hearing damage; such a measure is the frequency spectrum which we shall encounter later. What is initially required is some average measure of the pressure variation over an interval of time. We cannot simple average the pressure itself because the pressure increases will tend to cancel out the decreases and we would end up with the static value, which has nothing to do with the "strength" of the sound. We thus square the sound pressure and measure the average value over a period of time; the resulting quantity is called the *mean square sound pressure* (*see* Fig. 9). The value will depend upon the time period over which the average is taken but for most reasonably steady, continuous sounds a suitable period is of the order of a few seconds. We conventionally write the mean square

sound pressure as $\overline{P^2}$. The square root of this quantity is called the root mean square (rms) sound pressure.

The hearing mechanism has a non-linear response to sound and it has been found that the response is approximately logarithmic. Partly in consequence of this fact, and partly because of the enormous range of magnitudes of mean square sound pressures normally encountered, a large number of quantities in applied acoustics are measured in logarithmic units. The logarithm of a number is the power to which a chosen base (number) must be raised to produce that number. In acoustics the base 10 has been chosen. For example, 100 equals 10 raised to the power 2, which is written as 10^2. Hence the logarithm (to the base 10) of 100 is 2. Similarly, $\log_{10} 1000 = 3$, $\log_{10} 1 = 0$, $\log_{10} 2 = 0.3010$, etc.

The logarithmic unit of mean square pressure is defined to be the decibel, abbreviated dB. The quantity so defined is called the *sound pressure level* (SPL) which is defined as follows:

$$\text{SPL} = 10 \log_{10} (\overline{P^2}/P_0{}^2) \text{ dB} \qquad (6.5)$$

where P_0 is a reference quantity incorporated to make the quantity in brackets a pure number (without units). The International Standard reference quantity is defined to be $P_0 = 2 \times 10^{-5}$ Pa ($P_0{}^2 = 4 \times 10^{-10}$ Pa^2), which requires $\overline{P^2}$ to be measured in units of Pa^2. The SPL corresponding to a particular sound depends, of course, upon the averaging time chosen for $\bar{p}^2$. It does not, however, rely in any way, or give any information about, upon the frequency content of the sound.

SPL is normally measured with a *sound level meter*. The sound level meter is an instrument for measuring sound levels as:

    (a) An unweighted, overall SPL.

    (b) An SPL weighted according to various networks, of which the most important, the A-network, is described below.

    (c) A 1/1 octave SPL spectrum.

Example 1. $\bar{p}^2$ is measured to be 300 Pa^2: what is the corresponding SPL?

$$\text{SPL} = 10 \log_{10} (300/(4 \times 10^{-10}))$$
$$= \log_{10} (7\cdot5 \times 10^{11})$$
$$= 10 \log_{10} (7\cdot5) + 10 \log_{10} (10^{11})$$
$$= 10 \times 0\cdot875 + 10 \times 11$$
$$\text{SPL} = 118\cdot75 \text{ dB}$$
$$\simeq 120 \text{ dB}$$

Example 2. $\bar{p}_1{}^2$ from one source is 150 Pa^2: $\bar{p}_2{}^2$ from another source of unrelated (incoherent) time dependence is 200 Pa^2 at the same point. What is the resulting total mean square pressure and the corresponding SPL?

The mean square pressures can be added arithmetically because the sources are incoherent and no interference effects occur in a time-average sense. Hence $\bar{p}_t{}^2 = \bar{p}_1{}^2 + \bar{p}_2{}^2 = 350 \text{ Pa}^2$.

$$\text{SPL} = 10 \log_{10} (350/(4 \times 10^{10})) = 119\cdot4 \text{ dB}$$
$$\simeq 120 \text{ dB}$$

Note that SPL$_1 = 115\cdot7$ and SPL$_2 = 117$ dB. Sound pressure levels *cannot be added arithmetically*. There are various ways of adding (or subtracting) SPL's of which one is presented in Fig. 15. A doubling of loudness corresponds *approximately* to an increase in 10 dB, i.e. ten times in $\bar{p}^2$, or in energy.

Addition of two equal SPL's from incoherent sources adds 3 dB ($10 \log_{10} 2$) to the value of either one, i.e. 75 dB + 75 dB = 78 dB. Similarly, a halving of mean square pressure corresponds to a reduction of 3 dB. The inverse square law of spreading of energy from a point source corresponds to a reduction of $10 \log_{10} (2^2) = 20 \log_{10} 2 = 6$ dB for each doubling of distance from the source. Sources which take the form of a long line, such as a traffic stream, do not produce spherically spreading fields and the reduction of SPL per doubling of distance is less than 6 dB (typically 3–4 dB), except for positions very near to the sources where individual components (vehicles) dominate.

Sound Power Level

This is the logarithmic measure of the acoustic power radiated by a continuous source. It is defined as follows:

$$\text{PWL} = 10 \log_{10} (W/10^{-12}) \tag{6.6}$$

where W is the radiated acoustic power in watts. (N.B. Some older books use 10^{-13} watt as a reference). Most sources radiate less than 1 watt of acoustic power and hence have a PWL of less than 120 dB.

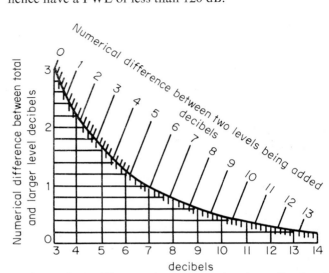

FIG. 15. Chart for addition of decibels (from G.R. Handbook).

Transmission Coefficient and Sound Reduction Index (Transmission Loss)

The transmission coefficient relates to the insulating property of a partition independent of its environment. It is defined as follows:

$$\text{transmission coefficient } (\tau) = \frac{\text{transmitted intensity}}{\text{incident intensity}} \tag{6.7}$$

The transmission loss is a logarithmic measure of τ defined thus

$$\text{TL} = 10 \log_{10} (1/\tau) \text{ dB} \tag{6.8}$$

If a partition transmits 1/1000th part of the incident energy, its TL is 20 dB. Good partitions have a TL of 40–50 dB.

Strictly, the form of the incident field corresponding to the quoted TL should be specified, e.g. normal incidence, diffuse incidence.

The standard measurement of transmission loss is specified in BS 2750; 1956, Amendment PD5065, or ISO R/140. It is measured and quoted in 1/3 *octave bands* between 100 and 3150 Hz to produce a transmission loss curve, examples of which are given in Chapter 11 on the performance of typical noise control systems.

Attenuation

The attenuation produced by a noise control system (or by natural effects such as spherical spreading, ground absorption or wind or temperature gradients) is the difference in SPL between two observation points, one on the source side and one on the observer side of the system, e.g. SPL difference between two rooms. *Note*: this is not the same as transmission loss, because a partition of given transmission loss subjected to a given incident intensity, or

SPL, from a source in one room, can produce different SPL's in the other room, depending upon the area of the partition and the total absorption of that room.

Insertion Loss

The insertion loss produced by application of a noise control system to a noise situation is given by the SPL difference at an observer position before and after the application. It is different from the attenuation because the application of a system such as a barrier affects source side SPL's, as well as observer side SPL's. Only the latter are accounted for by insertion loss.

Frequency Spectrum Measurements

As discussed earlier, it is important to be able to obtain a measure of the relative contributions to the total mean square pressure at a point in a sound field of the various frequency components. This is performed by passing the voltage from a microphone, which is an electrical analogue of the sound pressure, i.e. it imitates the variations of sound pressure, through electrical filters. The following sections describe the various standard methods used.

Frequency Spectra: Spectrum Level

As previously mentioned, sources of sound can to some extent be classified according to how the energy they produce is distributed with respect to the audiofrequency range from 20–12 000 Hz. The frequency content of the radiated sound to some extent reflects and characterizes the frequency content of the source vibrations, but the variation of radiation efficiency with frequency (wavelength) usually excludes a linear relationship. A knowledge of the frequency distribution or *spectrum*, of the mean

octave band and 1/3 octave band analysis. The audio frequency range is divided up into contiguous frequency bands centred on internationally agreed frequencies. These are listed in Table 3. The bandwidths are 70 and 26

TABLE 3

1/3 OCTAVE BAND CENTRE FREQUENCIES (Hz)

25	250	2 500
31·5	315	3 150
40	400	4 000
50	500	5 000
63	630	6 300
80	800	8 000
100	1000	10 000
125	1250	12 500
160	1600	16 000
200	2000	20 000

per cent of the centre frequencies respectively. The mean square pressures associated with frequencies lying in each band are added to give the total contribution to that band. Thus SPL-frequency graphs can be drawn. Other more narrow bandwidths are often used in research and diagnostic analysis, e.g. 6 per cent, 10 Hz. This can be used to ferret out the details of the SPL variation within the wider bandwidths, which often allows detection of the dominant sources of noise in a complex situation. Some typical spectra are shown in Figs. 16 and 17.

It is sometimes useful to be able to estimate the amount of energy of a complex noise which exists in the unit bandwidth, 1 Hz. This energy is rarely measured directly with 1 Hz bandwidth filters, but is estimated from the level in

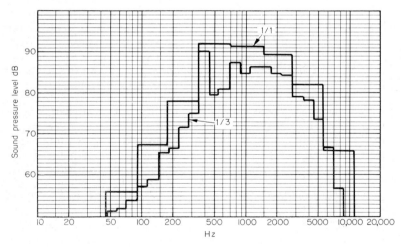

Fig. 16. 1/1 and 1/3 octave bandwidth analyses of a noise containing narrow band components.

square pressure, or sound power, is very important because (a) the ear is not equally sensitive at all frequencies in the radio range, and (b) a knowledge of the frequency spectrum of noise is useful in noise source identification.

There are many ways of presenting this information—known as frequency analysis. The most common are 1/1

a wider, usually constant bandwidth analysis band (e.g. 10 Hz) which contains the unit band of interest. The SPL in the 1 Hz band is termed the *spectrum level*. The relationship between spectrum level, band level and bandwidth $\triangle f$ is:

$$\text{Spectrum level} = \text{SPL}_{\text{band}} - 10 \log \triangle f \, \text{dB} \quad (6.9)$$

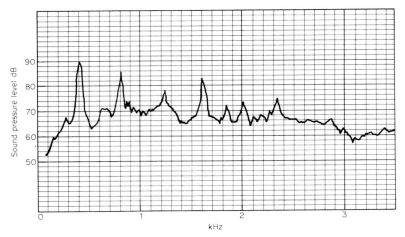

FIG. 17. 10 Hz bandwidth analysis of same noise as Fig. 16.

Discontinuous or unsteady noises, e.g. those of drop forges, explosive tools, individual vehicles passing, can also be frequency analysed. This is discussed in Chapter 11.

A-weighting curve: dB(A)

Because the ear is not equally sensitive to all audio frequencies, the SPL measured in dB, without reference to its frequency content, which is sometimes called the "*overall SPL*", or *dB (Lin)*, does not correlate well with subjective response to noise in terms of annoyance, or loudness. This variation of sensitivity is taken into account fairly satisfactorily by electrically modifying (weighting) the sound pressure signals in the different 1/3 octave bands. The A-weighting network is given in Table 4. The resulting

TABLE 4

dB(A) WEIGHTING, RELATIVE RESPONSE

Frequency (Hz)	Weighting (dB)	Frequency (Hz)	Weighting (dB)
20	−50·5	500	−3·2
25	−44·7	630	−1·9
31·5	−39·4	800	−0·8
40	−34·6	1000	0
50	−30·2	1250	+0·6
63	−26·2	1600	+1·0
80	−22·5	2000	+1·2
100	−19·1	2500	+1·3
125	−16·1	3150	+1·2
160	−13·4	4000	+1·0
200	−10·9	5000	+0·5
250	− 8·6	6300	−0·1
315	− 6·6	8000	−1·1
400	− 4·8	10000	−2·5

measure is termed dB(A). The dB(A) is the unit around which is based B.S. 4142: 1967.

NR and NC Curves

The noise rating (NR) and noise criterion (NC) curves are alternative methods of rating noise to the dB(A) measurement. They also serve, like the dB(A), as the basis of criteria for the assessment of community noise problems, and for noise control design. It should be pointed out that the NC curves are primarily for application to architectural spaces such as auditoria. The NR curves are more generally acceptable as industrial noise design criteria. ISO R/1996 (1970) describes the use of the NR curves, which include corrections for such factors as impulsive nature, tonal quality, duration and time of occurrence of the noise, together with location and *background noise*.

IMPEDANCE

The concept of impedance is familiar to electrical and electronic engineers. Input impedance refers to the ratio of voltage to current flowing in a circuit. Various types of impedance are defined in acoustics. The most common forms are specific acoustic impedance and the analogous acoustic impedance. The former is defined as the ratio of acoustic (sound) pressure to the associated velocity (or speed) of motion of the air particles in a sound field. The latter is used in the analysis of acoustic transmission lines, such as pipes, and is defined as the ratio of acoustic pressure to the product of particle velocity and cross sectional area (volume velocity). The specific acoustic impedance at any point in a fluid medium is a function of the type of wave field and of the conditions at every part of the field. It is common to restrict attention to the simplest types of sound field, of which the plane, progressive, unreflected wave, and the freely spreading wave far from a concentrated source, are the most commonly chosen examples. In these cases, the ratio of pressure to particle velocity, i.e. the specific acoustic impedance, are both equal to the product of the mean fluid density and the speed of propagation of sound waves (ρc); the impedance is independent of the frequency content of the wave. Comparing air ($\rho c = 410$ kg. m^{-2}. s^{-1}) and water ($\rho c = 1 \cdot 5 \times 10^6$ kg. m^{-2}. s^{-1}) we see that the rms particle velocity associated with a given SPL in air is greater by a factor of about 37 000 than that associated with the same SPL in water. This leads to almost complete reflection of sound at an interface between air and liquid, so that, for example, it is very difficult to transmit sound into and out of human tissue via a layer of air.

In general, because of reflections, frequency-dependent diffraction and scattering effects, and the complex nature of sources, the specific acoustic impedance in most real sound fields is far from ρc, except at great distances from compact sources. However, impedance measurements do form the basis of experimental evaluation of the absorption properties of materials and, when applied to the external ear canal, can also give an indication of the state of the middle ear (see Chapter 19).

FURTHER READING

Burns, W. (1968), *Noise and Man*, 2nd edition. London: John Murray.
Stephens, R. W. B. and Bate, A. E. (1966), *Acoustics and Vibrational Physics*. London: Arnold.

7. ELECTROACOUSTICS

W. TEMPEST

INTRODUCTION

Electroacoustics comprises the study of transducers—devices which provide an electrical output when subjected to an input of acoustic energy—and devices which provide an acoustic output for an electrical input.

The first category consists of microphones and vibration pick-ups (i.e. accelerometers etc.) while the second includes loudspeakers and earphones. Apart from a classification according to the direction of transduction (electrical to acoustic or vice-versa) transducers may, alternatively be classified according to whether or not they are reversible with respect to the directions of transduction. However, from the user's point of view it is probably more convenient to make a classification according to principles of operation; and having described each principle, to discuss applications and practical considerations. On this basis five classifications have been chosen: electrostatic (capacitative), piezoelectric, electrodynamic, magnetic, and "other"; this last section is needed to accommodate a growing variety of new and old principles which have found special application in particular circumstances.

TRANSDUCER SENSITIVITY AND CALIBRATION

Microphone Sensitivity

It is convenient to consider microphones first since they are themselves needed in the process of calibrating loudspeakers and earphones.

The sensitivity of a microphone is the relationship between the magnitude of its acoustic input and electrical output, this can be described in various ways, but the commonest in current use is to specify the output in volts for a standard sound pressure level. The actual numerical specification is now in dB relating to 1 volt per pascal. This gives a sensitivity equation of the form:

$$n = 20 \log_{10} \frac{(E)}{(P)} \qquad (7.1)$$

where E = voltage output (r.m.s.)
          P = sound pressure level (r.m.s.)

For certain types of microphones (particularly electrodynamic, and some magnetic types) it is possible to use a transformer which increases the output voltage, although, at the same time, it must increase the output impedance of the microphone. For this reason it is essential for comparison purposes to specify both voltage response and internal impedance. Table 1 gives some typical values for a number of microphone types.

TABLE 1

Type	Internal Impedance	Voltage Response (dB re 1 V. Pa^{-1})
Carbon	100 Ω	−25
Piezo-electric	2,000 pF*	−50
Electrostatic (condenser)	60 pF*	−26
Electrostatic with pre-amplifier	25 Ω	−26
Moving coil (dynamic)	10 Ω	−65
Moving coil (dynamic) with transformer	100 kΩ	−25
Velocity ribbon	≃1 Ω	−85
Velocity ribbon with transformer	100 kΩ	−35

* Capacitive output.

Since the presence of the microphone disturbs the sound field, it is important to define exactly the conditions under which the rms pressure P is specified, and to this end there are several definitions in use for different situations.

(a) *Free field* response of a microphone.

This is the ratio of the output voltage to sound pressure existing in a free field (plane sound waves) at the microphone location, with the microphone removed. (A condition which would apply in the open air away from reflecting surfaces, or inside an anechoic chamber.)

(b) *Pressure response* of a microphone.

This is the ratio of the output voltage to the sound pressure uniformly applied over the microphone diaphragm. (A condition which would apply, for example in an artificial ear.)

For a negligibly small microphone the two definitions coincide at all frequencies, but for a 2·5 cm electrostatic (1 in condenser) microphone a significant difference arises above about 1500 Hz.

A third definition of sensitivity is the "random incidence" or "diffuse field" response defined as the sensitivity in a sound field where the mean acoustic power flow per unit area is the same in all directions. (A condition which would apply in a normally reverberant room.)

Microphone Calibration—Absolute Methods

Microphones can be calibrated either by absolute methods (based on measurements of distances and electrical quantities), or by secondary methods which depend on comparison with other known microphones or sound sources.

The primary calibration procedure, which can take several forms, is the *reciprocity technique*, and can be performed either in free-field (in an anechoic chamber) or by means of a *"coupler"* which joins two transducers by means of a small enclosed volume. The method is discussed in detail elsewhere (*see* I.E.C. publications 327, 402 and Doc. 29c; Nielson (1952); and Bruel and Kjaer (1967)), it will be merely outlined here.

A reciprocity calibration depends on a basic principle of electro-acoustics, that for certain reversible transducers, there is a known and fixed relationship between the sensitivity of the transducer when used as a transmitter and its sensitivity when used as a receiver.

A free-field reciprocity calibration normally requires three transducers.

(i) A loudspeaker (not necessarily a reversible transducer).
(ii) The microphone to be calibrated.
(iii) A reversible transducer (for example an enclosed back dynamic loudspeaker).

The loudspeaker is used to produce a specific sound field which in turn produces an open circuit voltage at the terminals of the reversible transducer, which is at this stage used as a microphone.

The transducer is then replaced by the microphone to be calibrated, and the microphone open circuit voltage is measured. This procedure then gives the relationship between the sensitivity of the transducer and the microphone.

The third stage in the calibration is to replace the loudspeaker by the reversible transducer, and to measure the microphone output voltage for a given input current to the transducer.

Since the relationship between the sensitivity of the transducer in its two modes, speaker and receiver, is known, it is then possible to combine the results of the various measurements to obtain the microphone sensitivity.

As a technique, reciprocity can provide results of a high accuracy, but to undertake it satisfactorily, adequate facilities are required, and the method is not widely used outside acoustic laboratories.

Microphone Calibration—Secondary Methods

Secondary methods of calibration make use of known stable sources of sound, the most widely used being probably the piston-phone. This is a portable device in which a battery-driven electric motor operates a piston inside a small cavity. The cavity is designed to fit a specific type of (usually condenser) microphone, and when coupled to the microphone provides a standard sound pressure level (SPL).

One widely used pistonphone provides 124 ± 0.2 dB at 250 Hz. The pistonphone is an excellent stable calibrator but operates at only a single frequency.

Simpler alternatives to the pistonphone include the "falling ball" calibrator in which a stream of tiny ball bearings falls on to a diaphragm; and an electronic calibrator which utilizes a battery driven oscillator to drive a piezo-electric sound source.

The pistonphone, falling ball calibrator, and similar devices, measure sensitivity at one frequency, or band of frequencies only. In the case of the electrostatic (condenser) microphone there exists a relatively simple procedure to extend this single frequency to other frequencies. This is the electrostatic actuator, which operates by applying an alternating force to the microphone by means of an electrostatic field from an electrode close to the diaphragm, and measuring the corresponding microphone output. Since the actuating force is applied electrically, all the complications of acoustic inputs are avoided and the calibration can be extended to the whole frequency range of the microphone. Since the electrostatic method is not particularly accurate as a measure of absolute sensitivity, it is normally used in conjunction with a pistonphone or similar device to provide the basic sensitivity.

ELECTROSTATIC TRANSDUCERS

Electrostatic (Capacitor) Microphones

The electrostatic (capacitor or condenser) microphone depends for its operation on the variation in electrical capacitance between a fixed and a moving electrode. The moving electrode is commonly a taut stainless steel diaphragm mounted close to a fixed backplate, but carefully insulated from it. Figure 1 shows a (very much simplified) cross-section of a condenser microphone . A sound wave reaching the microphone will deflect the stretched diaphragm alternately towards and away from the fixed plate, causing an alternating change in the capacitance between the two. The "output" of the microphone is derived from the connection +, but in order to obtain an electrical signal from this point it is necessary to apply a polarizing voltage, typically in the region of 200 volts. Figure 2 shows a simple polarization circuit deriving its supply from a battery.

If it is assumed that the incident sound pressure is of a sinusoidal form, and that the diaphragm moves in response to this pressure, then the microphone capacitance will have the value:

$$C = C_o + C' \sin \omega t \qquad (7.2)$$

where C_o = static capacitance

C' = magnitude of capacitance change due to sinusoidal pressure

ω = angular frequency of sound

t = time

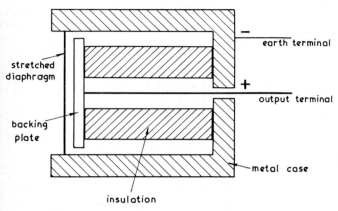

FIG. 1. Simplified section of an electrostatic microphone.

It can be shown that, for the circuit shown above, the microphone will now behave as a voltage generator, with an open circuit output voltage E_c given by:

$$E_c = \frac{E_o C'}{C_o} \qquad (7.3)$$

where E_o = polarization voltage

and an internal impedance of:

$$\frac{1}{j\omega C_o} \qquad (7.4)$$

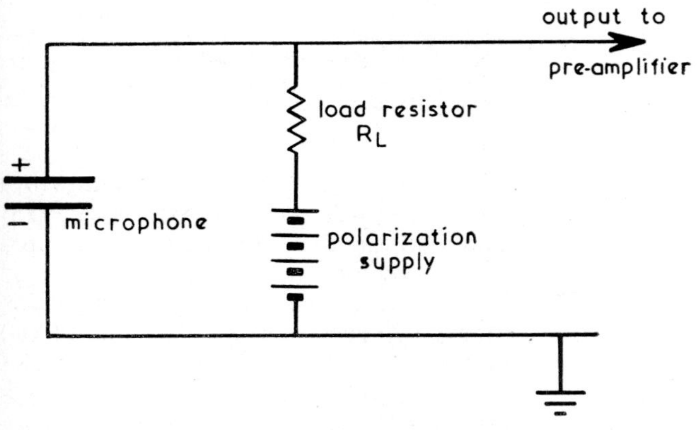

FIG. 2. Polarization circuit of an electrostatic microphone.

It is possible to calculate the extent of the capacitance change in response to a given acoustic pressure, with the result that the microphone sensitivity can be in turn evaluated. This leads to the expression:

$$E_c = \frac{E_o P a^2}{8 d T} \qquad (7.5)$$

where P = pressure amplitude (pascals)

T = diaphragm tension (newton per metre)

a = radius of circular diaphragm (metre)

d = electrode separation (metre)

This equation indicates immediately that the output voltage is proportional to the pressure amplitude (P), the polarizing voltage (E_o) and the area of the diaphragm, while being inversely proportional to the diaphragm tension and the electrode separation. In practice, the various factors are inter-related, and the final design is a compromise between the conflicting requirements of sensitivity, frequency response and distortion levels. As an example of current practice, one may quote the widely-used Bruel and Kjaer 2·5 cm microphone, which finds extensive application in acoustic and audiological measurements.

This unit (see Fig. 3) has a sensitivity of approximately 50 mV. Pa^{-1} at the normal polarization of 200 V, a dynamic range from 26 to 148 dB and frequency response from 2·6 to 18 500 Hz. The above limitations arise from the essential compromises of the design, for example the lower limit to the measurement range of 26 dB is the level at which the internal electrical noise of the microphone and its associated pre-amplifier is comparable with the electrical output. The higher limit of 148 dB is fixed by the fact that at that level the microphone generates 3 per cent harmonic distortion. The lower frequency limit (at which output is 3 dB below the mid-frequency value) is due to the necessity of having a "leak" to allow atmospheric pressure changes to reach the rear of the diaphragm; the upper limit is determined by the diaphragm resonance. It is of course possible to produce microphones with improvements in certain parameters, but these are invariably bought at the price of a deterioration in other factors. For example, smaller condenser microphones normally give an improved performance at high frequencies and at high sound pressure levels, but at the cost of a reduction in performance at the lower ends of the respective ranges.

The over-riding advantage of the electrostatic microphone is its stability in performance over a long period. This, coupled with its smooth frequency response, has lead to its dominating the field as a precise microphone for acoustic measurements and research purposes and, more recently, to its widespread use in radio and television broadcasting.

Against this must be set a number of disadvantages. Due to its very high output impedance it requires a pre-amplifier which must be mounted close to the microphone cartridge, its high polarizing voltage makes it susceptible to breakdown or damage in conditions of elevated humidity, and it is not particularly robust mechanically. In terms of its sensitivity, it is fairly good, but some other types of microphone can be used at slightly lower sound pressure levels if required.

Electrostatic Loudspeakers and Earphones

The electrostatic microphone is, in principle, a reversible transducer, and this fact is used in some reciprocity calibration procedures, however, in its "microphone" form,

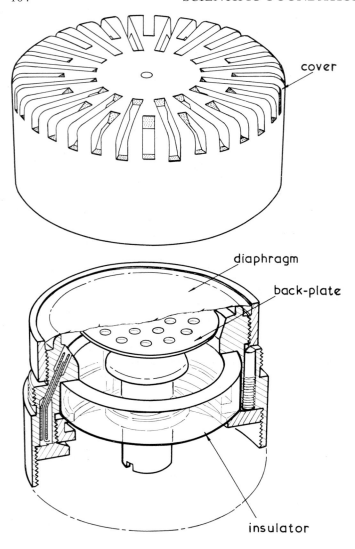

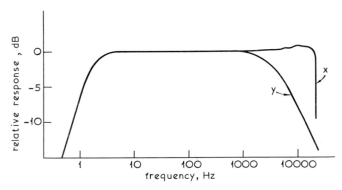

Fig. 3(a). 2·5 cm electrostatic microphone (Bruel and Kjaer).

Fig. 3(b). Frequency response of electrostatic microphone and pre-amplifier: (x) free field response, (y) pressure response measured by electrostatic actuator.

it can only produce very modest sound pressure levels, and only at fairly high frequencies. There are however, other electrostatic sound generators, which although perhaps not yet used in clinical audiology, have already found application in research work. These are the electrostatic loudspeakers and earphones.

The principle of the *electrostatic loudspeaker* is simple. If an electrically charged diaphragm is mounted between two perforated electrodes (Fig. 4), then the application of a

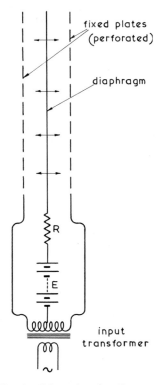

Fig. 4. Schematic of a "constant-charge" electrostatic loudspeaker: E = Polarizing voltage, R = High resistance feed to diaphragm.

"push-pull"* alternating potential to the fixed plates will deflect the diaphragm towards one plate or the other; it will thus radiate sound via the holes in the perforated plates. The practical development, however, has presented many difficulties and most of the real progress with this device appears to stem from the analysis by Hunt (1954) of the "constant-charge" method of operation. In this method the moving electrode (i.e. the sound radiator) is connected to the polarizing voltage via a large resistance so that, for the duration of one cycle of the sound frequency, it operates under a condition of constant electrostatic charge, rather than the constant voltage state that would obtain if the resistor were not present. Hunt shows (and it has been amply supported experimentally) that "constant-charge" operation greatly reduces distortion and makes the electrostatic speaker a practical device.

* In "push-pull" operation equal amplitude alternating voltages, but with a phase difference of 180°, are applied to the two fixed electrodes.

Due to its extremely light diaphragm, the electrostatic loudspeaker has excellent transient and high frequency response and it appears to be generally the best type of loudspeaker for the reproduction in free field of short tone bursts and clicks. It has found application in laboratory work in experiments involving the audibility of short duration signals of various types (Hempstock *et al.*, 1966). A good description of the practical aspects of electrostatic loudspeaker development and performance has been given by Walker (1955).

Electrostatic Earphones

The principles of the electrostatic loudspeaker have been successfully applied to the construction of *electrostatic earphones*. These have the property of providing an exceptionally good high-frequency performance, earphones with a uniform response to 20 kHz being currently available. These earphones have been used in audiological research in situations where excellent frequency response (and associated transient response) are needed, but they have certain features which must be taken into account in such applications. The first of these is the limited maximum output sound pressure level, normally specified by the manufacturers, which cannot be exceeded without distortion and/or possible damage to the earphones. The second problem arises because some of these units can derive their polarizing voltages from the signal. This leads to variations in sensitivity with changes in signal level, and, if any audiometry is intended, then it is essential to use external polarization.

PIEZO-ELECTRIC DEVICES

Piezo-electricity

The piezo-electric effect is the most modern of the long-established principles of transduction, and was discovered in 1880 by Jacques and Pierre Curie, who found that certain crystals would develop spontaneous electrical polarization under the action of mechanical forces. Since the relationship between deformation and electric polarization operates in both directions, both sound receiving and sound generating devices are possible.

Piezo-electric Microphones and Earphones

The operation of a piezo-electric microphone is simple, in that the sounds wave deflects a diaphragm, the movement of which deforms the piezo-electric element which generates the electrical output voltage. Figure 5 shows one possible arrangement in which the piezo-electric element is bent by the diaphragm movement. A basically similar design can be used to provide an earphone, and the simplicity of the system means that it can be used to provide very small transducers (although usually at some cost in sensitivity or quality of reproduction).

The simplicity of piezo-electric transducers would suggest that they might perhaps usurp most of their competitors. However, consideration of the available piezo-electric materials shows that the ideal piezo-electric substance does not exist (or, at least, has not yet been discovered or developed).

The piezo-electric effect is inherent in some natural crystals including quartz, tourmaline, and Rochelle salt (sodium potassium tartrate). A second class of piezo-electric materials is that of the "ferro-electric ceramics", a range of manufactured polycrystalline substances, in

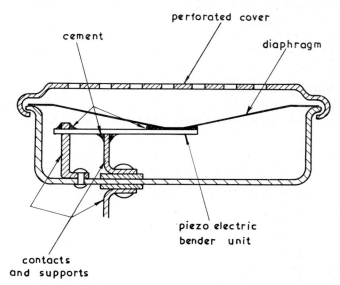

FIG. 5. Schematic of a simple piezo-electric microphone.

which piezo-electric properties can be artificially induced by the application of an electrostatic polarizing field. The best known of these are barium titanate and lead zirconate titanate.

All these materials have practical limitations. Quartz is stable, but provides only a small output, Rochelle salt gives a much larger output, but operates only within the temperature range 255 K (−18°C) to 297 K (+24°C) and must be protected from both low and high relative humidities. The ceramic materials provide properties which can to some extent be controlled during manufacture, and come nearer to an ideal combination of electrical properties and resistance to the environment, however they suffer from ageing effects, and in some cases are rather sensitive to changes in temperature.

In practice, Rochelle salt, and, more recently, the ceramic piezo-electric materials, have found very wide use in fairly low cost microphones and record player pick-ups. Their main use in the audiology and noise fields has been in low-cost sound level meters, and in hearing aid transducers.

ELECTRODYNAMIC TRANSDUCERS

Principles

The electrodynamic transducer consists essentially of an electrical conductor in a magnetic field so arranged that, when the conductor moves, it cuts lines of force. Its operation depends on the fundamental laws of magnetic induction in that a moving conductor in a magnetic field generates an electromotive force (hence acting as a microphone) while a current-carrying conductor in a magnetic field experiences a force and will therefore move if free to do so.

Electrodynamic Microphones, Earphones and Loudspeakers

There are two practical configurations for an electrodynamic transducer, namely moving coil and ribbon. Of these the moving coil finds the wider application, but both are used in microphones, loudspeakers and earphones, the ribbon being confined mainly to applications where the highest fidelity is aimed at.

Moving Coil Microphones

Figure 6 shows a diagrammatic version of a moving coil microphone, in which the moving coil is of aluminium and

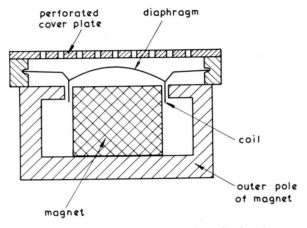

FIG. 6. Section of a (simplified) moving-coil microphone.

moves in the annular gap of a permanent magnet. The microphone diaphragm, of the order of 25 μm thick, may be of aluminium or plastic material. The basic electrodynamic principle is a good one, the microphones give an adequate output level, are reasonably robust and stable, and it is not difficult to achieve a low level of harmonic distortion. However, there are difficulties in design due to resonances which can give rise to a peaky frequency response. These difficulties can be largely overcome by means of careful damping. Figure 7 shows the construction of a moving coil microphone which provides a very satisfactory combination of robustness, performance and cost, and has been widely used in applications where high fidelity is required. Due to its complex construction, and its dependence on a permanent magnet, the moving coil microphone cannot quite match the stability and smooth frequency response of the electrostatic one, and is not normally used for precision measurement work.

Moving Coil Earphones and Loudspeakers

The most widespread use of the moving coil system is in loudspeakers, where, in order to achieve a better coupling to the air, the coil is mounted at the centre of a cone (Fig. 8). As a transducer, the moving coil loudspeaker is one of the most efficient ($\simeq$ 5 per cent) but it suffers from one

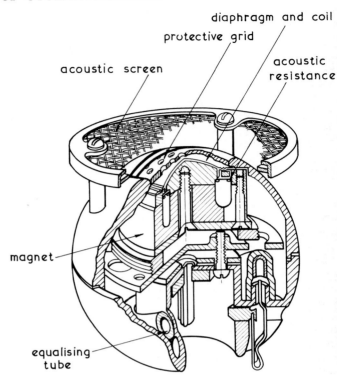

Spherical Omnidirectional Microphone

FIG. 7(a). High quality moving-coil microphone (STC).

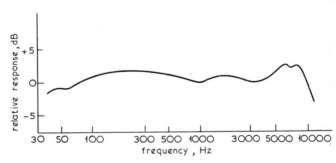

FIG. 7(b). Frequency response of microphone shown in Fig. 7(a) for sound incident normal to the diaphragm.

main resonance (due to the mass of the cone restrained by the total compliance of the suspension and any air loading), and subsidiary resonances due to the failure of the cone to move as a piston at the higher frequencies. The result of these limitations is that a speaker can provide a moderate performance over a wide frequency range (say 80–8000 Hz for a 20 cm (8 in.) diameter unit) or, for applications where a more uniform frequency response is required, a series of specially designed units is used, each covering a part of the frequency range. For example a high quality loudspeaker might use a 30 cm diameter cone "bass" unit for frequencies from 40–1000 Hz, a 7·5 cm diameter cone "mid-frequency" unit for 1000–5000 Hz, and a 2 cm diameter diaphragm "tweeter" for the range 5000–20 000

Hz, the last mentioned being similar to a rather robust earphone in its design.

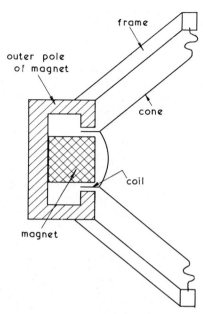

FIG. 8. Schematic section of a moving coil loudspeaker.

Ribbon Transducers

The ribbon transducer overcomes most of the disadvantages, and some of the advantages as well, of the moving coil unit by combining conductor and diaphragm into a single aluminium ribbon mounted between the poles of a magnet. Figure 9 illustrates one arrangement of such a microphone.

All the microphones discussed so far (condenser, piezoelectric and moving coil) are essentially responsive to sound pressure on one side of the diaphragm, the other side being in some way enclosed. Such pressure microphones have an omni-directional response and are not affected by the distance from the sound source. The ribbon however, is exposed to the sound field on both sides, and thus responds, not to the sound pressure directly, but to the pressure gradient. This construction has two effects, firstly the polar response (response as a function of direction in space) of the microphone is in the form of a figure of eight, being greatest for sounds arriving perpendicular to the plane of the ribbon and least for sounds originating in the plane of the ribbon. Its second characteristic is the "proximity" effect (a rise in sensitivity at low frequencies for sound sources close to the microphone). To summarize, the ribbon microphone is relatively free from resonances, giving a smooth frequency response and low distortion, its output is low, and it is rather fragile, being mainly suited to studio and indoor use.

The ribbon principle has also been successfully applied to loudspeakers. The limited size of the ribbon and its excursion mean that it can only be used on a high frequency unit (typically 2–35 kHz) and needs to be loaded by a small horn to improve the efficiency; however, it can, within its limits, provide excellent performance.

MAGNETIC (MOVING IRON) TRANSDUCERS

Like the electrodynamic transducer, the magnetic or variable reluctance (the quantity in a magnetic circuit which

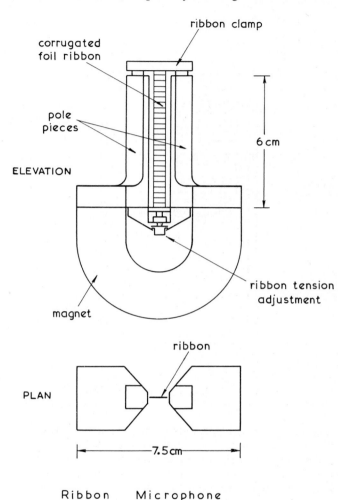

Ribbon Microphone

FIG. 9. Ribbon microphone.

is analogous to resistance in an electrical circuit) type relies on electromagnetism for the generation of e.m.f. or mechanical force. It is, however, the converse of the electro-dynamic transducer in that the conductors remain stationary while the magnetic flux is varied by the movement of an element in a magnetic circuit which involves a permanent magnet and one (or more) air gaps.

Figure 10 illustrates one application of the moving-iron principle to a microphone. Movement of the diaphragm in response to sound pressure varies the gap in the magnetic circuit; this in turn causes a variation in magnetic flux which induces e.m.f. in the coil. There are in practice many different ways of applying this principle, and, in theory, all can be used for both microphones, earphones and loudspeakers. In fact the predominant application has been in telephone ear-pieces, where the main criteria are high sensitivity, low weight and low cost. For this use, moving-iron devices have usually been preferred to moving-coil, since the latter need a larger permanent magnet.

However, as happens so often in engineering, an advantage in one aspect of performance must be paid for by a loss elsewhere. In this case it is in smoothness of response

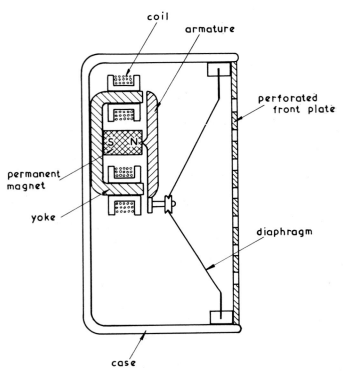

Fig. 10. Section of a rocking armature type moving-iron telephone receiver.

and harmonic distortion that the magnetic transducers fall below the standards of the electrodynamic types.

Two areas where moving-iron systems are of particular interest are record player pick-ups and sub-miniature hearing aid transducers. In this latter case complete receivers of less than 1 cm overall diameter are widely used. To attain this miniaturization some sacrifices in quality have to be made and the resulting earphone does not have a particularly flat frequency response or low distortion.

OTHER TYPES OF TRANSDUCER

Any known principle for the conversion of electrical to mechanical energy or vice-versa, can, in theory, be used in an electro-acoustic transducer. The following comprise a number of those which have been, are, or may become, of some importance.

Variable Resistance

Of all the variable-resistance type microphones the only type to achieve wide usage is the carbon type. Its operational principle depends on the fact that when a quantity

of carbon granules is contained between two conducting walls which subject them to a varying pressure, then the granules exhibit relatively large changes in resistance. The device is non-reversible, and, in order to utilize the change in resistance, it must be provided with an external source of polarizing current. It can provide a very high level output and is cheap and robust; hence its widespread use for many decades in telephones, but it is noisy, relatively unstable in sensitivity and tends to produce a high level of distortion. As a device it does not nowadays have much place in audiology.

The Electret

The term "Electret" is attributed to Heaviside who coined it in 1885 to describe a solid dielectric which could be electrically stressed and, in some way, hold the electrical stresses "locked" into the material when the external stressing was removed. An electret is analagous to a permanent magnet in the sense that it is a source of a permanent electrostatic field.

The practical development of the electret into a useful device began in the 1920's, but has only recently been applied to electroacoustics in the form of the electret polarized electrostatic (condenser) microphone (Carlson, 1973). Figure 11 shows an electret microphone in which polarization is provided by means of a permanent electret layer, which consists of a plastic material with appropriate dielectric properties. The main application of electret microphones is in situations such as hearing aids where a small, light device is required and a high voltage supply to polarize a normal electrostatic microphone is not available.

The Piezo-junction Microphone

The piezo-junction transducer is relatively new in principle, and is based on the behaviour of a semiconductor (germanium or silicon) which is subjected to a mechanical stress on the line of the *pn* junction (*see* Chapter 5). It is found that, if pressures is applied to the correct point by means of a small radius stylus then this pressure can cause a variation in the current through the junction. In its basic behaviour this device resembles the carbon microphone, but it would appear to have potentially much better qualities of stable performance, low noise and wide frequency response. In its present form it is rather fragile and has not yet reached commercial application.

DIRECTIONAL MICROPHONES

Microphones which are sensitive to the pressure of the incident sound are, in principle omnidirectional, although they show some directionality at the higher frequencies where the wavelength of sound is of the order of, or smaller than, the diaphragm. For many applications it is desirable that a microphone should have a directional response at all frequencies and a number of systems have been devised to achieve this.

The principle of operation of all the directional microphones is their sensitivity to the pressure gradient of the incident sound wave, rather than to its pressure at a single

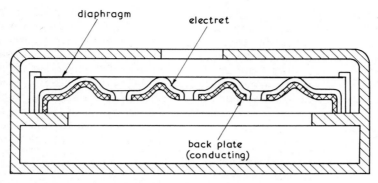

FIG. 11. Schematic of an electret microphone.

point. One type (already mentioned) is the ribbon micro-phone which is a symmetrical device and has a figure of eight response with equal maxima in sensitivity on the axis perpendicular to the plane of the ribbon (Fig. 12a).

The other widely used directional microphone is the cardioid type, so-called because of the shape of its polar

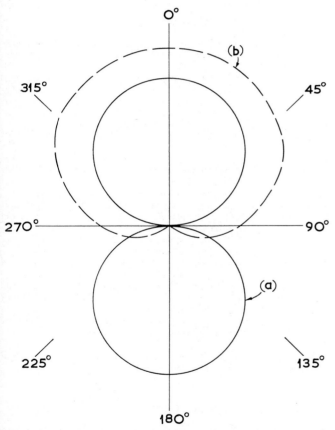

FIG. 12. Microphone polar diagrams. (a) Figure-of-eight ribbon type. (b) Cardioid type.

response source (Fig. 12b). A cardioid polar response can be obtained from a diaphragm type of microphone by providing an acoustic input to both sides of the diaphragm, the front receiving the sound directly while the rear is fed through an acoustic phase shifting network. The phase shift to the rear of the diaphragm is such that for sounds

arriving in the rear of the microphone the response is greatly reduced and such microphones are very valuable in conditions of high background noise.

The principle of the unidirectional pressure gradient microphone has been applied to moving coil, ribbon, piezo-electric and capacitor types, and recently to the electret microphone. This latter application is of particular interest since it has provided a subminiature directional microphone only 16 mm long, 6 mm wide and 2·3 mm thick, a unit small enough to be incorporated in a hearing aid (Carlson and Killion, 1973).

LOUDSPEAKER AND EARPHONE CALIBRATION

Loudspeaker Sensitivity and Performance

The sensitivity of a loudspeaker is usually defined in terms of the sound pressure level it produces for a given input, under specified acoustic conditions. A typical example being the SPL at 1000 Hz, measured 1 m from the loudspeaker along its axis of symmetry, (normally perpendicular to the radiating surface) for an input of 1 volt r.m.s., under anechoic conditions.

However, this absolute sensitivity is not usually of great significance, since in any experimental situation the SPL would normally be monitored by a calibrated microphone. Of much greater interest are the other features of the res-ponse i.e. variation with frequency, variation with direction, and level of harmonic distortion. These measurements are normally made inside an anechoic chamber, or sometimes on the edge of the roof of a fairly high building, the micro-phone in either case being suspended from a boom which permits it to be moved in three dimensions. Since both the loudspeaker sensitivity and its polar diagram are frequency dependent it will be clear that a complete measurement of the full frequency range in all directions will be rather time-consuming. In practice it may be partially automated by means of such features as a sweep frequency oscillator coupled to a level recorder, and the mounting of the loud-speaker on a turntable to facilitate polar response measure-ment.

Earphone Calibration

By contrast with the loudspeaker, the calibration of an earphone presents considerable technical difficulties, since, in use, the earphone is always coupled to the subject's ear, a situation which, due to inter-individual variations, makes standardization impossible. Moreover, due to the small volume of the coupling this makes direct measurements difficult. To overcome these difficulties three approaches to the problem have been developed: biological calibration, probe tube calibration, and the artificial ear.

Biological Calibration of Earphones

If an earphone is to be used in the measurement of the human hearing threshold, then there is no need to determine the actual sound pressure which it produces, provided one can establish the electrical input, in volts, corresponding to the "normal" hearing threshold at that frequency.

In order to do this it is necessary to make a hearing threshold determination on a group (usually 20 or more in number) of young persons all believed to have unimpaired hearing. A separate determination at each frequency is made and the input voltage at the hearing threshold is calculated on the assumption that the hearing level of the group corresponds to the normal level of the population as a whole. The method is fundamentally a good one, but is very time-consuming and expensive in practice, and it does not give any direct measure of the actual sound pressure level at the subject's ear.

Probe-tube Calibration of Earphones

The nearest approach to the direct measurement of the SPL produced at the entrance to the ear canal by a particular earphone is given by the use of a probe-tube microphone. This consists of a normal microphone mounted outside the earphone, and coupled by a small bore tube to the desired measuring point. Such an arrangement can give accurate calibration over the lower part of the audio-frequency range, but the sensitivity at the higher frequencies is affected by resonances in the tube; such a system is difficult to use above about 4 kHz. Another deficiency of the probe-tube technique (and one which applies equally to artificial ear methods) is that in order to eliminate errors from noise, the calibration must take place at a level above background noise and microphone noise. Calibration is therefore usually undertaken at about 60 dB or higher, and it is assumed that the linear relationship between input voltage and SPL applies at lower levels.

The Artificial Ear

The artificial ear is the basic device used in the laboratory calibration of earphones, and hence, indirectly, of audiometers. It consists essentially of a microphone (almost invariably electrostatic) in an open ended cavity which, to some extent, represents the human ear canal. If the artificial ear provided a perfect acoustic equivalent to the ear, then it could be used directly to calibrate earphones, by simply measuring the sound pressure produced in the artificial

ear by a given voltage, in the knowledge that it would behave in the same way when applied to the human ear.

In practice, the situation is less simple, since the sensitivity of the earphone, when mounted on the artificial ear is, at some frequencies, significantly different from that of the human ear. The result of this is that for a particular earphone and artificial ear combination a frequency dependant correction is required to relate the results to those obtained on human ears. A further complication is that, for a given artificial ear, the correction is dependent on the type of earphone used. This situation has led to the development and use, in various parts of the world, of a number of artificial ears. Only in 1970 was an internationally acceptable design published. This I.E.C. artificial ear (I.E.C. Publication 318) aims to represent the human ear more closely than a single cavity, and consists of three cavities acoustically coupled. It is designed for use in the frequency range 20–10 000 Hz, and is claimed to provide closer agreement with subjective ratings (on human subjects) than the relative sensitivities obtained using other existing types of artificial ear (Delany et al., 1967).

REFERENCES

Bruel and Kjaer (1967), *Instructions and Applications, Microphone Calibration Apparatus Type* 4142. Anon. Naerum, Denmark: Bruel and Kjaer.

Carlson, E. V. (1973), "A Subminiature Condenser Microphone," in *The Hearing Dealer*, April.

Carlson, E. V. and Killion M. C., (1973), "Subminiature Directional Microphones," Paper presented at the 46th Audio Engineering Society Convention, New York, September.

Delany, M. E., Whittle, L. S., Cook, J. P. and Scott, V. (1967), "Performance Studies on a New Artificial Ear," *Acustica*, **18**, 231–237.

Hempstock, T. I., Bryan, M. E. and Tempest, W. (1964), "A Redetermination of the Quiet Threshold as a Function of Stimulus Duration," *J. Sound Vib.*, **1**, 365–380.

Hunt, F. V., (1954), *Electroacoustics*. New York: John Wiley.

I.E.C. (International Electrotechnical Commission) Publication 318 (1970), *An I.E.C. Artificial Ear of the Wide-band Type for the Calibration of Earphones Used in Audiometry*.

I.E.C. Publication 327, *Precision Method for Pressure Calibration of One Inch Standard Microphones by the Reciprocity Technique*.

I.E.C. Publication 402, *Simplified Method for Pressure Calibration of One Inch Standard Microphones by the Reciprocity Technique*.

I.E.C. Draft Publication (Doc 29c Secretariat 15), *Precision Method for Free-field Calibration of One Inch Standard Condenser Microphones by the Reciprocity Method*.

Nielson, A. K. (1952), "A Simplified Technique for the Pressure Calibration of Condenser Microphones by the Reciprocity Method," *Acustica*, **2**, 112.

Walker, P. J. (1955), "Wide-range Electrostatic Loudspeakers," *Wireless World*, May, June and August.

FURTHER READING

Gayford, M. L. (1970), *Electroacoustics*. London: Newnes Butterworths.

Kinsler, L. E. and Frey, E. R. (1962), *Fundamentals of Acoustics*, 2nd edition. New York: John Wiley.

Robertson, A. E. (1963), *Microphones*, 2nd edition. London: Iliffe.

8. PHYSICS OF HEAT

DUNCAN D. LINDSAY

INTRODUCTION

In What Areas of Otolaryngology is Heat a Relevant Factor?

We must subdivide this question into three parts, (a) that relating to normal function of the ear, nose and throat (b) that relating to pathological conditions (c) that relating to clinical techniques, either diagnostic or therapeutic. It is the aim in this chapter to describe the physics of heat underlying these areas of relevance, thus laying a foundation for an understanding of the applications and indicating their nature, even though the detailed study of these biophysical and technological applications will be left for later consideration.

(a) Looking first at the relevance of heat to the normal function of the ear, nose and throat, we realize that we are in the realm of biophysics rather than of clinical physics, a realm that can be considered either as a branch of physics or of physiology. The physiologist will accentuate the bio-components whereas the physicist will accentuate the physics components and each will be able to deal with some realms outside the other's compass. Here we approach the matter from the physics side.

We might find ourselves concerned with temperature distribution in a volume of otolaryngological tissue, especially in regard to any variation amongst recognizable structures, variation of these temperatures with time and with environment, in regard to the generation, conversion and use of energy within these tissues, in regard to change of state between liquid and vapour in any part of this realm, in regard to the influence of body temperature or environmental temperature on functions such as nasal air conditioning, and, finally, in regard to the study of relative humidity in the respiratory tract and its relationship to speech, exercise and environmental conditions.

(b) Looking next at the relevance of heat to pathological states of the ear, nose and throat, one might be concerned with changes in temperature distribution throughout the region, due either to local inflammatory conditions or to localized neoplasms. We might also be concerned with changes in any of the circumstances mentioned in (a), but particularly with the effect of inflammation of the respiratory tract on liquid-vapour equilibrium.

(c) Looking finally at the relevance of heat studies in clinical techniques, both diagnostic and therapeutic, we notice several fields in which the physics of heat is not merely relevant, but is the controlling factor. Those that spring to mind on the diagnostic side are the use of the floor of the mouth as standard practice for the assessment of body core temperature, and the use of infra-red radiation emitted by the body in the practice of thermography, especially in the detection of near-superficial malignancies. On the therapeutic side, obvious applications are the use of hot filament cautery, the use of surgical diathermy for

coagulation or cutting, the use of cryosurgery and the occasional use of medical (therapeutic) diathermy, e.g. for the treatment of infected paranasal sinuses.

Which Aspects of the Physics of Heat are Relevant to Otorhinolaryngology?

Now that we have noted the areas of otorhinolaryngology which involve a knowledge of the physics of heat, we are in a position to choose the particular aspects of heat physics which need to be understood by a practising otorhinolaryngologist. Fortunately, the areas are fairly restricted and none need to be studied in any depth. While many massive text-books are written on heat and thermodynamics, particularly relating to quantitative aspects of energy conversion and heat flow, the need of the clinician can be adequately met by comparatively superficial qualitative study of a few restricted areas. From the above list of potential applications, one may identify the areas of interest as (i) the kinetic nature of heat, (ii) definition of quantity of heat, (iii) definition of temperature scales, (iv) measurement of temperature, (v) the convertibility of heat and other forms of energy, (vi) the concept of specific heat, (vii) thermal capacity, (viii) heat transfer mechanisms of special relevance e.g. conduction, forced convection and radiation, (ix) expansion of gases and, finally, (x) liquid–vapour equilibrium, including latent heat of vaporization and the concept of relative humidity.

Nature of Discussion

It is intended here to simplify the issues, attempt to clarify the fundamental principles and avoid unnecessary mathematics. The object is to provide a clear understanding of the physical principles so that the clinician will be able to use these in all his thinking about normal and abnormal function and about technology and techniques, without conscious reference.

The Kinetic Nature of Heat

Heat is not a nebulous concept. Its nature is well understood and its quantity can be measured. Heat is nothing more nor less than the kinetic energy (KE) of the particles that comprise matter. It so happens that the human organism has the faculty of assessing a facet of kinetic energy in external matter, relative to that in itself, by registering the sensations "hot" and "cold". If we consider two otherwise identical pieces of metal, one at room temperature, the other much hotter, the only relevant difference between these two pieces of metal ("bodies") is that the total kinetic energy of all the particles (free electrons, atoms, molecules, groups of molecules) in the second body is greater than that in the first. This is the objective reality. That you or I find the second "hotter" to the touch is a subjective sensation and is simply a name given to the sensation. If the external body is solid, the kinetic energy of its particles will be mainly in the form of vibrations of its atoms and molecules about their mean positions, though there may be a little random migration of free electrons in metals. If the external "body" is gaseous, the kinetic energy of its particles will be entirely in the form of random migration with changes of direction imposed only by collisions. If the external "body" is liquid, the kinetic energy of its particles will be partly in the form of atomic and molecular vibration, partly in the form of their migration. We ought carefully to distinguish between the concepts of "quantity of heat" and "temperature". They are distinguished from each other in the same manner as are "quantity of water" in a lake and "levels of the water" in the lake. A body such as a lump of iron, or a human being, at any chosen moment, will contain a vast number of particles with a wide range of kinetic energies. If we add together all the kinetic energies of the individual particles, we have a measure of the total quantity of heat in the body, analogous to the total volume of water in the lake. It is possible to derive an expression for this in the exceedingly simple case of a perfect gas. If we assess the square of the mean velocity of the individual particles, we have a measure of the temperature of the body, analogous to the depth of water in the lake. If the particles of the body lose kinetic energy there is a loss of quantity of heat (Q) i.e. heat has flowed from the body to its environment just as water may be lost from the lake by an effluent stream, by soakage into the soil and by evaporation. In the case of our hot body the loss of KE by particles will, *ipso facto*, involve a new, lower mean level of velocity of the particles, i.e. a lower temperature. In the case of our lake, the loss of water will result in a smaller depth.

Quantity of Heat

Though it would be logical to define and measure quantity of heat in terms of total particle KE it was historically practical to define a unit in terms of temperature change of a common substance. The unit was called the calorie and, with provisos about starting temperature and pressure, was defined as the quantity of heat required to change the temperature of 1 gm of pure water by 1°C. By the same token, we have no direct reading instrument for measuring calories, but must do experiments in which heat loss is minimized, water is weighed and temperature change is noted. However, modern practice is to quote quantities of heat directly in units of energy, i.e. joules, as specified in the International System of Units.

Temperature

The detecting system not only tells you that an external body is hot or cold, but gives you an estimate of how hot or cold it is. The organism relates the velocity parameter qualitatively to sensory signals to give a rough estimate of temperature, but we can relate it quantitatively to expansion of mercury, alcohol, etc. to make measuring instruments. The way in which the absolute temperature scale is related to the objective reality is a matter of great concern to physicists, but no concern at all to clinicians. It is only necessary to notice that thermometers can be constructed to measure the temperature accurately and the human body has a mechanism for estimating it roughly. If thermometers were constructed to read on an absolute scale, they would read zero in the unattainable state when particle energy was zero and we would be free to choose the size of unit by which we could make steps up the temperature scale from there. In fact, we have to choose an attainable datum point (the triple point of pure water*) and we choose the size of the unit so that 273·16 steps would take us from absolute zero to that point. Using this datum point and this size of unit, we can take the temperature of melting ice as about 273° and that of boiling water as about 373° on the absolute or thermodynamic scale. Values on that scale are designated in kelvins (K). In everyday usage, as we all know, we move the zero to make the fixed point for practical purposes 0°, the boiling point of pure water becomes 100° and temperatures are denoted by °C, which stand for degrees centigrade or degrees Celsius. The size of the unit, or degree, is exactly the same as that of the thermodynamic or absolute scale. The only important point on that scale for the otorhinolaryngologist is the mean temperature of the human body core, averaged over many healthy subjects and over 24 hours and taken to be 37·0°C (310 K). Core temperature can be measured accurately by a rectal thermometer, but readings from the floor of the closed mouth give a reasonable approximation.

There was another scale with its zero chosen by reference to weather conditions in the Baltic and its unit chosen to make 180 steps between freezing water and boiling water. This (Fahrenheit) scale was very arbitrary and its fixed points of 32°F for freezing water and 212°F for boiling water are not easy to remember or use, but it did have the advantage of a smaller unit, so that small variations appeared more clear. Thus mean human core temperature was 98·4°F and the clinician would obtain floor of mouth readings commonly ranging from 96°F to 104°F. On the centigrade scale the patient's condition has to be judged between 35°C (308 K) and 40°C (313 K).

The use of calories and degrees Fahrenheit is not recommended in the International System.

Thermometers

We have no more need to study the physics of the design of temperature measuring devices, or their engineering construction, than we have to study the theory of temperature scales. What we do need is a note of the types of thermometer that are of practical use in otolaryngology. These are (a) the common mercury-in-glass clinical thermometer and (b) electrical thermometers.

The first of these is quite accurate enough for clinical purposes and its only disadvantages lie in its slow speed of response and its bulk. It has special features, compared with ordinary mercury thermometers. First, it is a "maximum reading" thermometer, a characteristic necessitated by the

---

* The point at which the three phases, ice, water and vapour, coexist in equilibrium. It corresponds to a particular temperature and pressure.

fact that it is almost impossible to read it *in situ*. We must therefore be able to leave it in place for a minute or two, withdraw it and rely on the mercury still indicating the maximum temperature reached during the period of insertion. As we all know, this is achieved by the simple device of a constriction between the bulb and the capillary. The expansion process produces plenty of force to push the mercury past the constriction, but the weight of the mercury is quite insufficient to force it back again: it will maintain a maximum reading until it is shaken down. In the shaking process the whole momentum given to the mercury and glass is transferred to the mercury when the glass is abruptly stopped, so that a large force becomes available to push the mercury back through the constriction. Secondly, it is a short range thermometer, commonly graduated from 35°C (308 K) to 42°C (315 K). Thirdly, it is a sensitive thermometer, compared to other mercury in glass thermometers, giving a movement of about 10 mm for 1°C (1 K) temperature change. This is achieved by using a large volume of mercury in the bulb and a very narrow capillary. Fourthly, it is designed for bulb-only immersion; although it is calibrated by total immersion, the discrepancies are quite negligible. Fifthly, it is fairly slow to equilibrate with the temperature of its environment —mouth, axilla or whatever—because of the large mass of mercury. In fact, a few trials will readily establish that an insertion of about two minutes is needed to equilibrate within 0·1°C (0·1 K) with most of these thermometers. Times marked on clinical thermometers should be treated sceptically. It may be inconvenient to leave a clinical thermometer in place for two minutes as a matter of routine. If this is so, it is probably best to use the same insertion time in all cases: results will then be comparable amongst themselves. Sixthly, it is specially shaped to enable one to observe the very fine thread of mercury in the capillary. This is achieved by making the cross-section of the glass lenticular. Finally, an accuracy of ±0·01°C (±10 mK) is common.

Electric thermometers have several striking advantages, but there are also noticeable disadvantages. Their biggest virtue is the ability to attain an accuracy of ±0·000 000 1°C (0·1 μK) but this is quite valueless in clinical work. A worthwhile advantage is the ability to produce remote readings which can be continuously observed and, if desired, automatically recorded. Another advantage is that they can be more effectively sterilized than can mercury-in-glass thermometers. The main disadvantages are the cost, the need for maintenance and repair, and the fact that the patient has to be "wired up" from the transducer (where temperature is sensed and converted into an electrical signal), to the remote station where the signal is processed, displayed and recorded. Except in the operating room, this wiring is not well tolerated. A particular disadvantage associated with the transducer and wiring is the danger of burns at the transducer site if surgical diathermy is in use. This particular hazard will be dealt with later.

There are three principal types of electric thermometer available. These are dependent respectively on the change of resistance of a conductor with temperature, the generation of a thermo-electric electromotive force (emf) at the junction of two conductors and the change of resistance of a semiconductor with temperature.

The first effect is used in the simple resistance thermometer in which a coil of wire enclosed in a suitable insulating tube is the sensing element. The resistance of the coil, commonly made of platinum, may increase by a fraction of one ohm for each 1°C (1 K) temperature rise. It is reasonable to expect that the greater random motion imposed on the free electrons in the metal at raised temperature will in general reduce their freedom to flow in any particular direction and thus increase resistivity, though it is possible to produce special alloys with a negative temperature coefficient. The change of resistance is detected and measured by means of a Wheatstone bridge type of circuit. Ideally, the bridge would be balanced at all times to give zero current in the galvanometer, but it is common practice to take the "out-of-balance" current as a measure of temperature, the meter being calibrated accordingly. However, this type of instrument is not so commonly used as the others, because the size of the coil is liable to be bigger than the bulb of a mercury thermometer. The other two types have potentially much smaller sensing elements, and are therefore more attractive for clinical or biophysical needs.

The electric thermometers which use the Seebeck effect involve a circuit of the kind shown in Fig. 1, although in

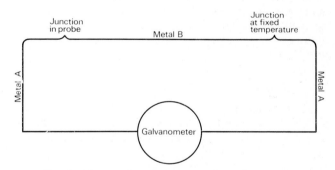

FIG. 1. Measurement of temperature by thermocouple.

practice an amplifier may be incorporated, to enable the tiny current to be registered on a robust meter. A thermoelectric emf is generated at any one junction, due to diffusion of electrons from one metal to the other as temperature rises, but of course, completion of the circuit involves an oppositely oriented junction of the same kind. If both were at the same temperature, equal and opposite emf's would be generated and current flow would be zero. If the junctions are at different temperatures, the net emf and hence the current flowing round the circuit will be dependent on the temperature difference. If therefore we intend to use the technique to measure variation of temperature at one junction, we must be sure that the other junction remains at a constant temperature throughout a reading. In elementary physics teaching, the other junction is generally maintained in melting ice and is referred to as the "cold" junction, but there is no need for it to be cold; the only requirement is that it should be at a constant temperature. There are various possible ways of achieving this in convenient and portable fashion. The most common is to sink the other junction in a block of metal whose temperature will not be affected appreciably by environmental changes during any one period of use. Another way is to maintain the other junction at a controlled high temperature in an electrically heated jacket.

The third type of electric thermometer, using the resistance change in a semiconductor, is perhaps the most popular at present. In this case the resistance generally falls with temperature increase and the effect is very much greater than in the case of a conductor. Materials giving positive temperature coefficients are available. The actual piece of semiconductor will commonly be a tiny chip of cerium, manganese or barium oxide and the sensitive element may be very small. The change of resistance is detected and measured by a bridge circuit on the same principle as that used for the older resistance thermometer.

All three types of electric thermometer are available commercially with their sensitive elements on the ends of probes of convenient size and shape for the particular application. Probably the most useful application in otolaryngology is during surgery, when a tissue temperature at any chosen location may be continuously indicated on a conveniently positioned meter and recorded on a paper chart for visual inspection, or on magnetic tape for subsequent computer analysis. Special precautions must be taken if surgical diathermy is to be used. Portable instruments involving only probes, leads, "black box" and indicating meter can, of course, be used to indicate mouth temperature, oesophageal temperature or any other special need.

Convertibility of Different Forms of Energy

It is very readily seen, from the molecular nature of heat described above and the single example of the production of heat by friction that mechanical energy may be converted into heat. Clearly rubbing at the surface of a body will stimulate the superficial molecules into more energetic motion and raise the temperature of both participants locally. It is not so obvious that the conversion of heat into mechanical work is possible, although we are all familiar with it in the internal combustion engine, where the sequence of combustion, heating, expansion and movement is easily understood. The complete conversion of mechanical energy into heat is possible and in this case the number of joules of mechanical energy needed to produce 1 calorie is 4·2. If we consider the general case of a body on which mechanical work is done, we notice that in any real circumstances there may independently be simultaneous flow of heat to or from the body from or to its environment and it is therefore necessary to take account of this in any equation we may write i.e. the total gain of internal energy equals the external work done on the body (i.e. the mechanical energy supplied) plus the heat flowing to the body from its environment, taking due account of signs for each term. This statement, so obvious when the nature of heat is understood, was historically glorified by the name of the First Law of Thermodynamics. It may, of course, be broadened to include gain of internal energy from other forms. However, although conversion between heat and mechan-

ical energy or "work", and vice versa, is deeply studied by physicists and engineers, we should here look at the wider implications of the convertibility of one form of energy into another. We are nowadays very conscious of the fundamental nature of energy in the scheme of the universe. Scientists of any discipline must be aware of the fact that energy is displayed in atomic form, chemical form, electric, magnetic, gravitational, mechanical, radiation forms, as well as heat, and that even mass is another form of energy. Probably all scientists are aware that energy is the one indestructible entity of the physical universe. The old principle of conservation of mass has been disproved; in nuclear reactions there is a loss of mass, but, in all physical changes, the total amount of energy is conserved. We thus see energy as the most fundamental of all concepts and appreciate that heat is just a particular form of energy, indeed a particular form of mechanical energy, which is detectable by the human nervous system, as is sound, which is another form of mechanical energy, and light, which is a form of radiant energy. Any and every form of energy can be converted by nature to any other form, although it may sometimes be necessary to pass through other forms on the way and there will rarely be conversion of the whole of one type of energy to one other type, but generally a conversion from one form to several others: in particular, heat will often be a by-product, sometimes wanted, sometimes unwanted, and classified as a "loss". Which of these conversions is pertinent to otolaryngology? On the biophysical side, the most obvious one is surely the conversion from chemical energy to heat by combustion of fuel within the tissues, but this is in no way peculiar to the ear, nose and throat. On the technological side, surgical diathermy is a very good example of conversion of electric energy to heat energy.

Specific Heat

This is a concept which no-one can ignore entirely if he is thinking about the applied physics of heat in otolaryngology or any other field. It should perhaps be dealt with only briefly, however, as one can see little need for the otolaryngologist to be concerned with detail, except perhaps in connection with cryosurgery.

The specific heat of a substance is the ratio of the amount of heat taken up by a substance to the rise of temperature produced. It is thus a measure of the ability of a substance to take in heat without appreciable rise in temperature. The higher the specific heat, the less temperature rise will result from the injection of a given number of joules. Quantitatively, number of joules, Q = mass of substance × specific heat of substance × temperature rise = $m \times c \times \Delta\theta$. Alternatively, we can say that a substance with a large specific heat is one that needs a lot of joules to produce a given temperature rise in a given mass. Specific heat is sometimes defined as the ratio of the number of joules needed to heat unit mass of the chosen substance by 1 K to the number of joules needed to heat unit mass of water by 1 K, in which case it is a dimensionless quantity, a pure number, without units. If it is defined as the former quantity of heat, it must be expressed in J. kg^{-1}. K^{-1} using SI units. It is a remarkable thing that water has the highest value of specific heat found amongst commonly available substances. On the ratio definition, this value is, of course, exactly equal to 1·0. Values of specific heat for biological materials are difficult to specify. In vitro measurements are bound to be from modified and dried samples, most forms of tissue are extremely complex mixtures, probably governed by their fluid content. It is just worth noticing, therefore, that numerical values of specific heat for common solids lie in the region of 0·1, for common liquids in the region of 0·5 (blood 0·9), for gases in the region of 0·3 (air 0·24, water-vapour 0·4). In the case of gases, there is some doubt about the value to be attached to the specific heat, on the basis of the simple definition above, because the heating of the gas would be accompanied by expansion if the external pressure were constant, but one could choose to keep the volume constant by changing the external pressure suitably. Measuring specific heat of a gas by these two techniques, one obtains two different results commonly designated as c_p (the specific heat at constant pressure) and c_v (the specific heat at constant volume). One would expect this difference, because in one case part of the heat energy is going into the form of external mechanical work. These niceties are fun for physicists postulating perfect gases, but bring little joy to practising otolaryngologists concerned with mixtures of real gases and vapours varying in both pressure and volume.

Thermal Capacity

Whereas specific heat relates to a substance, thermal capacity relates to a particular body. It is the number of joules that the body needs to be given to raise its temperature 1 K. This concept is probably more important to the otolaryngologist than the concept of specific heat. The thermal capacity of a particular organ may well have significance, especially in cryosurgery. Quantitatively, it is clear that thermal capacity is given by $m \times c$. Merely to get one's bearings, it is perhaps worth noting some order of magnitude estimates: the thermal capacity of a human body will be of the order of magnitude 200 000 J.K^{-1} ($\sim$50 nutritional Calories per °C) while the thermal capacity of a scalpel blade will be about 0·5 J.K^{-1}.

This is perhaps an opportune moment to observe that the Calories used in nutrition studies are in fact kilocalories.

Heat Transfer

Problems in this field are of vast importance to engineers and physicists, but somewhat less vital to clinicians. We will, however, look at those aspects that can be relevant either in the biophysical applications or the technology of otolaryngology.

The modes of heat transfer are conduction, convection and radiation and it is worth taking a brief look at each of these forms from the point of view of our kinetic concept of the nature of heat.

In the case of conduction, heat spreads slowly through a body from a warmer region to a cooler region and the mechanism can be clearly seen on the kinetic picture. The

molecules in the hot region will jostle their neighbours and so give kinetic energy to them, thus raising the temperature of the adjoining regions and in time this process will extend throughout the body. Any real biological case is, of course, extremely complex compared with the ultra-simple, artificial examples studied in elementary physics, but the mechanism conducting energy through tissue and leading to slow rise of temperature in connected regions is just the same. It is clear that because each substance has different molecular mass and different arrangements and behaviour patterns of molecules, each will be able to conduct heat with varying degrees of effectiveness. We can define this only in terms of an idealized example, as shown in Fig. 2. In

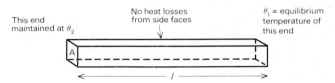

FIG. 2. Idealized concept for purpose of defining thermal conductivity.

these circumstances, the number of joules conducted along the bar is given by

$$Q = \frac{kA(\theta_2 - \theta_1)t}{l} \tag{8.1}$$

where A is the cross-sectional area of the bar, θ_2 and θ_1 are the end temperatures, l is the length of the bar and t is the time considered, if and only if there are no heat losses from the surfaces of the conductor and a steady temperature distribution has been reached. The equation will not apply during the build-up period.

The dependence on cross-sectional area, temperature gradient and time is clearly seen and the coefficient k is introduced to allow for the dependence on the nature of the substance. It is called the coefficient of thermal conductivity and it is quoted in units of watts per metre per degree (W . m^{-1} . K^{-1}). The numerical values for metals lie mostly in the range from 50–500. For other solids and liquids, values around 0·5 or less are common and for gases values of the order 0·01 or less are common. The high values of thermal conductivity for metals are, of course, due to the preponderence of "free" electrons which transfer kinetic energy to their neighbours very quickly. This structure also gives rise to the high electrical conductivity of metals. Blood can be expected to be a moderately good conductor, fat a poor conductor, while air is a good thermal insulator. The significance of these facts in normal and diseased states of the ear, nose and throat can be worked out for any individual state, the most obvious examples being inflamed conditions of the respiratory tract and the ear. The significance of heat conduction in cautery and cryosurgery is obvious, but it might be noted that, in the case of diathermy, there is actual heat generation, throughout the tissue, as well as spread of heat by conduction and any other mechanisms that happen to be relevant.

Passing to the second mechanism of heat transfer, convection, we find it to be of a totally different and much simpler nature. In convection, a whole stream of a fluid, either gaseous or liquid, is carried from one region to another and takes its energy with it. We are not concerned with kinetic theory or molecular behaviour, only with the crude movement of a hot fluid en masse. Convection is normally classified into two categories, natural and forced, natural convection being due to the lower density of a warm fluid, causing it to rise above its cooler parts, forced convection being due to any independent force producing circulation. Thus in normal or diseased functioning of the ear, nose and throat, we can see the possibility of natural convection arising due to the lower temperature of the skin compared to that of core tissue and to the lower temperature of the upper respiratory tract mucosed surfaces, when inhaling cold air, especially with the mouth open. However, this will only be effective in conditions where the subject maintains a particular posture and the hotter region is lower than the cooler, a rare circumstance. Forced convection, however, in the form of the blood and lymph circulations, is clearly of controlling significance, in normal function, diseased function and in thermal technology, where blood and lymph may be much heated or cooled before passing to other regions.

Passing to the third mechanism of heat transfer, we find that thermal radiation, both in its emission and its absorption, does involve the kinetic picture of the nature of heat. The radiation itself is in the infra-red (IR) waveband and is, of course, electromagnetic radiation and not a form of heat. It does, however, carry energy from one place to another in the form of electromagnetic waves or photons and when it is absorbed into any matter, solid, liquid or gaseous, it gives up its energy partly to increased kinetic energy of the molecules of the matter. Similarly, its formation and emission is by loss of energy in the molecules of the matter from which it emanates. Thus, as shown pictorially in Fig. 3, some of the heat energy in body A is converted to infra-red radiation, travels out in straight lines at

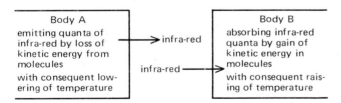

FIG. 3. Conversion of heat energy to electro-magnetic radiation and back again.

the speed of light and some of it may be absorbed into body B, where it is partially converted back into kinetic energy of the molecules i.e. heat. The infra-red will travel most readily through a vacuum, a little will be absorbed if it travels through gases or vapours, but it will penetrate only a few millimetres into a liquid or tissue. Infra-red wavelengths cover the range from the red end of the spectrum to the beginning of the microwave band, i.e. about 700 nm (nanometres) to about 100 000 nm. Notice that the longer wavelength limit is almost macroscopic; it is 0·1 mm. The different wavelengths differ greatly in their power of penetration into human tissue. The greatest penetration is

achieved at about 1100 nm, i.e. in the "near" infra-red, not far from the visible. So far as emission is concerned, we must remember that every body at any temperature above absolute zero is emitting radiation, though the higher the temperature, the shorter the wavelengths emitted. The qualitative relationship between emitted wavelengths and

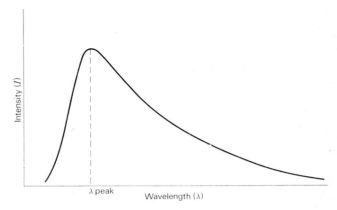

FIG. 4. Typical spectrum of an infra-red emitter.

intensity is shown in Fig. 4. It is seen that the spectrum shows three main features

    (a) a minimum wavelength, λ_{min}, where the emission is negligible
    (b) a wavelength at which the intensity of infra-red emission is greatest, λ_{peak}
    (c) a slow fall towards zero at long wavelengths.

The whole curve moves upwards and to the left if the temperature of the emitting body is raised. The short wavelength end of the spectrum begins to encroach significantly on the visible at less than 1000°C (1273 K). Our interest, however, lies in the gas-filled tungsten filament therapy lamp, which is effectively a source at 3000°C (3273 K) and has its peak emission at about 1100 nm (1·1 micrometres) and in the human body whose surface is at about 32°C (305 K) with peak emission in the region of 7700 nm (7·7 micrometres). More generally, there are three quantitative relationships that are worth noting.

The total amount of radiant energy emitted by a body at absolute temperature θ, i.e. the area under the spectrum, is proportional to θ^4.

The amplitude of the spectrum at its peak is proportional to θ^5.

The wavelength of the peak decreases as the temperature increases and the change is governed by Wien's displacement law ($\lambda_{peak} \times \theta$ is constant). It is also worth noting that the efficiency of emission of infra-red depends on the nature of the surface emitting, a matt black body being theoretically the best, as it is also for absorption of infra-red.

All of this has little applicability in normal or abnormal function of ear, nose and throat, but a great deal of applicability in clinical technology. The comparatively new diagnostic technique of thermography uses the IR radiation from a human subject obtained by scanning his surface for infra-red intensity as in a television picture, but using a specialized IR detector camera. Inflamed regions, superficial regions of high metabolic activity and other thermal abnormalities can be detected. It is worth noting that this is a diagnostic technique which subjects the patient to no invasion at all.

Expansion of Gases

Whereas the expansion of solids and liquids are much taught in pure physics studies, they have little significance in our present context, but expansion of gases is relevant in some cryosurgical instrumentation.

We can readily define a coefficient of thermal expansion as the change in volume produced per unit volume by unit change of temperature. Calling this e, we can write $V_2 = V_1[1 + e(\theta_2 - \theta_1)]$ where the other symbols have the usual meanings. In order to establish such a relationship we must assume that any other factor which could influence the volume is unchanged throughout the heating.

In most real circumstances the pressure is changing as well as the temperature. If we apply the first law of thermodynamics (see earlier) we see that the internal energy gain of the gas sample during a compression will be equal to the heat energy supplied plus the external work done. Even if no heat energy is supplied, the internal energy, and thus the temperature, will rise. More pictorially, we can see that the compressing piston or other object will give extra energy to many of the molecules as it moves among them. Conversely, during an expansion in which there is no heat exchange with the environment, the temperature of the gas will drop. Such expansions and compressions are known are adiabatic changes and in practice they occur when the change takes place so quickly that no heat can flow to or from the environment. A typical application is in cryosurgery where nitrous oxide under pressure is allowed to expand through an orifice into the region of the probe, where the pressure is much lower and there is thus a sudden temperature drop.

At the other extreme we can execute the compression so slowly that the mechanically generated heat flows to the environment and there is no rise in temperature i.e. the change is isothermal. Conversely during an expansion we may wait for heat flow from the environment to maintain a constant temperature. We could define a coefficient of pressure change analogous to that of thermal expansion.

Liquid-Vapour Equilibrium and Change of State

As we noted at the beginning of this chapter, the change of state between liquid and vapour and the equilibrium between these two phases is clearly important in the whole of the respiratory tract, extending to the auditory tube and the middle ear. Solid-liquid change seems to be irrelevant and the applications of liquid-vapour equilibrium seem to be entirely in the field of function rather than of clinical technology, so we will look at the physics of liquid-vapour equilibrium with special reference to water at around body temperature. An understanding of the concept of relative humidity is implicit in this field.

We will look at this topic, as others, from the molecular point of view, taking first the idealized case of Fig. 5 in which we have a space at a fixed temperature containing liquid water (H_2O), which initially had no water vapour above it. Some of the vibrating and migrating molecules in

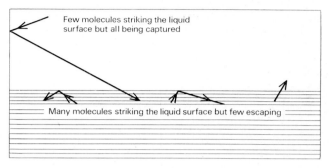

FIG. 5. Dynamic equilibrium between a liquid and its vapour.

the liquid will move towards the surface with sufficient energy to overcome the attraction of their fellows and escape: as time passes, a population of H_2O molecules in the vapour phase will build up in the space above the liquid. At this stage, some of the molecules in the vapour space will be striking the liquid surface and being attracted in, so that a two-way traffic will be established. At first, because of the vastly greater numbers in the liquid phase, more molecules will be leaving the surface per second than will be re-entering it. Thus the population density in the vapour space will go on increasing until the number of molecules re-entering per second is equal to the number leaving per second i.e. until there is a state of dynamic equilibrium. Most molecules striking the surface from the vapour side will enter the liquid, while only a proportion of those reaching the surface from the liquid side will have enough energy to escape. The existence of a population density in the vapour space implies a pressure of vapour, which clearly has a maximum value, or saturated vapour pressure (SVP) when the dynamic equilibrium is reached. If the vapour pressure is less than SVP there will be a net loss from the liquid to the vapour every second, and an observer will say that evaporation is taking place.

In this idealized picture, we have simply assumed a constant, unspecified temperature. If, however, we now consider the whole thing again at a higher temperature, we realize that the number of molecules in the liquid phase which have enough energy to escape from the surface will be greater and a greater number of faster moving molecules in the vapour phase will collide with the liquid surface and enter it. A new dynamic equilibrium will be established in which the new SVP will be higher. Clearly for each temperature there will be a particular value of SVP. There is no simple relationship between SVP and temperature as there is between pressure, volume and temperature for a permanent gas, but of course, the values are well known and are shown in Fig. 6, over the range from 0°C (273 K) to 100°C (373 K). It was traditional to express such values in "practical" pressure units—mm Hg—but in SI units we label the y-axis in pascals (newtons per square metre). In our idealized case, there is nothing but water-vapour above the liquid, whereas in real life there will be atmosphere as well. However, the behaviour of the gas molecules from the atmosphere entering and leaving the liquid can be ignored for our purposes, and the dynamic equilibrium achieved by the H_2O molecules can be considered independently.

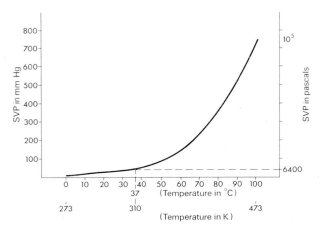

Fig. 6. Variation of SVP of water with temperature.

Notice that we are considering liquid-vapour equilibrium at temperatures between freezing and boiling. The phrase "changes of state" is most often used in connection with the process of boiling at atmospheric pressure, which does not interest us at all in the case of water for it takes place at a temperature far outside the range of body temperatures. We are, however, interested in boiling nitrogen at $-196°C$ (77 K) under normal atmospheric pressure as used in some cryosurgical techniques. It is just worth noting that ebullition occurs when the temperature of the liquid is such that its SVP equals the external pressure. Thus a liquid can be made to boil at any temperature above its freezing point, by reducing the external pressure appropriately. This has obvious applications in cryosurgery, where a suitable liquid could be made to boil at a chosen temperature by reducing the pressure.

Latent Heat of Vaporization

So long as we are considering a condition of dynamic equilibrium between liquid and vapour, there is no energy gain or loss by either phase and therefore no temperature change. In practice, the puddle on the ground, or the sweat on the skin, will have a region of atmospheric pressure above it, but the water vapour pressure will nearly always be less than the SVP for the prevailing temperatures. There will therefore not be a state of dynamic equilibrium, but there will be more molecules leaving the liquid per second than reaching it per second from the vapour. Thus there will be a net loss of liquid and the observer will say that evaporation is taking place. In fact, of course, both evaporation and condensation are always taking place, but the observer sees only the net effect and describes the process accordingly. In the case of the puddle or the skin a measurable mass of liquid water is being converted to vapour each second and in order to do this energy has to be provided. For each gram

of liquid that is converted to vapour without change of temperature, enough energy has to be provided to take some 33×10^{21} molecules from their state of vibration and minor migrations, to a state of random free flight and this amounts to about 2420 joules at 37°C (310 K). This is known as the latent heat of vaporization of the liquid and the energy has to be provided from the environment or from the bulk of the liquid itself. Hence the cooling of the skin during sweating. In the case of the mucosal surfaces that are involved in liquid-vapour equilibrium in ear, nose and throat, we clearly have an especially interesting situation where the space "above" the liquid surface is largely refilled with air from the atmosphere at each inspiration and this air will normally be much less than saturated with water vapour and at a temperature well below body temperature. It will rise a little in temperature and in percentage of saturation before being exhaled. Some parts of the system such as a closed mouth, may contain saturated vapour part of the time. Pressure will also be varying a little on each side of atmospheric during inspiration and expiration. Clearly net evaporation in some regions will lead to cooling of tissue which has to provide the energy for the necessary latent heat of vaporization. Examination of any one circumstance on a quantitative basis is of course a matter for biophysical study and may be exceedingly complex, though it is hoped that these notes will give useful pointers to the behaviour that may be expected.

Relative Humidity

This is a concept much used in meteorology and to some extent in pure physics. It simply expresses quantitatively the degree of saturation of any air sample i.e. the ratio

$$\frac{\text{(No. of molecules of the vapour actually present in a sample)}}{\text{(No. of molecules that would be present in the same sample if it were saturated)}}$$

and is usually multiplied by 100 to yield a percentage measure. Expressed in terms of pressure, the relative humidity (RH) becomes

$$\% \, RH = \frac{\text{(pressure of water vapour actually present in sample)}}{\text{(saturated vapour pressure of water at the same temperature)}} \times 100$$

The importance of the concept in the biophysics of the ear, nose and throat is in its indication of the rate at which evaporation will occur from a mucosal surface. There will be no net evaporation if the RH is 100 per cent: the smaller the value of RH in the body cavity, the greater the rate of evaporation will be, the greater risk of dry mouth and throat and greater cooling of the mucosal surfaces that do remain moist.

As will be seen from our graph of SVP against temperature, the denominator of the fraction goes up rapidly with temperature i.e. a sample of air can hold more water vapour as temperature rises. In our case, the temperature is always within narrow limits, say 35°C (308 K) to 40°C (313 K), although inspired air may be considerably colder. The short section of the graph of SVP against temperature, for this region, might almost be taken as linear. Although the situations with which we are concerned are complicated by flow and continual change of sample, they are simplified in that we can confine our attention to water, to a very restricted temperature range and neglect the effect of pressure variation.

SECTION III

GENETICS

9. GENETICAL BASIS FOR OTOLARYNGOLOGICAL DISORDERS

PAGE
121

9. GENETICAL BASIS FOR OTOLARYNGOLOGICAL DISORDERS

GEORGE ROBERT FRASER

THE NATURE OF MENDELIAN INHERITANCE

As is generally known, the modern science of genetics began with the work of the Augustinian monk Gregor Mendel in the second half of the nineteenth century. He was able to demonstrate in a bisexual organism, the pea, that the nature of the contribution passed from parent to offspring through the germ cells was particulate. Thus, he showed that the laws of heredity did not involve a blending

yy the yellow pea) are known as the *parental generation*. The pea is a *diploid* organism meaning that its chromosomes exist in homologous pairs, and the parental generation are homozygous meaning that the pair of genes they possess (their *genotype*) are the same. These genes exist in alternative forms *G* and *y* and these are known as *alleles*; they are located at a particular point or locus on one of the pea chromosomes where the biochemical processes leading to the colour of the pea are determined. The gametes formed by the parents contain only one of each pair of these

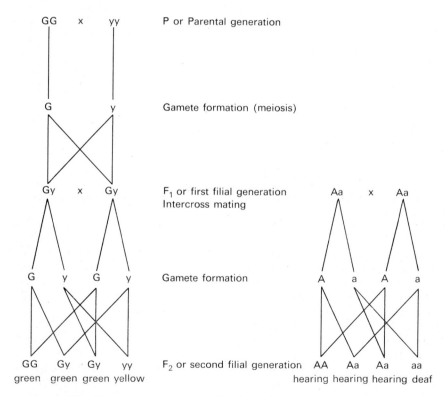

FIG. 1. Mendelian autosomal recessive inheritance. For further explanation see text.

of certain characteristics of the parents but conformed to a probabilistic expectation of a segregation of these characteristics in a dichotomous or polychotomous manner. Mendel's basic contribution can best be illustrated by a diagram drawn according to his original experiments with the pea and compared to an example more relevant to otology as such (Fig. 1).

There are a number of features in this diagram that need explanation. The original parents (*GG* the green pea and

chromosomes and are therefore said to be haploid (single). The process of reduction of the chromosomes from the diploid to the haploid state during gametogenesis is known as *meiosis*.

The offspring of these parents, known as the first *filial* or F_1 generation, are not of a colour intermediate between green and yellow but are all green. This is because of the phenomenon now known as *dominance*. This means that even one gene for the green trait is sufficient to assure this colour despite the presence of an allele for the yellow trait at the same locus on the paired homologous chromosome. We call this dominance of the green trait over the yellow. The F_1 generation are heterozygotes, meaning that the two paired alleles at the chromosomal locus under discussion are different rather than being the same as in the homozygous parental generation. When new matings take place within the F_1 generation, it will be seen that the offspring, known as the F_2, or second filial, generation, will consist of three green and one yellow pea since the two heterozygotes will be green like their parents. This is known as *recessive inheritance* and the yellow colour is a recessive trait because it was hidden in the F_1 generation and reappeared (having been present originally in the parental generation) in the F_2 generation. Thus, the well known Mendelian ratio of 3:1 (3 green; 1 yellow) is explained.

exist in allelic forms and this allelism consists in a difference which often involves only a single nucleotide pair in the pathological or mutant form. This however results in a difference in a particular triplet and the substitution of a different amino acid at a particular position in the specific protein. Such a substitution may seem numerically insignificant since each protein may be made up of several hundred amino acids but in fact it may have drastic effects as is evidenced by the case of S (sickle-cell) haemoglobin. Here the substitution of the amino acid valine, for glutamic acid at position 6 of the beta chain of haemoglobin, alters its function in such a fundamental manner that *SS* homozygotes suffer from a lethal disease, sickle-cell anaemia.

Unfortunately we are as yet very far from such a complete understanding of any form of hearing disorder or

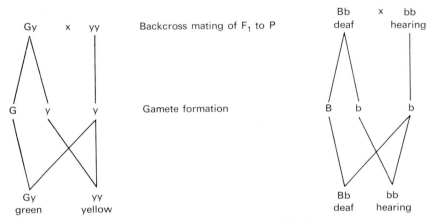

FIG. 2. Mendelian autosomal dominant inheritance.

These considerations may very simply be related to the field of otology as the second part of Fig. 1 shows. In this case the first filial generation is simply replaced by a couple who are heterozygous for one of the numerous alleles (*a*) responsible for the various types of recessive hearing loss. Their hearing is perfect because the normal allele *A* compensates for the effects of the abnormal allele *a* at the particular chromosomal locus at which the particular type of deafness is determined. One in four of their children however will be of the genetical constitution (genotype) *aa* and will therefore be deaf.

These very simple principles of particulate hereditary transmission which arose from the work of Mendel, are of paramount importance in otolaryngology, and indeed in all branches of medicine, today. The main progress which has been made since Mendel's day is that the particulate units which he hypothesized have now been defined as segments of deoxyribose nucleic acid (DNA) in a specific configuration at a locus on one of the chromosomes. Moreover, we now have at least a partial understanding of the chain of events by which this particular segment of DNA, or gene, exercises its final effect, whether this is to cause greenness in the pea or deafness in a child. Briefly, a genetical code exists which ensures that each triplet of nucleotide pairs constituting the DNA results in the insertion of a particular amino acid in a protein. Genes

other otolaryngological disease but, by this analogy, we may suppose that some recessive forms of hearing impairment, for example, are due to a single amino acid substitution in an enzyme vital to the development of normal hearing. This substitution affects the enzyme to such an extent that impaired hearing results from birth (or at least from earliest infancy since it is conceivable that the developing fetus may be shielded from this defect by maternal metabolism).

While this type of hereditary transmission is operative in most of the conditions for which Mendelian inheritance is responsible in otolaryngological practice, different but still basically simple patterns may be seen. Dominant transmission is seen when an abnormal allele causes disease even in the presence of a normal allele, and Fig. 2 is an extension of Fig. 1 which explains this type of transmission. To take Mendel's original experiments, we can perform a backcross of the F_1 generation to the recessive parent rather than an intercross between members of the F_1 generation. If now greenness is regarded as a disease it will be seen that half the offspring will be affected. The second part of Fig. 2 shows the corresponding situation in terms of human deafness; the pathological allele in this case is denoted as *B* to distinguish it from the *a* of Fig. 1. Thus, the hallmark of dominant inheritance is the vertical nature of the transmission from one generation to the next in contrast to the horizontal type in recessive inheritance, where only one generation is affected. The segregation ratio of affected to unaffected offspring is 1:1 rather than the 1:3 characteristic of recessive inheritance.

At this stage two further genetical concepts must be introduced. The situation does not always reflect a simple dichotomy between greenness and yellowness or complete deafness and normal hearing. Intermediate stages may exist in that the hearing loss may be unilateral, mild or both. This variation in the effect of the mutant or abnormal allele we call *expressivity*. Sometimes an individual may have apparently normal hearing despite the fact that he is carrying an allele which is sufficient to cause profound deafness in other members of the same family. This lower extreme of expressivity we term *failure of penetrance*.

transmission and, therefore, are presumably related to changes at a single locus or small segment of a chromosome. The latest edition of a catalogue of such traits (McKusick, 1974) contains brief details of 1142 conditions, mostly diseases or pathological states, presumably determined at distinct gene loci which are well documented as being inherited in a Mendelian manner. They are broken down as follows: 583 autosomal dominant, 466 autosomal recessive and 93 X-linked. In addition, a further 1194 conditions are included (635 autosomal dominant, 481 autosomal recessive, 78 X-linked) where the evidence of Mendelian inheritance is not entirely convincing, but it is probable that in the large majority this is in fact the correct explanation.

This is simply the total of recognized conditions of this

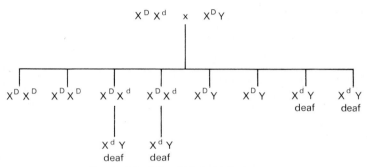

FIG. 3. Mendelian X-linked inheritance.
D is the normal and d the pathological allele situated at a locus on the X-chromosome. Thus $X^D X^D$ is a normally hearing homozygous female, $X^D X^d$ is a normally hearing heterozygous female, $X^D Y$ is a normally hearing male and $X^d Y$ is a deaf male. The stage of gametogenesis is omittted and a sibship of eight children is shown to illustrate the types of relationship between persons affected with a condition inherited in an X-linked manner, i.e. brothers, maternal nephews, uncles and male first cousins.

The third and last of these simple mechanisms of Mendelian inheritance to be discussed is that which involves traits determined on the X chromosome. The complement of man's 46 chromosomes is made up of 22 pairs of homologous autosomes (and the previous discussion has referred to these) and a pair of sex chromosomes which are homologous (XX) in females but not in males. The latter have only one X chromosome and a small Y chromosome which seems to contain few or no gene loci of the type under discussion. Figure 3 shows the pattern of inheritance to be expected of a type of deafness determined on the X chromosome; it may occur in several generations and is transmitted to males through unaffected females. This type of inheritance is of course very well-known; and colour blindness is determined in this way. In addition, even in biblical times, these peculiarities of the transmission of haemophilia were understood because of their relevance to the operation of circumcision.

THE RELEVANCE OF MENDELIAN INHERITANCE AND OTHER GENETICAL MECHANISMS TO OTOLARYNGOLOGY

There is a vast variety of disorders and diseases in the human race which follow these simple Mendelian laws of

nature, and of course the real number of possible aberrations of this type may be much larger. Of these conditions, a large proportion may present in otolaryngological practice for two main reasons:

(1) The development and maintenance of normal hearing is a process of very great complexity and, therefore, susceptible to a vast variety of disturbances. Thus, quite apart from Mendelian forms of deafness which do not involve lesions in other systems, hearing loss of all degrees may be implicated in a very large number of syndromes associated with a wide variety of concomitant disorders.

(2) A substantial proportion of conditions inherited in a Mendelian manner lead to malformations which are often of a complex nature. Quite apart from any influence such malformations may have on hearing, other structures within the purview of an otolaryngologist may be involved. There would be little point in attempting to enumerate here the various Mendelian conditions which may come to the attention of the otolaryngologist. For a simple list with minimal details, reference may be made to the catalogue already mentioned, while a review such as that of Schwarz and his associates (1964) may be consulted for a description of the hereditary aspects of anomalies and malformations

in this region. The more specific topic of deafness, especially profound deafness in childhood, is extensively discussed in various publications (Fraser, 1964; Konigsmark, 1969; Fraser, 1975). Instead of an enumeration, what will be done is to discuss in brief detail some characteristic types of these conditions which may come to the attention of an otolaryngologist.

Profound Childhood Deafness

Undoubtedly the most common type of serious condition of this sort is profound childhood deafness. The reviews of Fraser (1964, 1975) and of Konigsmark (1969) give some idea of the astonishing biological heterogeneity of those forms of this condition which are not determined primarily by exogenous factors which may be operative in pre-natal life (rubella), peri-natal life (kernicterus) or in infancy or childhood (meningitis). After such exogenous causes have been excluded (and this is often no easy matter especially retrospectively), the remainder of cases, with only a few exceptions, are inherited in a Mendelian manner. In the majority, the mechanism of transmission is autosomal recessive but autosomal dominant and X-linked forms are also found. This heterogeneity is further manifested by the fact that, within each of these categories, many different forms may occur. Thus, within the autosomal recessive group, at least some dozen quite distinct entities exist determined at different gene loci. The evidence for this statement is threefold. First, clinical, in that profound childhood deafness is a component of several syndromes in which the very disparate nature of the accompanying features makes it certain that quite different entities are involved. Among the more common of these syndromes are those of Pendred (hearing loss with goitre), of Usher (hearing loss with retinitis pigmentosa), and of Jervell and Lange-Nielsen (hearing loss with attacks of cardiac syncope which may terminate fatally, characterized by a unique abnormality of the electrocardiogram). A large number of rarer syndromes exist in this autosomal recessive group. In most of these syndromes the hearing loss is sensorineural but occasionally it is conductive and associated with actual malformation of the outer, middle or internal ears.

The second type of evidence for the genetical multiplicity of autosomal recessive types of profound childhood deafness comes from the results of matings between persons so afflicted. Because this condition tends to lead to educational and social segregation throughout life, it is natural that marriages should take place almost entirely within the deaf community. Since autosomal recessive inheritance accounts for a large proportion of cases in this group, many of these marriages are between persons with this type of deafness. The laws of simple Mendelian inheritance predicate in such cases that, if the children are all deaf, the same genetical entity is involved in the two parents whereas if, as often happens, all the children are normally hearing, the types of autosomal recessive deafness in the two parents must be different (*see* Fig. 4).

The third type of evidence concerning the multiplicity of genetical forms of autosomal recessive hearing loss is somewhat more technical. Autosomal recessive conditions in general are more common among the offspring of related parents (i.e. first cousins) than among those of unrelated persons. This is simply because the abnormal or mutant alleles causing these conditions are rare in the general population and since first cousins share two of their four grandparents it is somewhat more likely that they would each carry one of these rare abnormal alleles, both being derived from a common grandparent, than would unrelated marriage partners who would have to

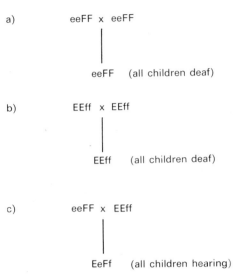

FIG. 4. Matings between persons with autosomal recessive deafness.

Two distinct loci at which pathological alleles e and f cause deafness in homozygotes ee and ff are depicted. Double heterozygotes (EeFf) enjoy normal hearing.

carry two quite independent mutant alleles. A simple mathematical relationship exists between the size of this excess of consanguineous matings between the parents of children with a particular autosomal recessive condition and its frequency in the general population. In the case of autosomal recessive deafness, this relationship deviates strongly in a direction which suggests that this is not a homogenous group but is made up of many component entities. In fact, this consanquinity rate among parents is much higher than would be expected suggesting that the condition is made up of many sub-classes, each naturally much lower in population frequency then the whole.

The same degree of biological heterogeneity is seen among forms of dominant profound childhood deafness. Once again forms exist where the deafness seems to be an isolated phenomenon, while in others it is associated with concomitant clinical features in other systems. A particularly well-delineated group of such syndromes is that in which impaired hearing occurs together with pigmentary anomalies. In the classical form of this condition, known as *Waardenburg's syndrome*, a hearing loss coexists with hypopigmentation which may affect large patches of skin, the hair, eye lashes, the irides and ocular fundi. Since the hypopigmentation is segmental, the very striking phenomenon of *heterochromia* of the irides may occur meaning that different colours may be found in the two irides. This heterochromia may be total in that each iris may be of a different colour (usually blue and brown), or segmental, indicating that segments of different colouration may occur in one or both irides. This is of course a very striking phenomenon and together with the leucism or partial depigmentation of skin and hair serves to identify such children easily. In addition, they show a most unusual morphological anomaly of the facial structure known as *telecanthus*, involving a lateral displacement of the medial canthi of the eyelid. While Waardenburg's syndrome is inherited in a dominant manner, the concepts of variable expressivity and penetrance alluded to above are of the utmost importance in this condition. Thus, only a few persons who possess the abnormal allele show all the features of the syndrome and only a small minority are in fact affected with profound bilateral deafness which is the sole detrimental feature of the condition. Many may in fact escape hearing loss altogether.

There seems to be some basic connection between the development of pigmentation and of hearing during embryogenesis, since Waardenburg's syndrome is by no means the only condition in which disorders of the two are associated. Two or even possibly three such distinct autosomal dominant conditions exist and in one apparently unique family the association seems to be inherited in an X-linked manner (Margolis, 1962; Ziprkowski *et al.*, 1962). It is not at all clear whether the autosomal dominant associations of hearing loss with pigmentary anomalies are determined at the same or at different gene loci but a very important discriminating feature is that the morphological anomaly of the eyelid occurs in most members of some families but not at all in affected members of other families. This suggests that at least two genetically quite distinct entities may be involved.

The hearing disorder in these conditions in which pigmentary anomalies are associated is of the sensorineural type but many autosomal dominant types of hearing loss exist in which the osseous part of the auditory apparatus is involved in a malformation affecting a wider area of the facial skeleton, thus giving rise to a primarily conductive form of hearing loss. The best known of these is the *Treacher Collins syndrome* (mandibulo-facial dysostosis). This consists of abnormalities of the outer, middle, and, occasionally, the internal ear, associated with anti-mongoloid palpebral fissures, coloboma of the lower eyelids, hypoplasia of the malar bone and mandible, macrostomia, high palate and malformed teeth, blind fistulae between the angles of the mouth and the ears and abnormal implantation of the facial hair. These deformities may occur in any combination and with varying degrees of severity. They may often be unilateral. Because of this marked variability, the mandibulo-facial dysostosis does not often lead to profound childhood deafness.

Apart from these syndromes, as in the case of autosomal recessive hearing loss, forms of autosomal dominant hearing loss exist in which this represents an isolated lesion without evidence of involvement of other body systems. Again, variable expressivity and lack of penetrance are rather common though the extent seems to vary from family to family, probably because, as in the case of autosomal recessive inheritance, different gene loci are involved. Thus, in some families, expressivity and penetrance are complete and profound bilateral childhood deafness is transmitted in a regular Mendelian manner to half the offspring of affected persons while, in others, the pattern is for more irregular and some persons carrying the abnormal allele may be unilaterally, or mildly affected, or both.

In the case of X-linked hearing disorders also, forms exist which are uncomplicated by other clinical features while others form part of syndromes. One such disorder has already been mentioned above (sensorineural hearing loss with pigmentary anomalies). Another is a fixation of the stapes base (Nance, *et al.*, 1971). A characteristic feature of this condition is abnormal patency of the cochlear aqueduct which tends to result in a profuse flow of perilymphatic fluid if surgery is attempted to correct the malformation.

So far, a wide variety of genetically determined conditions has been discussed which usually lead to profound childhood deafness. Although this is not, in population terms, a very uncommon condition, in that perhaps one person in a thousand is affected (half of these cases being due to the Mendelian mechanisms discussed above) such persons do not of course constitute a large proportion of an otolaryngological practice. The condition has, however, been discussed in some detail since it illustrates particularly well the mechanisms of simple inheritance.

Adult Hearing Disorders: Mendelian and Quantitative Inheritance

Milder types of hearing loss which may arise in adult life form a far greater part of otolaryngological practice. These may be sensorineural in nature and, in such cases, are often determined in a simple Mendelian manner, but, in contrast to the profound childhood variety, are more frequently autosomal dominant than recessive. A particularly well known type of autosomal dominant hearing loss of moderately severe type is Alport's syndrome (impaired hearing with nephritis). It is of course difficult in any given case to define a sharp dividing line between profound and mild forms of hearing impairment and, as already pointed out above, the same abnormal genotype can cause either form in members of the same family. Rather, the range of hearing loss is continuous in nature and it is the age of onset as well as the degree which will determine whether problems occur with the learning of speech and whether or not educational and social segregation will take place. Simple genetical factors are definitely proportionately more important in the category of profound childhood deafness then in the adult varieties of sensorineural hearing loss where many other causes may be operative. Indeed, ageing itself is an important cause and many older people are seriously inconvenienced by what must be regarded in some sense as a natural and inescapable deterioration of hearing.

Among the genetically determined autosomal dominant

forms of sensorineural hearing loss some may be distinguished by audiometric patterns. Thus a constant mid-tone hearing loss among affected members of the same family would suggest the presence of an abnormal allele which is distinct from those causing less specific types of hearing loss in other families.

The situation is precisely the same with milder types of conductive loss. In fact conductive hearing loss very rarely leads to impairment sufficiently profound to require educational segregation, and this applies to most cases of the syndromes mentioned in the preceding section. Thus, cases of these conditions are only infrequently seen among educationally segregated children. A well-known syndrome of this type which only very exceptionally leads to profound deafness in childhood is *osteogenesis imperfecta*. The most common type of conductive hearing loss of adult life is of course otosclerosis and the hereditary basis of this condition is far less simple than that of the forms of sensorineural hearing loss discussed thus far. Some investigators, for example Morrison (1967), consider that this is an autosomal dominant condition of variable expressivity with frequent failure of penetrance, thus accounting for the very irregular patterns of familial incidence which are observed. The situation, however, is likely to be far more complicated. First, otosclerosis is probably a biologically and genetically heterogeneous entity and, while such an explanation may apply in some families, in many cases more complex mechanisms are likely to be operative.

A condition is said to be transmitted in a Mendelian manner, as in the examples discussed above, if abnormal alleles at a single chromosomal locus are sufficient to cause it (with the reservation that variable expressivity and failure of penetrance may modify the effects of the abnormal genotype). However, in the case of many pathological conditions (and these include such common diseases as diabetes, hypertension, atherosclerosis and cancer), the genotype of the individual usually determines only a predisposition to the disease and in such cases multiple alleles at multiple gene loci may be involved. Naturally, the mathematical formulation of the pattern of inheritance to be expected under such conditions is very complex and this pattern is further profoundly influenced by environmental factors involving the mode of life of the individual. Nevertheless, since members of a family naturally tend to resemble each other in their total genetical endowment, it is not surprising that such diseases tend to show familial aggregation, though this does not follow any of the simple patterns of Mendelian inheritance discussed above. This type of mechanism is often known as *quantitative inheritance*, implying that many genes are involved in the synergistic determination of a quantitative trait. The operation of this kind of inheritance may most clearly be seen in the case of a trait such as height, and of course it is a matter of common observation that tall parents tend to have tall children and the converse is equally true for shortness. The same kind of mechanism may well operate in determining the predisposition to diseases such as those mentioned above and also possibly to the processes which can lead to otosclerosis. Thus, in the case of

height, it is supposed that the trait is determined by the additive action of many genes each of small effect, but this stipulation need not always apply. Some of these many genes may play a relatively large role in comparison to the others in the causation of otosclerosis and the other diseases mentioned.

In these cases, aetiology is said to be *multifactorial*, implying the interaction not only of many genes but also of exogenous influences. In the case of diabetes, these would involve the mode of life such as diet, degree of exposure to stress and degree of physical activity. In the case of otosclerosis, such factors are more difficult to define, but they probably exist. One factor which certainly seems to be of importance is sex, and presumably the hormonal milieu connected with such events as pregnancy and the menopause increases the genetically determined predisposition with the result that more females are affected than males.

In fact, every disease is to some extent genetically determined in that persons will vary in their susceptibility or predisposition because of their genotype. Thus the smoking of cigarettes cannot be regarded as the sole cause of carcinoma of the lung; clearly among persons whose exposure to cigarette smoke is very similar only a proportion will acquire the disease and these will do so after varying lengths of exposure. This variation is largely controlled by the genetically determined degree of susceptibility of the persons involved and it might be argued that everyone would eventually have carcinoma of the lung if they live long enough and if they do not die of other diseases first. This kind of reasoning implies that the sensorineural variety of hearing impairment associated with ageing is also under the influence of complex multi-genic mechanisms of this sort. This genetically determined predisposition may be aggravated by exogenous influences. In accordance with the analogy of carcinoma of the lung mentioned above, hearing may be expected gradually to fail with age in everyone if they live long enough and it is the rate of this gradual failure which may be influenced by such genetical factors.

Unfortunately, in the case of hearing loss we are at present largely ignorant of the environmental circumstances which will precipitate* adult hearing impairments, whether sensorineural or conductive; nor do we have any laboratory methods of identifying persons who are genetically exceptionally susceptible. Clearly, when our knowledge of these questions is more complete, we could take steps to persuade persons who are genetically susceptible to take precautionary measures to avoid the exogenous precipitating factors. It should be noted that, even in the absence of any laboratory parameters which could be used to measure genetically determined susceptibility, the existence of one or more affected close relatives does afford some indication that an individual is at greater than average risk.

To turn to the other extreme of life, i.e. childhood rather than old age, we may suppose that susceptibility to otitis media may be determined in the same complex manner. Thus, some genes may act synergistically to cause an

* Constant exposure to noise is a well-recognized factor of this type.

unusual degree of susceptibility to infection by the organisms which cause this condition, while other genes may determine minor anomalies of structure which make it easier for these organisms to gain access to the middle ear.

Thus, whether we are dealing with chronic otitis media, with presbyacusis or possibly, with otosclerosis, a tendency to familial aggregation of cases may be seen due to complex genetical influences even though simple Mendelian mechanisms may not be operative. As we have seen, many less common types of hearing disorder exist which are determined by simple Mendelian inheritance.

Other Conditions in Otolaryngological Practice

Great emphasis has been laid on genetical aspects of hearing impairment but, of course, as pointed out in the introduction, genetically determined conditions may occur in otolaryngological practice in which hearing is not involved. In a sense this is a truism since what has been said above concerning the complex genetical basis of otitis media applies equally to tonsillitis, for example, so that even a common condition of this type is strongly influenced by genetical factors.

Ménière's disease is, of course, another very common otological problem in some parts of the world and the situation is likely to be analogous to that applying to otosclerosis. Thus, it is probable that this is a heterogeneous entity and that it is determined by a complex interplay of environmental precipitating factors with an underlying susceptibility determined by the synergistic effect of many genes.

In addition, other conditions which may occur in otolaryngological practice may be inherited in a simple Mendelian manner. These include several distinct types of malformations of the auricle involving the structure of the cartilage and the presence of fistulae or appendages. Such simple Mendelian inheritance may apply also to some malformations of other structures of the head and neck region such as the nose and the larynx.

CHROMOSOMAL ABERRATIONS

Mendelian inheritance may result not only from changes in a single nucleotide base pair, leading to a substitution of a single amino acid in a particular protein; it may also be due to changes in larger segments of chromosomal material. It has become possible within the last 20 years to examine the chromosomes of an individual. The normal chromosomal constitution of an individual (the *karyotype*) consists of 46 chromosomes. It has already been described in connection with the mechanisms of X-linked inheritance. Gross deviations from this normal karyotype occur, and these can be detected by modern microscopic methods. Within the very recent past, refinements of staining techniques have been introduced (fluorescence and Giemsa banding) which can be used to define such abnormalities more accurately. Gross chromosomal aberrations are in fact probably very common in the early zygote at the moment of fertilization but fortunately most of them lead to early miscarriage. Nevertheless, perhaps as many as 0·5 per cent of all infants born are affected by a major chromosomal aberration. The most serious of these are the autosomal trisomies, where one particular pair of autosomes is present in triplicate, and such a condition is usually lethal, the only exception being Down's syndrome (mongolism) due to trisomy of chromosome 21. Such trisomies are associated with major malformations of virtually every organ system including the auditory apparatus and the larynx. In mongolism, these malformations of the auditory system are rather minor though mild hearing loss of a conductive nature is common in this condition.

Anomalies of the sex chromosomes lead to less serious results and monosomy (XO or Turner's syndrome) as well as trisomies (XXX, XXY, XYY) can occur; an even higher number of sex chromosomes (tetra and pentasomies) may be found in some individuals. Most of these conditions are compatible with a relatively normal life but mild hearing loss may often be found perhaps due to minor malformations of the auditory apparatus. A whole host of other chromosomal anomalies has been detected which do not involve the loss or gain of an entire chromosome. These can consist of deletions or inversions of segments of a chromosome or of translocations of material from one chromosome to another. In general, familial aggregation of pathological conditions due to overt chromosomal anomalies of this type, often involving the auditory apparatus as part of a complex malformation syndrome, is unusual but exceptions occur. Thus, a person with mongolism due to trisomy 21 will produce a proportion of gametes with two 21 chromosomes rather than one and a mongol child will occasionally result, simulating Mendelian dominant inheritance, though in general, such persons are too retarded to procreate.

Translocations, inversions and deletions may also lead to the production of abnormal gametes, and familial aggregation may occur in such circumstances though not in any regular Mendelian manner. A detailed consideration of the mechanism of familial aggregation in such situations would be out of place in such a text as this but an important point which should be made is that such gross chromosomal anomalies and point mutations due to changes in a single nucleotide pair are the two extremes of what is probably a continuous range of size of chromosomal changes. Thus, conditions which are apparently inherited in a Mendelian manner and are not associated with overt chromosomal aberrations may be due to smaller structural changes beyond the power of modern microscopic techniques to detect. Since it has already been stated that such anomalies do not lead to regular patterns of Mendelian inheritance, this may provide an explanation of some pedigrees in which very irregular patterns of dominant inheritance with frequent failure of penetrance occur.

CONGENITAL MALFORMATIONS

Congenital malformations may be inherited in a simple Mendelian manner as, for example, the dominant Treacher Collins syndrome (*see* earlier). They may also be due to chromosomal aberrations, as discussed in the preceding section, or to exogenous factors as in the rubella syndrome. A substantial proportion of cases, however, do not seem to be determined in a simple manner but are presumably due to the synergistic effects of multiple genes possibly interacting with environmental factors, in much the same way as was postulated for otosclerosis. An example of this group of conditions may well be Wildervanck's syndrome which combines hearing loss, associated with malformations of the outer, middle and/or internal ear, with the Klippel-Feil anomaly of the spine. Although the Klippel-Feil malformation itself seems to occur with equal frequency in the two sexes, its association with impaired hearing occurs much more often in girls, in a ratio of ten or more to one boy. The reason for this is not clear but a predilection for one or the other sex is a characteristic feature of congenital malformations as a whole, though it is usually less pronounced. Presumably, this phenomenon is due to the fact that one sex has a lower threshold of resistance to the combination of genetical and environmental factors determining a particular defect of embryogenesis. Since embryogenesis takes a substantially different course in the two sexes, such variations in resistance would not be surprising.

GENETICAL COUNSELLING: (THE PRACTICAL APPLICATION OF GENETICS IN OTOLARYNGOLOGY)

The main practical problem in which a knowledge of simple genetical principles is of importance to the otolaryngologist is that of profound deafness in childhood since this is a much more serious handicap than most forms of adult deafness, and therapy is not possible apart from management by educational measures. In this situation, special stress must be laid on the possibility of prevention. About half of all cases of profound childhood deafness are due to simple Mendelian inheritance, and it is only with this half that the ensuing discussion deals. The question of preventing hearing disorders due to exogenous causes is one which pertains to general medical care and involves such questions as avoidance of rubella in pregnancy through immunization programs and improved management of perinatal problems, and of meningitis in infancy and childhood.

Prevention of genetically determined hearing loss comes within the province of genetical counselling. Broadly defined, this involves detection of persons at risk of giving birth to a child defective for genetical reasons, and giving them advice which can be supported by ancillary measures for avoiding such risks. Of all cases of impaired hearing determined by Mendelian inheritance, about two-thirds are due to autosomal recessive mechanisms. Unfortunately, it is not possible to detect the heterozygous state of the parents and, therefore, in such a situation counselling can only be retrospective, that is after the birth of an affected child. Clearly, if the condition is recessive, in such a case the parents run a risk of 25 per cent that each subsequent child born to them will be affected (*see* Fig. 1). However, there is only a limited number of situations in which such

recessive inheritance can be unequivocally detected in view of the extreme biological heterogeneity of profound childhood deafness. These circumstances include situations in which there are two or more affected sibs at the time the couple in question comes for counselling, situations in which the parents are consanguineous and cases where a defined autosomal recessive syndrome can be identified. In other circumstances, it may be equally clear that, in an isolated case (that is to say when there is a deaf child without affected sibs or other relatives), the deafness is due to exogenous causes. This may be because the child shows other evidence of rubella embryopathy or because there is good evidence that he heard normally before an attack of, say, meningitis in infancy. In other cases, the evidence for an exogenous cause may be strong but not unequivocal as, for example, when the child passed through a particularly turbulent perinatal period perhaps with extreme prematurity and/or jaundice as complicating factors. When the cause of a hearing loss can be identified as being exogenous, the risk of recurrence in subsequent children is essentially zero and, therefore, it is extremely important to be able to distinguish between this situation and recessive inheritance, whether X-linked or autosomal, with its risk of recurrence of 25 per cent. In many instances, however, when the hearing impaired child is an isolated case it is quite impossible to make this distinction. Fraser (1975) has shown that, in such cases, the risk for subsequent children is about 10 per cent indicating that about 40 per cent of such isolated cases owe their deafness to recessive inheritance. The remaining 60 per cent include cases of dominant hearing loss due to fresh mutation and cases of loss due to exogenous causes which have not been identified. The risk of recurrence in these situations is very low.

These empirical risk figures can be somewhat modified by partial or circumstantial evidence. Thus, increased parental ages (especially paternal) at the birth of a hearing impaired child are suggestive of a mutation for autosomal dominant hearing loss since it is known that the incidence of some mutations of this type increases with paternal age. Again, total deafness without any residual hearing is very suggestive of an infection such as meningitis which may not have been diagnosed as such in infancy. In both these cases, the chance of recurrence would essentially be zero but such evidence is of course inconclusive. However, the chance of recessive inheritance is somewhat greater if an only child is deaf; the more hearing children there are, the smaller is the relative risk of autosomal recessive inheritance. This can readily be seen by an extreme example of a deaf child who is the 15th of a family, all his sibs having normal hearing. Clearly, recessive inheritance is relatively unlikely to have affected only 1 of 15 children, in view of the 25 per cent chance that each one has of being deaf.

This discussion applies equally to recessive inheritance, whether autosomal or X-linked. In the latter case, however, further evidence of the true nature of the condition may be provided by involvement of other relatives such as maternal uncles or first cousins (*see* Fig. 3).

The situation with regard to genetical counselling in connection with autosomal dominant hearing loss is also complex since, as pointed out above, the degree of expressivity and the proportion of cases of failure of penetrance vary from family to family. In the simplest case, i.e. in families where transmission is regular and expressivity is marked, a risk figure of 50 per cent can be given, while in others, where irregular dominant transmission seems to be involved, the risk of transmission of the abnormal gene remains 50 per cent but the risk of a hearing loss may be considerably less. Furthermore, the loss may be unilateral and/or mild rather than profound and bilateral. Thus, the advice regarding risks of recurrence if a hearing impaired child is born and dominant inheritance seems to be implicated must depend on the family history and on estimates of the expressivity and penetrance of the particular allele involved.

The last section involves consideration of the transmission of a hearing loss from parent to child and, in fact, this is a common problem in the field of genetical counselling even when no affected child has been born. Because of their educational and social segregation from early life and because of their isolation from the outside world on account of difficulty with communication, it is not surprising that those affected by profound childhood deafness very often marry within their own community (assortative mating). Such marriages only give rise to a small minority of deaf children but the problem of counselling such couples is a complex one. Deaf children are to be expected in two main classes of such marriages. In the first, one of the partners has a dominant hearing disorder and the counselling situation is exactly the same as previously discussed for such families even when the spouse has normal hearing. In the second class, both partners have the same type of autosomal recessive hearing disorder and, as discussed earlier, all their children may be expected to be deaf. Even though autosomal recessive inheritance accounts for about one-third of all cases of profound childhood deafness, such marriages are rare because there are so many different types determined at different gene loci so that, even within the group of autosomal recessive deafness, marriages are much more frequent between partners with different types (with the children expected to have normal hearing) than with the same type.

One of the most typical situations coming to the attention of a genetical counsellor is that where a couple has a child with an autosomal recessive disorder which in the context of the present discussion could be Pendred's syndrome of a hearing loss with goitre. Until very recently, the only advice which could be given to such couples to obviate the risk of 25 per cent that each subsequent child be affected was adoption, or, in a few cases, artificial insemination by an unrelated donor who would, of course, be extremely unlikely to be a heterozygous carrier of the rare allele responsible for Pendred's syndrome. In the last few years, techniques have been developed in the case of a great variety of autosomal recessive diseases to make a diagnosis in fetal life by ante-natal examination of the amniotic fluid. Abortion may then be considered if the fetus is of the affected genotype. Unfortunately as mentioned earlier we have insufficient knowledge of the biochemical basis of any form of auditory disorder to be able to use this technique of ante-natal diagnosis at present in this condition but this situation may change in the future. The ethical and moral basis of this technique of selective abortion is outside the purview of this presentation but it does allow a couple by monitoring of each pregnancy to achieve their desired number of normal children. Of course, this technique and, indeed, genetical counselling in general could be far more effective if advice could be prospective, that is if couples at risk could be identified before the birth of the first affected child. However, as pointed out earlier, at the present time we have no methods available for identifying heterozygotes. This is of course another aspect of our ignorance of the biochemical basis of any type of autosomal recessive hearing loss.

POSSIBILITIES OF TREATMENT

When such understanding comes it will open up perspectives of treatment as well as of prevention. The model for this is the disease phenylketonuria for which screening at birth is practised in many populations. Affected children are given a special diet which is free of phenylalanine. This avoids the accumulation of toxic metabolites of this amino acid which is presumed to be responsible for the pathological features of this condition. We may expect that, in the not too distant future, we will gain some knowledge regarding the exact nature of the biochemical defects determining at least some types of auditory disorders. Garrod's term of inborn error of metabolism is now generally applied to such diseases as phenylketonuria and galactosaemia, where the nature of the enzymatic defect is relatively well understood. These are autosomal recessive conditions and, in general, such enzymatic defects are likely to be associated with recessive inheritance.* Possibly in these future attempts at the unravelling of the aberrant pathways of metabolism involved in recessive hearing loss, the existence of autosomal recessive syndromes in which hearing loss coexists with conditions such as goitre (Pendred's syndrome), retinitsi pigmentosa (Usher's syndrome) and unique abnormalities of cardiac conduction (syndrome of Jervell and Lange-Nielsen) may provide clues. Thus, for example, if our understanding of the biochemical basis of hearing and of cardiac conduction were more complete, we should be able to pin-point the error which would lead to the syndrome of Jervell and Lange-Nielsen. With such understanding might come possibilities of mitigating the effects of the abnormal gene after birth, especially since it seems that, in such conditions as phenylketonuria and galactosaemia, the damage is mainly postnatal, presumably because the fetus is largely protected by maternal metabolism.

In the case of some autosomal dominant syndromes, the presence of disorders of pigmentation at birth suggests that the damage to hearing may be pre-natal in origin, though the work of Bosher and Hallpike (1965) in cats affected with an analogous condition indicates that this may not in fact be so. Whether the damage is pre-natal or not, however, the existence of multiple examples of

* This is because, in heterozygotes, the presence of the normal allele will usually compensate sufficiently for that of the abnormal one.

failure of penetrance with respect to the auditory component in such syndromes may eventually provide knowledge concerning a natural mechanism of escape from the effects of the pathological allele which might help in devising an analogous treatment, whether pre- or post-natal, for infants known to be at risk.

It seems that we are perhaps not making sufficient use of these syndromes, regarded as experiments of Nature, in the study of the aetiology and possible treatment of auditory disorders, and it is fitting to conclude with a remarkably prescient reflection written by Harvey in 1657:

"Nature is nowhere accustomed more openly to display her secret mysteries than in cases where she shows traces of her workings apart from the beaten path; nor is there any better way to advance the proper practice of medicine than to give our minds to the discovery of the usual law of Nature by careful investigation of cases of rarer forms of disease. For it has been found, in almost all things, that what they contain of useful or applicable nature is hardly perceived unless we are deprived of them, or they become deranged in some way."

REFERENCES

Bosher, S. K. and Hallpike, C. S. (1965), *Proc. roy. Soc. B*, **162**, 147.

Fraser, G. R. (1964), *J. Med. Genet.*, **1**, 118.

Fraser, G. R. (1975), *The Causes of Profound Deafness in Childhood. A Study of 3535 Individuals with Severe Auditory Handicaps Present at Birth or of Early Onset.* In Press. Johns Hopkins Press, Baltimore.

Konigsmark, B. W. (1969), *New Engl. J. Med.*, **281**, 713, 774 and 827.

Margolis, E. (1962), *Acta genet. (Basel)*, **12**, 12.

McKusick, V. A. (1974), *Mendelian Inheritance in Man. Catalogs of Autosomal Dominant, Autosomal Recessive, and X-linked Phenotypes* 4th edition. Baltimore: Johns Hopkins Press.

Morison, A. W. (1967), *Ann. roy. Coll. Surg. Engl.*, **41**, 202.

Nance, W. E., Setliff, R. C., McLeod, A., Sweeney, A., Cooper, C. and McConnell, F.(1971), *Birth Defects: Orig. Art. Ser.*, **7**(**4**), 64.

Schwarz, M., Becker, P. E. and Jorgensen, G. (1964), "Anomalien, Missbildungen und Krankheiten der Ohren, der Nase und des Halses," in *Humangenetik*, Vol. IV, p. 248 (P. E. Becker, Ed.). Stuttgart: Thieme.

Ziprkowski, L., Krakowski, A., Adam, A., Costeff, H. and Sadé, J. (1962), *Arch. Derm.*, **86**, 530.

SECTION IV

ENVIRONMENTAL SCIENCES

PAGE

10. EPIDEMIOLOGY   133

11. HEARING CONSERVATION AND NOISE REDUCTION   151

10. EPIDEMIOLOGY AND OTOLARYNGOLOGY

R. HINCHCLIFFE

INTRODUCTION

As Acheson points out (1971), epidemiology is now widely understood to be the science that deals with the prevalence, distribution and control of disease in a population, whether or not the disease in question is epidemic or communicable. The most important thing about epidemiology is measurement, since it depends upon a consideration of environmental and genetic factors and an ability to identify and measure relationships (Pickering, 1970). Clinicians in general have thus come to appreciate the value of this particular science in the application of whatever specialty with which they are concerned. Indeed, speaking as a clinician, Arnott (1954) has referred to the extension of the epidemiological approach beyond the infectious fevers as the most exciting feature of current medical science. However, epidemiology is not new. Hippocrates clearly appreciated the need to study disease in relation to environmental factors. Four and a half centuries ago, Paracelsus, who urged doctors to travel to study disease (Sigerist, 1941), noted the high prevalence of lung cancer in miners of the Erzgebirge. Over 200 years ago, Nils Skragge in Scandinavia was studying occupational hearing loss in coppersmiths and blacksmiths.

USES

(1) Elucidating the Nature of Diseases

In the nineteenth century, when epidemiology was endeavouring to elucidate the nature of the communicable fevers, Snow was able to deduce the nature of cholera. Later in that century, Takaki, conducting epidemiological studies in the Japanese navy, demonstrated that beri-beri was due to the lack of some essential nutritional factor. The initial observations of Moore and of Clark some 40 years ago on the Nigerian oto-neuro-ophthalmological syndrome have been extended, using epidemiological techniques, by Osuntokun and his associates (1969). In another African venture, the initial observation of Cook at the beginning of the century on "a little Mohammedan child with a large malignant tumour of the jaw" has been brilliantly extended by Burkitt in connection with the neoplasm which now bears his name. Indeed such have been the advances in the application of the epidemiological method to medicine in general, and otolaryngology in particular, over the past 20 years, that there is now scarcely a single major—or minor—disorder which has escaped the scrutiny of the epidemiologist.

However, it must be emphasized that the ultimate elucidation of these disorders has been due to a combination of the epidemiological method with the various laboratory sciences. Koch's bacteriological studies provided the necessary proof for Snow's hypothesis regarding the cause of cholera. The biochemical studies of Eijkman, of Funk and of Peters eventually confirmed Takaki's observation that beri-beri was due to lack of a nutritional factor. The indications from epidemiology that the Nigerian oto-neuro-ophthalmological syndrome is due to chronic cyanide poisoning consequent on cassava consumption has been confirmed by the biochemical studies of Monekosso and Wilson (1966) and of Osuntokun's group themselves (1968; 1970). More recently, the auditory pathophysiological basis of the disorder has been clarified by Evans' (1974) experimental neuro-physiological studies. Burkitt's epidemiological studies led to the virological investigations of Epstein and his associates (1964). These investigations themselves led to the discovery of the herpes-type EB (Epstein-Barr) virus and the role it plays in the aetiology of African malignant (Burkitt's) lymphoma. The EB virus is the cause of infectious mononucleosis (Henle et al., 1968; Niederman et al., 1968) and its oncogenic properties have given rise to fresh concepts in medicine. On the one hand, there has been the suggestion of a predisposition to develop the malignant lymphoma because of chronic infection (Cook and Burkitt, 1971) and, on the other hand, an interaction between DNA (e.g. a herpes-type virus) and RNA viruses—"tumour viruses in tandem" (Peters et al., 1973). Indeed, much of what has been mentioned has been associated with fresh concepts (Takaki's concept of epidemic non-communicable disease; Funk coined the word "vitamine" and Peters the phrase "biochemical lesion"). Thus, as well as contributing directly to the aetiology of disease in its own right, epidemiology has contributed by acting as a catalyst for other sciences whose contributions have been no less important.

(2) Elucidation of Syndromes

A syndrome is the occurrence of an association of certain specified symptoms and/or signs, the aetiology of which is unknown, diverse or multifactorial. It is implicit that the association is not a chance one, but epidemiologists are increasingly enquiring whether or not this is so in the various reputed syndromes. As Berkson (1946) has pointed out on statistical grounds, for conditions likely to bring a patient to hospital, the ratio of patients with several diagnoses to those with a single diagnosis, for example, will be greater than for people in the community from which these patients were drawn. Moreover, clinical experience indicates that syndromes are not so clear cut as the literature might suggest.

One syndrome that has recently been brought into question by epidemiologists is that of sideropenic dysphagia (Paterson-Kelly or Plummer-Vinson syndrome). Populations studies in South Wales have shown no evidence for a greater prevalence of anaemia in subjects with dysphagia than in controls. Both the mean haemoglobin level and the mean corpuscular haemoglobin concentration were in fact significantly higher in the group with dysphagia. Moreover, there was no difference in the serum iron and the total iron-binding capacity of serum between those people with dysphagia and those without. There was, however, some evidence, albeit inconclusive, that the occurrence of a post-cricoid web or stricture was associated with iron deficiency, mostly mild (Elwood et al., 1964).

(3) Determination of the Health Needs of a Community

As Kostrzewski (1970) has pointed out, the objective of social medicine is to secure the health of the population at large. To do this, the community physician requires to know from his epidemiological colleague the size and the nature of the health problems in his community. For example, a Health Ministry may need to know the prevalence of hearing impairments in excess of a certain level in order to provide the requisite number of hearing aids for that community. In this respect, and based on available data from the U.K., U.S.A. and Scandinavia, Jauhiainen (1968) has developed a statistical model for predicting the prevalence of hearing impairments of varying degrees in various age groups.

Thus epidemiology must be considered in relationship to community medicine in the same way that physiopathology is related to clinical medicine (Lobo and Jouval, 1973). Moreover, one is being made increasingly aware that health care must be evaluated in terms of cost as well as effectiveness. Only epidemiological studies, as Elwood and Weddell (1971) point out, can provide a valid basis for these cost-effectiveness decisions. These have yet to be applied to otolaryngology.

(4) As a Basis for Public Health Legislation

Epidemiological studies contributed to decisions as to which infectious diseases should, or should not, be listed in the U.K., for example, as "notifiable" diseases under the Public Health Act, 1936, and which occupational disorders should be "prescribed" diseases under the National Insurance (Industrial Injuries) Act, 1946. The recent extensive epidemiological study by Burns and Robinson (1970), quantifying the relationship between noise and hearing levels in industry, has formed the basis for the Report by the Industrial Injuries Advisory Council of the Department of Health and Social Security (U.K.) on the question of whether or not there are degrees of hearing loss due to noise which satisfy the conditions for prescription under that 1946 Act. The Report recommended that occupational hearing loss should be a prescribed disorder.

(5) Assessment of Effectiveness of Health Care

The Institute of Medicine of the National Academy of Sciences (U.S.A.) proposed a strategy for evaluating ambulatory health services. The method involves the use of a set of specific health problems, termed tracers. Middle ear infection is one of these.

(6) Screening

This is the procedure for surveying a population for unrecognized or presymptomatic disease, or for its precursors.

McKeown (1968) defines screening as a medical investigation which does not arise from a patient's request for advice regarding specific complaints. It encompasses people who:

(i) Have not sought medical assistance at all, e.g. in hearing surveys of the general population.
(ii) Have sought medical assistance but only for a screening test which they believe to be of value for them (health "check-up").
(iii) Have sought assistance for a condition unrelated to a screening procedure, e.g. a patient who presents with hay fever and is screened for vestibulocochlear nerve tumours by zonography and/or tests of abnormal auditory adaptation.

The aims of screening are also threefold:

(i) It may be used for research, e.g. the validation of a screening procedure.
(ii) The protection of community health, e.g. the detection of carriers of certain pathogenic bacteria.
(iii) The early detection of disease in individuals on the assumption that this enables earlier treatment and consequent better prognosis (prescriptive screening).

Whatever the type of screening programme, it will need to meet certain biological, economic and ethical criteria. In respect of prescriptive screening, Morrison and Last (1970) have pointed out that there is not much evidence that early detection of some chronic diseases materially influences their course, although complications may be reduced. Moreover, the screening test may be so expensive and the condition sufficiently rare that finding a case may be prohibitive. Knox (1968) has reviewed the evidence for prescriptive screening for severe hearing impairment in childhood and Fisch (1973a) has similarly reported on hearing disorders in the elderly.

(7) Study of Human Biology—Measurement of the "Norm"

In this respect, the scope of epidemiology has widened beyond the definition cited initially, since the epidemiological method has now been extended to encompass measurements on predominantly normal people. As Elwood and Weddell (1971) point out, almost all biological variates (measurements) are continuously distributed between wide limits. Few, if any, of these distributions provide any justification for a purported dichotomy between normals and abnormals. Thus, both hearing levels and taste thresholds in the general population are continuously distributed.

Few, if any, measurements are age-independent so that epidemiologists will want to investigate changes of a given variate as a function of age. This applies not only to changes in the parameters of central tendency (mean, median or mode) but also to measurements of dispersion (spread of values) and of the form of this distribution, i.e. whether normal (Gaussian) or otherwise. Figure 1 shows the median threshold of hearing for otoscopically normal women as a

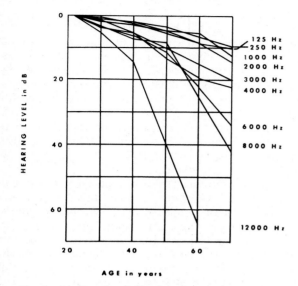

FIG. 1. Median threshold of hearing for otoscopically normal women as a function of age in a random sample of a rural population in Britain. (After Hinchcliffe, 1959.)

function of age. Not only do the "average" values change with age, but the dispersion also increases with age. Moreover, although the values may be normally distributed (Gaussian) for young age groups, the character of the distribution curve changes with increasing age, being skewed to the left.

With any measurement, there is always a certain amount of error. Some of this resides in the equipment, some in the technique and the rest in the observer (the person who does the measuring). Since it if often impossible to determine which observer's decision is correct, it is better to use the term "observer variation" instead of "observer error" (Yerushalmy et al., 1950). Differences between observers are spoken of as "inter-observer variation". This may be large. Thus differences in blood pressure measurements between two observers may be as much as 2 kPa (15 mm Hg) (Eilertsen and Humerfelt, 1968). Variability of results obtained by a single observer on different occasions is referred to as "intra-observer variation". Studies of the interpretation of radiographs of even the paranasal sinuses show that both inter-observer and intra-observer variation can be appreciable (Hinchcliffe, 1961a)

EPIDEMIOLOGICAL TERMINOLOGY

A distinction must be made between incidence and prevalence. *Incidence* refers to the number of new cases of a disease occurring within a specified period. *Prevalence* refers to the number of cases of a disease presenting in a population at a given time.

Incidence (attack rate) is a measure of the rate at which fresh cases are added to the total of affected individuals

and is dependent on the balance between resistance of the population and the factors that produce the disorder. The prevalence of a disease will depend not only on the incidence of the disease but also on its duration and the mortality rate. A disease such as acute otitis media has an incidence in children of the order of 100 per 1000 population per annum. However, the duration of this disorder is only of the order of 1 week so that the prevalence will be of the order of 2 per 1000 population.

The value of a test (screening or otherwise) depends on its sensitivity and on its specificity. The *sensitivity* of a test is the ratio of the number of diseased individuals detected by the test to the total number of diseased subjects in the sample studied. The *specificity* of the test is the ratio of unaffected subjects who give negative responses to the total number of unaffected subjects, whether they give negative or positive responses to the test. (Thorner and Remeim, 1961).

METHODOLOGY

Epidemiology may be divided into descriptive epidemiology and analytical epidemiology. Descriptive epidemiology would concern itself with, for example, differences in the incidence of diseases with time, either shorter time periods (seasons) in respect of epidemic diseases, or longer time periods (secular changes) in respect of chronic disease. It would also concern itself with differences in, say, prevalence in relationship to place (if on a larger space scale, geographical medicine) or persons (e.g. age—merging with gerontology, or occupational—merging with occupational medicine). Thus descriptive epidemiology could indicate a group of people who have a higher risk of developing a particular disorder. It could also provide clues to the aetiology of a disorder and lead to the formulation of hypotheses which could be tested by analytical epidemiology or by other sciences using laboratory methods. In analytical epidemiology, one would design epidemiological investigations to isolate particular factors that may be involved in the aetiology and then measure their importance.

Epidemiological studies may be *retrospective* or *prospective*. As Morrison and Last (1970) point out, the retrospective approach may be considered as an extension of the clinician's history-taking into the field of population studies. Retrospective (prevalence or cross-sectional) surveys have been critized on the basis that, being *ex post facto* studies, they are unable to determine a cause-effect relationship (Underwood, 1957; High, 1965). However, research workers in population medicine are cognizant of these shortcomings. As Fletcher and Oldham (1964) remark, prevalence surveys do not provide us with a means for their own interpretation. Berkson (1955) goes even further to contend that it is unwarranted to conclude that an observed association between two variates (measures) in a survey is a meaningful one. Selection may be the source of such an observed association, as was demonstrated to be the case for an observed association of hypertension and neuroticism (Robinson, 1962). It is therefore mandatory that one studies entire, non-hospitalized populations, or what is more practical, a random sample of these populations. Even then, research workers in this field tended originally rather to despise cross-sectional studies and considered them only as a base line for follow-up studies. This was an underestimate. Point prevalence surveys have been of considerable value (Cochrane, 1965). We tend to forget that all explanations in science must be in terms of established relationships of dependency. Moreover, although the actual survey itself does not produce evidence for a cause-effect relationship, the use of inductive inference will frequently indicate the cause-effect relationship of two intercorrelated measures. As Feigl (1953) declares, science is not a mere collection of miscellaneous items of information, but a well connected account of the facts. Because of what Feigl terms this coherence criterion of the scientific method, one is frequently able to adduce the cause-effect relationship of two intercorrelated measures.

Prospective (longitudinal or follow-up) studies resemble a planned experiment except that the occurrence of a suspected cause is determined by nature (Doll, 1964). In practice, however, and in contrast to retrospective studies, follow-up studies have, in general, been less productive than retrospective studies. This has been for a variety of reasons, including self-selection (Cochrane, 1965).

The three principal epidemiological *methods for acquiring* data depend on;

> (1) Direct examination of random or total samples of a population.
> (2) Interviewing techniques.
> (3) Registration of disease and of death.

The *direct examination* of random or total samples is of value in respect of biological variates (e.g. blood pressure, hearing level, taste threshold) and of relatively common disorders, i.e. those which occur in at least about 1 per cent of the population (e.g. otitis media, otosclerosis). The success of these population studies depends upon being able to examine a representative sample of that population. This entails first selecting the subjects by using random sampling tables and then ensuring a maximum yield, i.e. a minimum lapse rate. Lapse rates may be reduced to as little as 1·2 per cent of the sample studied (Kell *et al.*, 1970). Lasagna and Felsinger (1954) and others have shown that volunteers have different personality characteristics compared with those individuals in the general population. Since relationships have been indicated between personality and somatotype (Wretmark, 1953) and between, for example, noise-induced hearing loss and somatotype (Kristensen, 1946), it is possible that volunteer samples may exhibit different characteristics in these particular population studies than would the general population. Moreover, we often wonder, when, for example, hearing tests are being done, whether those who volunteer are individuals who suspect, and are subsequently shown to have, defective hearing. These individuals would bias the results in a direction that would not be counterbalanced by those who suspect that they have "supernormal" hearing. Cochrane (1965) has shown that the prevalence of disease is different in the last individuals in a sample to come forward compared with those who came forward to begin with. This "order of coming up" effect, which was originally noted

by Kayser-Petersen in 1931, has been confirmed by Refsum (1952) in Norway and by Palchanis (1952) in the U.S.A. In one survey conducted by the author, none of the cases of chronic middle ear disease that were responsible for a conductive hearing loss came up until more than two-thirds of the sample had been examined.

The feasibility of using both bacteriological and radiological, as well as clinical and audiometric examinations, for ascertaining the prevalence of the commoner ear, nose and throat disorders by direct examination of random or total samples has been amply demonstrated (Hinchcliffe, 1961b).

The *interviewing technique* is best exemplified by its use in relating smoking to the aetiology of lung cancer, using both retrospective (Doll and Hill, 1950) and prospective (Doll and Hill, 1956) studies.

Although *registration* of death, together with its cause, was introduced into Britain in 1838, this has proved of limited value to the epidemiologist. Morbidity statistics have been of more value. In Britain, the Public Health Act, 1936 and the National Insurance Acts have been the means of providing data on the incidence of specified infectious diseases (notifiable diseases) and of non-infectious disorders respectively. Statistics are also available for the incidence of occupational disorders which are prescribed diseases under the National Insurance (Industrial Injuries) Act, 1946. Thus miners' nystagmus in coal-miners and nasal cancer in nickel workers are prescribed disorders. Some occupational disorders, such as chrome ulceration, are also termed notifiable, in the sense that a doctor who discovers such a case must notify it to the Chief Inspector of Factories. The purpose of this is for the Factory Inspectorate to investigate the case with a view to preventing further cases. Cancer registration has been introduced into a number of countries to obtain data on the incidence and fatality rate of malignant neoplasias (*mortality* refers to the number of deaths per thousand or other unit of the population; *fatality* refers to the number of deaths per 100 cases). With the possible exception of skin malignancies, such registration based upon both hospital diagnoses and death certification information should provide a valid measure of the incidence of a particular cancer in a population. The establishment of Cancer Registries can thus be viewed as a valuable step in the epidemiological approach to the study of these diseases.

A more recent development in the acquisition of data for epidemiological purposes is that of *record linkage* (Acheson, 1967). Data relating to many measures of health and of disease in respect of one given individual are assembled and analysed by computer-based procedures. The Oxford Record Linkage Study has already shown an association between nasal cancer and woodworking occupations.

The method of *analysis of data* on the incidence of various disorders is again dependent upon the rarity, or otherwise, of the condition. The most useful indices are *age-specific incidence rates*, i.e. the frequency with which a particular disease occurs at each age in a given population in a specified period of time. Crude incidence rates may be grossly misleading because of the different age structure of various populations. Consequently Segi (1960) has advocated the use of the world population as a standard population for presenting data on cancer incidence. Unfortunately, since cancer incidence may show different patterns in the way it varies with age, this method is again not entirely satisfactory. It has therefore been suggested that a more valuable index would be the incidence between the ages 35–64 years (Doll and Cook, 1967). This index would be more meaningful in assessing the influence of possible carcinogenic factors; in younger age groups, incidence rates are generally too low, and, in older groups, so many other factors are operating.

In the absence of absolute incidence rates, *comparative incidence* figures (*proportional morbidity* rates) may be used. This method has been used to study the incidence of malignant disease of the ear, nose and throat in Uganda (Martin, 1967). Unfortunately, as Doll (1968) points out, the real difficulty with proportional rates is that the proportion attributed to one type of disease is affected by an increase or decrease in other types. However, there are fortunately so many different types of malignancies, for example, that the incidence of all taken together varies very much less than the incidence of any one type alone. It is thus better, when presenting comparative incidence figures, to express the frequency of, say, a cancer, as a proportion *of all other cases*, rather than as a proportion of the total number of cases.

In the absence of morbidity statistics, mortality statistics may be used. The value of *absolute mortality* rates is limited by the validity of diagnoses on death certificates and is inversely related to the curability of the condition. However, even with conditions as infrequent as nasal carcinoma (crude death rates in U.K. are of the order of 5 per million of the population), this index has been used to estimate the expected mortality rate in nickel workers and so demonstrate an occupational risk (Doll, 1958). *Proportional mortality* rates, analogous to proportional morbidity rates, may be used in the study of commoner disorders. Thus Doll (1958) has used such figures (ratio of deaths attributable to lung cancer to deaths from causes other than cancer of the respiratory tract) to demonstrate that nickel workers also run a greater risk of lung cancer (crude death rate in British males is normally of the order of 500 per million of the population).

The statistical methods that we have just mentioned are relatively simple, conventional ones aimed at determining exactly how common certain disorders are, with a view to ascertaining whether or not there is an association with differences in person, place or time. Over the past 15 years, new statistical techniques have been developed to ascertain whether or not there is any space-time clustering in respect of disease occurrences. This is always the fundamental question in epidemiology. Sayers (1974) has recently applied the techniques of the analysis of biological signals to epidemiology. The occurrence of a disorder in an individual is a point event signal of a special kind. The distance between successive events can be considered in the time domain as well as in the spatial domain. Knox (1959; 1964) has shown that satisfactory statistical tests may be developed to demonstrate clustering in respect of diseases so infrequent as congenital oesophagotracheal fistula (crude

incidence of the order of 5 per million population). The time intervals between not only successive pairs of events but also all other possible pairs are examined. For both Birmingham (U.K.) and the north-east of England, there was an excess of short intervals compared with those to be expected on the basis of a random distribution in time.

Knox's methods have been developed by Pike and his colleagues (1967) in a study of Burkitt's tumour in Uganda. In a subsequent study, Pike and Smith (1968) extended these methods to test more complex and specific epidemiological models, accounting for specified radii of movement, incubation periods and periods of infectiousness. A more generalized mathematical model of epidemicity has subsequently been developed by Abe (1969).

SYSTEMATIC EPIDEMIOLOGY

Ear

Wax

In a 1958 survey in Dumfriesshire, Scotland, it was found that 23 per cent of males had one or both meatuses occluded by wax, compared with 13 per cent of females (Hinchcliffe, 1961b). Corresponding values of 23 per cent and 16 per cent were reported by Kell and his associates (1970) for their 1968 survey of the Orkney island of Westray. By contrast, the prevalence of occluding wax in Dundee (Scotland) school teachers is only 2 per cent (Taylor *et al.*, 1967). A 1970 survey of Israeli schoolchildren showed that wax occluded one or both ears in 9 per cent of a sample of Arab children in the Negev Desert, compared with about 20 per cent of either Druze children in the mountains or Jewish children in the Mediterranean littoral (Hinchcliffe and Sadé, 1971). The reasons for these apparent sex and ethnic differences are not clear but almost certainly reflect exposure to different environmental conditions. Nevertheless, the frequency of this common aural state emphasizes the need for otological examinations in hearing surveys. Of course, much of the wax can be removed by either a wax curette and/or syringing. In the Mid-Annandale (Dumfriesshire) survey, only 5 per cent of meatuses which were initially occluded by wax could not be cleared by olive oil drops for 1 week in conjunction with syringing.

Otitis Externa

Jaffe (1969) mentions that external otitis is uncommon amongst the Navajo Indians. However, when it does occur, it is either secondary to chronic suppurative otitis media or due to the bite of the spinose ear tick, *Otobius megnini*. This argasid tick is known locally as the "sheep tick". Because the Navajos live in close contact with sheep and because they sleep on untreated sheepskins, this sheep tick can easily change hosts and reside in the external acoustic meatus of the Navajo. A wide spectrum of disease occurs, ranging from mild inflammation to severe perichondritis involving the auricle.

Otitis Media

The epidemiology of otitis media has recently been reviewed by both McEldowney and Kessner (1972) and by Jordan (1972). McEldowney and Kessner conclude that the overall impression is that both purulent (and probably secretory) middle ear disease and the associated hearing loss, are sensitive to variations in socio-economic and environmental factors. One particular difficulty in comparing various statistics to determine prevalances of otitis media is that, frequently, data relate only to cases causing a hearing loss. Otological examination of sample populations has been restricted to individuals failing an auditory screening test. Jordan and Eagles (1961) have clearly demonstrated that measurement of hearing is an insensitive indicator for the detection of middle ear disease. Nevertheless, it would appear that the prevalence of chronic otitis media ("perforated tympanic membrane as a cause of conductive hearing loss") in children of various countries is a power function of the *per capita* G.N.P. (gross national product) (Hinchcliffe, 1972). This is in contrast to chronic otitis media in adults. For example, although chronic otitis media is very common in children in Jamaica, chronic otitis media in one sample of an adult population on that island and in the age range 35–74 years, showed a prevalence about one-fifth of that for a comparable population in the U.K. It would thus appear that not only does the prevalence of otitis media vary with age, but, like the incidence of the many cancers, the way it varies with age may be different in different populations. More epidemiological investigations are required to look into this aspect by using populations covering the whole age range and including longitudinal as well as point-prevalence studies. Studies similar to those conducted on the Navajo Indians need to be extended. Jaffe and his colleagues (1970) showed that delayed ventilation of the middle ear cleft after birth predisposed to the later development of otitis media in affected individuals. Moreover, this delayed ventilation was correlated with prematurity and maternal complications during pregnancy. There is also the need to look into the question of the relationship in many populations of ear diseases to other, general medical disorders. Three out of four cases of chronic otitis media picked out of one tropical (Jamaican) otolaryngological survey also showed evidence for general disorders which could have influenced the hearing, if not the middle ear condition. The index of chronic otitis media frequently used in prevalence studies is the occurrence of "perforated tympanic membranes". Because of the influence of the duration of the disorder on prevalence rates, acute otitis media, although having a high incidence, would account for only a small fraction of measured prevalences of otitis media. Other causes of perforation, such as blast injury, are insufficiently common to influence these measured prevalence values in the general population.

Because of its short duration (of the order of 1 week), epidemiological studies of acute otitis media are best done by incidence studies. Notable amongst these was that conducted on British general practices in 1955 by the Medical Research Council (Medical Research Council, 1957). Such studies are appropriately done in general practice since, as the survey showed, 99 per cent of cases of acute otitis media in Britain are seen only by general practitioners. The longitudinal study of acute otitis media, where the condition is persisting, i.e. entering a chronic

phase, is, however, appropriately done in conjunction with otologists, as was done in a more recent investigation by Fry and his colleagues (1969). The latter follow-up study showed that 17 per cent of cases had a subsequent hearing loss (compared to 4·5 per cent of controls) and that this hearing loss was commoner in those children with a family history of ear disease. The 1955 M.R.C. survey showed that the incidence of acute otitis media rose rapidly with age to a maximum of about 200 cases per 1000 population at the age of 6 years, thereafter falling off rapidly to a level of the order of 50 per 1000 population in the teens. Of particular interest was the observation that there was a marked seasonal variation. Figure 2 shows the moving average* (3-monthly periods) incidence of acute otitis

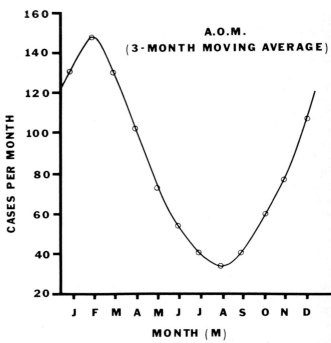

FIG. 2. Three-monthly moving (running) average monthly incidence of acute otitis media in Britain in 1955. Standardized on 1000 cases per annum. (After Medical Research Council, 1957.)

media (AOM) throughout the year studied (1955). The pattern is that of a sinusoid with a period of 1 year. It is to be noted that similar seasonal patterns can be seen in the data reported by Suehs (1952) for secretory (seromucinous) otitis media (Fig. 3). (Some otologists would perhaps refer to the latter as acute non-suppurative otitis media). Moreover, when the data for the two studies are standardized on 1000 cases per annum, the amplitudes of the two sinusoids are equal. In other words the coefficient of variation, i.e. the relative variability, is the same for the two sets of data. Furthermore, there is a phase difference (i.e. a difference for when the peak occurrences take place) of only 1 month between the two sets of data. The similarity of the two sets of data is shown in Fig. 4 where the time scale for the acute otitis media data has been shifted by 1 month. Note

* *See* Chapter 2.

not only how well the two sets of data agree, but how well they conform to a sinusoid whose equation is:

$$N_M = 51 \sin (30\,M) + 87 \qquad (10.1)$$

where N_M = total number of cases in month M.

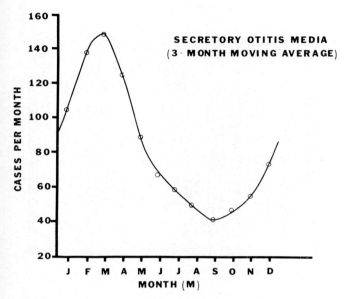

FIG. 3. Three-monthly moving average monthly incidence of "secretory otitis media" (acute non-suppurative otitis media) in one otological practice in Texas. Standardized on 1000 cases per annum. (After Suehs, 1952.)

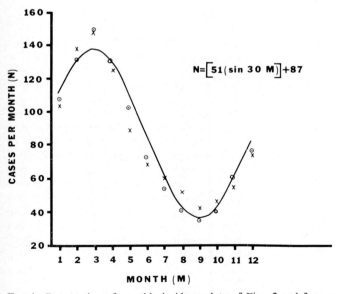

FIG. 4. Presentation of monthly incidence data of Figs. 2 and 3 on a single set of co-ordinates, but with the data for acute otitis media shifted by one month. Standardized on 1000 cases per annum. N = number of cases per month, and M = ordinal number of month (January = 1).

Since, for the purpose of this comparison, we have shifted the phase of the acute otitis media by 1 month, the appropriate expression for the acute otitis media data would be:

$$N_M = 51 \sin [30\,(M + 1)] + 87 \qquad (10.2)$$

The similarity of the two sets of data is the more remarkable when we realize that not only do the data apply to what are considered to be two different diseases but to two locations nearly 8000 km apart on the globe. (The acute otitis media data was obtained from 13 medical

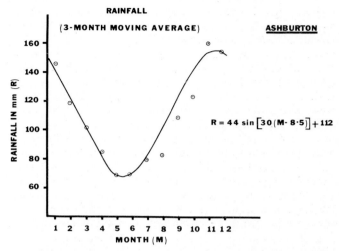

FIG. 5. Three-monthly moving average monthly rainfall for Ashburton, Devon, UK.

practices in various parts of Britain; the secretory otitis media data from an otological practice in Austin, Texas.) This again poses questions when one attempts to relate the seasonal fluctuation in otitis media incidence to climate. The 3 month moving average rainfall often conforms to a

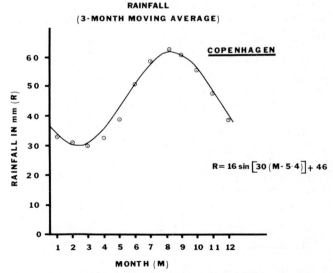

FIG. 6. Three-monthly moving average monthly rainfall for Copenhagen, Denmark.

conspicuous sinusoidal function, as Figs. 5 and 6 show for Ashburton (England) and Copenhagen respectively. The rainfall fluctuations in England and Texas are, however, about 180° out of phase. It would therefore appear that one should look elsewhere for the cause of these marked seasonal fluctuations in the occurrence of these middle ear conditions. As data for deaths from arteriosclerotic heart disease indicate, seasonal fluctuations by no means imply an infective aetiology (Begg, 1966). Nevertheless, in this context of middle ear infections, it would be appropriate to look at fluctuations in the seasonal incidence of various pathogens. It is unlikely that the answer will be found in bacteriological epidemiological studies since bacteriological patterns of otitis media vary in different parts of the world. *Streptococcus pyogenes, Staphylococcus pyogenes* and *Streptococcus pneumococcus* have been shown to be the predominant organisms in acute otitis media in Britain (Wright, 1970), Poland (Szcypiorski *et al.*, 1969) and the U.S.A. (Feingold *et al.*, 1966; Halsted *et al.*, 1968) respectively. Whatever clue is found to the aetiology of acute otitis media, it will also be expected to be that in respect of other common respiratory infections, with the exception of acute pharyngitis and tonsillitis which show little seasonal variation. As the M.R.C. report on acute otitis media observed, the seasonal incidence pattern for this condition is strikingly similar to that for the other respiratory infections. Consequently, the virological studies of acute otitis media are more important than the bacteriological one in elucidating the aetiology. Of note are Yoshie's (1955) isolation of the influenza A virus from the ear in Japan and Berglund and Halonen's (1970) isolation of RS (respiratory syncytial) virus from the ears of 22 children during two outbreaks of infection with this virus in Finland. It is therefore of note that seasonal fluctuations in the incidence of acute otitis media are in phase with seasonal fluctuations in the incidence of RS virus isolations (Fig. 7).

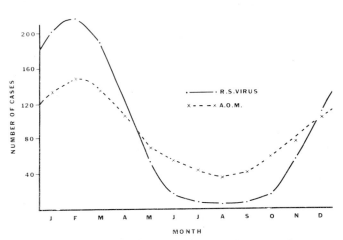

FIG. 7. Three-monthly moving average monthly incidence of RS virus isolations (averaged over period 1968–1972) superimposed on the three-monthly moving average incidence of acute otitis media shown in Fig. 2. (Data for RS virus isolations by courtesy of Public Health Laboratory Service, UK.)

Other evidence for a viral aetiology for otitis media is also available. Tilles and his colleagues (1967) have demonstrated antibody rises both to adenovirus and to parainfluenza virus in patients with acute otitis media.

Moreover, RS virus (Gronroos *et al.*, 1968) and parainfluenza virus (Halsted *et al.*, 1968) have been isolated from the middle ears of patients with otitis media. Finally, a viral otitis media may complicate a generalized viral infection, such as measles and smallpox, as Bordley and Kapur (1972) have reported (*see* Fig. 8).

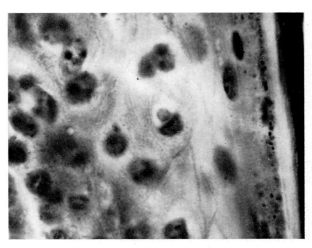

FIG. 8. Tympanic membrane of three-month old child who died of smallpox in India. A typical Guarnieri body can be seen in the cuticular layer of the membrane. This is an acidophilic intracytoplasmic inclusion body which lies close to the nucleus of the cell, with clear cytoplasm around it. The findings strongly suggest that the origin of the middle ear changes was the invasion by smallpox virus. (After Bordley and Kapur, 1972.)

Otosclerosis

About 1 per cent of the population of the U.K. are afflicted with clinical otosclerosis (Hinchcliffe, 1961b). This figure is somewhat higher than many estimates, but it is based upon direct examination of random samples of the general population. There is no evidence that the prevalence of this disorder differs significantly over Europe and North America. In fact, the prevalence seems remarkably constant throughout the white races. One possible exception is that of the Todas, an isolate in South India. The prevalence of what appears to be otosclerosis (there is no histological confirmation) in these people is about 17 per cent (Kapur and Patt, 1967). By contrast, otosclerosis is infrequent in the black and the yellow races. Examination of 11 000 Amerinds in Bolivia, Paraguay and Peru indicate that the prevalence of the disorder amongst these people is of the order of 3 per 10 000 population (Tato and Tato, 1969). The condition is rare in Japan (Nakamura, 1968).

Hearing Impairment

The epidemiology of hearing loss in general has recently been reviewed by Surján and his associates (1973). They conclude that significant degrees of loss affect about 10 per cent of the population. This value probably applies at least to Australasia, Europe and North America. In the U.K., 4 per cent of the adult population are considered to be sufficiently hard of hearing that they cannot hear more than tête-à-tête conversation (Wilkins, 1949).

Censuses to determine the prevalence of hearing loss

by questioning individuals or their relatives as to whether or not they think they are "deaf" or "hard of hearing" are no substitute for the direct examination of individuals in a given population. The threshold of subjective auditory

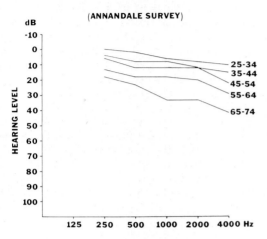

FEMALE

LEVELS AT WHICH HEARING SUBJECTIVELY CHANGES FROM "NORMAL" TO "NOT AS GOOD AS IT USED TO BE"

(ANNANDALE SURVEY)

Fig. 9. Threshold of subjective auditory handicap for women in a random sample of a British rural population. Figures against each curve refer to relevant age group. (After Merluzzi and Hinchcliffe, 1973.)

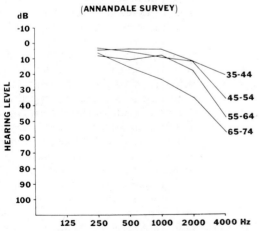

MALE

LEVELS AT WHICH HEARING SUBJECTIVELY CHANGES FROM "NORMAL" TO "NOT AS GOOD AS IT USED TO BE"

(ANNANDALE SURVEY)

Fig. 10. As for Fig. 9 but for men. (After Merluzzi and Hinchcliffe, 1973.)

handicap is age-dependent and there are provably considerable inter-individual differences (Merluzzi and Hinchcliffe, 1973). The thresholds of subjective auditory handicap for different age groups are shown in Figs. 9 and 10 for females and males respectively. An equivalent speech hearing loss for each of the curves was derived and the logarithm of the mean value for the two sexes plotted as a

function of age (Fig. 11). The data conformed to a straight line plot, i.e.

$$y = 0.0185\,x + 0.145 \qquad (10.3)$$

where y = logarithm of speech hearing level in dB HL corresponding to threshold of subjective auditory handicap

and x = age in years.

These results thus indicate that the commonly accepted value of 26 dB HL (ISO) for the "low fence" (threshold

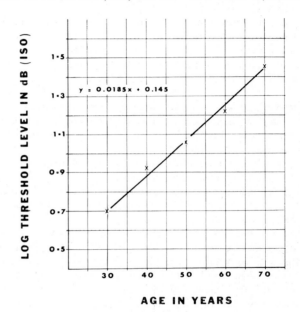

Fig. 11. Threshold of subjective auditory handicap as a function of age. Threshold is given in terms of the logarithm of a single value which is the equivalent hearing level for speech. y = logarithm of threshold of subjective auditory handicap in dB (ISO), x = age in years. (After Merluzzi and Hinchcliffe, 1973.)

at which a handicap commences) could be applicable to a 70-year-old person only. Values of 18 dB HL (ISO) and 10 dB HL (ISO) would also be appropriate to 60- and 45-year-old subjects respectively. However, it is unlikely that the actual (objective) threshold of auditory handicap is age dependent. It is much more likely that the gradual change in this subjective threshold with increasing age reflects the insidious onset and progression of presbyacusis. Thus it can be argued that the true "low fence"—the actual threshold of auditory handicap—is actually 0 dB HL.

In a review of the epidemiology of *congenital* hearing loss, Fisch (1973b) points out that the prevalence of profound hearing loss of congenital origin is of the order of 1:1000 population. Some countries, such as Peru, Honduras and Japan, may have appreciably higher prevalences (World Health Organization, 1953).

A study on Swedish *children* reported by Barr and his colleagues (1973) indicated that, although the prevalence of sensorineural hearing loss in 7-year-old children remains remarkably constant over the years, the prevalence of conductive hearing loss shows definite secular changes.

These secular changes involved not only fluctuations from year to year but, fortunately, a downward trend over the period 1958–71. Whereas conductive hearing loss in children showed a drop in prevalence with increasing age, sensorineural hearing loss showed an increase, more marked in boys than in girls. Because of this sex difference and the absence of significant noise exposure, Barr and his colleagues argued for an important genetic factor in the aetiology of high frequency hearing loss in children. In observations on the epidemiology of hearing loss in children, Chung and Brown (1970) have also argued that the most important factors are genetic.

The determination of the prevalence of sensorineural hearing loss in general, or of a specific sensorineural hearing disorder in particular, presents a problem that is not encountered with respect to conductive hearing loss. This is because of the absence, except with respect to the rarer types of sensorineural disorders, of qualitative tests to identify either sensorineural hearing losses in general or of sensorineural hearing disorders in particular. Epidemiological studies of sensorineural hearing loss therefore resolve themselves into measuring the hearing levels of ears which have been otologically screened to exclude conductive hearing losses, and then calculating "average" values for these measures and their dispersion, together with endeavouring to determine factors which are influencing these values.

Noise is the one environmental factor above all others which has been conclusively demonstrated as of importance in the aetiology of hearing loss. Following an extensive survey of noise and hearing levels in industry in the U.K., Burns and Robinson (1970) showed that the damaging effect of noise to hearing can be expressed in terms of a single, but composite, measure of exposure, which they termed the *noise emission level*. This level is proportional to the total sound energy received by the ear over the exposure period. It is usually expressed in terms of what is spoken of as the A-weighted noise emission level (E_A), where

$$E_A = L_A + 10 \log (T/T_0) \qquad (10.4)$$

where L_A = A-weighted sound pressure level of the noise, i.e. measured with a sound level meter with a particular (A) frequency response, in dB (A). (*See* Chapter 11)

T = duration of exposure in calendar years

and T_0 = reference duration (1 year).

When this equation is used in conjunction with a nomographic chart and an ageing correction added, it is possible to specify what hearing level at a given frequency will be attained by a given proportion of subjects who have been working for a certain number of years in a particular noise environment. Recently, using selected data, Scheiblechner (1974) has questioned the particular formulation given to the energy principle by the British workers and has suggested a multifactorial logistic model to relate noise exposure and hearing level.

The importance of *endemic oto-neuro-ophthalmological syndromes* in influencing the hearing levels in the general population has been demonstrated in both Jamaica (Ashcroft *et al.*, 1967; Hinchcliffe, 1968; Hinchcliffe and Jones, 1968) and in Nigeria (Hinchcliffe *et al.*, 1972). In Nigeria, the fully developed syndrome, termed Nigerian nutritional ataxic neuropathy (NAN) comprises myelopathy with predominant involvement of the posterior columns of the spinal cord, bilateral optic atrophy, sensorineural hearing loss and symmetrical peripheral polyneuropathy (Money, 1958; Osuntokun, 1968). The condition is more prevalent in the areas with a high cassava (*Manioc utilissima*) consumption (Osuntokun *et al.*, 1969). The disorder is associated with high plasma thiocyanate levels (Monekosso and Wilson, 1966; Osuntokun, 1968), and high blood free cyanide levels (Osuntokun *et al.*, 1970). Cassava contains high concentrations of a cyanogenetic glycoside, linamarin. The presumption is, therefore, that the disorder is primarily due to *chronic cyanide intoxication* consequent on high cassava consumption. An epidemiological study in Epe, a large fishing village 64 km east of Lagos, showed that the low frequency hearing levels of affected individuals correlated with the overall score of clinical neurological deficit (Hinchcliffe *et al.*, 1972). The data were fitted with a curve conforming to a power function, i.e.

$$y = 25x^{0.57} \qquad (10.5)$$

where y = overall score of neurological deficit

and x = hearing level in right ear at 500 Hz in dB HL (ISO).

Sudden hearing loss has recently been shown to exhibit seasonal fluctuations (Rowson *et al.*, 1975). Consequently, despite negative investigations in respect of a number of upper respiratory viruses, mumps and varicella-zoster viruses, a virus aetiology must still be entertained in respect of this condition. It is of note, however, that, in contrast to acute otitis media, the peak incidence occurs around October/November.

In the tropics, one may find a whole gamut of sporadic outbreaks of fever associated with neuro-otological symptoms, and which may be attributed to what one might term "hit and run" viruses. Lassa fever, so called because it was first reported from Lassa in north-eastern Nigeria, is characterized by a severe headache, fever, pharyngitis, hearing impairment and a bleeding tendency (Frame *et al.*, 1970; Henderson *et al.*, 1972). Outbreaks have occurred in both Nigeria and Sierra Leone (Woodruff *et al.*, 1973). The causative virus is related to the virus of lymphocytic choriomeningitis, forming a new group for which the name arenovirus has been proposed. A 1955 epidemic on the River Guana in Pará, Brazil, 200 km east of Belém, was characterized by fever, severe frontal headache, epigastric pain and vertigo (Causey and Maroja, 1957). The causative virus, termed the Mayaro virus was an arbovirus related to the Semliki Forest virus (Casals and Whitman, 1957).

Studies on random samples of the general population have shown that, by the time we have reached the age of 60 years, a third of us have experienced *tinnitus* and/or *vertigo* at one time or another. Most of the episodes were, however, transient and not troublesome. Nevertheless, it would appear that *Ménière's disorder* affects about one per cent of the population in Britain. In this context, the criteria for such a diagnosis was a low frequency sensori-neural hearing loss in association with at least a year's history of recurrent vertigo associated with nausea and vomiting, and the occurrence of such symptomatology in the presence of imperforate tympanic membranes (Hinchcliffe, 1961b).

Nose

Thomson and Buxton (1923) have pointed out that the platyrrhine type of nose, e.g. that of the Negro, is characteristic of the inhabitants of hot, moist climates, and the leptorrhine, e.g. that of the Eskimo, of the inhabitants of cold, dry climates. Weiner (1954) has shown that the nasal index correlates with the absolute humidity of the climate in which a people live.

Deviated nasal septa are rare in the Central African Negro (Manson-Bahr, 1956). In one European sample which was examined, there was only one undeviated septum. This had been surgically corrected (Moe, 1942).

Anomalies

Certain congenital anomalies in the region of the nose show a greater prevalence in certain areas of the world and for, as yet, unknown reasons. Thus *fronto-ethmoidal encephaloceles* show a relatively high prevalence in Thailand (Suwanwela and Hongsaprabhas, 1966), in the Uttar Pradesh region of India (Tandon, 1973), in Morocco and in Nigeria.

Specific Infections

Two particular nasal disorders show peculiar geographic restrictions for again, as yet, unknown reasons. Rhinoscleroma, due to *Klebsiella rhinoscleromatis*, has three autochthonous areas, Central America, Galicia and Indonesia. Rhinosporidiosis is endemic in Southern India and Ceylon. It is caused by *Rhinosporidium seeberi* (*see* Chapter 47).

Sinusitis

Studies in Britain by direct clinical and radiological examination of a random sample of a rural population indicated that active chronic suppurative sinusitis affects about 5 per cent of that population (Hinchcliffe, 1961b). As was pointed out in the report, the actual value depends so much on the criteria adopted for such a diagnosis. There is thus a need, for epidemiological purposes at least, to adopt criteria for such a diagnosis. Meer and his associates (1957) reported that, at least in Romania, the prevalence of sinusitis is low in agricultural workers so that a higher figure than 5 per cent may obtain in urban areas in the U.K. Coal miners are reported to show a higher prevalence of sinusitis (Hoffman and Worth, 1958). The particular geogens (environmental factors) influencing the prevalence of chronic sinusitis are difficult to identify, partly because of some uncertainty regarding the changes, if any, associated with different climatic zones. Both Jaffé (1951) and Manson-Bahr (1956) reported that sinusitis is rare in hot, wet

tropical climates, whereas, by contrast, Proctor (1963) found that over a third of 600 schoolchildren studied in Jordan (a hot, dry climate) had chronic sinusitis. It is to be noted that a particular vasomotor nasal disorder afflicts subjects who have come from cool areas to hot, dry climates and this non-infective condition must be differentiated from sinusitis (King, 1949; Manson-Bahr, 1956). The various aspects of nasal dysfunction in relation to environmental air have been reviewed previously (Hinchcliffe, 1961c).

Cancer

Doll (1958) has collected data from records of death held by Medical Officers of Health for districts in which workers at a nickel refinery lived. He found that the risk of nickel workers dying from *nasal cancer* was 150 times the normal risk. However, there were secular changes indicating that the hazard has largely, if not completely, been removed in the last 35 years.

Studies following an initial observation by Esme Hadfield in High Wycombe, England, have confirmed that there is a high prevalence of *ethmoidal adenocarcinoma* in woodworkers. (Acheson *et al.*, 1968). The risk is such that the occupation makes what is otherwise an extremely rare tumour a common one (incidence comparable to lung cancer in men or breast cancer in women) for that restricted group of people. This particular occupational risk of woodworkers, including furniture makers, has also been demonstrated in Belgium (Debois, 1969), in Denmark (Mosbeck and Acheson, 1971) and in France (Gignoux and Bernard, 1969).

Acheson and his colleagues (1970) have also been able to demonstrate an occupational risk for nasal cancer in the footwear industry. Since there were broadly two types of tumour concerned (*nasal adenocarcinoma* and *squamous carcinoma* of the nasal cavity and paranasal sinuses), the authors suggested that possibly two carcinogens were involved.

Acheson's group also suggested that snuff taking should be considered a possible contributory factor in both occupational and non-occupational cancer. Harrison (1964) has previously commented on this point. About 80 per cent of Bantu patients with carcinoma of the *maxillary sinuses* admitted to prolonged use of snuff, which contains 3:4 benzpyrene, a carcinogen. The incidence of carcinoma of the paransal sinuses is about 20 times greater in the Bantu than in the European (May, 1949). Reynaud (1968) studied epidemiological features of carcinoma of the paranasal sinuses in Senegal. Although relatively small (less than 200 000 km², i.e. smaller than Great Britain), this country is populated with a variety of ethnic groups, ranging from the Maure, who are of Hamitic stock, to the Banyun, Diola and Serere who are of Negritic stock. The combined incidence of cancer of the paranasal sinuses and the nasal part of pharynx (post-nasal space) was 25 times greater in the Maure than in the latter ethnic groups. The Fulani (Peuhl and Toucouleur), who are ethnically intermediate between the Hamitic and Negritic peoples, showed an incidence which corresponds to the geometric mean of the other two values. This finding should therefore support the thesis that there are ethnic factors in the aetiology of

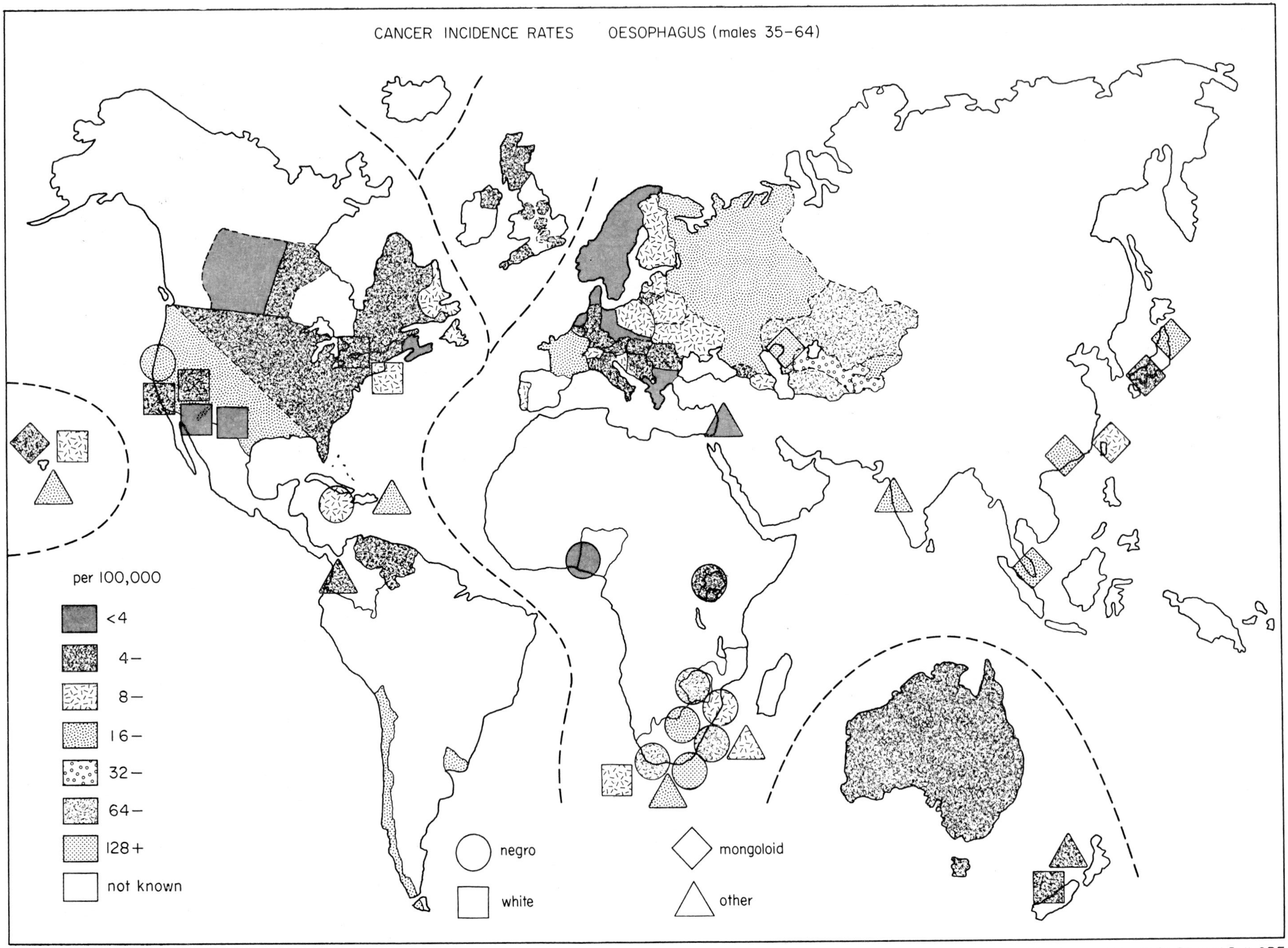

CANCER INCIDENCE RATES   OESOPHAGUS (males 35–64)

Map by courtesy of Sir Richard Doll OBE

per 100,000

<4
4–
8–
16–
32–
64–
128+
not known

negro   ○
white   ☐
mongoloid   ◇
other   △

Fig. 13. Map showing worldwide distribution of cancer of the oesophagus.

along the Caspian littoral have not yet been observed with other gastro-intestinal cancers.

Head and Neck—General

African Malignant (Burkitt's) Lymphoma

The first definitive description of this tumour—in Ugandan children (Burkitt, 1958) also pointed out an association between these jaw malignancies and similar tumours of the abdominal viscera. The tumour, which most commonly presents as a unilateral maxillary swelling, is found not only in a belt ($\pm 15°$ latitude) across tropical Africa (Burkitt, 1962), but also in the island of New Guinea (ten Seldam et al., 1966), where it is the most common tumour of childhood (Booth et al., 1968). The relatively recent history of this disorder eloquently illustrates the contribution that epidemiological studies can make to the elucidation of recently recognized diseases. The observation that the tumour was rarely seen in the mountainous regions was the starting point of Burkitt's epidemiological studies. This lymphoma belt of Africa corresponds to the tropical rain forest lowlands (less than 1500 m above sea-level), but with the notable exception of Zanzibar and the urban areas of the continent. This is in contrast to other types of malignant lymphoma in African children, which are not climatic dependent (Wright and Roberts, 1966). These areas of the world, Dalldorf and his associates (1964) observed, correspond to the areas where malaria is holo-endemic (this implies a palpable spleen rate of >75 per cent in children of 2–9 years of age, with a low spleen rate in adults). The tumour-free areas in the African lymphoma belt (urban areas and Zanzibar) are those that have been essentially cleared of malaria by successful eradication schemes. Space-time clustering of the tumour was subsequently demonstrated in Uganda (Pike et al., 1967). Pike and his colleagues said that the disease possessed the epidemiological character of what they termed "drift", i.e. patients whose dates of onset were close together tended to live closer than could be expected on the basis of chance alone. Following the isolation of a virus from tumour cells (Epstein et al., 1964), sero-epidemiological studies by Levy and Henle (1966) showed that 100 per cent of sera from patients with the lymphoma had high titres of antibodies to the EB (Epstein-Barr) virus. Burkitt (1969) then modified a previous vectored virus hypothesis. He now suggests that the tumour develops when a person whose cells have been previously altered by a chronic infection, specifically malaria, is infected by the EB virus. Experimental studies by Jerusalem (1968) on mice support this hypothesis. Repeated infection of these animals with *Plasmodium berghei* produced a high incidence of leukaemia. Consistent with this present hypothesis is the finding by Pike and his colleagues (1970) that the presence of the sickle-cell trait, which confers some protection against malaria, was only half the rate in affected individuals than in controls.

Lymphadenoma (Hodgkin's Disease)

A discussion of Burkitt's tumour cannot fail to bring to mind the question regarding the aetiology of that other malignant lymphoma, Hodgkin's disease. This tumour, which commonly presents as a swelling in the neck, has been reported as showing a higher than average incidence in children both in the Lebanon (Azzam, 1966) and in Peru (Solidoro et al., 1966). In the U.S.A., the tumour is responsible for a slightly higher mortality rate in white compared with non-white individuals (Miller, 1966). A study by Chopra (1968) in Zanzibar showed a much greater incidence in Arabs than in Negroes. Since the environmental factors are basically the same for these two ethnic groups on this 80 km long island, it would appear that Arabs have a greater genetic predisposition to develop the tumour. However, an infective aetiology and a relationship to the ornithoses has previously been suggested. More recently, epidemiological studies in the U.S.A. (Vianna and Polan, 1973) have again suggested the possibility of an infective aetiology. In view of the bimodal distribution of the condition as a function of age, perhaps the first start should be to attempt a better nosography of the disease.

Idiopathic Multiple Haeomorrhagic (Kaposi's) Sarcoma

Since 1872, when Kaposi described five patients with multiple pigmented tumours of the skin, in association with similar lesions of the gastro-intestinal tract, larynx and trachea, the disease has always excited a certain curiosity, despite (but perhaps because of) its rarity. Because of the possibility of head and neck involvement, the tumour may be met with in otolaryngological practice (Abramson and Simons, 1970), although it is usually only in children that it presents as a lymphadenopathy. It may also involve the ears (Gibbs, 1968; Naunton and Stoller, 1960). Although it was first considered to be a disease of Ashkenazi Jews, it is now known to be common in the African Negro (but not in the American Negro). The highest incidence is in north-east Zaire (formerly known as the Belgian Congo), where it accounts for about 10 per cent of all malignancies, radially diminishing in incidence in all directions (Oettlé, 1962). Williams and Williams (1966) have pointed out that the geographical distribution of Kaposi's disease in Africa is similar to that for onchocerciasis. They therefore suggest that the Simuliidae (Black Flies) are vectors for Kaposi's disease also.

Thyroid Gland

Like the Himalayan region (Srinivasan et al., 1964) in particular, north-east Zaire also shows a high prevalence of endemic *cretinism* and "deaf mutism". This condition is localized to the Uele region (Bastenie et al., 1962).

Mention was made previously of the role of cassava in the causation of the endemic oto-neuro-ophthalmological syndrome in Nigeria. Nwokolo and Ekpechi (1966) have reported that there is a high prevalence of *goitre* in the Nsukka division of Eastern Nigeria. In the village of Ette, the prevalence of visible goitre attains 32·5 per cent of the population. In general, the endemic area for goitre corresponds with that for the neuromyelopathy (Oluwasanmi and Alli, 1968). Experimental studies on rats show that cassava is goitrogenic (Ekpechi, 1967). It is suggested that cassava contains a thionamide-like compound, i.e.

like thiouracil. Cassava is also deficient in iodine so that this would reinforce the goitrogenic effect.

It is commonly held that the prevalence of thyroid *cancer* is related to the availability of dietary iodine. However, data available for Iceland, where there is a very high iodine content in the food and where endemic struma does not occur, show that there is a relatively high incidence of this malignancy, at least for women (Bjarnason, 1967). For the older age groups, the rate is about 5 times that for Sweden.

Facial Nerve

El-Ebiary (1971) reported that Bell's palsy is 20 times as prevalent in Alexandria as it is in London. Figure 14 shows the smoothed (3-monthly moving average) incidence data expressed per 1000 cases per annum. The author says that

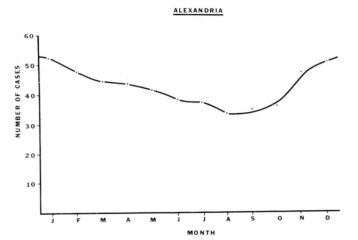

FIG. 14. Three-monthly moving average monthly incidence of Bell's palsy seen in Physical Medicine Department of Alexandria University Hospital, Egypt, between May 1966 and June 1967. (After El-Ebiary, 1971.)

the seasonal fluctuations are statistically significant. If Kettel's (1959) data for Denmark are similarly presented, they also show a seasonal fluctuation (Fig. 15). It is interesting to observe, however, that neither of these curves shows the pure sinusoidal annual fluctuation that was demonstrated for otitis media (Figs. 2 and 3). Moreover, the phase relationships for the two sets of data for Bell's palsy are dissimilar. An inspection of available climatic data, such as rainfall, for Alexandria and Copenhagen, fails to show any correspondence with the seasonal incidence data. Thus, although the available epidemiological evidence gives credence to an infective aetiology for "Bell's" palsy, at the same time it suggests a different aetio-pathogenesis in Denmark and in Egypt, with more than one causative factor probably in each country.

Speech Disorders

The prevalence of speech defects (articulatory, voice or rhythm difficulties) in schools in the U.S.A. has been

reported to exceed 20 per cent (Carhart, 1939). The high prevalence recorded may have been due to assessment being made by teachers and not trained speech scientists. A recent population study of 7-year-old children, conducted by Butler and his associates (1973) in the U.K.,

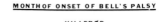

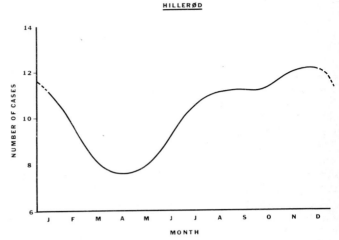

FIG. 15. Three-monthly moving average monthly incidence of Bell's palsy in a Danish series. (After Kettel, 1959.)

showed that between 1 and 2 per cent had a marked speech defect despite normal hearing. These affected children were more often male and of poor family background and were more likely to have been born towards the end of a long family. They also showed more clumsiness, defects of vision and of visual motor co-ordination, and were more likely to have educational difficulties. The lesson to be learned from this epidemiological study is that a speech defect in a child is not something to be brushed aside and relegated to a speech therapist working in isolation. It requires a full investigation by the various medical specialists, psychologists and teachers.

CONCLUSIONS

From this all too brief and patchy narrative, it is clear that epidemiology has contributed, and is continuing to contribute, to the scientific foundations of otolaryngology. It has passed beyond the study of the communicable fevers, to the study of congenital anomalies, neoplasias, neuro-otolaryngological disease and nutritional disorders. It has even passed beyond disease itself to the study of the "normal" ear, nose and throat and its senses. The role of the epidemiological method is, to use Acheson's (1971) own words, "very pervasive indeed". As Himsworth (1970) has said, the epidemiological approach is one of the most powerful research methods that we have and it has not yet been properly developed. In view of increasing restrictions on animal and human experimentation, the epidemiological method will assume even greater importance in the future.

REFERENCES

Abe, O. (1969), *Ann. math. Statist.*, **40**, 144.

Abramson, A. L. and Simons, R. L. (1970), *Arch. Otolaryng.*, **92**, 505.

Acheson, E. D. (1967), *Medical Record Linkage.* London: Oxford University Press.

Acheson, E. D. (1971), *Brit. med. Bull.*, **27**, 1.

Acheson, E. D., Cowdell, R. H., Hadfield, Esme and Macbeth, R. G. (1968), *Brit. med. J.*, **2**, 587.

Acheson, E. D., Cowdell, R. H. and Jolles, B. (1970), *Brit. med. J.*, **1**, 385.

Ahmed, N. (1966), *E. Afr. med. J.*, **43**, 235.

Arnott, W. M. (1954), *Brit. med. J.*, **2**, 887.

Ashcroft, M. T., Cruickshank, E. K., Hinchcliffe, R., Jones, W. I., Miall, W. E. and Wallace, J. (1967), *W. Ind. med. J.*, **16**, 233.

Azzam, S. A. (1966), *Cancer Res.*, **26**, 1202.

Babbott, J. G. and Ingalls, T. H. (1962), *Amer. J. pub.. Hlth.*, **52**, 2009.

Barr, B., Anderson, H. and Wedenberg, E. (1973), *Audiology*, **12**, 426.

Bastenie, P. A., Ermans, A. M., Thys, O., Beckers, C., Schrieck, H. G. van den and Visscher, M. de (1962), *J. clin. Endocr.*, **22**, 187.

Begg, T. B. (1966), *Brit. med. J.*, **2**, 815.

Berglund, B. and Halonen, P. (1970), *Eye, Ear, Nose Thr. Digest*, **32**, 37.

Berkson, J. (1955), *Proc. Staff Meet. Mayo Clinic*, **30**, 119.

Bjarnason, O. (1967), *Racial and Geographical Factors in Tumour Incidence*, (A. A. Shivas, Ed.). University Edinburgh Pfizer Medical Monogr. 2.

Booth, Kathleen, Cooke, R., Scott, G. and Atkinson, L. (1968), *Cancer in Africa* (P. Clifford, C. A. Linsell and G. L. Timms, Eds.). Nairobi: East African Publishing House.

Bordley, J. E. and Kapur, Y. P. (1972), *Laryngoscope*, **82**, 1477.

Burkitt, D. P. (1958), *Brit. J. Surg.*, **46**, 218.

Burkitt, D. P. (1962), *Brit. J. Cancer*, **3**, 379.

Burkitt, D. P. (1969), *Lancet*, **ii**, 1229.

Burkitt, D. P., Williams, E. H. and Eshleman, L. (1969), *Brit. J. Cancer*, **23**, 269.

Burns, W. and Robinson, D. W. (1970), *Hearing and Noise in Industry.* London: H.M.S.O.

Butler, N. R., Peckham, Catherine and Sheridan, Mary (1973), *Brit. med. J.*, **1**, 253.

Carhart, R. (1939), *J. Speech Hear. Dis.*, **4**, 61.

Casals, J. and Whitman, L. (1957), *Amer. J. trop. Med.*, **6**, 1004.

Causey, O. R. and Maroja, O. M. (1957), *Amer. J. trop. Med.*, **6**, 1017.

Chopra, S. A. (1968), "Chapter 4," in *Cancer in Africa* (P. Clifford, C. A. Linsell and G. L. Timms, Eds.). Nairobi: *East African Publishing House.*

Chung, C. S. and Brown, K. S. (1970), *Amer. J. hum. Genet.*, **22**, 630.

Clifford, P. (1970), *Int. J. Cancer*, **5**, 287.

Cochrane, A. L. (1965), *Milbank mem. Fd. Quart.*, **43**, 326.

Cook, Paula J. and Burkitt, D. P. (1971), *Brit. med. Bull.*, **27**, 14.

Dalldorf, G., Linsell, C. A., Barnhart, F. F. and Martin, R. (1964), *Perspect. Bio. Med.*, **7**, 435.

Daoud, E. H., El Hassan, A. M., Zak, F. and Zakova, N. (1968), *Cancer in Africa* (P. Clifford, C. A. Linsell and G. L. Timms, Eds.) Nairobi: *East African Publishing House.*

Debois, J. M. (1969), *Tjdsr. v. Geneesk.*, **25**, 92.

Denues, A. R. T. and Munz, W. (1968), "Chapter 13," *Cancer in Africa* (P. Clifford, C. A. Linsell and G. L. Timms, Eds.). Nairobi: East African Publishing House.

Doll, R. (1958), *Brit. J. industr. Med.*, **15**, 217.

Doll, R. (1964), *Medical Surveys and Clinical Trials*, p. 86 (L. J. Witt, Ed.). London: Oxford University Press.

Doll, R. (1967), *Prevention of Cancer: Pointers from Epidemiology.* London: Nuffield Provincial Hospitals Trust.

Doll, R. (1968), "Chapter 14," *Cancer in Africa* (P. Clifford, C. A. Linsell and G. L. Timms, Eds.). Nairobi: East African Publishing House.

Doll, R. and Cook, P. (1967), *Int. J. Cancer*, **2**, 269.

Doll, R. and Hill, A. B. (1950), *Brit. med. J.*, **2**, 739.

Doll, R. and Hill, A. B. (1956), *Brit. med. J.*, **2**, 1071.

Eilertsen, E. and Humerfelt, S. (1968), *Acta med. scand.*, **184**, 145.

Ekpechi, O. L. (1967), *Brit. J. Nutr.*, **21**, 537.

El-Ebiary, H. M. (1971), *Rheum. phys. Med.*, **11**, 100.

Elwood, P. C., Jacobs, A., Pitman, R. G. and Entwistle, C. C. (1964), *Lancet*, **ii**, 716.

Elwood, P. C. and Weddell, J. M. (1971), *Brit. med. Bull.*, **27**, 32.

Epstein, M. A., Achong, B. G. and Barr, Y. M. (1964), *Lancet*, **i**, 702.

Evans, E. (1974), *Sound Reception in Mammals* (R. J. Bench, Ade Pye and J. D. Pye, Eds.). London: Academic Press.

Feigl, H. (1953), *Readings in the Philosophy of Science*, p. 12 (H. Feigl and M. Brodbeck, Eds.). New York: Appleton Century-Crofts.

Feingold, M., Klein, J. O. and Haslan, G. E. (1966), *Amer. J. Dis. Child.*, **3**, 361.

Fisch, L. (1973a), "Prescriptive Screening for Auditory Disorders in the Elderly," Report of Working Group, Department of Health and Social Security, London.

Fisch, L. (1973b), *Audiology*, **12**, 411.

Flamant, R., Hayem, M., Lazar, P. and Denoix, P. (1964), *Cancer*, **17**, 377.

Fletcher, C. M. and Oldham, P. D. (1964), *Medical Surveys and Clinical Trials*, p. 57 (L. J. Witts, Ed.). London: Oxford University Press.

Frame, J. D., Baldwin, J. M., Gocke, D. J. and Troup, J. M. (1970), *Amer. J. trop. Med. Hyg.*, **19**, 670.

Fry, J., Dillane, J. B., McNab Jones, R. F., Kalton, G. and Andrew, Eileen (1969), *Brit. J. prev. Soc. Med.*, **23**, 205.

Gibbs, R. (1968), *Arch. Derm.*, **98**, 104.

Gignoux, M. and Bernard, P. (1969), *J. Med. Lyon*, **50**, 731.

Grönroos, J. A., Vihma, Leena, Salmivalli, A. and Berglund, B. (1968), *Acta oto-laryng.* (*Stockh.*), **65**, 505.

Halsted, C., Lepow, M. L., Balassanian, N., Emmeroch, J. and Wolinsky, E. (1968), *Amer. J. Dis. Child.*, **115**, 542.

Harrison, D. F. N. (1964), *Brit. med. J.*, **2**, 1649.

Henderson, B. E., Gary, G. W. Jr., Frame, J. D., Carey, D. E. and Kissling, R. E. (1972), *Trans. roy. Soc. trop. Med. Hyg.*, **66**, 409.

Henle, G., Henle, W. and Diehl, V. (1968), *Proc. Nat. Acad. Sci.*, **59**, 94.

High, W. S. (1965), "Ch. 4," in *Audiometry: Principles and Practice*, p. 93 (A. Glorig, Ed.). Baltimore: Williams and Wilkins.

Himsworth, H. (1970), *Proc. CIOMS Round Table Conf. on Medical Research—Priorities and Responsibilities*, p. 57. Geneva: WHO.

Hinchcliffe, R. (1958), *Acta oto-laryng.* (*Stockh.*), **49**, 453.

Hinchcliffe, R. (1959), *Acustica*, **9**, 303.

Hinchcliffe, R. (1961a), *J. Laryng.*, **75**, 101.

Hinchcliffe, R. (1961b), *Brit. J. prev. Soc. Med.*, **15**, 128.

Hinchcliffe, R. (1961c), *Ann. Occup. Hyg.*, **3**, 6.

Hinchcliffe, R. (1968), *Indian J. Otolaryng.*, **20**, 52.

Hinchcliffe, R. (1972), "Ch. 5," in *Otitis Media* (A. Glorig and K. S. Gerwin, Eds.). Springfield, Ill.: Chas. C. Thomas.

Hinchcliffe, R. and Jones, W. I. (1968), *Int. Audiol.*, **7**, 239.

Hinchcliffe, R., Osuntokun, B. O., and Adeuja, A. O. G. (1972), *Audiology*, **11**, 218.

Hinchcliffe, R. and Sadé, J. (1971), *Sound*, **5**, 97.

Hoffman, H. and Worth, G. (1958), *Beitr. z Silikose-Forschung.*, No. 56.

Hsu, M-M., Chiou, J-F. and McCabe, B. F. (1974), *Ann. Otol.*, **83**, 19.

Institute of Medicine (1973), *A Strategy for Evaluating Health Services.* Washington, D.C.: National Academy of Sciences.

Jaffe, B. F. (1969), *Laryngoscope*, **79**, 2126.

Jaffe, B. F., Hurtado, F. and Hurtado, E. (1970), *Laryngoscope*, **80**, 36.

Jaffé, L. (1951), *Z. Laryng.*, **30**, 295.

Jauhiainen, T. (1968), *J. Laryng.*, **82**, 1109.

Jerusalem, C. (1968), *Tropenmed. med. Parasitol.*, **19**, 94.

Jordan, R. E. (1972), "Ch. 4," in *Otitis Media* (A. Glorig and K. S. Gerwin, Eds.). Springfield, Ill.: Chas. C Thomas.

Jordan, R. E. and Eagles, E. L. (1961), *Ann. Otol., Rhin. and Laryng.*, **70**, 819.

Kaposi, M. (1872), *Arch. Derm.*, **4**, 265.

Kapur, Y. P. and Patt, A. J. (1967), *Arch. Otolaryng.*, **85**, 400.

Kayser-Petersen. Quoted by Cochrane, 1954.

Kell, R. L., Pearson, JC. G. and Taylor, W. (1970), *Int. Audiol.*, **9**, 334.

Kettel, K. (1959), *Peripheral Facial Palsy*, p. 114. Oxford:Blackwell

King, P. F. (1949), *J. Laryng.*, **63**, 501.
Kmet, J. and Mahboubi, E. (1972), *Science*, **175**, 846.
Knox, E. G. (1959), *Brit. J. prev. Soc. Med.*, **13**, 222.
Knox, E. G. (1964), *Appl. Stat.*, **13**, 25.
Knox, E. G. (1968), "Ch. 5," in *Screening in Medical Care*, Nuffield Provincial Hospitals Trust. London: Oxford University Press.
Kostrzewski, J. (1970), *Proc. Round Table Conf. on Medical Research —Priorities and Responsibilities*, p. 52. Geneva: WHO.
Kristensen, H. K. (1946), *Acta oto-laryng. (Stockh.)*, **34**, 82.
Kučera, J. (1966), *Čslká Pediat.*, **20**, 873.
Kuang-Heng, Li, Jen-Ch'uan, Kao and Ying-Kai, Wu (1962), *A Survey of the Prevalence of Carcinoma of the Oesophagus in North China*. Shanghai: Scientific and Technical Publishers.
Lasagna, L. and von Felsinger, J. M. (1954), *Science*, **120**, 359.
Leading Article (1973), *Lancet*, **2**, 1365.
Levy, J. A. and Henle, G. (1966), *J. Bact.*, **92**, 275.
Lobo, L. C. G. and Jouval, H. E. (1973), *Int. J. Epidem.*, **2**, 359.
Mahboubi, E., Kmet, J., Cook, P. J., Day, N. E., Ghadirian, P. and Salmasizadeh, S. (1973), *Brit. J. Cancer*, **28**, 197.
Manson, Bahr, P. (1956), *J. Laryng.*, **70**, 175.
Martin, J. A. M. (1967), *J. Laryng.*, **81**, 1079.
May, J. M. (1949), *Acta Un. int. Cancr.*, **7**, 136.
McEldowney, Diane and Kessner, D. M. (1972), "Ch. 3," in *Otitis Media* (A. Glorig and K. S. Gerwin, Eds.). Springfield, Ill.: Chas. C Thomas.
McKeown, T. (1968), "Ch. 1," in *Screening in Medical Care*, Nuffield Provincial Hospitals Trust. London: Oxford University Press.
Medical Research Council (1957), *Lancet*, **2**, 510.
Meer, P., Andrassy, L., Bodo, A., Codrea, A., Foldessy, Z. and Sirban, I. (1957), *Oto-rino-laring (Bucuresti)*, **2**. 115.
Merluzzi, F. and Hinchcliffe, R. (1973), *Audiology*, **12**, 65.
Miller, R. W. (1966), *Cancer Res.*, **26**, 1201.
Moe, J. (1942), *Acta oto-laryng.*, Suppl. 65.
Monekosso, G. L. and Wilson, J. (1966), *Lancet*, **1**, 1062.
Money, G. L. (1958), *West Afr. med. J.*, **7**, 58.
Morrison, S. L. and Last, J. M. (1970), "Ch. 35," in *A Companion to Medical Studies* (R. Passmore and J. S. Robson, Eds.). Oxford: Blackwell.
Mosbeck, J. and Acheson, E. D. (1971), *Danish med. Bull.*, **18**, 34.
Muir, C. S. and Shanmugaratnam, K. (1967), *Cancer of the Nasopharynx*. Copenhagen: Munksgaard.
Nakamura, S. (1968), *Arch. Otolaryng.*, **87**, 544.
Naunton, R. F. and Stoller, F. M. (1960), *Laryngoscope*, **70**, 1535.
Niederman, J. C., McCollum, R. W., Henle, G. and Henle, W. (1968), *J. Amer. med. Ass.*, **203**, 205.
Nwokolu, C. and Ekpechi, O. L. (1966), *Trans. roy. Soc. trop. Med. Hyg.*, **60**, 97.
Oettlé, A. E. (1962), *Acta Un. int. Cancr.*, **18**, 17.
Oluwasanmi, J. O. and Alli, A. F. (1968), *Trop. geogr. Med.*, **20**, 357.
Osuntokun, B. O. (1968), *Brain*, **91**, 215.
Osuntokun, B. O., Aladetoyinbo, A. and Adeuja, A. O. G. (1970), *Lancet*, **2**, 372.
Osuntokun, B. O., Monekosso, G. L. and Wilson, J. (1969), *Brit. med. J.*, **1**, 547.
Palchanis, W. T. (1952), *Amer. Rev. Tuberc.*, **65**, 451.
Peters, W. P., Schlom, J., Frankel, J. W., Prickett, C. O., Groupé, V. and Spiegelman, S. (1973), *Proc. Nat. Acad. Sci.*, **70**, 3175.
Pickering, G. (1970), *Proc. Round Table Conf. on Medical Research— Priorities and Responsibilities*, pp. 50, 58. Geneva: WHO.
Pike, M. C., Morrow, R. H., Kisuule, A. and Mafigiri, J. (1970), *Brit. J. prev. Soc. Med.*, **24**, 29.

Pike, M. C. and Smith, P. G. (1968), *Biometrics*, **24**, 541.
Pike, M. C., Williams, E. H. and Wright, B. (1967), *Br. med. J.*, **2**, 395.
Proctor, D. F. (1963), *The Nose, Paranasal Sinuses and Ears in Childhood*. Springfield, Ill.: Chas. C Thomas.
Refsum, E. (1952), *Acta tuberc. scand.*, **27**, 288.
Reynaud, J. (1968), "Ch. 35," in *Cancer in Africa* (P. Clifford, C. A. Linsell and G. L. Timms, Eds.). Nairobi: East African Publishing House.
Robinson, D. W. (1960), *Ann. Occup. Hyg.*, **2**, 107.
Robinson, J. O. (1962), *Brit. J. soc. clin. Psychol.*, **2**, 56.
Rowson, K. E. K., Gamble, D. R. and Hinchcliffe, R. (1975), *Lancet*, **1**, 471.
Sayers, B. McA. (1974), unpublished data.
Scheiblechner, H. (1974), *Audiology*, **13**, 93.
Segi, M. (1960), *Cancer Mortality for Selected Sites in 24 Countries (1950–7)*. Sendai, Japan: Department of Public Health, Tohoku University School of Medicine.
Shedd, D. P., von Essen, C. F., Ferraro, R. H., Connelly, R. R. and Eisenberg, H. (1968), *Cancer*, **21**, 89.
Sigerist, H. E. (1941), *Four Treatises of Theophrastus von Hohenheim*. Baltimore: Johns Hopkins Press.
Solidoro, A., Guzmán, C. and Chang, A. (1966), *Cancer Res.*, **26**, 1204.
Srinivasan, S., Subramanyan, T. A., Sinha, A., Deo, M. G. and Ramalingaswami, V. (1964), *Lancet*, **2**, 176.
Suehs, O. W. (1952), *Laryngoscope*, **62**, 998.
Surján, L., Dévald, J. and Pálfalvi, L. (1973), *Audiology*, **12**, 396.
Suwanwela, C. and Hongsaprabhas, C. (1966), *J. Neurosurg.*, **25**, 172.
Szcypiorski, W., Wroblewska, E., Tomaszewska, E. and Zmudzka, B. (1969), *Otolaryng. Pol.*, **23**, 183.
Tandon, P. N. (1973), "Ch. 9," in *Tropical Neurology*, (J. D. Spillane, Ed.). London: Oxford University Press.
Tato, J. M. and Tato, J. M. (1969), *Acto oto-laryng. (Stockh.)*, **67**, 277.
Taylor, W., Pearson, J. and Mair, A. (1967), *Brit. J. industr. Med.*, **24**, 114.
Ten Seldam, R. C. J., Cooke, R. and Atkinson, L. (1966), *Cancer*, **19**, 437.
Thomson, A. and Buxton, L. H. D. (1923), *J. Roy. Anthrop. Inst.*, **53**, 92.
Thorner, R. M. and Remein, Q. R. (1961), *Publ. Hlth Mongr. No. 67*.
Tilles, J. G., Klein, J. O., Jao, R. L., Haslam, J. F., Jr., Feingold, M., Gellis, S. S. and Finland, M. (1967), *New Engl. J. Med.*, **277**, 613.
Underwood, B. J. (1957), *Psychological Research*, p. 97. New York: Appleton-Century-Crofts.
Vianna, N. J. and Polan, A. K. (1973), *New Eng. J. Med.*, **289**, 499.
Weiner, J. S. (1954), *Amer. J. physical Anthropol.*, **12**, 1.
Wilkins, L. T. (1949), *Survey of Deafness in the Population of England, Scotland and Wales*. The Social Survey.
Williams, E. H. and Williams, P. H. (1966), *E. Afr. med J.*, **43**, 208.
Woodruff, A. W., Monath, T. P., Mahmoud, A. A. F., Pain, A. K. and Morris, C. A. (1973), *Br. med. J.*, **3**, 616.
World Health Organisation (1953), "The prevalence of blindness and deafmutism in various countries," *Epidem. Vital Stats. Rpt.*, **6**, 1.
Wretmark, G. (1953), *Acta Psychiat. Neurol. Scand.*, Suppl. 84.
Wright, D. H. and Roberts, M. (1966), *Br. J. Cancer*, **20**, 469.
Wright, I. M. (1970), *J. Laryng.*, **84**, 283.
Yerushalmy, J., Harkness, J. T., Cope, J. H. and Kennedy, B. R. (1950), *Amer. Rev. Tuberc.*, **61**, 443.
Yoshie, C. (1955), *Jap. J. Med. Sci. Biol.*, **8**, 373.

11. HEARING CONSERVATION AND NOISE REDUCTION

A. M. MARTIN

INTRODUCTION

Modern technology has created many environmental pollutants of which noise is an immediate and identifiable example. Many industrial processes generate noise of sufficient sound levels to cause impairment of hearing and many of these processes have existed since the industrial

impulse noise, although in practice both types often occur together. In general, industrial noise has a broadband frequency spectrum as illustrated in Fig. 1. Although there are instances where this spectrum may have superimposed upon it discrete pure tones or occasionally the basic source of noise may produce sounds of purely tonal quality. There are several industrial sources of impact

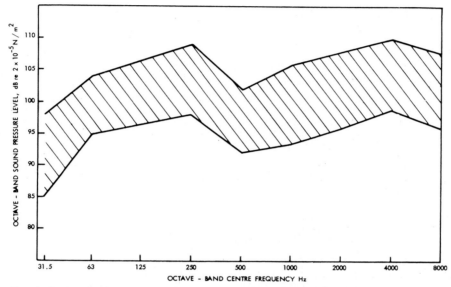

FIG. 1. Range of noise spectra measured at operator's position generated by several light-metal riveting operations.

revolution. Occupational hearing loss is not a new phenomenon. "Boilermakers' deafness", for example was well known among foundry workers in the nineteenth century and explosions are reported to have caused deafness amongst gun-crews in the Battle of Trafalgar.

Even though it has long been recognized, occupational hearing loss has generally been accepted until recent times as part of the price to be paid for full employment and technological progress. Fortunately a growing awareness of this problem in industry, changing attitudes to employment and the availability of noise reduction techniques and hearing protectors have resulted both in the quantification of the noise hazard and the reduction of the risk of hearing damage in many instances.

This chapter is concerned with the general subject of industrial hearing conservation and noise control, and describes methods for the measurement of noise, the evaluation of the hazard to hearing, personal hearing protection and the general requirements of a hearing conservation programme.

INDUSTRIAL NOISE HAZARD

Industrial noise may be divided for convenience into two separate types: steady-state noise and impact or

noise, such as drop forges, pneumatic hammers and stamping machines and these often represent a serious hazard to hearing. Figure 2 illustrates the sound pressure –time envelope of typical drop-forging noise. More

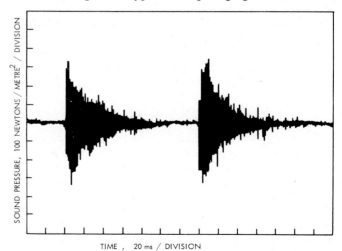

FIG. 2. Typical sound pressure-time waveform envelopes of drop-forging noise, measured at operator's position. The peak sound pressure level is about 144 dB(P).

common are processes which generate steady-state noise, although in these cases the noise levels vary considerably depending upon the actual process involved. To assess the hazard to hearing from industrial noise, it is necessary to establish a relationship between the noise parameters and the degree of hearing loss so produced.

A great deal of effort has been spent over the past three decades in an attempt to formulate methods for quantifying the relationship between noise exposure and hearing loss. Initially much of the work was based on laboratory

form the basis for the assessment of the majority of occupational noises. A-weighted sound energy and the equal-energy principle may be considered to be the unifying factors in what up to the present time has been a somewhat confused area of knowledge.

The concept of A-weighted sound energy is embodied in an equivalent-continuous sound level, L_{eq}, which may be defined as the level of continuous noise in dB(A), which in the course of a working day would cause the same sound energy to be received as that due to the actual noise

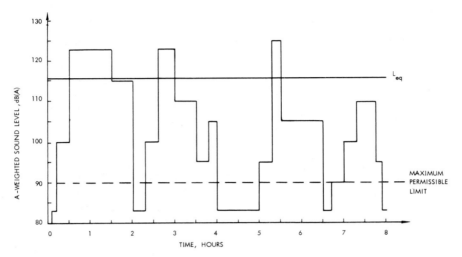

FIG. 3. Examples of A-weighted sound level history for an 8-hour day with its equivalent continuous sound level. $L_{eq} = 116$ dB(A) in this case.

experiments involving short-term hearing losses. However, the relationship between temporary hearing loss and persistent hearing loss caused by long-term exposure to noise in industry has since been doubted. In the last few years data have become available that have enabled persistent hearing losses to be correlated directly with long-term noise exposure. Much of the impetus for this work derived from the Medical Research Council and the National Physical Laboratory in Britain and a report by Burns and Robinson (1970) has since formed the basis for a method of assessing potential hazard to hearing from noise. A number of national and international bodies have based their standard methods of assessment on this type of information.

The Equal-Energy Principle

Burns and Robinson have shown for steady-state noise that a relationship exists between A-weighted sound energy and persistent hearing loss. This is known as the "equal-energy principle". Subsequent research by Atherley and Martin (1971) and Guberan *et al.* (1971) has shown that this principle may also be extended to include types of industrial impact noise. More recently Rice and Martin (1973) have concluded that the equal-energy principle may also be applied to the assessment of risk to hearing from high-level transient noises such as gunfire. Consequently a single and relatively simple principle may now be said to

over a typical day. Figure 3 illustrates the description, in terms of L_{eq}, of a complex noise exposure which fluctuates in level over a period of 1 working day of 8 h. The parameter L_{eq} may thus be considered as a measure of *noise dose*, a concept familiar to many other aspects of occupational medicine but relatively new to the field of noise.

A-weighted sound energy received during a noise exposure may be deduced from the product of the noise level in dB(A) and the duration of exposure. A doubling of energy represents an increase in noise level of 3 dB. Thus, for example, exposure to 90 dB(A) for a given period is equivalent in terms of sound energy, and therefore hazard, to an exposure of 93 dB(A) for half that period. Table 1 gives examples of values of sound level and exposure duration which, when considered together, represents an L_{eq} of 90 dB(A) for 8 h. These figures are considered at the present time to be maximum permissible limits for exposure to noise.

Standard Procedures for the Assessment of Hazard

In Britain at the present time there are three authoritative documents available that describe methods for the assessment of hazard to hearing from occupational noise exposure based upon an energy concept. These are:

(1) "The Code of Practice for Reducing the Exposure of Employed Persons to noise," prepared in 1971 by the

Industrial Health Advisory Committee's Sub-Committee on Noise, and published in 1972 by H.M.S.O. on behalf of the Department of Employment.

(2) The British Occupational Hygiene Society (BOHS) "Hygiene Standard for Wide-Band Noise," published in 1971.

(3) The International Organisation for Standardisation (ISO). Recommendation R1999. "Assessment of Occupational Noise Exposure for Hearing Conservation purposes," published in 1971.

TABLE 1

PERMISSIBLE EQUIVALENT CONTINUOUS SOUND LEVEL

(L_{eq}) FOR AN 8-H WORKING DAY

Sound Level dB (A)	Permissible Duration of Exposure per Day
90	8 h
93	4
96	2
99	1
102	30 min
105	15
108	7½
111	225 s
114	112
117	56
120	28
123	14
126	7
129	3½
132	1¾
135	less than 1 s

The Code of Practice is perhaps the most suitable document for application to the industrial situation in the United Kingdom at present. This specifies a limit for exposure to noise of an L_{eq} of 90 dB(A) and describes methods of measurement which can be used to determine whether the limit is exceeded. The Code makes the assumption that steady-state noise, fluctuating, intermittent and impact noise may all be described in terms of L_{eq}. Furthermore, it recommends overriding limits for the unprotected ear, these being a sound pressure level of 135 dB for steady-state noise and 150 dB for impulse noise. The Code is important in Britain because it specifies safe conditions of work. Although it is only advisory in nature at the present time, H.M. Factory Inspectorate relies upon its recommendations to define the auditory safety of a working environment.

However, the Code of Practice gives only a single demarcation between acceptable exposures and those which are unacceptable. Whereas the ISO and BOHS standards provide more detailed information regarding the percentage of persons who would be expected to exceed specified hearing losses after a given noise exposure.

The BOHS and ISO documents both set down values for noise exposure that will result in no more than specified

proportion of the exposed population suffering no more than a specified amount of hearing loss. The number of persons who will suffer these hearing losses is expressed as a percentage of the total exposed population, since it is impossible at the present time to predict accurately the effect that noise will have upon an individual prior to the noise exposure.

The British Occupational Hygiene Society's document refers solely to steady-state noise and is intended to restrict occupational exposure to noise so that handicap does not occur in more than 1 per cent of persons exposed during their working lifetime. This objective is considered to be achieved if the noise-induced impairment to hearing at the end of a 30-year working lifetime does not exceed levels of 40 dB, calculated as an average of audiometric test frequencies 0·5, 1, 2, 3, 4 and 6 kHz in 1 per cent of the persons exposed. To meet this criterion, noise levels should not exceed an L_{eq} of 90 dB(A). The BOHS Hygiene Standard also states that it must not be used for impulse noise or if there are significant pure tones present in the noise (the BOHS is at present considering a hygiene standard for impulse noise).

ISO recommendation R1999 does not quantify absolute levels which must not be exceeded. Rather, it gives a practical relationship between occupational noise exposure, expressed in terms of noise level and duration within a normal working week of 40 h, and the risk of increase in percentage of persons in specified age groups that may be expected to show hearing impairment as a result of specified amounts of occupational noise exposure. Hearing is considered to be impaired for conversational speech if the arithmetic average of hearing levels for the audiometric test frequencies 0·5, 1 and 2 kHz is 25 dB or more. Although the Recommendation does not set down actual limits for habitual noise exposure, levels of 90 dB(A) are mentioned as ones commonly found in legislation in those countries having laws prohibiting hazardous noise exposure. Impulse noises of less than 1 s. duration or single high-level transients such as gunfire are excluded.

Although the definitions of handicap and impairment are different in the BOHS and ISO documents, they may be assumed to be equivalent in terms of hazard to hearing. That is, the same noise level assessed by the two methods will probably result in the prediction of the same hearing losses.

THE MEASUREMENT OF EQUIVALENT CONTINUOUS NOISE LEVEL

Whichever standard specification is employed, the fundamental measure of the noise required is L_{eq}. This in turn entails the measurement of both sound level and time.

This section describes briefly the instrumentation necessary for the measurement of different types of industrial noise and the techniques of measurement to be applied in practice (Martin, 1974). Measurement techniques are categorized in terms of the necessary instrumentation as opposed to the types of noise measured. This approach is designed to provide a brief guide for the measurement of noise for those laboratories which already possess certain types of measurement equipment. A block diagram summarizing the basic approach to the problem and the essential equipment required is given in Fig. 4. The ability of different types of equipment to measure both steady-state and impact noise will be considered.

Sound Level Meter

The measurement of L_{eq} for steady-state noise may be made simply with a precision sound level meter (SLM)

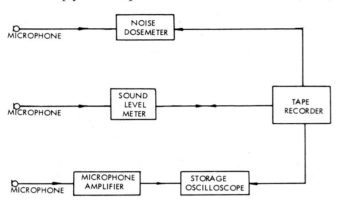

FIG. 4. Block diagram of basic equipment for the measurement of L_{eq} for industrial noise.

conforming to the specification recommended by the International Electrotechnical Commission (IEC 179, 1965) and a timepiece. The meter should be set to the A-weighting network and "slow" dynamic characteristic. Measurements of the sound level and exposure time should be made in close proximity to the ears of the personnel exposed to the noise. When the noise is steady in level and of unbroken duration, a few measurements of the level should provide a value of L_{eq}. Short-term fluctuations in sound level of no more than 10 dB, can be dealt with by "eye-averaging" the meter reading. However, if the sound level varies by more than 10 dB or varies more slowly with time, such as the noise produced by many cyclic industrial processes, the individual values of A-weighted sound level and "on" time should be recorded for each particular sound level. These components may then be summed to give a composite value for L_{eq} using one of the standard techniques, such as those described in the BOHS Hygiene Standard (1971) or the Code of Practice (1972).

In many practical situations, noise levels fluctuate considerably as various industrial processes, possibly operating in the same area, generate noise with different temporal patterns. It may be necessary in such cases to carry out work-study procedures with a SLM to establish a reliable estimate of L_{eq}. The situation may be further complicated by the requirement to obtain a measure of the noise dose received by an individual. If an individual remains in the same location during the working day, then noise dose may be assessed relatively simply. However, if he moves around from quiet to relatively noisy surroundings in a random fashion, both during the day and from day to day (such as maintenance workers for example),

the measurement of L_{eq} with a SLM for that individual becomes an extremely complicated procedure. The need to monitor a number of individuals' noise dose probably makes the use of a SLM impractical in such circumstances.

The measurement of L_{eq} for impulse noise is not easily achieved with a SLM. This is because measures are required of both sound level and time and it is not usually possible to measure both the true peak sound level and the duration of an impulse with a SLM and a simple clock or watch.

The Noise Dosemeter

This is a relatively new development in the noise field which promises to simplify the measurement of L_{eq} considerably. The dosemeter measures both A-weighted sound level and duration simultaneously and hence can provide a direct measure of L_{eq}. In principle it should be able to deal with any type of noise, both steady and impulse, having any type of temporal pattern and therefore should provide a relatively simple measure of L_{eq} in any industrial situation. Care should be taken that the dosemeter used complies with the energy concept, and not the present American Specification of 5 dB per doubling of exposure time.

The dosemeter relies upon long-term integration techniques for the measurement of L_{eq}. That is, it sums over a period of time all the A-weighted sound energy incident upon it, irrespective of the temporal characteristics of the noise. It should not possess limiting dynamic meter characteristics such as "fast" or "slow", and therefore should not in this respect modify the incoming signal. Consequently it should in theory be equally capable of measuring L_{eq} for steady-state noises or for impulses having fast rise times.

The dosemeter is available in two forms: a relatively large static device and a small personal monitoring instrument worn by the exposed person. The larger instrument usually has a slightly better technical specification than the personal device and may be used to measure the L_{eq} of noise generated by a particular machine or in a particular area. However it suffers from a similar drawback to the SLM in that it does not easily provide a measure of the noise dose received by an individual if that individual moves around a factory from day to day in a random fashion. It is in this type of situation that a personal noise dosemeter has an advantage. Being worn in a pocket, it monitors directly all the sound energy reaching the ears of an individual, wherever he may be, and thus greatly facilitates the measurement of total personal noise dose.

The measurement of L_{eq} for steady-state noises, even with complex variations in sound level and temporal pattern, is a relatively simple matter with a dosemeter. However, care should be exercised to ensure that the duration of the measurement period is sufficient to provide a representative measure of a complete day's exposure. Similarly in the case of many types of impulse noise, L_{eq} may be measured simply and directly. However, certain types of industrial noise contain both steady-state and impulse noise components where the peak sound levels of the impulses are considerably greater than the background noise-levels, although both may be hazardous. In this situation care should be taken that the peaks of the impulses do not overload the dosemeter, thereby introducing errors. A dynamic range of at least 60 dB is necessary for a dosemeter to give reliable results in such circumstances.

Tape Recorders

The use of a precision tape recorder in the field can greatly facilitate the determination of L_{eq} for industrial noise. Tape recordings allow noises having complex sound level and temporal characteristics to be analysed in the laboratory using a dosemeter or other analytical equipment, such as a graphic level recorder or oscilloscope, *see* Fig. 4.

The measurement of steady-state noise by this technique is straight-forward provided that the usual safeguards and standards are maintained. In the case of impulse noise, even greater care is needed. Walker and Behar (1971), have shown that the measurement of impulse noise by this method introduces an error of about 1 dB in the peak values of the impulses. Provided that care is taken to ensure that neither microphones nor tape recorders clip the peaks of the impulses and possible signal-to-noise ratio limitations are noted, a reliable measure of L_{eq} should be obtained.

Oscilloscopic Techniques

An oscilloscope can be used to advantage for the measurement of those impulse noises not adequately catered for by a dosemeter or where a dosemeter is not available. However it is not usually convenient for the measurement of steady-state noise.

The basic requirement is a storage oscilloscope and camera, so that recordings of the pressure-time waveform of the impulse noise can be obtained (*see* for example Fig. 2). The impulse signal may come directly from a SLM or microphone and amplifier, or may be tape recorded and analysed in the laboratory, as illustrated in Fig. 4. Measurements are made of a number of parameters of the waveform of the noise and L_{eq} is deduced from these parameters. Martin and Atherley (1973) have described a simple method for the measurement of equivalent continuous noise level of impulse noise from oscilloscopic recordings of the impulse waveform.

Oscilloscopic techniques, like the SLM, become rather complex when attempting to assess the individual noise dose of a person who moves around a factory. A number of measurements of the waveform may be required, together with work study procedures, if the noise is generated by several different machines or by a varying cyclic manufacturing process.

Calibration

The calibration of all measurement equipment is essential for reliable results. All instrumentation should be calibrated prior to making the measurements and this should be checked at regular intervals during its use.

Equipment such as the SLM and dosemeter can be calibrated relatively simply following the manufacturer's instructions with the standard acoustic source normally provided. Recording a calibration signal on tape requires due regard being paid to the problems of recording level, overloading and possible maximum peak sound level of the noise to be recorded. The use of a random acoustic source in this respect may add problems of peak clipping owing to the relatively high crest factors involved and therefore a non-random source is preferable. The calibration of an oscilloscope using a standard non-random source such as a pistonphone is essential, as the signal waveform itself is used to calibrate the graticule. The oscilloscope graticule should be calibrated in terms of the linear sound pressure units: pascals (newtons per square metre).

REDUCTION OF HAZARD TO HEARING

Having established the values of L_{eq} for a particular factory area or a group of individuals and assessed the hazard to hearing by comparison with the recommended limit of 90 dB(A), it is necessary to consider methods for reducing the noise level so that the hazard may be removed.

The classic description of an industrial noise problem may best be summarized as follows:

$$\text{Source} \rightarrow \text{Path} \rightarrow \text{Receiver}$$

Noise is radiated from the source (the offending machinery) via the path (the air and the structures of the machinery and the building) to the receiver (the person at risk). In theory the problem should always be approached in that specific order, so that reduction at source is the optimum solution, with reduction of the transmission of sound via the path as second best. Both approaches may be necessary, however, while personal protection of the receiver should be considered ideally as a last resort. In practice where reduction at source is not feasible for technological or economical reasons, some form of acoustic and/or vibration barrier should be inserted between the source and the receiver. However there are many situations where this latter approach is also not a practical possibility and resort must then be made to the use of personal hearing protection.

Planning for Noise Control

The most desirable method of noise reduction and that which provides by far the best and most efficient solution, is tackling the problem of industrial noise at the planning and design stages. Where a new factory or an extension to an existing plant is under consideration or where the purchase of new or replacement machinery is contemplated, consideration should be given to the noise levels likely to be introduced, so these and the number of persons exposed can be kept to a minimum. Thus, in planning the layout of a new factory or an extension to an existing one, noisy processes should be kept separate from relatively quiet processes where possible. Similarly, the specification of maximum noise levels should be included in the design of new plant or in the specification of machinery likely to be purchased from a manufacturer. In this way, many potential noise hazards can be eliminated at the design stage before they reach the factory floor, and hence the need for *ad hoc* noise control procedures after the machinery has been installed can be removed. If reduction of noise is found necessary after equipment has been designed and manufactured it may well prove to be expensive and often not entirely satisfactory.

Control of Noise at Source and in Transmission

The principles involved in the reduction of noise at source and in transmission will be outlined briefly in this Section. However, although some of the physical principles of noise attenuation and absorption are described elsewhere in this book, the reader is referred to other specialized publications on the topic of engineering noise control, given in the bibliography, which discuss in greater detail the practical problems likely to be faced in dealing with this widely diverse and somewhat complex subject. Nevertheless, the topic of personal hearing protection and the approach to a successful hearing protection programme are discussed in detail later in this chapter.

Reduction of Noise at Source

In the industrial situation the main concern is with noise generated by such prime movers as the internal combustion engine, moving machinery, aerodynamic and hydrodynamic flow and also by impact between two or more masses. However, there will often be other subsidiary noise sources present besides the item of main interest. In many complex situations a detailed analytical noise survey may be required to establish precisely which is the most important noise source, and hence indicate the initial point of attack. For the purpose of this section, a noise source is defined as a complete machine.

In general, procedures for noise control at source can be divided into two categories:

(1) Alteration of the duty or operating procedures of a machine.
(2) Alteration of the design of the machine.

In general noise levels may vary considerably with the running speed of a machine, and less so with the load. Hence it is undesirable to operate a machine in regions where the noise level is particularly sensitive to changes in operating conditions. However, appropriate adjustment of the speed and loading of a machine, compatible with production requirements, may be made so that noise levels are minimized. Considerable reduction in noise levels may be obtained by the replacement of a machine by a larger one which provides the equivalent power or number of processes being carried out at a lower speed. Similarly where possible, the operating times of particularly noisy processes should be arranged so that a minimum number of personnel are present in the hazardous area.

Adjustment of operating conditions in this way can in some instances result in significant reductions in noise exposure without recourse to more basic changes in the design of a machine and are obviously well worth considering as a first step.

If alteration of the duty of a machine is impossible or provides insufficient noise reduction, improving the machine design should be considered. The re-design of complex modern industrial machinery with noise reduction as the primary object is a task really only for the experienced engineer; and the reader is referred to the bibliography for publications describing the principles and techniques involved. Suffice it to say here that the main aim is to modify the exciting forces within a machine so that less acoustic energy is generated; and to alter the response of the machine structure to such forces so that less energy is radiated. Acoustic excitation can result from such sources as impulsive forces, frictional forces, electrical and magnetic forces and out-of-balance forces, so that reduction of these may result in a reduction in noise level. Appropriate alteration of the structural response of a machine by changing the mass, stiffness or damping of parts of its structure will also result in the reduction of the amount of sound or vibration radiated from the machine.

Reduction of Noise in Transmission

The fact that a noise control problem exists implies that there is a path via which the noise will reach the receiver from the source. Acoustic energy may be transmitted through the air as noise or through a solid structure as vibration, and the latter path may also result in the radiation of acoustic energy as noise at points away from the main source. In practice noise will often reach a receiver by a number of different paths, as illustrated in Fig. 5. Here acoustic energy is transmitted directly from the source as noise and via a number of flanking paths in the form of vibrational energy which is then re-radiated as noise by various surfaces. Noise control procedures involve, as a first step, the determination of the relative importance of each path for a particular situation, so that the predominant path may be ascertained and the appropriate measures then taken.

There are usually a number of alternative methods of controlling noise in transmission and the decision as to which is most appropriate may well also depend upon non-acoustic factors, such as the constraints of possible interference with industrial processes and economics.

(1) *Siting of a Source and Receivers*
If the source is some distance from the receiver or is outside the building containing the receiver, each doubling of the distance between the source and receiver reduces the noise level by between 3–6 dB. Hence the noisiest parts of a factory should be situated as far as possible from those areas where a quiet environment is important. Due regard should also be paid to the relation between the site of the source and those boundaries of the factory which border on other sites likely to find excessive noise objectionable.

Similarly all noisy processes should be grouped together as far as possible so that personnel not involved in such processes are not needlessly exposed to the noise.

(2) *Use of Radiation Pattern*

Some noise sources radiate sound more effectively in certain directions than in others; so that, in certain situations, careful siting and orientation of the source may result in a reduction of the noise level at the receiver. This approach is most effective under approximately free-field conditions when the reverberant component of the sound field is relatively small.

(5) *Noise Control by Enclosure*

The placing of a properly designed acoustic enclosure around either the source or the receiver is an effective means of noise reduction and should provide a considerable degree of attenuation. The attenuation of an enclosure is, in general, dependent upon the surface mass of the material from which it is constructed, including the floor and ceiling. Furthermore, comparatively small gaps in the enclosure may seriously impair its effective attenuation, so that attention should be paid to the details of both its construction and maintenance; particularly doors, windows and points

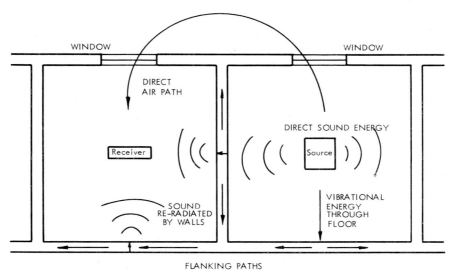

FIG. 5. Illustration of the transmission of sound from a source to a receiver via direct and flanking paths.

(3) *Building Design*

The careful design of room locations within a building, with respect to the relative positions of those areas where quiet conditions are required and the noise sources, will often result in efficient and economic noise control. Likewise, the position of rooms whose function is not particularly susceptible to noise may be arranged so that they act as a screen between the source and the receiver. Heavy vibrating machinery and other large sources of structure-borne sound should be sited low in a building, preferably in the basement, where the fabric of the building is likely to be heaviest. Where this is not possible, consideration should be given to the installation of the vibration isolation equipment at the design stage.

(4) *Path Deflection by Barriers*

Noise control by the use of barriers is only usually effective when they are large in relation to the wavelengths of the sound being transmitted. Furthermore, reflections from the barrier may increase the noise levels on the source side. They are of particular help where either the source or the receiver are close to the barriers. Under certain circumstances buildings could be employed as an effective screen where a simple barrier is impracticable.

where cables, ducts, pipes and other services emerge through it. The presence of an enclosure around a noise source may also increase the noise level within the enclosure due to reverberant sound, so that its inside surfaces should be treated with sound absorbent materials to reduce the reverberant sound level. Due consideration should also be given to the flanking transmission of acoustic energy from the source via the ground and via ducts or pipework connected to the source. Enclosure of the source is a common means of noise reduction. However, its use is limited when the source is mobile or hand-held and where large articles are processed on a production line.

(6) *Noise Control by Absorption*

In general, the application of sound absorbent materials alone to the surfaces of a room containing a noise source is not a particularly efficient method of noise reduction as only the reverberant sound field is affected. In practice a reduction in noise level of only about 6 dB is possible from such action. Although noise levels may be reduced at some distance from the source, little reduction is obtained near a machine where the operator is likely to be situated in the direct sound field. However, in certain industrial situations, such as workshops, functional or space absorbers may be suspended above or close to a noise source and receive more than the reverberant sound energy, hence providing a certain degree of noise reduction. Absorption is effective, however, in attenuating noise travelling along ventilation ducts, particularly if the duct is divided along its length by splitters covered with absorbent material.

(7) *Vibration Isolation*

The transmission of structure-borne energy from a source to a receiver via other radiating surfaces can be considerably reduced by mounting the source on resilient pads, thus isolating the source from the floor. Anti-vibration mounts should be designed to suit a specific machine, paying due regard to its mass, operating frequency and the resonant frequencies of the system. A machine when mounted on resilient pads may itself vibrate more, thus radiating higher sound levels, although these are generally lower than in the non-isolated case. Furthermore, rigid pipework, ducts, etc., connected to the machine may by-pass the effectiveness of the mounting if these are not also modified with flexible connectors.

(8) *Acoustic Filters and Mufflers*

Exhaust and inlet noise from internal combustion engines, fans and blowers and pneumatically operated machinery may be reduced effectively by the use of acoustic silencers. These devices are readily available in many sizes and provide a relatively economic means of noise reduction in a number of industrial situations.

In approaching a noise-control-in-transmission problem it is necessary to consider all possible energy paths, as reduction of one path alone, for example by enclosure, may not result in effective control if energy is still transmitted via other paths, for example by vibration or by a rigid connection to the source. Nevertheless, it is important in the first instance to establish the weakest link in a noise transmission problem.

Noise Control: General Summary

In practice, it may be necessary to tackle a noise control problem at a number of points. The application of techniques for reducing the noise at source by minimizing the exciting forces generating the energy is often not practical; and procedures for reducing the transmission of energy from the source to the receiver may have to be applied. If neither of these remedies reduces the noise sufficiently, then resort must also be made to personal hearing protection.

Figure 6 illustrates a general noise problem and the major paths by which airborne- and structure-borne sounds are transmitted from the source to the receiver. General points in the transmission pathways at which noise control may be effected are also shown and these are as follows:

A. Reduction at source
B. Control by enclosure of source
C. Control by vibration isolation of source
D. Control by barriers
E. Control by absorption
F. Reduction of radiated sound
G. Reduction by personal hearing protection
H. Control by isolation of receiver.

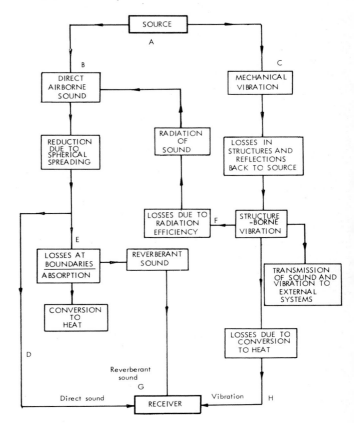

Fig. 6. A general noise control problem. Major paths by which airborne and structureborne sounds are transmitted from the source to the receiver and points at which noise control may be effected, see text.

In conclusion, it should be apparent that many noise control techniques involve no more than good engineering practice and commonsense, and these are perhaps the keynote of noise control in the industrial environment.

PERSONAL HEARING PROTECTION

As has been discussed above the most efficient means of reducing exposure to noise is to prevent the generation of the noise in the first place and where existing machinery represents a hazard to hearing, engineering noise control procedures should be instigated. There are many situations, however, where such noise control techniques are either impractical or not sufficient. In these cases personal hearing protective devices must be worn.

Where a hazard to hearing exists, the onus is on the employer to provide hearing protectors that attenuate noise sufficiently to remove the hazard. In the eyes of the law, as it stands at the moment in this country, it is not good enough merely to supply hearing protection. The devices provided must be capable of removing the hazard to hearing from the noise environment in which they are being worn. Consequently, knowledge is required of the physical characteristics of the offending noise as well as the acoustic attenuation characteristics of the hearing protectors provided. Furthermore, there is a certain degree of responsibility placed on the employer to educate the employee about noise and the need to wear hearing protection, and to persuade him to do so. Hence other non-acoustical properties such as comfort and wearer-acceptability may also have to be taken into account. Employers and other persons responsible for providing hearing protection should therefore have a good working knowledge of the many aspects and requirements of a hearing conservation programme.

Types of Hearing Protector

There are many brands and types of hearing protectors available on the market and there are several factors to be considered in addition to the protection they provide when selecting the most suitable type for any given situation. Some of these are comfort, cost, durability, chemical stability, availability, wearer acceptance and hygiene. Different hearing protectors will possess varying amounts of these properties, both good and bad, so that the requirements of the wearer and his environment must also be taken into account when considering the selection of a particular type.

Prefabricated Earplugs

Ear canals differ widely among individuals in size, shape and position and even between ears of the same individuals. Ear canals vary in cross-section from 3 to 14 mm, but most fall in the range 5 to 11 mm. The majority of ear canals are elliptical in cross-section but some are round and others have a small slit-like opening. Some ear canals are directed towards the centre of the head in a straight line while most bend in various ways and are usually directed towards the front of the head. It is immediately apparent from this that where prefabricated earplugs are chosen, they must be readily adaptable to a wide variety of canal shapes and sizes.

The best prefabricated earplugs for general industrial use are available in at least five different sizes. They are made from soft, flexible material that will conform readily to the many different ear canal shapes, thus providing a snug, airtight and comfortable fit. Earplugs must be non-toxic and should be made of a material that retains its shape and flexibility over extended periods of use and is not affected by the presence of earwax. There are a large number of different types of prefabricated earplugs available on the market. One of the most versatile and efficient types is the V-5IR. This is asymmetrically shaped and carries a single flexible flange that will adapt to a large number of differently shaped ear canals. It provides reasonable protection when fitted correctly combined with a certain amount of comfort. It is available in five sizes from the majority of manufacturers.

There are also a number of symmetrically shaped

earplugs available which provide sufficient protection and comfort under certain circumstances. However the round and straight types of earplugs do not adapt well to sharply bending or slit-shaped canals.

The correct fitting of earplugs is extremely important as the protection provided will be dependent to a large extent upon this factor. In many cases there is only a small space available in the ear canal to accommodate an earplug. However almost all entrances to ear canals can be opened and straightened by pulling the external ear directly away from and towards the back of the head so that an earplug may be seated securely. For comfort and retention of the earplug, the ear canal must return to its approximately normal shape once the protector has been fitted. The percentage distribution of sizes used by a large male population will be approximately as follows:

Earplug Size	% Male Population
Extra Small	5
Small	15
Medium	30
Large	30
Extra Large	15
Larger than normally supplied	5

The range of sizes, showing an equal percentage of wearers for medium and large sizes, is selected to provide the best fit for reasonable comfort and maximum attenuation. If an individual is permitted to fit himself with a particular set of earplugs, he will pay more attention to comfort than to the attenuation provided and hence the distribution of sizes will tend to shift towards the smaller plugs. Furthermore, some ear canals tend to enlarge slightly when earplugs are worn regularly; therefore, if a given ear falls between two sizes of earplug, it is advisable to choose the larger of the two. For this reason the fitting of earplugs should be checked periodically. Similarly, if earplugs are lost, care should be taken that the replacements fit correctly and a smaller size is not chosen for reasons of comfort.

Disposable and Malleable Earplugs

These types of earplugs are usually fashioned from low-cost materials such as cotton, wax, glass wool and mixtures of these and other substances. Typically, a small cone of the material is handformed and the apex of the cone is inserted into the ear canal with sufficient force so that it conforms to the shape of the canal and holds itself in position. In general, malleable and disposable earplugs made of non-porous and easily formed materials are reasonably comfortable and capable of providing attenuation values similar to those afforded by prefabricated plugs. Obviously they must be correctly made and inserted to obtain this level of performance.

The protection provided depends upon the material used and how firmly the plug is seated. Ordinary cotton wool by itself is extremely porous and provides very little attenuation (*see* Table 2). Indeed cotton wool is not recommended at all because of its inefficiency and the false sense of security which it engenders. Wax-impregnated cotton wool on the other hand provides a useful amount of protection; although it is often messy to use and lacks elasticity so that jaw movements may often cause such plugs to come loose. This requires that they are removed, reshaped and reinserted periodically which may cause problems of hygiene.

Glass wool (sometimes called glass down) is a practical and efficient form of disposable hearing protection. It is made from extremely fine glass fibres about 1 μm in thickness and provides good attenuation when folded and inserted according to the manufacturer's instructions. However, if not made correctly some of the material may stick in the ear canal, particularly if the plug is reinserted after being removed.

Although disposable earplugs are sometimes more comfortable to wear than prefabricated plugs and also have the advantage of universal fit, they require a greater standard of cleanliness from the wearer. Such earplugs should be formed and inserted with clean hands because any dirt or foreign bodies inserted into the ear may cause irritation or infection. This means that disposable and malleable earplugs should be carefully inserted at the beginning of a work shift and not removed or reinserted during the work period unless the hands are clean. As mentioned above, glass wool should never be reinserted into the ear, as the fibres tend to break up and thus be retained in the ear canal. Thus this type of earplug (and to a lesser extent all types of earplug) may be a poor choice for use in dirty areas having intermittent high noise levels or in other locations where it is necessary to remove and reinsert protective devices during the work period.

Individually Moulded Earplugs

These are usually made from some form of silicone rubber and are actually moulded in a permanent form within the ear canal. Usually the earplug material is supplied with a curing agent and the two are mixed to a putty-like consistency and then this is inserted into the ear canal of the person to be fitted. The material usually takes about 10 min to cure, during which time the subject must not move his jaws otherwise the ear canal is compressed and a sufficiently tight fit will not be achieved. Having cured, the earplugs are in a permanent form and may be removed and reinserted any number of times without affecting their performance. Some types are covered with a thin flexible coating after being cured to protect the surface and extend the plug's useful lifetime.

This type of earplug possesses the advantage of both prefabricated and malleable earplugs. It is comfortable and usually provides a high degree of protection if correctly made. When fitted with small handles, they can be removed and reinserted without getting dirty although, as with any type of earplug, problems of hygiene may still occur if the plugs are not kept in a clean place when not being worn.

The main advantage of individually moulded earplugs is their greater appeal to the wearer. In situations where difficulty is encountered in persuading men to wear hearing protection, the provision of an individually moulded device that will only fit the person for whom they are intended (like spectacles or false teeth!) is a psychological advantage. The word "personalized" is sometimes used to describe this earplug and comfort and wearer acceptability are its main assets.

Semi-insert Protectors

These are also called concha-seated hearing protectors or canal caps. They usually consist of two conical soft rubber caps attached to a narrow headband which presses them against the entrance to the external ear canal.

Semi-insert protectors have the advantage that one size will fit the majority of ears, unlike prefabricated plugs. As they are captive and may be reinserted hygienically at any time, they are suitable for industries where the loss of an earplug must be avoided, such as the food industry, and for people who must frequently enter noisy environments for short periods.

However, this type of plug is often not as comfortable as other forms of hearing protection, as they must be pressed firmly against the ear canal entrance to be effective. Such relatively high pressures exerted over a small area of the concha means that they may become uncomfortable, especially if worn for long periods of time. Nevertheless, semi-insert plugs may still be acceptable in hot environments as they do not cover the pinna and hence do not exacerbate the effects of perspiration.

Earmuffs

Most types of earmuffs are of similar design and are made from rigid cups specially designed to cover the external ear completely. They are held against the sides of the head by a spring-loaded adjustable band and are sealed to the head with soft circumaural cushions.

For maximum attenuation of sound, protector cups should be made from a rigid, dense non-porous material. The volume enclosed within the muff is proportional to the attenuation provided at low frequencies. Each cup should be partially filled with an absorbent material to reduce the high frequency resonances that may otherwise occur within the shell.

Earmuff seals may be liquid-filled or plastic foam-filled. Liquid-filled seals usually provide marginally better protection with only slight headband tension, all things being equal, but suffer from the additional problem of leakage of fluid if treated roughly. Also, certain early types of liquid seal became progressively more stiff as the liquid gradually absorbed the plastiser in the cushion skin, although this problem has been overcome now by many manufacturers. Modern foam-filled seals are almost as good as the liquid seals and have the additional advantage of robustness. These seals should have a small hole in the skin to allow them to distort to the shape of the side of the head. They usually require slightly higher headband pressures to provide a satisfactory seal.

All earmuffs should be provided with seals that are easily and separately replaceable in the factory environment. Seal materials that are placed against the skin should be non-toxic and non-irritant. They should not be affected by skin and hair oil, or by perspiration. Some earmuffs are provided with detachable muslin or linen seal covers that absorb perspiration, these may be either disposable or washable.

The acoustic seals on earmuffs will provide maximum protection when placed on a relatively smooth surface. Therefore less protection should be expected when muffs are worn over long hair, spectacle frames or other objects. Average-sized spectacle frames may cause a reduction of about 5 or 10 dB in the attenuation provided, although this loss may be much greater if the frames are thick or do not fit closely to the sides of the head. The loss of protection is dependent upon the size of the acoustic leak caused by the obstruction, hence smaller reductions may be achieved if the frames are made from thin wire, e.g. "gas mask" spectacles. Anti-perspiration covers over the seals may also reduce the attenuation afforded as they are porous and introduce acoustic leaks. If long hair over the ears or other obstructions cannot be avoided, it must be realized that the claimed attenuation of earmuffs may not actually be provided. This should be taken into account when deciding which type of hearing protector is most suitable for any particular situation.

Some earmuffs have an aperture that is asymmetrical or is curved beneath the seal so that it fits the contours of the head around the ear and thus can only be worn one way, i.e. only one cup will fit the left ear and only one the right. In these cases the correct way of wearing the muffs should be prominently marked and this pointed out to the wearer.

The attenuation provided by earmuffs is related to the force with which they are pressed against the sides of the head. Maintenance of the correct headband pressure is therefore important and care must be taken that this is not reduced by deliberately bending the headband so that they are more comfortable. The suspension force is usually chosen by the manufacturers as a compromise between performance and comfort and this should not be altered.

Earmuffs have the advantage over other hearing protectors of providing the greatest protection. Also, one size usually fits most people and they are easily removed and replaced in a hygienic fashion. This makes them eminently suitable for dirty and high-level noise areas and for people who frequently move in and out of noisy environments. They can also be worn by people who may suffer infections or skin disorders of the external ear canal or in other circumstances when earplugs cannot be worn.

The disadvantages of earmuffs lie in their bulkyness, initial cost and the fact that they tend to make the ears hot. However, their bulk has the advantage that it can easily be seen that they are being worn correctly. They are also usually more susceptible to damage than other forms of hearing protection.

A further problem may occur when earmuffs are worn with other safety equipment such as goggles and helmets. Not all types of earmuff are compatible with these safety appliances. Some earmuffs are provided with an adjustable headband which may also be worn under the chin or behind the nape of the neck, so that a safety helmet can be worn as well. One problem which sometimes occurs in these cases is that the weight of the muffs makes them slip down, so that they are actually supported by the auricles and are therefore more likely to leak. This obviously makes them uncomfortable and they cannot be worn for any length of time in this fashion. Some earmuffs are provided with an additional strap to get over this particular problem, the extra strap being worn over the top of the head (and under the helmet), thus supporting the weight of the earmuffs. There are also safety helmets available that carry earmuffs which may be swung down on to the ears.

Special Types of Hearing Protector

There are a number of earplugs and earmuffs designed for special purposes such as improved communication and the selective attenuation of high-level transient noises.

Frequency-selective Devices. All hearing protectors attenuate some frequencies more than others. Some are designed to augment this effect, especially certain types of earplug. These are usually fitted with an acoustic low-pass filter which ensures that the attenuation below about 2 kHz is relatively small. This filter enables the lower speech frequencies to be passed and this allows easier speech communication between wearers in the quiet.

However, improved speech communication in noise will only result if all the external noise is at a higher frequency. This is not the case in the majority of industrial situations and consequently the noise below 2 kHz is insufficiently attenuated and the communication advantages of this type of hearing protector are not realized. Although frequency-selective devices are often unsuitable for use on the factory floor when noise is continuously at a high level, they would provide some advantage in communication during the quiet periods if the noise is intermittent; provided, of course, that they give sufficient protection against the noise.

Amplitude-sensitive Devices. This type of hearing protector is designed to attenuate loud sounds more than quiet ones. One type of earplug, which is a modified version of the V-5IR plug, has a hole through its longitudinal axis in which is inserted a metal disc. There is a very small aperture in the centre of the disc which acts as an amplitude-sensitive device. At low sound levels, sound waves may pass easily through the hole, but high sound levels are progressively attenuated due to increased turbulence in the air flow through the aperture. Thus normal speech and other sounds may be heard with little impairment, but high-level transient noises, such as gunfire, will be attenuated to a much greater extent. These plugs are only useful for protection against gunfire and explosive-type noises, such as that generated by cartridge-operated tools. The main application of this type of earplug lies in the military and sporting aspects of impulse noise.

Earmuffs are available which incorporate an electronic peak-limiting amplifier in each cup. These have a microphone situated on the outside and an earphone on the inside of each shell which are connected by the amplitude-sensitive circuit. Such a device will allow all sounds to a level of, say, 85 dB(A) to pass through normally, but sound levels higher than this will not be transmitted by the electronic circuit, so that the basic earmuff then provides the attenuation. Such hearing protectors can be extremely valuable in situations where people are exposed to impulse noise, or any high-level intermittent noise, but wish to communicate easily during the quiet periods between noise bursts. The disadvantages of this type of earmuff

is unlikely that these limits will be realized in practice for the majority of hearing protectors.

The following rules should be observed to minimize losses due to acoustic leaks:

(1) Hearing protectors should be made of imperforate materials. If it is possible for air to pass freely through a material, noise will also be able to pass through with little attenuation. (There are exceptions to this rule in the case of non-linear devices for specialist purposes, such as the attenuation of high-level gunfire noise.)

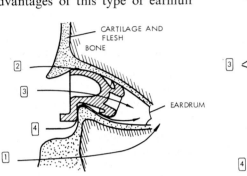

Fig. 7. Noise pathways through (a) an earplug and (b) an earmuff to the internal ear.

are that they are relatively expensive, require batteries, are heavy and must be handled with greater care than ordinary earmuffs.

Protector Performance Limitations and Requirements

An effective personal protective device serves as a barrier between noise and the internal ear and the protection afforded by such a device depends upon its design and upon several physiological and anatomical characteristics of the wearer.

Sound energy may reach the internal ears of persons wearing hearing protectors by four different pathways, as shown in Fig. 7.

(1) By passing through bone and tissue around the protector (bone conduction).

(2) By causing vibration of the protector which in turn generates sound into the external ear canal.

(3) By passing through leaks in the protector.

(4) By passing through leaks around the protector. Any one of these factors may severely limit the sound attenuating properties of a protector and therefore each should be minimized at all times.

Even if the protector should have no acoustical leaks through or around it, which is most difficult to achieve in practice, some noise will reach the internal ear by one or both of the first two pathways if the sound levels are sufficiently high. Therefore bone and tissue conduction thresholds set a practical limit to the attenuation provided by any hearing protector. These limits will vary considerably with the design of the protector and the wearer's physical make-up, but approximate values for both plugs and muffs are shown in Fig. 8. Due to effects such as acoustic leaks, it

(2) The protector should be designed to conform readily to the head or ear canal configuration so that an efficient acoustic seal may be achieved and, equally

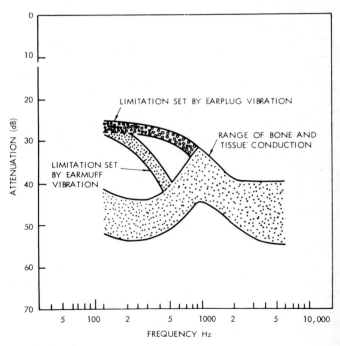

Fig. 8. Approximate attenuation limits for hearing protectors due to bone conduction and protector vibration.

important, so that the protector can be worn with reasonable comfort.

(3) The protector should have a means of support and

seal compliance that will minimize protector vibration when worn.

(4) Muff-type protectors should not be worn over long hair, poorly fitted spectacle frames or other obstacles.

These points should be borne in mind when selecting appropriate hearing protection for use in any situation or environment from the large number which are commercially available.

Attenuation Characteristics

The prime function of hearing protectors is to reduce noise level at the wearer's ears to within safe limits. Information on the ability and consistency of hearing protectors to attenuate sound should be closely examined when considering which type is most suitable for a particular noise environment.

The acoustic attenuation of hearing protectors is usually expressed in decibels mean attenuation at various test frequencies and is usually described in graphical form, as for example in Figs. 9 and 10, or in tabular form as given in Table 2. A second, but equally important measure associated with attenuation, is the degree of scatter of the attenuation data as measured on different subjects. This is usually expressed as the standard deviation about the grand mean, or as the interquartile range about the median. This figure should accompany each attenuation datum point when expressing the attenuation, *see* for example Table 2. Depending upon the measurement

TABLE 2

TYPICAL MEAN ATTENUATION AND STANDARD DEVIATION CHARACTERISTICS, IN dB, OF DIFFERENT TYPES OF HEARING PROTECTION

Test Frequency Hz.	125	250	500	1,000	2,000	4,000	8,000
Dry cotton wool	2	3	4	8	12	12	9
plugs: (S.D.)	(2)	(2)	(3)	(3)	(6)	(4)	(5)
Waxed cotton wool	6	10	12	16	27	32	26
plugs: (S.D.)	(7)	(9)	(9)	(8)	(11)	(9)	(9)
Glass down plugs:	7	11	13	17	29	35	31
(S.D.)	(4)	(5)	(4)	(7)	(6)	(7)	(8)
Personalized							
earmould plugs:	15	15	16	17	30	41	28
(S.D.)	(7)	(8)	(5)	(5)	(5)	(5)	(7)
V-51R type plugs:	21	21	22	27	32	32	33
(S.D.)	(7)	(9)	(9)	(7)	(5)	(8)	(9)
Foam-seal muffs:	8	14	24	35	36	43	31
(S.D.)	(6)	(5)	(6)	(8)	(7)	(8)	(8)
Fluid-seal muffs:	13	20	33	35	38	47	41
(S.D.)	(6)	(6)	(6)	(6)	(7)	(8)	(8)
Flying helmet:	14	17	29	32	48	59	54
(S.D.)	(4)	(5)	(4)	(5)	(7)	(9)	(9)

technique used, this figure tends to give among other things a measure of the hearing protector's ability to fit different individuals. The smaller the spread, the better the hearing protectors adapt to different head or ear canal shapes and sizes. It also provides a measure of the

accuracy with which the attenuation measurements were carried out.

Figure 9 shows an example of the mean attenuation characteristics of an earmuff, plotted with one and two standard deviations representing a spread of 67 and 95 per cent of the attenuation data respectively. Thus at a frequency of 4·0 kHz, 67 per cent of the people wearing the muff will be supplied with 40–50 dB protection and 95 per cent with 35–55 dB protection. In other words there will be 2·5 per cent of persons who will receive less

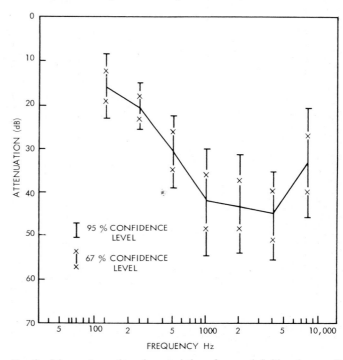

FIG. 9. Mean attenuation characteristics of a good fluid-seal earmuff with 67 per cent (mean minus one standard deviation) and 95 per cent (mean minus two standard deviations) confidence limits.

than 35 dB protection and 16·5 per cent who get less than 40 dB protection at this frequency for this particular earmuff. Figure 10 shows similar attenuation characteristics for an earplug. As can be seen, the spread of the attenuation data in this case is greater than that for earmuffs. These examples make the point that, when introducing a hearing protection programme, a decision has to be made as to the percentage of the population it is appropriate to consider and the hearing protector chosen accordingly.

Figures 9 and 10 give typical values for the attenuation to be expected from well designed and well fitted earmuffs and earplugs. However, if adequate protection cannot be provided by a single earmuff or earplug, both types may be worn at the same time to provide additional protection. The effect of earmuffs and earplugs being worn separately and both together is illustrated in Fig. 11. The combined attenuation provided by any two protectors cannot be deduced by simple addition and cannot be predicted accurately owing to complex coupling factors between them. However, the resultant attenuation from two good protectors may be estimated to average about 6 dB greater than the higher of the two individual attenuation values at most test frequencies.

The use of a good hearing protector can provide sufficient protection in a large majority of work environments where engineering control measures cannot be used successfully. For those relatively few persons exposed over long periods of time to noise levels in excess of about a 115 dB (A), special care should be taken to ensure that the

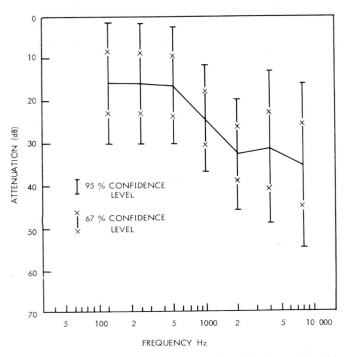

Fig. 10. Mean attenuation characteristics of a well-fitting earplug with 67 per cent and 95 per cent confidence limits.

best protectors are used correctly and hearing thresholds are monitored regularly. For higher exposure levels over extended periods of time, it may be necessary to use a combination of insert- and muff-type protectors and also limit the time of exposure. Hearing protectors will provide adequate protection for only a very small percentage of wearers when worn in sound levels greater than about 125 dB(A) over long periods of time.

Methods for the Evaluation of Hearing Protectors

The only certain method of evaluating the effectiveness of personal hearing protection is to measure periodically the hearing levels of all persons exposed to noise. If no hearing losses are observed beyond those expected due to the ageing process, the hearing protection may be considered to be successful. However, an audiometric monitoring programme may take some time to become meaningful and, due to the variations associated with such measurements, may not necessarily give an accurate indication of the start of a hearing loss until it has reached certain proportions. Although monitoring audiometry will detect a hearing loss in a normally-hearing person long before it becomes large enough to represent a significant social

handicap, hearing losses smaller than may be reliably detected by this method may be of importance to those who are already much impaired. A practical and immediate indication of the effectiveness of hearing protectors is required.

The only effective procedure for the measurement of the attenuation of hearing protectors available at the moment relies upon subjective measurements of threshold shift.

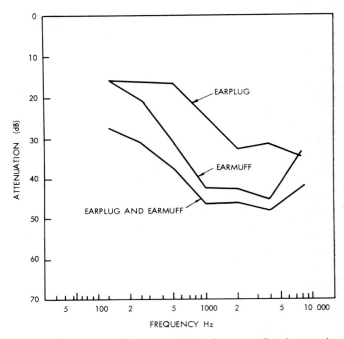

Fig. 11. Mean attenuation characteristics of an earmuff and an earplug worn separately and together.

Because the size and shape of peoples' heads and ears vary considerably and it is extremely difficult to simulate accurately the many physical characteristics of the human head, objective techniques using artificial heads or ears do not at the present time provide an absolute measure of the attenuation provided in practice. However, such methods may be extremely useful for the development and optimization of hearing protectors and for production testing during manufacture.

The subjective measurement procedure is based upon the differences between the thresholds of hearing of subjects measured with and without the hearing protection being worn. Each subject is seated in a quiet and usually anechoic room and the minimum sound pressure level which can be heard is determined at several test frequencies. The subject then puts on the hearing protection and his threshold is redetermined. The difference between the two threshold measurements is taken as a measure of the attenuation provided by the protector.

There are a number of national standard methods of measurements of attenuation available, published by different countries, as for example that specified in the American Standard ASA Z 24.22 (1957). This requires that threshold measurements are carried out 3 times on 10 subjects under free-field conditions, using a single loud-speaker to generate a pure-tone audiometric signal. However, it has been found that measurements carried out by different laboratories on the same protector, following this same procedure, can produce widely differing results (Martin, 1971). The American National Standards Institute is currently rewriting this standard.

The British Standard Institution is at present considering a standard method of measurement which, although based on the threshold shift technique, attempts to provide a more consistent evaluation of attenuation. This is attained by improvements in experimental technique such as a more diffuse test sound field, ⅓-octave bands of random noise as

Percentage of Time Worn

If hearing protectors are not worn all the time, their effective protection is severely reduced. As Else (1973) has pointed out, even if they are not worn for only a few minutes in a day, their effective attenuation may be halved. Figure 12 illustrates the maximum protection to be expected from hearing protectors providing differing amounts of attenuation as a function of the percentage of the time they are worn. As can be seen, even an "infinite" protector, which allows no sound to reach the ears at all, is effectively reduced in efficacy to about 20 dB(A) protection if worn for 99 per cent of the time. In the case

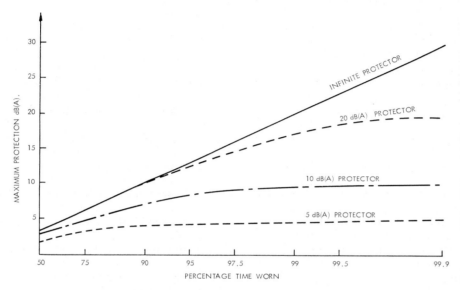

Fig. 12. Maximum protection, in dB(A), as a function of percentage time worn for different hearing protectors. (After Else, 1973.)

the test signal, rigorously specified fitting procedures and the revised estimate of the number of measurements required.

When using attenuation data as one of the guidelines for deciding upon the type and make of hearing protector required, the method by which this information is obtained and the laboratory carrying out the measurements should be carefully noted. It should be ensured that the attenuation data published by manufacturers are measured following a recognized standard procedure.

Amount of Protection Provided in Practice

To be able to estimate the degree of attenuation required of a hearing protector, a knowledge of the physical characteristics of the noise is required. This data may then be compared with the current criterion for noise-induced deafness and the amount by which the noise must be reduced to comply with the criterion estimated. A method for the calculation of the degree of protection needed in any particular situation is given in the Factory Inspectorate's Code of Practice for Reducing the Exposure of Employed Persons to Noise (1972).

of protectors encountered in practice this effect is even worse. For example, if hearing protectors with an effective attenuation of 30 dB(A) are worn in a noise environment of 115 dB(A), the sound level at the wearer's ears will be 85 dB(A), which may be considered as a non-hazardous exposure. If, however, the user fails to wear them for a total of only 2 per cent of the working day, i.e. about 10 min in 8 h, he will be exposed to 115 dB(A) for 10 min, which is equal to an equivalent continuous noise level of about 98 dB(A) for 8 h. Consequently, the effective protection has been reduced from 30 dB(A) to 17 dB(A) merely because the user failed to wear the hearing protection for a total time of 10 min in one working day. Furthermore, he is now exposed to an effectively hazardous noise.

These calculations make the most important point that, to be effective, all hearing protectors must be worn 100 per cent of the time the user is exposed to noise. Even a few minutes a day of unprotected exposure to noise very severely reduces the protection provided for the rest of the time. Remember the adage: "The only effective hearing protector is the one that is worn."

Practical Problems

Hygiene

Of the various types of hearing protector available, earplugs are obviously the type most likely to cause problems of hygiene. Before any form of earplug is issued, the user should be asked about and be examined for any ear troubles such as irritation of the ear canal, earache, discharging ears, or is under treatment for any ear disease.

Obviously earplugs should be kept absolutely clean and free from any chemicals or oil or grease when being inserted into the ear canal. Occasionally sensitization of the skin of the ear canal may occur. This could be due either to the nature of the material of the earplugs or to dirt or chemical substances handled by the wearer. Some ear canals are more sensitive to the presence of earplugs than others.

Earmuffs rarely cause infection in or sensitization of the ear canal and are a good alternative where this does occur with earplugs. However, if earmuffs are to be transferred from one person to another, because they tend to encourage perspiration they should be cleaned and disinfected before reissue.

Discomfort

The majority of earplugs are (and in fact should be) a little uncomfortable when worn correctly for long periods of time, although the wearer does become used to them after a time. Indeed if the user reports that the plugs are very comfortable, it is possible that they are not fitting correctly and hence will not be effective. Some types of earmuffs have headbands that tend to become uncomfortably tight when worn for any length of time. Again, this sensation will become less as the wearer becomes used to the muffs.

The main problem that could occur if hearing protectors are too uncomfortable is that the users may wear them in such a fashion that, although they appear to be worn correctly, they do not effectively attenuate noise. Thus, if the headband tension of a pair of muffs is too great, the user may bend the muffs' suspension so that they are more comfortable. This may mean that they do not form an effective seal with the sides of the head and hence will not protect the wearer. It is extremely difficult to ascertain whether earmuffs form an effective seal merely by external inspection in this case.

Similarly, earplugs that are too uncomfortable may not be worn correctly. They may be partially removed or readjusted to a more acceptable position within the ear canal and consequently may not provide the wearer with adequate protection. Again, it is very difficult to tell visually whether earplugs are completely or only loosely inserted into the ear canal.

It should be noted that there is only a fine dividing line between those types of hearing protectors that are effective and acceptable and those that are effective and unacceptable to the wearer. Consequently, those properties of hearing protectors that affect their comfort should be considered as equally important as those that provide protection.

Cost

Where hearing protectors must be supplied in large quantities, cost becomes an important factor. The total cost of providing hearing protection to a group of personnel may be divided into four basic parts: expenditure due to initial purchase, cost of supplying spare parts and replacements, the cost of time spent in administering the hearing protection and education.

Initial Expenditure. The majority of earplugs are cheaper to buy than the majority of earmuffs. Also it is probable that the cost per item will be reduced the larger the number purchased. However, the cost per year will depend upon the loss rate or the number of replacement parts required.

Prefabricated plugs, such as the V-51R type, may cost about 15p a pair when bought in small quantities, while other types may cost between 10 and 50p a pair. Glass wool may cost 15–25p per man per week for small quantities, but these figures will probably reduce with bulk purchase and the use of dispensers. Other types of malleable and disposable earplugs may cost more than glass down. Individually moulded earplugs are usually more expensive than other forms of insert device and may cost £1.50 a pair, depending upon the number purchased. Earmuffs usually cost from about £1.60 a pair depending upon their manufacture and the quantity purchased.

Replacements. The cost of replacing lost and broken hearing protectors is as equally important a consideration as the initial purchase price. It is probable that earplugs will be lost more easily and more often than earmuffs, particularly when they are removed from the ear canal several times a day. However, due to their size and construction, earmuffs are usually more susceptible to damage than earplugs.

Disposable earplugs which are replaced at least every day will cost much more per year than other types of earplug and even more than earmuffs. The number of replacement prefabricated earplugs required will depend upon a number of factors such as their inherent comfort, the type of container they are supplied in, the attitude of the employer and, most important of all, the attitude of the user. In any case earplugs must be replaced at regular intervals as they usually harden gradually with age and usage. Because of these factors the replacement rate will vary quite considerably between different industrial conditions, so that it is not possible to specify a typical figure.

Individually moulded earplugs usually have a lower loss rate than other types. Owing to their personal nature and greater psychological appeal to the wearer, they may be treated in a different and usually more preservative manner than other forms of earplug. In certain situations their loss rate may be so small that they may be effectively cheaper to supply than conventional earplugs.

Earmuffs are more likely to be broken than lost. The most susceptible part of the muff to damage is the seal. Replacement cushion seals are available for most types of earmuff and usually cost less than £1 per pair. Spare seals should be available at all times and the users of earmuffs should be encouraged to replace broken seals immediately. Other parts, such as headbands, also require replacement occasionally and suitable stocks of these items should be kept available.

Administration. The cost of administering a hearing protection programme will depend upon a large number of factors. Some of these are: the type(s) of hearing protection supplied; the number of replacements required; the time spent away from work by employees when being fitted and refitted; whether the person dispensing the hearing protection is a medical officer, industrial nurse or safety officer; and the amount of education and propaganda carried out during the protection programme.

If, for example, hearing protection is administered by a nurse situated in a first-aid room or medical centre, time would be spent by employees travelling to the centre to be fitted. Hearing protection may also be part of a larger hearing conservation programme in which audiometry is carried out regularly. In this case it is obviously beneficial for both audiometry and the administration of hearing protectors to be carried out at the same time.

Some earplugs, such as glass wool, can be dispensed automatically once the wearers have been instructed thoroughly in the correct procedure for making and inserting the plugs. In any case the external ear canals of all wearers of earplugs should be examined regularly for possible diseases by a medically qualified person.

In general, administrative costs in the case of earmuffs may be less than with earplugs. Less time should be spent in explaining their usage and fitting, and also in medical check-ups and obtaining replacements. These factors may mean that it could be cheaper to supply earmuffs than earplugs under certain circumstances, even though they may be more expensive initially.

Education. The cost of educating employees to wear hearing protection will depend for the most part on the time spent away from work. Educative films on noise and hearing protection may be hired quite cheaply and posters and notices will probably cost relatively little. In situations where screening audiometry is also carried out, the personal contact and encouragement from a nurse to wear hearing protection may be one of the most effective and cheapest methods of persuasion. Education is a most important aspect of the administration of hearing protectors and should not be neglected.

Communication

Workers must be able to communicate with each other and to hear warning sounds. The effect of hearing protection upon the wearer's ability to communicate in different high noise environments is obviously important.

Effects of Noise on Communication. The effect of noise on the ability of persons to communicate with each other depends to a large extent upon the spectrum of noise. It is most significant when the noise has high-level components in the speech frequency range from about 300–3000 Hz. It is known that conversational speech starts to become difficult when the speaker and listener (not wearing hearing

protection) are separated by about 60 cm in noise levels of about 88 dB(A). There are many such environments in places of work and the additional complication of hearing protectors is often imposed at higher levels.

Effects of Hearing Protection on Communication. Wearing hearing protection obviously interferes with conversational speech when worn in quiet environments. However, wearing conventional earplugs or earmuffs in noise levels above about 85 dB(A) should not interfere and indeed may improve speech intelligibility and the identification of warning signals for normally-hearing ears (Kryter, 1946; Howell and Martin, 1974). Figure 13 shows the relationship between percentage intelligibility scores and speech sound pressure level in various levels of noise for occluded and unoccluded ears. As can be seen, for the lower ambient noise levels intelligibility scores are greater in the unoccluded condition. However, as the noise level increases, intelligibility scores become progressively larger in the occluded case and eventually equal to or greater than the unoccluded situation for noise levels above 90 dB(A). Wearing protectors in high-level noise environments, therefore, can improve communication and the discrimination of warning sounds because their presence reduces both noise and speech about equally, thus maintaining the speech or signal to noise ratio. They also remove distortion in the ear which may be produced because of over-loading due to high speech and noise levels.

The concept of blocking up the ear to improve communication or reception of other important sounds is sometimes a difficult concept for the worker to accept. This is often given as a reason for resisting or refusing to wear hearing protection, and is further encouraged when protectors are first tried in a quiet environment. Such arguments sometimes lead to the choice of a "filter" type device that allows low frequencies in the speech range to reach the ear. Although such devices can provide better communication scores in quiet environments, this is not so in continuous noise levels above about 85 dB(A).

Existing Noise-induced Hearing Loss. Unfortunately, persons with noise-induced hearing losses may incur an added impairment when wearing hearing protection. Although the effects are not precisely known, it is probable that speech communication may be slightly impaired by the presence of protectors in such cases. This may be due to the fact that the level of the high-frequency components of the signal reaching the ears are reduced to below the wearer's (raised) threshold of hearing. The situation is aggravated by the following three points: much of the useful information in speech is contained in the higher frequency components, the majority of commercially available protectors attenuate these higher frequencies more than the low, and noise-induced hearing loss also often occurs maximally at these frequencies. Whilst the slight additional impairment may not be great for speech in a moderately affected person, it could cause certain warning sounds with mainly high-frequency components to lose their attention-arresting quality. Such effects could have serious consequences in certain industrial situations.

Presbyacusis, which mainly affects the higher frequencies, may also add to such difficulties as the wearer gets older.

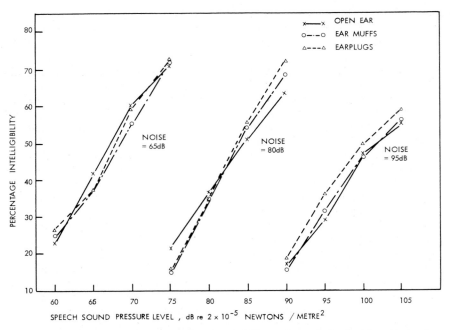

FIG. 13. Relationship between percentage intelligibility and speech level with noise level as parameter for earplugs and earmuffs. (After Howell and Martin, 1974.)

Persons with other forms of hearing disorder may also have additional problems when wearing hearing protectors.

In conflict with these arguments is the greater need to protect the hearing of a person who already has a hearing loss. He has, so to speak, less hearing to lose than normally-hearing persons and therefore requires greater protection. Although a worker may have experienced many years in a noise environment without wearing hearing protection and thus adapted gradually to a hearing loss and the needs of his work and social life, his hearing should still be protected to prevent further increase in any social handicap he may have.

Requirements of a Hearing Protection Programme

An effective hearing protection programme is not assured merely by making good and properly fitting hearing protectors available to those persons exposed to high-level noise. Management, medical, industrial hygiene and safety personnel must all be made aware of the problem as well as those habitually exposed to the noise. They must all support the programme to the full if it is to be effective. In addition, the programme will be much more efficient if a responsible member of the organization is designated as a co-ordinator to initiate the programme and follow it through; thereby sustaining both management's and worker's support.

The co-ordinator must determine the noise exposure patterns, both in terms of sound level and duration of exposure, for all persons under his responsibility and hence to pinpoint those areas where hearing protection is necessary. He must evaluate other existing environmental factors such as temperature, humidity, and possible communication and warning signal requirements. Also

he should ascertain the need for other personal safety equipment such as goggles, helmets and gloves in that these may affect the choice of hearing protector. With such information and by personally experimenting with different types of hearing protection in the various environments, he will be able to decide upon the most suitable types of protector required for the different situations existing in his organization. However, it is doubtful whether either earplugs or earmuffs alone can satisfy all the needs of a hearing protection programme in any one organization. The obvious advantages of each should be utilized wherever possible, so that a hearing protection programme may be made as acceptable as possible to the potential wearers. Furthermore it is often helpful initially to offer a personal choice of hearing protector from a range of potentially adequate devices and then allow trial periods with a number of different types until the wearer has chosen the model most suited to him. In this way individual wearers may feel that their chosen model is personal to them and hence may be further encouraged to wear them at all times.

Having started a hearing protection programme it is important that all efforts are made to maintain it. Education of the worker about the need to wear hearing protectors is paramount. This should take the form of films and lectures on the hazards of noise, personal issues of leaflets, posters and prominent warning signs, such as that recommended by the Department of Employment's Code of Practice (1972), should be displayed in the vicinity of all noise hazardous areas and on all noisy machinery, including hand-held tools. Management should set a good example by always donning hearing protection when entering a designated noise hazardous area. The possibility of introducing monitoring audiometry must be considered as a most useful medium for education and propaganda and also as a check upon the workers' hearing and thus the effectiveness of the hearing protection supplied. A close relationship must be maintained by the co-ordinator with management, medical staff and employees in order to be aware of reactions to various stages of the programme. In this way any problems will become evident early on and corrective measures can be taken before any serious damage to the programme results.

A HEARING CONSERVATION PROGRAMME

The application of a hearing conservation programme should be initiated the moment it is suspected that a noise hazard exists in part or all of a factory. The basic principles involved in the instigation of a successful hearing conservation programme have been discussed and may be summarized as follows:

(1) *Measurement of Noise:* a detailed noise survey should be carried out in those areas thought to present a possible hazard to hearing.

(2) *Evaluate the Hazard:* measured A-weighted equivalent continuous noise levels (L_{eq}) should be compared with the current criterion of 90 dB(A) and all machines, workshops and noisy areas where this level is exceeded should be designated "noise hazardous areas".

(3) *Noise Reduction*: all hazardous noise sources should be reduced to a level below the recommended limit following engineering noise and vibration control procedures. If reduction of the noise at source or in transmission is neither economic nor practical, then as a last temporary resort, a hearing protection programme should be instigated.

To be successful, each part of this programme should be considered in conjunction with the rest, as the results of any action taken should be considered in the light of the ultimate aims of the whole programme. If noise measurements indicate that a potential hazard to hearing does exist, then noise control techniques should be applied if possible. If these are successful the basic problem is solved and, apart from the regular monitoring of noise levels to ensure that these do not increase, that should be the end of the matter. However, if engineering noise control is neither economic, practical nor sufficient, a hearing protection programme, with its attendant problems of education and administration, should be undertaken.

Monitoring Audiometry

Because hearing protection is seldom used to its best advantage by exposed persons, and because current damage risk criteria cover only a certain percentage of a group of people and not individuals, it is desirable to monitor the hearing of all personnel habitually exposed to noise. Although this type of measurement is often imprecise, regular monitoring audiometry acts as a valuable check to ensure that hearing protection is being used efficiently and that noise exposures have not increased significantly.

Moreover it has several medico-legal advantages, not least being the detection of hearing loss on entry to a particular employment so that it cannot subsequently be attributed to noise exposure in that employment.

A good hearing conservation audiometric programme might consist of:

(1) Pre-employment audiogram, preferably measured over a wide range of audiometric frequencies including 250, 500, 1000, 2000, 3000, 4000, 6000 and 8000 Hz. A detailed pre-employment noise history and description of present work and noise environment. Individual education by the audiometrician or nurse about the hazards of noise and the need to wear hearing protection followed by individual fitting of the appropriate protectors.

(2) Monitoring audiograms after 6 months, 1 year and then every year, together with further education and individual discussion about the noise environment and the need for hearing protection.

The initial pre-employment hearing tests must be done at the beginning of a working day, preferably after a week-end's rest away from the noise. Otherwise the hearing levels recorded are liable to include temporary changes in threshold due to noise exposure. A practical compromise for monitoring retests is to ask the worker to wear well-fitting good-quality earmuffs during *all* noise exposure in the 24 h preceding the retest. If no significant deterioration relative to the initial audiogram is detected, the test result is accepted; if an apparent deterioration is found, he is tested again at the beginning of another working day. Owing to the relatively large sources of variation often associated with individual audiometry, an apparent change in the measured hearing level at any one test frequency of the order of 15 dB should be recorded before this loss can be considered as indicative of a significant deterioration in hearing acuity. If hearing losses are found to have developed or advanced by this amount since the initial test, stricter enforcement of the wearing of hearing protection or a change of working environment is necessary.

CONCLUSION

A hearing conservation and audiometric programme, if carried out with enthusiasm and perseverance and given full backing by management, trade unions and medical staff, should drastically reduce the incidence of occupational noise-induced hearing loss within an industry. Perseverance and propaganda are often required to overcome the reluctance to wear hearing protection *properly* that is shown by some employees and this must be achieved if such a programme is to be effective.

It should be apparent that the cost and effort required to ensure successful hearing conservation by hearing protection may be equal to or even greater than that involved in other engineering noise control measures. Furthermore, a hearing protection programme should not be considered as an easy or cheap alternative to the more desirable elimination of the noise from the working environment.

REFERENCES

American Standards Association (1957), "Measurement of Real Ear Attenuation of Ear Protectors at Threshold," ASA Z24.22 1957. ASA, New York.

Atherley, G.R.C. and Martin, A.M. (1971), *Ann. Occup. Hyg.*, **14**, 11.

British Occupational Hygiene Society (1971), *Hygiene Standard for Wide-Band Noise*. Oxford: Pergamon Press.

Burns, W. and Robinson, D. W. (1970), *Hearing and Noise in Industry*. London: H.M.S.O.

Department of Employment (1972), *Code of Practice for Reducing the Exposure of Employed Persons to Noise*. London: H.M.S.O.

Else, D. (1973), *Ann. Occup. Hyg.*, **10**, 415.

Guberan, E., Fernandez, J., Cordinet, J. and Terrier, G. (1971), *Ann. Occup. Hyg.*, **14**, 345.

Howell, K. and Martin, A. M. (1974), *J. Sound Vib.* In press.

International Electrotechnical Commission (1965), IEC 179, IEC, Geneva.

International Organization for Standardization (1971), ISO Recommendation R1999.

Kryter, K. D. (1946), *J. acoust. Soc. Amer.*, **18**, 413.

Martin, A. M. (1971), *Proc. Brit. Acoust. Soc.*, **1**(3).

Martin, A. M. (1974), *Ann. Occup. Hyg*, **16**, 353.

Martin, A. M. and Atherley, G. R. C. (1973), *Ann. Occup. Hyg.*, **16**, 19.

Rice, C. G. and Martin, A. M. (1973), *J. Sound Vib.*, **28**, 359.

Walker, J. G. and Behar, A. (1971), *J. Sound Vib.*, **19**, 349.

FURTHER READING

Beranek, L. L. (Ed.) (1954), *Acoustics*. New York: McGraw-Hill.

Beranek, L. L. (Ed.) (1971), *Noise and Vibration Control*. New York: McGraw-Hill.

Broch, J. T. (1971), *Acoustic Noise Measurements*. Naerum, Denmark: Brüel and Kjaer.

Diehl, G. M. (1973), *Machinery Acoustics*. New York: John Wiley.

Harris, C. M. (Ed.) (1957), *Handbook of Noise Control*. New York: McGraw-Hill.

Longmore, D. K. and Petrusewicz, S. A. (Eds.) (1974), *Noise and Vibration Control for Industrialists*. London: Paul Elek.

Parkin, P. M. and Humphreys, H. R. (1958), *Acoustics, Noise and Buildings*. London: Faber and Faber.

Peterson, A. P. G. and Gross, E. E. (1972), *Handbook of Noise Measurement*. Mass.: General Radio Company.

Sharland, I. (1972), *Woods' Practical Guide to Noise Control*. Colchester: Woods of Colchester Ltd.

Warring, R. M. (Ed.) (1972), *Handbook of Noise and Vibration Control*. Surrey: Trade and Technical Press.

Woods, R. I. (Ed.) (1972), *Noise Control in Mechanical Services*. Essex: Sound Attenuators Ltd.

SECTION V

EAR STRUCTURE

	PAGE
12. ORGANOGENESIS OF EAR	173
13. COMPARATIVE ANATOMY OF EAR	184
14. ULTRASTRUCTURE OF EAR	202
15. APPLIED MORPHOLOGY OF EAR	211

12. ORGANOGENESIS OF THE EAR

THOMAS R. VAN DE WATER and R. J. RUBEN

The mechanisms of organogenesis which act during the formation of the components of the ear will be presented and the embryological relationships of these components to each other will be discussed.

OUTER EAR

The outer ear consists of the auricle (pinna), external acoustic meatus and cuticular (epithelial) layer of the tympanic membrane. These structures of the external ear are formed by the ectodermal and mesodermal tissues of the first branchial groove and the surrounding first (mandibular) and second (hyoid) branchial arches.

The external acoustic meatus is formed by two successive mechanisms. The first stage of development consists of the invagination and medial growth of the first branchial groove to form a narrow funnel-shaped pit, the primary external acoustic meatus. This occurs in man at approximately the fourth gestational week. It is at this time that the ectoderm of the primary auditory pit comes in close contact with the entoderm of the dorsal division of the first pharyngeal pouch. This close relationship between the inpocketing branchial groove and outpocketing pharyngeal pouch is transient. Secondary to this interaction is the growth of a solid core of epithelial cells in a medial direction from the base of the primary external auditory pit. This strand of epithelial cells terminates in a round disclike swelling near the lower wall of the developing tympanic cavity. The formation of this core of epithelial cells occurs around the eighth week of fetal development and is the anlage of the secondary external acoustic meatus. At about the twenty-eighth week of development, a lumen is formed in this secondary auditory meatal plate by degeneration of a central core of cells and this now becomes a medial extension of the lumen of the primary external acoustic meatus. The disclike swelling that is found at the end of the secondary external acoustic meatus will become the epithelial layer of the developing tympanic membrane. The primary external acoustic meatus is the anlage of the cartilaginous portion of the meatus and the secondary external acoustic meatus corresponds to the bony portion of this structure. Information drawn from articles of Hammar (1902), Altmann (1950) and Arey (1954) was employed in formulating the above description.

The development of the auricle from six hillocks arising equally from the hyoid and mandibular arches on either side of the first branchial cleft was described by His in 1885. Hammar in 1902 designated these hillocks of His as ridges and reported his modified version of the genesis of the auricle. Using congenital anomalies of the outer ear in conjunction with embryological studies, Wood-Jones and Wen (1934) asserted that the entire auricle, except the tragus, is of hyoid arch origin. In their description the hillocks of the hyoid arch fuse and form the posterior auricular fold which extends beyond the dorsal limit of the first branchial cleft and then extends in a ventral direction depressing the growth of the anterior fold formed by the fusion of the mandibular arch hillocks. The suppressed anterior fold contributes only to the formation of the tragus.

Arey (1954) describes the formation of the auricle using a modified view of His (1885). This description includes the six hillocks of His with the added feature of an anterior fold. The mandibular arch contributes to the formation of the tragus and helix (partial) and the hyoid arch contributes to the formation of the helix (partial), antihelix, antitragus and auricular lobule. Streeter in 1922 observed in a report that the hillocks of His had been described for mammals with varying types of auricles and also reported them present during embryonic development in reptiles, amphibians and birds, all of which never acquire a distinct auricle. It was Streeter's (1922) opinion that too much significance had been placed on the hillocks which are transitory and incidental in nature rather than fundamental to the formation of the auricle. He stated that the auricle may be entirely of hyoid origin but since his human material did not corroborate such a supposition, Streeter continued to describe the tragus to be of mandibular arch origin. Boas (1912) developed a method of flattening the auricular cartilage and in a comprehensive comparative study he demonstrated that the tragus is a part of the posterior border of the ear cartilage which is rolled so that the proximal portion lies over the anterior edge. Using the techniques developed by Boas in a study of the development of the auricle in the Dachs rabbit, Crary in 1964 demonstrated that the entire auricle, which in cartilage preparations of adults appears as a single continuum, arises from an intact and continuous primordium as had been previously suggested by Streeter (1922) with the tragus arising from the mandibular arch and migrating to the hyoid arch during the course of organogenesis.

MIDDLE EAR

The middle ear is comprised of the middle fibrous layer and inner mucosal layer of the tympanic membrane, the ossicular chain (malleus, incus and stapes), auditory (pharyngotympanic or Eustachian) tube and middle ear cleft. The middle fibrous layer of the tympanic membrane is derived from the mesodermal cells that are present between the epithelial (outer) layer of the tympanic membrane and the entodermal (inner) layer of the development tubotympanic cavity. The presence of this middle fibrous layer is limited to the area of the tympanic annulus known as the pars tensa. The portion of the tympanic membrane where the middle fibrous layer is missing is the pars flaccida and develops at a later embryonic stage. The formation of the tympanic membrane of the frog depends upon the presence of the annular tympanic cartilage (Helff, 1940). Other visceral cartilages, especially the quadrate, have been demonstrated to possess the ability to induce the formation of a membrane when in contact with the skin of the frog. Cartilage of the appendicular skeleton is also effective but much less active in the induction of tympanic membrane formation in the frog. This induction of the tympanic membrane is probably mediated by some chemical quality of the cartilage, because cartilage that has been killed by various chemical and physical treatments still retains its inductive influence. The annular cartilage of the frog may be analogous to the tympanic annulus of man.

The inner layer of the tympanic membrane is entodermal in origin and originates from the entodermal cells of the inpocketing dorsal division of the first pharyngeal pouch. Studies by Senturia and his associates (1962), Sadé (1966), Hertzer (1970), Marovitz and Porubsky (1971) and Lim, and his associates (1973) have confirmed the entodermal nature of the ciliated, columnar cells that form the inner layer of the tympanic membrane.

The middle ear cleft and auditory tube was described by Hammar in 1902 to develop solely from the dorsal division of the first pharyngeal pouch. This concept was widely accepted until Frazer in 1910 and in later publications (1914, 1922) contended that the middle ear and auditory tube received entodermal contributions from not only the first pharyngeal pouch but also from the second arch entoderm and the dorsal division of the second pharyngeal pouch. Proctor in 1964 presented his theory that the middle ear spaces have developed from the dorsal division of the first pharyngeal pouch which splits into four separate compartments during development. Altmann (1950) in his review article on developmental mechanics of the ear also gave credence to Hammar's theory. Kanagasuntheram (1967) investigated the development of the human tubotympanic recess and concluded that migration of the first arch tissues into the area of the first pouch occurs during the 10–20 mm stages and that during this stage of human development there is a gradual and consequently total reduction in the contributions from the second arch and second pouch so that the tubotympanic recess and tube are formed solely from the first pouch.

The contention by most studies on the development of the middle ear cleft has been that this space is formed solely by the outpocketing entodermal tissues. The first report to the contrary of the above stated thesis was by Schwartzbart (1959). He suggested that the first pouch entoderm was responsible solely for the membranocartilaginous portion of the auditory tube and that the intra-osseous segment and middle ear cleft was formed by separations in the mesodermal mesenchyme which surrounded the otocyst. This concept of Schwartzbart was not widely accepted until Marovitz and Porubsky (1971) studied middle ear cleft development in the rat and concluded that due to early embryological rupture of the first pharyngeal pouch, it was highly probable that cells lining the rat middle ear are derived from mesoderm as well as first pharyngeal pouch entoderm. They suggested that areas of ciliated, pseudostratified, columnar epithelium and goblet cells correlate to the areas of entodermal origin and the remainder of the otic capsule and epitympanum are lined with cells of mesodermal origin. Lim and his associates (1973) reinforced Schwartzbart's observations with a report on the distribution of mucus-secreting cells and ciliated, columnar, epithelial cells in normal middle ear mucosa.

If an overall look is taken at the development of the middle ear cleft and the current reports by Schwartzbart (1959), Marovitz and Porubsky (1971) and Lim and his associates (1973) are considered in this analysis, then the following concept of middle ear cleft development emerges. The major entodermal contribution to the developing middle ear space is the dorsal division of the first pharyngeal pouch as was stated by Hammar in 1902, and the second pharyngeal pouch is a transient contributor to the tubotympanic cavity and tube. There is a growing body of evidence that a major role is played by mesodermal mesenchyme tissue in the formation of the lining of the developing middle ear space and that this tissue probably forms the epithelium that lines the mastoid antrum and much of the epi- and hypo-tympanic cavities.

The origin of the bones of the middle ear that comprise the mammalian ossicular chain has aroused great interest in both the biologist and otolaryngologist. The number of reports trying to define the embryological and phylogenetic origin of the auditory ossicles number in the hundreds and come from such diverse sources as classic anatomists, comparative zoologists, embryologists, morphologists, pathologists and surgeons.

Goodrich (1958) gives a classic review and analysis of the formation of the ossicular chain through the eyes of the comparative morphologist. He cites the original theories of Carus (1818), Meckel (1820) and Reichert (1837) and gives an excellent review of the contributions of the many many comparative zoologists that have approached this problem. The modern version of Reichert's theory states that the mammalian stapes was derived from the reptilian columella auris, the incus from the quadrate, and the malleus from the articular bone. This would support the contention that the malleus and incus are derived from first arch mesenchyme and that the stapes is derived from the mesenchyme of second arch, with the auditory capsule contributing to the formation of the stapedial base (footplate). An equally comprehensive view with greater medical orientation is presented by Strickland, Hanson and Anson (1962) in their historical review of the branchial sources of the auditory ossicles in mammals. The following facts concerning the origins of the auditory ossicles of man are evident in both of these presentations. These facts are:

(1) The major source of the ossicles and their associated structures is the mesenchyme of the first (mandibular) and second (hyoid) branchial arches.

(2) The auditory capsule plays a role in the formation of the stapedial base and oval window.

Controversy still exists as to the definitive origins of the tissues that form these auditory ossicles and their related structures. Hanson and his associates (1959), using the wax reconstruction technique of Broman (1899), stated that the head of the malleus and main body of the incus are derived from the first arch (Meckel's) mesenchyme and that the manubrium of the malleus, long process of the incus and the stapes are derived from second arch (Reichert's) mesenchyme. The lamina stapedius and the annular ligament were described as originating from the degeneration of cartilaginous tissues of the otic capsule. Development of the ear ossicles in the mouse was reported by Jenkinson (1911). His study stated that the stapes is formed by the dorsal medial portion of the hyoid arch and the only contribution that the auditory capsule makes to the formation of the stapes is the lamina stapedius. The incus and malleus were said to form in the upper part of the blastema of the mandibular arch. Fuch's (1905) observation on the formation of the ossicles in the rabbit reports that the stapes is a part of the auditory capsule. Reagan in 1917 studied the role that the auditory vesicle epithelium plays in the formation of the stepedial base and concluded that the auditory capsule formed the stapedial base while the second branchial arch formed the rest of this ossicle. Hanson and his colleagues in 1962 reiterated their previously published reports that the head of the malleus and body of the incus, including the short process, are derived from first arch mesenchyme. The manubrium of the malleus and long process of the incus, as well as the entire stapes with the exception of the lamina stapedius portion of the base, are of second branchial arch origin. These anatomical observations were backed up by some congenial anomalies of the middle ear observed by these investigators (i.e. frequent partial insertion of the stapedial tendon into the long process of the incus). A more extensive study of congenital malformations of the middle ear reported by Hough (1963) supports the branchial arch origins of the ossicles and their related structures as put forth by Hanson and his associates (1959, 1962). Alberti in 1964 described in detail the blood supply of the incudostapedial joint and the lenticular process. This work also supports the branchial arch derivations of the ossicular chain as put forth by Hanson and his colleagues (1959, 1962).

INTERNAL EAR

Huschke in 1824 was the first to accurately describe the development of the embryonic anlage of the membranous labyrinth from a placode of surface ectoderm. Boettcher in 1869 made further contributions to the understanding of the developmental anatomy of the human internal ear. Bartelmez in 1922 made observations on the origins of otic primordium in man and confirmed the early observa-

tions of Huschke (1824). A large part of the body of information on early stages of developmental anatomy of the human auditory vesicle was reported by Streeter in a series of publications (1906, 1918, 1942, 1945 and 1951). O'Rahilly (1963) in a more recent publication has re-examined some of the embryological anatomy that was done by Streeter. O'Rahilly placed special emphasis on the development and integrity of the otocyst's basement membrane during organogenesis. Bast and his colleagues (1947) and Bast and Anson (1949) have made a major contribution by describing in detail the anatomical changes that occur during organogenesis of the internal ear of man.

Tello (1931) and Ramon y Cajal (1960) reported the development of the internal ear in rodents with special notations on the developing patterns of innervation. Larsell and his colleagues (1944) reported the developmental anatomy of the membranous labyrinth of the opossum. Wada (1923) and later contributions of Belanger (1956) and Weibel (1957) presented morphological features that occurred in the development of the internal ear of rodents. In a more recent and detailed presentation, Sher (1971) described the embryonic and postnatal development of the internal ear of the mouse. Kikuchi and Hilding (1965) have described some of the postnatal ultrastructural features of the developing spiral organ (of Corti) of the mouse internalf ear.

Spemann (1918), working with amphibian embryos of the gastrula stage, found that the dorsal lip of the blastophore gives rise to the primary embryonic organizers. One of these primary organizers is the organizer of the head which induces the differentiation of the head area, brain and sense organs. During organogenesis of a specific sense organ, a succession of lower grade organizers might be produced which act in a more limited and specific manner. They are thought to exert an inductive influence on organ and tissue differentiation of the ear region. The presumptive ear ectoderm area has been determined by experiments employing vital dyes (Harrison, 1945) or extirpation (Rudnick, 1948) techniques. This original ear anlage (presumptive area) of the auditory placode occupies an area larger than the actual area of head ectoderm that forms the otocyst. The presumptive auditory area appears to be determined at the stage when the auditory placode is formed. This determination can be changed only by a very potent inductive force, such as a transplanted portion of the otic cup which may produce a lens vesicle instead of an auditory placode (Kawakami, 1952). The determination of the otocyst occurs gradually, not at any one particular stage.

Harrison's studies (1938, 1945) have shown that the formation of a normal ear results from the interplay of several factors; the ectoderm, mesoderm and rhombencephalon are involved as well as the position of the otocyst. Two relations of these tissues were especially noted:

(1) The chordamesoderm comes to lie under the presumptive auditory field during gastrulation.

(2) The folding of the neural tissue during neurulation brings the rhombencephalon in close relationship to the ear ectoderm (Yntema, 1946).

A complete analysis of induction of the internal ear in amphibians was reported in 1950 by Yntema. Yntema explains induction as a two factor process with activation on the part of the environment and response on the part of the tissue influenced. The ability of the environment to influence is termed inductor effect, and the readiness of the target tissue to respond to the influence of the environment is termed competence. Yntema's experiments showed that the maximal competence response of a target area always preceded the maximal production of an inductor substance (activation) by the immediate environment and that the competence of an area does not always exceed the period during which the inductor substance is produced (see Fig. 1). A progressive change in the differentiation of the

in Fig. 3 symbolizes the interval of maximal competence of the donor tissue to respond to mesodermal induction. Ridge C of Fig. 3 illustrates the stage of maximal competence of the donor tissue response to neural induction by the host. Areas E and F illustrate the inability of the donor tissues to react to induction by the host. Area E is an inability of the early stage donor tissues to respond to the induction forces of the later stage hosts. Area F represents the inclination of prospective ectoderm of the gastrulae to form central nervous tissue. It may be concluded from Yntema's study, which represented approximately 1500 animals in various confirmations of donor/host, that two overlapping cycles in the induction system of the amphibian internal ear occur. In order of occurrence these inductors are:

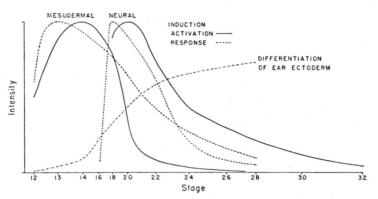

FIG. 1. A graphic representation of relative intensities of various components of ear induction in amphibia starting with the yolk plug stage of embryonic development. The maxima are placed at the same level arbitrarily. The differentiation of the ear ectoderm is represented according to the development obtained with dorsodorsal anterioposterior (ddap) transplants of prospective gill ectoderm into the region between the eye and ear of a host at the head process stage of development. (Yntema, 1950.)

internal ear is indicated by the forming of the otic placode and can be correlated with the migration of chordamesoderm beneath the area of the prospective ear ectoderm. A relationship similar to this has been established for the induction of neural tissue. The mesodermal inductor grows in intensity until the neural folds begin to form. At this stage of development, mesodermal induction has reached its peak and now begins to diminish. At the head process stage of embryonic development the mesodermal inductive action has nearly disappeared. During this period when the intensity of the mesodermal inductor is waning, a second inductive event is occurring. This second induction is qualitatively different from mesodermal induction and is localized in the developing neural folds. The rapidly proliferating ear ectoderm comes to lie adjacent to the neural folds during neurulation. Neural induction reaches its peak at about the time when the neural folds close to form the neural tube and then gradually diminishes but persists for a greater period of time than the mesodermal induction system. Figures 2 and 3 represent a three dimensional graphic presentation of the results obtained by Yntema. Ridge A of Fig. 2 represents the period of maximal induction by the mesoderm tissue of the host. Ridge B of Fig. 2 is caused by the period of maximal neural induction by the host neural tissue. The D ridge that is best visualized

(1) A mesodermal induction that begins during late gastrular and persists until early neurular stages.

(2) A neural induction beginning during late neurular stage and persisting past the early head process stage of development.

A graphic representation of this concept was taken from Yntema (1950) and is seen in Fig. 1. The maximal production of an inductor substance is always preceded by the period of maximal tissue competence. The period of mesodermal induction is limited by the production of the inductor substance whereas the neural induction period appears to be limited by the competence of the target tissue.

Yntema's (1950) findings give substance to the conclusion of Harrison (1945) who stated that "the differentiation of the ear is not a sudden action but one that is long drawn out and involves several different factors acting in succession".

Toivonen and Saxén (1968) experimented with amphibian cells of the presumptive forebrain region and axial mesoderm, which were disaggregated and combined in varying ratios, and then allowed to develop *in vitro*. An increase of mesodermal cells resulted in a corresponding increase in the frequency with which caudal structures of the central nervous system developed and a gradual loss of

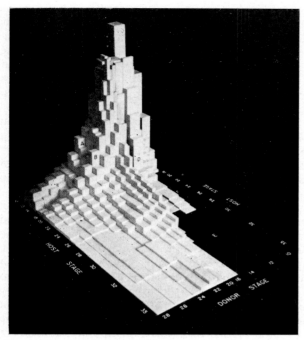

FIG. 2. Photograph of a three dimensional graph representing the normality of ears induced from prospective gill ectoderm grafted ddap into the ear region. The two horizontal axes represent donor and host stages of development at the time of transplant; the vertical axes represent the normality of labyrinths induced from various combinations of donor and host stages. This view of the graph represents to advantage the results obtained when older embryo donors are used with hosts ranging from yolk plug to motile stages of development. (Yntema, 1950.)

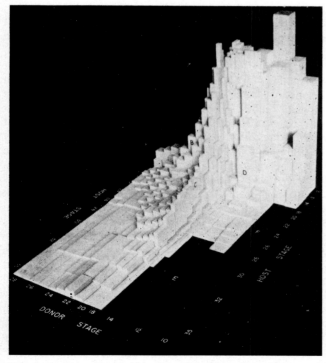

FIG. 3. Another photographic view of the three dimensional graph of Fig. 2. This view best represents the more complicated results obtained when younger donor stages are used in the embryonic transplantation experiments. (Yntema, 1950.)

forebrain formations (in a series in which an equal number of neuroepithelial and mesodermal fragments were combined, hindgrain and otic vesicles were seen in all explants). These observations point to the importance of the role of the mesodermal inductor in internal ear induction. Holtfreter (1933) observed that mesoblast implantation in the blastocele of young amphibian gastrula induced the formation of otic vesicles. Harrison (1935) was first to demonstrate the role of mesoderm in the absence of any other inductor. He excised the rhombencephalon and replaced it with a graft of ventral ectoblast in young neurula of *Amblystoma punctatum*. The graft produced an ear probably by mesodermal induction but partial reconstitution of the rhombencephalon by the contralateral side left the experiment open to doubt. Harrison in 1938 carried his experimentation further by bilateral excision of the rhombencephalon. Since he had bilaterally excised the brain from the presumptive otic region, there was no chance for reconstitution of the brain and the mesoblasts were the only possible inductor. The internal ears of these embryos were formed, giving definite proof to the existence of a potent mesodermal inductor. Albaum and Nestler (1937) obtained xenoplastic induction of ear rudiments between *Rana pipens* and *Amblystoma punctatum* and an induction by cephalic mesentoderm of an ear vesicle when transplanted in the flank of a recipient. Kogan (1944) also obtained induction of ear vesicles with impaired chordamesoderm when transplanted in a heterotypic ventral position in hosts of the same age.

Detwiler and Van Dyke (1950) stated that the neural influence was most important and with transplantation experiments showed that mesentoderm interaction with the otocyst does not alone produce a normal ear. In another article in 1951, Detwiler and Van Dyke illustrated that after the initial neural induction of the ear ectoderm, a continuing influence is exerted on the orderly development of the otocyst by the rhombencephalon. Garcia in 1961, working with the chick embryo, investigated this phenomena of a continuing influence of the rhombencephalon on the development of the internal ear. His results, using the technique of unilateral surgical extirpation of rhombencephalon, reinforced the findings of Detwiler and Van Dyke (1950). Garcia found that in the chick embryo the rhombencephalon exerted both a qualitative influence on the development of the internal ear.

The orderly organogenesis of the mammalian otocyst may be influenced by the same factors that affect the organogenesis of the internal ear in amphibians and birds. There are strong indications that the neural factor is very important in the organogenesis of the mammalian internal ear. The short-tailed shaker mouse (Bonnevie, 1936) has a hypoplasia of the rhombencephalon which leads to a thickening of the mesenchymal layer between the rhombencephalon and the otocyst. The brain anomaly of this mutant first becomes manifest during the ninth day of gestation and up to that time the development of the otocyst is normal. On the ninth gestational day the course of development of the short-tailed shaker mouse otocyst is altered. The endolymphatic ducts fail to develop and there is only an abortive subdivision of the otocyst into separate chambers and canals. Hertwig in 1942 produced and reported the abnormalities of the kreisler mouse. The invagination of the homozygotic kreisler otic pit occurs more laterally than it does in its heterozygotic litter mate or in a normal CBA–J/CBA–J embryo. There is a malformation of the fourth to sixth rhombomere in the homozygotic kreisler brain that can be detected on the ninth day of gestation. This produces a double effect on neural induction because:

(1) A more laterally placed otocyst is separated from the neural inductive influence of the brain by a thicker layer of mesenchyme than normal.

(2) A malformation of the otic area of the rhomben-cephalon probably affects the neural inductive ability of this brain area.

These two factors act to produce a severely malformed internal ear that never develops an endolymphatic duct or sac.

Deol (1966) examined four mutant strains of mice (kreisler—kr, dreher—dr, looptail—Lp and splotch—Sp) and noted that all of the internal ear malformations of these mutants had been preceded by malformations of the brain involving the otic area of the rhombencephalon. Deol suggested that the malformations of the labyrinths of the four mutant strains of mice that he had examined may have been caused through the agency of the rhombencephalon and that neural induction was not a singular event but rather a continuing influence of the brain on the orderly development of the internal ear.

Synotia dorsalis has been experimentally produced in mice by X-ray treatment of the fetuses of gravid females on their eighth gestational day. In these experiments by van der Borden (1967), the range of abnormalities was noted and the relationships between parachordal mesoderm, otic placode and rhombencephalon was observed. It was concluded that in the early development of the mouse embryo internal ear there are two mechanisms of induction; first, the influence of the parachordal mesoderm (including neural crest) and, second, the neural inductive influence of the associated area of rhombencephalon.

Harrison (1936) produced cystic ears in *Amblystoma punctatum* embryos by creating a faulty neural induction and he suggested that perhaps a functional endolymphatic sac may be required to regulate the hydrostatic pressure of the endolymph during development. Detwiler and Van Dyke (1950, 1951) also produced cystic ears in *Amblystoma punctatum* by manipulating neural induction. These cystic ears lacked an endolymphatic duct and sac but the authors maintained that the presence of an intact endolymphatic sac and cartilaginous capsule did not in themselves assure normal development. Van der Borden (1967) found in the X-ray abnormalities of the internal ear that he produced in mice a possible correlation between faulty neural induction and the lack of an endolymphatic sac. Hertwig (1942) in her original report on the kreisler mutant noted that this mutant lacked an endolymphatic duct and sac. Ruben (1973) confirmed the findings of Hertwig (1942). Van De Water and Ruben (1974) cultured homozygous and heterozygous kreisler otocysts *in vitro* and also observed the lack of development of the endolyphatic duct and sac

system in the homozygotic otocyst *in vitro*. They suggested that the lack of development of the endolymphatic duct and sac of the homozygotic kreisler *in vitro* may be one of the consequences of faulty neural induction. At present there is strong circumstantial evidence from the above cited reports that the formation of the endolymphatic projection (duct) of the developing otocyst is under the control of neural induction.

The relationship between the stato-acoustic ganglion and the developing sensory hair cells of the labyrinth is still an unresolved question. Kaan (1926) stated that her observation in amphibians indicated that contact with the auditory ganglion stimulates the formation of macular epithelium. Knowlton (1967) in her analysis of the development of sensory structures in the chick reported a relationship between the time of occurrence of neural innervation and maturation of sensory structures in the chick ear. Friedmann (1956) found that the inclusion of neural elements in explants of chick embryo otocysts enhanced the development of sensory structures in these otocysts as they developed *on vitro*. Orr (1968) performed dissociation/reaggregation experiments with extirpated chick embryo otocysts and she observed in the organ cultures of the reaggregated chick otocysts that there was a relationship between areas of sensory epithelia and nerve fibres. These observations led her to conclude that there was a definite relationship between the degree of differentiation of sensory structures *in vitro* and their association with neural elements. Thornhill (1972) studied the development of the labyrinth of the lamprey with light and electron microscopy. His observations were that individual sensory cells appeared autonomous and apparently intrinsically polarized with respect to orientation within the sensory structure and differentiation to the ciliary bud stage, but at this stage neuronal contact was necessary to stimulate further differentiation of the individual sensory cells.

The above observations support the hypothesis that neuronal contact is essential for the complete differentiation of sensory hair cells. The following articles reinforce the opposite theory. Fell (1928) in her original experiments with extirpation and culture of the chick embryo otocyst *in vitro* reported excellent differentiation of sensory structures but made no mention of the inclusion of the eighth nerve ganglion or nerve fibres in her explants. Hoadely (1924) explanted 4-day chick otocyst to chorioallantoic membranes and reported differentiation of chick internal ear sensory structures with no mention of neural elements. Evans (1943) repeated some of Hoadley's original work and reported development of sensory structures with no mention of neuronal elements. Evans specifically employed a Bodian protargol stain to detect neuronal elements. Waterman (1938) explanted 10- and 11-day rabbit embryo otocysts to chick chorioallantoic membranes. He claimed to have obtained differentiation of sensory areas independent of neural innervation. In all of these above articles, there was no mention of a specific effort to exclude the eighth nerve ganglion from the explants but, instead, the reports are based on microscopic observations of sensory areas that appeared to develop with no apparent neural elements.

Speidel (1948; 1964) studied the development of the lateral line in regenerating tails of frog tadpoles in which he repeatedly sectioned the lateral line nerves. He observed that a specific nerve supply was not necessary for the regeneration and early growth of the lateral line organs but that lateral line organs which had been kept nerve free for periods longer than three months began to show early regressive changes in the sensory hair cells. He concluded that neuronal elements were not essential to differentiation of the sensory structures of the lateral line system but were essential for long term maintenance of these sensory structures. The work of Speidel has recently been repeated in salamander tadpoles by Flock, Jorgensen and Russell (1973). Electron microscopic observation of regenerated lateral line hair cells in preparations where the nerve was repeatedly sectioned, showed that the sensory hair cells had arranged themselves in the proper doublet orientation. It was concluded from these results that the development of normal hair cells in lateral line organs does not depend on the presence of afferent or efferent nerve fibres in the vicinity of the developing organ. The hair cells of the lateral line organ appear to have the capacity of autonomous different-iation and spatial orientation, independent of neuronal contact. Recent observations by Van De Water and Ruben (1973) on quantification of development of sensory struc-tures in organ cultures of mouse embryo otocysts showed an uncoupling of the relationship between the presence of neuronal elements and the differentiation of sensory structures. Sensory structures occurred with 30 per cent greater frequency in the organ culture specimens than did stato-acoustic ganglion cells and/or neural elements associated with sensory hair cells.

Work in our laboratory performed by a student trying to reaffirm the work of Kaan (1926) in fate mapping the otocyst of the chick, duplicated a series of partial extirpation on the otic anlage of chick embryos. In some cases the acoustic-facial ganglion was inadvertently destroyed during the surgical manipulations. These specimens (see Fig. 4) were stained with Bodian's protargol method, and well formed areas of sensory epithelia with associated neural elements were observed on the unoperated side (Fig. 4A) while the contralateral operated side also possessed well formed areas of sensory epithelia but with no apparent neural contacts present (Fig. 4B). These observations confirm the findings of Waddington in amphibia (1937). A naturally occurring human malformation was reported by Altmann (1933) who observed a human temporal bone where the posterior ampullar nerve was absent and the posterior ampulla had developed normally.

When all of the evidence that currently exists is examined. it supports the theory that neuronal contact may not be required for the initial differentiation of the sensory struc-tures of the internal ear. This does not mean that neural contact is not required for the maintenance of these differentiated sensory structures. The establishment of functional neural contact is of probable importance in maintenance but this may not enter into the scheme of embryonic organogenesis of sensory epithelia of the in-ternal ear.

It is important when assessing the role of neuronal

contact in differentiation to examine the origins of the acoustic ganglion. Several early investigators examined early developmental stages in mammalian embryos and concluded that the acoustic ganglion arose from neural crest cells (Bartelmez, 1922; Adelman, 1925). Larsell et al. (1939) also studied the anatomical development of the acoustic ganglion in opossum embryos and concluded that this ganglion originated from a proliferation of neural crest cells and not from the cells of the otic placode. Deol (1967, 1970) in two later studies employed mutant strains of mice that were known to be deficient in neural crest. He examined their internal ears for abnormalities. He found internal ear pathology that was confined to the macula of the saccule and the spiral organ sensory hair cells. Deol hypothesized that the neural crest contributes to the forma-tion of the acoustic ganglion and that an abnormal neural crest produced an abnormal ganglion primordium which manifested itself as the pathological changes he had observed in the internal ears of the mutants. Deol (1970) on the basis of his observations maintains that the acoustic ganglion has a dual origin with contributions from both neural crest and otic placode. Deol further defined that the cochlea and macula of the saccule are innervated by the neural crest moiety and thereby a deficiency of the neural crest limits the pathology to these areas of the internal ear. Horstadius (1950) states in his book on the neural crest that the sheath cells of the seventh and eighth cranial nerves arise partially from the neural crest.

Several early investigators (Dalcq, 1933; Holtfreter, 1933) studying embryological stages in amphibia noted that the otic placode always preceded the development of the acoustic ganglion. Van Campenhout (1935) performed transplantation and extirpation experiments on the origin of the acoustic ganglion in amphibian embryos. His exten-sive investigations showed that in amphibian embryos the acoustic ganglion has its origins from the otic ectoderm. Later experimental studies in amphibia by Yntema (1937) concurred with the conclusions of van Campenhout (1935). Toerian (1965), working with turtle embryos and studying the relationship between the otic primordium and the otic capsule, observed that surgical extirpation of the otic placode resulted in absence of the acoustic ganglion and the otic placode resulted in absence of the acoustic ganglion and the membranous labyrinth.

Anatomical studies in embryonic mammalian species by Politzer in 1956 and Batten in 1958 concluded that the stato-acoustic ganglion did not develop from the neural crest. They observed the ganglion to arise from the rostral wall of the otocyst.

The overall view of the origins of the acoustic-facial ganglion that may be taken from a synthesis of all of the studies presented above is that this ganglion complex may have its origin from several sources. There is strong evidence that the otocyst makes a major contribution to this ganglionic moiety and there is a growing amount of evidence that neural crest cells participate in some aspect of the acoustic-facial ganglion complex.

The activator role of the otocyst in the induction of the ear capsule from the mesenchyme tissue that surrounds it

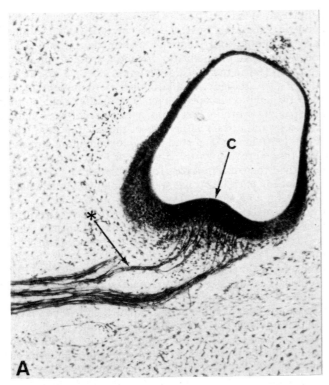

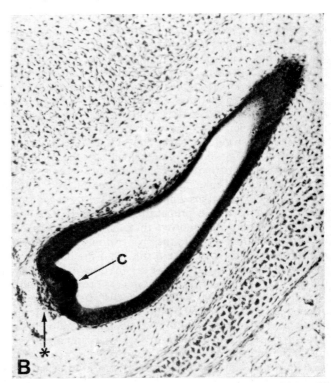

(A) Control side (Right)—the cristae (C) of the posterior semi-circular canal showing a bundle of fibres of the vestibular portion of the VIII nerve (arrow with asterisk) innervating the sensory hair cells.

(B) Contralateral operated side (Left)—the cristae (C) of the superior semicircular canal showing that no neuronal elements of the VIII nerve were present (arrow with asterisk).

FIG. 4. Photomicrographs of a 9-day chick embryo specimen that had the left otic cup partially destroyed and then was allowed to continue development until day 9.

was first demonstrated by Lewis in 1907. Lewis experimented with *Rana sylvatica* embryos and determined that if the otocyst is removed, the ear capsule does not develop. He also observed that if a foreign otocyst is transplanted xenoplastically between the ear and the eye, then local cephalic mesenchyme cells will aggregate around it and produce an additional cartilaginous ear capsule. Lewis concluded from these experiments that the otocyst had exerted a stimulatory effect on the associated mesenchyme cells and induced their differentiation into capsular cartilage. Spemann in 1910 repeated these experiments and agreed with the initial finding of Lewis (1907). Filatow (1927) on the basis of incomplete observations tried to demonstrate the action of foreign bodies in the role of inductors of cartilaginous capsules from cephalic mesenchyme. Ichikawa (1936) repeated Filatow's series of experiments in amphibian embryos and invalidated this hypothesis. These negative findings were confirmed and supplemented to include various allotransplanted organ rudiments by Kaan in 1938.

In studies by Detwiler (1948, 1951) and Detwiler and Van Dyke (1950, 1951) on the inductor role of the medulla in the formation of the otic vesicle, many cystic membranous labyrinths were induced and it was a frequent observation that the cartilaginous capsules of these cystic labyrinths were either incomplete or absent. This variability in the production of otic capsules suggests that more is required

than just the mere presence of the auditory epithelium for determining the formation of the otic capsule cartilage.

Kaan (1930, 1934, 1938) studied the competence of various mesenchymal tissues to react to transplanted otocysts and found that only the cephalic mesenchyme responded to this inductor in amphibians. Yntema (1933) noted in his studies several cases where sclerotome mesenchyme reacted to contact with a heterotypic otocyst by either the formation of a cartilaginous capsule or by hypertrophy of a vertebra. Persistent contraindications in this field of research led Ichikawa (1936) to reinvestigate the transplantation techniques employed in amphibian experimentation. When he transplanted otic placodes that had been freed of their underlying mesentoderm to different heterotypic positions, a cartilage capsule was never obtained but when these transplanted otic placodes were not freed of their adhering cephalic mesenchyme, then otic capsules were noted without regard to the localization of the implanted otic placode. Ichikawa concluded from his results that in amphibians the cephalic mesenchyme alone was capable of reacting to the influence of the otocyst inductor. Toerien in 1965 studied the development of the otic capsule, using surgical extirpation of the otic placode in turtle embryos, and he concluded that the formation of the cartilaginous ear capsule, with the exception of part of the floor which is of basal plate origin, is dependent upon the otocyst for its induction. He also noted that the full development of the stapes base is inhibited by the absence of the ear capsule. Kaan in 1938 performed surgical excision of otic mesentoderm in *Amblystoma punctatum* to show that these cells participate in the formation of the otic capsule. Her results were affirmative. Yntema (1939, 1950) showed that branchial ectoderm could also participate in the formation of the otic capsule but it did not appear to be a major source of capsular cartilage. Reagan (1917) destroyed the otocyst of chick embryos with a heated

embryo otocysts. There is also circumstantial evidence provided by Fell (1928) and Friedmann (1956) in their *in vitro* studies of chick otocysts and by the chorioallantoic membrane explants of otocysts by Hoadley (1924), Waterman and Evans (1940) and Evans (1943). These studies all demonstrated that the associated cephalic mesenchymal tissue included with the explanted otocyst formed a cartilaginous capsule. De Vincentis and Marmo (1965) used histochemical procedures for the detection of

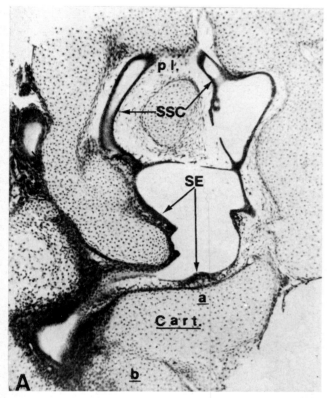

(A) Heterozygotic (+/kr) otocyst; areas *a* and *b* of the cartilaginous otic capsule show normal development. Sensory epithelium (SE), a developing semicircular canal (SSC) and a perilymphatic space (pl.) are labelled.

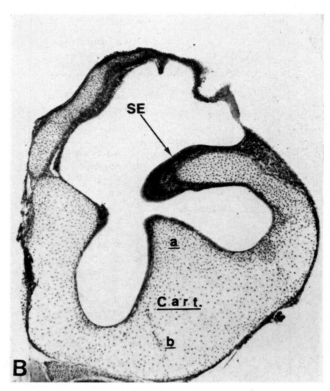

(B) Homozygotic (kr/kr) otocyst; area *a* of the cartilage capsule is normal but the more distal area, *b*, shows abnormal development of the cartilaginous otic capsule. An area of sensory epithelium (SE) is labelled.

FIG. 5. Kreisler mouse otocysts that were explanted into identical organ culture systems on their 12th day of gestation and allowed to develop for 9 days *in vitro*.

platinum needle. His results demonstrated in avian embryos that otic mesenchyme produces a cartilaginous capsule only in the presence of the auditory vesicle. Reagan also noted that complete formation of the stapedial base is dependent upon formation of a complete otic capsule. Yntema (1944) repeated the work of Reagan and observed after ablation of the otic placode the absence of the membranous labyrinth, acoustic ganglion and otic capsule. Benoit in 1955 performed extirpation experiments of the otocyst in chick embryos and concluded that the otic mesenchyme was induced by the otocyst to form the otic capsule and complete formation of the base of the stapes was dependent on the complete formation of the otic capsule. Benoit (1960) extended his studies and demonstrated that cephalic mesoderm cultivated *in vitro* could be induced to form cartilage by an extract of 3- and 4-day chick

RNA to study the development of the chick embryo otocyst *in vivo*. They observed an accumulation of RNA in the basal cytoplasm of the cells of the otocyst on the second through fourth day of development of the chick. The basal stratum RNA accumulation disappeared by the fifth day of development and it was noted that the days of occurrence of this accumulation of RNA within the basal stratum of the cells that comprise the otocyst concurs with the time sequence of induction of mesenchyme to become otic cartilage by the otocyst as demonstrated by Benoit (1964) *in vitro*. The authors suggested that this RNA is involved in the induction process of the otic capsule.

Grobstein and Holtzer (1955) in an *in vitro* series of experiments demonstrated the inductor role of the mammalian otocyst. They explanted 11-day mouse embryo otocysts that had been freed of adhering mesenchyme by trypsin and interacted these otocysts with somite mesoderm. The somite mesoderm cultivated by itself evolved into loosely organized mesenchymous tissue whereas the mesoderm that was interacted with the otocysts evolved into cartilage. This demonstrated an inductor-reactor coupling in a pure state and illustrated that, in mammals, somite mesoderm as well as cephalic mesoderm is competent to react to the inductor substance produced by the isolated otocyst.

mitoses. The exact period when the different cell types that compose the membranous labyrinth underwent their terminal mitoses was determined. Figure 6A, B are histograms that demonstrate the time of occurrence of the terminal mitoses of the cells of the spiral ganglion and the outer hair cells of the spiral organ respectively. These observations were employed as a basis for advancing a hypothesis concerning the growth and cytological differentiation of the cochlea. Ruben (1969) in a later report

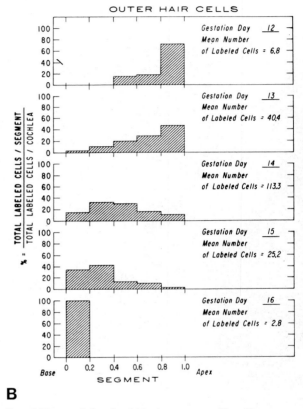

FIG. 6. Histograms depicting the position of labelled (A) spiral ganglion cells and (B) outer hair cells within the mature cochlea. The gestation day is the day of injection of tritiated thymidine. The cells of the spiral ganglion (A) were labelled from base to apex while the pattern of labelling of the outer hair cells of the spiral organ (B) was from apex to base.

Van De Water and Ruben (1974) explanted homozygotic and heterozygotic kreisler otocyst into organ culture (*see* Fig. 5) and observed aberrant development of the cartilaginous capsule of the homozygotic kreisler otocysts (Fig. 5B) when compared to the cartilaginous capsule produced by its heterozygotic litter mate (Fig. 5A) and/or the cartilaginous capsule formed by the normal (CBA–J) mouse *in vitro* (Van De Water, Heywood and Ruben, 1973). It was suggested that this malformation of the homozygotic kreisler cartilaginous capsule *in vitro* may be due to faulty induction of the otocyst by the rhombencephalon, which in turn produces a malformed otocyst which then acts as a weak or faulty inductor of the associated otic mesenchyme to form an aberrant cartilaginous otic capsule.

The development of the mouse internal ear during organogenesis was studied by Ruben (1967) utilizing pulse labelling of DNA in cells under-going their terminal

studied the production of RNA in the spiral organ in postnatal and adult mice. He found that as the spiral organ matures postnatally, its ability to synthesize RNA diminishes and in the adult spiral organ the ability to synthesize new RNA is greatly diminished. These findings suggested a hypothesis for a mechanism of deafness. Ruben, Van Water and Polesky (1971) and Ruben (1973) studied the cell kinetics of the otocysts of 11- and 12-day normal (CBA–J) and a mutant strain (kreisler) of mice. A significant difference was found between the cell cycle times of the otocysts of the homozygotic kreisler mouse and its heterozygotic litter mates (*see* Fig. 7). The cell cycle times of the heterozygotic kreisler otocysts were similar to those generated for the CBA–J (normal) mouse. The significance of these differences was discussed in relationship to the findings of Deol (1966).

Balinsky (1970) has stated that the middle ear, consisting of the auditory tube, ossicles and tympanic membrane,

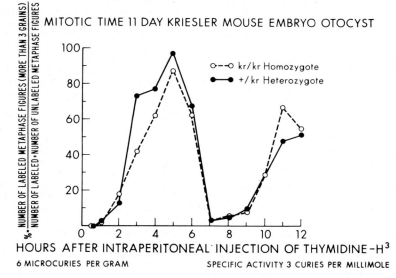

FIG. 7. A 12-hour graphic plot of the percentage of labelled mitoses in the cells that compose the otocysts of homozygotic (kr/kr) and heterozygotic (+/kr) eleven day kreisler mouse embryos. This graph illustrates the differences found in the cell cycles of these cells in the homozygote (kr/kr) and heterozygote (+/kr).

develop normally after removal of the ear vesicle. He suggested that this may be due to the different origins of the outer and middle ear in comparison to the internal ear. The outer and middle ear are derived from the branchial apparatus which is deeply rooted in the basic mechanisms of vertebrate development and, therefore, may not need stimulation from the internal ear for normal development. Yntema (1955) in a chapter on development of the ear suggested that the organ of hearing is made up of two parts not causally connected in development but linked together only through the medium of their definitive functioning.

REFERENCES

Adelman, H. B. (1925), *J. comp. Neurol.*, **39**, 19.
Ahlvin, R. C., Carr, C. D. and Senturia, B. H. (1962), *Ann. Otol.*, **71**, 632.
Albaum, H. G. and Nestler, H. A. (1937), *J. exp. Zool.*, **75**, 1.
Alberti, P. W. R. M. (1964), *J. Laryng.*, **78**, 808.
Altmann, F. (1933), *Mschr. Ohrenheilk.*, **67**, 765.
Altmann, F. (1950), *Arch. Otolaryng.*, **52**, 725.
Arey, L. B. (1954), *Development Anatomy*, 6th edition. Philadelphia and London: W. B. Saunders Co.
Balinsky, B. I. (1970), *Embryology*, 3rd edition. Philadelphia-London-Toronto: W. B. Saunders Co.
Bartelmez, G. W. (1922), *J. comp. Neurol.*, **34**, 201.
Bast, T. H. and Anson, B. J. (1949), *The Temporal Bone and the Ear*. Springfield, Ill., U.S.A.: Chas. C. Thomas.
Bast, T. H., Anson, B. J. and Garden, W. G. (1947), *Anat. Rec.* **99**, 55.
Batten, E. H. (1958), *J. Embryol. epx. Morph.*, **6**, 597.
Belanger, L. F. (1956), *Ann. Otol.*, **65**, 1060.
Benoit, J. A. A. (1955), *C. R. Soc. Biol.* (Paris), **149**, 998.
Benoit, J. A. A. (1960), *Ann. Sci. nat. Zool.*, **12**, 326.
Benoit, J. A. A. (1964), *C. R. Acad. Sci.* (Paris), **258**, 334.
Boas, J. E. V. (1912), *Ohrknorpel und äusseres Ohr der Säugetiere*, Copenhagen.
Boettcher, A. (1869), *Uber Entwicklung und Bau des Gehörlabyrinths*, Dresden: Blockman, Soba and Schultze.
Bonnevie, K. (1936), *Genetica*, **18**, 105.

Broman, I. (1899), *Anat. Hefte*, **11**, 509.
Crary, D. D. (1964), *Anat. Rec.*, **150**, 441.
Dalcq, A. (1933), *Arch. Anat.*, **29**, 389.
Deol, M. S. (1966), *Nature*, **209**, 219.
Deol, M. S. (1967), *J. Embryol. exp. Morph.*, **17**, 533.
Deol, M. S. (1970), *J. Embryol. exp. Morph.*, **23**, 773.
Detwiler, S. R. (1948), *J. exp. Zool.*, **108**, 45.
Detwiler, S. R. (1949), *J. exp. Zool.*, **110**, 321.
Detwiler, S. R. (1951), *J. exp. Zool.*, **116**, 45.
Detwiler, S. R. and Van Dyke, R. H. (1950), *J. exp. Zool.*, **113**, 179.
Detwiler, S. R. and Van Dyke, R. H. (1951), *J. exp. Zool.*, **118**, 389.
de Vincentis, M. and Marmo, F. (1965), *Naturwissenschaften*, **12**, 348.
Evans, H. J. (1943), *Biol. Bull.*, **84**, 252.
Fell, H. B. (1928), *Arch. exp. Zellforsch.*, **7**, 69.
Filatow, D. (1927), *Roux Arch. Entw. mech.*, **110**, 1.
Flock, A., Jorgensen, M. and Russell, I. (1973), "The Physiology of Individual Hair Cells and Their Synapses," In *Basic Mechanisms in Hearing* (A. R. Møller, Ed.). New York: Academic Press.
Frazer, J. E. (1910), *Brit. med. J.*, **1**, 1148.
Frazer, J. E. (1914), *J. Anat.*, **48**, 391.
Frazer, J. E. (1922), *J. Anat.*, **57**, 18.
Friedmann, I. (1956), *Ann. Otol.*, **65**, 98.
Fuchs, H. (1905), *Arch. Anat. Entwicklung*, suppl., pp. 1–178.
Garcia, F. M. (1961), *X Reunion de la Sociedad Español de Otorrino-laringologica*, **59**, 230.
Goodrich, E. S. (1958), *Studies on the Structure and Development of Vertebrates*, Vol. 1, Chap. 8, p. 449. New York: Dover Pub., Inc.
Grobstein, C. and Holtzer, H. (1955), *J. exp. Zool.*, **128**, 333.
Hammar, J. A. (1902), *Arch. mikr. Anat.*, **59**, 471.
Hanson, J. R., Anson, B. J. and Bast, T. H. (1959), *Quart. Bull. Northw. Univ. med. Sch.*, **33**, 358.
Hanson, J. R., Anson, B. J. and Strickland, E. M. (1962), *Arch. Otolaryng.*, **76**, 200.
Harrison, R. G. (1935), *Anat. Rec.*, **64**, suppl. 1, 38.
Harrison, R. G. (1936), *Proc. nat. Acad. Sci.* (*Wash.*), **22**, 238.
Harrison, R. G. (1938), *Anat. Rec.*, **70**, suppl. 3, 35.
Harrison, R. G. (1945), *Trans. Conn. Acad. Arts Sci.*, **36**, 277.
Helff, O. M. (1940), *J. exp. Biol.*, **17**, 45.
Hertwig, P. (1942), *Z. indukt.*, **80**, 220.
Hertzer, E. (1970), *Ann. Otol.*, **79**, 825.
His, W. (1885), *Anatomie menschlicher Embryonen*, Part III, p. 211.
Hoadley, L. (1924), *Biol. Bull.*, **46**, 281.
Holtfreter, J. (1933), *Arch. EntwMech. Org.*, **127**, 619.

Horstadius, S. (1950), *Neural Crest*. London: Oxford University Press.

Hough, J. V. D. (1963), *Arch. Otolaryng.*, **78**, 127.

Huschke, E. H. (1824), "Uber die Sinne," In *Beitrage zur Physiologie und Naturgeschichte*. Weimar.

Ichikawa, D. (1936), *Bot. Zool.*, **4**, 1211.

Jenkinson, J. W. (1911), *J. Anat.*, **45**, 22.

Kaan, H. W. (1926), *J. exp. Zool.*, **46**, 13.

Kaan, H. W. (1930), *J. exp. Zool.*, **55**, 263.

Kaan, H. W. (1934), *Anat. Rec.*, **58**, 72.

Kaan, H. W. (1938), *J. exp. Zool.*, **78**, 159.

Kanagasuntheram, R. (1967), *J. Anat.*, **101**, 731.

Kawakami, I. (1952), *Ann. Zool. Jap.*, **25**.

Kikuchi, K. and Hilding, D. (1965), *Acta oto-laryng.*, **60**, 207.

Knowlton, V. Y. (1967), *Acta anat.*, **66**, 420.

Kogan, R. (1944), *C. R. Acad. Sci. U.R.S.S.*, **45**, 39.

Larsell, O., McCrady. E. and Larsell, J. R. (1944), *Arch. Otolaryng.*, **40**, 233.

Larsell, O., McCrady, E. and Zimmerman, A. A. (1939), *J. comp. Neurol.*, **63**, 95.

Lewis, N. H. (1907), *Anat. Rec.*, **1**, 42.

Lim, D. J., Shimada, T. and Yoder, M. (1973), *Arch. Otolaryng.*, **98**, 2.

Livingstone, G. (1965), *Proc. roy. Soc. Med.*, **58**, 493.

Marovitz, W. F. and Porubsky, E. S. (1971), *Ann. Otol.*, **80**, 384.

O'Rahilly, R. (1963), *J. Embryol. exp. Morph.*, **11**, 741.

Orr, M. F. (1968), *Develop. Brol.*, **17**, 39.

Politzer, G. (1956), *Acta anat.*, **26**, 1.

Proctor, B. (1964), *J. Laryng.*, **78**, 631.

Ramon y Cajal, S. (1960), *Studies on Vertebratee Nurogenesis* (Trans. by Lloyd Guth). Springfield, Ill.: Chas. C. Thomas.

Reichert, C. (1837), *Arch. Anat. Physiol. wiss. Med.*, **8**, 120.

Reagan, T. D. (1917), *J. exp. Zool.*, **23**, 85.

Ruben, R. J. (1967), *Acta oto-laryng.*, Suppl., **220**, 1.

Ruben, R. J. (1969), *Laryngoscope*, **79**, 1546.

Ruben, R. J. (1973), *Laryngoscope*, **83**, 1440.

Ruben, R. J., Van De Water, T. and Polesky, A. (1971), *Laryngoscope*, **81**, 1708.

Rudnick, D. (1948), *Ann. N. Y. Acad. Sci.*, **49**, 761.

Sade, J. (1966), *Arch. Otolaryng.*, **4**, 137.

Schwartzbart, A. (1959), *J. Laryng.*, **73**, 45.

Senturia, B. H., Carr, C. D. and Ahlvin, R. C. (1962), *Ann. Otol.*, **71**, 632.

Sher, A. (1971), *Acta oto-laryng.*, suppl., **285**, 1.

Spemann, H. (1910), *Roux Arch. Entw. mech.*, **30**, 437.

Spemann, H. (1918), *Arch. Entw.Mech. Org.*, **43**.

Speidel, C. C. (1948), *Sci. Monthly*, **67**, 178.

Speidel, C. C. (1964), *Internat. Res. Cytol.*, **16**, 174.

Spirt, B. Unpublished data.

Streeter, G. C. (1906), *Amer. J. Anat.*, **6**, 159.

Streeter, G. C. (1918), *Contr. Embryol. Carneg. Instn.*, **14**, 111.

Streeter, G. C. (1922), *Contr. Embryol. Carneg. Instn.*, **14**, 111.

Streeter, G. C. (1942), *Contr. Embryol. Carneg. Instn.*, **30**, 211.

Streeter, G. C. (1945), *Contr. Embryol. Carneg. Instn.*, **31**, 27.

Streeter, G. C. (1951), *Contr. Embryol. Carneg. Instn.*, **34**, 165.

Strickland, E. M., Hanson, J. R. and Anson, B. J. (1962), *Arch. Otolaryng.*, **76**, 100.

Tello, J. R. (1931), *Tran. de lab. de recherches Biol. de l'univ. de Madrid*, **27**, 151.

Thornhill, R. A. (1972), *Proc. roy. Soc. (Lond.)*, **181**, 175.

Toerien, M. J. (1965), *J. Embryol. exp. Morph.*, **13**, 141.

Toivonen, S. and Saxén, L. (1968), *Science*, **159**, 539.

Van Campenhout, E. (1935), *J. exp. Zool.*, **72**, 175.

Van Der Borden, J. (1967), *Ann. Otol.*, **76**, 129.

Van De Water, T. R., Heywood, P. and Ruben, R. J. (1973), *Ann. Otol.*, **82**, suppl. 4, 1.

Van De Water, T. R. and Ruben, R. U. (1973), *Ann. Otol.*, **82**, suppl. 4, 19.

Van De Water, T. R. and Ruben, R. J. (1974), *Laryngoscope*, **84**, 738.

Wada, T. (1923), *Anat. Biol. Memoirs*, **10**, 1.

Waddington, C. H. (1937), *J. exp. Biol.*, **14**, 232.

Waterman, A. J. (1938), *Amer. J. Anat.*, **63**, 161.

Waterman, A. J. and Evans, H. J. (1940), *J. exp. Zool.*, **84**, 53.

Weibel, (1957), *Acta anat.*, **29**, 53.

Wood-Jones, F. and Wen, I. C. (1934), *J. Anat.*, **68**, 525.

Yntema, C. L. (1933), *J. exp. Zool.*, **65**, 317.

Yntema, C. L. (1937), *J. exp. Zool.*, **75**, 75.

Yntema, C. L. (1939), *J. exp. Zool.*, **80**, 1.

Yntema, C. L. (1944), *J. comp. Neurol.*, **81**, 147.

Yntema, C. L. (1946), *Collect. Net.*, **19**, 30.

Yntema, C. L. (1950), *J. exp. Zool.*, **113**, 211.

Yntema, C. L. (1955), "Ear and Nose," in *Analysis of Development* (B. A. Willier, P. A. Weiss and V. Hamburger, Eds.). Philadelphia and London: W. B. Saunders Co.

13. COMPARATIVE ANATOMY OF THE EAR

ADE PYE and R. HINCHCLIFFE

INTRODUCTION

A study of the comparative morphology of the mammalian ear provides a basis for an understanding not only of the structure but also of the function of the human ear.

The foundations of the comparative morphology of the ear in general were laid towards the end of the sixteenth century and the beginning of the seventeenth century by Casserius (1601). This anatomist was first the domestic servant, then the pupil and finally the successor, at Padua, of Fabricius, who was himself the successor of Fallopius and the teacher of Harvey (Cole, 1944). The foundations of the comparative morphology of the internal ear in particular were established in the nineteenth century, principally by Hyrtl (1845) and by Retzius (1881). Hyrtl used metal alloys to obtain casts of the periotic (osseous) labyrinth. It is, however, Hyrtl's student, Corti, who is best known to otologists for his micro-anatomical studies which demonstrated the spiral receptor organ that now bears his name (Corti, 1851).

Much of the comparative morphological work conducted in the twentieth century has been based on the use of decalcified bone sections of the ear, a technique which was probably perfected by Politzer in the late nineteenth century (Wright, 1971). The studies that we report have been based primarily on this technique.

Material

The material that we have studied comprized over 300 specimens drawn from over 100 species of mammals.

These species represented the following orders: Marsupalia, Insectivora, Edentata, Pholidota, Chiroptera, Rodentia, Carnivora and Primates.

The specimens were collected by one of us (AP) during surveys within a ten-year period following 1961 and covering Europe, North America, the Caribbean and Central America, as well as Africa. For the convenience of readers, Table I shows a classification of the animals referred to in this text.

Methods of Study

Thin (8 μm–10 μm in thickness) serial horizontal sections of intravitally fixed specimens were examined by light microscopy. In a small number of animals, the observations on the middle ear were supplemented by its dissection under the stereo-dissecting microscope. Similarly, observations on the cochlea were supplemented by microdissection using the surface specimen technique, with examination using phase contrast microscopy.

EXTERNAL EAR

Auricle (Pinna)

The auricle is a mammalian characteristic. However, it is absent in both aquatic and in burrowing mammals. In contrast, the auricle of *Cardioderma cor* (an East African false vampire bat) illustrates the complexity which this structure may achieve in some mammals such as bats

TABLE 1A

A. SHOWING THE GENERAL CLASSIFICATION OF THE ANIMALS REFERRED TO IN THE TEXT.

Phylum	Sub-phylum	Super-class	Class	Order	Genus
Chordata	Vertebrata	Agnatha			*Myxine*—hagfish *Petromyzon*—lamprey
		Gnathostomata	Pisces		*Chimaera*—ratfish *Gadus*—cod
			Reptilia		*Pachydactylus* *Hemidactylus*—geckos *Tarentola* *Crotalus*—rattlesnake
			Aves		*Gallus*-chicken *Aquila*—eagle *Otus*—owl *Procellaria*—petrel *Corvus*—crow
			Mammalia	Monotremata	*Ornithorhynchus*—platypus
				Marsupialia	*Didelphis*—opossum *Trichosurus*—phalanger
				Insectivora	*Crocidura* *Sorex* shrews *Talpa*—mole
				Chiroptera	*see* Table 1B
				Primates	*see* Table 1B
				Edentata	*Choloepus*—sloth
				Pholidota	*Manis*—pangolin
				Rodentia	*see* Table 1C
				Cetacea	*Phocaena*—porpoise
				Carnivora	*Panthera*—leopard *Felis*—puma *Nasua*—coati *Mustela*—weasel
				Proboscidae	*Elephas*—elephant
				Artiodactyla	*Sus*—pig

TABLE 1B

B. SHOWING THE CLASSIFICATION OF THE ORDERS CHIROPTERA AND PRIMATES.

Order	Sub-order	Super-family	Genus
Chiroptera	Megachiroptera		*Pteropus*—flying fox
	Microchiroptera	Emballonuroidea	*Taphozous*—tomb bat
		Rhinolophoidea	*Cardioderma*—false vampire *Rhinolophus*—horse-shoe bat *Hipposideros*—leaf-nosed bat *Asellia* *Triaenops* } trident bats
		Phyllostomatoidea	*Pteronotus*—moustache bat *Centurio*—Centurion bat
		Vespertilionoidea	*Natalus*—long-legged bat *Eptesicus* *Myotis* } common brown bats *Pipistrellus*—pipistrelle bat *Plecotus*—long-eared bat *Tadarida* *Otomops* } free-tailed bats
Primates	Anthropoidea	Ceboidea	*Saimiri*—squirrel monkey *Callithrix*—marmoset *Marikina*—tamarin
		Cercopithercoidea	*Cercopithecus*—common African monkey *Macaca*—Rhesus monkey
		Hominoidea	*Pan*—chimpanzee *Gorilla*—gorilla *Homo*—man

TABLE 1C

C. SHOWING THE CLASSIFICATION OF THE ORDER RODENTIA.

Order	Sub-order	Super-family	Genus
Rodentia	Sciuromorpha	Geomyoidea	*Heteromys* *Liomys* ——Spiny pocket mice *Perognathus* *Microdipodops*—kangaroo mouse *Dipodomys*—kangaroo rat
	Myomorpha	Muroidea	*Sigmodon*—cotton rat *Clethrionomys*—vole *Neotoma*—wood rat *Tatera* *Meriones* } gerbils *Mastomys*—rat *Mus*—mouse
		Gliroidea	*Glis*—dormouse
		Erethizontoidea	*Coendou*—tree porcupine
		Cavoidea	*Cavia*—guinea-pig *Galea*—cuy *Dasyprocta*—agouti
		Chinchilloidea	*Chinchilla*—chinchilla
		Octodontoidea	*Octodon*—degu *Ctenomys*—tuco-tuco *Proechimys*—spiny rat

(Fig. 1). This enlargement may also, as in *Cardioderma*, involve the tragus.

In conjunction with the external acoustic meatus, the auricle acts as a funnel at higher frequencies to bring about a pressure transformation making the pressure at the tympanic membrane greater than the pressure in the free sound field. This is equivalent to lowering of the threshold

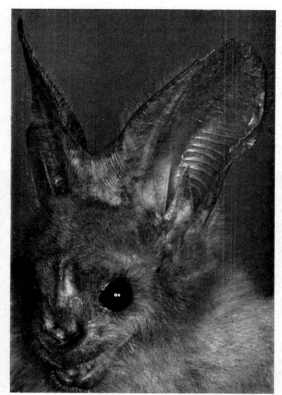

FIG. 1. *Cardioderma cor* showing enormously enlarged and complicated auricle connecting with the opposite auricle across the midline. Note the ribbed appearance. There is also a prominent tragus and an antitragus can also be discerned posterior to the tragus. A complex dermal structure, termed the nose-leaf, is seen surrounding the nostrils, through which the high frequency sounds used in echo-location are emitted.

of hearing for a certain band of frequencies. Indeed, Hayashi and Hagino (1963) have shown that auriculectomy in the cat impairs the auditory threshold by up to 15 dB in the range around 4000 Hz. Gardner (1962) has also shown experimentally that exaggerated auricles in man can improve the detectability of mid-high frequency signals in noise. This improvement in threshold is most marked for directions antero-lateral to the subject.

The auricle also has a role in sound localization (Batteau, 1969). Because of this, imperfect otoplasties can produce a 20° error in sound localization, compared with a normal error of about 4°. Moreover, the subject may be unaware of this dysstereoacusia.

In some animals, muscles in the auricle enable it to change shape to a greater or lesser degree and in bats, such as *Rhinolophus ferrumequinum* (the horseshoe bat), the ears can turn independently to wide angles and do so

rapidly. These movements, as Schneider and Möhres (1960) have shown, are essential for echo-location in this bat. These auricular alternating movements in this bat are synchronous with the pulse emission up to the maximum rates involved (80 s^{-1}) (Griffin *et al.*, 1962; Pye *et al.*, 1962). Similar observations have been made for hipposiderids by Pye and Roberts (1970) and for *Pteronotus parnellii* (a phyllostomatid bat) by Schnitzler (1970). These high speed movements, which occur only concurrent with ultrasound production, act as echo reflectors for the meatus, introducing an artificial velocity factor and causing a varying Doppler shift. A Doppler shift is the effect upon the observed frequency of a wave train produced by either motion of the source toward or away from a stationary observer, or motion of the observer toward or away from a stationary source, the motion in each case being with reference to the supposedly stationary medium.

The auricle may also have other functions in some mammals. For example, the long eared bat *Plecotus*, which hunts among bushes and hedgerows, emits sound through nostrils that open upwards under the auricles, which are held forward in flight. As Pye (1960) points out, this may be a mechanism for reflecting outgoing sound from the animal.

In animals such as the elephant and the rabbit, where the auricles are so large, they may subserve a secondary function of heat regulation.

External Acoustic Meatus

Kirikae (1960) measured the dimensions of the external acoustic meatus in some 30 animals. He noted that the length, but not the width, was proportional to the size of the skull. Small ratios of length to width were found in small animals like bats or the rat (values of about 1·0). In larger animals, values of the order of 10 were found, e.g. 13·7 for *Sus sp.* (pig). Even larger ratios were found in aquatic mammals, such as Pinnipedia (seals and sea lions). Owing to its resonant properties, the meatus contributes (together with the auricle) an additional pressure transformation and also a small load effect upon the tympanic membrane (Tonndorf and Khanna, 1967). The resonant frequency is inversely related to the size of the meatus. In the species recorded by Kirikae, the value ranged from 1100 Hz for the ox to 71 000 Hz for a bat. For man, this resonance effect is about 10 dB at 3000 Hz. Kirikae considered that there was a close relationship between the resonant frequency of the meatus and the dominant frequency of the animal's sound emissions.

The meatus offers protection of the middle and internal ear against foreign bodies and helps to isolate them from fluctuating ambient temperatures.

MIDDLE EAR

Tympanic Membrane

The membrane is not flat, but has the appearance of a shallow cone. This is best seen in *Tatera* (large naked soled gerbils) (Fig. 2). The cone is much shallower in man where the axial height of the cone is about 2 mm. Helmholtz likened the shape to that of an exponential horn and Kirikae (1960) likened it to the mathematical function known as the witch of Agnesi (effectively, a flattened normal error curve). As Wever and Lawrence (1954) point out, this form adds rigidity to the structure and makes

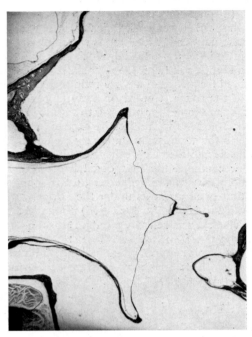

FIG. 2. *Tatera valida* showing external acoustic meatus projecting into the middle ear and the exponential horn appearance of the tympanic membrane. (×18)

it possible for the central portion to work as a unit and so adds considerably to the effective area. The acoustic impedance matching mechanism of the middle ear is primarily due to the pressure transformation achieved by the tympano-ossicular chain (specifically, the tympano-stapedial base area ratio) and only to a minor degree to the ossicular lever ratio. Thus, in considering the adequacy of these impedance transformations by the middle ear, we must take into account the anatomical ratio between the area of the tympanic membrane and the area of the stapes base. Kirikae (1960) measured the areas of the tympanic membrane and the fenestra vestibuli in over 20 animals and found that the ratio was within the range 10–20 for the majority of mammals. However, in reptiles and amphibians, the tympanic membrane changed in size in proportion to the size of their heads, whereas the size of the fenestra vestibuli remained essentially constant. Consequently, these area ratios varied from less than 6 for the toad to nearly 60 for the bull frog. In any case, Kirikae comments that the tympanic membrane in these animals seems to be too thick to be an effective receptor of sound waves. It is interesting to note that Tumarkin (1968), in developing his theory of the evolution of the various vertebrate auditory apparatuses, hypothesized that these animals that use their ear in a "reversed" role, "perfected" their ear by increasing the mass of the ossicles.

Mastoid Process and Pneumatization

The mastoid process i.e. the downward mammillary projection of the mastoid temporal bone behind the external acoustic meatus is not an exclusively human characteristic. As Ashton and Zuckerman (1952) have pointed out, it is seen also in *Pan troglodytes* (the chimpanzee) and in *Gorilla gorilla* (the gorilla) (Fig. 3). In fact, in some respects, mastoid development may be more marked in the great apes. It has been asserted that the shape of the mastoid depends upon the pull of splenius capitis and not on the sternocleidomastoid muscle. Howell (1932) however, has advanced the explanation that, in many mammals having the use of an efficient balancing mechanism in the form of a large tail, e.g. *Neotoma* (the wood rat), there is a hard thin shell of mastoid completely filled by the paraflocculus of the cerebellum. He argues that evolutionary loss of the tail is followed by regression of the paraflocculus and a cancellous mastoid bone thus arises.

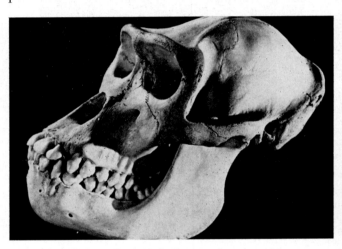

FIG. 3. *Gorilla gorilla* skull showing prominent mastoid process.

Although a pneumatized mastoid process is the naturally occurring condition in man, pneumatization of the bone surrounding the ear in mammals may exist in the absence of a mastoid process, e.g. in *Macaca irus* and other monkeys (Fig. 4). Indeed, in some monkeys, e.g. *Saimiri sciureus* (the squirrel monkey) it may, as Igarashi (1964) points out, be tremendous, extending anterior, and even medial, to the cochlea. Extensive pneumatization may also occur in the bone surrounding the semicircular canals not only in anthropoids, such as *Cercopithecus* and *Saguinus*, but also in prosimians, such as the Lemuroidea (Werner, 1960).

Many mammals that we have studied exhibit air spaces in the soft tissues adjacent to the medial portion of the external acoustic meatus. These spaces may subserve the same function as the bony air spaces surrounding, and connected with, the middle ear cavity. We have termed these air spaces the perimeatal air spaces. A biloculated perimeatal air space is found in *Sigmodon* (the cotton rat) (Fig. 5).

Pneumatization provides a series of air cells in the bone surrounding the ear. The cells are connected to the middle

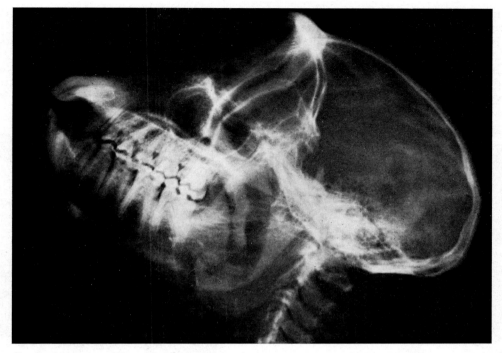

FIG. 4. *Macaca irus* (Cynomolgus monkey) showing pneumatisation in bone surrounding ear but absent mastoid process.

ear cavity, providing a reservoir of air on the medial side of the tympanic membrane, ensuring against the development of a pressure gradient across the membrane due to auditory tubal block. The phylogeny of pneumatization has been discussed at length by Tumarkin (1957).

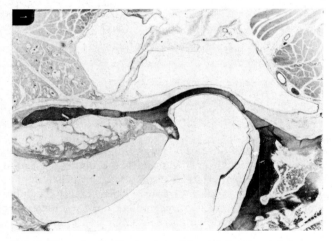

FIG. 5. *Sigmodon hispida* showing a biloculated perimeatal air space adjacent to the medial part of the external acoustic meatus. (×15)

It should be noted that, in birds, the entire skull is pneumatized and these air cells communicate with the middle ear cavity. Other bones, e.g. the humeri, may also be pneumatized. Pneumatization of the humeri in birds originates from an unpaired clavicular air sac which connects with both lungs. In both structure and mode of development, pneumatization of the chick humerus resembles that of the human mastoid. Moreover, permanent

occlusion of the foramen pneumaticum in the chick in association with slight inflammatory processes arrests the process of pneumatization (Ojala, 1957).

Middle Ear Cavity

Comparative anatomical studies of the middle ear of mammals have been conducted by Hagenbach (1835), by van Kampen (1905) and, more recently, by Henson (1961). Henson studied three genera of Insectivora and eight genera of Chiroptera and concluded that the size of the middle ear structures was related (inversely) to the predominant frequency of sound emission by the animal.

Our own studies (Pye and Hinchcliffe, 1968; Hinchcliffe and Pye, 1969) have shown that there is a considerable variation in the size of the middle ear cavity in the Mammalia. The largest cavities are found in some of the Insectivora, e.g. *Crocidura* (the shrew) and *Talpa* (the mole), in the Heteromyidae (the kangeroo rats) such as *Microdipodops pallidus* (Fig. 6), in Gerbillinae (gerbils), in Octodontoidea and in *Mustela* (the weasel). All these animals are fossorial (burrowing) so that this enlargement could be related to their mode of life. De Balsac (1936), having studied the middle ears of Saharan mammals, showed that there was a high correlation between bullar volume and environmental dessication. A subsequent study by Petter (1953) showed that the bullar volume was also correlated (inversely) with the population density for these animals. It was hypothesized that enlargement of the bulla would enable the animals to hear social signals at greater distances and so help them find mates. In the gerbilline rodents, Lay (1972) has shown that the effective tympanic membrane area increases concomitantly with the volume of the middle ear cavity. For low frequencies, the acoustic impedance of the tympanic membrane is greatly influenced by the cushion of air in the middle ear. Electrophysiological experiments conducted by Lay showed that gerbilline rodents were most sensitive to sounds in the range 500–2800 Hz. Experimental studies by Legouix and Wisner (1955) showed that reduction of

have a thick skull wall, such as man, the cochlea is embedded in the petrous bone.

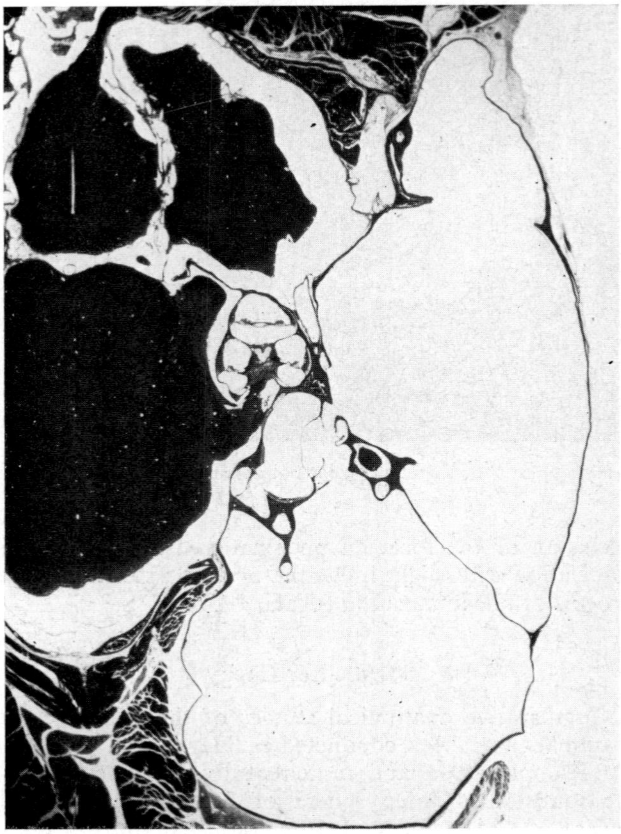

Large tympanic cavities are also associated with the presence of interlacing bony partitions, termed trabeculae. Figure 7 shows the moderately trabeculated middle ear cavity of *Liomy pictus* (the spiny pocket mouse). Trabeculation is also found in all the other Heteromyidae, but

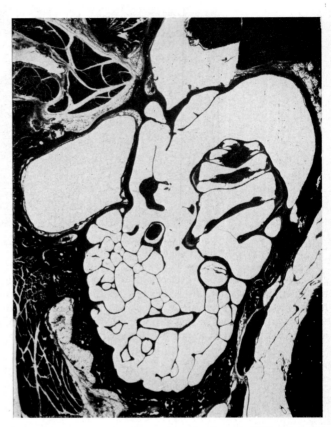

FIG. 6. *Microdipodops pallidus* showing enormously enlarged right middle ear cavity, especially posterior to the cochlea. The stapes base can also be seen opening into the junction of the vestibule and the basal turn of the cochlea. (×8)

FIG. 7. *Liomys pictus* showing moderately enlarged middle ear cavity, posterior part of which is trabeculated. The cochlea, facial nerve and parts of the ossicles are also seen. (×15)

the bullar volume of *Meriones crassus* (the gerbil) resulted in an appreciable reduction in cochlear potentials. Webster (1962) showed that all the sample of *Dipodomys sp.* (the kangeroo rat) with experimentally reduced middle ear volumes were, in contrast to control animals, quickly caught by predators, either *Otus assio* (an owl) or *Crotalus cerastes* (a rattle snake). The attack flight of *Otus assio* is associated with the production of sound containing energy for frequencies below 1200 Hz. The strike of *Crotalus cerastes* is associated with the production of weak bursts of sound containing energy frequencies below 2200 Hz.

Another function of the bulla, according to Békésy (1960), is to minimize bone conduction by locating the cochlea in a stressless zone of the skull wall. "Suspension" of the cochlea in a bulla is observed in many mammals that do not have a thick skull wall. In mammals which

the larger the middle ear cavity in this family, the less the degree of trabeculation. Marked trabeculation is found in the mole *Talpa*. Here it exists to such an extent that not only do the two enormously enlarged trabeculated tympanic cavities meet in the midline but the intervening partition is broken down and one single continuous cavity is formed. Other animals having trabeculated middle ear cavities are the hystricomorphs *Proechimys* (spiny rats of Central America), *Octodon* (a rodent of the Chilean and Peruvian coastal regions) and *Ctenomys* (the tuco-tuco of South America), the myomorph *Clethrionomys* (vole) and the carnivore *Mustela*. Trabeculae may provide mechanical strengthening of the middle ear cavities, or they may serve to divide the middle ear cavity into a number of Helmholtz resonators. "Flying buttresses" have also been described in man by Sammut (1967), where they may represent an atavistic trait.

Auditory Tube

The aeration of the middle ear of mammals is dependent on the auditory tube. This is of variable length and may be very short, as in *Taphozous* (tomb bat) and other bats. Bats also frequently show diverticula of the tube, as in *Molossus ater* (velvety free-tailed bat of Trinidad) (Fig. 8). Tubal diverticula are also said to occur in other mammals,

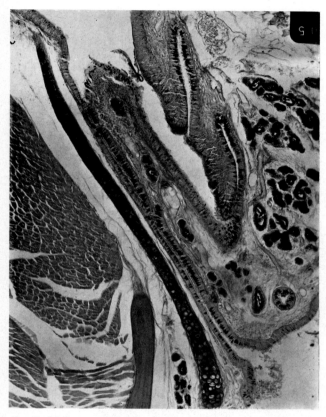

FIG. 8. *Molossus ater* showing diverticula of auditory tube. Note that the tube is lined with numerous mucous glands. (×88)

e.g. in the Hyracoidea (conies) and the Perissodactyla (odd-toed hoofed mammals), such as the Equidae (horses) and the Tapiridae (tapirs). These mammalian tubal diverticula may be so pronounced as to be termed air sacs. Diverticula of the auditory tube in man, referred to as Kirchner's diverticula, are rarely found. As Altmann (1951) points out, these diverticula usually originate from the floor of the tube near the pharyngeal ostium and expand between the tensor palati and levator palati muscles. Although Peters (1909) considered that these were pure malformations, von Kostanecki (1887) thought that they represented pulsion diverticula developing in a congenitally weak area. Finally, Stupka (1938) denied that they were homologous with the naturally occurring diverticula in other mammals.

Muftic and Loutfi (1955) reported what they considered to be an infected tubal diverticulum in man, although it has been questioned whether this might not have been a simple abscess cavity.

Stapedial Artery

A persistent stapedial artery occurs normally in most bats, e.g. *Tadarida thersites* (the free-tailed bat) (Fig. 9), in Insectivora and in the Myomorpha, a sub-order of rodents which contains the rats and mice. Although it persists in some species only, the artery is present in all mammalian embryos, including man (Fisher, 1914). As Goodrich

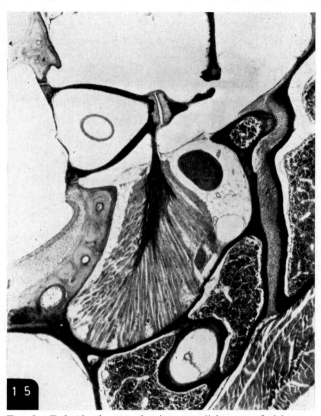

FIG. 9. *Tadarida thersites* showing stapedial artery, facial nerve, stapedius muscle and tendon, and complete stapes with stapedovestibular and incudo-stapedial joints. Note facial nerve and stapedius muscle are in the same bony cavity. (×50)

(1930) and others have pointed out, the artery can be traced from man down to the lowest fishes, where it is represented by the orbital artery. In gnathostomes in general, an artery arises from the dorsal end of the second (hyoidean) aortic arch or from the lateral dorsal aorta in front of that arch. It passes forwards to the orbit to give three main branches, i.e. the supraorbital, the infraorbital (to the upper jaw) and the mandibular (to the lower jaw) (Tandler, 1902). In certain geckonids, e.g. *Pachydactylus*, *Hemidactylus* and *Tarentola*, it pierces the columella, and in some birds, e.g. *Procellaria* and *Aquila*, it may do so also (Doran, 1878). Goodrich (1930) also pointed out that the perforated fossil stapes of the Stegocephalia (Embolomeri and Rhachitomi—primitive amphibians) and *Cynognathus* as well as *Thrinaxodon* (primitive reptiles), indicates that these ancestral vertebrates also possessed a stapedial artery.

Rarely, the stapedial artery persists in man, such a condition having been first described by Hyrtl (1836).

Since this report, there have been a dozen or so other reports of such an anomaly in man. More recent reports have been by House and Patterson (1964), by Maran (1965) and by Baron (1967). Hogg and his associates (1972) have reviewed the ontogeny and phylogeny of the artery. This anomaly may be associated with other anomalies, as in the recently reported Patau's (trisomy 13–15) syndrome (Sando *et al.*, 1972). A persistent stapedial artery in man invariably follows the same course (Altmann, 1951). The artery arises from the internal carotid, perforates the floor of the tympanic cavity, passes upward over the promontory (usually enclosed in a bony canal), passes through the obturator foramen of the stapes, enters the facial canal and finally divides into branches in the extradural space in the area of distribution of the middle meningeal artery.

Ossicles

An account of the comparative anatomy of the mammalian ossicles was published by Casserius in 1601. A more definitive study was reported by Doran in 1878. As Goodrich (1930) pointed out, few problems in morphology have aroused more interest than that of the origin of the auditory ossicles. Mammals differ from all other vertebrates in two respects. First, they have a lower jaw composed of a single dermal bone, the mandible (dentary) articulating with another dermal bone, the squamosal (squamous temporal in man) fixed to the skull. Secondly, they have a chain of three ossicles (malleus, incus and stapes) serving to convey airborne vibrations from the tympanic membrane to the internal ear. In explaining these two characteristics, the Reichert-Gaupp theory inter-relates them. The mammalian stapes derives from the reptilian columella auris, the incus from the quadrate of the upper jaw and the malleus from the articular of the lower jaw of ancestral vertebrates, whilst the dentary (mandible) has acquired a new articulation with the squamosal (Reichert, 1837; Gaupp, 1904). In man, the squamosal, as the squamous temporal bone, has fused with other bones to form the temporal bone.

A link between these reptilian and mammalian forms is seen in the fossil *Diarthrognathus*. Here there is a double articulation between the skull and the lower jaw, i.e. both a quadrato-articular and a squamoso-dentary articulation (Crompton, 1958, 1963). However, we must not be deluded into thinking that there has been a single evolutionary line, with the aim of producing a single type of air-conduction sound receptor. In Tumarkin's (1968) own words, such "can only be regarded as anthropocentric prejudice". Tumarkin has cogently argued for the evolution of a number of sound-conducting apparatuses in terrestrial vertebrates, including both "forward" and "reversed" bone conduction mechanisms. He suggests, moreover, that pelycosaurs, such as *Dimetrodon*, had two "reversed" sound conduction routes to the internal ear. One route was for air, using the "dorsal sail" (the membrane stretched across the specially elongated vertebral spines), and the other was for ground-conducted vibrations. The "sail" would be analogous to the acoustic fan

type of hearing aid. Tumarkin considers that the present day mammalian vestibulo-ossicular (perhaps more appropriately termed "labyrintho-ossicular") mechanism is developed from the therapsid (reptilian group ancestral to the mammals) vestibulo-quadrate (labyrintho-quadrate) mechanism. The therapsid stapes was in a deep recess surrounded by other skull bones. In a need to reach the surface, Tumarkin hypothesized that this stapes developed

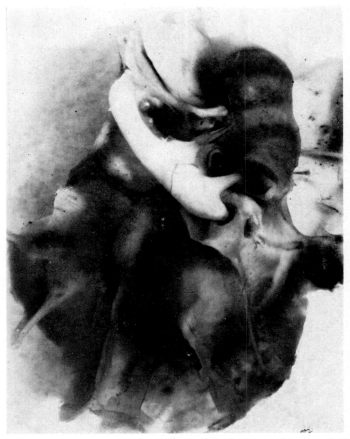

FIG. 10. *Chinchilla sp.* showing interior of left middle ear after removal of dorsal wall of bulla. Note bony trabeculae posteriorly, fused malleus and incus, anterior crus, and base of stapes, fenestra cochleae and cylindrically shaped cochlea.

a connection between the articular and quadrate bones which were no longer needed for mastication.

As Doran (1878) and subsequently others have pointed out, there is considerable variability in shape and size of the mammalian ossicles. The shape of the human ossicles may be compared with those of the chinchilla in Fig. 10. At a first glance, it would also appear that there is no relation between the size of ossicles and the size of the animal. For example, the stapes base in the elephant, which is about 100 times heavier than man, measures 5·3 mm times 3·8 mm. (Békésy, 1960). The comparable measurements for man are 3 mm and 1·4 mm (Bast and Anson, 1949). However, inspection of the data indicates that, as with the basilar membrane, ossicular size may be proportional to the square root of the animal size (Hinchcliffe and Pye, 1976).

Fusion of the malleus with the bony wall of the middle

ear occurs normally in a number of mammals, e.g. *Pteropus* (the flying fox—a fruit bat) (Fig. 11), and it may also be seen in the cat (Ritter, 1971). This may provide a phylogenetic explanation for the congenital fixed malleus syndrome. Most cases of the fixed malleus syndrome in man are, however, associated with previous inflammatory conditions of the middle ear cleft (Goodhill, 1966). Where congenital bony fixation does occur, it is due to a

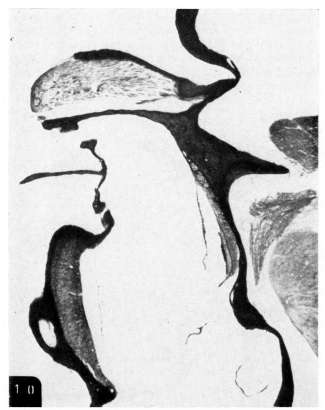

FIG. 12. *Octodon degus* showing unicrurate stapes and its base opening into the junction of the vestibule and the basal turn of the cochlea. Note the synovial type stapedo-vestibular joint. The tensor tympani is also seen. (×40)

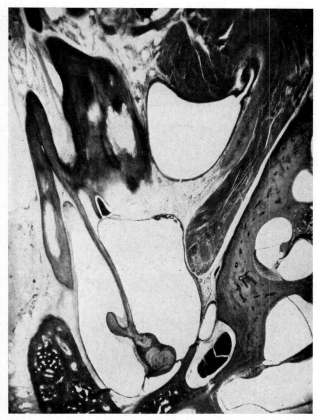

FIG. 11. *Pteropus giganteus* showing fusion of malleus to bony wall of the biloculated tympanic cavity. A large tensor tympani, the facial nerve and parts of the auditory tube, cochlea, and vestibular apparatus are also shown. (×40)

bony bar 120–180 μm in diameter, extending from the epitympanic wall to the head of the malleus. Audiometrically, this may show as a high frequency conductive type hearing loss, (Ritter, 1971). The so-called acquired type of fixed malleus syndrome may still have a congenital factor in its aetiology. Davies (1968) says that, in the normal temporal bone, a fine bony spur is frequently found to extend from the lateral aspect of the anterior epitympanic wall towards the head of the malleus. If well developed, this projection results in this ossicle being "at risk" to fixation.

A unicrurate stapes is not infrequently seen as a normal occurrence in mammals. As Goodrich (1930) points out, in many marsupials and in the monotremes, the stapes is imperforate and columelliform. The condition appears to be secondary since, in *Ornithorhynchus* (the duck-billed platypus) and *Trichosurus* (the flying phalanger) at

least, it surrounds the stapedial artery in the blastematous stage. Figure 12 illustrates a unicrurate stapes in *Octodon degus*. Stapedial structures intermediate between the unicrurate and the classical bicrurate stapes of man and most other mammals (Fig. 9), have also been observed. Thus Fig. 13 illustrates the condition in *Mustela nivalis*, the weasel. As the figure also illustrates, the plane of section goes through both fenestrae. During normal sound stimulation, there is a column of vibratory motion between the two windows and this figure demonstrates that this vibratory path cuts across the basilar membrane at a point near the basal extremity, but not at the very end. This provides an explanation for the occurrence of noise-induced hearing loss at a point in the mid-frequency range and not for the highest detectable frequency for an animal (Littler, 1965).

Joints and Fenestrae

As we previously reported (Hinchcliffe and Pye, 1969), all specimens that we examined of the orders Edentata and Primates showed a synovial type incudo-mallear joint. This was also the usual condition in the Order Chirontera, Fibrous, cartilaginous or bony fusion of the joint is found in many hystricomorph rodents (*see* Fig. 10).

In contrast to the synovial type incudo-mallear joint which prevails amongst the mammals, the stapedo-vestibular joint is characteristically a fibrous one, with an

annular ligament (Fig. 9). However, in a number of
rodents, e.g. *Mastomys* (a rat), *Perognathus* (pocket mice),
Heteromys (spiny pocket mice of the tropical rain forests
of Central Americas), *Proechimys* (spiny rats of Central
America) and *Octodon* (Fig. 12), a synovial joint is found.

The site of opening of the fenestra ovalis into the internal
ear is variable. Thus it may open into the basal turn of the

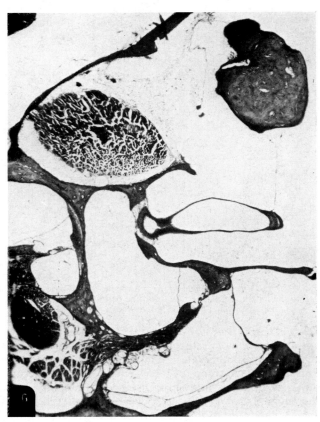

FIG. 13. *Mustela nivalis* shows a pattern of stapes development intermediate between the unicrurate type shown in Fig. 12 and the
classical bicrurate type shown in Fig. 9. Note that in contrast to
Fig. 12, the stapedo-vestibular joint here is the more commonly
found fibrous type, i.e. with an annular ligament. In this instance,
the stapes opens into the base of the cochlea. The plane of section
passes through both fenestra, this plane also passes through the
spiral organ near its basal extremity. (×35)

cochlea, as in man, into the vestibule as in the sloth,
Choloepus hoffmanni and other edentates, or into the
junction of these two structures, as in *Mustela nivalis*
(Fig. 13).

The fenestra cochleae (round window) is present in all
mammals, in most birds and in some reptiles, such as the
crocodile. As Békésy (1960) and Kirikae (1960) have
pointed out, a dynamic relationship between the two
fenestrae is of importance in optimizing sound stimulation
of the cochlea. Except for man, the monkey and the mole,
Kirikae found that the area of the fenestra cochleae was
larger than that of the fenestra vestibuli by a factor of up
to 3·2.

Intratympanic Muscles

The middle ear muscles exist in varying degrees of
development in the Mammalia. The greatest development
of both middle ear muscles is seen in the Microchiroptera
as illustrated in *Eptesicus rendalli* (Fig. 14), some of the
shrews (Insectivora), and some of the sloths (Edentata)
e.g. *Choloepus*. In contrast, it appears that the stapedius
muscle is normally absent in a number of rodent species
e.g. some of the Heteromyidae (*Heteromys, Liomys* and
Perognathus), the dormouse (*Glis glis*) which belongs to the
Myomorpha, and some of the hystricomorphs (*Proechimys, Octodon* and *Ctenomys*). As we have previously
commented (Hinchcliffe and Pye, 1969), all the species
where the stapedius muscle was absent are fossorial.
There appears to be some association between an absent
stapedius muscle, a trabeculated tympanic cavity and a

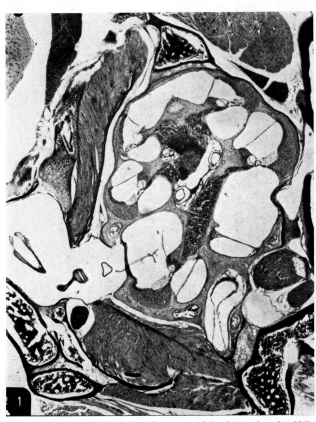

FIG. 14. *Eptesicus rendalli* showing parts of the internal and middle
ear, including the stapedial artery, enormously developed tympanic
muscles and parts of the ossicles, including the incudo-stapedial
joint. Note association of stapedius muscle with the underlying
muscle sheet. The section through the cochlea is a mid-modiolar
one with the five half-turns clearly seen. (×32)

burrowing habit. A possible explanation lies in an adaptation to receive ground-borne, as opposed to air-borne
vibrations. Changes in middle ear muscle tonus modulate
the frequency spectrum of external acoustic signals. The
modulation provides a means whereby an air-borne
auditory signal can be separated from a background noise.
These modulations may also eliminate middle ear resonances without sacrificing the sensitivity of transmissions.

Where the animal is concerned with ground-borne vibrations, this function of the middle ear muscles may be obviated. The effect of the trabeculations in forming sub-cavities in the middle ear might also eliminate middle ear resonances or at least eliminate sharp peaks, a role which would otherwise be filled by the middle ear muscles.

It would appear that an absent stapedius muscle, unassociated with other congenital anomalies, may occur in about 1 per cent of human beings (Hoshino and Paparella, 1971).

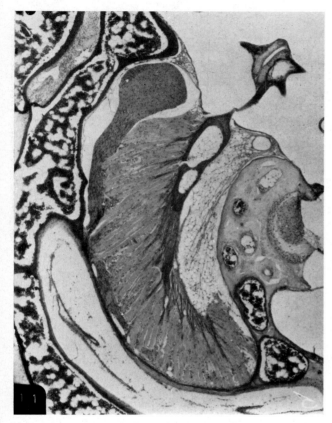

FIG. 15. *Otomops martiensseni* showing very large stapedius muscle being innervated by the adjacent facial nerve. A calcified Paaw's cartilage is seen in the muscle at the point of attachment of the tendon. An area of fatty tissue is seen medial to Paaw's cartilage, separating it and the muscle from the bony medial wall. Also note the incudo-stapedial joint. (×50)

In most mammals, the stapedius muscle does not lie in a bony cavity separate from the trunk of the facial nerve (Fig. 15). In man and some other mammals, e.g. the Gerbillinae, *Octodon*, *Ctenomys* and *Mustela*, the stapedius muscle is contained in a bony cavity.

In *Eptesicus* (Fig. 14) and some other mammals the stapedius muscle is clearly part of an underlying muscle sheet. As McClain (1939) has pointed out, the stapedius anlage first attaches to the ear at the stylohyal bone. It subsequently shifts its attachment by degeneration of its ventral fibres and formation of new dorsal fibres attaching it to the stapes. This, McClain maintains, is in complete agreement with Edgeworth's (1914) view that the stapedius muscle is really a levator hyoidei. It is thus probably

homologous with the extrastapedial muscle of crocodiles and birds (Killian, 1890), being thus derived from the same source as the sauropsid (bird-like reptiles) depressor mandibulae. The columella of the Anura (the order of amphibians containing the frogs) has, it should be noted, a quite different origin from the avian columella. It derives partly from the chondrocranium and partly from a local condensation of mesoderm (Gaupp, 1904). Correspondingly, the opercular middle ear muscle of anurans is not homologous with the stapedius muscle of mammals. It is assumed to be derived from the levator scapulae and is innervated by cervical spinal nerves (Kirikae, 1960).

In a number of mammals, the stapedius muscle contains what appears to be a sesamoid bone, or, more frequently, the cartilaginous equivalent. This structure, termed Paaw's cartilage (van der Klaauw, 1923) occurs at least in all Microchiroptera, e.g. *Otomops martiensseni* (Fig. 15), in Marsupialia, e.g. *Didelphys* (the Virginia opossum), in Edentata (ant-eaters, armadillos and sloths), in Pholidota, e.g. *Manis tricuspis* (the pangolin) and in some carnivores, e.g. *Nasua narica* (the coati). In some mammals, the tensor tympani may show a double origin, one origin from the bony semicanal, and the other from the medial wall of the middle ear. It is of note that Wright and Etholm (1973) have recently described a bifurcated tensor tympani as an anomaly in man. The condition was found in two trisomy syndromes (13–15 and 18).

Pathology

Our own survey of mammalian ears impressed us with the rarity of spontaneously occurring middle ear disease in feral mammals. One specimen only showed disease of the middle ear. Bilateral chronic otitis media was observed in *Coendou prehensilis* (the Trinidad Tree Porcupine). The histological picture was not dissimilar to the pattern that had been described in man with the exception that a spirochaetal type organism was seen in the sections (Pye and Hinchcliffe, 1970).

In contrast to the rarity of spontaneously occurring aural pathology in feral mammals, middle ear infections are common in laboratory animals, whether they be anthropoids (Keleman, 1966, 1968), cats or rodents.

INTERNAL EAR

Cochlea

The cochlea is not only the acoustic analyser of the mammalian auditory system but also, as Harris and van Bergeijk (1962) have pointed out, a mechanical impedance matching device complementing the tympano-ossicular mechanism. Throughout the mammals, we find the cochlea as a coiled bony structure (hence the name) containing the sensory neuroepithelium, i.e. the spiral organ of Corti. This coiling, as Békésy (1960) has pointed out, protects the structure against deformation. In birds, however, the cochlea is a short, curved tube only, e.g. in *Gallus domesticus* (chicken), where it is only 5 mm long.

Conventional light microscopic techniques are adequate to demonstrate many differences in cochlear structure in the various mammals. We have found that the following measures may show appreciable variability in the Mammalia:

(1) Shape
(2) Attachment
(3) Number of turns
(4) Dimensions
    (a) Height and width of cochlea
    (b) Width and thickness of basilar membrane
    (c) Height of cells of Claudius
    (d) Size of spiral ligament.

Three basic types of mammalian cochlear shape exist; the truncated cone, the polyhedron and the cylinder. The truncated cone shape is most common and is found in man and many other mammals, especially rodents. The polyhedron is found infrequently, e.g. *Clethrionomys*. The cylindrical type is commoner than the polyhedron and is found principally in the Chinchilloidea, in the Gerbillinae, and in the Heteromyidae.

In the vast majority of our specimens, we found that the cochlea was essentially suspended in the bullar space by an abutment from the dorsal surface of the cranium. This attachment to the cranium may be fibrous only, as in bats. It helps to insulate the cochlea against body-borne (bone conducted) vibrations, as illustrated for *Natalus tumidirostris* (funnel-eared bat) (Fig. 16). Fraser and Purvis (1959) and Reysenbach de Haan (1956) have pointed out that, in the whale, tissue conduction is also reduced by isolating the petrous bone from the rest of the body by air spaces.

The degree of coiling of the cochlea ranges from 550° (just over 3 half-turns) to over 1600° (9 half-turns). Most primitive mammals, as the mole, *Talpa*, and the shrew, *Sorex*, have 3–4 half-turns (A. Pye, 1972). The Megachiroptera and some rodents have 4, the Microchiroptera have 5–7, whilst some of the specialized rodents, e.g. the Heteromyidae and burrowing hystricomorphs, have 7–9 half-turns. It is interesting to note that, amongst the echo-locating bats (Microchiroptera), the ones emitting principally constant frequency pulses, e.g. *Pteronotus* (moustache bats of the Caribbean), *Hipposideros* (the Old World leaf-nose bats) and *Rhinolophus* (horse-shoe bats) have more half-turns than those, e.g. *Myotis*, which use frequency-modulated pulses (A. Pye, 1971).

In our series, the height of the cochlea ranged from 1·4 mm, in *Eptesicus rendalli* (a small bat) to 5·4 mm in *Dasyprocta punctata*, an agouti, a rodent found on the plains of countries bordering the Caribbean (Table 2).

A principal component analysis of cochlear dimensions in species of the Order Chiroptera, showed that there was a general size factor and a factor of structural type. The latter factor differentiated a type with tall cells of Claudius and a narrow basilar membrane, at one extreme, from a type with short cells of Claudius and a broad basilar membrane at the other extreme. It was also found that, the higher the frequency of the emitted sound of a species,

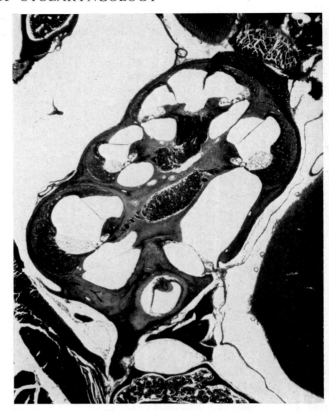

Fig. 16. *Natalus tumidirostris* showing mid-modiolar section of cochlea which is virtually suspended within the tympanic cavity. Note the tall cells of Claudius and the thickening of the basilar membrane at the first half-turn. These two cochlear characteristics become less prominent as one approaches the apex. (×35)

the narrower the width of the basilar membrane, especially that of more basal portions (Hinchcliffe and Pye, 1968).

Basilar Membrane

The length of the basilar membrane is a function of the size of the animal, ranging from 7 mm in the mouse (*Mus musculus*) to nearly 60 mm in the "elephant" (probably *Elephas maximas*) (Békésy, 1960). The lengths are not linearly related to body size but are a power function of body size (Hinchcliffe and Pye, 1976).

Usually the width of the basilar membrane is least at the basal end, widening out to the apical end. This increase may be anything from twofold, as in rodents, to fivefold as in man (*see* Table 2). Exceptions to this occur. Constant frequency pulse emitting bats often have the narrowest part of the basilar membrane in the second half-turn, e.g. *Rhinolophus* (A. Pye, 1966, 1970). In other mammals, e.g. *Eptesicus* and some hystricomorphs, e.g. *Galea* (a guinea pig) and *Octodon*, the width of the basilar membrane varies little or not at all along its length. The animals possessing the narrowest basilar membrane at the base are the echo-locating bats. In the non-echo-locating bats and in many rodents, the width at the base is at least twice that of the echo-locating bats.

TABLE 2

SHOWING SOME COCHLEAR MEASUREMENTS FOR SIX SELECTED MAMMALS. NOTE THE DIFFERENCES IN THE HEIGHTS OF THE COCHLEAE AND THE WIDTHS OF THE BASILAR MEMBRANE ALONG THE COCHLEAR SPIRAL

Species		Dasyprocta punctata	Octodon degu	Praeomys tullbergi	Roussettus aegyptiacus	Rhinolophus ferrumequinum	Eptesicus rendalli
Height of cochlea		5·4 mm	2·8 mm	2·0 mm	2·8 mm	2·7 mm	1·4 mm
Width of cochlea at every half-turn	1	2525 μm	1 364 μm	1 142 μm	1 715 μm	1 819 μm	10 56 μm
	2	2400 μm	1 199 μm	892 μm	1 164 μm	1 543 μm	823 μm
	3	1775 μm	980 μm	925 μm	1 168 μm	1 157 μm	767 μm
	4	1800 μm	995 μm	764 μm	996 μm	1 056 μm	745 μm
	5	1350 μm	939 μm	642 μm		760 μm	510 μm
	6	1225 μm	832 μm			506 μm	532 μm
	7	1050 μm	774 μm			450 μm	
	8	925 μm					
	9	950 μm					
Width of basilar membrane at every half-turn	1	160 μm	169 μm	100 μm	120 μm	99 μm	125 μm
	2	180 μm	195 μm	119 μm	153 μm	98 μm	103 μm
	3	200 μm	173 μm	139 μm	176 μm	82 μm	98 μm
	4	225 μm	166 μm	143 μm	184 μm	82 μm	92 μm
	5	240 μm	175 μm	144 μm		109 μm	106 μm
	6	230 μm	184 μm			120 μm	106 μm
	7	240 μm	164 μm			114 μm	
	8	220 μm					
	9	230 μm					
Thickness of basilar membrane at every half-turn	1			9 μm		24 μm	6 μm
	2			9 μm		21 μm	10 μm
	3						

Hyaline Mass

A specialized intracochlear structure, to which we have previously drawn attention in the heteromyid rodents (Pye, 1965), is a hyaline mass within the basilar membrane. A small structure of this type was first reported by Iwata (1924) in *Myotis* (mouse-eared bat). More pronounced structures were subsequently described in odontocete whales (Reysenbach de Haan, 1956) and in gerbilline rodents (Lay, 1972). The structure is here illustrated in a bat, *Hipposideros caffer* (Fig. 17), and in a rodent, *Microdipodops pallidus* (Fig. 18). The two figures show where the structure is most prominent in the two species, i.e. in the first half-turn for *Hipposideros* and in the fifth half-turn for *Microdipodops*. These specialized intracochlear structures are absent in the Primates, the cochlear architecture of which is illustrated by *Marikina geoffroyi* (a tamarin of South America) (Fig. 19). Amongst the bats, *Asellia tridens*, *Natalus tumidirostris*, *Triaenops persicus* and all the species of *Rhinolophus* and *Hipposideros* possess this hyaline mass, which is confined mainly to the basal turn. Except for *Natalus*, all of these bats emit constant frequency pulses only. Again, apart from this one exception, no bats emitting frequency-modulated pulses possesses any significant hyaline mass. Some Megachiroptera have a thickening of the basilar membrane to an extent not amounting to a hyaline mass and at the apical turn only.

In gerbilline and heteromyid rodents, the cells of Hensen demonstrate specialization. In such cases, the cells are most prominent not at the base, but in the middle and at the apical end of the cochlea, as seen in *Microdipodops* (Fig. 18). These cells of Hensen are flask-shaped with long cytoplasmic processes, not resting on the basilar membrane but upon a cup which is probably formed of the supporting cells of Deiter and of Claudius.

Lay points out that there appears to be a general correlation between the thickness of the hyaline mass and the height of the Hensen's cells along the cochlear partition with the frequency of maximum sensitivity as measured by cochlear potentials. Maximum cochlear potentials for the Gerbillinae occur in the range 1200–3000 Hz and maximum development of the hyaline mass and Hensen's cells occur in the central three half-turns of the cochlea. Lay showed that *Tatera indica* (a gerbil) and *Meriones hurrianae* (a jird or sand rat of Central Asia) have similar transformer ratio/middle ear volume ratios but markedly different cochlear potentials over all frequencies. *Meriones hurrianae* possesses this hyaline mass within its cochlea, but *Tatera indica* does not. This should indicate that the pronounced difference in spiral organ structure between these two species may be responsible for the different cochlear sensitivities, rather than the slight differences in middle ear structure which theoretically would favour a greater sensitivity for *Tatera indica*. Lay conjectures that the hyaline mass weights the basilar membrane, and so alters the vibratory characteristics of the cochlear partition, since weighting the centre of circular diaphragms in liquid effectively narrows the resonance frequency without decreasing sensitivity. Although, of course, the basilar

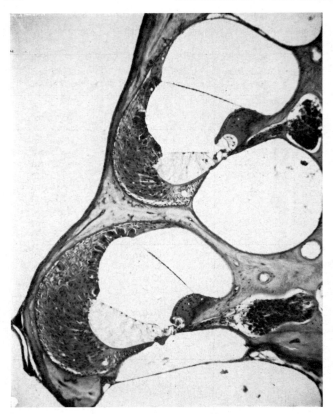

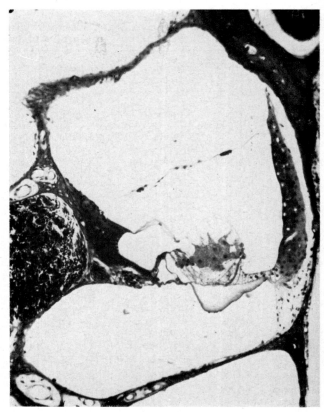

FIG. 17. *Hipposideros caffer* showing first and third half-turns of the cochlea. Note the enormous spiral ligament, the thickening (hyaline mass) of the basilar membrane and the tall cells of Claudius, all of which are more prominent in the first half-turn. (×80)

FIG. 18. *Microdipodops pallidus*. Section through fifth half-turn of cochlea showing a small spiral ligament (compare with Fig. 17), a prominent hyaline mass projecting from the under surface of the basilar membrane and flask-shaped cells of Hensen resting on a cup formed of the cells of Claudius and Deiter. (×130)

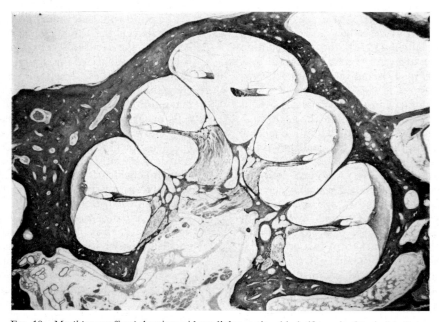

FIG. 19. *Marikina geoffroyi* showing mid-modiolar section (six half-turns) of typical anthropoid cochlea, i.e. a notable absence of specialised features which characterise so many other mammals. (×21)

membrane is not circular, it vibrates in a sinusoidal manner as does a diaphragm. Previously, J. D. Pye (1968) had suggested that the hyaline masses were responsible for narrowly tuned responses. Moreover, it is also tempting to speculate that these masses accentuate the non-linearity of the ear. That aural non-linearity does reside in the cochlea, as Wever and Lawrence (1954) have previously argued, was demonstrated by Rhode's (1971) study of the vibration patterns of the basilar membrane in *Saimiri sciureus* (squirrel monkey) using the Mössbauer technique. In contrast, the vibration of the malleus showed a linear function over the entire intensity range studied.

Cells of Claudius

The cells of Claudius are extremely tall in some bats at the cochlear base, attaining heights of 100 μm above the basilar membrane. This characteristic seems to be associated with the emission of constant frequency, or directed frequency-modulated pulses. This is shown for *Hipposideros caffer* in Fig. 17 (A. Pye, 1970).

Spiral Ligament and Stria Vascularis

The spiral ligament and the stria vascularis are very prominent at the base in many of the echo-locating bats, extending, in the case of the spiral ligament, well into the scala vestibuli, as in Figs. 16 and 17. Compare this with the condition in the rodent, *Microdipodops* (Fig. 18). It is possible that this great development of the stria vascularis in these mammals is related to the greater functional demands on the internal ear in animals employing a sound navigating system.

Cells of Böttcher

Webster (1961) has suggested that the cells of Böttcher, which are seen in the guinea pig but are absent in man, are displaced cells of the external spiral sulcus.

Cochlear Aqueduct

Although the cochlear aqueduct is certainly duct-like in man, in many mammals it is so short as to constitute a foramen, as in *Centurio senex*, the wrinkle-faced bat of Trinidad and Central America (Fig. 20).

Vestibular Labyrinth

Early in this century, A. A. Gray (1907) reported an extensive study of both avian and mammalian labyrinths. Gray used a paraffin technique to demonstrate the otic (membranous) labyrinths of his specimens. His son, Oliver Gray, subsequently extended the study to encompass also the vestibular apparatuses of invertebrates, which are analogous to, but not homologous with, those of vertebrates (Gray, 1955).

The basic pattern of the vertebrate vestibular labyrinth is that of three semicircular canals, together with a saccule, a utricle and a lagena (Fig. 21). The lagena is absent in

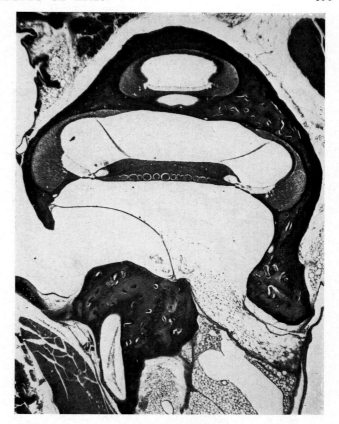

FIG. 20. *Centurio senex* showing a cochlear aqueduct of the foramen type which is more commonly found than the duct type in mammals. (×35)

mammals. An additional strip of sensory neuro-epithelium, the macula neglecta, lying on the roof of the saccule, has also been demonstrated in certain amphibians, reptiles and birds, but never in mammals. Lowenstein (1956) showed that, whereas the utricle functions as an "out-of-level" receptor, the lagena functions as an "into-level" receptor.

In contrast to gnathostome fishes, the agnatha demonstrate a different (possibly primitive, possibly specialized) labyrinthine structure. *Petromyzon* (the lamprey) possesses only two semicircular canals in each labyrinth. *Myxine* (the hagfish) has only one semicircular canal in each labyrinth, but each canal has an ampulla at each end. The arrangement of the vestibular labyrinth in *Chimaera*, the only survivor of primitive Selachian fishes termed Holocephali, is on a simpler plan (reminiscent of the arrangement in mammals) than that in birds, reptiles or any other fish (Gray, 1951). With the exception of *Corvus corone* (the carrion crow), the superior semicircular canal in all birds is much longer than either of the other two canals. There are some variations in the form of the semicircular canals in mammals. In both *Felis concolor* (puma) and in *Panthera pardus* (leopard), the posterior limb of the lateral semicircular canal enters the posterior ampulla, instead of joining the utricle directly. In *Callithrix jacchus* (common marmoset), the lateral semicircular canal enlarges at its medial end to form a pseudo-ampulla. In contrast to the large size of the vestibular labyrinth in seals and other Pinnipedia, the semicircular canals are degenerate in the Cetacea, being of smaller calibre in *Phocaena phocaena* (porpoise) than in *Mus musculus*.

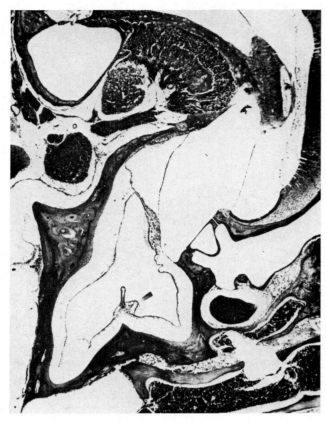

Fig. 21. *Carollia perspecillata*. Vertical section through base of cochlea and vestibular labyrinth, showing complete stapes base opening into junction of vestibule and basal turn of cochlea, maculae of saccule and utricle and two cristae with their cupulae. (×45)

In contrast to the labyrinths of Mammalia, which reach maximum size before birth, the labyrinths of fishes continue to increase in size with the general growth of the fish. Thus the span of the semicircular duct of *Gadus callarius* (cod) may be as much as 30 mm, compared with a value of less than 5 mm for man.

The endolymphatic duct is absent in the Crossopterygii (lung fish) and rudimentary in other fish except the Selachians (shark group), where it runs vertically from the saccule to open to the outside on the surface of the head near to the midline. In frogs and some other amphibians, the sacculae of both sides are connected with fine endolymphatic spaces above the spinal cord, from where intercommunicating channels pass through the intervertebral foramina and end in sacs containing otoliths.

OTHER TECHNIQUES

Although the conventional light microscopic technique on serial sections is adequate to demonstrate much variation in the structure of the mammalian ear, more refined techniques are required for studying variations in the structure of, for example, the spiral organ. The surface specimen technique can provide much additional information in this case. The method used by Retzius over a hundred years ago has been further employed by Engström and his associates (1966) in more recent years. The technique entails fixation with osmic acid, followed by microdissection, as illustrated in Fig. 22 for *Cavia*. The spiral organ is then removed and examined under phase contrast microscopy. One of us (A.P.) has used this technique on seventeen species of mammals and observed that there are differences in the cytoarchitecture of the spiral organ at least at the taxonomic level of the order and also according to location along the basilar membrane in a given cochlea.

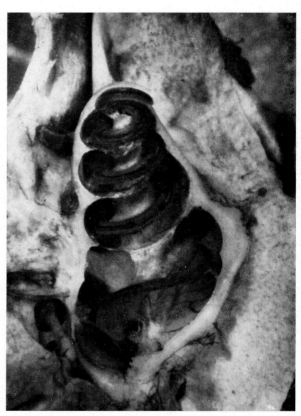

Fig. 22. *Cavia porcellus*. Microdissected specimen of right cochlea showing the basilar membrane and its associated structures coiling around the modiolus. The spiral ligament is shown at the right hand side of the basal turn, and the vestibular membrane at the left-hand side of the two apical turns. A segment of the dark staining tectorial membrane has been removed from a midsection of each of the two lowermost turns of the spiral organ. The membrane of the fenestra cochleae as well as the head, anterior crus and base of the stapes are also shown in the bottom left-hand corner of the figure.

The technique is also eminently suitable for experimental studies of the effects of drugs and of noise on the cochlea of animals, since every hair cell can be studied separately, as in *Cavia* (Fig. 23). Here, the inner row of hair cells is intact whilst some cells are missing from all the three rows of outer hair cells due to sound exposure.

The introduction of transmission electron microscopy by Engström and his associates (1953), and others, to the study of the ear has introduced a powerful additional technique to study structural differences between animals. Already, differences at the ultramicroscopic level have been shown between various groups of animals. Only one (Type II) of the two types of vestibular hair cells that Wersäll (1956) and others have demonstrated in man and other mammals, occurs in birds and fishes.

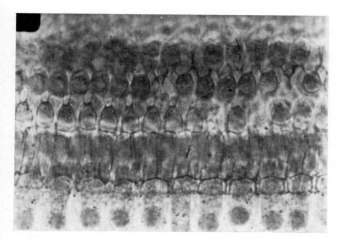

FIG. 23. *Cavia procellus*. Surface specimen view under phase contrast microscopy of the sensory cells of part of the spiral organ of a guinea pig subjected to an intense pure tone. Note intact row of inner sensory cells, compared with evidence for destroyed cells in all three rows of the outer sensory cells. (×600)

CONCLUSIONS

There is clearly considerable variation in the structure not only of the middle ear but also of the labyrinths of vertebrates. In many ways, the ear of man is a very unspecialized, unremarkable structure, its auditory component being surpassed by the chiropteran ear and its vestibular component by the selachian labyrinth. One can go further and say that not only is man's ear unspecialized, but, in some respects, it is degenerate. This occurs to such a degree that surgical operations on the external ear of man need take into account only cosmetic and not functional considerations. Such operations could be fatal in Chiroptera, and labyrinthectomy fatal also in Selachia. However, lest we take too otocentric view of hearing, let us remind ourselves that the computer which man possesses to process, *inter alia*, the information he derives from his ears has enabled him to forge ahead of all other animals and develop that communication code known as language.

ACKNOWLEDGEMENTS

We are grateful to Prof. J. D. Pye for Fig. 1. We are also indebted to Mr. D. J. Connolly of the Department of Clinical Photography, Institute of Laryngology and Otology, for technical assistance with the photographic reproductions.

REFERENCES

Altmann, F. (1951), *Arch. Otolaryng.*, **54**, 241.
Ashton, E. H. and Zuckerman, S. (1952), *Amer. J. phys. Anthrop.*, **10**, 145.
Balsac, H. Heim de (1936), *Bull. biol.*, suppl. 21.
Baron, S. H. (1967), *Laryngoscope*, **73**, 769.
Bast, T. H. and Anson, B. J. (1949), *The Temporal Bone and the Ear*. Springfield, Ill., U.S.A.: Chas. C. Thomas.
Batteau, D. W. (1969), *Proc. roy. Soc. B*, **168**, 158.
Békésy, G. von (1960), *Experiments in Hearing*. New York: McGraw-Hill.
Casserius, G. (1601), *De Vocis Auditusque Organis*. Ferrara.
Cole, F. J. (1944), *A History of Comparative Anatomy*. London: Macmillan.
Corti, A. (1851), *Ztschr f. wissen. Zool.*, **3**, 109.
Crompton, A. W. (1958), *Proc. zool. Soc. Lond.*, **130**, 183.
Crompton, A. W. (1963), *Evolution*, **17**, 431.
Davies, D. G. (1968), *J. Laryng.*, **82**, 331.
Doran, A. H. G. (1878), *Trans. Linn. Soc. Lond.*, **1**, 371.
Edgeworth, F. H. (1914), *Quart. J. micr. Sci.*, **59**, 573.
Engström, H., Sjostrand, F. S. and Wersall, J. (1953), *Proc. intern Congr. oto-rhino-laryng. (Amsterdam)*, **1**.
Engström, H., Ades, H. W. and Andersson, A. (1966), *Structural Pattern of the Organ of Corti*. Stockholm: Almquist and Wiksell.
Fisher, A. G. T. (1914), *J. Anat. Physiol.*, **48**, 37.
Fraser, F. C. and Purvis, P. E. (1959), *Endeavour*, **18**, 93.
Gardner, M. B. (1962), *J. acoust. Soc. Amer.*, **34**, 1824.
Gaupp, E. (1904), *Anat. Hefte, Ergeb.*, **14**, 808.
Goodhill, V. (1966), *Acta oto-laryng. (Stockh.)*, suppl. 217.
Goodrich, E. S. (1930), *Studies on the Structure and Development of Vertebrates*.
Gray, A. A. (1907), *The Labyrinth of Animals*. London: Churchill.
Gray, O. (1951), *J. Laryng.*, **65**, 681.
Gray, O. (1955), *J. Laryng.*, **69**, 151.
Griffin, D. R., Dunning, D. C., Cahlander, D. A. and Webster, F. A. (1962), *Nature, Lond.*, **196**, 1185.
Hagenbach, E. (1835), *Die Paukenhöhle der Säugetiere*. Leipzig: Weidmannsche Buchhandlung.
Harris, G. G. and Van Bergeijk, W. A. (1962), *J. acoust. Soc. Amer.*, **34**, 1831.
Hayashi, M. and Hagino, T. (1963), *Yokohama Med. J.*, **13**, 3.
Henson, O. W. (1961), *Kans. Univ. Sci. Bull.*, **42**, 151.
Hinchcliffe, R. and Pye, A. (1968), *Int. Audiol.*, **1**, 259.
Hinchcliffe, R. and Pye, A. (1969), *J. Zool., Lond.*, **157**, 277.
Hinchcliffe, R. and Pye, A. (1976). To be published.
Hogg, I. D., Stephens, C. B. and Arnold, G. E. (1972), *Ann. Otol.*, **81**, 860.
Hoshino, T. and Paparella, M. M. (1971), *Arch. Otolaryng.*, **94**, 235.
House, H. P. and Patterson, M. E. (1964), *Trans. Amer. Acad. Ophthal. Otolaryng.*, **68**, 644.
Howell, A. B. (1932), *Proc. Amer. Acad. Arts Sci.*, **67**, 2.
Hyrtl, J. (1836), *Med. Jahrb. k. k. osterr. staates.*, **10**, 421, 457.
Hyrtl, J. (1845), *Vergleichend-anatomische Untersuchungen über das Gehörorgan des Meuschen und der Säugetiere*. Prague.
Igarashi, M. (1964), *The Inner Ear Anatomy of the Squirrel Monkey*. Florida: U.S. Naval School of Aviation Medicine, Pensacola.
Iwata, N. (1924), *Aitchi J. exp. Med. Nagoya.*, **1**, 41.
Kampen, P. N. van (1905), *Morph. Jb.*, **34**, 321.
Kelemen, G. (1966), *Acta oto-laryng. (Stockh.)*, **61**, 236.
Kelemen, G. (1968), *Acta oto-laryng. (Stockh.)*, **66**, 399.
Killian, G. (1890), *Anat. Anz.*, **5**, 226.
Kirikae, I. (1960), *The Structure and Function of the Middle Ear*. University Tokyo Press.
Klaauw, C. J. van der (1923), *Z. Anat. Entw Gesch.*, **69**, 32.
Kostanecki, C. von (1887), *Arch. mikr. Anat.*, **29**, 539.
Lay, D. M. (1972), *J. Morph.*, **138**, 41.
Legouix, J. P. and Wisner, A. (1955), *Acustica*, **5**, 208.
Littler, T. S. (1965), *The Physics of the Ear*. London: Pergamon.
Lowenstein, O. (1956), *Brit. med. Bull.*, **12**, 110.
Maran, A. G. D. (1965), *J. Laryng.*, **79**, 971.
McClain, J. A. (1939), *J. Morph.*, **64**, 211.
Muftic, M. K. and Loutfi, S. D. (1955), *Brit. med. J.*, **1**, 1010.

Ojala, L. (1957), *Acta oto-laryng.* (*Stockh.*), suppl. 133.
Peters, F. (1909), "Die Pathologie der Kiernenspaltenresiduen mit besonderer Berücksichtigung der Divertikel der Recessus pharyngeus," Thesis. Rostock.
Petter, F. (1953), *C. R. Acad. Sci.*, **237**, 848.
Pye, A. (1965), *J. Anat.*, **99**, 161.
Pye, A. (1966), *J. Morph.*, **118**, 445.
Pye, A. (1970), *J. Zool.*, London, **162**, 335.
Pye, A. (1971), *Bijdr. Dierk.*, **40**, 67.
Pye, A. (1972), *Sound*, **40**, 67.
Pye, A. and Hinchcliffe, R. (1968), *Med. biol. Ill.*, **18**, 122.
Pye, A. and Hinchcliffe, R. (1970), *J. comp. Path.*, **80**, 243.
Pye, J. D. (1960), *J. Laryng.*, **74**, 718.
Pye, J. D. (1968), *Hearing Mechanisms in Vertebrates*, p. 66 (A.V.S. de Reuck and J. Knight Eds.), Ciba Foundation Symposium. London: Churchill.
Pye, J. D., Flinn, M. and Pye, A. (1962), *Nature* (*Lond.*), **196**, 1188.
Pye, J. D. and Roberts, L. H. (1970), *Nature* (*Lond.*), **225**, 285.
Reichert, C. (1837), *Arch. Anat. Physiol. wiss. Med.*, **8**, 120.
Retzius, G. (1881), *Das Gehörorgan der Wirbeltiere*. Stockholm: Samson and Wallin.
Reysenbach de Haan, F. W. (1956), *De Ceti Auditu*. Utrecht: Schotanus and Jens.
Rhode, W. S. (1971), *J. acoust. Soc. Amer.*, **49**, 1218.

Ritter, F. N. (1971), *Laryngoscope*, **81**, 1304.
Sammut, J. J. (1967), *J. Laryng.*, **81**, 137.
Sando, I., Baker, B., Black, F. O. and Hemenway, W. G. (1972), *Arch. Otolaryng.*, **96**, 441.
Schneider, H. and Möhres, F. P. (1960), *Z. vergl. Physiol.*, **44**, 1.
Schnitzler, H-U. (1970), *Z. vergl. Physiol.*, **68**, 25.
Stupka, W. (1938), *Die Missbildungen und Anomalien der Nase und des Nasenrachenraumes*. Vienna: Springer.
Tandler, J. (1902), *Morph. Jb.*, **30**, 275.
Tonndorf, J. and Khanna, S. M. (1967), *J. acoust. Soc. Amer.*, **41**, 513.
Tumarkin, A. (1957), *J. Laryng.*, **71**, 65.
Tumarkin, A. (1968), *Hearing Mechanisms in Vetebrates*, p. 18 (A. V. S. De Reuck and J. Knight, Eds.), Ciba Foundation Symposium. London: Churchill.
Webster, D. R. (1961), *Amer. J. Anat.*, **108**, 123.
Webster, D. R. (1962), *Physiol. Zool.*, **35**, 248.
Werner, C. F. (1960), *Das Gehörorgan der Wirbeltiere und des Menschen*. Leipzig: Thieme.
Wersäll, J. (1956), *Acta oto-laryng.* (*Stockh.*), suppl. 126.
Wever, E. G. and Lawrence, M. (1954), *Physiological Acoustics*. Princeton University Press.
Wright, J. L. W. and Etholm, B. (1973), *J. Laryng.*, **87**, 281.
Wright, M. I. (1971), *The Pathology of Deafness*. Manchester University Press.

14. ULTRASTRUCTURE OF EAR IN NORMAL AND DISEASED STATES

I. FRIEDMANN

INTRODUCTION

The delicate and somewhat complicated structures of the ear are exposed to a wide range of adverse effects either from agents in the normal environment or those occurring under pathological conditions. These may cause serious disorders of the neuroepithelium of the internal ear; the middle ear may also be affected. An exact knowledge of the aetiology, mechanism and effect would provide a firmer basis for the prevention and treatment of hearing loss.

The causes have been intensively studied and range from some comparatively trivial microbiological or inflammatory conditions to neoplasms and obscure developmental factors. The investigation of the lesions requires the application of all available scientific methods and it is interesting to note how promptly most of the recently developed highly sophisticated methods have been adopted for this purpose.

Electron microscopy has been intensively used and transmission electron microscopy (TEM) has been impressively complemented by scanning electron microscopy (SEM), to be followed by field-ion microscopy, electron probe analysis and other developing methods.

Conventional transmission electron microscopy, pioneered by Engström, Iurato, Catherine Smith, Spoendlin, Wersäll and others, has contributed greatly to our knowledge of the ultrastructure of the mucosa of the middle ear and of the neuroepithelium of the internal ear in health and in disease.

Scanning electron microscopy has added new insight into the surface pattern of the mucosa of the middle ear and of the spiral organ of Corti. It has the great advantage of visualizing three dimensional features that have only

previously been seen in the reconstructions of the histologist.

Ades, Bredberg, Engström, Lim and Wersäll form, with a few others, the group of workers who have applied this new technique to considerable advantage.

Scanning electron microscopy is best suited to the study of surface topography because the process of preparation may produce artifacts. For instance, the cytoplasm is condensed and retracts so that vacuoles are formed. The nerve fibres present as hollow tubes or cylinders since the axoplasm perishes and only the myelin sheath is preserved. Such artifacts may impair the value of scanning electron microscopy but methods are bound to improve.

High-voltage electron microscopy (750 000–5 000 000 volts) is even more difficult but permits the examination of intact cells. It has not yet been used in the study of the ear.

The electron probe analyser estimates the amounts of certain elements at their site in the cell and field-ion microscopy is used to probe individual atomic particles.

It is clear that no single method can be expected to stand alone and deliver all the answers. All methods have to be used in a concerted and systematic manner aimed at the solution of the various relevant problems of cellular morphology and cellular pathology of the ear.

MIDDLE EAR

Middle Ear Mucosa

The structure and cytology of the middle ear mucosa has remained a controversial issue. A thorough understanding of its normal morphology is essential to any consideration of pathological changes (Tos and Bak-Pedersen, 1973).

The healthy middle ear lining consists of a thin layer of

fibrous tissue covered by flattened endothelium-like cells. There are areas where columnar epithelium normally occurs as on the medial wall, near the orifice of the auditory (Eustachian) tube and on the promontory. The entire epithelial lining is, essentially, of respiratory epithelial character and its true nature is revealed in pathological circumstances, as, for instance, in the experimentally infected tympanic bulla of the guinea pig, in chronic otitis media, and in the "glue ear".

Kaneko and his associates (1971) have studied the anatomical characteristics of the epithelium of the normal middle ear in the squirrel monkey which the authors considered comparable to man.

Auditory Tube

According to Lim (1972), the epithelium of the auditory tube and of the middle ear forms a mechanical defence system composed mainly of ciliated columnar cells (about 80 per cent) and of secretory cells (about 20 per cent). Other defence systems include:

The mucociliary transportation system.
The enzyme defence system.
The immunological defence mechanisms.
The phagocytic system.

Various stimuli may induce a general inflammatory reaction activating some or all these defence systems. The failure of the mucociliary transportation system causes an accumulation of the secretory products in chronic catarrhal otitis media often resulting in "glue ear".

The production of IgA and other locally produced immunoglobulins in the middle ear mucosa has been demonstrated by Bernstein and his associates (1972).

Increased amounts of gammaglobulins have been noted in middle ear effusions by Juhn and his associates (1971).

Phillips and his colleagues (1974) found increased amounts of IgE in samples of middle ear secretions in secretory otitis media.

Biopsy specimens from catarrhal otitis media patients show the surface to be covered by secretory epithelium and the underlying inflamed stroma is infiltrated by lymphocytes, plasma cells and a small number of polymorph leukocytes, macrophages and similar cells. The inference drawn from these findings is that they are the result of an enhanced activity of the defence systems involved in infections of the middle ear cleft.

Epidermoid Cholesteatoma

The cellular lining of the middle ear cavity may be replaced by stratified keratinizing squamous epithelium. This usually results in the development of an epidermoid cholesteatoma, complicating chronic and acute infections of the middle ear cleft.

The morphological characteristics and the mode of epidermal migration in the advancing front of cholesteatoma was investigated by Lim (1972) with the electron microscope. Sixty specimens from patients formed the basis of this important study. Microscopically, the matrix was formed by keratinizing squamous epithelial cells and the advancing front was recognized by the presence of the epidermic-mucosal junction. Here, the basement membrane, as seen under the electron microscope, was often displaced and was pulled down by some delicate anchoring fibres underneath the branching basal cells. This anchoring fibre system may act, according to Lim, as "contact guidance" for the epidermis migrating into the middle ear.

The basement membrane may be damaged by the underlying inflammatory granulation tissue. It is noteworthy that Lim found no evidence of metaplastic transformation and points to the presence of abundant microvilli on the surface of the epithelial cells of epidermoid cholesteatoma.

There is no evidence of keratinization in metaplastic squamous epithelium (Friedmann, 1959; Lim and Saunders, 1972). This was confirmed by Karma (1972) who, in his recent thesis, concludes that "the cholesteatomatous aetiology cannot be explained on the metaplastic basis".

According to Ordman and Gillman (1966), there are two requisites for the immigration and spread of squamous epithelium:

(i) Intradermal epithelial elements must be injured.
(ii) The injury must be kept patent (as in the tympanic membrane).

The maintenance for a short period of time, say 24 h, of even a tiny tear in the tympanic membrane would suffice to encourage epidermal invasion; its advancing edge is secreting some proteolytic enzymes capable of degrading both fibrin and denatured collagen (Gillman and Penn, 1956).

As noted by Abramson (1969), the ground substance in the perimatrix of bone-resorbing epidermoid cholesteatoma contains fewer collagen fibres owing to enhanced collagenase activity.

Epithelial-mesenchymatous interaction is an important factor in the entire process and enhanced collagenase activity may further the expansion of epidermoid cholesteatoma at the cost of the surrounding bone and other tissues of the middle ear cleft.

The interaction of the epidermis with various types of mesenchyme has been widely studied and its significance emphasized.

Moreover, more experimental studies have shown that even disintegrated epidermal cells injected into the tongue of rats, for example, would reaggregate and produce an irregular epidermal cyst (Billingham and Silvers, 1968).

Activation of displaced embryonic epithelial cell rests has been suggested in the development of the so-called congenital cholesteatomas. This theory has attracted renewed attention but is based entirely on clinical evidence and is not supported by any histological evidence. Indeed, none of the major temporal bone laboratories has ever provided illustrations of such cell rests in their abundant histological material.

The epithelial cell rests of Malassez and their role in the formation of dental cysts may have some bearing on this problem. Malassez's cell rests can easily be identified as small clumps of epithelial cells close to the surface of the dental cementum or forming a network similar to a fishnet surrounding the root (Orban, 1971). The ultrastructure of the cell of the epithelial rests was described by Valderhaug and Nylén (1966): the cells have a high nuclear cytoplasmic ratio, sparse granular endoplasmic reticulum, no neutral lipid but some glycogen. The activation of the rests was studied by Ten Cate (1972) in experimentally produced apical granulomas in monkeys. Ten Cate concluded that the activation of the cell rests involved a switch in their metabolism and the utilization of the hexose-monophosphate shunt. Furthermore "it is perhaps the unique location of the cell rests of Malassez rather than the possession of any distinctive morphologic or chemical properties which gives them their potential for cyst formation". There remain some problems which require further elucidation concerning the role of these cell rests (Ten Cate, 1972). Not all apical granulomas lead to dental cyst formation. Could they be overwhelmed by the severity of the inflammatory process? The same question might be asked in connection with the, in any case, very rare congenital cholesteatoma of the ear.

Otosclerosis

Electron microscopy has contributed greatly to our knowledge of the constituents of bone, the collagen fibres, hydroxyapatite crystals, cement and cells (Prichard, 1969).

Transmission EM (Reydon and Smith, 1968) and scanning EM have been used (Lim, 1970; Clarke and Salisbury, 1971) in the study of otosclerotic specimens and elegant pictures were obtained of the entire surface of the spongified bone.

Chevance and his associates (1972) and Causse and his associates (1972) suggest that the active destructive phase of otosclerosis (otospongiosis) could best be explained on the basis of their concept of an enzymatic disease initiated by the hydrolytic enzymes released from histiocytes and their lysosomes. Lysosomal activity may be enhanced by "active congestion". The authors refer to a variety of non-specific factors causing the apparently critical "active congestion" e.g. obesity, trauma, puberty and inflammation. It is well recognized that lysosomes are closely associated with, and indeed responsible for, cell injury and necrosis. This activity may be enhanced by various processes and it is suggested that the attacks of vertigo are caused by the release of proteolytic enzymes into the perilymph (Causse et al., 1972). Nevertheless the pathogenesis of otosclerosis remains obscure.

INTERNAL EAR

Spiral Organ of Corti

Electron microscopy has given a new impetus to the study and, indeed, reinvestigation of this all important sensory organ. A vast literature exists based on the investigations of Bredberg, Engström, Friedmann, Iurato, Kimura, Lim, Catherine Smith, Spoendlin, Wersäll and others who have established the morphological baseline, confirming some of the observations of Hensen, of Kolmer and of Retzius, whose powers of analytical observation have not been surpassed by the present generation of electron microscopists.

Scanning electron microscopy (SEM) has added some admirable pictures in three dimension and the reader is referred to the book by Ades and Engström (1972), which is an excellent review of their own SEM studies, to Thalmann (1972) and to Lim (1973).

Outer Hair Cells

In most of the mammals studied the characteristically tall, almost columnar, outer hair (sensory) cells form three rows. In man, there are often four rows in the middle turn and five rows in the apical turn (Ades and Engström). The outer cell membrane is flanked by multiple, smooth-walled cisternae which may increase both in size and numbers when exposed to adverse conditions such as toxic agents.

Outer hair cells possess an average of 120 sensory hairs, which are structureless. Occasionally, rudimentary kinocilia (basal corpuscles) occur. These are a more regular feature of these cells during embryonic development (Nakai and Hilding, 1968) or in tissue cultures of the isolated fowl otocyst (Friedmann, 1960; 1969).

Engström has confirmed the presence of rudimentary kinocilia in the outer hair cells of the middle turn in some monkeys and in a 3-month-old human fetus.

The sensory hairs are arranged in a W or M shape which is brilliantly demonstrated in SEM pictures. The base of every W points laterally and its open angle is widest at the base of the cochlea, diminishing towards the apex. The stereocilia are arranged in three or more rows of various length. The outermost hairs are the longest ones and the length of the hairs diminishes gradually in the subsequent rows. Only the outer rows are firmly attached to the tectorial membrane (Lim, 1972).

Inner Hair cells

The bulkier flask-shaped inner hair (sensory) cells also differ from the outer hair cells by having fewer sensory hairs and a simple outer cell membrane.

The distribution and significance of lysosomal enzymes in the normal internal ear has been studied by Ishii and Balogh (1966) and it was found that the activity of lysosomal enzymes was localized in the subcuticular portion of outer hair cells and in the supranuclear portion of the inner hair cells. Thalmann (1972) has reviewed the results of quantitative histochemical analysis of single hair cells by means of his elegant method.

Supporting Cells

The most essential supporting cells are the pillar cells and the phalangeal cells of Deiters. In addition to their lending mechanical support and stability to the neuro-epithelium, some of the supporting cells, such as Hensen's cells, may have some absorptive function. Most of these cells are endowed with microvilli.

Tectorial Membrane

The exact mechanism of the initial excitation of the hair cell has remained obscure in spite of a great amount of work including electron microscopy. It has been rightly assumed that the physical structures in contact with the sensory hairs and the chemical materials surrounding them must play an important role in initiating the excitation of the hair cell. A great deal seems to depend on the morphological structure of the tectorial membrane (Dohlman, 1971).

Iurato's (1967) work has now been followed by some interesting investigations by Dohlman (1971) and by Lim (1972) of the structure of the tectorial membrane under TEM and SEM. Lim has shown that there exists a fixed attachment between the tectorial membrane and the spiral organ established in two anatomical ways. First, there is a close attachment of the membrane to the hairs of the outer hair cells. Secondly, the membrane is closely attached to Hensen's stripe and to the inner phalangeal cells and some other structures. Lim's observations support Tonndorf's theory that a travelling wave moves along the basilar membrane and causes displacement of the spiral organ followed by a shearing movement against the attached tectorial membrane. It is interesting to mention that the stiff stereocilia may soften during acoustic stimulation due to an apparently reversible process of protein denaturation (Vinnikov and Titova, 1963).

The Interdental Cells of the Spiral Limbus

In view of the role they seem to play in the attachment of the tectorial membrane, the structure of the spiral limbus and, in particular, of its interdental cells is of some importance (Friedmann, 1962; Voldrich, 1967; Lim, 1970). Voldrich noted a goblet cell type secretory activity and Lim (1969 and 1970) described a cytoplasmic duct between the interdental cells and the attached tectorial membrane.

Arnold and Vosteen (1973) have confirmed that the cytoplasm of the interdental cells shows features typical of secretory type cells: an amorphous electron-dense substance is produced in the endoplasmic reticulum and is condensed in the Golgi complex into vesicles of different sizes which are to be delivered into the endolymphatic space, where they disappear among the fibres of the tectorial membrane. Neutral glycoproteins form the main component of the pinocytotic vesicles and of the tectorial membrane.

Comparison may be made with the subcommissural organ which also produces neutral glycoproteins to be discharged into the cerebrospinal fluid. A fibrous structure, Reissner's fibre, is formed which passes through the third ventricle and the Sylvian aqueduct of the mid-brain to reach the central canal. It is present in all vertebrates.

The function of all these structures is unknown but the tectorial membrane may have ion-stabilizing properties and participate in fluid exchange.

It is interesting that the subcommissural organ of the rat contains some laminated cellular inclusions similar to the crystalline laminated inclusions described in the vestibular neuroepithelium of patients operated on to cure Ménière's disease (Friedmann et al., 1963). This is also a fairly consistent finding in some neurogenic neoplasms. One can only speculate on its origin from the secretory products mentioned or on their presence in the degenerated neuroepithelial cells of the macula in Ménière's disease.

The chemical composition of the endolymph is governed by the function of the vestibular membrane and of the vascular stria. It is therefore not surprising that electron microscopy has been applied to the reinvestigation of these two structures with a view to determining their functional significance.

Vestibular (Reissner's) Membrane

The membrane consists of two layers of flat elongated cells endowed with microvilli (Friedmann, 1962). The transport of ions is of great importance and Rauch and his associates (1963) were among the first investigators to establish that, following the injection of sodium and potassium compounds into the lymphatic system of the internal ear, the vestibular membrane is engaged in the active transportation of ions from the perilymph into the endolymph.

Electron microscopic studies by Ilberg and Hinojosa and by others by means of more sophisticated methods have greatly enhanced our knowledge of these transport mechanisms. Ilberg (1968) found that a colloidal suspension of thorium dioxide crossed the vestibular membrane in both directions by a combination of diffusion and active transport. Hinojosa (1971) employed a more biological, and less toxic, electron-opaque tracer (ferritin) followed by prompt fixation of the membrane by intracochlear in vivo perfusion. Ferritin was transported in one direction only (from perilymph to endolymph).

Vascular Stria

The ultrastructure of the vascular stria was first described by Catherine Smith in 1957. Subsequent studies by Iurato, by Hinojosa and by others have confirmed that the vascular stria is composed of three types of cells: marginal, intermediate and basal cells. Smith noted the greatly increased basal cell membrane of the marginal cells, its infolding and projections, especially around the numerous capillaries of the vascular stria.

Tight junctions exist between the marginal and basal cells and Spoendlin and Balogh (1964) regard them as diffusion barriers between the interior of the vascular stria and underlying spiral ligament and the cochlear duct. Such a diffusion barrier might be an important factor in the maintenance of the composition and of the pressure of the endolymph.

Various tracer substances have been used in the study of transportation through the vascular stria. Iron dextran has been used by Yamamoto and Nakai (1964), thorium dioxide by Ilberg (1968) and, more recently, the enzyme, horse-radish peroxidase by Graham and Karnousky (1966, 1967), by Duvall and his associates (1971) and by Winther (1971). Some of the conclusions are however contradictory and much yet remains to be re-examined by means of electron microscopic techniques. Following the injection of thorium dioxide into the peri- and endo-lymphatic spaces, it freely diffuses through the spiral ligament. Interepithelial movement was, however, obstructed by tight junctions.

Studies using the horseradish-peroxidase method showed that it passed through the vessel walls of the vascular stria by vesicular transport and not through intercellular clefts or spaces (Quick and Duvall, 1970; Duvall *et al.*, 1971). The basal cells formed a barrier preventing passage into the spiral ligament as also noted by Ilberg. Horseradish peroxidase entered the intermediate cells by micro-pinocytosis. None of it was observed within the marginal or basal cells. Hinojosa (1972) injected ferritin into the peri- and endo-lymphatic spaces of the cat. There was no transport of the tracer through the cytoplasm. Ferritin, as mentioned above, passed through the vestibular membrane into the endolymph and then it could be found in the marginal cells of the vascular stria. Only after perilymphatic injection, and not after endolymphatic injection, did ferritin pass into the spiral ligament, thus partly confirming Ilberg's observations of the unity of the peri-lymphatic spaces.

Schuknecht (1974) and his colleagues have furnished further convincing evidence for a causative link between atrophy of the vascular stria and sensorineural hearing loss in older people.

Microvilli

Microvilli are an important feature of the outer cell membrane of a great variety of cells (Friedmann and Bird, 1971) and participate in the nutrition of the cell as well as in its absorptive and secretory activities. Sensory cells, supporting cells, and the cells of the vestibular membrane possess microvilli.

The surface of microvilli is covered by a layer or coat, the glycocalyx, composed of carbohydrates and muco-polysaccharides (Küttner and Geyer, 1972). This is a largely unexplored field and might yield some valuable information.

Innervation of the Spiral Organ

An outstanding discovery in this field—based on Spoendlin's investigations on the cat—is the fact that about 95 per cent of afferent cochlear neurones are associated with the inner hair cells and only about 5 per cent with the outer hair cells. There is thus a great preponderance of innervation of the inner hair cells. Catherine Smith and her associates, however, have studied the afferent and efferent innervation in the guinea pig and in the chinchilla and find an equal distribution of afferent and efferent nerve endings in the basal turn and a preponderance of afferent nerve endings in the apical turn.

Development of the Cochlea

Electron microscopic studies of the development of the internal ear *in vivo* or *in vitro* have been rewarded with considerable success.

Nakai and Hilding (1968) have studied the development of the internal ear in rabbit fetuses removed by Caesarian section at varying stages from 22 to 30 days after mating. Here they have first noted the full differentiation of the hair cells before their nerve endings had established synaptic contact with the hair cell. They believe that the stereocilia and the cuticle are developed prior to innervation.

Hilding (1969) developed this investigation further on specimens obtained from a large number of animals of different species, including the rabbit, mink, mouse and guinea-pig, at various stages of development. The first cells he was able to identify were the pillar cells, followed by the hair cells. Ubiquitous nerve fibres make their appearance influencing differentiation. The first synaptic structures, however, did not appear until later, as reported by Nakai and Hilding.

We are now in a more favourable position to study the development of nerve processes and the establishment of contact *in vitro*. Friedmann (1959, 1969) and Friedmann and Bird (1961) have been able to develop further the method first described by Fell and Robison (1929) and have achieved notable results with tissue cultures of the isolated fowl embryo otocyst. Similarly, the elegant work of Mary Faith Orr has contributed greatly to our knowledge of the development of vestibulocochlear neurones.

Van De Water and Ruben (1971; 1974) have successfully grown the mammalian (normal and Shaker mouse) embryonic internal ear in tissue culture.

The establishment of synaptic contact is of fundamental significance and in nerve tissue it plays a "spectacular" role, as suggested by Szentágothai. The formation of synaptic contact might depend on natural stimuli: their deprivation during growth may prevent their formation (Szentágothai, 1968).

The development of the acoustic ganglia, as studied by the author and Mary Faith Orr in tissue culture (1965) reaches the stage of full differentiation of the Nissl substance. Peripheral nerve tissue development depends on the cytodifferentiation of the neurones. It has been thought that the growth of nerve fibres was non-selective, depending on mechanical or other unknown, mostly chemical, forces.

Various influences may be at work in protein synthesis. Nerve growth factors contained in the embryonic extract used by us in contrast to synthetic media and other nutrient materials are transported along the nerves which are protected by the surrounding supporting cells acting as Schwann cells. The micellar orientation of the medium in which the nerves grow, and the guiding surfaces of the supporting cells, are of great assistance.

VESTIBULAR APPARATUS

Neuroepithelium

The neuroepithelial structures of the vestibular apparatus have yielded some exciting observations ever since the medical student Jan Wersäll, working in Hans Engström's team, discovered the unique chalice-type nerve endings around the Type I hair (sensory) cells of the ampullary crista (Wersäll, 1956). This and the presence of a kino-cilium have long become textbook knowledge and have engendered a great deal of research. None of this would have been possible without the aid of the modern electron microscope, although we find that Ramon y Cajal had noted the clear spaces around the cells of the macula and had suggested that they were in fact nerve endings.

Comparative anatomical studies have contributed greatly to our knowledge of the ultrastructure of the sensory epithelial structures. Attention should be drawn to the scanning EM studies of Miller (1973) on the papilla basilaris of lizards and other reptiles.

The effect of ageing on the vestibular sensory cells and nerves has been intensively studied by Engström and his colleagues (1974) who noted a marked reduction in the numbers of both sensory cells and nerve fibres by the age of 40 years.

Rosenhall and Rubin (1975) have described degenerative changes in the human vestibular neuroepithelium; in some patients these changes were associated with vertigo.

More recent observations include those of certain cells which appear to be much darker than the hair cells (Iurato, 1967), and have been disregarded as degenerated cells by some observers including the present writer. Kimura (1969), however, noted these cells as a constant feature at the base of the crista on the canal side and surrounding the lumen on the utricular side. Furthermore, almost the entire posterior wall and the marginal area of the anterior wall of the utricle are covered by these dark cells. There are no dark cells in the saccule, saccular duct, ductus reuniens or main parts of the semicircular canals. As regards their function, it has been suggested that the high potassium and low sodium content of the endolymph might be the result of the metabolic activity of the dark cells. Active pinocytosis and vacuoles on the luminal surface of these cells is indicative of water transport facilitated by the increased surface of the cells created by the delicate infolding of the outer cell membrane, the large mitochondria providing the energy required.

The function of the dark cells may be absorptive, as suggested by Dohlman (1960), or secretory (secreting the endolymph), as suggested by Kimura (1969). Dark cells of a similar pattern occur in the lining of the semicircular canals in Ménière's disease (Friedmann, unpublished).

Striola

The striola was first described by Werner in 1933, and has been studied in greater detail by Lindeman (1969). It is a central curvilinear area of the macula where the otolithic membrane is of a different consistency and structure. Lindeman has added a great amount of additional information about the distribution, size and shape of the hair cells. The highly differentiated structural organization of the vestibular sensory regions is reflected in the regional differences in reactions to ototoxic agents.

The polarization of the kinocilia, as recognized by Flock and Wersäll (1962) and by Flock (1964 and 1965), was confirmed by Lim (1971) using the scanning electron microscope. Polarization of the kinocilia is also a feature of the striola (Lindeman, 1969). In the utricle, the two oppositely polarized groups of kinocilia face each other in contrast to the condition in the saccule.

Vestibular Neurones

The vestibular neurones of higher mammals are myelinated but the myelin layer may vary from one area to another (Ballantyne and Engström, 1969). This applies to the large neurones (15–40 μm in diameter). There are also smaller neurones not unlike those of the spiral ganglion of the cochlea (Kellerhals, 1967).

Statoconia (Otoconia)

The formation and the changing structure of the statoconia in normal mammalian and non-mammalian species and in pathological conditions has been studied under the transmission and under the scanning electron microscope by Lim (1973; 1974). The statoconia are composed of an organic matrix containing a crystalline component, calcium carbonate. In the decalcified, or chelated statoconia, a well organized matrix "and even a nucleus" can be seen and the organic matrix appears to be similar to the gelatinous matrix of the statoconial (otolithic) membrane.

The vestibular dark cells play a definite role in the absorption of calcium ions from the statoconia attached to their surface (Lim, 1973).

EXPERIMENTAL PATHOLOGY

The effect of various toxic agents, including the ototoxic antibiotics and hydrocyanic (prussic) acid, and of noise trauma have been studied by a large number of authors under the electron microscope and the number is growing as new methods and microscopes are developed.

Ototoxic Drugs

It is now well recognized that the so-called ototoxic antibiotics may damage the vestibulo-cochlear (eighth) nerve. Most of these belong to the "useful but unruly family of basic streptomyces antibiotics" (Hawkins, 1959) and include streptomycin, dihydrostreptomycin, neomycin and kanamycin. Their effect on the internal ear has been widely studied with the light microscope and the relevant literature reviewed in detail (e.g. Wersäll and Hawkins, 1962; Tyberghein, 1962; Leach, 1962; Ostyn and Tyberghein, 1968).

The effect of streptomycin on the ultrastructure of the neuro-epithelium of the internal ear was investigated in the cat by Wersäll and Hawkins and in the guinea pig by Duvall and Wersäll (1964); kanamycin was investigated by Farkashidy and his associates (1963). The action of various antibiotics, including neomycin, on the ultrastructure of the sensory areas of the isolated fowl embryo otocyst in tissue culture has also been studied (Friedmann and Bird, 1961; Friedmann et al., 1966).

As has been demonstrated in animals and in tissue culture, ototoxic antibiotics are mitochondrial poisons. They also affect the outer cell membrane and, in the outer hair cells, produce a hyperplasia of the cisternae lining the outer cell membrane. This may lead to the formation of multiple concentric, or irregularly arranged, cisternae overflowing into the cell body. Similar changes have also been described after exposure to noise, leading to the formation of multiple Hensen bodies. These may play a significant role in cell metabolism or defence.

The effect of hydrocyanic (prussic) acid on neurones has clearly been demonstrated by Friedmann (1971) on tissue cultures of the isolated fowl embryo otocyst exposed to sodium cyanide. The degenerative changes observed are comparable to those observed in patients with Nigerian Ataxic Neuropathy. This condition is due to the consumption of large quantities of cassava. The root of cassava (*Manioc utilissima*) is a widely consumed food in Africa. It contains a cyanogenic compound linamarin and it has been recognized that a multiple neuropathy associated with a hearing loss might ensue in persons consuming this otherwise simple food.

Such experiments offer an opportunity to follow up in detail the gradual deterioration of the endoplasmic reticulum whose cisternae may become enormously dilated and so rupture. There occur similar lesions in other organelles, in particular in the mitochondria and in the lysosomes, and the cytoplasm of the cells of the internal ear undergoes increasing autophagic vacuolation, necrosis and ultimate lysis.

In the vestibular apparatus, attention has previously been drawn to the highly differentiated structural organization as described by Lindeman (1969). This is also reflected in regional differences in reaction to ototoxic antibiotics. Degeneration may be confined to relatively small areas, such as the striola of the macula, or the central parts of the cristae. These features have to be taken into account when assessing the results of toxicological or other experimental investigations.

Lysosome activity is affected by cell injury. In the normal spiral organ, several important lysosomal enzymes are localized in the subcuticular part of the outer hair cells and in the supranuclear zone of the inner hair cells (Ishii and Balogh, 1968). In the cochlea of animals exposed to ototoxic antibiotics, for instance kanamycin, there is a temporary increase of enzyme activity, but it soon weakens. The basal turn is first affected and the lesion ascends until all hair cells are destroyed by this ascending process.

The effect of kanamycin on the neurones of the spiral ganglion runs in a descending fashion from the apical turn downwards. Ishii and Balogh suggest that these changes occur independently of damage to the outer hair cells.

Noise

The effect of noise or any acoustic trauma is of immense industrial and public health importance. The work of Engström and Ades (1960), Beagley (1965 a, b), Ward and Duvall (1971) and Lim and Melnick (1971) is representative of the great effort spent on this important problem in which electron microscopy has played an increasingly helpful role.

Ward and Duvall (1971) carried out an extensive study, comprising four experiments, on using behavioural responses to measure thresholds of chinchillas' hearing. The four experiments were:

(1) Severe exposure (125 dB SPL for two hours).

This caused nearly total destruction of the spiral organ. The spiral prominence of the vascular stria and the spiral ligament showed little ultrastructural change. The vestibular membrane was intact and there was no evidence of healed ruptures. Lysosome activity was enhanced. The limbus and the tectorial membrane were

intact although an occasional "rolled-up" tectorial membrane, surrounded by a thin layer of cells, is mentioned. The number of spiral neurones was reduced. There was no convincing correlation between the audiometric and electron microscopic findings.

(2) Four exposures of equal energy, ranging from 123 dB SPL for half an hour to 114 dB SPL for four hours.

Here there was equally severe damage to the spiral organ for the four groups. It may be mentioned here that Eldredge and Miller (1969) observed extensive hair cell damage in a chinchilla with only a 20 dB hearing loss.

(3) The chinchillas were exposed to 114 dB SPL for three hours and allowed to recover for varying periods of time.

A moderate degree of degeneration occurred and there were enlarged or fused "ghost" stereocilia present. The laminated multiple outer cisternae were swollen and the mitochondria showed degenerative lesions. The contents of the necrotizing outer hair cells spilled over into Nuel's space and into the intercellular spaces.

(4) In this experiment, animals that had apparently recovered from a temporary threshold shift caused by a 15 min exposure to a 123 dB SPL sound nevertheless suffered widespread loss of outer hair cells. There were distorted ballooned hairs and the Hensen bodies were enlarged; there was an increase of large osmiophilic inclusion bodies. The vestibular membrane was intact.

Lim and Melnick's (1971) and Spoendlin's (1971) observations under the transmission and scanning electron microscope confirmed the extensive changes in the stereocilia ("giant stereocilia"), the cytoplasmic changes, the multiplication of the smooth cisternae and the hyperplasia of Hensen bodies. The vacuolation of the cytoplasma eventually lead to rupture of the degenerated cells. The cuticular plate was softened and lifted up, or depressed, in the process.

In earlier extensive studies by Beagley (1965), gross sensory cell damage was noted. Tight junctions along the border of the Hensen cells and Deiters cells were separated but those of the reticular lamina appeared to be more resistant.

Lindeman and Bredberg (1972) exposed various animals to the effect of high intensity pure tones and examined the spiral organ by both light and scanning electron microscopy. There was derangement of the hairs of both outer and inner hair cells and fusion of stereocilia, forming giant hairs, especially in cats exposed to low frequency sounds. The cuticular plate was often deformed and the number of microvilli increased following intense acoustic stimulation.

The effect of ultrasonic irradiation is of interest in relation to the ultrasonic treatment of Ménière's disease. Lundquist and Igarashi (1971) treated guinea pigs with ultrasound for 2·5–15 min. The observed lesions consisted of ruptured cytoplasmic membranes, absence of ribosomes and mitochondria and the formation of intracytoplasmic vacuoles 1 or 2 min after applying the ultrasound. These lesions were limited to the vestibular system and no cochlear damage occurred in these acute experiments. The nuclei remained at first unaffected but later became pyknotic and, at high intensity irradiation, the nuclear membrane was ruptured.

The prime factor in the ability of ultrasonic irradiation to cause cell damage lies in its physical properties. We have noted vacuolation and cystic degeneration of the cells lining the membranous semicircular canal following treatment of Ménière's disease by ultrasonic irradiation.

Ménière's Disease

"Many otologists have engaged in the popular pastime of trying to develop an explanation for the dramatic symptoms which characterize Ménière's disease" (Schuknecht, 1968).

The enormous distension of the endolymphatic system, together with the disruption and displacement of anatomical structures, herniation, rupture and collapse are all a matter of fact, according to Schuknecht, who believes that the paroxysmal attacks of vertigo can logically be related to ruptures of the membranous labyrinth. This leads to:

a shift of the position of the sensory receptors coupled with dumping of potassium into the perilymph which has a paralyzing effect on the vestibular nerve fibres (Dohlman, 1971).

Experimental observations have confirmed the role of endolymphatic hydrops and provided material for electron microscopic analysis (Kimura, 1967). Hydrops was usually associated with atrophy of the neuro-epithelial structures and of the vascular stria of the apical turns.

Electron microscopy showed proliferation of the smooth endoplasmic cisternae, a sensitive indicator of cell injury as has been pointed out previously.

The structure of tissues from patients suffering from Ménière's disorder have been reported by Friedmann, Cawthorne and Bird (1965). The macula of the human vestibule has a structure similar to that of other mammals and two types of sensory cells can be identified, together with chalice-type nerve endings. In these patients, crystalline inclusions and broad banded collagen fibres can be seen. Whilst almost certainly non-specific in character, they indicate some metabolic disorder.

In another specimen, obtained from a patient previously treated with ultrasonic irradiation, there were two interesting findings. First, there was extensive vacuolation of the endothelial lining of the semicircular duct and some of these vesicles seem to have burst and emptied their contents into the duct, which contained some darkly stained granular matter. Secondly, there was the presence of many well developed cilia. It has been noted that cilia may develop from a multiplicity of cells whose centrioles might have been exposed to some activating factor. This may have been the cause in the peculiar development in this case (Friedmann et al., 1972).

As in other fields of otopathology, there is ample material but little is being used in a systematic manner for clinico-pathological analysis due often to the lack of appreciation of the importance of these diseases.

NEOPLASMS OF THE EAR

Vestibulocochlear Nerve Tumours (Schwannoma of the VIIIth Nerve)

The ultrastructure of tumours of the vestibulocochlear nerve is of great interest and studies have been concluded in some detail. Cravioto and Lockwood (1969) examined under the electron microscope specimens from 50 VIIIth nerve tumours.

About 40 specimens from such tumours have been examined by us (Friedmann and Bird, unpublished observations). Two interesting structures, similar to those observed in specimens from patients operated on to cure Ménière's disease are, in fact, present. First there is a crystalline proteinaceous structure and, secondly, long strips of broad-banded fibres in the intercellular spaces with a macro-period of about 120 nanometres (nm) (1 nm = 10 Å units). They seem to be more frequent in well differentiated schwannomas, and might be called Luse bodies after the late Sarah Luse who first described these structures in VIIIth nerve tumours.

Cravioto (1968) cultured VIIIth nerve tumour tissue *in vitro*. Similar inclusions and fusiform fibres of tropocollagen developed also in these cultured tissues. There seems to be a constant relationship, both *in vivo* and *in vitro*, between the increased amounts of fibrillary material and of basement membrane material, a characteristic component of Schwann cells (Cravioto and Lockwood, 1968).

Paragangliomas (Chemodectomas)

Paragangliomas or chemodectomas are comparatively common neoplasms of the ear and occasionally cause diagnostic difficulty. Under the electron microscope, the principal epithelioid cells mingle with smaller cells and pericytes. The principal cells have a rich cytoplasm which contains large numbers of neuro-secretory granules. This may be helpful in difficult cases where the diagnosis might be uncertain under the light microscope.

Similarly, Friedmann and his associates (1963) have shown that electron microscopy may be helpful in the identification of *rhabdomyosarcomas*.

There is no doubt that further systematic study of the ultrastructure of neoplasms of the ear would yield a great amount of useful information.

REFERENCES AND FURTHER READING

Abramson, M. (1969), *Ann. Otol.*, **78**, 112.
Ades, H. W. and Engström, H. (1972), *Acta oto-laryng.*, suppl 301.
Arnold W. and Vosteen, K. H. (1973), *Acta oto-laryng.*, **75**, 192.
Ballantyne, J. and Engström, H. (1969), *J. Laryng.*, **83**, 19.
Balogh, K. and Ishii, D. (1968), *Acta oto-laryng.*, **66**, 282.
Beagley, H. A. (1965a), *Acta oto-laryng.*, **60**, 437.
Beagley, H. A. (1965b), *Acta oto-laryng.*, **60**, 429.
Bernstein, J. M., Hayes, E. R. and Ishikawa, T. (1972), *Trans. Amer. Acad. Ophth. Otolaryng.*, **76**, 1305.
Billingham, R. E. and Silvers, W. K. (1968), *Epithelial—Mesenchymatous Interactions* (Fleischmajer and Billingham, Eds.). Baltimore: Williams and Wilkins.
Bredberg, G. (1968), *Acta oto-laryng.*, suppl. 236.
Bredberg, C., Lindeman, H. H., Ades, H. W., West, R. and Engström, H. (1970), *Science*, **170**, 861.

Cajal, *see* Ramon y Cajal, S.

Causse, J., Chevance, L. G., Bel, J., Michaux, P. and Tapon, J. (1972), *Ann. Oto-laryng.*, **89**, 563.

Chevance, L. G., Causse, J., Jorgensen, M. B. and Bretlay, P. (1972), *Ann. Oto-laryng.*, **89**, 5.

Clarke, J. A. and Salisbury, A. J. (1971), *Glaxo*, **35**, 7.

Cravioto, H. (1968), *Acta neuropath.*, **12**, 116.

Cravioto, H. and Lockwood, R. (1968), *J. Ultrastruct. Res.*, **24**, 70.

Cravioto, H. and Lockwood, R. (1969), *Acta neuropath.*, **12**, 141.

Dohlman, G. F. (1960), *Neural Mechanisms of the Auditory and Vestibular Systems*, p. 258 (Rasmussen and Windle, Eds.). Springfield, Ill., U.S.A.: Chas C. Thomas.

Dohlman, G. F. (1971), *Acta oto-laryng.*, **71**, 89.

Duvall, A. J. and Quick, C. A. (1973), *Otolaryngology*, p. 506 (M. M. Paparella and D. A. Schumrick, Eds.). Philadelphia: Saunders & Co.

Duvall, A. J., Quick, C. A. and Sutherland, C. R. (1971), *Arch. Otolaryng.*, **93**, 304.

Duvall, A. J. and Wersäll, P. (1964), *Acta oto-laryng.*, **57**, 581.

Eldredge, D. H. and Miller, J. D. (1969), *Noise as a Public Health Hazard*, p. 110. ASHA Reports No. 4.

Engström, H. and Ades, H. W. (1960), *Acta oto-laryng.*, suppl. 158.

Engstrom, H., Bergström, B. and Rosenhall, U. (1974), *Arch. Otolaryng.*, **100**, 411.

Farkashidy, J., Black, R. G. and Briant, T. D. R. (1963), *Laryngoscope*, **73**, 713.

Fell, H. B. and Robinson, R. (1929), *Biochem. J.*, **23**, 767.

Flock, Å. (1964), *J. Cell Biol.*, **22**, 413.

Flock, Å. (1965), *Acta oto-laryng.*, suppl 199.

Flock, Å. and Wersäll, J. (1962), *J. Cell Biol.*, **15**, 19.

Friedmann, I. (1956), *J. clin. Path.*, **9**, 229.

Friedmann, I. (1959a), *Ann. Otol.*, **68**, 57.

Friedmann, I. (1959b), *J. biophys. biochem. Cytol.*, **5**, 263.

Friedmann, I. (1960), *Acta oto-laryng.*, **67**, 224.

Friedmann, I. (1962), *Brit. med. Bull.*, **18**, 209.

Friedmann, I. (1968), *J. Laryng.*, **82**, 185.

Friedmann, I. (1969), *Acta oto-laryng.*, **67**, 224.

Friedmann, I. (1971), *Ann. Oto-laryng.*, **80**, 390.

Friedmann, I. (1972), *Acta oto-laryng.*, **73**, 280.

Friedmann, I., Angell-James, J. and Bird, E. S. (1972), *J. Laryng.*, **86**, 807.

Friedmann, I. and Bird, E. S. (1961), *J. Path. Bact.*, **81**, 81.

Friedmann, I. and Bird, E. S. (1967), *J. Ultrastruct. Res.*, **20**, 356.

Friedmann, I. and Bird, E. S. (1971), *Laryngoscope*, **81**, 1852.

Friedmann, I. and Bird, E. S. (1972), *Acta oto-laryng.*, **73**, 280.

Friedmann, I., Cawthorne, T. and Bird, E. S. (1965), *J. Ultrastruct. Res.*, **12**, 92.

Friedmann, I., Dadswell, J. W. and Bird, E. S. (1966), *J. Path. Bact.*, **92**, 415.

Friedmann, I., Harrison, D. F. N., Tucker, W. N. and Bird, E. S. (1965), *J. clin. Path.*, **18**, 63.

Gillman, T. and Penn, J. (1956), *Med. Progr.*, **2**, suppl., p. 121.

Graham, R. C., Jr., and Karnousky, M. J. (1966), *J. Histochem. Cytochem.*, **14**, 29.

Hawkins, J. E. (1959), *Ann. Otol.*, **68**, 698.

Hilding, D. A. (1969), *Laryngoscope*, **79**, 1691.

Hinojosa, R. (1971), *Acta oto-laryng.*, suppl. 292.

Hinojosa, R. (1972), *Acta oto-laryng.*, **74**, 1.

Ilberg, Ch. (1968), *Arch. klin. exp. Ohr.-, Nas-, u. Kehlk. Heilk.*, **190**, 415.

Ilberg, Ch. and Vosteen, K. H. (1969), *Acta oto-laryng.*, **67**, 165.

Ishii, T. and Balogh, K. (1966), *Acta oto-laryng.*, **62**, 185.

Ishii, T., Ishii, D. and Balogh, K. (1968), *Acta oto-laryng.*, **65**, 449.

Iurato, S. (1967), *Submicroscopic Structure of the Ear*, p. 160. New York: Pergamon Press.

Juhn, S. K., Huff, J. S. and Paparella, M. M. (1971), *Ann. Otol.*, **80**, 347.

Kaneko, Y., Hiraide, F. and Paparella, M. M. (1971), *Acta oto-laryng.*, **72**, 85.

Karma, P. (1972), *Acta oto-laryng.*, suppl. 226.

Karnousky, M. J. (1965), *J. Cell Biol.*, **27**, 137.

Karnousky, M. J. (1967), *J. Cell Biol.*, **35**, 213.

Kellerhals, B. (1967), *Acta oto-laryng.*, suppl. 226.

Kimura, R. S. (1966), *Acta oto-laryng.*, **60**, 55.

Kimura, R. S. (1967), *Ann. Otol.*, **76**, 664.

Kimura, R. S. (1969a), *Ann. Otol.*, **78**, 1.

Kimura, R. S. (1969b), *Ann. Otol.*, **78**, 542.

Kuttner, K. and Geyer, G. (1972), *Acta oto-laryng.*, **74**, 183.

Leach, W. (1962), *J. Laryng.*, **76**, 774.

Lim, D. J. (1969), *Acta oto-laryng.*, suppl. 255.

Lim, D. J. (1970a), *Acta oto-laryng.*, **69**, 32.

Lim, D. J. (1970b), *Acta oto-laryng.*, **70**, 176.

Lim, D. J. (1970a), *Ann. Otol.*, **79**, 82.

Lim, D. J. (1970b), *Ann. Otol.*, **79**, 780.

Lim, D. J. (1970c), *J. Laryng.*, **84**, 1241.

Lim, D. J. (1971), *Arch. Otolaryng.*, **94**, 69.

Lim, D. J. (1972), *Arch. Otolaryng.*, **96**, 199.

Lim, D. J. (1973a), *Ann. Otol.*, **82**, 23.

Lim, D. J. (1973b), *Otolaryngology*, p. 527 (M. M. Paparella and D. A. Shumrick, Eds.). Philadelphia: Saunders & Co.

Lim, D. J. (1974), *Brain Behav. and Evol.*, **10**, 37.

Lim, D. J. and Melnick, W. (1971), *Arch. Otolaryng.*, **94**, 294.

Lim, D. J. and Saunders, W. H. (1972), *Ann. Otol.*, **81**, 2.

Lim, D. J., Saunders, W. H. and Abramson, M. (1969), *Ann. Otol.*, **78**, 112.

Lim, D. J., Viall, J., Birck, H. and St. Pierre, R. (1972), *Laryngoscope*, **82**, 1625.

Lindeman, H. H. (1967), *Acta oto-laryng.*, suppl. 224.

Lindeman, H. H. (1969a), *Acta oto-laryng.*, **67**, 177.

Lindeman, H. H. (1969b), *Advances in Anatomy, Embryology and Cell Biology*, p. 42.

Lindeman, H. H. and Bredberg, G. (1972), *Arch. Klin. exp. Chr.-, Nas.- u. Kehlk. Heilk.*, **203**, 1.

Lundquist, P. G., Igarashi, M., Wersäll, J., Guildford, F. R. and Wright, W. K. (1971), *Acta oto-laryng.*, **72**, 68.

Miller, M. R. (1973), *Am. J. Anat.*, **138**, 301.

Nakai, Y. and Hilding, D. (1968), *Acta oto-laryng.*, **66**, 369.

Orban, B. (1971), *Oral Histology and Embryology*, p. 194 (H. Sicher and S. N. Bhaskar, Eds.). St. Louis: C. V. Mosby & Co.

Ordman, L. J. and Gillman, T. (1966), *Arch. Surg.*, **93**, 857, 883 and 991.

Orr, M. (1965), *Exp. Cell Res.*, **40**, 68.

Ostyn, F. and Tyberghein, J. (1968), *Acta oto-laryng.*, suppl. 234.

Phillips, M. J., Manning, Helen, Knight, N. J., Abbott, A. L., and Tripp, W. G. (1974), *Lancet*, **2**, 1176.

Platt, H. (1966), *Proc. roy. Soc. Med.*, **59**, 151.

Pritchard, J. J. (1969), *The Biochemistry and Physiology of Bone*, 2nd edition, Vol. 1, p. 1 (G. H. Bourne, Ed.). London: Academic Press.

Proctor, C. A. and Proctor, B. (1967), *Arch. Otolaryng.*, **85**, 45.

Quick, C. A. and Duvall, A. J. (1970), *Laryngoscope*, **80**, 964.

Ramon y Cajal, S. (1960), *Studies on Vertebrate Neurogenesis*. Springfield, Ill., U.S.A.: Charles Thomas.

Reydon, J. L. and Smith, C. A. (1968), *Laryngoscope*, **78**, 95.

Rosenhall, U. and Rubin, W. (1975), *Acta otolaryng.*, **79**, 67.

Schätzle, W. (1971), *Histochemie des Innenohres*. Vienna: Urban and Schwartzenberg.

Schuknecht, H. F. (1968), *Oto-laryng. Clin. N. Amer.*, p. 433.

Schuknecht, H. F. (1974), *Pathology of the Ear*. Cambridge: Harvard University Press.

Smith, C. A. (1957), *Ann. Otol.*, **66**, 521.

Spoendlin, H. (1966), *Adv. Oto-rhino-laryng.*, **13**, 77.

Spoendlin, H. (1971), *Acta oto-laryng.*, **71**, 166.

Spoendlin, H. and Balogh, K. (1964), *Pract. oto-rhino-laryng.*, **26**, 159.

Szentágothai, J. (1968), *Growth of the Nervous System*, p. 3 (S. E. W. Wolstenholme and Maeve O'Connor, Eds.), Ciba Foundation Symposium. London: Churchill.

Ten Cate, A. R. (1965), *Arch. oral Biol.*, **10**, 207.

Ten Cate, A. R. (1972), *Oral Surg.*, **34**, 956.

Thalmann, R. (1972), *Acta oto-laryng.*, **73**, 160.

Tos, M. and Bak-Pedersen, K. (1973), *Acta oto-laryng.*, **75**, 55.

Tyberghein, J. (1962), *Acta oto-laryng.*, suppl. 17.

Valderhang, J. and Nylén, M. (1966), *J. Periodont. Res.*, **1**, 51.

Van De Water, T. R. and Ruben, R. J. (1974), Personal Communication.

Van De Water, T. R. and Ruben, R. J. (1971), *Acta otolaryng.*, **71**, 303.

Vinnikov, J. A. and Titova, L. K. (1963), *Int. Rev. Cytol.*, **14**, 157.

Voldrick, L. (1967), *Acta oto-laryng.*, **63**, 503.

Ward, W. D. and Duvall, A. J. (1971), *Ann. Otol.*, **80**, 881.

Werner, C. F. (1933), *Anat. entw.-gesch.*, **99**, 696.

Wersäll, P. (1956), *Acta oto-laryng.*, suppl. 126.

Wersäll, J. and Hawkins, J. E., Jr. (1962), *Acta oto-laryng.*, **54**, 1.

Winther, F. O. (1971), *Z. Zellforsch.*, **121**, 499.

Yamamoto, K. and Nakai, Y. (1964), *Ann. Otol.*, **73**, 332.

15. APPLIED MORPHOLOGY OF THE EAR

D. GARFIELD DAVIES

As a matter of convenience, this chapter is divided into five sections: Historical Introduction, Techniques and Normal Findings, Pathological Aspects, Surgical Anatomy and Conclusions. Inevitably, there will be some degree of overlap.

HISTORICAL ASPECTS

Over two thousand years ago, Hippocrates compared the tympanic membrane to a spider's web. One hundred years after Hippocrates' description, Aristotle noted the similarity in morphology of the internal ear and the shell of a snail. However, it was Galen who later first used the term labyrinth to describe the internal ear. Galen, having dissected many different animals, noted the presence of the vestibulocochlear nerve, suggested the introduction of drainage in cases of otitis and stated that "carious" bone should be removed after making an incision behind the ear. Thus, this is likely to have been the earliest record of any mastoid operation.

Andreas Vesalius was the first to describe the malleus and he likened the incus to a molar tooth. He gave an account of the vestibulocochlear nerve and was aware of the existence of the auditory tube but not of the stapes. Phillippus Ingrasia, Professor of Anatomy at Palermo, was the first to describe the stapes in the mid-sixteenth century and he also noted the tensor tympani muscle which Vesalius had imagined to be a nerve. Ingrasia was also the first to demonstrate that teeth could conduct sound (Weir, 1974). Fallopius, who followed Vesalius at Padua, noted the semicircular canals as part of the labyrinth but did not appreciate their function. He is probably best remembered for his description of the canal of the facial nerve, which he likened to an aqueduct.

Bartholomeus Eustachias (1520–74) held the Chair of Anatomy in Rome. Although the majority of his work was lost and not published until over 150 years after his death, his *Epistola de Auditus Organis* was printed in 1563 and is probably the earliest work relating exclusively to the ear. Although he was not the first to describe the auditory tube, he likened it to a "quill pen". Its function was established a hundred years later by Joseph Duverney as a channel through which the air of the tympanic cavity (tympanum) was renewed.

Thomas Willis, although best known for his description of the circle of arteries at the base of the brain, con-

tributed to the theory of hearing and made the observation that certain people hear better in a noisy environment (*paracusis*). He quoted an example of a deaf woman whose husband, when he wished to converse with his wife, always instructed a servant to beat a drum.

Joseph Duverney, Professor of Anatomy in Paris, published in 1683 the first textbook of otology not to be written in Latin. It contained many new ideas including a description of the labyrinth and he ventured a theory of hearing. Duverney, through work in the post-mortem room, suggested that the presence of pus in the ear did not necessarily signify an overflow from the brain, a belief that was still held by some, including Antonio Valsalva (1665–1723).

Valsalva applied the name "Eustachian" to the auditory tube in honour of Bartholomeus Eustachias whose works had been rediscovered about this time and he was the first to notice ankylosis of the stapes at post-mortem examination, but he did not appreciate the significance of this finding. Politzer a century later introduced the term otosclerosis. Although the manoeuvre for which Valsalva is best known was originally suggested as a means of expelling pus in the cases of otitis, it was later used for introducing air into the middle ear when the auditory tube was obstructed.

The first operation for the evacuation of pus from the mastoid is attributed to Jean Louis Petit of Paris who described three cases in 1740. James Yearsley in the early nineteenth century founded the Metropolitan Ear Institution, Piccadilly, London. Yearsley believed strongly in the inter-relationship of diseases of the ear, nose and throat and was aware of the presence of adenoids and the benefit of hearing achieved by their removal, many years before they were described by Meyer of Copenhagen (Weir, 1974). Joseph Toynbee, however, established otology on a sound pathological basis. He noted a number of cases of molluscous tumour which is now recognized as cholesteatoma, and described otosclerosis as "ankylosis of the stapes to the fenestra ovalis". William Wild pioneered otology in Ireland in the early nineteenth century and is best remembered for his incision for acute mastoiditis. However, it was not until the 1870's that von Tröltsch and Schwartze established mastoidectomy on a firm pathological basis. Stack and Zaufal, in 1889, introduced the radical mastoidectomy but during the first few years many patients were subjected to it unnecessarily. However, in

1904 Heath introduced his conservative operation, exteriorizing the disease but leaving the bridge intact.

Postoperative infection thwarted many early attempts at stapedectomy and stapes mobilization by Kessel and others in the late nineteenth century. A new approach to the treatment of otosclerosis was made in 1913 by Jenkins of King's College Hospital who described the operation to by-pass the fixed stapes by making an opening into the lateral semicircular canal. However, the initial improvement achieved in the hearing was unfortunately not sustained. Nylén in 1921 first suggested the use of the microscope in otological surgery. This early instrument was monocular and it was Holmgren who popularized the operating microscope and working with Zeiss developed the first binocular instrument for ear surgery. Littman developed an optical design for changing magnification without altering the focal length. Working with Zöllner and Wullstein in 1951, Littman developed the operating microscope as we use it today. The development of the modified radical mastoidectomy by Bondy and others led to the concept that mastoid disease could be eradicated in certain selected cases without disturbing the hearing. When sulphonamides and antibiotics were introduced they revolutionized the treatment of the acute infections of the middle ear. Complications of acute otitis media and hence acute mastoiditis and its *sequelae* then became uncommon. Otologists' thoughts then turned to reconstructive surgery and it was Zöllner (1951, 1963) and Wullstein (1952, 1956) who applied the concepts of basic physiology to surgical principles and greatly advanced the course of reconstructive surgery in chronic ear disease. In the field of otosclerosis, Julius Lampert of New York introduced his classical one-stage fenestration operation in 1938. This had an unrivalled popularity for over a decade. Rosen then revived a permeatal operation for mobilization of stapes and reported this in 1952. This delicate procedure removed the necessity of a potentially troublesome mastoid cavity but was only successful in one-third of cases. In 1958 John Shea of Memphis introduced stapedectomy and covered the oval window niche with a vein graft restoring ossicular continuity by interposing a piece of fine polyethylene tubing between the graft and the lentiform process of the incus. Modifications of this technique have evolved over the years. In the late 1950's and early 1960's William House broadened the horizons of otology by carrying out pioneering work on the microscopic removal of vestibulocochlear schwannomas ("acoustic neuromas")(House, 1964, 1968) and more recently has introduced the concept of a cochlear implant (*see* Chapter 54).

TECHNIQUES OF EXAMINATION AND NORMAL FINDINGS

The various techniques for examining the structure of the ear are shown in Fig. 1. Whilst everyone is well aware of the conventional techniques of microdissection and microscopy (light or electron), fewer people appreciate the contribution which is now made by radiography. The advent of tomography (body section radiography) has indeed produced a technique of "bloodless dissection" (Kane, 1953).

It will be convenient to discuss the techniques of examination of the ear's structure in the order in which they were evolved, i.e. dissection, microscopy (light, then electron) and, finally, radiography, particularly tomography.

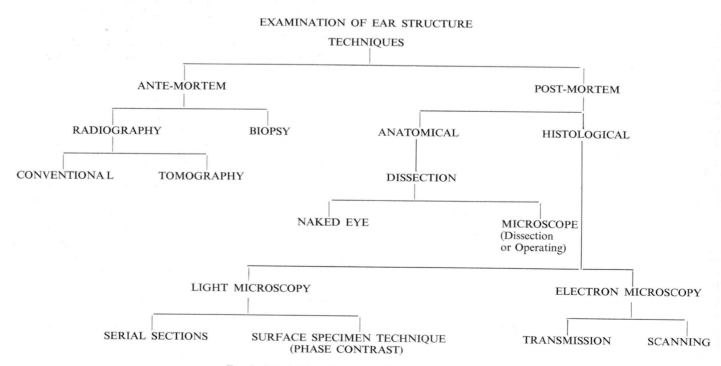

FIG. 1. Examination of structure of ear: techniques available.

Dissection

It is not feasible or practical to examine the finer points of the anatomy of the temporal bone in the cadaver. Because of rigor mortis it is virtually impossible to position the head for a complete dissection of the mastoid bone and the usual surgical instruments and operating microscopes are not readily available in the anatomy rooms of medical schools. Thus human temporal bones are removed at autopsy and can then be used for a pathological study or for anatomical dissection by the student of anatomy or the trainee otolaryngologist. The specimen that is removed contains part of the external acoustic meatus, middle ear, mastoid and petrous pyramid which are important structures for surgical dissection. The trainee otolaryngologist must dissect a minimum of ten temporal bones using modern surgical equipment and the operating microscope before he is allowed to assist in surgical operations on the ear.

A portion of the temporal bone adequate for dissection or histological study can be obtained at autopsy without any disfigurement of the head after the brain has been removed. The facial (VII) and vestibulocochlear (VIII) cranial nerve should be severed with a sharp knife rather than avulsed from the internal acoustic meatus when removing the brain. Refrigeration inhibits post-mortem autolysis very effectively and temporal bones removed from a refrigerated body as long as 15 h after death may show only a moderate post-mortem change. Where refrigeration facilities are not available injection of 10 per cent formalin into the middle ear soon after death reduces the speed of autolysis. Removal of the stapes and injection of formalin into the internal ear has been tried, but tears of the membranous labyrinth are so frequent that this method is not recommended.

A block of temporal bone can be removed with a mallet and osteotome or, more effectively, with an electrically operated vibrator saw. A smaller and neater bone plug method is also available so that the saw is centred over the arcuate eminence and the specimen encompasses all the important anatomical structures required for either surgical dissection or histological study. This also has the advantage that it does not require further trimming or redundant bone as in the "block" technique.

A temporal bone specimen may be prepared for anatomical-surgical dissection by embedding it in Plaster of Paris in a suitable container. A temporal bone holder is commercially available (Fig. 2), but various metal and plastic containers can be utilized for this purpose. In order to make the most use of the anatomical material the trainee must have first acquired a detailed knowledge of the anatomy of the temporal bone and this is assisted by examining serial sections of the microscopic anatomy.

Anatomy

Many important structures lie within the temporal bone and are crowded together in a very confined space. The problems encountered by the surgeon in this "narrow exposure" are further complicated by the variability of anatomical relationships among the structures within temporal bone. The risk to the delicate structures within the temporal bone are great in the hands of an incompetent operator because of their fragile construction and minute size. Surgical technique and the mastery of a difficult area of anatomy cannot be acquired from a book nor solely in the dissecting room. Painstaking temporal bone dissection in a fully equipped section laboratory is the only preliminary safe path to be followed through a maze of problems that can exist in temporal bone surgery. It is impossible in just a few pages to delve into the full surgical anatomy of the temporal bone but an outline will be given of the surgical landmarks and points that arise during basic

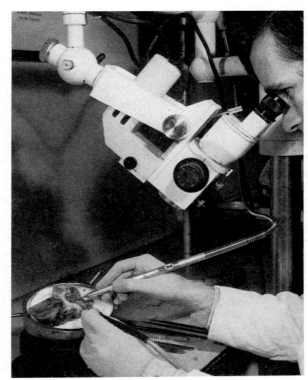

Fig. 2. Dissection of the temporal bone.

mastoid surgery. For a more detailed account the reader is referred to the book by Anson and Donaldson (1973) and the various papers by Proctor (1964, 1967, 1969).

When the lateral surface of the temporal bone is exposed by either a postaural or endaural incision, examination of the upper posterior angle of the meatus usually reveals a small spine, the *suprameatal spine* (of Henle) and about 10 mm behind this there is a shallow pitted depression perforated by numerous blood vessels known as the cribriform area (suprameatal triangle of Macewen). The suprameatal spine is frequently used as a guide to the *mastoid (tympanic) antrum* but, in poorly pneumatized mastoids or in certain anomalies, the sigmoid venous sinus, facial nerve or middle cranial fossa dura may be encountered by the surgeon who proceeds directly inwards from the spine to the antrum. The structure which in the past has kept the general surgeon out of the ear is the facial nerve and it is essential that young otologists should be thoroughly familiar with the normal course of this nerve and its abnormalities.

The posterior root of the zygomatic process of the temporal bone (zygoma) forms the outermost limit of the antero-superior osseous meatal wall. When this is traced backwards, there is a ridge, the *supramastoid crest*, which is continuous posteriorly with the *temporal line*, to which, superiorly, the temporal fascia is attached. The supramastoid crest is sometimes used as a rough guide to the level of the middle fossa dura but this landmark is variable. When the periosteum is elevated far posteriorly the mastoid emmisary vein that passes from the scalp to the sigmoid sinus will be encountered running through the mastoid foramen.

As the periosteum is raised from the superior and posterior bony meatal wall two fissures are revealed. The *squamotympanic suture* lies at the anterosuperior angle of the meatus and a band of fibrous tissue from the periosteum enters into this suture line. At about the middle of the posterior bony meatal wall a similar but weaker band of tissue from the periosteum enters the *tympanomastoid suture* between the mastoid process and the tympanic bone. The surgeon must remember that the infant has no external bony meatus and no mastoid process. Thus, the facial nerve emerges from the stylomastoid foramen onto the lateral surface behind the tympanic membrane and can be cut by the usual type of postauricular incision. Not until the second year of life does the mastoid process begin to develop and the osseous meatus begin to form by growth of the tympanic bone which was in earlier life an incomplete ring.

The anterior wall of the bony meatus forms the posterior wall of the mandibular (glenoid) fossa. Removal of the anterior bony wall does not usually cause any major incapacity to the joint as the posterior half of the mandibular fossa is filled with loose connective tissue and is non-articular. The close relationship of the mandibular joint to the meatus and tympanic membrane and their common innervation by the mandibular division of the trigeminal nerve account for the referred pain so common in diseases of the molar teeth or of the joint.

In a well pneumatized temporal bone nearly all of its middle fossa surface from the squamous part to the petrous tip may be occupied by the middle ear air spaces, including the epitympanic recess (attic), antrum and air cells, their mucoperiosteum being separated from the dura only by a thin plate of bone. Two small areas not usually pneumatized are the arcuate eminence produced by the arch of the superior semicircular canal on the middle fossa surface and the bone over the *facial (genicular) ganglion* posterior to the *hiatus for the greater petrosal nerve*. The posterior surface of the petrous portion of the temporal bone is partially occupied by the sigmoid sinus, jugular bulb, endolymphatic sac and internal acoustic meatus. Air cells may also extend close to the posterior cranial fossa dura from as far laterally as the sigmoid sinus to as far medially as the petrous tip and thus it is not surprising that most cases of bacterial meningitis (apart from meningococcal) as well as the majority of brain abscesses, are of otitic origin.

In surgical operations, the middle fossa dura elevates quite easily from the squamous part of the temporal bone and from the tegmen tympani above the epitympanic recess and the mastoid antrum and medially as far as the arcuate eminence where it is more tightly adherent. The posterior fossa dura medial to the sigmoid sinus is more adherent to the bone and therefore more vulnerable to accident when exposed. There is no dependable surface landmark for the location of the sigmoid sinus. The position of this large venous sinus in relation to the mastoid cortex and the posterior osseous meatal wall is so extremely variable that the surgeon must be ever alert for the unusually far forward or superficially lying sinus.

The roughly triangular area of the posterior fossa plate behind the mastoid antrum and bounded by the sigmoid venous sinus, superior petrosal venous sinus and bony labyrinth is called *Trautmann's triangle*. As Palva and his colleagues (1964) have pointed out, special attention has to be paid to Trautmann's triangle and the perilabyrinthine cells in cortical mastoidectomy. The solid bone medial to the antrum in the angle formed by the three semicircular canals is known as the *solid angle*. The angle between the middle fossa above and the posterior fossa and sigmoid sinus behind the antrum is called the *sinodural angle (of Citelli)*.

The *tympanic* (middle ear) cavity, fully developed and of approximately adult size at birth, includes the mesotympanum just medial to the tympanic membrane, the epitympanic recess (epitympanum or attic) above the tympanic part of the facial nerve canal, the hypotympanum below the lower edge of the tympanic sulcus and the mastoid antrum lying behind the epitympanic recess. The aditus to the mastoid antrum is the opening from the recess to the antrum. The middle ear contains the ossicular chain with its ligaments and the tendons of the tensor tympani and stapedius muscles. Along with the chorda tympani nerve, these structures may be considered as the "viscera" of the tympanic cavity.

To understand the structure of the *tympanic cavity* (tympanum), and especially the variations in configuration of its posterior wall (Fig. 3), it is essential to bear in mind its development. This is important for an appreciation of the various subdivisions of the tympanic cavity which may be responsible for the loculation of disease, or its persistence in spite of surgical treatment, due to continuing infective foci in recesses of the cavity.

The general aspects of aural organogenesis are discussed in Chapter 12. In the development of the tympanic cavity, the first pharyngeal pouch splits into four separate compartments, which Hammar (1902) termed the anterior, medial, superior and posterior sacs. The *anterior sac*, according to Proctor's (1964) interpretation, extends anteriorly to the tendon of tensor tympani to form the *anterior recess* of *the tympanic membrane (anterior pouch of von Tröltsch)*. This recess is a cul-de-sac, open inferiorly, which lies anterior to the handle of the malleus. Laterally, the recess is bounded by the tympanic membrane. Medially, it is bounded by the anterior mallear fold which is a reflection of the mucous membrane over the anterior part of the chorda tympani nerve, the anterior process and the anterior ligament of the malleus. This ligament extends from the neck of the malleus to the anterior wall of the

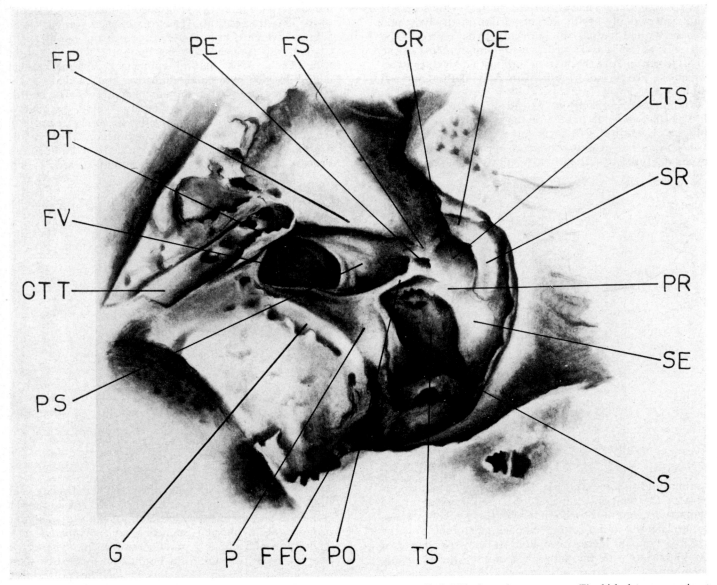

FIG. 3. View of posterior tympanus and medial wall of tympanum showing the fenestra vestibuli (FV) above the promontory (P) which shows a prominent groove (G) for the tympanic branch (Jacobson's nerve) of the glossopharyngeal nerve. The canal for the tensor tympani (CTT) together with the processus trochleariformis (PT) is seen superior to the promontory. The fossula for the fenestra cochleae (FFC) lies postero-inferior to the promontory. The facial prominence (FP) lies above the posterior tympanic sinus. A ponticulus (PO) separates a large posterior tympanic sinus (PS) above from the principal tympanic sinus (TS) below. The pyramidal eminence (PE) is short and is seen below the facial sinus (FS). The pyramidal (PR), styloid (SR) and chordal (CR) ridges connect the pyramidal, styloid (SE) and chordal (CE) eminences to surround the lateral tympanic sinus (LTS). The support (subiculum) of the promontory (S) extends from the styloid prominence to the posterior lip of the fossula fenestrae cochleae (after Proctor, 1969).

tympanic cavity, with some of its fibres being prolonged through the *petrotympanic (Glaserian) fissure* to reach the spine of the sphenoid. On occasion, an elongated anterior process of the malleus (Fig. 4) may itself extend into the fissure (Davies, 1968b). This may be related to the morphological findings in some species of bats (*see* Chapter 13). The anterior mallear ligament together with these prolongations in the sphenomandibular ligament is held to be the persistence of the sheath of the intermediate part of the ventral (*Meckel's*) cartilage of the first branchial arch.

The *medial sac* forms the epitympanic recess. In more detail, this sac splits up into three saccules. The *anterior*

saccule forms the anterior compartment of the epitympanic recess. The *medial saccule* forms the superior incudal space by growth over the superior extremities of the malleus and incus as far as the *posterior ligament* of the *incus* (which connects the short process of the incus to the *fossa incudis*), and to a *lateral incudal fold*. This medial saccule sends an offshoot forward between the lateral incudal fold and the lateral ligament of the malleus (a curved triangular band passing from the posterior border of the *tympanic incisure** and the head of the malleus) to form the *superior recess* of

---

* The tympanic incisure (*notch of Rivinus*) is the superior deficiency in the tympanic ring (anulus tympanicus). It forms the superior attachment of the flaccid portion (*pars flaccida*) of the tympanic membrane.

the *tympanic membrane* (*Prussak's space*). This recess is bounded medially by the flaccid portion of the tympanic membrane and laterally by the neck of the malleus. The *posterior saccule* passes medial to the long process of the incus to pneumatize that part of the mastoid air cell system which is derived from the petrous part of the temporal bone.

Hammar's *superior sac* extends posteriorly in the interval between the handle of the malleus and the long process of the incus to form the *posterior recess of the tympanic membrane* (*posterior pouch of von Tröltsch*), before extending further posteriorly to pneumatize that portion of

muscle (*see* Chapter 18), is situated immediately posterior to the fenestra vestibuli. The apex of the pyramid has an aperture which transmits the tendon of the muscle. The cavity of this eminence may be continuous with that of the facial canal. The chordal eminence (prominence) lies lateral to the pyramidal eminence and medial to the posterior border of the tympanic membrane. The chorda tympani nerve enters the tympanic cavity through a foramen (*apertura tympania canaliculi chordae tympani* or *iter chordae posterioris*) in the eminence. The styloid prominence corresponds to the root of the styloid process. Proctor points out that three ridges may be seen to link

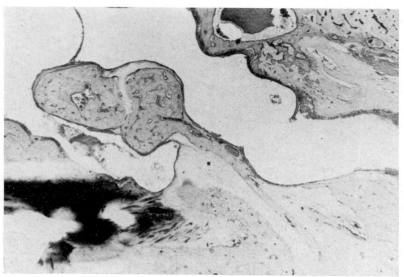

FIG. 4. Ossified anterior ligament of malleus extending into the petrotympanic fissure.

the mastoid process which is derived from the squamous part of the temporal bone. The posterior recess of the tympanic membrane is bounded by the tympanic membrane laterally and a fold of mucous membrane over the chorda tympani nerve medially. It may or may not communicate with the superior recess of the tympanic membrane. The demarcation between the superior sac and the posterior saccule of the medial sac may persist and be evident in the adult as the *petrosquamosal lamina* (*Koerner's septum*). This is a bony partition in the mastoid antrum and air cells.

The *posterior sac* forms the *fossula fenestrae cochleae* (round window niche), the *tympanic sinus*† and the greater part of the *fossula fenestrae vestibuli* (oval window niche). It may also form the *posterior tympanic sinus*.

These sinuses, i.e. depressions, of the posterior part of the tympanic cavity are formed because of the impingement of these primitive pouches (sacs and saccules) on to the remnants of the upper portion of the second branchial arch (*styloid complex*). These remnants ossify to form three permanent projections, i.e. the *pyramidal eminence*, the *chordal eminence* and the *styloid prominence* (Fig. 3). The pyramidal eminence, which contains the stapedius

these three posterior tympanic wall eminences; he suggests that these be termed the *chordal ridge* (chordal eminence to pyramidal eminence), *styloid ridge* (styloid prominence to chordal eminence) and *pyramidal ridge* (styloid prominence to pyramidal eminence). The *lateral tympanic sinus* lies within the boundaries formed by these eminences and ridges. The *tympanic sinus* lies posterior to the promontory and medial to the styloid complex. Inferiorly it is limited by the *support of the promontory* (*subiculum promontorii*), a bony ridge which extends from the styloid prominence to the posterior lip of the fossula fenestrae cochleae. Superiorly, this sinus is limited by the *facial prominence* (prominent bone around the facial canal as the latter crosses the medial wall of the tympanic cavity and turns downward along the mastoid wall). The ampulla of the posterior semicircular canal lies medial to the sinus. Sometimes, a bony ridge (*ponticulus*) extends from the pyramidal eminence to the promontory, so transecting the tympanic sinus. In this case, the upper part is termed the *posterior tympanic sinus*.

The depression in the posterior tympanic wall lying between the styloid complex and the upper descending portion of the facial canal is termed the *facial sinus* (*facial* or *suprapyramidal recess*), or *antrum threshold angle*. Superiorly, it is limited by the *fossa incudis* (this is a depression in the lower part of the posterior wall of the

---

† Since two other tympanic sinuses have been described and named, it might be advisable to further specify this sinus by the prefix "principal" or "inferior".

epitympanic recess; it contains the short process of the incus connected to the fossa by the *posterior ligament* of the incus) (Fig. 5). This sinus is formed during the development of the canal, constituting a cul-de-sac between the cartilaginous element of the second branchial arch (*Reichert's cartilage*) and the adjacent membrane bone. This sinus is invariably involved in chronic middle ear infections and is frequently responsible for continuing otorrhoea following surgical treatment of the diesase. Its importance in this respect has been emphasized by Smyth and his associates (1969), Sheehy (1970) and others.

deposits, exudates will accumulate above the level of obstruction.

The otologist can operate safely only if he is aware of the complexity of the relationship of the *facial nerve* to its bony canal, the pattern of its blood supply, and the progress of developmental changes whose arrest or distortion results in anomalies. Chapter 30 is devoted to the facial nerve and its disorders. However, some of the more important aspects of its anatomy which are relevant to ear surgery must be mentioned here. The facial nerve surpasses all other nerves in the human body in respect

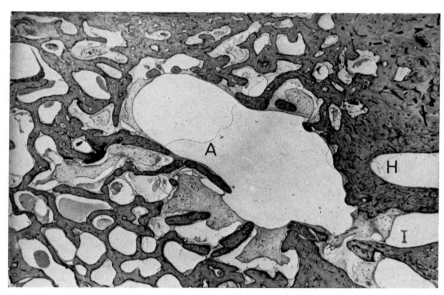

FIG. 5. Relationship of the mastoid antrum (A) to the lateral semicircular canal (H) and the short process of incus in its fossa incudis (I).

Mucosal folds are clearly seen in the fresh temporal bone and they disappear or disintegrate rapidly if the bones are permitted to dry or are immersed in fixative solutions. They may be considered as "the mesenteries" of the tympanic cavity (Proctor, 1964). They are important in the blood supply of the ossicles (Yates, 1936; Hamberger *et al.*, 1963). These folds and their remnants are often considered as residues of inflammations or adhesions but it must be stressed that they occur in fairly constant anatomical positions which can be explained by the embryological development of the middle ear. Subdivision of the tympanic cavity into compartments ("trabeculation") is a notable feature of some other mammals (*see* Chapter 13). Thus the mucosal or muco-osseous partitions in man which are variable in the degree of development (Sammut, 1967) may represent a persistence of an atavistic trait. This anatomical variability is also most certainly a factor, perhaps an appreciable one, in the persistence of middle ear infection in man, with or without medical or surgical treatment. By dividing the middle ear into various spaces, the folds may limit disease for a considerable time to one or more compartments. If the small openings from one compartment or middle ear space to another is blocked by swollen mucosa, cholesteatoma or tympanosclerotic

of the length and tortuosity of its intraosseous course, but the student of temporal bone anatomy who learns the nerve's route and variation and who approaches the nerve with respect, and not fear, realizes that the facial nerve is a friend and a useful guide.

The facial nerve having originated in the facial nucleus and having left the brain stem at the inferior border of the pons in the recess between the olive and the inferior cerebellar peduncle, enters the porus of the internal acoustic meatus accompanied by the nervus intermedius (sensory division of the facial nerve), the cochlear and vestibular divisions of the vestibulocochlear nerve together with the internal auditory artery and vein. As it traverses the relatively short internal acoustic meatus, it lies in an anterosuperior position remaining essentially anterior to the superior vestibular nerve and superior to the cochlear nerve. As it leaves the internal acoustic meatus, the nerve is superior to the transverse crest and anterior to a vertical bar of bone known as House's bar which provides a useful guide to identification of the facial nerve in surgical approaches to the internal acoustic meatus in the removal of vestibulocochlear nerve tumours. As the facial nerve leaves the internal meatus, it curves gradually inferiorly around the basal turn of the cochlea. It then expands at the genicular ganglion and proceeds abruptly in a posterior route. The greater petrosal nerve leaves the facial nerve at the anterior edge of the genicular ganglion and proceeds through the hiatus for the greater petrosal nerve. As the facial nerve proceeds in its horizontal portion it is first overlapped by the *trochleariform process* (*formerly, cochleariform*), just slightly in a superoinferior direction and by the full width of the trochleariform process in an anteroposterior direction. The facial nerve is particularly liable to damage in this horizontal segment (Fig. 6). It is important to remember this relationship in cases in which the trochleariform process is removed so that a fracture is

from the facial nerve. It is very important that the cells be cleared since residual disease is frequently found in this area in revision mastoid surgery. After leaving the facial nerve, the chorda tympani runs in its own canal (canaliculus chordae tympani) to the posterior aperture (iter chordae posterioris) from which it escapes and passes lateral to the long process of the incus and medial to the handle of the malleus towards the anterior canaliculus at the end of the petrotympanic fissure.

The facial nerve itself continues to the stylomastoid foramen passing lateral to the retrofacial cells. The bony canal widens considerably at the stylomastoid foramen,

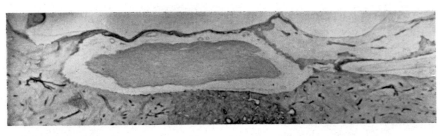

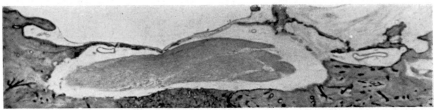

FIG. 6. Normal facial nerve covered by its thin bony wall in the horizontal segment (upper figure). The lower figure illustrates the in-fracture caused by manipulations during stapes surgery and an ensuing neuropraxia.

not rotating into the facial nerve. Through most of its horizontal course the facial nerve forms the superior boundary of the fossula fenestrae vestibuli. Leaving the fossula the facial nerve turns more gently to its vertical portion related at first to the prominence of the lateral semicircular canal to which the nerve is anterior and inferior. It then passes lateral to the tympanic sinus and to the stapedius muscle.

At this stage, the nerve is, however, medial and inferior to the short process of the incus. When the short process is viewed end on, an important triangular relationship exists between the tip of the short process, the facial nerve and the lateral semicircular canal (Donaldson and Anson, 1965). The authors term this the *triple S* (seventh nerve, semicircular canal, short process of incus) *triangle*. The median distance from the tip of the short process of the incus to the nearest part of the lateral semicircular canal, which lies medially, is given as 1·25 mm (range 0·9–1·7 mm). The median distance of the short process to the facial nerve is 2·4 mm (range 1·4–3·0 mm). The median distance from the lateral canal to the facial nerve is 1·8 mm (range 1·0–2·3 mm). This triangular relationship provides the easiest landmark for the identification of the facial nerve. The facial sinus cells are located lateral to the facial nerve and inferior to the tip of the short process of the incus and may extend as far inferiorly as the exit of the chorda tympani

accounting for the fact that some surgeons prefer to identify the nerve within the foramen.

Dehiscences (gaps) in the facial nerve (fallopian) canal are the result of arrested development in the bony wall. Exposure of the nerve at these points increases the possibility of injury to the nerve from the pathological or surgical point of view. The most common site of dehiscence is in the region of the fenestra vestibuli. Dehiscences can also be present (in order of decreasing frequency) at the processus trochleariformis, the vertical segment and lateral to the *geniculum*.*

Dehiscences in the region of the fenestra vestibuli are most often limited to one wall of the facial canal, and, in order of frequency, the nerve may be exposed on its anterior, lateral and medial aspect. Occasionally, a marked protrusion of the facial nerve from a gap in the bony wall may result in it overhanging the fenestra (Fig. 7). The facial nerve does not always follow the course described above and Fowler (1961) collected from the literature, and made comparative drawings of, the best known exceptions to the normal course of the nerve. The nerve may be found anywhere in the temporal bone since it has been located in the anterior osseous wall of the

* This is not to be confused with the *genu* of the facial nerve which is the intrapontine segment of the nerve which curves forward and laterally around the upper pole of the abducent nucleus.

external acoustic meatus and as far back as the region of the sigmoid sinus. The facial nerve has been described as lying below the fenestra vestibuli and, on occasions, being bifid. Splitting of the vertical segment of the nerve into two or three branches each in a separate bony canal has also been recorded. It was not until the introduction of the microscope for stapes surgery that it was realized how often dehiscences occur in the facial canal, especially in the horizontal (tympanic) segment.

(j) Clearing in Oil of Origanum.

(k) Mounting on glass slides.

The sections are usually cut at a thickness of 20 μm resulting in about 400 sections from each temporal bone. Three representative sectioning planes exist for the investigation of the temporal bone and the internal ear:

(1) A horizontal section—parallel to the superior surface of petrous portion of the temporal bone.

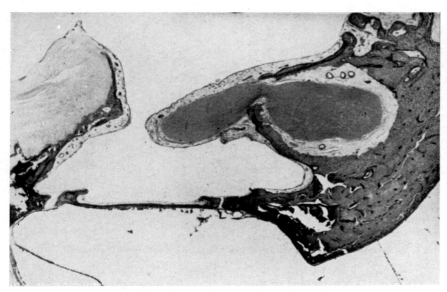

FIG. 7. Dehiscence in the facial canal so that nerve protrudes and overhangs the fenestra vestibuli

Light Microscopy

The internal ear end organs are structurally fragile with the membranous labyrinth weakly supported within the bony labyrinth. The technique of histological preparation must be directed towards preserving the anatomical relationships of the internal ear structures and also minimizing post-mortem changes. The densely ossified petrous portion of the temporal bone must be decalcified and the internal ear spaces uniformly infiltrated with celloidin, all the while maintaining the histological integrity of the membranous labyrinth. Temporal bone laboratory technicians are trained to handle the specimens in a very careful manner and ideally each technician should be responsible for each individual temporal bone specimen from the beginning to the very end of the procedure. The steps in the histological examination are:

(a) Fixation with a Heidenhain's (1916) Susa solution.

(b) Decalcification using trichloroacetic acid solution.

(c) Washing and neutralization using sodium sulfate solution.

(d) Dehydration using a series of alcohols of increasing concentration.

(e) Embedding in celloidin.

(f) Hardening and mounting.

(g) Cutting the temporal bone on a sliding microtome.

(h) Staining with haematoxylin and eosin.

(i) Counterstaining in eosin.

(2) Vertical—perpendicular to the long axis of the petrous portion (frequently called "vertical section").

(3) Vertical—parallel to the long axis of the petrous portion.

The most frequently used planes for study are the horizontal and the vertical sections.

In 1921, Stacy Guild described a technique for graphic reconstruction of the spiral organ (of Corti) and this resulted in a significant improvement in the methods for studying the pathology of the internal ear by spatially orientating structures within the cochlea; it is an essential and simple method for interpreting pathological changes. The student of pathology should acquaint himself with the steps in graphic reconstruction by studying routine histological horizontal preparations of the cochlea cut at 20 μm with every fifth section mounted and stained for study. The sections should be numbered consecutively, beginning at the superior aspect of the cochlea.

The trainee in the speciality should study both horizontal and vertical sections in order to appreciate the anatomy and, later, pathology of this region. Both the horizontal and the vertical planes have advantages and disadvantages and these will be outlined.

Horizontal Plane

The *advantages* of horizontal sections (Fig. 8) are:

(1) The posterior and anterior margins of the fenestra vestibuli (oval window) appear together in the same

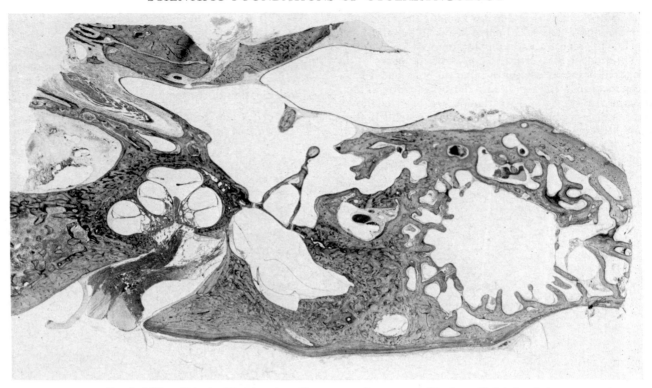

FIG. 8. Mid-modiolar horizontal section of human ear. (By courtesy of Professor H. Schuknecht.)

slide and the stapes base (footplate) is presented so that an area of fixation by otosclerosis is easily appreciated.

(2) The stapes base, macula of the saccule and the major part of the cochlea appear in the same section, also a more thorough study of the saccular macula is permitted.

(3) More accurate hair cell counts are permitted in the upper, middle and basal turn of the cochlea which is important if the temporal bone has been obtained from a patient who has had a history of stimulation hearing loss, i.e. due to noise or head injury.

(4) The internal acoustic meatus and major cochlear and vestibular structures appear in the same section.

(5) The upper portion of the utricular macula and the crista of the lateral semicircular canal as well as the basal turn of the cochlea appear in the same section (this is of great help in cases that are thought to have ototoxic lesions).

(6) The relationship between the tympanic cavity, mastoid cells, auditory tube, carotid canal and apex of the petrous pyramid can be investigated in one slide.

(7) Horizontal sections are fewer in number than vertical sections and less time and materials are utilized in sectioning, staining and mounting.

However, the *disadvantages* of horizontal sections are:

(1) It is difficult to investigate the major horizontal portion of the utricular macula and the superior and posterior semicircular cristae, as these end organs will be sectioned more or less tangentially.

(2) The vertical relationship of the tympanic cavity to the tegmen tympani and jugular fossa cannot be examined.

Vertical Plane

The *advantages* of vertical sections are:

(1) It is possible to investigate the vertical relationship of the middle ear cavity to the tegmen tympani and to the jugular fossa in cases of inflammatory disease and tumours.

(2) The fenestrae vestibuli and cochleae (oval and round windows) appear together in vertical sections.

(3) The major part of the utricular macula is sectioned so that it can be adequately studied.

The *disadvantages* of vertical sections are:

(1) The major part of the cochlea, except for the vestibular caecum and the vestibular apparatus will not appear in the same section.

(2) The saccular macula will be cut tangentially making investigation of this end organ difficult.

(3) The vertical series requires almost twice as many slides as the horizontal series and is more time consuming and more expensive in preparation.

Normal Histology

The normal histology of the *middle ear* cleft is adequately described in current texts, and it can be easily studied by the sectioning technique just described. It will therefore not be discussed further here. The histology of the *internal ear*, however, is more intricate and more subject to *post-mortem* change. Further discussion will therefore be required of this topic; it is impossible in just a few pages to outline the histology of the internal ear but some of the more important points will be mentioned here.

Sense Organs

Auditory: The receptor organ (end-organ) of hearing is the spiral organ (of Corti) and it consists of a continuous collection of hair cells and supporting elements extending the length of the cochlea ($2\frac{1}{2}$ turns in man, extending 30–33 mm). The sense organ is contained in the cochlear duct (endolymphatic space or scala media). It has cortilymph (possibly identical with perilymph) within it in the tunnel of Corti (inner tunnel), outer tunnel and space of Nuel. The nerve fibre terminations are based in this cortilymph. There are 3–4 rows of outer hair cells but the inner hair cells form a single row. Each hair cell has about 140 cilia protruding from its top on to the rather stiff tectorial membrane. The cilia are arranged in an orderly fashion but have one more obvious cilium, the kinocilium, on the spiral ligament side of all the stereocilia. This polarity in the arrangement of cilia has functional significance in that electrical stimulation occurs in the hair cell when the stereocilia are bent towards the kinocilium. There are structural and nerve terminal differences between the inner and outer hair cells which suggest functional differences. The outer hair cells are generally more sensitive than the inner hair cells; their threshold stimulus is less than that of the inner hair cells and they are more susceptible to trauma—for example, acoustic trauma and noxious agents such as ototoxic drugs and anoxia. The hair cells have been classified into types I and II, mainly on the basis of nerve endings connecting them. These hair cells are surrounded by supporting elements (Deiters' cells and pillar cells) which apparently play more than just a supporting role in the metabolism of the spiral organ.

Schuknecht (1953) established in both human temporal bone material and by experimental animal work that the high frequencies localize at the most basal end of the cochlea, low frequencies at the apex and intermediate frequencies in orderly fashion between these ends.

Descriptions of surface architecture of the internal ear employing the scanning electron microscope can be found in the accounts by Lim (1969, 1971).

The mechanism of the auditory apparatus is discussed in Chapter 16.

Vestibular: The vestibular sense organs are also located within the endolymphatic space. They are of two types:

(1) The ampullary crests (crista) located in the ampulla of each of the three semicircular ducts.
(2) The maculae of the utricle and of the saccule.

The ampullary crests being located in the ampullary ends of the semicircular ducts thus represent the three planes of rotation. Each crest is composed of supporting cells and hair cells. These hair cells also have cilia, including a kinocilium and many stereocilia. These cilia are embedded in a gelatinous cupula which extends up the roof of the ampulla. These cilia are also orientated in a definite way

so that the bending of the cilia towards the kinocilium by movement of endolymph provides the natural stimulus. In the vertical canals this direction is away from the ampullated end of the canal (ampullo-fugal); in the horizontal canal the direction is towards the ampulla (ampullo-petal). This is reflected in Ewald's second law.

The maculae of the utricle and the saccule are flat sense organs lying in horizontal and vertical planes within their respective endolymphatic compartments. They are gravity receptors. As in other parts of the labyrinth, these hair cells have a kinocilium and stereocilia all of which are embedded in a gelatinous blanket (otolithic membrane), which contains otoliths (otoconia). These consist of calcium carbonate crystals with a specific gravity of 2·7. The hair cells appear to arrange themselves in groups according to the orientations of the cilia. These groups have their polarity in many different directions on the macula. It is well known that the utricular macula will respond to stimulation in any rectilinear direction. Stimulation of these position receptors takes place when the otoliths are moved in one direction or the other by gravity after the macula has been tilted or by inertia in the case of sudden movement in a linear direction. The physiology of the labyrinth is discussed in Chapters 26 and 27.

Innervation

The labyrinth is supplied by the vestibulocochlear (VIII) cranial nerve, formerly termed the stato-acoustic nerve. It is divided into a cochlear and a vestibular component which consist of sensory neurones forming the afferent nerve supply of the sense organs and the end organs are also reciprocally innervated by a system of efferent nerve fibres whose cell bodies are located in the central nervous system.

Afferent Nerves: The sensory neurones of the vestibulocochlear nerve are true bipolar neurones derived from the neural crest cells. In the human, the cochlear nerve contains about 40 000 myelinated neurones and the vestibular nerve about 18 000. The cells of the cochlear neurones are located in the spiral ganglion which is lodged in the spiral (Rosenthal's) canal of the modiolus. The dendrites of these cells extend out through the habenulae perforata (canaliculi of the osseous spiral lamina), where they lose their myelin sheaths, to enter the spiral organ where they terminate on both inner and outer hair cells. The dendrites that innervate the inner hair cells do so in a very straightforward manner, that is each dendrite ends on one or two cells by means of large calyx-like endings. The innervation of the outer hair cells is more diffuse and complex for unmyelinated extensions of these dendrites cross the tunnel of Corti to assume a spiral course between the supporting Deiters' cells and the outer hair cells and terminate on many hair cells over an extensive length of the basilar membrane. The axons of the cochlear neurones form the cochlear nerve and terminate in the cochlear nucleus in a very orderly arrangement of frequency orientated fibres.

The vestibular nerve cells are found in the vestibular

(Scarpa's) ganglion which lies within the internal acoustic meatus. The nerve splits on the distal (sometimes proximal) side of the ganglion to form the superior, inferior and posterior branches of the nerve. The superior branch supplies the ampullary crests of the superior and lateral ducts, the utricular macula and a small portion of the saccular macula. The inferior division supplies the main portion of the saccular macula and the posterior branch runs through the foramen singulare to supply the ampullary crest of the posterior semicircular duct. The precise neural ending on the hair cells of the vestibular neural epithelium has not been studied so extensively as the cochlear hair cells but in general terms there are two modes of afferent termination giving rise to the type I and type II hair cell situations similar to those occurring on the cochlear cells.

The axons of the vestibular neurones enter the medulla to terminate in the vestibular nuclei (superior, medial, lateral and descending) or in the cerebellum, passing along the inferior cerebellar peduncle.

Efferent Nerves: A system of efferent nerve fibres has been clearly demonstrated in detail in all end organs of the labyrinth. The efferent cochlear system has been extensively studied. The efferent olivo-cochlear neurone to the spiral organ has its cell body in the superior olivary complex of the medulla and actually represents the final link in the chain of two or three efferent or descending neurones originating in the auditory cortex and paralleling the classical afferent auditory pathway down to the hind brain area. The olivo-cochlear bundle to one cochlea has both homolateral and contralateral limbs. Although the efferent system is small numerically (about 500–600 fibres), these fibres ramify greatly within the cochlea and actually form as many, if not more, nerve terminals on the hair cells in the spiral organ as the afferents. The efferents end directly on the outer hair cells adjacent to the afferent endings (type II hair cell) after crossing the tunnel spaces as bare fibres. The efferent nerve endings are larger than the afferent and have many small vesicles similar to those in the presynaptic terminals elsewhere in the central nervous system. Very few, if any, efferents end on the inner hair cells but some appear to make contact with the afferent nerve fibres or endings associated with the inner hair cells (type I hair cells). Electrophysiologically, the efferent cochlear system seems to produce an inhibition of the action potential in the afferent nerve fibres at the neurone-hair cell junction. High acetylcholinesterase activity has been found to be one of the biochemical characteristics of this efferent system.

Efferent neurones to all parts of the vestibular labyrinth have also been clearly demonstrated. They appear to be about as numerous as cochlear efferent neurones and probably end as vesiculated endings on the vestibular neurone terminals (type I) or on the vestibular hair cells directly (type II). Although the vestibular efferent system is also associated with high acetylcholinesterase activity, its physiological role has not been as clearly elucidated as that of the efferent cochlear system. It is likely that its function here is also of an inhibitory nature and may play an important part in the characteristic adaptation or habituation that the vestibular system displays.

Surface Specimen Technique

A surface preparation technique using osmic acid fixed temporal bones recently employed in the light microscopic investigation of the internal ear has added a new dimension to otological research. The best results were initially derived from animal and from fetal human specimens but with constantly improving techniques similar methods are being applied to adult specimens. The guinea pig is the easiest of all the smaller animals to work with and it is enlightening for the trainee otolaryngologist to carry out the surface preparations on this animal; good specimens for study can be obtained routinely once the technique has been mastered. Damage to a specimen may occur but this is a matter of individual skill and care. The greatest problem with the human material is that of obtaining sufficiently fresh specimens. Descriptions of the technique and the results obtained can be found in the accounts by Engström and his colleagues (1966) and by Johnsson and Hawkins (1967a, b). However, these studies are also limited by the resolving power of the light microscope.

Electronmicroscopy

The development of phase microscopy set the limit of resolution of the light microscope. This resolution is about $0\cdot2\ \mu m$, a limit imposed by the wavelength of light, precluding adequate resolution at magnifications over 1 100 times. With increasing knowledge it became evident that there were definitive structures smaller than those visualized by light microscopy and many of these features have been investigated by the electron microscope which utilizes a beam of electrons instead of light waves. The first practical electron microscope appeared over 30 years ago and soon came into use in metallurgy. The electron microscope allows a resolution in the order of 100–200 pm (1–2 Å) and consequently magnification of over a million times. Electrons pass through thin sections of a specimen and through systems of magnetic lenses and are finally made to impinge upon a fluorescent screen or a photographic plate. This electron beam is influenced to such an extent by its environment that it must be produced in a vacuum. Sections must be extremely thin to allow clear penetration without scattering of the electrons. Producing sufficiently thin sections (25 nm) without folds is the chief technical stumbling block of biological electron microscopy. Electron microscopy has made new demands on fixation and preparation of specimens, for post-mortem changes can be very misleading.

Distinguishing the normal from the abnormal is difficult. Only by many hours of patient scanning with the electron microscope will ability be acquired. The reader is referred to individual publications and electron microscopic texts on the internal ear for more detailed descriptions (Engström *et al.*, 1966; Iurato, 1967; Spoendlin, 1969).

The electron microscope may have raised as many questions as it has answered for morphology alone cannot delineate function but can only suggest it. Thus the combination of electron microscopy (*see* Chapter 14) with the tools of histochemistry, biochemistry (Chapter 20) and electrophysiology (Chapter 21) will together further our knowledge of the internal ear.

Scanning Electronmicroscopy

The scanning electronmicroscope (SEM) which is widely used in the metallurgy industry, is now available for biomedical use. Three-dimensional views of the ear at an ultrastructural level obtained with the scanning microscope have added a new dimension to the understanding of this complex organ. These new views help to bridge the gap between information obtained by light microscopy and that provided by transmission electron microscopy.

Unlike the conventional transmission electron microscope which uses thin sections, the scanning electron microscope can examine most biological tissue without sectioning. It thus provides a surface view of the cells. In the scanning electron microscope, a narrow, constant electron beam, about 20 nm in diameter, is focused on cell surfaces which have been coated with a thin layer of conductive metal. As the electrons bombard the surface of the metal-coated tissue in a vacuum tube, they cause emission of secondary electrons which are collected, electronically amplified and projected on a cathode ray tube. The result is a picture similar to the image produced on a television screen.

Biopsies

Although the *biopsy* is considered as a technique used to provide a pathological diagnosis, it has also proved of value in elucidating some aspects of normal aural structure. In particular, there have been the *light microscopic* studies of Palva and his associates (1964), of Sadé (1967) and of Ferlito (1974) on specimens of both *mucous membrane* and *bone* removed from the *tympanic* and *mastoid cavity*. Using cupped forceps, Sadé removed mucosal tissue from every topographic site in the tympanic or mastoid cavities of chronically infected ears. The biopsies were fixed in formaldehyde solution and the sections stained with a variety of stains, i.e. Alcian blue, colloidal iron, haematoxylin eosin, periodic acid Schiff (PAS) and tolonium chloride (toluidine blue). Both Palva and his associates and Ferlito studied mucosal and bone fragments (bone chips). Palva and his colleagues stained their sections with haematoxylin eosin. Ferlito also used haematoxylin eosin as well as Alcian blue, tolonium chloride and van Gieson's stain.

Electron-microscopic studies of the *internal ear* have been reported by Hilding and House (1964) and by Friedmann and his colleagues (1972). Hilding and House studied the ultrastructure of the utricle removed from patients who were not primarily suffering from internal ear disease. Friedmann and his colleagues studied the ultrastructure of a portion of the lateral semicircular duct of a patient who was undergoing surgical treatment for Ménière's disorder. In each case, immediately after removal, the specimens were placed in fixative, osmic acid in one case (Hilding and House), glutaraldehyde in the other (Friedmann *et al.*).

Radiography

As Welin (1955) pointed out, there are many who consider that the most important task of radiology in the otological examination is to produce a detailed description of the anatomy of the ear. There is a concensus that the anatomy of the temporal bone plays a considerable part in determining the course of an inflammatory process; it is obviously of great importance to the surgeon to know, before he operates, the extent of pneumatization, possible low lying middle fossas, anterior displacements of the sigmoid venous sinus and elevations of the bulb of the internal jugular vein. All these anatomical features can be demonstrated by *conventional* (*straight* or *plain*) radiography, using one or other views. The easiest and best view for the otologist in training to comprehend is the film that looks most like the temporal bone as exposed at operation. Radiographic examination is a matter of interpreting overlapping shadows of a structure which is in essence translucent to X-rays. The effort of the radiologist is to direct the X-ray beam in such a manner and to position the patient in respect of the X-ray film so that there will be as few confusing overlapping shadows as possible. The lateral view the otologist would like to see cannot be achieved by passing the ray directly laterally through the skull since the side under examination would be hopelessly obscured by the shadow of the opposite temporal bone. The X-ray tube is therefore moved to a position above the opposite ear and the incident beam directed 20° caudally and 15° anteriorly (*Law's lateral oblique view*) so as to avoid the overlapping shadows of the petrous portion of the temporal bone on the examined side. From the anatomical viewpoint all lateral radiographic views of the temporal bone provide good visualization of that part of the bone most accessible to surgery—the mastoid process, the squamous part of the temporal bone and part of the tympanic bone. The petrous bone and the tympanic cavity are superimposing on each other. From the pathological point of view the X-ray films taken in these projections indicate directly the condition of the cell system and the anatomical location of some important structures such as the sigmoid sinus and the tegmen tympani, together with the sinodural angle cells (Figs. 9 and 10). Note that this view, as well as showing the extent and translucency of the mastoid air cells, also shows the external and internal acoustic meatuses superimposed, the lateral venous sinus, mastoid antrum and the temporo-mandibular joint. Other radiographic views used in British hospitals for visualizing the mastoid and petrous portions of the temporal bone are as follows:

Half-axial (Townes) view (Figs. 11 and 12): The patient sits with the occiput resting on the X-ray table, the orbito-meatal line in the horizontal plane. The X-ray tube is tilted 30° caudally, centering through the petrous portion of the temporal bones on each side. The Townes' view shows both sides of the petrous bones on the one projection, the mastoid antrum, its aditus, the superior and lateral semicircular canals, the cochlea and the internal acoustic meatuses.

Submentovertical (Hirtz) view (Figs. 13 and 14): The patient sits facing the X-ray tube and the head is placed so that the vertex of the skull is resting on the X-ray table; the patient is looking up towards the ceiling. The X-ray beam is directed through the base of the skull in the midline at a point midway between the mandibular angles, bisecting the petrous bones at the level of the external

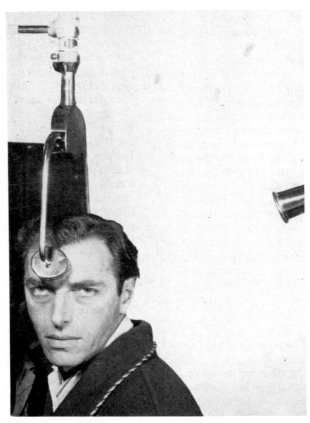

FIG. 9. Positioning for Law's lateral oblique view.

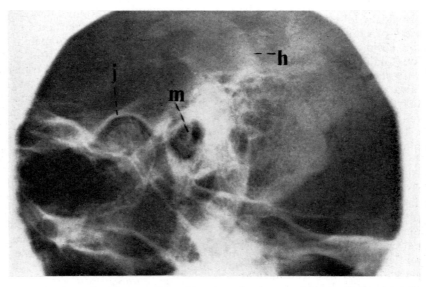

FIG. 10. Lateral oblique radiographic view showing temporo-mandibular joint (j), superimposed internal and external acoustic meatuses (m) and helix of auricle (h).

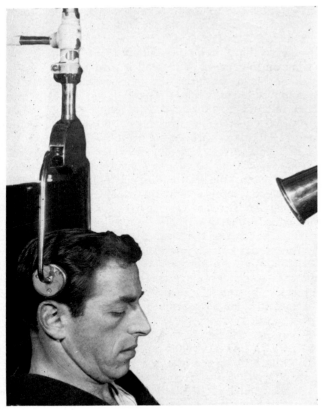

FIG. 11. Positioning for Towne's view.

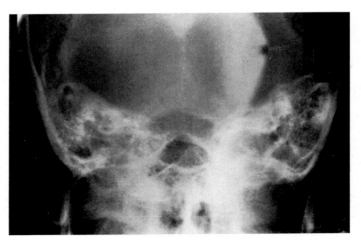

FIG. 12. Towne's radiographic view.

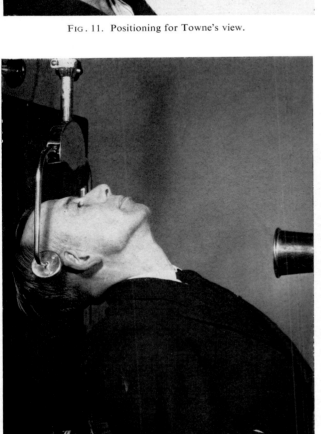

FIG. 13. Positioning for Hirtz's submento-vertical view.

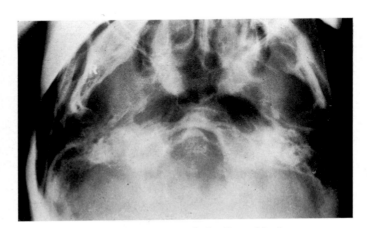

FIG. 14. Submento-vertical radiographic view.

acoustic meatus. The submentovertical view demonstrates both the external and internal acoustic meatuses as well as the bony part of the auditory tubes. A view of the cochlea and the semicircular canals is also obtained but one of its main functions is to show the middle ear with its ossicular chain clear of the other structures. The carotid canals, petrous apices and the foramina ovale, spinosum and stylomastoideus are also shown on each side.

Modified Stenvers (Figs. 15 and 16): The patient sits facing the X-ray table with the forehead and nose resting on the centre. The head is then rotated approximately 35° away from the side under examination and the head moved laterally until the ear being examined is at the centre of the X-ray table and X-ray beam. The X-ray beam is projected just below the petrous bone, centering just lateral to the external occipital protuberance.

The true Stenvers view demonstrates the internal ear; this modified Stenvers view will demonstrate the external acoustic meatus, the mastoid tip, mastoid antrum, cochlea, superior and lateral semicircular canals and petrous apex. Although the Stenvers view for the internal meatus was condemned thirty-five years ago by Camp and Cilley because the axes of the meatus run perpendicular to the sagittal plane, the use of this view has persisted. This Stenvers projection has even been used for tomographic studies (*see below*) of the meatus where it may give a false impression of widening of the meatus. The latter artefact is frequently due to suprameatal pneumatization of the petrous apex (Vergau, 1973).

Anteroposterior projection through the orbits (Figs. 17 and 18): In this perorbital position the patient's head is tilted anteriorly so that the horizontal plane crossing the superior aspect of the external acoustic meatus also crosses the upper third of the lateral orbital wall. This view projects the internal acoustic meatuses through the orbits and allows comparison of the two sides on the one film.

Tomography

Conventional radiography has the intrinsic defect of producing a picture that is the summation on a single plan of multiple structures located in different planes so that small structures under investigation are more or less

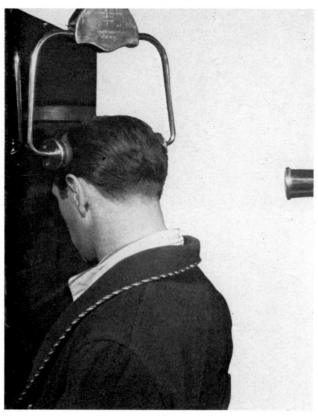

FIG. 15. Positioning for modified Stenvers view.

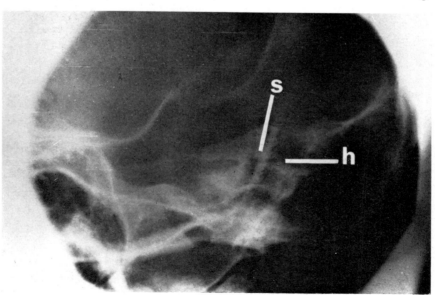

FIG. 16. Modified Stenvers radiographic view showing lateral semicircular canal (h) and superior semicircular canal (s).

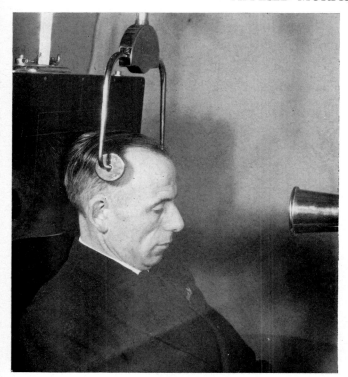

FIG. 17. Positioning for perorbital view.

X-ray source and the film. This adjustable fulcrum enables the selection of a particular body plane to be radiographed. Any object not in the plane of the fulcrum is displaced relative to that plane and thus deliberately obscured by the blurring action. In the simplest tomographic systems, the X-ray source (tube) and the film move relative to one another in one fixed plane (*linear tomography*). Linear (unidirectional) tomography as used initially in the development of tomography proved unsatisfactory for the study of the small structures of the temporal bone. This was because the short scanning movement produced inadequate blurring and those structures whose long axes were parallel to the longitudinal axis of the trajectory were not effaced but merely elongated.

Polytomography (*multidirectional body section radiography*) overcame these obstacles. The advantage of the polytome (radiographic equipment to conduct polytomography) over previous tomographic apparatus lies in its ability to produce tomograms by elliptical, circular or hypocycloidal movement of the X-ray tube in addition to the linear movement normally used. Thus this eliminates the linear blurring pattern characteristic of unidirectional tomography and produces greater blurring of structures outside the plane of focus. The polytome is also capable of producing thick section tomograms or zonograms.

The term *zonography* is used by radiologists to denote tomograms which employ a narrow arc of swing of the

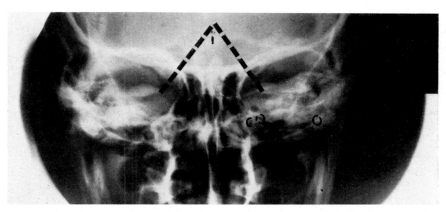

FIG. 18. Perorbital radiographic view showing internal acoustic meatus (i) on each side.

obscured. By moving the X-ray tube and film in opposite directions simultaneously but synchronously, an X-ray picture is obtained in which the area of the focal plane is shown clear of surrounding structures. The level of the focal plane can be varied and the temporal bone, for example, can be sectioned at various depths. Hence, the use of the term *body section radiography*. *Tomography* is the term recognized by the International Commission on Radiological Units and Standards to designate all systems of body section radiography (previously termed *laminography* or *planigraphy*). Depending on the technique used (there are various tomographic techniques), the thickness of the section analysed, i.e. the width of the sharp plane (a layer giving a sharp image), is in the order of 1–10 mm. The synchronization in tomography is done by a mechanical coupling, with an adjustable fulcrum (pivot point), of the

X-ray tube. It should be understood that in any tomograph the wider the arc of swing during the X-ray exposure, the *thinner* will be the layer of tissue in sharp radiographic focus and the greater will be the blurring of images of structures outside that plane. Zonography usually results in radiographs of better contrast than thin section tomography and may be extremely useful diagnostically in certain anatomical sites—the petrous tip and the internal acoustic meatus (Fig. 19). The polytome is also fitted with an attachment for enlargement of the radiographic image to 1·6 times the true anatomical size. This has distinct advantages when dealing with small structures such as those found in the middle ear (Lloyd, 1973). Polytomography is thus extremely useful in detecting *anatomical variations*, such as a low lying dura, and a forward lying sigmoid sinus, extension of the jugular bulb into the hypotympanum, and any unusual congenital anomalies such as displacement of the carotid artery.

Lloyd and Wylie (1971) point out that the ideal situation for zonography exists when one wishes to study a comparatively dense structure which is isolated on either side by a *free zone* of soft tissue between it and the nearest parts producing disturbing shadows. By careful positioning, the petrous portion of the temporal bones may be made to conform to these criteria. During zonography in the coronal plane, the petrous is isolated from other bony structures by ensuring that the patient's chin is tucked well into his chest. This places the soft tissues of the middle fossa in front of the petrous with the soft tissues of the posterior fossa behind it. A 12° angle of swing has been found to be convenient for circular zonograms of the petrous temporal.

6 mm. Although unilateral enlargement of the antrum has been described (Tillitt *et al.*, 1970), the antra are almost always bilaterally symmetrical, despite considerable inter-individual variability in size (Brunner, 1969).

Although Valvassori and Pierce stated categorically that a difference of more than 2 mm in the vertical diameter of the two internal meatuses is definitely abnormal, Camp and Cilley found this difference in 2 per cent of skulls. Valvassori and Pierce also stated that, while the meatuses showed considerable inter-individual variation in shape, intra-individual variation occurred in only 10 per cent of subjects. Other points mentioned were as follows:

(1) The concave medial lip of the posterior wall should always be distinct and smooth.

(2) Any meatus with a vertical diameter less than 2 mm or greater than 9 mm should be considered abnormal.

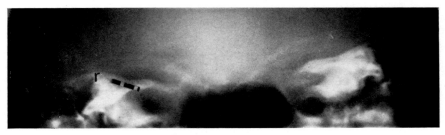

Fig. 19. Circular zonograms howing expansion and erosion of the right internal acoustic meatus (r).

Base zonograms may be used, *inter alia*, to demonstrate the incudo-mallear joint (Lloyd and Wylie, 1971. However, since ossicular joint measurements are of the order of a millimetre, and these structures are surrounded by relatively dense bone, wide angle hypocycloidal tomography is the preferred technique for their demonstration. The use of hypocycloidal polytomography with a multi-section cassette allows five separate tomographic cuts to be obtained simultaneously. This reduces the amount of radiation received by the patient (Lloyd, 1973). In view of the report by Chin and his colleagues (1970) that full hypocycloidal tomography of the temporal bones in the antero-posterior position delivers a dose of 10·5 R to the corneas, the postero-anterior projection is preferred. (Upton and his colleagues (1953) had previously demonstrated lens opacities in experimental animals following single exposures of the eyes to 15 R)

A considerable amount of work has now accrued on the *normal radiographic anatomy* of the ear. François and Barrois (1959) have described the tomographic anatomy of the normal temporal bone. Other authors have studied the normal radiographic anatomy of particular structures which are of clinical importance. Thus the radiographic anatomy of the normal *mastoid antrum* has been described by Waltner (1949) and both Camp and Cilley (1939) and Valvassori and Pierce (1964) have described the anatomy of the normal *internal acoustic meatus* in regard to conventional radiography and tomography respectively.

Waltner reported that the normal antrum appears radiographically as a cone with a maximum vertical diameter of 11 mm and a maximum transverse diameter of

(3) The length of the posterior wall varies from 4 to 11 mm.

(4) The length of the anterior wall is difficult to evaluate but varies from 9 to 27 mm.

(5) The *transverse crest* (*crista falciformis*) is never situated below the midpoint of the fundus of the meatus.

(6) This crest, usually about 3 mm long, may vary from 1 to 7 mm in length.

Contrast Radiography

Studies of the cerebello-medullary cistern and of the subarachnoid space within the internal acoustic meatus can be accomplished by use of negative or positive *contrast media*. Air has the advantage of being the most innocuous contrast material and of being rapidly absorbed. However, because of the superimposition of bony structures and of the smaller spaces under investigation, especially within the internal acoustic meatus, air does not provide a differential contrast sufficient for the detection of small masses. To detect small tumours, a positive contrast medium, such as iofendylate 2·5–5 ml, introduced by lumbar puncture should be used. By careful positioning of the patient under fluoroscopic control, the cerebello-medullary cisterns are filled in turn, radiographs obtained in two planes and the two sides compared. Provided that the contrast material does not rise above the tentorium cerebelli, severe headaches will be avoided. Extrameatal tumours produce a filling defect within the column of iofendylate. Intrameatal tumours obstruct the entry of contrast medium into the internal acoustic meatus on the affected side. The diagnostic accuracy of this investigation is high for the extrameatal tumours but less so for the intrameatal lesions. The tumour detection rate increases when the positive contrast cisternography is combined with hypocycloidal tomography. However, it must be pointed out that occasionally non-filling of the internal acoustic meatus may be caused by arachnoidal adhesions. At the end of this study, the contrast material is removed with the lumbar puncture needle. This is in an endeavour to obviate any possible arachnoidal reactions.

Angiography

Angiography (Olsson, 1953) is used most frequently to demonstrate tumours in the region of the cerebello-pontine

jugulare tumour it is necessary to fill the *external carotid artery* because of the frequent supply of these tumours by the ascending pharyngeal artery. Jugular *venography* is also a useful aid in this condition. Subtraction methods, which cancel out bone shadows that obscure vascular detail, have in recent years proved a valuable adjunct to the standard angiographic techniques.

Computerized Tomography

The concept of *computer applications* to diagnosis by roentgenography has been studied by many investigators in the past but the ultimate development in the application of the process to clinical medicine is due to the work of

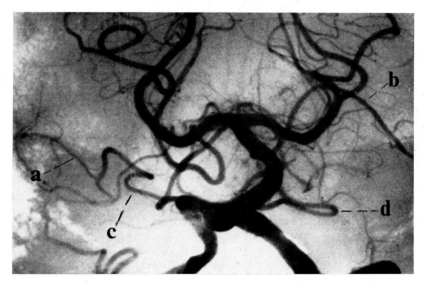

FIG. 20. Vertebral angiogram showing normal hemispheric branch of right anterior inferior cerebellar artery (a), hemispheric branch of left anterior inferior cerebellar artery (b) displaced postero-superiorly by a tumour, normal floccular loop of right anterior cerebellar artery (c), and slightly displaced floccular loop of left anterior inferior cerebellar artery (d).

angle and of the jugular fossa and to detect possible vascular lesions such as saccular aneurysms or arteriovenous malformations. Cerebello-pontine angle tumours may be either vestibulocochlear schwannomas ("acoustic neurinomas"), meningiomas or, less commonly, metastatic deposits or tumours such as ependymomas arising from the lateral recesses of the fourth ventricle.

Vertebral angiography is carried out via a catheter inserted through the femoral artery and up the aorta into either vertebral artery. In the arterial phase of the examination the vessels that might be affected by a cerebello-pontine angle tumour are the anterior inferior cerebellar artery (Fig. 20) and the superior cerebellar arteries. In very large tumours other vessels may be compressed or displaced. Tumours in the same area may compress the petrosal veins which fail to fill on the affected side (Fig. 21).

The tumours in the region of the jugular fossa and hypotympanum may be glomus jugulare tumours or schwannomas arising from the ninth, tenth and eleventh nerves. To help in establishing the diagnosis of a glomus

Ambrose and Hounsfield (1973) and EMI. The EMI *scanner* has made it possible to analyse the brain in depth without danger of discomfort to the patient and to diagnose brain tumours, hydrocephalus, cerebral atrophy and cerebral infarcts without contrast agents or radioactive material. This ingenious application of computer techniques permits analysis of the variations in X-ray absorption through multiple sections of brain substance. The picture produced displays the structure and configuration of the soft tissues of the brain. Undoubtedly computerized axial tomography (CAT*) will have a very significant impact on the conventional approach to the diagnosis and treatment of neurological conditions. The EMI system is an X-ray unit in the pure sense of the word in that it emits photons that pass through the skull in a narrow beam to sensitive crystal detectors. The transmission of the X-ray photons can be measured and analysed by the computer where it demonstrates the internal architecture of the

* Unfortunately, owing to the proliferation in abbreviations, this abbreviation may also refer to *combined approach tympanoplasty* or a *computer of averaged transients.*

brain. The computer is programmed to recover and analyse the enormous quantity of information which in the past would have been lost by conventional radiography. By solving equations of absorption coefficients, a display is produced on a cathode ray tube which is a picture of the intervening brain tissue. A black and white record permits analysis of densities ranging from black (air) to white (bone) and permitting polaroid photography to provide a permanent record. The system utilizes the principle of tomography and examines the head in a series of brain slices extending from the base of the skull to the top of the

chondral, as well as the endochondral, layers (Hanson and Anson, 1962). This process of remodelling may begin during the second decade of life, or it may be observed in elderly patients. The central marrow cavity is, however, obliterated and the basic pattern of perichondral and endochondral bone occurs throughout the ossicles except at the site of attachment of the ligaments and at the tip of the manubrium of the malleus. The extent of the remodelling varies and is manifest by the presence of tertiary lamellae and accompanying destruction of the primary pattern. Occasionally, an ossicle may show little

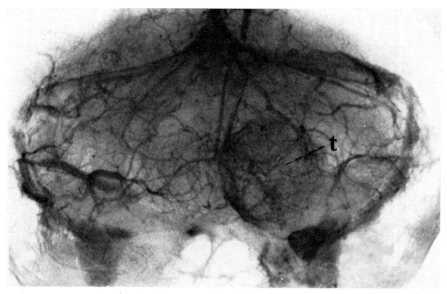

FIG. 21. Vertebral angiogram showing "tumour blush" (t) due to congestion and displacement of petrosal vein tributaries.

calvaria. A single passage of the X-ray beam results in two contiguous slices approximately 13 mm in width. The tomographic recording is caused by the fixed alignment of sodium iodide crystals to the X-ray source and the movement of the source and the detectors around the patients. High density tumours, vestibulocochlear schwannomas and meningiomas can be picked up in the cerebello-pontine angle by this technique.

PATHOLOGICAL ASPECTS

Abnormal Histology

For an authoritative, definitive account of this topic, the reader is referred to Friedmann's (1974) and to Schuknecht's (1974) texts on aural pathology.

As the author has previously pointed out (Davies, 1968b) a proper understanding of normal ossicular bone remodelling is essential to interpreting the histological appearances of the auditory ossicles. In the neonatal period, the ossicles undergo a series of changes in structure. Areas of bone are locally eroded and, after resorption of the primary osseous layers, new lamellae of bone are deposited. This irregular form of secondary lamellae alters the primary pattern of ossification and this involves the peri-

evidence of remodelling and may be mistaken for that of a young patient even though the individual may be in the seventh or eighth decade of life. The presence of cartilage in the zone beneath the periosteal layers may be taken to represent the fetal characteristic of an ossicle. Failure to recognise these changes in ossicular structure may lead investigators to label findings as pathological and, occasionally, to link these observations with otosclerosis.

The author has previously reported on the histopathology of Paget's disease. A correct understanding of the changes that Paget's disorder can produce in the ossicular mechanism is important to a rational surgical treatment of the condition. The conductive hearing loss in this disorder could well be related to causes other than stapedo-vestibular joint fixation. Increased ossicular mass and epitympanic fixation of the malleus may well be a contributory factor (Davies, 1968a, 1970).

Sadé's study showed that chronically infected *tympanic mucosa* contains many glandular structures that produce mucus. The glands are more numerous and frequently much greater in size than those found in the normal tympanic mucosa. As he points out, this change is not surprising since hypertrophy and hyperplasia of mucous glands is the usual reaction of any mucosa to infection.

The study of Palva and his colleagues (1964) of bone

chips and granulations removed from the mastoid process during cortical mastoid operations for acute mastoiditis confirmed the early findings of Krainz (1926) and others. This is to the effect that *progressive new bone formation* is a common observation in *acute mastoiditis*. Thus the fundamental pathology of the condition has not been altered with the advent of the antibiotics. Moreover, in *subacute mastoiditis*, thickened mucosa was often covered by fibrinous exudate. This may become organized, forming permanent adhesions between the ossicles and the tympanic membrane, leading to *tympanosclerosis* (Davies,

study is required before the light microscopic alterations are fully defined. (Figs. 22 and 23 show the histopathological appearances in a case of temporal bone fracture and of Paget's disease respectively.)

In 1910, Nager and Yoshii called attention to postmortem changes and to the fact that they appear in the internal ear before being observed in other structures. Autolysis is initiated immediately after death. Thus, research workers dealing with experimental animals have found that it is essential to adopt methods of intravital fixation as the best procedure for histological preparations.

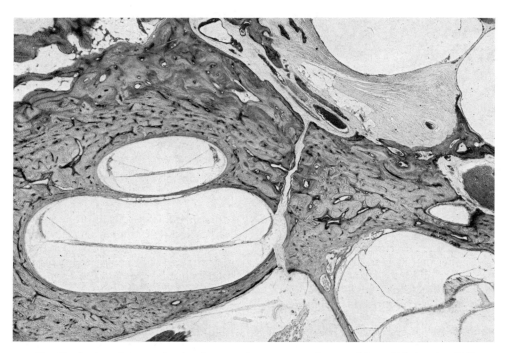

Fig. 22. Section of the ear showing fracture of petrous part of temporal bone (Schuknecht, 1974).

1968b; Friedmann, 1971). In later adult life, "chalk patches" in the tympanic membrane may provide otoscopic evidence for the existence of this latter condition.

Ferlito (1974) conducted both histological and histochemical studies on mucosa and bone structure in *chronic suppurative otitis media*, basing it on 826 specimens. Ferlito sought to emphasize the severity and extent of the lesions not only of the mucosa but also of the bone, whether of the mastoid process or of the ossicles. He therefore pointed out that it would be more appropriate, as others have done previously, to talk about *chronic otomastoiditis*.

The need for a better understanding of ear pathology, especially that of the *internal ear*, has resulted in the formation of "temporal bone banks" in many countries. These centres are able to acquire temporal bones from individuals with ear disorders on whom auditory and vestibular function tests have been carried out. However, there is great difficulty even in the most modern university hospital, in acquiring temporal bones in a good state of preservation from individuals who have had previous auditory and vestibular function tests and much more

Nevertheless, confusion about what is meant by "normal internal ear structure" still exists. In addition to two *artefacts* (agonal and post-mortem change), the position, size and shape of cells and membranes in living and fixed tissue have been the centre of many debates. Not an inconsiderable number of papers have been published describing changes which have since been correctly attributed to post-mortem autolysis.

Fernandez (1958) completed an excellent study under light microscopy of the sequence of histological changes of the vestibular and cochlear receptors in 82 guinea pigs as autolysis progressed. This paper is essential reading for the otolaryngologist who is rotating through the department of pathology during his training.

In very general terms certain principles of pathological reactions of the internal ear can be summarized, depending on the various types of pathological injury.

(1) When the labyrinth suffers a severe insult, this usually affects both the auditory and vestibular portions. This is especially true in inflammatory conditions (fibrinous or suppurative labyrinthitis), hydrops and severe trauma, such as a transverse fracture of the temporal bone. There are no

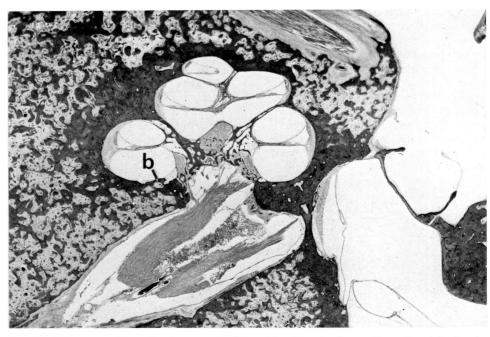

FIG. 23. Right temporal bone showing a more active variety of Paget's disease. The region of the fenestra vestibuli is clear but breaching (b) of the endosteum can be seen in the basal turn of the cochlea.

physical boundaries for the spread of noxious agents within the bony labyrinth.

(2) Whilst both halves of the labyrinth are affected by severe trauma, the pars inferior (cochlea and saccule) is definitely much more susceptible to lesser degrees of trauma than is the pars superior (utricle and semicircular ducts). This is very evident in forms of physical (mechanical or acoustic) trauma, some forms of hereditary ear pathology, ageing and both pre-natal (rubella) and acquired (mumps) viral infections. Degeneration of this pars inferior, which is the phylogenetically newer half of the labyrinth, to such agents, has been classified as "cochleo-saccular" degeneration.

(3) The vestibular organs, while generally exhibiting resistance to most form of injury, show a distinct pre-dilection to degeneration from the administration of streptomycin. The effect of streptomycin is selective on the ampullary crests and is so selective that the effect can be titrated to the point where the maximum degenerative effect can be obtained while preserving cochlear function completely. All other ototoxic drugs derived from the streptomycins affect the auditory labyrinth before the vestibular.

(4) Neurone degeneration: The primary bipolar neurones of the two divisions of the vestibulocochlear nerve behave very differently to injury. The cochlear neurones will consistently undergo complete retrograde degeneration to almost any lesion of its axons (cochlear nerve) such as transection or severe compression. They similarly undergo retrograde degeneration when the end organ (spiral organ) is involved in a severe enough injury to effect the dendritic terminals of the cochlear neurone. This degree of severity is indicated by involvement of the supporting elements in the spiral organ. The vestibular bipolar neurone, on the other hand, is so resistant to injury that neither transection of the axon (vestibular nerve) nor severe end organ injury (even labyrinthectomy) will cause complete retrograde degeneration of the neurone. Only direct injury to the cell bodies in the vestibular (Scarpa's) ganglion will cause the neurone to degenerate.

(5) Internal ear pathology is usually expressed clinically in terms of three symptoms—hearing loss, vertigo and tinnitus. Auditory function has been well correlated with certain degrees and locations of pathology in both the end organ and the primary auditory neurone. Vestibular dysfunction is very difficult to precisely correlate with pathology in the labyrinth because basic neuroanatomy and neurophysiology of the vestibular end organs and neurones have not been as well elucidated as in the cochlea (but *see* Chapter 26). Tinnitus is extremely difficult to evaluate and there is no auditory pathological correlate of this clinical sign, although there have been some inferences from experimental studies on animals (Kiang *et al.*, 1970). Presumably, neurophysiology or biochemistry will uncover the reason for this very frequent accompaniment of cochlear pathology.

Abnormal Radiographic Anatomy

Various disease processes can be detected because of the production of secretions which are (compared with air) relatively radio-opaque, or by the particular changes that they produce in the aural structure. For example, in inflammatory middle ear processes, the lumina of the mastoid air cells are filled with swollen mucosal lining, mucus and other secretions. On radiographic examination, the normal translucency due to the air content in the mastoid cellular system then disappears. As a result of progressive acute infection, the normally sharply delineated trabeculae become less defined and decalcified both because of the inflammatory process and because of mechanical compression by the secretion filling the mastoid cells. Radiologically, chronicity of infection is characterized by a small number of opaque cloudy cells and thickened bony walls. This may be interpreted pathologically as destruction of the cell walls, the presence of granular mucosal lining and osteoid tissue development. In chronic infection, the surgeon wishes to know where there is any bony erosion. The study of the lateral wall of the epitympanic recess has the greatest clinical importance since this wall is usually the first to be involved in a cholesteatoma. Large areas of erosion of the lateral wall are usually detected by the views previously mentioned. Using conventional radiography, cholesteatoma may first be detected by enlargement of the aditus to the mastoid antrum (seen just lateral to the lateral semicircular canal in a Townes' view) (Welin, 1947). However, conventional radiography can demonstrate only about two-thirds of aural cholesteatomas (Winderen and Zimmer, 1954). Hypocycloidal polytomography can detect nearly 95 per cent of these lesions (Brunner et al., 1966). In outlining the anatomical and pathological features of a temporal bone affected by a cholesteatoma, polytomography can demonstrate (a) the size and extent of the cholesteatoma sac and any associated reaction, (b) erosions of the facial canal, (c) fistula or erosions of the semicircular canals, (d) erosions of the lateral wall of the epitympanic recess, of the postero-superior wall of the external meatus, of the mastoid and of the dural plates and (e) the state of the ossicles and the ossicular chain, including lesions that might fix the ossicles in the epitympanic recess.

Base zonograms are invaluable not only for detecting abnormalities in the foramina of the base of skull (e.g. enlargement of the *jugular foramen* in glomus jugulare tumours) but also for detecting *incudo-mallear* dislocations (Lloyd and Wylie, 1971). However, hypocycloidal tomography is the preferred radiographic technique for investigating ossicular abnormalities (Lloyd, 1973). This technique is invaluable in demonstrating normal middle and internal ear structures in atresia of the external acoustic meatus.

Fractures of the temporal bone, either longitudinal or transverse, can be accurately depicted and ossicular chain injuries can also be delineated.

It must be stressed that minimal bony erosion produced by very small *tumours* involving the temporal bone cannot be detected by a routine conventional radiological examination. Some malignant tumours such as glomus jugulare tumours and carotid aneurysms may reach a considerable size before the bony changes produced by the expanding lesions become visible on conventional views. A zonogram of the internal acoustic meatus is eminently suitable for screening the meatus for abnormalities. The particular abnormality which one has in mind is, of course, a *vestibulocochlear nerve tumour* (exclusively a schwannoma). Widening of the porus of the internal acoustic meatus is a characteristic sign of a vestibulo-cochlear tumour but occasionally the intra-meatal location

of the tumour may result in widening of the mid-portion of the meatus. Any suspected abnormality of the zonogram may then be elucidated using thin section hypocycloidal polytomography with postero-anterior views and, if necessary, lateral views.

Polytomography may also provide evidence for *otosclerosis* by demonstrating narrowing of the fenestra vestibuli (Jensen et al., 1966). Valvassori (1969) has also reported both osteolytic and sclerotic (according to the stage of otosclerotic process) changes in the labyrinthine capsule in otosclerosis.

SURGICAL ANATOMY

There are now a variety of surgical procedures that may be conducted on the ear. A knowledge of the relevant anatomy is a *sine qua non* to their proper and faultless execution.

Cortical (Simple) Mastoidectomy

This operation, although now rarely necessary by itself alone in the antibiotic era, is performed as an approach in other surgical procedures. It exposes the mastoid antrum, posterior edge of the short process of the incus and varying amounts of the epitympanic recess, depending upon the extent of the disease and the preference of the surgeon. This approach is useful in the treatment of acute mastoiditis, for decompression of the facial nerve and as an approach to the saccus endolymphaticus. The relationship of the tip of the short process of the incus, the lateral canal and the facial nerve as mentioned previously should always be borne in mind. Identification of the nerve is considerably easier at the level of the tip of the short process of the incus than it is at the anterior end of the *mastoid notch* (*digastric groove*), where it is frequently, quite indistinct.

Modified Radical Mastoidectomy

For several years the modified radical mastoidectomy has been used quite successfully in the treatment of choleasteatoma. It combines preservation of the ossicular chain with eradication of disease and should still be considered as a useful form of tympanoplasty. However, the most frequent cause of failure of the operation was the failure of the operator to open all infected cells. Occasionally, the sinodural angle was inadequately cleaned because of the surgeon's trepidation or the limitation placed on his exposure by an endaural incision. Not infrequently the residual disease could be found in the facial sinus cells. Another disadvantage to be mentioned in this type of operation was the creation of a bony mastoid cavity. While most patients requiring a modified radical mastoidectomy had sclerotic or diploic mastoids, there was a surprising number who had well pneumatized mastoids. Provided that the mastoid process was removed lateral to the digastric ridge and the cortical bone was extensively bevelled over the middle fossa dura and sinus plate, the size of the cavity was reduced. A variety of obliterative techniques are available using muscle or soft tissue pedicle and also bone chips. Reconstruction of the posterior meatal wall by means of cartilage and/or bone has been developed in the past few years.

Radical Mastoidectomy

For many years radical mastoidectomy has been successful in the treatment of secondary acquired cholesteatoma. Essentially, a careful, complete anatomical dissection was carried out under adverse conditions with a minimum of landmarks. The long process of the incus is readily eroded by chronic middle ear disease but not infrequently the whole incus may disappear. In these instances of minimal landmarks, the surgeon should immediately locate the trochleariform process which can be located by finding the junction of the anterior wall of the middle ear with the tegmen and proceeding posteroinferiorly. Once the trochleariform process has been identified, the surgeon is now aware of its relationship to the facial nerve, which can be safely followed posteriorly.

Tympanoplasty

A variety of tympanoplastic techniques have arisen in the past 20 years but only a few have stood the test of time. Failures have been due to inadequate clearance of disease, infection and rejection of graft materials (see Chapter 65) and poor selection of patients for reconstructive surgery. It is not my brief to dwell on the more modern and more successful types of tympanoplasties, but it should be mentioned that the trainee otologist should not undertake reconstructive middle ear surgery unless he is fully familiar with the methods used and also satisfied with his ability to eradicate disease in the temporal bone before embarking upon improving sound conduction. During the past 10 years, because of the necessity to clean out mastoid cavities left after early surgery, intact wall tympanoplastic procedures have been developed and the middle ear space can be viewed from behind via a posterior tympanotomy (Jansen, 1958, 1968; Smyth et al., 1967). The tympanotomy is made after an extended cortical mastoidectomy has been completed; a trough is cut from the tip of the short process of the incus in an inferior direction towards the mastoid tip parallel to the facial nerve. It is essential to gain exposure on a broad base and to avoid a narrow pothole as the facial nerve lies immediately medial to the bone. When the posterior wall of the facial sinus has been removed it is then possible to visualize the upper and posterior part of the mesotympanum. The breadth of the surgical exposure here is related to the height of the chordal eminence and the chordal ridge. These structures form a rigid bone lying obliquely across the inferior edge of the tympanotomy aperture. Once removed, the pyramid and stapes superstructure are clearly seen. The view, inferiorly and medially, may be restricted by the styloid eminence and subiculum, which should be removed to gain access to the hypotympanum. Bone removal can then be continued inferiorly to bring the lower edge of the tympanotomy aperture flush with the floor of the hypotympanum. It is essential to realize that a full exposure of the middle ear must be obtained otherwise cholesteatoma and residual disease may remain. Details of the surgical anatomy are given by Smyth and his colleagues (1969).

Stapedectomy

In operations on the stapes (House, 1967; Schuknecht, 1971), the distance between the base of the stapes laterally and the utricle and saccule medially is of paramount importance. This intervening space will change from one transverse level to another in the same specimen owing to the vesicular form of the two membranous chambers. Hanson and his colleagues (1965) found that, at a transverse level near the superior margin of the fenestra vestibuli, the distance between the stapedial base and the saccule varies between 1 and 1·4 mm. The corresponding distance for the utricle was 0·7–1·4 mm. At a level passing through the stapes base at its maximum width, the shortest intervening distance was 1·4 mm for both the saccule and utricle. The distances are slightly greater at a more inferior level near the lower margin of the fenestra vestibuli.

Labyrinthine Surgery

A plethora of procedures is now available for operations on the membranous labyrinth in cases of Ménière's disorder. The decompressive type of operation began with the pioneering work of George Portmann (1927) nearly half a century ago. The value of the subarachnoid shunt in endolymphatic hydrops has been emphasised in more recent years by House (1965) and others. Destructive procedures have either been total, e.g. membranous labyrinthectomy (Cawthorne, 1943), or partial, e.g. vestibular labyrinthine destruction by ultra-sound (Arslan, 1962; Angell-James, 1969) or by cryosurgery (House, 1966).

Vestibulocochlear Neural Surgery

An approach to the internal acoustic meatus through the middle cranial fossa has been used by William House in sectioning the vestibular branch of the vestibulocochlear nerve, removing facial nerve tumours and decompressing the facial nerve after injury (House, 1964; House and Hitselberger, 1969). The procedure is based on the identification of the greater petrosal nerve which is carefully followed through its hiatus to the genicular ganglion. Once the genicular ganglion has been located, the internal meatus can be unroofed safely and the appropriate procedure performed. In the translabyrinthine microscopic removal of vestibulocochlear nerve tumours, an extended cortical mastoidectomy is carried out and the facial nerve is defined just below the lateral canal. The superior, posterior and lateral semicircular canals are opened and removed and then the posterosuperior aspect of the vestibule is opened. The superior vestibular nerve is identified where it enters the vestibule to supply the ampullary crests of the superior and lateral ducts and the utricle. With a diamond drill the superior vestibular nerve is followed and House's bar is located. The petrous segment of the facial nerve canal is thus identified just anterior to the canal for the superior vestibular nerve where they both enter the lateral end of the internal acoustic meatus. The bone inferior and posterior to the meatus is then removed. This exposes the entire posterior fossa dura, from the sigmoid sinus posteriorly and the superior petrosal sinus above to the jugular bulb below. Thus the entire internal meatus is exposed extradurally. Finally, the dura of the internal meatus overlying the tumour is incised and the tumour is removed by careful dissection.

More recently, Gacek (1974) has introduced transection of the posterior division of the vestibular nerve in the foramen singulare for relief of intractable paroxysmal vertigo (*see* Chapter 28). The distal half of the posterior division of the vestibulocochlear nerve parallels the superior segment of the *secondary tympanic membrane* (round window membrane). In this region, the foramen singulare lies 1·5–2 mm beneath the floor of the fossula fenestra cochleae.

CONCLUSIONS

The most complex anatomy in the human body is that of the ear. This involves a plethora of minute, delicate structures, damage to which could almost certainly be irreparable. A knowledge of the relevant anatomy is therefore of vital importance to the aural surgeon; in fact perhaps much more than it is to his other surgical colleagues. It is therefore important that he acquire this information and that it be based on the practical knowledge which can be gained only from persistent and painstaking temporal bone dissections.

REFERENCES

Ambrose, J. (1973), *Brit. J. Radiol.*, 46, 1023.
Ambrose, J. and Hounsfield, G. (1973), *Brit. J. Radiol.*, 46, 148.
Angell-James, J. (1969), *Arch. Otolaryng.*, 89, 95.
Anson, B. J. and Donaldson, J. A. (1973), *Surgical Anatomy of the Temporal Bone*, 2nd edition. Philadelphia: Saunders.
Anson, B. J., Donaldson, J. A., Warpeha, R. L. and Winch, T. R. (1967), *Laryngoscope*, 77, 1269.
Arslan, M. (1962), *Acta oto-laryng. (Stockh.)*, 55, 467.
Brunner, S. (1969), *Semin. Roentgenol.*, 4, 129.
Brunner, S., Petersen, O. and Sandberg, L. E. (1966), *Amer. J. Roentgenol.*, 36, 747.
Camp, J. D. and Cilley, I. L. (1939), *Amer. J. Roentgenol.*, 41, 713.
Cawthorne, T. E. (1943), *Proc. roy. Soc. Med.*, 27, 663.
Chin, F. K., Anderson, W. B. and Gilbertson, J. D. (1970), *Radiology*, 94, 623.
Davies, D. Garfield (1968a), *Acta oto-laryng. (Stockh.)*, suppl. 242.
Davies, D. Garfield (1968b), *J. Laryng.*, 82, 331.
Davies, D. Garfield (1970), *J. Laryng*, 84, 553.
Donaldson, J. A. and Anson, B. J. (1965), *Ann. Otol. (St. Louis)*, 74, 59.
Engström, H., Ades, H. W. and Anderson, A. (1966), *Structural Patterns of the Organ of Corti*. Baltimore: Williams and Wilkins.
Ferlito, A. (1974), *ORL*, 36, 257.
Fernandez, C. (1958), *Arch. Otolaryng.*, 68, 460.
Fowler, E. P., Jr. (1961), *Laryngoscope*, 71, 937.
François, J. and Barrois, J. (1959), *Ann. Radiol.*, 11, 71.
Friedmann, I. (1971), *Otol. (St. Louis)*, 80, 411.
Friedmann, I. (1974), *Pathology of the Ear*. Oxford: Blackwell.
Friedmann, I., Angell James, J. and Bird, E. S. (1972), *J. Laryng.*, 86, 807.
Gacek, R. R. (1974), *Ann. Otol. (St. Louis)*, 83, 596.
Guild, S. R. (1921), *Anat. Rec.*, 22, 141.
Hamberger, C. A., Marcuson, G. and Wersall, J. (1963), *Acta oto-laryng. (Stockh.)*, suppl. 183, p. 66.
Hammar, J. A. (1902), *Arch. mikr. Anat.*, 59, 471.
Hanson, J. R. and Anson, B. J. (1962), *Quart. Bull, Northw. Univ. med. Sch.*, 36, 119.

Harper, D. G. and Anson, B. J. (1962), *Quart. Bull, Northw. Univ. med. Sch.*, 36, 144.
Heidenhain, M. (1916), *Z. wiss. Mikr.*, 33, 232.
Hilding, D. A. and House, W. F. (1964), *Laryngoscope*, 74, 1135.
Hounsfield, G. (1973), *Brit. J. Radiol.*, 46, 1016.
House, H. (1967), *Laryngoscope*, 77, 1410.
House, W. F. (1964), *Arch. Otolaryng.*, 80, 617.
House, W. F. (1965), *Laryngoscope*, 75, 1547.
House, W. F. (1966), *Arch. Otolaryng.* 84, 616.
House, W. F. (1968), *Arch. Otolaryng.*, 88, 571.
House, W. F. and Hitselberger, W. E. (1969), *Acta oto-laryng. (Stockh.)*, 67, 413.
Iurato, S. (1967), *Submicroscopic Structure of the Inner Ear*. Oxford: Pergamon.
Jansen, C. (1958), *Sitz. Ber. Fortbild. Arztek.*, Ob. v. 18 Febr.
Jansen, C. (1968), *J. Laryng.*, 82, 779.
Jensen, J., Rovsing, H. and Brunner, S. (1966), *Brit. J. Radiol.*, 39, 669.
Johnsson, L-G. and Hawkins, J. E., Jr. (1967a), *Arch. Otolaryng.*, 85, 599.
Johnsson, L-G. and Hawkins, J. E., Jr. (1967b), *Science*, 157, 1454.
Kane, I. (1953), *Sectional Radiography of the Chest*. New York: Springer.
Kiang, N. Y. S., Moxon, E. C. and Levine, R. A. (1970), *Sensorineural Hearing Loss*, p. 241 (G. E. W. Wolstenholme and Julie Knight, Eds.), Ciba Foundation Symposium. London: Churchill.
Krainz, W. (1926), *Z. Hals-, Nasen- u. Ohrenheilk.*, 13, 361.
Lim, D. J. (1969), *Acta oto-laryng. (Stockh.)*, suppl. 255.
Lim, D. J. (1971), *Arch. Otolaryng.*, 94, 69.
Lloyd, G. A. S. (1973), *Recent Advances in Otolaryngology*, Chap. 25 (Joselen Ransome, H. Holden and T. R. Bull, Eds.). Edinburgh and London: Churchill Livingstone.
Lloyd, G. A. S. and Wylie, I. G. (1971), *Brit. J. Radiol.*, 44, 940.
Nager, F. and Yoshii, V. (1910), *Z. Ohrenheilk.*, 60, 93.
Olsson, O. (1953), *Acta radiol. (Stockh.)*, 39, 265.
Palva, T., Friedmann, I. and Palva, A. (1964), *J. Laryng.*, 78, 977.
Portman, G. (1927), *Arch. Otolaryng*, 6, 309.
Proctor, B. (1964), *J. Laryng.*, 78, 631.
Proctor, B. (1967), *Arch. Otolaryng.*, 84, 503.
Proctor, B. (1969), *Ann. Otol. (St. Louis)*, 78, 1026.
Rosen, S. (1952), *Arch. Otolaryng.*, 56, 610.
Sadé, J. (1967), *Isr. J. med. Sci.*, 3, 479.
Sammut, J. J. (1967), *J. Laryng.*, 81, 137.
Schuknecht, H. F. (1953), *Arch. Otolaryng.*, 58, 377.
Schuknecht, H. F. (1971), *Stapedectomy*. Boston: Little Brown & Co.
Schuknecht, H. F. (1974), *Pathology of the Ear*. Cambridge, Mass., U.S.A.: Harvard University Press.
Schuknecht, H. F. and Woellner, R. C. (1955), *J. Laryng.*, 69, 75.
Shea, J. (1958), *Ann. Otol. (St. Louis)*, 67, 932.
Sheehy, J. L. (1970), *J. Laryng.*, 84, 1.
Smyth, G. D. L., England, R. M., Gibson, R. and Kerr, A. G. (1967), *J. Laryng.*, 81, 69.
Smyth, G. D. L., Kerr, A. G., Dowe, A. C. and Khajuria, K. C. (1969), *J. Laryng.*, 83, 1143.
Spoendlin, H. H. (1969), *Acta oto-laryng. (Stockh.)*, 67, 239.
Tillitt, R., Wilner, H. I., Conner, G. H. and Eyler, W. R. (1970), *Radiology*, 94, 619.
Upton, A. C., Christenberry, K. W. and Forth, J. (1953), *Arch. Ophthal.*, 49, 164.
Valvassori, G. E. (1969), *Radiology*, 92, 449.
Valvassori, G. E. and Pierce, R. H. (1964), *Amer. J. Roentgenol.*, 92, 1232.
Vergau, W. (1973), *Fortschr. Röentgenstr.*, 119, 112.
Waltner, J. G. (1949), *Amer. J. Roentgenol.*, 62, 674.
Weir, N. (1974), *Brit. J. Audiol.*, 8, 113.
Welin, S. (1947), *Brit. J. Radiol.*, 20, 192.
Welin, S. (1955), *J. Laryng.*, 69, 515.
Winderen, L. and Zimmer, J. (1954), *Acta radiol. (Stockh.)*, suppl. 3.
Wullstein, H. (1952), *Arch. Ohr.-, Nas.- u. Kehlkheilk.*, 161, 422.
Wullstein, H. (1956), *Ann. Otol. (St. Louis)*, 65, 1020.
Yates, A. (1936), *Proc. roy. Soc. Med.*, 29, 837.
Zöllner, F. (1951), *Arch. Ohr.-, Nas.- u. Kehlkheilk.*, 159, 358.
Zöllner, F. (1963), *Arch. Otolaryng.*, 78, 301.

SECTION VI

EAR-FUNCTION

PAGE

16. MECHANICS OF THE AUDITORY APPARATUS 237

17. AUDITORY TUBAL FUNCTION 252

18. INTRATYMPANIC MUSCLES 257

19. ACOUSTIC IMPEDANCE 281

20. LABYRINTHINE FLUIDS 290

21. COCHLEAR ELECTROPHYSIOLOGY 303

22. AUDITORY NERVOUS SYSTEM 312

23. APPLICATION OF AUDITORY ELECTRONEUROPHYSIOLOGICAL TESTS 334

24. PSYCHOACOUSTICS 344

25. APPLICATION OF PSYCHOACOUSTICS TO CENTRAL AUDITORY DYSFUNCTION 352

26. VESTIBULAR SYSTEM—EXPERIMENTAL PATHOPHYSIOLOGY 361

27. VESTIBULAR PHYSIOLOGY 371

28. NEURO-OTOLOGY 383

SECTION VI

16. MECHANICS OF THE AUDITORY SYSTEM

J. TONNDORF and S. M. KHANNA

INTRODUCTION

Sound is a form of radiated *physical* energy. It is represented by the transmission of small vibratory changes in air pressure. The sensation of hearing is evoked when sound is directly transmitted to its specific receiver, the ear ("air conduction"), and also when the head is set into vibrations either by high-intensity sounds or by contact with vibrating structures ("bone conduction"). The present chapter will be exclusively concerned with the reception of airborne sound by the ear.

The sound energy taken up by the tympanic membrane is converted into mechanical vibrations. After transmission through the middle ear, this mechanical energy is utilized by the internal ear to elicit nerve impulses, a process that is carried out in the hair cell/nerve junction. The ear is an extremely sensitive detector of acoustic energy. Such sensitivity can be achieved only if the energy received by the tympanic membrane is transmitted to the hair cells with a minimum of loss. This condition demands efficient transmission from air to the fluids of the internal ear and then onto the semi-solid structures of the spiral organ of Corti. The internal ear performs a complicated analysis on acoustic signals before their actual detection by the hair cells.

The present chapter will discuss (1) how energy transmission through the ear is maximized and (2) how the analysis is carried out by the internal ear.

Past studies have provided us with a good understanding of the function of the ear as a whole as well as of its parts. The ear is essentially a mechano-acoustic device. Therefore, its responses are governed by the laws of Acoustics and/or Mechanics. A clear understanding of function, both under normal and pathological conditions, can best be achieved by direct application of acoustical and mechanical principles.

IMPEDANCE MATCHING

Vibratory energy is transmitted poorly from one medium to another, e.g. from air to water, and vice versa; most of it is reflected at the interface. The reason for such poor transmission lies in the difference in *impedance* between the two media.

Impedance is defined as the ratio of the applied sound pressure to the resulting velocity. In other words, the lower the velocity for a given sound pressure the higher the impedance. The impedance of fluids is higher than that of gases by a factor of at least 100, and the impedance of solids is in turn higher than that of fluids by an additional factor of approximately 30.

Maximal power transfer between two systems of different impedances can be accomplished by the interposition of an *impedance-matching transformer*. If we refer once more to the transmission of energy from air (low impedance) to water (high impedance), the required transformer should increase force and decrease velocity proportionally. A simple example of a transformer is given by an ideal lever (Fig. 1). Its lever ratio k changes the force by a factor of k and changes the velocity by $1/k$. Therefore, an impedance attached to one end of the lever appears at the other end changed by a factor of k^2. Ideal matching is achieved if the ratio of two simple (purely resistive) impedances is equal to k^2.

In actual physical systems the impedances are usually *complex*. That is to say, they possess both *resistive* and *reactive* parts. The former represents dissipative effects, the latter result from effects of the inertial and elastic components of the system. In such cases the matching transformer is also more complex than the simple lever system of Fig. 1. Impedance and impedance matching is

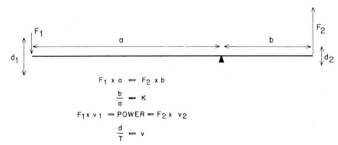

$$F_1 \times a = F_2 \times b$$

$$\frac{b}{a} = K$$

$$F_1 \times v_1 = POWER = F_2 \times v_2$$

$$\frac{d}{T} = v$$

FIG. 1. A lever of the first class. Functional relationships as shown. An ideal, i.e. *massless*, lever would be the equivalent of a transformer in a purely resistive system. (Adapted from Tonndorf and Khanna, 1970.)

more fully discussed by Guillemin (1963) and by Ware and Reed (1949).

Real transformers cannot be made without mass and elasticity; these two factors generally limit the useful frequency range. There is also friction present with its resultant losses. A full understanding of such transformer systems can only be gained by *network analysis*. Its description is beyond the scope of the present chapter. Such analyses pertaining to the middle ear were performed by Onchi (1961), Zwislocki (1962) and Møller (1963).

Since the impedance of the internal ear is very high compared to that of air, impedance matching is necessary for maximal transfer of energy to the internal ear. This impedance matching is accomplished in many stages taking place in all three parts of the ear. The transformer function of the outer ear was first described by Wiener and Ross

(1946); that of the middle ear was first recognized by Weber (1851)—it might have been known earlier; and finally that of the internal ear became evident from Békésy's* studies (1953).

TRANSFORMER MECHANISM—OUTER EAR

The transformer action starts even before the ear canal is reached. Diffraction around the head and the auricle increases the sound pressure at the entrance of the ear canal slightly over that in a free field (Wiener and Ross,

TRANSFORMER MECHANISM—MIDDLE EAR

Sound, after entering the ear canal is received by the tympanic membrane (TM) and the *manubrium mallei* and thus converted into mechanical vibrations, which are then transmitted through the ossicular chain to the oval window.

Three Transformers

The transformer action of the middle ear takes place in three stages: (1) the curved membrane mechanism of the TM, (2) the ossicular lever and (3) the area ratio: TM/

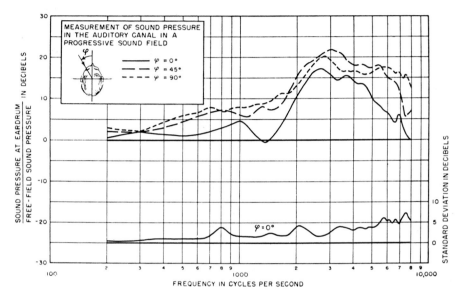

FIG. 2. Ratios of sound pressure at the tympanic membrane to those in a free-field at a place in the centre of an observer's head. Average values for 6 to 12 observers as functions of frequency. The difference between azimuths enables a person to discriminate between fore and aft in order to resolve the ambiguity when listening to broad-band (click) signals. (From Wiener and Ross, 1946.)

1946; Wiener *et al.*, 1966). The auricle (pinna) collects sound in the manner of a horn. However, each of its many convolutions has filter characteristics of its own, and because of the highly asymmetrical form of the auricle these characteristics change sharply with the angle of incidence in a predictable manner (Shaw, 1972).

Like any tube-like structure the external canal has a resonance point which for human ears (canal length of approximately 3·5 cm) happens to be at 4 kHz. Due to this resonance, the ear canal acts as a transformer over a limited frequency range.

Figure 2 shows the combined effects of head, pinna and canal resonances for three different angles of incidence. In front of the tympanic membrane, there is a slight gain in sound pressure over that in a free field at the expense of velocity. Maximal gain is approximately 20 dB at 3 kHz, but it varies widely both with frequency and angle of incidence.

stapes base (footplate). Their contributions are integrated in a complicated manner.

Curved Membrane Mechanism (Helmholtz)

Due to the curvature of the TM the force acting on the malleus is increased over that acting on the TM. That is to say, larger displacements in the centre of each membrane section on both sides of the manubrium are exchanged for smaller displacements of the manubrium itself (Fig. 3).

This principle was originally proposed by Helmholtz (1868). It was thought to be invalidated by the experimental findings of Békésy (1941) and of Wever and Lawrence (1954). However, in recent holographic experiments performed in cats, it was reconfirmed in both living and fresh cadavers, and in human cadavers (Khanna, 1970; Khanna and Tonndorf, 1972; Tonndorf and Khanna, 1970; Tonndorf and Khanna, 1972).

Figure 4 shows a series of displacement profiles across the TM at a low frequency. Consider especially profile no. 2. The displacement amplitude of the malleus is seen to be smaller than that of the membrane on either side, as had been predicated by Helmholtz. (For actual

---

* Békésy's contribution are too numerous to be listed individually. References will therefore be made to his book: *Experiments on Hearing*, a compilation of all his papers up to 1960. The reference number refers to the numerical listing of his own bibliography in that book.

holographic records cf. Fig. 7 below.) This part of the transformer ratio is small. For cats it was estimated to be equal to 2·0.

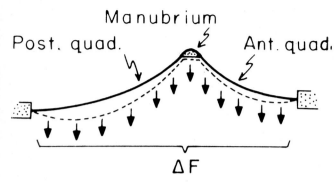

FIG. 3. The Helmholtz concept of TM displacement (schematic). A cross-section through the TM shows greater displacements of lesser force in the centre of each membrane section and smaller displacements of greater force of the manubrium. (Adapted from Tonndorf and Khanna, 1970.)

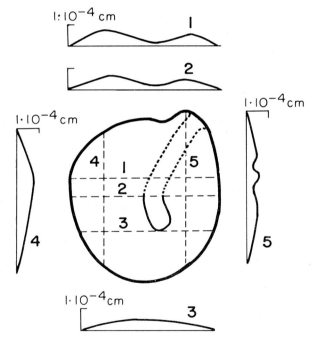

FIG. 4 Displacement profiles of the right tympanic membrane of a fresh human cadaver, measured by time-averaged holography (991 Hz, 111 dB SPL). The outline of the malleus as indicated. The profiles shown around the tympanic membrane were measured along the interrupted lines of corresponding numbers. Displacements in the posterior segments were invariably larger than those in the anterior one. Note the difference in displacement between the membrane, in both segments, and the malleus along profile no. 2, which confirms Helmholtz's concept of Fig. 3. The present schematic outline disregards the curvature of the tympanic membrane. (From Tonndorf and Khanna, 1972.)

The two-dimensional presentation of Fig. 4 might give the misleading impression that the areas of maximal displacement of the TM carry the main burden of the transformer process. The TM is curved in a complex manner (Fig. 5A), and the transformer ratio of a curved membrane varies with inverse curvature. Figures 5B and C then suggest that there is a reciprocal relationship. For each place along the manubrium the product of the curved membrane lever and of the ossicular lever might be constant—or nearly so. Hence the entire TM should contribute to the transformer process.

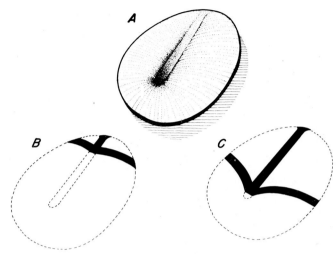

FIG. 5. *Pars tensa* of a cat's left tympanic membrane. Drawing A: Due to its cone shape, the curvature, both anteriorly and posteriorly, increases systematically along the malleus, becoming largest in the inferior quadrant. Drawings B and C indicate, somewhat schematically, the reciprocal relationship between the curved-membrane transformer and the ossicular one (as given below) for two different points along the manubrium. (From Tonndorf and Khanna, 1970.)

Ossicular Lever

At audiofrequencies, the malleus and incus vibrate as a unit around a common axis as shown in Fig. 6 (Bárány, 1938); they stay in phase (Tonndorf and Khanna, 1967), moving the stapes in and out of the oval window.

Traditionally, the ossicular-lever ratio was measured from the tip of the manubrium to the lenticular process (Wever and Lawrence, 1954; Guinan and Peake, 1967; Tonndorf and Khanna, 1967). This concept implies that the centre of the force acting on the TM lies at the umbo. In reality the transfer of force from the TM onto the manubrium is distributed along its entire length (cf. Fig. 5). Hence each point along the manubrium had its own lever ratio. In cats, where more precise data were at hand, the "effective" lever ratio was calculated; it turned out to be a "mere" 1·2 instead of the "full" value of 2·2 or 2·5 (Khanna, 1970; Khanna and Tonndorf, 1972). In man even the "full" ossicular-lever ratio is very small i.e. only 1·3 (Dahmann, 1929–30). Thus, the effective lever ratio must be expected to be even smaller—possibly smaller than one.

Area Ratio: Tympanic Membrane/Stapes Base (Footplate)

Pressure equals force per unit area. Therefore, in the transmission of force from the larger TM to the smaller stapes base the pressure is increased. However, the

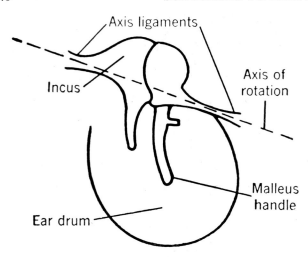

FIG. 6. The two major ossicles and their common axis of rotation. This concept, revival of that of Ed. Weber (1851), was presented by Barany (1938). It replaced Helmholtz's (1863) notion, according to which malleus and incus would operate in phase opposition due to a cog-like action of the incudo-mallear joint. The masses of the mallear head and the incudal body counterbalance the long processes of both ossicles. Therefore, their common centre of gravity is very close to their axis of rotation and the moment of inertia is small, a fact that extends high-frequency transmission.

The recent holographic findings demonstrated that the TM does not vibrate like a stiff plate. Hence, the area ratio had to be re-evaluated. As Fig. 5 indicated, the entire TM contributes to the ossicular displacement; consequently the full area ratio must be taken into account (Khanna and Tonndorf, 1972). Its value for cats, according to anatomical measurements of Wever and Lawrence (1954), is 34·6.

High frequency Responses

Patterns of the TM vibration at higher frequencies were first recorded with the aid of the holographic method. Figure 7 shows that, at low frequencies, the vibratory pattern of the TM is uniform; above a frequency of approximately 3 kHz the pattern breaks up and increases in complexity with further increases in frequency (Khanna, 1970; Khanna and Tonndorf, 1972; Tonndorf and Khanna, 1972). Similar changes in pattern occur in all vibrating membranes at higher frequencies (Rayleigh, 1877).

For a given volume displacement of the TM the mallear displacement becomes smaller and smaller above 3 kHz, indicating that the malleus becomes gradually decoupled from the TM. It appears that, above 4 kHz, only the manubrium and the area immediately around it is effective in transmitting the received energy onto the ossicular chain. The remainder of the TM may then act merely as a baffle (Tonndorf and Khanna, 1970).

These changes with frequency affect the numerical values of all three transformer ratios. For low frequencies Table 1 summarizes their values as assessed in cats. However, the point must be made that these values represent nothing more than current best estimates. The quantities in ques-

pressure increase would be proportional to the area ratio only if the TM and stapes base were both vibrating in a piston-like manner. If this is not so corrections have to be applied to take the exact modes of vibrations into account.

Until recently the TM had been considered to vibrate like a stiff plate rotating around a hinge, the axis of ossicular

TABLE 1

A summary of the concepts of the middle-ear transformer action.

Component of the middle-ear trans-former ratio	Author	Earlier concept		Numerical value	Present concept		Numerical value
		Definition			Definition		
Area ratio	von Békésy (1941) Wever and Lawrence (1954)	$\frac{2}{3}$ Area of TM / Area of footplate		24.3	Area of TM / Area of footplate		36.5
Ossicular lever ratio	Wever and Lawrence (1954)	Displacement mallar tip / Displacement stapes		2.5	Force acting on malleus / Force acting on stapes		1.2
Curved membrane ratio	Helmholtz (1868)	Force acting on TM / Force acting on malleus		Not determined	Force acting on TM / Force acting on malleus		2.0
Force transformation ratio	Wever and Lawrence (1954)	Force acting on footplate / Force acting on TM		Orig. value 60.7 Revised value 31.5 (see text)	Force acting on footplate / Force acting on TM		87.6

rotation, located superiorly (cf. Fig. 6). This mode of vibration required a loose "lower fold". Since the latter would not be coupled to the stiff portion of the TM, it could not contribute to the ossicular displacement (Békésy, 1941). Therefore, the concept of an "effective" area ratio was introduced. Its magnitude was given as approximately 2/3 of the total area ratio (Békésy, 1941; Wever and Lawrence, 1954).

tion are not directly measurable, especially at high frequencies. The clinical implications of this concept have previously been discussed (Tonndorf et al., 1971).

Middle ear Transformer Ratio in Man

The only quantitative assessment of the middle ear transformer ratio in man is that by Békésy (1941). The results of an experiment conducted in a cadaver ear are

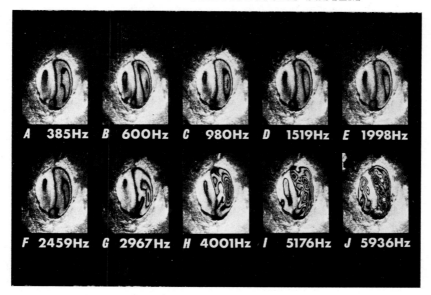

FIG. 7. Time-averaged holography: Vibration patterns of a left feline tympanic membrane at ten different frequencies. This technique generates alternating bright and dark *fringe lines*, each of them representing a *iso-amplitude contour*. These patterns must be read like geodesic maps. The relation between fringe lines and amplitude is not a linear one; it is given by a zero-order Bessel function. For a helium–neon laser, as was used here, the first dark fringe represents a displacement amplitude of 1.92×10^{-5} cm. In order to know the exact order of fringe lines, one has to take a series of about 8 to 12 holograms in each situation, i.e., for each frequency in the present case, at intervals of 2 dB or less. On the tympanic membrane, the lowest-order fringes are of course located at the periphery. Present photographs were selected with the first dark fringe just reaching the tip of the manubrium, the blank strip running vertically down from the top a little left, off-centre. (Note that 600 Hz falls slightly short in this respect.) At low frequencies, there are two broad displacement maxima, anteriorly and posteriorly of the manubrium, in line with the findings of Fig. 4. Above 3 kHz, the tympanic membrane starts breaking up into sectional vibrations: their complexity increases with further increases in frequency. (From Khanna and Tonndorf, 1972.)

given in Fig. 8. The ratio was 20 dB at low frequencies, rising gradually to a maximum of 26 dB just above 2 kHz.

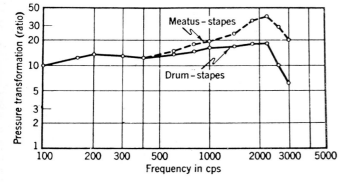

FIG. 8. Pressure transformation in the middle ear for various frequencies in a human cadaver specimen. The ratios given represent the gain in pressure at the stapes over that at the entrance of the ear canal or the tympanic membrane, respectively. The divergence of the two curves at higher frequencies is due to the canal resonance shown above in present Fig. 2. The latter was said to contribute to the transformer action of the external ear. In the actual experiment, sound pressure was applied spontaneously to the ear canal and the backside of the stapes through the vestibule opened for that purpose. Amplitudes and phases were adjusted until the ossicles came to a standstill ("cancellation"). Then, the pressure ratio was read. (From Békésy, 1941.)

Middle ear Network

If the middle ear consisted of nothing but the three transformers described above, and if all three were ideal transformers, then the internal ear impedance, when seen from the middle ear side, should appear smaller, in proportion to the square of the transformer ratio, k^2.

Under such conditions, a stapedial fixation should produce at least a tenfold increase in the measured middle-ear impedance. An ossicular discontinuity ought to reduce the middle ear impedance to a mere fraction of its normal value.

Zwislocki (1961), using an impedance bridge of his own design, obtained such measurements (Fig. 9). Changes occurred in the right direction, but, surprisingly, they were much smaller than those which were to be expected from the above argument. Such measurements, in combination with anatomical considerations led to the design of equivalent networks of the middle ear (Onchi, 1961; Zwislocki, 1961; Møller, 1963). These are complicated networks, a fact which implies that changes in impedance of only one component, namely that of the internal ear as seen from the middle ear side, are masked by the fixed values of the other components.

The network representation also shows that the middle ear dissipates part of the energy received by the TM. This latter portion of the energy is not delivered to the internal ear.

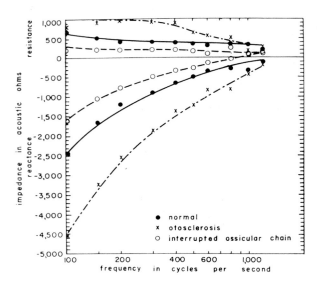

FIG. 9. The resistive and reactive components of middle ear impedances presented separately: (a) in a normal ear; (b) in the presence of stapedial fixation (otosclerosis); and (c) in the presence of an ossicular discontinuity. Results were obtained in absolute terms, i.e., in acoustic Ohms (dynes × sec × cm⁻⁵) by means of the Zwislocki impedance bridge. (From Zwislocki, 1961.)

Middle ear Transfer Function and Their Relation to the Auditory Threshold

Displacement Transfer Function

The middle ear function is most conveniently assessed by measuring the displacement of any given structure for a constant sound pressure. Results assessed for various frequencies are then expressed as a *displacement transfer function*. Several examples of such functions pertaining to the middle ear are presented in Fig. 10. The displacement is seen to be frequency independent in the low frequency range, but decreases with the frequency squared above approximately 1·5 kHz.

These curves are generally accepted as indicating that the middle ear lets low frequencies pass unattenuated, but that it attenuates high frequencies. In other words, the middle ear is held to act as a low-pass filter. In contrast, the auditory threshold curve has a downward slope at low frequencies, a fact that cannot be explained on the basis of the above displacement transfer functions.

Power Transfer Function

The purpose of the middle ear, as will be recalled, is to transfer the maximum of the power it receives to the internal ear. The acoustic power at any frequency is given as the product of sound pressure, velocity and the cosine of the phase angle between them at that frequency. Displacement by itself is not a measure of power. [See Khanna and Tonndorf (1969) *Arch Klin. Exp. Ohr, Nas-Kehlk.,* **193,** 78.] An example of a power transfer function for a human ear is given in Fig. 11; it was calculated

from data collected by Zwislocki (1962). Results are plotted onto the human auditory threshold curve. The fact that the agreement is reasonably good shows that the middle

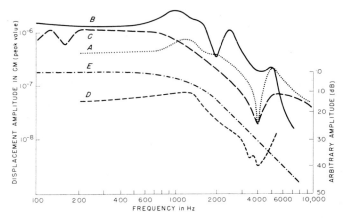

FIG. 10. *Displacement transfer functions* representing peak displacement amplitudes as a function of frequency in response to a r.m.s. sound pressure of 0·1 pascal (one dyne/cm²). The five curves, which show essentially good agreement, were obtained by various authors using different methods of assessment. Curve A: Guinan and Peake (1967)—direct observation; Curve B: Tonndorf and Khanna (1967)—substitution method; Curve C: Tonndorf and Khanna (1968a)—laser interferometry; Curve D: Møller (1963)—condenser probe; Curve E: Flanagan (1962)—data computed from Zwislocki's (1962) impedance measurements. With the exception of curve D and E, all are plotted in absolute terms. (From Tonndorf and Khanna, 1968a.)

ear is largely responsible for the shape of the threshold curve. It also argues for the contention that hair cell stimulation depends upon the power delivered to their sites.

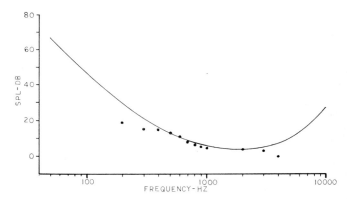

FIG. 11. *Power transfer function* calculated from Zwislocki's (1962) impedance data and inverted to fit the human auditory threshold curve. The systematic deviations at low frequencies were due to the fact that the underlying calculations did not take account of the low-frequency attenuation caused by the oval window (cf. Fig. 12). (From Khanna, unpublished, 1972.)

Internal ear Impedance

Since the external and middle ears serve to match the impedance of air to that of the internal ear, it is essential to know the impedance of the latter.

In addition to obtaining the results given in Fig. 8, Békésy (1941) measured the displacement amplitude of the stapes for a constant sound pressure at the TM. However, the latter amplitudes are too high, since in order to do these experiments he had to drain the fluid from the internal ear. From these results of Békésy's, Wever and Lawrence (1954) calculated the internal ear impedance of the human ear. Their results are given in Fig. 12, curve A. These values are too small for the reasons just given.

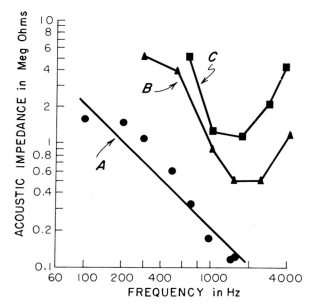

FIG. 12. Acoustic impedance of the internal ear. Curve A: Calculated by Wever and Lawrence (1954) from human data of Békésy's (1941[38]) such as those given in present Fig. 2. The line approximating these values has a slope of two to one per octave. Curves B and C: Measured by means of time-averaged holography of round-window displacements in two live cats (data from Khanna and Tonndorf, 1971); the sound was applied to the oval window in a closed system.

In cats, internal ear impedances were assessed in a direct manner with the aid of two different techniques: condenser probe (Tonndorf *et al.*, 1966) and holography (Khanna and Tonndorf, 1971). The low frequency slope of the resulting curves (Fig. 12 curves B and C) was similar to that of the curve obtained by Wever and Lawrence, but absolute values were higher by about one order of magnitude.

These results, together with data on the middle ear impedance in cats (Møller, 1963), were utilized to calculate the middle ear transformer ratio (Table 2). These calculations are only approximate. They rest upon two simplifying assumptions: (1) that the system is purely resistive and (2) that perfect matching occurs at all frequencies.

The negative slope of the impedance curves B and C of Fig. 12 was obtained only when the stapes base (footplate) was left intact. After its removal the low frequency slope became inverted, but the values at frequencies between approximately 2 and 4 kHz were hardly affected (Tonndorf *et al.*, 1966). These findings indicate that, at low frequencies, the internal ear impedance is dominated by the reactive component, stiffness controlled with the stapes base intact, and mass controlled after its removal.

TABLE 2

Inner ear impedance of cat, its middle-ear impedance, and ideal transformer ratio for matching.

Frequency (Hz)	Inner-ear impedance $\times 10^6$ (cgs units)	Middle-ear impedance (cgs units)	Impedance ratio	Ideal transformer ratio
200	6.0	1585	3.8×10^3	62
400	4.2	767	5.4×10^3	73.5
800	2.1	422	5.0×10^3	71.0
1000	1.7	422	4.2×10^3	65.0
2000	1.2	380	3.2×10^3	57.0
3000	1.9	485	3.9×10^3	63.0
4000	1.3	317	4.1×10^3	64.0

The low frequency data of Fig. 11 appertaining to the power entering the ear deviated systematically from the threshold curve. This deviation is due to the fact that the low frequency attenuation caused by the oval window (cf. Fig. 12) was not taken into account. The functional significance of this low-frequency slope may be in preventing low frequency sounds from masking high-frequency signals.

INTERNAL EAR PROTECTION

Protection of the delicate internal ear is another important function of the sturdier middle ear.

Middle ear Muscles

A dynamic protection of this kind is provided by the middle ear muscles. Their reflex contraction on exposure to sound—mainly those of the stapedius—attenuate the transmission of energy through the middle ear (Simmons, 1963). Evidence for the contraction of the *tensor tympani*, long a controversial subject, was recently obtained in human subjects after surgical removal of the stapedius (Weiss *et al.*, 1962). For further details on the entire subject, reference must be made to representative monographs (Klockhoff, 1961).

Variable Internal ear Impedance

Another form of internal ear protection was suggested by the holographic studies on internal ear impedance (Khanna and Tonndorf, 1971). Data were assessed at high SPLs, beyond 140 dB at the oval window—for cats this is the equivalent of approximately 100 dB at the TM. Especially at low frequencies, the impedance appeared to increase in some proportion to the applied sound pressure. The phenomenon was only observed in *living* animals. The underlying mechanism is not understood at this time. Nevertheless, this induced increase in internal ear impedance ought to impair the power transfer across the middle ear temporarily by affecting the impedance match ordinarily provided.

Slippage in the Incudo-mallear Joint

A third function of this kind is provided by the incudo-mallear joint. At low frequencies, i.e. below 60 Hz, this joint begins to slip (Fig. 13), thereby reducing the energy flow to the internal ear (Tonndorf and Khanna, 1967). A similar slippage was observed to occur in the incudo-stapedial joint upon contraction of the stapedius muscle (Zwislocki, 1962).

All three forms of internal protection described here are most effective at low frequencies.

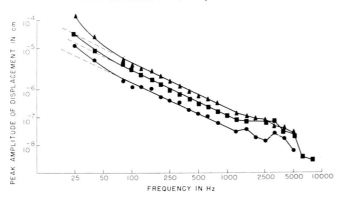

UMBO DISPLACEMENT FOR 10 μV MICROPHONICS

FIG. 13. Displacements of the feline manubrium mallei (in cm) required for a constant cochlear–microphonic response of 10 μV at the round window; frequencies between 25 and 10 000 Hz; results from three animals. The malleus was driven *mechanically* by means of a driving rod cemented firmly to its (denuded) tip. When the same drive system was used on the incus, directly over its lenticular process, the curves, although running at different levels remain perfectly straight down to the lowest frequency tested. Therefore, the deviation from a straight line, starting for all three animals at about 60 Hz and shown in this figure, indicates *slippage* in the incudo-mallear joint. There was a concommitant phase shift (not shown). This phenomenon was observed only in young cats (less than 2·5 kg), but not in older ones (more than 3 kg). (From Tonndorf and Khanna, 1967.)

The Key Properties of the Outer and Middle Ears and Their Implications

The outer and middle ears have three primary functions:

(1) To deliver a maximum of energy to the internal ear for achieving high sensitivity.

(2) To shape the overall frequency response of the ear.

(3) To protect the delicate internal ear against excessive energy inputs.

These tasks are accomplished in the following manner:

(1) (a) The outer and middle ears act as a series of transformers, matching the low impedance of the surrounding air to the higher one of the internal ear. These transformers were artificially separated for the purpose of describing the principles of their operation. However, they function as an integrated system.

(b) In the outer ear the transformer action takes place due to the resonance of the ear canal; in the middle ear it occurs in three stages: (i) the curved membrane mechanism, (ii) the ossicular lever action, (iii) the function of the area ratio, TM to stapes base.

(c) The true representation of the middle ear is that of a complex mechanical network in which optimal matching is only achieved over a limited frequency band (1–3 kHz).

(2) The crucial measure in any detector system is the energy delivered to it. The auditory threshold curve follows closely the power function of the middle ear.

(3) The middle ear must match efficiently at low signal levels. At higher levels the internal ear must be protected against overload. Such protection is accomplished by mismatching or partial decoupling. The protection is largest for low frequencies.

INTERNAL EAR

Place/Resonance Theory (Helmholtz)

The first serious attempt to formulate a hypothesis on mechanical cochlear functions was made by Helmholtz (1863). He based his *Place/Resonance Theory* on the fact that the transverse fibres of the basilar membrane increase systematically in length with distance from base to apex; he postulated that these fibres should be under some tension, and that each of them could be tuned to a different frequency. The resonant frequency would then be roughly an inverse function of the distance from the base. Expressed differently, basal fibres should resonate for high frequencies, whereas low frequencies should produce such resonances closer to the apex.

First support for the place principle came from cochlear histopathology. The absence of hair cells in the basal turn was found to be well correlated with high frequency hearing loss (Habermann, 1890; Crowe *et al.*, 1934). For apical lesions and low frequencies the correlation was less clear. (A more extensive list of other supporting pieces of evidence will be presented in Fig. 15 below.)

Helmholtz's theory can therefore be divided into two parts: (1) The *Place Principle* and (2) the *Resonance Mechanism*. The latter was not supported by later findings.

Travelling wave Concept (Békésy)

Békésy was the first to employ an experimental approach (Békésy, 1928). In the *first direct measurements* on the cochlea he confirmed the elastic nature of the membrane postulated by Helmholtz—but he did not find any tension in the transverse fibres, as required by Helmholtz's theory. Instead, he found that its stiffness varies from the base, where it is high, to the apex, where it is low: the *stiffness gradient* of the basilar membrane.

He incorporated these propoerties into mechanical cochlear models. Observation in such models led to a first understanding of the *travelling wave* phenomenon, which was then confirmed in further studies on cadaver ears from humans as well as from several different animals (Békésy, 1944) and finally in the ears of living guinea pigs (Békésy, 1952; Perlman, 1950).

According to Békésy's observations (1928) the travelling wave phenomenon is mainly determined by the properties of the basilar membrane. Therefore, the term *cochlear partition* was introduced.

The travelling waves (Fig. 14) represent displacements of the cochlear partition. They invariably progress from base to apex. For sine wave inputs, all points along the basilar membrane vibrate at the input frequency. The travel speed of these waves *decrease* continuously with distance, while the displacement amplitude gradually *increases*. After reaching a maximum, amplitude decreases rather abruptly.

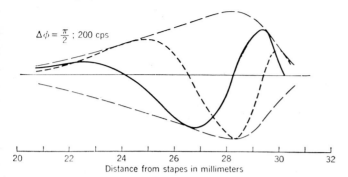

FIG. 14. Travelling-wave patterns in response to a frequency of 200 Hz observed in the cochlea of a human cadaver; displacements: arbitrary scale and overstated for the sake of presentation. The dotted outline occurred half a period after the solid one; thus waves travel from base to apex. Note the gradual decrease of wavelength with distance. The outline (*envelope*) shown by the interrupted lines, gives the long-time average of wave crests, positive or negative one, at each point. It forms a maximum—in the present case slightly beyond 28 *mm*. Later observations (Békésy, 1954[71]; Tonndorf, 1970b) have indicated that the point of termination of the wave pattern at its apical end (on the right of this figure) depends upon the resolving power of the method of observation. Waves continue to become smaller and shorter with distance of travel. (From Békésy, 1947[47].)

The location of amplitude maxima in response to sine-wave signals were found to be frequency dependent in accordance with the place principle (Fig. 15). That is to say, the location of the maxima varied systematically from base to apex as the frequency was lowered. In this

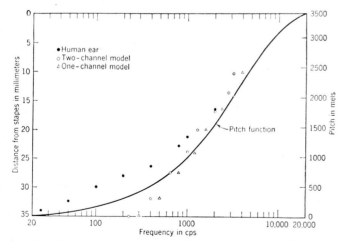

FIG. 15. Place *vs* frequency for the amplitude maxima of travelling waves. Data obtained in different situations (models and cadaver ears) are plotted on the "pitch function" (pitch *vs* frequency) developed by Stevens and Volkmann (1940). This map is in essential agreement with a number of independent findings derived from other fields of inquiry: (1) maximal cochlear–microphonic responses (Tasaki *et al.*, 1952; Dallos *et al.*, 1971); (2) correlation between audiometric high-tone losses and post-mortem findings (Crowe, Guild and Polvogt, 1934); (3) integration of pitch jnds (Stevens *et al.*, 1935); (4) critical band data (Fletcher, 1951; Scharf, 1970); (5) contributions of various frequencies to total loudness (Fletcher, 1951); (6) contributions of various frequencies to speech intelligibility (French and Steinberg, 1947). (From Békésy, 1951[51].)

respect Helmholtz's original hypothesis was upheld, but the mechanism upon which it was based, the resonance mechanism, was replaced by the travelling wave mechanism.

So far, the travelling wave phenomenon was described here in terms of basilar membrane displacements, occurring as a function of distance and time. There is another way of looking at the same phenomenon. Measurements of displacement may also be taken at a given place, while the frequency is being varied. The results are expressed as *resonance* or *tuning* curves. Several examples are presented in Fig. 16.

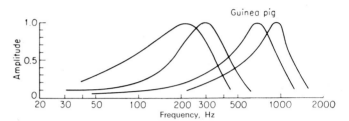

FIG. 16. Tuning curves along the cochlear partition of a guinea pig. In contrast to the *envelope* of Fig. 14, which gave long-term-average amplitude *vs distance*, these curves represent amplitude *vs frequency* for given places of observation. Maximal amplitudes were arbitrarily set to unity. Note the gradual "sharpening" of the curves from left (low-frequency region) to right (higher-frequency region). (From Békésy, 1944[45].)

Travelling Waves: Supporting Evidence

Because of technical limitations Békésy's observations required very high sound pressure levels and were limited to the apical cochlear turn. That travelling waves occur also at lower, physiological levels was first shown by recording cochlear microphonic responses at several places along the cochlea (Tasaki *et al.*, 1952). Such responses, obtained at sound pressure levels (SPL) of about 60 dB, displayed the pertinent aspects of mechanical travelling waves.

Békésy's measurements were recently confirmed with the aid of two new techniques applying (1) the Mössbauer effect (Johnstone and Boyle, 1967; Johnstone *et al.*, 1970; Rhode, 1971) and (2) the speckle pattern of a laser beam (Kohllöffel, 1972). Resonance curves thus obtained at higher frequencies (Fig. 17) were narrower than Békésy's low frequency curves (cf. Fig. 16). It must be emphasized, however, that this "sharpening" was already evident in Békésy's own data (Tonndorf and Khanna, 1968b).

For the discussion on the analysis of the travelling wave phenomenon reference should be made to the publications of Békésy (1956), of Zwislocki (1965) and of Tonndorf (1970, 1973).

Shearing Displacements Between the Spiral Organ and the Tectorial Membrane

Displacements of the basilar membrane do not stimulate the hair cells directly. Hair cells generally respond to a lateral deflection of their hairs (von Holst, 1950).

While the basilar membrane is fixed along both rims, the tectorial membrane is fixed only at its medial rim. The hairs of cochlear hair cells are attached to the underside of the tectorial membrane. Therefore, a *vertical* displacement of the basilar membrane must produce a net *sliding*

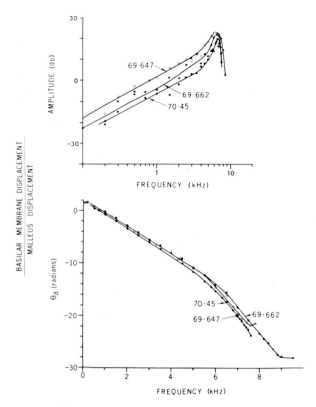

FIG. 17. Tuning curves measured with the aid of the Mössbauer effect for three different squirrel monkeys at a basal place that responded maximally to about 8 kHz and was located a few mm from the stapes. Data were taken at 85 dB SPL and are expressed in terms of uniform amplitude of the malleus. Note the "sharpness" of the maximum compared to those of Fig. 16 which had been obtained at more apical places (from Rhode, 1971). For the guinea pig similar findings had been reported (Johnstone *et al.*, 1970); the increase in "sharpness" was shown to be a simple function of distance (Tonndorf and Khanna, 1968b).

displacement between the spiral organ and the tectorial membrane, as is schematically shown in Fig. 18. Békésy (1953a) referred to this as a *shearing displacement*.

The above concept (Békésy 1953a; Hilding, 1953) is supported (1) by the fact that the tectorial membrane lies close to the spiral organ (de Vries, 1949; Hilding, 1952) and (2) by the mode of attachment of the sensory hairs to the tectorial membrane (Kimura, 1966; Lim, 1972a; Johnsson, 1973). Only the very tips of the longest hairs, which constitute the outermost row of hairs on each cell, are attached to the underside of the tectorial membrane. On surface preparations, bundles of hairs, both from inner *and* outer hair cells, are occasionally seen clinging to the tectorial membrane (Johnsson, 1973). Scanning electron-microscopy has so far demonstrated such attachments for the hairs of *outer* hair cells only (Lim, 1972a).

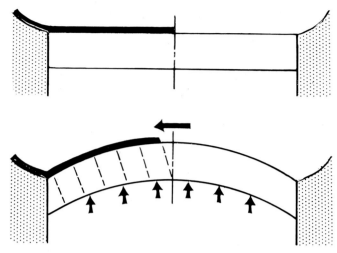

FIG. 18. Above: Cross-sectional "model" of the spiral organ and the tectorial membrane. A soft pad, the basilar membrane and the organ is fastened at both ends and covered by a stiff layer; the tectorial membrane that is fastened on one end only. Below: Upon displacement of the whole structure in an upward direction, shearing displacements occur as indicated. Upon downward displacements, they occur in the opposite direction. Note the increase in force (indicated by the length of the arrow) in the conversion of vertical displacement to shearing displacement to shearing) displacement. From Békésy, 1953[67].)

Two Modes of Shear: Radial and Longitudinal

In the ears of living guinea pigs, Békésy (1953a) observed displacements of the Hensen cells (Fig. 19). Displacements in the plane of the basilar membrane were found to occur in two directions: (1) radial (i.e. transverse) and (2) longitudinal. (The mechanism underlying the radial shear was shown in Fig. 18.) The maximum

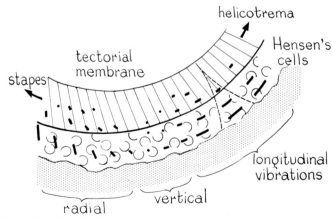

FIG. 19. The distribution of vertical (i.e., travelling-wave) as well as radial and longitudinal shear vibrations along a section of the spiral organ of a guinea pig for a low-frequency tone, as seen through the vestibular (Reissner's) membrane. (From Békésy, 1953[67].)

displacement in the radial direction occurred in the region proximal to that of the travelling wave and the maximum displacement in the longitudinal direction just beyond that point.

Why were there different modes of shear in two separate locations? Figure 20 shows that, in the region *proximal* to the travelling-wave maximum, the dominant curvature runs in the *radial* direction, whereas in the region distal to that point it runs in the longitudinal direction. Since shear is proportional to the underlying curvature, Fig. 20 accounts for the prevalence of each mode in its particular region (Tonndorf, 1960).

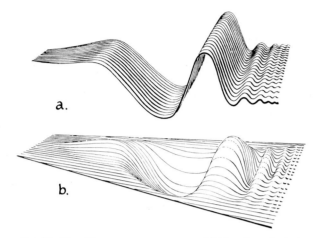

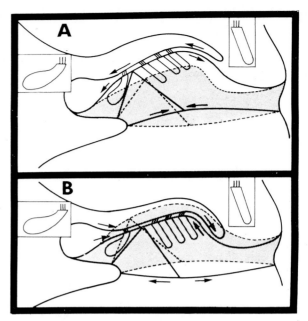

Fig. 20. Travelling-wave pattern executed (a) by a hypothetical ribbon-like partition and (b) by one restained along both of its rims. Scales are arbitrary and magnitudes are greatly exaggerated. (From Tonndorf, 1960.)

Fig. 21. Schematic cross-section of the spiral organ, illustrating shearing stresses (indicated by arrows) in the transverse direction and the displacement of the sensory hairs thus produced. In (A) the basilar membrane is displaced upward, in (B), downward. In both instances, the opposite position of the organ is indicated by overlays. Note the different tendency in shearing stresses across the reticular membrane/tectorial membrane discontinuity in the region of the *outer* hair cells (opposite tendency) and of the *inner* hair cells (*same* tendency). This difference is due to the different types of suspension of the two structures as commented on in Fig. 18 above. Consequently, the effect of radial shear is *maximal* upon the hairs of the *outer* hair cells, but *minimal* upon the hairs of the *inner* hair cells. The experiment underlying the construction of the present figure revealed that the shearing displacement on either side of the displacement maximum of the whole structure were in phase opposition. This was to be expected from considerations of Fig. 18. In an experiment performed by D. J. Lim (1972b) at the request of the present authors, fixation of the organ in the state of downward deflection, induced by hydrostatic pressure, showed phase-opposite deflections of the sensory hairs on inner and outer hair cells as indicated in the present figure. Another similar set of schematic figures presented earlier by Davis (1960) did not reveal this differential effect upon outer and inner hair cells. The reason is that the different kinds of suspension of the basilar membrane and tectorial membrane (cf. Fig. 18) had not been taken into account. (From Tonndorf, 1970c.)

Two Shear Modes: Electrophysiological and Anatomical Considerations

In cochlear microphonic experiments Békésy (1953b) obtained maximal outputs in response to radial shear at the outer margin of the tectorial membrane and in response to longitudinal shear at its inner margin. This evidence indicates that, most likely, the *outer* hair cells respond to *radial* shear and the *inner* ones to longitudinal shear. Considerations based on a mechanical model that illustrates the fact that radial shear stimulates mainly the outer hair cells (Fig. 21) supports this viewpoint (Tonndorf, 1970b).

However, this view is hard to reconcile with other findings: (1) Vestibular hair cells could only be excited by a deflection of their sensory hairs toward, or away from, their kinocilia (Löwenstein and Wersäll, 1959; Flock, 1971)—the basal body of cochlear hair cells—and (2) all cochlear hair cells are polarized in the *radial* direction (Fig. 22) (Held, 1902). Consequently, *all* hair cells, outer as well as inner, should respond only to radial shear, although in opposite phases (cf. Fig. 21). Nevertheless, Békésy's cochlear microphonic findings (1953) are experimental *facts*. Consequently, the mode of stimulation of inner hair cells is currently an open question.

Hair cell stimulation due to shearing displacements

The height of the sensory hairs on each hair cell decreases systematically in a lateral to medial direction; that is, the tallest hairs are attached to the underside of the tectorial membrane, and then only at their very tips (Kimura, 1966; Spoendlin, 1966). The attachment of the hairs of *inner* hair cells is still being disputed, viz. Lim (1972a) is against attachment; L. G. Johnsson (1973) and

W. Arnold (1974) are in favor of attachment. The experiment of Lim described briefly in the legend to Fig. 21 could also be cited in favor of such an attachment; but then again, their mode of shearing stimulation is not yet understood either (cf. above). Therefore, the following comments are limited to the stimulation of *outer* hair cells.

The above cited structural findings have led to two alternative hypotheses concerning the ultimate mechanical stimulation of hair cells. There are *pro* and *con* arguments with respect to both of them.

The first hypothesis assumes that the hairs are being bent in the shearing displacement, and that such bending will lead to a longitudinal stress in the cell membrane which covers all hairs tightly (Flock, 1973). Such bending has actually been demonstrated by means of slow-acting, hydro-static displacements of the cochlear duct (Lim, 1972a). According to this view, then, the hairs serve merely to enlarge the cell membrane, and to make it more sensitive to such stresses. However, no enzymes have so far been demonstrated in the hairs that could serve the

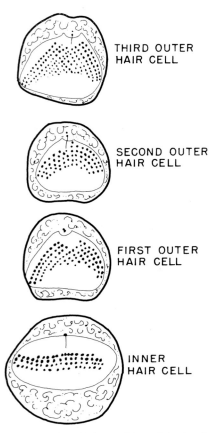

FIG. 22. The relative position of the basal body and the sensory hairs in the four rows of hair cells of the second turn (man). Although the pattern formed by the hairs varies between the outer and inner hair cells (V-, W-, or U-shaped on outer hair cells, but in straight rows on the inner ones), all of them are polarized in the radial direction. (From Held, 1902.)

reception and further transmission of a signal thus generated. Furthermore, Engström and his associates (1962) found the hairs to be rather stiff (actually, brittle) which would make their bending in response to fast-acting audio-frequency signals rather unlikely.

The second hypothesis is based on the anatomical finding that the roots of the sensory hairs are deeply implanted in the cuticular plate. This plate has a sizeable thickness and extends over most of the top of each hair cell (Engström and Wersäll, 1953). It has therefore been suggested (initially by Engström *et al.*, 1962) that the whole tuft of hairs together with the cuticular plate form a rigid lever that is hinged medially, *i.e.*, opposite the "soft" area around the basal body. As is schematically shown in Fig. 23, the hinged displacement of the cuticular plate should *distort* the cytoplasm, especially around the basal

body. According to this view then, it might be the basal body which is the ultimate receptor of mechanical energy in hair cells. [A similar notion was expressed by Hilman and Lewis (1971) with respect to the stimulation of *vestibular* hair cells, a problem that is somewhat different due to the existence of the kinocilium.] Displacements of the basal body region such as those of Fig. 23, *B* and *C* are occasionally observed in electron microscopic pictures (L. G. Johnsson, 1973). The second hypothesis is further supported by the presence of large clumps of mitochondria around the basal body, which would make it suitable for the conversion of the incoming mechanical energy into a receptor potential. The task of the shorter sensory hairs would then be to support and stiffen the tall hairs where they need it most, *i.e.*, just above their roots where the bending moment and the transverse shearing stress should be largest (Tonndorf, 1971). However, Spoendlin (1966) failed to find basal bodies in the hair cells of cats. He also stated that each cuticular plate is very tightly connected by desmosomes to the surrounding phalangeal end plates of Deiters' cells. Thus, he considers the occurrence of such hinged displacements as unlikely.

At present, there is no convincing evidence which would clearly favor one of these hypotheses over the other.

Figure 24 shows that the spatial sharpening takes place mainly on the *proximal* side of the envelope. A computer simulation of longitudinal shear indicated that tuning curves become also more restricted, but only on their *low frequency* sides (Khanna *et al.*, 1968). In other words, the conversion process has the properties of a *high-pass* filter.

On the basis of a comparison between mechanical tuning curves of the basilar membrane, which are relatively broad, and eighth nerve tuning curves, which are narrower, the existence of such a high-pass filter was recently postulated (Evans and Wilson, 1973).

It appears that the mechanical sharpening due to the shear conversion may be sufficient to account for the sharp tuning curves observed in the eighth nerve fibres.

The Key Properties of the Internal Ear and Their Implications

(1) The properties of travelling waves may be summarized as follows:

(a) The cochlear displacement waves travel from base to apex.

(b) Their travel speed slows down continuously from base to apex; for sine wave inputs this can be expressed as a progressive phase delay.

(c) For sine wave responses there are two kinds of envelopes that can be measured—(i) *spatial* (time/distance); they build up gradually with distance and decay sharply; furthermore they are narrow for high frequencies and wide for low frequencies; (ii) *resonance* or *tuning* curves; their low frequency slopes are invariably less steep than their high frequency slopes; they are also narrower for high frequencies and wider for low frequencies.

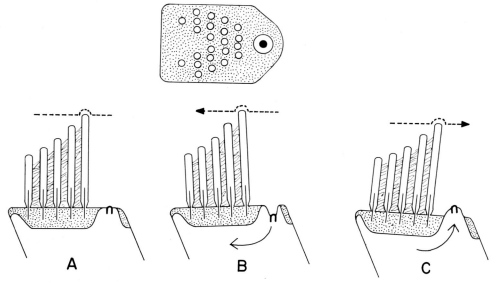

FIG. 23. The lever-like deflection of the sensory hairs and the cuticular plate and the resulting mechanical distortion of the basal body (second hypothesis). Amplitudes are grossly overstated. A: Situation at rest; B: deflection toward the modiolus; C: deflection in the lateral direction. Note the resulting cytoplasmic displacements away from or toward the area around the basal body (arrows). The hairs are interconnected by an amorphous (Lim, 1972a) or fibrous (Flock, 1973) material, facilitating the displacement shown in C. The drawing on top is a surface view of the cuticular plate (schematic after Spoendlin, 1966). Note that the "soft" area around the basal body is completely surrounded by the cuticular plate.

(2) The properties of shear waves may be summarized as follows:

(a) In the conversion from travelling waves to shear waves, an internal ear transformer action becomes apparent; it magnitude is approximately ten, and it contributes to the impedance matching between the basilar membrane and the hair cells.

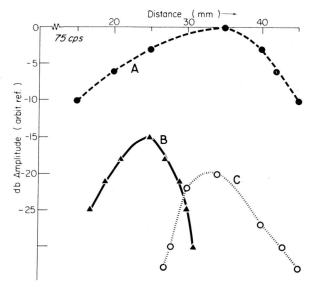

FIG. 24. Envelopes over (a) the travelling wave; (b) radial shear; and (c) longitudinal shear in a cochlear model. The amplitude is given in log terms, and that of the travelling wave is arbitrarily set to unity. The amplitude of both modes of shear is seen to be reduced by 15 to 20 dB (transformer action!). Moreover, the shear envelopes are restricted in length, i.e. made "sharper", due to the change in slope of their proximal legs (Tonndorf, 1960).

(b) Compared to the travelling wave envelopes the shear wave envelopes are much more localized spatially, and the resonance curves are sharpened in frequency.

(c) The travel direction of shear waves is the same as that of travelling waves.

(d) The significance of the two modes of shear is not clear, except that the results of Békésy's microphonic experiments (1953b) argue for a different effect on inner and outer hair cells.

(3) These phenomena taken together have the following consequences for the stimulation of hair cells and the triggering of nerve impulses by them:

(a) The fact that spatial envelopes become narrower with frequency may explain (i) the good correlation between localized lesions in the basal turn and high-frequency hearing losses and (ii) the much poorer correlation between apical lesions and low frequency hearing losses (Schuknecht, 1953).

(b) The fact that mechanical displacement varies, under the shear envelope means that the cells undergoing the largest displacements will cause higher neural firing rates than do those undergoing smaller displacements. Near threshold, this implies that hair cells in only a narrow range around the place of maximum displacement have large enough displacements to trigger nerve firings and that this area will broaden as intensity increases.

(c) The direction of wave travel both in the travelling wave and the shear wave, means that, in response to a click, basilar hair cells evoke nerve firings invariably earlier than cells in more apical regions.

(d) The consequence of the variations in travel speed along the partition is that the sequence of neural firing evoked by a row of basal hair cells is faster than that evoked by a comparable row of apical hair cells; consequently, neural responses from basal fibres sum up to a higher value than those from apical fibres.

THE EAR AS A DETECTOR

Time/Frequency Analysis

Sound was said to consist of small vibratory changes in air pressure, varying as a function of time. In some such *waveforms*, for example of sine waves, the long term average amplitude does not change with time (*steady-state* events). In others, for example, of short lasting speech sounds, there are characteristic changes of the waveform with time: *time varying* events. Hidden in either type is information that a receiver must *detect*. The are two basic methods for such a detection, i.e. methods of *signal analysis:* (1) The receiver may look at the amplitude changes of the signal with *time* or (2) it may look at its *frequency spectrum*. In the case of a simple steady-state event, both methods are equally good for analytic purposes. With time-varying events, however, either method alone is of limited value—both of them are needed.

Ohm (1843) and Helmholtz (1863) had postulated that the cochlea acts like a frequency analyzer, a notion that became widely accepted with the discovery of the Place Principle. Later psychophysical (Seebeck, 1843; Schouten, 1938; Backhaus, 1932) and physiological findings (Wever, 1949) indicated that the ear may also make use of time analysis—in fact it employs both methods side by side. For a formal discussion of this *Time/Frequency Analysis* reference should be made to Gabor (1946). An analysis of the responses of mechanical cochlear models confirmed this general concept (Tonndorf, 1962).

The point is occasionally made that the cochlea was not "designed", as it were, to respond to sine-wave signals, since it evolved as a receiver of animal sounds, e.g. speech in the case of man. This comment is not really pertinent. Sine-wave signals are a convenient means for the systematic exploration of the acoustic properties of *any* communication channel. If the responses to sine waves are known, and if the system is linear, the responses to any other signals can be calculated.

A further point must be made here: The messages a given acoustic signal (e.g. speech) may contain are completely unimportant from the standpoint of the function of a receiver such as the cochlea. The message content does only become important in *central* auditory processing—but that was not the subject of the present chapter.

Cochlear Nonlinearities

Psychophysical experience has shown that the ear produces harmonic distortion, and that it detects beats, difference tones, "missing fundamentals", periodicity pitches, etc. Such phenomena can only originate in a *nonlinear* system. Helmholtz was of the opinion that such nonlinearities should arise in the middle ear. Yet, the latter turned out to be a much better device than he had

thought. Its range of linearity extends up to, at least, 140 dB (Guinan and Peake, 1967; Tonndorf and Khanna, 1972).

Evidence accrued over the years pointed strongly to the *cochlea* as the place of origin of some nonlinearities. (Others occur apparently in the neural domain.) Potential sources of internal ear distortion have been recognized in (a) cochlear hydrodynamic processes (Tonndorf, 1970a, 1973); (b) the deflection process of the sensory hairs (Lowenstein and Wersäll, 1959; Flock, 1971) and (c) the process underlying the cochlear microphonics (Dallos and Sweetman, 1969).

In man-made devices the occurrence of distortion is commonly considered a shortcoming, limiting the dynamic range of the system. However, this may not apply to the cochlea in the same manner.

(1) Harmonic distortion resulting from high sound intensities is instrumental in spreading the energy along the cochlear partition, instead of keeping it concentrated in one place, i.e. that of the original frequency (Beck and Michler, 1960; Tonndorf, 1970a, 1973). This mechanism serves to protect the spiral organ.

(2) The nonlinearity may well be an essential part of the encoding process that translates the acoustical signals into nerve impulses.

Sensitivity of the Ear

In the mid-frequency range, where the sensitivity of the ear is maximal, an intensity of only 1 pW.m^{-2} is

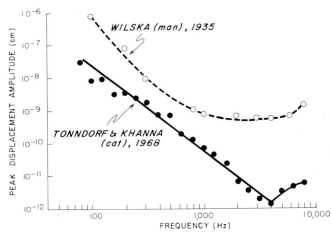

FIG. 25. Displacement amplitude of the tympanic membrane at the threshold of hearing. Wilska (1935) determined thresholds in human observers by means of an electrodynamic mechanism that drove the tympanic membrane. The device had been calibrated at an amplitude of about 10^{-3} cm. Tonndorf and Khanna (1968a) employed laser interferometry, took readings at 10^{-7} cm, and then converted results by using the threshold data of Miller *et al.* (1963). Input/output functions had been found to be linear down to 10^{-9} cm. A previous study in cats (Tonndorf and Khanna, 1967) that had employed a condenser probe on the mallear tip had given very similar results (cf. Fig. 10).

sufficient to evoke a sensation of hearing (Licklider, 1951). Calculations of appropriate noise power levels that were based upon the critical band concept indicated signal-to-noise ratios of approximately 20 dB (Khanna, unpublished, 1972). De Vries (1952) made similar calculations, but they were based upon displacement data. The results of both calculations are in good agreement.

Displacement data for human ears were obtained by Wilska (1935) and by Békésy (1951). In the mid-frequency range displacements of the TM at threshold are of the order of 10^{-9} cm and those of the basilar membrane (for a 200 Hz tone) about 10^{-11} cm. Because of the experimental limitations then existing, it was repeatedly argued that these results might have been much too small, possibly by several orders of magnitude.

In cats direct measurements of TM displacements were recently obtained at very low SPLs (Tonndorf and Khanna, 1968a). Displacements at the cat threshold were calculated with the aid of data provided by Miller et al. (1963). Only small extrapolations were required. Results are shown in Fig. 25, together with those of Wilska. Figure 25 indicates that the magnitudes of displacement of the tympanic membrane at threshold are indeed very low.

This work was supported by NINDS grants Nos. 5 K06 NS 21691 and 2 R01 NB 03654.

REFERENCES

Arnold, W. (1974), Personal Communication.
Backhaus, H. (1932), Z. tech. Phys., 13, 31.
Bárány, E. (1938), Acta oto-laryng., suppl. 26.
Beck, C. and Michler, H. (1960), Arch. Ohr.-, Nas.-u. Kehlk Heilk., 174, 496.
Békésy, G. von (1960), Experiments in Hearing. New York: McGraw-Hill.
Crowe, S. J., Guild, S. R. and Polvogt, L. M. (1934), Johns Hopk. Hosp. Bull., 54, 315.
Dahmann, H. (1929–30), Ztsr. f. Hals usw Heilk., 24, 462; 27, 329.
Dallos, P. and Sweetman, R. H. (1969), J. acoust. Soc. Amer., 45, 37.
Dallos, P., Schoeny, Z. G. and Cheatham, M.A. (1971), J. acoust. Soc. Amer., 49, 1144.
Davis, H. (1960), Neural Mechanisms of the Auditory and Vestibular Systems, p. 21 (B. U. Rasmussen and W. L. Windle, Eds.). Springfield, Illinois, U.S.A.: Chas. C. Thomas.
Engström, H. and Wersäll, J. (1953), Acta oto-laryng., 43, 323.
Engström, H., Ades, H. W. and Hawkins, J. E., Jr. (1962), J. acoust. Soc. Amer., 34, 1356.
Evans, E. F. and Wilson, J. P. (1973), in Basic Mechanisms in Hearing. Møller, A. (Ed.), Academic Press, New York.
Flanagan, J. L. (1962), J. acoust. Soc. Amer., 34, 1370.
Fletcher, H. (1951), Speech and Hearing. New York: Van Nostrand.
Flock, Å. (1971), Handbook of Sensory Physiology, Vol. I, p. 396 (W. R. Loewenstein, Ed.). Heidelberg: Springer.
Flock, Å. (1973), J. acoust. Soc. Amer. 54, 293.
French, N. R. and Steinberg, J. C. (1947), J. acoust. Soc. Amer., 19, 90.
Gabor, D. (1946), J. Inst. elect. Engrs, 93 (3), 429.
Guillemin, E. A. (1963), Theory of Linear Physical Systems. New York: Wiley & Sons.
Guinan, J. J., Jr. and Peake, W. T. (1967), J. acoust. Soc. Amer., 41, 1237.
Habermann, J. (1890), Arch. Ohrenheilk., 30, 1.
Held, H. (1902), Abh. Sachs. Akad. Wiss. Leipzig. Math. Phys. Kl Abh. I., 28, 1.
Helmholtz, H. (1863), On Sensations of Tone. New York: Dover Reprint, 1954.
Helmholtz, H. (1868), Pflügers Arch. ges. Physiol., 1, 1.
Hilding, A. C. (1952), Ann. Otol., Rhinol., Lar., 61, 354.
Hilding, A. C. (1953), Ann. Otol., Rhinol., Lar., 62, 757.
Hilman, D. E. and Lewis, E. R. (1971), Science, 174, 416.
Holst, E. von (1950), Z. vergl. Physiol., 32, 60.
Johnsson, L. G. (1973). Personal Communication.
Johnstone, B. M. and Boyle, A. J. F. (1967), Science, 158, 389.
Johnstone, B. M., Taylor, K. L. and Boyle, A. J. F. (1970), J. acoust. Soc. Amer., 47, 504.
Khanna, S. M. (1970), Ph.D. Thesis. New York: City University.
Khanna, S. M. (1972). Unpublished data.
Khanna, S. M., Sears, R. E. and Tonndorf, J. (1969), Arch. Klin. exp. Ohr.-, Nas.- Kehlk. Heilk., 193, 78.
Khanna, S. M. and Tonndorf, J. (1971) (J. acoust. Soc. Amer., 50, 1475.
Khanna, S. M. and Tonndorf, J. (1972), J. acoust. Soc. Amer., 51, 1904.
Kimura, R. S. (1966), Acta oto-laryng., 61, 55.
Klockhoff, I. (1961), Acta oto-laryng., suppl. 164, 1.
Kohllöffel, L. U. E. (1972), Acustica, 27, 40, 66, 82.
Licklider, J. C. R. (1951), Handbook of Experimental Psychology (S. S. Stevens, Ed.). New York: Wiley & Sons.
Lim, D. J. (1972a), Arch. Otolaryng., 96, 199.
Lim, D. J. (1972b). Personal Communication.
Lowenstein, O. and Wersäll, J. (1959), Nature, 184, 1807.
Miller, D. J., Watson, C. S. and Covell, W. P. (1963), Acta oto-laryng., suppl. 176, 1.
Møller, A. R. (1963), J. acoust. Soc. Amer., 35, 1526.
Ohm, G. S. (1843), Poggendorfs Ann. Phys. Chem., 59, ser. 2, 497.
Onchi, Y. (1961), J. acoust. Soc. Amer., 33, 794.
Perlman, H. B. (1950), Laryngoscope, 60, 77.
Rayleigh, Lord (1877), Theory of Sound. New York: Reprinted by Dover, 1945.
Rhode, W. S. (1971), J. acoust. Soc. Amer., 49, 1218.
Scharf, B. (1970), Foundations of Modern Auditory Theory, Vol. I, p. 157 (J. V. Tobias, Ed.). New York: Academic Press.
Schouten, J. F. (1938), Proc. kon. ned. Acad. Wet., 41, 1086.
Schuknecht, H. F. (1953), Trans. Amer. Acad. Ophthal. Otoloaryng., 57, 366.
Seebeck, A. (1841–43), Poggendorfs Ann. Phys. Chem., 53, Ser. 2, 41; 60, Ser. 2, 449.
Shaw, E. A. G. (1972), J. acoust. Soc. Amer., 51, 150.
Simmons, F. G. (1963), Ann. Otol., Rhinol., Lar., 72, 528.
Spoendlin, H. (1966), Ultrastructure of Ear. Karger, Basel.
Stevens, S. S., Davis, H. and Lurie, M. H. (1935), J. gen. Psychol., 13, 297.
Stevens, S. S. and Volkmann, J. (1940), Amer. J. Psychol., 53, 329.
Tasaki, I., Davis, H. and Legouix, J.-P. (1952), J. acoust. Soc. Amer., 24, 502.
Tonndorf, J. (1960), J. acoust. Soc. Amer., 32, 238.
Tonndorf, J. (1962), J. acoust. Soc. Amer., 34, 1337.
Tonndorf, J. (1970a), J. acoust. Soc. Amer., 47, 579.
Tonndorf, J. (1970b), Foundations of Modern Auditory Theory, Vol. I, p. 203 (J. V. Tobias, Ed.). New York: Academic Press.
Tonndorf, J. (1970c), in Sachs, M. B.: Natl. Educ. Consultants, Baltimore, p. 69.
Tonndorf, J. (1973), in Basic Mechanisms in Hearing. Møller, A. (Ed.). Academic Press, New York.
Tonndorf, J. and Khanna, S. M. (1967), J. acoust. Soc. Amer., 41, 513.
Tonndorf, J. and Khanna, S. M. (1968a), J. acoust. Soc. Amer., 44, 1546.
Tonndorf, J. and Khanna, S. W. (1968b), Science, 160, 1139.
Tonndorf, J. and Khanna, S. M. (1970), Ann. Otol., Rhinol., Lar. 79, 743.
Tonndorf, J. and Khanna, S. M. (1972), J. acoust. Soc. Amer., 52, 1221.
Tonndorf, J., Khanna, S. M. and Fingerhood, B. (1966), Ann. Atol., Rhinol., Lar., 75, 752.
Tonndorf, J., Khanna, S. M. and Greenfield, E. C. (1971), Ann. Otol., Rhinol., Lar., 80, 861.
de Vries, H. L. (1949), Acta oto-laryng., 37, 334.
de Vries, H. L. (1952), J. acoust. Soc. Amer., 24, 527.
Ware, L. A. and Reed, H. R. (1949), Communication Circuits. New York: John Wiley & Sons.

Weber, Ed. (1851), *Verh. k. Sächs. Ges. d. Wiss., Leipzig. Math.-Phys., Kl.*, p. 29.

Weiss, H. S., Mundie, J. R., Cashin, J. L. and Shinbarger, E. W. (1962), *Acta oto-laryng.*, **55**, 505.

Wever, E. G. (1949), *Theory of Hearing*. New York, N.Y., U.S.A.: John Wiley & Sons.

Wever, E. G. and Lawrence, M. (1954), *Physiological Acoustics*. Princeton, N.J., U.S.A.: Princeton University Press.

Wiener, F. M., Pfeiffer, R. R. and Backus, A. S. N. (1966), *Acta oto-laryng.*, **61**, 255.

Wiener, F. M. and Ross, D. A. (1946), *J. acoust. Soc. Amer.*, **18**, 401.

Wilska, A. (1935), *Skand. Arch. Physiol.*, **72**, 161.

Zwislocki, J. J. (1961), *Ann. Otol., Rhinol., Lar.*, **70**, 599.

Zwislocki, J. J. (1962), *J. acoust. Soc. Amer.*, **34**, 1514.

Zwislocki, J. J. (1965), *Handbook of Mathematical Psychology*, Vol. III, p.1 (R. D. Luce, R. R. Bush and E. Galanter, Eds). New York

17. AUDITORY TUBAL FUNCTION

JÖRGEN HOLMQUIST

INTRODUCTION

This chapter is not a comprehensive and in-depth review of everything published about auditory tubal function. Instead, the attempt here has been to define broadly the limits of this area, and to specify some of the more interesting problems of current concern. The author has also tried to point out some of the questions that, hopefully, will stimulate the reader to a working interest in the area of auditory tubal function.

Historical Aspects

The anatomical tubal connection between the nasal part of the pharynx (nasopharynx) and the middle ear was recognized as early as 580 B.C. by Alcmaeon of Sparta (Stevenson *et al.*, 1949). In 1563, the auditory tube was described in detail by the Italian anatomist, Bartolomeus Eustachius, who said, "The knowledge of this passage could be of great use to doctors for the proper use of medicines." However, the important role which the tube plays in maintaining the normal function of the middle ear has only been emphasized as recently as the last four decades.

Variations in the barometric environment experienced by aviators and marine divers in the early 1940's led to the recognition of otitic barotrauma (McGibbon, 1942; Shilling *et al.*, 1942) and drew attention to the complications of disorders of auditory tubal function. The introduction of middle-ear surgery in the early 1950's also increased the demands for accurate and detailed knowledge of auditory tubal function under normal and pathological conditions. It is now generally accepted that an adequately functioning auditory tube is one of the vital factors for the maintenance of a normal middle-ear cleft.

ANATOMY

Excellent detailed descriptions of the anatomy of the auditory tube have recently been published by Proctor (1967; 1973). Particular attention is drawn here to the following facts, which are relevant to the discussion of auditory tubal function.

Gross Structure

The auditory tube is 31–38 mm in length (Graves *et al.*, 1944) and is described as having two portions: the osseous and the cartilaginous (Fig. 1). The osseous portion, also called the protympanum, must be considered as an extension of the middle ear cleft (Schwartzbert, 1958). Therefore, inflammatory changes of the middle ear easily extend into this portion of the tube. Pneumatized cells may sometimes surround the osseous portion. It is possible that tubal infections may lodge in these cells for a long time in a manner similar to residual infection in the air cells of the mastoid process. It has also been observed that this portion of the tube may be obstructed by polypoid mucosa, fibrosis tissue, or new bone formation as a response to inflammatory ear disease (Schuknecht *et al.*, 1967). Therefore, radiological investigation of this portion might be considered in certain cases (Welin, 1947; Compere, 1960; Parisier *et al.*, 1970).

The lumen of the cartilaginous portion is enclosed by cartilage and soft tissue. Figure 2 shows a schematic cross-section of this portion of the tube. Elastic fibres in the concavity of the cartilage are purported to maintain the shape of the cartilage and ensure its shape after displacement (Aschan, 1955; Holborow, 1962).

The junction between the two portions of the tube is the narrowest part, known as the isthmus. At this point the diameter is less than 2–3 mm, but may vary over a wide range even in people of the same age (Eggston *et al.*, 1947).

Microscopic Structure

The mucous membrane in the osseous portion of the tube is firmly adherent to the bony walls and consists of low columnar ciliated epithelium. In contrast, that of the cartilaginous portion is taller with pseudostratified, columnar, ciliated cells and with a marked submucosa, similar to that in the nasal part of the pharynx (Lim *et al.*, 1967; Hentzer, 1970). Goblet cells and seromucinous glands are abundant, especially towards the nasopharyngeal end. They provide the tube with a mucous blanket, which, dependent on the ciliary stream, moves towards the nasal part of the pharynx. A surface tension lowering substance has recently been found in the tube of dogs (Birken *et al.*, 1972). It is suggested that in humans a similar substance may be found playing a role in the ventilation of the middle-ear cavity. The presence of a mucociliary transportation system from the middle ear to the nasal part of the pharynx has been acknowledged, but the importance of this in disease and health is yet to be elucidated.

Auditory Tube Muscles

In this review, two muscles related to the auditory tube will be briefly described: the tensor palati and the tensor tympani muscles. These muscles are sometimes found to be continuous parts of the same muscle group (Lupin,

tube. Its head passes posteriorly, forming a tendon which turns at a right-angle at the processus trochleariformis, and after, crossing the tympanic cavity, is inserted in the neck of the malleus as shown in Fig. 1.

Besides the two muscles described, the levator veli palatini and the salpingopharyngeus muscles are also involved in the auditory tubal opening and closing mechanism. A detailed description of these muscles is given by Proctor (1973).

Lymphatics

A lymphatic plexus around the auditory tube has been demonstrated (Arnould, 1927). The plexus, which is more

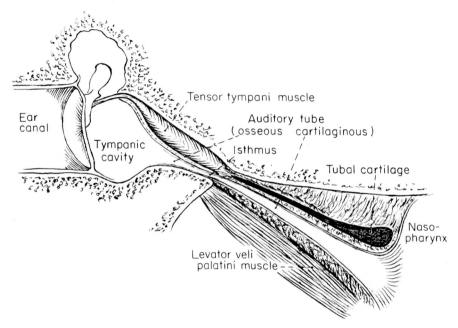

Fig. 1. A schematic anatomical diagram of the auditory tube.

1969). They have also been demonstrated to have a common embryological origin and a common nerve supply from a branch of the fifth cranial nerve. Presumably, their action in relation to the auditory tube is synergistic.

Tensor Veli Palatini Muscle

This muscle is situated on the lateral aspect of the cartilaginous portion of the tube. It has been demonstrated to originate: (1) from the spine of the sphenoid, (2) from the scaphoid fossa, and (3) from the lateral lamina of the tubal cartilage and the adjacent membranous part of the tube. The flattened triangular muscle runs downward and forward and becomes tendinous. The tendon winds around the pterygoid hamulus to be radially inserted into the soft palate and the palatine bone (Ross, 1972).

Tensor Tympani Muscle

This muscle originates: (1) from the cartilaginous portion of the tube, (2) from the adjoining part of the sphenoid, and (3) from its own bony canal. The muscle is contained in a bony canal, situated above the osseous part of the

dense toward the nasopharyngeal end, drains into the cervical nodes via different routes. It has been suggested that blockage of these lymphatic channels may be the etiological factor in serous otitis media (Senturia, 1960; Reiner *et al.*, 1969). Since 1874, when Gerlach described a lymphoid mass in the cartilaginous tube, the presence of lymphatic tissue around the auditory tube has been widely discussed. It is now obvious from many investigations (Farrior, 1943; Eggston *et al.*, 1947; Aschan, 1954) that such a tissue does not exist in or around the auditory tube, but is restricted to the nasal part of the pharynx.

Changes in the Auditory Tube with Age

At birth, the auditory tube is shorter, with a less well defined isthmus compared to that in the adult. The direction of the tube is almost horizontal in childhood, but inclines to an angle of 30–40° with the horizontal plane in the adult. This also means that the nasopharyngeal opening of the tube is close to the level of the soft palate and more widely exposed compared to that in the adult. While the medial lamina of the tubal cartilage is vertical on cross-section in the adult, it lies in a horizontal plane in the infant (Holborow, 1970). These age differences in anatomy also mean age differences in tubal opening and closing mechanisms, which have to be taken into consideration when discussing auditory tubal function.

PHYSIOLOGY

The most important function of the auditory tube is to maintain air pressure equality across the tympanic membrane. The continuous absorption of air through the mucosal lining in the middle ear space together with the variations of the ambient barometric pressure constitute the

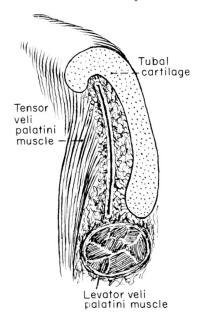

Fig 2. A schematic cross-section of the auditory tube in its cartilaginous portion. The relationship to the levator and tensor veli palatini muscles are shown.

basic need for intermittent air exchange through the auditory tube. This is accomplished by opening the tube to permit air to pass either from or into the middle ear space.

Besides air flow, drainage of mucous, produced in the middle ear or in the auditory tube itself, is also part of proper function of the auditory tube (Fig. 2).

Middle ear Pressure

Due to the different partial pressures of oxygen in the middle ear and in the surrounding tissue, a small amount of gas is continually absorbed through the mucosal lining (Riu *et al.*, 1966). This corresponds to a decrease of the middle-ear pressure of approximately 50 mm H_2O (490 Pa).h^{-1} if the tube is closed. The greater part of this gas absorption takes place through the mucosa of the promontorial wall (Tumarkin, 1957; Flisberg *et al.*, 1963; Flisberg, 1966). This nonuniform gas absorption is supported by the less vascularized mucosa in the mastoid cells compared to that of the middle ear. The mastoid air cell system must therefore be looked upon as a reservoir of air. Depending

on the normal distribution of the mastoid air cell sizes (Diamant, 1940), the volume of this air reservoir varies between ears. This means that the speed of air pressure drop increases as the volume of the reservoir decreases. It is not known how the auditory tube meets these differences between ears. Further research in this field is necessary to elucidate all the interacting factors, including the mobility of the tympanic membrane, the volume of the middle ear, the gas absorption, and the auditory tubal function.

The Collapsed Auditory Tube

Depending on the construction of the cartilaginous support, the loose arrangement of the peritubal tissue, and the rugose mucosa, the lumen of the cartilaginous portion is collapsed. The closure force is influenced by a series of so-called tissue factors: the elasticity of the cartilage, the venous pressure, the properties of the mucous membranes, and others. The magnitude of these factors may be evaluated by calculating the least overpressure able to keep the mucosal walls separate. Only a few data have been published indicating pressure values in the range of 50–75 mm H_2O (490–735 Pa) (Ingelstedt *et al.*, 1967). Rundcrantz (1969) elegantly demonstrated the influence of venous pressure and posture on tubal function. He found that air volumes passing through the tube were drastically reduced during compression of the neck veins or in the horizontal compared to a 20° body elevation position. However, a great lack of knowledge still exists both regarding the exact composition of these tissue factors and their quantitative meaning and significance.

Tubal opening Mechanism

As a result of muscular activity, the cartilaginous portion of the tube will open. The tensor palati muscle is considered the main dilator, while the levator veli palatini muscle, forming part of the bottom of the tube, supports the opening. The tensor tympani muscle may also play a role in the tubal opening mechanism. As stated previously, the tensor tympani is attached to the neck of the malleus and contraction of the muscle may slightly increase the middle-ear pressure by medial displacement of the tympanic membrane. The origin of this muscle from the cartilage of the tube as well as from the adjoining bone may well influence the opening of the tube at this point (Ingelsted *et al.*, 1967; Holmquist *et al.*, 1973). This is also supported by the fact that the tube begins to open from the middle ear end. Thus, contraction of the tensor tympani may facilitate tubal opening.

Another mechanism for opening the auditory tube must also be taken into account. If the intratympanic pressure, for some reason, exceeds 100–150 mm H_2O (981–1471 Pa), above the ambient pressure, the auditory tube may open spontaneously without any muscular activity involved. This holds also for overpressure applied from the nasopharyngeal end of the tube, exemplified in tubal catheterizing or in applying overpressure in the nasal part of the pharynx as in Valsalva's manoeuvre.

The importance of small air pressure differences across the tube for a complete separation of the mucous surfaces and a breaking of the mucous film is discussed in the literature (Perlman, 1967). Using a sound transmission technique (Guillerm *et al.*, 1966), it was found that only one-third of normal individuals had "perfect permeability" of the tube on swallowing. If, however, a pressure difference across the tube was used, almost all tubes opened completely upon swallowing. In pressure-chamber experiments performed by Ingelstedt and his associates (1963, 1967) it was shown that the tube did not open upon swallowing until the chamber reached $+150\ mm\ H_2O$ (1471 Pa) relative to the ambient pressure. The importance of air pressure difference across the tube for proper opening is also shown in Fig. 3. This demonstrates the

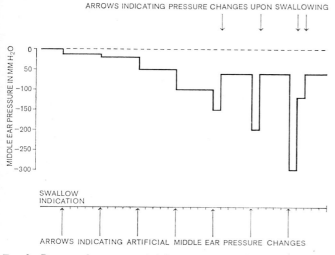

FIG. 3. Pressure changes recorded from one case. The artificial middle ear pressure has been changed stepwise. Not until the pressure reaches $-150\ mm\ H_2O$ is the patient able to change the pressure upon swallowing. (From Holmquist, 1969.)

effects of step-by-step increases of negative pressure in the middle ear. Not until the pressure reaches $-150\ mm\ H_2O$ is the patient able to change the pressure by swallowing. This means that it is easier to equalize a pressure of $-150\ mm$ than that of $-100\ mm.\ H_2O$. This has been shown repeatedly when testing auditory-tube function in ears with chronic otitis media (Flisberg, 1966; Miller, 1965; Holmquist, 1969) and this presumably holds for normal ears also.

Tubal closing Mechanism

In contrast to opening of the tube, closure is exclusively a passive phenomenon. When the muscles relax or when a static pressure no longer keeps the tubal walls separated, the tubal lumen collapses. Using radiographic techniques, Aschan (1954) showed that the closure of the tube starts at the nasopharyngeal end. In this way it is possible that small air volumes are forced into the middle ear during closing of the tube. This may explain the presence of a slight overpressure in many ears under normal conditions, as shown by Holmquist and his associates (1973) (*see* Fig. 4).

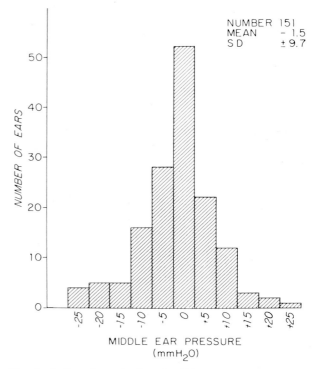

FIG. 4. Indirect determination of middle ear pressure using an acoustic impedance bridge. (From Holmquist and Miller, 1973.)

Tubal Opening Time

The equalization capacity of the tube is influenced by many factors, among which the time the tube stays open as a result of muscular activity seems to be the most critical. According to many investigators (Perlman, 1951; Aschan, 1955; Miller, 1965; Flisberg, 1966), the opening time varies between $0.1–0.9\ s$. Depending on the pressure difference across the tube, the width, and length of the narrowest part together with the opening time, the air volumes passing through the tube may vary, explaining the great difference in tubal equalization capacity even between normal individuals (Elner *et al.*, 1971).

Testing Ventilating Function

Testing the ventilating function of the auditory tube is a problem which has not been completely solved. Many tests have been designed but, as the basic physiology of the tube is not clearly understood and as the variations in normal function seems to be wide (Elner *et al.*, 1971), it is premature to present a list of the available testing methods. It is suggested that tests of tubal function should minimally include measurements of:

1. Least positive and negative air pressure difference across the tube which permits passage upon swallowing.
2. Tubal opening time upon swallowing at different pressures across the auditory tube.
3. The least positive pressure necessary to maintain the tubal walls separate.
4. The air volumes passing through the tube upon opening at different pressures across the tube.

5. The capacity of the tube to meet variations in middle ear pressure.

At the present time, measurement of these parameters is complicated and time-consuming. Hopefully, future research in this field will provide us with a simple technique for auditory tube testing permitting adequate prediction in health and disease.

Draining Function of the Tube

Recently, the importance of the mucociliary system for proper draining function of the tube has been emphasized (Sadé *et al.*, 1970). The action of the cilia beating towards the nasal part of the pharynx will cause a mucous flow in the same direction. Furthermore, the moving of mucous plugs by the cilia may cause slight negative pressure to occur in the middle ear space (Hilding, 1932). This might play a role in the development and persistence of middle ear disease. The undesirable effect of different agents and diseases on the cilia, as well as on the mucus, of the respiratory tract has been extensively studied (Dalhamn, 1956; Ballinger *et al.*, 1965). It seems logical to assume that the results of these studies also apply to the auditory tube.

Testing Draining Function

Compere and his associates (1958) suggested injection of contrast media into the middle ear, followed by repeated radiographs of the ear, to evaluate the clearance capacity of the auditory tube. Rogers and his associates (1962) injected fluorescent dye into the middle ear and subsequently inspected the nasopharyngeal opening of the tube for fluorescence. These techniques have certain merits, but have not been generally accepted for clinical routine. The need for simple, valid and reliable measures of the draining function still exists.

Auditory tubal Function at Changing Ambient Pressure

The response of the auditory tube to changes in the ambient pressure as occasioned by flying, has been studied by many authors (Armstrong, 1961; Flisberg *et al.*, 1963; Thomsen, 1958; Ingelstedt *et al.*, 1967, and others.) There is a general agreement that, during ascent, which causes a relative increase in middle ear pressure, tubal opening is facilitated upon swallowing; or the tube may even open spontaneously as graphically shown in Fig. 5 (Donaldson, 1973). The situation is more complex during descent, however, when the relative middle ear pressure is decreasing. As indicated above, increased negative middle-ear pressure up to at least −200 to −300 mm. H_2O (−1961 to −2942 Pa) facilitates tubal opening as illustrated in Fig. 3. At higher negative middle ear pressure levels, more complicated conditions occur, which influence tubal opening. It seems clear that negative middle ear pressure impairs tubal opening by a suction effect on the mucosal surfaces in the tube (Flisberg, 1966). It has also been shown that a negative middle ear pressure already of about −1100 mm H_2O (−10787 Pa) may make it impossible for the muscles to overcome the collapsing force (Armstrong, 1961). These

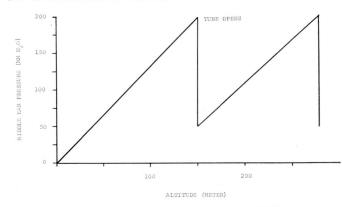

FIG. 5. An increase in altitude causes an increase in middle ear purpose. At about +200 mm H_2O (Armstrong, 1961), the tube opens spontaneously and the intratympanic pressure is reduced to +50 mm H_2O. (From Donaldson, 1973.)

observations are especially relevant for divers and pilots exposed to great and rapid changes in ambient pressure.

In order to evaluate the response of tubal function to pressure variations, functional tests predicting difficulties arising in individuals who are engaged in flying or diving obviously need to be assessed using a pressure chamber.

REFERENCES

Armstrong, H. G. (1961), *Aerospace Medicine*. Baltimore: Williams and Wilkins Co.

Arnould, P. (1927), *Contribution à l'étude des lymphatiques de l'appareil auditif*. Paris: Thesis.

Aschan, G. (1954), *Acta oto-laryng*. (Stockh.), **44**, 295.

Aschan, G. (1955), *Acta Soc. Med. upsalien*. **60**, 131.

Ballinger, J. J., Dawson, F. W., De Ruyler, M. G. and Harding, H. B. (1965), *Ann. Otol.*, **74**, 303.

Birken, E. A. and Brookler, H. K. (1972), *Ann. Otol.*, **81**, 268.

Compere, W. E., Jr. (1958), *Trans. Amer. Acad. Ophthal. Otolaryng.*, **62**, 444.

Compere, W. E., Jr. (1960), *Arch. Otolaryng.* (*Chicago*), **71**, 386.

Dalhamn, T. (1956), *Acta physiol. scand.*, suppl. 123.

Diamant, M. (1940), *Acta oto-laryng*. (Stockh.), suppl. 41.

Donaldson, J. A. (1973) *Arch. Otolaryng.*, **97**, 9.

Eggston, A. A. and Wolff, D. (1947), *Histopathology of the Ear Nose and Throat*. Baltimore: Williams and Wilkins Co.

Elner, Å., Ingelstedt, S. and Ivarsson, A. (1971), *Acta oto-laryng.*, **72**, 320.

Farrior, J. B. (1943), *Arch. Otolaryng.* (*Chicago*), **37**, 609.

Flisberg, K., Ingelstedt, S. and Örtegren, U. (1963), *Acta oto-laryng.* (*Stockh.*), suppl. 182.

Flisberg, K. (1966), *Acta oto-laryng.* (*Stockh.*), suppl. 219.

Graves, G. O. and Edwards, L. F. (1944), *Arch. Otolaryng.* (*Chicago*), **39**, 359.

Guillerm, R., Riu, P., Badre, R., Le Den, R. and Le Mouel, C. (1966), *Ann. Oto-laryng.* (*Paris*), **83**, 523.

Hentzer, E. (1970), *Ann. Otol.*, **79**, 1143.

Hilding, A. C. (1932), *Ann. Otol.*, **52**, 58.

Holborow, C. (1970), *Arch. Otolaryng.* (*Chicago*), **92**, 624.

Holborow, C. A. (1962), *J. Laryng.*, **76**, 762.

Holmquist, J. (1969), *Acta Otolaryng* (Stockh.), **68**, 391.

Holmquist, J. and Strothers, G. (1973), *Mayo Clinic Symposium on Middle Ear Impedance*. Rochester, Minn. (U.S.A.): Mayo Clinic.

Holmquist, J. and Miller, J. M. (1973), *Mayo Clinic Symposium on Middle Ear Impedance*. Rochester, Minn. (U.S.A.): Mayo Clinic.

Ingelstedt, S. (1963), *Acta oto-laryng.* (Stockh.), suppl. **188**, 19.

Ingelstedt, S., and Jonson, B. (1967), *Acta oto-laryng.* (Stockh.), suppl. **224**, 452.

Ingelstedt, S., Ivarsson, A. and Jonson, B. (1967), *Acta oto-laryng.* (*Stockh.*), suppl. **228.**

Lim, D. J., Paparella, M. and Kimura, R. (1967), *Acta oto-laryng.* (*Stockh.*), **63,** 425.

Lupin, A. J. (1969), *Ann. Otol.,* **70,** 792.

McGibbon, J. E. G. (1942), *J. Laryng.,* **57,** 14.

Millier, G., Jr. (1965), *Arch. Otolaryng.* (*Chicago*), **81,** 41.

Parisier, S. C. and Khilnani, M. T. (1970), *Laryngoscope,* **80,** 1201.

Perlman, H. B. (1951), *Arch. Otolaryng.* (*Chicago*), **53,** 370.

Perlman, H. B. (1967), *Arch. Otolaryng.* (*Chicago*), **86,** 632.

Proctor, B. (1967), *Arch. Otolaryng.* (*Chicago*), **86,** 503.

Proctor, B. (1973), *Arch. Otolaryng.* (*Chicago*), **97,** 2.

Reiner, C. E. and Pulec, J. L. (1969), *Ann. Otol.,* **78,** 880.

Riu, R., Flottes., L., Bouche, J. and Le Dene, R. (1966), *La physiologir de la trompe d'Eustache.* Paris: Librairie Arnette.

Rogers, L., Kirschner, F and Proud, G. O. (1962), *Laryngoscope,* **72,** 456.

Ross, M. A. (1972), *Arch. Otolaryng.* (*Chicago*), **93,** 1.

Rundcrantz, H. (1969), *Acta oto-laryng.* (*Stockh.*), **68,** 279.

Sadé, J. and Eliezer, N. I. (1970), *Acta oto-laryng.* (*Stockh.*), **70,** 351.

Schuknecht, H. and Kerr, A. (1967), *Arch. Otolaryng.* (*Chicago*), **86,** 497.

Schwartzbart, A. (1958), *Ann. Otol.,* **67,** 241.

Senturia, B. H. (1960), *Trans. Amer. Acad. Ophthal. Otolaryng.,* **64,** 60.

Shilling, C. W. and Everly, J. A. (1942), *U.S. Navy Bulletin,* **40,** 664.

Stevenson, R. S. and Guthrie, D. (1949), *A History of Oto-Laryngology.* Edinburgh: E. & S. Livingstone.

Thomsen, K. A. (1958), *Acta Otolaryng.* (*Stockh.*), suppl. **140,** 269.

Tumarkin, A. (1957), *J. Laryng.,* **71,** 65, 137, 211.

Welin, S. (1947), *Acta radiol.* **28,** 95.

18. THE INTRATYMPANIC MUSCLES

S. D. ANDERSON

INTRODUCTION

In all mammals, except for certain fossorial forms, the middle ear contains two muscles, the stapedius and the tensor tympani, which are attached to the ossicular chain. These muscles constitute the effectors of an input control system of the ear. Contraction in response to loud sounds in an acoustic reflex, and in conjunction with certain motor activities, affects the transmission properties of the middle ear. An understanding of the extent of this regulatory activity, its dynamic and static properties, and the threshhold for such activity, are essential for an improved understanding of the auditory system as a whole.

In turn, these properties of the middle ear muscles are best viewed in the context of, and with an appreciation of, the interspecies differences in the structure and physiology of the muscles. There are interspecies differences both in the general morphology, size and arrangement of the supporting tissues, and in terms of the types of muscle fibres present. It may be inferred that the properties of the middle ear muscles are reflected in these differences, and this would seem to indicate at least differences in the extent of activity, if not differences in function in different animals.

The advent of the use of the acoustic impedance bridge for testing the acoustic reflex response in the diagnosis of auditory dysfunction, and the protective effect of the muscle activity against certain intense sounds, further emphasizes the need for an adequate understanding of the properties of the middle ear muscles. Information on the function of the middle ear muscle system in animals and man has been obtained from neuroanatomical, neurophysiological, behavioural and psychoacoustic experiments.

GENERAL AND COMPARATIVE MORPHOLOGY

Derivation

There are muscles attached to the transmission system of the ear in both amphibia and birds (*see* Kirikae, 1960).

In amphibia, an opercular muscle attaches to the operculum, and another muscle to the columella. Similarly, in birds there is a muscle which attaches to the tympanic membrane. The stapedius muscle is a derivative of the second branchial (hyoid) arch and is innervated by the facial nerve. The tensor tympani muscle, however, is ontogenetically and phylogenetically related to the pterygoid musculature, and receives its innervation from the motor root of the trigeminal nerve.

The Stapedius Muscle

The tendon of the stapedius muscle inserts at the neck and the head of the stapes (Fig. 1) and the muscle pulls the stapes sideways on contraction in the direction of greatest flexibility of the incudostapedial joint. Occasionally a fine branch of the tendon reaches the lenticular process of the incus. The stapedius is a bipennate muscle, which in man is approximately 8 mm long and is contained in the canal of the pyramidal eminence.

In terms of topography and shape, there are only minor differences between the stapedius muscle of various mammals (Kobayashi, 1956). Often, variations seem to be due to differences in the form of the pyramidal eminence (Platzer, 1961), with variations in the extent of the bony sheath surrounding the muscle particularly apparent. In man, only the tendon of the stapedius muscle is exposed to the tympanic cavity, whereas in the guinea-pig the very small stapedius muscle is almost entirely exposed, arising from a somewhat spoon-shaped concavity (Fig. 2A).

In a comparative study of the middle ear, Hinchcliffe and Pye (1969 and unpublished observations) commented on the variability of several features of the stapedius muscle in various mammalian species. The stapedius muscle is absent in a number of rodent species, all of which are fossorial and have trabeculated middle ear cavities. These authors suggested that this condition is probably an adaptation for the reception of structure-borne vibrations.

When present, the stapedius muscle was found to vary considerably in size from one species to another, but since there was also considerable intra-species variability it was suggested that size has little taxonomic significance. However, the middle ear muscles are much better developed in microchiropteran bats, especially in the Molossidae, and other bats which emit intense orientation cries (Henson, 1961; Pye, 1970), than in the megachiropteran bats and

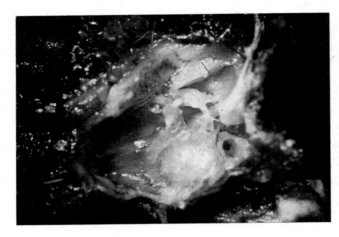

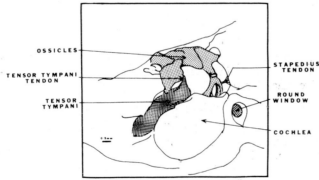

FIG. 1. Dissection of the middle ear of the cotton rat (*Sigmodon hispida*) to show the large tensor tympani muscle. The stapedius muscle tendon is also visible. The malleus has been deflected to show that the tensor tympani muscle is situated in a semicanal. The diagram is drawn to scale.

other mammals. For example, in the bat *Myotis lucifugus* each of the middle ear muscles has a mass almost equal to that of the ossicular chain.

Hinchcliffe and Pye also linked the absence of a Paaw's cartilage in the stapedius muscle with the presence of separate cavities for this muscle and for the facial nerve. The cartilaginous or osseous skeletal element of Paaw is found within the stapedius muscle of species of several mammalian orders, but not in the Insectivora (Henson, 1961) and rarely in the Rodentia. In addition, although generally present in the Microchiropteran bats, it is absent from the Megachiroptera that have been studied (Wassif, 1948; Pye, 1966). Paaw's cartilage has been described as functionally equivalent to a sesamoid bone (McCrady, 1938) and as representing a homologue of the reptilian extra-stapes (van Kampen, 1915). Analysis of function on purely comparative grounds is very difficult because there

is considerable intra-species variability in the presence or absence of this cartilage. Indeed, in a single specimen of the primate *Tupaia* a cartilage was found in the stapedius muscle of one ear only.

The Tensor Tympani Muscle

The tensor tympani muscle in man is spindle-shaped, 20–25 mm long, and is contained in a canal that is partly osseous and partly membranous. This muscle is attached to the malleus, the tendon inserting on the upper third of the ossicle immediately below the anterior long process. The tendon begins in the canal at the level of the oval window, and as it emerges it bends around a small hook-like process on the promontory, the processus trochleariformis.

Gross structural differences in the tensor tympani have however been described in comparative studies. Basically the muscle consists of two portions, one inserted on the temporal bone (temporal portion) and the other on the auditory tube (tubal portion). In some species both portions are present but completely separate, e.g. *Capra hireus* and *Ovis aries* (Malan, 1934a; Fumagalli, 1949), whilst in others one of the two parts may be reduced or completely absent. The latter is commonly the case, resulting in a spindle-shaped muscle when only the tubal part is present (e.g. man, horse, rabbit, guinea-pig and rat); and a round-shaped muscle when only the temporal portion remains (pig, cow, dog and cat). The round-shaped tensor tympani is housed in a scaphoid fossa and the spindle-shaped muscle in a semicanal, e.g. as in the cotton rat (shown in Fig. 1); although the latter may be partly closed over by a thin body lamina belonging to the tympanic bone as in man and guinea-pig (Fig. 2B). When both parts are present the muscle is contained in a cavity of intermediate shape (Malan, 1934a). The spindle-shaped muscle is pennate (bi- or semipennate) and its apical tendon ends partly inside the muscle, and partly extends along it to form a lamina on its outer surface, with the muscle fibres inserting on both parts. The apical tendon of the round-shaped muscle similarly extends into the muscle, but here there are radial fibres between it and the epimysium (circumpennate).

Both Wassif (1948) and Henson (1961) have described four different insertion patterns for the tensor tympani in microchiropteran bats. These patterns may illustrate an evolutionary progression. Indeed, three of the patterns of insertion have been described in only a few other mammals (some monotremes and marsupials), and are usually evident only in the embryos of these animals.

The tensor tympani has not been observed in *Scalopus*, an insectivore (Henson, 1961). It has been suggested that, in this animal, and in other fossorial mammals where there is a general decrease in size of the intra-aural muscles, this arises because of an adaptation to enhance low frequency auditory acuity.

Connective and Other Supporting Tissues

The total encasement for the entire length (in bony cavities or sub-cavities), of both intratympanic muscles in man, has been viewed as an arrangement to avoid muscular vibrations interfering with sound transmission (Békésy, 1936). Similarly, the varied arrangement of

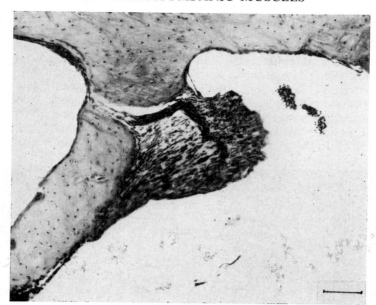

FIG. 2A. Transverse section of the stapedius muscle of the guinea pig (*Cavia porcellus*) to show how the muscle is almost totally exposed to the middle ear cavity. The entrance of the stapedial nerve into the muscle may also be seen. (Van Gieson stain. Scale 83·5 μm)

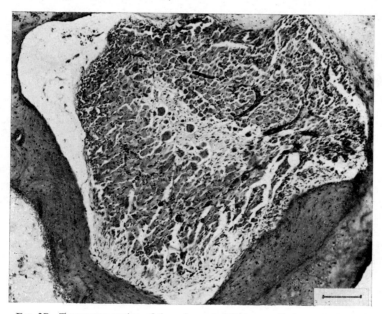

FIG. 2B. Transverse section of the guinea-pig (*Cavia porcellus*) tensor tympani muscle to show the thin bony lamina enclosing the muscle in its semicanal. The section is at the level at which the tendon first appears in the centre of the muscle and the nerve bundles branch out to supply the muscle fibres. The nerve fibres have been stained by a silver cyanate method. (Scale 0·1 mm)

supporting and connective tissues of the middle ear muscles may provide a kind of acoustic insulation.

In man, the tendons of both middle ear muscles contain elastic fibres (Davies, 1948), which may form a network around each muscle fibre of the stapedius muscle in older individuals. There is also abundant stroma of connective tissue in the stapedius muscle, with septa dividing the muscle into numerous bundles. Both arrangements probably facilitate a smooth contraction.

Between the periotic bone and the epimysium of the tensor tympani, there is a layer of adipose tissue, the perimuscular fat; but what has excited interest for many years has been the presence of large amounts of intrafascicular adipose tissue (Zuckerkandl, 1884). The intrafascicular adipose tissue is found at the junction of the muscle and tendon, and also interposed between both bundles of muscle fibres and individual fibres (Fig. 3). In some animals however, this tissue is not present (e.g. guinea-pig), complicating attempts to explain its function. It was first proposed that this tissue occurred as a result of degenerative processes involving the contractile matter (Zuckerkandl, 1884). Indeed, in man the appearance is somewhat reminiscent of certain myopathic conditions. However, it is present at an early age in the cat, 45 days after birth (Candiollo, 1965a, b) and in the cotton rat, one week after birth, which suggests it is not due to degenerative processes. Its function may be mechanical, as an elastic support for the fibre bundles (Spiesmann, 1927). In the laboratory rat

Contractile Tissues

Smooth Muscle Fibres

It is clear that the intratympanic muscle fibres are predominantly striated. However, smooth muscle cells have been reported within the tensor tympani (Byrne, 1938; Erulkar *et al.*, 1964). Some authors have refuted this (e.g. Blevins, 1963), and if these cells are present they are clearly few in number. Fine bundles of smooth muscle fibres in association with skeletal muscle fibres can occur

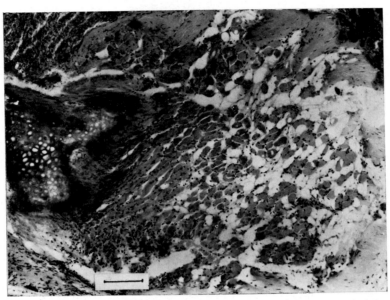

FIG. 3. Fresh frozen transverse section of the tensor tympani muscle of the fruit-bat *Rousettus aegyptiacus*, to show areas occupied by intrafascicular adipose tissue. The muscle is mounted in liver, and is still attached to a fragment of bone. Stain tolonium chloride (toluidine blue, Scale 0·1 mm.

and the cotton rat, the adipose tissue virtually forms a core around which parts of the muscle and tendon pass and which also might be deduced to smooth the contractile action. Certainly the adipose tissue is a substantial part of the mass of the tensor tympani muscle in these animals. Another possibility is that the adipose tissue serves as an energy source for sustained contraction, much as heart muscle derives energy from fatty acid metabolism. "Red" skeletal muscle fibres with high oxidative enzyme content have also been shown to derive energy in this way and many fibres of the tensor tympani muscle have a comparable high enzyme content in the cat and rabbit (Hayata, 1963), rat and cotton rat (Anderson, 1973). However, Wersäll (1958), doubts that the intramuscular fat has any functional significance, in particular because he found the stapedius muscle to be practically devoid of fat. It is nevertheless difficult to explain such large quantities of adipose tissue in the tensor tympani muscle of some animals and its absence in other animals without assigning some significance to the presence of the tissue. Adipose tissue is in fact found in the stapedius muscle of some animals, although in smaller amounts than in the tensor tympani. It is sometimes only ascribed to the muscle-tendon junction (Brzezinski, 1962).

in vertebrate muscle, but such associations are difficult to distinguish with light microscopy and their function is obscure. Alternatively, these cells may have been embryonic fibres as described in electronmicroscopy studies of the stapedius muscle (David *et al.*, 1966).

Atypical Striated Fibres

Another anomaly reported in the middle ear muscles of various mammals and man are the so-called atypical striated muscle fibres in which the myofibrils follow a spiral or annular course around the longitudinal axis of the fibres (Malan, 1934b; Filogamo, 1940). The proportion of myofibrils affected within individual muscle fibres is progressive and it was originally tentatively suggested as being due to ageing (Malan, 1934b). However, since it was found that this progressive change appears at an early age in the rat, it was later proposed that this arrangement may enable finer adjustments of contraction (Candiollo, 1965b).

Muscle Fibre Diameter

The muscle fibres of both the tensor tympani and the stapedius muscles characteristically show a large variation in fibre diameter. In the tensor tympani muscle two types of fibres can usually be distinguished with different maximal diameters, the mean values of which vary from species to species. The maximum diameter of the thinnest muscle fibres is often no more than 4–5 μm, whereas the maximum diameter of the thickest fibres may range from approximately 20–30 μm to approximately 50–60 μm. In the stapedius muscle of man a range of fibre diameters from 2·9–35·4 μm has been reported (Brzezinski, 1962). There is also a decrease in the number of muscle fibres from the stapedius muscle of the fetus and newborn to that of the adult (Blevins and Noble, 1965).

Recently, muscle fibre diameter has been related to histochemical enzyme staining of the fibres in the middle ear muscles. In the cat tensor tympani muscle, staining for myofibrillar adenosine triphosphatase (ATPase) reveals two populations, termed ATPase strong (diameter 5–30 μm, mean greater than about 10 μm), and ATPase weak (5–17 μm, mean below 10 μm) (Teig and Dahl, 1972). Similarly, in the cat stapedius muscle, ATPase weak staining fibres have a range of 5–22 μm (mean approximately 12 μm), and ATPase strong, 5–40 μm (mean approximately 18 μm). These authors did not distinguish any subgroups on the basis of fibre size, but in various other mammals the present author has distinguished at least three "types" of fibres according to histochemical staining properties which characteristically bear a relationship to fibre diameters (Anderson, 1973, 1974).

Muscle Fibre Types

The suggestion that the variation in muscle fibre diameter might reflect functional differences between fibres of the middle ear muscles first arose on the basis of electromyographic studies of the tensor tympani muscle of the cat (Okamoto et al., 1954). Two types of motor units were distinguished; units with a tonic activity, a low contraction threshold, and small amplitude action potentials, and a second type with phasic properties, large action potentials, and a high contraction threshold. Later, the results of micro-electrode penetrations in conjunction with electron microscopic studies (Erulkar et al., 1964) in the tensor tympani muscle of the cat were assessed to indicate a "slow striated muscle fibre type" and a "fast striated muscle fibre type", corresponding to the "Fibrillen Struktur", and "Felder Struktur" types of Krüger (1949). However, more recent work on vertebrate striated muscle has clarified distinctions between fibres beyond the work of Krüger. Basically, extrafusal skeletal muscle fibres can now be divided into fibres that are focally innervated with propagated action potentials and "all or none" twitch responses, and those that are multiterminally innervated and characteristically respond with a slow and graded contraction (for reviews of the latter, see Peachey, 1968 and Hess, 1970). A further classification of the "twitch" fibres into three principal types of fibre that differ in their outer structure, the activities of oxidative and glycolytic enzymes, myoglobin content, and certain properties of the myosin, is now commonly accepted (see Close, 1972). Within the framework of this classification the problem posed by the "tonic" units of the middle ear muscles is: do these reflect the presence of multi-terminally innervated slow fibres, or the presence of the "slower" type of "twitch" fibres?

Multi-terminally Innervated Fibres

The case for the presence of multi-terminally innervated fibres rests mainly on the afore-mentioned work of Erulkar and his associates (1964), and another study of the middle ear muscles of the cat by Fernand and Hess (1969). The latter work involved both electron microscope and cholinesterase stained light microscope preparations. It revealed muscle fibres with typical end-plates and fibres with "elongated" nerve terminals seen as a series of small dots or lines running along the muscle fibres in the cholinesterase preparations. Both the stapedius and tensor tympani muscles possessed the latter fibres, but there were fewer in the stapedius muscle. Unfortunately, the electronmicroscopic description of these fibres differed considerably from that of the slow fibres of the previous work. Moreover, a recent study of the middle ear muscles in man, cat, rabbit, guinea-pig and albino rat, also with preparations stained for cholinesterase, failed to find any multi-terminally innervated fibres despite their presence in extra-ocular muscle used as controls (Mayr and Mayr, 1973). Cholinesterase positive sites in myomyous junctions (as described in bird skeletal muscle: Mayr et al., 1967) were found, and these might bear some relation to the "elongated" nerve terminals of Fernand and Hess. Alternatively, these latter endings might be concerned with a proprioceptive efferent innervation. Certainly, whatever the derivation of the structures reported by Fernand and Hess, attempted correlation with the innervation of the slow fibres of extraocular muscle, both by cholinesterase staining (Mayr and Mayr, 1973) and by silver impregnation (Barker, 1967; Anderson, 1972), has otherwise failed in middle ear muscle studies.

Focally Innervated Muscle Fibres

The different types of focally innervated "twitch" muscle fibres may be distinguished by histochemical staining of transverse sections. The intensity of staining of certain oxidative enzymes and Sudan black B was found to be high in one type of fibre and low in another, in both middle ear muscles of the cat and the rabbit (Hayata, 1963). This is similar to the previously mentioned division into two populations of muscle fibres made by Teig and Dahl (1972) by staining of cat middle ear muscles for myofibrillar ATPase. Unequivocal histochemical identification of the three principal types of twitch muscle fibres was reported by Anderson (1973) in the middle ear muscles of the fruit bat, Rousettus aegyptiacus. Recently a comparative histochemical study has been made of the middle ear muscles of the cotton rat, guinea-pig and rabbit (Anderson, 1974). To enable a coherent description of results it was necessary to propose a histochemical classification of muscle fibres based on a concept of transformation between fibre categories. The middle ear muscles were shown to be heterogeneous in their fibre composition, but there are differences in the types of fibres found in different species. Slow twitch, "intermediate" fibres are present in quite large numbers in the middle ear muscles of the guinea-pig and the fruit bat. This is especially so in the guinea-pig stapedius muscle and appears to be so in the middle ear muscles of the rabbit.

However, in the guinea-pig tensor tympani muscle, the percentage of cross-sectional area represented by the "intermediate" fibres is relatively low and this therefore indicates a very small slow component in contractions. No such fibres were found in the middle ear muscles of the cotton rat.

Conversely, all the middle ear muscles studied have a large percentage of fibres staining intensely for myofibrillar ATPase, indicating that, as a group, they are fast muscles. This is especially so for the cotton rat middle ear muscles. The usefulness of the exercise of distinguishing different histochemical fibre types is apparent when one considers that the dynamic characteristic of a muscle as a whole is dependent upon "fibre composition" of the muscle (Edgerton and Simpson, 1971), and also that the

or disproved forthwith, to avoid further confusion in the literature. In an ultrastructural study of the stapedius muscle of the rabbit, Hirayama and Daly (1974) distinguished a morphologically slow muscle fibre type and two types of twitch fibres. The two twitch fibre types were described as similar to white and red fibres of skeletel muscle, but the slow muscle fibre type was compared to the slow muscle fibres found in extraocular muscle. A slow muscle fibre type has similarly been described in the tensor tympani muscle of the rabbit (Hirayama et al., 1974) and the guinea-pig (Seiden, 1971). However, in all three papers, the ultrastructural characteristics of the slow fibres, poorly delineated myofibrils and sparse sarcoplasmic reticulum, have simply been related to the description of "Felder

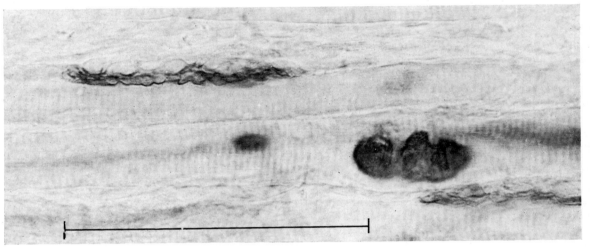

FIG. 4. A long motor ending on a small muscle fibre and a broad but shorter type of motor ending on a large muscle fibre of the stapedius muscle of the cat. Parts of the broad ending which are in focus show synaptic folds. (Fixation: Perfusion with buffered paraformaldehyde under pentobarbital anaesthesia; Koelle incubation of muscle fibre bundle for four hours in a medium containing ISO-OMPA[1].) (From D. Mayr and R. Mayr, 1973.) Scale = 0·1 mm.

"fibre profile" has been shown to be the same in homologous limb muscles of different species (Ariano et al., 1973). This permits conclusions to be drawn by a relatively simple histochemical procedure regarding not only the dynamic activity of particular muscles, but also inferred differences of function.

A higher intensity of oxidative enzyme staining was observed in the stapedius muscles than in the tensor tympani muscles. This suggests a more tonic or repetitive activity and a greater resistance to fatigue in the stapedius muscle. In the guinea-pig stapedius muscle, the substantial intermediate fibre population together with heavy oxidative enzyme staining of the majority of the other fibres suggest both tonic and repetitive activity. However, in the cotton rat stapedius muscle, fast repetitive contractions would seem to be clearly indicated.

In the light of the need for further indications of the presence of multiterminally innervated fibres, it is likely that the tonic motor units distinguished by electromyographic and tension studies are composed of "intermediate" twitch fibres. It is important that this conclusion is accepted

Struktur" fibres. No evidence for multi-terminal innervation of these fibres was obtained, although the myoneural junctions were described. It is more appropriate to compare these muscle fibres with the slow twitch intermediate fibre types rather than the multi-terminally innervated extraocular slow muscle fibre type.

Further support for the presence of different types of focally innervated fibres, is the finding, in the cat stapedius muscle, of long type nerve endings and broad type nerve endings (Mayr and Mayr, 1973). The long type endings (70–110 μm in length) show less synaptic folds, are thin and are situated on smaller muscle fibres than the broad endings (30–70 μm in length) (see Fig. 4). These authors did not distinguish different types of endings in the stapedius or in the tensor tympani muscles of the rat, rabbit, guinea-pig and man, but in these animals the range of absolute values of motor end plate length is smaller than in the cat, being lowest in the guinea-pig and man (10–20 μm). A factor of greater importance is probably the relationship between the area of motor end-plate and muscle fibre volume. The "relative innervationsgroße" ratio of Anzen-

[1] OMPA is octamethylpyrophosphoramide. ISO-OMPA is diisopropylpyrophosphoramide.

bacher and Zenker (1963) is always higher in stapedius than in tensor tympani muscle, but varies in the same muscle of different species (Mayr and Mayr, 1973, Table 1).

TABLE 1

Animal	Stapedius Muscle	Tensor Tympani Muscle
Cat	Long endings: 7500 Broad endings: 2400	800
Guinea-pig	5600	1250
Rat	2200	500
Man	1500	240

The "relative innervationsgrosse" ratio of Anzenbacher and Zenker (1963) of number of μm² of motor end plate area per 1 million μm³ of muscle fibre volume in the middle ear muscles of several mammals (Mayr and Mayr, 1973).

According to Zenker, the higher this ratio, the more finely regulated and rapid the activity of a muscle. These figures for the middle ear muscles are extremely high in comparison to other striated muscles, including extra-ocular muscle. They support earlier data of high innervation ratios of the number of nerve fibres to muscle fibres in suggesting that the middle ear muscles are finely controlled.

Fibre Arrangement

The distribution of the different types of twitch muscle fibres within the individual middle ear muscles may be characteristic for a species (Anderson, 1974). A clearer understanding of the fibre arrangements observed (*see* Fig. 5A) may prove useful for anticipating the effect of middle ear muscle contractions on the ossicular chain in different animals.

Innervation

General

The stapedius muscle is innervated by a branch of the facial nerve, and the tensor tympani muscle by a branch of the trigeminal nerve. Both muscles may often receive minor nerve branches from other sources. These minor nerve connections and several associated ganglia have been reviewed by Filogamo and his colleagues (1967). Their function is as yet unknown.

In man, the nerve of the stapedius muscle originates from the descending portion of the facial nerve, at the level of the pyramidal eminence. It courses forwards, crosses the anterior wall of the facial canal, reaches the canal of the pyramidal eminence and finally enters the stapedius muscle, after splitting up into two or three branches.

In both muscles the diameters of the intramuscular nerve fibres are very small. The nerve of the tensor tympani reaches the muscle in its lower third, courses for a short distance in the perimysium and then enters the muscle proper, splitting up into numerous branches, the fibres of which

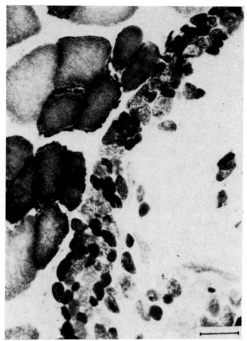

FIG. 5A. Fresh frozen transverse section of cotton rat (*Sigmodon hispida*) tensor tympani muscle stained for the enzyme reduced nadide (coenzyme I) diaphorase. Distinct groups of muscle fibres staining heavily for this oxidative enzyme can be seen around the periphery of the section. Scale 62 μm.

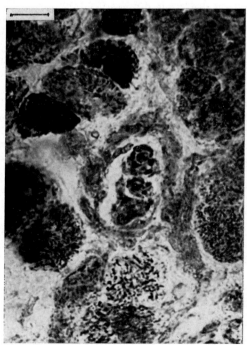

FIG. 5B. A group of very thin muscle fibres within a well defined connective tissue capsule, in a fresh frozen transverse section of the cotton rat (*Sigmodon hispida*) tensor tympani muscle. The section has been stained for reduced nadide diaphorase, so that the fibre boundaries are not distinct and spiralling nerve fibres are difficult to distinguish. Comparable to a limb muscle spindle although considerably smaller. Scale 16 μm.

have a maximal diameter of 5 μm in the rabbit (Malmfors and Wersäll, 1960). In fact, in the rabbit, 75 per cent of these fibres are within the range 2–4 μm, and, in the cat, the majority are between 2 and 2·9 μm in diameter. Similar values have been reported for stapedial nerve fibre diameters.

Innervation Ratios

The nerve fibres, although small, are numerous in relation to the size of the middle ear muscles, and it is the consensus in the literature that the motor units in both muscles are composed of only a few muscle fibres. Estimates of the motor innervation ratio cannot be considered to be very accurate because of variations with age (Blevins and Noble, 1965) and the fact that the proportion of nerve fibres that are sensory is unknown and may be as high as 90 per cent (Teig, 1972a, b).

Sensory Innervation

There has been some controversy as to the presence or absence of sensory nerve endings in the middle ear muscles, but there would seem little doubt that there are at least simple spindle-like structures in the intratympanic muscles of most mammals (e.g. Fig. 5B). Typical neuromuscular spindles occur in the human tensor tympani muscle (Winkler, 1959; Candiollo, 1965a). Filogamo, Candiollo and Rossi (1967) conclude that the middle ear muscles have a self-controlling mechanism, regulating the muscular tonus, but physiological proof in the form of the recording of afferent impulses has not yet been obtained. Since the muscles shorten only slightly, their contraction might be considered almost isometric, with some of the sensory information obtained from typical limb muscles spindles seemingly redundant. However, the force of contraction of both middle ear muscles, particularly the stapedius muscle, is very dependant upon initial muscle length (Teig, 1972a). Thus a proprioceptive mechanism for regulating muscle length, and consequently the force of contraction, would seem likely, especially when middle ear muscle activity is not elicited by acoustic stimuli. In this case, feedback information on the effects of contraction from changed acoustic inflow to the cochlea is limited.

Central Pathways

The course of the acoustic stapedius muscle reflex arc in man is not known but the pathway of the acoustic reflex arc in rabbits, as determined by Borg (1973a), is depicted in Fig. 6. A probably parallel, but slow, polysynaptic pathway is not shown, nor are the input pathways for non-acoustic stimuli. It is known that the reticular formation can influence the activity of the middle ear muscles of the cat, particularly the stapedius muscle (Hugelin *et al.*, 1960a, b, c) and that higher auditory centres, including the auditory cortex, can also exert control of these muscles (Baust and Berlucchi, 1964). The superior olivary complex, which also contains elements of the reflex pathways of the outer ear muscles and the efferent innervation of the spiral organ, possibly regulates the conduction of centrifugal impulses along the reflex circuit of the middle ear muscles

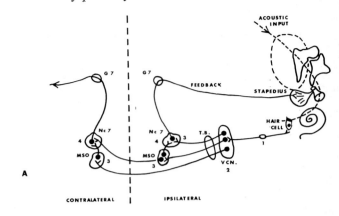

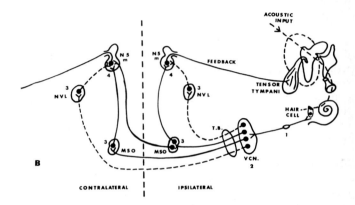

Fig. 6A. Stapedial Acoustic Reflex: Acoustic input via the ossicles stimulates cochlear hair cells resulting in afferent impulses via the primary acoustic neurones (1), to second order neurones (2), in the ventral cochlear nucleus (VCN). Axons of the second order neurones pass, via the trapezoid body (TB), mainly to interneurones (3) *in or near* the medial superior olivory nucleus (MSO) of both sides, but a few pass *directly* to the motor neurones (3) of the facial motor nucleus (Nc7). Axons of the contralateral MSO pass to the motor neurones (4) of the contralateral Nc7, and those of the ipsilateral MSO to the Nc7 of both sides. The axons of the motor neurones pass in the facial nerve via the genu of the facial nerve (G7) to the stapedius muscle, thus effecting a feedback input control. B. Tensor Tympani Acoustic Reflex: The same input pathway is followed up to and including second order neurone axons passing through the TB but there is no *direct* pathway to the motor neurones of the trigeminal motor nucleus (N5M). There are again similar pathways via the interneurones (3) in or near the MSO of both sides, to the motor neurones. The ventral nucleus of the lateral lemniscus (NVL) receives fibres from the TB of both sides; and third order neurones in the NVL, with fibres passing to the N5M on the same side are a further possibility (dotted). Axons of the motor neurones of the trigeminal motor nucleus follow the mandibular branch of the trigeminal nerve to the tensor tympani muscle, again affecting modification of the input to the cochlea. (Drawn from data of Borg, 1973a.) Possible polysynaptic reflex pathways parallel to the trapezoid body are not represented.

and these two other regulatory systems. The resultant effects on middle ear muscle activity of interaction between the auditory pathways and the cortex via the centrifugal extra-reticular auditory control system (CERACS), the cortex and the reticular substance, and between the reticular substance and the auditory pathways, are difficult to predict and remain to be resolved. Activity patterns are further complicated by direct control exerted by fibres descending from non-auditory cortical areas (pyramidal tract, gamma system), the possible proprioceptive control mechanisms of the middle ear muscles, and reflex interconnections between afferent fibres from some other motor systems and cutaneous receptors of the external ear canal and the face. For example, electrical stimulation of the internal branch of the superior laryngeal nerve in the cat results in reflex contraction of the stapedius and tensor tympani muscles (McCall and Rabuzzi, 1973). Thus, there is a reflex interconnection between the middle ear muscles and the afferent nerve supply of the larynx.

MUSCLE CONTRACTION AND ITS EFFECTS

Motor Units

The electromyographic and histochemical evidence for the presence of fast and slow motor units in the middle ear muscles has been substantiated by myographic recordings.

As predicted by the histochemical evidence, both the stapedius and the tensor tympani muscles have mean twitch contraction times in the cat and rabbit within the range of fast muscles (Teig, 1972a) e.g. cat stapedius muscle 21·2 ms, tensor tympani muscle 29·2 ms. However, prolongation of the last part of the relaxation phase of the tensor tympani muscle was noted in both species, and this was attributed to a slow component. Then, in a subsequent paper, Teig (1972b), when recording the all-or-none contraction of individual cat tensor tympani motor units in response to threshold stimulation of their motorneurones, distinguished a slow and a fast twitch type of motor unit. The two types of motor unit could be distinguished by their contraction times, half-relaxation and tetanic fusion rates. Also, the twitch tension of the slow units were all weak in comparison to the overall range of tensions recorded and considerably smaller than the mean tension of the fast units. The two groups could not be separated from each other by differences in tension alone, since there was an overlap in the tension ranges of the groups. Nevertheless, the strongest motor units had a faster contraction time than the average of the units recorded, and the slowest units were all weak.

A working hypothesis to explain these results in terms of the histochemical findings and muscle fibre types is not difficult. However, the finding in Teig's (1972b) tension studies of only one type of motor unit in the stapedius muscle of the cat conflicts with histochemical findings. It has already been mentioned that Teig and Dahl (1972) found two fibre populations in both middle ear muscles of the cat when staining for myofibrillar ATPase. In the tension studies, only fast units were distinguished in the stapedius muscle. This may have been due to the biasing of the method of threshold stimulation in favour of stimulating the motor neurones of faster motor units. Another possibility, however, is that the slow units are served by motorneurones in the lateral group of the facial nucleus as opposed to the dorsomedial group which was stimulated.

It has already been mentioned that the tensions produced by the middle ear muscles vary with the resting length of the muscles (Teig, 1972a). Initial length is particularly critical in the stapedius muscle. This probably reflects the highly isometric working conditions of the stapedius muscle, because intact ossicular chain movements of the stapes due to the stapedius contraction have been recorded as maximally 50 μm (Philip, 1932).

In Teig's experiments, deviations of a little more than this from the optimum length, gave a large reduction in tension of the muscle as a whole. However, Teig's careful control of muscle length enabled him to show that the middle ear muscles are capable of producing much larger tensions than those indicated by earlier studies. Supramaximal electrical tetanic stimulation of the stapedius muscle of the cat and rabbit produced tensions equivalent to 136·5 and 151 mN respectively. Similarly the tensor tympani muscle of the same animals gave tensions equivalent to 532·5 and 317 mN respectively.

Teig estimated that the cat stapedius muscle has approximately 87 fast motor units, and the cat tensor tympani muscle 92 fast and 40 slow motor units.

These estimates of the number of twitch motor units suggest that only about 12 per cent of the nerve fibres supply twitch motor units. As Teig points out, in the absence of non-twitch multi-terminally innervated muscle fibres, and with few, if any, intrafusal muscle fibres, nearly 90 per cent of the nerve fibres would be sensory. This seems rather high, although the proportion of afferent fibres in the nerves to various hind-limb muscles has been found to vary as much as from 34 to 95 per cent (Boyd and Davey, 1966). In the event of polyneuronal innervation of individual muscle fibres the estimate of sensory fibres would be too high, but there is little basis for such an assumption.

Assuming that the units sampled in Teig's study were representative, there was in both middle ear muscles a predominance of units which develop small tensions. When plotted as a histogram of unit tension against number of units, a plot that was typically skewed to the left (i.e. towards weaker units) was obtained and this corresponds to the plot one obtains when the distribution of fibre diameters is represented (Anderson, 1974). Large numbers of weak units as opposed to a few strong units once again suggest a fine control of tension and a smoother contraction. This is to be expected for a finely tuned input control system, and manifests itself in the effects of middle ear muscle contraction on transmission.

Transmission Effects of Contraction

Differential Effects of Graded Contraction

Recently Teig followed his tension studies with a study of the differential effects of graded contractions of middle ear muscles on the sound transmission of the ear (Teig, 1973). He measured the change in amplitude of cochlear microphonic (c.m.) potentials of pure tones from 250–7000 Hz resulting from middle ear muscle contractions elicited by electrical stimulation of their motor nuclei in the brain stem. This was later compared with muscle tension (measured myographically) elicited by stimuli of comparable strength. The strongest contractions elicited had tensions only 10–20 per cent of maximal muscle tension, and yet weak contractions were far more selective in their effect on transmission than the strongest tensions used. In Fig. 7 data from Teig's paper has been re-drawn to show attenuation effects at three tensions. Weak contractions of the stapedius muscle are seen to affect frequencies below 2 kHz, most markedly at the lowest frequencies tested. Stronger contractions produce an additional modest reduction equally pronounced for all frequencies. The most marked attenuation produced by the tensor tympani muscle is at frequencies below 750 Hz, although tensions up to 57 mN (equivalent to 5.84×10^{-3} kg) give a reduction in the sound transmission of most frequencies below 4 kHz. However, there are peaks of absolutely or

weakest motor units present, and thus contribute especially in a fine gradation of effect on sound transmission of frequencies below 1500 Hz, at weak muscle contraction. The reductions of transmission for a given amount of tension were much greater for the stapedius muscle than for the tensor tympani, as observed in earlier studies (Wever and Bray, 1937, 1942). One explanation offered for this difference is that the distance from the rotational axis of the ossicular chain to the insertion of the stapedius muscle is considerably longer than the distance to the insertion of the tensor tympani muscle, thus giving shorter leverage for the tensor tympani muscle.

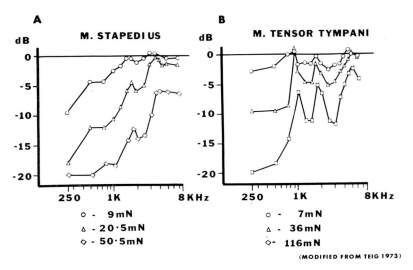

FIG. 7. The effects of contraction of the middle ear muscles of the cat on the transmission of pure tones of various frequencies, as registered by cochlear microphonic potentials. The extent of attenuation or slight enhancement is plotted in dB against the frequencies tested at three levels of stimulation for each muscle. The tension exerted (measured later and originally expressed in terms of a muscle load) at each level of stimulation is indicated.

relatively increased transmission in certain frequency ranges. In individual ears these peaks have a very narrow range (e.g. Fig. 7), but the frequencies at which the peaks occur varies somewhat from ear to ear. The three peaks are in the ranges 750–1200 Hz, 1500–2500 and 4000–6000 Hz. Again, stronger contractions of the tensor tympani muscle gave a nearly equal effect upon all frequencies up to 4 kHz. The amount of attenuation per unit (10 mN) of muscle tension decreases relatively with increases in tension beyond about 50–60 mN (Fig. 7). For example, an increase in tension of 58.5 mN added to a tension of 57 mN gave an increase in attenuation of only 3–5 dB whilst an initial increase in tension from the inactive state gave a maximal sound reduction of more than 15 dB (although only at frequencies below 250 Hz).

Teig suggested that the slow twitch motor units of the tensor tympani muscle, when maximally activated, should together be capable of producing a tension of approximately 39 mN, within the range in which relatively selective reduction of low frequency tones below 750 Hz occurred. Similarly, he suggested that the supposedly slow muscle fibres in the stapedius muscle, with smaller diameters than the fast twitch fibres, may constitute the

Degree of Muscle Contraction

Comparison of Teig's data with other experiments is difficult because none of the previous investigators have included measurements of the muscle tension developed. In most studies correlating muscle contractions with the effect on sound transmission through the middle ear, it would appear that relatively large tensions have been elicited, and a certain degree of reduction of sound transmission has been noted (Wever and Bray, 1937, 1942; Neergaard et al., 1963; Cancura, 1970). Usually, reduction of the lower frequencies has been emphasized, as in impedance studies in both cats and rabbits, in which contraction of either or both middle ear muscles attenuated frequencies below 2 kHz, leaving higher frequencies practically unaffected (Møller, 1965).

Selective Enhancement of Certain Frequencies

The enhancement of certain frequencies caused by small contractions has also previously been reported, although certain inconsistencies are apparent. Spontaneous contractions of the guinea-pig middle ear muscles were found to reduce transmission of frequency components below 1 kHz, but to slightly enhance frequencies from 1 kHz up to 2·5 kHz (Wiggers, 1937). In man small improvements of sound transmission have been observed for components between 2 and 3 kHz (Cancura, 1970). Conversely, during weak reflex activation of the middle ear muscles, enhancement of a 450 Hz test tone has been reported both in cats and in rabbits (Wever and Vernon, 1956; Price, 1963). It has been suggested that this low frequency enhancement is the by-product of the change in muscle tension (Stevens and Davis, 1938).

Acoustic Impedance Experiments

Borg's use of unanaesthetized, unrestrained rabbits under the closely controlled stimulation conditions of his impedance studies provide perhaps the most accurate assessment of the effects of the acoustic reflex on transmission through the middle ear (as opposed to the potential effects of muscle contraction elicited by electrical stimulation as in Teig's experiments). However, it must be remembered that the effect of muscle contraction is probably not solely a simple increase in the stiffness of the middle ear system. Thus, when comparing the change in impedance with the change in transmission upon stapedial contraction in rabbits and cats, Møller (1965) obtained a larger change in transmission than in admittance.

Figure 8 is a summary of the results of Borg's impedance studies on the rabbit. In order to describe the magnitude

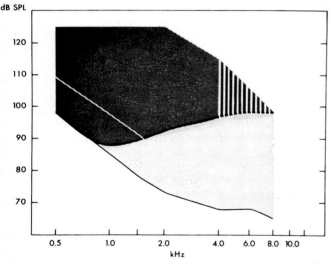

FIG. 8. Static properties of the acoustic middle ear reflex of the rabbit. The threshold of the total reflex (stapedius muscle in conjunction with the tensor tympani muscle) is shown by the thin black line and it is identical to the stapedius muscle reflex threshold. The threshold of the tensor tympani muscle is shown by the thin white line. The reflex threshold was defined as the intensity at which 10% of the maximal obtainable impedance charge was obtained. The dark shaded area shows the region where single pure tones are attenuated by the middle ear muscle contraction elicited by the pure tone itself. (From Borg, 1972a.)

of the influence of middle ear muscle activity on sound transmission Borg introduced a concept of "efficiency of regulation", being the slope of the curve showing the relation between sound pressure level in dB (relative to ipsilateral reflex threshold) and the attenuation of sound expressed

in equivalent decrease in sound pressure level (re: stimulus sound pressure). In the rabbit, the regulatory efficiency above the threshold for attenuation was about 0·7 (i.e. 0·7 dB attenuation per dB increase in sound pressure level in the ear canal). This value was nearly independant of the frequency of the stimulus tone; and at 0·5 kHz above tensor tympani threshold, the stapedius muscle provided about 0·5, and the tensor tympani muscle 0·2, of the total regulatory efficiency of 0·7. Only the stapedius muscle contributed to attenuation of sound above 2 kHz, but did so at least up to 8 kHz. In man the stapedius muscle alone has a regulatory efficiency of 0·7 at 0·5 kHz (Borg, 1968) which may mean that any acoustic reflex tensor tympani muscle activity would be superfluous in man. All degrees of stapedius muscle activity in man attenuate low frequency sounds (below about 1 kHz) at a fairly constant rate above reflex threshold; but, in contrast to other animals, frequencies higher than about 2 kHz are only attenuated, if at all, at intensities far above reflex threshold (Borg, 1968). Limiting attenuation to components below 2 kHz is in accordance with Cancura's observation on temporal bones (1970), and experiments involving non-acoustic stimulation of middle ear muscle activity in humans (Reger, 1960; Pichler and Bornschein, 1957). However, the data of Pichler and Bornschein resemble Teig's results with weak contractions in the cat. Thus, it is possible that, in man, very high levels of stapedial activity might also influence frequencies well above 2 kHz.

Attenuation of High Frequencies

It is indicated quite clearly by a number of sources that the middle ear muscles can attenuate higher frequencies in animals other than man. The attenuation effects in the cat with large contractions (Teig, 1973) and in the rabbit (Borg, 1972d), at least up to 8 kHz, have already been mentioned. Indirect evidence for attenuation of frequencies as high as 16 kHz, has been obtained in the rabbit with observation of reflex responses with oscillations at this frequency (Lorente de Nó, 1935). Further evidence for high frequency attenuation has been obtained in studies involving anaesthetized cats (Gisselsson et al., 1957) and rabbits (Price, 1966); but particularly startling are the results obtained with unanaesthetized bats. In Fig. 9B the attenuating capacity of the middle ear muscles in the bat, *Pteronotus p. parnellii* (Gray) is plotted as a function of frequency. The data has been redrawn from Pollak and Henson (1973). In this study the possibility of attenuation due to the crossed olivocochlear bundle and movements of the auricle, were not entirely excluded (although immobilization of the auricle did not influence the attenuation attributed to the middle ear muscles). However, in earlier work on the Mexican free-tailed bat, *Tadarida brasiliensis*, attenuation of 12–22 dB of high frequency tones was abolished by removal of the stapedius muscle in one animal (Henson, 1965). Moreover, in the latter study, electromyograms of the stapedius muscle were found to correlate muscle contraction with the cochlear microphonic attenuation. If the contraction of the tensor tympani muscle should be, in this particular function, dependent upon prior contraction of the stapedius muscle (*see later*), involvement of the tensor tympani muscle might not be excluded and certainly merits further investigation. There is a sharp decrease in attenuating capacity for frequencies above 57 kHz, which in some preparations was even more pronounced than in the example shown. As with the weak contractions of the tensor tympani muscle of the cat, the attenuation attributable to the middle ear muscles is highly selective.

Acoustic Response of the Tensor Tympani Muscle

In man, it is generally agreed that only the stapedius muscle consistently responds in an acoustic reflex as such, (Jepsen, 1955; Salomon and Starr, 1963). The tensor tympani muscle contractions in man elicited by sound stimuli have a long latency (90–300 ms) compared with that of the stapedius muscle (*see later*), and the activity has

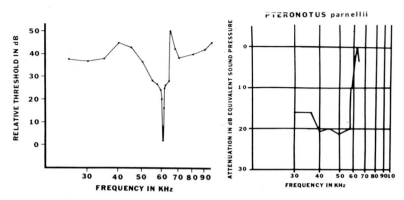

FIG. 9. Middle ear muscle activity in the bat, *Pteronotus parnellii*. A. Cochlear microphonic audiogram from an awake bat. The thresholds are expressed in decibels above the threshold at the "best" frequency (60·6 kHz). (From Pollak and Henson, 1973.) B. The attenuating capacity of the middle ear muscles as a function of frequency. This curve was derived by measuring the maximum attenuation of CM potentials elicited by tone bursts 20 ms in duration. The bursts were 30 dB above the CM "threshold" and the interstimulus interval was 200 ms. The ordinate represents the decrease in sound pressure required to elicit a CM response equal in amplitude to the attenuated portion of a tone burst response. Note the sharp decrease in middle ear muscle attenuating capacity for frequencies above 57 kHz. (Modified after Pollak and Henson, 1973.)

Although there seem to be differences between man and animals with regard to the frequency range of sounds influenced by the middle ear muscles, the threshold for significant influence on sound transmission is about the same (90–100 dB SPL for pure tones). Weaker sounds will, of course, be attenuated if they coincide with or appear shortly after an intense sound.

EXCITABILITY OF THE ACOUSTIC REFLEX

Sound is the most consistently effective stimulus for middle ear muscle activation, and there is quantitative information concerning the magnitude, consistency and dynamic properties of the acoustic reflex. Such information is lacking for middle ear muscle activity evoked by non-acoustic stimuli, so such activity will not be discussed until the final section on middle ear muscle functions.

To elicit contractions of the middle ear muscles in both ears, sound need only be presented to one ear. Usually, the sound intensity required is well above the hearing threshold, but at a higher level the reflex threshold as a function of frequency largely parallels the cochlear microphonic sensitivity function. This in turn reflects the behavioural sensitivity curve. The acoustic reflex seems to occur when the neural output of the cochlea reaches a certain level, and, in most animals, both the stapedius and the tensor tympani muscles respond.

been interpreted as part of a general reflex pattern in a startle reaction to both acoustic and non-acoustic stimuli (Klockhoff, 1961; Djupesland, 1967). Lidén and his colleagues (1970) have, however, shown that in a small percentage of individuals (13 per cent of sample) it is possible that the tensor tympani muscle contracts selectively in response to sound. Also, recently, an acoustic impedance response within the normal range, has been obtained from a patient who had earlier had a stapedectomy with section of the stapedial tendon (Prasansuk and Hinchcliffe, 1972). Although stapedial tendon reattachment is a possibility, it is interesting to consider that, in the rabbit, the isolated tensor tympani threshold (after section of the stapedial tendon) is on average only 3 dB higher than the total reflex threshold at 0·5 kHz, compared with 10 dB when working with the stapedius muscle (Borg, 1972b). The presence of two muscles in a reflex system, one with a low threshold and fast response and the other with a higher threshold and slow response, can enhance the stability of the system (Borg, 1973b). This could certainly apply to the acoustic reflex in animals, where it has long been recognized that the tensor tympani threshold is usually higher than that of the stapedius and that the latency is often longer. Moreover, in impedance studies with rabbits, Borg (1972b, d) found that oscillations in response that were frequently observed in both ears were increased in amplitude when the tensor tympani muscle was cut in the stimulated ear. Could the same apply to the human acoustic reflex with the comparatively higher stapedius threshold resulting in an even higher tensor tympani threshold at a level at which a general muscle startle response also occurs? Unfortunately, data from stapedectomized patients must be treated with great caution since it must be a difficult task to relate the properties of a diseased ear with the normal. However, some of the first studies investigating the human acoustic reflex by measuring acoustic impedance did compare the threshold of the reflex with the threshold of hearing in normal and pathological subjects (Metz, 1952; Jepsen, 1955).

Investigations in Man

Reflex excitability has been extensively investigated in man (for reviews *see* Jepsen, 1963; Møller, 1972). Most experiments have been on unanaesthetized subjects by measuring changes in the acoustic impedance of the ear (e.g. Metz, 1946; Klockhoff, 1961; Møller, 1961; Zwislocki, 1963), especially those associated with changes in the air pressure in the outer ear canal (Terkildsen, 1957; Weiss *et al.*, 1962; Holst *et al.*, 1963; Mendelson, 1966). More direct measurements, recording electromyographically from the actual muscles, have also been performed, although usually in connection with operations on the ear (Perlman and Case, 1939; Fisch and Schulthess, 1963; Salomon and Starr, 1963; Djupesland, 1967). In general, the stapedius reflex threshold is about 80 dB above the hearing threshold for the 250–4 000 Hz range (Jepsen, 1955; Møller, 1962a) and somewhat lower for noise (e.g. Møller, 1962a; McRobert *et al.*, 1o68). The thresholds for noise stimuli are also significantly more stable than those for pure tones.

Animal Experiments

Precise stimuli were not used until Lorente de Nó and Harris's (1933) myographic study of acute, anaesthetized rabbits. Later, anaesthesia was avoided by the implantation of electrodes within the muscles (e.g. Galambos and Rupert, 1959; Simmons, 1959; Hilding, 1960). The most striking results of these studies were the low thresholds, and the variability of the acoustic reflex responses observed (also the frequent non-acoustic activity). One reason for the variability in response is undoubtedly the relation between acoustic reflex activity and fluctuations in the state of wakefulness of the animals (Baust and Berlucchi, 1964). However, as emphasized by Borg (1972a), other experimental factors were also probably involved, such as the difficulty in controlling stimulus conditions and measurement, without the ability to determine sound pressure levels in the ear canal close to the ear drum. Similarly, activity may have been influenced by the very presence of the metallic implants, just as electrodes in the stapedius tendon of man give rise to a noise sensation (Salomon and Starr, 1963).

Threshold Differences in Man and Animals

It now seems most unlikely that the higher reflex thresholds obtained by impedance measurements in man compared to those obtained with chronically implanted electrodes in cats are mainly due to methodological shortcomings in the human experiments.

The results of Borg's impedance measurements on the rabbit have already been mentioned (Fig. 8). The average threshold for the ipsilateral reflex in the rabbit is 98 dB SPL at 0·5 kHz but decreases by about 12 dB per octave until about 2 kHz. Above 4 kHz it averages 70 dB SPL. These figures show a lower threshold than that obtained for man by the order of 10–20 dB over a wide frequency range (Møller, 1961, 1962a, 1962b; Borg, 1968). The lowest threshold observed in Borg's study with rabbits was 44 dB SPL (at 4 kHz). Although the reproducibility for individual rabbits was very good (Borg, 1972c), the interindividual variability was large, with a range in threshold of about 40 dB at 2 kHz.

Near the actual reflex threshold, as opposed to an arbitrary intensity giving 10 per cent of maximal impedance change, the relation between stimulus strength and reflex activity is relatively inconsistent compared to that obtained a little above threshold in both rabbits and man. This presumably reflects background activity in the nervous system.

Contralateral versus Ipsilateral Thresholds

In man, stimulation of the contralateral ear is required to be 2–14 dB greater than that necessary to obtain the same response ipsilaterally (Møller, 1961). Bilateral stimulation is even more efficient than ipsilateral stimulation by a difference of about 3 dB (Møller, 1962a). In Borg's study on rabbits, a similar higher sensitivity to sound for the ipsilateral reflex than the crossed reflex was observed both for the total reflex and in the bilaterally isolated tensor tympani reflex. However, differences in the threshold of the total reflex were small (less than 2 dB) though significant at 0·5 and 2 kHz ($p = 0·0001$). At 80 per cent of maximal response amplitude at 0·5 kHz the difference in stimulus level required was about 5 dB, which corresponded to a difference in response amplitude of nearly 20 per cent (i.e. with an 80 per cent ipsilateral response, the crossed response corresponds to a 60 per cent ipsilateral response). The maximum response amplitude of the contralateral ear was, however, at most a few per cent below that of the ipsilateral response, and the possibility could not be excluded that it would reach the same level if a higher intensity sound had been available. Probably because of non-linearities in the auditory system, the difference in sensitivity between bilateral and ipsilateral stimulation increases when repetitive signals (like band pass filtered pulses) are repeated at less than 50 per second, as opposed to above 50 per second, when results agree with those for noise (Møller, 1962a). Anaesthesia also increases the differences between the excitability of the crossed and ipsilateral reflexes (Borg and Møller, 1967).

TEMPORAL AND DYNAMIC ASPECTS OF THE ACOUSTIC REFLEX
Dynamic Range

Once the reflex threshold is passed, the strength of contraction as reflected by impedance change increases roughly in proportion to the magnitude of the stimulus over a range of approximately 30 dB, above which it levels off in man (Møller, 1962). There is thus a relatively narrow dynamic range between the reflex threshold and the level of saturation. In the rabbit (Borg, 1972b, d), the dynamic range, arbitrarily defined as the sound levels between which response amplitudes of 10–80 per cent of the maximum are obtained, is dependent on stimulus frequency. The range is smaller at low frequencies (e.g. 15 dB for the total reflex at 0·5 kHz) than at higher frequencies (e.g. 28 dB at 4 kHz). Whereas the isolated stapedius reflex does not differ from the total reflex with respect to the dynamic range and shape of the stimulus response curve, the tensor tympani reflex (when in conjunction with the stapedius reflex) has a less steep stimulus-response curve, especially at low frequencies. This stimulus-response curve for the tensor tympani reflex also failed to consistently reach 80 per cent of the maximal response obtained for the tensor tympani in isolation, within the stimulus intensity range available in Borg's study, emphasizing again the influence of the stapedius muscle on the tensor tympani muscle response.

Latent Period

With contralateral stimulation using a high amplitude sinusoid, the stapedius muscle in man has a latent period of 10 ms (Perlman and Case, 1939). A value some 10 times greater than this was later confirmed for the tensor tympani muscle (Salomon and Starr, 1963). Measured to the onset of an impedance change, latencies of 35 and 25 ms for the highest intensity sounds investigated, were obtained by Metz (1951) and by Borg (1968), respectively. Near reflex threshold the latent period can be as long as 150 ms.

The latent period of the tensor tympani muscle in animals seems similiar to that of the stapedius muscle in man. For example, in rabbits under superficial penta-barbitol anaesthesia, a mean latency to contralateral stimulation of 14 ms for the stapedius muscle and 18 ms for the tensor tympani muscle have been obtained (Wersäll, 1958). An even closer agreement between the stapedius muscle response latency 6 ± 0.5 ms and the tensor tympani muscle response latency 7 ± 0.7 ms, was obtained myographically in cats (Eliasson and Gisselsson, 1955).

Dynamic Properties

It is clear that, since the acoustic reflex modifies the input to the cochlea, and is elicited by the output of the cochlea reaching a certain level, it is acting as a feedback system. If contraction is assumed to decrease transmission through the middle ear, then the reflex will act as a servo-system tending to keep the output of the middle ear constant. The efficiency of such a system depends on the magnitude of the change in transmission and, when time varying signals are concerned, on the dynamic properties of the system. Since both the intensity and frequency characteristics of the acoustic environment are rapidly varying functions of time, an analysis of the dynamic properties of the reflex is essential for describing and under-

standing the role of the middle ear muscles as regulators of the sound input to the internal ear.

Experimental Methods

Electromyographic analysis of the system (Salomon, 1966) is only of limited value for describing the feedback function of the reflex, and descriptions of the dynamic properties of the acoustic reflex have been based almost solely upon the results of impedance studies. The dynamic properties of the human reflex have been the subject of several studies including those by Møller (1962a) and by Dallos (1964).

The amplitude and phase characteristics of a linear system may be described by its frequency transfer function. This function is usually produced as a *Bode plot* and can be used to determine the output corresponding to any arbitrary input signal. Unfortunately, the acoustic reflex shows certain non-linearities, one dependent on stimulus amplitude and another dependent on the direction of change of stimulus amplitude, so that an overall description of the reflex cannot be obtained in this way. However, like most biological systems which are not linear, the reflex can be described by linear methods under certain restricted circumstances (Møller, 1962a; Dallos, 1964; Borg, 1971, 1972e). First though, the non-linearities of the system must be described.

Amplitude Dependent Non-linearity

The amplitude dependent non-linearity manifests itself as a longer rise-time for response to weak stimuli than for intense ones. Just as the rise time of the response decreases with an increase in stimulus amplitude, so there is a concomitant decrease of latency. The decrease of latency is probably the result of an exponential build-up of the level of excitation in synapses involved in the reflex arc, while the decrease in rise time will be predominately due to the eliciting of responses from faster, more phasic motor units with higher thresholds.

The time course of the contraction which follows the latent period depends, in fact, upon both the intensity and frequency content of the stimulus (viz. the frequency dependence of threshold and feedback gain). The amplitude dependence alone may be demonstrated by measuring responses to wide-band random noise stimuli, thus effectively eliminating the frequency dependence by having all important frequencies represented in the acoustic input and by plotting the responses on an amplitude-normalized basis (Fig. 10A). An orderly progression of curves representing the various signal intensities is seen.

Directional Non-linearity

If, however, the corresponding "off" responses are plotted in this way (Fig. 10B), the curves overlap indicating a linear process. Thus, the characteristics of the middle ear muscle acoustic reflex system depend upon the direction of change of the input (increase or decrease).

There is no inverse relationship between the cessation of response and stimulus strength. In man, the "off"-latency ranges between 75 and 100 ms and is largely independent of stimulus strength. The latency of decay in the rabbit is shorter than that of onset and values range from 5 to 10 ms (Borg, 1972e). This is probably a better expression of pure transport delay of the reflex arc than the latency of onset in that the latter includes the time taken for the neurones to reach threshold levels and time in which slack is taken up in the mechanical parts of the system. Similarly, at every stimulus level in the human reflex the actual "on" response is faster than the corresponding "off" response to wide-band noise stimuli. A more rapid contraction than relaxation is common to many other skeletal muscles, and the relaxation is generally considered

The character of the response is also determined by the amplitude dependent non-linearity of the system producing a faster response as the intensity increases. In the high gain region the response becomes more and more oscillatory as the intensity increases, while in the low gain region there is simply a decrease in rise-time with increasing stimulus intensity without the response ever becoming oscillatory.

Linear Analysis

How then can linear analysis help in the description of the acoustic reflex properties? In Fig. 11 the frequency

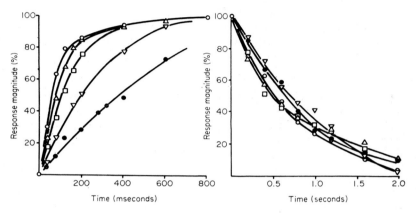

Fig. 10. Normalised on-(left) and off-(right) responses of a subject computed from impedance changes in response to noise bursts. The steady-state response magnitude is taken as 100% at each intensity and the relative size of the responses at an given instant of time beyond the latent period is plotted. Parameter is stimulus SPL. Left graph: 0, 112; △, 107; □, 102; ▽, 97; ●, 92 dB. Right graph:●, 112; ○, 107; △, 102; □, 97; ▽, 92 dB. (From Dallos, 1973.). Note the different time scales and that the same symbols do not relate to the stimulus intensities for both graphs.

to be dependent solely upon the physico-chemical properties of the contractile material.

Stability of Response

In a feedback system not only the speed of response, but the stability of the response, is important. The impedance responses from which the data for Fig. 10 were taken, all appeared over-damped. With wide-band noise stimuli, the human acoustic reflex never shows overshoot or oscillatory responses (Dallos, 1973), although these can occur when the stimulus is an intense pure tone of the appropriate frequency.

For low frequency sounds, damped oscillation in the response of the acoustic reflex occurs in man (Møller, 1958, 1962a) and in animals (Lorente de Nó, 1933; Okamoto et al., 1954). This is related to the larger effective feedback gain at low frequencies where the attenuation produced is maximal. In high frequency regions, where the gain is low, the response is overdamped and monotonic (Møller, 1962a; Hung, 1972). Some results have also indicated that the response becomes overdamped at the lowest frequencies (Hung, 1972). Thus, at a given frequency there is apparently a given feedback gain that determines the basic nature of the response. Dallos (1973) likens the frequency dependence of this gain factor to a band-pass filter.

transfer function for the onset of an open-loop step response to contralateral stimulation with 2 kHz stimuli of the rabbit acoustic reflex is shown (from Borg, 1972a). Because of the amplitude non-linearity of the reflex, it must be treated as a different linear system at each reflex response amplitude (Borg, 1971, see later). This assumption is valid providing the stimuli are rapidly changing in amplitude and the onset and decay properties are analysed separately. In this example, tone bursts of three different intensities are plotted. First, it can be seen that the amplitude decreases as the frequency increases, that is to say, the system has a low pass characteristic. The cut-off frequency in this rabbit's acoustic reflex increased from 2·5 to 9·4 Hz with an increase from 16 to 34 dB above reflex threshold. Secondly, the slope of the amplitude transfer function at high frequencies is a measure of the complexity of the system. Here the slope is −12 dB per octave which implies that a second-order differential equation can be expected to describe the reflex system adequately.

The right hand graph of Fig. 11 is the phase-transfer function. The frequency where there is a phase shift of 180° may be used to characterize the stability of a system. Here, this frequency varied with stimulus intensity in a similar way to the cut-off frequency, increasing from 7·2 to 20·6 Hz. (Note that this frequency refers to that of the stimulus envelope not that of the carrier tone.) Also, instead of measuring the latency of response directly, it can be determined from the slope of the phase-transfer function at high frequency, thereby utilizing information from the response curve as a whole.

In Borg's study of the rabbit, he showed that the properties of the isolated tensor tympani reflex can be described in the same way as the total reflex, but with smaller parameters and also less dependence on intensity. Differences still exist when allowances are made for the dissimilarities in excitability between the total and isolated tensor tympani reflex. Moreover, onset and decay differ less for the isolated tensor tympani reflex than for the total reflex. In rabbits, in terms of a frequency transfer function, the decay of the response is of the same general type as the onset. However, the decay is slower and the time constants become longer when there are increases in the sound level.

resonance peak at about 5 Hz (Møller, 1962a). In the rabbit it is at about 18–22 Hz (Borg, 1972e), and is intensity dependent. A resonance peak is seen only in responses of about 80 per cent of the maximal impedance change for 2 kHz stimuli, whereas with tones of 0·5 kHz it is clearly distinguished above about 30–40 per cent of the response level. As the stimulus level is increased, so the frequency of the resonance peak increases up to about 20 Hz, from lower limits of 15 Hz at 2 kHz stimulus frequency and about 8 Hz at 0·5 kHz stimulus frequency. Borg found good agreement between the oscillation frequency in the closed-loop system and the frequency for which the phase shift of the open-loop system was −180°.

Oscillations in the response appear more regularly with the stapedius muscle than with the tensor tympani muscle (Wersäll, 1958). In the rabbit, when one of these resonance peaks occurs in the tensor tympani reflex transfer function,

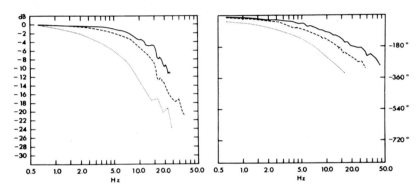

Fig. 11. The frequency transfer function for the onset of the open-loop step response of the middle ear reflex of a rabbit to contralateral stimulation with 2 kHz stimuli (Bode plot). The amplitude (in dB relative to the highest value) of sinusoidal components as a function of frequency is shown to the left and phase shift to the right, for tone bursts at three different intensities. ———— : 112 dB SPL, 99% of maximal impedance change response amplitude. — — — — : 102 dB SPL, 89% of maximal impedance change response amplitude. . . . . : 94 dB SPL, 50% of maximal impedance change response amplitude. (From Borg, 1972a.)

Obviously the open-loop dynamic properties are most easily studied in animals such as the rabbit, where the muscles may be experimentally deactivated. However, the open-loop transfer characteristics can be estimated in a normal human by two methods (Møller, 1962a). First, measurement of impedance responses when the stimulus is shorter in duration than the latency period may be performed. The muscles are not then active during the stimulus presentation and thus do not influence the transmission of sound. Secondly, a stimulus frequency may be used for which transmission is unchanged or only slightly changed by muscle contraction. With a stimulus frequency of 1450 Hz, Møller (1962a) then estimated that the open-loop transfer function of the acoustic reflex in man has a cut-off frequency of from 2 to 4 Hz. However, the servo-system's absolute gain cannot be determined in this way, because the magnitude of the impedance changes obtained are not equivalent to the amplitude regulation.

Direct comparisons between man and animal may be made for the closed-loop frequency transfer function. The dynamic properties of the reflex in the rabbit differ markedly from that in man. In man the closed-loop system has a

it does so at a frequency of about 10 Hz. A frequency of oscillation of about 15–20 Hz has been observed in the cat responses (Okamoto et al., 1954; Eliasson and Gisselsson, 1955). However, in the cat they seemed more pronounced in the tensor tympani than the stapedius muscle response.

When stimuli are prolonged for periods of 10 s to 1 min, at a constant level of intensity, the reflex response in a rabbit maintains a constant amplitude (Borg and Møller, 1968). Conversely, above 1 kHz, the reflex responses in man (Anderson et al., 1969, Tietze, 1969) and in the cat (Simmons, 1963) fail to show this constant amplitude. A similar decay in the reflex responses can be produced in the rabbit, but only with excessive stimulation of 130–140 dB SPL (Wersäll, 1958).

Differences also occur in the degree of habituation exhibited by the reflex in different animals. When repeated stimuli are presented to the cat, the reflex threshold may increase by as much as 50 dB during a 2 h testing session (Simmons and Beatty, 1964). In contrast, the response of non-anaesthetized rabbits is very stable, giving a difference in threshold of only 1·2 dB over a period of 1 h. Returning to cats, the tensor tympani response is fully habituated quite rapidly within 5–20 min (Baust and Berlucchi, 1964). It is of interest to note that such a rapid change in response is very similar to the habituation of the startle response to sound in cats (Hoffman and Searle, 1968).

Models of the Acoustic Reflex

Frequency Transfer Functions

It is clear that the frequency transfer functions of the acoustic reflex provide a convenient description of the system, albeit with certain limitations, and a useful basis for the derivation of mathematical models. Thus, Møller (1962a) calculated frequency transfer functions for the human acoustic reflex using 1450 Hz stimulus tones. Similarly, Dallos (1964) computed transfer functions to represent the impedance change due to activation and deactivation of the acoustic reflex when stimulating with wide-band noise of 100 dB SPL. However, these functions do not adequately describe the reflex generally, because of the non-linear amplitude dependence of the reflex response characteristics and the frequency-dependent feedback gain.

A Non-linear Mathematical Model

Dallos (1973) has also described another model that takes the magnitude dependent effects of the reflex into consideration. Basically a feedback configuration, as shown in Fig. 12, is assumed, with the muscle motors being modelled along the lines of the simple and effective model of skeletal muscle by Green (1964). A second-order non-linear differential equation with parametric excitation is then derived. Analogue computation of the step responses of this model were in good agreement with the onset step responses of the middle ear muscle reflex to wide-band noise and low frequency tone bursts. However, this representation may not necessarily be appropriate for providing the proper simulation of different types of time varying responses, such as those generated by amplitude-modulated tones. This is a basic property of non-linear systems.

Linear Representation of Each Amplitude Level

Similarly, the limitation of Borg's (1971) linear analysis of the acoustic reflex at each reflex response amplitude, to stimuli that are rapidly changing in amplitude and with the onset and decay properties analysed separately, has already been mentioned. Borg (1972e) has described the open-loop transfer functions of the acoustic reflex response of the rabbit by a second-order system with transport delay. The parameters were determined at several input amplitudes by approximating the model transfer function to the values calculated from experimental recordings by using the least mean square criterion of best fit.

A Piece-wise Linear Model

Recently, another model has been presented by Borg (1973) to simulate the two prominent non-linearities of the open-loop responses of the acoustic middle ear reflex, and to investigate their significance for stability of the closed-

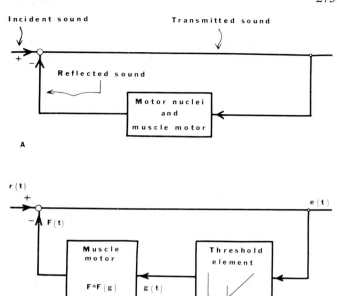

FIG. 12. Schematic representation of the acoustic reflex as a feedback system, A. The assumed feedback loop, B. The equivalent model with a feedback gain represented by the function F = F(g), where g(t) is the input to this block. A threshold element is included, represented by E. The input signal is r(t) where the time function denotes amplitude variations of the carrier. The output signal is e(t), representing the transmitted sound and again the time variation refers to the envelope. The reflected sound is considered directly proportional to muscle tension (F), the proportionality for simplicity being unity, giving a feedback signal of F(t). (Modified from Dallos 1973).

loop feed-back system. This piecewise linear model, depicted in Fig. 13, is most interesting because the pool of "reflex units" bear an indirect relation to the motor units of the middle ear muscles discussed earlier. The "reflex units" in this model were regarded as including both motor-neurone and inter-neurone properties, and in themselves were linear systems. Thus, they cannot be thought of as having any simple anatomical counterpart, but the concept of phasic and tonic units with different thresholds bears obvious comparison with motor units. Each unit had an individual threshold and independently specified properties. Models were investigated which had tonic reflex units with various time constants, as well as combinations of tonic and phasic units. Direction sensitive properties were simulated by including phasic units in the pool or having different time constants for an increase and a decrease in amplitude. Amplitude dependent non-linearity was simulated when low threshold reflex units were made slow and tonic, and high threshold units fast and tonic, or when some of the high threshold units were phasic. Those models with more than one type of reflex unit exhibited smaller amplitudes of oscillation and faster damping of the oscillation when responding to step stimuli, than a model composed of only one type of unit, although the rise time to 50 per cent was the same. In other words, the stability of the response was improved without affecting the system band-width (speed of response). Similarly, stability was improved when the time constants for decreases in amplitude were made greater than the time constants for increases in stimulus amplitude (i.e. direction dependent properties of the closed-loop system).

Oscillations also decreased significantly when a model system was composed of low threshold tonic units and high threshold phasic units, both of which had the same decay constants, compared with a model with equal time constants of onset. At high input amplitude, the band-width of the system was the same, or even slightly increased in the non-linear system of mixed units, compared to the system with all units equal. However, at low input ampli-tude the non-linear systems were slower. Another system, where the low threshold tonic units were fast and the high

fast motor units may be utilized at the expense of stability (compare oscillations in the stapedius muscle responses). If a maintained, but stable, response is required at all intensities, then, as in the model, speed of response at low intensities may be sacrificed for stability and slow tonic units may be utilized. Although Borg's model involves simplifications in the fundamental assumptions on the physiological origins of the non-linearities (e.g. the ex-clusion of properties relating to firing frequency of the motor-neurones, inhibition and the variations in contractile strength of the motor units), comparison with the varia-tions in the fibre composition of the muscles would seem

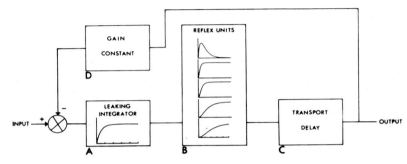

FIG. 13. A block diagram of a piecewise linear model of the acoustic middle ear reflex. Block A the "leaking integrator" represents smoothing in the lower auditory system of excitatory input to a pool of "reflex units" in block B. The curve shows a step response; full time scale 50 ms. The "reflex units" are triggered at different levels of output from the "leaking integrator". In block B the time courses of step responses of a phasic unit (top), two fast tonic units with high thresholds (middle) and two slow tonic units with low thresholds (bottom) are represented (full scale 500 ms). The time course of each reflex unit was described by second-order differential equations, and had the same properties, independently of how much thresholds were exceeded Peak amplitudes of all units were assumed to be the same and were defined as 1·0. The output after a "transport delay" in block C is fed back, via a feedback gain constant in block D, to be subtracted from the input. This gain constant was zero for the open-loop conditions and generally taken as equal to 1 in the closed-loop conditions. (From Borg, 1973b.)

threshold units were slow, had increased stability over an all-units-equal system, yet the response was not slower at low input amplitudes. It was suggested that this system and its consequent advantages is comparable to the parallel action of the two middle ear muscles; the stapedius muscle having a fast response and a low threshold, while the tensor tympani muscle has a slow response and a high threshold. Finally, it was shown that a decreased latency increased the stability of the response, but that the amplitude of oscillation also decreased when the system was made slower with tonic units with longer time constants for onset.

In a polysynaptic reflex arc, such as the middle ear acoustic reflex, a transport delay is inevitable. Borg suggested that since a transport delay may decrease stability, the non-linearities may counteract this effect and be important in system stabilization. It can be inferred further that if the reflex system is required to perform differ-ent functions, or under different conditions in different animals, the various physiological counterparts represented by the factors of this model will differ to obtain the optimum performance for the particular function. For example, if a fast response at low intensity stimulation is required,

justified. Thus, the presence of intermediate fibres in the fruit-bat middle ear muscles may be related to slow tonic "units". However, before attempting to infer system pro-perties from muscle fibre composition, two points must be considered. First, although histochemical fibre types reflect the properties of the motor-neurones, inter-neuronal properties must also be taken into account. Secondly, a compromise may be effected within a system between sta-bility and speed of response. For example, the fact that the cotton rat middle ear muscles contain only phasic motor units (as inferred from histochemical typing) could mean that stability of response has been sacrificed for speed of response. Alternatively, perhaps stability is achieved not by tonic units but by firing patterns i.e. the onset of contrac-tion is fast and strong (with white muscle fibres) but the contraction is maintained by repetitive firing and contrac-tion of red muscle fibres, with a gradual decay of response.

The fact that differences in fibre composition of the middle ear muscles do occur between species, and that the presence of tonic and phasic "reflex units" can be expected to influence the feedback stability of the system, indicates the usefulness of such studies. They may serve as a basis for further models, and as our knowledge of the reflex increases (particularly in regard to neuronal properties), as a basis for predicting the optimal performance, and indeed probable function, in various animals.

FUNCTION

The strategic position of the middle ear muscles, attached as they are to the ossicular chain, would seem to indicate that the muscles are primarily concerned with modification of the auditory input to the cochlea. We have seen that the muscles have been shown to be capable of selectively attenuating, and to a lesser degree enhancing, certain sounds. There is both a frequency specificity and a dynamic specificity. The latter arises from the transport delay before response and the amplitude non-linearity of the system. Fast changing and short duration sounds are relatively unaffected by the muscles, compared to slower and more maintained sounds, but the more intense the sound the faster the response. If the middle ear muscles are triggered acoustically a transport delay is inevitable, and the beginning of the sound will not be affected by the contraction. However, if the sound is anticipated, it may be affected by the contraction. It appears that the middle ear muscles contract in order to affect the transmission into the ear of self-produced sounds. This allows anticipation of sound and muscle contraction immediately prior to it.

Since the middle ear muscles are acting as an input control system, presumably modifying the input to the cochlea for optimal processing, some correlation may be expected between their properties and those of the neural elements of the auditory system. One example of this is the relatively constant difference, across the frequency spectrum, between the acoustic reflex threshold and the auditory threshold. The accommodation theory which is discussed later suggests that the middle ear muscles are responsible for tuning middle ear transmission for the optimal characteristics of the internal ear. It has been suggested that the introduction of the accentuated masking effect of low frequencies on high frequencies, by the mechanism for frequency analysis, is a weakness in cochlear functioning. Since the middle ear muscles predominantly attenuate low frequencies in many animals, this may be expected to partly compensate for these masking effects. Reduction of masking by low frequency self-produced sounds is probably a major effect of middle ear muscle contraction during motor activities.

The middle ear muscles have been implicated with activity in several motor-controlled arrays within the central nervous system. In both animals and man, the middle ear muscles contract during certain movements and vocalization (Kato, 1913; Carmel and Starr, 1963; Salomon and Starr, 1963; Simmons, 1964a, 1964b; Henson, 1965 and Djupesland, 1967).

Non-reflex contractions of the middle ear muscles are also associated with bursts of phasic motor activity in rapid eye movement (REM) sleep (Baust and Berlucchi, 1964; Dewson et al., 1965).

Simmons (1964a) has shown electromyographically in cats that the middle ear muscles contract with head movement. Brief, unsustained middle ear muscle contraction

associated with novel or otherwise unexpected sounds when accompanied by an auricular twitch and other orienting reflexes, could be useful for distinguishing between internal physiological and neural noise and external environmental signals. Attenuation of the external signal would distinguish it from neural and bone-conducted internal noise. Such middle ear muscle responses are especially prominent when the sound is a relatively high frequency transient, one that, if continuous, would not ordinarily cause sustained acoustic reflex activity. If such sounds are repeated and the animal becomes habituated to them, the acoustic reflex response diminishes and disappears (Simmons and Beatty, 1964).

Conversely, middle ear muscle activity associated solely with head movements does not appear to habituate (Simmons, 1964a). A major function of this type of contraction would seem likely to be to reduce both air- and bone-conducted low-frequency sounds produced by this activity. This is probably a prime function of middle ear muscle contractions during other inherently noisy activities such as chewing, teeth clenching, vocalization and swallowing.

In man, Djupesland (1967) found that a number of complex movements such as tight closure of the eyes, swallowing, opening of the mouth, and clenching of the teeth, were accompanied by acoustic impedance changes attributable to the effects of middle ear muscle contractions. It was also suggested that perhaps such contractions were associated with these activities because several of the muscles of the head and neck are innervated by the same motor nerves (facial and trigeminal) as the tympanic muscles. Voluntary movements involving contraction of muscle not innervated by these nerves, did not cause impedance changes. Thus, no impedance change was observed on rotation of the head or lifting of arms or legs. When middle ear muscle activity is elicited by surprise or by painful stimuli it probably occurs as an integral part of an extensive muscle contraction which does include head and neck muscles innervated by the facial and trigeminal nerves.

The reflex interconnection between ear muscles and the afferent nerve supply of the larynx in the cat (McCall and Rabuzzi, 1973) has already been mentioned. This reflex may be part of a protective mechanism such as the cough reflex, or it may have a function in vocalization.

Middle ear muscle activity in association with vocalization has been reported in the waking cat (Carmel and Starr, 1963) and in man (Salomon and Starr, 1963; Djupesland, 1967). Salomon and Starr (1963) showed that this activity precedes the production of sound, and lasts throughout the period of sound production and for some time afterwards. This was substantiated by Djupesland (1967), who found that the activity started 30–450 ms before the speaking voice was recorded, and persisted for up to 300 ms after the sounds of speaking had ceased. These contractions do not appear to habituate and their magnitude is proportional to the intensity of the following vocalization (Simmons, 1964a). It thus seems that the middle ear muscles are activated relatively concurrently with the speech musculature (Shearer and Simmons, 1965) perhaps by neural impulses direct from the motor cortex.

A similar pattern of activity occurs in the bat, *Tadarida*, during production of sounds other than frequency modulated (FM) pulses. However, when this bat is producing FM pulses during echolocation, although the stapedius muscle begins to contract 10 ms prior to each pulse emission, the maximum state of contraction occurs as the pulse begins, and the muscle relaxes over the duration of the pulse.

The tympanic muscle contractions (possibly only the stapedius muscle) attenuate the pulsed emissions reducing fatigue and/or possible acoustic trauma. At low rates of pulse emissions, the attenuation also has the effect of maintaining the sensitivity of the ear at frequencies of emission up to 50 kHz which facilitates the reception of weak echoes which will not be attenuated between pulses. At pulse rates higher than 50–62 per second, the muscles do not relax between pulses and are tonically contracted throughout, attenuating both pulse emissions and echoes. However, this rate of emission occurs in the terminal phase of echolocation when echoes are loud and travel only a short distance. At such intensities, attenuation may reduce distortion and be beneficial to the analysis of the echoes. In this activity then, attenuation of high frequency sounds is important. Middle ear muscles may in fact act as a very sharp filter at high frequencies, as in the bat *Pteronotus parnelli*. In this bat there is a sharp decrease in the attenuating capacity of the middle ear muscles for frequencies above 57 kHz (Fig. 9B) and this shows a distinct correlation with the frequency characteristics of the orientation pulses. During pulse emission, the contracted middle ear muscles can protect the ear from most components of the pulses, but not a loud (at least 100 dB SPL) 60 kHz constant frequency (CF) component. Protection of the ear at this frequency is not necessary because of the bat's relatively higher threshold in this region (Fig. 9A). The maximum sensitivity peak is approximately 1·5 kHz higher than that of the emitted pulse, and this peak corresponds to the frequency predicted for echoes from calculation of the Doppler shift due to the flight speed of *Pteronotus* (Pollak *et al.*, 1972). These echoes are probably never loud enough that protection is required. Thus, even during periods of pulse-echo overlap, reception of echoes is facilitated by a combination of a sharply tuned auditory system and the high pass filter characteristics of the middle ear muscles. Action potential (AP) first negative peak (N_1) audiograms also exhibit a relatively high threshold to 60 kHz CF components, but, in contrast to the CM audiogram, low thresholds for the lower frequency components of the pulses (Pollak and Henson, 1973). Thus, the attenuating properties of the middle ear muscles in this animal are finely adapted to the characteristics of the internal ear.

It is in a perceptive role, of helping to distinguish external sounds when one is talking oneself, that Borg (1974) concludes probably lies the greatest significance in man of stapedius muscle activity during vocalization and when listening to speech. In subjects with unilateral stapedius muscle paralysis (Bell's palsy), Borg and Zakrisson (1973) had earlier determined articulation scores and stapedius reflex responses to the same speech phrases before and after treatment. A significantly poorer articulation score occurred for intensities of the test word at and above 100 dB SPL prior to treatment. The lowered score during paralysis was considered due to masking produced by the low frequencies of the speech on the high frequency components. This conclusion was supported by the finding that masking produced by 0·5 kHz narrow-band noise on pure tones in the range 1–8 kHz rose up to 50 dB in the absence of the stapedius reflex. When subjects listened to speech, the stapedius muscle was activated in normal ears by phrases at levels above 92 dB SPL, which was close to the reflex threshold for a 0·5 kHz pure tone. The stapedius reflex threshold in normal ears is at and above the intensity level where the discrimination of complex sounds was found to decline when the stapedius muscle was paralysed. It was therefore concluded by Borg and Zakrisson that the stapedius muscle extends the dynamic range of the ear by 15–20 dB. The role of the stapedius muscle may be to prevent a large increase in the generation of distortion products at high sound intensities.

Stevens and Newman (1936) showed that contraction of the tensor tympani muscle decreases the amplitude of harmonics in cochlear microphonics recorded in the guinea-pig. One source of non-linearity in the guinea-pig cochlea occurs at about 80–90 dB SPL (Worthington and Dallos, 1971), which, as Borg (1972a) points out, is close to the threshold for the middle ear muscle reflex. The increased rigidity of stiffening of the ossicular chain by middle ear muscle contraction may serve to reduce excessive movement of the ossicles (Békésy, 1960). Prevention of changes in the articulation between the ossicles during high acceleration has been described as the fixation theory. The relatively high sound levels at which the acoustic reflex is activated support these contentions.

The dynamic range of the ear is extended because of the high regulatory efficiency of the reflex. The animal experiments of Wever and Vernon (1955), using decerebrate unanaesthetized cats, indicated a near perfect regulation of cochlear input over a limited intensity and frequency range (Fig. 14). When the intensity of a contralateral stimulus increased above reflex threshold an orderly decrease in the cochlear microphonic response to a steady test tone occurred. With both muscles active the cochlear microphonic decreased proportionally from its pre-reflex value for a range of about 20 dB above reflex threshold. The input was potentially held constant with virtually perfect regulation, the decrease being equivalent to almost 20 dB for a 20 dB stimulus. Significant, but less perfect, regulation has been demonstrated in man. In man and the rabbit, Borg (1968, 1972d) found that, above reflex threshold, only about 3 dB of a 10 dB increase in sound level over a wide frequency range reaches the cochlea. This considerably decreases the slope of the stimulus-response curve which has the disadvantage that it decreases the sensitivity for small differences in intensity. However, discrimination of high level sound is increased and performance below reflex threshold may be indirectly improved.

The increase in dynamic range effected by this feedback attenuation has usually been described in terms of protection from fatigue or structural damage to the cochlea (protection against overloading of the analysing system). This role has been reviewed by Wever and Lawrence (1954) and by Cancura (1970). It is well established that, in both animals and man, the ear suffers less damage and fatigue from sound exposure if the muscles are contracting during the stimulation (e.g. Taruya, 1953; Hilding, 1961; Fletcher and Riopelle, 1960).

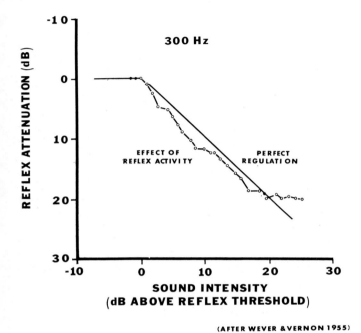

FIG. 14. The near perfect regulation of cochlear input over a 20 dB intensity range is a result of the contraction of both middle ear muscles in decerebrate unanaesthetised cats. The attenuation of the cochlear microphonic response to a steady 300 Hz tone is shown plotted against the intensity of contralateral stimulation. (From Wever and Vernon, 1955.)

However, the relatively long latency of the acoustic reflex means that it is not effective in dealing with single brief pulses from an external source. For example, the cry of the bat *Tadarida*, mentioned earlier, is of 3–4 ms duration with a peak sound pressure level occurring with 1 ms of the beginning of a pulse. The ear of another bat would be maximally stimulated before the middle ear muscles would begin to contract, but, in a large colony, perhaps a degree of tonic activity is present. Cancura (1970) stressed the fatigueability of the reflex as another limitation of any protective function. However, Guzman-Flores and colleagues (1960), Alcaraz and colleagues (1962a, b) and Bogacz and colleagues (1962) found that the monotonous repetition of an acoustic stimulus enhances the reflex activity of the middle ear muscles. Comparing these results with the work of Simmons and Beatty (1964), in which middle ear muscle contraction became habituated to repeated high frequency sounds, it appears that habituation effects may depend upon the frequencies involved and of the relevance of the stimulus to the animal.

Yet another criticism of the protective theory has been that the greatest damage to hearing caused by acoustic trauma occurs around 4 kHz in man. This frequency is usually considered to be outside the range of frequencies influenced by the tympanic muscles in man. In this respect it is interesting to note the results of a recent conditioning experiment with cats (Sokolovski, 1973). In Sokolovski's experiments, cats with the stapedius muscle tendon cut (tenotomized) and stapedius muscle intact (non-tenotomized) were exposed to white noise. Their hearing thresholds were measured by behavioural audiometry and the permanent threshold shift (PTS) studied three months after the noise exposure. In Fig. 15 the median PTS of three non-tenotomized, and three tenotomized cats, for the three exposure conditions are plotted. In the non-tenotomized animals at the lower intensity (C) damage is mainly limited to the frequency range 2–4 kHz but spreads to include low and high frequencies with a greater noise

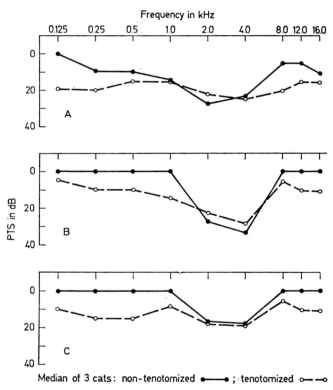

FIG. 15. The median permanent threshold shift (PTS) of three-tenotomized and three tenotomized cats, in each of three groups, each given a different noise exposure. A—105 dB SPL white noise continuously for 8 hours. B—105 dB SPL white noise continuously for 4 hours. C—95 dB SPL white noise continuously for 8 hours. (From Sokolovski, 1973.)

exposure. However, in the tenotomized animals although there is no essential difference in PTS under each of the three noise conditions and in the frequency range 2–4 kHz, at frequencies below and above this frequency band, the PTS is greater than for the non-tenotomized animals. Sokolovski refers to the frequency band of 2–4 kHz as the *site of election* for noise-induced permanent hearing loss in the cat. The effect of tenotomy was to produce a widening of this so-called traumatic notch, and to produce PTS that shows less frequency dependance. It might be inferred from this that the influence of an intact stapedius muscle is to confine the noise-induced hearing loss to the mid-high frequency region and to protect the frequencies below and above this region. It is not however clear, as to what extent the passive presence of the stapedius muscle might have been responsible for this effect. For frequencies below 2 kHz, protective action was assessed as equivalent to a reduction of intensity of up to a maximum of 20 dB, and slightly less over 4 kHz. Sokolovski proposed that these findings in the cat might be extended to man. The stapedius muscle could then be considered incapable of reducing the noise-induced hearing loss at the site of election of such a loss, i.e. about 4 kHz, but providing protection at frequencies below this point. In fact, Lehnhardt (1960) found that, when the stapedius is paralysed, a maximal post-exposure shift of hearing threshold occurs within the range of frequency most essential for the understanding of speech, but mainly above these frequencies when its function is normal. If Sokolovski's suggestion is correct, this partly explains the failure of studies in stapedectomized ears to demonstrate a difference from normals in their temporary threshold shift (TTS) when exposed to noise. Many experiments have measured TTS at 4 kHz (e.g. Ferris, 1965), at which frequency no difference from normals would be predicted. It must also be appreciated that patients with stapedectomized ears are not suitable for making strict comparisons between normal ears and demuscled ears.

There is little doubt that both middle ear muscles in animals and the stapedius muscle alone in man are potentially capable of providing a measure of protection against maintained low frequency sounds (for example Zakrisson and Borg, 1974). Borg (1972a) discusses the suggestion that there may in fact be a causal relationship between the great resistance of the cochlea to fatigue to low frequency stimulation and the attenuation provided by the middle ear muscles in this frequency range. A significant increase in susceptibility to low frequency sound exposure has been observed in human subjects with decreased or abolished stapedius muscle contraction (Lehnhardt, 1959, 1960; Mills and Lilly, 1971). Similarly Price (1972) found a greatly increased sensitivity to low frequency sound exposure in deeply anaesthetized cats in which the middle ear muscle reflex was depressed. Protection can even be provided in humans against impulsive noise when the acoustic reflex is elicited with a stimulus of appropriate intensity about 150 ms prior to the arrival of the impulsive noise (Ward, 1962). Anticipatory activity of the middle ear muscles has also been shown to reduce TTS (Coles and Knight, 1965; Simmons, 1959).

Middle ear muscle activity in relation to auditory habituation and orientating reactions has been reviewed by Filogamo, Candiollo and Rossi, (1967). During both activities there is a decrease in acoustically evoked potentials. When the mesencephalic reticular formation of an "encéphale isolé" cat is stimulated there is a decrease in the cochlear microphonics and the responses evoked by acoustic clicks at the level of the dorsal cochlear nucleus (Hugelin et al., 1960a, b). This effect does not occur in curarized cats nor when the stapedius and tensor tympani muscles are severed. Because the reflex arc of the stapedius

muscle is more sensitive to impulses from the reticular substance than is that of the tensor tympani muscle, it is believed that it is mainly the contractions of the former that are involved (Hugelin et al., 1960c). Nevertheless, Alcaraz and his associates (1962) reported that the characteristic electrophysiological phenomena of "habituation" could not be observed in animals after the tensor tympani tendon had been cut. In the same animal, however, the electrophysiological phenomena, elicited by diverting the animal's attention, did persist.

The involvement of higher auditory centres is an implicit part of some of the perceptive functions attributed to the middle ear muscles by Simmons (1964a). He proposed that constant changes in middle ear muscle tonus provide minute amplitude modulations of ambient sounds, as a most effective background for auditory perception. He compared this activity with that of the extraocular muscles, which constantly change the position of the retinal image. The middle ear muscles are thus envisaged as performing a role in the maintenance of attention. In the cat, Simmons showed that the oscillations in middle ear muscle activity occur as long as the animal is alert to the environment. The activity is, however, accentuated by the introduction of an above threshold tone. Simmons (1964a) proposed that this activity may enable the auditory system to distinguish between physiological and neural noise in the ear, and external stimuli. He emphasized the particular difficulties in the perception of a constant low-frequency sound or a slowly changing stimulus, and compared the proposed function of the middle ear muscles with the activity of a "chopper" amplifier.

Another possible consequence of changes in intratympanic muscle tonus is to cause a continual shift of the resonant loci of the middle ear. In contrast to previous accommodation theories, Simmons did not propose a tuning of transmission of particular frequencies through the middle ear. He postulated that the inevitable resonances and nulls in the transmission system could be shifted continually so that the sensitivity at any one frequency is never permanently affected. Simmons measured the round window CM response at several frequencies at constant SPL in awake and anaesthetized cats that were either normal or had inactive middle ear muscles (tendons cut or animal anaesthetized). In all the situations where the muscles were inactive, a deep notch in the response curve was found around 4 kHz, whereas, in the normal awake cat, the transmission function was relatively smooth. Middle ear muscle contractions might therefore detune the middle ear antiresonance and average out its effect. The selective peaks of attenuation found by Teig and discussed earlier, may be relevant to this proposed function. However, Teig did not find any evidence for a shift in these peaks of attenuation, to compare with Simmons' proposed shift of the resonance loci of the middle ear.

Unfortunately, it does not seem clear to what extent fluctuations in the tonus of the middle ear muscles occur in man. Some electromyographic recordings have indicated very little activity in the absence of sound stimuli (Fisch and Schulthess, 1963; Salomon and Starr, 1963). Conversely Djupesland (1967) recorded changes in impedance and electromyographic activity in both intratympanic muscles in association with anxiety or other mental factors causing contraction of various muscles. He commented that man is seldom completely mentally and physically relaxed. He therefore concluded that the intratympanic muscles are in continuous activity for the greater part of the day. This assumption corresponds with the electromyographic recordings of the middle ear muscles in conscious cats (Carmel and Starr, 1963; Simmons, 1964a). From histochemical findings on the middle ear muscles of several other animals Anderson (1974) concluded that the stapedius muscle is better adapted for maintained activity than is the tensor tympani muscle.

A considerable degree of spontaneous tonic activity of the middle ear muscles is a prerequisite of a function proposed for the muscles by Wigand and Borucki (1965). They observed a deterioration in the ability of patients who had been stapedectomized or had Bell's palsy, to separate double clicks. They envisaged an increase in the duration of the clicks when the middle ear muscles are paralysed.

Simmons (1964a) pointed out that the precise exposition of the role of the middle ear muscles in auditory perception is difficult because of the plastic nature of the nervous system and the capacity for redundancy of function. The effects of middle ear muscle contractions in man may be subtle and compensations for the impairment of functioning of the muscles probably exist. Head and auricle movements (in animals) may modulate incoming sounds especially those of high frequency. The olivocochlear efferent fibres also probably decrease noise masking, although mainly affecting weak sounds of frequencies above 2–3 kHz (Wiederhold, 1970). The exact relationship between the various input control systems of the ear remain to be resolved. However, it is clear that the intratympanic muscles have a significant role to play in the control of afferent auditory activity. The significance of various properties of the acoustic reflex in regard to the testing of normal and pathological ears is also an area of continuing research, although one that is outside the scope of this chapter. In the case of pathological ears it is hoped that it will be concluded from this chapter that the functional integrity of the middle ear muscles should be maintained whenever possible.

REFERENCES

Alcaraz, M., Salas, M., Pacheco, P. and Guzman-Flores, C. (1962a), *Bol. Inst. Estud. méd. biol. (Méx.)* **20**, 287.

Alcaraz, M., Pacheco, P. and Guzman-Flores, C. (1962b), *Acta physiol. lat-amer.*, **12**, 1.

Anderson, S. D. (1972), *Reports—Institute of Laryngology and Otology*, **20**, 487.

Anderson, S. D. (1973), Paper given at the 10th International Meeting on Inner Ear Biology, Graz.

Anderson, S. D. (1974), In *Sound Reception in Mammals, Symposium of the Zoological Society of London*, No. 37. London: Academic Press. In press.

Anderson, H., Barr, B. and Wedenberg, E. (1969), *Nobelsymposium 10, Disorders of the Skull Base Region*, p. 48. Stockholm: Almqvist and Wiksell.

Anzenbacher, H. and Zenker, W. (1963), *Z. Zellforsch.*, **60**, 860.

Ariano, M. A., Armstrong, R. B. and Edgerton, V. R. (1973), *J. Histochem. and Cytochem.*, **21**, 51.

Barker, D. (1967), Comment in CIBA Foundation Symposium, *Myotatic, Kinesthetic and Vestibular Mechanisms*, p. 38.

Baust, W. and Berlucchi, G. (1964), *Arch. ital. Biol.*, **102**, 686.

Békésy, G. von (1936), *Akust. Z.*, **1**, 13.

Békésy, G. von (1960), *Experiments in Hearing*. New York, Toronto and London: McGraw-Hill Series in Psychology.

Blevins, C. E. (1963), *Amer. J. Anat.*, **113**, 287.

Blevins, C. E. and Noble, B. (1965), *Anat. Rec.*, **151**, 325.

Bogacz, J., Vanzulli, A. and Garcia-Austt, E. (1962), *Acta neurol. lat-amer.*, **8**, 244.

Borg, E. (1968), *Acta oto-laryng. (Stockh.)*, **66**, 461.

Borg, E. (1971), *Brain Res.*, **31**, 211.

Borg, E. (1972a), *Acta oto-laryng.*, suppl., **304**.

Borg, E. (1972b), *Acta physiol. scand.*, **85**, 374.

Borg, E. (1972c), *Acta oto-laryng. (Stockh.)*, **74**, 240.

Borg, E. (1972d), *Acta physiol. scand.*, **86**, 175.

Borg, E. (1972e), *Acta physiol. scand.*, **86**, 366.

Borg, E. (1973a), *Brain Res.*, **49**, 101.

Borg, E. (1973b), *Acta physiol. scand.*, **87**, 15.

Borg, E. (1974), In *Sound Reception in Mammals, Symposium of the Zoological Society of London*, No. 37 London: Academic Press: In press.

Borg, E. and Møller, A. R. (1967), *Acta oto-laryng. (Stockh.)*, **64**, 415.

Borg, E. and Møller, A. R. (1968), *Acta oto-laryng. (Stockh.)*, **65**, 575.

Borg, E. and Zakrisson, J. E. (1973), *J. acoust. Soc. Amer.*, **54**, 525.

Boyd, I. A. and Davey, M. R. (1966), *Nobel Symposium I, Muscular Afferents and Motor Control*, p. 59. Stockholm: Almqvist and Wiksell.

Brzezinski, D. K. (1962), *Arch. Ohr.-, Nas.- u.Kehlk Heilk.*, **179**, 550.

Byrne, I. G. (1938), *Studies on the Physiology of the Ear*. London: Lewis and Co.

Cancura, W. (1970), *Mschr. Ohrenheilk.*, **19**, 3.

Candiollo, L. (1965a), *Z. Zellforsch.*, **67**, 34.

Candiollo, L. (1965b), *Atti. Accad. Sci. Torino*, **99**, 517.

Carmel, W. P. and Starr, A. (1963), *J. Neurophysiol.*, **26**, 598.

Close, R. I. (1972), *Physiol. Rev.*, **52**, 129.

Coles, R. R. A. and Knight, J. J. (1965), *J. Laryng.*, **79**, 131.

Dallos, P. J. (1964), *J. acoust. Soc. Amer.*, **36**, 2175.

Dallos, P. (1973), *The Auditory Periphery, Biophysics and Physiology*. New York and London: Academic Press.

David, H., Gerhardt, H. J. and Uerlings, I. (1966), *Z. Zellforsch.*, **70**, 334.

Davies, D. V. (1948), *J. Laryng.*, **62**, 533.

Dewson, J. A. III, Dement, W. C. and Simmons, F. B. (1965), *Exp. Neurol.*, **12**, 1.

Djupesland, G. (1967), *Contractions of the Tympania Muscles in Man*. Oslo: Universitetsforlaget.

Edgerton, V. R. and Simpson, D. R. (1971), *Exp. Neurol.*, **30**, 374.

Eliasson, S. and Gisselsson, L. (1955), *Electroenceph. clin. Neurophysiol.*, **7**, 395.

Erulkar, S. D., Shelanski, M. L., Whitsel, B. L. and Ogle, P. (1964), *Anat. Rec.*, **149**, 279.

Fernand, V. S. V. and Hess, A. (1969), *J. Physiol. (Lond.)*, **200**, 547.

Ferris, K. (1965), *J. Laryng.*, **79**, 881.

Filogamo, G. (1940), *Boll. Soc. ital. Biol. sper.*, **15**, 742.

Filogamo, G., Candiollo, L. and Rossi, G. (1967), Translations of the Beltonian Institute for Hearing Research No. 20.

Fisch, U. and Schulthess, G. von (1963), *Acta oto-laryng. (Stockh.)*, **56**, 287.

Fletcher, J. L. and Riopelle, A. J. (1960), *J. acoust. Soc. Amer.*, **32**, 401.

Fumagalli, Z. (1949), *Arch. ital. Otol.*, **60**, suppl., 1.

Galambos, R. and Rupert, A. (1959), *J. acoust. Soc. Amer.*, **31**, 349.

Gisselsson, L., Löfström, B. and Metz, O. (1957), *Acta oto-laryng. (Stockh.)*, **47**, 233.

Green, D. G. (1964), Unpublished Doctoral Dissertation, Northwestern University, Evanston, Illinois. Cited by Dallos, 1973.

Guzman-Flores, C., Alcaraz, M. and Harmony, T. (1960), *Bol. Inst Estud. méd. biol. (Méx.)*, **18**, 135.

Hayata, T. (1963), *Otologia Fukuoka*, **9**, 91.

Henson, O. W., Jr. (1961), *Kans. Univ. Sci. Bull.*, **42**, 151.

Henson, O. W., Jr. (1965), *J. Physiol. (Lond.)*, **180**, 871.

Hess, A. (1970), *Physiol. Rev.*, **50**, 40.

Hilding, D. A. (1960), *Ann. Otol. (St. Louis)*, **69**, 57.

Hilding, D. A. (1961), *Trans. Amer. Acad. Ophthal. Otolaryng.*, **65**, 297.

Hinchcliffe, R. and Pye, A. (1969), *J. Zool., London*, **157**, 277.

Hirayama, M. and Daly, J. F. (1974), *Acta oto-laryng.*, **77**, 13.

Hirayama, M. Davidowitz, J. and Daly, J. F. (1974), *Acta oto-laryng.*, **77**, 171.

Hoffman, H. S. and Searle, J. L. (1968), *J. acoust. Soc. Amer.*, **43**, 269.

Holst, H. E., Ingelstedt, S. and Örtegren, U. (1963), *Acta. oto-laryng. (Stockh.)*, suppl., **182**, 73.

Hugelin, A., Dumont, S. and Paillas, N. (1960a), *Electroenceph. clin. Neurophysiol.*, **12**, 797.

Hugelin, A., Dumont, S. and Paillas, N. (1960b), *Science*, **131**, 1371.

Hugelin, A., Paillas, N. and Dumont, S. (1960c), *C. R. Soc. Biol. (Paris)*, **154**, 30.

Hung, I. J. S. (1972), Doctoral Dissertation, Northwestern University, Evanston, Illinois.

Irvine, D. R. F. and Webster, W. R. (1972), *Brain Res.*, **39**, 109.

Jepsen, O. (1955), Thesis, Universitets forbget, Aarhus.

Jepsen, O. (1963), In *Modern Developments in Audiology*, p. 193. New York: Academic Press.

Kampen, P. N. van (1915), *Ned. Tijdschr. Geneesk.*, **59**, 2444.

Kato, T. (1913), *Arch. Ges. Physiol.*, **150**, 569.

Kirikae, I. (1960), *The Structure and Function of the Middle Ear*. Tokyo: University Tokyo Press.

Klockhoff, I. (1961), *Acta oto-laryng. (Stockh.)*, suppl., 164.

Kobayashi, M. (1956), *Hiroshima J. med. Sci.*, **5**, 63.

Krüger, P. (1949), *Anat. Anz.*, **97**, 169.

Lehnhardt, E. (1959), *Arch. Ohr.-, Nas.-u.KehlkHeilk.*, **175**, 383.

Lehnhardt, E. (1960), *Acta oto-laryng. (Stockh.)*, **52**, 438.

Lidén, G., Peterson, J. L. and Harford, E. R. (1970), *Acta oto-laryng. (Stockh.)*, suppl., **263**, 208.

Lorente De Nó, R. (1933), *Laryngoscope (St. Louis)*, **43**, 327.

Lorente De Nó, R. (1935), *Laryngoscope (St. Louis)*, **45**, 573.

Lorente De Nó, R. and Harris, A. S. (1933), *Laryngoscope (St. Louis)*, **43**, 315.

Malan, E. (1934a), *Z. Anat. EntGesch.*, **103**, 409.

Malan, E. (1934b), *Arch. Biol. (Liège)*, **45**, 355.

Malmfors, T. and Wersall, J. (1960), *Acta morph. neerl. -scand.*, **3**, 157.

Mayr, D. and Mayr, R. (1973), Paper given at the 10th International Symposium on Inner Biology and Personal Communication.

Mayr, R., Zenker, W. and Gruber, H. (1967), *Z. Zellforsch.*, **79**, 319.

McCall, G. N. and Rabuzzi, D. D. (1973), *J. Speech Hear. Res.*, **16**, 56.

McCrady, E., Jr. (1938), *Amer. anat. Mem.*, No. **16**, 1.

McRobert, H., Bryan, M. E. and Tempest, W. (1968), *J. Sound Vib.*, **7**, 129.

Mendelson, E. S. (1966), *Acta oto-laryng. (Stockh.)*, **62**, 125.

Metz, O. (1946), *Acta oto-larnyg. (Stockh.)*, suppl., 63.

Metz, O. (1951), *Acta oto-laryng. (Stockh.)*, **39**, 397.

Metz, O. (1952), *Arch. Oto-laryng.*, **55**, 536.

Mills, J. H. and Lilly, D. J. (1971), *J. acoust. Soc. Amer.*, **50**, 1556.

Møller, A. R. (1958), *Laryngoscope (St. Louis)*, **68**, 48.

Møller, A. R. (1961), *Ann. Otol.* **70**, 735.

Møller, A. R. (1962a), *J. acoust Soc. Amer.*, **34**, 1524.

Møller, A. R. (1962b), *Ann. Otol.*, **71**, 86.

Møller, A. R. (1965), *Acta oto-laryng. (Stockh.)*, **60**, 129.

Møller, A. R. (1972), In *Foundation of Modern Auditory Theory II*. New York and London: Academic Press.

Neergaard, E. B., Andersen, H. C., Hansen, C. C. and Jepsen, O. (1963), *Acta oto-laryng. (Stockh.)*, suppl., **188**, 280.

Okamoto, M., Sato, M. and Kirikae, I. (1954), *Ann. Otol.*, **63**, 950.

Peachey, L. D. (1968), *Ann. Rev. Physiol.*, **30**, 401.

Perlman, H. B. and Case, T. J. (1939), *Ann. Otol.*, **48**, 663.

Philip, R. (1932), *Rev. Laryng. (Bordeaux)*, **53**, 695.

Pichler, H. and Bornschein, H. (1957), *Acta oto-laryng. (Stockh.)*, **48**, 498.

Platzer, W. (1961), *Mschr. Ohrenheilk.*, **95**, 553.

Pollak, G. and Henson, O. W., Jr. (1973), *J. comp. Physiol.*, **84**, 167.

Pollak, G., Henson, O. W., Jr. and Novick, A. (1972), *Science*, **176**, 66.

Prasansuk, S. and Hinchcliffe, R. (1972), *J. Laryng.*, **86**, 637.

Price, G. R. (1963), *J. Aud. Res.*, **3**, 221.

Price, G. R. (1966), *J. Aud. Res.*, **6**, 175.

Price, G. R. (1972), *J. acoust. Soc. Amer.*, **51**, 552.

Pye, A. (1966), *J. Morph.*, **119**, 101.

Pye, A. (1970), In Proceedings 2nd International Bat Research Conference.

Reger, S. N. (1960), *Ann. Otol.*, **69**, 1179.

Salomon, G. (1966), *Proc. roy. Soc. Med.*, **59**, 966.

Salomon, G. and Starr, A. (1963), *Acta neurol. scand.*, **39**, 161.

Seiden, D. (1971), *Amer. J. Anat.*, **132**, 267.

Shearer, W. M. and Simmons, F. B. (1965), *J. Speech Hear. Res.*, **8**, 203.

Simmons, F. B. (1959), *Ann. Otol.*, **68**, 1126.

Simmons, F. B. (1963), *Ann. Otol.*, **72**, 528.

Simmons, F. B. (1964a), *Ann. Otol.*, **73**, 724.

Simmons, F. B. (1964b), *Int. Audiol.*, **3**, 136.

Simmons, F. B. and Beatty, D. L. (1964), *Electroenceph clin. Neurophysiol.*, **17**, 332.

Sokolovski, A. (1973), *Arch. klin. exp. Ohr.-, Nas.- u. Kehlk Heilk.*, **203**, 289.

Spiesmann, I. G. (1927), *Mschr. Ohrenheilk.*, **61**, 971 (*cited after* Wersall, R.).

Stevens, S. S. and Davis, H. (1938), *Hearing*. New York: Wiley and Sons.

Stevens, S. S. and Newman, E. B. (1936), *Proc. nat. Acad. Sci.*, **22**, 668.

Taruya, T. (1953), *Hiroshima J. med. Sci.*, **2**, 245.

Teig, E. (1969), *Acta physiol. scand.*, **76**, 16A.

Teig, E. (1972a), *Acta physiol. scand.*, **84**, 1.

Teig, E. (1972b), *Acta physiol. scand.*, **84**, 11.

Teig, E. (1973), *Acta physiol. scand.*, **88**, 382.

Teig, E. and Dahl, H. A. (1972), *Histochemie*, **29**, 1.

Terkildsen, K. (1957), *Arch. Otolaryng.*, **66**, 484.

Tietze, G. (1969), *Arch. Ohr.-, Nas.-u. KehlkHeilk.*, **193**, 43.

Ward, W. D. (1962), *J. acoust. Soc. Amer.*, **34**, 234.

Wassif, K. (1948), No. 27, Fouad I University 177.

Weiss, H. S., Mundie, J. R., Cashin, J. L. and Shinabarger, E. W. (1962), *Acta oto-laryng. (Stockh.)*, **55**, 505.

Wersäll, R. (1958), *Acta oto-laryng. (Stockh.)*, suppl., 139.

Wever, E. G. and Bray, C. W. (1937), *Ann. Otol. (St. Louis)*, **46**, 947.

Wever, E. G. and Bray, C. W. (1942), *J. exp. Psychol.*, **31**, 35.

Wever, E. G. and Lawrence, M. (1954), *Physiological Acoustics* Princeton, New Jersey: Princeton University Press.

Wever, E. G. and Vernon, J. A. (1955), *Acta oto-larung. (Stockh.)*, **45**, 433.

Wever, E. G. and Vernon, J. A. (1956), *Ann. Otol. (St. Louis)*, **65**, 5.

Wickelgren, W. D. (1968), *J. Neurophysiol.*, **31**, 769.

Wiederhold, M. L. (1970), *J. acoust. Soc. Amer.*, **48**, 966.

Wigand, M. E. and Borucki, H. J. (1965), *Arch. Ohr.-, Nas.-u. KehlkHeilk.*, **185**, 655.

Wiggers, H. C. (1937), *Amer. J. Physiol.*, **120**, 771.

Winckler, G. (1959), *Arch. Anat. path.*, **7**, 170.

Worthington, D. W. and Dallos, P. (1971), *J. acoust. Soc. Amer.*, **49**, 1818.

Zakrisson, J. E. and Borg, E. (1974), *Audiology*, **13**, 231.

Zuckerkandl, E. (1884), *Arch. Ohrenheilk.*, **20**, 104 (*cited after* Wersäll, R., 1958).

Zwislocki, J. (1963), *J. Speech Res.*, **6**, 303.

19. ACOUSTIC IMPEDANCE

DENZIL N. BROOKS

INTRODUCTION

Otoscopic examination has been practiced for many years as a means of obtaining information regarding the tympanic membrane and the middle ear. In conditions such as acute otitis media or where there is a perforation of the tympanic membrane, direct observation is invaluable, but considerably less assistance is obtained in middle-ear disorders where the tympanic membrane is imperforate, such as otosclerosis, discontinuity of the ossicular chain or secretory otitis media. Some indication of the mobility of the tympanic membrane may be obtained by the use of a Siegle pneumatic speculum, but the pressures employed considerably exceed the pressures of even the loudest sounds and consequently valid conclusions regarding normal tympanic membrane function cannot be drawn (Coles, 1972). Pure tone audiometry by both air and bone conduction, even when performed under ideal conditions and with the careful employment of masking noise to the non-tested ear, provides only indirect information regarding middle-ear function. It is of limited value in the diagnosis of specific middle-ear conditions. The value of pure tone audiometry is further limited by its subjective nature. Accurate results are often not possible with young children, the mentally retarded, and non-co-operating patients.

Acoustic impedance measurements offer a third approach to the examination of the middle ear. As currently carried out, the vibration amplitudes fall within the physiological range and consequently give a much more realistic assessment of the efficiency of the middle-ear sound transmission system. Information obtained with an impedance bridge may be specifically or differentially diagnostic. The test is almost completely objective, and is generally practicable with the very young, the mentally subnormal and the non-co-operating patient, as well as with normal subjects.

Furthermore, acoustic impedance measurements give information not only about the middle ear but also about the internal ear and the higher levels of the auditory system.

ACOUSTIC IMPEDANCE—PRINCIPLES

The function of the middle ear is to transform, with the maximum efficiency, the pressure variations in air within the auditory frequency range into hydrodynamic waves in the cochlea. A sound wave entering the external acoustic meatus progresses inwards until it reaches the tympanic membrane. Thence, if the middle ear is normal, the majority of the energy is transmitted to the cochlea through the mechanical movement of the ossicles. A small part of the incident energy is inevitably lost in overcoming friction, and a small fraction is reflected. If the middle-ear mechanism is in any way abnormal, the relationship between the transmitted, reflected and frictional loss components will probably be disturbed. For example, in secretory otitis media the mobility of the tympanic membrane is greatly reduced owing to fluid filling the middle-ear space. A much greater proportion of the incident energy is reflected than occurs normally. Frictional loss is increased and consequently the amount of energy transmitted to the cochlea is greatly reduced. Conversely, in ossicular discontinuity, where the tympanic membrane mobility is likely to be higher than normal owing to the restraint of the stapes base being removed, the reflected component is diminished.

It can be seen that the wave reflected at the tympanic membrane carries information about the state of the middle ear, and if the properties of the incident and reflected sound are both known, it should be possible to obtain information about the mechanical condition of the middle-ear system. The relationship between sound transmission, sound reflection and frictional loss is governed by the acoustic impedance of the ear.

The concept of acoustic impedance is probably easier to appreciate by first considering mechanical impedance. Figure 1A shows a simple mechanical system having three basic elements, i.e. mass, stiffness and resistance (friction). If an alternating force is applied to the mass it will oscillate along the line of application of the force. The amplitude of the oscillation will depend on the magnitude of the applied force, on the mass, on the stiffness and on the resistance. The mechanical impedance is defined as the ratio between the applied force and the resultant velocity. It is a complex quantity having both real and imaginary components. The real component is that due to the resistance in the system; it is the loss due to friction. The imaginary component is reactive, that is, the energy is not lost as in the resistive part, but is converted into kinetic or potential energy. The reactive part itself has two elements. The first of these is the mass or inertial reactance. This is directly proportional to the frequency of excitation. At higher frequencies, more of the applied force is taken up in moving the mass than in overcoming the stiffness. At high frequencies the system is therefore said to be mass controlled. The second reactance element is that due to the stiffness and this is inversely proportional to the excitation frequency. At low frequencies, more energy is taken up in overcoming the stiffness than in moving the mass. The system is then said to be stiffness controlled. Figure 1B illustrates how the three impedance elements are related as vector quantities. Expressed in mathematical terms, the reactance is the sum of two parts, inertial reactance $2\pi f M$ and stiffness reactance $S/2\pi f$. The two parts are 180° out of phase, and hence of opposite sign. Therefore,

$$\text{Reactance} = 2\pi f M - S/2\pi f$$

The total impedance is the vector sum of the reactive and resistive parts:

$$\text{Impedance} = Z_m = \sqrt{R_m{}^2 + (2\pi f M - S/2\pi f)^2}$$

Where Z_m = the mechanical impedance
$\quad\quad R_m$ = the mechanical resistance
$\quad\quad M$ = the mass
$\quad\quad S$ = the stiffness
$\quad\quad f$ = the frequency

From mechanical impedance to acoustic impedance, certain changes are necessary. The applied force is due to an alternating pressure in the air, and the resultant movement is more easily determined in terms of a volumetric change because the different portions of the tympanic membrane are displaced through differing distances.

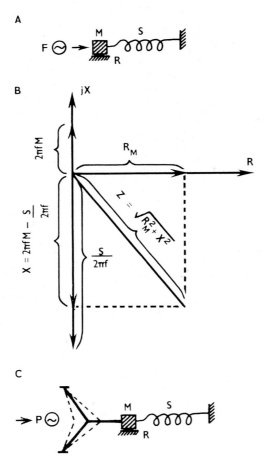

FIG. 1. A. Simple mechanical system comprising mass (M), stiffness (S) and friction (R). B. Vector relationship between the different impedance elements and the frequency (f). C. Acoustical equivalent of simple mechanical system in 1.A.

Acoustic impedance is thus defined as the ratio between the applied sound pressure and the volume displacement (Fig. 1C). In considering the acoustic impedance of the middle ear from a pathological standpoint, we are more interested in the mobility of the system than in its stiffness,

and so compliance (the inverse of stiffness) is substituted in the impedance formula which now becomes:

$$\text{Acoustic impedance} =$$
$$Z_a = \sqrt{R_a{}^2 + (2\pi f M_a - 1/2\pi f C_a)^2}$$

Where R_a = the acoustical resistance
$\quad\quad M_a$ = the acoustical mass
$\quad\quad C_a$ = the acoustic compliance

HISTORY

Just over one hundred years ago, Lucae (1867) reported attempts he had made to study middle-ear conditions by comparing the sound reflections from left and right ears using an "Interference Otoscope" of his own design. In collaboration with Helmholtz, he attempted to develop the method into a clinically practicable system, but technical facilities were not adequate at that time. Furthermore, the results were of limited use, because the method was comparative; no absolute standards existed, nor could they be established at that time.

In 1928, West reported a series of measurements of the impedance at the eardrum. Stationary waves were studied in a pipe which was first closed with a rigid disc, and then terminated with the unknown impedance of the ear. The acoustical properties of the ear were determined by calculation. This method was time consuming and complex, and the necessary calculations extremely difficult. These factors alone ruled out this method as a practicable clinical method for examining the function of the ear.

A somewhat simpler method of determining acoustical impedance was devised by Schuster in 1934. His bridge consisted of two tubes, identical in length and bore, mounted end-to-end with a symmetrical transducer between them. One tube was terminated with the unknown impedance and the other with an adjustable impedance calibrated in terms of resistance and reactance. This was adjusted until the wave patterns in the two tubes were identical, at which point the acoustical characteristics of the "unknown" termination could be calculated. Metz (1946) worked with the Schuster bridge for a number of years, testing both normal and pathological ears. His monograph, *The Acoustic Impedance Measured on Normal and Pathological Ears*, was the starting point for acoustic impedance measurement as a clinically valuable and practicable method of examination. One of the main objects that Metz set out to achieve was the differential diagnosis between conductive hearing loss and sensorineural hearing loss, which still presented difficulty at the time when the monograph was written. In the conclusion to his paper, Metz stated: "The results here obtained show with certainty a difference between mean values for the impedance measured on ears with conductive affections and on ears with perceptive affections (and normal ears). This difference is so great that the areas which include twice the standard deviation and so comprise 95 per cent of the cases, overlap each other but very slightly. The original aim—to examine if the impedance measuring could be used in the diagnosis of conduction affections—

may be looked upon as attained with a positive result." In his studies, Metz noted the change in impedance produced by contraction of the middle-ear muscles, and also drew attention to the possibility of measuring the middle-ear pressure, and the function of the auditory tube by observing the changes in the acoustic impedance with air pressure loading applied to the drum, or during performance of the Valsalva manoeuvre. The work of Metz did not receive immediate recognition, possibly because the bridge was still difficult to manipulate and required fairly complex calculations.

Zwislocki (1957a, b) investigated three different methods of measuring the impedance at the eardrum. Two of these were psycho-physical and were used only in an exploratory way. The third method was entirely physical. The fundamental components of the acoustic impedance of the ear were measured on normal subjects, and in a few selected pathological cases. An electrical analogue of the middle ear was derived from the data.

Thomsen (1955) has described the changes in impedance that could be observed when the middle-ear muscles were made to contract. He also suggested a method of testing the function of the auditory tube by observing the changes in impedance that occur when the tube opens and equalizes the middle-ear pressure to the external pressure. Thomsen showed that, by observing the impedance changes during artificial variations of the pressure on the outside of the drum, the middle-ear pressure could be determined.

After experimenting with four different models of electro-acoustic impedance bridge, Terkildsen and Scott Nielsen (1960) developed an instrument which was reasonably simple to operate, did not require any complex calculations, and was sufficiently sensitive to detect very small changes of impedance.

At present, there are two types of impedance measuring instruments in use. First, there is the mechanical-acoustic impedance bridge which is designed primarily to determine absolute values of acoustic resistance and compliance. Secondly, there is the electro-acoustic impedance bridge. This is more frequently used to detect changes in impedance elicited either by contraction of the middle-ear muscles or by application of a pressure differential across the tympanic membrane. It is possible, however, to use either type of instrument for all three types of observation.

THE ELECTRO-MECHANICAL IMPEDANCE BRIDGE

Zwislocki (1963) adopted the principle of the Schuster bridge, eliminated the unstable elements and produced an instrument which has the appearance of a clinical syringe some 20 cm in length. Being manufactured completely out of inoxidizable metal to a high standard of precision it can, once calibrated, be used to obtain absolute values of the resistive and reactive parts of the acoustic impedance. Figure 2 is a schematic diagram of the Zwislocki bridge. There is however an obstacle to the measurement of absolute acoustic impedance with this, or any other type of impedance measuring device, in that there is a space between the tip of the measuring instrument and the tym-

panic membrane. The column of air in this space has an acoustic impedance which is primarily dependant on its volume and so the impedance measured at the tip will be a composite value made up of the true impedance of the middle ear and the impedance of the enclosed portion of the ear canal. If the true impedance of the middle ear alone is to be determined a correction must be made for the ear canal volume between the tip of the instrument and the tympanic membrane. Prior to measuring with the Zwislocki bridge, a speculum is inserted into the ear canal of

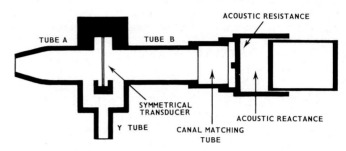

FIG. 2. Schematic diagram of the Zwislocki acoustic impedance bridge.

the patient whose head has been placed in such a position that the ear to be examined is uppermost. The volume of the canal between the tympanic membrane and the speculum tip is determined by filling the canal with alcohol from a calibrated syringe. This measured volume is then offset on the instrument. The acoustic resistance and reactance are adjusted until a null is achieved in the Y tube (either by listening or using a microphone detector). At this point, the resistance and reactance of the comparison impedance are exactly equal to that of the middle ear being examined, and may be read off from the bridge. In skilled hands, the Zwislocki bridge is capable of producing information of considerable diagnostic value (Zwislocki, 1963; Zwislocki and Feldman, 1969; Feldman, 1963, 1964, 1967; Nixon and Glorig, 1964; Tillman et al., 1964; Priede, 1970). Resistance and reactance can be measured in standard physical units. The middle-ear muscle reflex responses can be detected. There are, however, some limitations in the adoption of the instrument for routine clinical use. First, although assessment of the ear canal volume by filling with alcohol is a practicable procedure with intelligent, co-operative adult patients, it is much less likely to meet with success when the patient is a child, temperamentally difficult or otherwise un-co-operative. Secondly, measurements are taken only with normal atmospheric pressure in the ear canal. Where there is a retracted eardrum secondary to auditory tubal malfunction, this produces diminished compliance, raised resistance and generally an absence of reflexes; this condition may not be readily distinguishable from massive middle-ear adhesions or secretory otitis media (Zwislocki and Feldman, 1969). Thirdly, recording of the reflex responses although not impossible, is difficult. Since the bridge is a tuned mechanical circuit the microphone output is not linearly related to the detuning of the bridge and hence not linearly related to the stimulus. This non-linearity may be disadvantageous if one wishes to examine the relationship between stimulus and response of the middle-ear muscles. Fourthly, the bridge requires a high degree of skill and understanding in its use.

THE ELECTRO-ACOUSTIC IMPEDANCE BRIDGE

Terkildsen and Scott Nielsen (1960) devised an electro-acoustic impedance bridge which was an electronic equivalent of the Schuster bridge. A tone of 220 Hz produced by an electronic generator and a transducer was led into the tightly sealed ear canal through a long narrow tube (Fig. 3). The reflected wave from the tympanic membrane was

IMPEDANCE MEASURING BRIDGE

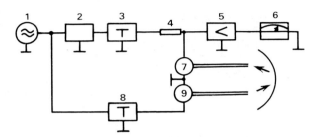

FIG. 3. Block diagram of the Madsen Z0 61 acoustic impedance bridge. 1. Oscillator (220 Hz). 2. Variable phase shifter. 3. Attenuator. 4. Fixed attenuator. 5. Selective amplifier. 6. Voltmeter. 7. Microphone. 8. Attenuator. 9. Telephone.

sampled through an identical tube leading to a microphone. The microphone voltage after selective amplification was counterbalanced to a zero state with a voltage from the original generator which had passed through regulable phase and amplitude controls. The phase control setting was found to have little significance at this probe frequency but the amplitude control setting related to the impedance of the middle ear. With a stiff tympanic membrane, the reflected wave would be of greater amplitude than normal and consequently the counterbalancing voltage required would be of greater magnitude. Similarly, with a reduced impedance of the middle ear a lower voltage to effect the zero state would be needed. It was possible to calibrate the amplitude control setting in terms of the compliance at the tip of the probe. The same problem was however present as with the Zwislocki bridge i.e. that posed by the volume of air enclosed between the tympanic membrane and the measuring point. An elegant solution to this problem was proposed by Terkildsen (1964). The ear canal and close fitting probe together constitute an airtight space. Both Békésy (1932) and Geffken (1934) had demonstrated that the meatal walls can be considered as acoustically rigid, hence the tympanic membrane is the only structure within the enclosure that is to any degree susceptible to variations of pressure. Even small pressure differentials across the normal tympanic membrane cause considerable changes in its stiffness. A difference of 500 pascals (Pa) between the middle ear and the meatus reduces the compliance of the drum by 40–50 per cent. This pressure difference is equivalent to a column of water only 5 cm in height

(1 mm water pressure is approximately equivalent to 10 Pa). Normal atmospheric pressure is equivalent to a column of water about 1000 cm in height, and so the pressure difference of 500 Pa, sufficient to reduce the compliance by 40–50 per cent is equivalent only to a change in pressure of one half of one per cent of the normal atmospheric pressure. If the pressure load is increased to 2000 Pa (equivalent to 2 per cent of atmospheric pressure) the tympanic membrane is so loaded that it becomes effectively acoustically rigid. A third tube was therefore added to the probe inserted into the ear canal. This tube is connected to a small air pump and pressure gauge by means of which small, accurately measured variations of pressure, within the normal physiological range of pressure variation, could be introduced into the cavity. With a load of 2000 Pa the acoustic probe is working into a cavity with rigid walls and a rigid termination. In this situation, the measured compliance is that of the air contained within the cavity and so a knowledge of the ear canal volume at the probe tip is obtainable without recourse to filling the canal with liquid. The original impedance bridge designed by Terkildsen and Scott Nielsen and commercially marketed as the Madsen ZO 61 had some features which limited its routine use as a clinical instrument; balancing the voltage to the "zero" condition was complicated by the need to manipulate two interdependent controls for phase and amplitude; the amplitude scale was an arbitrary one, and, if it was desired to measure compliance in standard units, it was necessary to calibrate the instrument against a series of standard cavities, and the rigid metal probe was difficult to insert into the meatus with comfort.

More recent electro-acoustic impedance meters (Madsen ZO 70; Peters AP 61) are considerably simpler to use, and operate on somewhat different principles. In Fig. 4 we

SCHEMATIC DIAGRAM OF ELECTRO–ACOUSTIC IMPEDANCE METER
(MADSEN ZO;70 PETERS AP61)

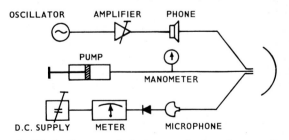

FIG. 4. Block diagram of electro-acoustic impedance meter. (Madsen ZO 70; Peters AP 61.)

have a schematic diagram of such an impedance bridge. A low frequency tone from an oscillator, variable gain amplifier and telephone transducer is fed into the ear canal through a narrow flexible tube terminating in a lightweight probe. The sound pressure level in the sealed ear canal cavity is monitored through a second tube attached to a miniature microphone. The microphone signal is filtered, amplified, rectified and finally conducted to one side of a centre-balancing voltmeter. To the opposite side of the meter is supplied a constant, stabilized voltage, the level of which is such that it exactly equals the microphone voltage when the sound pressure level in the cavity is precisely 95 dB SPL (65 dB above the threshold for normal hearing at that frequency). Higher or lower sound pressure levels in the meatus will produce out-of-balance readings on the indicator meter. The level of the sound in the meatal cavity is determined by two factors:

(1) The amount of sound energy supplied by the telephone transducer which is determined by the gain of the oscillator amplifier.

(2) The absorbtion and reflection of the sound energy which occurs within the cavity, which, since the walls of the cavity are acoustically rigid, is determined primarily by the condition of the tympanic membrane.

To maintain a constant sound pressure of 95 dB SPL in the cavity, less acoustical energy will be required (low gain setting on amplifier) for a stiff tympanic membrane (high impedance) than for a normal one. There is then an inverse relationship between the amplifier gain setting and the acoustic impedance of the middle ear as seen at the tympanic membrane. Low gain is required to maintain a level of 95 dB SPL with a high impedance termination; higher gain setting is required to maintain the same SPL with a low impedance termination. As on the earlier model of the impedance bridge, there is a third tube in the probe through which the pressure load variations can be introduced. The study of the relationship between acoustic impedance and applied pressure load is known as tympanometry.

TYMPANOMETRY

In normal circumstances, the pressure in the middle ear is virtually the same as the external ambient pressure, the auditory tube having the function of equating the middle-ear pressure to atmospheric pressure. If, for any reason, there exists a pressure differential across the tympanic membrane there will be a stress applied to it and this will result in an increased stiffness, i.e. a diminished compliance. Two per cent excess pressure (2000 Pa) is sufficient to render the membrane effectively acoustically rigid and hence reduce the middle-ear compliance to zero. As the pressure differential is reduced the compliance rises, reaching a peak at the point where the pressure in the external acoustic meatus is exactly equal to the pressure in the middle ear. If the pressure in the meatus is further reduced, the tympanic membrane is now drawn out into the meatus and again subjected to stress. The compliance will fall, reaching a minimum when the pressure load is approximately 2000 Pa. Figure 5A shows the way in which the middle-ear compliance varies as a function of the pressure differential across the membrane for a normal middle ear. Where there is simple auditory tubal block with tympanic membrane retraction but no fluid in the middle-ear cleft, the tympanometry curve (tympanogram) has the same basic shape as for the normal middle ear but the point of maximum compliance is displaced towards the side of negative pressure (Fig. 5B). The tympanic membrane attains maximal compliance only when free from stress, and this will occur when the pressure in the

external canal is reduced to the same degree as that pressure existing within the middle-ear cleft. The degree of retraction can be measured from the manometer reading at maximum compliance. However, some error is present in this method of determining reduced middle-ear pressures since no account is taken of the tympanic membrane displacement (Flisberg et al., 1963). Nevertheless, this error is probably not of clinical significance. Tympanograms of greater than normal height may be obtained where the tympanic membrane has atrophic scarring or is abnormally flaccid, as well as in cases of ossicular discontinuity (Fig. 5C). The diagnostic significance of such a tympanogram is however limited due to the wide distribution of

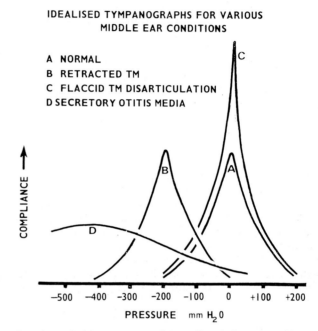

FIG. 5. Typical tympanograms for specific middle ear conditions.

compliance values obtained on normal ears. The same reservation applies also to tympanograms with reduced height (but normal middle-ear pressure). This pattern may be associated with otosclerosis, but there is a considerable overlap in the distribution for an otosclerotic population and that for a normal population. The most clearly distinctive tympanogram is that obtained where fluid is present in the middle ear, as in secretory otitis media (Fig. 5D).

There are three marked differences between this curve and the normal:

(1) The height of the curve (the compliance of the middle ear seen at the tympanic membrane) is markedly reduced.

(2) The point of maximum compliance is appreciably displaced towards the side of negative pressure—an indication of auditory tubal block.

(3) The curve no longer has a definite peak, as in the other tympanograms illustrated. Instead it is considerably flattened. It is this feature which most

clearly differentiates the tympanogram of secretory otitis media from all other tympanograms.

Tympanometry with the electro-acoustic impedance bridge has proved to be a highly satisfactory method for detecting the presence of fluid in the middle-ear cavity, especially in young children. Other methods (otoscopic or audiometric) are not sufficiently sensitive. Brooks (1968, 1969), employing a tympanometric technique, established a high correlation between the presence of fluid in the middle ear and the shape of the tympanogram. In 1950, Hoople drew attention to the problem of otitis media with effusion and termed it "a challenge to otolaryngology". The impedance bridge is a tool especially suited for the early detection of this condition (Brooks, 1971).

An imperforate tympanic membrane is, of course, a *sine qua non* for application of a pressure differential across the membrane. Where a perforation exists, a straight line function is obtained with attempted pressure change. The line gives an appearance of rising compliance with decreasing pressure. This is due to the increase in compliance of air with reduction of pressure which occurs at the rate of approximately 1 per cent for each change of 1000 Pa.

Lidén (1970, 1972) has developed an acoustic impedance device for tympanometry with a working frequency of 800 Hz. For normal middle ears and those with reduced compliance, the tympanograms are virtually identical with those obtained with the lower probe frequencies (Madsen: 220 Hz; Peters: 275 Hz). However, very different curves are seen in patients where the ear has an increased compliance, particularly in cases of ossicular discontinuity. On such conditions, a curve is obtained having two or more peaks. The reason for the difference in shape lies in the proximity of the 800 Hz tone to the resonant frequency of the tympano-ossicular mechanism. In the normal ear this is about 1000–1200 Hz. With increasing stiffness, e.g. with otosclerosis, the resonant frequency is raised and with diminished stiffness (i.e. disarticulation; flaccid tympanic membranes) the resonant frequency is lowered. It is difficult, if not impossible, to explain in detail the specific variations in curve shape when the probe frequency is close to the resonant frequency, but observation of certain tympanograms may alert one to the possibility of such conditions as ossicular discontinuity. It should be noted that the ear canal can be regarded as a simple compliance arithmetically added to that of the middle ear, only with low frequencies of the probe signal. For frequencies greater than 500 Hz, this assumption is not valid (Pinto and Dallos, 1968). Consequently, if any reasonable form of uncomplicated measurement is to be made with the tympanogram, as opposed to simple observation of curve pattern, it is necessary to use a low frequency probe signal. In a very small number of instances, the author has observed tympanograms having two distinct compliance maxima when using an impedance bridge with a low frequency probe tone. Other similar cases have been reported in personal communications. In every instance to date these most unusual tympanograms have been obtained with children who have had a history of secretory otitis media. Physical examination of the drum frequently reveals a normal or near normal membrane, except that the pars flaccida, where this can be visualized, is darkened and retracted. According to Proctor (1964) "The attic or epitympanum is almost completely separated from the mesotympanum by the ossicles and their folds except for two small but constant openings . . . the isthmus tympani anticus and the isthmus tympani posticus." If these small openings are occluded, the normal aeration of the epitympanic recess will be prevented. It is hypothesized that such a situation may arise after an episode of secretory otitis media whereby the isthmi are occluded. The situation in the mesotympanum may apparently return to normal with normal restoration of auditory tubal function, but in the epitympanic region there may still be reduced air pressure and secretion. The communication between the epitympanic recess and the external acoustic meatus is the pars flaccida of the drum. The tympanogram of the epitympanic section will, in such circumstances, be typical of secretory otitis media having a compliance maximum at some negative pressure relative to normal. (The tympanogram for the mesotympanic section will have the characteristics of a normal tympanogram, with maximum compliance at approximately normal atmospheric pressure.) The resultant tympanogram of the two parallel systems will then be double peaked.

TYMPANOMETRY AND ABSOLUTE MEASUREMENT OF ACOUSTIC IMPEDANCE

In the past there has been a tendency to regard the electro-acoustic bridge as capable of giving information only about the variation of impedance of the middle ear due either to changes in the pressure load (tympanometry) or to the contraction of the middle-ear muscles. The compliance parameter of the absolute impedance can, however, be measured with electro-acoustic bridges possessing low frequency probe tones as the difference between the indicated compliance value with the tympanic membrane fully stressed and that with it fully unstressed.

Feldman and his associates (1971) tested 11 normally hearing subjects with both the Zwislocki bridge and the Madsen ZO 70. A high correlation was reported between both compliance and absolute impedance measurements for the two instruments, but stress was laid on the fact that this related only to normal ears. Brooks (1971) used an electro-acoustic impedance bridge to measure the compliance factor in the acoustic impedance in 697 children with ages ranging from 4–11 years and who were considered to have both normal hearing and normal middle-ear function. Jerger (1972), using the same equipment and technique, tested 825 adults whose middle ears were considered to be "reasonably normal". Using the Zwislocki bridge only, Feldman (1967) and Burke and his associates (1970) measured both compliance and resistance for 33 and 25 adults respectively. Table 1 shows the distributions for compliance obtained in each of these studies. There is good agreement between the two instruments. The slightly lower median value with the

Zwislocki bridge may be due to there being no provision for compensation for differences between middle-ear pressure and atmospheric pressure. Even in normal middle ears, very small underpressures may be present, dependent on the threshold of function of the auditory tube. If a slight underpressure is present in the middle ear, the measured compliance without compensation will be lower than the true compliance measured after equalization of the pressure, as is performed with the electro-acoustic type of bridge.

TABLE 1

DISTRIBUTION OF STATIC COMPLIANCE

Study	Type of Bridge	No.	Percentile		
			10	50	90
Jerger (1972)	Madsen ZO 70	825	0·39	0·67	1·30
Brooks (1971)	Madsen ZO 70	697*	0·45	0·70	1·05
Feldman (1967)	Zwislocki	33	0·45	0·65	0·90
Burke et al. (1970)	Zwislocki	25	0·45	0·65	1·00

* Children aged 4–11 years.
Note: Madsen probe tone 220 Hz; Zwislocki probe tone 250 Hz. Measurements of compliance are in terms of the equivalent volume of an air-containing cavity.

High test-retest correlation coefficients for the Zwislocki bridge have been reported by Nixon and Glorig (1964), by Tillman and his associates (1967) and by Feldman and his associates (1971). Similar information for the electro-acoustic bridge was reported by Feldman (1971) and by Brooks (1971). The repeatability for this second method of measurement was shown to be of the same order.

MIDDLE EAR MUSCLE REFLEX MEASUREMENTS

In subjects with a normal middle ear, a change in acoustic impedance is observable with contraction of one or both middle ear muscles in response to acoustic, tactile, electrical or pneumatic (? equivalent to tactile) stimuli. The consensus of opinion is that, except when very intense stimuli are used, the stapedius muscle is principally involved in the impedance change elicited by acoustic stimulation though the tensor may contract without producing an impedance change (Jepsen, 1955; Terkildsen, 1960; Klockhoff, 1961; Holst et al., 1963; McRobert, 1968; Lidén et al., 1970). Prasansuk and Hinchcliffe (1972) have reported an apparently typical acoustic stapedius reflex elicited in an ear following stapedectomy. It is a matter of conjecture as to whether or not fibrous tissue had reconnected the severed tendon to the prosthesis or one of the remaining ossicles. Stapedius muscle contraction can also be registered in a middle ear free from conductive lesions by electrical stimulation of the wall of the external acoustic meatus (Klockhoff, 1961). This method of elicitation is, however, frequently uncomfortable and so it has not attained any appreciable degree of acceptance. Pneumatic stimulation with a puff of air to the orbital region produces a transient impedance change attributed to contraction of both tympanic muscles (Klockhoff, 1961; Lindstrom and Lidén, 1964; Djupesland, 1967). Tactile stimulation by touching the skin of the anterior part of the auricle with a twist of cotton wool may be used to produce a stapedius reflex (Djupesland, 1964: Lidén et al., 1970).

Examination of the middle-ear muscle reflexes has a number of clinical applications:

(1) Determination and Investigation of a Conductive Component in Hearing Impairment

Klockhoff (1961) stated that a recordable stapedius reflex was proof of the absence of a conductive component. Brooks (1969) qualified this statement by defining the level of contralateral acoustic stimulation necessary to elicit the response as not greater than 95 dB hearing level. If, in a given ear, a stapedius muscle reflex can be obtained when the contralateral ear is stimulated with a tone (500–2000 Hz) of no more than 95 dB hearing loss, then there is a very low probability that there is a conductive lesion in that ear. If a higher level of contralateral stimulus is required to elicit a response then there may be a slight conductive lesion on the probe ear, or, of course, some hearing loss on the stimulus ear. If no response is obtained to contralateral acoustic stimulation, there may be a lesion of either ear or a defect in the reflex arc. Non-acoustic reflex stimulation can aid in determining which of the three possibilities is responsible for the absence of response. A puff of air to the ipsilateral orbit produces a tensor tympani response. A puff of air to the contralateral external ear produces a combined acoustic and non-acoustic stapedius response (Coles, 1972). Djupesland (1969) tabulated the anticipated muscle responses for a number of different pathological conditions (Table 2).

(2) As An Objective Test of Loudness Recruitment

Metz (1952) first showed that the measurement of stapedius muscle reflex thresholds could be used as an objective test of loudness recruitment. For normal ears, the modal hearing level for elicitation of the reflex is 85 dB HL (Jepsen, 1955; Jerger, 1970), with individual values rarely lower than 70 dB HL. For patients with sensorineural hearing losses, recruitment is considered to be present when the difference between pure-tone threshold and reflex threshold is less than 65 dB. The value of the Metz test has been confirmed by many researchers and shown to correlate well with the Fowler ABLB (alternate binaural loudness balance) test and the Hood LDL (loudness discomfort level) test, i.e. measurement of the threshold of uncomfortable loudness, (Thomsen, 1955; Ewertsen et al., 1958; Lidén, 1970; Djupesland and Flottorp, 1970).

TABLE 2
(After Djupesland)
IMPEDANCE CHANGE IN RELATION TO TYPE OF STIMULUS IN VARIOUS MIDDLE-EAR LESIONS
Size of Impedance Change: 0 = Absent; + = Small; ++ = Normal; +++ = Large

Stimulation			Middle Ear Lesion
Tactile (stapedius)	Acoustic (stapedius)	Lifting the Upper Eyelids (stapedius and tensor tympani)	
0	+	+ or ++	Reduced middle ear pressure of moderate degree
0	0	0	Fixation of malleus
0	0	+++	(a) Absence of the long process of incus or total incudo-stapedial joint separation
		+	(b) Paralysis of the stapedius muscle
0 to ++	+ to +++	+++	Abnormal incudo-stapedial joint (fibrous connection between incus and stapes)
0 or +	++	++ or +++	Abnormal stapedial crura (fractured or fibrotic)
0	0	+	Fixation of the stapes (otosclerosis, advanced stage)
		(Frequently diphasic)	
0 or diphasic	Diphasic	Diphasic	Reduced mobility of the stapes (Otosclerosis, early stage)

(3) In the Investigation of Neuronal Lesion

A feature of the reflex response in normally hearing subjects is its persistence with concomitant sustained acoustic stimulation. With tones of frequencies of 1000 Hz. or below, and a stimulus level 10 dB above the threshold of response, no fatigue is normally observed in the muscle response over a period of 10 s. However, Anderson and his associates (1970) reported that, in 10 cases of surgically or radiologically confirmed neuronal lesions, a rapid and marked decay of the response was observed. Alberti and Kristensen (1970) report a similar finding in a patient with a neuronal lesion. It is suggested that a decay of more than 50 per cent of the initial contraction in a period of 6 s, while the stimulus remains constant, is indicative of a neuronal lesion.

(4) To Indicate Non-organic Hearing Loss

Contraction of the middle-ear muscles in the presence of loud sounds appears to be a totally involuntary reaction. Response to pure tone audiometry depends, however, on the readiness of the patient to co-operate in the test. Normal acoustic stapedius reflex thresholds in a person with a hearing loss implies that the loss exhibits recruitment and/or it is non-organic. Jepsen (1953) first drew attention to this as a means of alerting a tester to the presence of a non-organic hearing loss, and several authors have since confirmed the value of this test (Thomsen, 1955; Terkildsen, 1964; Lamb and Peterson, 1967; Lamb et al., 1968).

(5) As An Indicator of Hearing Sensitivity for the Very Young

Inferences regarding the hearing level of infants can be drawn from the presence of middle-ear muscle reflex responses. If, for example, normal reflex thresholds are obtained across the frequency range, the probability is that the hearing is also within normal limits, if the occurrence of a recruiting ear can be excluded. When the reflex thresholds are elevated, however, much less certainty can be attached to pure tone threshold extrapolations. The elevation of reflex thresholds may be due to a slight hearing loss without recruitment, or to a much greater loss with recruitment. Both McRobert and his associates (1968) and Flottorp and his associates (1971) have shown that reflex response is related not only to the intensity and loudness of the stimulus, but also to its bandwidth. Lower thresholds were obtained for reflex thresholds when broad band stimulation was used than when pure tones were used. Niemeyer and Sesterhenn (1972) suggest that some estimate of hearing loss can be made by observing the differences between reflex response thresholds to pure tones and to broad band noise (or a complex tone). They report that white noise thresholds in normal hearing subjects are 30–35 dB lower (more sensitive) than pure tone thresholds, but in children with sensorineural hearing loss the difference between the two thresholds diminishes to as little as 10–15 dB. Using 1156 subjects with either normal hearing or with sensorineural hearing loss, Jerger and his colleagues (1973) have tested the hypothesis that severity of hearing loss may be predicted from the acoustic reflex thresholds for pure tones and for white noise. Predictions were usually quite accurate. Serious errors occurred in only 4 per cent of cases, and the majority of these proved to be over-estimations, rather than under-estimations, of the degree of loss. In view of the simplicity and objectivity of this test, it is suggested that these findings have important implications for the auditory evaluation of babies and young children. Olivier (1972) studied the slope of the stapedius thresholds as a function of frequency, the detectability of the reflex at 125 Hz, and the number of frequencies (125–4000 Hz at octave intervals) for which reflexes could be obtained using a conventional audiometer. He concluded that, if a reflex response is obtainable at 125 Hz with a stimulus of 70 dB or less, the probability is that the hearing loss is not greater than 30 dB at that frequency. If a reflex response is obtainable with only one stimulus frequency, the overall hearing loss is probably severe, with two frequencies less severe, with three frequencies the hearing loss is probably only moderate, and, if responses are obtained to four or more stimulus frequencies, the hearing is probably within normal limits.

A major limitation to the use of reflex measurements for assessing hearing in the very young, apart from the present uncertainty, is the common occurrence of a conductive component in addition to the sensorineural loss. In this condition, reflexes are unobtainable and it is impossible to draw conclusions regarding the characteristics of the sensorineural loss. Nevertheless, this particular use of acoustic-impedance bridges appears to be a promising area for further research.

(6) Functional Tests for the Facial Nerve

The stapedius muscle is innervated by a fine branch (nerve to stapedius) of the facial nerve which leaves the trunk of the facial nerve at the point nearest to the muscle. Consequently, contraction or non-response of the muscle provides information about the site of lesions involving the VIIth nerve. In the absence of a ossiculo-tympanic disorder on the side of the facial palsy and a non-recruiting hearing loss on the contralateral side, absence of a recordable stapedius reflex response points to a suprastapedial facial nerve lesion. The presence of a reflex under the same circumstances points to an infrastapedial lesion (Jepsen, 1955). Return of stapedial muscle contraction may be one of the first signs of recovery from facial palsy (Feldman, 1964).

(7) Other Applications

Muscle reflex measurements have been employed for various other purposes:

(a) In the identification of normal hearing carriers of genes responsible for inherited auditory disorders transmitted in a recessive manner (Anderson and Wedenberg, 1968). An abnormally high reflex threshold, frequently coupled with an abnormal Békésy audiogram (using a sustained test tone) showing dips in the mid-frequency range, was observed as an audiological feature in a number of carriers who had normal hearing as measured by conventional pure tone audiometry.

(b) To determine the presence or absence of a conductive element in patients with a profound hearing loss of apparently sensorineural type (Farrant and Skurr, 1966). In residential schools for severely and profoundly deaf children, a higher prevalence of conductive hearing loss has been noticed (Brooks, 1970). This was attributed to a greater difficulty in detecting middle-ear disorders in this group.

(c) To differentiate between normally hearing and sensorineural hearing impaired children by observing the middle-ear reflex responses to pulsed-tone stimuli (Norris et al., 1972).

CONCLUSION

Acoustic-impedance measurement is a relative newcomer to the audiological field. In the space of a short time, it has shown that it can provide much diagnostic information. Investigations using the acoustic-impedance bridge can produce valuable clinical information not only in conductive hearing losses but also in sensorineural losses, as well as in cases where there is no hearing loss at all. Future developments in equipment and technique will almost certainly lead to even more information about the normal and disordered auditory system.

REFERENCES

Alberti, P. W. R. M. and Kristensen, R. (1970), *Laryngoscope*, **80**, 735.
Anderson, H., Barr, B. and Wedenberg, E. (1970), *Acta oto-laryng.*, suppl. **263**, 232.
Anderson, H. and Wedenberg, E. (1968), *Acta oto-laryng.*, **65**, 535.
Békésy, G. (1932), *Ann. d. Physik*, **5**, 51.
Brooks, D. N. (1968), *Int. Audiol.*, **7**, 280.
Brooks, D. N. (1969), *Int. Audiol.*, **7**, 563.
Brooks, D. N. (1970), *Int. Audiol.*, **9**, 141.
Brooks, D. N. (1971), *Audiology*, **10**, 334.
Brooks, D. N. (1971), *J. Speech Hear. Res.*, **14**, 247.
Burke, K., Nilges, T. and Henry, G. (1970), *J. Speech Heat Res.*, **13**, 317.
Coles, R. R. A. (1972), *J. Laryng.*, **86**, 191.
Djupesland, G. (1964), *Acta otolaryng.*, suppl. **188**, 287.
Djupesland, G. (1967), *Universitetsforlaget*. Oslo.
Djupesland, G. (1969), *Int. Audiol.*, **8**, 570.
Djupesland, G. and Flottorp, G. (1970), *Int. Audiol.*, **9**, 156.
Ewertsen, H. W., Filling, S., Terkildsen, K. and Thomsen, K. A. (1958), *Acta oto-laryng.*, suppl. **140**, 116.
Farrant, R. H. and Skurr, B. (1966), *J. Otolaryng. Soc. Austral.*, **2**, 49.
Feldman, A. S. (1963), *J. Speech Hear. Res.*, **6**, 315.
Feldman, A. S. (1964), *Int. Audiol.*, **3**, 156.
Feldman, A. S. (1967), *J. Speech Hear. Res.*, **10**, 165.
Feldman, A. S., Djupesland, G. and Grimes, C. T. (1971), *Arch. Otolaryng.*, **93**, 416.
Flisberg, K., Ingelstedt, S. and Ortegren, U. (1963), *Acta oto-laryng.* Suppl. **182**,
Flottorp, G., Djupesland, G. and Winther, F. (1971), *J. acoust. Soc. Amer.*, **49**, 457.
Geffken, W. (1934), *Ann. d. Physik*, **5**, 829.
Holst, H. E., Ingelstedt, S. and Ortengren, U. (1963), *Acta oto-laryng.*, suppl. **182**, 73.
Hoople, G. (1950), *Laryngoscope*, **60**, 315.
Jepsen, O. (1953), *Acta oto-laryng*, suppl. **109**, 61.
Jepsen, O. (1955), Thesis. Denmark: University Aarhus.
Jerger, J. (1970), *Arch. Otolaryng.*, **92**, 311.
Jerger, J., Burney, P., Mauldin, L. and Crump, B. (1973) Personal Communication.
Jerger, J., Jerger, S. and Mauldin, L. (1972), *Arch. Otolaryng.*, **96**, 513.
Klockhoff, L. (1961), *Acta oto-laryng.*, suppl. **164.**
Lamb, L. E. and Peterson, J. L. (1967), *J. Speech Hear. Dis.*, **32**, 46.
Lamb, L. E., Peterson, J. L. and Hansen, S. (1968), *Int. Audiol.*, **7**, 188.
Lidén, G. (1970), *Ciba Foundation Symposium on Sensorineural Hearing Loss.* London: J. & A. Churchill.

Lidén, G., Bjorkman, G. and Peterson, J. L. (1972), *J. Speech Hear. Dis.*, **37**, 100.

Lidén, G., Peterson, J. L. and Bjorkman, G. (1970), *Arch. Otolaryng.*, **92**, 248.

Lidén, G., Peterson, J. L. and Harford, E. R. (1970), *Acta oto-laryng.*, suppl. **263**, 208

Lindstrom, D. and Lidén, G. (1964), *Acta oto-laryng.*, suppl. **188**, 271.

Lucae, A. (1867), *Arch. Ohrenheilk*, **3**, 186.

McRobert, H. (1968), *Sound* **2**, 71.

McRobert, H., Bryan, M. E. and Tempest, W. (1968), *J. Sound. Vib.*, **7**, 129.

Metz, O. (1946), *Acta oto-laryng.*, suppl. **63**.

Metz, O. (1952), *Arch. Otolaryng.*, **55**, 536.

Niemeyer, W. and Sesterhenn, G. (1972), *Audiology.* In press.

Nixon, J. and Glorig, A. (1964), *J. Aud. Res.*, **4**, 261.

Norris, T. W., Stelmachowicz, P. G. and Taylor, D. J. (1972), *Audiology.* In press.

Olivier, J. C. (1972), Pub. by Compagnie Francais d'Audiologie, Paris 8.

Pinto, L. H. and Dallos, P. J. (1968), *IEEE Trans. Biomed. Engng. BME.*, **15**, 10.

Prasansuk, S. and Hinchcliffe, R. (1972), *J. Laryng.*, **86**, 637.

Priede, V. M. (1970), *Int. Audiol.*, **9**, 127.

Proctor, B. (1964), *J. Laryng.*, **78**, 631.

Schuster, K. (1934), *Physik. Ztsr.*, **35**, 408.

Terkildsen, K. (1960), *Acta oto-laryng.*, suppl. **158**, 230.

Terkildsen, K. (1964), *Int. Audiol.*, **3**, 147.

Terkildsen, K. and Scott Nielsen, S. (1960), *Arch. Otolaryng.*, **72**, 339.

Thomsen, K. A. (1955a), *Acta oto-laryng.*, **45**, 82.

Thomsen, K. A. (1955b), *Acta oto-laryng.*, **45**, 159.

Tillman, T. W. and Dallos, P. (1976), *J. acoust. Soc. Amer.*, **36**, 582.

West, W. (1928), *Post Office Elect. Eng. J.*, **21**, 293.

Zwislocki, J. (1957a), *J. acoust. Soc. Amer.*, **29**, 349.

Zwislocki, J. (1957b), *J. acoust. Soc. Amer.*, **29**, 1312.

Zwislocki, J. (1963), *J. Speech Hear. Res.*, **6**, 303.

Zwislocki, J. and Feldman, A. S. (1969), Special Report LSC-S-5, University Syracuse, N.Y.

20. PHYSIOLOGY OF THE LABYRINTHINE FLUIDS

S. K. BOSHER

INTRODUCTION

Since the reports of the unique character of the endolymph, namely the association of its large positive dc potential (Békésy, 1952a) with a high K^+, low Na^+ electrolyte composition (Smith, Lowry and Wu, 1954), there has been little doubt about the importance of this fluid's physiological role in the cochlea. There have also been frequent suggestions that alterations in its physico-chemical constitution were a major feature in the pathogenesis of Ménière's disease and many other conditions resulting in sensorineural hearing loss.

Although a variety of human and experimental histopathological evidence has been advanced in support of such a concept, it must be admitted that much of this has been circumstantial in nature. Nevertheless, experimental changes in the composition and dc potential of the endolymph do produce loss of cochlear function (Konishi *et al.*, 1966), together with morphological abnormalities in the hair cells and the stria vascularis (Duvall and Rhodes, 1967; Duvall, 1968). Moreover, a number of drugs and pathological conditions appear to cause similar endolymphatic disturbances and these may be more common than previously thought. For example, kanamycin, an amino glycoside antibiotic, in addition to its well-documented direct effect upon the hair cells, also produces concomitant alterations in the endolymph, which alone could have a deleterious action on the sensory end organ (Mendelsohn and Katzenberg, 1972).

Initially, disorders of the stria vascularis were believed to be the main source of these anomalies, but this view has now been extended to include the cochlear duct membranes. As a result, the part played by the endolymphatic system in the pathological processes responsible for sensorineural hearing loss is undeniably complex and a detailed knowledge of its physiology accordingly essential.

COCHLEAR ENDOLYMPH

Normal Composition

The normal composition of the cochlear endolymph is shown in Table 1 and, although derived from the rat (Bosher and Warren, 1968, 1971), it is considered typical for man and other mammals. The unique high K^+, low Na^+ content has already been emphasized but the anion structure is extra-cellular in type and so analogies to intracellular fluid are best avoided, particularly as the dc

TABLE 1

THE ELECTRO-CHEMICAL CONSTITUTION OF THE COCHLEAR ENDOLYMPH AND PERILYMPH

		Range	Mean
Endolymphatic	potential (mV)	+88–+96	+92
	sodium	0·4–1·4	0·9
	potassium	140–163	154
	chloride	122–132	128
	bicarbonate	25–29	27
	pH*	7·3–7·5	7·4
Perilymphatic	sodium	115–180	138
	potassium	4–9	7
	chloride	122–133	127

Ionic concentrations in mequiv./1. Since the above ions are monovalent, these quantities are numerically identical with quantities in millimoles per litre.

* From Misrahy *et al.*, 1958.

potential is positive in nature. The bicarbonate figures represent the residual non-Cl⁻ anion concentration. The pH range calculated from these figures, however, does correspond to that found experimentally (Misrahy *et al.*, 1958). An early investigation also suggested that the Ca⁺⁺ and Mg⁺⁺ levels corresponded to extra-cellular fluid but contamination with perilymph was almost certainly present.

Direct examination has revealed the glucose concentration to be very low, 0·833 millimoles per litre (15 mg per cent) (Silverstein, 1966a) and the ionic constituents to account completely for the osomolality of the fluid (Bosher and Warren, 1971). In consequence, the total content of all metabolites must be exceptionally low, another unusual feature of this fluid and one which seems to preclude it from any major metabolic role.

Despite some initial reports to the contrary, the endocochlear potential decreases progressively along the length of the cochlear duct by 5–12 mV per turn, depending on the species (Änggård, 1965; Bosher and Warren, 1971). While it is tempting to correlate this with similar changes in the stria vascularis enzymes, many other relevant factors, such as membrane resistance, have yet to be investigated and both the underlying cause and functional significance (if any) of the gradient remain obscure. No comparable differences in the chemical composition have been found (Bosher and Warren, unpublished observations), thus excluding complications which would arise if longitudinal ionic gradients were present.

Because it is concerned with hair cell stimulation, the relationship between the tectorial membrane and the endolymph has provoked much speculation. Current pilot studies by X-ray spectroscopy of freeze-dried specimens indicate the K⁺ and Cl⁻ concentrations to be identical in the two situations (Flock, 1973), unlike the results of earlier and less accurate chemical methods.

However, there is still a great deal of controversy over the magnitude of the dc potential within the membrane. Early investigators thought the positive endocochlear potential persisted as the membrane was traversed and only disappeared at the level of the reticular lamina, a conclusion challenged in 1967 by Lawrence, whose results indicated the absence of any significant potential in the tectorial membrane. Such a feature is of great importance for it means the membrane could act as a mechano-electric transducer in the same way as a polarized crystal. Attempts to confirm this finding by other workers have been unsuccessful but Lawrence has recently presented preliminary observations of values identical to his original ones obtained by means of a vastly improved technique. The problem is not an easy one for the tectorial membrane is almost certainly a water structured gel which appears to lack the requisite biophysical, high resistance barrier for the maintenance of a large potential difference at its endolymphatic interface, and it accordingly seems prudent to await the publication of detailed information on this matter.

The details of the chemical composition not only indicate that the endolymph is a most unusual fluid but they also provide a great deal more information about the nature of the endolymphatic system. Each ion is subject to two main forces, the one arising from the chemical and the other from the electrical gradients present between the endolymph and the surrounding fluids. These forces, which may be mutually complimentary or antagonistic, can be compared by means of the appropriate derivative of the Nernst equation, and thus the net force acting on any individual ion in the endolymph can be determined.

Na⁺ will be examined in detail since its extremely low concentration (confirmed by Johnstone *et al.*, 1963; Mendelsohn and Konishi, 1969; Sellick and Johnstone, 1972a) implies the occurrence of a gross error even when control values of only 5 mmol. l⁻¹ (millimoles per litre), a not unusual figure, are obtained and it is worthwhile considering whether this is, in fact, a serious defect in accuracy. In Table 2, the endolymphatic Na⁺ concentration which

TABLE 2

THE RELATIONSHIP BETWEEN THE ACTUAL AND EQUILIBRIUM SODIUM CONCENTRATION (IN mmol. l⁻¹) IN A CONSECUTIVE SERIES OF EXPERIMENTS

Equilibrium concentration	4·74	3·83	3·54	4·68	5·33	4·61	3·90
Physiological concentration	1·10	0·81	0·68	1·44	1·02	0·41	0·91

would arise from the physico-chemical forces alone has been calculated from the Nernst equation in a consecutive series of experiments and, in every case, the actual concentration found was substantially below the equilibrium concentration (Bosher and Warren, 1968). Such a feature can only be explained by the presence of some additional biological force removing Na⁺ from the endolymph, i.e. by the presence of active Na⁺ transport out of the scala media.

In the same way, it is possible to establish that K⁺ is actively transported in the reverse direction into the endolymph, while Cl⁻ is actively removed (Fig. 1). Bicarbonate ions, too, are not in equilibrium, but active transport cannot necessarily be inferred as nothing is known about the possible presence of H⁺ and OH⁻ exchange.

Effect of Anoxia

Electro-chemical examination of the endolymph, therefore, is sufficient to reveal that the ionic constitution is controlled entirely by active mechanisms. Confirmation of this exceptional state of affairs was provided quite simply by investigation of the endolymphatic changes produced by anoxia. As predicated, there was a progressive increase in the Na⁺ (Fig. 2) and a concomitant decrease in the K⁺ concentrations due to the inactivation of the mechanisms concerned, which were clearly dependent on oxidative metabolism (Bosher and Warren, 1968).

In addition to the chemical effects, anoxia also abolished the normal positive endocochlear potential (Békésy, 1952b), suggesting this to be likewise produced by one or more of the active transport mechanisms. Recent evidence from enzyme studies described later has confirmed this initial impression but the matter was in question for some years, the alternative proposed being a modified Na⁺ diffusion

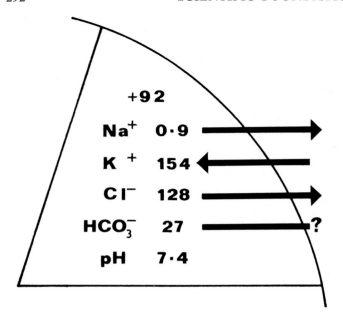

FIG. 1. Active ionic transport in the cochlea. Mean values in mV or mmol. l^{-1}. (Since these ions are monovalent, these quantities are numerically identical with quantities in milliequivalents per litre.)

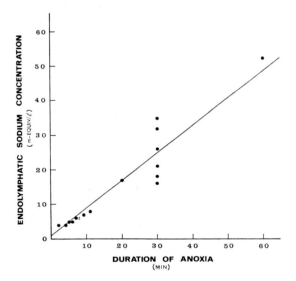

FIG. 2. The effect of anoxia upon the cochlear endolymphatic sodium concentration. (From the results of Bosher and Warren, 1968; Mendelsohn and Konishi, 1969.)

potential (Johnstone *et al.*, 1963). In fact, the positive potential is not merely abolished but replaced by a negative potential of about 40 mV (Fig. 3), which is a K^+ diffusion potential rather than a depolarization potential, i.e. it is a chemical potential arising from the K^+ concentration gradient in the presence of selective permeability to K^+ of some portion of the cochlear duct membranes (Johnstone, 1965; Kuijpers and Bonting, 1970b). This selective permeability is not the consequence of the anoxia but is present under normal conditions (Kuijpers and Bonting, 1970b) and, as the physico-chemical forces all tend to accentuate K^+ diffusion from the endolymph, marked

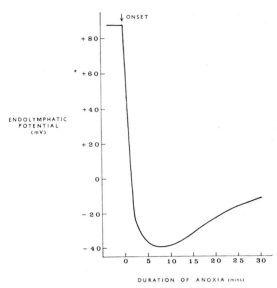

FIG. 3. The effect of anoxia upon the endocochlear potential.

activity of the inward K^+ transporting processes consequently seems likely.

Coupled Ionic Transport

A widespread phenomenon in physiology is obligatory coupling between individual active ionic fluxes, and abundant evidence now exists from enzyme studies of coupling between Na^+ and K^+ transport in the cochlea. It has also been suggested, by analogy to other systems, that Cl^- movement, too, may be associated with Na^+ transport and experimental evidence of such a linkage has recently been found (Bosher *et al.*, 1973). Nevertheless, the whole question of interdependent ionic fluxes is extremely complex and a great deal more information is required about this aspect of the endolymph system. Indeed, methods for the quantitative determination of these various active and passive fluxes are urgently needed if this enigmatic system is to be characterized satisfactorily. Attempts at direct measurements have, as yet, been unsuccessful, while indirect calculations involve so many assumptions as to be of little value.

COCHLEAR DUCT ENZYMES

Ion Transporting Enzymes

Active transport processes in a biological situation are formed by enzyme systems and the complex commonly associated with Na^+ and K^+ transport is Na^+ K^+-activated, ouabain-inhibited ATPase. Consequent search for this enzyme has confirmed that it is present in high concentration in the cochlear duct but, significantly, it is confined almost entirely to the stria vascularis (Kuijpers and Bonting, 1969; Thalmann, 1971). Here, its concentration is slightly greater in the basal region than in the apex, and its mean activity is about 8 mols/kg dry wt. per h, a level as high as in renal tubules. By contrast, the enzyme's concentration in the remaining cochlear tissues is very low (less than 0·5 mol/kg dry wt. per h), apart from the external spiral sulcus where a level of 1·6 mol/kg dry wt. per h is reported. Furthermore, the ratio of activity in stria vascularis compared to the vestibular (Reissner's) membrane, calculated on the basis of the total amount of tissue present, is 68:1. The characteristics of the strial ATPase were similar to those described for this enzyme system in other tissues concerned with ion transport, and its ouabain inhibitory function was in outstanding agreement with that for the endocochlear potential, a finding which strongly indicated a close relationship between the two (Kuijpers and Bonting, 1970a).

The concentration, 5·5 mol/kg dry wt. per h of Mg^{++} activated ATPase, the principal ATPase of the spiral organ of Corti, is also high in the stria vascularis (Kuijpers and Bonting, 1969). Its significance, however, remains conjectural, as does the function of the reported high activity of carbonic anhydrase (Erulkar and Maren, 1961), although this enzyme may be related to the possible H^+ and OH^- exchange mentioned earlier. Other ATPases, especially anion activated ATPases, have been isolated elsewhere in recent years, but no information is available to date about their likely presence in the cochlea.

Energy Producing Enzymes

Active processes are ultimately dependent on the energy producing enzyme systems and their investigation has been oxidative metabolism and eventually, therefore, upon an adequate and continuous supply of oxygen from the blood.

Representative enzymes of the three relevant metabolic pathways have subsequently been investigated in great detail and energy production in the stria confirmed to be respiratory in nature (Thalmann et al., 1970), while the pentose—P pathway was unexpectedly more prominent in the cochlea than in the brain, a feature shared by the retinal photoreceptor cells. The capacity to phosphorylate glucose, however, was calculated to be only 20 per cent of stimulated cerebral cortex and the enzyme activity in the vestibular membrane was merely 10–30 per cent of the strial levels. The authors concerned were forced to conclude, after careful consideration, that previous direct estimations of the oxygen consumption of the stria vascularis, and more especially of the vestibular membrane, were over-estimated due to technical difficulties.

Histochemical Studies

Classical histochemical staining methods are, of necessity, greatly lacking in quantitative accuracy compared to enzyme assay studies and provide little additional information about the endolymphatic homeostatic mechanisms. Discussion of such methods will consequently be omitted as excellent reviews by Vosteen (1961) and Schätzle (1971) are available.

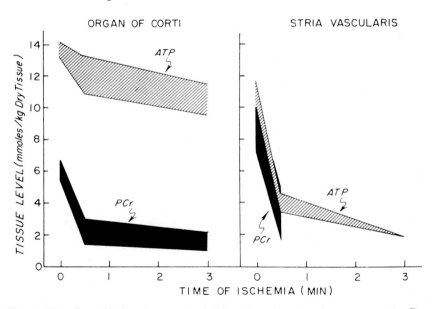

FIG. 4. The effect of ischaemia upon the A.T.P. and creatine phosphate concentrations in the stria vascularis compared with the spiral organ of Corti. (Matschinsky and Thalmann, 1967.)

vital in advancing our knowledge of the endolymph system. The ATP concentration in the stria vascularis (Fig. 4), the substrate for the ATPases previously described, was early found to fall precipitously to negligible levels after only 30 s of anoxia (Matschinsky and Thalmann, 1967). This was a finding of the utmost importance for it revealed that the ion transporting, potential producing enzyme systems in the stria vascularis were entirely dependent upon

Enzyme Inhibitors

An essential and complementary approach to the direct methods just described is investigation of the effects produced by enzyme inhibitors. The demonstration of the high concentration of Na^+ K^+-activated ATPase in the stria thus led to the study of the changes brought about by its specific inhibitors, ouabain and other cardiac glycosides.

The progressive increase in Na$^+$ and decrease in K$^+$ content, at a rate comparable to that found in anoxia (Konishi and Mendelsohn, 1970), firmly established this ATPase complex to be the principal agent controlling the endolymphatic concentration of these ions. In addition, ouabain completely abolished the normal endocochlear potential, which demonstrated it was undeniably a secretion potential due to the activity of the Na$^+$ K$^+$ activated ATPase (Kuijpers and Bonting, 1970a; Konishi and Mendelsohn, 1970). Furthermore, a negative potential (Fig. 5), identical to the anoxic endolymphatic potential, was revealed in

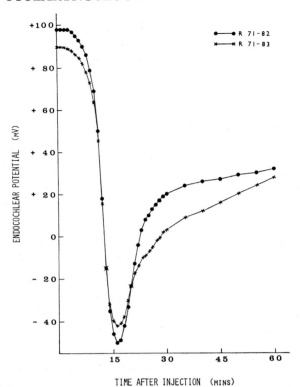

FIG. 6. The effect upon the endocochlear potential of an injection of etacrynic acid (60 mgm/kg body weight) in two typical experiments. (Bosher *et al.*, 1973.)

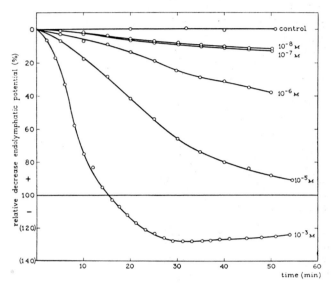

FIG. 5. The effect upon the endocochlear potential of continuous perfusion of the scala vestibuli with various concentrations of ouabain. (Kuijpers and Bonting, 1970a.)

these circumstances. Since ouabain does not inhibit respiratory enzymes nor alter membrane permeability, this negative K$^+$ diffusion potential must normally be present but hidden by the positive secretion potential and reducing its apparent magnitude, a revolutionary discovery (Kuijpers and Bonting, 1970b).

Because of the irreversible nature and relatively slow rate of action of ouabain, the possibility that some secondary abnormality had a role in the abolition of the secretion potential could not be completely excluded. Etacrynic (ethacrynic) acid, a diuretic, also inhibits Na$^+$ K$^+$ - activated ATPase and, although it has many other complex effects currently under investigation, these are now known to be delayed until after the early potential alterations, as are gross deviations in the endolymphatic electrolyte concentrations (Bosher *et al.*, 1973). In this case, the endocochlear potential is quickly replaced by a typical negative potential, and recovery, too, is initially rapid (Fig. 6). The time course of the changes, being comparable with that found in anoxia, accordingly provides appropriate support for Kuijpers and Bonting's concept of the dual nature of the endocochlear potential.

Full investigation of a number of other metabolically active compounds, in particular tetrodotoxin, tetrylam-

monium (tetra-ethyl ammonium) bromide and procaine, has revealed these to have little or no effect upon the cochlea; while others, such as furosemide, have yet to be adequately studied. Although often difficult to interpret, such research will undoubtedly considerably increase our knowledge in due course. In this respect, mention must also be made of inhibitors of oxidative metabolism, e.g. cyanide and dinitrophenol, which, as expected, mimic the effects of anoxia.

STRIA VASCULARIS

The foregoing discussion of the enzymic complexes ultimately responsible for endolymphatic homeostasis leads naturally to the question of the anatomical structures concerned with this function. Here, the evidence overwhelmingly indicates the stria vascularis to have the dominant, if not the sole, role. Apart from being the only cochlear structure to possess the necessary high concentrations of ion transporting and energy producing enzymes, its morphological organization is also ideally suited for this purpose (Engstrom *et al.*, 1955; Smith, 1957; Spoendlin, 1957).

The stria vascularis is composed of three types of cells, of which the marginal cells at the endolymphatic surface comprise the main bulk of the tissue (Fig. 7A). These cells are connected by zonulae occludentes (tight junctions) around their entire circumference, an arrangement which

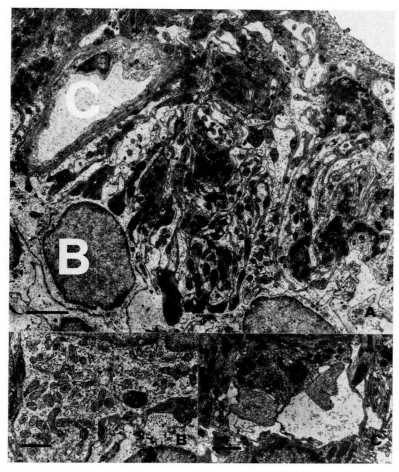

FIG. 7A. The main bulk of the stria vascularis is formed by the intermingling marginal (dark) and intermediate (light) cell processes. The latter are virtually absent from an adjacent area (top left). B, basal cells. C, capillary. Marker, 2 μm. B. Normal intermediate cell body. Marker, 1 μm. C. Shrunken intermediate cell body after etacrynic acid administration. Marker, 1 μm.

appears to form an effective barrier to any communication between the endolymphatic and intercellular spaces, and their most distinctive feature consists of the extremely large number of intertwining processes, containing many mitochondria, that extend from their deep aspect. Ultrastructural examination reveals significant amounts of ATPase to be bound to the plasma membrane of these processes, although some doubt over the exact interpretation of this finding exists (Nakai and Hilding, 1966). The marginal cells, therefore, closely resemble those cells in other situations which are known to be engaged in water and electrolyte transport, except for the absence of the numerous superficial villous processes present in cells associated with large scale fluid reabsorption, such as those in the small intestine and in the proximal renal tubule.

In other respects, however, the stria vascularis presents a number of major features not found elsewhere. Firstly, its deep aspect consists of several layers of flattened basal cells, which separate the stria proper from the connective tissue of the spiral ligament. The spaces between these cells are largely obliterated by extensive zonulae occludentes and no tracer so far studied, whether histochemical or ultra-

structural, has been found to pass across this layer (Vosteen, 1961; Spoendlin and Balogh, 1963; Ilberg, 1968a; Winther, 1971b). It thus appears to form a diffusion barrier isolating the remainder of the stria vascularis from the surrounding tissues, a barrier whose purpose is highly puzzling.

Secondly, another cell type of mesenchymal origin (Kikuchi and Hilding, 1966), the intermediate cell, is present with relatively robust processes radiating amongst those of the marginal cells from a centrally situated body (Fig. 7B). These cells do not form a continuous layer but are distributed sporadically, intervening areas occurring where virtually only marginal cell processes are to be found, and it is consequently difficult to attribute a primary role in endolymph homeostasis to them. Ultrastructural tracers which escape into the strial intercellular spaces are taken up by the intermediate cells (Winther, 1971a, b) and after exposure to etacrynic acid (Fig. 7C) they appear markedly shrunken (Quick and Duvall, 1970). Little else is known about them and the significance of such observations remains completely obscure, as does the general function of the cells.

Finally, the strial capillaries are not separated from the cells by connective tissue but only by the usual basement membrane and intercellular spaces. The blood flow through these capillaries was thought to be rather sluggish until recent investigation revealed it to be about 1 mm.s^{-1}, i.e. unusually fast (Costa and Brånemark, 1970a). Neither contractile elements nor nerve endings are present and vasoactive drugs have been shown to exert no direct action on the vessels (Costa and Brånemark, 1970b). Therapeutic attempts to locally influence internal ear disorders by their use therefore seem likely to be of little avail, any effect merely being secondary to changes in the general circulation. The capillaries are freely permeable to horseradish peroxidase (Duvall et al., 1971; Osaka and Hilding, 1971; Winther 1971a), so resembling those in other active tissues but, unexpectedly, histamine appears to decrease and not increase their permeability (Osaka and Hilding, 1971).

Another unrelated observation that cannot easily be explained is the atrophy which follows the electro-chemical changes arising from rupture of the vestibular membrane (Duvall, 1968). Since it is now possible to obtain specimens of human stria vascularis (Kimura and Schuknecht, 1970) for ultrastructural examination, the correlation of such experimental strial abnormalities with the co-existing functional derangements becomes particularly important; yet little has so far been achieved. Etacrynic acid administration results in the accumulation of excess fluid in the intercellular spaces (Quick and Duvall, 1970), which seems to arise from an increase in membrane permeability (Bosher et al., 1973). A similar appearance is found after the application of NaCl crystals to the round window membrane, a procedure advocated for the relief of Ménière's disease, and, while it is tempting to attribute this to increased fluid movement due to the rise in osmotic pressure (Arslan, 1969), proof is still lacking.

By contrast with the stria vascularis, the cells of the vestibular membrane are relatively undifferentiated and, in the absence of the requisite enzymes, can hardly have an active role in endolymphatic homeostasis. Evidence has been deduced in the past suggesting they may play a subsidiary part in this process (Vosteen, 1970) but such a view lacks support from recent experimental investigation. A stronger case could be made for the involvement of the cells lying deep to the external spiral sulcus, although these have been shown to be concerned with the fluid in the interstices of the spiral ligament rather than with the endolymph (Ilberg et al., 1968).

It is nevertheless extremely difficult to provide a detailed explanation of strial function in this respect and the two main models proposed (Fig. 8) on theoretical grounds indicate the urgent need for further experimental investigation.

COCHLEAR MEMBRANE CHARACTERISTICS

Indirect Studies

The nature of the cochlear duct membranes is another extremely important factor in maintaining the endolymphatic constitution in the presence of the large concentration and electrical gradients, and changes in the charac-

teristics of these membranes are thought today to have a place in the pathology of sensorineural hearing loss.

An approach, widely used for the determination of membrane characteristics, is observation of the chemical and electrical effects produced by alteration of the fluid composition on one aspect of the membrane. Despite the

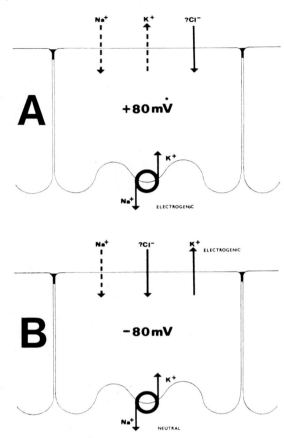

FIG. 8. Schema of strial marginal cell activity as proposed by (A) Johnstone (1964) and (B) Keynes (1969), showing the hypothetical sites of active (solid arrow) and passive (dotted arrow) ionic movements. Note the difference in polarity of the intracellular potential.

large number of such investigations performed utilizing perilymphatic, endolymphatic and vascular perfusion, the advance in our positive knowledge (as opposed to the accumulation of negative data) has been disappointingly small, apart from the inhibitor studies described earlier. Two relatively early experiments worthy of note were the demonstrations that endolymphatic perfusion with solutions of perilymphatic composition had no catastrophic effect on the endocochlear potential (Konishi et al., 1966) and that a potential still persisted at the surface of the stria vascularis after the endolymph had been removed by suction (Tasaki and Spyropoulos, 1959); both of which suggest the endocochlear potential is dependent on strial activity.

More recently, increases in the endocochlear potential have been reported after either scala media perfusion with a solution containing a slight excess of Na^{+} (Sellick and Johnstone, 1972a) or perilymphatic perfusion with a high

K^+ fluid (Kuijpers and Bonting, 1970b), providing the concentrations in each case are not so high as to produce cellular damage. Elevation of endolymphatic Na^+ would be expected to increase the activity of the strial ATPase, while increase in perilymphatic K^+ should reduce or abolish the negative K^+ diffusion potential, and both findings thus support Kuijpers' and Bonting's (1970b) concept of the dual nature of the endocochlear potential.

With regard to the chemical composition, attention in the cochlea has been restricted to Na^+ and the ability to attain the high K^+ composition has been investigated in the vestibular labyrinth. A small rise in endolymph Na^+ produced by perfusion or transitory anoxia is eventually reduced to the normal very low level, but whereas the decrease from 20 mmol. l^{-1} to the equilibrium concentration occurs in about 6 min, that from this concentration to 2 mmol. l^{-1} takes a further 15 min or more (Sellick and Johnstone, 1972a). The impression given is of some possible insensitivity of the endolymphatic homeostatic mechanisms to slight increases in the sodium concentration. Such a conclusion would certainly be in accord with Kuijpers and Bonting's (1969) activation values for the $Na^+ K^+$- activated ATPase and the time course is in agreement with that of the action of the $Na^+ Cl^-$ coupled system in preventing a rise in endolymphatic Na^+ following etacrynic acid administration (Bosher et al., 1973). Nevertheless, much obviously remains to be discovered about the sensitivity and inter-relation of these transport mechanisms.

Direct Investigations

Attempts to investigate the properties of the cochlear membranes by direct means have been greatly hindered by the enormous technical problems arising from their inaccessibility and delicate nature. The electrical resistances of the individual walls of the cochlear duct have been very ably determined by Johnstone and his colleagues (1966), who found the stria vascularis to have the lowest resistance, 48 ohm/cm², as might be expected from its ion transporting function. The vestibular membrane had the highest resistance, 368 ohm/cm², a surprisingly low value (c.f. nerve and muscle membranes which also maintain a potential difference of about 80 mV and have resistances of 700–5000 ohm/cm²) suggesting that considerable passive ion diffusion occurs across the membrane.

Radioactive labelled elements have naturally been used in an attempt to estimate the rate of such ion movement, particularly by Rauch (1964), although the heterogeneous and complex nature of the cochlea has made it impossible to assess the results with accuracy. In so far as they can be interpreted, the findings suggest that the vestibular membrane, and possibly other structures, have a relatively high permeability to both sodium and potassium, a conclusion in keeping with the electrical resistance measurements and one latterly proposed by Rauch (1970), who has abandoned his original concept of active transport across the vestibular membrane.

The equivalent pore size of these various membranes is also under investigation but no reports are available at present. However, some portion of the membranes bounding the endolymphatic space is relatively freely permeable to water (Bosher and Warren, 1971), a fundamental property of especial significance with regard to the problems of the endolymph circulation, the pathogenesis of labyrinthine hydrops, and the treatment of Ménière's disease by alteration of internal ear fluid osmolality. As a consequence, both the osmotic and hydrostatic pressures of the endolymph and perilymph must be identical under normal circumstances, and this has been confirmed (Bosher and Warren, 1971; Beentjes, 1972) despite initial reports to the contrary. Osmotically induced water movements have been shown not to be accompanied by any major ionic shunts, another relevant feature.

ENDOLYMPH CIRCULATION

The endolymph circulation has been the subject of considerable attention over the years and has provoked a vast amount of speculation and controversy. A great deal of experimental work and many ingenious ideas have been reported in the large number of papers devoted to this problem and, as a result, two main types of concept have emerged. One is the longitudinal flow theory attributed principally to Guild (1927b) following his studies on dye dispersion in the endolymph system. According to this hypothesis, endolymph is secreted by the stria vascularis and passes along the length of the cochlea, first to the saccule and then to the endolymphatic sac, where it is reabsorbed. The other is the radial flow theory, probably best exemplified by the proposals advanced on theoretical grounds by Naftalin and Harrison (1958). Perilymph formed as an ultrafiltrate of plasma, these authors postulated, flows freely across the vestibular membrane, to be reabsorbed by the stria, where there is an exchange of Na^+ for K^+.

Unfortunately, a better understanding of the techniques previously employed has brought the realization that none of the methods utilized can be considered really satisfactory for the purpose of demonstrating fluid circulation. Indeed, this was realized at the time, for only the inadequacies of the scientific evidence could permit the wide variety of opinions advanced. Even such meticulous and valuable investigations as the confirmation of the ability of the basal turn of the cochlea to function normally despite destruction of the apical portions (Lawrence et al., 1961), the demonstration of the absence of any longitudinal spread of injury to localized toxic endolymphatic changes (Duvall and Rhodes, 1967) and the finding of cochlear hydrops following obliteration of the endolymphatic sac (Kimura, 1967), must be considered inconclusive as they provide no positive evidence about the underlying movement of water.

Still more recently, hopes were raised by the first use in this field of inert electron-dense tracers for electron microscopy, e.g. dextriferon (iron dextran) (Yamamoto and Nakai, 1964), thorium dioxide sol (thorotrast) (Ilberg, 1968a, b), iron albuminate (ferritin) (Rudert, 1968) and lanthanum (Duvall and Quick, 1969), but the results obtained from other situations, particularly the choroid plexus (Tennyson and Pappas, 1968), have proved beyond doubt that these substances cannot be relied upon for accurate determination of endolymph flow. An adequate experimental method for this purpose is consequently still lacking and progress thus blocked.

The term circulation implies the bulk movement of fluid from a place of secretion to an anatomically distinct site for reabsorption and there is no evidence to suggest such active water movement (as opposed to passive diffusional exchange) is essential in the endolymph system, where such movement would undeniably be a most severe handicap for an organ concerned with the transduction of physical movements of the order of 10^{-10}m.

across these cells to be discharged into the endolymph and subsequently re-pinocytosed by the strial and other cells (Fig. 9). This type of movement does not occur in the reverse direction, nor does it take place anywhere else in the cochlea where, for example, no tracer has been found in the intercellular spaces of the stria vascularis following its insertion into the endolymph. Although the exact significance of this finding has yet to be explored, it appears to be one route whereby macro-molecular toxic agents, which would otherwise be excluded, could gain access to the endolymphatic space and stria vascularis.

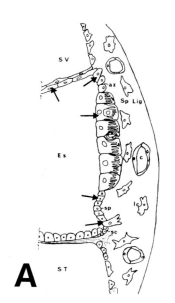 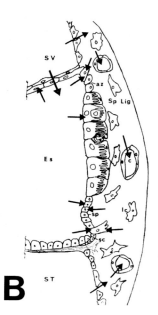

FIG. 9. The movement of iron albuminate (ferritin) after its injection into (A) the endolymphatic space and (B) the perilymphatic space, where transfer across the vestibular (Reissner's) membrane is followed by secondary removal from the scala media: az, attachment zone of the vestibular membrane; c, capillary; Es, endolymphatic space; lc, spiral ligament cell; Sc, external spiral sulcus; sp, spiral prominence; Sp Lig spiral ligament; ST, scala tympani; SV, scala vestibuli. (Hinojosa, 1972.)

What the distribution of electron-dense tracers, following their injection into the fluid spaces of the internal ear, has been valuable in revealing is the fate of macro-molecular substances in these spaces. In general, the lining cells take up and retain such substances by the process of pinocytosis, although nothing is known about the functional significance of this feature. In the perilymphatic spaces, the most active cells in this respect are those of the vestibular membrane and of the spiral ligament, especially at the attachment of this membrane and deep to the external spiral sulcus; the perilymph clearly having free access to these regions (Ilberg, 1968a; Lim, 1969). In the cochlear duct, the cells chiefly concerned are the marginal cells of the stria vascularis, together with those of the spiral prominence, external spiral sulcus and the vestibular membrane.

However, there is one important exception to the usual pattern. In a very extensive study using iron albuminate, Hinojosa (1972) has conclusively confirmed that perilymphatic tracer material is not merely taken up by the cells of the vestibular membrane, but it is actually transported

ENDOLYMPH FUNCTION IN THE COCHLEA

Physiologically, endolymph is undoubtedly a quite unique fluid, for not only is its constitution extremely unusual, but it is controlled in all its major aspects by active mechanisms entirely dependent on oxidative metabolism. It must, therefore, surely play a vital and irreplaceable role in cochlear function and, since the fluid is now known to be unable to supply the metabolic needs of the spiral organ of Corti, this function can only be concerned with the mechano-electric transduction processes of the hair cells.

Of the ideas advanced, Davis' (1957) mechano-electrical concept of modulation of a standing current passing through the hair cell, by changes in the electrical resistance of its apical membrane which arise from the mechanical stresses associated with sound stimulation, is probably the best attested. Should this electrical current be carried by K^+ ions, then such a theory would explain the need for the endolymphatic positive potential and low Na^+ content. Certainly, stimulation by sound does alter the basilar membrane resistance, does increase the standing current through the spiral organ and is associated with endolymphatic potential and composition changes. However, investigation has also shown the correlation between the induced current changes and the basilar membrane displacement to preclude a simple regulating mechanism such as direct variation in pore size of the hair cell apical membrane (Johnstone and Sellick, 1972). This finding, accordingly, directs attention to the more complex suggestions that have been advanced, in particular to the proposals of induced alterations in the membrane configuration at a

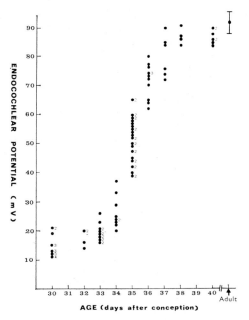

FIG. 10. The change in the endocochlear potential with age. Numericals indicate the number of experiments giving the same result and the range and mean of the adult potential is also shown. The average length of gestation was 22 days. (Bosher and Warren, 1971.)

molecular level (Vinnikov and Titova, 1964; Naftalin, 1968).

The other groups of theories, the displacement potential and piezo-electric concepts (e.g. Christiansen, 1964), together with those involving frequency analysis by the tectorial membrane (Naftalin, 1968; Tiedemann, 1970) seem unable in their present forms to provide an adequate explanation of the experimental findings (Johnstone and Sellick, 1972). Nevertheless, further ideas will undoubtedly be advanced as more information becomes available, but an explanation of the role played by the endolymphatic composition and potential must now be considered an essential part of any account of cochlear transduction.

Some evidence of the possibly differing function of these two features was provided by a report of the endolymphatic changes during the neonatal period in the rat (Bosher and Warren, 1971). The endocochlear potential developed substantially between the 12th and 14th day after birth (Fig. 10) at precisely the time when the inception of hearing occurred. This association can hardly be fortuitous

and the potential thus appears to be vitally concerned with the hearing processes, possibly increasing the sensitivity of hair cell transduction sufficiently to enable the threshold of the nerve-activating mechanisms to be overcome for the first time. Unexpectedly, the electrolyte composition of the endolymph was already completely mature several days before the dramatic increase in the potential. Histological examination of these same animals revealed the spiral organ was fully developed and the low Na^+, high K^+ constitution, therefore, seems necessary for the integrity of the hair cells once they have acquired their adult character. The exact role of the endolymph in this respect remains obscure, although it is clearly related to the toxic effect of a high endolymphatic Na^+ content in adults.

The attainment of the characteristic endolymphatic constitution implies the presence of considerable activity of the strial, ion transporting ATPases in these younger animals, an implication supported by the mature morphological appearance of the stria vascularis. It does, however, raise the question of the nature of the mechanism subsequently responsible for the increase in the endocochlear potential. The most likely explanation is that some change in the cochlear duct membranes, probably a developmental alteration in the zonulae occludentes between the cells, resulted in an increase in their electrical resistance during the period concerned. Recently, comparable changes in zonulae occludentes have been discovered in other situations, such as the mammary gland at the onset of lactation (Linzell and Peaker, 1973), and the findings in the neonatal animals again indicate the importance of the cochlear membranes in endolymph homeostasis.

VESTIBULAR LABYRINTH

Utricle and Semicircular Canals

The utricular endolymph (Table 3) has the same high K^+ content (Smith et al., 1954) as cochlear endolymph, but its sodium content, 12 mmol. 1^{-1}, is very much greater

TABLE 3

THE ELECTRO-CHEMICAL CONSTITUTION OF THE VESTIBULAR
ENDOLYMPH SHOWING RANGES AND MEAN VALUES
(After Sellick et al., 1972; Sellick and Johnstone, 1972b)

	Utricle	Saccule
Potassium (mmol. 1^{-1})	144*	144†
Sodium (mmol. 1^{-1})	2–22 (12·6)	2·3–4·0 (3·2)
Potential (mV)	−10–+7 (1·8)	−8–+2·5 (−2.8)
Resistance (kohm)	0·9–3·8 (2·0)	4·2–40 (16)

* Smith et al., 1954.
† Rauch, 1968.

(Sellick et al., 1972). In addition, the values reported for the dc potential vary only a few millivolts about zero (Smith et al., 1958; Schmidt, 1963; Sellick et al., 1972). Anoxia, however, reveals a K^+ diffusion potential of approximately −15 mV and indicates that a positive secretion potential of the same order must normally be present (Sellick *et al.*, 1972). The nature of the utricular dc potential is therefore more complex than appears at first and resembles that of the endocochlear potential.

Na$^+$ K$^+$ activated ATPase is present in this situation and, although the reported concentrations have not been substantial, the values obtained to date are certainly underestimated due to the large amount of inactive tissue in the gross specimens analysed (Thalmann, 1971). The effects of ouabain and other inhibitors have yet to be determined, but evidence of the active transport of potassium, at least into the semicircular canals, is now available (Dohlman and Radomski, 1968). The access resistance is considerably below the 7 kohm found in the basal turn of the cochlea (Sellick *et al.*, 1972) and this may be related to the low endolymphatic potential. Continued investigation will nevertheless be necessary to establish whether the differences in the utricular endolymph arise from variations in the ion transporting enzyme systems, the limiting membranes, or both.

Specialized cells closely resembling the strial marginal cells, except that their height is only 4–7 μm compared to approximately 18 μm and their basal processes project into the underlying connective tissue spaces, are widely distributed in the walls of the utricle, the ampullae and semicircular canals (Smith, 1956; Iurato, 1967; Kimura, 1969). They are termed dark cells, after their osmium-staining character, and are almost certainly responsible for maintaining the endolymphatic constitution. These dark cells are associated in the ampullary juxta-crista regions with so-called light cells, which appear to lack the necessary morphological differentiation for their proposed secretory function (Dohlman, 1967).

No such reservations exist about the cells in the ampullary plana semilunata and utricular peri-macular regions. Their secretion product, possibly a sulphur containing mucopolysaccharide or a mucoprotein, becomes intimately related to the cupulae and otolith membrane, before it is in turn displaced by freshly elaborated material (Dohlman *et al.*, 1959). The function and exact nature of this material is not known, while the relationship between the cells described and the interdental cells of the spiral limbus in the cochlea, which may also be secretory in nature (Iurato, 1967; Ilberg, 1968c), remains entirely conjectural.

Earlier observations that the utricular endolymphatic system persisted unaltered after destruction of the cochlea have recently been completely substantiated (Sellick *et al.*, 1972), and the function of Bast's utriculoendolymphatic valve in preventing loss of endolymph from the utricle thus confirmed. There can accordingly be no doubt about the complete independence of the utricular endolymphatic system from the cochlea. In addition, caution must be observed in the extrapolation of findings between the two systems in view of the significant differences in endolymphatic homeostasis and their, as yet unexplored, effect on hair cell transduction.

Saccule

The endolymph in the saccule, unlike the utricle, has a Na$^+$ content only slightly in excess of the very low cochlear level, as well as a high K$^+$ content. The dc

potential, of the usual composite nature, again varies a few mV either side of zero, but the access resistance is considerably greater than the utricular value and the resistances of the saccular and vestibular (Reissner's) membranes seem equivalent (Sellick and Johnstone, 1972b).

Despite their superficial resemblance, the utricular and saccular systems thus exhibit marked differences and this conclusion is confirmed by the finding, on ultrastructural examination, of a complete absence of any specialized cells capable of active ion transport (Smith, 1970; Kimura, 1969). Furthermore, the saccular dc potential has recently been shown to depend primarily upon the potential in the basal turn of the scala media (Sellick and Johnstone, 1972b) and the endolymphatic constitution in the saccule must therefore be maintained essentially by the stria vascularis in the cochlea. This is a most unusual situation, even if the cochlea is phylogenetically an outgrowth of the saccule, and one which is clearly quite different from the state of affairs in the utricle. The resistance of the ductus reuniens, however, can be calculated to be 181 kohm, a value which precludes any bulk flow of fluid and hence the presence of gross circulation of endolymph from cochlea to saccule. Presumably, saccular homeostasis must depend primarily on ionic diffusion and the transfer of electrical energy, allied to extremely low permeability and high resistance of its limiting membranes.

ENDOLYMPHATIC SAC

The final portion of the endolymphatic system, the endolymphatic sac, is an appendage connected by a series of narrow ducts to the utricle, to the saccule and, indirectly, to the cochlea. In recent years a number of surgical procedures upon this structure have been devised in an attempt to alleviate Ménière's disease, and its relationship to the endolymphatic system as a whole is consequently of topical interest.

Guild's (1927a) classical studies revealed that, although the sac had three morphological divisions, only the rugose epithelium of the intermediate portion showed evidence of marked activity. With the electron microscope, two main epithelial cell types were identified in this situation, again termed light and dark cells after their relative osmium-staining characteristics. The light cells seemed comparable to the vestibular dark cells and concerned with electrolyte and possibly water transfer, while the dark cells were actively phagocytic in nature. In addition, the free cells in the sac's lumen were confirmed to be mainly macrophages and cellular debris was found to be a prominent feature of its fluid contents (Lundquist, 1965). Subsequent investigation demonstrated that this portion of the sac had a high protein turnover (Koburg *et al.*, 1967) and was rich in enzymes concerned with protein degradation (Ishii *et al.*, 1966), and that the luminal fluid possessed a very high concentration of protein, namely 5g/100 g fluid (Silverstein, 1966b).

The distribution of a wide variety of substances injected into the endolymphatic space of the cochlea and of the vestibule has been studied, in an attempt to define the origin of the sac's contents. These substances have subsequently been demonstrated in the endolymphatic sac in every case, although some variation in detail has been observed. For example, phagocytosis of colloidal silver by the lining cells was reported 5 h after its injection into the basal turn of the cochlea (Lundquist et al., 1964), but horseradish peroxidase injected into the third cochlear turn did not appear in the sac until two days later and was taken up largely by the free macrophages. When radioactive labelled protein was introduced directly into the sac itself, however, it was ingested within 5 min by the lining cells, followed shortly afterwards by the luminal cells (Ishii et al., 1966). A finding of a more physiological nature was the discovery that the sulphur-containing compound secreted by the plana semilunata cells (see above) travelled from the ampullary cupulae to the endolymphatic sac (Dohlman et al., 1959), and cochlear degeneration is often followed by increase in the sac's content and activity, as is Ménière's disease (Rauch, 1968).

A major, if not the principal, function of the endolymphatic sac is accordingly considered to be the removal from the endolymph of cellular debris and macro-molecules arising elsewhere. What remains at issue is whether such material is brought to the sac simply by diffusional processes, aided by random fluid oscillations, or not; for its movement has often been taken as proof of fluid flow and the concept of considerable endolymph reabsorption in the sac has thus arisen.

Nevertheless, evidence of this nature is quite inconclusive and the effects of obliteration of the sac are therefore of much interest. This procedure is followed, under appropriate circumstances, by endolymphatic hydrops and cochlear hair cell damage (Kimura, 1967; Schuknecht et al., 1968). Unhappily, the changes induced are most complex and are not invariable (Lindsay et al., 1952), so other possibilities, such as the accumulation of osmotically-active substances, cannot be excluded and nothing definite can be concluded about the possible circulation of endolymph. The endolymphatic sac, it is also noteworthy, persists unaltered after complete cochlear degeneration (Bosher and Hallpike, 1965). In this respect, Silverstein's report (1966b) that the endolymphatic sac endolymph had a Na^+ content of 153 mmol. l^{-1} and a K^+ content of only 8 mmol. l^{-1} is of great importance. Such values are vastly different from those found in either the vestibular labyrinth or the cochlea and it is extremely difficult to conceive how such concentration differences could be maintained in the face of a large and continuous flow of endolymph towards the endolymphatic sac. Here again local water interchange and the absence of any active circulation seem more than distinct possibilities.

Finally, the endolymphatic sac appears likely to have a role in the pressure regulation of the endolymph system, compensating for any sudden variations in fluid pressure. Disturbance of this function, say due to peri-saccular fibrosis, has been thought to be a possible feature in Ménière's disease and forms the rationale for various decompression procedures, but direct experimental evidence is completely lacking due to the enormous technical difficulties involved.

PERILYMPH

This review has been largely concerned with the endolymph system because of its intimate involvement with hair cell transduction and integrity, but the perilymph cannot be entirely neglected, although no attempt will be made to discuss its physiology in detail.

The composition of this fluid closely resembles extracellular fluid in general (Table 1) but opinions differ regarding its origin. Two possibilities exist, namely exchange of the usual tissue fluid type with blood in the capillaries lining the perilymphatic spaces and replenishment by bulk flow of cerebrospinal fluid along the cochlear aquaduct. The problem has been investigated by studying the equilibration between perilymph and blood, by following tracers introduced into the cerebrospinal fluid, by comparing perilymphatic protein and enzyme composition with other fluids, and by elucidating the effect of cochlear aquaduct obstruction. It is unfortunate, in view of the great bulk of evidence thus provided, that the most recent comprehensive assessment (Schnieder, 1970) is not readily available. However, the composition of the perilymph appears, despite some fluid flow from the cerebrospinal space (which probably varies with the species involved), to be almost entirely determined by its interchange with the perilymphatic capillaries, a feature of importance clinically in connection with the distribution of therapeutic agents.

The turnover rate has been estimated independently in two laboratories to be 0·8 μl. min^{-1} (Schnieder, 1970; Moscovitch and Laszlo, 1972), and free communication between the perilymph and the fluid spaces of the spiral organ has been demonstrated, principally from the speed with which electron-dense tracers (Ilberg, 1968d) and drugs acting upon neural transmission (Konishi and Kelsey, 1968; Konishi, 1972) enter these spaces when they are introduced into the scala tympani.

The internal ear fluids are, of course, essential for the hydrodynamic processes responsible for hair cell activation but, in addition, the perilymph in the cochlea appears to have another important function. Calculations reveal that the fluid could meet the entire metabolic needs of the spiral organ, and in animals in whom the spiral vessel has involuted, the nutrition of the hair cells must depend entirely on the perilymph. Where the spiral vessel persists, the spiral organ can survive unimpaired in experimental situations where the perilymph is completely removed, at least in the short term (Lawrence and Nuttall, 1972). What is controversial is whether this vessel can maintain the supply of metabolites indefinitely without perilymphatic support and also the relative importance of the two sources where they co-exist. In the vestibular labyrinth, any possible nutritive function remains entirely speculative.

CONCLUSION

Although much obviously remains to be achieved in the investigation of the endolymphatic and perilymphatic systems, their general nature now seems firmly established. Furthermore, our understanding of their physiology continues to increase as new information becomes available and experimental work is also progressing which will substantially add to our knowledge of their pathological derangements. Such studies have had little impact, as yet, on investigation and treatment in the human situation but they will undoubtedly make a vital contribution in the future to the alleviation and prevention of sensorineural hearing loss and labyrinthine-induced vertigo.

REFERENCES

Änggård, L. (1965), *Acta oto-laryng.*, suppl. 203.

Arslan, M. (1969), *Acta oto-laryng.*, **67**, 360.

Beentjes, B. I. J. (1972), *Acta oto-laryng.*, **73**, 112.

Békésy, G. v. (1952a), *J. acoust. Soc. Amer.*, **24**, 72.

Békésy, G. v. (1952b), *J. acoust. Soc. Amer.*, **24**, 399.

Bosher, S. K. and Hallpike, C. S. (1965), *Proc. roy. Soc. B*, **162**, 147.

Bosher, S. K., Smith, C. and Warren, R. L. (1973), *Acta oto-laryng.*, **75**, 184.

Bosher, S. K. and Warren, R. L. (1968), *Proc. roy. Soc. B*, **171**, 227.

Bosher, S. K. and Warren, R. L. (1971), *J. Physiol.*, **212**, 739.

Christiansen, J. A. (1964), *Acta oto-laryng.*, **57**, 33.

Costa, O. and Brånemark, P.-I. (1970a), *Adv. Microcirc.*, **3**, 96.

Costa, O. and Brånemark, P.-I. (1970b), *Adv. Microcirc.*, **3**, 108.

Davis, H. (1957), *Physiol. Rev.*, **37**, 1.

Dohlman, G. F. (1967), *Myotatic, Kinesthetic and Vestibular Mechanisms* (A. V. S. de Reuck and J. Knight, Eds.). Churchill: London.

Dohlman, G. F., Ormerod, F. E. and McLay, K. (1959), *Acta oto-laryng.*, **50**, 243.

Dohlman, G. F. and Radomski, M. W. (1968), *Acta oto-laryng.*, **66**, 409.

Duvall, A. J. (1968), *Ann. Otol., Rhinol., Lar.*, **77**, 317.

Duvall, A. J. and Quick, C. A. (1969), *Ann. Otol., Rhinol., Lar.*, **78**, 1041.

Duvall, A. J., Quick, C. A. and Sutherland, C. R. (1971), *Arch. Otolaryng.*, **93**, 304.

Duvall, A. J. and Rhodes, V. T. (1967), *Ann. Otol., Rhinol., Lar.*, **76**, 688.

Engström, H., Sjöstrand, F. S. and Spoendlin, H. (1955), *Pract. oto-rhino-laryng.* (*Basel*), **17**, 69.

Erulkar, S. D. and Maren, T. H. (1961), *Nature* (*Lond.*), **189**, 459.

Flock, Å. (1973), *J. acoust. Soc. Amer.*, **54**, 293.

Guild, S. R. (1927a), *Amer. J. Anat.*, **39**, 1.

Guild, S. R. (1927b), *Amer. J. Anat.*, **39**, 57.

Hinojosa, R. (1972), *Acta oto-laryng.*, **74**, 1.

Ilberg, C. v. (1968a), *Arch. Klin. exp. Ohr.-, Nas.- u. Kehlk. Heilk.*, **190**, 415.

Ilberg, C. v. (1968b), *Arch. Klin. exp. Ohr.-, Nas.- u. Kehlk. Heilk.*, **190**, 426.

Ilberg, C. v. (1968c), *Arch. Klin. exp. Ohr.-, Nas.- u. Kehlk. Heilk.*, **192**, 163.

Ilberg, C. v. (1968d), *Arch. Klin. exp. Ohr.-, Nas.- u. Kehlk. Heilk.*, **192**, 384.

Ilberg, C. v., Spoendlin, H. and Vosteen, K. -H. (1968), *Arch. Klin. exp. Ohr.-, Nas.- u. Kehlk. Heilk.*, **192**, 124.

Ishii, T., Silverstein, H. and Balogh, K. (1966), *Acta oto-laryng.*, **62**, 61.

Iurato, S. (1967), *Submicroscopic Structure of the Inner Ear* (S. Iurato, Ed.). Oxford: Pergamon.

Johnstone, B. M. (1964), *Transcellular Membrane Potentials and Ionic Fluxes* (F. M. Snell and W. K. Noell, Eds.). New York: Gordon and Breach.

Johnstone, B. M. (1965), *Acta oto-laryng.*, **60**, 113.

Johnstone, B. M., Johnstone, J. R. and Pugsley, I. D. (1966), *J. acoust. Soc. Amer.*, **40**, 1398.

Johnstone, B. M. and Sellick, P. M. (1972), *Quart. Rev. Biophys.*, **5**, 1.

Johnstone, C. G., Schmidt, R. S. and Johnstone, B. M. (1963), *Comp. Biochem. Physiol.*, **9**, 335.

Keynes, R. D. (1969), *Quart. Rev. Biophys.*, **2**, 177.

Kikuchi, K. and Hilding, D. A. (1966), *Acta oto-laryng.*, **62**, 277.

Kimura, R. S. (1967), *Ann. Otol., Rhinol., Lar.*, **76**, 664.

Kimura, R. S. (1969), *Ann. Otol., Rhinol., Lar.*, **78**, 542.

Kimura, R. S. and Schuknecht, H. F. (1970), *Acta oto-laryng.*, **70**, 301.

Koburg, E., Haubrich, J. and Kernbach, B. (1967), *Acta oto-laryng.*, **64**, 146.

Konishi, T. (1972), *Acta oto-laryng.*, **74**, 252.

Konishi, T. and Kelsey, E. (1968), *J. acoust. Soc. Amer.*, **43**, 471.

Konishi, T., Kelsey, E. and Singleton, G. T. (1966), *Acta oto-laryng.*, **62**, 393.

Konishi, T. and Mendelsohn, M. (1970), *Acta oto-laryng.*, **69**, 192.

Kuijpers, W. and Bonting, S. L. (1969), *Biochim. biophys. Acta*, **173**, 477.

Kuijpers, W. and Bonting, S. L. (1970a), *Pflügers Arch. ges. Physiol.*, **320**, 348.

Kuijpers, W. and Bonting, S. L. (1970b), *Pflügers Arch. ges. Physiol.*, **320**, 359.

Lawrence, M. (1967), *Ann. Otol., Rhinol., Lar.*, **76**, 287.

Lawrence, M. and Nuttall, A. L. (1972), *J. acoust. Soc. Amer.*, **52**, 566.

Lawrence, M., Wolsk, D and Litton, W. B. (1961), *Ann. Otol., Rhinol., Lar.*, **70**, 753.

Lim, D. J. (1969), *Acta oto-laryng.*, suppl. 255.

Lindsay, J. R., Schuknecht, H. F., Neff, W. D. and Kimura, R. S. (1952), *Ann. Otol., Rhinol., Lar.*, **61**, 697.

Linzell, L. J. and Peaker, M. (1973), *J. Physiol.*, 230, 13P.

Lundquist, P. -G. (1965), *Acta oto-laryng.*, suppl. 201.

Lundquist, P. -G., Kimura, R. S. and Warsäll, J. (1964), *Acta oto-laryng.*, suppl. 188.

Matschinsky, F. M. and Thalmann, R. (1967), *Ann. Otol., Rhinol., Lar.*, **76**, 638.

Mendelsohn, M. and Katzenberg, I. (1972), *Laryngoscope* (*St. Louis*), **82**, 397.

Mendelsohn, M. and Konishi, T. (1969), *Ann. Otol., Rhinol, Lar.*, **78**, 65.

Misrahy, G. A., Hildreth, K. M., Clark, L. C. and Shinabarger, E. W. (1958), *Amer. J. Physiol.*, **194**, 393.

Moscovitch, D. H. and Laszlo, C. A. (1972), *J. acoust. Soc. Amer.*, **52**, 144.

Naftalin, L. (1968), *Progr. Biophys. mol. Biol.*, **18**, 1.

Naftalin, L. and Harrison, M. S. (1958), *Proc. Roy. Soc. Med.*, **51**, 624.

Nakai, Y. and Hilding, D. A. (1966), *Acta oto-laryng.*, **62**, 411.

Osako, S. and Hilding, D. A. (1971), *Acta oto-laryng.*, **71**, 365.

Quick, C. A. and Duvall, A. J. (1970), *Laryngoscope* (*St. Louis*), **80**, 954.

Rauch, S. (1964), *Biochemie des Hörorgans.* Stuttgart: Thieme Verlag.

Rauch, S. (1968), *Oto-lar. Clin. N. Amer.*, **1**, 369.

Rauch, S. (1970), *Biochemical Mechanisms in Hearing and Deafness* (M. M. Paparella, Ed.). Springfield: Thomas.

Rudert, H. (1968), *Arch. Klin. exp. Ohr.-, Nas.- u. Kehlk. Heilk.*, **191**, 783.

Schätzle, W. (1971), *Histochemie des Innenohres.* Munich: Urban and Schwarzenberg.

Schmidt, R. S. (1963), *J. gen. Physiol.*, **47**, 371.

Schneider, E. A. (1970), *Die Entstehung des Schalltraumas: Ein Beitrag über die Physiologie der Perilymphe.* Thesis, University of Würzburg.

Schuknecht, H. F. and Kimura, R. S. (1953), *Laryngoscope* (*St. Louis*), **63**, 1170.

Schuknecht, H. F., Northrop, C. and Igarashi, M. (1968), *Acta oto-laryng.*, **65**, 479.

Sellick, P. M. and Johnstone, B. M. (1972a), *Pflügers Arch. ges. Physiol.*, **336**, 11.

Sellick, P. M. and Johnstone, B. M. (1972b), *Pflügers Arch. ges. Physiol.*, **336**, 28.

Sellick, P. M., Johnstone, J. R. and Johnstone, B. M. (1972), *Pflügers Arch. ges. Physiol.*, **336**, 21.

Silverstein, H. (1966a), *Ann. Otol., Rhinol., Lar.*, **75**, 48.

Silverstein, H. (1966b), *Laryngoscope* (*St. Louis*), **76**, 498

Smith, C. A. (1956), *Ann. Otol., Rhinol., Lar.*, **65**, 450.

Smith, C. A. (1957), *Ann. Otol., Rhinol., Lar.*, **66**, 521.

Smith, C. A. (1970), *Biochemical Mechanisms in Hearing and Deafness* (M. M. Paparella, Ed.). Springfield: Thomas.

Smith, C. A., Davis, H., Deatherage, B. H. and Gessert, C. F. (1958), *Amer. J. Physiol.*, **193**, 203.

Smith, C. A., Lowry, O. H., and Wu, M. L. (1954), *Laryngoscope (St. Louis)*, **64**, 141.

Spoendlin, H. (1957), *Submicroscopic Structure of the Inner Ear* (S. Iurato, Ed.). Oxford: Pergamon.

Spoendlin, H. and Balogh, K. (1963), *Laryngoscope (St. Louis)*, **73**, 1061.

Tasaki, I. and Spyropoulos, C. S. (1959), *J. Neurophysiol.*, **22**, 149.

Tennyson, V. M. and Pappas, G. D. (1968), *Progr. Brain Res.*, **29**, 63.

Thalmann, I., Matschinsky, F. M. and Thalmann, R. (1970), *Ann. Otol., Rhinol., Lar.*, **79**, 12.

Thalmann, R. (1971), *Laryngoscope (St. Louis)*, **81**, 1245.

Tiedemann, H. (1970), *Acta oto-laryng.*, suppl. 277.

Vinnikov, J. A. and Titova, L. K. (1964), *The Organ of Corti*. New York: Consultants Bureau.

Vosteen, K. -H. (1961), *Arch. Klin. exp. Ohr.-, Nas.- u. Kehlk. Heilk.*, **178**, 1.

Vosteen, K. -H. (1970), *Arch. Klin. exp. Ohr.-, Nas.- u. Kehlk. Heilk.*, **195**, 226.

Winther, F. Ø. (1971a), *Z. Zellforsch.*, **114**, 193.

Winther, F. Ø. (1971b), *Z. Zellforsch.*, **121**, 499.

Yamamoto, K. and Nakai, Y. (1964), *Ann. Otol., Rhinol., Lar.*, **73**, 332.

21. APPLIED COCHLEAR ELECTROPHYSIOLOGY

J.-M. ARAN AND M. PORTMANN

INTRODUCTION

In seeking some objective means of studying auditory function, the scientist as well as the clinician has remained fascinated by the cochlea and the vestibulocochlear (eighth) nerve. Indeed the end-organ is the key to the auditory system and its function determines the basic auditory capabilities of the patient. Moreover this end-organ is the only specific acoustical mechanism if one considers that, as soon as the acoustic signal has been transposed into nerve impulses, it is involved in the general processes of the central nervous system and can be dealt with in the scope of general neurophysiology.

Since the work of Wever and Bray (1930), electrophysiological studies of the cochlear receptor have been performed for various purposes—from the verification of the effectiveness of functional middle ear surgery to verifications of mechanical theories about the travelling wave—from fundamental studies of the function of the sensory epithelium, to studies directed more towards the damaging effects of noise and of ototoxic drugs. All these goals have been considerably interwoven.

These basic topics are dealt with elsewhere in this book. Here, the clinical applications of such electrophysiological measurements will be considered. This considerably narrows the field to be covered since all the attempts to find, for the patient, a successful application of such an approach have suffered, until the past few years, from tremendous technical difficulties together with some reluctance, on the part of the research worker, to appear to use the human being as a guinea pig.

Because of the paucity of such human recordings it is possible to present here an extensive chronological survey of the attempts made during the past forty-three years, with reference to the main steps of the on-going experimental studies on animals.

HISTORICAL SURVEY

Wever and Bray (1930) reported electrical activity recorded from the eighth nerve in animals.

Adrian (1931), Saul and Davis (1932) showed evidence that this activity arises in the spiral organ of Corti and that the neural response is a different signal (Derbyshire and Davis, 1935).

The first attempts to record the cochlear microphonic (CM) in humans, during surgery, were presented by Fromm *et al.* (1935). Other similar attempts followed (Gersuni *et al.*, 1937; Andreev *et al.*, 1939; Perlman and Case, 1941).

Lempert and his colleagues published, six years later, interesting recordings from the round window niche during surgery (Lempert *et al.* 1947). However three years later, while seeking a clinical application, they reported their unsuccessful attempts at recording the cochlear microphonic in a non-surgical way, using a needle electrode introduced through the tympanic membrane and pushed onto the promontory (Lempert *et al.*, 1950). They failed essentially because of the small amplitude of the microphonic response recorded in such a way.

Human cochlear microphonic records were presented again (Krejci, 1949; Krejci and Bornschein, 1950).

Davis *et al.* (1958) described the summating potential in animals. Recordings of eighth nerve single fibre activity in animals were presented by Tasaki (1954).

Ruben and his colleagues at the Johns Hopkins Hospital in Baltimore, undertook extensive studies in humans of the cochlear microphonic and, for the first time, of vestibulocochlear (eighth) nerve compound action potential (AP) responses to click stimulation. They investigated either adults or children with various pathological conditions (Bordley *et al.*, 1964; Ruben *et al.*, 1959 to 1967). However the recordings were still performed during surgery or through a surgical approach to the round window and, most of the time, without the new averaging technique developed during the same period and applied to the recording of evoked electroencephalic responses. However many of the characteristics of human CM and AP were clearly described (Fig. 1), and their work emphasized the possible interest of such recordings if the approach could be simplified and the quality of the signals improved.

Some further studies of the human cochlear microphonic

have since been presented (Brinkman and Tolk, 1961; Flach and Seidel, 1968; Fink *et al.*, 1969). One particular non-surgical approach was presented by Gavilan and Sanjuan (1964): they recorded the cochlear microphonic from the tympanic membrane. Owing to the very small amplitude of this response, as already reported when recorded from the round window, this technique inevitably encountered difficulties.

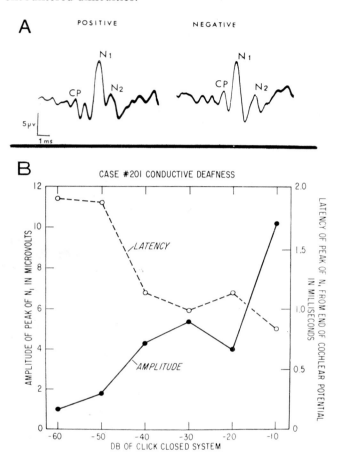

FIG. 1. A: Single responses to clicks of opposite polarities recorded from the round window in a patient with a conductive hearing loss. (CP: Microphonic; N₁, N₂: Action Potential.) (Negativity upwards.) B: Input–output functions of the action potential response (amplitude ●——— and latency ○– – –) measured on single responses to clicks recorded from the round window in a patient with a conductive hearing loss. Thus, without the averaging technique, the records were already sometimes very clear. (After Ruben, 1967.)

The averaging technique was then introduced for such recordings, and Ronis (1966) presented very clear averaged responses to clicks (Fig. 2). However, the recordings at this time were still obtained during surgery (in cases of otosclerosis), the aim of this particular work being: "monitoring the cochlea during surgery and thus providing an immediate index of success . . ."

Finally, in 1967, Yoshie, Ohashi and Suzuki presented successful non-surgical recordings of averaged vestibulocochlear nerve AP responses to clicks in humans, using an electrode placed in the external acoustic meatus near the annulus tympanicus (Fig. 3).

Since then many different non-surgical techniques have been presented. Besides the Bordeaux technique based on averaged recordings from the promontory—which returned to the method proposed by Lempert (Aran and Le Bert, 1968), and which was decided upon after different approaches (Portmann *et al.*, 1967, 1968)—other solutions have been proposed, notably the techniques of Sohmer and Feinmesser and of Spreng and Keidel.

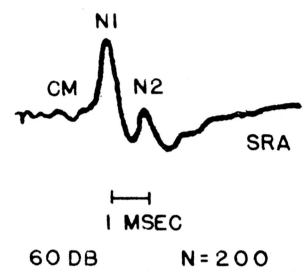

FIG. 2. Averaged response recorded per-operatively from the round window in a case of otosclerosis immediately following stapedectomy. (CM: cochlear microphonic; N1, N2: action potential.) (Negativity upwards.) (After Ronis, 1966.)

Sohmer and Feinmesser (1967) recorded from an active electrode placed on the ear lobe and were able to observe successive waves thought to originate in the vestibulocochlear nerve and the successive relays of the auditory pathway (Fig. 4). With such a technique they can record both the earliest eighth nerve AP and the cortical evoked response some 200 ms later (Sohmer and Feinmesser, 1970). They applied their method to diagnostic procedures in adults as well as in children and are satisfied with its clinical usefulness (Sohmer *et al.*, 1972; Lieberman and Sohmer, 1973a, 1973b). Although the amplitude of the signal recorded in such a way is so small that they cannot obtain the same information that can be obtained from the transtympanic approach, their particular procedure gives some interesting specific information on the function of the auditory nervous system.

Spreng and Keidel obtained similar information using mastoid or palatal electrodes (Fig. 5), covering the whole field from vestibulocochlear nerve AP to sustained dc responses from the brain references should be made to Keidel, 1971, 1972).

During the past few years other recordings have been presented according to the method of Yoshie (electrode in the external acoustic meatus). If the results of Coats and Dickey (1970, 1971) are quite similar to those of Yoshie, the recordings by Salomon and Elberling (1971) (Fig. 6) differed in that the stimuli were different: they used half sine waves of different frequencies in a closed acoustical

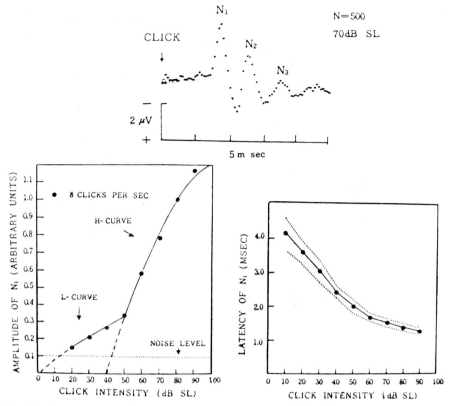

Fig. 3. A: Averaged response recorded from the external acoustic meatus to clicks presented to a normal subject. (Negativity upwards.) B: Input–output functions amplitude and latency measured on eight normal subjects in this manner. (After Yoshie, 1968.)

system rather than free field unfiltered or filtered clicks (tone pips) from unfiltered and filtered rectangular electrical pulses. Their method of placing the electrode is also different in that they introduce the wire electrode from behind the auricle under the skin of the external acoustic meatus (Elberling and Salomon, 1971). However Yoshie now uses the promontory as well as ear canal electrode, the promontory electrode being most convenient to record the cochlear microphonic (Yoshie, 1968, 1971, 1972; Yoshie and Ohashi, 1969, 1971; Yoshie *et al.*, 1967; Yoshie and Yamaura, 1969).

The technique of recording from the promontory is now in use in a few places and it is very satisfactory to see that the results are consistent (Kupperman, 1971; Tybergheim, 1972; Eggermont and Odenthal, 1972).

METHODOLOGICAL CONSIDERATIONS

While the reader can consult the references for the various approaches proposed by different authors, the main points of the technique that has been developed in Bordeaux and used as a routine clinical test in the audiological department for more than four years will be described here.

The particular options concerning the method are orientated towards the clinical use of such recordings which implies the reliability of the method and its simplicity. It can then be handled by otolaryngologists not necessarily trained in electronics, electrophysiology or physics.

It was thus decided:

(a) To record only the vestibulocochlear nerve action potential response to transient stimulation.

(b) To place the recording electrode on the promontory.

AP versus CM Responses

The human cochlear microphonic, which has been looked for in numerous studies and is still under investigation in some research centres, gives valuable information on the function of the hair cells alone but not on the function of the nerve fibres which are activated by the hair cells. These fibres have to transpose the information contained in the acoustic signal into a coded sequence of unit spikes. This is the signal which enters the central nervous system and is the output of the peripheral receptor which we prefer to study. There are additional advantages:

(a) The amplitude of this nerve response is larger than that of the cochlear microphonic.

(b) There is a precise threshold.

(c) Its pattern is quite different from that of the sound waveform and the response cannot be confused with electrical or electromechanical artefacts; it can be recognized very easily.

Promontory versus External Ear Electrode

Recordings from the ear-lobe, the mastoid, the palate or the scalp permit some degree of investigation of the

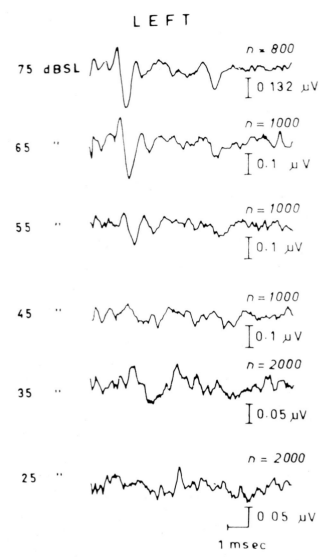

FIG. 4. Averaged responses, recorded between the earlobe and the vertex to clicks presented to the normal ear of a child. (After Sohmer *et al.*, 1972.)

high reliability and, on the other hand, the best quality recordings. This quality, as will be shown later, enhances considerably the clinical use of this method which goes much further than mere threshold determination. Although there is some reluctance to "invade" the middle ear and to

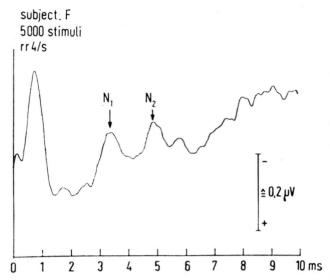

FIG. 5. Averaged response recorded between the hard palate and the ipsilateral earlobe. (After Keidel, 1971.)

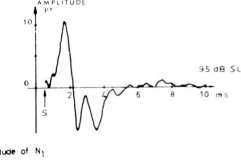

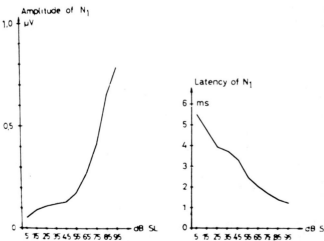

FIG. 6. A: Averaged response recorded from the external acoustic meatus to half-sine-waves (2 ms). Normal subject. (Negativity upwards.) B: Input–output functions amplitude and latency measured in 17 normal subjects in this manner. (After Elberling and Salomon, 1971.)

auditory system. However, the information which they provide does not have the same scope as the more specific and precise recordings from the external acoustic meatus or the promontory. If it is decided that electrocochleography must focus on peripheral events such as the cochlear microphonic and vestibulocochlear nerve action potential responses, only these two electrode locations are suitable.

If cochlear microphonic recordings are possible only with an electrode on the promontory, as Yoshie has shown (Yoshie and Yamaura, 1969), this is not the reason which led the Bordeaux group to record from this place, since, up to the present time, there has been little interest in this response. On the other hand, the main reason for the adoption of this technique was that it gives on the one hand "violate" the tympanic membrane, in practice, there have been problems. As in any medical procedure, the disadvantages must be weighed against its usefulness for the patient.

From our experience it appears that as soon as audiologists and otolaryngologists come to understand the nature and the quality of the information which is made available by this method, they consider that such results justify the use of this procedure. This is, of course, only in cases where such information cannot be obtained by any other means.

The same considerations apply to the problem of the general anaesthesia which is used for infants and babies for conveniently running the test (Aran *et al.*, 1969, 1971). This anaesthesia is not practiced to provide analgesia of the child's tympanic membrane which may be conveniently obtained in adults and in older children (over around eight years of age) with simple local anaesthesia with a lidocaine jelly or spray. The general anaesthesia is necessary only to keep the child at rest during the test which can then be performed rapidly and completely on both ears. In this respect, anaesthesia or sedation is necessary no matter what the position of the electrode. Since the anaesthesia is worthwhile only when the results of the test can be safely guaranteed, it implies also the use of the transtympanic electrode.

If some other treatment of the electrophysiological signal, other than and better than simple averaging, could provide the same information from a noisier and a weaker signal, it would be better to avoid perforating the tympanic membrane and to use an external electrode. However such a new electronic technique (such as correlation techniques, for example,—Charlet de Sauvage *et al.*, 1973) would also improve the recordings from the promontory. It is thus possible that, from there again, new and more precise information would be available.

Click and Tone Pips

The choice of stimuli used for electro-cochleography is quite limited since, as is explained later, only very short sounds (transients) can evoke a clear compound nerve action potential.

The stimulus which is most commonly used and which is the most convenient is a click produced by a rectangular electric pulse, usually of 0·1 ms duration, fed into a loudspeaker or an earphone. This electrical excitation gives a very short sound whose frequency spectrum is broad (from 100 Hz to 20 kHz) but much dependent on the acoustical properties of the transducer and of the room or the closed system where it is produced.

The click will stimulate the whole cochlea and, *a fortiori*, no indication of the frequency sensivity of the tested ear can be expected. The use of transients covering a narrow band of frequencies is necessary. They can be obtained either by gated short duration pure tones with fast rise and decay times (tone pips) or, more easily, with rectangular pulses filtered by a passive band-pass filter (filtered clicks). The filtered clicks used in Bordeauax according to the specifications of Davis (1970), have been described elsewhere (Aran, 1972).

Other stimuli which have been used are tone bursts (Kupperman, 1971; Eggermont and Odenthal, 1972) and half-sine-waves (Salomon and Elberling, 1971).

Standardization is difficult and is not desirable until the effects and the usefulness of the different parameters of the stimuli have been explored. Until then, it can only be recommended that each time a response is described, the stimulus be carefully described too. This is very important because the pattern of the response is strictly dependent on the structure and function of the ear *and* on the stimulus parameters. Indeed filtered clicks or tone pips are intended to give separate information on the sensitivity of the cochlea for the different frequencies, at least as far as threshold determinations are concerned. Owing to the precise specificity of the response, this information must be latent in the pattern of the response to the broad frequency spectrum click. It could be retrieved by a precise analysis of this pattern. It is already possible, without a sophisticated analysis, to infer, in many cases, from the pattern of the response to the click (its amplitude, latency, input-output functions), the pattern of the audiometric curve.

GENESIS OF THE VESTIBULOCOCHLEAR (EIGHTH) NERVE COMPOUND ACTION POTENTIAL

The cochlea may be regarded as quite a sophisticated transducer. It can be considered as a "black box" transforming an acoustical waveform carried by the air, into a complex sequence of neural electrical signals carried by the 50 000 myelinated nerve fibres inside the internal acoustic meatus. Experimentally a known acoustical signal may be fed into this black box. Looking at the output as much information as possible on the events and mechanisms which take place inside this system should be obtainable. Moreover, from the study of this signal which then enters the central auditory system, it is important to be able to infer many characteristics of the auditory function up to the level of auditory sensation.

Such information is available only through a detailed analysis of this signal with reference to actual knowledge of the structure and function of the ear and the nerve fibres.

It is first necessary to take into account the conditions under which the activity of the vestibulocochlear nerve may be observed, remembering that the compound vestibulocochlear nerve response is only an image of this activity and that it is not the specific signal in the nerve.

Recording some distance from the nerve, from the promontory for instance, the active electrode is placed at one point in a complex electrical potential field and is simultaneously influenced by the individual response of each of the 50 000 fibres. All these responses are mixed and give a global signal which, expressed mathematically by Teas, Eldredge and Davis (1962), is the product of the *convolution* of two functions of time: (1) the waveform of each unit response, $f(t)$; and (2) the number of newly activated fibres in time, $N(t)$. These same authors have accurately determined the pattern of the unit response recorded between a cochlear electrode and a reference electrode placed farther away on the head or neck. Thanks to the narrow bony tube in which the nerve travels from the cochlea to the brain, the two segments on each side of this tube are electrically isolated from each other. One electrode on the cochlea can be considered as connected to the cochlear side of the nerve while an electrode placed farther away records mainly the activity on the central side of the nerve. Thus the depolarization, as it travels along the fibre, appears at the cochlear electrode first, and later at the other electrode. This results in a diphasic pattern of the signal recorded between these two electrodes.

Since all the afferent fibres of the auditory nerve have about the same diameter, one can consider that the pattern of the unit response is similar and, no matter how complex this pattern $f(t)$ may be, it is consistant. The only other parameter which determines the development of the whole nerve action potential is the sequence of firing of the fibres, and at once it may be understood why this firing must be synchronous. If the firing of the different fibres was occurring at randomly distributed times, such as when the ear is stimulated by white noise, at each instant there would be statistically the same number of spikes and nothing would be seen at the tip of the electrode. On the contrary if it were possible that all the fibres responded only once and at the very same time, $N(t)$ would be O except for the moment when it would be equal to the total number of activated fibres. At this time, a very clear signal, whose pattern would be $f(t)$ and whose amplitude would be directly proportional to this number should be recorded. The use of very short transients (such as the sudden onset of a sound) is intended to approach this ideal condition. However, if the stimulus is the first factor which determines $N(t)$, other factors intervene between the time the stimulus arrives at the oval window and the time at which the different nerve fibres are stimulated. These make $N(t)$ a complicated function which is indeed the "function" of the internal ear. The ultimate goal of the analysis of the pattern of the compound vestibulocochlear (eighth) nerve response is to retrieve this function $N(t)$ and then to obtain some insight into the normal or abnormal function of the ear.

Anatomical Factors

According to well established anatomical and electro-physiological data, as well as to the subsequent hypothesis, it is possible to consider some of the processes which occur in the internal ear when it is stimulated by an acoustic transient.

Mechanical Processes

First, there are those processes arising from the mechanical properties of the basilar membrane and the spiral organ both in the longitudinal (or spiral) and the radial direction.

With respect to the travelling wave theory it is known that the transient, as it starts from the oval window, will travel towards the apex and will thus stimulate successively differents parts of the basilar membrane. It is also known that the waveform of the mechanical vibration will progressively lose its high frequency components, starting as it does with a broad spectrum at the base; only the lowest frequencies remain when it reaches the apex. $N(t)$ will thus be a function of the speed of the travelling wave and of the frequency spectrum of the click with respect to the frequency sensitivity of the different parts of the basilar membrane.

In the radial direction, Davis and subsequent authors have suggested that the outer hair cells, which are lightly supported in the middle of the basilar membrane, are highly susceptible to mechanical excitation and are thus sensitive to low intensities. By contrast the inner hair cells, situated on the inner edge of the basilar membrane, above the osseous spiral lamina, are less sensitive to mechanical vibration and are stimulated only at high intensities. Very schematically, and only on the basis of mechanical considerations, it is well established that there is a mechanical system which can analyse the acoustical input both in the time-frequency and in the intensity domains, this deriving respectively from its longitudinal and radial organization.

Neurophysiological Processes

The organization of the cochlear receptor is oriented toward the required type of analysis. Anatomical studies, up to the latest ultrastructural observations of Spoendlin (1966, 1973), demonstrate that there are two populations of nerve fibres, related respectively to the outer and inner hair cells. Very few afferent fibres (5 per cent) innervate the outer hair cells, but since each of these fibres is connected to about 10 outer hair cells, it is thought that the principle of spatial summation applies here, bringing down the threshold of excitation of the neurone. By contrast, the fibres innervating the inner hair cells are very numerous (95 per cent), but one fibre innervates only one inner hair cell, each inner hair cell receiving in turn several neurones. Thus the threshold of excitation of each neurone is much higher, but when it is reached, many fibres are simultaneously stimulated and respond synchronously.

These so called "two populations" of neurones have not yet been recognized in the numerous microelectrode studies of the activity of individual fibres which demonstrate, to the contrary, that the various fibres have a very homogenous sensitivity (at their best frequency) (Kiang, 1965). However it must be emphasized that many experiments, as well as considerable experience in normal and pathological human whole nerve responses and experimental studies on animals strongly support the theory that, whether or not there are two populations of nerve fibres, there are undoubtedly two different mechanisms of stimulation of the fibres, one for the low intensities and related to the outer structures (outer hair cells and/or associated nerve fibres) and the other for the high intensities and related then to the inner structures of the spiral organ.

These problems are very schematically presented here, but they are discussed in more detail elsewhere in this book. Only the basic theory has been mentioned, through which an attempt can be made to understand the normal and pathological patterns of the vestibulocochlear (eighth) nerve response as observed in man. Other more complicated and incompletely understood factors have been excluded. There is, for instance, the activity of the efferent system which is thought to control the activity of the hair cells and the afferent fibres. There are also general factors such as the metabolism and the biochemistry of the hair cells and nerve fibres, the electrochemical problems and so on, all of which can indirectly affect the function of the receptor.

THE NORMAL AND PATHOLOGICAL RESPONSES

The different patterns of responses which can be observed in disordered human hearing have been described many times (Aran, 1971, 1972). Here the interpretations

and high intensities is very clear (Figs. 7 and 8) (Charlet de Sauvage and Aran, 1973).

In the normal responses, the two parts of the input-output amplitude function (the L and H curves of Yoshie, 1968), with the plateau intervening (around 50–60 dB), can be attributed to the stimulation of the outer hair cells at low intensities and of the inner hair cells at high intensities for the whole basilar membrane (as long as the frequency spectrum of the click covers the entire frequency domain of the basilar membrane). In the dissociated responses (Figs. 7 and 8), since it is accepted that a high frequency hearing loss corresponds to lesions of the outer hair cells of the base of the cochlea, the late response observed near

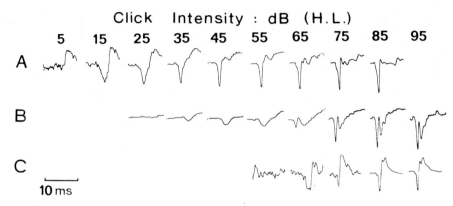

FIG. 7. Typical A: "Normal", B: "Dissociated" and C: "Recruiting" averaged responses recorded between the promontory and the earlobe. (Negativity downward.) See Fig. 8 for the corresponding input–output functions.

which relate to the above mentioned theory with respect to the corresponding changes in the auditory sensation are considered.

The normal and pathological responses can be classified into two very different groups. The first group includes the responses which are normal or near-normal and which reflect normal function in either all the sensorineural structures, or part of them, the other part being either inactive or destroyed. The second group consists of all the other responses which are more or less severely abnormal and which seem to reflect, besides the destruction of part of the sensorineural structures as in the first group, a dysfunction of the remaining, responding, elements.

Normal and Para-normal Responses

The first group consists of the responses recorded from normal internal ears (that is normal ears or ears with pure conductive hearing loss), and in cases of cochlear sensorineural hearing loss with recruitment, either limited to the high frequencies (dissociated responses) or spread over the entire frequency spectrum (recruiting responses). This group clearly demonstrates the theory of the two mechanisms of stimulation of the auditory nerve fibres. Looking at all the components of the responses (their pattern, amplitude and latency) for all clicks intensities from 0–80 or 100 dB, this differentiation between responses to low

threshold would be the response of the external structures of the more apical portions of the basilar membrane,

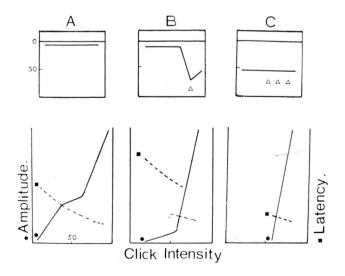

FIG. 8. Typical input–output functions (amplitude ●—— and latency ■ – – –) from a "Normal" ear (A), and in cases of sensorineural hearing loss of cochlear origin, with recruitment (△) limited to the high frequencies (B, "Dissociated" responses) or spread over the frequency range (C, "Recruiting" responses), recorded from the promontory in response to clicks.

which would be effectively stimulated by the low frequency components of the click, while the faster responses at high levels would be the response of the inner structures mainly from the base. This absence of low level responses from the base (thus lack of function of the outer structures there) is evident when one uses a high pass filtered click instead of the broad frequency spectrum unfiltered click. The threshold is much higher for the filtered click, the latency is short, the increase in amplitude with intensity very marked, and the pattern of the response is fast and diphasic. It is thus obvious that only the H part of the input-output function is being observed. Moreover, the same pattern is observed (recruiting) in response to the broad frequency spectrum click in ears where the hearing loss is somehow the same for low and high frequencies (Portmann *et al.*, 1973a) (Figs. 7 and 8). That is, the outer structures are inactive from the base to the apex, and here only the high (H) responses from the inner structures can be observed, either with the high pass filtered click or with the unfiltered click.

Distorted Responses

If the first group appears quite clear and simple on the basis of the theory, the situation is very different for the *broad* and *abnormal* responses which constitute the second group (Fig. 9). However some characteristics which are

Click   Intensity :   dB   (H.L.)
45   55   65   75   85   95

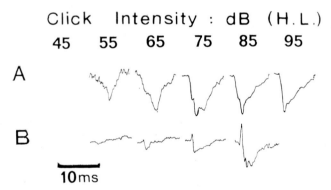

10ms

Fig. 9. A: "Broad "responses recorded from the promontory in a vascular disorder. B: "Abnormal" responses (with an early positive peak), recorded in a patient with a facial nerve schwannoma inside the internal acoustic meatus. (Click stimulation, negativity downwards.)

commonly found in these cases can be pointed out. First, there are the responses observed in patients presenting with Ménière's disorder, which are broad, the width of the negative peak ranging from 3 ms up to more than 8 ms. The width of this response seems to be related to the degree of the Ménière's attack, but many more cases have to be investigated before the relationship between the disorder and the response can be specified exactly. It seems that the raised endolymphatic pressure can affect the mechanical properties of the basilar membrane and/or the processes through which the nerve fibres are stimulated (Aran and Negrevergne, 1973). In all other cases of distorted responses, there is, when confirmed clinical cases only are considered, a retro-labyrinthine disorder due to vascular

problems or tumours inside the internal acoustic meatus (Portmann and Aran, 1972). These responses, (mainly the abnormal ones presenting with a marked positive peak prior to the slow negative wave) are also observed in children efflicted with kernicterus.

Up to the present time it is difficult to propose any interpretation for these cases. But it is clear that they all reflect a retro-cochlear lesion and it is interesting to note that both Daigneault and his associates (1970) and Kupperman (1972) have recently observed similar patterns in experimental animals after section of the efferent fibres of the cochlear nerve. These responses thus reflect a lesion of the nerve itself (perhaps in its efferent part) rather than of the cochlea. However, the cochlea may also be affected, especially in cases of vascular disorders.

One remark which seems very important is that in such cases: (1) there is sometimes a discrepancy between the auditory threshold and the objective threshold of the response, the latter being more sensitive, and this indicates that the lesion responsible for the hearing loss is situated central to the cochlea; (2) the speech discrimination is very poor and this is quite understandable since, owing to the distorted pattern of the compound response, it is obvious that the coding in the nerve is much disturbed.

CLINICAL APPLICATIONS

The emphasis which has been put so far in this chapter on the nature and possible interpretation of the normal and pathological compound vestibulocochlear nerve response is intended to explain its use in its clinical applications and to show how its analysis can be helpful in the differential diagnosis of hearing loss. For instance, if, in a patient, the response presents the characteristics described for the first group, it can be ascertained that the disorder is located inside the internal ear, at the level of the hair cells and associated nerve fibres; its location can eventually be defined along the basilar membrane, and the characteristics of the hearing of the patient objectively estimated (pattern of the pure tone audiogram, recruitment). However, if the response is classed in the second group, the diagnosis will automatically be oriented towards Ménière's disorder, a vascular problem, or a retro-labyrinthine disorder. Indeed it is to be expected that, within the next few years, such differential diagnosis through electrocochleographic recordings will be refined, on the one hand by a more detailed analysis of the pattern of the response and the study of related phenomena such as fatigue and adaptation and, on the other hand, by the increasing amount of clinical experience and the study of well established pathological groups.

At the present time, and perhaps for many years to come electrocochleography has a considerable clinical application in the diagnosis of auditory disorders in very young children. In this particular application, the advantages of the method can be listed as follows:

The investigation can be made very early, starting at one month, and the results are equally dependable whatever the age of the child.

The threshold of function of each ear is determined very precisely and separately, without any problem of lateralization, and so without the problems of masking the contralateral ear.

The response characteristics of each ear are carefully studied and the same differential diagnostic information as is found in adults is available.

Thus the application of hearing aids and the organization of a suitable educational procedure can be very precisely defined.

All this information is now available at any time in any child. Thus electrocochleography is a worthwhile procedure when dealing with very young and apparently autistic, psychotic, or mentally retarded children. In such cases the discovery of either an impaired ear or, on the other hand, normal function of the end-organ, is absolutely decisive in the establishment of an overall medical diagnosis involving much more than solely the otological diagnosis For example, in the University ENT Clinic of Bordeaux, a recent statistical survey (Portmann et al., 1973b) has revealed that, out of the overall number of children who pass through the audiological department for hearing evaluation, 12 per cent are tested by electrocochleography. In more than one-third of these children, this procedure was the only way of obtaining a clear assessment of peripheral auditory function. In the other cases, the test confirmed the diagnosis but gave more precise information which has been very important in the subsequent management of the child.

In conclusion it must be emphasized that, although such recordings do not permit one to say whether or not the patient hears, they give a very clear indication of the function of the cochlea and of the vestibulocochlear nerve, which determine the basic functioning of the auditory system. Each time there is a discrepancy between these results and the results of the classical audiometry (always in the direction of the objective peripheral response being better than subjective response) it is an indication that the disorder, if any, is either psychological or central, as it has been often observed in children and on a few occasions in adults (Aran and Negrevergne, 1973).

REFERENCES

Adrian, E. D. (1931), *J. Physiol.*, **71**, 28

Andreev, A. M., Arapove, A. A. and Gersuni, S. V. (1939), *J. Physiol. S.S.R.R.*, **26**, 205.

Aran, J.-M. (1972). *Cahier C.F.A.*, Paris, **14**.

Aran, J.-M. and Le Bert, G. (1968), *Rev. Laryng. (Bordeaux)*, **89**, 361.

Aran, J.-M. and Negrevergne, M. (1973). *Audiology*. In press.

Aran, J.-M., Pelerin, J., Lenoir, J., Portmann, Cl. and Darrouzet, J. (1971), *Rev. Laryng. (Bordeaux)*, **92**, 601.

Aran, J.-M., Portmann, Cl., Delaunay, J., Pelerin, J. and Lenoir, J. (1969), *Rev. Laryng. (Bordeaux)*, **90**, 615.

Bordley, J. E., Ruben, R. J. and Lieberman, A. T. (1964), *Laryngoscope*, **74**, 463.

Brinkman, W. F. B. and Tolk, J. (1961), *Pract. oto-rhino-laryng.*, **23**, 325.

Charlet de Sauvage, R., Anderson, D. J. and Pugh, J. E. (1973), *J. acoust. Soc. Amer.*, **54**, 284 (Abstract).

Charlet de Sauvage, R. and Aran, J.-M. (1973), *Rev. Laryng. (Bordeaux)*, **94**, 93.

Coats, A. C. and Dickey, J. R. (1970), *Ann. Otol.*, **79**, 844.

Coats, A. C. and Dickey, J. R. (1971), *J. acoust. Soc. Amer.*, **52**, 1607.

Daigneault, E. A., Brown, R. D. and Blanton, F. F. (1970), *Acta oto-laryng. (Stockh.)*, **70**, 254.

Davis, H. (1970). Personal communication.

Davis, H., Deatherage, B. H., Eldredge, D. H. and Smith, C. A. (1958), *Amer. J. Physiol.*, **195**.

Derbyshire, A. J. and Davis, H. (1935), *Amer. J. Physiol.*, **113**, 476.

Eggermont, J. J. and Odenthal, D. W. (1972), *XIth Congress of Audiology*, Budapest, October.

Elberling, C. and Salomon, G. (1971), *Rev. Laryng. (Bordeaux)*, **92**, 691.

Fink, A., Ronis, M. L. and Rosenberg, P. E. (1969), *J. Speech and Hear. Res.*, **12**, 156.

Flach, M. and Seidel, P. (1968), *Arch. Klin. exp. Ohr.-, Nas.- u. Kehlk. Heilk.*, **190**, 229.

Fromm, B. Nylen, R. D. and Zotterman, Y. (1935), *Acta oto-laryng.*, **22**, 477.

Gavilan, C. and Sanjuan, J. (1964), *Ann. Otol.*, **73**, 101.

Gersuni, G. V., Andreev, A. M. and Arapova, A. A. (1937), *Proc. Acad. Sci. S.S.S.R.*, **16**, 429.

Keidel, W. D. (1971), *Rev. Laryng. (Bordeaux)*, **92**, 709.

Keidel, W. D. (1972), *J.F.O.R.L.*, **21**, 153.

Kiang, N. Y.-S. (1965), *M.I.T. Res. Monograph No 35*. Boston.

Krejci, F. (1949), *Mschr. Ohrenheilk.*, **83**, 224.

Krejci, F. and Bornschein, H. (1950), *Mschr. Ohrenheilk.*, **84**, 1.

Kupperman, R. (1971), *Rev. Laryng. (Bordeaux)*, **92**, 739.

Kupperman, R. (1972), *Acta oto-laryng. (Stockh.)*, **73**, 130.

Lempert, J. Meltzer, P. E., Wever, E. G. and Lawrence, M. (1950), *Arch. Otolaryng. (Chicago)*, **51**, 307.

Lempert, J., Wever, E. G. and Lawrence, M. (1947), *Arch. Otolaryng. (Chicago)*, **45**, 61.

Lieberman, A. and Sohmer, H. (1973a), *Arch. Klin. exp. Ohr.-, Nas.- u. Kehlk. Heilk.*, **203**, 267.

Lieberman, A. and Sohmer, H. (1973b), *Develop. Med. and Child Neurol.*, February 1973.

Perlman, H. B. and Case, T. J. (1941), *Arch. Otolaryng. (Chicago)*, **34**, 710.

Portmann, M. and Aran, J.-M. (1972), *Acta oto-laryng. (Stockh.)*, **73**, 190.

Portmann, M., Aran, J.-M. and Lagourgue, P. (1973a), *Ann. Otol. (St. Louis)*, **82**, 36.

Portmann, M., Aran, J.-M. and Le Bert, G. (1968), *Acta otolaryng. (Stockh.)*, **65**, 105.

Portmann, M., Le Bert, G. and Aran, J.-M. (1967), *Rev. Laryng. (Bordeaux)*, **88**, 157.

Portmann, M. Portmann, Cl., Negrevergne, M. and Aran, J.-M. (1973b), In preparation for the 3rd Symp. of the Int. Electric Response Audiometry Study Group (Bordeaux, September 1973).

Ronis, B. J. (1966), *Laryngoscope*, **76**, 212.

Ruben, R. J. (1967), *Sensorineural Hearing Processes and Disorders*, 313 (A. B. Graham, Ed.). Boston: Little-Brown.

Ruben, R. J., Bordley, J. E. and Lieberman, A. T. (1961), *Laryngoscope*, **71**, 1141.

Ruben, R. J., Knickerbocker, G. G., Sekula, J., Nager, G. T. and Bordley, J. E. (1959), *Laryngoscope*, **69**, 665.

Ruben, R. J., Lieberman, A. T. and Bordley, J. E. (1962), *Laryngoscope*, **72**, 545.

Ruben, R. J. Sekula, J. Bordley, J. E., Knickerbocker, G. G., Nager, T. G. and Fisch, U. (1960), *Ann. Otol.*, **69**, 459.

Ruben, R. J. and Walker, A. E. (1963), *Laryngoscope*, **73**, 1456.

Salomon, G. and Elberling, C. (1971), *Acta oto-laryng. (Stockh.)*, **71**, 379.

Sohmer, H. and Feinmesser, M. (1967), *Ann. Otol.*, **76**, 427.

Sohmer, H. and Feinmesser, M. (1970), *Israel J. med. Sci.*, **6**, 219.

Sohmer, H., Feinmesser, M., Bauerberger-Tell, L., Lev, A. and David, S. (1972), *Ann. Otol.*, **81**, 72.

Spoendlin, H. (1966), *Advances in O.R.L.*, **13**, (S. Karger, Ed.). Basel, New York.

Spoendlin, H. (1972), *Acta oto-laryng. (Stockh.)*, **73**, 235.

Tasaki, I. (1954), *J. Neurophysiol.*, **17**, 97.

Teas, D. C., Eldredge, D. H. and Davis, H. (1962), *J. acoust. Soc. Amer.*, **34**, 1438.

Tyberghein, J. (1972), *Acta oto-rhino-laryng. belg.*, **26**, 664.

Wever, E. G. and Bray, C. W. (1930), *Proc. nat. Acad. Sci. (U.S.A.)*, **16**, 344.

Yoshie, N. (1968), *Laryngoscope*, **78**, 198.

Yoshie, N. (1971), *Rev. Laryng.* (*Bordeaux*), **92**, 646.

Yoshie, N. (1972), 11th Congres of Audiology, Budapest October. In press in *Audiology*.

Yoshie, N. and Ohashi, T. (1969), *Acta oto-laryng.* (*Stockh.*), suppl. **252**, 71.

Yoshie, N. and Ohashi, T. (1971), *Rev. Laryng.* (*Bordeaux*), **92**, 673.

Yoshie, N., Ohashi, T. and Suzuki, T. (1967), *Laryngoscope*, **77**, 76.

Yoshie, N. and Okudaira, T. (1969), *Acta oto-laryng.* (*Stockh.*), suppl. **252**, 89.

Yoshie, N. and Yamaura, K. (1969), *Acta oto-laryng.* (*Stockh.*), suppl. **252**, 37.

22. AUDITORY NERVOUS SYSTEM

W. D. KEIDEL AND S. KALLERT

Since Seebeck's controversy with Ohm and with von Helmholtz in the nineteenth century regarding the mechanism of hearing, considerable progress has been made in our understanding of the basic function of the auditory system, either as a spectral analyser and/or as a time-resolving device. As Møller (1972) points out, in formulating his resonance theory of hearing, von Helmholtz (1863) was influenced by Ohm's (1843) Law of Auditory Analysis. This stated that the ear analyses a complex periodic sound wave by separating it into a series of sinusoidal waves corresponding to the Fourier components of the sound. Wien (1905) objected to this spectral analysis explanation on the grounds that the fine pitch discriminability of the human ear could not work with the same damping factor that was necessary for the fast time resolution of transients as occurs, for example, in speech analysis. Von Békésy measured this damping factor and found it to be relatively great. Since that time, physiologists have looked carefully for some possible explanation for this much better frequency analysis of the auditory system having regard to the known hydrodynamics of the ear. Since it is accepted that the central nervous system had something to do with hearing, and since the ear itself performs a frequency analysis, the conclusion was: It must be the nervous system which makes this improvement in our overall capability of pitch discrimination. The only question was: "To what degree?" This made the entire story of the function of the auditory nervous system so interesting during the last decades. Temporal information could be handled by the auditory nervous system whose spatially arranged anatomical organization also provides the morphological basis for the place theory of hearing. The latter theory is consistent with Johannes Müller's doctrine of specific nervous energies. This was the notion that the nature of a sensation is determined by the particular nerve fibres which are stimulated.

Detailed knowledge of the workings of the auditory system has come from studies of the hydrodynamics of the internal ear and microelectrode studies of single cell units in the spiral ganglion, the cochlear nucleus, the olivary complex, the trapezoid body, the inferior colliculus, the medial geniculate body and at the auditory cortical level.

With the present (1973) state of knowledge, including an application of the Mössbauer effect (Johostone and Boyle, 1967) Wien's objection has finally been brought to an end.

The number of receptors, i.e. the sensory or hair cells, is of the order of 15 000–18 000. Seventy-five per cent of them are outer, the rest inner, hair cells. Spoendlin (1970) could demonstrate, in the cat, that, out of about 50 000 primary auditory nerve fibres, nearly 90 per cent originate at inner, and only about 10 per cent at the outer, hair cells. This means that one-quarter of the receptor cells has nine-tenths of all afferent fibres and three-quarters of the total number of sensory cells is linked to only one-tenth of the primary neuron population (Fig. 1). This aspect makes clear the important role that the *inner* hair cell population plays within the auditory nervous system. This organization is somewhat comparable to the cell distribution in the receptor layer of the retina, with the fovea bearing only cones, whilst the periphery contains proportionately more rods as the distance from the fovea is increased. However, experiments to separate electrophysiologically two populations of first order neurones in a clear-cut manner, as was possible for the eye, have so far failed. It seems to be the set of conditions under which one or other population of hair cells responds to sound that makes the functional difference. Moreover, the influence of the efferent fibre tract upon the afferents should not be neglected. If, on the one hand, the innervation of the outer hair cells indicates that large numbers of outer hair cells are connected with one single afferent fibre, on the other hand, there exists a similar problem with respect to the efferents: as few as 500 efferent fibres within the bundle of Rasmussen branch into about 40 000 efferent terminals (*see* Fig. 1). These efferent terminals are to be found, as presynaptic endings, particularly on the outer hair cells, especially in the basal turn. Efferent connections with the inner hair cells seem to be post-synaptic in character, consequently influencing the afferent axons.

Kiang considers the influence of the efferent inhibition to be a suppression of the spontaneous activity rather than an excitatory effect upon the hair cells or the first order neurons (Fig. 2). This seems to be in good agreement with the principle of anatomical structure as demonstrated in this figure. The question as to whether or not a lateral inhibition, in addition to that afforded by the efferents, is

realized in the neuronal system of the cochlea, has still not been clearly decided. Since the inhibition phenomenon

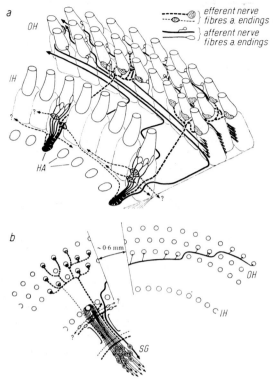

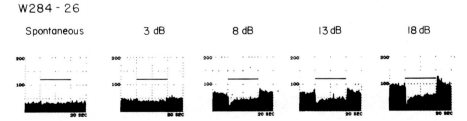

FIG. 1. (*a*) Schema of the general innervation pattern of the spiral organ of Corti. OH: outer hair cells; IH: inner hair cells; HA: habenula openings. (*b*) Schematic outline of the fibre distribution of the spiral organ. Continuous thick lines: afferent fibres from the outer hair cells. Continuous thin lines: afferent fibres from the inner hair cells. Interrupted thick lines: efferent nerve fibres from the contralateral olivo-cochlear bundle. Interrupted thin lines: efferent nerve fibres from the homolateral olivo-cochlear bundle. SG: spiral ganglion. (From Spoendlin, 1970.)

observed at that level either has an extremely short latency and appears nearly instantaneously or shows up a very great latency of the order of 8 ms to more than 150 ms

it is unlikely that the lateral inhibition of the type observed in the *Limulus* eye could play a role in the first order neuronal set.

A very clear outline of the neuronal *auditory network* has recently been given by Møller (1972). As indicated in his diagram (Fig. 3), he summarizes his ideas as follows:

Usually, three main regions of the cochlear nuclear complex are recognized in connexion with electro-physiological investigations, namely the dorsal, the anterior ventral and the posterior ventral. The cochlear nerve fibres terminate both in the ventral and the dorsal part of the cochlear nucleus and no primary fibres reach higher centres. The ascending projection leaves the cochlear nuclear complex via three main tracts, the corpus trapezoideum, the intermediate acoustic stria of Held and the dorsal acoustic stria of Monakow. The trapezoid body contains several fibre types originating in the different sub-groups of the cochlear nucleus. The trapezoid body connects ipsilaterally to the lateral superior olive (LSO), bilaterally to the medial superior olive (MSO), contralaterally to the nucleus of the trapezoid body (NTB), and ascends in the contralateral lateral lemniscus (LL) to the inferior colliculus (IC). The stria of Held originates in a cell group in the posteroventral cochlear nucleus and terminates in the periolivary nuclei of both sides. The stria of Monakow, the most dorsal tract, has been studied less extensively, but it has been shown that it originates mainly in the dorsal cochlear nucleus (DCN) with possible connexions to the contralateral superior olive and reaches the contralateral inferior colliculus. Cells of the lateral superior olive connect bilaterally via the lateral lemniscus to the inferior colliculi. The medial superior olive connects mainly to the cells of the homolateral, but also to the contralateral, inferior colliculus. The inferior colliculus cells give rise to fibre tracts that terminate in the medial geniculate, the thalamic auditory relay, from which the primary auditory cortical area receives its input. In addition, there are more diffuse pathways from the cochlea to the cortex, probably through more medial brain stem structures. Connexions between the left and

FIG. 2. Histograms on a 20s time scale showing the effects of COCB (crossed olivo-cochlear bundle) stimulation on a single auditory nerve fibre as a function of tone level. The visually detected "threshold" of this fibre for tone bursts at its CF (characteristic frequency) was 8 dB SPL. Each histogram represents 200s of data. The first histogram shows the effects of 10s shock trains delivered at 1 shock train/20s on spontaneous activity. In the other histograms, a tone at CF was presented together with the shock trains. Tone level in dB SPL is indicated above the histograms. The times during the shock trains are indicated by the horizontal bars. Shocks were 400/s. Unit W 284–26. CF is 8·66 kHz. (From Wiederhold and Kiang, 1970.)

right sides occur at the level of the dorsal nucleus of the lateral lemniscus and the level of the inferior colliculus. Numerical estimates of the number of neurons and the cell density at various levels in the ascending auditory pathway in the monkey were made. Running in parallel

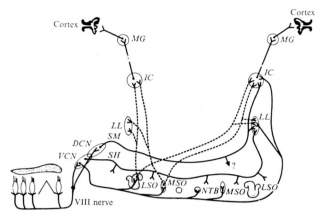

FIG. 3. Main ascending auditory pathways. DCN: dorsal cochlear nucleus; VCN: ventral cochlear nucleus; LSO: S-Segment of superior olive; MSO: medial superior olivary mucleus; NTB: trapezoid body; LL: lateral lemniscus; IC: inferior colliculus; MG: medial geniculate body; SH: intermediate acoustic striae of Held; SM: dorsal acoustic striae of Monakow. (From Møller, 1972.)

with the ascending pathways is the descending or efferent auditory system. The most peripheral portion of the system is the olivo-cochlear efferent system (Rasmussen), the fibres of which originate in the superior olivary complex and terminate on the haircells in the cochlea. It is

tem can be found, e.g. in von Noort (1969) and in Harrison and Feldman (1970).

Frequency Domain

Studies of the tuning curves in mammals were performed as early as 1943 by Galambos and Davis. Nevertheless, considerable progress has been made in the evaluation of data obtained by means of the micropipette and microelectrode technique when the application of electronic computers was introduced into neurophysiology. The most elaborate experimentation has been done by Kiang, Goldstein, Rose, Hind, Pfeiffer and others. One classical example is shown in Fig. 4. It is obvious that the high-frequency steepness of those tuning curves is very great, at least in units with high characteristic frequencies (CF), the characteristic frequency of a unit being the frequency which needs the least energy to evoke a just detectable difference of its firing rate compared to its spontaneous activity. Slopes of 200 dB/octave have been extrapolated from Kiang's data for the cat. In guinea pigs, greater slopes (200–500 dB/octave) have been found (Evans, 1970). The lower-frequency skirt may be considerably flatter (down to 12 or even 6 dB/octave for the long tails). Figure 4 also clearly shows the shape of the threshold curve of hearing recorded by means of other techniques, e.g. psychophysical or behavioural. This figure also shows that a marked difference (20 dB or more) in absolute thresholds for adjacent units may occur. Whether or not this is a result of injury incurred by the experimental procedure is another question. We have to touch on this point later in discussions of the "intensity range of primary neurons".

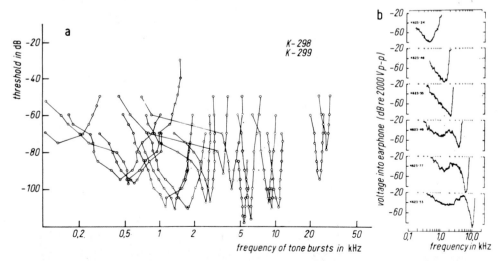

FIG. 4. Sample of tuning curves of single fibres in the vestibulocochlear nerve in anaesthetised cats. Data from two cats are shown (a from Kiang, 1965b; b from Kiang and Moxon, 1972).

known that there is also a rich efferent system at higher levels of the nervous system. Our present knowledge of the anatomy of this part of the efferent system is, however, sparse and the functional organization of the system is practically unknown. A more detailed description on the neuroanatomy of the auditory nervous sys-

Whilst the tuning curves are well suited to describe the near-threshold behaviour of single units, they are rather unsatisfactory for stimulus intensities above threshold but within the physiological dynamic range. Here, two further techniques have been developed. First, curves (iso-intensity curves) describing firing rates at constant sound

levels as a function of tone frequency may be used (Hind *et al.*, 1967, 1970; Greenwood and Maruyama, 1965) secondly, stimulus intensities that evoke a constant average rate of discharge (iso-rate curves) may also be determined. These latter curves are nearly identical with the tuning curves for sound intensities near threshold. The advantage of both (iso-intensity and iso-rate) curves, however, is their

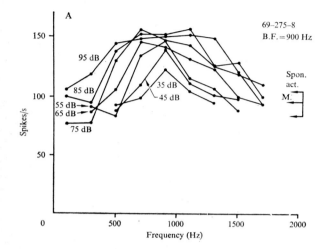

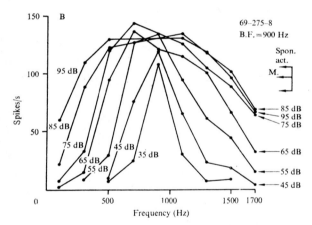

FIG. 5. A. Iso-intensity contours of a fibre having a high rate of spontaneous activity. B. The number of discharges per sec. that occur synchronously with the stimulus waveform. (From Rose *et al.*, 1971.)

applicability to the physiological range of sound intensities. A set of iso-intensity curves is shown in Fig. 5. Considerably broader tuning (bandwith) for "normal" intensities occurs when compared to the narrow ones for the tuning curves. Note that both sets of curves in Fig. 5 are the inverse of tuning curves. Only a combination of tuning curves and iso-intensity curves gives a representative picture of the activity of a single fibre within the first order neurons.

Another important aspect in the frequency domain is that, for units having a relatively low characteristic frequency, the intervals between peaks in the PST (post-stimulus-time) histograms are the inverse of the unit's CF (*see* Fig. 6).

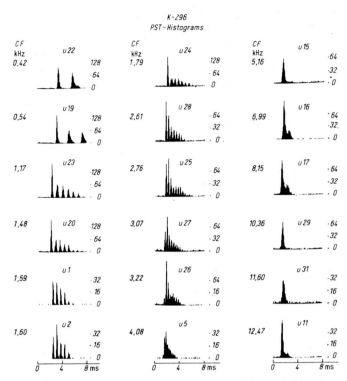

FIG. 6. PST (post-stimulus time) histograms of the responses of 18 units in the vestibulo-cochlear nerve of a single cat to stimulation with clicks. The CFs of the units ranged from 0·42 kHz to 12·47 kHz. (From Kiang, 1965b.)

Frequency Tuning at First Order Level

The classical concept of the relation between the shape of the envelope of the basilar membrane's vibrations and the tuning curves at first neuron level is shown in Fig. 7. This shows a discrepancy between the sharp tuning curves

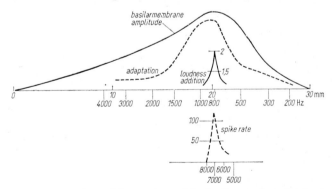

FIG. 7. Comparison of the envelope of the basilar membrane's vibrations with the frequency dependence of the cochlear fibres excitation. (From Keidel, 1966b.)

of first order auditory neurons and the flat tuning curves of the basilar membrane. Has this now been resolved?

Using ears from human cadavers, von Békésy determined tuning curves for the basilar membrane at very low frequencies. He found a low-frequency slope of 6dB/octave and a high-frequency slope of 20 dB/octave. This was done at sound intensities of as much as 140 dB above human threshold, and for pure tones of 200–300 Hz. Steeper slopes have now been demonstrated by means of the Mössbauer effect (*see* Chapter 16). The technique was first employed on guinea pigs, using very high-frequency sounds (Johnstone and Boyle, 1967; Johnstone *et al.*, 1970). The lower-frequency limb of the tuning curve was shown to have a slope of 12 dB/octave and the high-frequency limb 95 dB/octave. These high values were confirmed by Rhode (1971) on squirrel monkeys. For a sound of 7 kHz, the low-frequency limb of the tuning curve had a slope increasing from 6 dB/octave to 24 dB/octave, and the high-frequency limb a slope of 100 dB/octave. Møller (1972) quotes Rösler in regard to the abrupt high-frequency losses which not infrequently may be seen in sweep frequency audiograms of some patients with hearing defects. When this cut-off occurs above, 2000 Hz, the slope may be greater than 200 dB/octave. That these slopes are greater than those observed by means of the Mössbauer effect is not surprising since here not only the cochlear hydrodynamics, but also the neuronal information processing has been included in the procedure of measurement. This then leads us to the values obtained at the primary neuron level. Wilson (1970) calculated a symmetrical low- and high-frequency slope of the order of 200 dB/octave based on Kiang's data in the cat. Evans (1970), for the guinea pig, found an even greater steepness for both low- and high-frequency slopes, amounting to as much as 500 dB/octave. Frishkopf (1964) investigated the little brown bat (*Myotis l. lucifugus*) and arrived at values ranging from 100 dB/octave for a 10 kHz CF and 300 dB/octave for higher CF's (up to 85 kHz). Although the cochlear nucleus will be discussed systematically later on, a comparison for this particular problem is appropriate here. Møller demonstrated low-frequency slopes ranging from 15–25 dB/octave in the flat part of the tuning curve in the rat. When the curve reaches the symmetrical portion, steepnesses of 700 dB/octave are found (*see* Fig. 8).

Time Domain

We shall now deal with the manner in which temporal coding is performed at the first neuron level. If one looks at the PST (post-stimulus-time) histograms of the auditory nerve when the cat's ear is stimulated by clicks, it should be possible to determine whether the upward or the downward deflection of the basilar membrane provides the excitation of the nerve fibre. This problem was investigated by Kiang (1965b) by means of a comparison of the temporal patterns of: (a) a rarefaction- and (b) a condensation-click. In the case of the rarefaction-click (in which the stapes is pulled out of the oval window by the first peak of the sound pressure level of the click), the maximal hydrodynamic displacement would correspond to an upward motion of the basilar membrane (toward the scala vestibuli), while a condensation-click originates a downward movement of the cochlear partition first (Fig. 9). Kiang describes the results as follows:

> The interleaving of peaks for condensation- and rarefaction-clicks . . . lends strong support to the idea that increased and decreased neural activity can result

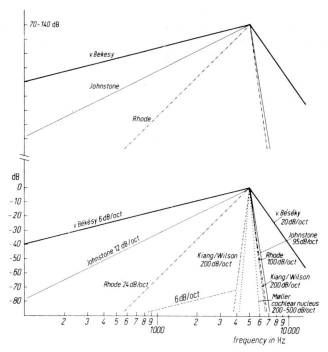

Fig. 8(a). Synopsis of the slope values of the envelope of the basilar membrane's vibrations described in the literature and comparison with the tuning curve of a fibre of the cochlear nerve.

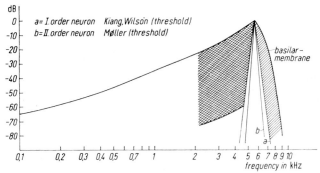

Fig. 8(b). Comparison of the ratio between displacement of a narrow segment of the basilar membrane and that of the malleus and tuning curves of first order neuron and of second order neuron.

from opposite directions of movement of cochlear structures. Since at high click levels the earliest peak always occurs for rarefaction-clicks, it is likely to be the *rarefaction-phase . . .* of the cochlear motion that corresponds to *increased* neural activity. This conclusion is in agreement with suggestions from earlier experiments with gross potentials (Rosenblith and Rosenzweig, 1952; Peake and Kiang, 1962).

However, in 1972, Pfeiffer reported a different result in that he detected, at intensities between 65 and 105 dB, the first peak in the PST histogram being related to the *condensation*-click. This is shown in Fig. 10. Now, if one looks carefully at Kiang's records, it can be seen that, at low intensities, the first peak of a rarefaction PST histogram is leading in time, at middle intensities that for condensation- and, at high intensities (as Kiang himself describes) again the rarefaction-click is leading in latency. However, at relatively high intensities, Pfeiffer and Kiang have shown conflicting results. Further studies are therefore required to clear up this very important theoretical question of the way in which the auditory coding takes place between the hydrodynamics of the internal ear and the first auditory neurons.

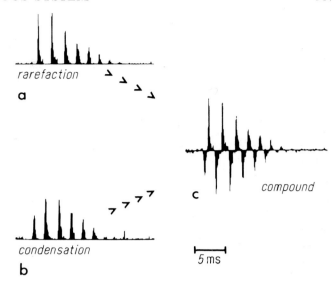

FIG. 10. PST histograms of responses to click stimuli. (a) PST histogram of responses to rarefaction clicks. (b) PST histogram of responses to condensation clicks for the same nerve fibre and for the same stimulus amplitude as for part (a). (c) A combination of parts (a) and (b) (compound PST histogram), except that the histogram for condensation clicks (b) has been inverted and put in time registration with the histogram for rarefaction clicks (a). (From Pfeiffer and Kim, 1972a.)

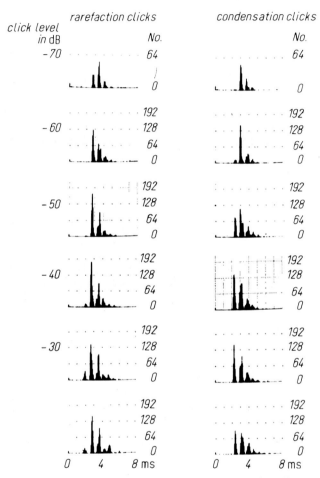

FIG. 9. Response patterns to rarefaction and condensation clicks as functions of click level. CF 1·65 kHz. Stimuli: 10/s clicks. (Reference level in this experiment was 2·5 V into dynamic earphone.) (From Kiang, 1965b.)

Pfeiffer also demonstrated that two different types of fibres could be separated when he counted the number of peaks in the PST histograms to clicks (Fig. 11). In one group (5 per cent of fibres, the number of peaks increased rapidly in comparison to the increase in the rest (95 per cent) of the fibres studied. He therefore concluded that these two populations could be related to the two populations of sensory cells separated histologically by Spoendlin. This interpretation is tempting. A relatively greater number of peaks could be regarded as indicating greater sensitivity for those neurons. This would accord with the concept of higher sensitivity for the outer hair cells. In addition, even

the innervation of many hair cells by one single-branched afferent fibre seems to have its counterpart in neurophysiological data. Beating of the envelope of the PST histogram's pattern could be explained by the innervation of the outer hair cells positioned along 0·3–1·1 mm of the basilar membrane (Pfeiffer and Kim, 1972a).

Another important aspect is the so-called "time-locking" or "phase-locking" which can be observed within the PST histogram of single auditory nerve fibres. This has been demonstrated most clearly by Rose and his associates (1966, 1967). If one plots the probability of discharge during the stimulus cycle of a sinusoidal tone ("cycle-histogram", "period-histogram" or "folded-histogram") it is evident that the discharge pattern is the rectified half-wave of the temporal pattern of the stimulus, whilst the interval-histogram reveals the distribution of the intervals between each successive pair of spikes independent of the phase relation. Thus the cycle-histogram proves to be very useful for this type of investigation. By analysing a long period of time, the spatial integration over an ensemble of neurons usually implicated in this part of the coding can be mimicked. By reversing the polarity of the stimulus, the other half-wave can be obtained and added to a full sinewave as in the original sound (Pfeiffer and Kim, 1972a). Rose and Hind have demonstrated that the time-pattern of cycle-histograms over a wide range of intensities (up to 50 dB) is practically identical with that of the complex sound, in time and in the relative phase of the constituent tones. Phase-locking was governed by the tone with the higher intensity, as indicated by inverting the relative intensities of the two tones to one another (Fig. 12).

Interestingly enough, the study of stimulation by two tones has its counterpart in the frequency domain in the

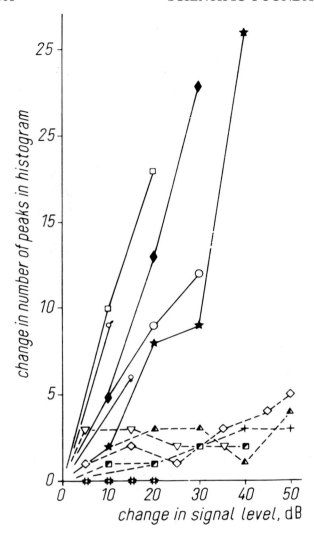

Fig. 11. Plot of the change in the number of peaks in the compound PST histogram versus change in the signal level for 12 different fibres, i.e. six from Population I (interrupted lines) and six from Population II (continuous lines). (From Pfeiffer and Kim, 1972a.)

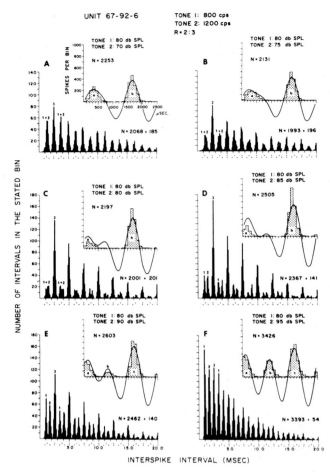

Fig. 12(a). Relation between interspike intervals and the distribution of spikes in the period histograms. A tone of 800 Hz was locked to a tone of 1200 Hz in a ratio of 2:3. A to F: interspike interval and period histograms obtained when the lower frequency was at 80 dB SPL while the strength of the higher frequency varied as indicated. Each sample is based on responses to two 10s presentations. Interspike interval histograms: abscissa: time in ms, each bin equals 100 μs Ordinate: number of interspike intervals in each bin. Period histograms: abscissa: time in μs; each bin equals 100 μs; period of the complex sound equals 2500 μs Ordinate: number of spikes in each bin. Each period histogram is fitted by a curve which is the sum of two sine functions. (From Rose, 1970.) (A bin is the time range within which the events encompassed by a particular bar of the histogram occur.)

so-called "two-tone-inhibition". This means that the tuning curve of a single auditory fibre can be changed by a simultaneously acting second tone. Usually, the activity elicited by the first tone is diminished and suppressed by the second one. This suppression belongs mostly to the frequencies in the neighbourhood of the CF of the fibre under study (*see* Fig. 13).

Since the spontaneous activity is usually not suppressed (in contrast to the effect of inhibition by efferent fibres), it is assumed (Sachs and Kiang, 1968) that the effect of suppression in the two-tone situation is not due to neural inhibition in the usual fashion (lateral inhibition, single or poly-synaptic inhibitions) but is more likely to have originated hydrodynamically by some sort of mechanical modulation, as is known in psychophysical and behavioural masking experiments. Pfeiffer (1970) described a model consisting of two band-pass filters and a non-linear connecting network. Whether this non-linearity is originated

by that type of non-linearity which was shown by Rhode (1971) is open to question.

Intensity Coding

Kiang (1965b) observed that the absolute threshold for fibres can vary as much as 30 dB. However, he claims that most primary neurons have a threshold corresponding to behavioural thresholds in the cat. If indeed 95 per cent of all fibres belong to the inner hair cells (Spoendlin, Pfeiffer), then this is difficult to understand. There is clear evidence in the rat (Fig. 14) that the range of threshold sensitivity within a population of units is of the order of up to 40 dB, whilst the dynamic range of all sorts of single units is of the order of 20–50 dB (Kiang, Rose), the maximum firing rate for the cat being of the order of 270–300 spikes . s^{-1} (Rose).

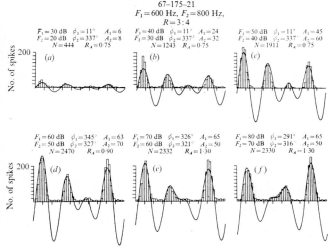

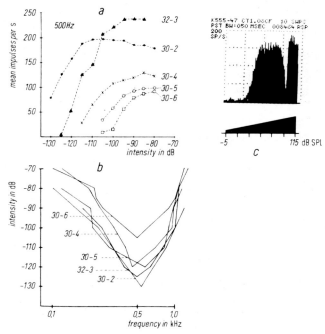

FIG. 12(b). Period histograms of the activity recorded from a fibre in the vestibulo-cochlear nerve of the squirrel monkey in response to stimulation with a complex periodic sound composed of two sinusoidal tones locked together with a frequency ratio of 3:4. The amplitude ratio between the two tones was kept constant at 10 dB while the overall intensity was varied in a 50 dB range. The amplitude and phase of the primaries used to construct the fitted waveforms are specified in each graph. (From Rose *et al.*, 1971.)

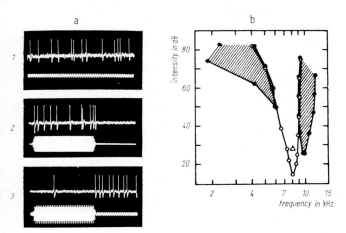

FIG. 13. An example of two-tone inhibition, (a) and excitatory and inhibitory areas (b). (a) A single primary auditory neuron responds to a 40 dB continuous tone at the best frequency of 360 Hz (a1), and also to a 60 dB tone burst at 720 Hz (a2). When these two tones are simultaneously delivered, inhibition is demonstrated (a3). The duration and rise-decay time of the tone burst are 100 and 2·5 ms respectively. (b) The ordinate represents sound pressure level (dB SPL) and the abscissa, stimulus frequency in kHz. The area above the tuning curve (open circles) is the excitatory region in which the discharge rate is more than 20 per cent above the spontaneous rate. The hatched areas are inhibitory ones in which the response to a continuous tone at the best frequency (triangle) plus a second tone is more than 20 per cent below the response to the continuous tone alone. (From Arthur *et al.*, 1971.)

By means of a spatial integration for an ensemble of neurons, this allows not more than 90 dB at the most to be covered. There is thus a deficiency of knowledge on this topic.

The intensity function for a single fibre, when plotted semi-logarithmically, is S-shaped and can be linearized only a little, if at all, by double-logarithmic plotting. This is different to the behaviour of the intensity functions for other sensory modalities. For example, in the somaesthetic system, the intensity functions are essentially linear in a double-logarithmic plot. This may have some relevance to the psychophysical overall behaviour (it is double-logarithmic). One can easily understand that the great dynamic range in audition needs non-linearity, whilst that for the somaesthetic modalities (intensity ranges of the

FIG. 14. (a) Rate-intensity functions for best frequency (500 Hz) stimulation of five ventral cochlear nuclear nuerons whose response areas are shown in part (b) of the figure. (From Moushegian and Rupert, 1970.) (b) Response areas of five units whose rate-intensity functions are shown in (a) of the figure. (From Moushegian and Rupert, 1970.) (c) Discharge rate of a single fibre as a tone at the CF (1·08 kHz) is swept in level. For the first 10 bins (0·5 s), the tone is off. For the next 180 bins (9 s) the level of the tone is swept from −5 dB SPL to 115 dB SPL. For the last 10 bins (0·5 s), the tone is again off. The histogram is computed from the responses to 10 successive sweeps. (From Kiang and Moxon, 1972.)

order of 35 dB) can be covered by linear system. Whether or not the synaptic transmission itself is associated with non-linearity in the auditory system requires more experimentation. Theoretically, in agreement with the facts elaborated for somaesthetic synapses, there is no need to invoke non-linearity in respect of auditory synapses (Mountcastle, 1961).

COCHLEAR NUCLEUS

When considering the *frequency domain* at the level of the cochlear nucleus, little change in the tuning curves of single neurons can be detected (Fig. 15) (*see also* Katsuki *et al.*, 1958; Kiang, 1965a). Three differences, however, should be mentioned. First, some tuning curves for cochlear nuclear cells have relatively broad peaks. This is due to some convergence phenomenon within the neuronal network, and deviates from older ideas according to which a continuously increasing steepness of the tuning curves occurs as one goes higher within the central neural pathway. Secondly, a small percentage of the neurons show up a second peak of appreciable size in their tuning curves. It will be demonstrated later on, that, at higher levels of the CNS (e.g. in the geniculate body), even multiple stimulus response curves can be obtained. Thus, there is a continuous change from clearly single-peaked curves in the auditory nerve, through two-peaked tuning curves in the cochlear nucleus to multiple-peaked response curves at

Maruyama (1965). The closed iso-rate-contours in Fig. 18 indicate, for a given stimulus frequency, two different intensities for the same firing rate of the unit. As a corollary, such units have a part of the intensity function which is increasing, and a part which is decreasing.

For the experiments so far described, static stimuli were used, i.e. both the frequency and the intensity of each single stimulus was constant. To determine tuning curves,

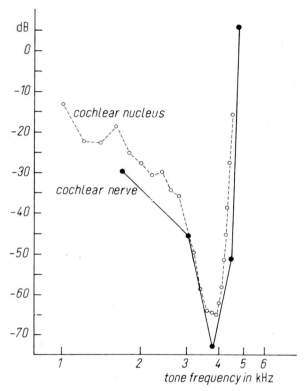

Fig. 15. Iso-rate function of a rat cochlear nuclear unit (open circles) (from Møller, 1969a) compared with a tuning curve of a cochlear nerve fibre (from Kiang, 1965b).

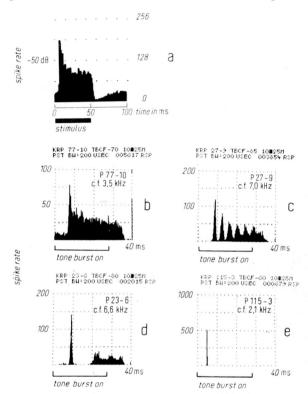

Fig. 16. (a) Typical response pattern of cochlear nerve fibres to tone burst stimulation. (From Kiang, 1965b.) (b)–(e) Typical PST histograms of the unit activity to tone burst stimulation for one unit of each of four classes of units in the cochlear nucleus. (From Pfeiffer, 1966.)

the geniculate. Thirdly, post-stimulus-time histograms do not have as many peaks as in the auditory nerve. The response is restricted to one single peak of increased firing probability after a given latency (Kiang, 1965b). Within the general principle of reduction of information from 10^9 bit.s^{-1} at receptor level to 10^2 bit.s^{-1} at conscious level this makes sense, because redundant information (about the single vibrations of the basilar membrane) is skipped even at levels as low as the cochlear nucleus.

As regards the *time domain*, four different types of temporal patterns (primarylike, chopper, pause and on-pattern) of single neurons in the cochlear nucleus can be observed in contrast to the single one for first order neurons (Fig. 16). Starting with the cochlear nucleus, sensitivity to the differential ratio df/dt (rate of frequency change) is characteristic of all levels of the auditory system above that of the auditory nerve (Fig. 17).

Some cochlear nuclear units have non-monotonic intensity functions, as has been shown by Greenwood and

a sequence of tone bursts with discrete frequency differences was given, but the frequency of each single stimulus of the sequence was kept constant. Experiments have also been reported using frequency-modulated (FM) and amplitude-modulated (AM) pips, or complex stimuli composed of several pure tones simultaneously with FM-tones. At the level of the cochlear nucleus, the majority of cells tested with complex stimuli have not shown major deviations in response characteristics from those expected from their responses to transient and steady state tones (Erulkar *et al.*, 1966, 1968; Evans and Nelson, 1966; Fernauld and Gerstein, 1972; Møller, 1969c, 1971, 1972). The responses to complex tonal stimuli can thus be explained in terms of responses to simple pure tones. A small minority of units, however, showed responses which are difficult to predict on the basis of pure-tone responses, showing critical dependance on modulation rate or exhibiting responses which are selective to the direction of the frequency modulation. Nevertheless, the rate of change of stimulus or of frequency does not seem to be the relevant parameter for the activation of the vast majority of units at this level.

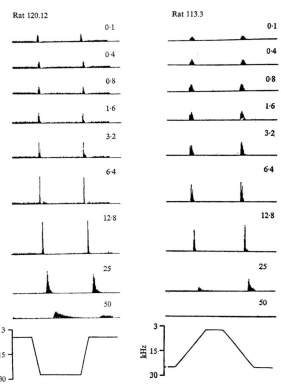

Fig. 17. Cycle histograms of the activity of two units in the cochlear nucleus of a rat in response to sweep tones. The shape of the frequency modulation is shown below. The sweep rate in sweeps per second is shown by legend numbers. The sound intensity at the unit's CF (22 kHz) was 45 dB SPL (left hand column) and 50 dB SPL (right hand column) at the unit's CF (15 kHz) (approximately 25 dB and 15 dB above threshold respectively). (From Møller, 1971.)

DORSAL NUCLEUS OF CORPUS TRAPEZOIDEUM (SUPERIOR OLIVE)

In general, the tuning curves of the dorsal nucleus of the corpus trapezoideum are similar to those for primary fibres of the first neuron and to those at the cochlear nuclear level. In iso-rate curves, however, a considerably greater flat region around the CF has been observed (Tsuchitani and Boudreau, 1967; Boudreau and Tsuchitani, 1970). Multiple-peaked tuning curves may also be demonstrated (Fig. 19a). This again seems to be due to some convergence of information within the neuronal network connections between the cochlear nucleus and the dorsal nucleus of the corpus trapezoideum. Interestingly enough, in contrast to the units within the cochlear nucleus and similar to the auditory nerve fibres in the dorsal nucleus of the corpus trapezoideum, the PST histograms reveal multiple peaks with intervals which are the inverse of the CF of the units (Moushegian et al., 1967). Since those units, however, do not have any relationship to the basilar membrane and its mechanical properties as the primary units do, the question arises as to what extent the CF of units in the

dorsal nucleus of the corpus trapezoideum is determined by the properties of the unit itself or by its connection with neighbouring elements. The problem of neuronal periodicities thus begins at this level, but will be discussed in more detail at collicular and geniculate level, where it plays

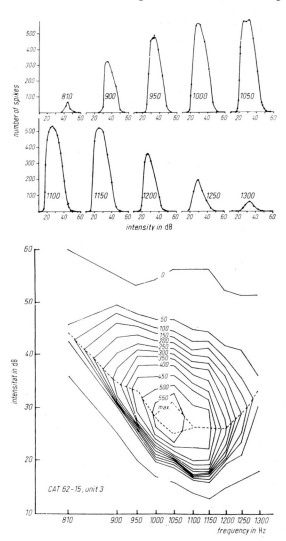

Fig. 18. Stimulus response curves (upper graphs) and various tone frequencies of a rat cochlear nuclear unit with non-monotone stimulus response curves. Total number of discharges occurring during twenty 200 ms tones are shown as a function of stimulus intensity. Lower graph shows successive contour lines representing spike counts of 50, 100, 150, etc., during 20 presentations of 200 ms long tone bursts. The curve at the bottom of the figure is the threshold curve (tuning curve). (From Greenwood et al., 1965.)

an even more important role including the concept of biological "clocks".

CORPUS TRAPEZOIDEUM

Time-delay detectors within the *trapezoid body*, especially within the two symmetrical accessory nuclei, have been carefully explored electrophysiologically. As shown in Fig. 19b, the firing rate of a unit at this level is a function of the interaural time difference that would be produced by different directions of the sound source (Galambos *et al.*, 1959). Interaural intensity differences are physiologically associated with time delays since latency of response increases non-linearly with decreasing intensity (Kemp *et al.*, 1937). As is shown in Fig. 19c, the neurophysiological results at that level are in good agreement with the psychophysical and behavioural studies involving

ceases to respond. If now the frequency of the tone pip is changed, the unit will again respond. The tuning curves of these units are broadly tuned (Aitkin *et al.*, 1972; Webster *et al.*, 1971). The broadening of the tuning curves may be associated with the observation of Moore and his associates (1963, 1966) that the external nucleus receives its afferents from the neurons of the central nucleus. However, one cannot exclude an habituation disturbing the

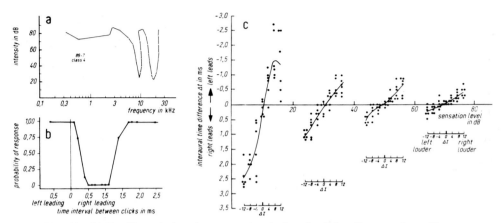

FIG. 19. (a) Double-peaked tuning curve of a single unit of the olivary nucleus. (From Guinan *et al.*, 1972.) (b) Effect of interaural time differences upon probability of unit response. (From Galambos *et al.*, 1959.) (c) Dependence of trading function on (i) absolute intensity level, and (ii) right-left intensity difference. (From Keidel, 1966a.)

trading experiments (time-delay and intensity difference).

INFERIOR COLLICULI

It was previously held that the inferior colliculi are concerned solely with auditory reflexes whilst the primary sensory pathway leads through the medial geniculate body to the cortex. It is now clear, from experiments on cats, guinea pigs, monkeys and rabbits, that very few of the lemniscal fibres reach the medial geniculate body directly. The vast majority of the lemniscal fibres terminate in the inferior colliculus, which, in turn, gives origin to the fibres reaching the medial geniculate body (Barnes, *et al.*, 1943; Moore *et al.*, 1963a, b, 1966; Powell and Hatton, 1969; Rasmussen, 1946; Woolard and Harpman, 1940). A more complex role for the inferior colliculi is thus suggested by these studies as well as behavioural (Neff, 1961) and numerous microelectrode studies (Aitkin *et al.*, 1972a, b; Benevento *et al.*, 1970; Bock *et al.*, 1972; David *et al.*, 1968, 1969a; Erulkar, 1959; Geisler *et al.*, 1969; Hind *et al.*, 1963; Katsuki *et al.*, 1958; Keidel, 1969, 1970b, 1971b, d; Nelson *et al.*, 1963, 1966; Rose *et al.*, 1963, 1966; Suga, 1964, 1969; Thurlow *et al.*, 1951).

There is a clear tonotopical localization of neurons in the inferior colliculus (Aitkin *et al.*, 1972; Rose *et al.*, 1963), especially in the central nucleus. The tuning curves of these neurons are relatively sharp but very similar to those for lower level neurons. Units in the external nucleus exhibit a form of habituation to tonal stimuli such that, after two to five repetitions of the same stimulus, the unit

determination of the tuning curve. These units may perhaps have a role in attentive behaviour, so that they are more sensitive to the presence, or absence, of sounds rather than their frequency content (Aitkin *et al.*, 1972).

Spontaneous activity becomes progressively less common and lower in frequency for the upper parts of the auditory pathway. For the inferior colliculi, a mean value may be 40–50 spikes . s^{-1} (Bock *et al.*, 1972). Discharge rates as a function of tone intensity show similar forms as at lower auditory levels, only that the number of spikes per time-interval is less. Both non-monotonic functions (David *et al.*, 1968; Erulkar, 1959; Rose *et al.*, 1963) and monotonic (Bock *et al.*, 1972) functions have been reported.

Individual neurons differ greatly in their firing patterns in response to tones. The patterns range from pure onset patterns, in which the onset burst is the only sign of activity throughout the duration of the tone, to sustained patterns, consisting of an onset, silent period and then sustained discharge; or merely a sustained discharge, as well as pure offset patterns. Finally, there are units which show only depression of the spontaneous discharge during application of the stimulus (Aitkin *et al.*, 1972; David *et al.*, 1968; Rose *et al.*, 1963). There are also response patterns which show, in their sustained discharge, period phase locking or time locking (Bock *et al.*, 1972; David *et al.*, 1968; Keidel, 1969, 1970a, 1971b; Rose *et al.*, 1966). For lower sound frequencies, the shortest discharge period is equal to the period of the tone (*see* Fig. 20); but for higher sound frequencies, the discharge period may be equal to an integral multiple of the tone period (Keidel, 1969, 1970a, b, 1971b; David *et al.*, 1969a; Kallert *et al.*, 1970).

This phenomenon is called demultiplication and it permits discharge periods of the order of 10–30 ms, whilst the corresponding tone period may be of the order, for instance, of 0·15 ms (Fig. 21). The inferior colliculus is the highest level in the auditory pathway where time locking has been demonstrated.

The response pattern of a single unit may dramatically change its form if the stimulus frequency is changed. Time

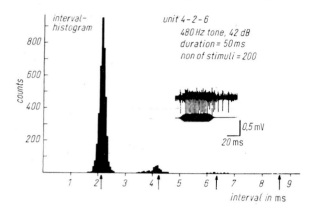

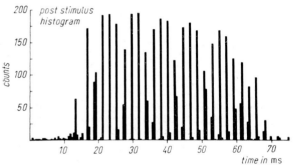

FIG. 20. Unit 4–2–6. 480 Hz tone. Interspike-interval histogram (top) and poststimulus histogram (bottom) for the same record. The small arrows on the interval histogram indicate integral multiples of the stimulus period. The inset shows a single sweep photographed from the oscilloscope screen, with amplifier output as the top trace and electrical input to the transducer as the bottom trace. Tone duration: 50 ms; repetition rate: 1/s; number of stimuli: 200. (From Bock *et al.*, 1972.)

locking may thus appear only for a narrow frequency range of the stimulus, other tone frequencies producing an aperiodic discharge. A typical onset-discharge pattern may be changed to an offset-discharge pattern if the stimulus frequency is changed and "pause" patterns may change to "primarylike" patterns (*see under* "Cochlear Nucleus").

If an early spike is consistently discharged, the latency of that first spike is a function of stimulus intensity or of stimulus frequency (Hind *et al.*, 1963). Typical changes in the latency period are shown in Fig. 22.

There are also binaural effects with EE or EI character (Hind *et al.*, 1963) or with different latencies for contralateral and ipsilateral stimulation. For neurons with best frequencies less than 3000 Hz, it is known that the number of spikes discharged is critically dependant upon the phase relationship of binaural sine-wave stimuli (Rose *et al.*, 1966). There are right-left delay times, for which the unit

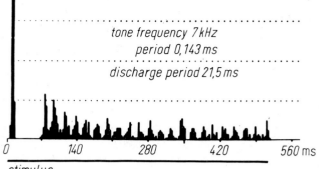

FIG. 21. PST histogram of the response pattern of a single unit of the inferior colliculus. Stimulus: tone-burst 500 ms, 7 kHz. (From David *et al.*, 1969.)

ceases to discharge altogether, even though stimulation of each ear alone produces a substantial number of spikes. The time delay which causes the first maximum or minimum of discharge rate may differ for different neurons, but, for a single unit, it is normally independent of stimulus frequency and intensity (characteristic delay time) and it is also the same if noise stimuli are used (Geisler *et al.*, 1969). In some cases, the second stimulus suppresses preferentially the sustained discharge, leaving the onset almost unaffected. In other cases, the reverse is true, or both responses may be equally affected. By contrast, a different group of cells has discharge characteristics which, although completely insensitive to interaural time delays, are very sensitive to interaural intensity differences. They usually discharge to a contralateral stimulus but the response is greatly reduced or abolished when stimuli of the same frequency are presented binaurally (Rose *et al.*, 1966). Using clicks, units could also be found which were sensitive to interaural time differences, units sensitive to interaural intensity differences, units sensitive to neither interaural time nor intensity differences and units sensitive to both interaural time and intensity differences (Benevento *et al.*, 1970). These binaural units may have a bearing on the problem of localization of a sound source. Results for these electrophysiological studies are consistent with the results of ablation experiments. Bilateral ablation of the inferior colliculus renders a cat incapable of using time or intensity cues for sound lateralization (Masterton *et al.*, 1968). But there are also binaural effects which cannot have localization functions because the effective interaural time delay is of the order of 4–120 ms. Erulkar (1959) found that, if the first stimulus precedes the second by an interval of more than 4 ms, a response to the second stimulus may be entirely suppressed.

At the level of the inferior colliculus, many more units respond selectively than in the cochlear nucleus to particular aspects of the amplitude- and frequency-modulated acoustic stimuli. Stimulus properties to which units are sensitive include the rate of change, the direction of change amd the magnitude of change of frequency and of amplitude of the stimulus. Nevertheless, it is conceivable that even these responses might be predictable from responses to pure-tone stimuli (Nelson *et al.*, 1966), especially if

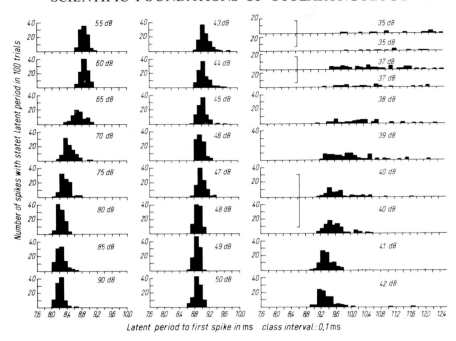

FIG. 22. Histograms of first spike latent period for unit 61–716–2. Stimulation of contralateral ear with clicks. Repetition rate: 2/s; intensity: dB SPL. Each histogram is based on 100 trials. Location near the border between the external and central nuclei of the inferior colliculus. (From Hind *et al.*, 1963.)

attention is paid to the existence of inhibitory areas on one or both sides of the excitatory area (Suga, 1968).

MEDIAL GENICULATE BODY

The medial geniculate nucleus consists of a small-celled pars principalis and a large-celled pars magnocellularis. Morest (1964) also recognized a number of more detailed sub-nuclei in the lateral division of the geniculate body. The pars principalis seems to be the actual auditory area of the nucleus. The pars magnocellularis does not appear to send fibres to the auditory areas of the cortex (Rose and Woolsey, 1949). In the pars magnocellularis, multimodal sensory activation of cells is described (Wepsic, 1966). Using acoustic, caloric, tactile, nociceptive, photic and vestibular stimulation, it is possible to record activation of units (Table 1). From the geniculate body, similar response patterns of single units to acoustic stimuli are described as for the inferior colliculus (Altman *et al.*, 1970; David *et al.*, 1968; Dunlop *et al.*, 1969; Keidel, 1971b; Starr and Don, 1972). Thus there are "onset", "primarylike", "pause" and "offset" responses, as well as binaural responses, i.e. sensitivity to time or intensity differences between ipsilateral and contralateral stimulation. Monotonic and non-monotonic intensity functions have also been described as well as variations in response patterns if stimulus parameters are changed. Spontaneous activity is, however, generally very low (1–20 spikes.s^{-1}) and the responses to static stimuli, e.g. tone bursts, is less than at lower levels in the auditory system, consisting nearly always of an onset effect only. Moreover, many units show

TABLE 1

TABULATION OF MAJOR* PATTERNS OF SENSORY INFLUENCE UPON MEAN DISCHARGE RATE IN MG UNITS
(From Wepsic, 1966)

No. of Units	Caloric inc.	Caloric dec.	Click inc.	Click dec	Touch inc.	Touch dec.	Nocicept. inc.	Nocicept. dec.
15	+		+		+		+	
4	+		+		+			
6	+		+				+	
10	+		+					
6	+				+			
9	+						+	
3	+							+
13	+							
3		+	+		+			
3		+			+		+	
4		+	+					
3		+			+			
4		+					+	
6		+						
7			+		+		+	
4			+		+			
4			+				+	
3			+					+
12			+					

* The above listing includes 80 per cent of units affected by sensory stimulation.

response patterns which are unknown for lower level units, and these differences seem to be of great importance. The most specific features of geniculate unit responses are:

(1) Occurrence of periodicity in spontaneous activity with periods of the order of 10–100 ms (Keidel, 1969, 1970a, b, 1971b; Aitkin *et al.*, 1966; David *et al.*, 1969a; Kallert *et al.*, 1970).

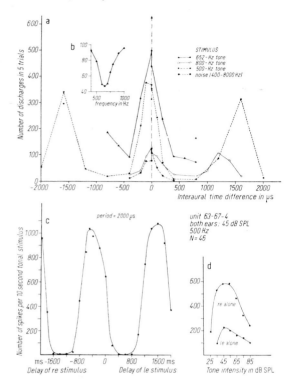

FIG. 23. Number of spikes discharged to binaural stimuli when the stimulus presented to one ear was delayed in time relative to the stimulus presented to the other ear.
(a) Different stimuli as indicated.

      Intensities: 500 Hz 87 dB (ipsilateral).
                 91 dB (contralateral).
          652 Hz 59 dB (ipsilateral).
                 62 dB (contralateral).
          800 Hz 84 dB (ipsilateral).
                 87 dB (contralateral).
      Noise 71 dB (ipsilateral).
                 74 dB (contralateral).

(b) Threshold curve of the same unit as (a) for monaural contralateral stimuli (monaural ipsilateral stimuli elicited no response at any frequency).
(c) All stimuli: duration 10 s, pure tone 500 Hz, intensity 45 dB SPL.
(d) Spike rate-intensity functions for the same unit as in (c). CF 500 Hz. Location: right inferior colliculus. re = right ear; le = left ear.
((a) and (b) from Geisler *et al.*, 1969.) ((c) and (d) from Rose *et al.*, 1966.)

(2) Appreciably longer excitation, inhibition and latency times (Aitkin *et al.*, 1966; Keidel, 1971b, 1972c, 1974) (Fig. 24). Units with short latency (8–20 ms) do, however, exist (Galambos, 1952; Gross and Thurlow, 1951).

(3) Occurrence of periodicity in firings during or especially after stimulation, with periods of the order of 100–200 ms (Fig. 25). (Aitkin *et al.*, 1966, 1968, 1969; Keidel, 1972b, 1972c, 1974.)

This is similar to findings in other thalamic nuclei (Andersen *et al.*, 1964; Andersen, 1966; Eccles, 1966).

In contrast to phase locking at lower levels, this periodicity does not reflect properties of the stimulus but must be endogenous.

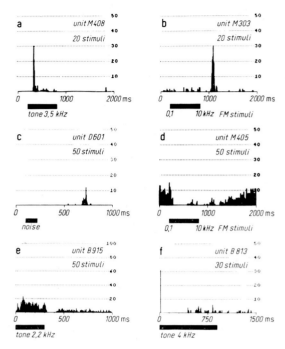

FIG. 24. PST histograms showing characteristic latency, inhibitory and excitatory times in geniculate units. (From Kallert, 1972.)

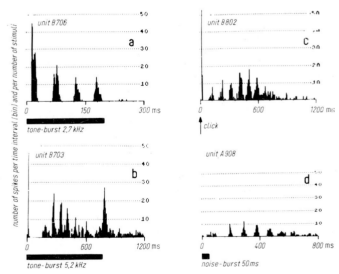

FIG. 25. Some examples of discharge periodicities representing specific response patterns of geniculate units. Each histogram is based on 50 stimuli. (From Kallert, 1972.)

(4) Although there are units with a single best frequency (CF), tuning curves and frequency response curves may show several prominent frequencies (Fig. 26) (David *et al.*, 1969a; Dunlop *et al.*, 1969; Galambos *et al.*, 1952; Keidel, 1969, 1970a, b, 1971b, 1972c, Kallert, 1972). Tonotopic organization therefore does

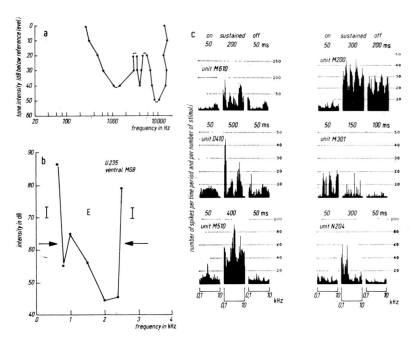

FIG. 26. Tuning curves (a, b) and frequency response curves (= iso-intensity curves) (c) of single units from geniculate body showing several characteristic frequencies instead of a single CF. The areas below the frequency response curves are filled black. Frequency response curves for different time intervals relative to the stimulus are taken from the same record, the different time-intervals are indicated ("on means that the first time-interval of the stimulus duration which was mostly 50 ms, "sustained' means the whole remaining duration of the stimulus, and "off" means the first time-interval immediately after the stimulus). ((a) from Galambos, 1952.) ((b) From Dunlop et al., 1969, and (c) from Kallert, 1972.)

not occur, or, at least, not in the same manner as that described for lower levels.

(5) Responses to static stimuli are relatively poor but dynamic (frequency modulated) stimuli are more effective (Fig. 27), and there are response patterns which are distinctly sensitive both to the direction and to the rate of frequency change (Keidel, 1971b, 1972c, 1974; Kallert, 1972). These response patterns to dynamic stimuli cannot be predicted from those to static stimuli (Fig. 28).

(6) There are units showing a marked response to complex stimuli (stimuli consisting of two or more simultaneous acoustic components) but with only poor or no response to each single component of the stimulus (Fig. 29) (Keidel, 1971b, 1972c, 1974; Kallert, 1972).

Although one cannot state the definitive functional significance of the geniculate body, the special features described above lead to some formulations. The relative ineffectiveness of static tone stimuli, the multi-peaked frequency response curves (and therefore missing tonotopic organization) suggest that the medial geniculate body is not concerned with tonal discrimination. This is in agreement with ablative studies of the auditory cortex (AI, AII, Ep, I, T) where retrograde degeneration of geniculate cells occurred but where frequency discrimination was preserved. (Goldberg and Neff, 1961; Neff, 1961; Thompson, 1960). (Incidentally, discrimination of sound intensity of changes in stimulation from right to left ears can

each be learned by cats with bilateral cortical lesions [Axelrod et al., 1963]). The phase-locked demultiplicated discharges at the inferior collicular level, together with the periodicity of spontaneous activity of geniculate units may allow a sort of coincidence measurement which may result in multi-peaked frequency response curves with equidistant peaks (Keidel, 1969, 1970a, b, 1971b; David et al., 1969a; Kallert et al., 1970). The frequencies of these peaks are in integral numerical ratios to each other. This may perhaps be the electrophysiological correlate of the sensation of consonance. Of course, it is also conceivable that multi-peaked frequency response curves are a result of convergence of units with single-peaked response curves.

Especially impressive is the sensitivity of geniculate units to frequency modulation and to complex stimuli. Because human and animal acoustic signals consist of such components as frequency modulation, intensity modulation and the simultaneous combination of several frequencies, the geniculate body may have a role in speech analysis. It is also suggested that the reverberation of discharges and the long times for excitation or inhibition may be related to short-term memory.

AUDITORY CORTEX

In contrast to lower levels of the auditory system, the extent and position of the auditory cortex cannot be un-

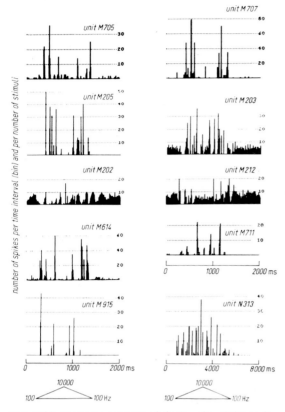

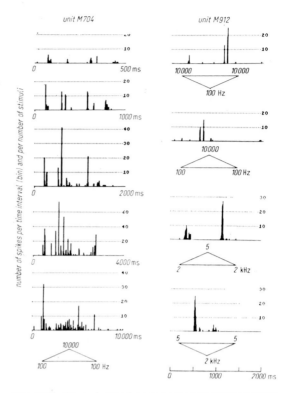

FIG. 27(a). Response patterns of single units of the geniculate body to frequency modulated stimuli. Each PST histogram is based on 20 stimuli. The stimuli are indicated in relation to the time-scale of the abscissa. The direction of modulation is indicated by the stimulus symbol, i.e. modulation first from 100 Hz to 10,000 Hz and then back from 10,000 Hz to 100 Hz. Note that there are frequency ranges without any response to 20 stimuli but others are sharply tuned with strong excitation. (From Kallert, 1972.)

FIG. 27(b). Dependance of the response pattern upon sweep rate (left) and direction of modulation (right). The sweep rate can be taken from the time scale of the abscissa, the direction of frequency modulation can be seen from the stimulus symbol below the abscissa. (From Kallert, 1972.)

equivocably stated. Nevertheless, one can delimit a small area which is overwhelmingly connected with other parts of the auditory system, with units responding exclusively to acoustic stimuli. Surrounding this area are extensive regions which are certainly not exclusively concerned with audition but have other additional inputs. For example, cats are able to learn discrimination of "dim-bright-dim" against "bright-dim-bright" light sequences after bilateral lesions of the visual cortex, but they cannot learn this discrimination after bilateral lesions of the insular-temporal region (Colavita, 1972).

The main features of single unit discharge patterns for the auditory cortex are as follows:

(1) Spontaneous activity is even less than in the geniculate body. In one study, about 40 per cent of the units had spontaneous discharge rates less than 1 spike.s^{-1} (mean values for the cochlear nerve are 200 spikes.s^{-1}). Rates of more than 35 spikes.s^{-1} are quite unusual (Goldstein et al., 1968). A few special units have thinner spikes exhibiting higher rates (de Ribaupierre et al., 1972). Consequently, the inhibitory effects of sound stimuli can be demonstrated only with two-tone

stimulation or by intracellular study (de Ribaupierre et al., 1972a, b).

(2) A multiplicity of tuning-curve types is seen. Some, with a single best-frequency and narrow shape, are similar to those for lower level units. Others are multi-peaked curves similar to those described for some geniculate units. Yet others are broadly tuned curves, so that it is impossible to assign any particular best-frequency to them. A tonotopic arrangement based upon single unit responses cannot therefore be upheld for the auditory cortex (Abeles and Goldstein, 1970; Oonishi and Katsuki, 1965; Whitfield, 1967).

(3) Binaural effects, similar to those for the geniculate units also occur (Hall and Goldstein, 1968). Time differences as well as intensity differences are effective and contralateral stimulation usually leads to excitation, whilst ipsilateral stimulation leads to inhibition (Brugge et al., 1969).

(4) A small minority only of cortical units respond vigorously in a sustained manner to static stimulation but, as at the geniculate level, frequency-modulated stimuli and complex stimuli are most effective (Bogdanski and Galambos, 1960; Evans and Whitfield, 1964; Evans et al., 1965; Feher and Whitfield, 1966; Whitfield, 1967). Figure 31 illustrates a special sensitivity to the direction of frequency change. Numerous units are especially sensitive to natural sounds. Some researchers

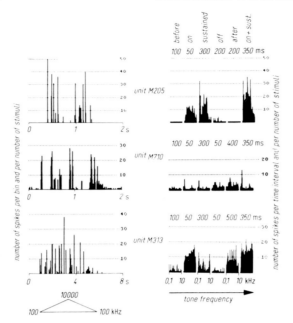

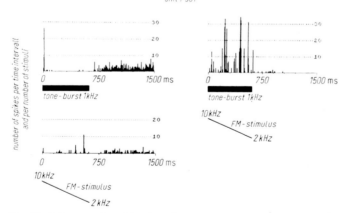

FIG. 28. Comparison between response patterns to frequency modulated stimuli and frequency response curves determined with a sequence of static tone bursts with discrete differences. For details of frequency response curves see Fig. 26. In addition, "before" means the time-interval before the stimulus begins and "after" means a time-interval directly after the "off" interval. It can be clearly seen that the principal frequency ranges for excitation and inhibition, which are demonstrated in the PST histograms to frequency modulated stimuli, do not have any correlate in the frequency response curves to static stimuli. (From Kallert, 1972.)

FIG. 29. Influence of combination of several stimuli (complex stimuli) on the response pattern of a single unit of the geniculate body. Each PST histogram is based on 50 stimuli. Left: upper part: tone bursts only; lower part: frequency modulted stimuli only. Right: tone bursts and frequency modulated stimuli presented simultaneously. (From Kallert, 1972.)

(Funkenstein *et al.*, 1970; Wollberg and Newman, 1972) have studied responses from units in the auditory cortex of awake squirrel monkeys to species-specific vocalizations. More than 80 per cent of all units responded to such tape-recorded vocalizations.

(5) Sometimes a lability of responses can be found, i.e. the response pattern of single units to the same

stimulus may change in type. Changes from excitatory to inhibitory response patterns, and vice versa, have been observed (Whitfield, 1967).

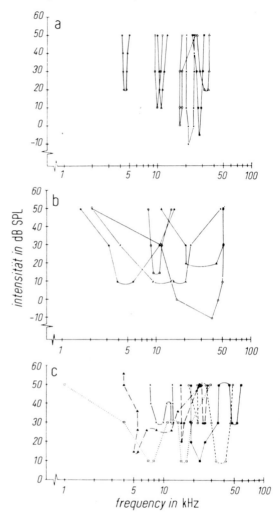

FIG. 30. Examples of three kinds of tuning curves observed in auditory cortical units: (a) narrowly-tuned curves, (b) broadly-tuned curves, and (c) multiple-peaked tuning curves. (From Abeles and Goldstein, 1970.)

Averaged Evoked Potentials

Averaged evoked potentials, as recorded from the human scalp in response to sound, are of special interest to audiologists, because they can be used for objective audiometry. These averaged evoked potentials can be divided into short-latency, middle-latency and long-latency groups, with latencies of less than about 50 ms, about 50–250 ms and more than 250 ms respectively (Davis, 1968; Davis and Zerlin, 1966). The components whose latencies lie between 130 and 170 ms can be linked more closely with stimulus parameters than can either earlier or later components (Keidel, 1965a, b; Keidel and Spreng, 1965a, b, c, 1970; Spreng and Keidel, 1970). And their amplitudes are related to the intensity of the stimulus by a power function, the slope of which is the same as that of Stevens' sensory magnitude plot, although the steepness can also be demonstrated as a function of latency (Keidel, 1971a; Finkenzeller, 1969). Recent investigations (Jerger *et al.*, 1969; Vaugham and Ritter, 1970) lead to the suggestion that the short- and the middle-latency groups of the averaged evoked potentials are from generators localized in the

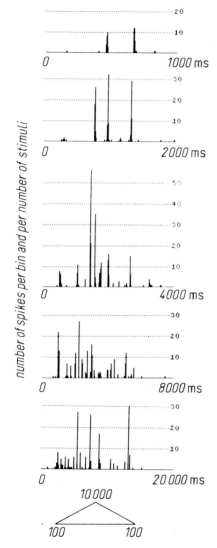

FIG. 31. Response patterns of a single unit of the auditory cortex to frequency modulated stimuli of different sweep rates. (For details see Fig. 27.)

primary auditory projection areas of the cortex, whilst the long-latency group is from generators diffusely located in the cortex, but the definite origin of cortical evoked potentials is still yet unknown.

In respect of the *predictability potential* ("expectancy wave") (Keidel, 1962, 1970b, 1971c, 1972b; Walter, 1964, 1967), it can be said that the evoked potential is the sum or the difference of two types of information, namely: (a) that previously stored, and (b) that actually processed (Keidel, 1971a).

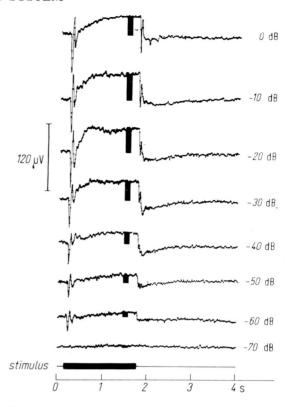

FIG. 32. DC-potentials and classical evoked potentials (on- and off-effect) in the unanaesthetised cat (Chronically implanted electrodes). Auditory stimuli: long-lasting sinusoidals. (From David *et al.*, 1969b.)

It seems convenient to distinguish between intramodal-specific and intramodal-nonspecific components in the total evoked response (Keidel, 1971a). Three possibilities are conceivable:

(1) An intermodal-nonspecific response
(2) An intramodal-nonspecific response
(3) An intramodal-specific response.

The first type is clearly that described by Bickford and others, i.e. the generalized motor reaction within the first 6–30 ms after stimulus onset. In this case, it is signalled only that "something" has happened, but it is not recognized whether the "something" was a visual, auditory, vibratory, somaesthetic or other event. This is followed by another event which is certainly related to a specific sensory system, for instance to the auditory one. Hence, this is an intermodal-specific response, but it must still be considered an intramodal-non-specific. This is the main part of the on-effect, and it is in essence what "objective audiometry" is concerned with up to the present time.

Quality recognition leads finally to the intramodal-specific phase, that is to say, the brain now recognizes what type of auditory stimulus was delivered to the ear. This event is represented by a dc-shift that lasts exactly as long as the auditory stimulus does. It is cut off almost immediately after cessation of the stimulus, and it is followed by an off-effect (Fig. 33). It is not surprising that this intra-modal-specific component is rather precisely localized (Fig. 34). Considerable intermodal interaction has also been

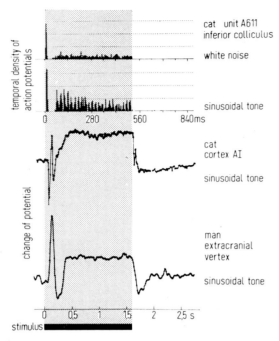

FIG. 33. Comparison of the temporal pattern of colliculus and cortical activity to auditory stimulation in cats and in man respectively. The three upper traces are recorded in the cat, the bottom trace is extracranially recorded from the vertex in man. Duration of all stimuli is indicated by the cross-hatched vertical strip and by the black line at the bottom of the figure. It can be seen that the on-effect in the PST histograms before a silent period precedes the intramodal non-specific auditory activation. This on-effect is somehow related to the V-potential, although this lasts during the silent period at colliculus-level and even a little longer. The specific activation at colliculus is indicated by the fact that noise and sinusoidal tone are clearly represented in the envelope of the main part of the histogram. During this time, in the cat as well as in man, the dc-potential can be observed which is cut off by the small evoked off-effect. (From Keidel, 1971a.)

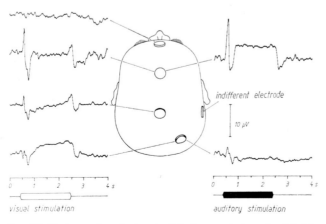

FIG. 34. Vertex and occiput potential changes during visual (white bar on the left hand side) and auditory (black bar on the right hand side) stimulation alternatingly applied at random The negative deflection is drawn upwards. 200 single tests are averaged for each curve. (From David et al., 1971.)

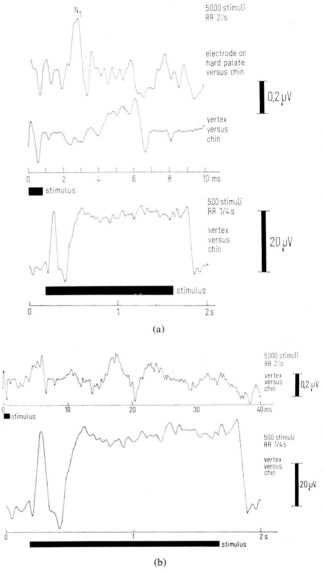

FIG. 35. Simultaneous recording of all components from the auditory nerve up to the cortical evoked potentials. (a) A 10 ms scale has been shown for the early responses which allows particularly the N_1N_2 and the responses of latencies of 6 to 8 ms to stand out. (b) same as (a) but with a 40 ms scale for the early responses, thus the responses with latencies between 15 and 30 ms are particularly clear. RR = repetition rate.

described (Keidel, 1971a; David et al., 1971). One may expect the dc-potential to assume more importance in the future with respect to objective audiometry.

It should be emphasized that it is possible to record simultaneously the events from the very beginning up to the very end of the neuronal train of the auditory channel (Keidel, 1972c). Since there are necessarily two time domains within the records, namely one of the order of 50 ms for the early response, and a second time domain of the order of 500–800 ms for the vertex potential, the dc-potential and the off-effect, two different averagers, amplifiers and special types of stimuli are necessary. Using,

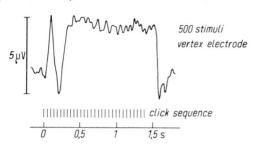

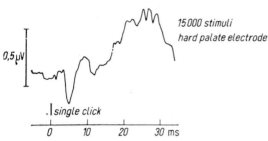

Fig. 36. Simultaneous record of all components from the auditory nerve up to the evoked potentials of the auditory cortex by using trains of clicks. (From Keidel, 1972e.)

for instance, long-lasting trains of clicks (alternating rarefaction- and condensation-clicks to avoid electrical artefacts and additional microphonic potentials) with high repetition rates, responses to each single click in the first time domain as well as responses to the train of clicks in the second time domain have been recorded (Figs. 35 and 36). This method may be of great importance to audiology in the future. It gives the additional advantage of the possibility of having a running cross-correlation between any pair of early, late or dc-deflections for longer periods of time. This allows one access to the influence of vigilance, attention, habituation, sedation and alertness upon size and latency of the single components in the complex responses and their relationship to each other. Thus, the state of a subject, or patient, can be measured objectively, so reducing the problem when recording of the classical V-potential has been done alone.

REFERENCES

Abeles, M. and Goldstein, M. H. Jr. (1970), "Functional Architecture in Cat Primary Auditory Cortex; Columnar Organization and Organization According to Depth," *J. Neurophysiol.*, **33**, 172–187.

Aitkin, L. M., Blake, D. W., Fryman, S. and Block, G. R. (1972b), "Responses of Neurones in the Rabbit Inferior Colliculus. II. Influence of Binaural Tonal Stimulation," *Brain Research*, **47**, 91–101.

Aitkin, L. M. and Dunlop, C. W. (1968), "Interplay of Excitation and Inhibition in the Cat Medial Geniculate Body," *J. Neurophysiol.*, **31**, 44–61.

Aitkin, L. M. and Dunlop, C. W. (1969), "Inhibition in the Medial Geniculate Body of the Cat," *Exp. Brain Res.*, **7**, 68–83.

Aitkin, L. M., Dunlop, C. W. and Webster, W. R. (1966), "Click-evoked Response Patterns of Single Units in the Medial Geniculate Body of the Cat," *J. Neurophysiol.*, **29**, 109–123.

Aitkin, L. M., Fryman, S., Blake, D. W. and Webster, W. R. (1972a), "Responses of Neurones in the Rabbit Inferior Colliculus. I. Frequency specificity and Topographic Arrangement," *Brain Research*, **47**, 77–90.

Altman, J. A., Syka, J. and Shmigidina, G. N. (1970), "Neuronal Activity in the Medial Geniculate Body of the Cat During Monaural and Binaural Stimulation," *Exp. Brain Res.*, **10**, 81–93.

Andersen, P. (1966), "Rhythmic 10/sec Activity in the Thalamus," in *The Thalamus* (D. P. Purpura and M. D. Yahr, Eds.). New York and London: Columbia University Press.

Andersen, P., Eccles, J. C. and Sears, T. A. (1964), "The Ventrobasal Complex of the Thalamus: Types of Cells, Their Responses and Their Functional Organisation," *J. Physiol.*, **174**, 370–399.

Arthur, R. M., Pfeiffer, R. R. and Suga, N. (1971), "Properties of 'Two-tone Inhibition' in Primary Auditory Neurones," *J. Physiol.*, **212**, 593–609.

Axelrod, S. and Diamond, I. T. (1965), "Effects of Auditory Cortex Ablation on Ability to Discriminate Stimuli Presented to the Two Ears," *J. comp. physiol. Psychol.*, **59**, 79–89.

Barnes, W. T., Magoun, H. W. and Ranson, S. W. (1943), "Ascending Auditory Pathway in the Brainstem of Monkey," *J. comp. Neurol.*, **79**, 129–152.

Békésy, G. von (1960), *Experiments in Hearing.* New York–Toronto–London: McGraw-Hill.

Benevento, L. A. and Coleman, P. D. (1970), "Responses of Single Cells in Cat Inferior Colliculus to Binaural Click Stimuli; Combinations of Intensity Levels, Time Differences and Intensity Differences," *Brain Research*, **17**, 387–405.

Bickford, R. G., Jacobson, J. L. and Cody, D. T. R. (1964), "Nature of Average Evoked Potentials to Sound and Other Stimuli in Man," *Ann. N.Y. Acad. Sci.*, **112**, 204–223.

Bock, G. R., Webster, W. R. and Aitkin, L. M. (1972), "Discharge Patterns of Single Units in Inferior Colliculus of the Alert Cat," *J. Neurophysiol.*, **35**, 265–277.

Bogdanski, D. F. and Galambos, R. (1960), "Studies of the Auditory System with Implanted Electrodes," in *Neural Mechanisms of the Auditory and Vestibular Systems* (G. L. Rasmussen and W. F. Windle, Eds.). Springfield, Ill., U.S.A.: Thomas.

Boudreau, J. C. and Tsuchitani, C. (1970), "Cat Superior Olive S-segment Cell Discharge to Tonal Stimulation," in *Contributions to Sensory Physiology*, Vol. 4 (W. D. Neff, Ed.). New York and London: Academic Press.

Brugge, J. F., Dubrovsky, N. A., Aitkin, L. M. and Anderson, D. J. (1969), "Sensitivity of Single Neurons in the Auditory Cortex of Cat to Binaural Tone Stimulation; Effects of Varying Interaural Time and Intensity," *J. Neurophysiol.*, **32**, 1005–1023.

Colavita, F. B. (1972), "Auditory Cortical Lesions and Visual Pattern Discrimination in Cat," *Brain Research*, **39**, 437–337.

David, E., Finkenzeller, P., Kallert, S. and Keidel, W. D. (1968), "Die mit Mikroelektroden ableitbare Reaktion einzelner Elemente des Colliculus inferior und des Corpus geniculatum mediale auf akustische Reize verschiedener Form und verschiedener Intensität," *Pflügers Arch. ges. Physiol.*, **299**, 83–93.

David, E., Finkenzeller, P., Kallert, S. and Keidel, W. D. (1969a), "Reizfrequenzkorrelierte 'untersetzte' neuronale Entladungsperiodizität im Colliculus inferior und im Corpus geniculatum mediale," *Pflügers Arch. ges. Physiol.*, **3–9**, 11–20.

David, E., Finkenzeller, P., Kallert, S. and Keidel, W. D. (1969b), "Reizkorrelierte Gleichspannungsänderungen der primären Hörrinde an der wachen Katze," *Pflügers Arch.*, **306**, 281–289.

David, E., Finkenzeller, P., Kallert, S. and Keidel, W. D. (1969c), "Akustischen Reizen zugeordnete Gleichspannungsänderungen am intakten Schädel des Menschen," *Pflügers Arch.*, **309**, 362–367.

David, E., Finkenzeller, P., Kallert, S. and Keidel, W. D. (1971), "Interaction Between Visually and Auditorily Evoked DC-Potentials in Man," in *Biokybernetik*, Band III (H. Drischel and N. Tiedt, Eds). Jena: VEB Gustav Fischer Verlag.

Davis, H. (1968), "Auditory Responses Evoked in the Human Cortex," in *Ciba Foundation Symposium Hearing Mechanisms in Vertebrates* (A. V. S. de Reuck and J. Knight, Eds.). London: J. & A. Churchill Ltd.

Davis, H. and Zerlin, S. (1966), "Acoustic Relations of the Human Vertex Potential," *J. acoust. Soc. Amer.*, **39**, 109–116.

Dunlop, C. W., Itzkowic, D. J. and Aitkin, L. M. (1969), "Tone-burst Response of Single Units in the Cat Medial Geniculate Body," *Brain Research*, 16, 149–164.

Eccles, J. C. (1966), "Properties and Functional Organization of Cells in the Ventrobasal Complex of the Thalamus," in *The Thalamus*," (D. P. Purpura and M. D. Yahr, Eds.).

Erulkar, S. D. (1959), "The Responses of Single Units of the Inferior Colliculus of the Cat to Acoustic Stimulation," *Proc. roy. Soc, B.*, 150, 336–355.

Erulkar, S. D., Gerstein, G. L. and Butler, R. A. (1966), "Transmembrane Potentials from Cat Cochlear Nucleus in Response to Pure and Frequency-modulated (FM) Tonal Stimuli," *Fed. Proc.*, 25, 463.

Erulkar, S. D., Nelson, P. G. and Bryan, J. S. (1968), "Experimental and Theoretical Approaches to Neural Processing in the Central Auditory Pathway," in *Contributions to Sensory Physiology*, Vol. 3 (W. D. Neff, Ed.). New York and London: Academic Press.

Evans, E. F. (1970), "Narrow 'Tuning' of the Responses of Cochlear Nerve Fibers Emanating from the Exposed Basilar Membrane," *J. Physiol. (Lond.)*, 208, 75–76.

Evans, E. F. and Nelson, P. G. (1966), "Behaviour of Neurones in Cochlear Nucleus Under Steady and Modulated Tonal Stimulation," *Fed. Proc.*, 25, 463.

Evans, E. F., Rosenberg, J. and Wilson, J. P. (1970), "Effective Bandwidth of Cochlear Nerve Fibres," *J. Physiol. (Lond.)*, 207, 62–63.

Evans, E. F., Ross, H. F. and Whitfield, I. C. (1965), "The Spatial Distribution of Unit Characteristic Frequency in the Primary Auditory Cortex of the Cat," *J. Physiol.*, 179, 238–247.

Evans, E. F. and Whitfield, I. C. (1964), "Classification of Unit Responses in the Auditory Cortex of the Unanaesthetized and Unrestrained Cat," *J. Physiol. (Lond.)*, 171, 476–493.

Feher, O. and Whitfield, I. C. (1966), "Auditory Cortical Units Which Respond to Complex Tonal Stimuli," *J. Physiol. (Lond.)*, 182, 39.

Fernauld, R. D. and Gerstein, G. L. (1972), "Response of Cat Cochlear Nucleus Neurons to Frequency- and Amplitude-Modulated Tones," *Brain Research*, 45, 417–435.

Finkenzeller, P. (1969), "Die Mittelung von Reaktionspotentialen," *Kybernetik*, 6, 22–44.

Frishkopf, L. S. (1964), "Excitation and Inhibition of Primary Auditory Neurones in the Little Brown Bat," *J. acoust. Soc. Amer.*, 36, 1016.

Funkenstein, H. H., Winter, P. and Nelson, P. G. (1970), "Unit Responses to Acoustic Stimuli in the Cortex of Awake Squirrel Monkeys," *Fed. Proc.*, 29, 394.

Galambos, R. (1952), "Microelectrode Studies on Medial Geniculate Body of Cat. III. Response to Pure Tones," *J. Neurophysiol.*, 15, 381–400.

Galambos, R. and Davis, H. (1943), "The Response of Single Auditory Nerve Fibers to Acoustic Stimulation," *J. Neurophysiol.*, 6, 39–58.

Galambos, R., Schwartzkopff, J. and Rupert, A. (1959), "Microelectrode Study of Superior Olivary Nuclei," *Amer. J. Physiol.*, 197, 527–536.

Geisler, C. D., Rhode, W. S. and Hazelton, D. W. (1969), "Responses of Inferior Colliculus Neurons in the Cat to Binaural Acoustic Stimuli Having Wide-band Spectra," *J. Neurophysiol.*, 32, 960–974.

Goldberg, J. M. and Neff, W. D. (1961), "Frequency Discrimination After Bilateral Ablation of Cortical Auditory Areas," *J. Neurophysiol.*, 24, 119–128.

Goldstein, M. H., Jr., Hall, J. L. II and Butterfield, B. O. (1968), "Single-unit Activity in the Primary Auditory Cortex of Unanaesthetized Cats," *J. acoust. Soc. Amer.*, 43, 444–455.

Greenwood, D. D. and Maruyama, N. (1965), "Excitatory and Inhibitory Response Areas of Auditory Neurons in the Cochlear Nucleus," *J. Neurophysiol.*, 28, 863–892.

Gross, N. B. and Thurlow, W. R. (1951), "Microelectrode Studies of Neural Activity of Cat. II. Medial Geniculate Body," *J. Neurophysiol.*, 14, 409–422.

Guinan, J. J., Jr., Guinan, S. S. and Norris, B. E. (1972), "Single Auditory Units in the Superior Olivary Complex. I: Responses to Sounds and Classifications Based on Physiological Properties," *Int. J. Neuroscience*, 4, 101–120.

Hall, J. L., II and Goldstein, M. H., Jr. (1968), "Representation of Binaural Stimuli by Single Units in Primary Auditory Cortex of Unanaesthetized Cats," *J. acoust. Soc. Amer.*, 43, 456–461.

Harrison, J. M. and Feldman, M. L. (1970), "Anatomical Aspects of the Cochlear Nucleus and Superior Olivary Complex," in *Contributions to Sensory Physiology*, Vol. 4 (W. D. Neff, Ed.). New York and London: Academic Press.

Helmholtz, H., von (1863), *Die Lehre von den Tonempfindungen als physiologische Grundlage für die Theorie der Musik*. Braunschweig: Vieweg.

Hind, J. E., Anderson, D. J., Brugge, J. F. and Rose, J. E. (1967), "Coding of Information Pertaining to Paired Low-frequency Tones in Single Auditory Nerve Fibers of the Squirrel Monkey," *J. Neurophysiol.*, 30, 794–816.

Hind, J. E., Goldberg, J. M., Greenwood, D. D. and Rose, J. E. (1963), "Some Discharge Characteristics of Single Neurons in the Inferior Colliculus of the Cat. II. Timing of the Discharges and Observations on Binaural Stimulation," *J. Neurophysiol.*, 26, 321–341.

Hind, J. E., Rose, J. E., Brugge, J. F. and Anderson, D. J. (1970), "Two Tone Masking Effects in Squirrel Monkey Auditory Nerve Fibers," in *Frequency Analysis and Periodicity Detection in Hearing*. (R. Plomp and G. F. Smoorenburg, Eds.). Leiden: A. W. Sijthoff.

Jerger, J., Weikers, N. J., Sharbrough, F. W., III and Jerger, S. (1969), *Acta oto-laryng.*, suppl. 258, 51.

Johnstone, B. M. and Boyle, A. J. F. (1967), "Basilar Membrane Vibration Examined with the Mössbauer Technique," *Science*, 158, 389–390.

Johnstone, B. M. and Taylor, K. (1970), "Mechanical Aspects of Cochlear Function," in *Frequency Analysis and Periodicity Detection in Hearing* (R. Plomp and G. F. Smoorenburg, Eds.). Leiden: A. W. Sijthoff.

Kallert, S. (1972), "Uber die Reizantwort einzelner Zellen in Corpus geniculatum mediale der Katze bei Untersuchung mit Mikroelektroden," Dissertation, University of Erlangen.

Kallert, S., David, E., Finkenzeller, P. and Keidel, W. D. (1970), "Two Different Neuronal Discharge Periodicities in the Acoustical Channel," in *Frequency Analysis and Periodicity Detection in* (R. Plomp and G. F. Smoorenburg, Eds.). Leiden: A. W. Sijthoff.

Katsuki, Y., Sumi, T., Uchiyama, H. and Watanabe, T. (1958), "Electric Responses of Auditory Neurons in Cat to Sound Stimulation," *J. Neurophysiol.*, 21, 569–588.

Keidel, W. D. (1962), *Nachrichtenübermittlung und Nachrichtenverarbeitung in Organismen*. Munich; Vortrag, gehalten auf Einladung der Carl-Friedrich-von-Siemens-Stiftung.

Keidel, W. D. (1965a), "Neuere Ergebnisse der Physiologie des Hörens," *Arch. klin. exp. Ohr.-, Nas.-u. Kehlk. Heilk.*, 185, 548–475.

Keidel, W. D. (1965b), "On the Neurophysiological Exponents of Steven's Power Functions Electronically Computed in Man," *6th Int. Conf. Med. Electron. Biol. Eng.* Tokyo.

Keidel, W. D. (1966a), "Das räumliche Hören," in *Handbuch der Psychologie*, Vol. 1; *Wahrnehmung und Bewusstsein* (W. Metzger, Ed.). Göttingen: Verlag für Psychologie, Dr. C. J. Hogrefe.

Keidel, W. D. (1966b), "Anatomie und Elektrophysiologie der zentralen akustischen Bahnen," in *Hals-Nasen-Ohren-Heilkunde*, Vol. 3 (J. Berendes, R. Link and F. Zöllner, Eds.). Stuttgart: George Thieme Verlag.

Keidel, W. D. (1969), "Informationsphysiologische Aspekte des Hörens," *Studium Gen.* 22, 49–82.

Keidel, W. D. (1970a), "Optische und akustische Zeichenerkennung beim Menschen," *Naturw. Rdsch.* 23, 491–498.

Keidel, W. D. (1970b), "Neuere Ergebnisse der akustischen Informationsverarbeitung," in *Ergebnisse der experimentellen Medizin*. *Präsidium der Deutschen Gesellschaft für experimentelle Medizin*, Vol. 3. Berlin: VEB Verlag Volk und Gesundheit.

Keidel, W. D. (1971a), "What Do We Know about the Human Cortical Evoked Potential After All?" *Arch. klin. exp. Ohr.-, Nas.-u. Kehlk. Heilk.*, 198, 9–37.

Keidel, W. D. (1971b), "Information Processing in the Higher Parts of the Auditory Pathway," *Proc. of the International Union of*

Physiological Sciences, Vol. VIII. Munich: XXV International Congress.

Keidel, W. D. (1971c), "D.C.-potentials in the Auditory Evoked Response in Man," *Acta oto-laryng.*, **71**, 242–248.

Keidel, W. D. (1971d), "Neuere Ergebnisse der akustischen Informationsverarbeitung," *Naturw. Rdsch.* **24**, 461–471.

Keidel, W. D. (1972a), "The D.C.-potential in the Human Cortical Evoked Response, a New Contribution to the Objective Audiometry," *J. Franc. d'Oto-Rhino-Laryng.*, **21**, 153–158.

Keidel, W. D. (1972b), "Temporal and Spatial Aspects of Sensory Pattern Recognition in Man," Paper given at the International Symposium: *Neurophysiological Mechanisms of Mental Activity.* 2–5 July, Leningrad.

Keidel, W. D. (1972c), "A New Technique for Simultaneous Recording of Auditory Early, Late and D.C.-evoked Responses in Man," Paper given at the *International Congress of Audiology.* 3–7 October, Budapest.

Keidel, W. D. (1974), "Human Biocybernetics," in *Advances in Cybernetic Systems* E. Rose (Ed.). London: Gordon and Breach.

Keidel, W. D. and Spreng, M. (1965a), "Audiometric Aspects and Multisensory Power Functions of Electronically Averaged Evoked Cortical Responses in Man," *Acta oto-laryng. (Stockh.)*, **59**, 201–8.

Keidel, W. D. and Spreng, M. (1965b), "Computed Audioencephalograms in Man. (A Technique of 'Objective' Audiometry)," *Int. Audiol.*, **4**, 56–60.

Keidel, W. D. and Spreng, M. (1965c), "Neurophysiological Evidence for the Steven's Power Function in Man," *J. acoust. Soc. Amer.*, **38**, 191–195.

Keidel, W. D. and Spreng, M. (1970), "Recent Status Results and Problems in Objective Audiometry," 1st Part, *J. Franc. d'Oto-Rhino-Laryng. Numero special d'audiophonologie*, **19**, 45–53.

Kemp, E. H., Coppée, G. E. and Robinson, E. H. (1937), "Electric Responses of the Brain Stem to Unilateral Auditory Stimulation," *Amer. J. Physiol.*, **120**, 304.

Kiang, N. Y-S. (1965a), "Stimulus Coding in the Auditory Nerve and Cochlear Nucleus," *Acta oto-laryng. (Stockh.)*, **59**, 186–200.

Kiang, N. Y-S. (Ed.) (1965b), *Discharge Patterns of Single Fibers in the Cat's Auditory Nerve.* Cambridge, Mass.: M.I.T. Press.

Kiang, N. Y-S. and Goldstein, M. H. (1962), "Temporal Coding of Neural Responses to Acoustic Stimuli," *I.R.E. Trans. Inf. Theory*, Vol. IT–8, 113–119.

Kiang, N. Y-S. and Moxon, E. C. (1972), "Physiological Considerations in Artificial Stimulation of the Inner Ear," *Ann. Otol.*, **81**, 714-731.

Masterton, R. B., Jane, J. A. and Diamond, I. T. (1968), Role of Brain-stem Auditory Structures in Sound Localization. II. Inferior Colliculus and its Brachium," *J. Neurophysiol.*, **31**, 96–108.

Møller, A. R. (1969a), "Unit Responses in Cochlear Nucleus of the Rat to Pure Tones," *Acta physiol. scand.*, **75**, 530–541.

Møller, A. R. (1969b), "Unit Responses in the Rat Cochlear Nucleus to Repetitive Transient Sounds," *Acta physiol. scand.*, **75**, 542–551.

Møller, A. R. (1969c), "Unit Responses in the Cochlear Nucleus of the Rat to Sweep Tones," *Acta physiol. scand.*, **76**, 503–512.

Møller, A. R. (1971), "Unit Responses in the Rat Cochlear Nucleus to Tones of Rapidly Varying Frequency and Amplitude," *Acta physiol. scand.*, **81**, 540–556.

Møller, A. R. (1972), "Coding of Sounds in Lower Levels of the Auditory System," *Quart. Rev. Biophys.*, **5**, 59–155.

Moore, R. Y. and Goldberg, J. M. (1963), "Ascending Connections of the Inferior Colliculus in the Cat," *J. comp. Neurol.*, **121**, 109–136.

Moore, R. Y. and Goldberg, J. M. (1966), "Projections of the Inferior Colliculus in the Monkey," *Exp. Neurol.*, **14**, 429–438.

Moore, R. Y. and Tarlov, C. E. (1963), "Ascending Projections of the Inferior Colliculus in the Rabbit," *Anat. Rec.*, **145**, 262.

Morest, D. K. (1964), "The Neuronal Architecture of the Medial Geniculate Body of the Cat," *J. Anat. (Lond.)*, **98**, 611–630.

Mountcastle, V. B. (1961), "Some Functional Properties of the Somatic Afferent System," in *Sensory Communication* (W. A. Rosenblith, Ed.). Cambridge, Mass.: M.I.T. Press.

Moushegian, G. and Rupert, A. L. (1970), "Response Diversity of Neurons in Ventra 1 Cochlear Nucleus of Kangaroo Rat to Low-frequency Tones," *J. Neurophysiol.*, **33**, 351–364.

Moushegian, G., Rupert, A. L. and Langford, T. L. (1967), "Stimulus Coding by Medial Superior Olivary Neurons," *J. Neurophysiol.*, **30**, 1239–1261.

Müller, J. (1826), *Zur vergleichenden Physiologie des Gesichtsinnes des Menschen und der Tiere, nebst einem Versuch über die Bewegungen der Augen und über den menschlichen Blick.* Leipzig: Cnobloch.

Neff, W. D. (1961), "Neural Mechanisms of Auditory Discrimination," in *Sensory Communication* (W. A. Rosenblith, Ed.). Cambridge, Mass.: M.I.T. Press.

Nelson, P. G. and Erulkar, S. D. (1963), "Synaptic Mechanisms of Excitation and Inhibition in the Central Auditory Pathway," *J. Neurophysiol.*, **26**, 908–923.

Nelson, P. G., Erulkar, S. D. and Bryan, J. S. (1966), "Responses of Units of the Inferior Colliculus to Time-varying Acoustic Stimuli," *J. Neurophysiol.*, **29**, 834–860.

Noort, J. von (1969), *The Structure and Connections of the Inferior Colliculus.* Assen: van Gorcum and Co. N.V.

Ohm, G. S. (1843), "Über die Definition des Tones, nebst daran geknüpfter Theorie der Sirene und ähnlicher tonbilden der Vorrichtungen," *Ann. Phys.*, **59**, 497–565.

Oonishi, S. and Katsuki, Y. (1965), "Functional Organisation and Integrative Mechanism on the Auditory Cortex of the Cat." *Japan J. Physiol.*, **15**, 342–365.

Peake, W. T. and Kiang, N. Y-S. (1962), "Cochlear Responses to Condensation and Rarefaction Clicks," *Biophys.J.*, 223–24.

Pfeiffer, R. R. (1966), "Classification of Response Patterns of Spike Discharges for Units in the Cochlear Nucleus: Tone-burst Stimulation," *Exp. Brain Res.*, **1**, 220–235.

Pfeiffer, R. R. (1970), "A Model for Two-tone Inhibition of Single Cochlear Nerve Fibers," *J. acoust. Soc. Amer.*, **48**, 1373–1378.

Pfeiffer, R. R. and Kim, D. O. (1972a), "Response Patterns of Single Cochlear Nerve Fibers to Click Stimuli: Descriptions for Cat," *J. acoust. Soc. Amer.*, **52**, 1669–1677.

Pfeiffer, R. R. and Kim, D. O. (1972b), "Anomalies of Response Patterns of Single Cochlear Nerve Fibers to Click Stimuli," *J. acoust. Soc. Amer.*, **51**, 93 (A)·

Powell, E. W. and Hatton, J. B. (1969), "Projections of the Inferior Colliculus in Cat," *J. comp. Neurol.*, **136**, 183–192.

Ranke, O. F. and Lullies, H. (1953), *Gehör-Stimme-Sprache.* Berlin-Göttingen-Heidelberg: Springer-Verlag.

Rasmussen, G. L. (1946), "The Olivary Peduncle and other Fiber Projections of the Superior Olivary Complex," *J. comp. Neurol.*, **84**, 141–220.

Rhode, W. S. (1971), "Observations of the Vibration of the Basilar Membrane in Squirrel Monkeys Using the Mössbauer Technique," *J. acoust. Soc. Amer.*, **49**, 1218–1231.

de Ribaupierre, F., Goldstein, M. H., Jr. and Yeni-Komshian, G. (1972a), "Intracellular Study of the Cat's Primary Auditory Cortex," *Brain Res.*, **48**, 185–204.

de Ribaupierre, F., Goldstein, M. H., Jr. and Yeni-Komshian, G. (1972b), "Cortical Coding of Repetitive Acoustic Pulses," *Brain Res.*, **48**, 205–225.

Rose, J. E. (1970), "Discharges of Single Fibers in the Mammalian Auditory Nerve," in *Frequency Analysis and Periodicity Detection in Hearing.* (R. Plomp and G. F. Smoorenburg, Eds.). Leiden: A. W. Sijthoff.

Rose, J. E., Brugge, J. F., Anderson, D. J. and Hind, J. E. (1967), "Phase-locked Response to Low-frequency Tones in Single Auditory Nerve Fibers of the Squirrel Monkey," *J. Neurophysiol.*, **30**, 769–793.

Rose, J. E., Greenwood, D. D., Goldberg, J. M. and Hind, J. E. (1963), "Some Discharge Characteristics of Single Neurons in the Inferior Colliculus of the Cat. I. Tonotopical Organization, Relations of Spike Counts to Tone Intensity and Firing Patterns of Single Elements," *J. Neurophysiol.*, **26**, 294–320.

Rose, J. E., Gross, N. B., Geisler, C. D. and Hind, J. E. (1966), "Some Neural Mechanisms in the Inferior Colliculus of the Cat which may be Relevant to Localization of a Sound Source," *J. Neurophysiol.*, **29**, 288–314.

Rose, J. E., Hind, J. E., Anderson, D. J. and Brugge, J. F. (1971), "Some Effects of Stimulus Intensity on Response of Auditory

Nerve Fibers in the Squirrel Monkey," *J. Neurophysiol.*, **34**, 685–699.

Rose, J. E. and Woolsey, C. N. (1949), "The Relations of Thalamic Connections Cellular Structure and Evokable Electrical Activity in the Auditory Region of the Cat," *J. comp. Neurol.*, **91**, 441–466.

Rosenblith, W. A. and Rosenzweig, M. R. (1952), "Latency of Neural Components in Round Window Response to Pure Tones," *Fed. Proc.*, **11**, 132.

Sachs, M. B. and Kiang, N. Y-S. (1968), "Two Tone Inhibition in Auditory Nerve Fibres," *J. acoust. Soc. Amer.*, **43**, 1120–1128.

Spoendlin, H. (1970), "Structural Basis of Peripheral Frequency Analysis," in *Frequency Analysis and Periodicity Detection in Hearing* (R. Plomp and G. F. Smoorenburg, Eds.). Leiden: A. W. Sijthoff.

Spreng, M. and Keidel, W. D. (1970), "Recent Status Results and Problems in Objective Audiometry," 2nd Part, *J. Franc. d'Oto-Rhino-Laryng. Numero special d'audiophonologie*, **19**, 55–60.

Starr, A. and Don, M. (1972), "Responses of Squirrel Monkey (Samiri Sciureus) Medial Geniculate Units to Binaural Click Stimuli," *J. Neurophysiol.*, **35**, 501–517.

Suga, N. (1964), "Single Unit Activity in Cochlear Nucleus and Inferior Colliculus of Echo-locating Bats," *J. Physiol. (Lond.)*, **172**, 449–474.

Suga, N. (1968), "Analysis of Frequency-modulated and Complex Sounds by Single Auditory Neurons of Bats," *J. Physiol. (Lond.)*, **198**, 51–80.

Suga, N. (1969), "Classification of Inferior Collicular Neurons of Bats in Terms of Responses to Pure Tones, FM Sounds and Noise Bursts," *J. Physiol. (Lond.)*, **200**, 555–574.

Thompson, R. F. (1960), "Function of Auditory Cortex of Cat in Frequency Discrimination," *J. Neurophysiol.*, **23**, 321–334.

Thurlow, W. R., Gross, N. B., Kemp, E. H. and Lowy, K. (1951), "Microelectrode Studies of Neural Activity of Cat. I. Inferior Colliculus," *J. Neurophysiol.*, **14**, 289–304.

Tsuchitani, C. and Boudreau, J. C. (1967), "Encoding of Stimulus Frequency and Intensity by Cat Superior Olive S-segment Cells," *J. acoust. Soc. Amer.*, **42**, 794–805.

Vaughan, H. G., Jr. and Ritter, W. (1970), "The Sources of Auditory Evoked Responses Recorded from the Human Scalp," *Electroenceph. clin. Neurophysiol.*, **28**, 360–367.

Walter, G. W. (1964), "Slow Potential Waves in the Human Brain Associated with Expectancy, Attention and Decision," *Arch. Psychiat. Nervenkr.*, **206**, 309.

Walter, G. W. (1967), "Electrical Signs of Association Expectancy and Decision in the Human Brain," *Electroenceph. clin. Neurophysiol.*, suppl. **25**, 258–263.

Webster, W. R., Bock, G. R. and Aitkin, L. M. (1971), "Sensory Coding in the Inferior Colliculus of the Alert Cat," *Proc. Int. Union Physiol. Soc.*, **599**. XXV Int. Congr., Munich.

Wepsic, J. G. (1966), "Multimodal Sensory Activation of Cells in the Magnocellular Medial Geniculate Nucleus," *Exp. Neurol.*, **15**, 299–318.

Whitfield, I. C. (1967), *The Auditory Pathway*. London: Edward Arnold.

Wiederhold, M. L. and Kiang, N. Y-S. (1970), "Effects of Electric Stimulation of the Crossed Olivocochlear Bundle on Single Auditory-Nerve Fibers in the Cat," *J. acoust. Soc. Amer.*, **48**, 950–965.

Wien, M. (1905), 'Ein Bedenken gegen die Helmholtzsche Resonanztheorie des Hörens," in *Festschrift für Wüllner*, pp. 28–35, Leipzig.

Wilson, O. (1970), In Discussion to B. M. Johnston and K. Taylor. "Mechanical aspects of cochlear function," in *Frequency Analysis and Periodicity Detection in Hearing* (R. Plomp and G. F. Smoorenburg, Eds.). Leiden: A. W. Sijthoff.

Wollberg, Z. and Newman, J. D. (1972), "Auditory Cortex of Squirrel Monkey: Response Patterns of Single Cells to Species-specific Vocalizations," *Science*, **175**, 212–214.

Woolard, H. H. and Harpman, J. A. (1940), "The Connexion of the Inferior Colliculus and of the Dorsal Nucleus of the Lateral Lemniscus," *J. Anat.*, **74**, 441–458.

23. ELECTROPHYSIOLOGICAL INVESTIGATION OF AUDITORY FUNCTION: APPLICATIONS

H. A. BEAGLEY

Electrophysiological methods have been widely exploited by physiologists investigating basic auditory physiology and it has proved a potent tool in the hands of these researchers. For example, the cochlear microphonic potential, known originally as the Wever and Bray (1930) phenomenon, has provided a convenient electrical indicator of cochlear function. In fact, the phase shift of the microphonic described by Tasaki, Davis and Legouix (1952) provided an independent confirmation of the travelling wave produced in the cochlear partition and described by von Békésy (1947) and by Ranke (1950). Békésy was able to make limited observations only when examining the cochlea by direct vision and to get a further insight into its dynamics he had to resort to the construction of cochlear models in which the behaviour of an artificial cochlear partition was studied. However, the electrophysiological observations of Tasaki, Davis and Legouix in 1952 made it possible to confirm these observations on the actual cochlea of a living animal. This gave a much more authentic insight into the phenomenon.

Similarly, electrophysiological procedures have been employed in the investigation of human subjects both in the normal and in the diseased state. While much of this investigative activity was orientated towards research, inevitably interest has turned towards the exploitation of these techniques in the investigation of patients suffering from disorders of the auditory system and an account will now be given of the techniques which have proved valuable for diagnostic purposes, as well as some speculations on the likely direction of future developments in this rapidly expanding field.

The methods at present incorporated into clinical practice may in some cases appear to have little in common with one another and indeed this is true. The common factors linking these very different tests together are: (1) the fact that an electrophysiological technique is involved as an indicator of an underlying physiological function, or dysfunction, and (2) the fact that some aspect of auditory function is the matter under scrutiny.

A. Reflex Responses

One of the earliest reflexes to be investigated in the context of auditory function was the sudomotor reflex which gave rise to the so-called electrodermal response (EDR) or psychogalvanic skin response (PGSR). This was in fact a form of classical Pavlovian conditioning where the innate sudomotor reflex—sweating induced by electric shock—was "generalized" by associating it with a simultaneous auditory stimulus. A subject rapidly became conditioned to associating the sound stimulus with the nocuous electric shock and would respond by sweating even if the sound stimulus were later used without the electric shock. This formed a basis of a test of hearing since the effect of the sudomotor activity in the skin, as shown by sweating, resulted in a reduced skin resistance to a direct electric current. Electrodes on the forearm could be used to monitor the drop in resistance. However, a simple drop in resistance of the skin is not the only factor involved, as there is also a skin potential change produced by the stimulation, and this potential is also detected by the electro-physiological monitoring system. The PGSR was investigated extensively as a method of testing hearing of young children by Bordley and Hardy (1949) and by Barr (1955) but the variability of the response proved to be too great a problem to overcome and it was finally abandoned. It is still used today, however, as a method for detecting malingerers claiming a hearing loss (Portmann, 1965) and it was for many years regarded as an essential investigation by the War Veterans (exservicemen) Administration in the U.S.A. when hearing-loss was claimed to result from war service.

The acoustic stapedial reflex (*see* chapter by Brooks) has been used considerably in recent years as a result of the introduction of the acoustic impedance bridge into otological practice as a result of the work of Terkildsen and Nielsen (1960); Zwislocki (1961); Klockoff (1961); Anderson and his associates (1970); Chiveralls and FitzSimons (1973) and others. The stapedial reflex is a bilateral consensual reflex, i.e. stimulation of one ear by an appropriate acoustic stimulus causes a reflex contraction of both the homolateral and contralateral stapedius muscles. It is simpler to use the crossed reflex by stimulating one ear and observing the effect in the opposite ear. However, by suitable refinements of the instrumentation, it is possible to stimulate and measure the effect of the stimulus on the one ear at the same time. That is to say, the homolateral reflex can be elicited and this has obvious advantages as a disorder of the opposite ear, e.g. a hearing loss, or a tympanic perforation, will not affect the reflex as it could do in the case of the crossed reflex. The effect of the stapedial reflex is to rock the stapes around its axis of rotation in such a way that it tends to move the stapes base (footplate) outwards. This has the effect of altering the impedance of the middle ear as shown by a fluctuation of the meter on the impedance bridge, or by a deflection of the pen on a strip chart recorder, which gives a written record of the reflex, its direction, duration, amplitude and decay or adaptation. The acoustic stimulus used in clinical applications is a tone from an audiometer and the threshold of the reflex is usually about 85 dB although it is occasionally elicited at intensities as low as 75 dB, or even 70 dB HL.

The acoustic stapedial reflex has a place in the assessment of hearing, as well as other clinical uses.

(1) In young children it indicates the presence of cochlear activity.

(2) In suspected non-organic hearing loss, its presence will also indicate cochlear activity.

(3) In known cases of sensorineural hearing loss a positive stapedial reflex at sensation levels less than the actual hearing level indicates the presence of loudness recruitment and is probably the simplest way of demonstrating this effect. For example, if the patient has a sensorineural hearing loss of 60 dB, but a positive stapedial reflex is elicited at, say, 100 dB, or even at normal levels around 85 dB, this is evidence for loudness recruitment.

(4) In ankylosis of the stapes (otosclerosis) the stapedial reflex cannot be elicited. In this respect, the paradoxical response described by Terkildsen in early otosclerosis is noteworthy. It is characterized by a Z-shaped trace when the impedance change is written out on the chart recorder.

(5) Other forms of ossicular fixation also prevent the reflex from being recorded, e.g. ossicular fusions of congenital origin, or intratympanic scarring following otitis media.

(6) Reflex "decay", or abnormal suprathreshold adaptation, is seen in cases of vestibulocochlear (eighth) nerve tumours when acoustic stimuli are administered. This is attributed to neural fatigue affecting the auditory nerve fibres and this is considered by Anderson and his associates (1970) to be a very sensitive test for early acoustic neuroma.

(7) In cases of facial paresis, the presence or absence of a stapedial reflex has some value in indicating the level of the lesion of the facial nerve which supplies the stapedius muscle.

(8) Ossicular discontinuity will result in inability to demonstrate the presence of the reflex except in those cases of disruption or discontinuity which occur at the level of the crura of the stapes, as in this case contraction of the stapes can still exert its effect on the tympanic membrane and thereby give rise to an impedance change. In (7) and (8), the problem is not one of auditory acuity and, if the reflex cannot be elicited on account of a hearing loss in the ear to be stimulated, a non-auditory stimulus will give the necessary information. A puff of air to the ear or to the deep meatus or to the side of the neck will often trigger this reflex, as will also a galvanic current applied to the skin of the deep meatus, as shown by Klockoff (1960).

The tensor tympani muscle can also contract and alter the middle ear impedance but it is not certain that sound will trigger this reflex in man. It is part of a mass reflex mediated through the motor division of the trigeminal nerve and it can be elicited by a puff of air to the eyeball or the orbit. It tends to be enhanced in ossicular discontinuity and depressed in otosclerosis. The written-out reflex response recorded on the X-Y chart recorder sometimes shows a deflection in the opposite direction to that shown by the acoustic stapedial reflex.

Another reflex of interest to those investigating auditory function is the so-called post-auricular response described by Kiang and his associates in 1963. It is a bilateral consensual reflex in that stimulating one ear causes a response on both sides and the effector agent of the response is the collection of vestigal muscles fibres attached to the posterior aspect of the auricle. A surface electrode placed on the body of the mastoid at the level of the external acoustic meatus will pick up the response, which has a latency of 15–18 ms. As it is a small signal buried in physiological "noise", electronic averaging must be used to extract it from the background noise. Interest in the post-auricular response has been re-awakened by Douek and his associates (1973), and these workers have developed it as an electrophysiological screening test of hearing for recalcitrant infants. Its value lies in the fact that increased muscle tone tends to enhance the response and the use of bilateral recordings means that if, due to head movements, the reflex on the one side is reduced, on the other side it is likely to be enhanced. The threshold of this response is about 30 dB, which makes it a potentially useful test for the identification of hearing loss in young children. As the reflex arc crosses at the brainstem level, it can be used to help indicate the level and extent of intracranial tumours and other lesions in this area. Douek has reported an example of an intracranial tumour which was successfully investigated by this means.

B. Peripheral Bio-electric Signals Related to the Cochlea

Physiologists are aware of several biological potentials that can be recorded in the vicinity of the cochlea, but for clinical purposes only two categories have any relevance at the present time, namely:

    (1) cochlear nerve compound action potential; and
    (2) the cochlear microphonic.

The Electrocochleogram. This is the term usually employed to describe the procedure whereby the compound action potential of the cochlear nerve is recorded as a clinical test of hearing. Basically, it depends upon picking up the action potential of the whole cochlear nerve, consisting of about 50 000 fibres, in response to a series of acoustic clicks, or, sometimes, of very short tone bursts. Basically, this can be done in two slightly different ways:

    (a) from electrodes placed a short distance from the cochlea (usually in the region of the external ear); or
    (b) from a transtympanic electrode which is in contact with the bony shell of the cochlea, a little anterior to the fenestra cochleae (round window).

The reader is referred to a very full account of these potentials in the chapter by Aran and Portmann, in which are described the physiological principles upon which electrocochleography is based, together with the clinical applications of the technique, which are reviewed in some depth. It is reviewed much more briefly in this chapter to indicate its application in relation to other electrophysiological techniques that may be used in the investigation of auditory disorders.

Using superficial electrodes (ear lobe-vertex), Sohmer and Feinmesser (1967) have been able to demonstrate the compound action potential of the eighth (vestibulocochlear) nerve. Although the amplitude is quite minute, well under 1 μV, the great interest of their method is the fact that a series of small waves which follow the compound cochlear nerve action potential appear to be related to synaptic activity in the various nuclei along the auditory pathways. These phenomenon appear to be closely related to the "far field" recordings of Jewett and Williston (1971) and the recordings of Terkildsen and his associates (1973). Although Sohmer and Feinmesser's method, which picks up biopotentials which have been volume-conducted a considerable distance through the tissues of the head, would appear to be mainly of research interest, there is equally no doubt that these authors have been able to exploit clinically the minute signals in the assessment of hearing in young infants, as well as in older subjects.

Most other superficial electrode placements are concerned with the application of needles or sharp wires inserted into the skin of the meatus (Elberling and Salomon, 1971), or in contact with the skin near the annulus tympanicus (Yoshie and Ohashi, 1969) or in contact with the tympanic membrane at the annulus tympanicus (Khcchinashvili *et al.*, 1974). Yoshie differs from most other investigators in that he has used both a superficial, as well as a penetrating, transtympanic electrode placement, and now tends to employ the latter more frequently. As Aran and Portmann state in their chapter, the transtympanic placement has many advantages, not the least being the large amplitude and unequivocal nature of the action potential recorded by this means and the precise information it yields concerning the peripheral auditory mechanism, as well as avoiding problems related to laterality which make masking of any sort unnecessary. In addition to these advantages can be added another, the fact that general anaesthesia can be employed without adversely influencing the action potential and this is a great advantage in dealing with some of the emotionally disturbed, or brain-damaged or multiply-handicapped children whose hearing must be tested by this method quite frequently, because of the absence of any practicable alternative. And, as Aran and Portmann also point out, the information obtained by their method, although restricted as far as frequency information is concerned (due to the fact that the site from which the recordings are taken is concerned mainly with events occurring in the basal cochlear turn), goes beyond a simple threshold determination.

Currently, the writer tends to use electrocochleography selectively in those children who cannot be tested by conventional methods, and who would need sedation. In such cases electrocochleography under ketamine anaesthesia seems an ideal solution and many children who are emotionally disturbed, hyperactive, brain-damaged, epileptic, or neurologically abnormal (e.g. due to gross cerebral palsy or athetosis) or multiply-handicapped (e.g. deaf and blind) have been successfully assessed by this method (Beagley *et al.*, 1974), and it seems unlikely that this technique will be displaced for many years to come.

The Cochlear microphonic is the other potential of interest when electrocochleography is being considered. Normally, it is usual to eliminate the microphonic by alternatively inverting the polarity of the acoustic signal. This has the effect of cancelling out the microphonic potential while leaving the compound action potential (AP) unaffected. However, in many cases where there is little or no AP present, if the acoustic stimulus is presented in one polarity only, a clearly defined cochlear microphonic can sometimes be observed (Beagley, 1973). This observation raises two possibilities: (1) that the microphonic is genuinely being generated within the cochlea, in which case it can be concluded that there is still a population of hair cells within the spiral organ (of Corti) and that these are producing the microphonic in response to the acoustic stimulation, or (2) that the microphonic is an artefact due to some unexplained mechanism such as vibration of the electrode by the acoustic stimulation, or by the vibration of polarized tissues in relation to the electrode.

While it is impossible to deny with complete certainty that the appearance of a microphonic potential under these circumstances is an artefact, nevertheless, repeated observation and examination of this phenomenon, when it is observed during clinical electrocochleography, suggest that it is a genuine cochlear microphonic generated by hair cells. In an ear which has a degree of function as revealed by the presence of a compound action potential—whether or not there is some loss of acuity—there is no difficulty in observing the cochlear microphonic. This satisfies the usual criteria for a microphonic potential, namely, that it follows the polarity and form of the acoustic stimulus. When the stimulus is alternatively inverted in polarity, the one microphonic is cancelled by the succeeding one in the "memory" of the averager due to the fact that it is also inverted in polarity. In this way the potential is routinely excluded during electrocochleography.

The case of interest is that in which no cochlear nerve action potential can be demonstrated, i.e. a non-functioning clinically "dead" ear. In cases such as this, it is reasonable to expect that there may be no cochlear microphonic either, if it is considered that the disease process has eliminated all cochlear hair cell function; and in fact this is the usual finding in such cases, the most florid examples being the patient who has become profoundly deaf following cerebrospinal meningitis, where suppuration has invaded the perilymphatic spaces and has destroyed all the neurosensory epithelium within the cochlea; and cases of profound deafness as a result of rubella embryopathy, where development of the spiral organ is completely inhibited.

The converse of this situation, however, is seen in the totally deaf with no evidence of a cochlear nerve action potential, but where there is a well marked microphonic potential. This can most readily be explained on the basis of a lesion affecting the fibres of the cochlear nerve, but sparing the cochlear hair cells, or many of them. The alternative explanation (that it is an artefact due to mechanical vibration) seems unlikely in view of the fact that the identical technique is used under the two different circum-

stances. One is therefore impelled towards the conclusion that the observation of a microphonic potential in a deaf ear with no evidence of a cochlear nerve action potential indicates that at least some of the hair cells of the spiral organ are capable of excitation, and that, in such cases, the crucial lesion is located within the fibres of the cochlear nerve. As it is unlikely that direct histological evidence will become available from such cases to prove the point, or refute it, it seems likely that continued collection and collation of data from cases of this type will give added support to an already perfectly plausible explanation.

C. Cortical Responses

From the early days of physiology at the end of the last century, it was discovered that sensory stimulation of the periphery caused a corresponding electrophysiological reaction in the cerebral cortex (Caton, 1875). The occurrence of a specific, if rather inconstant, response to auditory stimulation was observed in the EEG record, especially during sleep, by Davis and his associates in 1939. This was named the K-complex, so well known to EEG specialists. This has been revived from time to time as an audiometric method, but it was finally abandoned with the advent of electronic averagers. These averagers permit the cortical response evoked by peripheral stimulation to be extracted from the EEG background, as shown by Dawson (1954), by Geisler (1958), by Williams and his associates (1964), by Davis and Zerlin (1966) and by Keidel and Spreng (1965).

The Vertex Potential. The introduction of the recently developed small averaging computers lead to great interest in the auditory evoked cortical response as an indicator in a system of "objective" audiometry, now generally referred to as electric or "evoked" response audiometry, or ERA. The potential most widely studied is the rather slow electrical wave which occurs about 50 ms after the time of onset of the stimulus and has a duration of about 250–300 ms in adults and rather longer in young children and in infants. This is the well known V-potential, first described by Gastaut (1954), and which is recorded maximally from a scalp electrode placed on the vertex. It has been shown by Vaughan and Ritter (1970) that the V-potential is generated essentially within the primary auditory cortex. This explains why it is picked up maximally with an "active" electrode on the vertex and a reference electrode on the earlobe or mastoid, i.e. above and below the primary auditory area of the cortex, which is situated in the region of the superior temporal gyrus. The reader should consult the chapter by Keidel and Kallert for a review of this and other evoked potentials within the more comprehensive framework of the neurophysiology of the entire auditory system.

As a result of the ease with which the V-potential can be elicited with a small electronic averager from the EEG background, there has been a great deal of interest in adapting it, as a direct electrophysiological method, for testing the sensitivity of the auditory system in the hope of evolving an "objective" method of audiometry as an alternative to conventional subjective audiometry. The latter is sometimes unsuitable in some subjects, especially in some small children suspected of having a hearing loss. A great deal of

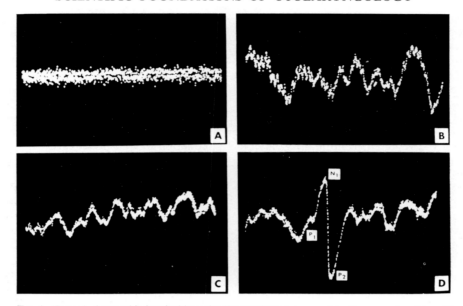

FIG. 1. Trace A shows wide-band white noise (20–20 000 Hz) averaged by the computer. Trace B shows the effect of passing the same white noise through the physiological amplifiers with a band-pass of 0.5–10 Hz, and thence to the computer. Trace C shows the effect of averaging the on-going EEG rhythms, without sound stimulation. Trace D shows the effect of averaging the on-going EEG rhythms while 1000 Hz sound pulses at 50 db HL stimulate the patient. There is a typical auditory evoked response. In each trace 60 one-second sweeps are averaged. (After Beagley and Kellogg, 1970.)

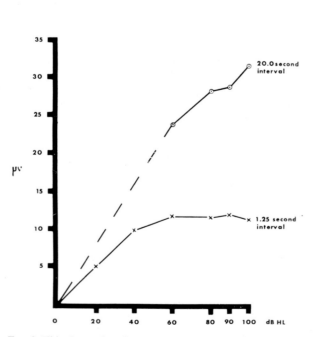

FIG. 2. This shows the effect on evoked response amplitude of a greatly prolonged interstimulus interval. (After Beagley and Kellogg, 1970.)

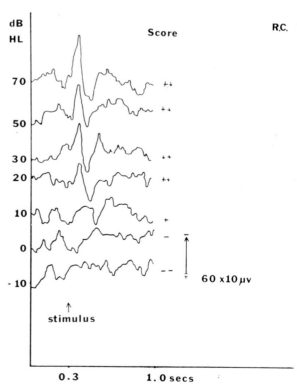

FIG. 3. Although this young patient claimed a moderately severe hearing loss, her evoked response threshold was within normal limits, as was her stapedial reflex threshold. In addition, she had a type V Békésy curve and a positive DSFB (delayed speech feedback) effect. Non-organic hearing loss was diagnosed. (After Beagley, 1974.)

research effort has been devoted to the investigation of the properties of the V-potential in an audiometric context and the following properties can be enumerated:

(1) An auditory stimulus with a sufficiently abrupt onset will evoke the V-potential. Clicks can be used, but, as they give no frequency information, "bursts" of pure tone with short rise-decay times (5–20 ms) and durations of at least 30 ms are generally employed. A

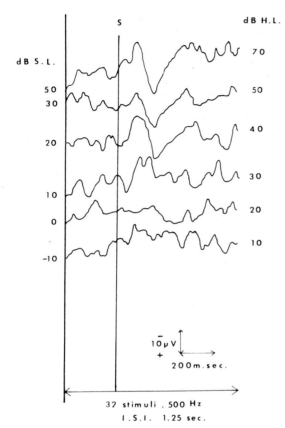

Fig. 4. A series of evoked response traces from a man aged 43 years who had suffered an extensive fracture of the vault of the skull. (After Beagley, 1974.)

series of such stimuli is always needed so that the averaging process can be employed and 30 to 60 presentations of the acoustic stimulus are generally employed. The evoked cortical response is a reaction to a change of state, either the onset of a stimulus or the cessation ("offset") of the same stimulus, if the stimulus has been steady for a a sufficient length of time. A change of frequency, as well as a change of intensity, will evoke a cortical response equally well (Antonelli, 1973). In the case of a long pure tone of 500 ms duration with an abrupt onset and offset, it is possible to obtain an evoked response as a result of the onset of stimulation, and a similar but smaller response as a result of the offset of the tone. For this reason, many people employ a tone of short duration (50 ms or thereabouts) so that the offset effect occurs when the onset response is already being generated and

when the cortical generators are relatively unresponsive to the second stimulus produced by the offset of the tone. Alternatively, a very long tone (1 s) may be used in which the offset response will fall outside the time of analysis of the averager and will therefore not affect the form of the response.

(2) The interval between successive stimuli has a marked effect on the amplitude of the V-potential. The longer the silent interval between successive auditory stimuli the greater will be the amplitude of the response. (Beagley and Kellogg, 1970; Antinoro et al., 1969). In practice, an inter-stimulus interval of 1–2 s is considered satisfactory for most clinical purposes (Fig. 1).

(3) The amplitude of the response is directly related to the intensity of the acoustic stimulus and grows steadily until about 50 dB above threshold, after which it tends to level off, except in cases where the inter-stimulus interval is very large (20 s) in which case continued growth of amplitude occurs up to levels of about 100 dB HL (Beagley and Kellogg, 1970) (Fig. 2).

(4) The latency of the principal negative wave of the V-potential, which is usually a little above 100 ms, begins to lengthen below 30 dB HL (Rapin, 1964; Beagley and Knight, 1967) when the averaged responses are arranged in descending order of stimulus intensity. Nearer subjective threshold, the reduced amplitude, combined with a variable increase in latency, makes the V-potential increasingly difficult to identify with precision, although in the majority of cases this can be done to within 10 dB of the subjective threshold, or even less (Beagley and Kellogg, 1969). The ability to trace the diminishing V-potential towards the subjective threshold is quite easily acquired once the observer has had a little practice and the opportunity of observing the behaviour of the response on some normal adult subjects as Fig. 3 shows.

(5) The V-potential can be produced by pure tones of any frequency used in conventional pure tone audiometry, although the rate of growth tends to be slower in the case of frequencies ranging from 6–8 kHz. Usually, as this is a time consuming test, it is sufficient to consider tones with a frequency of 500, 1000 and 2000 Hz, but 250 and 4000 Hz can also be checked if it is considered necessary.

In view of the above properties, the V-potential makes a a very suitable index of hearing for these cases where the conventional pure tone audiogram is inadequate. Cases for whom it is required include persons who give widely varying pure tone thresholds on conventional audiometry. An ERA will indicate which of the several curves obtained is the correct one. It can also be used for subjects who are too confused to carry out a valid pure tone audiogram, or in those cases where a non-organic hearing loss is suspected, regardless of whether this has an "hysterical" basis, or whether it is a case of deliberate malingering (Fig. 3).

To carry out the test, the passive co-operation of the patient is necessary and he must be prepared to sit reasonably still with head resting against the back of a high-backed chair in order to relax the neck muscles as the contraction

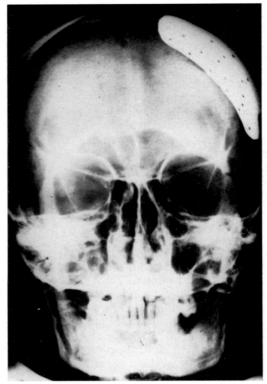
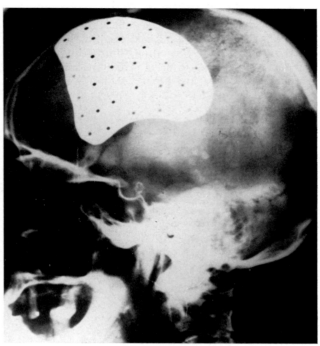

FIG. 5. Frontal and lateral views showing a metallic plate used to repair the skull defect. (After Beagley, 1974.)

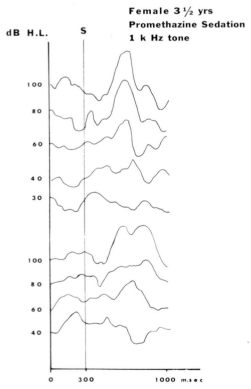

Female 3½ yrs
Promethazine Sedation
1 k Hz tone

dB H.L.   S

FIG. 6. This series of traces is from a 3½ year old child whose hearing was assessed by electric response audiometry (V-potential) while she was sedated with promethazine. Note that the late negative waves are dominant in the young child, especially during sleep.

of these can cause the record to be partly obscured by arte-facts of muscle origin. A series of 60 tone pulses 1 s apart means that the subject is expected to sit reasonably

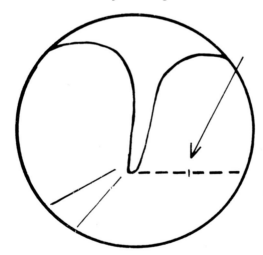

FIG. 7. This sketch shows the site of insertion of the penetrating electrode half-way between the umbo and the posterior part of the annulus tympanicus. (After Beagley, 1973.)

still for 1 min at a time in order to obtain records of good quality.

An obvious application of electric response audiometry (ERA) is in cases where legal action is being brought by the patient for alleged loss of hearing, as it gives an import-ant second check on the validity of the conventional audio-

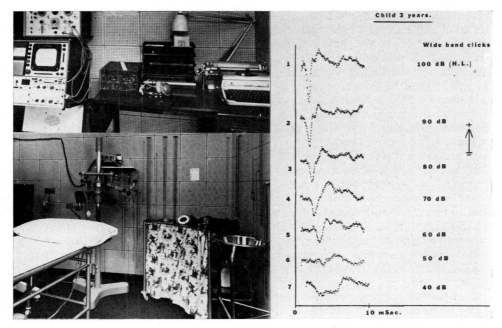

FIG. 8. This shows the recording apparatus (upper left) for electrocochleography and the room (lower left) where the patient is tested. On the right is a series of compound cochlear nerve action potentials from a 3 year old child. The threshold of this child for wide-band clicks was of the order of 45 dB above the normal threshold of hearing. (After Beagley *et al.*, 1974.)

grams as there should be reasonably close correspondence between the two. If the patient has been exaggerating his hearing loss, the objective test based on the V-potential

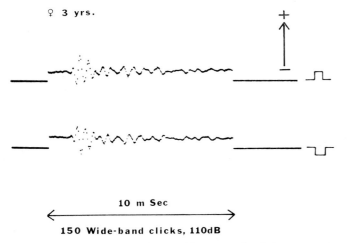

FIG. 9. This shows the trace of the cochlear microphonic in response to clicks in one polarity, above, and in the opposite polarity below. Note that, as the stimulus polarity is inverted, the cochlear-microphonic polarity is similarly inverted.

should allow this fact to be discovered, as in the case of non-organic hearing loss, or malingering (Figs. 4 and 5).

Young hyperactive children are often difficult to assess audiometrically and it was hoped that electric response audiometry would provide the answer to this problem. In fact this has been the case, in part, as it is possible to assess hyperactive children, if necessary under sedation or in natural sleep, but the interpretation of the results can be

difficult and testing rather tedious. In co-operative children, the V-potential, which differs somewhat from that of the adult by the presence of a frequently predominant second negative peak at about 250–300 ms, can be traced towards

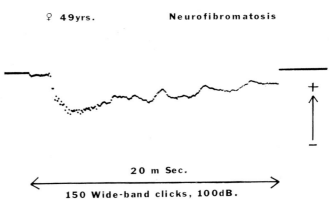

FIG. 10. This trace shows the compound action potential of the cochlear nerve in a patient with neuro-fibromatosis with probable involvement of the vestibulocochlear nerve. Vestibulocochlear (VIII) nerve tumours frequently show this wide trough-like nerve action potential with delayed recovery to the prestimulus level.

threshold as in adults, but it is not possible to identify the response as near to the audiometric zero as it is in adults. In pre-school children, a gap to 20 dB is not unreasonable and, for infants aged 1–2 years, a gap of 30 dB may be encountered. Thus, in many cases it is possible to determine the threshold of hearing only approximately. This would not be so bad except that, in the case of hyperactive children, the occurrence of large numbers of artefacts can make the interpretation even more difficult. Restlessness, if it cannot be allayed by careful handling of the child, must be overcome by the use of sedation and many different types of sedatives have been tried, including secobarbital (Davis, 1971), diazepam (Gestring, 1972), promethazine (Beagley et al., 1974; Stange, 1972) and pentobarbital (Morgon et al., 1971). Promethazine appears to be the most popular sedative for ERA at present (Burian, 1973). The ideal state of sleep for ERA is fairly deep, with large amplitude EEG. The rapid eye movement (REM) stage is generally considered unsuitable for ERA.

Using sedatives where necessary, it is usually possible to make an estimate of the hearing loss in children who are difficult to test. Long term follow-up has indicated that the assessment has been valid in the great majority of cases. It is essential for the tester to be a "non-enthusiast"—that is to say, he must adopt a sceptical view point which will lead him to accepting as a positive response only those traces which seem fairly definite. The tendency to give the patient the benefit of the doubt can lead to artefacts, which can be numerous in some children, being accepted as true responses. The sceptical attitude of the tester reduces this tendency and may be part of the reason that the thresholds by ERA tend to be higher than one would expect, i.e. that ERA seems less sensitive, especially in children. However, this fault is preferable to accepting a possible artefact as a true response. It is the difficulty of interpretation near threshold in children that makes the term "objective audiometry" somewhat objectionable as the interpretation is clearly very subjective from the tester's viewpoint at least. Nevertheless, if the tester works carefully, gross errors should be avoided. If the patient does not respond even to stimuli at very high intensities (100 dB or greater), one is either dealing with a very deaf subject, or the response is not being recognized. To some extent, this can be resolved by the use of an alternate stimulus through a different sense modality. For this purpose, it is possible to use a vibrator applied to the finger tips and actuated by 250 Hz electrical signal. This will make the vibrator vibrate at 250 Hz, as well as radiate an audible sound at 250 Hz. If the patient has not previously given an evoked response at high levels of sound stimulation, including 250 Hz, he may well respond to the 250 Hz vibratory stimulus. Or, alternatively, a flash of light from the stroboscope can be used as a stimulus. A subject who does not respond to high intensities of sound stimulation, but who does respond to a vibrator or a light stimulus will almost certainly be deaf.

Although ERA can be used successfully, if with some difficulty, in otherwise untestable, hyperactive young children, certain conditions make the test so difficult as to constitute an actual contra-indication. These conditions include epilepsy, athetotic cerebral palsy and spasmodic tics, all of which greatly impair the clarity of the ERA traces. Deaf-blind infants, on the other hand, can generally be tested successfully by ERA. In the hope of overcoming some of the problems associated with the signal analysis problems of identifying the V-potential in young children, Sayers, Beagley and Henshall (1974) have been examining the phase control mechanism that appears to be important in the generation of the V-potential. This is in the hope of being able to improve the signal extraction methods as an alternative to averaging. Averaging has a number of inherent disadvantages (in the mathematical sense) when the EEG background has frequency components in common with the evoked potential. It is hoped that this approach will be successful, as ERA does permit a typical audiogram to be constructed and this is a very attractive concept for the clinician. However, until some fundamental improvements can be achieved, the writer advocates, as a general working rule, that those children for whom sedation is thought to be essential should have their hearing assessed not by ERA, but by electrocochleography under ketamine anaesthesia and using a transtympanic electrode as described in the chapter by Aran and Portmann (Fig. 7–10).

In view of the decision to test the hearing of children who require sedation by electrocochleography instead of ERA, one may wonder whether or not there is any place for ERA in the assessment of hearing loss in young children, either now or in the future. However, it must be remembered that ERA, if it can be successfully applied, gives more information than does the electro-cochleogram.

Further refinements of this test are therefore desirable in general, and in one particular application which may well assume some importance in the future. This is the use of electronic cochlear implants for use in patients who are totally deaf. There is already a little experience in this field (House, 1973) although the physiological basis of the method still has many shortcomings (Kiang and Moxon, 1972). To date, it has been used on totally deafened adults whose deafness is purely sensory, i.e. with an intact cochlear nerve, e.g. after streptomycin-induced hearing loss. In adults, the history is often enough to indicate a case such as this, but in a young child one would need to be more circumspect if implanting an electronic prosthesis were contemplated as it would not be easy to decide whether or not the case is one of pure sensory (i.e. cochlear) deafness. It is clear that electrocochleography would not give sufficient information either, as only the first order neurone and the cochlear end-organ are assessed by this technique. A more comprehensive test might possibly be a form of ERA conducted at operation where the cochlea is stimulated by a series of electrical pulses to see whether or not cortical excitation followed. This would go some way towards ensuring that an intact neural pathway exists between the peripheral end-organ—the cochlea—and the cerebral cortex (Beagley, 1974). For this reason, further research into extraction of the auditory evoked cortical potential, possibly by monitoring the apparent phase control mechanism, as Sayers, Beagley and Henshall have suggested, seems desirable in this context.

The Early Vertex Potential. In the hope of avoiding some of the problems of determining the threshold of hearing by means of the V-potential, Davis and Hirsh (1973) have carried out careful trials of the early vertex potentials which occur in the 6–30 ms period following the onset of the stimulus. These small waves were described by Mendel and Goldstein (1969) and, in a small group of normal adults, they proved extremely stable. However, when tried by Davis and Hirsh on a series of children in various stages of sleep, they proved disappointing on account of the high false negative rate—that is to say where the early response was absent even though the classical V-potential could be positively identified. It therefore seems unlikely that in the immediate future a method of audiometry based on the early vertex responses will replace that based on the classical V-potential.

The Late Vertex Potentials (DC Responses). Under this heading are included two separate phenomena:

(1) the contingent negative variation (or expectancy wave) described by Grey Walter (1967) and others; and
(2) the dc shift discovered by Keidel and co-workers and described in Chapter 22.

The expectancy wave occurs under conditions of operant conditioning and attempts have been made, using words as stimuli, to associate this response with the semantic content of acoustic signals. This type of approach is described by Brix and Burian (1973) and, although difficult to evaluate, it is certainly of great interest as a potential method of evaluating the ability of the subject to appreciate differences in the semantic content of the signals employed. By contrast, the dc shift described by Keidel lasts for the duration of a long burst of a pure tone (i.e. about 1 s duration) and appears to be related to recognition of the quality or nature of the stimulus. Clearly, these dc shifts represent important physiological responses to various types of auditory stimulation and will no doubt lead eventually to better understanding of information processing by the central nervous system which will be valuable in audiological investigation. Keidel and Kallert also draw attention to the fact that, in experimental situations at least, it would be possible to use long trains of clicks, for example, to monitor all the currently recognized auditory evoked potentials from the very earliest to the latest, i.e. the compound action potential of the cochlear nerve (2–4 ms), the early vertex potential (6–30 ms), the V-potential (50–300 ms, or later in the case of children) and the long duration dc potentials. This would give a comprehensive electrophysiological view of the entire auditory system and it is an exciting concept. However, this is for the future; at the present time it can be stated that the only clinically valid neurophysiological tests in actual clinical use are the electrocochleogram, using the transtympanic electrode for preference (although superficial electrodes have some advantages), and ERA based upon recognition of the V-potential, as well as the acoustic stapedial reflex and the post-auricular response.

REFERENCES

Anderson, H., Barr, B. and Wedenberg, E. (1970), *Sensorineural Hearing Loss.* G. E. W. Wolstenhome and J. Knight, Eds.), pp. 275–289. Ciba Foundation Symposium. Churchill.
Antinoro, F., Skinner, P. H. and Jones, J. J. (1969), *J. acoust. Soc. Amer.*, **46**, 1433.
Antonelli, A. R. (1973), Paper read at X World Congress of Otorhinolaryngology, Venice.
Barr, B. (1955), *Acta oto-laryng.* (*Stockh.*), suppl. 121.
Beagley, H. A. (1973), *J. Laryng.*, **87**, 441,
Beagley, H. A. (1973), *Minerva O.R.L.*, **23**, 173.
Beagley, H. A. (1974), *Rev. Laryng.* In press.
Beagley, H. A., Gordon, A. G. and Fateen, A. M. (1972), *Sound*, **6**, 8.
Beagley, H. A., Hutton, J. N. T. and Hayes, R. A. (1974), *J. Laryng.* In press.
Beagley, H. A. and Kellogg, S. E. (1969), *Int. Audiology*, **8**, 345.
Beagley, H. A. and Kellogg, S. E. (1970), *Sound*, **4**, 86.
Beagley, H. A. and Knight, J. J. (1967), *J. Laryng.*, **81**, 861.
Békésy, G. (1947), *J. acoust. Soc. Amer.*, **19**, 452.
Bordley, J. E. and Hardy, W. G. (1949), *Ann. Otol.* (*St. Louis*), **58**, 751.
Brix, R. and Burian, K. (1973), *Audiology*, **12**, 481.
Burian, K. (1973), Paper read at X World Congress of Otorhinolaryngology, Venice.
Caton, R. (1875), *Brit. med. J.*, **2**, 278.
Chiveralls, K. and FitzSimons, R. (1973), *Brit. J. Audiol.*, **7**, 105.
Davis, H., Davis, P. A., Loomis, A. L., Harvey, F. M. and Hobart, G. (1939), *J. Neurophysiol.*, **2**, 500.
Davis, H. and Hirsh, S. K. (1973), *Rev. Laryng.* In press.
Davis, H. and Zerlin, S. (1966), *J. acoust. Soc. Amer.*, **39**, 109.
Dawson, G. D. (1954), *EEG Clin. Neurophysiol.*, **6**, 65.
Douek, E., Gibson, W. and Humphreys, K. (1973), *J. Laryng.*, **87**, 711.
Elberling, C. and Salomon, G. (1971), *Rev. Laryng.*, suppl. p. 691.
Gastaut, Y. (1954), *EEG Clin. Neurophysiol.*, **6**, 161.
Geisler, C. D., Frishkopf, L. S. and Rosenblith, W. A. (1958), *Science*, **128**, 1210.
Gestring, G. (1972). Personal communication.
Grey Walter, W. (1967), *EEG Clin. Neurophysiol.*, Suppl. **25**, 258.
Jewett, D. L. and Williston, J. S. (1971), *Brain*, **94**, 681.
Keidel, W. D. (1972), *J. Franc. ORL.*, **21**, 153.
Keidel, W. D. and Spreng, M. (1965), *Acta oto-laryng.* (*Stockh.*), **59**, 201.
Khechinashvili, S. N., Kevanishvili, Z. Sh., Khachidze, O. A. and Aphonchenko, V. S. (1974), *Br. J. Audiology*, **8**, 6.
Kiang, N. Y., Crist, A. G., French, M. A. and Edwards, A. G. (1963), *M.I.T. Quart. Rep.*, **68**, 218.
Kiang, N. Y. and Moxon, E. C. (1972), *Trans. Amer. otol. Soc.*, p. 72.
Klockhoff, I. and Andersen, H. (1960), *Acta Oto-laryng.* (*Stockh.*), **51**, 188.
Mendel, M. E. and Goldstein, R. (1969), *J. Speech Hear. Res.*, **12**, 344.
Morgon, A., Charachon, D. and Gerin, P. (1971), *Rev. Laryng.*, suppl., p. 765.
Portmann, M., Aran, J. M. and Le Bert, G. (1968), *Acta oto-laryng.* (*Stockh.*), **65**, 105.
Portmann, M. and Portmann, Cl. (1965), "Précis d'Audiométrie Clinique," Masson et Cie.
Ranke, O. (1950), *J. acoust. Soc. Amer.*, **22**, 772.
Rapin, I. (1964), *Acta oto-laryng.*, suppl. **206**, 113.
Sayers, B. McA., Beagley, H. A. and Henshall, W. (1974), *Nature.* **247**, 481.
Sohmer, H. and Feinmesser, M. (1967), *Ann. Otol* (*St. Louis*), **76**, 427.
Stange, G. (1972), *Arch. Klin. exp. Ohr.-, Nas.- u. Kehlk. Heilk*, **201**, 294.
Tasaki, I., Davis, H. and Legouix, J. P. (1952), *J. acoust. Soc. Amer.*, **24**, 502.
Terkildsen, K. and Nielsen, S. S. (1960), *Arch. Otolaryng.*, **72**, 339.
Terkildsen, K., Osterhammel, P. and Huis in't Veld, F. (1973), *Scand. Audiol.*, **2**, 141.
Vaughan, H. G. and Ritter, W. (1970), *EEG Clin. Neurophysiol.*, **28**, 360.
Wever, E. G. and Bray, C. W. (1930), *Psychol. Rev.*, **37**, 365.
Williams, H. L., Morlock, H. C., Morlock, J. V. and Lubin, A. (1964), *Ann. N.Y. Acad. Sci.*, **112**, 172.
Yoshie, N. and Ohashi, T. (1969), *Acta oto-laryng.*, suppl. 252, p. 71.
Zwislocki, J. (1961), *Ann. Otol.* (*St. Louis*), **70**, 559.

24. PSYCHOACOUSTICS

S. D. G. STEPHENS

Psychoacoustics is the branch of psychophysics concerned with auditory sensation and perception. The term psychophysics is generally attributed to Fechner (1860) and may be defined as "The science that investigates the quantitative relationship between physical stimuli and corresponding psychological events." Many of the phenomena which are generally considered under this umbrella term were, however, described long before the work of Fechner, although their detailed quantification has had to wait until the present century.

More important from the otologist's standpoint, psychoacoustics is the scientific basis of audiology. Most tests used in clinical audiology are based on the findings of psychoacoustics and the changes in psychoacoustical phenomena which may occur in different lesions or derangements of the auditory pathways.

Between the two disciplines, psychoacoustics and dia-

ance and speech perception. The former may be regarded in many ways as more psychological than acoustical, and is burdened with severe semantic difficulties, whereas the latter is afflicted with problems regarding accurate physical quantification, in addition to the inevitable problems arising with different languages and linguistic groups.

Each section will consist of a brief account of a particular psychoacoustical phenomenon and will include a section on actual or possible clinical applications.

Auditory Threshold and Detection Theory

The auditory threshold for a sound is customarily defined as the smallest intensity of that sound that could be consistently heard. In different studies "consistently" was variously defined usually as 50 per cent but sometimes as 75 per cent correct detection.

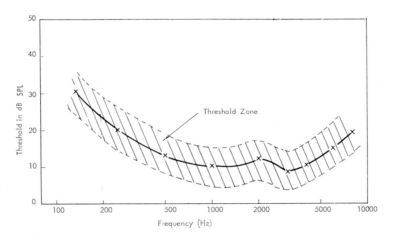

FIG. 1. Mean auditory threshold as a function of frequency.

gnostic audiology the main difference lies in the methodology employed. The psychoacousticist may spend hours or even days investigating a certain minor aspect of auditory function in a normal subject, and in order to study more subtle effects may need to look at the averaged results across a large number of experimental subjects. The audiologist, on the other hand, is looking for quick simple tests which he can use to define whether a particular patient shows normal or abnormal results and so to localize the site of his auditory lesion. The failure to recognize this distinction between priorities in the two disciplines has led to much confusion and many false trails being blazed by various workers trying to apply the techniques of one to the other.

In this account, I shall concentrate on the relatively simple perceptual phenomena of psychoacoustics and shall deliberately exclude the two phenomena of noise annoy-

Thresholds of hearing are defined in relation to some absolute acoustical measure. In experimental studies they are normally defined in terms of the sound pressure level (SPL) of the test tone which is expressed in decibels relative to 20 μPa. In a clinical context however, as the normal threshold varies in sound pressure level with the test frequency, the International Standards Organisation, as the result of studies on normal young adults in a number of different countries, has defined the normal average threshold in sound pressure level across the audiometric frequency range. This then acts as the standard for the calibration of audiometers (see Fig. 1).

Not every normally hearing person will have 0 dB hearing across his audiometric range. Some may hear better at some frequencies and worse at others, the normal curve being an average figure. Even normal people may show different results at different times. Thresholds can be influenced by the positioning of headphones on the head (low frequencies leaking out from loose fitting phones, and high frequency detection being influenced by their precise positioning), by the motivation and practice of the subject (Watson and Clopton, 1969), by the background noise in the test environment and by variations in the subject's detection threshold and judgement criterior (Robinson, 1960). The measured threshold can also be influenced by the technique used to measure it, whether a descending threshold approach (coming down from high intensities until the subject no longer responds), an ascending approach (coming up from below until the subject responds) or a bracketing approach around the threshold is used (Hirsh, 1952).

The application of the theory of signal detectability to psychoacoustics in the mid 1950's (Swets, 1964) led to a fresh consideration of the auditory threshold and even the question as to whether it actually existed at all (Swets, 1961). It was pointed out that the strategy adopted by the subject could have a considerable effect when threshold was defined in classical ways. For example if a subject was instructed to respond whenever he thought a signal might possibly be present, he detected considerably more signals than if he was instructed to respond only if he was absolutely certain that he heard the sound. In the former condition the subject also makes many "false positive" responses: That is, he responds that he thinks there is a signal present when in fact there is none. In the latter condition he would make very few, if any, false positive responses. The theory of signal detectability takes the incidence of these false positives into account in the definition of the detectability measure d′ (pronounced "d-prime") by comparing the results obtained in a trial when a signal is present with those obtained when no signal is present. This measure d′ may be defined as difference of the means of the two neural response distributions (X on Fig. 2) divided by the standard deviation

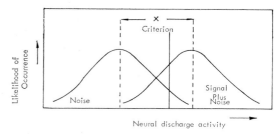

Fig. 2. Histograms showing the distribution of neural discharge activity in the presence of noise alone, and in the presence of signal plus noise.

(Green and Swets, 1966). The second measure commonly used in signal detection theory is that of β, which specifies the criterion adopted by the subject, and may be defined as the ratio of the ordinate of the signal and noise distribution to that of the noise distribution at the criterion point. For all purposes, the threshold is considered as a threshold-in-noise task, whether that noise is added, existing physiological acoustic noise arising from the blood vessels in the external acoustic meatus, or merely spontaneous neural activity.

The applications of these principles to audiometry are based on the attempts to reduce the variance of the threshold measures, particularly when the criterion adopted by the subject is of little interest to the experimenter. A study in which the threshold was determined either by a standard audiometric technique or by a detection theory method in which the threshold was expressed in terms of an arbitrary value of d′ = 1·00, gave a reduction in the median intra-subject variance of 2–3 dB^2 for the latter technique, although some subjects showed a larger variance in the detection part of the experiment (Stephens, 1969). The main problem here appears to lie in the considerably increased length of the test session necessary to obtain signal detection.

Difference Limens

Difference limens are based on Weber's concept of the just noticeable difference (JND). As its name implies, the JND is the smallest change in a certain parameter of a stimulus that can be detected. Weber formulated the concept of the Weber-Fechner law which states that the JND is a constant fraction of the test stimulus. Unfortunately this concept has been shown to be not strictly true for a number of auditory measures.

The difference limens normally considered in an auditory context are those for the intensity, frequency and duration of the acoustical stimulus. Of these, the intensity difference limen has been most extensively studied and applied in a clinical context. Two methods are normally used to determine the intensity difference limen. In the first the subject is required to detect a small change in an otherwise constant sound, and in the second he is required to indicate whether two successive sounds are of the same or different intensities. The intensity difference limen is greater just above the auditory threshold than at higher intensities (Miller, 1947), a fact that is used in the Denes-Naunton test (1950) in a clinical context, which compares the intensity difference limen at 4 dB sensation level with that at 40 dB sensation level. This was based on the premise that in normally hearing patients the difference limen at 40 dB should be smaller than that at 4 dB, whereas in patients with recruitment this difference was reputed to disappear. The idea that patients with cochlear lesions have a relatively smaller difference limen at just supra-threshold levels has been proposed as an application of Békésy audiometry in that these patients were thought to have shown a smaller excursion size with a continuous Békésy stimulus (Békésy, 1947).

Differences at a higher sensation level between recruiting and non-recruiting patients were proposed as a basis of the Lüscher-Zwislocki (1949) and SISI tests (Jerger et al., 1959), but, at equal sound pressure levels, the intensity difference limens for normal and cochlear damaged patients does not differ significantly. Some patients with neural lesions do, however, show larger difference limens.

The intensity difference limen is also dependent upon the frequency and the duration of the test stimulus. With increasing frequency at the same sensation level, the intensity difference limen becomes smaller. There has been much controversy about the effect of stimulus duration on the intensity difference limen. Some recent very careful studies involving pedestal experiments, in which the increment to be discriminated is an increase of variable duration in the intensity of a pure tone of fixed duration (the pedestal) presented in a background of noise, suggest that when the duration of the increment is decreased below 150 ms, its intensity must be increased by 6 dB/decade of shortening (i.e. changing from 150–15 ms) (Leshowitz and Wightman, 1971). This compares with about 10 dB/decade change in a simple threshold or noise-masked threshold task.

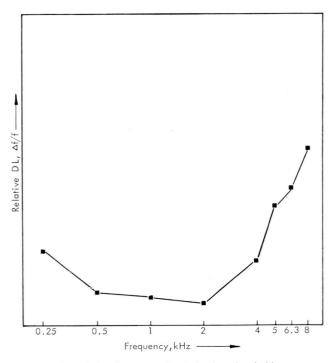

FIG. 3. Relative frequency discrimination thresholds as a function of frequency and sensation level.

Frequency discrimination has been proposed as a clinical tool, on the assumption that patients with cochlear lesions have larger frequency difference limens than normally hearing patients. However auditory pathology is only one of a number of factors which may influence a person's ability in this respect, others being the test frequency, the intensity and duration of the stimulus, and the training of the subject, so that musicians after training have smaller frequency difference limens than untrained listeners. Because of these sources of variability, this test has found relatively little favour as a diagnostic test for cochlear lesions. Figure 3 shows the complex relationship between intensity and frequency of the difference limen, which is expressed here as the relative difference limen df/f, which is more constant over frequency (Shower and Biddulph, 1931). The duration of the signal influences the frequency difference limen over durations shorter than about 200 ms. Thus as the duration of the stimulus is shortened below this point the frequency difference limen increases with shortening duration

(Turnbull, 1944). It has been suggested that the frequency difference limen for very short durations is selectively impaired in the ear contralateral to a lesion involving the auditory cortex on one side (Gersuni, 1971).

The duration discrimination of a signal is again dependent on the overall signal duration, even when expressed as a ratio dt/t. Thus, again for long sounds this value is relatively constant, but increases as the sound is shortened below about 100 ms (Small and Campbell, 1962). It is influenced by the stimulus intensity in that the difference limen becomes shorter with increasing intensity. The stimulus frequency, on the other hand, has no appreciable influence on duration discrimination. At the present time this has been little used in a clinical context, although physiological studies on animals suggest that it may have some relevance in the localization of lesions in the central auditory pathways (Neff, 1967).

Auditory Temporal Integration

This is the sensory phenomenon in which a sound becomes louder or more detectable when, within certain limits, its duration is increased. A typical example of the change in auditory threshold with tonal duration for a 1000 Hz tone is shown in Fig. 4.

From this figure it may be seen that as the duration of the tone is sortened below about 200 ms, the threshold increases with a slope of about 10 dB/decade shortening of duration. Thus constant energy tones of different durations over this range remain equally detectable. For the very short duration tones of less than about 15 ms this slope of increased threshold with shortening duration becomes even greater, so that the intensity of these very short sounds must be increased beyond the equal energy point for them to be equally detectable as the longer duration signals.

This same general pattern is found also in noise-masked thresholds and in loudness studies. In the latter, however, the results found are very variable and dependent on the exact methodology used, so that the detailed configuration is still very uncertain (Scharf, 1970).

The end-point of the increase in detectability with duration is known as the critical duration. This critical duration may be rather difficult to define, as the integration curve follows an exponential pattern, although it has been fitted with a series of straight-line components showing some increase in detectability with increasing duration even up to $1\frac{1}{2}$ s (Licklider and Green, 1959).

The critical duration varies considerably with different individuals although these all show a consistent effect of different stimulus parameters. Thus the critical duration shortens with increasing stimulus intensity (Miller, 1948) and with stimulus frequency (Watson and Gengel, 1969). The latter effect of the stimulus frequency is, however, even more complicated in that it appears to be a function of the test technique used, showing a marked shortening of the critical duration with increasing stimulus frequency in detection studies, whereas with Békésy audiometry and other tracking techniques there appears to be little frequency effect (Gengel and Watson, 1971).

In patients with cochlear lesions the slope of change in

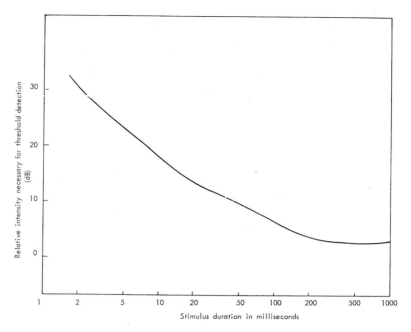

FIG. 4. Auditory temporal integration at 1000 Hz.

threshold with duration may be considerably reduced (as low as 3 dB/decade) and the critical duration shortened (Elliott, 1963). The slope may be reduced in potentially damaging conditions such as noise exposure even when there is no shift of the auditory threshold, so that it has been proposed as the most sensitive measure of cochlear function (Eisenberg, 1956).

It has also been suggested that in patients with a lesion in the auditory cortex there is a particular elevation of threshold to very short duration sounds in the ear contralateral to the lesion (Baru, 1966).

Loudness

Loudness is the subjective impression of the intensity of a sound. When the growth of loudness is plotted against increasing stimulus intensity, the results are best fitted by a power-law formulation (Stevens, 1956),

$$\psi = kI^n$$

where ψ = loudness, I = stimulus intensity and k and n are constants.

Thus, when the logarithm of the subjective rating of loudness is plotted against the logarithm of the stimulus intensity there is a straight line relationship with a slope of n, i.e. n is the exponent in the power function.

This straight line relationship breaks down at lower suprathreshold intensities, when the rate of growth of loudness with intensity is increased (*see* Fig. 5). This effect is greater at lower frequencies (e.g. 125, 250 Hz) where the auditory threshold is limited by physiological acoustic noise in the external acoustic meatus, than at higher frequencies, where the limiting factor is random neural "noise". This rapid growth of loudness at low frequencies is known as physiological recruitment, in distinction from the pathological recruitment found in

patients with damaged cochleae (Stevens, 1966). It has been proposed as a means of directly measuring the presence of recruitment, by comparing the growth of loudness at 250 Hz and 4000 Hz (Stephens, 1971). In the absence

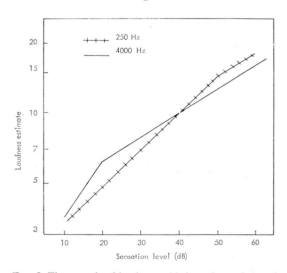

FIG. 5. The growth of loudness with intensity at 250 and 4000 Hz.

of pathological recruitment, the rate of growth of loudness is greater at 250 Hz, but with high frequency cochlear lesions, it is greater at 4000 Hz.

Two scales have been used for expressing the general loudness of a sound. The first of these is the phon scale (Fletcher and Munson, 1933) in which a tone is expressed as the sound pressure level of a 1000 Hz tone which is equally loud. This is referred to as the loudness level of the sound. Thus when a sound is considered equally loud to a

1000 Hz tone of 70 dB SPL it is said to have a loudness of 70 phons, or one of 40 dB, 40 phons.

The second scale commonly used in the sone scale (Stevens, 1936), which is a logarithmic scale based on the 40 phon tone which has a loudness of 1 sone. A tone of 50 phons is regarded as being twice as loud and thus has a loudness of 2 sones, one of 60 phons, 4 sones, etc. A number of complex formulae have been devised to calculate the loudness of complex sounds, based on the sound pressures of the components of different octave bands (Stevens, 1972).

The sensation of loudness has been subdivided into the two components of tonal volume and tonal density. The former is the sensation of "size" or enveloping sensation produced by the tone, particularly in a free-field situation. This component is marked at low frequencies, decreasing with increasing frequency. The tonal density or "compactness" of a sound, on the other hand, is particularly marked at the high frequencies, decreasing with decreasing frequency. Loudness has been shown to be a product of tonal volume and tonal density (Stevens *et al.*, 1965).

Critical Bands

It has been shown that around each tonal frequency there is a critical bandwidth of tones (e.g. about 160 Hz wide at 1000 Hz) within which the integration of loudness is complete (Scharf, 1970). That is to say that if the power of the sound is all concentrated at the centre frequency, or the same power is spread throughout the critical band, the sound will have the same loudness. This is true of narrow band noise and for combinations of pure tones. The critical bandwidths may be measured by gradually increasing the bandwidth of noise of constant sound pressure level and noting the point at which the loudness begins to increase. This point is taken as the critical bandwidth.

Likewise if a pure tone is masked by two narrow bands of noise on either side of it frequency-wise, when the separation of these bands of noise is increased there is no change in the threshold for the tone until the separation of the bands exceeds the critical bandwidth. When this happens, the noise threshold drops rapidly. It is obvious that the critical bandwidth can be easily measured this way and the results support those found in loudness experiments.

The magnitude of the critical band increases with frequency above 300 Hz, below which the results are less certain. The overall relationship to frequency is shown in Fig. 6.

Closely related to the critical bandwidth is the critical ratio, generally taken as 2/5 of the critical bandwidth. This is the bandwidth of the frequencies in white noise around a test tone which contribute to the masking of that tone. It was based on the assumption that the power in this band was equal to the power of the tone.

The change in critical bandwidth with frequency has been related to relative lengths of those sections of the cochlea representing those frequencies. The critical band corresponds to about 1·3 mm along the basilar membrane. It has thus also been related to the magnitude of the difference limen for pitch and to the mel scale of pitch.

On the basis of these analogies it is perhaps not surprising that in patients with cochlear pathology, critical bandwidths have been found to be abnormally wide or even absent (de Boer, 1959). This has been shown using narrow-band noise-masking techniques and in loudness studies. The analagous critical ratio effect has also been used as one of the bases of Langenbeck's "noise audiometry" (1965).

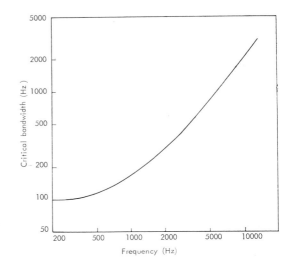

FIG. 6. Critical bandwidth as a function of centre frequency. (After Scharf, 1970.)

Masking

Masking is the phenomenon by which one sound impairs the perception of another. What is normally understood by masking in a general acoustical context is ipsilateral direct masking which occurs when the masker and test sound are both in the same frequency region and presented to the same ear. Masking used in a clinical context is, strictly speaking, contralateral direct masking due to the fact that the test-tone and the masker are applied to opposite ears. However, as its function is to mask out the sounds arriving by bone conduction at the ear to which it is applied, the exact terminological position is somewhat difficult.

Masking can, however, be of different frequency to the test tone, presented to the opposite ear, or even be presented before or after the test tone, yet still be effective.

As was seen in the previous section, for the direct masking to be effective, normally some of the masking noise must come within the critical bandwidth of the tone to be masked. However, at relatively high intensities (over 60–70 dB SPL) the phenomenon of "remote masking" may occur (Bilger and Hirsh, 1956), and a noise or tone distant in frequency from the test tone may produce a considerable shift in the threshold for that tone. This is thought to be due to a kind of distortion process occurring in the cochlea, perhaps related to the overload phenomenon (Deatherage *et al.*, 1957).

Of more relevance to the normal clinical context is the phenomenon of "central masking". This arises from the lack of neurological isolation between the inputs from the two ears, and is the means by which a tone or noise presented to one ear can shift the threshold of a tone of the same or near frequency in the opposite ear, despite the two ears being acoustically isolated from each other (Wegel and Lane, 1924). This effect has been shown to have similar critical bandwidth characteristics as direct masking, but to be very dependent on the difference in time of onset between the test tone and the masker. Thus if the masker and the test tone are switched on simultaneously there is a large central masking effect, which declines rapidly until there is a delay of about 200 ms between the onset of masker and test tone, when the effect reaches its minimal level (Zwislocki et al., 1967). In a clinical masking context, when effective masking noise is applied to the ear contralateral to the test tone, this may result in an abnormally elevated threshold in the contralateral ear as a result of central masking.

When a masker is terminated before a test tone begins, provided the separation between masker and tone is less than about 200 ms, it will still have a masking effect (Samoilova, 1959). This is known as forward (or post-stimulatory) masking. The time course of the decay of this masking effect from the masker offset is similar to that for central masking, and is shown in Fig. 7, which

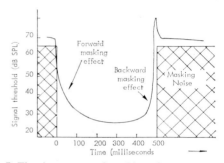

FIG. 7. The time course of masking of a pure tone signal during a gap in a noise masker. (After Elliott, 1969.)

illustrates both this and backward masking in the context of interruptions of the masking stimulus (Elliott, 1969).

Thus in contrast to forward masking, there is the phenomenon of backward (or pre-stimulatory) masking, by which a masking noise of sufficient intensity can mask a signal which has preceded it. The time course of this phenomenon is much shorter and the effect is not measurable if there is more than about 50 ms between the stimulus offset and the masker onset (Elliott, 1962). This phenomenon is less easily explained than that of forward masking which can be regarded as being a result of the time course of the decay of neural activity evoked by the masker. Backward masking, on the other hand, can be explained only by a mechanism which enables the later activity evoked by an intense masker to overtake the effects of a less intense test stimulus.

Adaptation and Fatigue

Adaptation is the reduced sensation of loudness which is experienced while an adapting stimulus is being presented, whereas fatigue or temporary threshold shift (TTS) is the shift in the threshold found after that fatiguing stimulus is

stopped. Adaptation may be demonstrated by matching the loudness of the adapting tone to an intermittent tone in the opposite ear at the beginning of the experiment. After the tone has been present for several minutes and the balance is repeated its subjective loudness will be found to have decreased.

In a clinical context, the degree of fatigue produced by a sound has been proposed as a measure of the likely danger of permanent hearing damage which would be produced by sustained exposure to that sound. Much work has been based on the relationship between the temporary threshold shift produced by a noise in the course of a short period of time, and the permanent hearing loss which would result from sustained exposure to that noise. The relationship between the two is still, however, far from clear (Ward, 1963).

One or other measure of the adaptation phenomenon is widely used in clinical audiology, where marked adaptation is held to be indicative of a neuronal lesion, especially that due to a tumour (Reger, 1965). Abnormal adaptation is usually sought at threshold, where it is also variously termed "tone decay" (Carhart, 1957), relapse or temporary threshold drift. At a supra-threshold level, abnormal adaptation may be investigated either subjectively or objectively. Subjective recordings may be done using Békésy audiometry and recording the patient's most comfortable loudness level for a sustained test tone. Objectively, one can measure the decay of the acoustic stapedius reflex (Anderson et al., 1970).

The detailed characteristics of adaptation and fatigue differ quite considerably from each other. The greatest adaptation occurs at the adapting frequency with the degree of adaptation at adjacent frequencies falling away steeply (see Fig. 8) (Small, 1963). Fatigue, on the other hand, characteristically produces its greatest effect at about $\frac{1}{2}$-octave above the peak frequency of the fatiguing stimulus (Ward, 1962).

The time courses of the two phenomena also differ quite considerably with most adaptation being complete within about 3 min of stimulus onset (Egan, 1955). Fatigue, however, will continue to increase with the stimulus duration over periods of hours (Ward et al., 1958). Likewise the recovery from adaptation will generally be complete within 2–3 min or even shorter, whereas recovery from auditory fatigue may continue over a period of days.

The effects of the intensity of the stimulus differ considerably in adaptation and fatigue with a fairly regular increase in the adaptation with stimulus intensity, perhaps even flattening off at the higher intensities. The fatiguing effect of a stimulus, on the other hand, is marked only at high intensities, above 80 dB SPL, after which it increases rapidly with increasing stimulus intensity.

The effects of adaptation are thought to occur at a neural level, with its time course and other effects closely paralleling those of neural activity in the auditory nerve. Fatigue on the other hand, occurs at a predominantly cochlear level with many of its psychophysical effects being analagous to changes found in the electrical potentials of the cochlea (Elliott and Fraser, 1970).

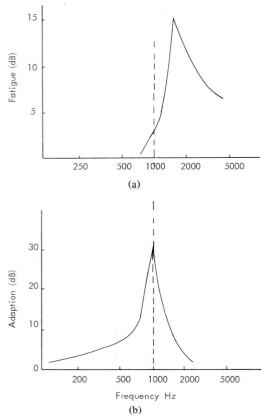

FIG. 8. (a) Fatigue produced by 1000 Hz tone. (b) Adaptation produced by a 1000 Hz tone.

Pitch

Pitch is the subjective impression of the frequency of a sound. It was traditionally expressed on a logarithmic scale as the basis of the musical octaves, each of which is twice the frequency of the octave below. However, when the mel scale of pitch was developed (1000 mels is the pitch of a 1000 Hz tone of 40 phons) by careful experimentation (Stevens and Volkmann, 1940), it was found that this logarithmic relationship did not strictly hold true, the actual results coming somewhere between a linear and a logarithmic relationship.

The term "absolute pitch" is reserved for the ability of certain individuals to identify or sing a specific note on demand. It is uncertain how much this is due to natural endowment and how much to training, and the ability to do this has been shown to fluctuate over periods of time (Wynn, 1972).

Pitch and frequency are not synonymous terms and the pitch of a tone of a given frequency may be altered by changing its intensity or duration. When low frequency sounds are presented at very high intensities, they appear to become even lower in pitch, and high frequency tones at high intensities appear higher in pitch (Ward, 1965).

With the increase of the duration of a tone, it goes through several stages of pitch development. Initially when very short, it sounds just like a click with no tonal quality. When the duration is increased it acquires the

quality known as "click-pitch" in which it still sounds like a click but has some quality of pitch. Finally, as the duration is increased still further, it may have a click onset and offset but there is a definite tonal quality in between. This stage is known as "tone-pitch" (Bürck *et al.*, 1935). The thresholds, in terms of duration at which these changes occur, have been referred to as the "click pitch threshold" and "tone-pitch threshold" respectively (Doughty and Garner, 1947). They are both very dependent on the frequency (Fig. 9) and the intensity of the tone, shortening with increasing intensity. In a clinical context this measure of tone-pitch threshold as a function of intensity has been proposed as a test for vertebrobasilar artery disease in which condition the threshold is reported to be increased (Broomsliter *et al.*, 1964). Analagous changes may be found by looking at the change in frequency discrimination with stimulus duration (Moore, 1972).

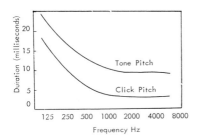

FIG. 9. The relationship between frequency and stimulus duration required for the establishment of "click pitch" and "tone pitch". (After Doughty and Garner, 1947.)

Localization and Lateralization

Auditory localization is the ability to identify the source of a sound in space. In the lateralization task, on the other hand, sounds are normally presented through headphones and the subject locates them within his head.

Conceptually the most difficult aspect of localization from a physiological standpoint is localization in the vertical plane. Here the subject does not have the advantage of different inputs from his two ears but is still able to locate with some degree of accuracy the source of the sound. Some studies have shown that predominantly high frequency sounds are necessary for this phenomenon (Roffler and Butler, 1968). The most careful studies in this field suggest that the auricle plays an important role in this phenomenon, with its different components acting as parabolic reflectors, reflecting the sound into the external acoustic meatus and producing echoes some 100–300 μs after the main component of the sound has entered the meatus (Batteau, 1967). The separation of the echoes depends on the elevation of the sound. A different suggestion proposes a "comb filter" mechanism again based on the shape of the auricle (Blauert, 1970). In a clinical context it has been found that certain patients with central auditory lesions are able to localize horizontally but not vertically (Walsh, 1957), but a problem in this respect is the difficulty which a number of apparently normal subjects experience in vertical localization.

Horizontal localization in which the two ears are used

has been far more extensively studied and the mechanisms are better understood. The subjective component of localization as opposed to lateralization is again considered to be dependent on the echoes or comb filter effects produced by the auricle, which enable even a patient with complete unilateral hearing loss to have some degree of localization ability.

However, in the normal person this component plays a minimal role, with most clues for horizontal localization and lateralization coming from three major components of the stimulus. These are the time difference between the stimulus onsets, the phase difference, and the intensity difference between the two ears. The time difference is important in the case of transient sounds and stimulus onsets, but not for sustained tones. The phase difference is important for the latter but applies only up to 1000–1500 Hz, beyond which the wavelength of the tone becomes too short in relation to the interaural separation for phase to be relevant (Nordlund, 1962). The intensity difference is important in the localization of high frequency tones in which the "head-shadow" effect occurs, and also in the lateralization of clicks. Physiological studies have shown a complex additive mechanism occurring for time and intensity difference cues (Hall, 1964).

Similarly, in experiments on the lateralization of clicks, it is possible to manipulate the apparent sound source through the head by trading-off the intensity difference between the ears with the time difference. For these studies on clicks a trading relationship of the order of 15 μs.dB^{-1} has been found.

Abnormal horizontal localization and lateralization is found in patients with lesions of the VIIIth nerve and is also reported in brain-stem lesions in which the integration of the information from the two ears is not possible (Nordlund, 1964). Most of these tests have used clicks presented with a time delay between the two ears, perhaps the most ingenious device being a stethoscope with the two earpieces connected together via a curved metal tube which could be tapped in different places to produce different time differences between the two ears (Groen, 1969). The position with regard to lesions in the auditory cortex is more complicated and controversial and a complex localization task is probably necessary to identify patients with such lesions.

Other Binaural Phenomena

Involved in lateralization is the phenomenon known in detection studies as the Masking Level Difference (MLD). This is the threshold shift which results from changes in the interaural phase relations. For example, consider the case when noise is presented in phase to the two ears and a tone has to be detected against this background noise. When the tone is presented in phase to the two ears its threshold is about 15 dB less sensitive than if it is presented 180° out of phase to the two ears (Hirsh, 1948). When the tone is presented monaurally, or the noise in the two ears is uncorrelated, intermediate results are found (see Fig. 10). It is thought that this interaction occurs in the olivary complex, so that it could be used as a test for the integrity of that part of the brainstem. Un-

fortunately, however, the universality of the effect is far from definite. It is also dependent on a number of stimulus factors, the maximal effects being found at about 200 Hz. As the stimuli are increased far above the threshold level the effect rapidly disappears (Townsend and Goldstein, 1972).

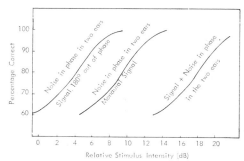

Fig. 10. Psychometric functions under different binaural conditions. Masking noise at constant level.

A related phenomenon is found in effects of contralateral stimulation on the intensity difference limen. It has been shown that the intensity difference limen for intensity modulated tones is increased by contralateral stimulation of the same frequency. Conversely, contralateral stimulation with a different frequency reduces the difference limen (Chocholle, 1959). In a clinical context the comparison of the intensity difference limen under conditions of contralateral stimulation of the same and different frequencies appears to provide a promising tool for the detection of brainstem lesions (Stephens, 1972).

A large number of other auditory phenomena have been described of various degrees of importance, some of which, such as the threshold of overload (Lawrence and Yantis, 1956) have been advocated as diagnostic tools. In a brief account of this nature it is inevitable that much selection must occur, but an attempt has been made to present the most important psychophysical phenomena and those with most current or potential use in a clinical diagnostic context.

REFERENCES

Anderson, H., Barr, B. and Wedenberg, E. (1970), *Sensorineural Hearing Loss* (G. W. Wolsthenholme and J. Knight, Eds.). London: Churchill.
Baru, A. V. (1966), *Zh. Vyssh. nerv. Deyat. I.P. Pavlova*, **16**, 655.
Batteau, D. W. (1967), *Proc. roy. Soc. B*, **168**, 158.
Békésy, G. von (1947), *Acta oto-laryng. (Stockh.)*, **35**, 411.
Boer, E. de (1959), *Proc. 3rd I.C.A.*, **1**, 100.
Bilger, R. C. and Hirsh, I. (1956), *J. acoust. Soc. Amer.*, **28**, 623.
Blauert, J. (1970), *Acustica*, **22**, 205.
Broomsliter, P. C., Creel, W. and Powers, R. J. (1964), *J. acoust. Soc. Amer.*, **36**, 1958.
Bürck, W., Kotowski, P. and Lichte, H. (1935), *Elek. Nachr. Techn.*, **12**, 278.
Carhart, R. (1957), *Arch. Otolaryng.*, **65**, 32.
Chocholle, R. (1959), *Acustica*, **9**, 309.
Deatherage, B. H., Davis, M. and Eldredge, D. H. (1957), *J. acoust. Soc. Amer.*, **29**, 132.
Denes, P. and Naunton, R. E. (1950), *J. Laryng.*, **64**, 375.
Doughty, J. M. and Garner, W. R. (1947), *J. exp. Psychol.*, **37**, 351.
Egan, J. P. (1955), *J. acoust. Soc. Amer.*, **27**, 111.

Eisenberg, R. B. (1956), "A Study of Auditory Threshold in Normal and in Hearing Impaired Persons," D.Sc. Thesis, Johns Hopkins University.

Elliott, D. N. and Fraser, W. (1970), *Foundations of Modern Auditory Theory*, Vol. 1 (J. V. Tobias, Ed.). New York: Academic Press.

Elliott, L. L. (1962), *J. acoust. Soc. Amer.*, **34**, 1108.

Elliott, L. L. (1963), *J. acoust. Soc. Amer.*, **35**, 578.

Elliott, L. L. (1969), *J. acoust. Soc. Amer.*, **45**, 1277.

Fechner, G. T. (1860), *Elemente der Psychophysik*. Leipzig: Breitkof and Härtel.

Fletcher, H. and Munson, W. A. (1933), *J. acoust. Soc. Amer.*, **24**, 80.

Gengel, R. W. and Watson, C. S. (1971), *J. Speech Hear. Dis.*, **36**, 213.

Gersuni, G. V. (Ed.) (1971), *Sensory Processes at the Neuronal and Behavioural Levels*. New York: Academic Press.

Green, D. M. and Swets, J. A. (1966), *Signal Detection Theory and Psychophysics*. New York: John Wiley.

Groen, J. J. (1969), *Acta oto-laryng. (Stockh.)*, **67**, 326.

Hall, J. L. (1964), MIT Electronics Research Lab. Tech. Rep. 416.

Hirsh, I. J. (1948), *J. acoust. Soc. Amer.*, **20**, 536.

Hirsh, I. J. (1952), *The Measurement of Hearing*. New York: McGraw-Hill.

Jerger, J., Shedd, J. and Harford, E. (1959), *Arch. Otolaryng.*, **69**, 200.

Langenbeck, B. (1965), *Textbook of Practical Audiometry*. London: Edward Arnold.

Lawrence, M. and Yantis, P. A. (1956), *Arch. Otolaryng.*, **63**, 653.

Leshowitz, B. and Wightman, F. L. (1971), *J. acoust. Soc. Amer.*, **49**, 1180.

Licklider, J. C. R. and Green, D. M. (1959), *Proc. 3rd ICA*, 114.

Lüscher, E. and Zwislocki, J. (1949), *Acta oto-laryng. (Stockh.)*, suppl. **78**, 156.

Miller, G. A. (1947), *J. acoust. Soc. Amer.*, **19**, 609.

Miller, G. A. (1948), *J. acoust. Soc. Amer.*, **20**, 160.

Moore, B. C. J., (1972), *Sound*, **6**, 73.

Neff, W. D. (1967), *Sensorineural Hearing Processes and Disorders* (A. B. Graham, Ed.). London: Churchill.

Nordlund, B. (1962), *Acta oto-laryng. (Stockh.)*, **55**, 405.

Nordlund, B. (1964), *Acta oto-laryng. (Stockh.)*, **57**, 1.

Reger, S. N. (1965), *Audiometry: Principles and Practice* (A. Glorig, Ed.). Baltimore: Williams and Wilkins.

Robinson, D. W. (1960), *Ann Occup. Hyg.*, **2**, 107.

Roffler, S. K. and Butler, R. A. (1968), *J. acoust. Soc. Amer.*, **43**, 1255.

Samoilova, I. K. (1959), *Proc. 3rd ICA*, 139.

Scharf, B. (1970), *Foundations of Modern Auditory Theory*, Vol. 1 (J. V. Tobias, Ed.). New York: Academic Press.

Shower, E. G. and Biddulph, R. (1931), *J. acoust. Soc. Amer.*, **3**, 275.

Small, A. M. (1963), *Modern Developments in Audiometry* (J. Jerger, Ed.). New York: Academic Press.

Small, A. M. and Campbell, R. A. (1962), *Amer. J. Psychol.*, **75**, 401.

Stephens, S. D. G. (1969), *Int. Audiol.*, **8**, 131.

Stephens, S. D. G. (1971), *Sound*, **5**, 73.

Stephens, S. D. G. (1972), *Audiology*, **11**, suppl. p. 138.

Stevens, S. S. (1936), *Psychol. Rev.*, **43**, 405.

Stevens, S. S. (1956), *Amer. J. Psychol.*, **69**, 1.

Stevens, S. S. (1966), *J. acoust. Soc. Amer.*, **39**, 725.

Stevens, S. S. (1972), *J. acoust. Soc. Amer.*, **51**, 575.

Stevens, S. S., Guirao, M. and Slawson, A. W. (1965), *J. exp. Psychol.*, **69**, 503.

Stevens, S. S. and Volkmann, J. (1940), *Amer. J. Psychol.*, **53**, 329.

Swets, J. A. (1961), *Science*, **134**, 168.

Swets, J. A. (Ed.) (1964), *Signal Detection and Regognition by Human Observers*. New York: John Wiley.

Townsend, T. H. and Goldstein, D. P. (1972), *J. acoust. Soc. Amer.*, **51**, 621.

Turnbull, W. (1944), *J. Exp. Psychol.*, **34**, 302.

Walsh, E. G. (1957), *Brain*, **80**, 222.

Ward, W. D. (1962), *J. acoust. Soc. Amer.*, **34**, 1610.

Ward, W. D. (1963), *Modern Developments in Audiology* (J. Jerger, Ed.). New York: Academic Press.

Ward, W. D. (1965), *Audiometry: Principles and Practice* (A. Glorig, Ed.). Baltimore: Williams and Wilkins.

Ward, W. D., Glorig, A. and Sklar, D. L. (1958), *J. acoust. Soc. Amer.*, **30**, 944.

Watson, C. S. and Clopton, B. M. (1969), *Perception and Psychophysics*, **5**, 281.

Watson, C. S. and Gengel, R. W. (1969), *J. acoust. Soc. Amer.*, **46**, 989.

Wegel, R. L. and Lane, C. E. (1924), *Physiol. Rev.*, **23**, 266.

Wynn, V. T. (1972), *J. Physiol.*, **220**, 627.

Zwislocki, J. J., Damianopoulos, E. N., Buining, E. and Glantz, J. (1967), *Perception and Psychophysics*, **2**, 59.

25. APPLICATION OF PSYCHO-ACOUSTICS TO CENTRAL AUDITORY DYSFUNCTION

S. D. G. STEPHENS

INTRODUCTION

The differential diagnosis of lesions in the middle ear, cochlea and cochlear nerve has become relatively easy with the development and refinement of audiometric tests over the past two decades. By contrast, the diagnosis of lesions affecting more central parts of the auditory pathway remains something of a morass. Figure 1 shows the main sections of the afferent central auditory pathways schematically.

The main factor in this difference between the diagnosis of central and peripheral lesions was succinctly put by Jerger (1964) when he contrasted the disastrous effects of severe or even total deafness which could arise if a tiny piece of wire is inadvertently dropped into the labyrinth during stapes surgery, with the minimal and subtle changes in hearing found when an entire temporal lobe is removed.

A second factor, arising partly from the first, is that most patients with central nervous system lesions affecting the auditory pathway generally suffer concomitantly from other neurological symptoms more serious to their general wellbeing than their minor auditory problems. Thus they present to neurological departments where they are rarely subjected to extensive audiological investigation.

However in the past 20 years some progress has been made in this field, stemming largely from the extensive work of Bocca and his colleagues in Italy with a great variety of speech tests (e.g. Bocca and Calearo, 1963).

The various approaches to the problems of lesions in the central auditory pathways may be divided into four main categories:

(1) The use of "classical" audiometric tests.

(2) The use of measures of the middle ear muscle reflexes (discussed in Chapter 19).

(3) The use of electrophysiological measures (discussed in Chapter 23).

(4) Specific tests of central auditory dysfunction.

A number of studies have applied tests from several of these different groups, and certain tests such as the alternate binaural loudness balance may be regarded as being in both the first and last groups, showing different patterns of results with cochlear and with cortical lesions.

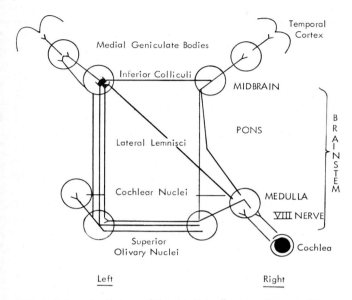

FIG. 1. Schematic diagram of the classical afferent auditory pathway (after Jungerts, Acta otolaryng. Suppl. 138, 1958).

CLASSICAL AUDIOMETRIC TESTS

This group of tests can be regarded as including the pure tone audiogram, the discrimination of normal speech signals, tone decay tests, the alternate binaural loudness balance, and the SISI test (see p. 354).

PURE TONE AUDIOMETRY

There has been more controversy surrounding the effects of central nervous system lesions on the pure tone audiogram than on almost any other audiometric measure. The claims range from total deafness to normal hearing in patients with temporal lobe lesions. Bramwell (1927) reported sudden bilateral hearing loss in a patient who had softening of both temporal lobes after embolic phenomena, and Jerger and his associates (1969) described a severe bilateral hearing loss which largely recovered over a period of 3 months, in a patient who apparently infarcted both temporal lobes. However even in a number of cases of presumed bilateral temporal lobe disorders and certainly in unilateral lesions the results are very variable and at best equivocal (Jerger *et al.*, 1969; Baru and Karaseva, 1972). It does seem, though, that the presence of bilateral damage is necessary for there to be pronounced effects on the pure tone threshold.

The nature of changes in the pure tone audiogram found in brainstem lesions is equally controversial. Pialoux

(1962) described a series of audiograms related to lesions in different parts of the auditory pathways, but this work has not been supported by other investigations. Parker *et al.* (1968) reported variable and generally mild hearing losses in pontine lesions, and Noffsinger and his associates (1972) found threshold elevation of over 25 dB in only 15 of 122 ears tested of patients with multiple sclerosis. They do however comment that in the majority of these patients with a hearing loss, the deficits were bilateral.

Similarly Dix and Hood (1973) have presented data showing a bilateral symmetrical hearing loss in 9 of 500 patients reviewed with brainstem lesions. They argue, that with bilateral representation of both cochleas above the level of the cochlear nuclei, any lesion producing a hearing loss must affect the fibres of the particular frequencies concerned coming from both ears, so producing a bilaterally symmetrical hearing loss. Unfortunately bilaterally symmetrical cochlear hearing losses from a variety of causes are relatively common and in the absence of a more detailed statistical evaluation of their results, together with the results of other tests of brainstem disorders, the question is far from resolved.

An apt resumé of the use of pure tone audiometry in central auditory dysfunction comes from Greiner and Conraux (1971) who stated that the profile of the audiometric curve contributes scarcely anything to the diagnosis of central auditory lesions.

SPEECH DISCRIMINATION

The discrimination of normal speech test material such as phonetically balanced word lists and spondaic word lists is normally little affected by lesions in the central auditory pathways. Thus Noffsinger and his associates (1972) found less than 90 per cent discrimination scores for tests comprising monosyllabic words in only 9 out of 121 ears tested of patients with multiple sclerosis. Similarly Parker and his associates (1968) found that in patients with pontine lesions over half had discrimination scores in excess of 80 per cent, whereas the figure for patients with cochlear nerve lesions was only 13 per cent. Jerger (1960a) on the other hand has argued that brainstem lesions produce a marked contralateral impairment in speech discrimination ability, even in patients with normal pure tone audiograms.

The same author concluded that in lesions in the auditory cortex the discrimination of standard phonetically balanced lists is normal, although he later (1964) reported reduced discrimination in the ear contralateral to a temporal lobe lesion. A number of similar cases have been reported subsequently by other authors (e.g. Lynn *et al.*, 1972) but it is a far from universal finding and other studies have failed to confirm this (e.g. Berlin and Lowe, 1972). A considerable bilateral impairment of speech discrimination has, however, been reported in a patient with bilateral lesions of the temporal lobes (Jerger *et al.*, 1969).

Interestingly, Goldstein and his associates (1956) studying speech discrimination in patients with infantile hemiplegia on which left hemispherectomies were performed, used several word lists and noticed impaired discrimination in the right ear to one of the lists in which they comment that the enunciation of the words was poor.

This is in accord with the concept of distorted or low redundancy speech tests designed specifically for testing patients with central lesions, and which will be discussed later.

In conclusion it seems reasonable to quote the conclusions of Lidén and Korsan-Bengtsen (1973) that, on the whole, there is relatively good speech discrimination in patients with brainstem lesions, and normal discrimination in those with temporal lobe lesions.

TESTS OF ABNORMAL AUDITORY ADAPTATION

A number of different tests of abnormal auditory adaptation ("tone decay") at threshold have been proposed at different times, but they all appear to measure the same phenomenon. Thus Stephens and Hinchcliffe (1968), and a number of other workers reported abnormal adaptation with both Békésy and Carhart techniques in patients with a variety of brainstem lesions.

Abnormal auditory adaptation in patients with brainstem lesions has been reviewed and discussed at some length by Eichel and his associates (1966), and indeed some of the earliest demonstrations of "tone decay" using Békésy audiometry were of patients with multiple sclerosis and one patient with a pinealoma (Kos, 1955). In their extensive study on the audition of patients with multiple sclerosis, Noffsinger and his associates (1972) found over 30 dB "tone decay" using the Carhart test in 38 of 120 ears tested, although they found types III or IV Békésy patterns in only 19 out of 115 ears tested. This is in accord with the widely reported finding that Békésy audiometry is a less sensitive measure of abnormal auditory adaptation than is manual testing. Of their patients who exhibited "tone decay", in the majority it was bilateral.

It is interesting to note in their study that there was least "tone decay" in patients with lower brainstem lesions, a result agreeing with the finding of Morales-Garcia and Hood (1972) that abnormal auditory adaptation was conspicuously absent in patients with medullary or midline lesions, although moderate abnormal adaptation was more common in pontine and mesencephalic lesions. Parker and his associates (1968) also found either bilateral abnormal adaptation or tone perversion (a change in the subjective quality of a sustained tone to a noise, lacking tonality) commonly in patients with pontine lesions.

There appears to be little evidence for abnormal adaptation in patients with lesions of the auditory cortex, and the bilaterally infarcted patient of Jerger and his associates (1969) gave a type I Békésy response from both ears, as did a patient of Hodgson (1967) following a unilateral hemispherectomy.

In conclusion it may thus be stated that a moderate degree of abnormal auditory adaptation is commonly found in pontine and mesencephalic lesions but in these cases it is usually less pronounced than in patients with cochlear nerve lesions.

THE ALTERNATE BINAURAL LOUDNESS BALANCE TEST

This test was developed as a measure of loudness recruitment but has been advocated by Jerger (1960) as a test for lesions in the auditory cortex in testing for the loudness reversal phenomenon. As such it will be considered later.

There has been considerable controversy as to the existence of the phenomenon of recruitment in patients with brainstem lesions. Parker and his associates (1968) found it present in the majority of their patients with pontine lesions and Lidén (1969) commented that it was often present in brainstem lesions. Dix (1965), on the other hand, in a series of 31 patients with multiple sclerosis and unilateral hearing loss found no recruitment in the majority of cases. In the series of patients with multiple sclerosis tested by Noffsinger and his associates (1972), 11 patients with asymmetrical thresholds were tested with the alternate binaural loudness balance technique, and of these, 8 showed recruitment. Of 12 such patients tested with simultaneous midplane lateralization technique, 10 showed recruitment.

It thus seems that the results of tests of recruitment are somewhat variable in brainstem lesions so that they would appear to have little diagnostic significance in this context.

SHORT INCREMENT SENSITIVITY INDEX (SISI) AND INTENSITY DIFFERENCE LIMEN TESTS

These tests were originally introduced as tests of recruitment with stimuli presented at 20 or 40 dB. sensation levels. Patients with end organ lesions were considered to have better discrimination of small changes in intensity than normally hearing patients or patients with conductive lesions. More recently, as a test for cochlear nerve lesions many workers have advocated presenting the stimuli at high intensity levels (e.g. 80–90 dB HL), when patients with end organ lesions and normally hearing patients show good discrimination of small intensity increments (e.g. 100 per cent SISI scores). It has been argued that under these conditions, patients with cochlear nerve lesions have poor scores. Using the test in this way, Noffsinger and his associates (1972) found reduced scores in 52 of the 117 ears tested of patients with multiple sclerosis, although the incidence of these low scores was least in the group of patients considered to have medullary lesions. Lidén and Korsan-Bengtsen (1973) likewise comment that low SISI scores are generally found in brainstem lesions.

In the patient with bilateral temporal lobe lesions presented by Jerger and his associates (1969) intensity discrimination was minimally impaired in one ear and severely impaired in the other. Hodgson (1967) found impaired SISI scores in the ear opposite to the side of a unilateral hemispherectomy, and Baru and Vasserman (1969) reported the same but only for very short duration signals. None of these groups of authors, however, were able to support the findings of Swisher (1967) who reported improved intensity discrimination following removal of the left temporal lobe.

In conclusion, it may be stated that simple intensity discrimination measures may be impaired in a variety of neural lesions, but that this is a far from universal finding.

This conclusion is true of most of the tests of classical audiometry, which explains some of the interpretative problems when these tests alone are used in the diagnosis of lesions in the central auditory pathways.

SPECIFIC TESTS OF CENTRAL AUDITORY DYSFUNCTION

Tests of central auditory dysfunction may be subdivided into two main categories, those using modified speech stimuli, and those using non-speech stimuli. These may be further subdivided into tests in which the stimulus or stimuli are presented monaurally and those in which there is binaural presentation of stimuli. The more widely described of these four classes of tests are illustrated in Table 1.

TABLE 1

TESTS OF CENTRAL AUDITORY DYSFUNCTION

	Speech	Non-Speech
Monaural	Filtered speech	Temporal integration
	Time compressed speech	Reaction time
	Low sensation-level speech	Vertical localization
	Masked speech	Duration discrimination
	Periodically interrupted speech	Temporal order perception
		Rhythm perception
		Bromsliter-Creel test
Binaural	Matzker	Lateralization
	Competing messages	Horizontal localization
	Staggered spondaic test	Chocholle test
	SWAMI	Masking level difference
	Swinging speech	Alternate binaural loudness balance
	Groen and Hellema test	Simultaneous midplane lateralization test
		Cross masking

TESTS USING SPEECH MATERIAL

Many people have argued that the perception of speech is the highest auditory function so that tests of central auditory dysfunction should be based on speech material. However, as was discussed in an earlier section, normal speech material contains a considerable amount of redundant information so that most patients with central auditory disorders have good speech discrimination. The first approach to reducing this redundancy came with the work of Bocca and his associates (1954) who passed bisyllabic speech material through a 500 Hz low-pass filter and found that discrimination of this speech material was impaired in the ear opposite to the lesion in a patient with a temporal lobe tumour. Unfiltered speech discrimination was, however, equally good in both ears.

The following year Bocca (1955) introduced a binaural test in which this low-pass filtered speech was passed to one ear and the same material, unfiltered but at a low sensation level (giving about 30 per cent discrimination) to the other ear. He showed that considerable binaural summation of the discrimination occurred in normally hearing subjects.

Since that time a plethora of monaural low-redundancy speech tests and a great variety of binaural tests embodying many different principles have been proposed by many different authors. These have been extensively reviewed by a number of authors (Korsan-Bengtsen, 1973; Berlin and Lowe, 1972; Bocca and Calearo, 1963) and will be described briefly below, but not discussed in great detail.

At this stage it might be opportune to consider to some extent the disadvantages of the use of speech material in testing for central auditory dysfunction. The first problem is one which these tests share with many of the non-speech tests to be described later and is that the results may be grossly disturbed by peripheral auditory dysfunction particularly in the cochlea and in the cochlear nerve.

The problems more characteristic of the speech material are several. They are based mainly on the fact that as the redundancy of the material is reduced the task of discriminating the signal becomes more difficult even for normally hearing subjects. Thus a variety of audiometrically irrelevant factors about the patient may influence his test results. Bocca (1965) has shown that the optimal discrimination obtained for filtered speech and time-compressed speech increases with the patient's Intelligence Quotient (IQ) as measured on the Wechsler scale, up to an IQ of about 107. The results of the periodically interrupted speech are even more dependent on IQ increasing with intelligence over the entire range tested (< 140).

The age of the patient has a considerable effect on speech discrimination scores. This has been discussed at some length by Palva and Jokinen (1970) who reviewed the results obtained with a variety of low-redundancy speech tests and presented their own results on a test using band-pass filtered speech material. Table 2 shows the results obtained in a similar study by Kastelanski (1974) which compares the discrimination in a group of subjects aged 60–70 years with normal pure tone thresholds with that of normally hearing subjects aged 20–30 years. It may be seen that in the elderly patients the unfiltered speech was discriminated normally, but the filtered speech, both low-pass and high-pass is discriminated significantly ($P < 0.01$) worse than in the young subjects. Binaural integration of the test material, with high-pass filtered speech

TABLE 2

SPEECH DISCRIMINATION IN YOUNG AND
ELDERLY SUBJECTS

Condition	Mean	Standard Deviation
Elderly Subjects		
ODS (L)	99·0	0·9
HP (L)	63·0	7·5
LP (L)	67·0	10·2
HP (L) + LP (R)	95·6	2·9
Young Subjects		
HP (L)	78·4	5·9
LP (L)	80·5	6·3
HP (L) + LP (R)	97·2	2·0

(ODS—Unfiltered speech optimal discrimination score; HP—High-pass filtered speech; LP—Low-pass filtered speech.)

presented to one ear and low-pass filtered speech to the other ear, was not significantly different from that found in the young subjects.

A further problem arises when the patient's native language is not that of the test material. Such patients are able to adequately discriminate normal speech material but experience considerable problems when its redundancy is reduced. Table 3 shows the results obtained by Kastelanski

TABLE 3

SPEECH DISCRIMINATION BY NATIVE ENGLISH SPEAKERS,
AND BY NORMALLY HEARING SUBJECTS WHO LEARNED
ENGLISH AS A SECOND LANGUAGE

Condition	Mean	Standard Deviation
Foreign Subjects		
ODS (L)	95·2	4·1
HP (L)	69·2	6·1
LP (L)	79·2	5·3
English Subjects		
HP (L)	78·4	5·9
LP (L)	80·5	6·3

(ODS—Unfiltered speech optimal discrimination score; HP—High-pass filtered speech; LP—Low-pass filtered speech.)

(1974) for a group of young people aged 20–30 years who had been using English as a second language over a period of 1–21 years, compared with those for whom it was their first language. It may be seen that their discrimination of unfiltered speech is only slightly reduced but that of high-pass filtered speech is considerably impaired when compared to the English speakers ($P < 0.01$).

These points illustrate just a few of the problems in the use of low redundancy speech tests from an interpretative

point of view. Other problems arise from the fact that speech material is difficult to quantify and calibrate, even in the context of simple undistorted clinical speech tests, and more so when its redundancy is reduced in one way or another. Other problems arise from the difficulty in directly comparing results obtained in different laboratories even within the same linguistic area because of differing dialects, a complication which obviously becomes more pronounced when the results obtained in different linguistic areas are compared.

However, despite these problems, a considerable number of speech tests have been described and are used in a limited number of audiological centres.

Monaural Speech Tests

(a) *Filtered Speech Tests.* The first of these tests in which standard speech material was passed through a filter was described by Bocca and his associates (1954) and used a low-pass 500 Hz filter to reduce the redundancy in the speech information. Since that time a variety of modifications of this procedure have used high-pass filtered speech, low-pass filtered speech and band-pass filtered speech with various cut-off frequencies and rejection rates. These have been reviewed extensively by Hodgson (1972), and the general conclusion would appear to be that in all the studies described, the discrimination of this filtered material is relatively poorer in the ear contralateral to a lesion in the auditory cortex than in the homolateral ear. Jerger (1964) however, reported similar results in the ear contralateral to a brainstem lesion. Other studies have suggested that the results are more variable in brainstem lesions (Bocca and Calearo, 1963).

(b) *Time Compressed Speech.* This approach has normally been restricted to speech test material using sentences in which the normal Italian speech rate was increased from 140 to 350 words per minute (Calearo and Lazzaroni, 1957). Since that time this procedure has also been used with a variety of other speech materials, even with monosyllabic words (Beasley *et al.*, 1972). The various results have been reviewed by Korsan-Bengtsen (1973) and by Kastelanski (1974) and although they support the general findings with filtered speech, of poorer discrimination in the ear contralateral to a temporal lobe lesion, impaired results are also obtained in a variety of rather non-specific intra-cranial lesions. Korsan-Bengtsen (1973), however, in her study found little difference between results obtained with this test and those with filtered speech testing in patients with lesions outside the auditory cortex.

(c) *Low Sensation Level Speech.* This has been used by Jerger (1960b, 1964) and by Hodgson (1972) both of whom used speech material at 5–10 dB sensation level. They reported impaired discrimination in the ear contralateral to a temporal lobe lesion. The main difficulty here arises with problems in consistently defining the critical stimulus level at a point where the discrimination score is extremely dependent on the stimulus level.

(d) *Masked Speech.* A number of authors (Dayal *et al.*, 1966; Morales-Garcia and Poole, 1972; Noffsinger *et al.*,

1972; Lafon, 1966) have used a test situation in which speech material is presented in a background of noise. Poor discrimination has been reported in the ear contralateral to a lesion in the auditory cortex, and generally reduced discrimination found in patients with brainstem lesions. Noffsinger and his associates (1972) found that good discrimination was given by patients with lower brainstem lesions, and variable, but generally impaired, results by patients with more central lesions. The results published by Morales-Garcia and Poole (1972) would suggest that this test may be useful in testing patients with cortical lesions, but that the variability of the results limits its diagnostic potential in patients with brainstem lesions.

(e) *Periodically Interrupted Speech.* In this test the speech material is periodically interrupted by an electronic switch. In this way parts of the speech message are cancelled.

Bocca (1958) introduced this approach to clinical testing with phonetically balanced lists interrupted ten times per second. Patients with temporal lobe lesions showed poorer discrimination in the ear contralateral to the lesion than in the homolateral ear. Bocca did, however, report that it discriminated less well between the ears than did the accelerated or filtered speech tests.

This test has been used subsequently by a number of other workers and reduced scores in one or both ears have also been reported in patients with brainstem lesions (Calearo and Antonelli, 1968). Korsan-Bengtsen (1973) reported that this test showed better differentiation between the homolateral and contralateral ears in patients with temporal lobe lesions that did either filtered or accelerated speech, but she also reported considerable inter-ear differences in patients with brainstem lesions.

Binaural Speech Tests

Whereas most of the monaural speech tests were developed to test for lesions in the auditory cortex, many of the binaural tests have been produced to evaluate interactive processes in the brainstem.

(a) *Matzker Test.* The test devised by Matzker (1959) involved passing speech material through a high frequency (1815–2500 Hz) band-pass filter to one ear and through a low frequency (500–800 Hz) band-pass filter to the other ear. The principle is that both bands of speech material presented independently are poorly discriminated but when they are presented simultaneously, the brain is able to integrate the information received from the two ears and reconstitute the speech, thus giving considerably increased discrimination scores. Rather contradictory results have been obtained subsequently by several authors and a number of these results are reviewed by Hodgson (1972). The recent work by Lynn and his associates (1972), however, supports Matzker's original contention that lack of binaural integration occurs only in patients with brainstem lesions, normal integration occurring in patients with pure cortical lesions.

Bocca (1955) had previously used a somewhat similar approach in which low-pass filtered speech was presented to one ear and low sensation level unfiltered speech to the other. This was also used by Jerger (1960a) who noted impaired integration of the two inputs by patients with lesions in the auditory cortex.

(b) *Competing Message Tests.* Jerger (1964) used a test in which a word list was presented to the test ear while unrelated speech was presented to the opposite ear. He found that in patients with temporal lobe and brainstem lesions, better discrimination was obtained when the test signal was presented to the homolateral ear than to the contralateral ear. These differences were more pronounced in patients with cortical than with brainstem lesions. Korsan-Bengtsen (1973) reported rather smaller differences between the two ears and Berlin and Lowe (1972) found a negligible difference. In their study on patients with multiple sclerosis, Noffsinger and his associates (1972) found reduced discrimination only in patients with lesions involving the higher parts of the auditory pathway.

(c) *Staggered Spondaic Tests.* This test was developed by Katz (1962) and involves overlapping spondees so that for example RAILWAY may be presented to one ear with "WAY" being presented at the same time as "DOWN" of DOWNTOWN being presented to the opposite ear. The results obtained by various workers on this and other comparable tests in which the patient is required to repeat both messages, have been reviewed by Brunt (1972). It would appear that impaired discrimination is found in patients with lesions in the auditory cortex. There seems to be little evidence available for the effects of brainstem lesions on the results of this test.

(d) *SWAMI Test.* The speech with alternate masking index (SWAMI) test was described by Jerger (1964). In this test speech material is presented simultaneously to the two ears, and at the same time a masking noise at an intensity level 20 dB greater than the words is alternated between the two ears at the rate of one oscillation per second. Jerger considered this to be a test of lower brainstem function, but his results showed the score to be more depressed in patients with temporal lobe lesions than in those with brainstem disorders. A similar reduced score in patients with temporal lobe lesions was reported by Berlin and Lowe (1972).

(e) *Swinging Speech Tests.* These involve the periodic switching of a speech message from one ear to the other so that each ear receives half of the message. Bocca and Calle010 (1963) have maintained that normal scores in this test are obtained by patients with lesions in the auditory cortex, and Calearo and Antonelli (1968) found abnormally low discrimination in 9 out of 22 patients with brainstem lesions.

(f) *Groen and Hellema Test.* This was described by Groen and Hellema (1960). The two authors based their test on a comparison of the monaural and binaural speech discrimination curves, and concluded that if the binaural curve is steeper than the monaural curve there was a lesion between the cochlea and superior olivary nucleus, whereas if the curves were parallel the lesion was more central. Van Zyl and Braiser (1973) have been unable to verify these results in children with various pathologies.

TESTS USING NON-SPEECH MATERIAL

As with the speech tests, these may be subdivided into two main groups, one involving monaural presentation of the stimuli and the other using binaural stimulus presentation. Again the former are generally considered to be sensitive to lesions in the auditory cortex and the latter to brainstem lesions, although important exceptions occur in both groups.

Monaural Non-speech Tests

(a) *Auditory Temporal Integration*. As the duration of a tonal stimulus is shortened below a certain limit (ca 200 ms at 1000 Hz) a larger stimulus amplitude is necessary for the tone-burst to remain detectable. For 1000 Hz signals Garner and Miller (1947), and a plethora of other authors, have shown that for every halving of duration the stimulus intensity must be increased by 3 dB for the signal to remain equally detectable. Miskolczy-Fodor (1953) and many subsequent authors have shown that this slope is reduced in patients with cochlear lesions. Baru and her associates (1964), Gersuni and his associates (1971) and a number of other studies from the U.S.S.R. have suggested that in patients with lesions in the auditory cortex the threshold for very short duration signals (less than 20 ms) is selectively impaired in the contralateral ear. Jerger and his associates (1969) in their patient with bilateral temporal lobe lesions found a considerable increase of slope in the temporal integration function in one ear of their patient. Baru and Karaseva (1972) reported essentially normal results in nine patients with brainstem lesions.

Unpublished results of Olsen *et al.* indicated occasional abnormally steep slopes of increasing threshold with shortening duration in some patients with cochlear nerve tumours. The present author has found abnormally steep results in one ear of a patient with a dermoid of the cerebellopontine angle, and also steep growth for the short duration stimuli in some patients with lesions in the cortex.

It would appear that considerably more data is required on auditory temporal integration in patients with lesions in the central auditory pathways, but that this test may be found to be diagnostically valuable.

(b) *Auditory Reaction Times*. The use of auditory reaction time measures in clinical testing was first suggested by Chocholle (1954) who proposed that it could be used as a measure of recruitment. It was applied in the context of clinical testing by Maspetiol and Semette (1968) who reported that the reaction time to tones presented to the ear contralateral to a lesion in the auditory cortex was prolonged relative to the reaction time to tones presented to the homolateral ear. In bilateral involvement of the auditory cortex, the reaction times to acoustical stimuli could be prolonged relative to reaction times to visual stimuli.

Karasseva (1972) has suggested that the difference between reaction times to homolateral and to contralateral acoustical stimuli in lesions of the auditory cortex may be more pronounced when short duration stimuli (1 ms) are used than with longer duration stimuli (120 ms). She comments that no systematic pattern of results was found in patients with lesions elsewhere in the cerebral cortex, and Maspetiol and Semette (1968) reported normal reaction times in patients with brainstem lesions.

Any conclusions based on the results of such a test must remain somewhat tentative at present, until more basic experimental work has been performed.

(c) *Auditory Localization in the Vertical Plane*. Walsh (1957) investigating the vertical localization ability of patients with cortical lesions, using a musical box as a sound source, reported that a number of such patients showed normal localization of sounds in the horizontal plane, but deficient localization in the vertical plane. Fritze and Glonig (1973) report that patients with lesions in the auditory cortex make more errors in localization in the vertical plane when they use the ear contralateral to the lesion.

One of the problems in such a task is that many normal subjects have considerable difficulty in localization in the vertical plane. Roffler and Butler (1968) have shown the importance of frequencies of over 8000 Hz for the performance of such a task, and Davis and Stephens (1974) the effects of stimulus intensity and the nature of the test material.

Butler (1970) has shown that patients with bilateral high frequency end-organ hearing losses are unable to localize in the vertical plane. It is thus perhaps not surprising that even the normal subjects of Fritze and Glonig (1973) make considerable errors when listening to a 2000 Hz narrow-band noise stimulus. Much further developmental work is needed on such a test before it can be used as a reliable clinical test.

(d) *Duration Discrimination*. The animal studies of Neff (1968) have suggested that the discrimination of sounds of different duration is impaired in animals following ablation of the auditory cortex. Very little work has been performed on the discrimination of sounds of different durations by humans with different lesions in the auditory pathways. Ruhm and his associates (1966) have shown that the ability to discriminate in this way is not impaired in cochlear lesions. Van Allen and his associates (1966) investigated duration discrimination in a series of brain damaged patients with a variety of cortical lesions. They reported that the brain-damaged patients showed poorer discrimination than non-brain damaged controls, but the lesions were not clearly defined in many of these cases.

It would thus appear that auditory duration discrimination cannot be regarded as a clinically useful task until considerably more patients with well defined lesions have been tested.

(e) *Temporal Order Perception*. Neff (1968) also reported considerable defects in the discrimination of the order of presentation of two or three short acoustical stimuli following ablation of the auditory cortex. These findings have been more extensively investigated in patients with a variety of auditory lesions and this general premise confirmed.

Efron (1963) found that the discrimination of the order of pulses at different frequencies was impaired following a cortical lesion, and Jerger and his associates (1969) in their patient with bilateral cortical lesions found a considerable impairment of order discrimination with a variety of stimulus paradigms. This has been further supported by Swisher and Hirsh (1972) and a number of other authors.

(f) *Rhythm Perception.* Abnormalities of musical rhythm perception as measured by the Seashore test have been reviewed by a number of authors (e.g. Williams, 1970) in patients with temporal lobe lesions. Russian work reviewed by Luria (1973) and by Baru and Karaseva (1972) also suggested abnormal perception of short simple rhythmic patterns in patients with lesions in the auditory cortex.

This aspect of auditory perception which is closely linked to the two preceding phenomena of duration and temporal order perception would appear to merit a more detailed exploration.

(g) *Broomsliter–Creel Test.* This test is based on the finding of Doughty and Garner (1947) that it takes a finite stimulus duration for a sinusoid to produce an impression of tonal quality, and that this duration shortens with increasing stimulus intensity. Broomsliter and his associates (1964) have shown abnormal results in this test in patients with vertebro-basilar insufficiency affecting the brainstem in that they may require abnormally long stimuli for the perception of tonality. Moore (1972) has, however, suggested that a frequency discrimination task involving short duration tones might be a more useful means of examining such a defect.

Binaural Non-speech Tests

(a) *Lateralization and Horizontal Localization.* Lateralization is the intracranial localization of a sound source presented to both ears, usually through earphones. Localization in the horizontal plane is the directionalization of a sound-source in space. Batteau (1967) has shown that the modifications of the sound source effected by the auricle are necessary for the apparent source of a recorded sound presented to the subject by headphones, to be perceived as being in space rather than within the subject's head.

Sanchez-Longo and his associates (1957) ,Walsh (1957), Nordlund (1964) and others have examined the ability of patients with a variety of central lesions to localize the source of sound in space. Rather variable results were obtained by Walsh (1957) although a number of his subjects showed impaired horizontal localization ability. Sanchez-Longo and his associates (1957) reported defective horizontal localization ability in a series of patients with temporal lobe lesions, the confusion being particularly marked in the auditory field contralateral to the lesion. Nordlund (1964), however, reported normal localization ability in patients with "brain lesions" the extent of which were not clearly defined, although he found markedly abnormal localization in patients with pontine lesions. Jerger and his associates (1969) found considerably impaired localization ability in their patient with bilateral lesions of the auditory cortex.

Matzker (1959) described a lateralization test with a time delay between tone-bursts presented to the two ears. He described abnormal lateralization ability in patients with a variety of cortical lesions, and later (1964) with a range of brainstem lesions. Groen (1969) further investigated this problem and described a simple stethoscope-device for testing lateralization ability. Recently, however, Nilsson and his associates (1973) and the present author have found that there is considerable intra- and inter-subject variability in the results obtained from normal subjects with this device, so limiting its diagnostic potential.

It would thus appear that in studies both on directionalization in the horizontal plane and in lateralization, more data is required from patients with a variety of CNS lesions before any categorical statements can be made as the exact diagnostic significance of such tests. Further caution is necessary as Nordlund (1964) and other workers have shown that horizontal localization may be impaired by lesions in the middle ear and more strikingly in the cochlear nerve.

(b) *Chocholle Test.* Chocholle (1959) described the effects of contralateral pure tone stimulation on intensity discrimination in the test ear. Contralateral stimulation with a tone of the same frequency as a test tone impairs intensity discrimination and contralateral stimulation with a tone of a different frequency improves discrimination.

Maspetiol and Semette (1968) have applied this in a clinical context and report a considerable impairment of this phenomenon in patients with brainstem lesions. Stephens (1974) studied the various experimental parameters involved in some detail and supported the finding of absent contralateral effects on intensity discrimination in patients in whom the lesions were restricted to the brainstem. Further studies by the present author have also supported Maspetiol and Semette's (1968) contention that in cortical lesions the effects of contralateral stimulation may be present when testing one side but absent when the test signal is presented to the opposite ear.

(c) *Masking Level Difference (MLD).* This is a phenomenon which occurs when the phase relationships of a signal presented to the two ears differs from that of a noise presented to the two ears. Thus when a masking noise is presented in phase to the two ears, a test tone will be detectable at a lower sound pressure level if it is presented 180° out of phase to the two ears than if it is presented in phase. This effect is maximal with low frequency tones in the range 200–300 Hz, and is also found when speech stimuli are used.

Noffsinger and his associates (1972) found abnormally small MLDs in the majority of their patients with multiple sclerosis regardless of which part of the central nervous system appeared to be affected. These results were supported by a larger unpublished series later reported by Noffsinger and Olsen (1973) who found that both the incidence of abnormally small MLDs was raised and the mean MLD was abnormally small in such patients.

It would appear that MLD tests whether speech or pure tone would merit further investigation in the context of central auditory pathology.

(d) *Alternate Binaural Loudness Balance (ABLB) and Simultaneous Midplane Lateralization (SML) Tests.* These two tests may be considered together. The ABLB requires no description as it is one of the most commonly used of all audiometric test procedures. The simultaneous mid-plane lateralization test involves essentially the same technique, but with the test-tones being presented simultaneously to the two ears of the patient who is required to indicate which stimulus level in the test ear results in the auditory image occurring in the middle of his head.

Jerger (1960) advocated the use of these two tests in parallel for the investigation of patients with suspected lesions in the central auditory pathways. He reported that in patients with unilateral cortical lesions there was a derecruitment phenomenon with an impaired growth of loudness in the ear contralateral to the lesion, which was shown by the ABLB test. Patients with brainstem lesions found difficulty in performing the SML test.

The findings with the ABLB were supported by Davis and Goodman (1966) and by Hodgson (1967), in patients following hemispherectomies, although Davis and Goodman (1966) reported that the derecruitment was followed by some recruitment at high stimulus intensities. Noffsinger and his associates (1972) found derecruitment in 11 out of 48 of the patients with multiple sclerosis and normal thresholds. All these patients had lesions in the higher auditory pathways. These authors also found abnormal results in SML task in 10 out of 48 patients with normal thresholds, but these were also in patients with lesions in the higher parts of the central nervous system.

(e) *Central Masking.* This is the phenomenon by which a masker presented to one ear may elevate the threshold to a signal presented to the opposite ear. This has been extensively studied in normally hearing subjects by a variety of authors (e.g. Ingham, 1959). Hopkinson (1971) has reported a greater masking effect in patients with multiple sclerosis involving the brainstem than in patients with peripheral lesions or normally hearing subjects.

CONCLUSIONS

In this review it has been possible to consider only some of the more important tests which have been applied to patients with a variety of lesions affecting the central auditory pathways. Other approaches are discussed by Bocca and Calearo (1963), Baru and Karaseva (1972) and in other reviews cited.

It is apparent from the foregoing account that knowledge of this field remains rather limited, although it is perhaps possible to decide which avenues are not worth further extensive exploration. In the context of the more specific tests of central auditory dysfunction it is the author's contention that in the long run, tests using non-speech stimuli may well be found to be of more ultimate diagnostic value than speech tests. Any evaluation of such tests must be conducted in parallel with electrophysiological investigations.

ACKNOWLEDGEMENT

This work was supported by Grant 970/512/C from the Medical Research Council.

REFERENCES

Baru, A. V. and Karaseva, T. A. (1972), *The Brain and Hearing.* New York: Consultants Bureau.

Baru, A. V. and Vasserman, L. I. (1969), *Trud. Leningrad. Naucho-Isseldor,* **46**, 90.

Baru, A. V., Gersuni, G. V. and Tonkonogii, I. M. (1964), *Zhurnal Neuropatol. Psikiatr.,* **64**, 481.

Batteau, D. W. (1967), *Proc. roy. Soc. B,* **168**, 158.

Beasley, D. S., Forman, B. S. and Rintelmann, W. F. (1972), *J. Auditory Res.,* **12**, 71.

Berlin, C. I. and Lowe, S. S. (1972), in *Handbook of Clinical Audiology* (J. Katz, Ed.). Baltimore: Williams and Wilkins.

Bocca, E. (1955), *Laryngoscope,* **65**, 1164.

Bocca, E. (1958), *Laryngoscope,* **68**, 301.

Bocca, E. (1965), in *Sensorineural Hearing Processes and Disorders* (B. A. Graham, Ed.). Boston: Little Brown & Co.

Bocca, E. and Calearo, C. (1963), in *Modern Development in Audiology* (J. Jerger, Ed.). New York: Academic Press.

Bocca, E., Calearo, C. and Cassinari, V. (1954), *Acta oto-laryng. (Stockh.),* **44**, 219.

Bramwell, E. (1927), *Brain,* **50**, 579.

Broomsliter, P. C., Creel, W. and Powers, S. R. (1964), *J. acoust. Soc. Amer.,* **36**, 1958.

Brunt, M. A. (1972), in *Handbook of Clinical Audiology* (J. Katz, Ed.). Baltimore: Williams and Wilkins.

Butler, R. A. (1970), *Int. Audiology,* **9**, 117.

Calearo, C. and Antonelli, A. R. (1968), *Acta oto-laryng. (Stockh.),* **66**, 305.

Calearo, C. and Lazzaroni, A. (1957), *Laryngoscope,* **67**, 410.

Chocholle, R. (1954), *Annales d'oto-laryng.,* **71**, 379.

Chochole, R. (1959), *Acustica,* **9**, 309.

Davis, R. and Stephens, S. D. G. (1974), *J. Sound and Vibration,* **35**, 223.

Dayal, V. S., Tarantino, L. and Swisher, L. P. (1966), *Laryngoscope,* **76**, 1798.

Dix, M. R. (1965), *J. Laryng.,* **79**, 695.

Dix, M. R. and Hood, J. D. (1973), *Acta oto-laryng. (Stockh.),* **75**, 165.

Efron, R. (1963), *Brain,* **86**, 403.

Eichel, B. S., Hedgecock, L. D. and Williams, H. L. (1966), *Laryngoscope,* **76**, 1.

Fritze, W. and Glonig, K. (1973), *Mschr. Ohrenheilk.,* **107**, 432.

Garner, W. R. and Miller, G. A. (1947), *J. exp. Psychol.,* **34**, 450.

Gersuni, G. V., Baru, A. V., Karaseva, T. A. and Tonkonogii, I. M. (1971), in *Sensory Processes at the Neuronal and Behavioural Levels* (G. V. Gersuni, Ed.). New York: Academic Press.

Goldstein, R., Goodman, A. L. and King, R. B. (1956), *Neurology,* **6**, 869.

Greiner, G. F. and Conraux, C. (1971), *Bulletin d'Audiophonologie,* **1**, 679.

Groen, J. J. (1969), *Acta oto-laryng. (Stockh.),* **67**, 326.

Groen, J. J. and Hellema, A. C. M. (1960) *Acta oto-laryng. (Stockh.),* **52**, 397.

Hodgson, W. R. (1967), *J. Speech Hear. Dis.,* **32**, 39.

Hodgson, W. E. (1972), in *Handbook of Clinical Audiology* (J. Katz, Ed.). Baltimore: Williams and Wilkins.

Hopkinson, N. T. (1971), *Proceedings of 7th International Congress on Acoustics,* p. 465. Budapest.

Ingham, J. G. (1959), *J. exp. Psychol.,* **58**, 199.

Jerger, J. (1960a), *Laryngoscope,* **70**, 417.

Jerger, J. (1960b), *Arch. Otolaryng.,* **71**, 797.

Jerger, J. (1964), in *Neurological Aspects of Auditory and Vestibular Disorders* (W. S. Fields, Ed.). Springfield, Ill.: C. Thomas.

Jerger, J., Weikers, N. J., Sharborough, F. W. and Jerger, S. (1969), *Acta oto-laryng. (Stockh.),* suppl. 258.

Karasseva, T. A. (1972), *Neuropsychologia,* **10**, 227.

Kastelanski, W. (1974), "Methodological Studies of the Matzker Test," Unpublished M.Sc. Dissertation, University of Southampton.

Katz, J. (1962), *J. Auditory Res.,* **2**, 327.

Korsan-Bengtsen, M. (1973), *Acta oto-laryng. (Stockh.),* suppl. 310.

Kos, C. M. (1955), *Laryngoscope,* **65**, 711.

Lafon, J. C. (1966), *The Phonetic Test and the Measurement of Hearing.* Einthoven: Centrex.

Lidén, G. (1969), *J. Laryng.*, **83**, 507.

Lidén, G. and Korsan-Bengtsen, M. (1973), *Scand. Audiology*, **2**, 29.

Luria, A. R. (1973), *The Working Brain.* Harmondsworth: Penguin Books.

Lynn, G. E., Benitez, J. T., Eisenbrey, A. B., Gilroy, J. and Wilner, H. I. (1972), *Audiology*, **11**, 115.

Maspetiol, R. and Semette, D. (1968), *Int. Audiology*, **7**, 66.

Matzker, J. (1959), *Annals Otol.*, **68**, 1185.

Matzker, J. (1964), *Acta oto-rhino-laryng. belg.*, **18**, 511.

Miskoiczy-Fodor, F. (1953), *Acta oto-laryng. (Stockh.)*, **43**, 573.

Moore, B. C. J. (1972), *Sound*, **6**, 73.

Morales-Garcia, C. and Hood, J. D. (1972), *Arch. Otolaryng.*, **96**, 231.

Morales-Garcia, C. and Poole, J. P. (1972), *Acta oto-laryng. (Stockh.)*, **74**, 307.

Neff, W. D. (1968), *Int. Audiology*, **7**, 12.

Nilsson, R., Lidén, G., Rasen, M. and Zoller, M. (1973), *Scand. Audiology*, **2**, 125.

Noffsinger, D., Olsen, W. O., Carhart, R., Hart, C. W. and Sahgal, V. (1972), *Acta oto-laryng. (Stockh.)*, Suppl. 303.

Nordlund, B. (1964), *Acta oto-laryng. (Stockh.)*, **57**, 1.

Olsen, W. O., Rose, D. E. and Noffsinger, D. (1973). Personal communication.

Palva, A. and Jokinen, K. (1970), *Acta oto-laryng. (Stockh.)*, **70**, 232.

Parker, W., Decker, R. L. and Richards, N. G. (1968), *Arch. Otolaryng.*, **87**, 228.

Pialoux, P. (1962), *J. franç. d'Oto-Rhino Laryng.*, **11**, 909.

Roffler, S. K. and Butler, R. A. (1968), *J. acoust. Soc. Amer.*, **43**, 1255.

Ruhm, H. B., Mencke, E. D., Milburn, B., Cooper, W. A. and Rose, D. E. (1966), "*J. Speech Hear. Res.*, **9**, 371.

Sanchez Longo, L. P., Forster, F. M. and Auth, T. L. (1957), *Neurology*, **7**, 655.

Stephens, S. D. G. (1974), *Audiology*, **13**, 260.

Stephens, S. D. G. and Hinchcliffe, R. (1968), *Int. Audiology*, **7**, 267.

Swisher, L. P. (1967), *Cortex*, **3**, 179.

Swisher, L. and Hirsh, I. J. (1972), *Neuropsychologia*, **10**, 137.

Van Allen, M. W., Benton, A. L. and Gordon, M. C. (1966), *Neuropsychologia*, **4**, 159.

Van Zyl, F. J. and Brasier, V. J. (1973), *Brit. J. Audiology*, **7**, 69.

Walsh, E. G. (1957), *Brain*, **80**, 222.

Williams, M. (1970), *Brain Damage and the Mind.* Harmondsworth: Penguin Books.

26. VESTIBULAR SYSTEM—EXPERIMENTAL PATHOPHYSIOLOGY

MAKOTO IGARASHI

Much of the information derived from animal vestibular experiments has a direct bearing on clinical problems, even though there are significant inter-species differences. This chapter presents experimental studies in the following order:

Ablation experiments
Experimental production of endolymphatic hydrops
Experimental labyrinthine destruction by ultrasound, cryosurgery and laser beam
Vestibular ototoxicity experiments
Vestibular trauma experiments
Motion sickness experiments

ABLATION EXPERIMENTS

The fundamental responsibility of the vestibular system is that of contributing to the maintenance of bodily equilibrium function under ordinary circumstances in daily life. In addition, the equilibrium system responds to several types of stimulation of the end organ or directly to its neural system. By means of an ascending pathway, information is sent to the oculomotor system and the effects of vestibular stimulation may be manifested by the eye movement (nystagmus). Therefore, in order to evaluate the vestibular system, it is necessary to investigate both bodily equilibrium and oculomotor function, first, in the natural state (without applying any bizzare stimulation) and, secondly, under conditions with stimulation.

The experimental ablation of a part of the equilibrium system results in systemic imbalance, which is manifested by changes in the bodily equilibrium system and the oculo-motor system. The severity of the imbalance depends upon the overall importance of the part involved. In addition, ablation of different parts of the equilibrium system may produce quite different effects upon systemic responses depending upon such variables as the following: the excitatory or inhibitory nature of the part, the modality used to produce the destruction, and the influence of compensatory activities from other remaining intact areas of the central nervous system.

Inasmuch as the equilibrium system is a multi-input, ascending and descending reflex system, vestibular symptoms may dynamically change in accordance with the state of the disease process or the influence of the central compensation activity. This fact makes the diagnosis of many vestibular disorders extremely difficult. Consequently, the vestibular examination must be repeatedly performed along a time span in order to understand the vestibular disorder. Investigations conducted at one fixed time have only limited value.

Comparison of changes in function after ablation of different areas and subsequent compensation of both the bodily equilibrium system and the oculomotor system along the time span indicate the relative importance of different segments within the system. The information obtained after experimental selective ablation contributes to clinical diagnostic information. Also, it is extremely important to have morphological confirmation of the extent of ablation in order to correlate the degree of disturbance and recovery in performance or reflexes.

The author developed the squirrel monkey rail test (1968, 1969) and the squirrel monkey platform runway test in order to measure dynamic body equilibrium function in subhuman primates. By using these techniques of measuring behaviourally conditioned equilibrium performance, it is possible to quantitate the degree and direction of bodily dysequilibrium during the dynamic phase (locomotion). While the squirrel monkey rail test measures physically trained maximum ability for maintenance of dynamic equilibrium function, the platform runway test provides data about ordinary walking gait without the influence of any physical training.

Selective or Total Ablation of Vestibular End Organs

Igarashi *et al.* (1970) reported that, after unilateral labyrinthectomy in squirrel monkeys, the preoperative level for dynamic equilibrium function was regained within an average of two months postoperatively; however, after bilateral destruction, no matter whether the labyrinthectomy was performed simultaneously or not, the performance ability declined severely and the preoperative status was never regained even though the postoperative studies were continued for three to four months (squirrel monkey rail test). It was concluded, therefore, that some part of the peripheral vestibular end organ is needed for animals to satisfactorily recover from dysequilibrium produced after end organ lesions.

Probably the most interesting finding after unilateral labyrinthectomy in squirrel monkeys was the balance sway or oscillatory type of directional compensation in some of the post-labyrinthectomy cases (Igarashi *et al.*, 1970). This tendency was noticed in both the squirrel monkey rail test and the platform runway test. Concomitant with gradual reduction of the percentage of falls, the falling direction changed from one side to the other along the postoperative time span. Probably the falls toward the operated side represent balance disturbance and the falls toward the opposite side represent coordination activity or an excess of compensation efforts. In oculomotor responses, the secondary phase of nystagmus after strong thermal or rotary stimulation displays a similar situation of acute and severe imbalance.

Cohen and his group (1973) studied optokinetic nystagmus and optokinetic afternystagmus in rhesus monkeys after unilateral and bilateral labyrinthectomy. The reduction in the maximum velocity of slow phase, frequency and total deviation of optokinetic nystagmus was found after the operation. Eventually, normal function resumed. However, after bilateral labyrinthectomy, optokinetic afternystagmus could no longer be evoked and the loss was permanent. These data demonstrated the importance of the vestibular contribution to optokinetic nystagmus and optokinetic afternystagmus. In 1971, Watanabe *et al.* conducted a study on the optic-vestibular coordination by utilizing simultaneous optokinetic and vestibular stimulation in squirrel monkeys. Concomitant subliminal rotatory stimulation facilitated the slow phase eye-speed of optokinetic nystagmus. In other words, the presence of simultaneous vestibular stimulation assisted in maintenance of the retinal image for a moving target.

In regard to the otolithic end organs, a significant difference between the effects of unilateral saccular macular ablation and unilateral utricular nerve section on the main-

tenance of dynamic bodily equilibrium was documented in a series of studies (Igarashi, 1965, 1970; Igarashi *et al.*, 1972) (Fig. 1). Together with step-by-step surgical controls, the contribution of the saccular macula to the

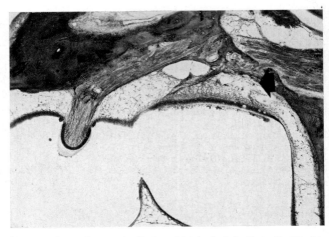

Fig. 1. Photomicrograph displays histological finding of utricular nerve section (arrow). A part of the utricular nerve adjacent to the lateral ampullar nerve remains. H. & E. staining. ×32·5. (From: Igarashi, M., Miyata, H. and Alford, B. R. (1972), "Utricular Ablation and Dysequilibrium in Squirrel Monkeys," *Acta otolaryng.*, **74**, 66–72.)

psychophysically-advanced locomotive performance was found to be minimal. Saccular ablation in the frog by McNally and Tait (1925) and in the rabbit by Versteegh (1927) and Jongkees (1950) did not create bodily dysequilibrium.

On the other hand, severe dysequilibrium was observed after unilateral utricular nerve section, and complete equilibrium compensation took place 3–4 weeks postoperatively (squirrel monkey rail test).

According to Igarashi and Miyata (1972), dynamic equilibrium function severely declined after unilateral lateral ampullary nerve section (previously studied in cats by Mair and Fernandez). However, the average degree of rail threshold decline on the eighth postoperative day was statistically insignificant when compared to the preoperative threshold. This study confirmed the relative importance of the input (spontaneous discharge) from the crista ampullaris of the lateral semicircular duct for the maintenance of dynamic equilibrium function. However, compared to the post-labyrinthectomy or post-utricular nerve section status, equilibrium compensation occurred more rapidly.

Experimental Neck Lesions

It is well known that balance disturbances occur after cervical lesions such as whiplash injuries in automobile accident victims. Abnormal proprioceptive input and circulatory alterations through either direct or sympathetic reflex mechanisms are considered to be major factors in producing these disturbances. The vascular alterations involve not only the peripheral labyrinthine system, but also the brain stem, which is especially sensitive to ischemia;

thus, cervical lesions often produce very complex symptomatology.

A study of dynamic bodily equilibrium function and evoked oculomotor function after lidocaine (xylocaine) injections into the unilateral deep neck or after unilateral C1, C2 dorsal root section, was performed by Igarashi *et al.* in squirrel monkeys (1969, 1972). A moderate degree of bodily dysequilibrium with no directional preponderance of the resultant ataxia was found in the subjects. Also, the relationship between cervical proprioceptive cues and the oculomotor system was reconfirmed in these studies.

Cerebellum and Brain Stem

A series of studies using squirrel monkeys confirmed that the cerebellar uvulo-nodular area is important for bodily equilibrium maintenance, probably as an inhibitor of vestibular evoked oculomotor function and a facilitator for optokinetic nystagmus. This type of experimental approach may assist in the topodiagnosis of vestibular-related diseases within the central nervous system.

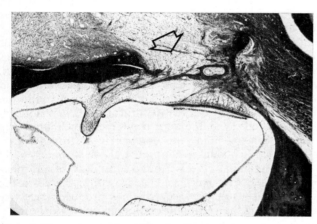

FIG. 2. Photomicrograph exhibits the histological condition of the crista ampullaris of the lateral semicircular duct and utricular macula from the lateral ampullar nerve sectioned ear. The arrow indicates the area of lateral ampullary nerve section. H. & E. staining. ×30. (From: Igarashi, M. and Miyata, H. (1972), "Effects of Lateral Ampullary Nerve Section in Squirrel Monkeys," *Arch. oto-laryng.*, **95**, 158–163.)

As far as bodily equilibrium function is concerned, the ablative effects eventually disappeared along the postoperative time course. Even after moderately extensive destruction of the nodulus and uvula, complete compensation took place. The dysfunction caused by a small, slowly-developing lesion in this area such as a tumor might be masked, however. Therefore, the clinical diagnosis of such conditions may be difficult. The repeated performance of a neuro-otologic test battery may provide possible clues for the diagnosis of this condition.

Repeated tests along the postoperative time course demonstrated that the severity and fate of all different kinds of nystagmus were not necessarily related to bodily equilibrium compensation. Oculomotor symptoms generally lasted longer as compared to the bodily dysequilibrium. Optokinetic nystagmus showed a fairly clear recovery tendency. The ablation of the cerebellar nodulus and uvula,

therefore, contributes in a different way to bodily equilibrium maintenance, vestibulo-oculomotor function, and optokinetic nystagmus.

Probably, the contribution by Cohen in 1971 is the most up-to-date, extensive survey of vestibulo-oculomotor investigations. The report covers oculomotor function after end-organ stimulation, after lesions of the medial longitudinal fasciculus and in the paramedian pontine reticular formation, etc. While studying the effects of vestibular nuclear lesions in rhesus monkeys (Uemura and Cohen, 1972), changes in bodily equilibrium were towards the ipsilateral direction after destruction of the lateral or caudal part of the vestibular nuclear complex, and were toward the contra-lateral direction after superior or rostral medial vestibular nuclear lesions. Optokinetic nystagmus was little affected by vestibular nuclear lesions. Convergent direction-changing positional nystagmus was found after caudal descending vestibular nuclear lesions. Positional nystagmus was also produced by superior vestibular nuclear lesions.

Visual Cue Alteration

The importance of visual cues for maintenance of bodily equilibrium has been known both clinically and experimentally. Using an ataxiameter, Edwards (1946) reported that an increase of sway was found when vision was eliminated by closing the eyes or by decreasing the illumination to the point of complete darkness. A very limited number of animal experiments, however, have been performed in this regard. Igarashi and Miyata (1971) examined body equilibrium maintenance ability in squirrel monkeys before and after the administration of cyclopentolate hydrochloride and homatropine eyedrops (squirrel monkey rail test). The maximum ability of dynamic equilibrium maintenance declined significantly after the cyclopentolate eyedrops; however, homatropine failed to produce any significant change. Thus, as far as cycloplegic eyedrops are concerned, a temporary and partial change in the visual cue will affect a subject's equilibrium performance when a physically advanced task in required.

EXPERIMENTAL PRODUCTION OF ENDOLYMPHATIC HYDROPS

Endolymphatic hydrops was described in 1938 by Hallpike and Cairns as the principal pathological finding in human temporal bones with Ménière's disease. In order to investigate the mechanism, many animal studies have been performed to create labyrinthine hydrops in different species. Lindsay (1947) performed obliteration of the saccus and ductus endolymphaticus on rhesus monkeys, but failed to produce hydrops after a survival time of $3\frac{1}{2}$ months. In 1952, he performed a similar experiment on cats and again failed to create hydrops after a survival time of 3–9 months. In a study by Schuknecht *et al.* (1968) an attempt was made to keep the animals alive for a maximum of 3 years. Probable endolymphatic hydrops, which was represented by ectasia or enlargement of the cochlear duct was present in 12 out of 15 experimental ears in which the saccus endolymphaticus had been destroyed. The hydrops consisted of mild to moderate displacement of the vestibular membrane toward the scala vestibuli throughout all coils of the cochlea; however, in none of these ears was there clear distension of the utricle, saccule, or semicircular ducts. Kimura (1968) also created endolymphatic hydrops in 100 per cent of his experimental guinea pigs and chinchillas. It is important to note that some of these hydropic guinea pigs' labyrinths had sensory hair cell lesions. Extensive saccular distension was demonstrated in these animals and, on certain occasions, the saccular wall was touched by the stapedial base. Probably, the endolymph reabsorption in the guinea pig is more dependent upon the endolymphatic sac while, in the larger animals, other areas of the membranous labyrinth are able to eliminate excess endolymph adequately. This might be one reason why inter-species difference exists in the creation of endolymphatic hydrops after saccus endolymphaticus obliteration. Squirrel monkeys, after saccus endolymphaticus obliteration, failed to demonstrate any hydrops and, in some of these, a fistula was found in the saccular wall.

It is well known that the enlargement of the endolymphatic space may be the result of many etiological factors including infection and vascular obliteration. In our dog microembolism experiments (1965; 1969), segmental ectasia of the cochlear duct was observed together with stria vascularis and sensory end-organ lesions. The extent of hydrops was moderate and there was no clear enlargement of the utricle, saccule or semicircular ducts. In these dog ears with peripheral vascular obliteration, the functional and morphological correlation was good.

EXPERIMENTAL LABYRINTHINE DESTRUCTION BY ULTRASOUND, CRYOSURGERY AND LASER BEAM

In order to relieve patients with Ménière's disease, which produces recurrent attacks of vertigo, many different surgical procedures have been developed in addition to the medical treatment of the disorders. Furthermore, in cases in which it is worthwhile to preserve hearing function in the affected ear, attempts have been made to destroy the vestibular end-organs selectively.

For this purpose, ultrasonic irradiation has been extensively studied and clinically used. Histological evidence of labyrinthine end-organ degeneration after this treatment was confirmed by many animal experiments. The biophysical effects of the ultrasonic beam are the following: agitation, rise of temperature, cavitation with the formation of bubbles in the cells, streaming with bubble formation in the cellular cytoplasm and blocking of the metabolic system, increased permeability of the cell membranes, chemical changes and change of enzymatic activity.

Recent electron microscopic investigations (Lundquist et al., 1971) of the guinea pig labyrinth after ultrasonic irradiation (acute experimentation) indicates that the biophysical effects of these ultrasonic irradiations such as agitation and streaming are the primary factors producing the destruction of the sensory cells. The basic pattern of degeneration is identical regardless of the duration of irradiation and whether the crus osseum is drilled; however, the thinner

the bone, the shorter the exposure time necessary to achieve the identical degree of destruction.

With the techniques used in this acute experiment, no cochlear involvement (morphological) was found even after 15 min of irradiation. The tops of the sensory hair cells looked intact and the epithelial cytoplasm exhibited normal cellular organelles; however, this merely indicates the very acute condition of the sensory epithelium after ultrasonic irradiation.

Cryosurgery has been used experimentally and clinically in order to destroy the vestibular end-organs without disturbing the spiral organ. In basic animal experiments, Cutt and Wolfson's group, using light microscopy, studied the effects of cryosurgery. In other electron microscopic investigations (Lundquist et al., 1972) different parameters of freezing techniques were studied. In the fast-freeze specimens, changes were always present in the crista ampullaris of the lateral semicircular duct even after immediate sacrifice. Formations of intracytoplasmic vacuoles were found in the hair cells, but no change was observed in sensory hairs or cuticular plates. The mitochondrial cristae had disappeared. After a long survival time, more changes were found in these fast-freeze specimens.

In the slow-freeze specimens, severely degenerated cells were present even after immediate sacrifice. Other findings were: mitochondrial damage or rupture, vesicle formation, cytoplasmic protrusions, etc. Some hair cells were found to be expelled into the endolymphatic space. Even in the supporting cells, some ultrastructural changes were noticed. In the animals with the very slow-freeze technique, the sensory epithelial lining was completely destroyed with a collapsed and condensed connective tissue stroma.

In all animals in this series, the cochlear duct was morphologically intact even by electron microscopy; therefore, the possibility exists that cryosurgery may produce a selective destruction of the vestibular end-organ apparatus, especially the cristae ampullares. When cryosurgery is used as an ablative procedure, the destruction of the neuroepithelium is probably due to the formation of ice crystals inside the cytoplasm. In the quick-freeze mode, the changes are more of a metabolic type due to the destruction of the internal crista of the mitochondria, which may attenuate the function of the sensory cells. It is also possible that these changes are enhanced by changes in the function of the secretory epithelia.

According to Stahle's experiments (1965, 1972), a ruby laser beam can produce focal lesions in the vestibular part of the pigeon labyrinth. He extended his experiments by using an argon laser beam to create a very fine local lesion within the guinea pig cochlea, thereby suggesting the possibility of selective ablation.

VESTIBULAR OTOTOXICITY EXPERIMENTS

A large number of publications in the field of antibiotic ototoxicity experiments exist, as antibiotics have been used extensively in clinical medicine and some of them have long been known to have an ototoxic effect. In this section, the animal experiments concerned with vestibular ototoxicity are presented. No studies of human patients or human temporal bones are included.

Streptomycin and Dihydrostreptomycin

With streptomycin, Hawkins (1947) was the first to experimentally produce vestibular disturbances in rabbits and cats. He continued his investigations from both a functional and morphological standpoint (1950, 1952, 1957). Postrotatory nystagmus, gait and posture were investigated in his studies. The cristae ampullares of the lateral semicircular duct showed definite degeneration of the sensory cells. There was also shrinking of the sensory epithelium (1952). Similar vestibular end-organ involvement after streptomycin administration was found in cats by Schuknecht (1957), McGee (1958), McGee and Olszewski (1962) and in guinea pigs by Ostyn and Tyberghein (1968). McGee and Olszewski (1962) and in guinea pigs by Ostyn and Tyberghein (1968). McGee and Olszewski confirmed that the ampullar cristae were more vulnerable than the maculae.

Wersäll and Hawkins (1962) were probably the first to utilize the electron microscope as a tool to investigate streptomycin vestibular ototoxicity. They found severe changes in the sensory epithelium of the cristae ampullares. In their experiment, nuclear degeneration, mitochondrial degeneration, and cytoplasmic protrusion were observed. In addition to the morphological study, bodily equilibrium function and postrotatory nystagmus were studied in these cats. McCabe (1964), by using a rhythmic vertical linear acceleration, reported that streptomycin damages mainly the cristae ampullares.

Winston and his group (1948, 1949, 1953) reported some evidence of damage to the vestibular-related central nervous system in cats after streptomycin or dihydrostreptomycin administration. Marked pathologic change was found in the flocculus and the nodulus; less marked but definite damage was noticed in the lateral vestibular nucleus. Floberg and his associates (1949) also demonstrated by cyto-chemical methods that streptomycin had a destructive effect on the vestibular ganglion and on the lateral vestibular nucleus.

In view of the above study, Hamberger and his associates (1949) suggested the possibility of using streptomycin as a therapeutical measure in Ménière's disease; this was also advocated later by Schuknecht (1957). Christensen *et al.* (1951) have reported some changes in the vestibular neural pathway of the guinea pig. In Cherkasov's study (1962) of the effect of streptomycin sulfate on cats, pathologic changes were found in the phylogenetically-older portions of the vestibular analyzer, namely the vestibular ganglion and the lateral vestibular nucleus. Probably the phylogenicity is an important factor in deciding the vulnerability in the vestibular or auditory system. In the study by McGee and Olszewski (1962), however, none of their cats had changes in the brain stem which could be attributed to the direct toxic action of streptomycin sulfate or dihydrostreptomycin. Their opinion was that streptomycin toxicity was due to peripheral lesions. In support of this contention, Vrabec *et al.* (1965) have found that the streptomycin level in the perilymph was well above that in the cerebrospinal fluid in the cat.

Caloric threshold, motion sickness in the slow-rotation room, and ataxia after streptomycin sulfate were studied by Igarashi and associates (1966) through the use of experimental subhuman primates. After a series of streptomycin injections, many subjects showed an ataxia, a complete or almost complete suppression of caloric response and no manifestation of emesis in the slow-rotation room. Subsequently, some of these functions recovered. The suppression of the vestibular function after streptomycin administration may represent mainly a biochemical effect and partly some other systemic involvement. The histopathological findings

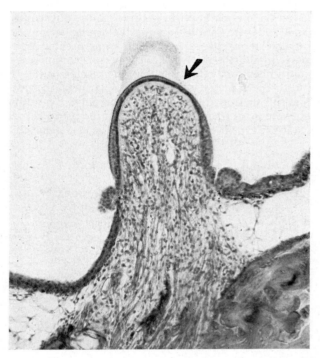

FIG. 3. This photomicrograph shows sensory (hair) cell loss in the crista ampullaris of the lateral semicircular duct from the squirrel monkey which received systemic injections of streptomycin sulfate (total doses: 1100 mg). The arrow indicates that the sensory cell loss is prominent on the summit (central area) of the ampullary crista. H. & E. staining. ×88. (From: Igarashi, M., McLeod, M. E. and Graybiel, A. (1966), "Clinical Pathological Correlations in Squirrel Monkeys after Suppression of Semi-circular Canal Function by Streptomycin Sulfate," *Acta oto-laryng.*, suppl. **214**, 1–28.

were largely confined to the cristae mpullares (Fig. 3) and the spiral organ. The maculae in all ears showed slight-to-moderate pathology.

Experiments in dihydrostreptomycin ototoxicity in cats were performed by Hawkins and Lurie (1953), Hawkins *et al.* (1957), and McGee and Olszewski (1962). All reported that intensive treatment with dihydrostreptomycin caused vestibular disturbance in cats associated with degeneration of the hair cells at the base of the cristae ampullares. In general, however, the dihydrostreptomycin ototoxic effect was later in onset and less severe than that after streptomycin sulfate administration. In 1970, Balogh *et al.* performed an experiment in guinea pigs which were injected with tritium-labelled dihydrostreptomycin, which was then localized autoradiographically in freeze-dried cochleae. It appeared that dihydrostreptomycin entered the perilymphatic space from the spiral ligament and then the antibiotic ultimately reached the endolymph either from the stria vascularis, the perilymphatic space, or both. Apparently the antibiotic could reach every cell, but did not show preferential localization. This, however, does not rule out the possibility of specific sensitivity or vulnerability of certain cells to this antibiotic.

Viomycin

In 1965, Daly and Cohen reported that, based upon cupulometry investigations, viomycin sulfate was more toxic to the vestibular apparatus than to the cochlea. Subsequently, Kanda and Igarashi (1969) studied the vestibular end-organs of squirrel monkeys and cats electron microscopically after viomycin sulfate administration. The crista ampullaris was found to be more vulnerable than the macula to this drug in both species. Vacuolization, vesicle formation, mitochondrial degeneration, nuclear chromatin aggregation, etc., were more frequently observed in the type I hair cells than in the type II hair cells (Fig. 4). The nerve chalice was

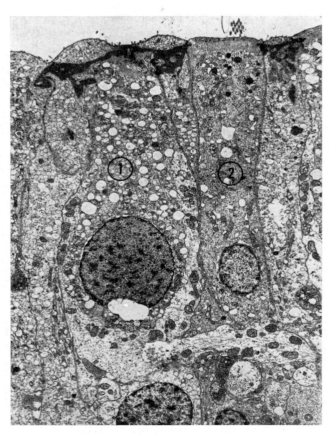

FIG. 4. Electron micrograph demonstrates a view of type I (1) and type II (2) sensory cells in the ampullary crista of the lateral semicircular duct from the cat which received 200 mg/kg daily systemic injections of viomycin sulfate. The animal was ataxic on the tenth day after a total dose of 4140 mg. The vacuolization in the cytoplasm of the type I sensory cell is marked. Lysosome-like electron-dense granules are found at the apical part of the type II sensory cells. ×2300. (From: Kanda, T. and Igarashi, M. (1969), "Ultrastructural Changes in Vestibular Sensory End-organs after Viomycin Sulfate Intoxication," *Acta oto-laryng.*, **68**, 474–488.)

swollen and cytoplasmic contents were decreased. Primary involvement of this area after viomycin may also occur inasmuch as an irregular cytoplasmic boundary was found where the sensory cells were least involved.

Neomycin

Hawkins and Lurie (1953) reported that small doses of neomycin had little or no effect upon vestibular function in the cat, but it caused complete degeneration of the cochlear hair cells and corresponding loss of microphonic and nerve-action potentials.

Kanamycin

Probably, the experiment by Hawkins (1959) is the first well-designed, basically auditory, kanamycin animal experiment. So far as the vestibular system is concerned, kanamycin is less toxic than either streptomycin or dihydrostreptomycin. The experiment suggested that the primary effect of kanamycin occurs in the spiral organ.

Functional and morphological studies in the guinea pig after kanamycin administration were performed by Ward and Fernandez (1961). These animals had loss of hearing and were also ataxic with staggering and falling. The histopathological studies revealed severe damage to the outer hair cells and the supporting elements; however, the vestibular receptors were considered to be morphologically normal. Some of the animals showed patchy disseminated rarified areas primarily involving the granular layer of the cerebellum (Klüver's strain).

The following several reports are not directly related to the vestibular end-organ toxicity; however, these works demonstrate important clues of ototoxic mechanisms. By utilizing electron microscopy, Lundquist and Wersäll (1966) studied cochlear hair cells in kanamycin-intoxicated guinea pigs. Some of the early changes were: clumping of the chromatin in the nucleus, swelling of the nuclear membrane and mitochondrial degeneration. The changes caused by kanamycin in the cytoplasmic membrane were a fairly late effect; the early changes occurred apparently in the RNA protein synthesis system and in the mitochondria.

By utilizing the differential type of ultramicrorespirometer, Mizukoshi and Daly (1967) observed that the kanamycin-damaged cochleae had a decreased rate of oxygen consumption.

Stupp and associates (1967), using 210 guinea pigs, observed that, at a low range of dosage, when the dosage was raised only slightly, the kanamycin contents of the labyrinthine fluid increased substantially. This increase could be explained not only by the delay in the elimination of the antibiotic, but also by the fact that accumulation seemed to be increased by the membrane-sealing effect of kanamycin. Their experimental findings indicated that high and maximum internal ear concentrations that have a toxic effect will arise within the low and narrow therapeutic dosage range.

Kaneko et al. (1970) also studied the change in the vestibular membrane after kanamycin. According to their results, after kanamycin administration, the vestibular membrane might cause perilymph and endolymph to lose their ability to maintain the normal biochemical composition.

In a histochemical study of guinea pigs after kanamycin injections conducted by Ishii and his associates (1968), there was a slight temporary increase in the intensity and area of enzyme activity prior to the structural changes that developed in the hair cells. Afterwards, the reaction became gradually weaker and finally was negative. Ultimately, all hair cells were destroyed. The histochemical changes in the spiral ganglion may have been independent of damage to the spiral organ.

Quantitative analysis of acid mucopolysacharrides in the kanamycin-intoxicated guinea pig cochlea was performed by Saito and Daly (1971). The decreased quantity of acid mucopolysacharrides in the stria vascularis and spiral ligament suggested that the main pathway of kanamycin into the endolymph is from the stria vascularis and the spiral ligament and that the change of ground substance in the connective tissues may affect a static equilibrium state and dynamic transport process between endolymph and stria vascularis. This situation might lead to high concentration and prolonged presence of kanamycin within the labyrinthine fluid. Further, it was assumed that the formation of kanamycin-acid mucopolysacharride complexes in the hair cells, without digestion, might be more serious than presence of kanamycin in the endolymph.

Gentamicin

Experimental vestibular damage due to gentamicin was first reported in cats and dogs by Black and his associates in 1963. Electron microscopic studies by Lundquist and Wersäll (1967) and Wersäll and associates (1969) in the guinea pig, demonstrated more damage in the vestibular than in the cochlear end-organ system. Early ultrastructural changes with hair swelling and fusion by protrusion of the cell surface, and mitochondrial degeneration were observed leading to complete degeneration. Type I hair cells were damaged first; later type II hair cells were involved.

Using the cat, McGee and associates (1969) and Webster and his associates (1971) studied hearing loss after gentamicin administration. According to them, the cochlea, the crista ampullaris of the lateral semicircular ducts and the saccules were the vulnerable end-organs. In Hawkins and others' study (1969), bodily dysequilibrium (ataxia) was investigated in cats after varying doses of gentamicin to confirm vestibular toxicity. They concluded that on a weight-to-weight basis, gentamicin was more than twice as toxic as streptomycin for the vestibular system. With reference to the time of the appearance of ataxia, Waitz and associates (1971), studying cats, ataxia after gentamicin, reported that total dosage and duration appear to be more important factors than peak levels of drug in the serum.

Our ototoxicity study of gentamicin in squirrel monkeys (Igarashi et al., 1971) revealed both vestibular and cochlear toxicity of this drug. The intermittant, rather than daily, administration of this drug produced less disturbance and the disturbance was slower in onset. Even considerably lower daily doses caused more severe and earlier loss of ability to maintain bodily equilibrium. Subsequent electron microscopic study of the vestibular end-organs demon-

strated the hair cell pathology (Fig. 5). The correlation of the morphological findings and the vestibular function alteration was not good. The considerable weight-loss in some animals that received a high daily dose probably reflected systemic involvement including renal tubular degeneration. This kidney pathology was observed histologically.

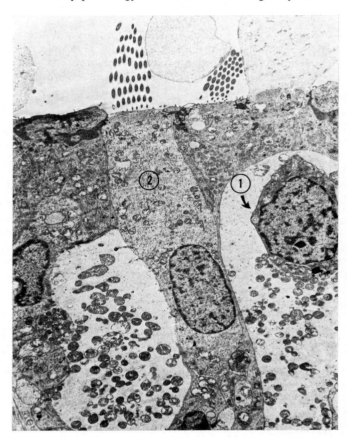

FIG. 5. This electron micrograph exhibits sensory cell pathology in the utricular macula from the squirrel monkey that received daily systemic injections of gentamicin, 60 mg/kg; total dose of 390·6 mg. Severe destruction of type I sensory cells (1) can be observed while the type II sensory cell (2) was better preserved. ×860. (From: Igarashi, M., Lundquist, P. G., Alford, B. R. and Miyata, H. (1971), "Experimental Ototoxicity of Gentamicin in Squirrel Monkeys," *J. infect. Dis.*, **124**, S114–S124, [The University of Chicago Pres).

All of the gentamicin animal experiments were performed by administering high doses. Gentamicin, in the recommended clinical dosage of $1-3$ mg.kg^{-1}, may have a reasonable margin of safety in man, as was suggested by Hawkins *et al.* (1969).

Salicylates

Using the cat, Silverstein and his associates (1967), experimentally produced salicylate ototoxicity; they studied the effects both electrophysiologically and biochemically. Two or three hours after the injection of sodium salicylate, the electrical activity of the cochlea, as recorded from the area of the fenestra cochleae, showed an elevation of threshold. Also, the N1 action potential was reduced by 70 per cent while the cochlear microphonic was reduced by 40 per cent of its original voltage. Salicylate intoxication produced biochemical changes in endolymph (including vestibular) and perilymph manifested by decreased malic dehydrogenase activity. There was hyperglycemia and elevation of glucose in the endolymph and perilymph. Sodium, potassium and total protein concentration of the internal ear fluids appeared to be unaffected.

Others

Reports exist on the ototoxicity in animals and humans of tobramycin, chloramphenicol (topical application), etacrynic acid, nitrogen mustard and chloroquine. However, in these reports, no detailed description of vestibular involvement is available.

General Comments

The surface preparation technique developed by Engström (1964) which provides a surface scanning view of individual end-organs is very useful in investigating the regional differences of the ototoxic end-organ involvement. In Lindeman's study (1969) of guinea pigs, clear regional differences in vulnerability were noticed after intratympanic or systemic applications of antibiotics. In general, the sensory cells of the crista ampullaris were more vulnerable than those of the utricular macula, which in turn was distinctly more vulnerable than the saccular macula. The degenerative changes primarily involved the central portion of the cristae ampullares and the striolae of the maculae.

Subsequent studies by Watanuki and Meyer zum Gottesberge (1971) also demonstrated similar findings. The morphological vulnerability was emphasized by a difference in degrees of sensitivity between type I and type II hair cells. Watanuki et al. (1972) further extended the ototoxicity study after gentamicin administration and found that the sensory epithelia of the cristae ampullares were more fragile than those of the otolithic end-organs. Among the otolithic end-organs, the utricular maculae were more vulnerable than the saccular maculae. In the striola, the type I hair cells with common nerve chalices were most vulnerable. With reference to type II hair cells, however, there were no differences in sensitivity between the striola and the peripheral parts of macula. We have utilized a similar surface preparation technique (succinic dehydrogenase staining) for the internal ear end-organs of the squirrel monkey after gentamicin injections. To date, similar regional differences and similar differences in vulnerability between the different end-organs were observed.

The reason for the difference in the vulnerability among different internal ear end-organs and among different regions within one single end-organ is not known. Probably the difference in end-organ vulnerability is dependent upon the condition of nutritional supply, oxygen consumption rate, phylogenesis, ecological validity, biological importance, etc. Assuming that the antibiotic is distributed to different end-organs evenly and diffusely, different rates of metabolic activity among the different internal ear end-organs or different cells, which may be decided by the functional necessity, determines the vulnerability.

The direct application of streptomycin solution to the lateral line organ was studied by Wersäll and Flock in 1964. Suppression and restoration of the microphonic output

from the lateral line organ after local application of streptomycin was observed. By using electrophysiological methods, the effect of streptomycin sulfate, dihydrostreptomycin, neomycin and kanamycin, on the ampullar receptor of the isolated posterior semicircular duct of the frog (Rana esculenta) was studied by Harada et al. in 1967. Both the spontaneous activity and the response to stimulus of the ampullar receptors were promptly and reversibly inhibited by the antibiotics tested. The depressant effect was higher for streptomycin and lower for the other antibiotics.

Hawkins (1970) described major sites of ototoxic action upon the secretory and reabsorptive tissues of the cochlea. Pericapillary elements of the external spiral sulcus and other cells throughout the spiral ligament were damaged by kanamycin and neomycin. The stria vascularis, limbus spiralis and vestibular membrane were also affected. It was postulated that the primary actions of these agents on the internal ear resemble those in the kidney tubules and affected membrane function and protein synthesis in tissues responsible for the active transport of ions. Therefore, destruction of the spiral may be the result of a disturbance at special homeostatic mechanisms upon which its normal function and integrity depend.

It is suspected that ototoxic mechanisms are similar in the vestibular end-organs, even though the end-organ architecture and endolymph circulation are not identical. Further advances in the application of electron microscopy, histochemistry, autoradiography and surface preparation techniques will answer many of the remaining questions.

In our recent studies of gentamicin ototoxicity in squirrel monkeys (1971), dysequilibrium occurred rapidly when high daily doses such as 30 or 60 mg.kg^{-1} of the drug were injected; however, the results obtained by the body-equilibrium function tests and the morphological findings were not necessarily in agreement. One possible reason for this is that body equilibrium function represents not only the internal ear condition, but also other systemic involvement concomitantly.

Many different factors must be considered regarding the ototoxic effects of the antibiotics. Much smaller doses of antibiotics are usually administered to humans when compared to the doses used in the experimental animal studies. It is, however, important to examine kidney function repeatedly during the long course of antibiotic treatment. In our primate experiments, kidney involvement was confirmed and it is well known that these changes will accelerate pathological involvement of internal ear end-organ apparatus. As far as the vestibular end-organs are concerned, the cristae ampullares are vulnerable in many instances after antibiotic injections; therefore, in addition to repeated hearing tests, repeated vestibular tests such as the post-rotatory nystagmus test, or the caloric test are recommended. The sensitivity of these vestibular tests is limited, however.

In addition, in the author's studies utilizing experimental animals, many animals demonstrated rather sudden onset of ataxia or sudden loss of the semicircular duct response. Prior to that time, the vestibular functions were normal; therefore, it was difficult to predict the occurrence of ototoxic vestibular disorders. Also, in some instances, the ototoxic involvement progressed even after cessation of administration of the drug. Another factor which could influence the vestibular symptomatology and findings is the rate of functional compensation.

VESTIBULAR TRAUMA EXPERIMENTS

Since the time of classic animal centrifuge experiments, only a limited number of traumatic experiments have been performed to create vestibular lesions in different animal species. Schuknecht and Davison (1956) applied intensive and repeated head blows to cats. They found a tear in the membranous wall of both the utricle and the saccule in one cat. The saccular membrane collapsed against the saccular macula and about 30 per cent sensory cell reduction was noticed. In 1967, Igarashi and Nagaba exposed 54 squirrel monkeys to different levels of high-intensity linear acceleration stimuli (by centrifuge) which were directed so as to produce a backward acceleration force. Functional studies were carried out at both pre- and post-exposure stages. Post-exposure ataxia and abnormal eye movement were definitely due to both peripheral and central involvement. The basic light microscopic change was dislocation of the otolithic (statoconial) membrane, which was consistently observed after 150 G for 1 min exposure or more. The possibility of preparation artifacts for otolithic membrane displacement was eliminated by processing simultaneously, many control animal temporal bones in an exactly identical preparation procedure to that of the experimental group. Also, the severity of the otolithic membrane dislocation was somewhat parallel to the level of applied G forces. Some of the membranes dislocated from the utricular macula were found within the posterior membranous ampulla (Fig. 6). This finding somewhat resembles

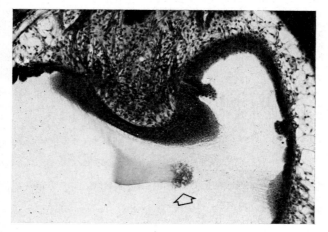

FIG. 6. This photomicrograph illustrates dislocated membrana statoconiorum from utricular macula (arrow) adjacent to the cupula of the crista ampullaris of the posterior semicircularis duct. This squirrel monkey was exposed to a peak G. of 400 G. linear acceleration force in a backward (−Gx) direction. H. & E. staining. ×93.

that of Schuknecht's cupulolithiasis (1969) condition. No light microscopic change was detected in either the cristae ampullares or the spiral organ. In monkeys which were exposed to 200 G for 1 min and to a peak G of 450 G,

the ultrastructural changes observed in the utricular macula were increased lysosomes and mitochondrial transformation in the nerve chalice, which might be the result of anoxia.

MOTION SICKNESS EXPERIMENTS

The purpose of the motion sickness experiment utilizing experimental animals is to study etiological factors, to analyze symptomatology, to investigate the effect of training and to study the effect of treatment. Inasmuch as this sort of experimentation has a very important application in aerospace and marine medicine, a large number of human experiments have been performed in the past. Probably the best summarization of these studies appears in the transactions of *Fourth Symposium of the Role of the Vestibular Organs in Space Exploration*, which was published by NASA (1968).

Dogs are the most commonly used motion sicknesssusceptible experimental animal species (Money, 1970). Wang and Chinn's group have used this species very extensively to investigate the role of the peripheral vestibular labyrinth, vestibular cerebellum and chemo-receptor trigger zone, etc., in the coordination of motion sickness. Money and Friedberg (1964) performed bilateral labyrinthectomies inactivation of all six semicircular ducts by canal plugging, and inactivation of fewer than six of the semicircular ducts. Dogs were restrained and swung along the floor. They found that the discreet inactivation of all six semicircular ducts was equivalent to bilateral labyrinthectomy in eliminating motion sickness in dogs, although the otolithic end-organs remained functional. Inactivation of fewer than six semicircular ducts reduced the susceptibility of dogs to motion sickness, but to a lesser degree than the inactivation of all six semicircular ducts. These findings were consistent with the hypothesis that stimulation of the ampullary cristae causes motion sickness.

Subhuman primates have been used extensively also for motion-sickness experiments by several investigators. In 1960, Graybiel *et al.* observed the "canal sickness" symptom and adaptation in chimpanzees in the Pensacola slow-rotation room. One of the animals demonstrated a form of "canal sickness" similar to that experienced by human subjects. After being exposed to slow speeds of rotation for 2 days, this animal tolerated exposure to higher speeds without signs of sickness; however, this adaptation seemed to be of short duration. Igarashi and his associates (1968) performed a series of experiments on motion sickness susceptibility using South American-born squirrel monkeys. The animals in a cage were rotated at 10 r.p.m. (about 1 rad. sec^{-1}) until either the subject actually vomited or 15 min had lapsed. Sound was given in order to keep the animal alert and active so that its head movement produced Coriolis forces to cause motion sickness. The test was repeated 5 or 6 times on different days. A total of 57 squirrel monkeys were tested over a period of 2 years. The approximate results were these: one-third of them were found to be very susceptible to motion sickness; one-third were moderately or slightly susceptible; the remaining one-third were not susceptible. This testing procedure could also be used to select motion sickness-susceptible animals for other studies such as streptomycin experiments. In these squirrel monkeys, other otolith (statoconia) function tests were not performed; therefore, the possibility of otolithic end-organ origin of motion sickness could not be excluded.

ACKNOWLEDGEMENTS

The present study is partly supported by the National Institute of Neurological Disease and Stroke—Research Career Development Award KO3NS38619; Program Project Grant PO1NS10940, Research Grant NS7237, the McFadden Charitable Trust Research Fund and the Schewing Corporation Research Fund.

Gratitude is extended to Dr. B. R. Alford, Dr. H. Miyata, Mrs. M. Lewis, Mrs. K. Cummings, Mrs. E. Marbley, Mr. V. Storey, Mr. J. Ledet and Mr. S. Christian for their support and encouragement.

REFERENCES

Alford, B. R., Shaver, E. F., Rosenberg, J. J. and Guildford, F. 1965), *Ann. Otol., Rhinol., Lar.,* **74**, 728.

Balogh, K., Jr., Hiraide, F. and Ishic, D. (1970), *Ann. Otol., Rhinol., Lar.,* **79**, 641.

Black, J., Calesnick, B., Williams, D. and Weinstein, M. J. (1963), *Antimicrobial Agents and Chemotherapy,* p. 138.

Cherkasov, V. S. (1962), *Zhurnal Ushnykh, Nosovykh i Gorlovykh Boleznei,* **4**, 51.

Christensen, E., Hertz, H., Riskaer, N. and Vra-Jensen, G. (1951), *Ann. Otol., Rhinol., Lar.,* **60**, 343.

Cohen, B. (1971), *The Control of Eye Movements,* p. 105.

Cohen, B., Uemura, T. and Takemori, S. (1973), *Equilibrium Res.* In Press.

Daly, J. F. and Cohen, N. L. (1965), *Ann. Otol., Rhinol., Lar.,* **74**, 521.

Edwards, A. S. (1946), *J. exp. Psychol.,* **36**, 526.

Engström, H., Ades, H. W. and Hawkins, J. E., Jr. (1964), *Acta oto-laryng.,* suppl. **188**, 92.

Floberg, L. -E., Hamberger, C. -A, and Hyden, H. (1949), *Acta oto-laryng.,* suppl., **75**, 36.

Graybiel, A., Meek, J. C., Beischer, D. E. and Riopelle, A. (1960), Research Report. U.S. Naval School of Aviation Medicine, Pensacola, Fla.

Hallpike, C. S. and Cairns, H. (1938), *J. Laryng.,* **53**, 625.

Hamberger, C. A., Hyden, H. and Koch, H. (1949), *Arch. Ohr.-, Nas.- u. Kehlk. Heilk.,* **55**, 667.

Harada, Y., Musso, E. and Mira, E. (1967), *Acta oto-laryng.,* **64**, 327.

Hawkins, J. E., Jr. (1947), *Fed. Proc.,* **6**, 125.

Hawkins, J. E., Jr. (1950), *J. Pharmacol.,* **100**, 38.

Hawkins, J. E., Jr. (1959), *Ann. Otol., Rhinol., Lar.,* **68**, 698.

Hawkins, J. E., Jr. (1970), *Biochemical Mechanisms in Hearing and Deafness,* p. 323.

Hawkins, J. E., Jr., Johnsson, L. -G. and Aran, J. -M. (1969), *J. infect. Dis.,* **119**, 417.

Hawkins, J. E., Jr. and Lurie, M. H. (1952), *Ann. Otol., Rhinol., Lar.,* **61**, 789.

Hawkins, J. E., Jr. and Lurie, M. H. (1953), *Ann. Otol., Rhinol., Lar.,* **62**, 1128.

Hawkins, J. E., Jr., Wilcott, H. and O'Shanny, W. J. (1957), *Antibiotics Annual* 9156–1957, p. 554.

Igarashi, M. (1965), *Laryngoscope,* **75**, 1048.

Igarashi, M. (1968), *Acta Otolaryng.,* **66**, 199.

Igarashi, M. (1970), *Proceedings Bárány Society—First Extraordinary Meeting, Amsterdam-Utrecht,* p. 169.

Igarashi, M., Alford, B. R., Konishi, S., Shaver, -E. F. and Guildford, F. R. (1969), *Laryngoscope,* **79**, 603.

Igarashi, M., Alford, B. R., Watanabe, T. and Maxian, P. M. (1969), *Laryngoscope,* **79**, 1713.

Igarashi, M., Alford, B. R., Watanabe, T. and Maxian, P. M. (1970), *Laryngoscope,* **80**, 896.

Igarashi, M., Graybiel, A. and Deane, F. R. (1968), N.A.S.A.—Navy Joint Report, Naval Aerospace Medical Institute, Pensacola, Fla.

Igarashi, M., Lundquist, P. G., Alford, B. R. and Miyata, H. (1971), *J. infect. Dis.,* **124**, S114.

Igarashi, M., McLeod, M. E. and Graybiel, A. (1966), *Acta Otolaryng.,* suppl., suppl. **214**, 1.

Igarashi, M. and Miyata, H. (1971), *Acta Otolaryng.,* **72**, 424.

Igarashi, M. and Miyata, H. (1972), *Arch. Otolaryng.,* **95**, 158.

Igarashi, M., Miyata, H. and Alford, B. R. (1972), *Acta oto-laryng.* **74**, 66.

Igarashi, M., Miyata, H., Alford, B. R. and Wright, W. K. (1972), *Laryngoscope,* **82**, 1609.

Igarashi, M. and Nagaba, M. (1967), *Third Symposium on the Role of the Vestibular Organs in Space Exploration,* p. 63.

Igarashi, M., Watanabe, T. and Maxian, P. M. (1970), *Acta Otolaryng.,* **69**, 247.

Ishii, T., Ishii, D. and Balogh, K., Jr. (1968), *Acta oto-laryng.,* **65**, 449.

Jongkees, L. W. B. (1950), *Acta oto-laryng.,* **38**, 18.

Kanda, T. and Igarashi, M. (1969), *Acta oto-laryng.,* **68**, 474.

Kaneko, Y., Kanagawa, T. and Tanaka, K. (1970), *Arch. Otolaryng.,* **92**, 457.

Kimura, R. S. (1968), *Ménière's Disease,* p. 457.

Lindeman, H. H. (1969), *Studies on the Morphology of the Sensory Regions of the Vestibular Apparatus.*

Lindsay, J. R. (1947), *Arch. Otolaryng.,* **45**, 1.

Lindsay, J. R., Schuknecht, H. F., Neff, W. D. and Kimura, R. S. (1952), *Ann. Otol., Rhinol., Lar.,* **61**, 697.

Lundquist, P. G., Igarashi, M., Wersäll, J., Alford, B. R. and Wright, W. K. (1972), *Arch. Otolaryng.,* **95**, 530.

Lundquist, P. G., Igarashi, M., Wersäll, J., Guildford, F. R. and Wright, W. K. (1971), *Acta oto-laryng.,* **72**, 68.

Lundquist, P. G. and Wersäll, J. (1966), *Ztsr. f. Zellforsch.,* **72**, 543.

Lundquist, P. G. and Wersäll, J. (1967), *Gentamicin First International Symposium, Paris,* p. 26.

Mair, I. W. S. and Fernandez, C. (1966), *Acta oto-laryng.,* **62**, 513.

Maxian, P. M. and Igarashi, M. (1969), *Percept. Motor Skill,* **29**, 959.

McCabe, B. F. (1964), *Laryngoscope,* **74**, 372.

McGee, T. M. (1958), *Henry Ford Hosp. Med. Bull.,* **6**, 182.

McGee, T. M. and Olszewski, J. (1962), *Arch. Otolaryng.,* **75**, 295.

McGee, T. M., Webster, J. and Williams, M. (1969), *J. infect. Dis.,* **119**, 432.

McNally, W. J. and Tait, J. (1925), *Amer. J. Physiol.,* **75**, 155.

Mizukoshi, O. and Daly, J. F. (1967), *Acta oto-laryng.,* **64**, 45.

Money, K. E. and Friedberg, J. (1964), *Can. J. Physiol. Pharmacol.,* **42**, 793.

Money, K. E. (1970, *Physiol. Rev.* **50**, 1.

Ostyn, F. and Tyberghein, J. (1968), *Acta oto-laryng.,* suppl. **234**, 1.

Saito, H. and Daly, J. F. (1971), *Acta oto-laryng.,* **71**, 22.

Schuknecht, H. F. (1957), *Acta oto-laryng.,* suppl. **132**, 1.

Schuknecht, H. F. (1969), *Arch. Otolaryng.,* **90**, 765.

Schuknecht, H. F. and Davidson, R. C. (1956), *Arch. Otolaryng.,* **63**, 513.

Schuknecht, H. F., Northrop, C. and Igarashi, M. (1968), *Acta oto-laryng.,* **65**, 479.

Silverstein, H., Bernstein, J. M. and Davies, D. G. (1967), *Ann. Otol., Rhinol., Lar.,* **76**, 118.

Stahle, J. and Högberg, L. (1965), *Acta. oto-laryng.,* **60**, 367.

Stahle, J., Högberg, J. and Engström, B. (1972), *Acta oto-laryng.,* **73**, 27.

Stupp, H., Rauch, S., Sous, H., Brun, J. P. and Lagler, F. (1967), *Arch. Otolaryng.,* **86**, 515.

Uemura, T. and Cohen, B. (1972), *Basic Aspects of Central Vestibular Mechanisms,* p. 515.

Versteegh, C. (1927), *Acta oto-laryng.,* **11**, 393.

Vrabec, D. P., Cody, D. T. R. and Ulrich, J. A. (1965), *Ann. Otol., Rhinol., Lar.,* **74**, 688.

Waitz, J. A., Moss, E. L., Jr. and Weinstein, M. J. (1971), *J. infect. Dis.,* **124**, S125.

Ward, P. H. and Fernandez, C. (1961), *Ann. Otol., Rhinol., Lar.,* **70**, 132.

Watanabe, T., Igarashi, M. and Wright, W. K. (1971), *Equilibrium Res.*, suppl. **1,** 99.

Watanuki, K. and Meyer Zum Gottesberge, A. (1971), *Pract. oto-rhino-laryng.*, **33,** 169.

Watanuki, K., Stupp, H. F. and Meyer Zum Gottesberge, A. (1972), *Laryngoscope*, **82,** 363.

Webster, J. C., Carroll, R., Benitez, J. T. and McGee, T. M. (1971), *J. infect. Dis.*, **124,** S138.

Wersäll, J. and Flock, A. (1964), *Life Science*, **3,** 1151.

Wersäll, J. and Hawkins, J. E., Jr. (1962), *Acta oto-laryng.*, **54,** 1.

Wersäll, J., Lundquist, P. G. and Bjorkroth, B. (1969), *J. infect. Dis.*, **119,** 410

Winston, J., Lewey, F. H., Parenteau, A., Marden, P. A. and Cramer, F. B. (1948), *Ann. Otol., Rhinol., Lar.*, **57,** 738.

Winston, J., Lewey, F. H., Parenteau, A., Marden, P. A. and Cramer, F. B. (1949), *Ann. Otol., Rhinol., Lar.*, **58,** 988.

Winston, J., Lewey, F. H., Parenteau, A., Spitz, E. B. and Marden, P. A. (1953), *Ann. Otol., Rhinol., lar.*, **62,** 121.

27. VESTIBULAR PHYSIOLOGY

T. D. M. ROBERTS

The sense organs of the labyrinth to some extent resemble those in the cochlea as a consequence of their common evolutionary history. In each case we have specialized receptor cells, the neuromasts, supported side by side in a sheet forming part of the membraneous wall of the endolymph cavity. The hair-like processes of the neuromasts project into the endolymph where they engage with the gels formed by the polysaccharides in the endolymph fluid. The stiffness of the gels varies in different places in the labyrinth and confers special selectivity to the sense organs in the different regions. In each case the process of generating a sensory discharge seems to depend on the development of shearing forces between the endolymph and the containing wall. The forces are detected in consequence of the displacement of the hairs produced by the tendency to relative movement of the gel over the surface of the sensory epithelium. To understand the significance of the resulting sensory discharge it is necessary first to examine the nature of the forces involved.

Let us start with a familiar example, such as a cup of coffee. We have a fluid supported within a rigid container. The notion of support is important. If we hold the cup in our hand while standing on firm ground, the fluid stays in place only so long as we hold the opening of the cup in a particular orientation, namely "up". If we tip the cup over, the coffee pours out. We explain this by saying that there is a force, called "gravity", that pulls the coffee toward the centre of the earth. However, if we repeat the experiment in an orbiting spacecraft, the coffee stays in place in the cup, so long as this is not shaken. There is a temptation to interpret this result and other related observations as indicating that, in orbit, there is an "absence of gravity". The expression "weightlessness" is based on this interpretation and it has crept into common parlance in the context of space flights.

Closer examination of the situation reveals, however, that there is a misunderstanding here. What we mean by the "force of gravity" is a force of attraction exerted between any two bodies by virtue of their mass. The magnitude of the force is related to the product of the masses of the two bodies under consideration, divided by the square of the distance separating them. Such a force acts on the cup as well as on the contained coffee, and both

are attracted towards the centre of the earth. The difference between the behaviour of the coffee on the ground and that in the spacecraft depends not on any difference in the action of gravity, but on the differing conditions of support. On the ground we push against the earth with our legs to prevent ourselves from falling, and we apply corresponding forces to objects held in the hand, such as the coffee cup. If we let go, the cup falls as well as the coffee. This is what is happening in the spacecraft. Cup, coffee and observer are all falling together, like Gallileo's pound of lead and pound of feathers. It is not gravity that is absent in orbital flight, it is the supporting force that is missing. In fact it is the force of gravity that keeps the spacecraft to its curved path in the orbit, and, if gravity were not acting, the spacecraft would move in a straight-line path through space indefinitely, or until it collided with some other body.

From the way that gravity acts on the cup as well as on the coffee we can conclude that gravity is not responsible for the relative movement of the coffee within the cup. It is true that the gravitational force on a particular volume of a denser material will be greater than the force on a similar volume of a less dense material. But the accelerations under gravity will be the same for each, because the relation between force and acceleration is also dependent on mass. It follows also that gravity does not produce any relative deformations within the sense organs of the labyrinth, so that the receptor apparatus is not stimulated by gravity itself.

When we stand on the ground and hold our coffee cup upright, the coffee stays in place because of the supporting force transmitted to the fluid from the rigid wall of the cup. The nature of the forces acting in these conditions of support precisely corresponds to the nature of the forces between the spoon and the coffee when we stir the coffee with a spoon. The hydrostatic pressure in the fluid exerts a force on the rigid wall in a direction at right angles to its surface and the wall exerts a reaction force on the fluid. When we move the hand that holds the cup, there is a difference between the forces transmitted to the coffee from the two sides of the cup. A difference in hydrostatic pressure is set up and the coffee is accelerated along the pressure gradient to keep up with the cup. If we look closely we will see differences in the level of the surface of the coffee corresponding to the gradient of hydrostatic pressure.

The situation may be analysed with the aid of a figure. Consider a U-tube partly filled with fluid of density ρ and subjected to a contact force in the direction of the arrow in Fig. 1 to produce an acceleration f in that direction. The

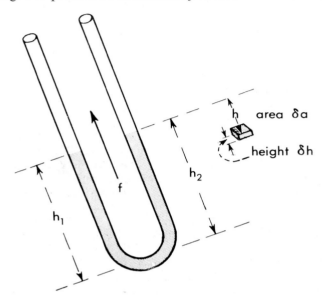

FIG. 1. U-tube partially filled with fluid, subjected to a contact force accelerating it in the direction of the arrow.

force needed to produce a corresponding acceleration in a small volume of the fluid will be the product of its mass times its acceleration, or $\rho . (\delta h \times \delta a) . f$, where δh is the depth of our sample measured in the direction of the arrow, and δa is the area measured at right angles to that direction. Thus the hydrostatic pressure at a distance h measured from the free surface along the direction of the arrow, will be

$$\int_0^h \frac{\rho . \delta a . f}{\delta a} \, \delta h, \quad \text{or} \quad \rho . f . h$$

If we measure the distances h_1 and h_2 from the free surfaces in the two arms of the U-tube to some reference plane normal to the direction of the arrow, then if $h_1 = h_2$, there will be no flow from one arm to the other round the bend of the U, because there will be zero pressure gradient normal to the direction of the arrow.

We may now make a second fluid-filled connection between the two arms of the U-tube (Fig. 2) and again there will be no flow along this connection either, if $h_1 = h_2$. The next step is to close off the open arms of the U-tube, leaving the tube as a closed ring completely filled with fluid (Fig. 3). With this system there is no tendency for the fluid to move within the tube when contact forces of any magnitude are applied in any direction. As we have made no stipulations about the diameter of the tube or of the shape of the ring, the argument can be seen to apply to any closed vessel completely filled with fluid of uniform density.

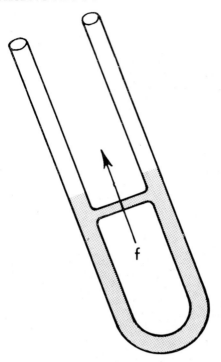

FIG. 2. U-tube with a second cross-connection.

We now consider the effects of inhomogeneous densities. Suppose that, in the U-tube of Fig. 4, the density of the fluid in the left hand arm is ρ_1 and of that in the right hand arm is ρ_2, the interface and the positions of the free surfaces being symmetrically disposed with respect to the direction

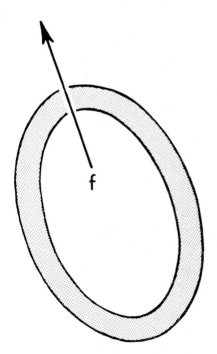

FIG. 3. Fluid-filled tube in the form of a closed ring.

of the applied contact force. The hydrostatic pressure on the left hand side of the interface will be $h \cdot \rho_1 \cdot f$, while that on the right hand side will be $h \cdot \rho_2 \cdot f$. This means that, if $\rho_1 > \rho_2$, the application of a contact force to produce an acceleration f will lead to movement of fluid from left to right through the connecting tube. Cor-

respondingly, in the closed ring of Fig. 5, the application of a contact force in the direction of the arrow will produce an anticlockwise rotation of the fluids.

Let us now apply the argument to the otolith organs. Each consists of a chamber completely filled with fluid (Fig. 6). These chambers are of somewhat complex shape with openings into the various ducts, which are also completely fluid filled. As we have seen from the earlier

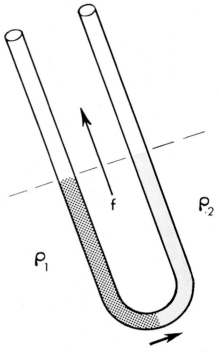

FIG. 4. U-tube with fluids of different densities in the two arms.

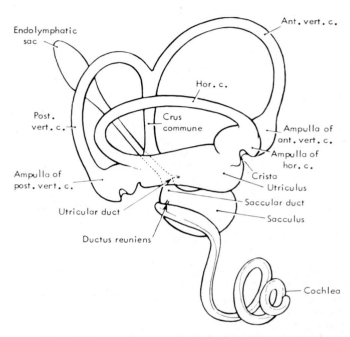

FIG. 6. Sketch of the membraneous labyrinth of the right ear of a guinea-pig, lateral view from below and slightly from behind. The viewpoint is that of the photograph (his figure 2) given by Lindeman (1969) with clarifications of detail based on Retzius (1884) and on Gray (1907).

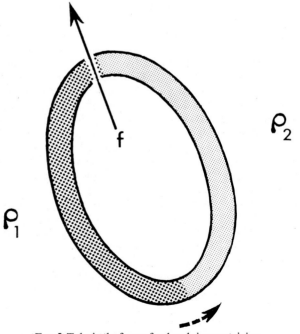

FIG. 5. Tube in the form of a closed ring containing fluids of different densities.

part of the argument set out above, the application of contact forces to the containing structure produces no tendency to movement of the fluid in those regions where the fluid density is uniform. In parts of the utricular and saccular cavities, however, the endolymph jelly is loaded with crystals of calcite, the otoconia. This part of the endolymph consequently has a higher mean density than the rest and we can expect behaviour like that of the system in Fig. 5. The similarity is illustrated in Fig. 7 which shows a diagrammatic view of a slice through the utriculus. A contact force applied to the skull in the direction of the arrow in this diagram will produce a tendency for the denser region of endolymph to slide round counter-clockwise.

This region of endolymph jelly contains, in addition to the otoconia, a network of fine elastic filaments whose ends are attached to the wall of the otolith organ (van Egmond, 1940). These filaments tether the loaded jelly so that it remains approximately in place over the underlying macula which contains the array of sensory hair cells. The combination of jelly, otoconia and restraining filaments is referred to as the otolithic membrane. When externally applied contact forces produce tendencies for the otolithic membrane to move, corresponding elastic forces are developed in the restraining filaments so that the displacement is limited to an amount dependent on the magnitude and direction of the contact force. The sliding of the otolithic membrane over the macula deforms the underlying hair cells and it is this deformation that gives rise to the neural signal sent to the central nervous system.

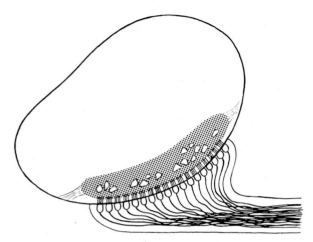

FIG. 7. Diagram of a section through the utricle.

The signal from each of the sensory units in the otolith organs consists of a stream of impulses at a frequency dependent on the degree of deformation of the hair cells connected to the afferent nerve-fibre in question. We must now consider what information is contained in this signal and how the nervous system can interpret such signals in terms of movements of the head.

It should be noticed that in the foregoing account of the mechanisms for generating neural signals in the otolith organs, it has not been necessary to make any mention of gravity. Nevertheless, the otolith organs have been traditionally regarded as "gravity receptors". This is because our notions of gravity are developed in a context of living on the earth's surface with the entailed necessity of continually pushing against the earth to keep from colliding with it as a result of falling under the action of gravity. The direction in which the supporting push is exerted does not have to be always precisely opposed to the pull of gravity, indeed it is by periodically altering the magnitude and direction of the support thrusts in the limbs in a systematic fashion that we perform acts of locomotion.

If the strategy of patterned limb thrusts is unsuccessful, the body will topple over and the head will strike the ground. It is interesting in this context to watch a newborn foal during the first few minutes after birth while it goes through the process of learning a successful strategy for standing. It quickly learns in which directions the skull should be accelerated to avoid the punishing experience of impact. After a few minutes, it gets the knack of keeping at least some of its feet between its body and the ground for at least some of the time. We might say that it is at this stage that it has learned which is the direction we call "up". Very soon the animal can also

recognize this direction from visual cues, if the environment is suitably structured, and thereafter it becomes difficult for an observer to disentangle what sensory cues an animal is using for orientation in any specific situation.

Usually there are four systems involved: the otolith organs, vision, proprioception from muscles and joints, and mechanoreceptors reporting the pressures of the supporting surfaces against the skin. The role of the otolith organs has been worked out from observation of the nature of the disturbances to standing and locomotion that follow acute damage to the labyrinths (de Kleijn and Magnus, 1921; Magnus, 1924). The effects are particularly pronounced if the damage is unilateral and they are most clearly demonstrated if the animal is blindfolded and deprived of cutaneous cues by being placed in water. A blindfolded labyrinthectomized animal will drown if placed in water, because it cannot find its way to the surface.

The other sensory modalities involved in orientation clearly serve other functions also, consequently it is the sensory apparatus of the labyrinth that has come to be labelled as the one specifically concerned with verticality. The otolith organs in particular have come to be spoken of as "gravity receptors" from the association of the vertical with the direction of the pull of gravity. However, as we have seen, the adequate stimulus for the receptors is not actually the pull of gravity itself but rather the contact force applied to the skull. It is true that, when the skull is stationary with respect to the earth's surface, the contact force must be equal and opposite to the gravitational pull. But the skull of a waking animal is very seldom at rest, and the contact force on the skull is continually varying both in direction and in magnitude. All these fluctuations affect the receptors in the otolith organs and contribute to the signal transmitted to the nervous system.

In an experimental study to analyse the patterns of sensory discharge generated in the otolith organs, it is convenient to use the special conditions of a stationary skull. The head is supported in a clamp that can be tilted in various ways and the firing frequency of single afferent units is recorded with the skull in different positions. It is found that, for each unit, there is a particular position of the skull in which the discharge frequency is at a maximum (Lowenstein and Roberts, 1949; Fujita et al., 1968; Beerens, 1969; Vidal et al., 1971; Fernandez et al., 1972; Loe et al., 1973). With the skull fixed, the direction of the supporting contact force is vertically upwards, and we note which direction, in a reference system attached to the skull, coincides with the vertical in this position of maximum discharge for the unit being studied. This direction is the "polarization vector" for that unit. It presumably corresponds to the orientation of the relevant hair cells.

The projections that characterize the neuromasts as "hair cells" consist of a set of stereocilia closely packed in a hexagonal array, together with a single kinocilium on one side of the bundle (see Fig. 8). The shearing motion of the endolymph across the face of the hair-cell produces an increase in firing frequency if the stereocilia are bent towards the kinocilium, and a decrease in frequency if the shearing motion is in the opposite direction. Other directions of motion produce intermediate changes in firing frequency according to the magnitude of the resolved component in the direction of the kinocilium. Each hair cell thus has its own polarization vector, determined by the structural arrangement of its cilia.

When we determine the direction of the polarization vector for a particular afferent fibre this does not tell us where the relevant hair cells are located in the maculae of the otolith organs. Indeed, for an idealized spherical otolith organ, hair cells with the same polarization vector directed towards one pole of the sphere could be located anywhere on the equator. The problem is further complicated by the fact that a single afferent fibre may serve several hair cells whose individual polarization vectors are not necessarily parallel, but which each contribute a component of directional sensitivity to the overall behaviour of the unit. In practice, the hair cells are not distributed over the whole surface of the walls of the otolith organs. They are confined to restricted regions known as maculae, where the structural polarization vectors are systematically distributed as shown in Fig 8.

Recording from a number of afferent fibres in turn, and taking both utricle and saccule together, it has been found

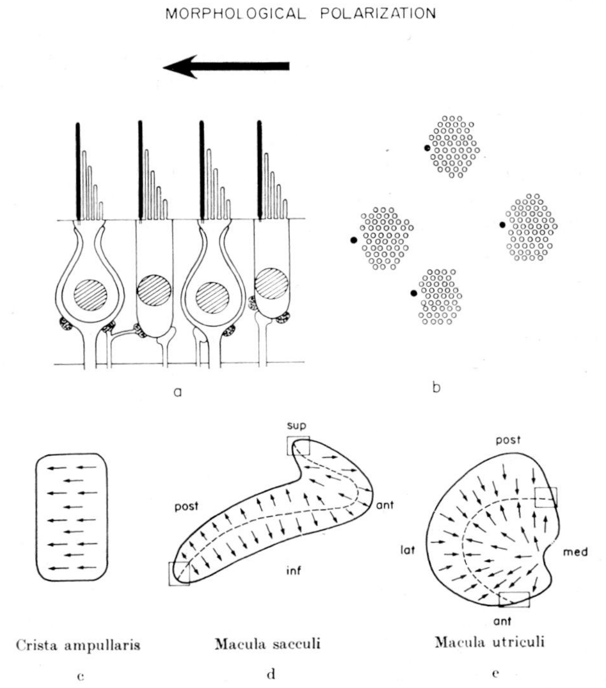

FIG. 8. Diagram illustrating the morphological polarization of the sensory cells and the polarization pattern of the vestibular sensory epithelia. The morphological polarization (arrow) of a sensory cell is determined by the position of the kinocilium in relation to the stereocilia. (a) Section perpendicular to the epithelium. Note increasing length of stereocilia towards the kinocilium. (b) Section parallel to the epithelial surface. (c) The sensory cells on the crista ampullaris are polarized in the same direction. (d) Macula sacculi and (e) macula utriculi are divided by an arbitrary curved line into two areas, the pars interna and the pars externa, with opposite morphological polarization. On the macula sacculi the sensory cells are polarized away from the dividing line, on the macula utriculi towards the line. Constant irregularities in the polarization pattern are found in areas corresponding to the continuation of the striola peripherally (rectangles in (d) and (e)). (From Lindeman, 1969.)

(Loe et al., 1973) that the directions of the functional polarization vectors are all grouped around the plane of the lateral (horizontal) canal. All directions in this plane are represented, with a slight preponderance towards the contralateral side. This means that the sensory units are well placed to indicate tilting around the normal position, and to contribute to adjustments of the directions of the support thrusts that keep the animal from falling. If the direction of the supporting contact force does not coincide with the polarization vector for a particular unit, the firing frequency will be less than the maximum for that unit. In some cases, the discharge can be silenced by turning the unit upside down but most units discharge continually in all positions at a frequency that is trigonometrically related to the deviation between the direction of the contact force and that of the appropriate polarization vector. The relationship is not precisely linear, but this is hardly surprising when one considers how many steps are involved in the transformation. First there is the elastic deformation of the restraining filaments in the otolithic membrane, then the displacement of the cilia, with the consequent changes in the membrane permeability of the hair cell and alterations in local circuit currents. This is followed by the intermittent liberation of transmitter substance alternating with recovery processes before the next threshold-crossing. Next comes the interaction between effects at individual hair cells in generating impulses in a common axon, and finally, the experimenter's conversion from impulse interval into firing frequency.

The reverse transformation is complicated by the fact that even if the signal indicates the amount of the angular deviation from the polarization vector, it cannot show its direction, because all directions of deviation right round the compass, produce the same neural signal if the angles of deviation are the same. Again, in the neurophysiological recording experiment, the magnitude of the support force is kept constant while its direction is varied by tilting the skull. In more normal conditions the support force varies in magnitude as well as in direction, and there is no way in which the discharge in a single afferent fibre can signal the difference between combinations of magnitude and direction of the contact force when these produce the same resolved component of deformation in the direction of the polarization vector. Yet a further complication arises from the fact that the response of many of the sensory units includes, as well as the static component related directly to the prevailing conditions of stimulation, an additional dynamic component related to changes in the stimulus (Lowenstein and Roberts, 1949). When the skull is tilted from one position to another, the firing frequency shows an exaggerated change during the movement, followed by an adaptation to the value appropriate to the new steady position.

We do not need to be dismayed by the task of computing the nature of the forces acting on the skull from the signals recorded from individual sensory units. The nervous system has at its disposal very many such units and the task of interpreting their combined discharges is comparable to the everyday recognition tasks that arise in any sensory modality. We need to know only what is the nature of the information on which the relevant judgements are based. We can then understand how these judgements are likely to be affected when the environment is manipulated to provide stimulating conditions outside the normal range.

The adequate stimulus for the otolith organs is the shearing motion of the otolithic membrane across the faces of the underlying hair cells. Such motion arises from the application of contact forces to the skull. In the neural signal, the magnitude of such a force is necessarily confounded with its direction and also to some extent with its recent history of change. Gravity does not come into the picture at all, except in so far as the contact forces are sometimes concerned with preventing the skull from falling. Other fields of force acting at a distance, such as magnetic and electrostatic forces, also play no part in generating sensory signals from the otolith organs.

It has been indicated already that the otolith organs have an important part to play in organizing the pattern of support forces that are used to keep the body from falling over. They may be taken to indicate the nature of the contact force currently being applied to the skull. Another signal needed is some indication of whether the current support strategy is successful or not. A suitable signal is available from another part of the vestibular labyrinth namely from the sense organs in the ampullae of the semicircular canals. To understand how these work let us take another look at our cup of coffee.

Consider the problem of stirring the coffee, that is, to generate a rotary motion of the fluid contained in the cup. If we rotate the cup around a vertical axis, the fluid at first tends to stay behind. Because the hydrostatic forces act at right angles to the surface of the container, they are unsuitable for imparting motion parallel to this surface. Accordingly, if the cup is circular in plan, it can be rotated about its axis of symmetry without altering the distribution of hydrostatic forces on the contained fluid. However, if there is relative movement of the fluid over the walls of the cup, viscous forces will come into play to resist shearing of the fluid near the wall. These viscous forces act parallel to the surface at which the relative movement is taking place, consequently they can impart angular acceleration to the fluid when the cup is rotated. If the cup is set on a turntable rotating at constant speed, the contained fluid will eventually come to rotate at the same speed as the cup, with no viscous force acting at the wall, because the magnitude of the viscous force is related to the velocity of the relative motion, and if there is no relative motion there is no viscous force. When the motion of the turntable is arrested, the fluid will, for a time, continue to rotate by virtue of the angular momentum corresponding to the previously prevailing constant-speed rotation. The fluid will then be brought to rest gradually by the action of viscous forces between the moving fluid and the now stationary walls of the cup.

The magnitude of the viscous forces depends on the rate of shearing and also on a property of the fluid called its "viscosity", or resistance to shearing. The polysaccharides dissolved in the endolymph give it a viscosity greater than that of water. In the neighbourhood of the patches of sensory epithelium, such as in the cupulae over the cristae of the ampullae in the semicircular canals, the endolymph has the consistency of a semi-rigid gel.

If the wall of the containing vessel is not truly circular, and particularly if there are paddle-like projections sticking out into the fluid, it becomes easier to impart rotary motion from the container to the fluid, just as the use of a spoon helps in stirring the coffee. To some extent the hair-like processes of the hair cells, together with the gell in which their free ends are imbedded, act as paddles to transmit forces from the wall of the labyrinth to the contained fluid. When they do so, they suffer elastic deformation, the hairs being bent back by the shearing force. It is the bending of the hairs that generates the signal in the afferent nerve.

Let us turn now to the semicircular canals. Anatomically speaking, the word "canal" should be reserved for the tunnel in the bone, while the membraneous tube within it is called a "duct". The essential features of the structure are that each duct is a curved tube opening at each end into the cavity of the utricle, which leads by further ducts in turn to the saccule and then to the cochlea (Fig. 6). Each of the semicircular ducts swells out at one region into an ampulla partly crossed by a ridge of the wall running at right angles to the general direction of the duct. The epithelium of the surface of this ridge (the ampullary crest or "crista") contains hair cells (neuromasts) whose hairs project into a mass of jelly, the cupula, that completely blocks the lumen of the duct at this point. The assembly of duct, ampulla, ampullary crest and cupula form a single sense organ with a single function. It is convenient to use the term "semicircular canal" to refer to the whole of this sense organ.

The precise shape of the ducts varies very slightly from one animal species to another. Usually the three ducts on each side of the head lie roughly in mutually perpendicular planes, so that one can distinguish them by the following names: horizontal, anterior vertical and posterior vertical. In human anatomy, these are called respectively: lateral, superior and inferior. The lateral canals of the two sides lie in approximately the same plane, and in most animals this plane is in fact horizontal when the animal is holding its head in its "characteristic" position (Girard, 1930). It is interesting that this should be true even of animals such as the camel and the bison which characteristically hold their heads in markedly different attitudes. In man, the "characteristic" attitude of the head is more difficult to define. If we take the plane of the canals as a guide, applying the argument in reverse, it corresponds to the pose in which a man scrutinizes something held in the hand, or looks at the ground two or three paces ahead, as when walking briskly over rough ground. The vertical canals are inclined to the midline at about 45 degrees so that the superior (anterior vertical) canal of one side is roughly parallel to the inferior (posterior vertical) canal of the other side. The ampullae of the vertical canals lie at their lower ends near to the utricular opening. The lateral canal has its ampulla at the anterior end. (It may have another dilatation at the posterior end but this second swelling is not innervated, and it is usually disregarded.)

To understand the function of the canals one must remember that the lumen of the semicircular ducts is continued into a full circle through the cavity of the utricle (Fig. 9). This means that, if an angular acceleration is applied to the skull about an axis through the centre of such a circle, the only structure suitably placed to transmit the acceleration to the endolymph of the canal is that made up of the cupula and crest of the ampulla. Were it not for

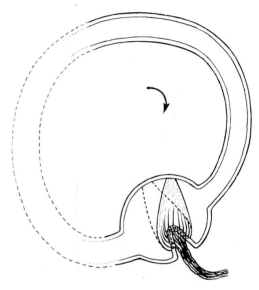

FIG. 9. Diagram to illustrate the mechanism of action of a semi-circular canal, showing the deflection of the cupula produced by clockwise angular acceleration in the plane of the paper.

the presence of this structure, the endolymph would stay behind, just as the coffee stays behind when we rotate the cup, until the viscous forces resulting from the relative motion between endolymph and duct wall gradually accelerated the fluid. However, the tendency to relative movement of the endolymph encounters the resistance of the cupula and crest, and this structure consequently develops elastic deformation and exerts a force on the fluid. The degree of deformation is related to the force, and this in turn is related to the acceleration required to keep the endolymph in place relative to the duct. Thus the deformation of the cupula is related to the angular acceleration applied to the skull.

The relation is complicated by two factors. Deformation of the cupula implies movement of the endolymph along the canal and this movement is resisted by viscous forces, whose magnitude depends on the speed of relative movement. Furthermore, when the acceleration is discontinued, the cupula cannot instantaneously return to the rest position because to do so requires a displacement of the endolymph, and such displacement is again resisted by viscous forces. If we consider the combined effects of the restoring force from the elastic deformation of the cupula, the inertia of the endolymph, and the viscous drag between the endolymph and the wall of the duct, we see that the system as a whole acts as a damped accelerometer, so that the signal transmitted by the neural discharge from the

receptors is not a faithful representation of the angular acceleration applied to the skull. The effects are illustrated in Fig. 10, which shows the time-courses of the relevant variables in a simple but comparatively unusual manoeuvre.

We consider a single lateral canal. We start with the skull at rest facing North. At the point A in time we apply

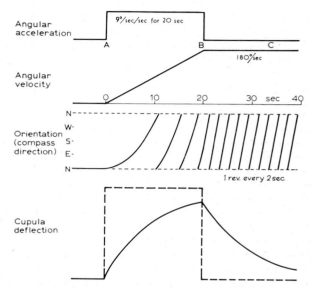

FIG. 10. Time courses of the changes in angular velocity, orientation of the skull in space, and cupula-deflection, arising from the application of a constant angular acceleration during the period from A to B. (From Roberts, 1967.)

an angular acceleration of $9°\,s^{-2}$ for a period of 20 s. This is indicated by the "square wave" in the upper line of the figure. The effect of the constant angular acceleration is to produce a steady increase in the angular velocity, or speed of turning, starting from zero and rising linearly to attain a value of $180°\,s^{-1}$ at the end of 20 s. The time-course of the orientation should be a parabola, as the speed of turning gets faster and faster. In the figure, the parabola has been broken into segments to correspond with the successive full-circle rotations. At B the angular acceleration is discontinued, and the head thereafter continues to turn at constant speed.

The lower part of the figure shows the relationship between the angular acceleration and the magnitude of the deflection produced in the cupula. At the onset of the applied acceleration, the cupula does not move instantaneously to the position appropriate to the new value of the applied acceleration, but approaches this with an exponential time course. At first the endolymph remains stationary while the skull begins to move. Thus the speed of development of the cupula deflection corresponds at first to the speed of rotation of the skull. But the relative movement of the endolymph within the duct is resisted by viscous forces as well as by the force of elastic deformation of the cupula. The relative movement of the cupula thus slows down as the endolymph begins to catch up with the movement of the skull. The viscous forces decrease as the elastic force takes over the function of accelerating the endolymph until, if the acceleration were continued long enough, the endolymph would keep its station within the duct without relative movement, all the acceleration of the endolymph being provided by the elastic force, and with the deflection of the cupula corresponding precisely to the magnitude of the applied acceleration.

In our example, the external acceleration is discontinued at the end of 20 s, at B. From this point onward, the skull continues to rotate at constant speed. The endolymph in the duct is however still subject to the accelerating force of the deflected cupula, so it will now begin to move ahead relative to the wall of the duct. As it does so, the cupula deflection declines, so the driving force decreases. At the same time the relative movement of the endolymph is resisted by viscous forces. In combination these factors lead to an exponential return of the cupula to the rest position. We then have zero acceleration and zero deflection of the cupula, yet the skull is continuously rotating at the speed of one complete rotation every 2 s.

It is clear from this example that the sense organs of the semi-circular canals are not ideally suited to signal the speed of turning, because the sensory discharge, which is related to the cupula deflection, necessarily declines to resting conditions during constant speed rotation. Nor is the sense organ suited to signal the applied accelerations, because of the sluggishness of its response. However, the conditions of this example are somewhat different from the conditions in which the sense organ is normally called upon to function, so let us examine a more realistic situation.

Constant speed rotations are not commonly encountered in everyday life, if we disregard the daily rotation of the planet on its axis. It is more usual for any angular acceleration in one direction to be followed very soon by a deceleration bringing the rotation to an end. Such a pattern is illustrated by Fig. 11. Here we consider a movement of the head from one position to another, the change in orientation being completed in rather less than a second. The traces have been generated electronically, for ease of computation, but the time course of the change in orientation has been made to mimic very closely the time course of a natural movement recorded from a human subject. We see that the acceleration waxes and wanes fairly smoothly and is followed after a small interval by a deceleration with a similar time course. The angular velocity rises with an S-shaped curve to a maximum, holds this value momentarily, and then declines along another S-shaped curve. The orientation moves smoothly from one direction to another and then remains constant.

To discover what the cupula would be doing during such a manoeuvre we make use of measurements made during experiments using the special conditions of Fig. 10. From such measurements we can derive a mathematical equation of motion for the cupula which can be used to predict the time course of the deflection in response to any pattern of imposed accelerations (van Egmond, Groen and Jongkees, 1949; Groen, Lowenstein and Vendrik, 1952; Melvill Jones, 1972). In Fig. 11 an analogue computer has been used to solve the necessary differential equations and

indicate the time course of the cupula deflection. This is shown on the bottom line. It is clear that this time course more closely resembles that of the angular velocity of the skull than it does that of the angular acceleration. Thus for the types of movement that occur in a normal environment, the sensory discharge from the semi-circular canals can be taken as indicating the speed of rotation, each canal

Canal response in a naturally-occurring movement.

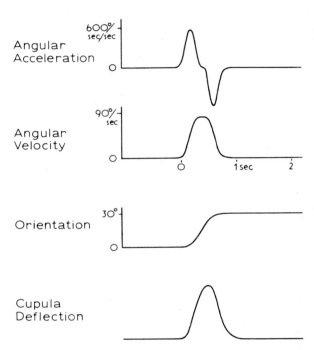

FIG. 11. Angular acceleration, angular velocity and cupula-deflection to be expected during a naturally occurring movement. The curve for acceleration (generated electronically) was chosen to give (by double integration) a time-course of displacement which closely matched an experimental record from a human subject. The cupula-deflection (y) is computed from the angular acceleration (x) of the skull, using the equation $\dot{y} + 10\ddot{y} + y = kx$, and an analogue computer. (From Roberts, 1967.)

reporting the resolved component of head movement in the appropriate plane.

The central interpretation of the sensory discharge is based on this correlation both for purposes of the reflexes of balance and for the perception of movement. An important subset of the reflexes of balance consists of reflex movements of the eyes in the skull. The behaviour of images in the visual field also contributes to the perception of movement and vestibular eye movements naturally affect the positioning of images on the retina. Decisions about movement thus involve information from the labyrinth and from the retina as well as information about what eye movements have been generated either voluntarily or by reflexes from the labyrinth. In such a complex situation it is not surprising that the perceptions of movement should be inappropriate in the special environmental conditions imposed by travel in the sophisticated high-speed vehicles of modern civilization, where the pattern of acceleration can be very different from that in which we have evolved. Many of the disturbances occurring in the perception of motion can be attributed to the physics of the semicicular canals, where the cupula deflection produced by unusual patterns of acceleration ceases to correspond to the speed of head rotation. The mechanism for central interpretation of the sensory signal continues to act as before, and it now generates sensations and reflex movements which are no longer appropriate to the environmental conditions.

As a first example of unusual conditions we may take those used for the examination of vestibular function in the Bárány chair. Here the subject sits in a chair that can be rotated about a vertical axis. After a short period of moderate angular acceleration, the chair is rotated at constant speed for a prolonged period, say 30 s. During this period the cupula deflection declines to zero by the mechanism already described (Fig. 10). If the subject has his eyes closed at this stage and if the chair moves fairly smoothly, the subject may report that he has no sensation of turning. The brakes are now applied and the chair is quickly brought to a standstill. The impulsive deceleration generates a cupula deflection whose magnitude depends on the speed of the previous constant speed rotation and not on the exact pattern of the deceleration (Fig. 12). This is because, in the range we are talking about, a large deceleration for a short period produces the same effect as a smaller deceleration for a longer period. In each case, the time integral of the deceleration must add up to the same change in angular velocity, i.e. from the original speed to zero.

The cupula deflection produced by the impulsive deceleration takes time to die away exponentially, just as the initial deflection took time to build up. While the cupula remains deflected, the central nervous system will still be receiving the corresponding sensory discharge. Accordingly we will see reflex movements of the eyes, and the subject will experience sensations of motion, even though he is at rest.

The manoeuvre is particularly useful for the examination of canal function just because the subject is at rest, giving the observer a chance to spot effects that cannot readily be seen when the subject is in motion. Comparisons can then be made between subjects to assess deficiencies in canal function. The most notable effect is that on the eyes.

When the head is moved, the signal from the canals produces a movement of the eyes in the skull in such a direction, and at such a speed, as approximately to cancel the effect of the head movement on the orientation of the visual axis, so that the gaze continues to be aimed at roughly the same spot in spite of the movement of the skull. This means that, for movements of the type normally encountered, the speed of eyeball movement is matched to the extent of the cupula deflection as signalled by the nervous message to the central nervous system. In the postrotatory phase, following impulsive deceleration in the Bárány chair, the nervous system carries out the same signal transformation and generates eye movements corresponding to cupula deflection as before. Thus, when the head is brought to rest, the eyes continue to rotate

round the axis of the chair, as though they were attached to a flywheel not affected by the brakes applied to the chair.

Of course the eyes cannot rotate indefinitely in their sockets. Their motion is interrupted at intervals by jerks directed toward the resting position of the eye in the skull. The nystagmic jerks are readily seen by an observer. It should be remembered, however, that it is the "slow" movement, not the nystagmic jerk itself, that reflects the influence of the labyrinth. The time course of the slow movements of the eyes can be recorded by taking advantage

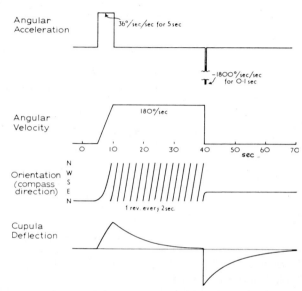

FIG. 12. Sequence of changes in angular velocity, orientation, and cupula-deflection, during the procedure for imposing an impulsive deceleration. Note that the cupula-deflection persists after the skull has been brought to rest. Note also that, if the deceleration were spread over one second, instead of occupying only 0·1, the force needed would be reduced to one tenth, yet the cupula-deflection reached in the rest position would have the same value as that shown here. (From Roberts, 1967.)

of the existence of an electrical potential difference between the corneal and retinal poles of the eyeball. As the eyeball moves, there is a change in the magnitude of the component of this corneoretinal potential that appears at electrodes placed near the borders of the orbit. The resulting electronystagmogram can be calibrated in terms of eyeball movement by asking the subject to direct his gaze voluntarily to two targets in turn set up at a known angle of separation. The speed of eyeball movement in the slow phases of the nystagmogram following impulsive deceleration exhibits the type of exponential decay illustrated in Fig. 12.

If we assume that there is a direct relationship between the slow phase velocity of the eye and the magnitude of the cupula deflection, we may obtain one of the two constants in the equation of motion for the cupula by calculation from the time course of the decay of eyeball velocity. The other constant may be obtained from estimates of the phase difference between eyeball movement and turntable movement during sinusoidally varying angular accelerations on a torsion swing using different values for the period of oscillation (Fig. 13). Although procedures of this kind give one some confidence in the validity of the theory, full confirmation would require that the canal data

cupulogram for the lateral canals of a particular subject may be different for the same type of rotation about the long axis of the body according as this axis is vertical, as in the normal erect posture, or horizontal, as in the "barbecue" experiment where the subject is strapped to a

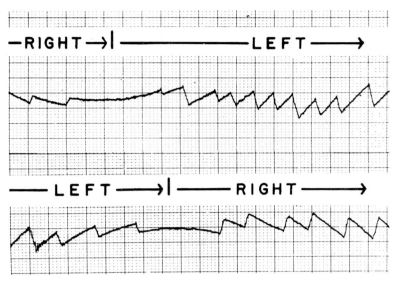

FIG. 13. Electronystagmogram from a human subject exposed to sinusoidally fluctuating angular accelerations of variable frequency and fixed amplitude in the Human Disorientation Device at the U.S. Naval School of Aviation Medicine. The subject is upright and the axis of rotation is vertical. The velocity of the slow phase of eye movement is related to the stimulating acceleration with a phase shift that depends on the period of the stimulus. (From Niven, Hixson and Correia, 1965.)

and the eye movement data be derived from the same animal, and this has not yet been achieved.

There is some evidence to suggest that the link between eye movements and the signals generated by the semicircular canals may be quite a complex one and it may be incorrect to think of the relation as a true reflex.

The mechanics of the canal suggest that an alternative derivation of the time-course of the decay of cupula deflection may be obtained by plotting the time to the end of a visible effect after an impulsive deceleration against the logarithm of the magnitude of the impulse, measured as the angular velocity before the brakes were applied. Such a plot is called a "cupulogram" and its slope is related to the time constant of the decay of the event that is being measured. This may be either eyeball movement or a subjective sensation of turning. Interestingly enough, although the mechanical event responsible for the phenomena is the same for eyeball movement as it is for the sensation of turning, the cupulograms often show different slopes (Fig. 14). Furthermore, these slopes may alter according to the training or experience of the subject, being shallower in test pilots or figure skaters than in others (Fig. 15).

It is not at all clear how a change in the slope of the cupulogram can be produced, because it implies that the signal received from the semicircular canals is acted upon by some central process whose effect is also time-dependent and related to the conditions of labyrinth stimulation. Another unexplained finding is that the slope of the

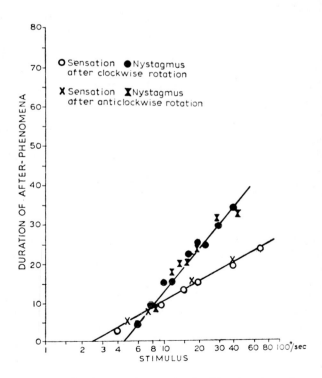

FIG. 14. Cupulograms for a normal subject based on the reported duration of the sensation of turning, and on the recorded nystagmus, after impulsive decelerations of various magnitudes. (From Groen, 1967.)

horizontal stretcher rotating about its long axis (Fig. 16). The mechanical conditions for canal stimulation should be

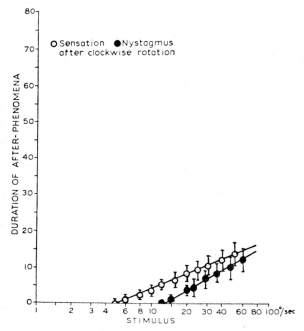

FIG. 15. Cupulograms for sensation and nystagmus in 18 experienced fighter pilots after 2000 hours of stunt flying. The slopes are considerably lower than normal but reverted to the normal type (Fig. 14) after 14 days holiday. (From Groen 1967; after Krijger, 1954.)

unaffected by tilting the skull, if the axis of rotation is similarly tilted. The possibility has been canvassed that the otolith organs may be implicated, but the question is still unresolved.

The mechanism by which the canals are stimulated leads to undesirable effects in certain special situations. It has been suggested that the inconvenience of having objects floating freely within the cabin of a spacecraft might be avoided by spinning the spacecraft like a gigantic centrifuge. The astronauts could then stand and walk about much as they do on the ground. However, problems would arise whenever an astronaut tilts his head, because of the Coriolis effects. During the rotation of the spacecraft parts of the endolymph lying further from the axis of rotation will have more momentum than corresponding parts lying closer in. If the head is tilted the distances from the axis will alter. Regions moving nearer to the axis will now have excess momentum and will therefore tend to move ahead. Regions moving out will tend to lag behind. The effect of these factors on the endolymph in the semicircular canals is to tend to rotate the fluid relative to the walls of the canal. This tendency is resisted by the cupula, which is deflected in precisely the same way as during an angular acceleration of the skull. Head tilting in a rotating environment thus produces signals like those generated during angular accelerations, leading to inappropriate reflex movements of the eyes and limbs together with spurious sensations of turning. All the canals are involved. The conflict of visual cues with the information from the labyrinth is such as readily to lead to motion sickness.

"Unphysiological" stimulation of the labyrinths also occurs in the caloric test used clinically to localize a defect to one ear or the other. Warm or cold water is run into the external acoustic meatus to set up temperature gradients in the temporal bone. The consequent changes in endolymph density interact with the contact forces on the skull, by the mechanism indicated in Figs. 4 and 5, to set up

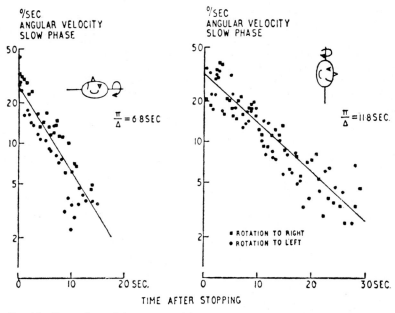

FIG. 16. Comparison of the patterns of decay of the slow phase velocity of nystagmus following impulsive deceleration from $60°.s^{-1}$ when the axis of rotation is vertical (left) and horizontal (right). Note logarithmic scale for ordinates. (From Benson and Bodin, 1966.)

convection currents. These may lead to cupula-deflection and the generation of neural signals. By setting the skull in a suitable orientation with respect to the support force it is possible to control which canal is likely to be most affected. The pattern of neural signals received by the central nervous system in conditions of caloric stimulation does not, however, mimic any naturally occurring situation because the temperature change is applied to one ear only while any head movement necessarily affects the labyrinths of both sides.

There is another aspect of vestibular function that should be mentioned although it is not yet fully explored. The receptors in the various parts of the vestibular apparatus, like receptors in many other sites in the body, may have their transducing properties adjusted by nerve fibres that carry impulses outwards from the central nervous system (Klinke and Galley, 1974). The precise function of these outgoing pathways is not yet experimentally verified but the indications are that they may serve to suppress the vestibular signals that are generated by the animal's own movements, such as those involved in the pursuit of a visual target (Klinke, 1970). There is much to be said for a system that allows voluntary movements to proceed without the constraint of too efficient a set of stabilizing reflexes. If the stabilization were 100 per cent effective, no voluntary movement would be possible.

REFERENCES

Beerens, A. J. J. (1969), *Stimulus Coding in the Utricular Nerve of the Cat. A Quantitative Study of the Response to Static Stimulation of the Utricle as Recorded from Primary Afferent Fibres*. Amsterdam: Drukkerij Cloeck en Moedigh.

Benson, A. J. and Bodin, M. A. (1966), "Interaction of Linear and Angular Accelerations on Vestibular Receptors in Man," *Aerospace Med.*, **37**, 144–154.

van Egmond, A. A. J. (1940), "Anatomie et Topographie des Elements Sensoriels du Labyrinth Vestibulaire," *Oto-rhino-Laryng. int.*, **24**, 46–63.

van Egmond, A. A. J., Groen, J. J. and Jongkees, L. B. W. (1949), "The Mechanics of the Semi-circular Canal," *J. Physiol.*, **110**, 1–17.

Fernandez, C., Goldberg, J. M. and Abend, W. K. (1972), "Response to Static Tilts of Peripheral Neurons Innervating Otolith Organs of the Squirrel Monkey," *J. Neurophysiol.*, **35**, 978–997.

Fujita, Y., Rosenberg, J. and Segundo, J. P. (1968), "Activity of Cells in the Lateral Vestibular Nucleus as a Function of Head Position," *J. Physiol.*, **196**, 1–18.

Girard, L. (1930), "L'attitude normale de la tête déterminée par le labyrinthe de l'oreille," *Oto-rhino-Laryng. int.*, **14**, 517–37.

Gray, A. A. (1907), *The Labyrinth of Animals* (2 vols). London: Churchill.

Groen, J. J. (1967), "Central Regulation of Vestibular Responses," in *Myotatic, Kinesthetic and Vestibular Mechanisms*, pp. 198–204 (A. V. S. de Reuck and Julie Knight, Eds.). London: Churchill.

Groen, J. J., Lowenstein, O. and Vendrik, A. J. H. (1952), "The Mechanical Analysis of the Responses from the End-organs of the Horizontal Semi-circular Canal in the Isolated Elasmobranch Labyrinth," *J. Physiol.*, **117**, 329–346.

de Kleijn, A. and Magnus, R. (1921), "Uber die Function der Otolithen: I. Mitteilung. Otolithenstand bei den tonischen Labyrinthreflexen. Labyrinthreflexe auf Progressivbewegungen. II. Mitteilung. Isolierte Otolithenausschaltung bei Meerschweinden," *Pflügers Archiv.*, **186**, 6–81.

Klinke, R. (1970), "Efferent Influence on the Vestibular Organ During Active Movements of the Body," *Pflügers Arch. ges. Physiol.*, **318**, 325–332.

Klinke, R. and Galley, N. (1974), "The Efferent Innervation of the Vestibular and Auditory Receptors," *Physiol. Rev.*

Krijger, M. W. W. (1954), Thesis, University of Utrecht.

Lindeman, H. H. (1969), "Studies on the Morphology of the Sensory Regions of the Vestibular Apparatus," *Ergebn. Anat. EntwGesch.*, **42**, 4–113.

Loe, P. R., Tomko, D. L. and Werner, G. (1973), "The Neural Signal of Angular Head Position in Primary Afferent Vestibular Nerve Axons," *J. Physiol.*, **230**, 29–50.

Lowenstein, O. and Roberts, T. D. M. (1949), "The Equilibrium Function of the Otolith Organs of the Thornback Ray (*Raja clavata*)," *J. Physiol.*, **110**, 392–415.

Magnus, R. (1924), *Körperstellung*. Berlin: Springer.

Melvill Jones, G. (1972), "Transfer Function of Labyrinthine Volleys Through the Vestibular Nuclei," in *Basic Aspects of Vestibular Mechanisms* (A. Brodal and O. Pompeiano, Eds.). *Prog. Brain. Res.*, **37**, 139–156.

Niven, J. I., Hixson, W. C. and Correia, M. J. (1965), "An Experimental Approach to the Dynamics of the Vestibular Mechanisms," pp. 43–56, in *Symposium on the Role of the Vestibular Organs in the Exploration of Space*. NASA SP-77, Washington: NASA.

Roberts, T. D. M. (1967), *Neurophysiology of Postural Mechanisms*, 354 pp. London: Butterworths.

Retzius, G. (1884), *Das Gehörorgan der Wirbelthiere II*. Stockholm: Samson and Wallin.

Vidal, J., Jeannerod, M., Lifschitz, W., Levitan, H., Rosenberg, J. and Segundo, J. P. (1971), "Static and Dynamic Properties of Gravity-sensitive Receptors in the Cat Vestibular System," *Kybernetik* **9**(6), 205–215.

28. NEURO-OTOLOGY

R. HINCHCLIFFE

INTRODUCTION

Neuro-otology encompasses not only audiology and vestibulology but also those aspects of neurology that are relevant to otology. The scope of neuro-otology, as has been previously indicated (Hinchcliffe, 1961; Greisen and Jepsen, 1973), is thus far-reaching. Audiology itself is a discipline with many ramifications and some of these are dealt with elsewhere in the book. The facial nerve itself is the subject of Chapter 30. The purpose here will therefore be to mention some aspects of vestibulology that have not previously been considered. This chapter will thus encompass those aspects of the neuro-otological examination which are listed in Table 1 and will supplement an account previously given by the author (Hinchcliffe, 1973).

It is said that the examination of vestibular function is essentially an examination for, or of, nystagmus. However, an examination for nystagmus must imply that consideration be given to eye movements other than nystagmus. The vestibulologist must have some knowledge of eye movements in general and of their physiological control. Indeed, with this concept, vestibulology straddles the area where neurology, ophthalmology and otolaryngology all meet.

EYE MOVEMENT CONTROL SYSTEMS

The subject of ocular kinetics is highly complex, with contributions coming from biomedical engineers, biophysicists, clinicians, physiologists and psychophysicists (Bach-y-Rita et al., 1971). There appear to be at least four

TABLE 1
ASPECTS OF THE CLINICAL VESTIBULO-OCULOMOTOR INVESTIGATION

Eye Movements

I. Spontaneous
   A. Pseudonystagmus
   B. Nystagmus

II. Induced
   A. Non-nystagmic
      Optic
         Command
         Following
      Vestibular
         Counterrolling
         Parallel swing
         Oculocephalic manoeuvre
   B. Nystagmus
      Optic
         Optokinetic (optomotor)
      Vestibular
         Provocation
         Rotational
         Caloric
         Galvanic
         Pneumatic
         Tullio

rapid type of eye movement (up to 700° s⁻¹) of which the oculomotor system is capable. It does, however, have a relatively long latency (about 200 ms) between stimulus and the response. Saccades of equal magnitude and direction

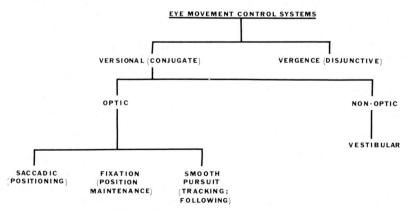

FIG. 1. Eye movement control systems.

main systems for the control of eye movements (Fig. 1). The slow phase of at least one component of optokinetic (optomotor) nystagmus is mediated by the pursuit eye tracking system and the quick phases of both optomotor and vestibular nystagmus are mediated by what is termed the *saccadic system*. Indeed, all fast eye movements are saccadic. As Fuchs (1971) points out, a saccade is the most

in the visual field are made simultaneously by both eyes. The appropriate stimulus for a saccade is an image of interest on the retina but distant from the fovea. Saccades are responsive to target displacement only (Rashbass, 1961). Displacements of < 0·3° do not result in a saccade. As Gay and Newman (1972) point out, once a saccade is triggered, the predetermined movement is executed despite subsequent changes in stimulus conditions. The maximum velocity of a saccade is a function of its magnitude. Studies by Young and Stark (1962) led them to propose a discrete control system which sampled the error created by a target step and which then became unresponsive to any subsequent target behaviour for 200 ms. After that, a movement was executed which was appropriate to the error that existed 200 ms previously. The saccadic response cannot therefore be modelled by a continuous system. Consequently, Young and Stark

horizontal and vertical gaze *only after passing* through the cerebellum (cortex and nuclei). Thus the so-called oculomotor decussation does not take place in the mesencephalic reticular formation but within the cerebellum. The supranuclear gaze centre for horizontal eye movements is part of the nucleus giganto-cellularis, which is in the paramedian zone of the pontine reticular formation (Goebel *et al.*, 1971). This comes to lie dorsal to the oculomotor and trochlear nerve nuclei and rostral to the abducent nerve.

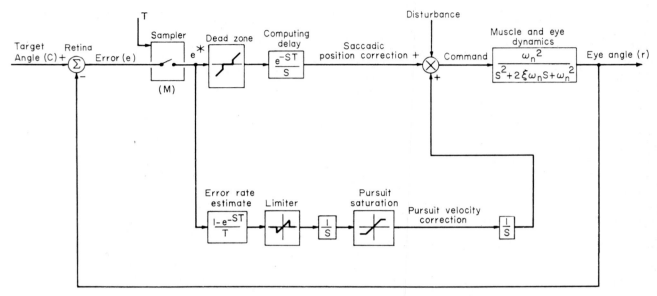

FIG. 2. Dual mode (saccadic and tracking) model for control of eye movements.

presented a *sampled-data* model for saccadic eye movement control, although such a possibility was mentioned by Vossius in the previous year. Modifications to this original model have subsequently been made by other workers. Young and Stark's original sampled-data model for the control of eye movements is shown in Fig. 2. (In this figure, S is the complex operator $j\omega$ which is described in Chapter 5.)

At the moment, ideas concerning the probable pathway for the saccadic system are controversial. A number of clinical and experimental studies have been interpreted as indicating that the centre for saccadic eye movement is in the frontal cortex (specifically, Brodmann's Cortical Area 8). However, such a hypothesis receives no support from single unit studies. Using the monkey, Bizzi (1968) failed to detect a single neuron in that area which fired *prior* to the saccadic eye movement. This applied to studies both in the light and in the dark. The balance of evidence available from anatomical and physiological studies at the present time indicates that saccadic eye movements are initiated in the association areas of the parietal and occipital lobes where visual and other inputs are integrated (Aschoff, 1974). Aschoff maintains that these visual and paravisual association areas project homolaterally on to the lateral nuclei pontis (in the ventral pons). This pathway terminates in the supranuclear gaze centres for

The supranuclear gaze centres for vertical and rotatory eye movements are located in the pretectal nuclei, such as the interstitial nuclei (of Cajal), which are situated near the rostral end of the oculomotor nucleus and mark the rostral extension of the medial longitudinal fasciculus (Mehler *et al.*, 1958). The input to the supranuclear gaze centres is from the more lateral parts of the cerebellum via the nucleus interpositus and the nucleus dentatus.

The supranuclear gaze centres mark the beginnings of the final common path for both saccadic and slow pursuit movements. For example, stimulation of the paramedian zone of the pontine reticular formation produces horizontal movements which may be either saccadic or slow pursuit in type, depending on the stimulus characteristics (Cohen and Komatsuzaki, 1972).

The cerebellar cortex participates solely in saccadic movements. In Wadia and Swami's (1971) heredofamilial spinocerebellar degeneration, all saccadic eye movements are abolished but smooth pursuit movements are normal.

As envisaged by Kornhuber (1971), the operation of the saccadic system is as follows. Saccadic movements are "ballistic" movements; once started, these fast movements cannot be modified before they terminate a preprogrammed movement. They are thus too quick to be regulated continuously. The duration of these fast preprogrammed movements must therefore be timed. The cerebellar cortex acts as this timing device, i.e. clock (Braitenberg and Onesto, 1962). The regular spacing of the Purkinje cells in relation to the parallel fibres of the cerebellar cortex and the convergence of a row of such cells on a neuron of the cerebellar nuclei could form the structural basis for this clock. Thus the cerebellar cortex could be considered to be what is termed a *function generator* in electronics. In contrast, the cerebral cortex is not a function generator. The role of the cerebral cortex is envisaged as that of data reduction. Sensory messages, processed in the primary and association areas of the cerebral cortex, give rise to motor commands that are transformed into spatio-temporal patterns for the function generators in the cerebellar cortex and in the basal ganglia. Whereas the cerebellar cortex can be considered as a *step function generator* for these voluntary fast movements, the basal ganglia are seen as *ramp generators* for voluntary slow movements. Such movements are, however, not possible in respect of the eyes, which show only involuntary, slow following movements. Thus the basal ganglia are not involved in the control of ocular movements.

The *smooth pursuit system* is the one responsible for following eye movements. The phrase "human eye tracking system" is sometimes restricted to this system or it may encompass both this and the saccadic systems. The time between stimulus and response for smooth pursuit movements is shorter (*c.* 125 ms) than that for saccadic movements. The velocity of a slow pursuit movement is linearly related to that of the target up to about $25° s^{-1}$. Since, as Young (1971) points out, target velocity is a signal which is not directly available it can only be re-created by the eye movement system on the basis of eye velocity and retinal slip velocity. It is to be noted that, in the rabbit, Barlow and his associates (1964) have demonstrated retinal ganglion cells responding selectively to the direction and speed of image motion. The extraocular muscle EMG (electromyogram) in smooth pursuit movements shows a gradually increasing contraction of the agonist and a gradually increasing relaxation of the antagonist. This is in contrast to the condition with saccadic movements, where the EMG shows abrupt contraction of the agonist associated with immediate silence of the antagonist.

Although slow pursuit movements are absent during the first few months of life (Kestenbaum, 1930), complete pursuit palsy only, i.e. total inability to pursue an object in one or both directions is extremely rare (Raff, 1967). Smooth pursuit movements to one side with jerky (saccadic) pursuit movements to the other side is characteristic of deep posterior hemisphere lesions to the latter side.

The slow pursuit system is subserved by an occipito-mesencephalic pathway. This projects from the striate (visuosensory) cortex, i.e. Brodmann's (1909) Area 17, to the interstitial nucleus (of Cajal) and other mesencephalic nuclei. The fibres lie medial to the optic radiation and then pass through the posterior end of the internal capsule (Mettler, 1935).

The *fixation* (position maintenance) *system* should be distinguished from the two eye control systems just mentioned. Its function is to hold the eye constant if required. According to Kornhuber (1971), this *holding function* is conducted by the cerebellar nuclei. Thus these nuclei not only participate in the timing function of the cerebellar cortex by integrating the output of a row of Purkinje cells, but they also have their own distinctive hold function. This function is similar to that of the vestibular nuclei which hold the position of the whole body as determined by the labyrinth. However, the cerebellar nuclei hold positions of only parts of the body, and as determined by the cerebral cortex. Although the output of this fixation system is by means of rapid eye movements, termed *microsaccades* ("flicks"), Robinson (1971) argues for it being considered as separate from the saccadic system. Certain drugs (diazepam and pentobarbital) can abolish an animal's ability both to make smooth pursuit movements and to maintain fixation away from the primary position, although saccadic movements remain unimpeded. Simultaneous loss of fixation and smooth pursuit movements may not be a coincidental one considering that fixation is a special case of pursuit where the target velocity is zero.

Vergence, i.e. disjunctive, eye movements are probably restricted to primates. These movements permit the fixation of points in visual space and at various distances from the organism. The appropriate stimulus for a vergence (convergence or divergence) movement is, of course, a stimulus that falls on non-corresponding retinal elements. *Squint* (strabismus) is the pathological condition of chronically misaligned visual axes. This is frequently genetically determined and is rare in coloured races. Minor degrees of squint may be recognized clinically from the asymmetric positions of the bright corneal light reflections relative to their respective pupil margins. There are two principal types of squint, i.e. concomitant squints and paralytic squints. *Concomitant squints* are so named because the eyes retain their relative positions in all directions; in *paralytic squints*, the difference in eye positions is greatest when gaze is in the direction of the normal action of the paralysed muscle. Concomitant squints are due to a disorder of the sensory component of the reflex arc or its central connections; paralytic squints are due to damage to the motor component of the arc. Persistent squints can result in an amblyopia ("lazy eye"). Experimental studies on monkeys have shown this to be due to shrinkage of cells in the lateral geniculate nuclei (von Noorden, 1974).

A vertical divergence of the optic axes (*skew deviation*) must be distinguished from squint (Smith *et al.*, 1964). This corresponds to the Magendie-Hertwig phenomenon in animals (Ohm, 1949). It is characterized by a maintained deviation of gaze of one eye above the other, the angle of which may or may not be fixed for all directions of gaze and is due to lesions other than those involving the extraocular muscles, their motor neurones or local mechanical factors in the orbit. The eye on the side of the lesion is usually hypotropic, i.e. the lower one. Skew deviation is seen in patients with acute asymmetrical cerebellar disease and represents a dysfunction of the vertical vergence mechanism. Although rare in demyelinating disease, it has been reported in cerebellar and pontine artery thromboses, in platybasias and in vestibulo-cochlear schwannomas ("acoustic neuromas"). It has also been produced experimentally in animals with lesions of the vestibular nuclei and their connections with the oculomotor nuclei (Oloff and Korbsch, 1926).

As was pointed out in the preceding chapter and by Melvill Jones (1971), the hydrodynamics of the *semicircular canal system* are such that the system performs an integration upon the angular acceleration to which the whole system is exposed. Thus, with a normal labyrinth

stretch receptor information. A model for the vestibulo-ocular reflex arch which was proposed by Sugie and Melvill Jones (1966) is shown in Fig. 3. In addition to the "primary" oculomotor response which passes through a first order lag system, there is a "secondary", saccadically generated, signal operating through the lag system which tends to restore correct phase and amplitude relations between the response and the original stimulus head movement. Thus, together with information from neck proprioceptors, the eye control system now appears as a

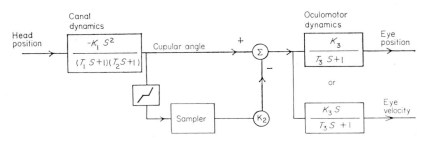

FIG. 3. Model of the vestibulo-ocular reflex arc incorporating the saccadic influence upon slow phase nystagmic response. (After Sugie and Melvill Jones, 1966.)

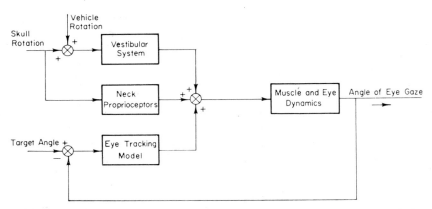

FIG. 4. Model for multi-imput eye control system incorporating information from vestibular receptors and neck proprioceptors. (After Meiry, 1971.)

and normally encountered head movements, endolymph displacement at any instant provides an accurate measure of instantaneous angular velocity. Experiments on cats have shown a close correspondence between the firing frequency of vestibular nuclear units and stimulus angular velocity (Melvill Jones and Milsum, 1967). Further studies on cats subjected to rotational acceleration showed firing frequency patterns in the abducent nerve nucleus almost indistinguishable from those obtained from the vestibular nucleus (Precht *et al.*, 1969). Thus the neural message transduced by the mechanical components of the canal end organ is conveyed, essentially unchanged, through the vestibular nucleus to the extraocular motor neurone system. A second integration would be required in the oculomotor system to convert an angular velocity signal to an angular eye position signal. This might be attributable to either ocular torque in the presence of high damping of the viscus in the orbit or to rate dependent negative feedback obtained from postulated rate dependent

multi-input one (Fig. 4). Consequently, in examining the vestibulo-ocular reflex, the clinical investigator should give consideration to the oculomotor system in general. Table 1 outlines what might be termed the vestibulo-oculomotor examination.

EYE MOVEMENTS

Spontaneous Eye Movements

The principal techniques in use for detecting and measuring abnormal eye movements comprise examination by the naked eye, with the ophthalmoscope, with Frenzel glasses and by means of electrophysiological techniques (*see later*).

As well as being of value in providing diagnostic information unrelated to disorders of ocular kinetics, the naked eye examination of the eyes may disclose nystagmus or other pathological eye movements. The distinction between these two groups, although customary, is to some extent artificial. There is indeed a continuum from the quasi-periodic, quasi-conjugate, essentially unidirectional eye movements with a basically periodic waveform that characterizes true nystagmus to the chaotic, multi-directional movements of opsoclonus. The various types of eye movements usually considered as pseudo-nystagmus (paranystagmus) are listed in Table 2. Those movements

TABLE 2

NON-NYSTAGMIC SPONTANEOUS EYE MOVEMENTS

Movement	Frequency
A. Physiological	
1. Slow rhythmic pendular eye-deviations	0·3 Hz
2. Square wave jerks	c. 1
3. Superior oblique myokymia	12–15
B. Pathological	
1. Oculo-gyric crises	c. 0·1 (usu. tonic)
2. Pendular macro-oscillations	c. 1
3. Ocular bobbing	
4. Random eye movements (of oculomotor apraxias)	
5. Opsoclonus	
6. Kippdeviationen	2·5
7. Ocular seizures	c. 3
8. Ocular flutter	3–11
9. Ocular myoclonus	1·5–26

classified as "physiological" are those which may be observed in otherwise normal subjects. Slow rhythmic pendular eye deviations, which are observed with the eyes closed, have a frequency of c. 0·3 Hz and amplitudes of up to 60°. They are associated with diminished vestibular excitability and are attributable to impaired alertness (to the extent of falling asleep) on the part of the subject. In contrast to these slow pendular deviations, *square waves* (*Gegenrucke*), which have a repetition rate of about 2 Hz and an amplitude of 2–10° may be observed when using Frenzel glasses or when recording electro-oculographically with the eyes closed. They are associated with mental alertness, particularly in apprehensive subjects. They are also to be found at the termination of caloric-induced nystagmus, following on the nystagmus. As such they can be used to determine the end point of the nystagmus. Higher amplitude square wave jerks that are recorded with the eyes closed are observed in certain cerebellar and brain stem syndromes. *Superior oblique myokymia* is manifest as monocular, intermittent, small amplitude torsional eye movements which appear spontaneously in otherwise normal subjects. The subject may experience diplopia or oscillopsia. One would therefore question whether or not this type of eye movement should be reclassified as "pathological".

Oculogyric crises (tonic eye fits) consist of conjugate spasmodic deviations of the eyes, usually upward. The eyes remain open and there are usually associated movements such as rhythmic contractions of levator palpebrae superioris and of orbicularis oculi, as well as head and neck movements. Although a sequel of post-encephalitic

Parkinsonism (Hohman, 1925), the phenomenon has also been reported in neurosyphilis (Krabbe, 1931; de Nigris, 1933) and following trauma (Kaslin, 1936). Ablation and electrical stimulation studies indicate that the motor and pre-motor cortex are involved in the generation of these crises (Klemme, 1941). The crises can be abolished by coagulative lesions of the posterior limb (pathway of the corticospinal tract) of the internal capsule (Gillingham and Kalyanaraman, 1965). These crises must be distinguished from the *ocular seizures* which may be observed in children with petit mal. The latter last for a few seconds only and tend to be clonic instead of tonic. In these cases, simultaneous electro-encephalographic recordings and ciné films of the eye movements show that the frequency of myoclonic jerking corresponds with the 3 Hz spike-and-wave discharges of the EEG (Bickford and Klass, 1964). Moreover, the eye movements commence at least 10 ms before the EEG spikes.

Pendular macro-oscillations (50°) of about 1 Hz frequency may be observed following an acute unilateral cerebellar failure for two to three weeks. The movements follow a saccade and have been likened to an underdamped control system.

Ocular bobbing (Susac *et al.*, 1970) is characterized by an abrupt, erratic spontaneous downward jerk of the eyes followed by a slow return to the mid-position. The condition may be associated with an ocular palsy but is more likely to be a sign of a brain stem lesion, such as an intrapontine haemorrhage.

Random eye movements are characteristic of the ocular motor apraxias (an apraxia indicates an impaired or absent purposeful movement despite the integrity of neural structures directly subserving that movement). The minimum expression of this group of disorders is characterized by saccadic paralysis in the horizontal plane. These ocular motor apraxias result from lesions disrupting cortico-cortical relationships and have been aptly referred to by Geschwind (1965) as the *disconnection syndromes*.

Opsoclonus consists of repetitive but non-rhythmic, multi-directional, quasi-conjugate eye movements ("saccadomania" or "dancing eyes"). The condition occurs particularly in encephalitis (Cogan, 1968) but also in subacute parenchymatous degeneration of the cerebellum (Ellenberger *et al.*, 1968). The morphological basis for this sign is damage to the dentate nucleus (Ross and Zeman, 1967) or to its connections (Gilbert *et al.*, 1963).

"*Kippdeviationen*" (sweep deviations) are high amplitude (10–50°) square waves with a repetition frequency of 1–3 Hz and which are suppressed by optic fixation (Kornhuber, 1966). This last feature is in contrast to non-vestibular spontaneous nystagmus which is suppressed by abolishing optic fixation and which, although termed "pendular", is characteristically non-sinusoidal. *Kippdeviationen* are associated with chronic cerebellar disease and myeloencephalitis but they have also been reported in otherwise normal subjects. Kornhuber attributes this type of eye movement to either normal or pathological disinhibition of the rostral mesencephalic reticular formation which appears when visual inhibitory controls are suspended. The movements thus correspond to underdamped, exaggerated microsaccades. They are more conspicuous with the eyes closed than when open in the dark.

Ocular myoclonus is an oscillation of the eyes, usually vertical, which is associated with synchronous rhythmical movements of other structures (particularly the soft palate but also the tongue, pharynx, larynx and facial muscles). The pathological basis of both ocular and palatal myoclonus is pseudohypertrophy of the inferior olivary nucleus, which follows on acute lesions of the dentate nucleus or its associated structures.

Ocular flutter consists of brief episodes of intermediate frequency (3–11 Hz) horizontal oscillations of the pendular type. If the subject also shows limb tremor, the frequency of the flutter is the same as that of the tremor (Brumlik and Means, 1969). The condition is commonly associated with ocular dysmetria (Higgins and Daroff, 1966).

A *spontaneous nystagmus* may be fixation, gaze or vestibular in type.

A *fixation nystagmus* may or may not be congenital and may or may not be pendular* but, characteristically, it either disappears or changes its direction or form with eye closure. The congenital nystagmus of Müller-Jendraskis is sex-linked and affects only males (Kestenbaum, 1947). A rapidly disappearing occupational disorder, Miner's nystagmus (Ohm, 1930), results from the subjects working in poorly lit conditions for long periods. This is similar to the darkness nystagmus which can be produced experimentally in animals (Raudnitz, 1902). The illuminance required to prevent the disorder is at least 4·3 lux (Sharpley, 1936). An acquired pendular nystagmus is not infrequently seen in demyelinating diseases and this may give sinusoidal recordings of eye movements. A *latent fixation nystagmus* uncovered by monocular fixation is, in view of its small amplitude, best observed by an ophthalmoscope. This type is very often associated with a squint and is hereditary.

A *gaze nystagmus*, which may be unilateral or bilateral, implies a disturbance of the mechanisms for the maintenance of eccentric positions of gaze. It must be distinguished from the slight degree of unsustained nystagmus (*Endstellungsnystagmus*) which is frequently present in otherwise normal subjects at the limits of conjugate gaze. It is probable, however, that this difference is one of degree only (Sauvineau, 1909). Nevertheless, Jung and Kornhuber (1964) distinguish two types of gaze nystagmus: *Blickparetischer* (gaze paretic) *nystagmus* and *Blickrichtungs* (gaze directional) *nystagmus*. The former accompanies partial gaze paresis in the direction of the quick phase and has a frequency of the order 1–2 Hz. The latter is not associated with voluntary gaze paresis and has a somewhat higher frequency, 3–5 Hz. Dix and Hallpike (1966) maintain that the spontaneous nystagmus associated with vestibulocochlear schwannomas is dependent not upon fixation *per se* but upon the maintenance of conjugate eye deviations. They therefore propose that this nystagmus be termed "deviation maintenance" nystagmus. Even with voluntary deviation of the eyes maintained, however, the

---

* The term "pendular" is a misnomer, since such a term would imply a sinusoidal waveform. Probably most cases of spontaneous nystagmus which do not exhibit a quick and a slow component, i.e. a saw-tooth waveform, are not sinusoidal. The waveform in such cases is usually of a variable composite saw-tooth sinusoidal-triangular character.

nystagmus, even though it persists, becomes slow and irregular. One wonders whether this might be due to there being more than one component in this nystagmus.

Hood (1967a) reported that a *congenital nystagmus* characteristically showed no difference in pattern or degree of activity whether recorded under conditions of optic fixation or with the eyes open in darkness. He also reported that a spontaneous nystagmus due to a lesion at or about the level of the vestibular nuclei showed enhanced amplitude but decreased velocity of its slow phase when recorded with eyes open in darkness; if the eyes were closed, this nystagmus was abolished.

Spontaneous vestibular nystagmus is commonly horizontal with a rotatory component. It is usually directed away from the involved ear but may be directed towards the involved ear if it represents either an irritant nystagmus or a recovery nystagmus (*Erholungsnystagmus*) (Stenger, 1959). A spontaneous vertical nystagmus is almost always due to a lesion of the central nervous system. A downward directed nystagmus is characteristic of lesions of the medulla oblongata. If this nystagmus is most marked during extremes of gaze instead of when looking straight ahead, a cervico-medullary lesion, such as an Arnold-Chiari malformation is most likely (Daroff, R. B.: at p. 209 in Bach-y-Rita *et al.*, 1971).

Recently, Hood and his colleagues (1973) have reported what they term a *rebound nystagmus*. This should not be confused with a rebound positional nystagmus, which is a nystagmus that is associated with resuming the upright position in patients who have a positioning (benign paroxysmal) nystagmus. The characteristic of rebound nystagmus is such that, in the initial examination of the eyes in a straight ahead gaze position, no nystagmus is observed. With a subsequent gaze deviation to, say, the right, a brisk nystagmus with its fast component to the right appears. After about 20 s, the nystagmus fatigues and may even reverse direction. If at this time the eyes are returned to the primary position, nystagmus to the left, not present initially, occurs and this too fatigues with time. It was reported that this type of nystagmus is associated with chronic cerebellar disease and was found in 6 per cent of neurological patients referred for a neuro-otological examination.

There are a number of rarer types of spontaneous nystagmus which are of interest because of the nature of the pathophysiology and the clues which they give to the aetio-pathological diagnosis. *Seesaw* nystagmus shows a conjugate torsional oscillation with a superimposed disjunctive vertical component which characteristically is such that, when one eye goes up, the other eye comes down, and vice versa. The condition is usually associated with bitemporal hemianopsia and parasellar tumours extending into the III ventricle but it has been observed in apparently exclusively ocular conditions (Slatt and Nykiel, 1964).

Nystagmus retractorius (Koerber, 1903; Salus, 1910; Elschnig, 1913) is characterized by irregular jerks of the eye backward into the orbit when the patient attempts to look in one direction or the other. It is usually associated with paralysis of upward gaze which is termed Parinaud's (1883) syndrome. These two signs, together with dissociated or total pupillary areflexia, make up the Koerber-Salus-Elschnig cerebral (Sylvian) aqueduct syndrome. The syndrome is commonly due to a pinealoma. The tumour may also show marked abnormal auditory adaptation, which may (Benitez *et al.*, 1966) or may not (Kos, 1955) be associated with a hearing loss. The retraction nystagmus is best elicited with the optokinetic drum; retraction jerks are associated with each upgoing fast component of the optokinetic nystagmus (Smith *et al.*, 1959). The abnormal adaptation is best demonstrated by recording auditory thresholds for a continuous test tone using Békésy type audiometry. Studies of the effects of stereotactic lesions (produced to treat intractable pain) on man (Nashold and Gills, 1967) and on monkeys (Pasik *et al.*, 1969) indicated that the ocular kinetic fators, at least, of this syndrome are due to a lesion of the posterior commisure. The posterior commisure is a complex fibre bundle which crosses the midline in the caudal lamina of the pineal stalk. The commisure is associated with various nuclei, including the interstitial nuclei of the posterior commisure and the interstitial nucleus of Cajal which is situated near the rostral end of the oculomotor nucleus. It would appear, from the study of Pasik and his associates, that neither the interstitial nuclei of Cajal nor the superior colliculi are essential for vertical eye movements.

Voluntary nystagmus is a rare type of pendular nystagmus where the subject can cause his eyes to make very fine, rapid (up to 10 Hz) horizontal oscillations (Westheimer, 1954). The nystagmus can be produced at will but cannot be sustained. It disappears when optic fixation is abolished.

Non-nystagmic Induced Eye Movements

Command eye movements provide for the clinician a means for not only calibrating apparatus used in the electrical recording of eye movements but also for detecting ocular *dysmetrias*. A slight undershoot when the subject looks from one point to another is normal but an overshoot, especially if associated with several oscillations, is not. This phenomenon constitutes *ocular dysmetria* and is characteristic of cerebellar dysfunction. The pathophysiology is probably the abolition or slowing of signals received by the cerebellum from the extra-ocular muscle stretch receptors (Fuchs and Kornhuber, 1969). Ocular motor dysmetria is best demonstrated by having the patient look from eccentric points of gaze to the midline (Cogan, 1970). Absence of eye movements on command but the presence of slow pursuit movements (dissociated paralysis), or absence both of command and slow pursuit movements, together with intact vestibular responses, is the pattern of the pseudo-ophthalmoplegic syndrome (Wernicke, 1889).

The *oculocephalic* (doll's head) manoeuvre is performed by (a) briskly turning the subject's head from side to side, and then (b) flexing and extending the neck. In each case, conjugate deviations of the eyes in the direction opposite to the direction of movement constitute a positive (normal) oculocephalic reflex. In such a case, the nuclear and infranuclear oculomotor pathways must be intact. When a conscious patient is examined, he should be told to fix his gaze on an object in the primary position of gaze. In

such a case, the manoeuvre tests the fixation (the position maintenance system) mechanism, the slow pursuit (following) mechanism and the vestibular mechanism. With comatose patients, only the last system is tested.

The neuro-otologist usually tests slow pursuit movements by asking the subject to fixate on a pendulum (Ohm, 1940). The mechanisms underlying this, however, are similar to those underlying optokinetic nystagmus. Corvera and his associates (1973) refer to this test as the PETT (*Pendular Eye Tracking Test*). These authors use a simple pendulum with a period of 2 s and an amplitude of 15–20°. Since the maximum angular velocity for the sinusoidal eye movement associated with this pendular tracking is given by

$$V_{max} = (2\pi/T) A_{max} \qquad (33.1)$$

where V_{max} = maximum angular velocity in degrees per second

A_{max} = maximum angular displacement of eyes in degrees

and T = period of sinusoidal movement,

then the maximum eye velocity with Corvera's method is about 60° s^{-1}. Although von Noorden and Preziosi (1966) found that the critical frequency at which saccadic movements begins to replace smooth movements is between 0·5 and 0·8 Hz with maximum amplitudes of stimulus displacement of 13° (corresponding to a maximum angular velocity of between 40° s^{-1} and 65° s^{-1}), Corvera and his colleagues reported no significant interference of saccades with the smooth sinusoidal pursuit curve. It should be noted, however, that Fender and Nye (1961) considered that this type of system behaves as a feedback mechanism in which the input is the movement of the retinal image and the output is the movement of the eye. With such a model, the feedback has a gain of 0·8. Thus the appropriate equation for the maximum velocity of the angular eye movement in these cases is

$$V_{max} = 0.8(2\pi/T)A_{max} \qquad (33.2)$$

Thus the maximum angular velocity of the eyes with Corvera's technique is about 50° s^{-1}. Corvera and his colleagues reported that a normal sinusoidal curve with superimposed fast movements is associated with cerebellar disease and a deformed curve occurs with more widespread brain lesions. In brain stem lesions with a gaze nystagmus, impairment of pendular following eye movements is usually more marked than optokinetic defects (Jung and Kornhuber, 1964). Conversely, in peripheral vestibular lesions with a spontaneous vestibular nystagmus, the pendular following eye movement is essentially normal. Disappearance of the sinusoidal curve is associated with lesions of the oculomotor pathways in the tegmentum of the mesencephalon and of the pons. The following movement is also impaired by drugs, e.g. barbiturates (Rashbass and Russell, 1961), chlordiazepoxide, ethanol and phenytoin (Corvera *et al.*, 1973). The obvious disadvantage of this pendular eye tracking test is the strong influence of the predictability of object motion (Dallos and Jones, 1963). This is an objection that may be relevant only to man, since the predictability of visual object motion is not present in monkeys (Fuchs, 1967). In man, the pursuit eye movement system is able to predict future positions of the target up to 300 ms ahead. It would thus appear that the present system for investigating eye tracking should be replaced by a more nearly random target movement in respect both of velocity and (at least in a two dimensional plane) of direction. This necessitates some type of large oscilloscope screen with a programmed target movement. Nevertheless such a technique would enable one to study both the saccadic and the slow pursuit eye control systems and to do this not only with the horizontal gaze directions but with all gaze directions.

Lateral inclination of the head on the shoulder provokes an ocular rotation in the opposite direction. This phenomenon of *counter-rolling* of the eyes was first observed by John Hunter in 1786, and subsequently described, under the name *Gegenrollung* by Bárány (1906a). In the French literature, this phenomenon is referred to as *la contre-rotation oculaire* and Nelson and Cope (1971) refer to it as the ocular countertorsion reflex (OCR). Bárány cited cases where the counter-rolling was augmented during vertiginous episodes. Normally, static head tilts of up to 45° produce compensatory counter-rolling of the order of only 5° both in monkeys (Cohen *et al.*, 1970) and in man (Miller, 1962). Dynamic compensatory counter-rolling, as induced in pilots by rapid rolls, can, however, attain values of up to 20° (Melvill Jones, 1958). However such a manoeuvre stimulates not only the otolith organ but also the vertical semicircular canals. In other words, whilst static compensatory counter-rolling is a statotonic reflex, dynamic compensatory counter-rolling is a combined statotonic and statokinetic reflex. Experiments on animals by Szentágothai (1964) and by Suzuki and his colleagues (1969) showed that stimulation of the utricular macula or utricular nerve respectively produced counter-rolling of the eyes. The animal experiments of Cohen and his colleagues indicated that neck receptors were unimportant in respect of counter-rolling. In man, ocular counter-rolling is absent in "deaf mutes" (Miller and Graybiel, 1963) but may be preserved in cases of streptomycin intoxication where both caloric and rotatory stimulae fail to elicit a vestibular response. Nelson and House (1971) reported that the degree of counter-rolling was halved in subjects who had undergone unilateral labyrinthectomy or a vestibular nerve section. At the present time the evidence relating head position to the degree of counter-rolling in these labyrinthectomized cases is conflicting. This may well relate to the degree of vestibular accommodation (or over-accommodation) that has occurred.

The otolith system may also be examined with the *parallel swing* (Walsh, 1960; Oosterveld, 1970). Oosterveld recorded eye responses with electro-oculographic techniques (*see later*). All of 35 subjects, each having complete unilateral loss of auditory and vestibular (to caloric testing) function, showed normal sinusoidal eye movements when swung sideways and tested in the supine position. However, when the subjects lay sideways to be tested, 27 subjects showed a difference in amplitude of the eye movements between the right and the left lateral positions.

The difference was such that a greater amplitude was registered when the normal labyrinth was undermost.

Induced Vestibular Nystagmus

Vestibular nystagmus may be induced by a variety of procedures. This induced nystagmus may or may not be pathological. In general, nystagmus produced by a variety of clinically applied static and kinetic mechanical stimuli applied to the head and neck is pathological. It is convenient to use the German term *Provokationsnystagmus* for this type of nystagmus.

Provocation Nystagmus

This term is used to encompass what we find referred to in the German literature as *Kopfschüttelnystagmus* (head-shaking nystagmus), *Lagenystagmus* (positional nystagmus) and *Lagerungsnystagmus* (positioning nystagmus). Provocation nystagmus is best studied with the aid of Frenzel glasses. The reason for this is that, with the exception of the cervical posture test, it is usually transitory and it is also frequently dominated by a rotatory component. On both these counts, electrophysiological techniques are unsuitable for its investigation.

Kopfschüttelnystagmus is provoked by rapid side-to-side movements of the head (Vogel, 1932). Twenty such movements provide a suitable stimulus. The eyes are then observed for nystagmus immediately after this manoeuvre. In the case of peripheral lesions, this nystagmus is usually directed to the contralateral side. This may be the case even when a recovery nystagmus is present (Frenzel, 1961). If such a discordance is evident, it may be due to the operation of neck proprioceptors (*see later*) in the head-shaking procedure. However, it is equally (perhaps more) likely that it can be explained on the basis of the operation, within the vestibular system, of something analogous to "recruitment" in the auditory system. The test is contraindicated in cases of raised intracranial pressure and retinal detachment.

In addition to the head-shaking test, there are a group of tests, sometimes referred to as the *positional tests for nystagmus*, in which the nystagmus is elicited by means of a variety of either cervical posture or head positioning tests. In the routine examination for a nystagmus, especially when using electro-oculographic (EOG) recordings, nystagmus should be sought not only with the head in the primary position but also when flexed, extended, laterally inclined or rotated. These constitute the *cervical posture tests*. Nystagmus produced by these manoeuvres is due to the operation of neck proprioceptors and/or vertebral artery compression. Since the nystagmus produced by the cervical posture tests usually has a predominantly horizontal component but is of relatively small amplitude, it is conveniently recorded by EOG. Greiner and his colleagues (1964, 1969) have in fact developed a particular test of *cervical torsion* nystagmus. The subject's head is fixed but the body is subject to alternating, partial (60° amplitude) rotations. This is accomplished by seating the subject in a rotating chair from which the drive has been disconnected. The nystagmus is recorded by EOG. A cervical torsion nystagmus can be elicited in labyrinthectomized rabbits, so that the response is not mediated by the peripheral vestibular apparatus (Philipszoon and Bos, 1963).

The positional test described by Dix and Hallpike (1952) to elicit a nystagmus consists of firmly grasping the head of the patient who is sitting on a couch and then briskly taking the patient back into the critical position (head rotated 30–45° to one side and extended 30° over the edge of the couch). The test has consequently been criticized in that at least three nystagmogenic factors are operating. These are what are referred to in the French literature as *l'élément cinétique* (kinetic factor), *l'élément cervical* (cervical factor) and *l'élément spatial* (truly positional factor). It is, however, precisely because of these multiple factors that the test, performed in this manner, is a convenient screening test for "positional nystagmus"; thus in the French literature it is referred to as *une épreuve de dépistage* (Aubry and Pialoux, 1957). It is nevertheless doubtful whether the cervical factor is important in the production of nystagmus under these conditions, especially when viewed by the naked eye or by Frenzel glasses. Dix and Hallpike retested a group of subjects who demonstrated a nystagmus with this procedure by examining them on a tilt table; this would abolish any cervical factor. There was no appreciable change in the findings. In any case, subsequent manoeuvres can be conducted to eliminate one or other potential nystagmogenic factors. One can, as Nylén (1950) and others have reported, perform the positional test by asking the subject to assume the critical position slowly of his own accord. Thus any nystagmus produced by this procedure would be truly *positional* (*Lagenystagmus*) and not *positioning* (*Lagerungsnystagmus*). The latter type of nystagmus broadly corresponds to the "benign paroxysmal positional nystagmus" of Dix and Hallpike, and the former type, to the "central type of positional nystagmus". The paroxysmal type is much more common than the central type. The term "benign" has been objected to by Lindsay (1962) and others because some of the cases, albeit a small proportion (probably less than 1 per cent), are associated with an intracranial tumour (Cawthorne and Hallpike, 1957; Riesco McClure, 1957; Harrison and Ozsahinoglu, 1972). Thus these cases are not representative of the clinical condition. Similarly because of the paucity of histological material available, it is doubtful if these are representative of positioning nystagmus in general. Moreover, there is disagreement amongst the experts regarding the interpretation of this histological material (compare Cawthorne and Hallpike, 1957; Schuknecht, 1962; Lindsay, 1962). We should therefore take a fresh look at the clinical picture. Tables 3a and 3b show the pattern of the paroxysmal nystagmus in 30 consecutive cases. The very fact that the eye movement is a vestibular nystagmus must imply that the phenomenon is being mediated by the semicircular duct, and not the otolith, system. The amplitude of the nystagmus is frequently in excess (i.e. > 5°) of that associated with the statotonic reflexes (*see previously*). Moreover, since, with this manoeuvre, the head is taken back in a position of 45° rotation, the movement is in a plane of a pair of vertical ducts (Stenger, 1955; Frenzel, 1960; Hallpike, 1967).

Specifically, the ipsilateral posterior and the contralateral superior (anterior vertical) ducts are implicated. Stimulation of this pair of ducts would be expected to produce a rotatory nystagmus which would appear elliptical when viewed by the observer facing the patient. This is the usual finding. (Incidentally, it is frequently forgotten that *all nystagmus is rotatory*; it merely appears non-rotatory when the axis of rotation is in the coronal plane, or thereabouts). The production of nystagmus by this manoeuvre might be considered to be analogous to the precipitation of nystagmus by head shaking. In the one case we have stimulation of the pair of horizontal ducts, and in the other, of a pair of vertical ducts. Both manoeuvres would temporarily "release" nystagmus when an imbalance exists with respect to the particular duct systems. Thus, one can postulate a *Nystagmusbereitschaft* (state of nystagmus "readiness") in respect of not only the horizontal duct system, but also the vertical duct systems. It is conceivable that this vertical duct imbalance might be sufficiently marked to enable a nystagmus to be provoked by certain head positions only and without vertical duct stimulation. In this respect, the transitory, predominantly rotatory nystagmus produced by slowly assuming the critical head position, as advocated by Nylén (1950) and others, could be considered to differ only in degree from that elicited by the rapid manoeuvre which gives vertical duct stimulation. Relevant to this are the results of the animal experimental studies by Ledoux (1958) and by Duensing (1967). Ledoux demonstrated that the resting action potential discharges in the nerves from the vertical semicircular ducts were appreciably affected by head positioning. Duensing found that cells in the lateral vestibular nucleus, which receive vertical duct signals, also show a marked interaction with gravity receptor mechanisms. The direction of this paroxysmal positional nystagmus must be commented on. Figure 3a shows that, where it is known which ear in a peripheral lesion is the site of the disease, this ear is the undermost ear in about 70 per cent of cases. Because of the size of the sample, this value is not statistically significantly different from values which would be expected if the involved ear had an equal chance of being undermost or uppermost. Nevertheless, in view of Dix and Hallpike's finding on a much larger series, one expects to find that the affected ear is undermost in the positive postional test in the majority of cases. This would imply that, of the pair of vertical ducts which are stimulated, the ipsilateral posterior duct is the faulty one. If this were so, then one would expect the provoked nystagmus to be in a clockwise direction for right posterior ampullary crest lesions and in an anticlockwise direction for left posterior ampullary crest lesions. (The plane of nystagmus is the same plane as that of the damaged duct. For horizontal ampullary crest lesions, the nystagmus is in an ampullopetal direction with respect to the damaged duct; for vertical ampullary crest lesions, the nystagmus is in an ampullofugal direction.) These predicted directions are both opposite to the findings in Table 3a and also to the observations of Dix and Hallpike. One must therefore postulate that, in these cases, the provoked nystagmus is a form of recovery nystagmus, i.e. a form of Stenger's (1959)

TABLE 3

THE PATTERN OF PAROXYSMAL NYSTAGMUS IN
THIRTY CONSECUTIVE CASES

(a) Cases in which nystagmus occurred following the head "going down" in the positioning manoeuvre (28 cases).

(b) Cases in which nystagmus was produced with the head "coming up" (2 cases).

RHDP refers to the right head down position manoeuvre, and LHDP refers to the left head down position manoeuvre. The symbol "R", "L" or an asterisk under either of the columns headed RHDP or LHDP signifies that the right ear was at fault, the left ear was at fault or it was not known which ear was at fault respectively.

$$\left(\begin{array}{c} \text{HEAD} \\ \text{GOING DOWN} \end{array}\right)$$

Table 3a

$$\left(\begin{array}{c} \text{HEAD} \\ \text{COMING UP ONLY} \end{array}\right)$$

Table 3b

Erholungsnystagmus. If such were true, then one would expect to find, in some patients, a change in the direction of the nystagmus during the course of the disorder. Only one of the cases included in Table 3 showed a change. This was a man who initially showed a counter-clockwise rotatory paroxysmal nystagmus in the "left head down" position and subsequently showed a clockwise nystagmus in the same "head down" position. This is consistent with a left posterior duct failure giving, initially, a paralytic *Nystagmusbereitschaft* and then, subsequently, a recovering *Erholungsnystagmusbereitschaft*. But what is the commonest pathological basis of paroxysmal positional nystagmus? We have previously indicated the difficulties in generalizing from the sparse histological material available, which material may be open to various interpretations. An analogy may be drawn with Bell's palsy. No one would suggest that, because there have been reports of monosymptomatic unilateral facial palsy due to tumours or to parasites that this represents the pathological basis for the majority of acute, isolated facial nerve paralyses. But can one draw on the analogy further? The answer is probably "yes". The ampullary crest of the posterior semicircular canal duct, and this structure only, is supplied by the posterior branch of the vestibular nerve. It is therefore conceivable that the monosymptomatic acute vestibular failures which subsequently exhibit a rotatory paroxysmal positional nystagmus are, in effect, posterior branch vestibular nerve palsies. In continuing to draw on the analogy with Bell's palsy, which might be considered to be a "facial canal" syndrome, we can suggest that the monosymptomatic paroxysmal positional nystagmus of sudden onset might well be a "foramen singulare" syndrome. If such a condition does exist, one would expect this to be its mode of presentation.

Just as a vestibular imbalance with respect of a pair of vertical semicircular ducts might be expected to give a predominantly rotatory provocation nystagmus, so an imbalance with respect to the pair of lateral ducts might be expected to give a predominantly horizontal nystagmus in the positional test. Thus a predominantly horizontal positional nystagmus might be "triggered off" by a critical head position in cases where a *Nystagmusbereitschaft* exists in regard to the horizontal duct system. Duensing and Schaefer's (1959) animal experimental studies would provide support for such a hypothesis. These workers showed an interaction of lateral semicircular duct and gravity receptor mechanisms in cells of the lateral vestibular nucleus. Finally, one should comment on reports by Barber and Wright (1973) and others that, with electrical recordings, not only might a positional nystagmus be found in otherwise normal subjects, but it is found in the majority of such subjects. Clearly, if we consider positional nystagmus to be a measure of a vestibular imbalance with respect to vertical canal pairs, then the detection of such would be a function of the sensitivity of the measuring device. No mechanism, whether vestibular or otherwise, is perfectly balanced, so that whether or not an imbalance exists cannot be in question. What is in question is only the degree of imbalance. The finding of a positional nystagmus with electrical recordings in otherwise normal

subjects may also be compared to the findings of spontaneous nystagmus or of a high tone audiometric notch in otherwise normal subjects. One must expect that a number of people are suffering from subclinical dysfunctions which might be congenital or the residua of previous, long forgotten, illness. Nevertheless, it would appear that a positional nystagmus detectable with the naked eye or by Frenzel glasses is pathological. This therefore provides another reason for testing for positional nystagmus by these techniques instead of by electrical ones, where the question of abnormality might be in doubt.

Many other hypotheses have been offered from time to time to explain positional nystagmus. Of particular note is the study of positional nystagmus by Bergstedt (1970) using a human centrifuge. He concluded that positional nystagmus could be viewed as a defective adaptation of the vestibular receptor system to gravity.

A vestibular imbalance can also be demonstrated by a variety of other procedures, e.g. *hyperventilation* (Adlersberg and Forschner, 1931; Hart, 1974) and the Valsalva manoeuvre (van Saane, 1970). Van Saane indicates that the production of a vestibular nystagmus by hyperventilation is a particular feature of vestibulocochlear schwannomas.

Rotatory Tests

The physical basis for these tests has been discussed in the previous chapter. Its clinical value lies in respect of (a) detecting subjects with bilaterally impaired vestibular function, and (b) detecting subjects with a vestibular imbalance. If the subject has a unilateral vestibular paresis to which he has accommodated (i.e. central compensation in the vestibular system itself has occurred), then this will go undetected. Thus, in clinical practice, rotatory tests, whether of the gyratory or of the pendular type, is used, should always be employed in conjunction with caloric tests of vestibular function, as indicated, for example, by Torok (1969).

It is usual to investigate only horizontal duct function with the rotating chair since a spontaneous vertical nystagmus can be recorded in the majority of normal subjects when optic fixation is abolished (Fluur and Mendel, 1963). Indeed, in a group of 25 normal subjects studied by Fluur and Mendel, all had either a spontaneous nystagmus or a directional preponderance (DP) in the vertical direction, i.e. the sagittal plane.

In respect of horizontal duct stimulation, it is convenient to define the threshold as that angular acceleration which, when sustained for a duration of 20 s, is just sufficient to produce a detectable nystagmus when recorded by electrical techniques. Normal threshold sensitivity is of the order of $0.15° \text{ s}^{-2}$ when measured with optic fixation abolished. Optic fixation exerts a strong inhibitory effect upon induced nystagmus so that the threshold measured under these conditions is of the order of $1.5° \text{ s}^{-2}$. The ratio of the threshold sensitivity measured under conditions of optic fixation to that measured with optic fixation abolished has been termed the *fixation index* (Hood, 1970). Thus, for normal subjects, the fixation index has a value of the order of 10. Ballet dancers and ice skaters as well as aerospace and marine personnel and others who have undergone some occupational vestibular habituation show much higher indices (up to 80 or more).

Wilmot (1970) has reported on the clinical application in the U.K. of the rotatory chair examination using equipment of the type developed by Montandon and Dittrich (1961) on the Continent.

In addition to the gyratory rotating method of stimulation just described, there exists the *pendular rotation* method of stimulation. Whereas the former method produces a single acceleration-deceleration rotatory stimulus, the latter method produces a repetitive to-and-fro rotatory stimulus. Although more recent machine-driven pendular chairs have been developed, the simplest is the torsion swing (Mach, 1875; de Boer *et al.*, 1964). Mach's torsion swing consisted of a chair suspended from the ceiling by a steel cable. Using himself and his assistant, Mach determined the threshold of rotatory sensation with this swing. The investigation was done with the eyes closed and he found that the threshold depended on the angular acceleration and not on the angular velocity of the swing. Mach found the threshold to be between $2° s^{-2}$ and $3° s^{-2}$. The movement of the torsion swing is an example of simple harmonic motion in which the amplitude of the sinusoidal movements undergoes an exponential decay with time. The period (τ), i.e. time required for one oscillation, of a torsion pendulum is given by

$$\tau = 2\pi \sqrt{(I/Q)} \qquad (33.3)$$

where I = moment of inertia of the body with respect to the axis of oscillation

and Q = torsion coefficient of fibre (torque required to twist it through an angle of one radian)

The amplitude of any given oscillation bears a fixed relationship to the amplitude of the initial oscillation (this is determined by the experimenter who manually twists the chair from its resting position),

i.e. $A_n = A_o e^{-nk\tau} \qquad (33.4)$

where A_n = amplitude at end of nth oscillation

 k = time constant for damping of pendular movements

and τ = period of pendulum

The commercially available, machine-driven pendular chairs do not appear to provide a torsion pendulum-type stimulus in that either there is no damping of the oscillation, or, if there is damping, this is linear and not exponential. For the undamped pendular rotating chair, the maximum angular acceleration (γ) in any given oscillation is given by

$$\gamma = (4\pi^2/\tau^2)A \qquad (33.5)$$

where A = amplitude of oscillation.

The pendular chair has been extensively used as a clinical tool by Greiner and his colleagues (1961), by Hennebert (1956) and others. Greiner draws attention to the tonic eye deviations which are of vestibular origin. They reflect the sinusoidal changes in acceleration of the mechanical stimulus and are always present in normally functioning vestibular labyrinths. More recently, Eviatar and his associates (1974) have used the torsion swing in studying the maturation of vestibular responses in 10–75 days old infants. More infants responded to this type of stimulus than to caloric testing with water at 0°C. However, Eviatar (1970) properly cautioned against the use of the torsion swing as the sole vestibular test in screening for vestibulocochlear schwannomas. Such a tumour, although showing both labyrinthine preponderance and a DP with the caloric test, may give normal responses with the torsion swing test.

Caloric (Thermal) Tests

The principal disadvantage of rotatory tests of all types is that they stimulate both labyrinths. The caloric test is an attempt to simulate a unilateral rotatory stimulus. Thermal stimuli applied to the ear under test tend to produce convection currents in the semicircular ducts, i.e. a tendency to move the fluid relative to the walls of the duct, so exerting a deflecting force on the cupula concerned. On each side, the lateral semicircular duct lies more laterally than the other ducts so it is convenient to attempt to stimulate this duct with thermal stimuli, i.e. fluids (usually air or water) above or below body temperature. Since this duct is inclined 30° to the horizontal plane, the head must be tilted back 60° to place the duct in the optimum (vertical) position for setting up convection currents. If the patient is recumbent, which is the usual position for conducting the conventional caloric test, this means that the head will be flexed 30° with the subject in the supine position. In order to have equally strong but opposite (i.e. equipollent ampullopetal and ampullofugal) stimuli, the temperature of the warm stimuli should be the same number of degrees above body temperature as the cold stimuli are below it. Since 44°C (317 K) is the threshold of uncomfortable warmth, this is usually used as the temperature of the warm stimulus; correspondingly, 30°C (303 K) is used as the temperature of the cold stimulus. The use of these two temperatures for caloric test stimuli forms the basis of the so-called bithermal caloric test which was first reported by Thornval (1917) and subsequently standardized for clinical use by Fitzgerald and Hallpike (1942). Schmaltz (1932) has considered the physics of the caloric test and concluded that the observations regarding the latency and time course of the nystagmic response agree with theoretical predictions. With the patient in the prone position, the warm stimulus becomes an ampullofugal, and the cold an ampullopetal, stimulus. There is no significant difference in the nystagmic response to the caloric test stimulus in the prone compared with the supine position (Lee, 1969).

Two principal patterns of caloric test response are recognized, i.e. "*canal paresis*" (CP) and "*directional preponderance*" (DP). A third principal pattern, i.e. "*response decline*" (RD), may also be observed. In addition to these three principal patterns of response, there are a number of mixed patterns (Fig. 5). A CP pattern of response, unassociated with a DP, occurs when one or both ears are completely, or partially, unresponsive to both the warm and the cold stimuli. A DP means that nystagmus is more easily elicited, or shows a more marked activity, in one direction than the other. A DP pattern of response shows, for each ear, a difference in response to the two thermal stimuli; for the one ear, the warm stimulus gives a better nystagmic response, for the other ear, the cold stimulus elicits a greater response. The particular ear which gives a better response to the warm stimulus depends on the direction of the DP; if the DP is to the right, a warm stimulus applied to that right ear elicits a better response than a cold stimulus applied to that same ear, or a warm stimulus applied to the opposite (left) ear. In practice, caloric response patterns indicate a mixture of CP and DP. For unilateral vestibular lesions, this combined pattern is characterized by little or no difference in response of the two ears in respect of one temperature, but a significant difference in the response of the two ears for the other temperature. For DPs away from the side of the paresis, the two ears show a significant difference in response to the warm stimulus, but little or no difference in respect of the cold reaction; for DPs directed towards the side of the paresis, the converse is true. Thus Fig. 5f shows a combined RCP (right canal paresis) associated with a DP to the left; 5g, a combined LCP and a DP to the right; 5h, a combined RCP and a DP to the right; and 5i, a combined LCP and a DP to the left. One should remember that, in the interpretation of these responses, a warm caloric stimulus produces nystagmus to the same side as the stimulus, a cold caloric stimulus, to the opposite side. A mnemonic which has been suggested to remember these directions is COWS (cold opposite; warm same). The direction of a nystagmus is always designated according to the direction of the fast phase. "Warm" and "cold" stimuli refer to caloric stimuli whose temperatures are above or below body temperature respectively.

The magnitude of nystagmic response (duration, total number of beats or maximum velocity of slow phase) in the caloric test can be specified by expressing either CP or DP as a percentage. Thus the percentage CP (C) can be expressed as

$$C = [\{(\beta + \delta) - (\alpha + \gamma)\}/(\alpha + \beta + \gamma + \delta)]\,100 \quad (33.6)$$

where α = response to warm stimulus applied to the right ear,

β = response to warm stimulus applied to the left ear,

γ = response to cold stimulus applied to the right ear,

and δ = response to cold stimulus applied to the left ear,

and the percentage directional preponderance, D, as

$$D = [\{(\alpha + \delta) - (\beta + \gamma)\}/(\alpha + \beta + \gamma + \delta)]\,100 \quad (33.7)$$

Thus, if C is positive, a RCP is the case, if negative, a LCP is the case. If D is positive, the DP is to the right, if negative, to the left.

Equation (33.6) is a measure of the preponderance of one vestibular labyrinth, or, more specifically, the lateral duct, ampullary crest and nerve, over the contralateral corresponding structure. Consequently, Jongkees (1973)

prefers to use the term *labyrinthine preponderance* instead of canal paresis. He also points out that the use of the term "canal paresis" might lead to irrational utterances in certain cases, e.g. in demyelinating disorders, where the patient may have completely normal labyrinths. Most importantly, a semicircular canal, being a bony structure, cannot be paralysed. However, the term "labyrinthine preponderance" is itself not free from criticism since "labyrinth" is a synonym for the internal ear, and cochlear function in so-called labyrinthine preponderance cases may be entirely normal. Objections would also arise in respect of the terms "duct preponderance" or "ampullary preponderance"; abbreviation of the former would give confusion with directional preponderance and the abbreviation of the latter would give confusion with action potential. The matter must therefore rest until vestibulometric terminology has been standardized. Nevertheless, the term *lateral ampullo-neural preponderance* (LAP)* might be suggested since the term would (a) emphasize a relative caloric response in respect of the two ears and (b) emphasize that the test is primarily one of the lateral semicircular duct and its sensor (ampullary crest) together with its pathway (nerve). The relative, rather than the absolute, response of the two ears is important; this is indicated by the animal experiments of McCabe and Ryu (1969). These authors showed that, after unilateral labyrinthectomy, cerebellar inhibition shuts down the resting activity of tonic neurons of the medial vestibular nuclei of the intact side. This would explain observations of diminished caloric reactivity of contralateral ears in a period subsequent to a unilateral vestibular labyrinthine damage.

Irrespective of whether we accept CP as an absolute or as a relative measurement, it is the sole measurement of vestibular function which can be used to lateralize the dysfunction. A DP due to a peripheral vestibular lesion may be directed away from or towards the involved side. A DP reflects the degree of vestibular imbalance so that, if a spontaneous nystagmus is present, it will be in the same direction as this nystagmus. If, during the course of recovery from a peripheral vestibular lesion, the spontaneous nystagmus disappears, then it will be replaced by a DP. This DP will, initially, at least, continue to be in the same direction as the antecedent nystagmus. Later, however, it may reverse direction and be directed towards the affected ear. This condition is not infrequently found in chronic vestibular disorders. This reversed DP is analogous therefore to Stenger's *Erholungsnystagmus* (recovery nystagmus). A further complication is that if the caloric test has been conducted under conditions of optic fixation a DP may have arisen as the result of a hemisphere lesion, especially of the posterior half of the temporal lobe. The DP is such cases is directed towards the side of the lesion (Fitzgerald and Hallpike, 1942).

The "carry over" effect in which a test can influence the behaviour to a subsequent test is of special application to vestibulometry. Here, the effect is known as RD (response

* An alternative term to lateral ampullo-neural preponderance would be lateral ampullo-neural hypoexcitability or hyperexcitability. Such a term would be more appropriate physiologically.

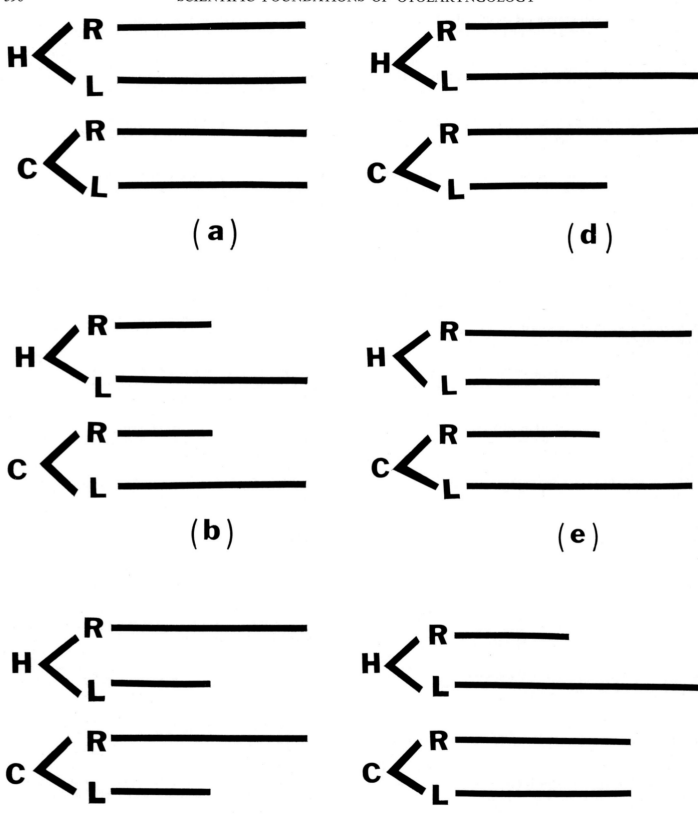

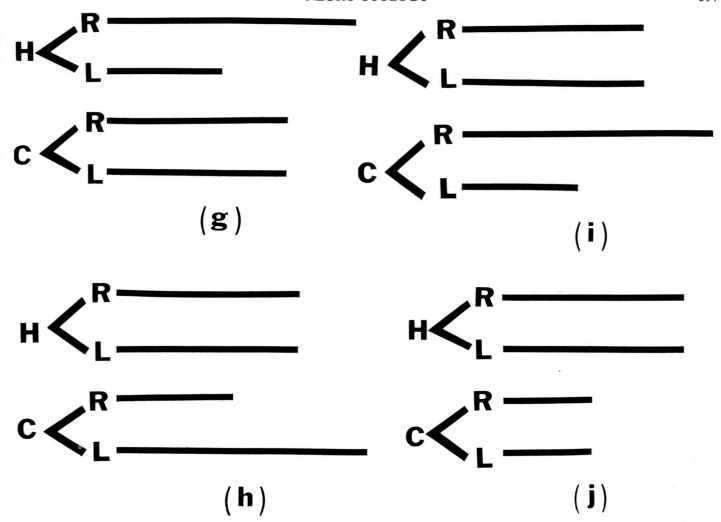

FIG. 5. Patterns of caloric test response: (a) normal; (b) right "canal paresis"; (c) left "canal paresis"; (d) directional preponderance to the left; (e) directional preponderance to the right; (f) combined right "canal paresis" with DP (directional preponderance) to the left; (g) combined left "canal paresis" and DP to the right; (h) combined right "canal paresis" with DP to the right; (i) combined left "canal paresis" and DP to the left; and (j) response decline.

decline) or *habituation*. It may occur to varying degrees, and may be appreciable in certain pathological conditions. Whether or not RD is said to be present depends very much on the index of response which is being used. For inter-test irrigation intervals of 5 min, marked RD occurs in subjective, but not in objective, measures of caloric response (Hinchcliffe, 1967a). In that investigation the nystagmic response was measured electro-oculographically under conditions where optic fixation was abolished. Even under conditions of optic fixation, as in the conventional Fitzgerald-Hallpike test, RD rarely occurs (Hallpike and Hood, 1953). Reports which have indicated some measure of RD under normal conditions of testing have been criticized by the authors themselves on the grounds of deficiencies in the experimental design. One would therefore consider that significant degrees of RD (objective measures) under the usual conditions of clinical testing are pathological. Halama's (1968) studies indicated that once the nystagmus induced by an irrigation has ceased, the next irrigation in the test may be given.

The importance of *testing sequence* is evident in data presented by Van der Laan and Oosterveld (1974). Caloric test responses were clearly much more age dependent when a cold-warm sequence of testing was used than when a warm-cold sequence was used.

Caloric Test Variations

The various methods for conducting the caloric test are discussed by Hamersma (1957). Broadly speaking, one may use one of two methods for applying the stimulus, two positions for the subject, three test conditions and two main methods for measuring the response.

Methods of *applying the stimulus* derive either from Bárány's (1906b) mass caloric or from Kobrak's (1918) *Schwachreizmethode*, a minimal stimulus method.

The *position* of the subject in the caloric test may be one of recumbency, or, as in the Fischer (1926)–Veits (1928) method, sitting with the head moved back only after 1 min has elapsed following the application of the stimulus.

The three *test conditions* are with the eyes open and

fixating, with the eyes open in darkness and not fixating, or with the eyes closed. Not only might these three conditions influence the relative *intensities* of the *observed nystagmus* (or even whether it is present or not) (Hood 1967; Hinchcliffe 1971; Haciska 1973) but the *pattern* of the *caloric test results* may also be different (Carmichael *et al.*, 1961; Dix and Leech, 1974). Consequently, caloric testing should, if possible, encompass these three conditions. The evidence which is now available suggests that abolishing optic fixation may reduce the chance of detecting an abnormal caloric pattern not only in cerebral hemisphere disorders, but also in peripheral vestibular disorders. It might therefore seem appropriate, until the matter is further elucidated (including measurement of the reliability of the various tests and of the ability of a test to differentiate normal from abnormal), to employ *screening caloric tests* under conditions of optic fixation.

The two principal methods of determining the *response* encompass either *subjective* procedures or *objective* procedures. Subjective procedures relate to the patient's sensation, and these may be quantified. For example, he may be asked whether or not he is "dizzy" and, if optic fixation is employed, whether or not the spot (or light) is moving; in the first case, the patient can be asked to express his vertigo on a subjective magnitude scale and, in the second case, he can be asked to indicate immediately the spot appears to have stopped moving. Objective procedures relate to measurement of the caloric response by the observer. The latter may observe the nystagmus directly by naked eye, with an infra-red viewer (Dix and Leech, 1974) or he may record it electrically (see later). The subject may also be wearing Frenzel glasses (also discussed later). Clearly, the methods of measuring the response will have a bearing on the test conditions which we have just discussed.

In addition to these variables, the stimuli may all be at the same *temperature*, or two, or more than two, temperatures may be used. Moreover, the stimuli may be administered either *consecutively* or, as in the so-called binaural (bilateral) caloric test, *concurrently* to the two ears. Finally, the degree of *mental alertness* as Sokolovski (1966) and others have shown, influences caloric response at least under conditions of eye closure. Mental arithmetic should therefore be required of the subject under this condition of examination.

Although a two-temperature (so-called *bithermal*) caloric test (Thornval, 1917; Fitzgerald and Hallpike, 1942) is in general use, indications do exist for a single temperature caloric test. The case for the bithermal caloric test is the observation, on occasion, of an interaction between a directional preponderance and a labyrinthine preponderance that results in little or no difference between the nystagmic responses to one particular temperature (*see above*). However, if preceding tests have been unable to demonstrate any vestibular imbalance, it is unlikely that there is any significant degree of directional preponderance. In these cases, a single temperature caloric test may be performed. Since the nystagmic response to a warm caloric stimulus appears to be a more valid measure of vestibular labyrinthine function than a cold

stimulus (Hinchcliffe, 1967b), this *monothermal* caloric test should use warm water. Part or whole of the explanation for this higher validity of the warm stimulus must be that it is an ampullopetal one. This, of course, refers to the condition which occurs in conventional caloric testing, i.e. with the subject supine. Thus, if the subject were to adopt a prone position, one would expect cold water to be a more valid stimulus. Kornhuber points out that hot caloric stimulation is more important than cold because non-specific activation of spontaneous nystagmus by cold irrigation may simulate a normal caloric response.

The use of stimuli at several temperatures provides the basis for *thermal vestibulometry* (Litton and McCabe, 1967; Halama 1969). In thermal vestibulometry, the ear is irrigated several times with water whose temperature becomes progressively more removed from body temperature. The test may or may not provide information of diagnostic value regarding the site of a vestibular system lesion.

Bithermal Caloric Test Procedures

In practice, the caloric test performed without electrical recording is a bithermal test which is usually one of two types. One of these, as in Britain, is the Cawthorne-Fitzgerald-Hallpike test (Cawthorne *et al.*, 1942; Fitzgerald and Hallpike, 1942). In that it uses a water volume of at least 0·25 l, given over 40 s, this test derives from Bárány's procedure. The reliability of this test is high. Product-moment correlation coefficients in respect of the reproducibility of nystagmic beats in a particular interval of time are of the order of 0·8 (Halama and Hinchcliffe, 1970). Reports of poor reliability of the test may be attributed either to inter- and intra-observer variation or, as Jongkees (1973a) points out, to changes in the subject's head position. Fluctuations in vestibular excitability may also be responsible for differences in test and retest results. Such fluctuations are particularly likely to be the case with endolymphatic hydrops, known or suspected cases of which are more likely than other disorders to be investigated with the caloric test.

The other principal clinical caloric test is the one which is used in many of the other European countries and which derives from the Kobrak method. Here a volume of water, which ranges from 10 to 50 ml, is injected into the external acoustic meatus with a syringe and the resulting nystagmus (if any) viewed with Frenzel glasses. The smaller volume of water in this procedure is less disturbing to the patient than the larger volume (at least 250 ml) which is associated with the other procedure. Moreover, the use of Frenzel glasses precludes visual fixation. This is an advantage if one is interested primarily in vestibular function and wishes to exclude the influence of a possible hemisphere lesion.

Singh (1974) has found a modification of the Fischer-Veits caloric test to be particularly suitable for clinical use. Here, 10 ml of water at the appropriate temperature are injected into the external meatus when the patient, who is wearing Frenzel glasses, is sitting head erect. The head is then extended to bring the lateral semicircular canal into the vertical plane and the resulting nystagmus (if any) observed. Using this procedure, patients experience little or no vertigo. The basis for this absence of ill effects is undoubtedly the observation, from rotating chair studies, that the objective threshold (for nystagmus) is below the subjective threshold (for vertigo). A criticism of procedures of the Fischer-Veits type is that extension of the head may bring neck reflexes or arterial compression mechanisms into operation. This, however, is of little import. A directional preponderance which is exhibited by a caloric test and any nystagmus which result from the particular cervical posture of this test both indicate a central tonus imbalance. The extent to which cervical factors are involved can be assessed by repeating the test with the patient recumbent and with a normal cervical posture.

If, with the subject supine, the two ears are *simultaneously irrigated* with water at the same temperature, a nystagmus will result which, at least in theory, will reflect the difference in response to the two stimuli given separately. Thus, if a response of the same magnitude is obtained with water at 30°C (303 K) when the ears are separately stimulated, then the responses will cancel out when the ears are simultaneously stimulated. No nystagmus would then be observed. If water at 30°C produces, when given monaurally, a greater response from the right ear than from the left ear, simultaneous (binaural) stimulation with water at the same temperature should produce nystagmus to the left. This technique of bilateral calorization was introduced into neuro-otology by Ruttin and by Brunner many years ago but it is only recently that Brookler (1971) has reported a satisfactory procedure where the test is performed and recorded electro-oculographically. For judging an abnormal response to binaural stimulation, Brookler now looks for three clearcut beats in a 3 s period and occurring within 30 s after the end of an irrigation. Unfortunately, the absence of any observable nystagmus following both warm and cold bilateral stimulation could mean not only that the labyrinth (specifically the lateral ampullary cristo-neural systems) was normal but also that there was no vestibular function whatsoever. Moreover, in the absence of any vestibular imbalance, the absence of any nystagmus following bilateral stimulation could also mean that the two labyrinths showed equal degrees of hyporeflexia (bilateral vestibular nerve or labyrinth lesion) or equal degrees of hyperreflexia (central release). In clinical practice, equal degrees of hyporeflexia or hyperreflexia without vestibular imbalance should be infrequent so that the only pathological condition to guard against would be bilateral non-functioning vestibular labyrinths.

In cases where a conventional bithermal caloric test gives a normal response, prolonged (about 3 min) simultaneous bilateral irrigation may produce nystagmus. This indicates vestibular fatigue and occurs in central vestibular disorders including vestibulocochlear schwannomas (Bauer, 1972).

Simultaneous bilateral caloric stimulation may also be used to test ampullary cristo-neural function in respect of the vertical semicircular canals. For such purposes, the subject's head is placed in the vertical position. Downward directed nystagmus occurs with binaural warm caloric stimuli; upward directed nystagmus occurs with binaural cold caloric stimuli. Dix (1970) has recently used this procedure to investigate neural mechanisms of nystagmus using patients with supranuclear ophthalmoplegias.

Galvanic Test

As Hennebert (1950) has pointed out, the galvanic test has remained "*l'enfant pauvre de la famille des épreuves vestibulaires*". The principal reason for this is that (1) the mode of action is unsolved, (2) a variety of methods are used in the test, (3) there is a divergence of opinion in interpreting results, and (4) there are difficulties in recording galvanic-induced nystagmus. Because of electrical interference of the stimuli with the response, electro-oculography using the corneo-retinal potential cannot be used to record the responses. Consequently, recording of galvanic induced nystagmus must rest on photo-electric techniques of recording eye movement (Pfaltz, 1965). It is usual to employ a bipolar technique where one of a pair of electrodes is placed on each mastoid region. Normally, a current of 1–2 mA is required to produce nystagmus (*le nystagmus pergalvanique*). This nystagmus is directed towards the negative electrode. Following the termination of the electrical stimulus, there is a nystagmus, *le nystagmus postgalvanique*, which is in the opposite direction. This reversal of nystagmus (*Pfaltz's phénomène d'inversion*) also normally occurs when an applied current is reversed. The nystagmus of this reversal phenomenon is characterised not only by a much shorter latency but also by a greater intensity than the pergalvanic nystagmus. The threshold of pergalvanic nystagmus is always normal in receptor organ (vestibular labyrinthine neuro-epithelial) lesions, unless secondary neural degeneration, for example 4–5 years following trauma, has occurred. The reversal phenomenon is also normal in these receptor organ lesions, except in cases of recent onset where there is a directional preponderance away from the affected side. In traumatic vestibulocochlear nerve lesions and intrameatal schwannomas of this nerve, the galvanic reaction is absent. With intra-medullary brain stem lesions, the galvanic response may be unimpaired or only slightly affected.

Pneumatic Test

In cases of chronic suppurative otitis media, especially when the subject complains of vertigo, compression of the air in the external acoustic meatus may produce nystagmus. It is generally accepted that, in such cases, mechanical movement of air in the external meatus is readily transmitted through the tympanic membrane perforation to the middle ear, and thence to the internal ear through an erosion of the bony wall of the periotic labyrinth. Such a phenomenon was first demonstrated by Lucae in 1881 and, in such cases, is known as a *fistula* sign or a positive fistula test. Such a term is, of course, a misnomer. Were a fistula, i.e. a channel, to exist between the middle and internal ears, then not only would fluids leak from the internal ear but infection would pass from the middle to the internal ear and immediately destroy the latter. Thus these so-called "fistulas" are sealed at least with the endosteum lining the bony labyrinth.

According to Eckel (1959), an ear which exhibits a positive fistula test in conjunction with a spontaneous nystagmus directed towards the opposite side frequently progresses to total loss of function.

The pneumatic tests may also produce nystagmus in patients with imperforate eardrums (Hennebert's sign); this occurs in labyrinthine lesions associated with congenital syphilis. The mechanism here is said to be the transmission of pressure changes via the vascular channels in the osteitic labyrinth.

Sono-ocular test

The Tullio phenomenon consists of the production of vestibular symptoms and/or signs by an acoustic stimulus (Tullio, 1926; Huizinga, 1935). The effect depends upon the functional integrity of the vestibular labyrinth only, and is reproduced in animals when the cochlea has been ablated. Bleeker and de Vries (1949) have shown that a microphonic (analogous to the cochlear microphonic) can be recorded from the crista of the fenestrated semicircular canal of the pigeon and the frequency response curve of this cristal microphonic parallels the frequency response curve for the Tullio phenomenon. This vestibular microphonic can be recorded from any of the vestibular end-organs (Huizinga et al., 1951). It has been observed in fishes (Pumphrey, 1939), reptiles and amphibians (Adrian et al., 1938).

Cawthorne (1956) considered that the Tullio phenomenon occurred in man only when more than one mobile window opened into the internal ear on the vestibular side of the vestibular membrane. The phenomenon has, however, been reported to occur in other conditions, such as congenital hearing loss, direct vestibular trauma and endolymphatic hydrops (Kacker and Hinchcliffe, 1970; Stephens and Ballam, 1974). There appears to be no doubt that the symptom is much more frequent than has hitherto been assumed. This is possible because the symptom is not sought and, when it is reported, it is confused with phonophobia. Moreover, it is possible that the phenomenon never occurs to a sufficient degree to be observed without recourse to electro-oculography, a technique which is still rather little used in the examination of patients with vestibular disorders.

Induced Optic Nystagmus

Optokinetic (Optomotor) Nystagmus

Optokinetic nystagmus is a physiological nystagmus which is produced when the subject looks at a succession of objects which pass in front of his field of vision. Purkinje is said to have observed it in bystanders watching passing cavalry in Berlin. It is also observed in passengers in railway trains who gaze at the passing countryside; hence the name, railway nystagmus. It is similar to vestibular nystagmus in that, although of optical origin, it shows a fast and a slow phase. However, optokinetic nystagmus differs from vestibular nystagmus in two respects. First, optokinetic nystagmus is associated with deviations of the eyes in the direction of the fast, and not the slow, component. Secondly, the reversal of the direction of optokinetic nystagmus begins with a change in the direction of the fast phase. Consequently, the fast phase is not simply a reflex return of the eyes to the mid-position (as had been held by some) but a manifestation of high order cortical activity involving the frontal centre for voluntary gaze (Hood, 1967b). However, the matter is not just as simple as that since, under conditions of liminal illumination, a different pattern is observed. Under conditions of poor (liminal) illumination, the deviation of the eyes and the phase in which the nystagmus reverses are precisely the same as in vestibular nystagmus, i.e. deviation of the eyes in the direction of the slow component and reversal in the slow phase. Moreover, similar features to those seen under conditions of liminal illumination are seen when the subject is instructed to follow the stripes of the optokinetic drum ("active" optokinetic nystagmus). Despite conscious efforts of the subject, this "active" nystagmic response repeatedly lapses into the "passive" type of response. The latter is therefore the type which is usually elicited in the clinical situation. Hood and Leech (1974) have discussed the implications of these observations but clearly different nervous mechanisms must subserve each of these types of optokinetic nystagmus.

In 1926, Fox and Holmes showed that a DP (directional preponderance) of optokinetic nystagmus occurred in lesions of the inferior part of the parietal lobe. In these subjects where the DP occurs, the fast phase of optokinetic nystagmus, which is directed towards the side of the lesion, is relatively more pronounced than that directed to the contralateral side. The actual change is a suppression of the optokinetic nystagmus away from the side of the lesion. Gassel and Williams (1963) considered that impaired slow pursuit function which is observed in deep posterior hemisphere lesions is the basic disturbance in the optokinetic DP which Fox and Holmes observed. The integrity of the slow pursuit system for objects going away from the side of the lesion would permit the fast phase of optokinetic nystagmus to be retained towards the side of the lesion.

The first and only sign of an internuclear ophthalmoplegia may be a *dissociated* optokinetic nystagmus (Smith and David, 1964). Bilateral internuclear ophthalmoplegias are virtually pathognomonic of multiple sclerosis.

TECHNIQUES OF INVESTIGATION

A number of techniques employed by the neuro-otologist in the investigation of nystagmus are designed to accentuate an already present, or to disclose an otherwise undetectable, vestibular nystagmus. The techniques therefore hinge upon the fact that vestibular nystagmus is enhanced by abolishing optic fixation. Bartels (1922) showed that this could be achieved by using + 20 dioptre* biconvex lenses. These not only interfere with fixation by the patient but also, by magnifying, assist observations by the observer. A source of illumination was added by Frenzel (1925), which further interferes with fixation by the subject and improves conditions for observing the subject's

---

* The dioptre is the unit of measurement of the power of a lens. It is given numerically by the reciprocal of the focal length expressed in metres. It is not an SI unit.

eyes. Mahoney and his associates (1957) indicate that the amplitude of vestibular nystagmus may be increased nearly fourfold with the use of Frenzel glasses.

An increasing number of reports are appearing in respect of electrical techniques for the registration of both spontaneous and induced nystagmus (Aschan *et al.*, 1956; Hallpike *et al.*, 1960; Aboulker *et al.*, 1963). The technique is frequently referred to as electronystagmography (ENG) but, in conformity with the terminology for other electrophysiological methods, it is more appropriately termed electro-oculography. There are two principal techniques for the electrical recording of eye movements. One is a photoelectrical technique whereas the other is a bioelectrical technique. The photoelectrical technique (Pfaltz, 1960), although in less widespread use, is the only one of these two techniques which can be used for recording galvanic-induced nystagmus (Pfaltz, 1970).

The more widely used bioelectrical technique depends on the fact that the eyeball behaves as a dipole, i.e. it is positively charged at one point with respect to a negative charge at another. In man, the posterior pole is negatively charged with respect to the cornea and, fortunately, the electrical axis coincides with the anatomical and optic axes. Thus a pair of electrodes placed on either side of an eye will register a difference in potential whenever there is a movement of the eye in the plane of the electrodes. Since the eyeball acts as a dipole, potential differences produced by rotation of the eyeball in the plane of the electrodes will be proportional to the sine of the angle of rotation. However, in practice, because of the relatively small angles associated with nystagmus, this relationship between the voltage produced and the angular eye deviation is not significantly different from a linear one.

Vertical movements of an eye will be registered with one electrode above, and one below, the eye. A pair of vertical electrodes across each eye will be required to register a see-saw nystagmus. The otologist, however, is usually concerned with detecting and registering horizontal nystagmus, so that he will probably be content with a pair of electrodes in the horizontal plane, each electrode of the pair being placed on the face just lateral to the lateral canthus. Such an arrangement assumes that the patient displays conjugate eye movements, at least in the horizontal plane. A patient with a spontaneous ataxic nystagmus shows a dissociated nystagmus on lateral gaze, where the abducting eye has greater amplitude. To detect and record this would require a *pair* of horizontal electrodes across each eye.

Controversy has raged over whether d.c. (direct current) or a.c. (alternating current) amplification should be used. If one requires to know the gaze position of an eye, when individual eye movements are registered, or the concomitant gaze position of the two eyes when their movement is recorded by a single pair of electrodes, then d.c. amplification must be used. As Cawthorne and his associates (1968) pointed out, vestibular nystagmus is enhanced by gaze in the direction of the quick phase, a law which was first enunciated by Gustav Alexander. Thus gaze deviations might account for variations in the activity of a recorded vestibular nystagmus. However, Alexander's law is more particularly applicable to conditions of optic fixation, where, in any case, the gaze position of the eyes is known. Vestibular nystagmus is usually recorded electro-oculographically where optic fixation has been abolished either by eye closure or by recording with the eyes open in darkness. Under these conditions, as the paper by Cawthorne and his associates shows, Alexander's law does not hold so well. Moreover, under conditions of eye closure, which are usually used by otologists, the eyes tend to adopt a straight-ahead gaze position. For these reasons, the otologist is inclined to be content with the simple and electrically more stable a.c. amplifying system for electro-oculography.

In certain disorders of the central nervous system, such as the supranuclear ophthalmoplegias occurring in Huntington's chorea and in the Steele-Richardson-Olszewski syndrome, there are abnormalities of the quick phase of both optokinetic and induced vestibular nystagmus (Dix, 1970). The quick phase of vestibular nystagmus is also suppressed by fentanyl, a morphine-like substance used as an adjuvant to local or general anaesthetics. If the quick phase is totally absent, a negative response of the electro-oculographically registered caloric test would be recorded if a.c. amplification were used. D.c. amplification only would be able to record the tonic deviation of the eyes in these cases. Consequently, a d.c. amplifying system is desirable for electro-oculographic machines used in neurological departments. For the purposes of detecting these cases of selective abolition of the quick phase of nystagmus, Janeke and his associates (1969) advocate testing patients with the torsion swing. In these cases, the response to the torsion swing would be a sinusoidal eye movement in phase with the stimulus, indicating the integrity of the peripheral vestibular organ.

A.c. amplifying systems have an electrical response characteristic which is termed the coupling time constant (*see* Chapter 5). A suitable time constant for electro-oculography is of the order of 10 s. This coupling time constant is sufficiently long to record nystagmus without distortion of its waveform, but, at the same time, sufficiently short to avoid appreciable drift in the recording which arises from slowly shifting d.c. levels anywhere within the pick up or recording system. Appreciably smaller coupling time constants (e.g. 0·03 s) will differentiate the electro-oculographic electrical signal so that the recording will be a measure of the velocity of eye movement. Additional circuitry (rectification and integration of the signal) for such an amplifying system provides recording of the average velocity of either the slow or the quick phase of nystagmus as a function of time (Hinchcliffe and Voots, 1962). Unfortunately, the characteristics of equipment for recording nystagmus in otological practice are far from being standardized but some desirable features are listed by Rubin (1968).

Further developments in electro-oculographic techniques to record nystagmus have been the use of vectornystagmography by Padovan and Pansini (1972) and others and the use of radiotelemetry by Fukuda and Tokita (1971). Vectornystagmography enables one to measure the resultant direction of nystagmus in the coronal plane.

Radiotelemetry permits the recording of electrical signals at a distance without the intervention of connecting wires. Using this technique, Fukuda and Tokita have shown that a physiological nystagmus occurs with normal body movements.

A logical development of the increased availability of computers has been the use of computers for electro-nystagmographic data reduction by Herberts and his associates (1968) and others. As a less expensive substitute for a computerized system, Voots (1969) has reported a "computerless" automatic data reduction system for use in conjunction with a standard nystagmus recording system. This "computerless system" gives an automatic printout of slow phase velocity. It functions completely automatically, has no complicated adjustment or maintenance procedures for the technician to learn and demands no technical background in handling instruments including computers.

CLINICAL PRACTICE OF NEURO-OTOLOGY

To bring this presentation on neuro-otology to a close, it would be appropriate to consider the application of the basic neuro-otological sciences to clinical practice. This is best done by presenting a flow chart (Appendix to this Chapter) that has been developed by the author over many years for the clinical investigation of auditory or vestibular function. Since the flow chart crystallizes a system of investigation which has evolved in clinical practice it shows a number of interesting features. In particular, tests for loudness recruitment and speech audiometry are conspicuous by their absence in the principal line of investigation. This is because information on these tests is of less value to the diagnostician (neuro-otologist or otological physician) than it is to others. These particular tests are of more value to the auditory prosthetician or the rehabilitative audiologist or even the aural surgeon who must decide on a particular form of surgical intervention, or even whether to operate or not. Appreciably different flow charts could therefore be developed by individuals who fill other roles. A different, or a modified, flow chart will also be followed when there is a special investigation of a particular symptom; this is instead of following the general theme of attempting to elucidate an aetiopathological diagnosis. Thus the investigation of tinnitus requires, for example, tinnitus masking (Ghose and Sardana, 1970; Feldmann, 1971) and tinnitus matching (Reed, 1960) tests. The construction of flow charts is always a valuable exercise in setting out logically the steps which are to be followed by a system of practice. In the context of otolaryngology in general the author believes they will form a prerequisite to developing a comprehensive computer-assisted diagnosis in the not too distant future.

APPENDIX

Flow chart for investigation of auditory and/or vestibular function. The aim of this flow chart is to ensure more efficient use of audiometric and vestibulometric facilities; it has not been extended to provide a diagnosis. Broadly speaking, as pointed out in Chapter 3, a flow chart, such as

this, encompasses two "happenings". First, a trapezoid indicates an action or, in computer terminology, an input–output operation, e.g. otoscopy. Secondly, a diamond-shaped box indicates a decision or, in computer terminology, an IF statement, i.e. where one chooses a different path according to whether the answer to a question is YES or NO (or DON'T KNOW). Thus, somewhere along the flow chart one requires a decision to proceed along one or other course of action dependent upon whether or not there was a perforation of the ear drum. A decision does not necessarily immediately follow the relevant action. Thus a decision on one or other of further courses of action, e.g. air or water caloric test, which is based upon whether or not there is a perforation of the ear drum, does not follow otoscopy (the "action") until much further along the chart. Circles indicate transfer points, i.e. where one can go from or come back to. Asterisks indicate DON'T KNOW or NOT KNOWABLE. In this flow chart, particular attention has been paid to the condition of the external acoustic meatus. Part of the reason for this is that, if tests are going to be conducted by personnel other than otologists, it is essential that the ears are in an "optimal testable condition". This particular first section of the flow chart has however an instructional purpose since, by its emphasizing a simple initial matter, it enables the user himself to flow easily and rapidly into the mechanism of the chart. Although appearing cumbersome on initial inspection, proficient use of the chart should ensue after a short time with individuals having the requisite very basic audiological and otological knowledge. Shortening flow charts does *not* make them more efficient—only more ambiguous. The meanings of the abbreviations in the chart is as follows:

A/ROM, acute or recurrent otitis media; AOE, acute otitis externa; ASVD, auditory, speech or vestibular disorder; CND, other cranial nerve deficits; ?ICT, intracranial tumour suspect; FW, forced whisper test; HL, hearing loss; BING, (occlusion phenomenon) test performed; <5, patients' age less than five years; PAU, Paediatric Audiology Unit; CV, conversational voice test performed; BTHL, bilateral total hearing loss; UTHL, unilateral total hearing loss; BARANY, Bárány box applied to contralateral ear; ABC, absolute bone conduction testing; UPTA, unmasked pure tone audiogram; USA, unmasked speech audiogram; ERA, electric response audiometry; U/B UBC, unilateral or bilateral unmasked bone conduction; ITHL, ipsilateral total hearing loss for air conducted sound; PTA, pure tone audiogram; SHADOW EXPECTED, shadow curve expected; POST-TR HTL, high frequency post-traumatic hearing loss; BCGM, bone conduction by graduated masking procedure; OKN, optokinetic nystagmus; HA, hearing aid prescribed; REHAB, auditory rehabilitation; SUDDEN, sudden hearing loss; HAEM, request for haemoglobin concentration and blood film, examination; $<\frac{1}{12}$, duration of disorder less than one month; VIROL, virological investigation; AB GAP, air-bone gap; PERF, perforation of tympanic membrane; AUTOINFL, autoinflation; BC HL, bone conduction hearing loss; SISI, short increment sensitivity index; SN(NE), spontaneous nystagmus

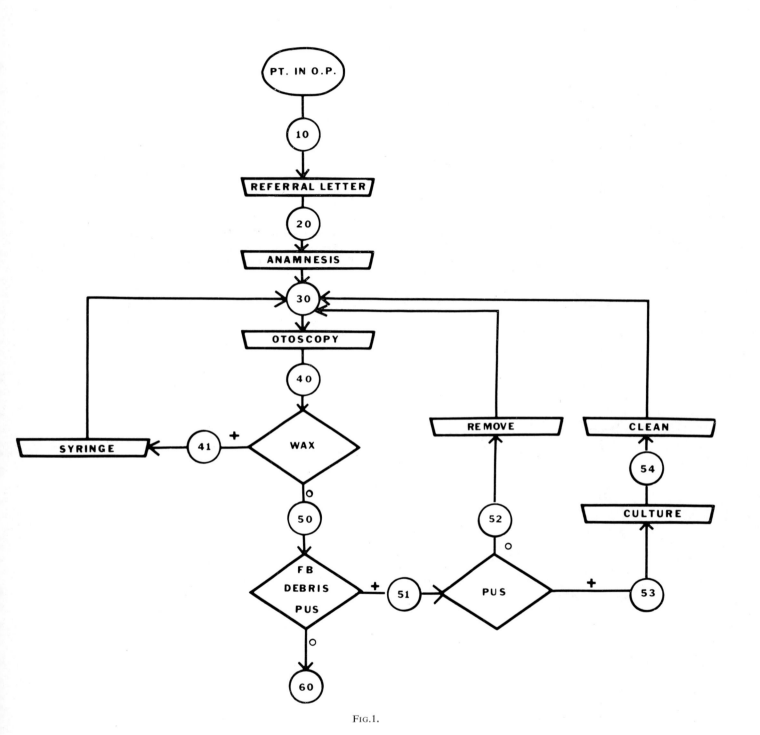

Fig.1.

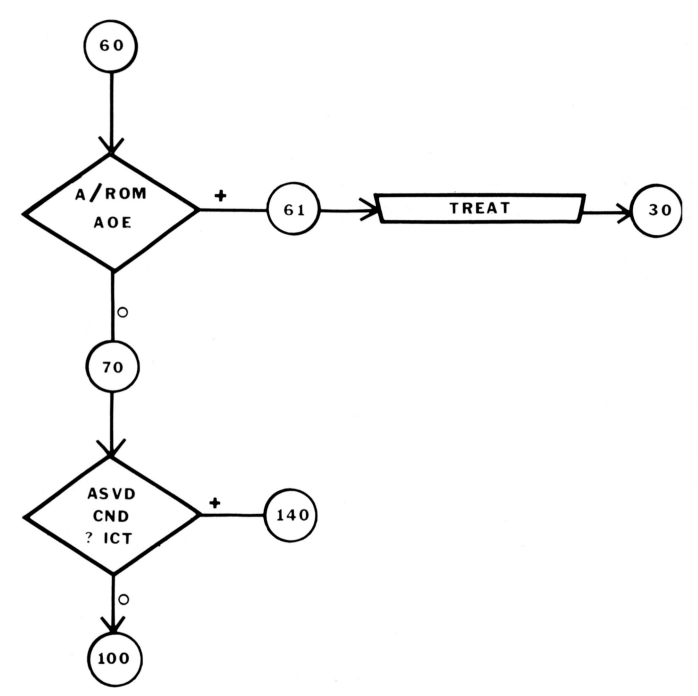

F<small>IG</small>. 2

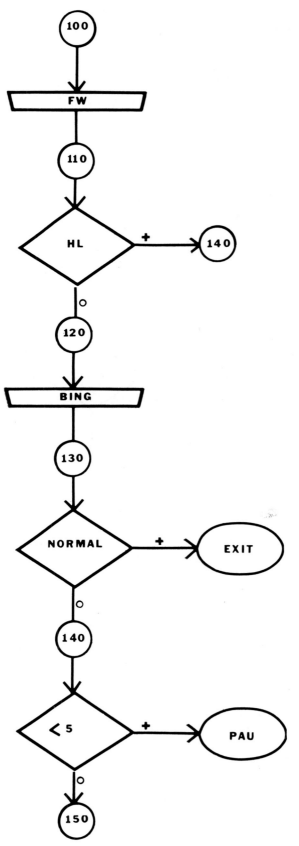

FIG. 3.

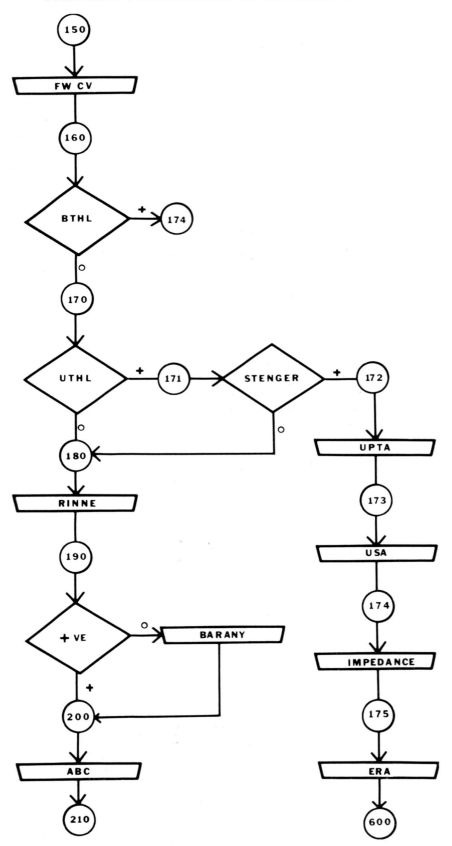

Fɪɢ. 4.

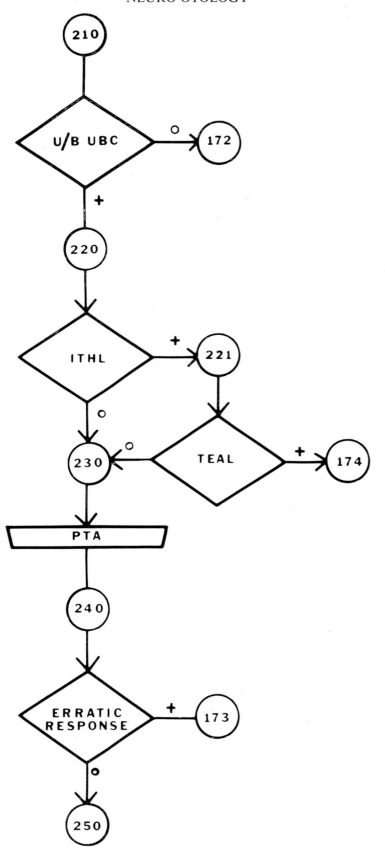

Fɪɢ. 5.

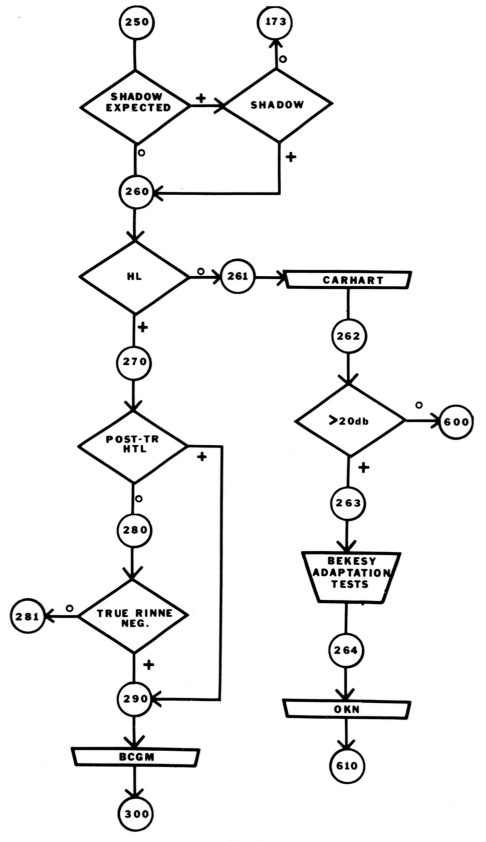

FIG. 6.

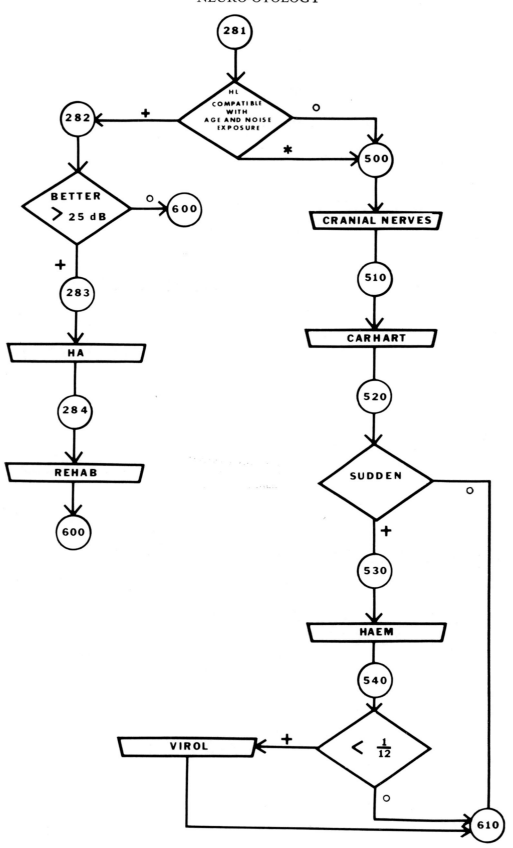

F<small>IG</small>. 7.

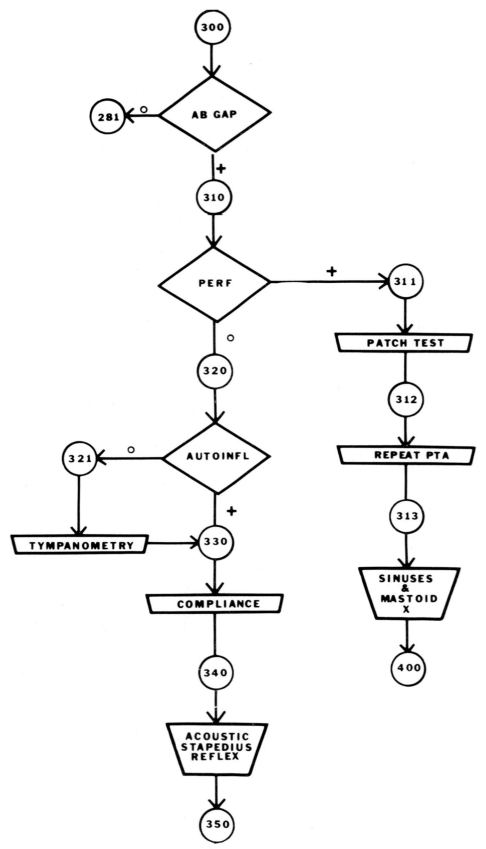

Fig. 8.

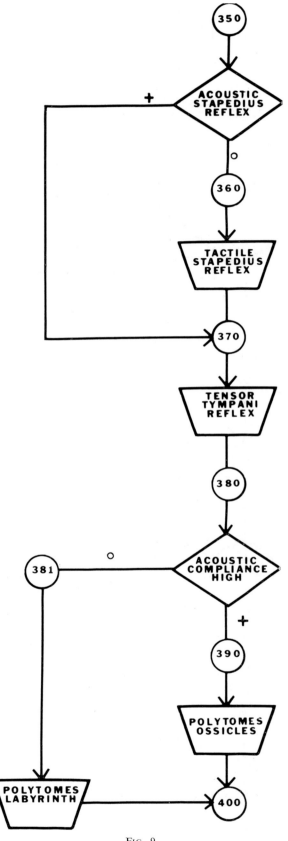

Fig. 9.

412   SCIENTIFIC FOUNDATIONS OF OTOLARYNGOLOGY

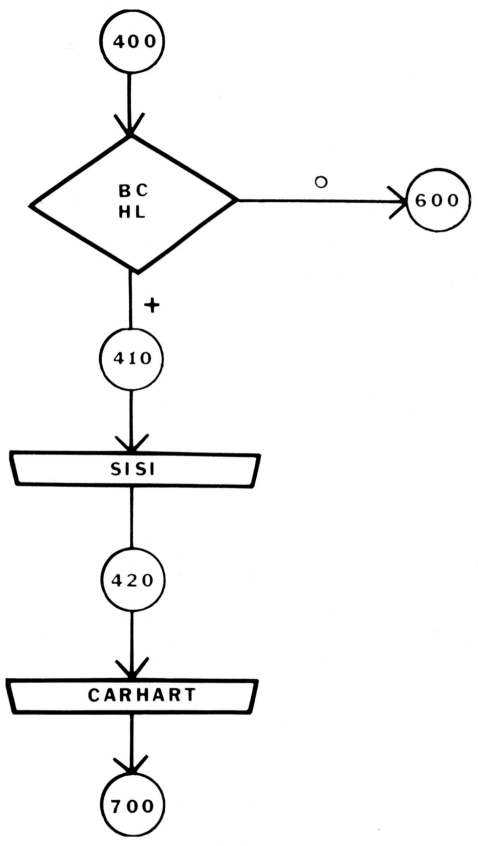

Fig. 10.

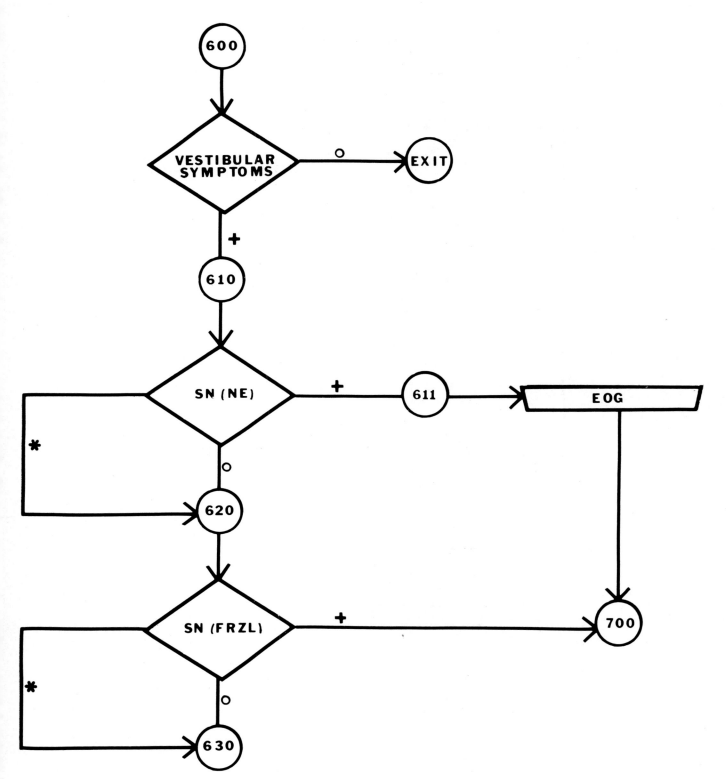

Fig. 11.

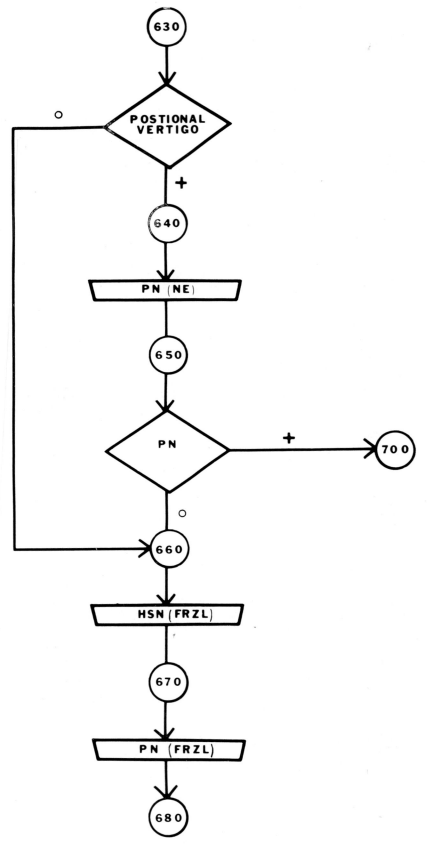

FIG. 12.

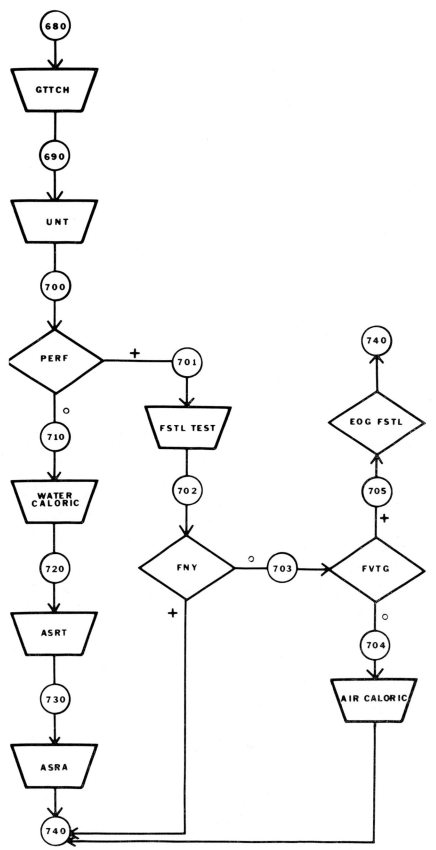

Fig. 13.

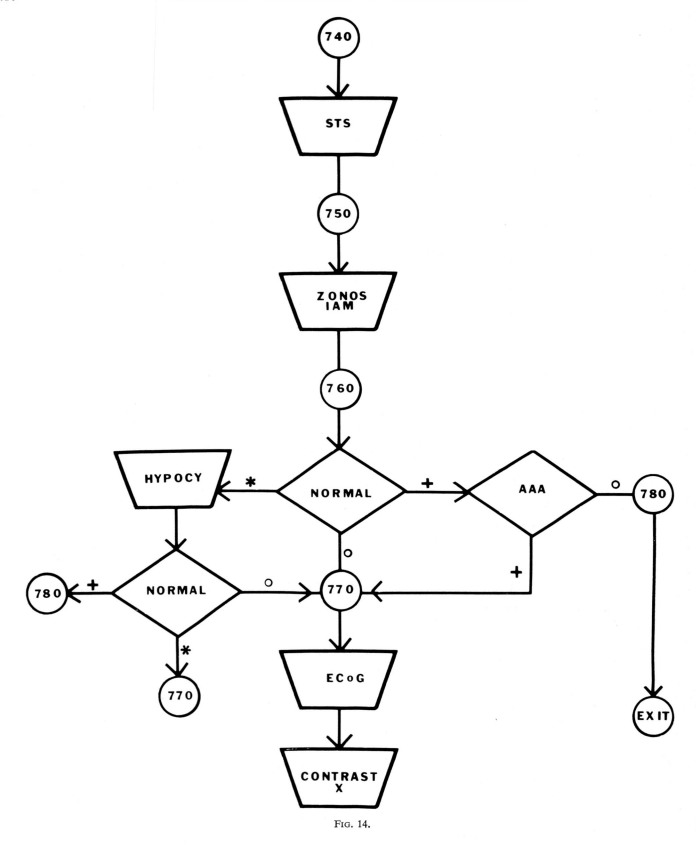

Fig. 14.

visible to the naked eye; SN(FRZL), spontaneous nystagmus visible with Frenzel glasses; EOG, electro-oculography; PN(NE), positional/positioning nystagmus visible to naked eye; HSN(FRZL), head-shaking nystagmus (Kopfschüttel-nystagmus) visible with Frenzel glasses; PN(FRZL), positional/positioning nystagmus observable with Frenzel glasses; GTTCH, Güttich extended arms' deviation test; UNT, Unterberger's stepping test for vestibulo-spinal reflex appraisal; ASRT, acoustic stapedius reflex threshold; ASRA, acoustic stapedius reflex adaptation; FSTL TEST, fistula test; FNY, fistula induced nystagmus; FVTG, fistula test induced vertigo; EOG FSTL, fistula test conducted with electro-oculographic recordings; STS, serological tests for syphilis; ZONOS IAM, radiographic zonography of internal acoustic meatus; HYPOCY, radiographic hypocycloidal examination; AAA, abnormal auditory adaptation; ECoG, electro-cochleography; CONTRAST X, contrast radiography.

REFERENCES

Aboulker, P., Pialoux, P., Neveu, M., Butruille, P. and Bouchet, J. (1963), *Syndromes vestibulaires et nystagmographie.* Paris: Arnette.

Adlersberg, D. and Forschner, L. (1931), *Klin. Wschr.,* **10**, 828.

Adrian, E. D., Craik, K. J. W. and Sturdy, R. S. (1938), *Proc roy. Soc. B,* **125**, 435.

Aschan, G., Bergstedt, M. and Stahle, J. (1956), *Acta oto-laryng. (Stockh.),* suppl. 129.

Aschoff, J. C. (1974), *The Neurosciences: Third Study Program,* Chapter 26 (F. O. Schmitt and F. G. Worden, Eds.). Cambridge, Mass.: M.I.T. Press.

Aubry, M. and Pialoux, P. (1957), *Maladie de l'oreille interne et otoneurologie.* Paris: Masson.

Bach-y-Rita, P., Collins, C. C. and Hyde, J. E. (1971), *The Control of Eye Movements.* New York and London: Academic Press.

Barany, R. (1906a), *Arch. Ohrenheilk.,* **68**, 1.

Barany, R. (1906b), *Mschr. Ohrenheilk.,* **40**, 193.

Barber, H. O. and Wright, Grace (1973), *Adv. Otolaryng.,* **19**, 276.

Barlow, H. B., Hill, R. M. and Levick, W. R. (1964), *J. Physiol,* **173**, 377.

Bartels, M. (1922), *Arch. Ophthal.,* **110**, 426.

Bauer, M. (1972). Personal Communication.

Benitez, J. T., Corvera, J. and Novoa, V. (1966), *Ann. Otol.,* **75**, 149.

Bergstedt, M. (1970), *Adv. Otolaryng.,* **17**, 67.

Bickford, R. G. and Klass, D. W. (1964), *The Oculomotor System,* p. 299 (M. B. Bender, Ed.). New York: Harper & Row.

Bizzi, E. (1968), *Exp. Brain Res.,* **6**, 69.

Bleeker, J. D. and De Vries, H. L. (1949), *Acta oto-laryng. (Stockh.),* **37**, 287.

Boer, E. de, Carels, J. and Philipszoon, J. (1964), *Acta oto-laryng. (Stockh.),* **56**, 457.

Braitenberg, V. and Onesto, N. (1962), "The Cerebellar Cortex as a Timing Organ. Discussion of a Hypothesis," *Proc. 1st. Congr. Int. Med. Cibernetica.* Naples: Giannini.

Brodmann, K. (1909), *Vergleichende Lokalisationslehre der Grosshirnrinde in ihren Prinzipien dargestellt auf Grund des Zellenbaues.* Leipzig: Barth.

Brookler, K. H. (1971), *Laryngoscope,* **81**, 1014.

Brumlik, J. and Means, E. D. (1969), *Brain,* **92**, 157.

Carmichael, E. A., Dix, M. R., Hallpike, C. S. and Hood, J. D. (1961), *Brain,* **84**, 571.

Cawthorne, T. E. (1956), *J. Laryng.,* **70**, 559.

Cawthorne, T. E., Dix, M. R. and Hood, J. D. (1968), *Neuro-ophthalmology,* **4**, 81.

Cawthorne, T. E., Fitzgerald, G. and Hallpike, C. S. (1942), *Brain* **65**, 138.

Cawthorne, T. E. and Hallpike, C. S. (1957), *Acta oto-laryng. (Stockh.),* **48**, 89.

Cogan, D. G. (1968), *Arch. Ophthal.,* **79**, 545.

Cogan, D. G. (1970), *Neurology of the Ocular Muscles.* Springfield, Ill., U.S.A.: Chas. C. Thomas.

Cohen, B. and Komatsuzaki, A. (1972), *Exp. Neurol.,* **36**, 101.

Cohen, B., Krejcova, H. and Highstein, S. (1970), *Fed. Proc.,* **29**, 454.

Corvera, J., Torres-Courtney, G and Lopez-Rios, G. (1973), *Ann. Otol.,* **82**, 855.

Dallos, P. J. and Jones, R. W. (1963), *I.E.E.E. Trans Automatic Control AC-8,* . p218.

Dix, M. R. (1970), *Adv. Oto-rhino-laryng.,* **17**, 118.

Dix, M. R. and Hallpike, C. S. (1952), *Proc. roy. Soc. Med.,* **45**, 341.

Dix, M. R. and Hallpike, C. S. (1966), *Acta oto-laryng (Stockh.),* **61**, 1.

Dix, M. R. and Leech, J. (1974), *J. Laryng.,* **88**, 199.

Duensing, F. (1967), Quoted by Hallpike, 1967.

Duensing, F. and Schaefer, K. P. (1959), *Arch. Psychiat. Nervenkr.,* **199**, 345.

Eckel, W. (1959), *Arch Ohr.-, Nas.- u. KehlkHeilk.,* **174**, 458.

Ellenberger, C., Jr., Campa, J. F. and Netsky, M. G. (1968), *Neurology,* **18**, 1041.

Elschnig, A. (1913), *Med. Klin.,* **1**, 8.

Eviatar, A. (1970), *Arch. Otolaryng.,* **92**, 437.

Eviatar, L., Eviatar, A. and Naray, I. (1974), *Develop Med. Child Neurol.,* **16**, 435.

Feldmann, H. (1971), *Audiology,* **10**, 138.

Fender, D. H. and Nye, P. W. (1961), *Kybernetik* **1**, 81.

Fischer, M. H. (1926), *Pflügers Arch. ges. Physiol.,* **213**, 74.

Fitzgerald, G. and Hallpike, C. S. (1942), *Brain,* **65**, 115.

Fluur, E. and Mendel, L. (1963), *Pract. oto-rhino-laryng.,* **23**, 319.

Foster, J. D. (1968), "Man Vehicle Control Lab. Rpt." Cambridge, Mass.: M.I.T.

Fox, J. C. and Holmes, G. (1926), *Brain,* **49**, 333.

Frenzel, H. (1925), *Klin. Wschr.,* **4**, 138.

Frenzel, H. (1960), *Acta oto-laryng. (Stockh.),* suppl. 159, p. 73.

Frenzel, H. (1961), *Zur Systematik, Klinik u. Untersuchungsmethodik der Vestibularisstörung.* Berlin: Springer.

Fuchs, A. F. (1967), *J. Physiol.,* **193**, 161.

Fuchs, A. F. (1971), "The Soccadic System," in *The Control of Eye Movements* (P. Bach-y-Rita, C. C. Collins and J. F. Hyde, Eds.). New York and London: Academic Press.

Fuchs, A. F. and Kornhuber, H. H. (1969), *J. Physiol.* **200**, 713.

Fukuda, T. and Tokita, T. (1971), *Acta oto-laryng. (Stockh.),* **71**, 282.

Gassel, M. M. and Williams, D. (1963), *Brain,* **86**, 1.

Gay, A. J. and Newman, N. M. (1972), "Eye Movements and Their Disorders," in *Scientific Foundations of Neurology* (M. Critchley, J. L. O'Leary and B. Jennett, Eds.). London: Heinemann.

Geschwind, N. (1965), *Brain,* **88**, 237.

Ghose, P. and Sardana, D. S. (1970), *Indian J. Otolaryng.,* **22**, 24.

Gilbert, G. J., McEntee, W. J. and Glaser, G. H. (1963), *Neurology,* **131**, 365.

Gillingham, F. J. and Kalyanaraman, S. (1965), *Confin. neurol.,* **19**, 237.

Goebel, H., Komatsuzaki, A., Bender, M. and Cohen, B. (1971), *Arch. Neurol.,* **24**, 431.

Greiner, G-F., Conraux, C. and Picart, P. (1961), *Confin. neurol.,* **21**, 438.

Greiner, G-F., Conraux, C., Picart, P. and Beyer, P. (1964), *Rev. Otoneuro-ophtal.,* **3**, 1.

Greiner, G-F., Conraux, C. and Collard, M. (1969), *Vestibulométrie Clinique.* Paris: Doin.

Greisen, O. and Jepsen, O. (1973), *Neuro-otologi.* Denmark: Århus Kommunehospital.

Haciska, D. (1973), *Acta oto-laryng.,* **75**, 477.

Halama, A. (1968). Unpublished data.

Halama, A. (1969), *Sound,* **3**, 102.

Halama, A. and Hinchcliffe, R. (1970), *J. Laryng.,* **84**, 149.

Hallpike, C. S. (1967), *Proc. roy. Soc. Med.,* **60**, 1043.

Hallpike, C. S. and Hood, J. D. (1953), *Proc. roy. Soc. B,* **141**, 542.

Hallpike, C. S., Hood, J. C. and Trinder, E. (1960), *Confin. neurol.,* **20**, 232.

Hamersa, H. (1957), *The Caloric Test*. Bergen op Zoom: Juten.

Harrison, M. S. and Ozsahinoglu, C. (1972), *Brain*, **95**, 369.

Hart, C. (1974). Personal Communication.

Hennebert, P. E. (1950), *Acta oto-rhino-laryng. Belg.*, **4**, 409.

Hennebert, P. E. (1956), *Acta oto-laryng. (Stockh.)*, **46**, 221.

Herberts, G., Abrahamson, S., Einarsson, S., Hofmann, H. and Liner, P. (1968), *Acta oto-laryng.*, **65**, 200.

Higgins, D. C. and Daroff, R. B. (1966), *Arch. Ophthal.*, **75**, 742.

Hinchcliffe, R. (1961), *J. Iowa Med. Soc.*, **51**, 697.

Hinchcliffe, R. (1967a), *J. Laryng.*, **81**, 875.

Hinchcliffe, R. (1967b), *Acta oto-laryng. (Stockh.)*, **63**, 69.

Hinchcliffe, R. (1971), *Acta oto-rhino-laryngol. belg.*, **25**, 770.

Hinchcliffe, R. (1973), *Recent Advances in Otolaryngology*, Chapter 7 (J. Ransome, H. Holden and T. R. Bull, Eds.). Edinburgh and London: Churchill Livingstone.

Hinchcliffe, R. and Voots, R. J. (1962), *Neurology*, **12**, 686.

Hohman, L. B. (1925), *J. Amer med. Assoc.*, **84**, 1489.

Hood, J. D. (1967a), *Myotatic, Kinesthetic and Vestibular Mechanisms*, p. 252. Ciba Foundation Symposium. London: Churchill.

Hood, J. D. (1967b), *Acta oto-laryng. (Stockh.)*, **63**, 208.

Hood, J. D. (1970), *Adv. Oto-rhino-laryng.*, **17**, 149.

Hood, J. D. and Leech, J. (1974), *Acta oto-laryng. (Stockh.)*, **77**, 72.

Huizinga, E. (1935), *Acta oto-laryng. (Stockh.)*, **22**, 359.

Huizinga, E., De Vries, H. L. and Vrolijk, J. M. (1951), *Acta oto-laryng. (Stockh.)*, **39**, 372.

Hunter, J. (1786), *Observations on Certain Parts of the Animal Oeconomy*. London.

Janeke, J. B., Jongkees, L. B. W. and Oosterveld, V. J. (1969), *Acta oto-laryng. (Stockh.)*, **68**, 468.

Jones, G. M. (1958), *Proc. roy. Soc. Med.*, **52**, 185.

Jones, G. M. (1971), "Organisation of Neural Control in the Vestibulocular Reflex Arc," in *Control of Eye Movements* (P. Bach-y-Rita, C. C. Collins and J. E. Hyde, Eds.). New York: Academic Press.

Jones, G. M. and Milsum, J. H. (1967), *Proc. 38th Ann. Sci. Meeting Aerospace Med. Assoc.*, p. 252.

Jongkees, L. B. W. (1973a), *Otolaryng. Clin. N. Amer.*, **6**, 73.

Jongkees, L. B. W. (1973b), *Arch. Otolaryng.*, **97**, 77.

Jung, R. and Kornhuber, H. H. (1964), *The Oculomotor System*, Chapter 19 (M. B. Bender, Ed.). New York: Harper & Row.

Kacker, S. K. and Hinchcliffe, R. (1970), *J. Laryng.*, **84**, 155.

Käslin, W. (1936), *Zbl. ges. Ophthal.*, **36**, 447.

Kestenbaum, A. (1930), *Arch. Ophthal.*, **124**, 339.

Kestenbaum, A. (1947), *Clinical Methods of Neuro-ophthalmologic Examination*. New York.

Klemme, R. M. (1941), *Amer. J. Ophthal.*, **24**, 1000.

Kobrak, F. (1918), *Beitr. Anat.*, **10**, 214.

Koerber, H. (1903), *Clin. ophthal.*, p. 147.

Kornhuber H. H. (1966), "Physiologie und Klinik des zentralvestibulären Systems," *Handbuch der Hals-Nasen-Ohrenheilkrunde*, Vol 3, Part 3, p. 2150. Stuttgart: Thieme.

Kornhuber, H. H. (1971), *Kybernetik*, **8**, 157.

Kos, C. M. (1955), *Laryngoscope*, **65**, 711.

Krabbe, K. H. (1931), *Acta psychiat. et neurol.*, **6**, 457.

Ledoux, A. (1958), *Les Canaux Semicirculaires*, p. 73. Brussels.

Lee, M. D. (1969), *J. Laryng.*, **83**, 797.

Lindsay, J. R. (1962), *Trans. Amer. Acad. Ophthal. Otolaryng.*, p. 331.

Litton, W. B. and McCabe, B. F. (1967), *Arch. Otolaryng.*, **86**, 445.

Mach, E. (1875), *Grundlinien der Lehre von der Bewegungsempfindungen*. Leipzig: Engelmann.

Mahoney, J. L., Harlan, W. L. and Bickford, R. G. (1957), *Arch. Otolaryng.*, **66**, 46.

McCabe, B. F. and Ryu, J. H. (1969), *Laryngoscope*, **79**, 1728.

Mehler, W. R., Vernier, V. and Nauta, W. (1958), *Anat. Rec.*, **130**, 430.

Meiry, J. L. (1971), "Vestibular and Proprioceptive Stabilization of Eye Movements," *Control of Eye Movements* (P. Bach-y-Rita, C. C. Collins and J. F. Hyde, Eds.). New York: Academic Press.

Mettler, F. A. (1935), *J. comp. Neurol.*, **61**, 509.

Miller, E. F. (1962), *Acta oto-laryng. (Stockh.)*, **54**, 479.

Miller, E. F. and Graybiel, A. (1963), *Ann. Otol.*, **72**, 885.

Montandon, A. and Dittrich, F. (1961), *Confin. neurol.*, **21**, 464.

Nashold, B. S. and Gills, J. P. (1967), *Arch. Ophthal.*, **77**, 609.

Nelson, J. R. and Cope, D. (1971), *Arch. Otolaryng.*, **94**, 40.

Nelson, J. R. and House, W. (1971), *Trans. Amer. Acad. Ophthal. Otolaryng.*, p. 1313.

Nigris, G. de (1933), *Riv. oto-neuro-oftal.*, **10**, 73.

Noorden, G. K. von (1974), *Brit. J. Ophthal.*, **58**, 158.

Noorden, G. K. von and Preziosi, T. J. (1966), *Arch. Ophthal.*, **76**, 162.

Nylén, C. O. (1950), *J. Laryng.*, **64**, 295.

Ohm, J. (1930), *Arch. Ophthal.*, **125**, 245.

Ohm, J. (1940), *Arch. Ophthal.*, **142**, 482.

Ohm, J. (1949), *Arch. Ophthal.*, **149**, 364.

Oloff, H. and Korbsch, H. (1926), *Klin. Mbl. Augenheilk.*, **77**, 618.

Oosterveld, W. J. (1970), *Arch. Otolaryng.*, **91**, 154.

Padovan, I. and Pansini, M. (1972), *Acta oto-laryng. (Stockh.)*, **73**, 121.

Parinaud, M. H. (1883), *Arch. Neurol.*, **5**, 145.

Pasik, T., Pasik, P. and Bender, M. B. (1969), *Brain*, **92**, 521.

Pfaltz, C. R. (1960), *Confin. neurol.*, **20**, 240.

Pfaltz, C. R. (1965), *Acta oto-rhino-laryng. belg.*, **19**, 367.

Pfaltz, C. R. (1970), *Acta oto-rhino-laryng. belg.*, **24**, 394.

Philipszoon, A. J. and Bos, J. H. (1963), *Pract. oto-rhino-laryng.*, **25**, 339.

Precht, W., Richter, A. and Grippo, J. (1969), *Pflügers Arch. ges. Physiol.*, **309**, 285.

Pumphrey, R. J. (1939), *Nature (Lond.)*, **143**, 898.

Raff, N. C. (1967), *New Engl. J. Med.*, **276**, 1432.

Rashbass, C. (1961), *J. Physiol.*, **159**, 326.

Rashbass, C. and Russell, G. (1961), *Brain*, **84**, 329.

Raudnitz, R. W. (1902), *Klin. Mbl. Augenheilk.*, **40**, 271.

Reed, G. (1960), *Arch. Otolaryng.*, **71**, 94.

Riesco McClure, J. S. (1957), *Rev. Otorrinolaring.*, **17**, 42.

Robinson, D. A. (1971), "Models of Oculomotor Neurol Organisation," *Control of Eye Movements* (P. Bach-y-Rita, C. C. Collins and J. E. Hyde, Eds.). New York: Academic Press.

Ross, A. T. and Zeman, W. (1967), *Arch. Neurol.*, **17**, 546.

Rubin, W. (1968), *Arch. Otolaryng.*, **87**, 266.

Salus, R. (1910), *Arch. Kinderheilk.*, **47**, 61.

Sauvineau, C. (1909), *Arch. ophthal.*, **29**, 416.

Schmaltz, G. (1932), *Proc. roy. Soc Med.*, **25**, 359.

Schuknecht, H. F. (1962), *Trans. Amer. Acad. Ophthal. Otolaryng.*, p. 319.

Sharpley, F. W. (1936), *Brit. J. Ophthal.*, **20**, 129.

Singh, G. (1974). Unpublished Observations.

Slatt, B. and Nykiel, F. (1964), *Amer. J. Ophthal.*, **58**, 1016.

Smith, J. L. and David, N. J. (1964), *Neurology*, **14**, 307.

Smith, J. L., David, N. J. and Klintworth, G. (1964), *Neurology*, **14**, 96.

Smith, J. L., Zieper, I., Gay, A. J. and Cogan, D. G. (1959), *Arch. Ophthal.*, **62**, 864.

Sokolovski, A. (1966), *Acta oto-laryng. (Stockh.)*, **61**, 209.

Stenger, H. J. (1955), *Arch. Ohr.-, Nas.- u. KehlkHeilk.*, **168**, 220.

Stenger, H. J. (1959), *Arch. Ohr.-, Nas.- u. KehlkHeilk.*, **175**, 545.

Stephens, S. D. G. and Ballam, H. M. (1974), *J. Laryng.*, **88**, 1049.

Sugie, N. and Jones, G. M. (1966), *Bull. Electrotechn. Lab.*, Japan, **30**, 598.

Susac, J. O., Hoyt, W. F., Daroff, R. B. and Lawrence, W. (1970), *J. Neurol. Neurosurg. Psychiat.*, **33**, 771.

Suzuki, J., Tokumasu, K. and Goto, K. (1969), *Acta oto-laryng. (Stockh.)*, **68**, 350.

Szentágothai, J. (1964), *The Oculomotor System*, Chapter 8 (M. B. Bender, Ed.). New York: Harper & Row.

Thornval, A. (1917), *Funktionsundersøgelser af Vestibularorganet og Cerebellum*. Copenhagen: Busck.

Torok, N. (1969), *Arch. Otolaryng.*, **90**, 52.

Tullio, P. (1926), Sulla funzione delle varie parti dell'orecchio interno.

Van der Laan, F. L. and Oosterveld, W. J. (1974), *Aerospace Med.*, **45**, 540.

Van Saane, C. J. (1970) Thesis, University of Amsterdam. Quoted by Jongkees, 1973b.

Veits, C. (1928), *Z. Hals.-, Nasen- u. Ohrenheilk.*, **19**, 542.

Vogel, K. (1932), *Z. Laryng.*, **22**, 202.

Voots, R. J. (1969), *Aerospace Med.*, **40**, 1080.

Wadia, N. H. and Swami, R. K. (1971), *Brain*, **94**, 359.

Walsh, E. G. (1960), *J. Physiol.*, **153**, 350.

Walsh, F. B. and Hoyt, W. F. (1969), *Clinical Neuro-ophthalmology*, 3rd edition. Baltimore: Williams and Wilkins.

Wernicke, C. (1889), *Arch. Psychiat.*, **20**, 243.

Westheimer, G. (1954), *Ophthalmologica*, **128**, 300.

Wilmot, T. J. (1970), *J. Laryng.*, **84**, 1033.

Young, L. R. (1971), "Pursuit Eye Tracking Movements," in *Control of Eye Movements* (P. Bach-y-Rita, C. C. Collins and J. F. Hyde, Eds.). New York: Academic Press.

Young, L. R. and Stark, L. (1962), *Quart. Progr. Rept. Res. Lab. Electr. M.I.T.*, **67**, 212.

SECTION VII

OROFACIAL STRUCTURES

PAGE

29. EMBRYOLOGY OF THE FACIAL STRUCTURES   421

30. FACIAL NERVE   429

31. THE SALIVARY APPARATUS   460

32. TASTE   468

33. PALATAL FUNCTION   484

29. EMBRYOLOGY OF THE FACIAL STRUCTURES

LESLIE BERNSTEIN

The young embryo is curled toward its ventral surface like the letter C, with the developing head flexed onto the cardiac prominence, or thorax, so that much of the interesting developmental changes that are going on in the facial region are not visible on external examination. Consequently, in order to assist the clinician with proper orientation of the various developing structures, the plane and directional terms used in this chapter will parallel those which are employed in post-natal life, although this may be at variance with terminology used in texts on embryology.

At about 16 days of intra-uterine life, the primitive gut exists as a blind tube. The foregut ends blindly at a shallow external depression, the primitive mouth or *stomodeum*, which forms the topographic centre of the developing facial structures. As the stomodeal depression deepens, its ectodermal covering comes to lie against the entodermal lining of the foregut. This double-layered partition, the *oro-pharyngeal (buccopharyngeal) membrane*, separates the primitive oral cavity from the developing pharynx. It breaks down toward the end of the 4th week to connect the oral opening with the foregut, or *primitive pharynx* (Fig. 1).

During the 5th week, all of the major primordia which are involved in the formation of the face and jaws become clearly distinguishable. Above the stomodeum is the large convexity of the forebrain known as the *forebrain (frontal) prominence*. On each side, near the lateral margins of the overhanging forebrain prominence, local thickenings of the ectoderm appear during the 4th week, which are called the *olfactory (nasal) placodes*. They are destined to form the lining of the olfactory (nasal) pits and, ultimately, the olfactory epithelium with its sensory cells. Posterior to each nasal placode, an optic vesicle appears at about the same time. This is the primordium of the eye (Fig. 2A).

The nasal placodes become bordered by rapidly growing horseshoe-shaped elevations, so that they appear to have sunk below the general surface and to lie at the bottom of depressions called the *olfactory (nasal) pits*. The medial limbs of these elevations around the nasal pits are known as the *medial nasal elevations (processes)* and the lateral limbs are called the *lateral nasal elevations (processes)* (Fig. 2B).

Growing toward the midline from the cephalolateral angles of the oral cavity are the *maxillary processes* which are destined to form the lateral parts of the upper jaw, and the *mandibular processes* which will form the lower jaw.

The *oral cavity* is not formed by invagination, but rather is deepened by the growth of the structures bordering it. At the time that the oropharyngeal membrane ruptures, the stomodeum is merely a shallow depression. Some idea of the extent of the forward growth of the structures about its margins may be gained from the fact that the tonsillar region

of the adult is approximately at the level which was occupied by the oropharyngeal membrane before it ruptured and disappeared. An even more helpful point of orientation is the position of *Rathke's pouch*. In a one-month embryo, it is just at the margin of the stomodeal depression (Fig. 1); by the 8th week it has come to lie far back in the rapidly

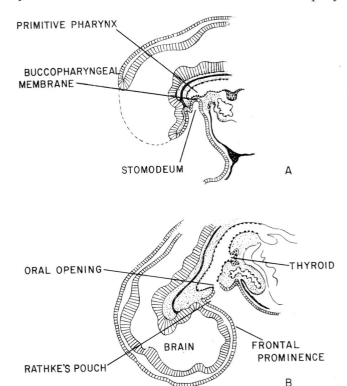

FIG. 1. Diagram of sagittal section of human embryos. (A) About three weeks. (B) End of fourth week. (Based on Carnegie Embryologic Collection, Davis, California.)

deepening oral cavity. The growth of the structures bordering the stomodeum, then, not only gives rise to superficial parts of the face and jaws, but actually builds out the walls of the oral cavity itself.

At 5 weeks (Fig. 2B), the structures which border the oral cavity cephalically are: (1) the unpaired forebrain prominence in the midline; (2) the paired nasal processes on each side of the frontal area; and (3) the paired maxillary processes at the upper lateral angles. These primitive tissue masses will develop into the upper lip, the upper jaw, the palate and the nose. The caudal boundary of the oral cavity is less complex, being constituted by the mandibular processes only. In very young embryos, the origin of the mandible from paired primordia is still clearly evident. Appearing first on each side of the midline are marked local

421

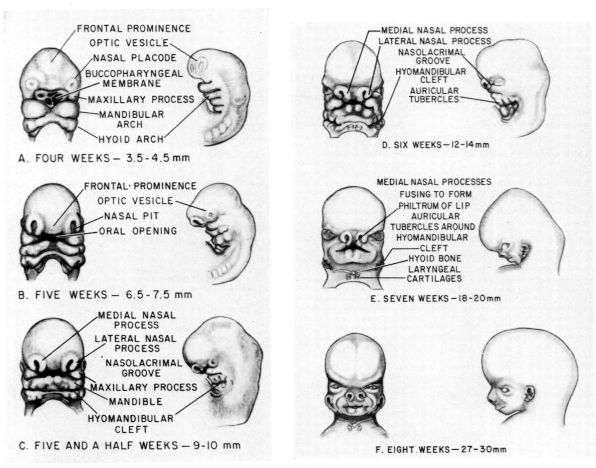

FIG. 2. Diagrammatic representation, in frontal and lateral views, of some of the important steps in the development of the face. (After Patten, 1953.)

thickenings due to the rapid proliferation of the underlying mesenchymal tissue. Until these thickenings have extended from each side to meet in the midline, there remains a conspicuous median notch. Once they merge, the arch of the mandible is completed (Fig. 2B, C).

UNDERLYING DEVELOPMENTAL MECHANISMS

The preceding discussion has dealt with the superficial configuration only. Thus, far, we have considered the various prominences on the future face as if they were distinct entities with definite boundaries. This is a misleading oversimplification. We should try to understand the underlying structures that have brought these prominences into existence.

Mesenchyme is the tissue which is found between the ectoderm and the entoderm, and is composed of aggregations of cells supported in a gelatinous ground substance. This primordial tissue has the ability to differentiate into specialized cells, as dictated by their inherent developmental potency. Gradually, within given areas, particularly dense accumulations of mesenchymal cells are formed and, by

imperceptibly subtle alterations within these cell aggregations, histogenetic changes begin to segregate specific areas of developing tissues.

Obviously, the most dynamic component of the facial primordia is mesenchyme. This is not a specific type of tissue, but rather one with pleuripotential abilities that can give rise to an amazing variety of adult tissues. Its derivatives range through the whole gamut of connective tissues, including cartilage and bone, and extend into such widely different tissue types as blood cells, vascular endothelium and smooth muscle.

As the head takes shape, the mesenchymal cells increase in number with great rapidity. It is these cells and their descendents which come to underlie the named elevations in the developing face. By their very numbers, and by the concurrent increase in the ground substance, they cause these elevations to increase in size and conspicuousness and change their relationship to each other. The same basic histogenetic processes go on in all of the various hillocks, but with each one the shape of the developing cartilage or bone is characteristic and the muscles are formed in a definite pattern with reference to the growing skeletal parts.

With this background concerning mesenchymal activity,

we may review the elevations involved in the formation of the face and some of the related substructures.

The region designated as the forebrain prominence is initially merely the gently rounded territory cephalic to the stomodeum, which follows the contour of the forebrain. There are relatively few mesenchymal cells between the brain and the overlying ectoderm. Moreover, there are no recognizable local concentrations of mesenchyme at these early stages, the scattered cells forming a continuous system all around the front of the head.

margin. Actually, the early pit is more like a groove, since it is deficient inferiorly where it communicates with the forming oral aperature, as it does in the shark (Fig. 2A, B). At this stage it is convenient to designate the raised peripheral wall on each side of the pit as the *medial* and *lateral nasal elevation*. By the middle of the 2nd month, the nasal pits have become much deepened, primarily by the growth of the nasal elevations around them. Close at hand laterally are the *maxillary processes* of the first branchial arches, while in the midplane is the tissue destined to become the

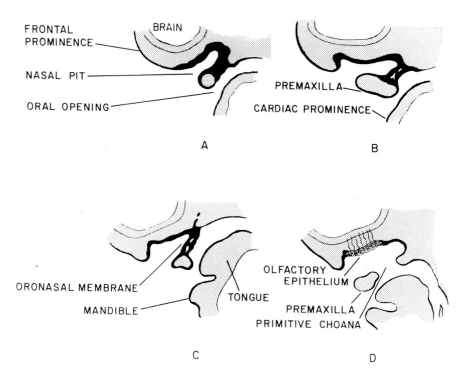

Fig. 3. Diagrammatic representation of parasagittal sections of a developing nasal pit. (A) Pit extending posteriorly until it is separated from oral cavity by oronasal membrane (B and C). (D) Nasal cavity communicates with mouth through primitive choana.

The first advance beyond this primordial condition is the development of concentrations of mesenchymal cells causing the nasal elevations to become elevated around the nasal placodes, converting them into pits. The forward growth of these processes then deepens the nasal pits.

THE NOSE

The development of the nose is bound up with the changes that produce the face and the palate. In primitive vertebrates, the olfactory organ is a blindly ending sac used solely for the sense of smell. However, as air breathing was adopted, these cavities opened into the mouth and they came to subserve respiration as well.

The first indication of the olfactory organ is an oval area of thickened ectoderm which forms on each ventrolateral surface of the head in an embryo of about 26 days. Each is an *olfactory (nasal) placode*, which is soon converted to an *folactory (nasal) pit* as it becomes bounded by an elevated

future *dorsum* (bridge) of the nose and *nasal septum* (Fig. 2C).

As the nasal pit deepens, it soon comes to be separated from the oral cavity by an epithelial plate, the *oronasal membrane*, which thins and ruptures during the 7th week (Fig. 3). Each nasal cavity now opens to the outside through a *naris* and communicates internally with the oral cavity through the *primitive choana*, as in amphibians. A thickened region between and beneath the two nasal pits constitutes the *intermaxillary segment*, or *primitive palate*. This will differentiate into the median part of the upper lip and the primary or premaxillary palate (Fig. 4). The incisive foramen remains as the vestige of the former primitive choanae.

Meanwhile, the head has been broadening, so that the nasal pits have shifted from their lateral locations to a more ventral position and they tend to approach the midplane. In accomplishing this, the deep frontonasal region between the two nasal pits becomes compressed and submerged to

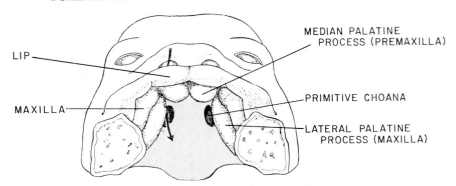

FIG. 4. Establishment of primitive nasal airway (arrow) after bilateral perforation of oronasal membrane. The premaxilla is fusing with the maxillary processes.

form the *nasal septum*. The alae of the nose arise from the lateral nasal elevations (Fig. 2D, E).

The extent and relations of cysts in the nose are very interesting from the embryologic standpoint. They may occur anywhere in the midline of the nasal dorsum or the columella and are accompanied by a skin pore. Frequently, they extend into the septum. This location of their occurrence coincides with the line of merging of the medial nasal elevations. The extension of the cysts to the nasal septum records the depth to which frontal tissue has been overgrown by that of the merging medial nasal elevations.

Extensions to the original nasal cavities are gained when the palatal processes of the maxillae unite to divide the primitive mouth into oral and nasal parts. The nasal septum extends ventrocaudally to fuse with the primary and secondary palates, thus completing the separation of the two nasal cavities (Fig. 5A). The permanent nasal cavities thus consist of the original nasal pits and a portion of the primitive oral cavity that has been separated-off secondarily by development of the (secondary) palate. This corresponds to the region occupied by the vomer. The nasal chambers open into the pharynx by secondary permanent choanae (Fig. 5B).

Anomalies. Atresia or stenosis of the nostril results from retention and organization of the temporary epithelial plug, which normally closes-off each naris from the 2nd to the 6th month. The more common atresia of the choanae is probably due to organization and persistence of a portion of the primitive oropharyngeal membrane, which is carried back with the secondary extension of the oral cavity and the vomer. The rare failure of the region between the nasal pits to consolidate into a normal septum, leads to a "doubling" of the nose which may range from a bifid lobule to a fully cleft nose. Other malformations may accompany cleft lip and palate.

THE EYE

Because the eye is highly organized even in the lowest groups of vertebrates, comparative anatomy fails to give any clue to its evolution. The constituents of the eye are derived from three sources: (1) the *optic nerve* and *retina*, from the forebrain; (2) the *lens*, from surface ectoderm of the head; and (3) the *accessory coats*, from adjacent mesenchyme.

By the 4th week, an *optic vesicle* has evaginated out of each side of the future forebrain, to which it is attached by a somewhat slender *optic stalk*. The optic vesicle soon becomes indented, forming the *optic cup*. This is destined

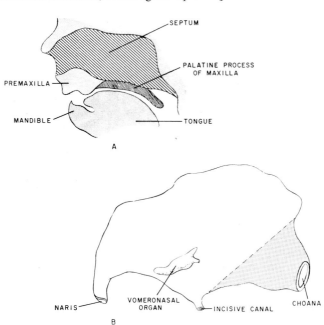

FIG. 5. (A) Fusion of lateral palatine processes and nasal septum. (B) Drawing from cast of right nasal cavity, in median view, at eleven weeks. Shaded area shows extent or oral addition. (From Arey, 1965.)

to become the *retina*, and fibres of the *optic nerve* will grow from it to the brain via its stalk.

During the 5th week, the optic vesicle begins to indent, forming an *optic cup*, and the ectoderm directly overlying it thickens into a *lens placode*. This plate immediately invaginates the deepening optic cup to form the *lens vesicle*, or lens primordium. Slightly later, the *accessory coats* of the eyeball organize from the surrounding mesenchyme.

The axes of the primitive eyes, in an embryo not yet 6 weeks old, are set at an angle of 180° to each other. As the head broadens, this divergence is gradually reduced. Like the brain, the eye grows precociously, so that it is three-fourths its final size at birth.

The Nasolacrinal Duct. Where the lateral nasal elevation and the maxillary process meet each other, there is formed for a time a well marked groove which extends to the medial angle of the eye. This is known as the *nasomaxillary (nasolacrimal) groove* or *naso-optic furrow.* It soon closes over superficially and its deep portion is converted into a tube, the *nasolacrimal duct.*

THE BRANCHIAL ARCHES

The construction of the jaws and neck is closely bound-up with the *branchial arches.* These are 5 bar-like ridges, separated by *branchial grooves,* which appear on each ventrolateral wall of the pharynx during the 4th week. As the paired ridges grow, they tend to merge with each other midventrally in such a manner that each pair of elevations comes to constitute an arch which embraces the pharynx laterally and ventrally. Each arch contains a cartilaginous core, a nerve, a main blood vessel and appropriate muscles. On the inside, corresponding to each of the grooves, there appear pharyngeal concavities, the *pharyngeal (branchial) pouches.* The ectoderm of the groove and the entoderm of its complimentary pouch then meet and unite. As a result, a typical arch is separated from its neighbour by a thin epithelial plate only.

The 1st branchial arch on each side, called the *mandibular arch,* bifurcates into separate *maxillary* and *mandibular processes.* Next behind the mandibular arch is the *hyoid arch,* Below the hyoid arch, the remaining arches are unnamed but are referred to as arches 3 and 4. There are also suggestions of a rudimentary 5th arch. During the 6th week, the 2nd arch overlaps the next 3 arches and obscures them. As development progresses, these caudal arches sink into a triangular depression called the *cervical sinus.* In this trasformation, branchial grooves 3 and 4 becomes drawn out into *branchial ducts.* That part of the cervical sinus which contains arches 4 and 5 closes-off, and the ectodermal-lined cavity obliterates. All this happens within 2 weeks, at the end of which the branchial arches largely disappear. Imperfect obliteration of a branchial groove leads to the formation of a branchial cyst.

The completion of these transformations marks the appearance of the *neck,* which is a characteristic of land vertebrates. This part of the body results from an elongation of the region between the 1st branchial arch and the body wall enclosing the heart. The 2nd and 3rd arches, at least, can be seen to contribute to its ventral and lateral surfaces and their deepest tissues give rise to such characteristically located structures as the hyoid bone and the laryngeal cartilages (Fig. 2E, F).

THE MOUTH

After breakdown of the oropharyngeal membrane, there are no exact landmarks to distinguish the junction between ectoderm and entoderm in the oral cavity. Considerable backward displacement has shifted this line in the roof region back into the nasal part of pharynx (nasopharynx), but keeping it in front of the palatine tonsils and the openings of the auditory tubes. Therefore, the nasal passages,

the palate, the free part of the tongue and the buccal cavity are considered to be lined with ectoderm. The enamel of the teeth and the salivary glands are likewise ectodermal derivatives. A further derivative of the ectodermal stomodeum is a dorsal inpocketing known as *Rathke's pouch,* which becomes the epithelial lobe of the hypophysis (Fig. 1).

THE UPPER JAW

During the 6th week, marked progress is made in the development of the upper jaw. The maxillary processes become more prominent and grow toward the midline, crowding the nasal elevations closer to each other (Fig. 2D). The lessening of the distance between the nasal pits is given added visual emphasis by the rapid expansion of the facial structures lateral to them. Meanwhile, the nasal elevations have grown so extensively that the lower part of the frontal area between them is completely overshadowed. The growth of the medial limbs of the nasal elevations has been especially marked and they come to lie almost in contact with the maxillary processes on each side. Inferiorly, the boundary zone between the medial nasal elevations is evident as the permanent *philtrum,* or median groove of the upper lip (Fig. 2F). The inferior edge of this median region often protrudes the central portion of the vermilion substance of the lip as a distinct *tubercle of the philtrum (labial tubercle).* In bilateral clefts of the lip, the fused medial nasal elevations are represented by the *prolabium.*

Patten (1961) suggested that all of the upper oral arch which is of medial nasal origin be designated as the *intermaxillary segment.* It would then be logical to recognize components of the intermaxillary segment: (1) the labial component—that is, the medial portion of the upper lip (the *philtrum* or *prolabium*); (2) the dental arch component, within which will develop the incisor teeth; and (3) the palatal component, or *primary medial palatal triangle,* which is continuous above with the anterior portion of the nasal septum.

The foundations for the formation of the upper jaw are now well laid. Its arch is completed by the merging of the two medial nasal elevations with each other in the midline and their fusion with the maxillary processes laterally. The external parts of these components contribute the primodial tissues from which the lips and cheeks will be formed. At deeper levels they give rise to the upper jaw and the palatal primordia.

THE TEETH

Teeth have a double source of origin: the enamel is from ectoderm; the dentine, pulp and cement are mesodermal. No essential difference exists between the development of the temporary, or deciduous, teeth and the permanent ones.

The first indication of oncoming development is an epithelial plate, the *dental lamina,* which arises during the 7th week near the crest of the forming jaw. The dental lamina soon becomes buried by the upgrowing primitive gum. At intervals along the lamina of each jaw there develop simultaneously 10 knob-like thickenings called the *enamel organs,* which will both produce the enamel and serve as the moulds for the future teeth. Early in the 3rd month, a dense accumulation of mesenchyme forms deep to the enamel organ. The epithelial surface of the enamel organ that is in contact with the mesenchymal aggregate invaginates into itself, until the whole enamel organ is hollowed like a cap. The concavity formed in this manner is occupied by the condensed mensenchymal tissue, or the *dental papilla*, which is destined to differentiate into dentine and pulp (Fig. 6). An enamel

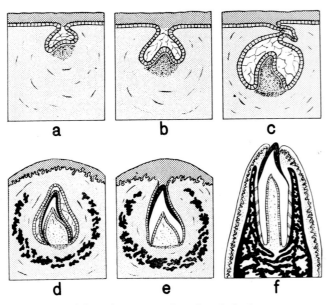

FIG. 6. Schematic representation of tooth development.

organ and its associated dental papilla are the developmental basis of each tooth. Although the original dental lamina breaks down, part of its free edge persists and gives rise to the primordia of the permanent enamel organs.

The Enamel Organ. During the 3rd month the enamel organ becomes a double-walled sac, composed of an outer convex wall and an inner concave wall. Between the two is a filling of looser ectodermal cells which transform into a stellate reticulum named the *enamel pulp*. The enamel organ first encases the crown portion of the future tooth, moulds its shape and deposits enamel there. Later, the enamel organ elongates and similarly models the root portion of the dental papilla, which organizes in response to its influence. This extension is called the *epithelial sheath* of the root.

The inner cells on the concave surface of the enamel organ become columnar and are designated *ameloblasts* (enamel formers). They produce enamel along their surfaces that face the dental papilla. The enamel is deposited in the form of parallel enamel prisms, one for each ameloblast.

The Dental Papilla. At the end of the 4th month, the superficial cells of the dental papilla which are in juxtaposition with the enamel organ begin to assume a columnar appearance. These are the specialized connective tissue cells which are named *odontoblasts* (*dentinoblasts*). They lay down the ground substance, which will become *dentine*, in a direction away from the enamel.

The more central mesenchyme of the dental papilla, internal to the odontoblast layer, differentiates into a soft substance composed of a reticular framework binding together blood vessels, lymphatics and nerve fibres. This constitutes the *dental pulp*, popularly known as the "nerve" of the tooth.

The Tooth Follicle. The mesenchymal tissue surrounding the developing tooth is continuous with that of the early dental papilla. Outside the tooth, it differentiates into ordinary connective tissue which constitutes the *tooth follicle* (*dental sac*). In the region of the future root, the tooth follicle takes on three important functions: (1) The layer of cells closest to the root differentiates into *cementoblasts*. These cells deposit upon the dentine an incrustation of specialized bone, known as *cementum*. (2) The external surfaces of the dental sacs become active in producing bone so that each tooth becomes surrounded with spongy bone, forming a *socket*, or *alveolus*, around the root of the tooth. (3) The intervening fibre sac itself, consolidates into the thin *periodontal ligament* (*membrane*), which is a specialized periosteum that suspends the tooth root in the socket by having its fibres embedded in the cementum on the one hand and the surrounding bone on the other.

THE PALATE

About the middle of the 2nd month, when the upper jaw has been established, the palatal shelves begin to make their appearance. The formation of the palate subdivides the more cephalic portion of the original stomodeal chamber. Since the nasal pits break into the primitive oral cavity in front of the secondary palate, completion of the palate in effect elongates the nasal cavities backward so that they eventually open into the pharynx.

As pointed out above, the intermaxillary component of the upper jaw is contributed to by the medial nasal elevations. From their deeper portions, the small, triangular, median part of the palate is formed anteriorly. The main part of the palate is derived from the portion of the upper jaw which arises from the maxillary processes. Shelf-like outgrowths of these processes arise on each side and grow toward the midline. When these *palatine processes* first start to develop, the tongue lies between them and they are directed obliquely downward so that their margins lie along the floor of the mouth on each side of the root of the tongue (Fig. 7A). At the 8th week, the position of the tongue shifts downward and the margins of the palatal shelves begin to swing upward and toward the midline. This elevation occurs as a wave from front to back. Further growth brings them into contact with each other and they fuse together from the anterior to the posterior direction, the fusion being complete by the 12th week (Fig. 7B).

It has been shown that, in rodents, the right palatal shelf reaches the horizontal position before the left one, thus leaving the left side vulnerable to interruption or interference in its normal development for a longer period of time than the one on the right. This may explain the more frequent occurrence of unilateral clefts on the left than on the right side in humans (Walker, 1961).

The more medial portion, which carries the incisor teeth,

arises from separate ossification centres formed in the part of the upper jaw that originated from the medial nasal elevations. It develops between the 4th and 7th weeks, by the end of which it fuses with the maxillary processes laterally. This independent origin of the incisor portion of the human maxilla emphasizes its homology with what is in lower forms a separate bone known as the *premaxilla*. Not infrequently, the sutures separating the incisive portion

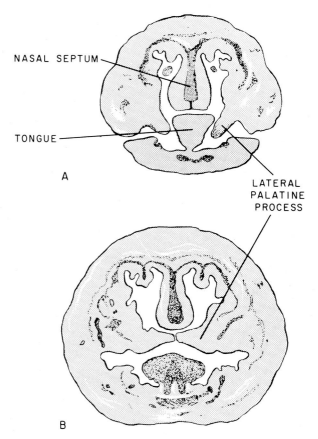

FIG. 7. Coronal sections showing the relationship of the palatine processes before (A) and after (B) retraction of the intervening tongue.

from the rest of the maxilla are evident in the skulls of human infants and occasionally traces of them may be made out in an adult skull.

At the same time that the palate is thus being formed, the nasal septum grows downward toward it and soon becomes fused to its cephalic surface. Thus, the separation of right and left nasal cavities from each other is accomplished at the same time that the nasal region as a whole is separated from the oral cavity. For some time after the palatal shelves make contact with each other and with the nasal septum, epithelial vestiges mark their original contours.

Anomalies

Maxillary Cysts. Figure 8 gives a schematic classification of cysts of the upper jaw. Their formation may be readily explained on the basis of our knowledge of fusion of the component parts involved.

Cleft Lip and Palate. Stark (1954) studied 6 human embryos with cleft lip and cleft palate. He found that the absence of mesenchyme in the lip and premaxilla coexisted with the presence of a cleft in each instance. On the other hand, it is noteworthy that, in the region of the hard and soft palate, mesenchyme was present on each side of the cleft in approximately equal amounts; but this may be explained on the basis that these are midline clefts. In each

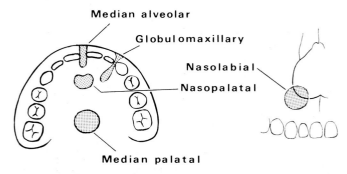

FIG. 8. Developmental cysts of the maxilla.

of the 6 embryos studied, some mesenchyme was always present in the lip-premaxillary region. However, when the mesenchyme was absent unilaterally, a single cleft resulted; when it was absent bilaterally, a double cleft ensued. It is suggested from these studies that a lack or even a diminution in mesenchyme will lead to the formation of a cleft in an area that is normally poor in mesenchyme.

THE TONGUE

While the formation of the palate has been roofing over the mouth, the tongue has been taking shape in the floor. The primordial areas which are to be involved in the formation of the tongue appear early in the 2nd month of development. In the 5th week of intra-uterine life, paired lateral thickenings may be distinguished on the internal face of the mandibular arch. These thickenings, which involve both the rapidly proliferating mesenchyme and the overlying epithelium, are known as the *distal tongue buds* (*lateral lingual swellings*). Between them is a small median elevation known as the *median tongue bud* (*tuberculum impar*) ("unpaired tubercle"). Behind and below the median tongue bud is another median elevation appropriately known as the *hypobranchial eminence* or *copula of His* (yoke), for it unites the 2nd and 3rd arches in a midventral prominence. This eminence extends cephalocaudally from the median tongue bud to the primordial swelling which marks the beginning of the epiglottis (Fig. 9A, B).

On each side of the hypobranchial eminence there is evidence of rapid growth in the adjacent tissues of the 2nd, 3rd and 4th visceral arches. These areas merge so early and so completely that any dogmatic statement as to exactly what part of the adult tongue comes from each of them is unwise. However, we do have one unmistakable point of orientation retained, which gives us the general picture sufficiently clearly for all practical purposes. This landmark is the *foramen cecum*, a small median pit in the dorsum of

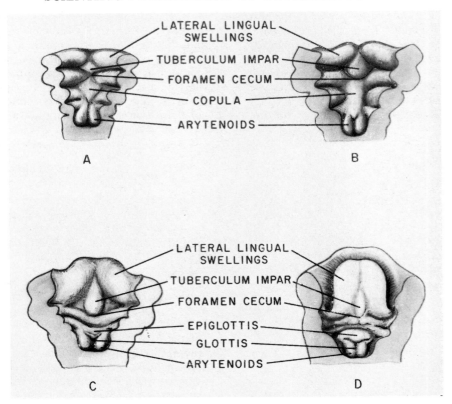

Fig. 9. Development of the tongue. (Adopted from Patten, 1953.)

the adult tongue, located at the apex of the V-shaped *sulcus terminalis* just behind the row of vallate papillae. Embryologically, the foramen cecum is a vestige of the invagination from the floor of the pharynx which gives rise to the thyroid gland (Fig. 1B). It is known that this invagination is formed at the cephalocaudal level where the 1st and 2nd branchial arches merge with each other. When the lingual primordia begin to take shape, this pit is situated between the median tongue bud and the hypobranchial eminence.

In adult anatomy, the sulcus terminalis with this same pit at its apex is regarded as the boundary between the "body" and "root" of the tongue. Thus, using the foramen as a landmark, it can be seen that the mucosal covering of the body of the tongue arises from 1st arch tissue. This makes its sensory innervation by the mandibular branch of the 5th nerve (tactile) and by the chorda tympani branch of the 7th nerve (gustatory) seem entirely natural in view of the primary relations of these nerves to the mandibular and hyoid arches.

The median tongue bud is soon overshadowed by the much more rapidly growing distal tongue buds and, at most, is responsible for only a small, median, thromboid area just anterior to the foramen cecum (Fig. 9C, D). It is difficult to state exactly the level of the adult tongue which represents the place where ectoderm and entoderm became continuous when the oropharyngeal membrane ruptured. There can be no doubt, however, that the greater part of the body of

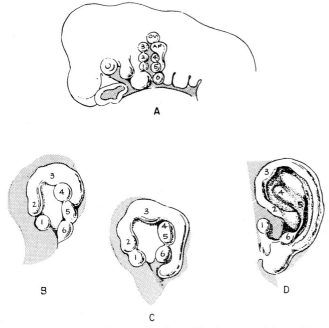

Fig. 10. Diagrammatic representation of development of the auricle. (After Arey, 1965.) OV-Otic vesicle; AF-auricular fold; 1–6-elevations on mandibular and hyoid arches which respectively become: 1-tragus; 2 and 3-helix; 4 and 5-antihelix; 6-antitragus.

the tongue is clothed with what was originally stomodeal ectoderm.

THE EXTERNAL EAR

While the above changes had been going on in the oro-nasal region, the early steps in the formation of the external ear have taken place. The auricle (pinna) of the ear is formed by the growth of the mesenchymal tissue flanking the 1st (hyomandibular) branchial groove of the young embryo. During the 2nd month, a group of nodular enlargements (hillocks) appear, some of them arising from mandibular-arch tissue cephalic to the 1st branchial groove and others from the hyoid arch along the caudal border of the groove (Fig. 2B and 10A). The coalescence and subsequent growth of these hillocks mould the auricle of the ear (Fig. 10B, C, D). In view of the number of separate growth-centres involved, it is not surprising that the configuration of the fully formed external ear exhibits a wide range of variations. These individual differences are easy to overlook until one begins to give particular attention to the details of ear shapes. A little critical observation, however, will soon make it apparent why police utilize the configuration of the ear as one of the very important features in the identification of individuals in whom they are interested.

REFERENCES AND FURTHER READING

Arey, L. B. (1965), *Developmental Anatomy*. Philadelphia: W. B. Saunders.

Patten, B. M. (1953), *Human Embryology*. New York: McGraw-Hill.

Patten, B. M. (1961), *Congenital Anomalies of the Face and Associated Structures* (S. Pruzansky, Ed.). Springfield, Illinois: Charles Thomas.

Stark, R. B. (1954), *Plast. reconstr. Surg.*, **13**, 20.

Walker, B. E. (1961), *J. Embryol. Exp. Morph.*, **9**, 22.

30. FACIAL NERVE

JOHN GROVES

INTRODUCTION

Otology could be a dull way of life without the seventh cranial nerve arrogantly swerving through the temporal bone to the muscles of facial expression. It is subject to all inflammatory, traumatic and neoplastic lesions of the region, subserves the vital functions of lacrimation, salivation, taste, and acoustical reflexes, and is vulnerable to almost every surgical operation in the otologist's repertoire. The exhortation to "make friends with the facial nerve" might well be made the first lesson in the art of otology. The gross anatomy of this nerve reveals the three-dimensional anatomy of the ear. Its neuro-physiology and neuro-pathology are a microsm of neurology. Its functional integrity protects the eye and cochlea, serves salivation and mastication, and, through the registration of facial expression, is essential to the human psyche. Such versatility may be rivalled only by the vagus, another maid-of-all-work phylogenetically derived from gill-slit nerves. The intricate relationship of the facial nerve (the nerve of the second branchial arch) to the middle ear and its diseases demands that otologists accept first responsibility for the facial nerve and for all cases of lower motor neurone facial palsy.

SURGICAL ANATOMY

"Surgeon's anatomy" may often be confined by the laudable aims of avoiding trouble and saving time. These are indeed prime considerations at operation. The most precise, instinctive, recognition of fine spatial relationships is the hallmark of experience and skill, and without it mere dexterity is a dangerous illusion which eventually will bring disaster. The surgeon must not cause facial palsies, and his studies must therefore combine anatomical texts with extensive dissection of the cadaver temporal bone. "Livic" adventures in the operating theatre must always be tempered with an obsessional degree of caution. Human and technical fallibility are very real enemies and wherever possible "fail-safe" manoeuvres must be cultivated and applied. For armchair study Anson and Donaldson's book *The Surgical Anatomy of the Temporal Bone* (1973) is recommended as a most valuable atlas from which the three-dimensional anatomy may be gleaned. In the assessment of established facial palsies the neuro-physiologist's approach is more appropriate and a sound working knowledge of the microstructure and functions of the nerve are necessary.

Gross Anatomy

Figure 1 represents the basic plan of the nerve in the temporal bone and may remind the reader of the levels of its various branches. The fibre composition, and the effects of a lesion at each succeeding level are implicit. Figure 2 shows how the pattern of branching in the face varies from one subject to another.

At each level, from the porus acousticus distally, there are basic anatomical relationships to be emphasized. In the internal acoustic meatus, as seen at operation through the middle fossa floor, the facial nerve runs laterally parallel to the superior vestibular nerve (Fig. 3). It is anterior to its companion, and conceals the cochlear nerve which lies inferiorly. Within the meatus the facial nerve has no separate "sheath", but shares the dural investment with the nervus intermedius and vestibulocochlear nerve and is bathed in cerebrospinal fluid. The internal auditory vessels also are related, but are discussed in detail later.

After entering the facial (Fallopian) canal above the crista falciformis the nerve is joined by the nervus intermedius at the genicular ganglion. The ganglion is but thinly covered by the bony middle fossa floor, and is identified by the greater (superficial) petrosal nerve which runs forwards and medially from it in the direction of the foramen lacerum. At the geniculum the nerve is "cradled" by

foramen. A well-defined "digastric ridge" provides a quicker landmark (Fig. 6), but in a non-cellular bone this area is difficult.

The vertical part of the nerve is closely related to the sinus tympani medially and the "facial recess" laterally (Fig. 7). The sinus and the recess are variable in depth. Just above the stylomastoid foramen an uncommonly large jugular bulb is a close medial relation of the nerve. In some dried skulls observed by the author there is a direct communication between the facial (Fallopian) canal and the jugular fossa.

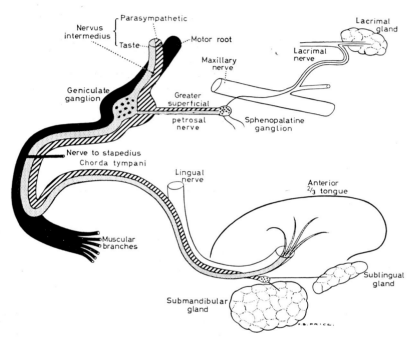

Fig. 1. Plan of the facial nerve showing its constituent fibres, their relay stations, and destinations. (Groves, 1971.)

the superior semicircular canal behind and the cochlea in front and below. Completing its right-angled backward turn, the nerve is land-marked by the processus trochleariformis immediately beneath it on the medial tympanic wall.

The horizontal course of the nerve, beneath the lateral canal and above the fenestra vestibuli (oval window), is familiar. Less well known is the surgical anatomy as seen from the medial (vestibular) aspect. Here the nerve is recognizable above the base (footplate) of the stapes, as described by Smyth (1973) in his posterior fossa approach designed to preserve the nerve during neurosurgical removal of vestibulocochlear nerve tumours ("acoustic neuroma") (Fig. 4).

In its vertical (mastoid) course, the facial nerve can be located surgically by the interval between the short process of incus laterally and the lower border of the horizontal canal medially (Fig. 5). The stylomastoid foramen can be found by the removal of air cells until the periosteum on the medial aspect of the mastoid process is reached. Followed medially this plane will be found to turn upwards at the

After its apperance in the neck the nerve lies below the tympanic plate and lateral to the base of the styloid. This is surgically a "non-vascular area", lateral to the carotid sheath and behind the parotid gland. The first major subdivision usually occurs within the parotid capsule, and the upper branch lies on the neck of the mandible. The plane of the "goose's foot" is superficial to the external carotid and its terminal branches.

Microanatomy

Facial nerve structure has been extensively studied by conventional dissection under magnification, and by serial sectioning and selective staining for histological examination in decalcified temporal bones. In addition to human cadaver material, experimental animals have included almost every relevant species, from Sir Charles Bell's donkey to the cat, rabbit and spiny ant-eater. Monkeys were extensively used by Ballance and Duel (1932).

Cross-section of the nerve trunk shows it to be histologically equivalent to a single fasciculus in the structure

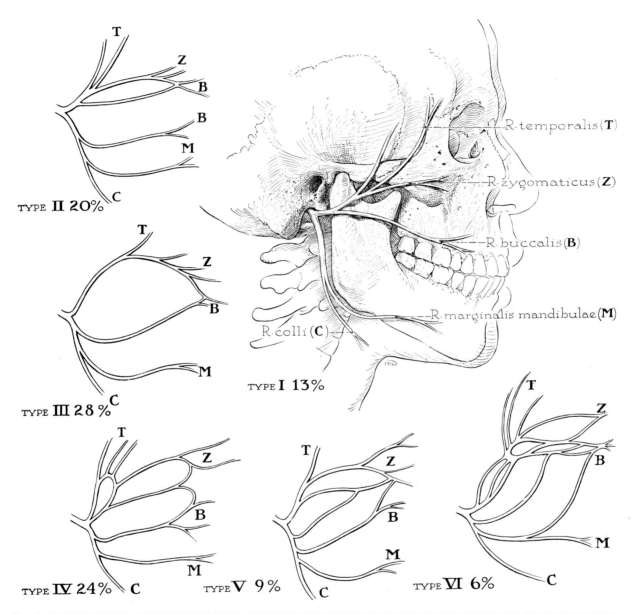

FIG .2. FACIAL NERVE: MAJOR TYPES OF BRANCHING AND INTERCOMMUNICATION, WITH PERCENTAGE OCCURRENCE OF EACH PATTERN. FROM RECORDS ON 350 CERVICOFACIAL HALVES. Schematically shown, as of the right side of the head. Note that types III, IV and V, and VI together represent almost 70 per cent of specimens. *Type I*—Absence of anastomosis between the branches of the two divisions (temporofacial and cervicofacial) of the facial nerve; although regularly pictured, actually a least common type. *Type II*—Anastomoses within the temporofacial division. *Type III*—Anastomosis between chief divisions. *Type IV*—Two anastomotic loops within the temporofacial part. *Type V*—Two loops from the cervicofacial division, intertwined with branches of the temporofacial. *Type VI*—Extensive intermixture. (From Anson and Donaldson, 1973.)

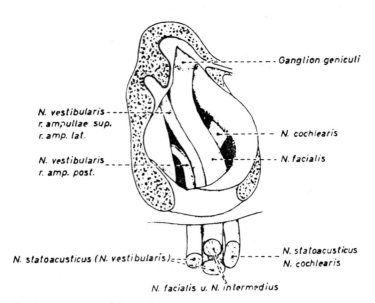

N. vestibularis
r. ampullae sup.
r. amp. lat.

N. vestibularis
r. amp. post.

Ganglion geniculi

N. cochlearis

N. facialis

N. statoacusticus (N. vestibularis)

N. statoacusticus
N. cochlearis

N. facialis u. N. intermedius

FIG. 3. Contents of left internal acoustic meatus as seen through floor of middle fossa. (after Fisch, 1969.)

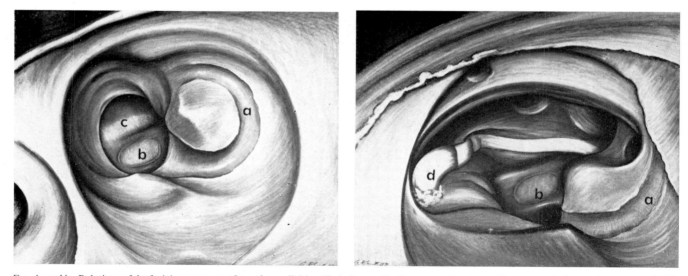

FIG. 4a and b. Relations of the facial nerve as seen from the medial (vestibular) aspect in the course of posterior fossa removal of acoustic neuroma. (a) The posterior semicircular canal (a) is followed to the vestibule. The medial surface of the stapes footplate (b) and the bone overlying the horizontal facial nerve (c) are not visible.
(b) The facial nerve is uncovered and followed to its point of exit from the internal acoustic meatus (d). (a) Posterior semicircular canal; (b) medial surface of the stapes footplate. (Smyth, 1973.)

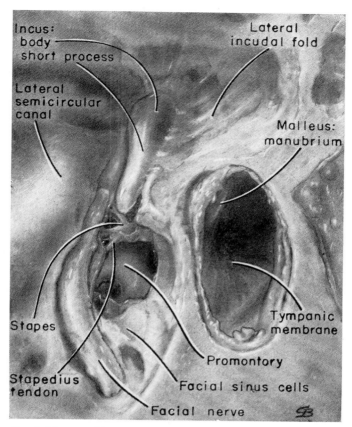

FIG. 5. The pyramidal course and relations of the right facial nerve. (From Anson and Donaldson, 1973.)

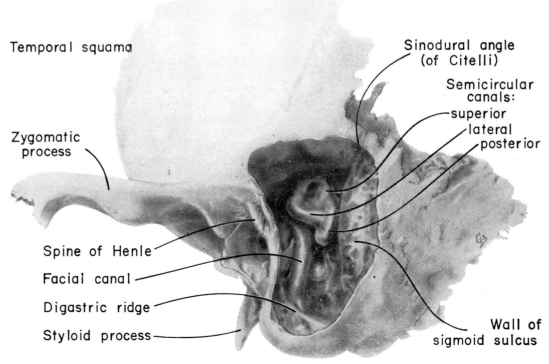

FIG. 6. The mastoid (vertical) course of the left facial nerve, and its relation to the digastric ridge. (From Anson and Donaldson, 1973.)

of a typical nerve (Anson *et al.*, 1973). This implies that epineurium and perineurium are one and the same. Individual nerve fibres are surrounded by neurolemmal

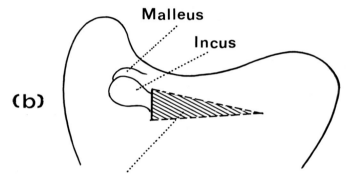

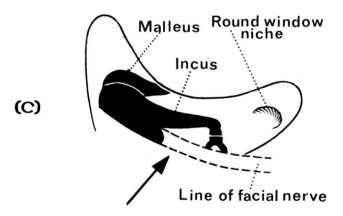

FIG. 7. The facial recess, sinus tynpani, and facial nerve, by the posterior tympanotomy (transmastoid) approach. (Adapted from Groves, 1971.)

sheaths, and supported by the endoneurium as in any other nerve. Myelinated nerve fibre counts give totals of around 5000–6000 in rabbits (Bowden and Mahran, 1960). The fibre diameters range from 1 to 12 micrometres with almost 50 per cent within the average range of 4–6 μm.

Attempts have been made to correlate the arrangement of particular fibres in the nerve trunk with their final muscular destinations. White and Verma (1973) dissected 15 human temporal bones and showed that there is a spiralling of the nerve fibre-bundles, so that fibres lying superficially at the stylomastoid foramen first become posterior, and then medial, as they are followed upwards. Dissection within the nerve showed superficial and deep divisions, both of which contribute to the two main branches of the nerve (Fig. 8). In addition numerous smaller communications between these intraneural divisions were found. White and Verma conclude from their findings that it is unlikely that a partial lesion would result in specific regional paralysis, and that effects would show in the distribution of all of the branches.

Interconnections of the Facial Nerve

The main trunk has one or more communications with the vestibular nerve (Fig. 3). The writer has found no indication in the literature as to the functional significance of this, but the fact is of surgical relevance, and may conceivably have bearing upon the occurrence of vestibular disturbances in Bell's palsy and the Ramsay Hunt syndrome.

At the periphery the many smaller branches have free anastomoses with one another, and equally freely with branches of the trigeminal nerve. It has been suggested (Bowden *et al.*, 1960) that the intercommunications allow the distribution of single parent axons to innervate simultaneously, by branching, motor units in more than one part of the face. Such a concept would provide an anatomical basis for the very complex normal variety of associated movements in facial expression. Another point of interest here is that, within the muscles, single fibres have been noted as receiving more than one axon approaching from different directions (Bowden and Mahran, 1956). The concept of such a "collateral" motor innervation would further account for elaborate expressive patterns, although it would complicate the classical simplicity of the conventional motor unit.

Muscle spindles (stretch receptors) are present in the facial musculature (Kadanoff, 1956) and from extensive animal studies it seems possible (Bowden, 1964) that the afferent pathways may be collected together in the trigeminal, rather than the facial, nerve. The large diameter axons (up to 22 μm) in the trigeminal support this hypothesis.

The Sheath

The fibrous sheath of the facial nerve is a blend of the periosteum of the facial bony canal with the dura proximally, and the cervical fascia distally. As exposed surgically in the temporal bone it is tough, shiny, well-defined, and easily uncovered by drill or curette. It seems to be a very effective barrier to middle ear disease, and, if not grossly abused, to surgical contact. Between the periosteal sheath and the epineurium is an extensive vascular plexus. The final integument, classically slit open in decompression operations is,

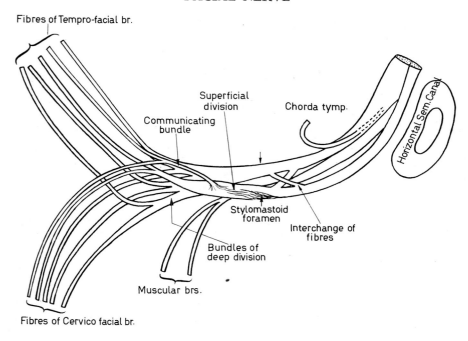

Fig. 8. Intraneural branching in the facial nerve. (after White and Verma, 1973.)

according to Anson and his colleagues, the epineurium itself.

Blood Supply

The arterial supply of the nerve has been studied by injection techniques (Blunt, 1954; Anson *et al.*, 1973) and may be summarized as follows:

Level	Artery
(1) Intracranially	Anterior inferior cerebellar
(2) In the internal meatus	Internal auditory
(3) Genicular ganglion	Petrosal branch of middle meningeal
(4) Geniculum to stylomastoid foramen	Petrosal and stylomastoid, anastomosing
(5) In the neck	Occipital and posterior auricular
(6) In the face	Occipital, posterior auricular, superficial temporal and transverse facial

The work of Fisch (1969) in relation to the internal auditory artery requires mention here. Injection studies in 22 human temporal bones showed some variability of the arterial arrangements. In general, it was found that two or more arteries enter the porus. These vessels arise from a cerebellar vessel (never from the basilar trunk) and are little larger than arterioles. They form an intricate network within the meatus, supplying its contents, and giving rise to one or two labyrinthine arteries.

A venous plexus surrounds the course of the nerve within the facial canal (Fig. 9). Both arteries and veins have frequent communications with the vessels of the surrounding bone, and of the middle ear mucosa. This degree of vascularity would seem to be far in excess of the metabolic needs of the nerve itself. Intraneurally there are no vessels of significant size, but it is supposed that the micro-circulation is adequate to allow surgical mobilization of adequate lengths of nerve.

The Facial (Fallopian) Canal

The bony tunnel for the nerve has been scrutinized carefully by many workers. It is not uniformly cylindrical, but in cross-section shows numerous irregularities of form at the places where vascular channels pass into the surrounding bone. There is a large aperture for the stapedius muscle, and the bony cavity for this muscle gives the appearance in section of two "semicanals", side by side, in the pyramidal course of the nerve. A smaller aperture, lower down, transmits the chorda tympani.

Ballance and Duel (1932) give some dimensions of interest for the human adult facial canal. The descending (mastoid) portion is 14 mm and the horizontal portion 6–7 mm in length. The diameter of the bony canal is 1–1·5 mm.

Lindeman (1960) measured the areal dimensions of the canal in 8 human temporal bones. He did not find the narrowest point was at any particular level, and specifically ruled out any anatomical constriction at the stylomastoid foramen. The nerve itself occupied from 10 to 45 per cent of the canal area. Sunderland and Cossar (1953) obtained similar results.

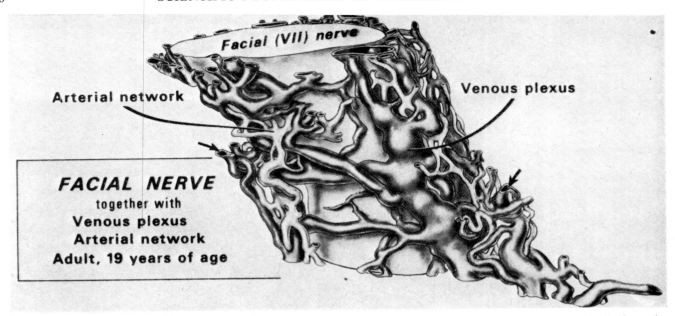

FIG. 9. Facial nerve, venous plexus, and arterial network. Reconstruction in lateral view, from 19-year-old male patient. Wisconsin collection, series 29, left ear, sections 215–450; original reconstruction × 100, reduced to × 20 in original print. The plexiform arrangement of the capacious veins and the complex system of intercommunicating arteries that surround the nerve are shown. (Anson *et al*, 1973.)

Anomalies of Facial Nerve Anatomy

Variations in the course and form of the nerve are of obvious surgical importance, and are, understandably, related to the developmental anatomy of the temporal bone. In the normal infant, with its absent mastoid and rudimentary tympanic ring, the stylomastoid foramen is on the lateral aspect of the skull. With normal development the foramen migrates to its more protected adult position. In its tympanic course, the nerve acquires its bony cover by progressive ossification of mesenchymal tissue. The bone formation enfolds the nerve progressively and so separates it from the developing middle ear cavity. This process may be uncompleted, and dehiscences in this part of the bony canal are comparatively common. In the mastoid part of the nerve, development of air cells may encroach upon the facial canal wall.

The writer, in operating upon cases of accidental surgical facial paralysis, has observed instances where the pyramidal segment has occupied a plane significantly lateral to the lateral semicircular canal. It could be said that the nerve swings a little "wide at the bend"—wider, that is, than would normally be expected, though only by one or two millimetres.

Several cases have been described in which the nerve has passed below instead of above the oval window (Hough, 1958). Fig. 10 shows an example. Bifurcation of the nerve has been noted in the mastoid portion, with a double stylomastoid foramen.

The point of origin of the chorda tympani, usually one or two millimetres above the foramen, may occasionally be found at a higher level, or sometimes much lower, so that the chorda arises outside the skull, and re-enters by a separate canal close to the stylomastoid foramen.

PHYSIOLOGICAL CONSIDERATIONS

In repose, the resting tonus of the facial mask maintains the palpebral fissure, with the lacrimal puncta in contact with the globe. The nostrils are patent, and the lips and cheeks are in contact with the teeth. The stapedius muscle maintains optimal middle ear impedance, and in animals with mobile auricles (pinnae) and vibrissae the natural posture of these organs is maintained. In infants and children, the buccal fat pad makes a major contribution to the facial contour. It effectively conceals the loss of tonus in facial palsy, a loss which in the adult is appallingly obvious as a total "landslide", with sagging lips, cheek and eyelids, the whole effect made more grotesque by drag over the midline by the muscles of the other side.

Voluntary movements are less important than reflex ones. One may grimace, wink, whistle, blow, smile, or frown at will. Actors, including poker players, have a remarkable facility of conscious facial control. For the majority, voluntary facial movement is a blend of social conditioning and well-practised mannerism. The "stiff upper lip", the placatory smile, and the admonitory frown or scowl are cultivated almost to the status of Pavlovian reflexes.

Purely reflex activity in the facial muscles is of the highest physiological importance. Eyelid closure in blinking and sleeping, nostrial dilation in respiration, and the control of the lips in biting and chewing are basic sphincter-like functions. Together with the tongue, the buccinator muscle holds food between the teeth for chewing, whilst the lips and buccinator play essential parts in sucking and in speech.

Horner's muscle (lacrimal part of the orbicularis oculi) reflexly dilates the lacrimal sac during blinking, and thus facilitates the removal of tears from the conjunctiva.

Although in man auricular movements are negligible, the auricular muscles of most mammals are reflexly controlled to maintain a scanning and sound-location mechanism. In those animals such reflex activity, and the reflex movements of vibrissae, are important tools of survival. The stapedius reflex, of greater otological interest,

Each lower motor neurone and its associated muscle fibres form a motor unit, and in the face the innervation ratio (proportion of muscle to nerve fibres) is low. For example, the ratio is 25 : 1 platysma, compared to nearly 2000 : 1 for gastrocnemius. The ratios of 2 : 1 for laryngeal, and 9 : 1 for external ocular muscles are interesting com-

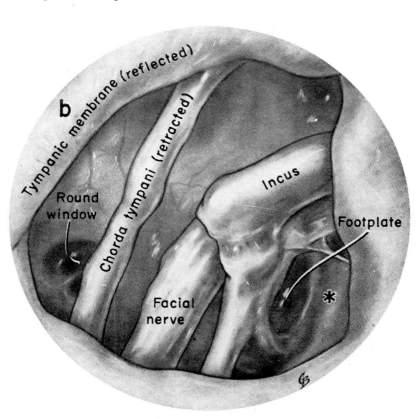

FIG. 10. Anomalous course of (left) facial nerve passing inferior to the oval window. (From Anson and Donaldson, 1973.)

regulates the impedance of the ear—a protective mechanism for the cochlea, and, according to some evidence (Simmons and Beatty, 1962) a regulator of aural sensitivity in maximum attentivity for listening.

Central Control of Facial Muscles

The facial nerve nucleus is activated by cortico-bulbar (pyramidal) fibres from the contralateral motor cortex of the brain. In the upper half of the face cortical representation is bilateral. In the dominant hemisphere the facial motor centres are closely linked with the speech area.

Penfield and Rasmussen (1950) found that stimulation of the lower parts of the pre- and post-central gyri at operation in man caused contralateral facial movements. The excitable area for the lips was the largest.

The facial nucleus in the medulla also receives connections from the medial longitudinal bundle, reticular formation, trapezoid body, nucleus of the spinal tract of the trigeminal, and ascending fibres from the spinal cord (Bowden, 1964).

parisons. Goodgold and Eberstein (1972) should be studied for a more detailed account of neuromuscular physiology, including the ultrastructure of the myoneural junction.

Electrical Activity

(a) *Electromyographic* observation of facial nerve activity may be made by means of skin electrodes, but this technique is less accurate than the conventional concentric needle electrode which is placed directly into the muscle being studied. Initially the electrode provokes a burst of action potentials—an artefact known as insertion activity. After this, normally innervated muscle at rest is electrically silent. When a weak contraction occurs motor unit action potentials—diphasic or triphasic waves—appear. Their duration is from 3–16 ms and amplitude from 300 μV to 5 mV. Electronic display techniques permit the response from single motor units to be studied (Fig.11). With stronger contractions the responses from large numbers of motor units are combined in the trace until an "interference pattern" of many spike potentials at high frequencies

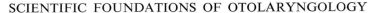

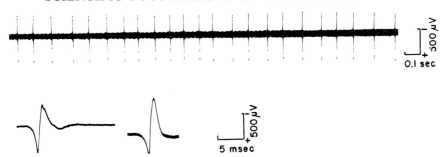

FIG. 11. Single motor unit action potentials recorded from biceps brachii. (From Goodgold and Eberstein, 1972.)

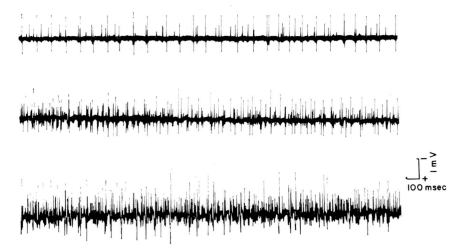

FIG. 12, Interference patterns. Single motor unit pattern is shown in *top* recording. With increased effort, frequency of discharge increases and additional motor units are recruited (*middle* and *bottom* recordings).

obscures the discrete individual motor unit components (Fig. 12).

(b) *Electrical Excitability.* Any motor nerve may be stimulated percutaneously by unipolar electrode and a visible muscle contraction will result. As the classical "faradic" (ac) and "galvanic" (dc) responses show, the nerve will respond to almost any electrical depolarization, whereas direct stimulation of muscle does not occur with very short duration stimuli. In electro-diagnosis the faradic-galvanic tests have long been superseded by the use of stimulators which can provide an electrical pulse of approximately square-wave form and known duration and intensity. A pulse of 1 ms duration is commonly used. This is too brief for direct stimulation of the muscles, and any observed contraction is therefore proof that the nerve itself is excitable.

In facial nerve work the trunk may be stimulated (between the mastoid and the ramus of mandible) or individual branches may be selected at will by more anterior placement of the active electrode. Normal threshold of excitability, that is the minimum stimulus which will just produce a visible twitch in any part of the face, is usually found for a current of between 2 and 5 mA. In most subjects the value is the same on the two sides of the face. Higher currents produce a stronger contraction and in wider areas, until at

the maximum tolerable intensity (10–15 mA) the whole hemiface will move vigorously. Some degree of observer-skill is needed not to mistake responses mediated through masseter and temporalis (trigeminal nerve) for facial nerve responses. The brief stimulus of 1 ms is well tolerated by most patients, but young children tend to resent even this, and in them essential testing may have to be done under anaesthesia.

Normal nerve excitability in the presence of a facial palsy proves that the nerve has not undergone degeneration, and that the lesion must lie above (centre to) the point of stimulation. A major difficulty in clinical practice is that there is an interval, even after complete transection of the nerve, of up to three days during which the distal part remains normally excitable. This was well shown by Gilliatt and Taylor (1959) who studied patients who had undergone operative section of the nerve for clonic facial spasm, or removal of vestibulocochlear nerve tumours.

(c) *Conduction Velocity.* The techniques of nerve stimulation and electromyography can be combined to measure the condition speed over a measured length of nerve. From the stylomastoid foramen to an electrode in the orbicularis oris the latency time is normally under 4 ms. This parameter is inversely proportional to conduction velocity in the largest (fastest-conducting) fibres. There has been some debate as to whether increased latency is due to slowed conduction in these fibres, or whether it represents the conduction time of slower (smaller) fibres when the faster fibres have lost their excitability. Although extensively studied, conduction velocity has not found much favour in clinical facial nerve work, thought it is, of course, widely applied to the investigation of peripheral neuropathies in the limbs.

Special Sensation—Taste

The innervation of the taste buds of the anterior two-thirds of the tongue has been shown by experimental work on animals and human subjects to pass in the chorda tympani and facial nerve. Relay is in the genicular ganglion, with the central axons passing in the nervus intermedius to the nucleus of the tractus solitarius. The earlier classical view was that the pathway was via the lingual and trigeminal nerves as well as by the facial nerve. It was Cushing who deduced from observations in patients who had undergone trigeminal (semilunar) ganglionectomy that the taste fibres, being unaffected, must travel via the seventh and not the fifth nerve. Lewis and Dandy consolidated this with conclusions drawn from the effects of intracranial division of isolated cranial nerves in patients.

Bull (1965) reported on the effects of chorda tympani section in patients undergoing stapes surgery and found homolateral loss of taste, with atrophy of the papillae in every case. Costen and his associates (1951) reported in detail the effects of chorda tympani stimulation in a patient whose nerve was exposed and accessible in a radical mastoid cavity. These workers also presented weighty evidence that the chorda carries afferent fibres for touch, pain and temperature, in addition to taste and autonomic pathways. It is of some historical interest to note that, from the very beginning, with Bell's own experiments on donkeys, the identification of the sensory functions of the facial nerve has been a halting, hesitant, research. As noted above, the proprioceptive fibres have been disputed until very recently, whilst the question of cutaneous supply in connection with the Ramsay Hunt syndrome is still unresolved.

The facial nerve also carries taste fibres from the palate, which travel in the greater petrosal nerve to the genicular ganglion. At the present time there has been no clinical exploitation of this sensory pathway, perhaps because it follows the same anatomical route as the parasympathetic fibres for lacrimation—a function more easily examined (*see* p. 440).

Clinical Testing. Although there are four recognizable modalities of taste—salt, sweet, sour (acid) and bitter (*see* Fig. 13)—clinical testing is usually restricted to the use of salt and sugar, in concentrated solutions. The protruded tongue is held, and dried with gauze, and the solution is then applied on a wool-dressed probe. The patient identifies his sensations as "salt", "sweet", or "nil" by pointing to the appropriate word on a chart. The technique, though simple, must be carried out as described to avoid false results due to taste perception in areas of the mouth and tongue not innervated by the chorda.

Renewed clinical interest in taste testing probably dates from the work of Krarup (1958) who explored quantitatively

the so-called "anodal galvanic response". Direct electrical current applied through anode upon the tongue and cathode remotely placed (e.g. on the back of the neck) induces an acidic sensation of taste. The minimum current detectable by the patient is the electrogustometric (ELG) threshold, and the normal range is from about 10 to 50 μA. In normal subjects the threshold is identical or nearly so on the two

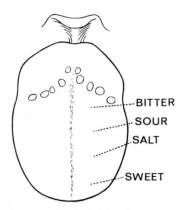

Fig. 13. The modalities of taste in the anterior 2/3 of the tongue. The areas indicated are not, of course, sharply demarcated from each other.

sides. In most of the clinical work published to date the absolute values in microamperes have been recorded, but it may well be that Krarup's original concept of a logarithmic scale of sensitivity (analogous to the decibel in audiometry) should be adopted. Clearly, the significance of a difference in threshold of, say, 10 μA between the two sides of the tongue cannot be the same if the absolute values are 10 and 20 μA, as it would be if the absolute values were 150 and 160 μA. Standardization of a decilog scale for taste has not as yet been attained, but the problems are discussed by Tomita and his associates (1972) and Fons and Osterhammel (1968). Alford and his associates (1973) record the ELG differences as a percentage of the sum of the thresholds of both sides (in μA), and further refine the test by averaging the results of five bilateral readings. From a study of 227 normal subjects they have adopted 22 per cent as the upper limit of normal difference between the two sides.

In general, electrogustometry may be considered a dependable test of the integrity of the taste fibres provided that the test is expertly done, and the patients responses are consistent and accurate. However, not a few subjects, especially the elderly and heavy smokers, fail to register valid thresholds.

Autonomic (Parasympathetic) Motor Function

From the superior salivary nucleus, the nervus intermedius brings secretomotor fibres for the lacrimal, nasal, sublingual and submandibular glands. The lacrimal (and nasal) fibres leave the facial nerve in the greater petrosal nerve, while the salivary fibres continue in the facial canal and exit by the chorda tympani. The functional integrity of these nervous pathways is clinically significant in any case of facial palsy, and in conjunction with other observations may help in localizing the level of the nerve lesion, or in assessing its severity.

Lacrimation. Schirmer's test is commonly used to compare lacrimal secretory activity on the normal and the affected sides. A strip of filter paper 5 × 0·5 cm is bent at one end and hooked over the edge of the lower eyelid. Spontaneous lacrimation produces visible wetting of the paper, and the length of the paper strip thus wetted can be measured and compared with an identical test-strip similarly placed in the other fornix. Zilstorff-Pedersen (1965) attempted to quantify what is, in essence, little more than a qualitative test. He utilized the nasolacrimal reflex, stimulating tear secretion by means of a measured dose of benzene vapour applied to the nasal mucosa. In the present state of knowledge it would seem as if lacrimation may only be usefully assessed as "unimpaired", "reduced", of "absent".

Salivary Flow. The rate of secretion from the submandibular duct, as stimulated by lemon juice, is measurable with a fine polyethylene tube into the duct on each side. The quantities of saliva collected from each side are compared, and any reduction on the affected side is expressed as a percentage of the normal contralateral secretion. Blatt (1965) advocated this test as clinically valid, and other workers (May and Harvey, 1971; Alford *et al.*, 1973) have pursued the proposition with varying conclusions. The present author is inclined to doubt the usefulness of the test insofar as submandibular cannulation can be a difficult and uncomfortable procedure. The salivary contribution of the numerous ducts of the sublingual gland may be outside the control of the experimenter, depending as it well may upon the length of penetration of the cannula on each side being exactly equal, and the anatomy exactly comparable on the right and the left.

An elegant solution to these problems is suggested by Bernard and his associates (1972) who demonstrated delayed clearance of technetium 99m from the submandibular salivary gland on the affected side in cases of Bell's palsy. As a possible prognostic sign this investigation clearly invites further assessment.

EFFECTS OF NERVE INJURY

Facial palsy of lower motor neurone type may result from compression, stretching, crushing, transection, excessive cooling, heat, ultrasonic energy, local anaesthetic and corrosives, as well as from disease processes more or less well-defined such as zoster, Bell's palsy, and direct involvement in inflammations and tumours.

The severity of the injury can be classified in terms of neurapraxia (reversible conduction block) or Wallerian degeneration. Commonly, peripheral nerve lesions are "mixed", having some neurapraxic and some degenerated fibres.

In *neurapraxia* the conductivity of the nerve fibres is blocked at the site of the lesion, but if the nerve is stimulated distal to the lesion a normal nerve action potential is evoked and the muscles contract. If a nerve is merely neurapraxic, removal of the cause is followed by complete restoration of function.

In degeneration the histological changes were first described by Waller (1862). Axon cylinders gradually disappear, and the myelin sheaths break up with the formation of fatty droplets. These changes occur throughout the nerve distal to the lesion, and proximally up to the nearest node of Ranvier. The neurilemmal (Schwann cell) sheath remains intact except where, in cases of neurotmesis, it is damaged or destroyed by the original injury. The time scale for these changes appears to vary widely in different experimental animals, and is of course difficult to estimate in man. It is probably a matter of days extending into weeks before the clearance of intraneural products of degeneration by macrophages is completed.

Regeneration begins very early by the downgrowth of axons from above the lesion. If there is continuity of the neurilemmal tubes with those in the distal part of the nerve most of the growing fibres will penetrate successfully and continue at an approximate rate of one millimetre per day until eventually some at least of the motor end-plates are re-innervated. Some fibres may be misdirected so that they innervate muscles other than those they served before the injury. If there is a breach in the continuity of the neurilemmal tubes at the site of the lesion the regenerating axons emerge from the proximal stump of the nerve and proliferate to form a bulbous swelling ("neuroma"). Only a comparatively small number of them succeed in entering the distal part of the nerve and reach the end-plates. The greater the gap between the two parts of the nerve, the smaller will be the percentage of successful fibres. This type of repair also results in a much greater degree of misdirection of those fibres which do succeed in bridging the gap. The rate of repair is such that a lapse of 10–14 weeks is usually required, after a lesion in the temporal bone, before voluntary movement returns to the paralysed muscles. Recovery that occurs sooner than this can only be attributed to relief of conduction block in fibres which have suffered merely from neurapraxia.

Electron microscope studies have contributed new information in recent years. Harkin and Skinner (1970) describe the changes observed in nerves taken from rats and mice at varying intervals after cutting and crushing injuries, and give useful references to the experimental work in this field. Basically their results accord with the earlier classical descriptions. The processes of regeneration are minutely observed, and the evolving relationships between the new axons and the Schwann cells are especially interesting.

Essential requirements of re-innervation are:

(a) The cell body (in the facial nucleus) must survive, as in most peripheral lesions. It may not do so in poliomyelitis, or in brain-stem vascular accidents.
(b) The initial cause of the paralysis must be either self-limiting, or amenable to therapy.
(c) The nerve trunk must be in gross continuity, or, it is not, the severed ends must be in apposition. When this condition is not met, only surgery, and possibly with nerve-grafting, can re-establish a possibility of re-innervation.

Defects of Re-innervation. Whereas recovery from neurapraxia is complete in every way, there are invariably defects in power, control, and co-ordination of facial movements if more than a small percentage of fibres degenerate and subsequently regenerate. These defects are due to a combination of some fibres failing to grow, and other ramifying peripherally to supply larger, randomly reassembled, motor units. Misdirection of axons within the disturbed neurilemmal architecture results in cross re-innervation with synkinesia between large muscle areas. Typically this

of the lesion. In clinical otology, this is obviously the commonest condition of testing. It can happen, however, that at operation, the nerve may be available for stimulation *above* the lesion, and then of course no muscle twitch occurs. Fisch and Esslen (1972) exploited this when exploring the palsied facial nerve in the internal acoustic meatus (Fig. 14).

Progressive loss of nerve excitability below the lesion occurs three days after total transection. Total inexcitability is proof that severe denervation is already certain, and that

Intraoperative electrical stimulation of the facial nerve in Bell's palsy.

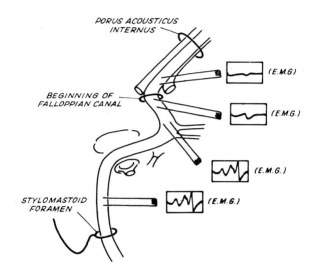

PORUS ACOUSTICUS INTERNUS

(E.M.G.)

BEGINNING OF FALLOPPIAN CANAL

(E.M.G.)

(E.M.G.)

STYLOMASTOID FORAMEN

(E.M.G.)

FIG. 14. Results of intra-operative electrical stimulation of the facial nerve following total intratemporal exposure for Bell's palsy. In three cases presenting at surgery with a conduction block (neuropraxia) in about 25 per cent of the fibres, the intra-operative electrical stimulation showed that the nerve impulses were blocked in a region situated proximally to the genicular ganglion and also extending within the internal acoustic meatus. (Fisch and Esslen, 1972.)

is seen as an oral movement during eye closure. Most reliably it is evidenced by asking the patient to blink repeatedly. Facial tics and involuntary spasms sometimes occur, so that the face becomes stiff and tightly drawn upwards between the eye and the angle of the mouth.

Secretory cross-reinnervation sometimes occurs, so that the eye waters excessively during meals. This "crocodile tear" phenomenon is thought (Golding Wood, 1962) to be due to new innervation developing from the tympanic plexus (IX) and spreading as collateral fibres into a degenerated greater petrosal nerve. The parotid secretomotor fibres thus gain control of the lacrimal (and nasal) glands. Even if tympanic neurectomy fails to cure crocodile tears, Vidian (nerve of pterygoid canal) neurectomy can still prove successful.

Electrical Changes in Nerve Lesions

Nerve excitability, as already stated, is retained in pure conduction block, if the nerve is stimulated below the level

it is too late to prevent it. Lesser impairments of nerve excitability are considered ominous by some workers, but it must be stressed that interpretation of this situation depends very much on the nature of the pathological condition causing the palsy, and other variable factors such as time elapsed since onset. Further discussion is therefore deferred (*vide infra*). Campbell (1963); Richardson (1962, 1963); Taverner (1955) and Laumans and Jongkees (1963) have written extensively on their clinical studies of this test, which has been much used—and somewhat ill-used—at times. The essential point to be grasped about this test is that it is extremely accurate in prognosis, but of no value in the selection of cases for treatment in the early stages *before* denervation has become unavoidable (Kristensen, 1968; Groves, 1973a).

After complete degeneration and recovery by regeneration, nerve excitability returns only very gradually over a period of months. In some cases it is never recovered, even in the presence of good movement, and caution is therefore needed in interpreting nerve excitability tests in cases of recurrent paralysis.

Strength-duration measurements (an extended test of nerve excitability which determines the differing intensities required for electrical stimuli to evoke muscle contraction) can be plotted graphically. They give an approximate estimation of the proportion of neurapraxic to degenerated fibres. Both the nerve excitability and strength-duration tests (if done more than three days after the onset of complete paralysis) can be accepted as evidence of gross continuity in the nerve, if any fibres show neurapraxia only.

Conduction Velocity. According to Taverner (1965) latency time measured below the level of the lesion is

though they cannot give a guide as to the final quality of recovery. Nevertheless, they should almost always be taken as a contra-indication to surgical interference.

With all facial nerve electrodiagnosis, the time elapsed has a bearing on the choice and interpretation of tests. Figure 15 is therefore reproduced here as a reference guide.

TOPOGNOSIS OF FACIAL NERVE LESIONS

As an academic exercise the notion of locating a given facial nerve lesion to a specific place anatomically has

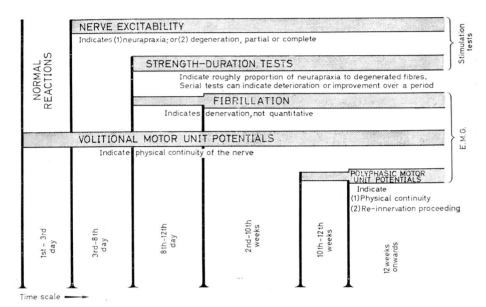

FIG. 15. Electrodiagnosis in cases of *complete* facial paralysis. The chart indicates the approximate times after onset of paralysis when the various tests may be expected to give helpful information. (Groves, 1971.)

prolonged during the period when degeneration is impending. As soon as degeneration is established this test is of course inapplicable.

Electromyography. Needle electromyography can reveal the presence of single or scattered residual normal motor units, even in the presence of total clinical paralysis, and absence of nerve excitability. Such residual units are most valuable proof that the nerve is still in gross physical continuity. They must be skilfully and patiently sought in any case where other omens are discouraging, and, if found, are a sound basis for conservative management.

Fibrillation potentials may be found from the 10th day onwards in the presence of degeneration, but the observation comes rather too late to be of help in selection for treatment. Absence of fibrillation is evidence that denervation is negligible, or that re-innervation (from 10 weeks onwards) is imminent. After a year or more of paralysis, absence of fibrillation implies wasting and fibrosis of the muscles.

Recovery potentials (polyphasic action potentials) are noted by EMG at, or after, three months following denervation, if there is impending re-innervation. They indicate a favourable prognosis in that re-innervation is progressing,

obvious intellectual appeal. It is a paradox therefore to realize that in daily clinical practice, after the essential differentiation between upper and lower motor neurone palsies, one is usually more preoccupied with trying to establish the severity of a lesion than with assessing its precise anatomical level. The level is, of course, usually evident from consideration of the diagnosis of pathological cause. Involvement of specific facial nerve branches will usually confirm or modify usefully such consideration.

Tschiassny (1953, 1955), Jepsen (1965) and other workers, have systematized topognosis as an anatomical exercise, utilizing clinical observation of facial movements, lacrimation, stapedius reflex, taste, and digastric muscle function (deviation of the chin when the mouth is opened). Table 1 from Tschiassny, gives details.

Neurologists, as well as otologists since the time of Erb himself (1876), have earnestly taught and emphasized these concepts, so it is as well to re-state Tschiassny's own very pertinent comment.

"The presented method has its limitations. It can be applied with reliability only to early lesions. In lesions of longer duration, partial recovery restricted to some functions may occur, or, by descending degeneration, some

TABLE 1

SIGNS CHARACTERISTIC OF FACIAL NERVE LESION AT EIGHT DIFFERENT LEVELS

(From Tschiassnyr, 1953)

Level	Upper Face Movement	Bell's Phenom.	Emotional Movements	Blinking Reflex	Stapedius Reflex	Orbicul. Oris Movements	Tears	Taste	Deviation of Chin on Mouth Open
Supranuclear	yes	no	yes	yes	yes	yes	yes	yes	yes
Nuclear	no	yes	no	no	no	yes	yes	yes	yes
Supragenicular	no	yes	no	no	no	no	no	yes	yes
Transgenicular	no	yes	no	no	no	no	no	no	yes
Suprastapedial	no	yes	no	no	no	no	yes	no	yes
Infrastapedial	no	yes	no	no	yes	no	yes	no	yes
Infrachordal	no	yes	no	no	yes	no	yes	yes	yes
Infraforaminal	no	yes	no	no	yes	no	yes	yes	no

(Note—Bell's phenomenon is the upward rolling of the eyeball which protects the cornea when the paralysed eyelids fail to close.)

functions may later be lost. Lacrimation may return very soon. Taste sensation may come back while the stapedius reflex may still be absent. In cerebellopontine angle tumours (suprageniculate lesion), taste sensation is frequently absent probably due to descending degeneration."

The present author (Groves, 1973b) pointed out that stapedius muscle paralysis can be present whether or not taste is (at the time) involved in Bell's palsy. And again, that lacrimation, stapedius function and taste may all recover at different times, so that, after a given interval, a transgenicular lesion, for example, may masquerade as an infrachordal one. The realization that one is dealing with a disease pattern that continually changes is essential not only to the interpretation of the clinical tests, but also to the evaluation of all the published literature.

It follows from these arguments that the topognostic exercise may well be valid for a localized lesion, such as a tumour, or a "once-for-all" insult such as localized trauma, but in diffuse "neuritic" conditions such as Bell's (idiopathic) facial palsy or Ramsay Hunt syndrome a more sophisticated view is necessary. Many workers today, whether from logic or practical necessity, assess the involvement of lacrimation, taste, stapedius and salivatory function as indicators of severity, rather than level, of the lesion. Taken in relation to time elapsed since onset such an assessment may be very significant (vide infra) and may reflect a selective vulnerability of the different types of nerve fibre we are studying.

GENERAL MANAGEMENT OF FACIAL PALSIES

Since diagnosis is the first and paramount part of management it follows that all cases should be seen and investigated by an otologist on the day of presentation. This doctrine still awaits general recognition, despite the urgent pleas of leading experts in every part of the world. Details of specific treatment are discussed in the following pages under specific aetiologies. Some aspects of management are common to all facial palsies, however, and the care of the unprotected eye, reassurance of the patient, and relief of pain are basic requirements. Ocular discomfort due to reduction of lacrimation is minimized by bland drops ("artificial tears") and any conjunctivitis, corneal abrasion or suspected foreign body should be attended to urgently by an ophthalmologist. Many such patients will require a lateral tarsorrhaphy if denervation indicates that recovery will be long delayed.

Complete paralysis with denervation also may warrant prosthetic support of the check by a hook, or by a "plumping bar" of plastic, attached to the upper teeth.

Physiotherapy is commonly advised, frequently demanded and yet sometimes condemned as futile by physical medicine specialists who are perhaps best qualified to judge. Mosforth and Taverner (1958) in a controlled trial failed to find any benefit from the use of galvanism. The theoretical expectation that patients with simple conduction block do not need this treatment was certainly confirmed by this work. Opinion is still divided however on the question of whether, in cases with denervation (which must last for at least three months) galvanic stimulation may be helpful in minimizing muscle wasting and fibrosis. It has been shown that in other areas (the hand for instance) frequent galvanic stimulation definitely maintains the bulk of denervated muscle, but similar direct proof of benefit in the small thin muscle sheets of the face would be hard to measure objectively.

Massage of the face can perhaps help morale and since it can be self-administered it places no burden on the patient (or on over-worked physiotherapy departments). There is one major exception to these somewhat nihilistic comments, in the situation where re-innervation is becoming apparent with its attendant defects. At this stage, galvanic stimulation skilfully combined with active exercises can help considerably in rehabilitation (Campbell, personal communication).

Surgical Rehabilitation

In any case where final recovery after denervation is unsatisfactory some, if not all, of the disabilities may be amenable to operation. It is axiomatic that the diagnosis of the cause of the palsy is beyond doubt, has been suitably treated to the fullest possible extent, and no further hope of facial nerve recovery can be entertained.

Plastic surgery is based on three principles:

(a) Static internal splinting by the insertion of fascial or wire slings, usually anchored to the zygomatic arch.

(b) Reanimation by local transplantation of masticatory muscles. The temporalis tendon may be detached, with the coronoid process of the mandible, and attached to fascial slings inserted round the mouth. The attachments of the masseter can be similarly transposed.

(c) Reanimation of free muscle transplants. In a new technique evolved by Thompson (1971), the transplanted muscle belly is laid into a bed of muscle prepared in the normal (unparalysed) side of the face, while its attached tendon passes in the subcutaneous plane across the midline to the paralysed side. The transplanted muscle receives reinnervation from sprouting axonal growth in its normally innervated muscle bed, so that, when the normal side contracts, a synchronous movement is transmitted by the tendon to the paralysed side. It has been shown that the muscle to be transplanted must be denervated surgically two weeks before it is moved to its new site. It is then in the most favourable condition to receive new axonal growth.

The palmaris longus, and the extensor digitorum brevis of the foot are suitable muscles. In practice they are split up and redeployed in the face so as to restore sphincteric action to the eyelids and the mouth. For eyelid reanimation, a muscle belly is laid into the normal orbicularis oculi of each lid on the normal side. The two tendons cross the midline and each other in a previously prepared tunnel behind the external nasal skeleton, and are passed subcutaneously in the paralysed lids to be finally anchored to each other and to the lateral palpebral ligament.

For the lips, another pair of muscle bellies is used with their tendons joined together at the paralysed corner of the mouth. This junction is then supported with another length of tendon securely tied to the zygomatic arch. Cosmetic and functional results have been highly rewarding in Thompson's series.

FACIAL NERVE SURGERY

Surgical awareness of the facial nerve certainly existed in the days of the pioneers of the nineteenth century. Ballance and Duel (1932) in their classical paper, which stands as a monumental landmark in our study, tell of records of nerve repair by direct suture dating from the fourteenth century. Flourens (1842) carried out successful nerve anastomoses in birds. In 1879 "Drobnik united in a man the peripheral end of the facial nerve to the central end of the external branch of the spinal accessory. After several months . . . the features had become more symmetrical." Ballance in 1895 performed an accessory (spinal)—facial anastomosis, closely followed by other surgeons, including Cushing. Other nerve anastomoses were subsequently tried clinically—facio-hypoglossal and facio-glossopharyngeal—in end-to-end and end-to-side variants. Even the cervical-sympathetic was joined to the facial nerve in animal experiments. Although some of these techniques continue in use to the present day, it is evi-

dent that gravely unsatisfactory results due to failure of cerebral re-education must have haunted the surgeons of the time. "It is an unnatural thing to anastomose one nerve to another, when the ideal surgical method of bringing the two ends of a divided nerve into contact, either directly or by means of a nerve graft, is both feasible and practicable. . . . We hold strongly that anastomosis operations for the cure of facial paralysis should be banished from future surgical practice." Thus declared Ballance and Duel, who went on to establish the concepts of nerve decompression and nerve grafting with such thoroughness and dedication that their teachings and dicta are still quoted by surgeons who have received them over four decades virtually by word of mouth. "The surgery of the temporal bone is no longer a field for legitimate and versatile experiment: certain fixed and useful laws and customs have been laid down by the dearly bought experience of great men; the Surgeon ought to begin fully equipped with such knowledge as has been gathered for him."

This advice was readily followed and the clinical application of nerve grafting and nerve decompression was keenly pursued, notably by Collier, by Bunnell, by Cawthorne, by Kettell and many others. These surgeons, accepting that "the operation cannot be done casually by the Light of Heaven" helped to move otology forward into the era of the operating microscope. Despite the technical difficulties and pitfalls stressed by Ballance and Duel, by 1949 Collier was able to say "Operations on the facial nerve are tedious more than difficult."

Another 25 years on, the otologist's skills with power driven burr and microscope are taken for granted and every part of the facial nerve is surgically accessible—in the best hands without unreasonable risk of life or hearing.

In their animal experiments, Ballance and Duel established the standards of facial nerve re-innervation which can be attained by the use of nerve autografts after surgically induced intratemporal lesions. They showed that any donor nerve, motor or sensory, would serve, reversed or or non-reversed, and the bony gutter of the facial canal provides adequate support without suturing. They tried, and abandoned, cavity obliteration by pedicled temporal muscle, and used gold leaf cover for the graft without conviction that it improved results.

Choice of donor nerve has an interesting history in that allogeneic and even xenogeneic grafts had been tried in other peripheral nerve injuries. Understandably, Ballance and Duel used autografts in their work, but very recent experimental work has shown that non-autologous tissue may in fact be accepted. Clearly there would be an advantage if stored cadaver nerves could be used with confidence.

Although the initial enthusiasm and claims for direct nerve repair proved excessive, there is no doubt that the principles laid down by Ballance and Duel have remained essentially unchanged and give better results than any others available to date. Some of their proposals have fallen, however; for example the use of "prepared" (i.e. degenerated) donor nerve (Collier, 1940). Their objection to grafting in the presence of sepsis has been largely overcome by antibiotics. Perhaps most disappointing, their belief in the virtues of decompression *per se* has proved a chimera which has decoyed all too many along an illogical pathway in the management of Bell's palsy.

In her later writings, Collier (1949, 1950, 1955) summarized the development of the classical transmastoid nerve repair techniques and the student is strongly urged to study these in detail. She particularly emphasized the value of the stabilizing effect upon anastomoses of the bony facial canal "gutter", and, with others, favoured a nerve graft lying in the normal course of the nerve, rather than mobilization and re-routing techniques which permit direct suture but leave the nerve exposed and devascularized.

From the early 1960's the middle cranial fossa approach has opened up a new field for research and operative management of lesions previously inaccessible. Decompression, direct repair, and grafting techniques in supragenicular lesions are now becoming standardized through the work especially of Miehlke (1973), of Fisch and Esslen (1972) and, of course, the "House Clinic" in Los Angeles, where the surgical approach was first developed (House and Hitzelberger, 1964).

Whatever therapy is undertaken it is essential to define the objective beforehand—to prevent denervation (the ideal) or to promote regeneration. In the latter situation, recovery is bound to be imperfect. If neurotmesis is found, though repair or grafting seldom fails to give *some* benefit, the *quality* of final recovery is to some degree a matter of chance. Even with the best results, synkinesis is usually marked, and emotional movements are often seriously distorted, but the patients, who have all experienced total paralysis, are usually very thankful for the relative normality finally achieved. Symmetry at rest, and adequate eyeclosure, are nearly always achieved (provided that treatment precedes too great a loss of muscle substance due to wasting). Collier believed that serious loss of muscle occurs from over-stretching of the paralysed fibres, and that this is a major cause of poor results. Surgical repair is justifiable even in late cases however, provided that fibrillation potentials, or a response to galvanic stimulation, can still be demonstrated.

Techniques

As the surgical exposure of the nerve is developed at operation it is necessary to observe certain principles of technique. Above all else the drill and the bone must be kept cool by irrigation. Glaninger and Mark (1967) measured in cadavers the temperatures when drilling at about 1 mm from the facial canal. They found that, with continuous irrigation for cooling, temperatures did not exceed 313·5 K (40·5°C). Without irrigation, temperatures up to 325 K (52°C) occurred. Locke's solution is advised rather than normal saline which can cause cellular damage (Kerth and Shambaugh, 1964). Diamond paste burrs should be used for thinning the canal wall prior to uncapping with a fine pick. The nerve sheath should be spared any unnecessary instrumental contact. Opening the sheath must be very delicately done with a sharp iridotomy knife, cutting outwards away from the nerve. The nerve itself when finally exposed is very vulnerable to injury. It should be disturbed from its bed as little as possible.

When it is necessary to excise damaged nerve (prior to grafting), both central and distal stumps must be cut back until all visible scar tissue has been cleared and the shiny cut ends of nerve bundles are seen. Guilford (1970) insisted on frozen histological sections of the excised scar to ensure that scar-free stumps are achieved. To allow for shrinkage the nerve graft must be slightly longer than the "gap". It is best stabilized in position after precise coaptation of the anastomoses by freshly precipitated human thrombin.

If a graft lacks an adequate bony groove for lodgement, one may be created for it with the burr, or it may be necessary to resort to suturing. It is perfectly possible to achieve accurate perineural stitching, without transfixing the nerve itself, under magnification, with a synthetic ophthalmic 10/0 (25 μm) suture on a 5 mm atraumatic needle. The latter must be closely watched, as it is extremely difficult to find again if mislaid outside the field of magnification.

It is the prevailing opinion that, given reasonable care, the above procedures do not injure the nerve (or make a bad case worse) but a recent paper by Devriese (1972) gives food for thought. He monitored facial nerve evoked action potentials in cats during exposure and slitting of the sheath (as in "decompression" in humans). In 7 out of 12 animals there was measurable impairment of nerve function. It was concluded that "in operations in the human the facial nerve will often be damaged. Also that it is possible to uncover the facial nerve in the mastoid portion of the temporal bone of the cat without damage to nerve function". Devriese adds "Experimental evidence justifies surgery on the facial nerve in a patient: if correctly done, this procedure can be performed on a healthy nerve without damage to its function". There is unintentional irony in this last sentence; it may be excusable to remove a healthy appendix, but healthy facial nerves are not fair surgical game. If they are tampered with, as Devriese shows, they are very liable to be injured.

There is no scientific evidence known to the writer on the question of whether some neuropathies may be aggravated by nerve exposure and decompression. In a great many so-called "entrapment syndromes" (e.g. carpal tunnel syndrome) there is not the slightest doubt that decompression is beneficial. To what extent similar arguments apply to individual facial palsies will be further discussed in the sections on idiopathic and traumatic paralysis.

The final cover of the nerve deserves mention. Amniotic membrane, gold leaf, middle ear mucosa and muscle have all been recommended to protect the decompressed or repaired nerve. Absorbable gelatin sponge soaked in hydrocortisone, or silicone rubber sheeting are contemporary suggestions. Campbell and Luzio (1964) advised on the basis of experimental work that foreign materials should not be used in the intratemporal course of the nerve. The present writer prefers to "encapsulate" the nerve in thrombin and leave it at that. Gibb (1970) suggested wrapping a length of vein round the anastomoses.

On Collier's advice, I forgo the use of BIPP* or any other "strong" chemicals so beloved of otologists trained in the

---

* Bismuth subnitrate and iodoform paste (BPC, 1954).

classical school, whenever facial nerve (or labyrinth, for that matter) are exposed.

INCIDENCE AND AETIOLOGY OF FACIAL PALSIES

The incidence of facial palsies is not known in relation to the population at large. From the literature it might be imagined that it is higher in some geographical areas than in others. El-Ebiary (1971), for instance, studied 580 cases (90 per cent of which were Bell's palsies) all of whom were seen in Alexandria (population 1·5 million) in one year. The following figures are taken from recent publications and serve to show the relative incidence of the various different causes. The discerning reader may also note the apparent bias towards neurology and away from otology in Jepsen's material, and the non-appearance of intratemporal neoplasms in three of the four series. Overall the figures serve to indicate the pattern of work in a Facial Palsy clinic.

TABLE 2

CAUSES DIAGNOSED IN THREE SERIES OF FACIAL PALSIES

	Adour and Swanson (1971)	Groves (1973)	Jepsen (1965)
Bell's (idiopathic)	308	206	149
Skull fracture	12	21	} 39
Surgical trauma	11	39	
Cephalic zoster	36	30	6
Otitis media	9	14	—
Encephalitis	—	—	16
Polyradiculitis	—	—	14
Sarcoidosis	3	14	12
Cerebello-pontine tumour	—	—	12
Chronic lepto-meningitis	—	—	5
Intratemporal neoplasm	—	5	—
Totals	379	329	253
Miscellaneous	24	11	63
Totals	403	340	316

The "miscellaneous" groups include a few cases of each of the following: cardiovascular accident, diabetic neuropathy, mononucleosis, chicken pox, mumps, histocytosis-X, leukaemia, poliomyelitis, multiple sclerosis, periarteritis nodosa, parotid tumours and congenital palsies. Vestibulo-cochlear and facial nerve tumours or neuro-fibrosarcoma have not appeared in these authors' series, and are of course very rare causes of facial paralysis.

Manning and Adour (1972) listed the aetiologies in a series of 61 children with facial paralysis (Table 3).

BELL'S (IDIOPATHIC) FACIAL PALSY

By general acceptance, Bell's name is attached to facial palsies having no detectable cause. Taverner (1955) listed the diagnostic criteria.

(1) Sudden onset of unilateral paralysis.

TABLE 3

DIAGNOSIS IN 61 CHILDREN WITH FACIAL PARALYSIS
(Manning and Adour, 1972).

Diagnosis		Patients (No.)
Bell's palsy		37
Otitis media		6
Birth trauma		5
Histiocytosis-X		2
Skull fracture		2
Known	1	
Probable (traumatic neuroma)	1	
Congenital		2
Hyperogenesis of facial nerve	1	
Otic capsule abnormalities	1	
Herpes zoster cephalicus		1
Varicella		1
Mumps		1
Postimmunization		1
Myxomatosis (probable)		1
Etiologic factor unknown		2

(2) Absence of symptoms or signs of other central nervous, posterior fossa, or ear disease.

(3) Absence of herpetic vesicles.

Today's basic facts about Bell's palsy can be briefly stated:

Aetiology: Unknown.

Prognosis: 80 to 90 per cent of cases recover satisfactorily without treatment.

Treatment: High-dose steriods and/or surgery (decompression). Both potentially hazardous.

The facts are harsh for doctors, but for the patients the news is good. Most of the latter are pleased to opt out of treatment, especially if the doctor cannot say with any confidence that without treatment the outcome will certainly be bad.

Perhaps it is the consequent professional sense of humiliation that directs so much research endeavour and so many surgical adventures. Miller (1967) is less charitable than this, and accuses surgeons of being influenced by pecuniary considerations—though not in Britain where the National Health Service, he suggests, undermines surgical *joie de vivre*. Not much has changed since Ballance and Duel complained that physicians protect their patients from surgeons, and if this is still so today, surgeons must bear the greater blame.

This sad picture has a brighter side as the following discussion will show. Dogmatism, especially about the pathology, is on the wane. Multi-disciplinary teams are at work, and prospective clinical studies with laboratory support are being published.

Pathology

It is quite remarkable to see how the dogma of "ischaemic" paralysis has been carried on from one publication to another. Its origin is obscure and any hard evidence in its support, if it ever existed, is lost in the mists of time, for it is never quoted. One may read that the increased bleeding from the bone around the nerve in decompression operations for Bell's palsy confirms the "vascular" nature of the disorder. In another paper one is informed that the reduced bleeding at operation endorses the ischaemic basis of the aetiology. Many distinguished authors support the hypothesis of primary ischaemia, concede that it is unproven, and then go on eloquently as though it were a fact, undeserving of further doubt or discussion.

Possible causes of primary ischaemia, such as a vasospasm, micro-embolism or thrombosis, do not seem very probable mechanisms to account for the frequency and common severity of Bell's palsy, nor for its incidence, equally in the young as in the elderly. The notion, in effect, proposes an infarct, highly unlikely in an area where collateral circulation is so free as it is in the facial canal. If it be conceded that the blood supply is more precarious in the internal acoustic meatus, clinical evidence of supra-geniculate involvement (reduced lacrimation) ought to be more frequently observed than it is. Philipszoon (1962) noted vestibular disturbances in 11 out of 12 cases of Bell's palsy, but cochlear disorders are seldom if ever coincident. If the site of hypothetical primary ischaemia is to be transposed thus, away from the mastoid segment, the classical "observations" and conclusions so long advanced in support of the "ischaemic" lesion at the classical site cannot be valid.

Secondary ischaemia—that is impaired blood supply—"strangulation"—could account for Bell's palsies. The hypothesis implies that swelling of the nerve (or of its sheath) due to whatever cause obstructs the blood vessels. Veins would be first engorged, giving increased swelling and oedema, while capillary compression would cause tissue anoxia. These secondary changes would only occur within the facial canal which allows only limited space for swelling.

It is usually at this point that the case for surgical decompression is made emphatically, but it is wise to pause and note that the entire fabric is based upon assumptions. Attempts to show that the pressure within the facial canal is in fact increased have not been fruitful. The pathological significance of bulging of the nerve when the sheath is slit is open to question. It is reported that in animals the normal nerve does the same. The fact that injection of saline into the canal in animals, and other techniques of experimental compression, result in facial paralysis is not proof that Bell's palsy is due to nerve compression or ischaemia.

To summarize, the arguments for primary and secondary ischaemia are purely hypothetical. The concept of nerve compression correlates the unique nature and frequency of Bell's palsy with the unique bony constraints of the facial canal, but impairment of blood supply is not an essential element in our theorizing. A "neuritis"—zoster for example—may cause inflammation and swelling of the nerve, and it is widely expected that eventually one or more neurotropic viruses will be identified for what is currently called idiopathic palsy.

Major obstacles in research of this field are the essentially benign nature of the condition, rendering biopsy and autopsy material almost unobtainable, and the fact that Bell's palsy seems to be confined to man. Its transmissibility to monkeys for example (by comparison with poliomyelitis) must presumably be attempted eventually, but will have to wait upon the unlikely and fortuitous availability of autopsy material from a prodromal or very early case.

Histopathology. Biopsy material has been restricted to fragments of sheath and of chorda tympani obtained during decompression operations. Sadé (1965) found no histological abnormalities in portions of nerve sheath in 4 cases. Jongkees (1954) found vascular engorgement of the chorda but no other inflammatory changes. Sadé described inflammatory changes in the chorda in cases of facial palsy associated with myringitis. Blatt and Freeman (1969) also described inflammation as well as axonal degeneration in chorda tissue. They specifically failed to find any vascular changes.

Autopsy material has been of dubious relevance. Fowler (1963) reviewed six earlier autopsy reports and added one of his own, the latter being the only one in which serial temporal bone sections had been made. Inconclusive findings of degenerative and fibrotic changes are listed. One case showed inflammatory changes. The histories of these cases are too fragmentary to establish what would today be acceptable as diagnoses of Bell's palsies. Reddy and his associates (1966) reported the autopsy findings in another case. Again, no certain evidence of inflammation of the nerve was found, but the mastoid air cells were abnormal. The ante-mortem (clinical) diagnosis of Bell's palsy seems open to question.

Operative Findings. Besides the bulging of the nerve when the sheath is split, intraneural haemorrhage, has been occasionally noted. Kettel (1959) commented on the presence of necrotic mastoid air cells in a few of his decompression cases.

One can only agree with Fowler that the paucity of pathological observations on Bell's palsy is a travesty of modern medicine. The practical difficulty of getting the material is too obvious, however, to require further comment.

Virology. The possibility of a virus causation for Bell's palsy has been well recognized since at least the turn of the century. The role of the varicella-zoster virus has received most attention. Pietersen and Caunt (1970) measured antibody titres in sera from 27 patients with facial palsy. Four of these were clinically cases of Ramsay Hunt syndrome, with skin vesicles, and showed the expected raised titres. Only one of the non-herpetic cases showed a significantly raised titre and this was strongly suspected on clinical grounds of homolateral abolished vestibular function. Two other cases with normal titres also had vestibulo-cochlear disturbances. These authors also tested the sera for evidence of influenza A, B and C, adenovirus, and herpes simplex with negative results.

Tomita and his colleagues (1972) found raised zoster titres in 11 out of 44 cases of Bell's palsy. It is of especial interest that 60 per cent of these cases of "zoster sine herpete" had pain, whereas only 10 per cent of the others had this symptom. In three cases only was evidence of herpes simplex found.

Kumagami (1972) reported a series of experiments on rabbits. He innoculated, through the stylomastoid foramen, herpes simplex virus and in 16 of 19 animals facial paralysis with denervation occurred. Five of them developed vestibular disorders. None of these animals developed a serological titre higher than 16, implying that serum complement fixation tests may be of questionable value in our present study. Kumagami also injected other animals with varicella-zoster, adenovirus and influenza virus without causing paralysis. Simplex virus given into the carotid artery, subarachnoid space and tympanic cavity likewise did not cause facial palsies.

Immunology. Coassolo (1952) showed that horse-serum sensitized rabbits are more liable to facial palsy from severe cooling of the face, and McGovern and his colleagues (1972a, b) developed this concept further. They induced facial palsies in horse-sensitized dogs by injection of epinephrine into the facial canal. In control nerves, saline injection produced similar changes, but in non-sensitized dogs the changes were much less marked. The same workers have shown that injection of vasoconstrictors into the nerve outside the canal produces only transient paresis or none at all.

Interpretation of these experiments by the authors is far-reaching, and they conclude "We have come to consider Bell's palsy as a polyneuropathy in which both facial nerves are often involved, although only one side may exhibit the paralysis: also Bell's palsy can have a concomitant trigeminal sensory neuropathy and is sometimes a familial, recurrent or alternating disease which in all suggests that Bell's palsy is a systemic disorder possibly immunologic in nature."

As to the "bilaterality" of Bell's palsy, these remarks are startlingly supported in a paper by Safman (1971). He found electromyographic abnormalities in the contralateral ("normal") side in 14 out of 18 cases studied. If this work is confirmed clinical tests which compare the paralysed with the "normal" side will obviously need re-assessment.

Prognosis of Bell's Palsy

The central issue in this condition is the outcome in untreated cases. The statistical likelihood of complete recovery is variously quoted as between 55 and 90 per cent. All the published figures, however, are based on hospital series and are therefore subject to uncontrollable effects of selection. The time elapsed since onset has a profound effect upon the apparent recovery rate. After the first week, increasingly gloomy results were evident owing to dilution by the severer cases showing no sign of early recovery, and the non-referral of milder cases already improving. This basic truth was identified by Matthews (1961) and has since been emphasized by Groves (1968a) and Campbell (1968).

Another reason for wide variation between untreated series is the fact that some authors for quite valid reasons report denervation rates—denervation however slight (and often insignificant)—while others report unsatisfactory outcome (about 10 per cent of all cases), allowing minor degrees of denervation to be acceptable.

The latter view of Bell's palsy is the practical one upon which considerations of treatment should be based, in view of the potentially hazardous nature of any of the currently available methods of treatment.

We cannot separate these issues of treatment and prognosis unless a completely innocuous and effective treatment becomes available. In that event, of course, every case could be treated and prognostic selection for treatment would be unnecessary. For the present, up to 90 per cent of patients must be protected from unnecessary treatment.

Prognosis and Selection for Treatment in Bell's Palsy

All of the variable aspects of the clinical picture have been scrutinized for prognostic significance and each will now be discussed.

Severity of Paralysis. It is not disputed that incomplete paralysis in the first 5 or 7 days is an absolutely favourable sign. Matthews (1961) pointed out, however, that partial paralysis observed after the first week can be misleading in that it may represent a slight improvement in what was previously a total palsy. Apart from this occasional difficulty, which does not influence decisions about early treatment, one may say with confidence that incomplete palsies will do well. In a personal series, all seen during the first 10 days of onset, he observed that, of 48 cases of incomplete paralysis, only 2 per cent showed denervation and none was dissatisfied with the final result. Of 78 cases of complete paralysis, 36 per cent showed denervation and 6 per cent were dissatisfied (Groves, 1973b).

The incidence of stapedius muscle paralysis was noted (*see* Table 4). If we regard this muscle as just one of the

TABLE 4

IDIOPATHIC FACIAL PARALYSIS: STAPEDIUS REFLEX, TESTED IN 36 CASES WITHIN TEN DAYS OF ONSET

Reflex	*No. of Cases*	*No. with Denervation*
Normal:		
Incomplete palsy	9	0
"Complete" palsy	3	0
Impaired or absent:		
Incomplete palsy	7	0
"Complete" palsy	21	8

many which may or may not be paralysed, rather than as an indication of the level of the lesion, the 3 cases in which "complete" clinical paralysis occurred while the stapedius reflex was retained are of special interest. All recovered without denervation. It is suggested that, in a prognostic sense, paralysis is not complete unless the stapedius is paralysed as well as all the other muscles.

If we exclude from treatment all cases presenting with incomplete paralysis we must consider what is the risk that they may later become complete and denervate badly. Figure 16 is a histogram showing the distribution of the time required to attain maximum paralysis in 97 cases. 44 per cent reached their worst within 48 h, and 84 per cent within 5 days. Figure 17 shows a similar distribution in respect of clinically complete Bell's palsies. One will discern the small proportion (who would thus miss treatment) becoming total after 5 days.

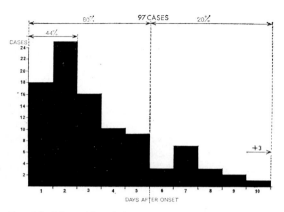

FIG. 16. Idiopathic facial paralysis: attainment of maximum paralysis in 97 cases. (Groves, 1973).

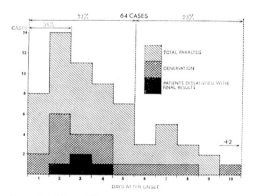

FIG. 17. Idiopathic facial paralysis: attainment of total paralysis in 64 cases. (Groves, 1973).

Nerve excitability thresholds were measured daily (Groves and Gibson, 1974) by the method described by Campbell (1963) and using a 1 millisecond stimulus (Table 5). Total loss of nerve excitability never occurred before

TABLE 5

NERVE EXCITABILITY THRESHOLD DIFFERENCES: DAILY TESTING IN 93 CASES

Nerve Excitability Threshold Differences (mA)	No. Recovered	No. Denervated
2 or more	17	10
3 or more	10	8
4 or more	6	5
5 or more	0	4

Rising threshold difference, 27 cases.
Progression to inexcitability and denervation, 10 cases.
Reversion to normal with complete recovery, 17 cases.

the fourth day. They did not find a "critical difference" of less than 5 mA to be a reliable precursor of denervation. Taking a difference of 3 mA as an indication for treatment, 10 out of 18 would have been treated unnecessarily. A difference of 5 mA was always significant, but was followed always within hours by total inexcitability; in other words, two or three days too late for treatment to prevent denervation. As is predictable on theoretical grounds, this test fails to select cases for early preventive treatment. This conclusion is at variance with earlier more hopeful views about the test as applied to idiopathic palsies.

Pain. Some workers have considered pain to be a sign of a bad prognosis (Kettel, 1959; Sardana *et al.*, 1971; Miehlke, 1973). Others deny any relevance. In the author's own series pain was a symptom in 89 of 119 cases. Table 6 shows that all the cases with bad result had total paralysis

TABLE 6

IDIOPATHIC FACIAL PARALYSIS: INCIDENCE OF PAIN IN 119 CASES

	No. of Cases	Percentage with Denervation	Percentage Dissatisfied
No pain:			
Partial paralysis	16	0	0
Complete paralysis	14	35	0
Pain:			
Partial paralysis	31	10	0
Complete paralysis	58	40	12

and pain. Severity of pain has been noted in the case records of 30 patients: of the 19 with slight pain one showed denervation and none was dissatisfied: of 11 with severe pain 7 showed denervation and 4 were dissatisfied. It would seem as if slight pain may be disregarded but that severe pain is a serious warning of denervation.

Hypogeusia. Interest in taste impairment has revived with the widespread use of electrogustometry, and the apparent correlation between ELG threshold differences and incidence of denervation. (Peiris and Miles, 1965; Taverner *et al.*, 1966). These workers did not however, publish results of repeated daily testing. Krarup's earlier observations that ELG thresholds are abnormal in 100 per cent of early Bell's palsies suggested that normal taste most probably represents restitution of function, not non-involvement, of the taste fibres. If taste involvement is to be considered as a prognostic sign, its measurable severity, and its duration must be studied.

Groves (1973a) and Groves and Gibson (1974) confirmed that virtually all cases presenting on the first day of paralysis have taste involvement, either subjectively, to salt and sugar testing, or to ELG. The incidence of taste involvement by any of these modes, or by ELG alone diminishes slowly in the first week, and markedly during the second week. Recovery of taste commonly precedes recovery of motor function and if it occurs within the first 8–10 days is a good prognostic sign. In Fig. 18, the duration of hypogeusia is related to denervation and the outcome of the palsy.

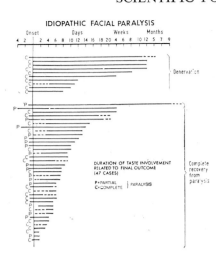

Fig. 18. Idiopathic facial paralysis: duration of taste involvement related to final outcome in 47 cases P = partial paralysis. C = complete paralysis. (Groves, 1973.)

The mere fact of taste involvement cannot, obviously, help in selection of cases for treatment in the earliest stages. The ELG threshold differences are the only available quantitative guide to the *severity* of taste fibre involvement and, in 46 cases, Groves and Gibson found that 4 out of 5 who had motor denervation had a threshold difference during the first week of 100 μA or more. Selection on this basis would have spared 72 per cent of the whole series from unnecessary treatment.

Lacrimation

Diminished or absent tear formation does not appear to have received as much attention as the other features mentioned above. This is unfortunate because the obligation to treat selected cases with steroids is now so strong that it is no longer ethical to study prospectively a wholly unselected and untreated series of cases. Fragmentary but statistically inadequate data suggest a poorer prognosis if lacrimation is impaired.

Submandibular Salivation

Blatt (1965) held that, if secretion on the involved side is 40 per cent or more of the normal side, full recovery can be expected. Ten per cent or less, he stated, required immediate decompression. May and Hawkins (1972) reported that 25 per cent or lower values gave an indication of poor prognosis earlier than nerve excitability tests.

Other Factors

It is generally agreed that denervation is more frequent and more severe in the elderly. Hypertension and diabetes are similarly adverse. Several writers have commented on the apparently poorer outcome in cases of recurrent or alternating palsy.

Summarizing the factors influencing prognosis and selection for treatment, it can certainly be said that partial palsies require no treatment. By no means all complete Bell's palsies need be treated; those with stapedius paralysis are more complete than the others in a valid prognostic sense. In total paralysis, *severe* pain and an ELG threshold difference of over 100 μA in the first week should each be seriously regarded as demanding treatment. ELG gives perhaps the most absolute indication if the patient's responses are consistent. Reduced submandibular salivary flow—certainly below 10 per cent, and possibly 25 per cent—must be taken seriously, but clinical judgement is still required to evaluate these many factors, one beside another. Impaired lacrimation and advanced age are of possible significance but by themselves do not firmly indicate a poor prognosis.

The aim is of course to identify within 24–48 h of onset those patients likely to have a poor recovery, and allow the majority to be spared unnecessary steroid therapy or (in some centres) decompression.

Treatment of Bell's Palsy

Intensive vasodilator therapy, including stellate ganglion block, has lost ground in recent years, no doubt because of the increasing polarisation of ideas between the extremes of steroid therapy and decompression surgery. Stellate block, urged by Swan (1952) and by Korkis (1961), does not satisfy the more critically-minded and sophisticated clinician of today. In a controlled trial, Fearnley and his colleagues (1964) observed no benefit from the treatment.

Hilger (1965) urges a aggressive medical regime, including procaine and nicotinic acid by intravenous drip, repeated 3 or 4 times daily, together with oral or intravenous steroids. He gives no results to substantiate these recommendation, and, although such treatment is widely used in some countries, there is no published evidence known to the present writer to show that it is beneficial.

Steroid Therapy

It has been widely assumed that steroid therapy is appropriate in Bell's palsy, and for some years cortisone derivatives have been given, usually in small dosage, without satisfactory evidence in favour. It is disturbing to note the unqualified statements of some drug manufacturers in this connection.

For a period of 20 years Taverner and his colleagues have sought to establish scientifically in controlled trials the efficacy or otherwise of steroid therapy. A trial by Taverner (1954) in which early cases treated with cortisone by mouth were compared with untreated randomly selected control cases showed no difference in the incidence of denervation in the two groups. He and his associates then went on to investigate the effect of ACTH gel injections (Taverner *et al.*, 1966, 1967), first in a controlled sequential analysis trial which failed to reach statistical significance, and then in a large series (383 cases) in which the overall final incidence of denervation was 13 per cent. Concurrent controls were not used, however, and the author compared his results with earlier series of untreated cases, unfortunately not similarly selected. The statistical presentation of this clinical trial has been criticized by Campbell (1968), by Groves (1968a, b), by Weiss (1968) and by Drachman (1969). The correct criteria in studies of treatment in Bell's palsy were clearly defined by Matthews (1961) who wrote "Most forms of treatment advocated for Bell's palsy are not based on satisfactory evidence. Control series in the assessment of any treatment must be matched for age, degree of paralysis and interval since the onset within quite narrow limits." Nevertheless, many embraced ACTH therapy as "the most important advance in the therapy of Bell's palsy" (Miller, 1967). The author's view is that the value of ACTH has not been satisfactorily demonstrated.

More recently, Taverner and his associates (1971) have compared the effects of intramuscular ACTH with oral prednisolone in 186 successive cases of Bell's palsy who were allocated at random to one or the other therapy. They concluded from a comparison of the results that oral prednisolone is the treatment of choice. The dose was 222 μmol daily in divided doses for 5 days, followed by a diminishing dose schedule for a further 4 days. They further concluded that the trial of oral cortisone in 1954 had been inadequate because of low dosage, starting treatment too late, and small numbers of patients. In this latest work the authors have scrupulously matched the comparability of the clinical material in the two groups of cases and their conclusion that prednisolone gave better results than ACTH, appears statistically unassailable. The brief and disputed vogue for ACTH in Bell's palsy must now surely be ended.

Given that high dose steroid therapy, commenced preferably within the first 2 days of the disease, appears to be beneficial, there remain decisions which must still be matters of clinical judgement. One may elect to treat all cases, discounting the possibility of side effects, or one may consider for treatment only cases with a bad prognosis based upon the criteria in the preceding section. Whereas the benefit of steroids was demonstrated when commenced in the first 4 days, it will often be necessary to consider starting treatment in cases presenting later. It is not known whether or not steroids will help if begun in the second or third week.

A final question remains, that of recognizing and evaluating contraindications. Very early pregnancy is the most difficult and potentially most serious, but tuberculosis, diabetes, hypertension, psychosis, epilepsy, cardiac conditions, concomitant infections, and peptic ulcer all require exclusion.

Decompression

The history of facial nerve decompression for Bell's palsy starts with Ballance and Duel, and relates to exposure of the mastoid segment from the stylomastoid foramen up to the lateral semicircular canal. In this format the operation stands indicated as of unproven value and potentially harmful. In former times it was performed only in late cases, and successes claimed for operations done at 12 weeks after onset of paralysis took no account of the natural history of Bell's palsy.

More recently the operation has, rightly, been put to the test as an *early* treatment, to determine whether it could improve results when performed immediately nerve excitability showed the probability of denervation. Groves (1965), reporting a "pilot" trial based on these principles, expressed serious doubts of the efficacy of surgery.

In pursuit of unscientific enthusiasm a large body of opinion has persisted in the advocacy of decompression, on the terms that aggressive treatment must be seen to be given. Operation has enjoyed unmerited encouragement from the spontaneous recovery which would happen in any case. Prominent authorities have urged surgery without sound logic, while conceding error in their views and policies of only yesterday or the day before. It is irrelevant to speculate about the nature or level of the lesion when we do not even know the aetiology. The only thing that matters is whether surgery can be beneficial. This too is not known, and the only justification for surgery lies in a planned, controlled experiment based ethically upon full explanations to the patients that an operation in Bell's palsy is only an investigation, without established therapeutic value. Such explanations must not be weighted by unfairly biased accounts of the prognosis without surgery. On reading "the indication for surgery was a relative one . . . to establish whether exposure of the nerve could influence in a positive way the regeneration of nerve fibres" one might imagine that an experimental animal lay upon the table, or that the surgical procedure was a minor one.

Properly controlled ethical trials of decompression have been reported by Mechelse and his colleagues (1971), and by May and Hawkins (1972). Both teams concluded that the conventional operation done promptly on the basis of lost nerve excitability showed no benefit. Adour and Swanson (1971) reached the same conclusion. Alford and his colleagues (1971) observed better results in cases decompressed, but nonetheless they emphasized that legitimate problems of selection remained unsolved.

Current efforts are exemplarized by May and Hawkins who performed decompressions with apparent benefit *before* the loss of nerve excitability, with selection based upon impaired salivary flow. Fisch and Esslen (1972) and others practice total exposure of the nerve from the internal meatus to the stylomastoid foramen, but as yet there appears to be no proof that this major intervention improves the statistical prognosis. The observation by Fisch of swelling and conduction block of the supragenicular part of the nerve is of enormous interest (Fig. 19) but we are discussing treatment, and to observe, even to "decompress", is not necessarily to cure.

A few authors have mentioned mishaps in facial nerve decompressions, quite apart from the obvious possibility that the nerve itself could be damaged. The writer has knowledge of a "dead" ear due to injury of the lateral canal. Multanen and Holopainen (1963) and others experienced accidental injuries to the ossicular chain. Olson and his colleagues (1973) refer to cochlear and vestibular sequelae in some cases. The natural hazards of surgery, and, in "total nerve exposures", of craniotomy, must further be measured against the overall good prognosis of Bell's palsy.

processing should clarify and standardized the management of these cases, but in a perfect world there would be no traumatic facial palsies anyway. As we must try to cope with the conditions of the moment, we must abandon philosophy and resort to rules of thumb, striving for consistency and logic as best we may.

Facial Palsy Complicating Head Injury

As far as we can know paralysis only occurs if there is a temporal bone fracture. Almost always there will be clinical evidence of damage to the middle or the internal ear besides the facial paralysis. There may be no radiological evidence of the fracture, and this part of the assessment depends largely upon the standards of radiographic technique available. The routine skull X-rays usually taken in emergency conditions are not adequate for the temporal bone. Lateral oblique mastoid films, and Stenver's views are essential when a fracture is suspected on clinical grounds. In the presence of a facial palsy only the highest quality tomography (anterior-posterior and lateral) is acceptable. Polytomography can define a fracture not visible by other means. The effort to define the precise relationship of a fracture to the line of the facial canal is all too often unrewarding; this is not too surprising when the described operative findings of a minute bony spicule pressing marginally upon the nerve are recalled. It must be admitted that clinical considerations are paramount and the X-ray findings, however interesting, offer little assistance in either prognosis or localization of the site of nerve injury.

Prognosis. Facial palsy is a rare complication of head injury according to the figures of Fleischer and Nockemann (1962), who reported 77 cases in 5047 patients with skull fracture. Eight of these cases had bilateral palsies. Sixty-eight patients were followed up and 46 (68 per cent) had recovered completely. Fourteen (21 per cent) had partial recovery, whilst 8 (12 per cent) did not recover at all. The 9 cases lost to follow up might or might not have altered somewhat the percentages given, but could not have altered the overall picture.

Turner (1944) observed 70 cases, reporting that of 36 with immediate palsy 75 per cent recovered completely. In 34 cases, palsy was delayed in onset and of these only 2 (less than 6 per cent) failed to recover completely. In a series of 23 cases, Groves (1973a) noted that, in delayed onset (11 palsies), and in immediate onset of incomplete palsy (4 cases), eventual recovery without surgery was always satisfactory. In 8 complete palsies of immediate onset the eventual outcome was unsatisfactory in 5, despite surgical exploration in 4 of them. Published data of this kind point clearly to an overall policy of conservatism, combined with energetic observation with a view to early recognition of the minority of cases with a poor prognosis. This process of selection, as in Bell's palsy, is worthwhile if it leads to valid prophylaxis or treatment.

If the preceding figures are representative, only 1·5 per cent of cases with skull fracture will develop facial palsy, and, of these, between 6 and 12 per cent (say 0·002 per cent of all cases of skull fracture) will eventually make an unsatisfactory recovery. Such calculations are very rough

but, even if there is an error of 10 times, only 1 in 50 skull fracture patients are at risk of this complication. It is unrealistic therefore to demand that otological assessment and observation should be invoked in every case. Such a view is confirmed by the figures of Briggs and Potter (1967) who found that, in 5000 consecutive admissions for head injury, only 70 patients had clinical evidence of temporal bone fracture. Twenty seven of the latter developed a delayed facial palsy.

Protocol for head injury managment should obviously therefore excuse the otologist unless there is bleeding from the ear, haemotympanum, apparent deafness, nystagmus and/or vertigo, facial weakness, or radiological evidence of temporal bone fracture. Any one of these manifestations should result in prompt consultation. Unfortunately they are commonly not sought or noted, let alone acted upon.

Management. The papers of Briggs and Potter (1967, 1971) show the possible value of early recognition of temporal bone fracture. These workers gave prophylactic treatment with ACTH to a series of cases with bleeding from an ear combined with X-ray evidence of fracture. They observed a significant reduction in the incidence of delayed facial palsy as compared to a retrospective untreated control group. It must be noted that this retrospective comparison is less convincing than a trial with concurrent control cases, identically investigated, would have been. The authors themselves summarized their work as follows: "Despite this demonstration of the effectiveness of corticotrophin in reducing the incidence of delayed post-traumatic facial weakness, we are not convinced that such prophylactic treatment need always be adopted as routine practice; for it is not entirely innocuous. Most patients who do develop this complication of head injury will recover completely, or to an acceptable degree, from their facial weakness without treatment, so the overall value of prophylaxis is relatively slight."

Early cases with known or suspected temporal bone fracture should certainly be observed at daily or twice daily intervals for any evidence of facial weakness. Cases in prolonged coma can be tested daily for nerve excitability threshold changes (Jongkees, 1965; Miehlke, 1973). Cases with total palsy of immediate onset who have lost nerve excitability should have electromyography in search of residual normal motor units. (The increasing portability of the equipment will bring this test to the bedside of the very ill or comatose patient.)

Preservation of taste, salivary flow (the technetium scan test is objective, safe and easy to perform), or lacrimation must be carefully interpreted, whether as indicators of level or severity of nerve injury. Loss of any these functions indicates a severe lesion at or above the origin of the nerve branch in question.

Any favourable observation drawn from the foregoing scheme should be accepted as supporting conservative management. In cases of doubt, the early use of corticosteroids such as dexamethasone, or of ACTH should be seriously considered. If every prognostic sign is bad, and especially if EMG reveals no motor unit action potentials, high doses of steroids should be commenced and surgical exploration undertaken as soon as the patient is fit for operation. However desirable it may be in theory to repair the lesion as soon as possible, it is scarcely conceivable that prudent management will precede actual denervation. If the nerve is severed nothing can prevent denervation. A delay of two or three weeks can therefore rarely be disadvantageous. If this time is utilized for precise topognosis of the likely level of the lesion, steroid therapy, repeated electrical tests and tomography, some unnecessary surgery will be avoided, and planning of actual operations can be more precise. Above all, proper assessment of middle and of internal ear function can be made. It is irresponsible to embark upon a serious facial nerve exploration without foreknowledge of the functional state of the hearing.

Scope of Surgery. If cochlear function has been totally destroyed by the injury, transmastoid exposure of the nerve can be extended by the translabyrinthine route if it is necessary to reach a supragenicular lesion. Total nerve exposure, with intact canal wall, and without craniotomy is perfectly feasible.

If cochlear function is normal and a conductive hearing loss is present posterior tympanotomy allows correction of an ossicular chain lesion as well as nerve exposure to the genicular level. For a supragenicular lesion, the middle fossa approach will have to be used but unless preoperative assessment has been very positive for the "high" lesion it seems prudent to explore the tympanic and mastoid sections first. Perhaps the majority of otologists, not trained in, or lacking facilities for, the middle fossa operation would need to transfer cases to suitable centres for the rare occasions when this technique is required.

Operation findings described in the literature include all degrees of contusion of the sheath and of the nerve, crushing, and even severance, of some or all fibres at a fracture site. Numerous instances of very small bone fragments driven into the nerve have been noted. Recent accounts (Miehlke, 1973; Fisch, 1969) would suggest that the genicular and supragenicular levels are often the site of injury. If this is confirmed the disappointing and negative transmastoid explorations of the past could be accounted for—we all have looked in the wrong places for the lesion. In successful cases, classical decompressions have been irrelevant, whilst "failures" of decompression have in fact been failures to look in the right place for torn nerves.

Nerve Repair. Decompression of the site of injury, removal of bone spicules, and, with total loss of continuity, autogenous nerve grafting have been performed at all levels, including the internal acoustic meatus. In this area a torn nerve can sometimes be sutured after excision of the genicular ganglion which allows approximation in some cases. Both Fisch and Miehlke advise ganglionectomy in these circumstances, believing that otherwise some regenerating axons are diverted from the face, wastefully along the greater petrosal nerve (Figs. 20, 21, 22).

Facial Palsy Complicating Middle Ear Surgery

The overall incidence of iatrogenic facial palsy can only be guessed at. Zuehlke (1956) noted 1·6 per cent facial nerve injuries in 1171 first operations on the ear. In repeat operations 8 of 72 (11·1 per cent) developed paralysis.

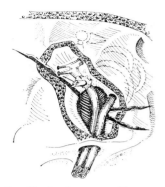

FIG. 20. Impingement of bone in intralabyrinthine course of facial nerve. (Miehlke, 1973.)

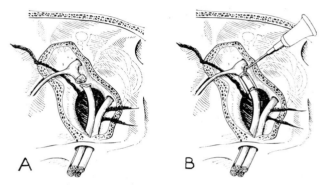

FIG. 21. Complete division of facial nerve in its intralabyrinthine course. (B) Repair of nerve by use of autogenous free graft. Collagenous cylinder is used to cover graft sites, over which Histacryl adhesive is used to seal anastomosis. (Miehlke, 1973.)

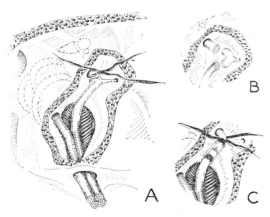

FIG. 22. Division of genicular ganglion, following fracture of base of skull. (B) Extirpation of geniculate ganglion. (C) Rerouting of facial nerve. Note collagenous cylinders covering nerve reanastomosis, as well as deliberate lysis of greater superficial petrosal nerve at ganglion. (Miehlke, 1973.)

Miehlke (1973) states that, in Germany at the present time, less than 1 per cent of ear operations are complicated by facial nerve injury. One may reasonably suppose that most of the cases occur in operations for cholesteatoma, especially when, during the posterior tympanotomy approach, the surgeon is "sailing close to the wind".

When the epitympanic recess (attic) is filled with granulation tissue, or cholesteatoma, the position of the nerve cannot be seen, nor can it be known whether it still has the protection of its bony canal. In this situation, the medial bony wall recess must be followed forwards from the lateral semicircular canal. As the diseased tissue is raised from the bone the horizontal part of the nerve comes into view. This stage is crucial because, if the bony covering has been destroyed, the nerve sheath is vulnerable, and it has been known to be removed, complete with the nerve, in the mass of diseased tissues.

To avoid damage to the nerve in the radical operation, no curettage is permissible in front of the plane of the lateral canal. Bone under the drill must be kept cool by irrigation. In the final lowering of the posterior meatal wall, sometimes regarded by the novice with apprehension, the risk to the nerve is small. By this time the landmarks are clearly defined. Provided that all bone cutting is parallel to the line of the nerve, a well-sculpted cavity can safely be made.

Ultrasonic treatment of Ménière's disease is a potential hazard but James (1969) reported only 1 (transient) palsy in 234 cases.

Permeatal operations may be complicated by facial palsy in the following ways:

(1) Diffusion of local anaesthetic from the external acoustic meatus. Such palsies recover completely within hours.

(2) Backward displacement of a wedge of bone during curettage of the postero-superior meatal wall and tympanic annulus. This may compress the nerve directly, or indirectly, by causing bleeding within the canal.

(3) Above the oval window the nerve should be safe during ordinary procedures on the stapes. "Drill-out" operations in obliterative otosclerosis or congenital abnormalities of the oval window are specially hazardous, however. Great care must be taken in cases where the nerve has no bony covering and overhangs the oval window niche.

The removal of bony hyperostoses of the deep meatal canal has been a cause of paralysis, due to a surgical fracture running backwards and medially from the point of impact of the gouge. This operation is much safer with modern burrs and magnification.

Unduly tight packing of mastoid cavities should be avoided. Indeed it is quite illogical to pack them at all, beyond the lightest dressing needed to hold meatal skin flaps in position.

In concluding any ear operation, as Dixon (1973) wisely observed, one should deliberately expose and inspect any possibly damaged section of facial nerve. In certain cases it is thus possible to decide at the first operation that the nerve is intact though perhaps bruised, and that, should facial palsy occur postoperatively, the correct treatment is conservative. Thus the need for, and worry about, further exploration might sometimes be avoided.

Management. As in other post-traumatic palsies, the aim of management is first to select those cases in whom gross nerve continuity has been destroyed. These cases have total palsy of immediate onset, and will not recover without surgery.

Incomplete palsies, and those of delayed onset, recover satisfactorily in most cases without specific treatment. The writer's own series (*see* Table 7) agrees with the general view that only complete palsies of immediate onset are likely to have a poor end result.

TABLE 7
POSTOPERATIVE FACIAL PARALYSIS: 39 CASES

	No. of Cases	Denervated	Dissatisfied
Delayed incomplete	6	1	0
Delayed complete	1	1	0
Immediate incomplete	5	2	0
Immediate complete	27	27*	7

* 6 cases were grafted, of which 3 remained dissatisfied.

In such cases, if electromyography shows any residual motor units, high dose steroid therapy (e.g. dexamethasone 10 μmol 8-hourly, "tapering" to conclude at 10 days) should be given. This policy is particularly appropriate if the nerve was reliably seen to be in gross continuity by an experienced surgeon at the end of the operation.

If there was real doubt about the integrity of the nerve at operation, or if EMG shows no motor units, a second operation must be faced, even if this means dismantling a tympanoplastic reconstruction, or disturbing a freshly stapedectomized ear. The timing of nerve exploration must depend on individual circumstances. To rush the half-anaesthetized patient back to the theatre merely adds bad judgement and policy to previous technical error or misfortune. The possibility of preventing denervation is very slight, if it exists at all. If the nerve is severed, there is no hurry whatsoever. In all circumstances the patient is entitled to a "breathing-space" of at least a few days, meticulous investigation and prognosis, full explanations, and a *planned* operation on the nerve, if any proves necessary.

Delayed paralysis, as already stated, does not require aggressive treatment, but some points of interest must be mentioned. Numerous authors (e.g. Collier, Jongkees and Kettell) have quoted cases in which later exploration revealed a totally severed nerve. Evidently "delayed onset" may be a figment of imagination—due to wishful thinking, or faulty observation. Facial movements must be observed and recorded *by the surgeon* at the end of the operation.

Occasionally, delayed post-operative palsies are associated with pain, and/or tenderness of the infratemporal course of the nerve. These findings, suggestive of coincidental Bell's palsy, are enough to exonerate direct nerve injury. As suggested previously, it is interesting to speculate on the possibility of traumatic activation of latent herpes in such a situation.

Management of Late Cases. Clinical and electrodiagnostic studies will usually indicate whether re-innervation is probable. It is not justifiable to intervene surgically in a case offered more than say 6–8 weeks after injury. Rather, myography should be repeated during the fourth month, by which time polyphasic (recovery) motor unit potentials may be detected. If paralysis remains total, and there is no electrical evidence of recovery at this time, the nerve should be explored. Though it is clearly desirable that nerve repair be done early whenever the indications are firm, nerve grafting gives acceptable results in these later circumstances (see Table 8). It should also be realized that

TABLE 8

FACIAL PARALYSIS: RESULTS OF NERVE GRAFTING.
ROYAL FREE HOSPITAL, 28 CASES

Time Elapsed Before Grafting	Outcome	
	Good or Fair	Poor or Nil
< 1 month	4	2
1–3 months	6	1
3–12 months	11	1
> 12 months	0	3

cases which recover spontaneously usually have a better result than is obtainable by nerve grafting. It is, furthermore, far from obvious in every case at operation whether a swollen nerve is capable of recovery. To resect and graft a nerve which could have recovered spontaneously is as bad an error as to leave in situ a mass of scar tissue through which new axons can never penetrate.

FACIAL PARALYSIS IN OTITIS MEDIA

Otogenic facial palsy has become rare since the advent of antibiotics, with the earlier detection of cholesteatoma and with the virtual extinction, at least in "developed" countries, of tuberculous otitis media. A satisfactory, but somewhat unsettling position has been reached in which a coincidental idiopathic (Bell's) palsy is more than an academic possibility in a patient presenting with otitis media and a facial weakness. This possible coincidence places a high premium upon the most painstaking correlation of history of onset of each of the two conditions. Mistaken conclusions can result in high-dose steroid therapy being given (with denial of antibiotics and/or essential operation). They can, at the other extreme, lead to unnecessary surgery on a perfectly safe ear which is quite irrelevant to the management of Bell's palsy.

Whenever doubt exists, expert otological assessment must be urgently obtained. Microscopical and audiometrical examinations of the ear should precede any decisions as to treatment. In some cases temporal bone X-rays and tomography will be required. Over and above other considerations, the utmost suspicion should be entertained about any facial palsy which, unlike Bell's, begins insidiously and develops gradually.

A diagnostic problem observed on several occasions by the author is facial palsy complicating unilateral (i.e. in children, non-symptomatic) secretory otitis media. The children were considered to have idiopathic palsies, until

otoscopy revealed suspicious-looking drums, and myringotomy yielded "glue". Facial nerve recovery promptly followed in all cases.

Management. In acute otitis, with or without mastoiditis, antibiotics and myringotomy are essential. Cortical mastoidectomy is indicated if clinical response is not rapid. The classical operation is adequate and there is no need to explore the nerve itself.

In chronic otitis media with facial palsy, cholesteatoma is usually responsible. Without treatment total interruption of nerve continuity is certain to occur. Early treatment may avert degeneration of nerve fibres. Late treatment may facilitate spontaneous regeneration. Too late treatment may still permit successful nerve grafting, but the results can never be as good as the recovery obtained when the nerve has been preserved by timely operation.

As soon as the cause of the paralysis is recognized the ear must be surgically explored and the appropriate procedure for eradicating the disease and making the ear safe must be completed. The lesion of the nerve is most likely to be in the horizontal (tympanic) portion and cholesteatoma or granulation tissue must be most carefully examined and removed from this region. Nerve sheath exposed by disease is gently defined under the microscope and necrotic bone edges are lifted away from it. If the bony covering is intact here, and there is extensive disease in the mastoid, then the vertical portion of the nerve must be approached and, if necessary, exposed. If any swelling or abnormality of the nerve sheath is found, the bony canal should be opened proximally and distally until healthy nerve sheath is exposed in both directions.

In early cases, and especially if pre-operative assessment showed incomplete paralysis or a mere neurapraxia, no more need be done. Whenever possible in the presence of infection it is preferable not to open the nerve sheath because infection is liable to result in intraneural fibrosis with a consequently poor functional result.

In cases of complete paralysis with electrical evidence of gross degeneration, it may be necessary to explore the nerve from the stylomastoid foramen to the genicular ganglion, and to open the sheath freely from below upwards until the entire problem can be exposed and assessed. Unless this is done, the possible need for insertion of a nerve graft may be overlooked. In a neglected case the gross continuity of the nerve may be destroyed, and in a mass of fibrous tissue there is no chance of spontaneous regeneration. Usually, because of the extent of disease in the middle ear, considerations of preservation of hearing do not hinder the surgeon. The ossicular chain is not worth preserving, and the nerve can be followed as far forward as the geniculum.

Decisions as to whether or not to open the nerve sheath, or to excise and graft a segment, or merely to "decompress" can be difficult. Except in very early cases and in cases with partial paralysis, it is most unwise to embark upon operation without the most careful electrodiagnostic assessment beforehand. Correlation of the information thus obtained with the appearances found at operation can often resolve the surgeon's dilemma of whether to go on or leave off at a given stage of exploration.

FACIAL PALSY DUE TO INTRA-TEMPORAL TUMOURS

Though a rare clinical manifestation, facial palsy may be caused by a wide variety of erosive "tumours"—true neoplasms and the so-called primary epidermoid cyst.

The common feature of most such cases is the insidious onset of facial weakness quite unlike the dramatic suddenness of Bell's palsy. Associated symptoms and signs of middle ear or labyrinth involvement may be evident on otoscopy, audiometry and tomography. Neurological examination may reveal evidence of posterior fossa or brainstem disorder, and in some cases lumbar puncture, air encephalography, or positive contrast (e.g. iofendylate) studies may be called for. In the differential diagnosis it is essential to realize that idiopathic palsies:

(1) Do *not* develop gradually.

(2) Are *not* associated with other otological or neurological disturbances.

(3) Invariably show *some* degree of spontaneous recovery, however imperfect, after 3–4 months at the latest.

Any case not conforming strictly to such criteria requires the most rigorous re-investigation. Many surgeons would urge that such untypical cases should have the nerve surgically explored as a diagnostic procedure in any case. This policy seems rational, provided that it is fairly certain that the lesion is in the temporal bone. Obviously great care is necessary to avoid a futile transmastoid procedure in cases where the lesion is retrolabyrinthine, in the internal meatus, cerebellopontine angle, or brainstem.

Any polypus or suspicious-looking granulations of the deep meatus or middle ear should be (cautiously) biopsied. Some tumours may be suspected behind an intact tympanic membrane by observation of redness or bulging, and permeatal tympanotomy may be necessary for final diagnosis.

Valuable reviews of these rare clinical problems have been published by Kettel (1959), who has discussed them from the facial nerve aspect, and by Fairman (1971) whose account of neoplasms of the middle ear is more broadly orientated. The otologist will be on his guard in any case of persistent or recurrent facial palsy. The patient's real danger lies in the insidiously undramatic course of his disease which all too often fails to evoke specialized investigation of the ear and temporal bone. Two of the present author's cases of middle ear carcinoma had been sent on by electrodiagnostician colleagues, as a direct result of their taking a history and looking inside the ear, before undertaking the electrical tests for which the patients had been innocently referred as "Bell's palsies".

Malignant tumours include primary and secondary carcinomas. Primary growth may be of the middle or external ear, usually squamous-cell in type. Occasional adenocarcinoma has been reported. Mesodermal tumours rarely reported are rhabdomyosarcoma, and neurofibrosarcoma.

"Benign" tumours described are chemodectoma (both tympanic and jugulare types), haemangioma, and schwannoma (neurinoma; neurofibroma) of facial or vestibulocochlear nerve.

In all these cases, and in the non-neoplastic "tumours" such as Wegner's granuloma, eosinophilic granuloma, and, most commonly, epidermoid cyst, the treatment is always that of the disease; the facial nerve is of secondary importance. In some carcinomas, for instance, successful radiotherapy may permit some degree of spontaneous facial recovery. If the nerve is irretrievably lost, and the causative disease cured or curable, then surgical nerve repair or plastic surgical rehabilitation can be usefully undertaken along the lines discussed earlier in this chapter.

REFERENCES

Adour, K. K. and Swanson, P. J. (1971), *Trans. Amer. Acad. Ophthal. Otolaryng.*, **75**, 1284.

Alford, B. R., Jerger, J. F., Coats, A. C., Peterson, C. R. and Weber, S. C. (1973), *Arch. Otolaryng.*, **97**, 214.

Alford, B. R., Sessions, R. B. and Weber, S. C. (1971), *Laryngoscope*, **81**, 620.

Anson, B. J. and Donaldson, J. A. (1973), *Surgical Anatomy of the Temporal Bone*, 2nd edition. Philadelphia: Saunders.

Anson, B. J., Donaldson, J. A., Warpeha, R. L., Rensink, M. J. and Shilling, B. B. (1973), *Arch. Otolaryng.*, **97**, 201.

Ballance, C. and Duel, A. B. (1932), *Arch. Otolaryng.*, **15**, 1–70.

Bernard, A. M., Durraffour, R., Mounier Kuhn, P. and Gaillard, J. (1972), *J. Françvoto-Rhino-Laryng.*, **21**, 416.

Blackley, B., Friedmann, I. and Wright, I. (1967), *Acta oto-laryng.*, **63**, 533.

Blatt, I. M. (1965), *Laryngoscope*, **75**, 1081.

Blatt, I. M. and Freeman, J. A. (1969), *Trans. Amer. Acad. Ophthal. Otolaryng.*, **73**, 420.

Blunt, M. J. (1954), *J. Anat (Lond.)*, **88**, 520.

Bowden, R. E. M. (1964), *Roy. dent. Hosp. Mag.*, **1**, 1.

Bowden, R. E. M. and Mahran, Z. Y. (1956), *J. Anat. (Lond.)*, **90**, 217.

Bowden, R. E. M. and Mahran, Z. Y. (1960), *J. Anat. (Lond.)*, **94**, 375.

Bowden, R. E. M., Mahran, Z. Y. and Gooding, M. R. (1960), *Proc. zool. Soc. Lond.*, **135**, 587.

Briggs, M. and Potter, J. M. (1967), *Brit. med. J.*, **2**, 464.

Briggs, M. and Potter, J. M. (1971), *Brit. med. J.*, **3**, 458.

Bruusgaard, E. (1932), *Brit. J. Derm.*, **44**, 1.

Bull, T. R. (1965), *J. Laryng.*, **79**, 479–493.

Campbell, E. D. R. (1963), *J. Laryng.*, **77**, 462.

Campbell, E. D. R. (1968), *Brit. med. J.*, **1**, 561.

Campbell, J. B. and Luzio, J. (1964), *Trans. Amer. Acad. Ophthal. Otolaryng.*, **68**, 1068.

Coassolo, M. (1952), *Minerva Otorinolaring.*, **2**, 444.

Collier, J. (1940), *Lancet*, **ii**, 91.

Collier, J. (1941), *Proc. roy. Soc. Med.*, **34**, 35.

Collier, J. (1949), *Am. Otol.*, **58**, 686.

Collier, D. J. (1950), *Proc. roy. Soc. Med.*, **43**, 746.

Collier, J. (1955), *Proc. roy. Soc. Med.*, **48**, 1.

Costen, J. B., Clare, M. H. and Bishop, G. H. (1951), *Ann. Otol.*, **60**, 591.

Denny-Brown, D., Adams, R. D. and Fitzgerald, P. J. (1944), **51**, 216.

Devriese, P. P. (1972), *Arch. Otolaryng.*, **95**, 350.

Dixon, J. W. (1973), *Proc. roy. Soc. Med.*, **66**, 558.

Drachman, D. A. (1969), *Arch. Otolaryng.*, **89**, 147.

Eaglstein, W. H., Katz, R. and Brown, J. A. (1970), *J.A.M.A.*, **211**, 1681.

El-Ebiary, H. M. (1971), *Rheum. phys. Med.*, **11**, 100.

Elliott, F. A. (1964), *Lancet*, **ii**, 610.

Erb, W. H. (1876), *Cyclopaedia of the Practice of Medicine*, Vol. 2 (H. von Ziemssen, Ed.). Translated by R. H. Fitz, C. P. Putman and others. New York: W. Ward & Co.

Fairman, H. D. (1971), *Scott-Brown's Diseases of the Ear, Nose and Throat*, 3rd edition, Vol. 2. London: Butterworths.

Fearnley, M. E., Rainer, E. H., Taverner, R. D., Boyle, T. M. and Miles, D. W. (1964), *Lancet*, **2**, 725.

Fisch, U. (1969), *Disorders of the Skull Base Region* (C. Hamberger and J. Wersäll, Eds.). Stockholm: Almqvist and Wiksell.

Fisch, U. and Esslen, E. (1972), *Arch. Otolaryng.*, **95**, 335.

Fleischer, H. and Nockemann, P. F. (1962), *Arch. klin. Chir.*, **302**, 60.

Flourens (1842), *Recherches expérimentales sur les propriétés et les fonctions dy système nerveux dans les animaux vertébrés*, 2nd edition. Paris: Baillière.

Fons, M. and Osterhammel, P. A. (1968), *J. Laryng.*, **82**, 85.

Fowler, E. P., Jr. (1963), *Trans. Amer. Acad. Ophthal. Otolaryng.*, **67**, 187.

Gelfand, M. L. (1954), *J.A.M.A.*, **154**, 911.

Gibb, A. G. (1970), *J. Laryng.*, **84**, 577.

Gilliatt, F. W. and Taylor, J. (1959), *Proc. roy. Soc. Med.*, **52**, 1080.

Glaninger, J. and Mark, H. (1967), *Mschr. Ohrenheilk.*, **101**, 209.

Golding-Wood, P. H. (1962), *J. Laryng.*, **76**, 683.

Goodgold, J. and Eberstein, A. (1972), *Electrodiagnosis of Neuromuscular Diseases*. Baltimore: Williams and Wilkins Co.

Groves, J. (1965), *Arch. Otolaryng.*, **81**, 486.

Groves, J. (1968a), *Brit. med. J.*, **1**, 508.

Groves, J. (1968b), *J. Laryng.*, **82**, 666.

Groves, J. (1971), *Scott-Brown's Diseases of the Ear, Nose and Throat*, 3rd edition (J. Ballantyne and J. Groves, Eds.). London: Butterworths.

Groves, J. (1973a), *Proc. roy. Soc. Med.*, **66**, 545.

Groves, J. (1973b), *Recent Advances in Otolaryngology* (J. Ransome, H. Holden and T. R. Bull, Eds.). Edinburgh and London: Churchill Livingstone.

Groves, J. and Gibson, W. P. R. (1974), *J. Laryng.* **88**, 581.

Guilford, F. R. (1970), *Ann. Otol.*, **79**, 241.

Harkin, J. C. and Skinner, M. S. (1970), *Ann. Otol.*, **79**, 218.

Hilger, J. A. (1965), *Minn. Med.*, **48**, 1463.

Hope-Simpson, R. E. (1965), *Proc. roy. Soc. Med.*, **58**, 9.

Hough, J. V. D. (1958), *Laryngoscope*, **68**, 1337.

House, W. F. and Hitselberger, W. E. (1964), *Arch. Otolaryng.*, **80**, 752.

Hunt, J. R. (1907), *Arch. Otolaryng.*, **36**, 371.

Hunt, J. R. (1910), *Arch. intern. Med.*, **5**, 631.

James, J. A. (1969), *J. Laryng.*, **83**, 771.

Jepsen, O. (1965), *Arch. Otolaryng.*, **81**, 446.

Jongkees, L. B. W. (1954), *Acta oto-laryng.*, (*Stockh.*), **44**, 336.

Jongkees, L. B. W. (1965), *Arch. Otolaryng.*, **81**, 518.

Jongkees, L. B. W. (1973), *Arch. Otolaryng.*, **97**, 220.

Juel-Jensen, B. E. (1970), *J. roy. Coll. gen. Practit.*, **20**, 323.

Kadonoff, D. von (1956), *Z. mikr.-anat. Forsch.*, **62**, 1.

Kerth, J. D. and Shambaugh, G. E., Jnr. (1964), *Arch. Otolaryng.*, **80**, 392.

Kettel, K. (1959), *Peripheral Facial Palsy*. Copenhagen: Munksgaard.

Koerner, O. (1904), *Münch. med. Wschr.*, p. 6.

Korkis, B. (1961), *Lancet*, **i**, 255.

Krarup, B. (1958), *Acta oto-laryng.* (*Stockh.*), **49**, 389.

Kristensen, H. B. (1968), *J. Laryng.*, **82**, 665.

Kumagami, H. (1972), *Arch. Otolaryng.*, **95**, 305.

Laumans, E. P. J. and Jongkees, L. B. W. (1963), *Ann. Otol.*, **72**, 307.

Lindeman, H. (1960), *Acta oto-laryng.*, suppl. 158. 204.

McGovern, F. H., Lewis, J. E. and Konigsmark, B. W. (1972a), *Arch. Otolaryng.*, **95**, 331.

McGovern, F. H., Konigsmark, B. W. and Sydnor, J. B. (1972b), *Laryngoscope*, **82**, 1594.

Manning, J. J. and Adour, K. K. (1972), *Pediatrics*, **49**, 102.

Matthews, W. B. (1961), *Brit. med. J.*, **2**, 215.

May, M. and Harvey, J. E. (1971), *Laryngoscope*, **81**, 179.

May, M. and Hawkins, C. D. (1972), *Laryngoscope*, **82**, 1337.

Mechelse, K., Goor, G., Huizing, E. H., Hammelburg, E., van Bolhuis, A. H., Staal, A. and Verjaal, A., (1971), *Lancet*, **ii**, 57.

Miehlke, A. (1973), *Proc. roy. Soc. Med.*, **66**, 549.

Miller, H. (1967), *Brit. med. J.*, **2**, 815.

Mosforth, J. and Taverner, D. (1958), *Brit. med. J.*, **2**, 675.

Multanen, I. and Holopainen, E. (1963), *Acta oto-laryng.*, suppl. 188, p. 402.

Netter, A. and Urbain, A. (1926), *C. R. Soc. Biol.*, **94**, 98.

Olson, N. R., Goin, D. W., Nichols, R. D. and Makim, B. (1973), *Trans. Amer. Acad. Ophthal. Otolaryng.*, **77**, 67.

Peiris, O. A. and Miles, D. W. (1965), *Brit. med. J.*, **2**, 1162.

Penfield, W. and Rasmussen, T. (1950), *The Cerebral Cortex of Man*. New York: Macmillan.

Philipszoon, A. J. (1962), *Pract. oto-rhino-laryng.*, **24**, 233.

Pietersen, E. and Caunt, A. E. (1970), *J. Laryng.*. **84**, 65.

Reddy, J. B., Jungching Liu, Balshi, J. F. and Fisher, J. (1966), *Eye, Ear, Nose Thr. Monthly*, **45**, 62.

Richardson, A. T. (1962), *Proc. roy. Soc. Med.*, **55**, 897.

Richardson, A. T. (1963), *Ann. Otol.*, **72**, 569.

Sadé, J. (1965), *Ann. Otol.* **74**, 94.

Safman, B. L. (1971), *Arch. Otolaryng.*, **93**, 55.

Sardana, D. S., Bassi, N. K. and Singh, D. P. (1971), *Indian J. Otolaryng.*, **23**, 124.

Simmons, F. B. and Beatty, D. L. (1962), *Science*, **138**, 590.

Smyth, G. D. L. (1973), *Arch. Otolaryng.*, **97**, 152.

Sunderland, S. and Cossar, D. F. (1953), *Anat. Rec.*, **116**, 147.

Swan, D. M. (1952), *J. Amer. med. Ass.*, **150**, 32.

Taverner, D. (1954), *Lancet*, **ii**, 1052.

Taverner, D. (1955), *Brain*, **78**, 209.

Taverner, D. (1965), *Arch. Otolaryng.*, **81**, 471.

Taverner, D., Cohen, S. B. and Hutchinson, B. C. (1971), *Brit. med. J.* **4**, 20.

Taverner, D., Fearnley, M. E., Kemble, F., Miles, D. W. and Peiris, O. A. (1966), *Brit. med. J.*, **1**, 391.

Taverner, D., Kemble, F. and Cohen, S. B. (1967), *Brit. med. J.*, **2**, 581.

Thompson, N. (1971), *Transactions of the Fifth International Congress of Plastic Surgery, Melbourne*, p. 66. Australia: Butterworths.

Tschiassny, K. (1946), *Ann. Otol.*, **55**, 152.

Tschiassny, K. (1953), *Ann. Otol.*, **62**, 677.

Tschiassny, K. (1955). *J. int. Coll. Surg.*, **23**, 381.

Tomita, H., Hayakawa, W. and Hondo, R. (1972), *Arch. Otolaryng.*, **95**, 364.

Tomita, H., Okuda, Y., Tomiyama, H. and Kida, A. (1972), *Arch. Otolaryng.*, **95**, 383.

Turner, J. W. A. (1944), *Lancet*, **i**, 756.

Waller, A. (1862), *Proc. roy. Soc. Lond.*, **2**, 89.

Weiss, A. D. (1968), *J. Laryng.*, **82**, 668.

Weller, T. H. and Coons, A. H. (1954), *Proc. Soc. exp. Biol.* (*N.Y.*), **86**, 789.

White, A. and Verma, P. L. (1973), *J. Laryng.*, **87**, 957.

Zillstorff-Pedersen, K. (1965), *Arch. Otolaryng.*, **81**, 457.

Zuehlke, D. (1956), *Dissertation*. Munich.

31. THE SALIVARY APPARATUS

H. DIAMANT

The saliva is produced by the parotid, submandibular and sublingual glands and by all the small salivary glands scattered over the mucous membranes of the oral cavity (Fig. 1). A thorough description was published as long ago as 1661 by the Danish scientist, Niels Steensen (Nicolaus Steno), in his book *Glandulis Oris, & nuper observatis inde prodeuntibus Vasis* (Figs. 2 and 3). Subsequent writings on this topic have added little to this account, and have been concerned largely with developments in microscopic technique.

cell. The striated ducts drain into interlobular excretory ducts, and finally into the parotid duct (Fig. 4).

The parotid gland has a single excretory duct, the parotid duct, also known as Stensen's duct. This runs from the antero-superior part of the gland outside the masseter muscle and curves round its border. It pierces the buccinator muscle and opens into the vestibule of the mouth opposite the upper second molar.

The submandibular gland is the second largest of the

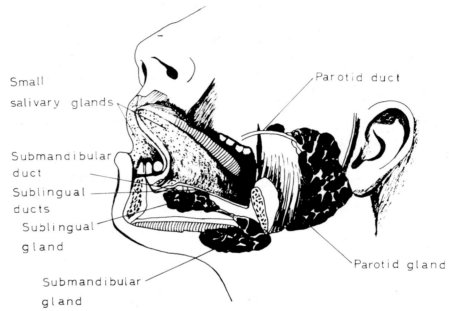

FIG. 1. Position of the salivary glands.

ANATOMY

The parotid gland is the largest of the three paired salivary glands. It is situated anterior to the external acoustic meatus and is delineated by dense fascia. The gland is covered by a layer of subcutaneous connective tissue and by skin. It weighs about 25 g and varies considerably in shape and size.

It is composed of glandular lobes of the first, second and higher orders connected by excretory ducts held together by connective tissue. The parotid gland is considered to be a purely serous gland, although some doubt about this has been expressed by Rauch and Emodi (1961). The alveoli consist of cylindrical or conical salivary cells supported by a basement membrane and arranged around a central lumen. Within the cells there are secretory capillaries and between the cells and the basement membrane there are regularly branched myoepithelial cells. The alveoli open into ducts lined with low cuboid epithelium and continue into striated ducts, lined with a special type of cylindrical

paired glands. It is sometimes called the submaxillary gland, a somewhat doubtful term, which is gradually becoming obsolete. Located below and partly medial to the mandible, the gland is enclosed in a fairly thin elastic capsule. It is about 2·5–3·5 cm in length and weighs 10–15 g.

A mixed gland with mainly serous elements, the submandibular gland is more complex in structure than the parotid. The serous part is alveolar, while the mucous part is alveolar and tubular. Both serous and mucous elements are found in gland alveoli. The serous cells are located in the most distal part of the alveoli, where in longitudinal section they are crescent-shaped—the demilunes of Gianuzzi—in the terminal end of the glandular elements. The duct system of the gland is essentially similar to that of the parotid gland (Fig. 4).

The excretory duct, named after Thomas Wharton, begins in the posterior part of the gland and is 5–6 cm long. It passes just below the submucosa and discharges into the floor of the mouth just lateral to the frenulum of

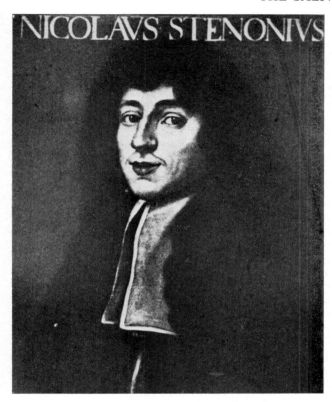

FIG. 2. Niels Steensen, Danish Scientist.

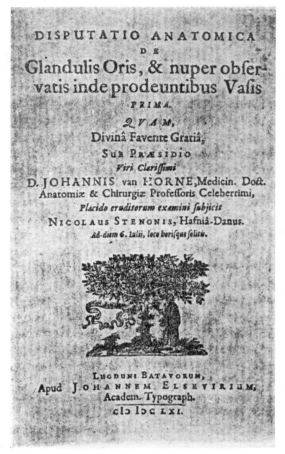

FIG. 3. The work of Niels Steensen.

the tongue. Part of the secretion of the sublingual gland empties into this duct, while the rest discharges through a row of orifices along the attachment of the tongue.

There are distinct differences between the excretory ducts of the large salivary glands. Whereas the parotid duct is fairly narrow, not particularly flexible and opens more or less funnel-shaped, the submandibular duct is wider and can tolerate considerable dilation (Fig. 5). However, its orifice close to the frenulum linguae is narrow and often difficult to enter with a probe.

PHYSIOLOGY

The salivary glands contain secretory fibres of both parasympathetic and sympathetic types. The parasympathetic fibres to the parotid gland originate in the inferior salivatory nucleus in the medulla oblongata. They leave the brain stem with the glossopharyngeal nerve and reach the otic ganglion via Jacobson's anastomosis (tympanic nerve, tympanic plexus and the lesser petrosal nerve). From here the postganglionic fibres lead to the parotid gland via the auriculotemporal nerve (Fig. 6).

The parasympathetic fibres to the submandibular gland are given off from the superior salivatory nucleus in the pons region. They pass via the nervus intermedius, the chorda tympani and lingual nerve to the submandibular ganglion, which lies close to the submandibular gland. Some preganglionic nerve fibres also enter the gland, the parenchyma of which contains ganglion cells. This means

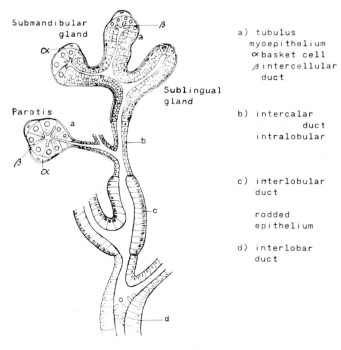

FIG. 4. A skeleton drawing of the salivary glands.

Stensen's duct

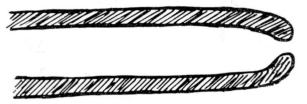

Wharton's duct

FIG. 5. The difference between the parotid (Stensen's) and the submandibular (Wharton's) duct.

that surgical parasympathetic denervation of the submandibular gland can be performed only proximal to the ganglion, whereas the parotid gland can be denervated both before and after the ganglion (Fig. 6).

The sympathetic nerve elements to the salivary glands originate in the superior cervical ganglion and reach the glands via the arterial plexus. Gustatory stimulation of the submandibular gland is still possible after division of the chorda tympani (Diamant, Enfors and Holmstedt, 1959). Reflex secretion is inhibited by injecting a local anaesthetic around the hypoglossal and/or the glossopharyngeal nerve. A careful description of the parasympathetic and sympathetic innervation is to be found in *Physiology of the Salivary Glands* by Burgen and Emmelin (1961). The authors point out the difficulty of extending to man the result of animal experiments; besides species differences there are intra-species variations in the autonomic nervous system. It has been found, for instance, that the chorda tympani in man contains secretory fibres to the parotid glands which probably run distal to the middle ear and which thus do not pass through Jacobson's anastomosis (Diamant and Wiberg 1965).

It is evident that there is a considerable difference in the effect of sympathetic stimulation of parotid and submandibular glands in man. The secretion of the parotid gland is extremely inconstant, sometimes lacking, whereas that of the submandibular gland is fairly constant. This resting secretion is not influenced by anticholinergic agents such

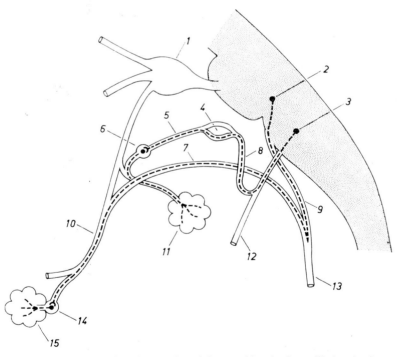

FIG. 6. Parasympathetic innervation of the parotid and submandibular glands (schematic representation). 1. Trigeminal (semilunar) ganglion. 2. Superior salivatory nucleus. 3. Inferior salivatory nucleus. 4. Tympanic plexus. 5. Lesser petrosal nerve. 6. Otic ganglion. 7. Chorda tympani. 8. Tympanic nerve. 9. Facial nerve and nervus intermedius. 10. Lingual nerve. 11. Parotid gland. 12. Glossopharyngeal nerve. 13. Facial nerve. 14. Submandibular ganglion. 15. Submandibular gland.

as atropine. The results of experiments in the cat concerning the effect of pre- and post-ganglionic division of efferent and afferent nerves are not applicable to man. It is thought that the paralytic secretion found in the cat by Emmelin and his associates (1957, 1958) does not occur in man.

Nor, would it seem, is increase in secretion induced by injecting a sympatheticomimetic agent in man due directly

our studies. In most studies, secretion was examined under normal and pathological conditions (Enfors, 1962; Ericson, 1969; Wiberg, 1971; Diamant, Ekstrand and Wiberg, 1972). The stimulated parotid secretion has also been used for measuring the inhibitory effect of anticholinergic drugs of the atropine type (Diamant and Zelezny, 1968; Diamant, Ekstrand and Rydnert, 1973). The secretion has also been

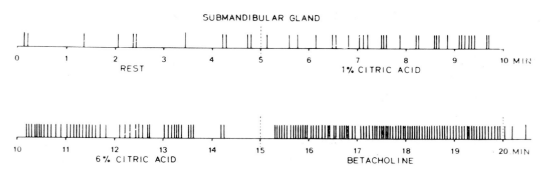

FIG. 7. The submandibular secretion at rest, after stimulation with 48 mmol. l^{-1} (1 per cent) and 286 mmol. l^{-1} (6 per cent) citric acid and after stimulation with methacholine chloride (acetyl-beta-methylcholine) intravenously

to the drug, but rather to a modification of blood supply; for the increase in secretion is moderate, in contrast to the large increase following injection of parasympatheticomimetics such as choline derivatives. Injection of a choline derivative is a practical means of inducing salivary secretion and in man methacholine chloride (acetyl-beta-methylcholine) is suitable for this purpose (Fig. 7). The stimulated secretion is directly proportional to dosage. Secretion can also be induced by electrical stimulation of the chorda tympani (Diamant, Enfors and Holmstedt, 1959). This has also been demonstrated in man, where a maximal secretory response has been obtained with a stimulus of 10 impulses per second at 3 volts (Fig. 8).

SALIVARY SECRETION UNDER NORMAL AND PATHOLOGICAL CONDITIONS

Under resting conditions—that is to say, in the absence of gustatory or any other type of stimulus—the total secretion of saliva is small. It suffices to keep the mucosa moist and thus maintain tolerable conditions in the mouth. At rest, there is a large difference between the volume produced by the large and small glands. The parotids secrete very little, the submandibular somewhat more and the small glands much more in relation to their size. In most persons, the parotid gland secretion is so low as to be difficult to measure. The small glands, on the other hand, have a constant resting secretion and obviously serve to keep the mouth moist.

All the salivary glands, the parotids in particular, respond strongly to stimulation and especially to physiological stimulation, that is, gustatory stimulus via the normal reflex pathways. Mechanical and chemical stimuli in the mouth produce secretory responses. The same applies to drug stimuli. As pointed out above, salivary secretion is subject to cholinergic regulation and is elicited by cholinergic agents such as pilocarpine and choline derivative. We have used methacholine chloride (Betacholine) to a large extent in

examined in functional impairment of the chorda tympani resulting from operations on the middle ear and in Bell's palsy (Wiberg, 1971; Diamant, Ekstrand and Wiberg, 1972).

EXAMINATION OF THE SALIVARY GLANDS

The various methods available for examining the salivary glands—for both scientific and clinical purposes—may be grouped as follows:

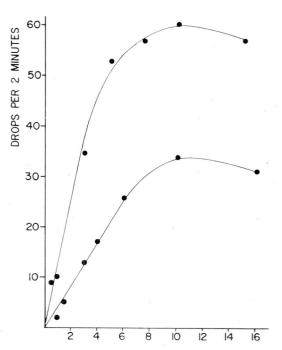

FIG. 8. Effect of increased impulse frequency on secretory response to the stimulation of the chorda tympani.

A. Anatomical methods
   (1) Sialography
   (2) Aspiration biopsy
   (3) Excision biopsy
B. Physiological methods
   (1) Sialometry
   (2) Scintigraphy
   (3) Radiosialometry
C. Chemical methods
   (1) Analytical
   (2) Histochemical
   (3) Radiohistological
D. Bacteriological methods

Particular attention will be devoted to three methods that have assumed increasing importance in both scientific and clinical contexts. One of these is the measurement of the salivary secretion. The other two methods are sialography and aspiration biopsy with a fine needle. From these examinations an extremely accurate picture of the state of the glands and the presence of pathological alterations can be obtained.

Sialometry

The secretory rate of the glands can be examined by direct measurement of the volume of saliva secreted; this is easy to perform for the parotid and submandibular glands since their excretory ducts are readily accessible. It is also possible to measure the total amount of saliva collected, but this method is less exact. Radiosialography and scintigraphy can also be used; the excretion of ^{131}I is then measured.

In the sialometric method, which has been described by a number of workers, including Diamant, Diamant and Holmstedt (1957); Enfors (1962); Ericson (1968) and Wiberg (1971), the saliva is collected in a sialometer, which is a steel or plastic collector attached firmly around the opening of the parotid duct by suction. From here it is led through a plastic (polythene) tube to a drop counter or a device for weighing or measuring the drops. The excretory duct of the submandibular gland, which drains the saliva from the submandibular gland and part of that from the sublingual gland, must be cannulated with a fine plastic catheter which leads to a drop counter. When resting secretion is measured, the catheter acts as a stimulus but the error so incurred has been shown to be negligible. The secretion is stimulated with citric acid. One per cent (48 mmol. l^{-1}) solution acts as a mild stimulus while a 6 per cent (286 mmol. l^{-1}) solution gives submaximum stimulation. For maximum stimulation, a 10 per cent (476 mmol. l^{-1}) solution is required, but in many subjects this produces marked soreness of the tongue, especially in the case of sensitive mucosa or a tendency to xerostomia. Among drugs used to stimulate secretion, methacholine chloride, given as an intravenous infusion 1–0.5–2 mmol. l^{-1} min^{-1} (0.1–0.4 mg. ml^{-1}. min^{-1})—is most suitable. The dose-rate results in a marked increase in pulse rate and a higher drop in blood pressure. Caution is indicated in the case of of elderly persons with hypertension. In none of the thousands of examinations performed over the years, how-ever, have any notable complications been observed (Diamant, Diamant and Holmstedt, 1957; Enfors, 1962; Wiberg, 1971). The dose rate of 1 mmol. l^{-1} min^{-1}(0.2 mg./ml^{-1}.min^{-1}) usually elicits a submaximal stimulus, and is of great value in determining secretory capacity. A typical result of complete sialometry performed on parotid and submandibular glands is illustrated in Fig. 9. There is a

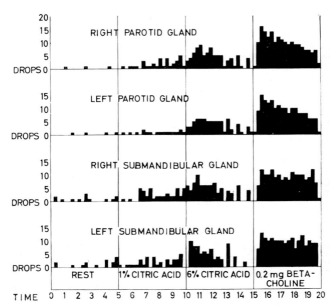

FIG. 9. Typical recording of salivary secretion during five-minute intervals with various stimuli. Normal innervation of the parotid and submandibular glands.

large inter-subject variation, and a considerably small left–right difference. Reproducibility is good for 286 mmol. l^{-1} citric acid and for infusion of methacholine chloride 1–1.5 mmol. l^{-1} (0.2–0.3 mg. ml^{-1}). For examination of the submandibular gland, a catheter must be used; this is inserted in the submandibular duct where the secretion is measured. There is some risk of swelling of the gland from irritation from the catheter. To measure the secreted saliva when secretion rate is low a fine pipette may occasionally be required, but it usually suffices to count the number of drops. The method is extremely sensitive, but the normal range is comparatively great. In cases where reduction is small or moderate it may then be difficult to decide whether abnormality is present. The left–right difference under normal circumstances is, however, quite small and the method is therefore much used in unilateral disorders such as facial palsy. Here the sensitivity of the method comes into its own and it is possible to determine prognosis for a case of Bell's palsy. Use is made not only of measurement of salivary secretion but also of another of the functions of the chorda tympani, namely the sense of taste (Diamant, Ekstrand and Wiberg, 1972).

Sialography

Though sialography, the radiographic examination of the salivary glands after injection of an opacifying medium into the excretory ducts, was introduced in 1926 by Barsony, it is only in recent years that thorough analyses have been made and standards of normality established (Ericson, 1968, 1970, 1973). Studies have also been made of the relationship between the sialographic findings, functional status and other parameters of the parotid and submandibular glands (Ericson, 1971; Ericson, Hedin and Wiberg, 1972).

Sialography has been developed as a standard method for clinical use. The procedure is essentially as follows. After probing the excretory duct, a plastic catheter is inserted in the duct orifice. A low viscosity water-soluble contrast medium is injected with a syringe graduated in tenths of a millilitre. Media containing oil should not be used as they can cause chronic tissue irritation and thus complicate diagnosis. The injection is fractionated and sialograms are exposed at three stages of filling. Suitable volumes of medium are 0·4–1·0 ml for the submandibular gland.

Lateral and frontal projections are used, with the patient supine and the side under examination nearer the film (Ericson, 1970). Examination is performed bilaterally. The criteria of normality applied in evaluating the sialograms are based on studies carried out by Ericson (1968, 1971, 1973).

With this method, the salivary glands of interest can be reproduced in detail (Fig. 10). It is also possible to determine the size of the glands (Ericson and Hedin, 1970). This has been found to be related to the rate of secretion. Size determinations will therefore play an important role in the investigation of the secretion rate under normal and pathological conditions.

Although sialographic examination of the parotid glands, in particular, is gaining in importance, it is realized that this method alone is insufficient to provide a reliable diagnosis, for radiographic appearances are nonspecific and not pathognomonic for particular pathological states. Of special interest, however, is the characteristic picture in sialectasis (Fig. 11).

Aspiration Biopsy

This method, a special feature of which is the use of a fine needle, is a purely cytological technique. Since it was developed it has been used increasingly in the diagnosis of salivary gland disorders. By means of aspiration through a needle, enough cell clusters can usually be obtained to provide a diagnosis. The method is of particular value in tumours of the salivary glands, but is also useful in other lesions of these organs. It calls for much experience and the stage to which the method has been developed is illustrated by Eneroth and Zajicek (1965) and by Franzen (1972). The specimens are taken with a very tight syringe, which can be held firmly so that cell clusters can be accurately aspirated from the region around its tip and stained. The differential diagnosis of some diseases calls for long experience while others—for example sarcoidosis—are much more easily recognized.

The three methods, sialometry, sialography and aspiration biopsy described here are certainly not the only ones available. They are, however, of crucial importance for making a clinical diagnosis. They are also valuable in research because of the information they provide on the

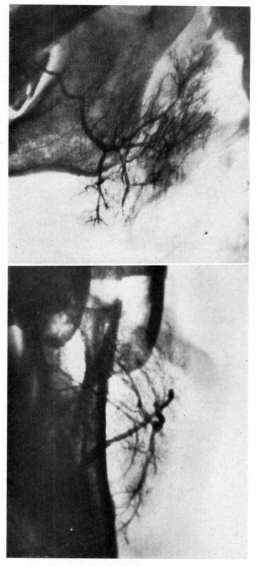

FIG. 10. Normal parotid sialogram in lateral and frontal projection.

pathological anatomy of the salivary glands and its bearing on their function.

PATHOLOGY

It is not the purpose here to give an account of the various lesions of the salivary glands, but rather to deal with two particular disorders that have been the subject of much discussion, namely xerostomia and sialectasis and two interesting methods of treatment, namely ligation of the parotid duct for recurrent chronic parotitis and a surgical method for drooling in children with cerebral palsy syndrome.

Xerostomia

Xerostomia has a number of causes. Nervous or functional xerostomia which occurs under conditions of stress is usually elicited centrally. Functional xerostomia is

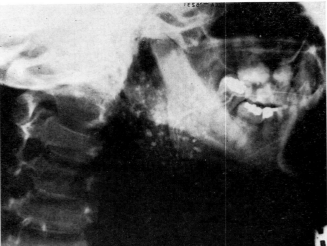

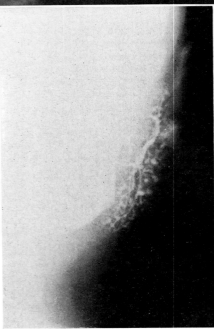

FIG. 11. Parotid sialogram with typical sialectasis.

enlargement has been described by Kelemen and Montgomery (1958).

It was formerly considered that xerostomia with arrested secretion was accompanied by irreversible changes of the salivary gland tissue so that salivary secretion could not recover. However, improvement has been observed to occur in Sjögren's syndrome though it is not usual (Ericson, 1973). In recurrent chronic parotitis, the secretion gradually decreases and may even be completely arrested. Even then the patient does not complain of dryness of the mouth, since both submandibular and the small salivary glands in the cheeks and palate are unaffected.

In persons complaining of xerostomia there is not always a reduction in secretion, but there may still be relative xerostomia due to certain systemic diseases or an impaired response to, for instance, gustatory stimulus. In persons where the gland function is not completely abolished, citric acid can stimulate enough secretion to produce adequate moistness of the mouth.

Sialectasis

The typical sialographic appearances in sialectasis have been dealt with in considerable detail in a number of studies (Rose, 1950; Ollerenshaw and Rose, 1951; Thackray, 1955; Patey and Thackray, 1956). It is particularly the views on the four types of sialectasis described by Ollerenshaw and Rose (1951) that will be discussed here. Whether these types represent different stages of development or whether they are stationary has not been easy to decide. It is true that in some patients the changes have been found to develop with time, but whether this is usual is not yet certain.

It was Thackray (1955) who strongly advanced the view that, in chronic parotitis and in chronic changes with lymphoid degeneration of the duct walls, the contrast medium injected in sialography tends to disperse. The medium used by Thackray was oil-soluble and collected in drops, the visualized structure resembling a bunch of grapes. This, according to Thackray, indicated that the cavities are not preformed but are lesions produced by the actual injection. Support for Thackray's theory has been voiced by Hemenway (1960) and by Ranger (1971). However, careful histological studies carried out by Ericson (1971, 1972) have shown that the appearance of the epithelium in the spaces is inconsistent with the changes having been produced by injection of contrast medium. Ericson used a water-soluble medium, and the injection pressure was low enough to minimize the risk of the ducts rupturing. Sialectasis in small children has been reported by Burczynski (1961). Using a very low injection pressure, he found that the cavities were preformed or possibly of congenital origin, in any case developing very early. He considered it remarkable that sialectasis could occur on both sides while the clinical symptoms were unilateral. This is consistent with our findings in a number of patients. In patients with severe changes and lymphocytic infiltration, no ectasia has been found even when a high injection pressure has been used. It is thus evident that the cavities must be preformed, and that they are perhaps of the same type as those in bronchiectasia.

In the evaluation of sialectasis, it must be borne in mind that the relationship between the appearance of the sialec-

governed by the autonomic nervous system. True xerostomia, which is due to reduced or arrested secretion of the salivary glands, usually affects all the glands, including the small ones. When the latter are not involved, the dryness is usually not severe, even if two, or even three, of the large glands are not functioning. Thus, persons who have undergone bilateral parotidectomy never complain of dryness of the mouth because the secretion from other glands suffices. The large glands may be intact while the small ones are completely dry. Persons with marked xerostomia often suffer from mucosal affections and a sialometric examination will disclose complete arrest of secretion. This is typical of Sjögren's syndrome, which when severe involves all glands. Xerostomia sometimes occurs as a physiological feature in elderly people; here diminished salivary secretion is due to involvement by fat with compensatory enlargement of, in particular, the submandibular glands. This tasis and the actual pathological changes is still obscure. Most authors agree that sialectasis occurs in a number of disorders. It may be an auto-immune reaction but, as in the case of chronic recurrent parotitis, it may also be an early development of a condition that is then either a cause or an effect of the chronic changes. It has also been proposed that sialectasis can be congenital (Burczynski, 1961). This should be a rewarding field for further investigation, and histological and immunological approaches should be examined in series with long follow-up.

THERAPEUTIC ASPECTS

Non-tumourous disorders of the salivary glands usually cause the patient little trouble. In chronic recurrent partitis, however, there may be intermittent severe pain. In salivary gland enlargement having other origins, tension may be set up, but the symptoms are otherwise moderate. The prognosis *quo ad vitam* is extremely good.

The medical therapy that is available in salivary gland disorders is limited. It is essentially symptomatic and, in principle, not focused on the gland disease as such. The same applies to surgical measures, but these can occasionally prove most beneficial. This is the case concerning treatment for chronic recurrent parotitis. In this condition, which is characterized by recurrent glandular swelling, accompanied by severe pain and often fever, the parotids display more or less marked changes with sialectasis. There is diminished secretion from the parotid but not from the submandibular glands.

This impairment of secretion would presumably provide an opportunity for infectious material to find its way up into the gland via the parotid duct and thus account for the recurrent infection. A logical counter-measure would be to block the duct by ligating it, thereby enabling the considerably reduced secretion to destroy the gland through intraductal pressure. One condition for the success of the ligation approach is that the secretion should not be more than moderate. A copious secretion can be diminished by irradiating the gland. A dose of about 5–7 J. kg^{-1} (500–700 rad) which incurs no risks will interrupt the secretion for about 14 days. Ligation is performed a few days after irradiation. (Diamant, 1958; Diamant and Enfors, 1965). In about one-half of cases where ligation of the parotid duct was carried out the symptoms cleared up entirely. One possible reason for failure is that the secretion pressure was too great for the often brittle duct, with the result that this ruptured, thereby opening-up a new flow path; it is then practically impossible to repeat ligation. In troublesome cases of chronic recurrent parotitis parotidectomy has been proposed (Beahrs, Devine and Woolner, 1961; Patey, 1965). This operation can be performed even after ligation has failed.

Another area in which surgery has been often used is in the treatment of drooling of saliva in children with cerebral palsy. The operation consists of extirpation of the submandibular gland on one side and division of the chorda tympani on the other. Gratifying results obtained in 12 children have recently been reported (Diamant and Kumlien, 1973). Another method that has been tried is to move the orifice of the submandibular duct to the back of the mouth so that the saliva is more easily swallowed (Laage-Hellman, 1969).

REFERENCES

Barsony, T. (1926), *Klin. Wschr.*, **4**, 2,500.
Beahrs, O. H., Devine, K. D. and Woolner, L. B. (1961), *Amer. J. Surg.*, **102**, 760.
Burczynski, E. (1961), *Otolaryng. pol.*, **15**, 355.
Burgen, A. S. V. and Emmelin, N. G. (1961), *Physiology of the Salivary Gland*. London: Edward Arnold.
Diamant, B., Diamant, H. and Holmstedt, B. (1957), *Arch. int. Pharmacodyn.*, **111**, 86.
Diamant, H. (1958), *Acta oto-laryng.*, **49**, 375.
Diamant, H., Ekstrand, T. and Rydnert, J. (1973), *Arzneimittel-Forsch.* In press.
Diamant, H., Ekstrand, T. and Wiberg, A. (1972), *Arch. Otolaryng.*, **95**, 431.
Diamant, H. and Enfors, B. (1965), *Laryngoscope*, **75**, 153.
Diamant, H., Enfors, B. and Holmstedt, B. (1959), *Acta physiol. scand.*, **45**, 293.
Diamant, H. and Kumlien, A. (1973), *J. Laryng.* To be published.
Diamant, H. and Wiberg, A. (1965), *Acta oto-laryng*, **60**, 255.
Diamant, H. and Zelezny, J. (1968), *Arzneimittel-Forsch.*, **18**, 1137.
Emmelin, N., Muren, A. and Strömblad, R. (1957), *Acta physiol. scand.*, **41**, 35.
Emmelin, N. and Strömblad, R. (1958), *J. Physiol.*, **143**, 506.
Eneroth, C. M. and Zajicek, J. (1965), *Acta cytol.*, **9**, 355.
Enfors, B. (1962), *Acta oto-laryng.*, **172**, 1.
Ericson, S. (1968), *Acta radiol.*, suppl. 275.
Ericson, S. (1969), *Arch. oral Biol.*, **14**, 591.
Ericson, S. (1970), *Acta oto-laryng.*, **70**, 294.
Ericson, S. (1971), *Arch. oral Biol.*, **16**, 9.
Ericson, S. (1972), *Acta radiol.*, **12**, 69.
Ericson, S. (1973), *Acta radiol.*, **14**, 17.
Ericson, S. and Hedin, M. (1970), *Oral Surg.*, **29**, 536.
Ericson, S., Hedin, M. and Wiberg, A. (1972), *Odont. Revy*, **23**, 411.
Franzen, S. (1972), *Sandorama*, **II**, 11.
Hemenway, W. G. (1960), *Laryngoscope*, **70**, 1508.
Kelemen, G. and Montgomery, W. W. (1958), *New Engl. J. Med.*, **258**, 188.
Laage-Hellman, J. E. (1969), *Nord. Med. 82*, **48**, 15.
Ollerenshaw, R. and Rose, S. S. (1951), *Brit. J. Radiol.*, **24**, 538.
Patey, D. H. (1965), *Ann. Roy. Coll. Surg.*, **36**, 26.
Patey, D. H. and Thackray, A. C. (1956), *Brit. Surg. Progress*, 115.
Ranger, D. (1971), *Diseases of the Ear, Nose and Throat*, Vol. 4 (Scott-Brown, Ed.). London: Butterworths.
Rauch, S. and Emodi, O. (1961), *Helv. med. Acta*, **28**, 270.
Rose, S. S. (1950), *Postgrad. med. J.*, **26**, 521.
Thackray, A. C. (1955), *Arch. Middx Hosp.*, **5**, 151.
Wiberg, A. (1971), Thesis, Umeå University, Sweden.

32. TASTE

R. I. HENKIN

INTRODUCTION

Taste may be defined broadly as detection and recognition of liquid phase stimuli. As such, this process in man may be divided rather arbitrarily into several component aspects as follows:

(1) stimulus characteristics,
(2) taste support systems,
(3) general taste bud characteristics,
(4) specific taste bud receptor characteristics,
(5) mechanisms of stimulus-receptor binding,
(6) transduction of the chemical binding energy to an electrically recognizable generator potential,
(7) neural transmission of the generator potential,
(8) formation of the action potential (i.e. true neural depolarization) and its axonal conduction,
(9) transmission of the action potential to those brain centers involved with taste detection and recognition, and
(10) central nervous system integration of the signals received. These steps have been divided, again for convenience, into two general processes: steps 1–5 have been termed the pre-neural events of taste [1-3], steps 6–10, the neural events of taste [1-3].

In order to define and evaluate the function of each of these steps in man, measurement techniques had to be developed by which consistent information about these taste processes could be obtained. These techniques will be discussed in relation to the manner by which taste detection and recognition occur.

Pathological processes affect the taste system in various ways at each of the steps in this system. These pathological processes are especially useful in the elucidation of the various pre-neural events of taste. Although the diverse nature and multiplicity of these pathological processes allow only representative examples of these processes to be presented they serve a useful purpose in the elaboration of the principles underlying each part of this complex system.

Taste altering substances are also important aspects of this system. The role they play in taste and nutrition and the role of the taste process in nutrition are important concepts of the functional significance of this sensory system.

TASTE STIMULUS CHARACTERISTICS

Present day dogma holds that taste stimuli represent four "primary" classes or qualities; salt, sweet, sour and bitter. This concept, promulgated by Fick[4] and reviewed by Ohrwall[5], was a condensation of earlier information in which a more extensive list of as many as ten taste stimuli or "primaries" was presented as representative of the capabilities of the taste system.

The limitations of our present, constricted view of taste stimuli is readily apparent when specification of the taste of a metal nail as salt, sweet, sour or bitter is requested or the taste of a peppermint drop is requested using the same nomenclature. The taste of metal or of mint obviously does not fit strictly within the limits of salt, sweet, sour or bitter. Although the present work does not justify a systematic investigation of this problem the limitations of our present dogma should be apparent.

Those characteristics of taste stimuli which are essential for their detection and recognition at a molecular level are not entirely clear for any taste stimulus. In general, salts are detected and recognized by their cation[6] but the counter ion, the molecular species of the cation and other factors[7] play influential roles in this process. For example magnesium sulfate (Epsom salt) tastes bitter not salty.

For sugars, stimuli which produce a sweet response are so diverse that the simple view of carbohydrates being equivalent to sweet cannot hold. Examples as diverse as amino acids[8], proteins[9], acids[10], salts[10] and many other substances such as lead and beryllium indicate the great diversity among sweet tasting stimuli. This suggested that an unifying concept common to all these different stimuli had to exist in order to allow each to produce a sweet taste. One such unifying concept was advanced by Shallenberger and his colleagues[8,10]. They reasoned that all stimuli which were sweet had a specific molecular structure and two component functional groups equivalent to a hard acid and a hard base. These latter groups were called AH and B, respectively. It was then reasoned that some form of complimentarity existed with the taste receptor such that hydrogen bonding or some other form of energy requiring process took place at a specific molecular distance of 0·3 nm (3Å) between the AH and B functions[10,12]. Although the validity of this theory remains to be established, it is of interest that only one form of complete taste blindness in man has been discovered and that in patients with a congenital lack of ability to recognize sugar, i.e., aglycogeusia[11].

The best correlation between taste stimulus and taste response relates to the sour taste for the hydrogen ion concentration and/or the degree of dissociation of the acid. In general, this correlates with the sour taste of the stimulus[7]. However, there are exceptions to this general rule for all acids are not sour (picric acid is intensely bitter, some amino acids are sweet).

Bitter substances, represented by alkaloids, ureas, nicotine, caffeine and similar stimuli represent a diversity of sensory stimuli which may be recognized by their bitter taste characteristics. Again, many anomalies exist which cannot be easily explained. For example, saccharin tastes sweet at low concentrations, bitter at high concentrations and, even at low concentrations, has a bitter after-taste. As with sweet, this diversity led to the formulation of a number of unifying concepts, including one similar to the AH-B concept used previously for sweet[12]. In this concept, the hard acid-hard base concept previously used for sweet was maintained but the molecular distance between these functional groups was reduced to 0·15 nm (1·5Å)[1,6].

Each of these theories of stimulus characteristics will require further testing prior to its acceptance as fully characterizing each specific taste stimulus. In addition, our knowledge of the characteristics of other taste stimuli not presently formally admitted as having a specific taste and how these relate to those stimuli presently emphasized must be investigated.

TASTE SUPPORT SYSTEMS

The major taste support systems are (1) secretions of glands of the oral cavity which come into continued direct contact with the taste system and (2) physical structures which house taste buds. Secretions which form the component parts of what is normally called saliva come from several oral glands in man. These include the parotid gland (the major serous secretory gland), the submandibular gland (the major mixed mucous and serous gland), the lingual and sublingual glands (the major mucous secreting glands), the palatine glands and various other small oral glands including von Ebner's glands. Little is known about the specific contributory role of any of these glands in the taste process. However, some generalizations about the role they play in the taste process may be made based upon clinical and pathophysiological observations. With the cessation or marked diminution of overall salivary gland function in man, as in Sjögren's syndrome[13], or following X-irradiation of the head and neck for treatment of a tumor in this area[14], taste acuity for all stimuli is either destroyed or markedly attenuated. Pathological changes which occur following these diseases reveal destruction or modification of taste buds[13,14]. Attempts to maintain the oral cavity moist through the use of water, saline or artificial saliva, made up of viscous liquids with or without added electrolytes have been ·uniformly unsuccessful in aiding the abnormal taste function[13]. Treatment of Sjögren's syndrome with chlormethine (nitrogen mustard) or with X-irradiation[13] and of post-irradiation hypogeusia with zinc ion[14] has been associated with the reinstitution of normal or near-normal salivary flow from these glands in some patients. With the return of salivary flow the gradual reappearance of taste buds has been observed. Subsequently, taste acuity returned to or toward normal in these patients[13,14]. These data support the hypothesis that there are, in saliva taste buds, stimulatory factors which may be necessary to maintain normal taste bud anatomy and function. The nature and function of these possible factors have not been clearly defined.

This hypothesis is supported by previous work carried out in animals. In the rat, surgical interruption of those nerves which innervate the major salivary glands, coupled with administration of agents which inhibit salivary gland secretion (e.g., pilocarpine or atropine) is uniformly associated with the production of decreased taste acuity for all tastants tested[15]. Unless these stringent measures are employed, taste acuity in the rat will be maintained for some tastants[16].

Taste buds in the oral cavity of man and of many animals are present in small hillocks or bumps called papillae (Fig. 1). On the tongue, taste buds which open up directly onto the lingual surface and into the oral cavity are present in fungiform papillae which cover the anterior two-thirds of the tongue (Fig. 1). These papillae, and buds, are innervated by the chorda tympani branch of the 7th or lingual nerve. These papillae are circular, sometimes red in color, and rather small, varying in diameter from 1–4 mm. In man they number between 20 and 60. They are not uncommonly slightly elevated above the lingual surface and are surrounded by smaller, more numerous spiny-like papillae called filiform papillae which do not contain taste buds. Taste buds in fungiform papillae vary in number from 0 to 8. They are usually multiple; i.e. a single bud within a papilla is less common than two or more buds. These papillae may contain specialized pressure, tactile and temperature receptors in addition to taste buds. They also usually contain myelinated and unmyelinated nerve fibres unrelated to the taste buds[17,18].

Over the posterior third of the human tongue, forming a somewhat V-shaped groove, are vallate (circumvallate) papillae (Fig. 1). These papillae are circular, about 2–4 times as large as the fungiform papillae, and 2–15 mm in diameter. They usually number between 7 and 20. These papillae are commonly elevated above the lingual surface but usually do not have any obvious coloration. Taste buds are normally present both in the papillary and contrapapillary surfaces of the crypts of these papillae (Fig. 1) and rarely come into direct contact with the lingual surface. These papillae and their buds are innervated by the second branch of the 9th or glossopharyngeal nerve. Taste buds in these papillae are present uniformly varying in number from 10 to 100. These papillae commonly contain specialized pressure, tactile and temperature receptors in addition to taste buds. They also contain many myelinated and unmyelinated nerve fibers unrelated to the taste buds[17,18].

Over the palate, mainly in the area near the junction of the hard and soft palate, are palatal papillae (Fig. 3) which house taste buds which open up directly into the oral cavity in a manner similar to the buds in fungiform papillae. These papillae are circular and small, varying in diameter from 1–3 mm. They number between 5 and 20. These papillae and buds are innervated by the 9th or glossopharyngeal nerve and also by the 10th or vagus nerve. These papillae may or may not be elevated above the palatal surface and are surrounded by small salivary glands which are difficult to differentiate from the taste bud bearing papillae by gross appearance. Taste buds in these papillae are commonly single (Fig. 1).

Characteristics of these papillae are summarized in Table 1.

Papillae and taste buds may appear in other oral and pharyngeal structures in man although they have been described mainly in infants[18]. These include the lips, the

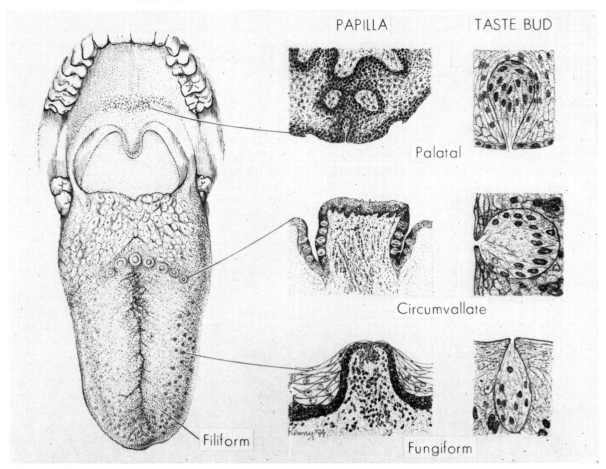

FIG. 1. Location and appearance of papillae and taste buds in the oral cavity of man. Filiform papillae are distributed over the anterior 2/3 of the tongue. Fungiform papillae are less common, appear over the anterior 2/3 of the lingual surface and are surrounded by filiform papillae. Vallate (circumvallate) papillae commonly form a V-shaped groove and appear only over the posterior 1/3 of the lingual surface. Palatal papillae appear on the epithelial surface near the junction of the hard and soft palate; papillae containing only salivary glands also appear in this same general area. The insets show a sketch of the light microscopic appearance of taste buds from fungiform, vallate and palatal papillae, respectively. ×450.

TABLE 1

ORAL PAPILLAE IN MAN

Papilla Type	Location	Number of Buds Per Papilla	Opening into Oral Cavity	Primary Taste Sensitivity
Fungiform	Tongue, ant. 2/3	0–8	Direct	Salt + Sweet
Vallate	Tongue, post 1/3	10–100	Indirect	Sweet
Palate	Junction, hard and soft palate	0–2	Direct	Sour + Bitter

inner surface of the lingual mucous membrane, the epiglottis and various areas of the pharynx. Some investigators have demonstrated taste buds in man to be present in the upper third of the esophagus[19,20]. Functioning of the taste buds in the pharynx of normal subjects has been previously demonstrated[20].

In addition to salivary glands and papillae other organelles are present in the oral cavity presumably to assist the taste system. Cilia encircle the opening of the von Ebner's glands in the bottom of the deep crypts of the vallate papillae[21]. These cilia which presumably propel the secretions from the von Ebner's gland into the crypt are consistent anatomical features in man.

Oral fungiform, vallate and palatal papillae also contain myelinated nerve fibers, muscles, blood vessels, small mucous and serous glands and various specialized receptors as noted above. These structures may serve in some way as specialized support structures for the taste buds.

GENERAL TASTE BUD CHARACTERISTICS

The function of taste buds in the several papillae found in the oral cavity differs. Although all buds are capable of responding to each taste quality, provided a sufficient concentration of tastant is provided, response characteristics are concentration dependent. Thus, differentiation of sensory discrimination may be observed. Taste buds in fungiform papillae appear to respond in a rather uniform manner to low concentrations of both salt and sweet tastants[20]. They also respond to sour and bitter stimuli but usually at relatively higher concentrations of these tastants[20]. Taste buds in vallate papillae appear to respond in a rather uniform manner to low concentration of sweet tastants and only in higher concentrations to salt, sour or bitter stimuli[22]. Taste buds in palatal papillae appear to respond in a rather uniform manner to low concentrations of both sour and bitter tastants[20]. They also respond to salt and sweet tastants but usually at relatively higher concentrations[20].

These observations indicate that the greatest number of taste buds in the oral cavity are involved with the response to sweet tastants, the fewest to sour or bitter stimuli. These observations correlate well with the clinical observations that the sweet taste quality is the best preserved and protected taste quality even in patients with pathological changes in taste, e.g. in taste loss secondary to metabolic or trace metal abnormalities[23], secondary to X-irradiation or to depressed salivary flow[13], sweet taste is least affected of those qualities normally measured. By contrast, the bitter taste quality is usually affected first and some effects which alter taste only slightly may be apparent in the measurement of a change in bitter taste only. Sour and salt taste losses occur in an intermediate degree between that of sweet and bitter.

Taste buds which comprise each type of taste papilla can be distinguished by their characteristic anatomical appearance. Whether or not these anatomical differences can be related to the functional significance of the buds is not presently apparent. However, most taste buds exhibit some anatomical similarities.

In general, taste buds in man are made up of between 20 and 50 cells. Taste buds in man differ somewhat in size, those from fungiform and palatal papillae being relatively long and slender, approximately 40–60 μm $\times$ 2–10 μm whereas buds from vallate papillae are more globular (Fig. 1). Cells in the bud have been divided, for convenience, into three major types (Figs. 2, 3). All cell types have processes which extend up into the tip or pore region of the bud. All cell types are tightly joined together at several levels of organization through a series of desmasomal attachments. No blood vessels or lymphatic channels are present in any portion of the taste bud proper. Mitotic processes are only rarely observed; although the cells of the taste bud of the rat[24], and presumably of man, undergo constant and rapid renewal. Present knowledge

suggests that epithelial cells adjacent to the outer membrane of the taste bud migrate into the bud and under the influence of neural and possibly salivary stimuli differentiate into the specialized cell types that make up the bud. Indeed, under appropriate conditions, previously nongustatory regions of tongue epithelium can form taste buds. The metabolic fate of the cells which comprise the taste bud is not known although the dense extracellular material (Figs. 2, 3) offers a possible repository for this material. Nerves enter and leave the taste bud through its base. These nerve fibers, once they appear within the taste bud proper, are unmyelinated. Nerve fibers generally do not extend more than halfway up into the taste bud proper although some fibers have rarely been observed to be present about 5 μm from the pore region. No nerve fibers have ever been observed normally in the pore opening of any bud. Adrenergic and cholinergic nerve fibers have been found in taste buds in man[2] whereas dopaminergic material has been found in buds in animals.

The cells within the bud in man, and in animals as well[25,26], have been divided into at least three major types. Type I cells constitute approximately 80 per cent of the cells of the bud, Type II cells approximately 15 per cent of the cells of the bud and Type III cells constitute approximately 5 per cent of the bud cells. Other cell types have also been observed on occasion in animals[25,26].

Type I cells exhibit the following major features which, in general, may be labeled anatomically from the pore region to the base of the bud:

(a) outer plasma membrane
(b) inner plasma membrane
(c) cell processes
(d) large dark core granules [occasionally called neurosecretory granules[13,27]]
(e) rootlet formation
(f) kinetosomes, usually in pairs
(g) cell nucleus
(h) neural synapse, the direction of which suggests an afferent transmission from nerve to bud[25 26].

Although the function of this cell type (Fig. 2) is not known, it is the only cell type in which large dark core granules are present close to the pore region. This, coupled with the afferent innervation of the cell, suggests that its function could lie in the production of neurotransmitter.

Type II cells consist of the following major features, which, in general, may be labeled anatomically from the pore region to the base of the bud:

(a) outer plasma membrane
(b) inner plasma membrane
(c) cell processes
(d) small and large vacuoles
(e) helical bundle(s) of tonofilaments
(f) cell nucleus
(g) neural synapse, the direction of which suggests an afferent transmission from nerve to bud as in the Type I cell[25,26].

Although the function of this cell type is not known, the presence of helical bundles which extend over the major

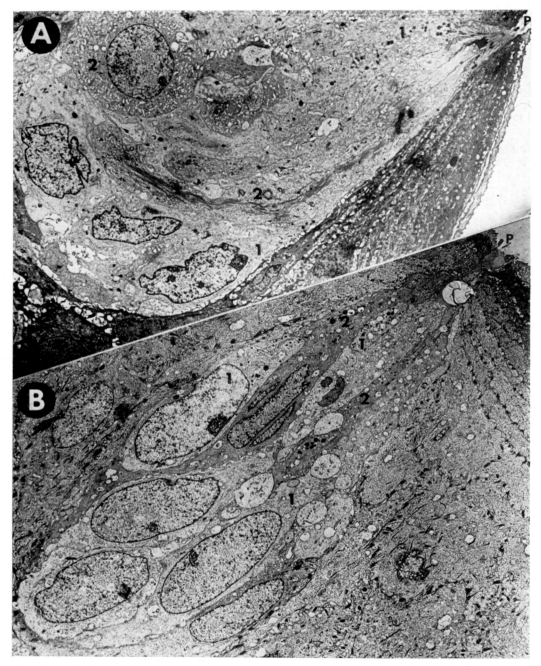

FIG. 2A and B. Electron microscopic appearance of a representative taste bud from a vallate papilla excised under general anesthesia from a human subject, (A) with normal taste acuity compared to that from a patient with post-influenzal hypogeusia, hyposmia, dysgeusia and dysosmia (PIHH) in (B). Open pore regions (P) may be observed in both figures. In (A) microvilli, finger-like projections from the taste bud cells, may be seen extending into the pore region, the dense extracellular material clearly observed near the pore. Numerous dark, dense core vesicles may be observed in Type I cells (1) whereas vacuoles and the bundle of tono-filaments may be observed in Type II cells (2). In (B) the immediate pore region is disrupted and the finger-like projections are not observed. Dense extracellular material is not commonly observed. Large vacuoles are seen both within Type I (1) and Type II (2) cells and extracellulary. The dark dense core vesicles of the Type I cells (1) appear disorganized.

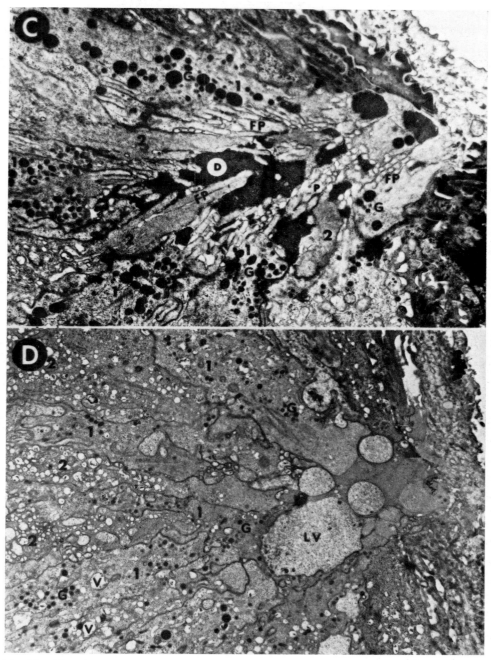

FIG. 2C and D. Electron microscopic appearance of the pore region, (C) of a representative taste bud from a vallate papilla excised under general anesthesia from a human subject with normal taste acuity compared to that, (D) from a patient with post-influenzal hypogeusia, hyposmia, dysgeusia and dysosmia (PIHH). ×4,500. In (C) the finger-like projections (FP) of the taste bud cells may be observed in the pore region, and the dense extracellular material (D) observed; the dense dark core vesicles or neurosecretory granules (G) may be observed in Type I cells (1), small and large vacuoles in Type II cells (2). In (D) there is marked disruption of the pore area. Small (V) and large vacuoles (LV) are commonly observed within and outside cells suggesting the degree of disruption of the pore area. Fewer and smaller dark core vesicles may be observed in Type I cells (1) which are still present. These granules appear less well organized than in C. Type II cells (2) may also be observed but increased numbers of intracellular vesicles are more commonly observed than in (C). Neither dense extracellular material nor microvillus projections are seen. The appearance of this bud suggests that degenerative changes have occurred.

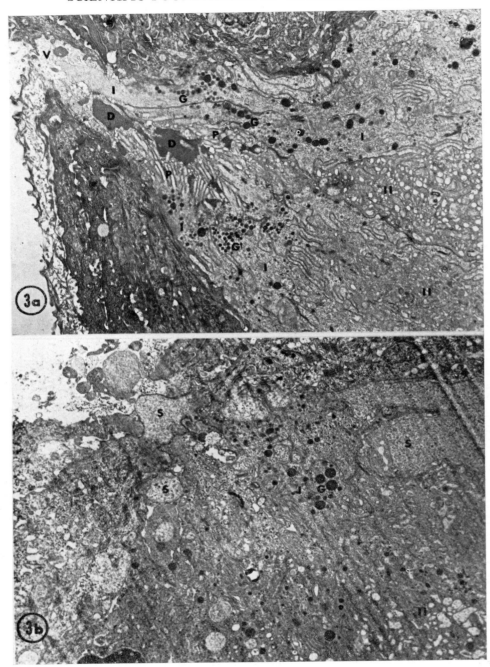

Fig. 3a and b. Comparison of electron microscopic appearance of a representative taste bud from a vallate papilla excised from a human subject with normal taste acuity, in (3a) with that a patient with Sjögren's syndrome, in (3b). Anatomical details of (3a) are similar to those observed in Fig. 2. Type I (1) and Type II (11) cells are easily observed in (3a) but not as well in (3b). Type I cells show numerous dark dense core vesicles (neurosecretory granules, G); Type 11 cells are characteristically vacuolated. Also observed in the pore region of (3a) is dense extracellular material (D), microvillus projections (P) and fine light core extracellular vesicles (V). In (3b) severe disorganization of the pore region (upper left) can be observed. Type 1 and Type 11 cells are identifiable, but their cytoplasm stains more homogeneously than normal making their differentiation difficult. There is a relative paucity of neurosecretory granules in Type 1 cells. Neither dense extracellular material nor microvillus projections are present. Pale-staining, membrane-bounded structures (S) containing finely granular material are observed in areas suggestive of degenerating cells or nerves, or both. The appearance of this bud suggests that degenerative changes have occurred.

length of this cell type (Fig. 2) and its afferent innervation suggests that this cell may play some contractile role in the function of the bud. These helical bundles have been previously observed by German anatomists in the 19th Century using light microscopy of the taste bud of the eagle and of the goat. Due to the tight desmosomal interconnections between all cells within the bud, contraction of the helical bundle could produce a contraction of all cells of the bud such as occurs with the folding of an umbrella. Such a contractile process was predicted[2] and has been suggested under direct vision in fungiform papillae of the mouse and rat upon direct stimulation with high concentrations of hydrochloric acid. Such contraction occurs relatively rapidly, within 1 to 3 seconds, whereas relaxation of this effect is relatively slow, requiring as long as 30 seconds. The presence of such a mechanism could serve as a very useful protective mechanism, protecting the bud receptors from noxious substances entering the oral cavity, much as the iris of the eye closes to protect the visual system from excessive light. Noxious stimuli may produce a reflex response by which the Type II cells contract and in so doing contract the entire taste bud, thereby protecting it from chemical and physical damage. Many electron micrographs from taste buds of man and animals show the taste bud with the pore open, the taste receptor membranes available to the oral environment; others show the pore area closed, the cell processes enclosed within the bud and covered with epithelium[2]. Although fixation artifacts, sampling problems and other technical considerations must be considered, these observations suggest that, for normal taste bud function, taste bud receptors may be exposed to the oral environment. Conceptually, taste bud receptors might function similar to a periscope on a submarine, allowing a continuous sampling of the oral environment.

Type III cells consist of the following major features, which, in general, may be labelled anatomically from the pore region down to the bud base:

(a) outer plasma membrane
(b) inner plasma membrane
(c) cell processes
(d) granulated cytoplasm with small dense core granules
(e) nucleus
(f) neural synapse, the direction of which suggests an afferent transmission from bud to nerve[25,26].

Although the function of this cell type is not known it is the only major cell type in which the synaptic direction is from bud to nerve suggesting that it might serve as the receptor cell in the taste bud.

In the pore area of the buds distal to the outer plasma membranes of the cell processes from all three major cell types there are clear core vesicles and granules which are uniformally present. The function and nature of the contents of these vesicles are not known.

TASTE BUD RECEPTOR CHARACTERISTICS

The taste bud receptor has not been well characterized in any species. However, recent work in the cow[28] has provided some insight into its specific anatomical and biochemical characteristics. Using special isolation techniques, bovine vallate papillae have been obtained free of the mucous and serous glands which exist in the center and beneath these papillae, respectively[28]. These papillae were then treated by hypotonic swelling, nitrogen pressurization and gentle homogenization such that the apical portions of the taste buds were extruded from their sites in the papillae and then amputated from the remainder of the bud[29]. This material was then filtered and treated by differential and sucrose gradient centrifugation to obtain purified membrane preparations[29]. The chemical characteristics of these taste bud receptor membranes are similar, in general, to membranes obtained from liver cells, red blood cells, intestinal villi or brush border of kidney. Thus, there is a proteolipid-rich membrane in which glycolipids are found. However, the enrichment of the receptor membrane in alkaline phosphatase and esterase suggests an important role for these enzymes in the taste process. Alkaline phosphatase has previously been demonstrated by histochemical techniques to be present in or near the taste bud pore. Its role is not entirely known but it is assumed that tastant-receptor interaction is a molecular process that requires a considerable expenditure of energy on the part of the receptor membrane either to maintain its molecular conformation and/or to return it to its normal conformation once the tastant-receptor interaction has taken place. The role of alkaline phosphatase in this process may be to supply these high energy phosphate bonds.

MECHANISMS OF STIMULUS-RECEPTOR BINDING

The initial event of the taste process presumably occurs with the binding of the tastant(T) to the taste bud receptor(R) on the exposed receptor membrane of the taste bud. This binding takes the general form of

$$T + R \rightleftharpoons [TR] \qquad (32.1)$$

and this has been the general hypothesis used by other investigators in this field of investigation[30]. However, examination of the taste responses of normal subjects (Fig. 4) and patients with various diseases suggests that equation (32.1) does not adequately describe physiological taste responses. Empirical examination of these responses (Fig. 4) suggests that tastant-receptor interactions follow the general form:

$$I/I_{max} = \frac{K[T]^2}{K[T]^2 + 1} \qquad (32.2)$$

where I is the intensity at the concentration [T], I_{max}, the maximum taste intensity (at highest [T]) and K is a constant (K_1/K_{-1}). These responses, which are shown both by normal subjects and by patients with several disorders of taste[3,27,31], can be best described mathematically by equation (32.2). The binding stoichiometry

$$R + 2T \underset{K_{-1}}{\overset{K_1}{\rightleftharpoons}} [RT_2] \qquad (32.3)$$

where $K = K_1/K_{-1}$, as before, and $[RT_2]$ the tastant-receptor complex, would lead to equation (32.2) if one

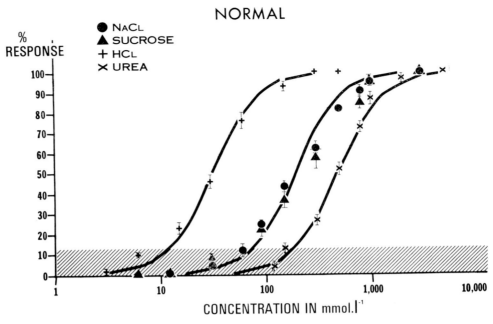

FIG. 4. Forced scaling responses in 21 normal subjects for varying concentrations of salt (Na Cl), sweet (sucrose), sour (HCl) and bitter (urea) tastants. Each point noted represents the mean ± 1 SEM of the responses of each of the subjects. Concentrations below recognition level are noted by the hatched area.

useful to obtain information about some aspects of some lingual receptors but they give little specific information about taste. Similarly cortical evoked potential techniques which involve complex, cumbersome and expensive equipment are not presently clinically useful or practical.

Whatever the measurement techniques that are used, several physiological and pathological factors must be kept in mind if adequate measurements are to be made and proper evaluation of the results obtained. The circadian variation in taste, dependent, in part, upon the circadian changes in adrenal cortical hormone secretion, indicates that taste detection acuity is greater in the afternoon and evening, when carbohydrate-active steroid secretion is lower, than in the morning[32,59]. If elevated thresholds are observed in the afternoon their pathological importance is enhanced. Tight fitting upper dentures severely attentuate normal taste responsiveness to sour and to bitter stimuli[60]. When testing taste, upper dentures should always be removed. However, subjects who have worn dentures for many years may exhibit elevated thresholds for sour and for bitter stimuli due to anatomical changes in palatal taste buds due to the persistent irritation produced in these structures by the wearing of the denture. Pipe smoking is uniformly associated with the lowering of taste acuity[22] and to a much lesser extent acuity is attenuated due to excessive smoking of cigars and cigarettes[22]. Taste detection acuity exhibits changes during the normal menstrual cycle[61] with maximum sensitivity occurring in the follicular phase just prior to ovulation. Taste acuity is also affected during the various stages of pregnancy[62].

Decreased taste acuity has been termed *hypogeusia* while total loss of all taste ability has been termed *ageusia*[63]. Pathological alterations in taste have been classified under the general term *dysgeusia*. *Cacogeusia* relates to the

obnoxious, unpleasant taste associated with the otherwise normally pleasant taste of food and drink; *phantogeusia* relates to the persistent presence of an unusual taste sensation in the oral cavity without the presence of a taste stimulus (this sensation is usually salty, bitter or metallic); *heterogeusia* relates to a persistent, consistent change in the taste of all food and drink (e.g., all foods taste sweet). Parageusia is a poorly defined term whose usage should be discontinued.

An attempt to relate the clinical abnormality observed by testing with the pathophysiological abnormalities found in the patient has been carried out. Within very general limits an increase in threshold for one or more tastants and associated alterations in forced scaling responses suggest that all those taste buds serving those tastants affected are functioning in a pathological manner. Preservation of normal thresholds with attenuation and/or abnormalities observed in forced scaling responses suggests that some buds are functioning in a normal capacity although the majority of buds serving those tastants affected are functioning in a pathological manner.

PATHOLOGICAL PROCESSES AFFECTING TASTE

Pathological processes can affect taste at most stages of the taste processes (Table 3). Although our present limited information does not allow for a systematic appraisal of pathology related to anatomy and/or function at each step of the taste process, these pathological processes serve to clarify and help define several of the steps in this entire process.

Oral stimuli which alter normal taste responsiveness are helpful in elucidating several of the concepts previously

TABLE 3
FACTORS PRODUCING TASTE ABNORMALITIES IN MAN

Infectious Diseases	Neurological Diseases	Metabolic Diseases	Drug or Device Induced	Other Disease Processes	Local Processes Involving Oral Structures	Genetic	Environmental Processes	Physiological Processes
Bacterial	Multiple Sclerosis	Goitre	Clofibrate	Malabsorption	Infection (Bacterial, fungal, viral)	Athyreotic cretinism	Pipe smoking	Menses
Fungal		Hypothyroidism	Colestyramine	Occult carcinoma		Glaucoma	Cigar, cigarette smoking	Pregnancy
Luetic	Myesthenic Syndrome	Addison's disease	Phenindione	Retinitis pigmentosa	Granulomatous			Circadian variation
Viral Post-influenza Viral hepatitis	Familial dysautonomia Type I	Panhypopituitarism	Antithyroid drugs	Idiopathic	Leukemic infiltration	Cystic fibrosis of the pancreas	Maxillary dentures	
Granulomatous Sarcoid Wegener's granuloma	Familial dysautonomia Type II	Congenital adrenal hyperplasia, non-salt losing variety	Antibiotics	Post-surgical procedures		Cranio-facial hypoplasia	Imbibing hot liquids or foods	
	Bell's palsy		Anticancer agents			Congenital	Chemical Exposure	
Rickettsial	Meningioma, other tumors	Cushing's syndrome	Tranquillizers (amitriptyline)	Post-anesthesia		Chromatin-negative gonadal dysgenesis	Jet Fuel Exposure	
Microfilarial	Cerebral vascular accidents	Acromegaly	Acetylsulfosalicylic acid	Sjögren's syndrome				
	Skull fracture	Metal Deficiencies (Zn, Cu)	Amino acids (histidine, cysteine, methionine)	Fatty parotid syndrome		Pseudohypoparathyroidism		
	Head Trauma (mainly contracoup)	Vitamin Deficiencies (retinol; cyanocobalamin)	Penicillamine			X-linked hypogonadism		
		Cystic fibrosis of the pancreas	Adrenal steroids (chronic usage)			Congenital taste blindness		
		Cirrhosis	Griseofulvin					
			X-irradiation (commonly to head and neck)					

stated. Miraculin, a glycoprotein of molecular weight 45 000[64–66] obtained from the berry of the African Shrub *Syncepalum dulcificum*,[64–67] in normal subjects, produces two taste changes, an attenuation or blocking of sour and bitter tastes[66] and the alteration of all sour tastes to a sucrose-like sweetness[66]. This glycoprotein binds tightly to the taste bud receptor and only agents which alter this binding, e.g. 350 μmol.l^{-1} sodium dodecyl sulfate, but not 5 mol. l^{-1} urea, produces a loss of either of these functions[66]. In patients with aglycogeusia[11], a congenital abnormality in which sweet recognition is absent, this glycoprotein has no effect and sour tastes are still recognized as sour albeit attenuated[11]. Gymnemic acid, a substance extracted from the leaves of the plant *Gymnema sylvestre* attenuates the taste of most sweet tastants[68,69]. These are only two examples of a growing number of stimuli which alter taste presumably through the interaction of the tastant with the taste receptor following an alteration in the taste receptor by introduction of a specific protein into the oral cavity.

Abnormalities in taste support systems usually produce decreased taste acuity. The xerostomia which commonly accompanies Sjögren's syndrome[13], fatty parotid syndrome[13], tumors or other processes of the salivary glands necessitating their removal, or following X-irradiation of the head and neck area[14,70,71] produce pathological changes of oral taste buds (Fig. 3), particularly in the pore region and subsequent abnormalities of taste. Taste alterations commonly follow Bell's palsy[72], sometimes transiently, of times persistent; taste may return to normal spontaneously following alleviation of the symptoms of the palsy. Taste changes also follow cerebral vascular insults which alter oral function. Deficiencies of cyanocobalamin (vitamin B$_{12}$), which result in a smooth, red beefy tongue, with the disappearance of the oral papillae has been associated with taste alterations as has deficiencies of

retinol (vitamin A) in man[73] and in animals[74]. The mechanisms by which these latter two changes occur are not clear although acuity usually returns to normal following appropriate vitamin replacement therapy.

Any process which produces pathological changes in taste buds or taste bud atrophy has been associated with alterations in taste. Surgical interruption of the seventh nerve following middle ear surgery can alter taste[75] as can surgical interruption of any of the major nerves supplying lingual or palatal taste buds[76]. Clinical confirmation of these changes can be observed by the disappearance of the neurally innervated papillae. In the rat, regeneration of papillae and their taste buds has occurred following neural reinnervation by several cranial nerves[77] and, in the frog, taste buds have been maintained following reinnervation by non-cranial nerves[78].

Other diseases which alter taste bud appearance without altering papillary appearance are more common than surgical interruption of nerves and require more clinical experience in diagnosis. These changes commonly follow coryza or influenza[23,27], surgery not involving the head or neck[23,27], post-partum, post general or local anesthesia[23,27] or post-head trauma[79], on occasion of such limited nature that medical help is not sought[79]. Other diseases which produce alterations of this type are hypothyroidism[34,35] hepatitis and cirrhosis[80,81], malabsorption of various types[22], Cushing's syndrome[3,33], zinc deficiency[23], infectious processes of various etiologies[82,83] granulomatous processes including sarcoid, Wegener's granulomatosis and midline granulomas of the face[22], collagen vascular diseases[84], malignancies of various types[22] including brain tumors[85], leukemia and lymphoma[22], or tumors involving various internal organs in either an advanced or an occult state[22]. Truly idiopathic changes in taste which alter taste bud appearance and function do occur and represent about 1/3 of the patients who suffer from taste abnormalities. However, over 50 per cent of patients with taste abnormalities suffer from post-influenzal hypogeusia and dysgeusia, a disease commonly associated with smell abnormalities as well[23,27]; in the United States alone estimates of these patients number about 500 000[23].

Drugs are among the most common agents which produce taste abnormalities in which papillae are intact but taste buds are altered[86]. These drugs include antibiotics, tranquilizing agents, frequently amitriptyline, and various drugs used as anticancer agents, including vincristine, vinblastine and doxorubicin (adriamycin). Drugs which alter cholesterol metabolism, e.g., colestyramine (cholestyramine), have produced taste abnormalities of this type, as have antithyroid drugs[87,88], the antituberculosis drug chlorambucil, and the amino acids histidine[89] in man and cysteine and methionine in rats[90]. Acetylsulfosalicylic acid has been reported to produce an attenuation of bitter taste[91] but complete studies have not been carried out with this agent. Penicillamine, a drug which produces copper deficiency, also produces the severe taste abnormalities of hypogeusia and dysgeusia[92].

Cranial nerve abnormalities may be associated with taste losses. Indeed, several of the diseases noted above are associated with alterations in axonal conduction and synaptic transmission. However, several neurological diseases, *per se*, may present or be associated with taste abnormalities. Multiple sclerosis[97], facilitating myesthenic syndrome[22] and some cerebellar syndromes fall into this category.

Types I and II familial dysautonomia are also associated with severe hypogeusia or ageusia[44,45,94]. In Type I familial dysautonomia, taste buds are apparently congenitally absent from the lingual and palatal epithelium[44,45] accounting for some aspects of the loss. However, parenteral administration of methacholine, an acetylcholine derivitive, returns taste responsiveness in these children for salt and sweet tastants to normal although the only anatomical structures capable of subserving taste in their oral cavity are unmyelinated free nerve endings[44,45]. Patients with Type II familial dysautonomia exhibit taste buds in fungiform, vallate and palatal papillae yet still exhibit ageusia unrelated to their mental retardation[94]. Parenteral administration of acetylcholine derivates, e.g., methacholine, does not restore their taste responsiveness[94] although it does in patients with Type I familial dysautonomia[44,45]. Similarly, methacholine administered parenterally to patients with Type II familial dysautonomia does not alter their abnormal triple response to injected histamine[94] whereas it does in patients with Type I familial dysautonomia[45,94]. In this sense, patients with Type II familial dysautonomia have what appears to be receptor unresponsiveness, a "pseudodysautonomia", similar in some ways to the relative lack of renal responsiveness to parathyroid hormone in patients with pseudohypoparathyroidism.

Untreated adrenal cortical insufficiency[3,32,33] non-salt losing virilizing congenital adrenal hyperplasia[3,33] and other diseases in which there is insufficient circulating carbohydrate-active steroid[3,33] are associated with an unusual taste abnormality; i.e., an extremely acute or increased taste detection acuity for all tastants coupled with an impaired taste recognition acuity[3,33]. These changes are associated with pathological changes in several aspects of neural activity including increased axonal conduction[95], prolonged synaptic transmission[95] and altered central nervous system activity[95]. A similar change in taste detection acuity has been observed in some patients with cystic fibrosis of the pancreas[96]. However, no taste changes have been observed in patients with excessively high secretion of sodium-potassium active adrenal corticosteroids[3,97] or with essential hypertension[97].

Patients with essential hypertension exhibit a significantly elevated appetite or drive for NaCl[98], an appetite which is apparently diminished somewhat following adequate treatment of their hypertension[99]. The relationship between this increased salt appetite, seen also for sodium and potassium salts in spontaneously hypertensive rats[100], and taste acuity, *per se*, is not readily apparent. However, this drive to excessive salt intake in these patients can contribute significantly to their hypertension.

About 20 per cent of patients with untreated adrenal cortical insufficiency also exhibit an increased salt appetite; this abnormality disappears following adequate replacement therapy with carbohydrate-active adrenocorticosteroids.

Various tastants have been discovered which are appreciated by one segment of the population in one manner and by another segment in a quite different manner. These genetic variations in taste perception have been useful as clues to medical diagnosis and to genetic mapping even though the physiological bases of these variations are unknown. Phenylthiourea is appreciated by about 80 per cent of the population as extremely bitter but by the remaining 20 per cent as having no taste at all[55,101]. This distribution which follows a simple Mendelian pattern is altered, with significant increases in non-tasters, among patients with athyreotic cretinism and goitre[102] and with glaucoma[103]. Another substance, an extract from the fruit of the tree *Antidesma bunius*, is appreciated by approximately 90 per cent of the population as sweet or sour, whereas 10 per cent consider this extract intensely bitter[104]. Of interest is that these 10 per cent are almost uniformly among the phenylthiourea non-tasters[104]. These differences in individual taste responsiveness have been correlated with individual differences in responsiveness to the administration of several drugs and may prove, in the future, to be a quick and simple approach to the individualization of administered drug dosages.

Genetic abnormalities, *per se*, with their associated anatomical correlates are commonly associated with taste and/or smell abnormalities. Patients with cranio-facial hypoplasia exhibit an unusual taste defect, recognition hypogeusia, wherein taste detection is apparently normal but tastant recognition is grossly deficient[105]. Patients with chromatin negative gonadal dysgenesis[106] and with pseudohypoparathyroidism[107] exhibit decreased acuity for sour and bitter tastants and exhibit anatomical abnormalities of their palates. Other forms of hypogonadism, many involving hyposmia of various types, have been observed to be associated with taste deficits, mainly involving bitter and sour tastants. Although patients with congenital and genetic abnormalities commonly exhibit taste loss, increased taste detection acuity has also been observed on a genetic basis[32].

Patients with taste defects commonly bring their complaints to their primary physicians (general practitioners) but these physicians are generally unaware of the myriad of metabolic and neurological factors that can produce altered taste sensations. Complaints which most commonly bring patients to their physicians are dysgeusia and hypogeusia of relatively sudden onset. However, patients commonly complain of taste loss when in reality they suffer from some abnormality of smell[23,27]. Differentiation between taste and smell abnormalities is important in order to provide an appropriate diagnosis and institute appropriate therapy.

Patients with taste and smell loss commonly lose their appetite once they realize that most or all foods taste alike or are without flavor. This can be associated with a severe weight loss which must be distinguished from the weight loss associated with malignancy. Patients with dysgeusia commonly state that their taste acuity is "too acute" due to the severity of their taste distortions. However, by test, most of these patients exhibit hypogeusia in addition to their dysgeusia. The dysgeusia forces many of the patients to alter their dietary habits in order to find some foods that they may eat without experiencing unpleasant sensations. Although foods such as meat, chicken, fish, fried foods, eggs, tomatoes, onions, chocolate and carbonated drinks are common offenders in the production of dysgeusia, bland foods such as rice, milk, noodles, and some fresh fruits have usually been well tolerated. In some patients only a very few foods may be tolerated. In these cases, this limitation of food intake has produced not only weight loss but also vitamin and mineral deficiencies. In addition, the inability to distinguish good from spoiled food by other than visual cues commonly causes episodes of food poisoning. In women this is particularly distressing causing many of them to give up their role as family cook or to seek assistance from other family members in the preparation of meals. Women are also unsure about the amount of perfume or bath powder to wear and are worried about their own body odor. These personal problems lead many of these patients to become depressed and failure to achieve understanding or help about their condition from their primary physician furthers this confusion and depression. Patients with olfactory defects fear their inability to smell escaping gas or the smoke from fire and indeed, patients with these defects have died from these causes, deaths which may have been averted had their taste and smell acuity been normal.

Many patients with these problems are referred by concerned, astute primary physicians to otorhinolaryngologists for further evaluation and potential therapy. When an obvious clinical change in papillary, taste bud support system or neural function is apparent, diagnosis itself may be readily apparent. However, in the majority of metabolic diseases which affect the taste system, these clinical signs are not readily obvious and the otorhinolarynologists must utilize specialized laboratory techniques to aid in the establishing of the appropriate diagnosis. This involves several steps:

(1) the measurement of taste detection and recognition thresholds and the measurement of, and interpretation of, forced-scaling responses in order to evaluate the functional status of the taste system;

(2) biopsy of lingual and palatal papillae and examination by electron microscopy in order to evaluate the anatomical status of the various taste buds[27];

(3) measurement of salivary flow rates, salivary zinc[108] and protein patterns in order to evaluate the functional status of the taste support systems; in patients with associated olfactory abnormalities;

(4) determination of olfactory detection and recognition thresholds[13,27];

(5) biopsy of the nasal mucous membrane and its examination by light microscopy[109] and

(6) determination of the presence of Rudolph's sign following intravenous injection of $^{99}Tc^m$ technetium pertechnitate[110]; this sign, seen on scanning the area of the face following injection of this radionuclide, is present in a significant number of patients with impaired olfactory function and is a manifestation of nasal accumulation of the radionuclide, probably due to inflammatory changes in the nasal mucous membrane[110]. On physical examination, the nasal mucous membrane can exhibit characteristic changes in some of the patients with abnormalities of both the taste and smell system; e.g., patients with post-influenzal hypogeusia and hyposmia exhibit widely patent nasal airways with pale, dry, nasal mucous membranes without the normally present thick mucus adhering to the membrane.

Since these local findings in the oral and nasal cavities may be manifestations of metabolic or other systemic changes, evaluation of hematological, hepatic, renal, collagen-vascular and endocrine system function is necessary. Infectious processes, including luetic, fungal and microfilarial infections should be considered. Sarcoid and malabsorptive processes should be evaluated. Malignancies must be considered and a detailed drug history must be taken. Neurological evaluation, including a careful history, physical examination, brain scan, skull films, and electroencephalogram is particularly important in patients with associated olfactory abnormalities where a central nervous system lesion may be responsible for the changes observed.

An important diagnostic consideration in some of these patients not commonly utilized in clinical conditions is the evaluation of zinc metabolism[23,27]. Zinc levels in blood, urine and saliva are important diagnostic factors. Patients suffering from post-influenzal hypogeusia and hyposmia[23,27] and taste and smell abnormalities following head injury[79] exhibit lower than normal levels of zinc in serum[23] and in saliva[22]. These findings are useful in order to distinguish these patients from those with other abnormalities.

Treatment of patients with taste abnormalities involves determination of the appropriate diagnosis and treating

33. PALATAL FUNCTION

BJÖRN FRITZELL

The palate separates the nasal and oral cavities. Its primary biological function is to keep everything but air away from the nasal pathways, the delicate respiratory and sensory epithelium of which must be protected from various noxious agents such as food and fluids. Situated at the cross-roads of the upper respiratory and alimentary tracts, the soft palate or velum plays a very important role in fulfilling this function. It acts like a valve, closing off the nasal cavities and nasal part of pharynx during deglutition, and closing off the mouth during the passage of air from the nose to the lower respiratory tract.

In man another important function has been added to this primary biological one. The soft palate participates in the production of articulate speech.

Historical Notes

The soft palate does not seem to have been identified by the ancients; remarks about the uvula only can be found in extant writings. In the manuscripts of Leonardo da Vinci (1452–1519), the soft palate was mentioned and, as far as we now know, drawn for the first time (Panconcelli-Calzia, 1943). Leonardo had no clear concept of its function, however, nor did the other early anatomists seem to have realized the rôle of the velum, in spite of the fact that they gave very accurate descriptions of the palatal muscles (Eustachio, 1552; Falloppio, 1561; Valsalva, 1704). It appears that the function of the soft palate in speech was first recognized in the seventeenth century, possibly by pioneers in the education of the deaf, such as Amman (1700).

In the first half of the nineteenth century, descriptions of the palatal movements as observed from above—through facial defects—were published (Hilton, 1836; Bidder, 1838). Debrou (1841) studied the palatal movements during swallowing by introducing a specially modelled iron wire along the floor of the nasal cavity and observing the deflections of its outer end. During the second half of the nineteenth century, a great number of other more or less ingenious methods were developed to study and record the palatal movements, as reviewed by Gutzmann (1899). With the discovery of X-rays at the end of the nineteenth century, a new era was started, and today very refined examination procedures are available, as will be described in a later section.

Muscles of the Soft Palate

Five pairs of muscles insert into the soft palate (*see* review by Fritzell, 1969), two of them arising from the base of the skull, two of them coming from below passing in the pillars of the fauces, and one coming from behind encircling the velopharynx (Fig. 1).

The *M. tensor veli palatini* is a flat muscle of triangular shape, with its base along the anterior wall of the cartilaginous auditory (Eustachian) tube, and its apex at the ptery-

goid hamulus. It descends almost vertically, and its tendon makes a right angle turn around the hamulus from where it spreads horizontally, or slightly upwards, forming the aponeurosis of the soft palate, to which the other palatal muscles are attached. The tensor is of paramount importance for the opening of the auditory tube. When contracting, it also makes the soft palate tense and presumably depresses its anterior part (Wardill and Whillis, 1936; Bloomer, 1953).

The *M. levator veli palatini* is a slender muscle of even dimensions along its course from a small area in front of the carotid canal at the base of the skull to the soft palate. The structure of the levator makes considerable shortening possible. The two levators form a sling, which pulls the velum upwards and backwards.

The *M. palatoglossus* muscle is small. It arises from transverse fibres within the tongue and ascends in the anterior pillar of the fauces to the palate. When the palatoglossus muscles contract the velum is lowered and drawn forwards.

The *M. palatopharyngeus* muscle is considerably larger than the palatoglossus. It has a wide origin from the back and side walls of the pharynx and from the thyroid cartilage. The vertically oriented, anterior fibres of the muscle constitute the stroma of the posterior pillars. When the palatopharyngeus muscles contract the velum is pulled in a dorso-caudal direction, the posterior pillars are stretched and adducted, the lateral walls of the upper pharynx are brought medially, and the larynx and pharyngeal walls are elevated.

The *M. constrictor pharyngis superior* constitutes the muscular coat of the upper pharynx. According to Whillis (1930) and Harrington (1944), in most subjects some of its fibres insert into the soft palate. When the superior constrictor contracts, the upper pharynx is narrowed and the velum is pulled backwards.

Variation exists between individuals in the muscle anatomy of this region (Bosma, 1957). There is also a divergence of opinions as to which fibres belong to what muscle at the velopharyngeal level of the pharynx, notably the palatopharyngeus or the superior constrictor, as pointed out by Bosma and Fletcher (1961, 1962).

The motor innervation of the tensor muscle is from the trigeminal nucleus and nerve. The other palatal muscles derive their motor innervation from the nucleus ambiguus, and the nerve fibres pass in the glossopharyngeus and vagus nerves to the pharyngeal plexus, from where the distal connections with the various muscles are made.

Topographic Changes During Growth

In newborn children, the palate is almost parallel to the base of the skull and situated well above the level of the anterior tubercle of the atlas. The nasal part of pharynx

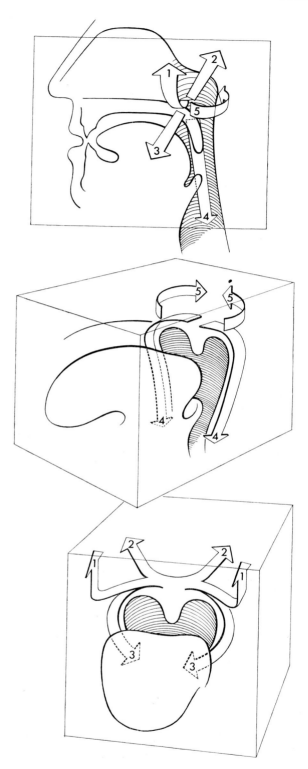

FIG. 1. Schematic presentation of the velopharyngeal muscles. The arrows indicate the approximate direction of their action and influence on the soft palate. (1) Tensor; (2) Levator; (3) Palatoglossus; (4) Palatopharyngeus; (5) Superior constrictor. (After Fritzell, 1969.)

(nasopharyngeal space) is small. During growth the vertical dimension doubles and there is also a general increase in sagittal depth, which leads to obvious changes of the structural relationships (Subtelny, 1957). The facial skeleton and the palate descend in relation to the cervical vertebrae. In the infant, palatal movements are predominantly cephalocaudal, whereas in the adult they are mainly antero-posteriorly directed (Fletcher, 1959).

Palatal Function During Respiration

In animals who rely heavily on olfaction, the palate is long and reaches all the way to the epiglottis. This arrangement ensures an uninterrupted respiration through the nose and no odour will be shunted through the mouth (Negus, 1949). In man this is not so. The human palate is shorter and there is a gap between the palate and the epiglottis. For this reason, when we are chewing or sucking liquid through a straw for instance (Moll, 1965), another mechanism is needed to keep the airway clear. This is accomplished by the apposition of the soft palate to the back of the tongue (Fig. 2).

During quiet nasal breathing, the soft palate usually has a similar position; it rests on the back of the tongue (Fig. 3). During forced respiration, when nasal breathing is not enough, the mouth is opened and the palate assumes an intermediate position to allow air to pass both ways. When, for some reason, nasal breathing is not wanted, the palate is raised to contact the posterior pharyngeal wall and velopharyngeal closure is accomplished.

The soft palate thus directs the air through the nose or through the mouth. This function of the velum as a respiratory valve is reflected in alternating activities of the palatoglossus and levator muscles, when a subject switches from nasal to oral breathing and then back again (Fig. 4).

Palatal Function During Food Intake and Swallowing

During oral preparation for swallow, the bolus is kept in the mouth by "velolingual closure", as indicated previously. The posterior portion of the tongue is elevated and the soft palate is lowered to make a firm contact.

When the bolus is passed from the mouth down to the pharynx, the soft palate and the maximally adducted palatopharyngeal folds form the dorsal wall of the channel by which food enters the pharynx proper, as emphasized by Bosma (1957) in his comprehensive review of the pharyngeal stage of deglutition. He has given this combination structure the term "palatopharyngeal partition", and points out that "it is particularly well demonstrated in lateral roentgenograms with the subject in supine position, in which circumstance the bolus is seen supported by the partition until it reaches the epiglottis". At this point of swallowing, there is an abrupt elevation of the pharyngeal walls and the larynx, and the soft palate is also quickly raised (Fig. 2.).

Electromyographic recordings from the palatal muscles indicate that all five pairs are highly active during swallowing, as demonstrated by Fritzell (1969). In his study, the intensity of the tensor and palatopharyngeus contractions

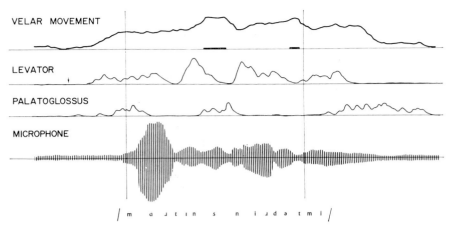

FIG. 5. Velar movement curve and velopharyngeal closure (broad black lines) plotted against tracings of levator and palatoglossus envelopes (rectified and averaged EMG) and microphone signal for the sentence, "Martin sneered at me" (American subject). The arrow indicates the first spike in the "raw" levator EMG. Levator activity and velar movement start before onset of phonation, and the velum is only partly elevated during the production of the first word. Velopharyngeal closure does not occur until the production of the s-sounds, and only two brief periods of closure occurred during the production of this sentence in this subject. Palatoglossus only moderately active. (After Fritzell, 1969.)

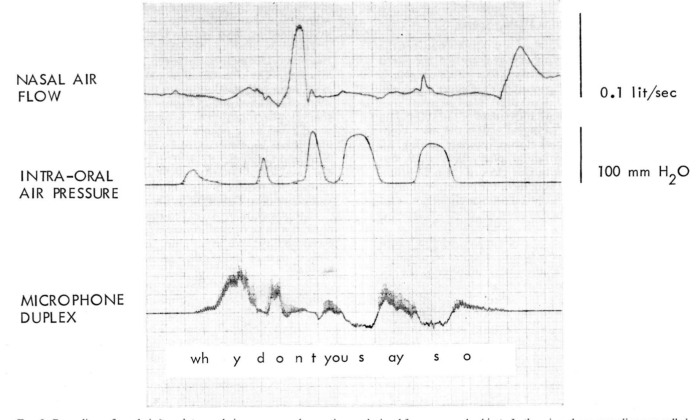

FIG. 6. Recordings of nasal air flow, intra-oral air pressure, and acoustic speech signal from a normal subject. In the microphone recording a so called "duplex" procedure has been used, by means of which high-frequency components are transformed into downward deflections, below the baseline. The air flow recording shows high peaks corresponding to the production of the n-sound and to the lowering of the velum after the utterance is finished, but there are also smaller peaks and deflections, presumably reflecting minor pumping movements of the velum. The pressure recording demonstrates high peaks for the t- and s-sounds and smaller ones for the wh- and d-sounds.

Electromyographic recordings from the palatal levators simultaneously with cinéfluorography have shown an increased muscle activity parallel to the increased elevation of the velum for closed vowel sounds (Lubker, 1968; Fritzell, 1969). A systematic variation in levator muscle activity for different oral consonant sounds has also been demonstrated (Lubker *et al.*, 1970)

elevation is preceded by levator activity and lowering of the velum is preceded by decrease or disappearance of levator activity. The superior constrictor acts in synchrony with the levator, and the palatopharyngeus muscles are also involved in the production of oral speech sounds. Podvineć (1952) elaborated on a theory already advanced by Luschka (1868), according to which the levator muscles

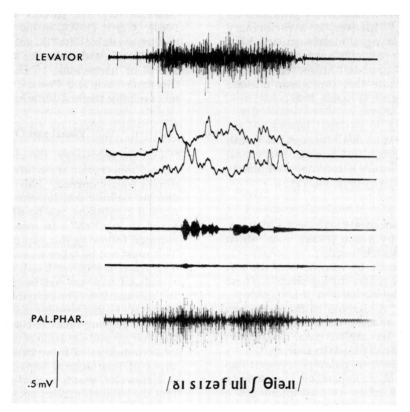

FIG. 7. A recording of the sentence "This is a foolish theory". The upper tracing is the "raw" electromyographic recording from the M levator veli palatini. The second tracing from top is the rectified and averaged EMG signal from the levator. The third tracing from top is the rectified and averaged EMG signal from the M palatopharyngeus, the "raw" electromyographic recording of which is the lowest tracing. The fourth tracing from top is the ordinary microphone signal, and the fifth is a recording from a small microphone placed in the nasal cavity. There is an increased activity in both muscles before the onset of the microphone signal, indicating participation in the production of velopharyngeal closure, which is maintained throughout the utterance. It can be seen from the average EMG tracings that the peaks for levator and palatopharyngeus activity do not coincide, which reflects a difference in the articulatory activity of the two muscles.

In cinéfluorographic films it can be seen that the velum does not have a fixed position during velopharyngeal closure. If a sentence with only oral sounds be spoken and there is continuous velopharyngeal closure, minor velar movements may still be observed. These movements may be indirectly demonstrated by recordings of the nasal air flow. During exaggerated articulation in particular, a certain amount of air flow may be recorded, which is obviously not coming from the lungs but presumably caused by pumping movements of the velum (Lubker and Moll, 1965) (Fig. 6).

The movements of the soft palate in speech are mainly determined by the action of the levator muscles. Velar

and the palatopharyngeus muscles act in synergism in speech. They form slings which pull the velum upwards-backwards and downward-backwards respectively, and the resultant force is directed backwards. Electromyographic studies have shown that this theory appears to be correct for some speech sounds but not for others. The activity of the palatopharyngeus muscle in speech differs from that of the levator (Fig. 7). Thus, in the production of vowel sounds, the palatopharyngeus is more active for *a* than for any other vowel. As previously mentioned, for the levator the opposite is true. This high degree of palatopharyngeus activity for *a* is no doubt related to the narrowing of the pharynx during the production of this

In some children, compensatory articulatory mechanisms develop. The sounds requiring a raised intra-oral pressure are produced in the larynx or pharynx, "before" the velopharyngeal insufficiency can exercise its influence. In this way, the plosives (*p, t, k, b, d, g*) are substituted by glottal stops, and oral fricatives (most often the *s*) are substituted by pharyngeal fricative sounds. This distorts speech and lowers the intelligibility even more. When well established through the years of growth, this compensatory articulatory behaviour is very difficult or impossible to change. For this reason it should be dealt with by speech therapy at an early age (Bzoch, 1971) and by early secondary surgical procedures.

It is well known that children with palatal dysfunction, notably children with cleft palate, have a higher incidence of otitis and otosalpingitis than the normal population. In adults with marked velopharyngeal incompetence, an atrophic type of nasopharyngitis is sometimes seen, with dried mucous and crusts glued to the mucous membrane of the posterior pharyngeal wall. In others, a very marked hypertrophy of the posterior end of the lower nasal conchae is observed, a finding which may be interpreted as nature's attempt to compensate for the failure of the palate.

Adenoids and Palatal Function

The adenoid takes up nasopharyngeal space. If it is very large, it will influence the production of nasal sounds and decrease the normal amount of nasalization in speech. This symptom is called *hyponasality*. An enlarged adenoid is what almost all parents suspect when they note nasal speech in their children.

A child with an enlarged adenoid may need only small velar movements to achieve velopharyngeal closure. For this reason, adenoidectomy sometimes causes a *temporary hypernasality*, which is heard for a certain period of time until the child has become habituated to use a wider range of velar movements.

However, an enlarged adenoid may also compensate, wholly or partially, for a short palate or a deep pharynx (Gibb, 1969; Calnan, 1971b). In these cases, adenoidectomy should, of course, be avoided. If the adenoid be removed, this will cause a *persisting hypernasality* or increase the nasal quality of speech, if present already before the operation. It might be argued that this would have happened at puberty anyway, since the adenoids tend to diminish and disappear at that age. This is of minor importance, however, because the ability to achieve velopharyngeal closure is very important at the early age, when our speech habits are formed and established.

Thus, when an otolaryngologist is consulted because of nasal speech, he must first find out whether it is a matter of hypernasality or hyponasality. If the speech quality of his patient is hypernasal, the surgeon should refrain from adenoidectomy. If the speech quality of his patient is hyponasal and an enlarged adenoid is present, adenoidectomy is justified. He should make it a rule, however, to be very cautious with adenoidectomy on patients in whom a latent palatal dysfunction might be suspected, e.g. children with an operated cleft palate, a bifid uvula, or signs of a neurological impairment of the head and neck (Lawson *et al.*, 1972). As to the possibility of making a preoperative diagnosis of a congenitally large pharynx in patients where there is no hypernasality, Calnan (1971b) is pessimistic. So far as we know, the condition is rare (Gibb, 1958).

In some children with velar dysfunction, e.g. because of cleft palate, recurrent or chronic otitis and otosalpingitis may make adenoidectomy imperative. When this is so, a partial adenoidectomy could be performed with removal of the lateral portions of the adenoid. They are more likely to interfere with the auditory tubes than the midline adenoid pad, which would thus be preserved (Lawson *et al.*, 1972). If it be deemed necessary for the conservation of hearing to carry out a complete adenoidectomy, the parents and the child should be informed about the possible influence on speech and prepared for surgical procedures to improve velopharyngeal closure.

REFERENCES

Amman, J. C. (1700), *Dissertatio de loquela*, Amsterdam (transl. Charles Baker; Sampson Low, Marston, Low, and Searle, London 1873. Reprinted by North Holland Publishing Co., Amsterdam, 1965.)

Bell-Berti, F. (1971), *Haskins Laboratories Status Report* 25/26, p. 117.

Bidder, F. H. (1838), *Neue Beobachtungen über die Bewegungen des weichen Gaumens und über den Geruchssinn.* Dorpat.

Bloomer, H. H. (1953), *J. Speech Hear. Dis.*, **18**, 230.

Bosma, J. F. (1953), *Ann. Otol.*, **62**, 529.

Bosma, J. F. (1957), *Physiol. Rev.*, **37**, 275.

Bosma, J. E. and Fletcher, S. G. (1961–62), *Ann Otol.*, **70**, 953, and **71**, 134.

Bzoch, K. R. (1970), *ASHA Report No. 5*, p. 248.

Bzoch, K. R. (1971), *Grabb-Rosenstein-Bzoch's Cleft Lip and Palate*, p. 825. Boston.

Calnan, J. S. (1954), *Brit. J. plast. Surg.*, **6**, 264.

Calnan, J. S. (1957), *Brit. J. plast. Surg.*, **10**, 89.

Calnan, J. S. (1971a), *Brit. J. plast. Surg.*, **24**, 263.

Calnan, J. S. (1971b), *Brit. J. plast. Surg.*, **24**, 197.

Curtis, J. F. (1970), *Cleft Palate J.*, **7**, 380.

Czermak, J. N. (1857), *Wiener Akad Sitzungsberichte.*

Debrou, T. (1841), *Des muscles qui concourent au mouvement du voile du palais.* Paris: Diss.

Eustachio, B. (1552), *Albinus' Explicato tabularum anatomicarum Barthol*, p. 1744. Leyden: Eustachii.

Falloppio, G. (1561), *Observationes Anatomicae.* Venetiis.

Fant, G. (1960), *Acoustic Theory of Speech Production.* 's-Gravenhage.

Fletcher, S. G. (1959), *Logos*, **2**, 71.

Fritzell, B. (1969), *Acta oto-laryng.*, suppl. 250.

Gibb, A. G. (1958), *J. Laryng.*, **72**, 433.

Gibb, A. G. (1969), *J. Laryng.*, **83**, 1159.

Gutzmann, H. (1899), *Encyclopädische Jahrbücher*, **8**, 74.

Gutzmann, H. (1913), *Arch. Laryng. Rhin.*, **27**, 59.

Hagerty, R. E., Hill, M. J., Pettit, H. S. and Kane, J. J. (1958), *J. Speech Hear. Res.*, **1**, 203.

Hardy, J. C. (1965), *ASHA Report No. 1*, p. 141.

Harrington, R. (1944), *J. Speech Dis.*, **9**, 325.

Hilton, (1836), *Guy's Hosp. Rep.*, **1**, 493.

Lawson, L. I., Chierici, G., Castro, A., Harvold, E., Miller, E. R. and Owsley, J. Q. (1972), *J. Speech Hear. Dis.*, **37**, 390.

Lermoyez, M. (1892), *Ann. Mal. Oriel. et Larynx.*, **18**, 161.

Lubker, J. F. (1968), *Cleft Palate J.*, **5**, 1.

Lubker, J. F. (1970), *ASHA Report No. 5*, p. 207.

Lubker, J. E., Fritzell, B. and Lindqvist, J. (1970), *Speech Transm. Lab—QPSR* 4/1970, **9** (Royal School of Technology, Stockholm).

Lubker, J. F. and Moll, K. L. (1965), *Cleft Palate J.*, **2**, 257.

Luschka, H. von (1868), *Der Schlundkopf des Menschen.* Tübingen.

Meskin, L. H., Gorlin, R. J. and Isaacson, R. J. (1964), *Cleft Palate J.*, **1**, 342.

Miles Foxen, E. H., Preston, T. D. and Lack, J. A. (1971), *J. Laryng.*, **85**, 811.

Minifie, F. D., Hixon, Th. J., Kelsey, C. A. and Woodhouse, R. J. (1970), *J. Speech Hear. Res.*, **13**, 584.

Moll, K. L. (1962), *J. Speech Hear. Res.*, **5**, 30.

Moll, K. L. (1964), *Cleft Palate J.*, **1**, 371.

Moll, K. L. (1965), *Cleft Palate J.*, **2**, 112.

Moll, K. L. and Daniloff, R. G. (1971), *J. Acoust. Soc. Amer.*, **50**, 678.

Moll, K. L. and Shriner, T. H. (1967), *Cleft Palate J.*, **4**, 58.

Morris, H. L. (1966), *J. Speech Hear. Dis.*, **31**, 362.

Negus, V. E. (1949), *The Comparative Anatomy and Physiology of the Larynx.* New York.

Osborne, G. S., Pruzansky, S. and Koepp-Baker, H. (1971), *J. Speech Hear. Res.*, **14**, 14.

Owsley, J. Q., Chierici, G., Miller, E. R., Lawson, L. I. and Blackfield, H. M. (1967), *Plast. reconstr. Surg.*, **39**, 562.

Panconcelli-Calzia, G. (1943), *Leonardo als Phonetiker.* Hamsburg: Wandsbek.

Pigott, R. W. (1969), *Plast. reconstr. Surg.*, **43**, 19.

Podvineć, S. (1952), *J. Laryng.*, **66**, 452.

Robin, L. G. (1968), *Proc. roy. Soc. Med.*, **61**, 575.

Sawashima, M. and Ushijima, T. (1971), *Ann. Bull. No.* 5, p. 25. Univ. Tokyo: Res. Inst. Logop and Phoniat.

Spriestersbach, D. C. and Powers, G. R. (1959), *J. Speech Hear. Res.*, **2**, 40.

Stewart, J. M., Ott, J. E. and Lagace, R. (1972), *Cleft Palate J.*, **9**, 246.

Subtelny, J. D. (1957), *Plast. reconstr. Surg.*, **19**, 49.

Subtelny, Joanne D., Worth, J. H. and Sakuda, M. (1966), *J. Speech Hear. Res.*, **9**, 498.

Valsalva, A. M. (1704), *Tractatus de aure humana.* Venice.

Wardill, W. E. M. and Whillis, J. (1936), *Surg. Gynec. Obstet.*, **62**, 836.

Warren, D. W. (1967), *Cleft Palate J.*, **4**, 148.

Warren, D. W. and Dubois, A. B. (1964), *Cleft Palate J.*, **1**, 52.

Whillis, J. (1930), *J. Anat.*, **65**, 92.

Willis, C. R. and Stutz, M. L. (1972), *J. Speech Hear. Dis.*, **37**, 495.

SECTION VIII

NOSE

		PAGE
34.	OLFACTION	495
35.	NASAL FILTRATION	502
36.	AIR CONDITIONING FUNCTION	513
37.	ACOUSTIC ASPECTS OF NASAL FUNCTION	523

34. OLFACTION

ELLIS DOUEK

Few aspects of animal function have attracted so much attention as the senses. Vision and hearing have been extensively studied, not only from the structural and physiological view-point, but also for their more complex artistic developments. The other senses have never been as clearly understood and there is no doubt that olfaction has remained the most mysterious. This sense has always retained certain mystical overtones because of the role of perfume and incense in religious ceremony from earliest times. It is worth noting that the tablet on the breast of the sphinx shows the Pharaoh Tothmes IV offering incense and fragrant oil to the Gods. The mystical aspect of olfaction has coloured research in the subject almost to the present time and has contributed to the formation of the most extraordinary theories over the years.

A scientific approach has been inhibited by the lack of a quantitative and qualitative method of measurement which could be rested on a valid theory. Even clinical opinions have rarely been based on properly recorded and documented pathological findings so that they can more often be placed in the realm of folklore than in that of scientific observation.

Recently however the picture has changed considerably, the impetus coming from chemists working in the perfumery and flavour fields and spreading towards the other specialities. The time is right therefore to consider the present position regarding the sense of smell, but no attempt can be made in a single chapter to review the whole subject. We will confine ourselves then to a few of the advances which may have a more direct clinical application.

The Structure of the Olfactory Organ

In man the olfactory organ consists of an area of specialized epithelium which is limited to a region which includes the upper part of the superior concha, a corresponding area of the adjoining nasal septum and the roof in between.

Although the classification which we use to describe the types of cells which constitute this organ was established by Schultz more than a century ago, electron microscopy has added so many features to the known structure that any description should be based on micrographs.

There are three types of cell: receptor, supporting and basal cells. Deep to them are found Bowman's glands (Fig. 1).

The receptor cell is a bipolar neuron. It has a cell body with a distal and a proximal process. The distal process or rod is 20–90 μm long and is rich in mitochondria, microtubules and vesicles. It ends as a *knob* which protrudes about 2 μm above the surface of the mucosa and bears 1–20 cilia which arise from basal bodies in the outer

cytoplasmic areas. There are also a number of centrioles. The cilia project into the nasal cavity and it is therefore assumed that they bear the receptor surface, but there is, as yet, no clear evidence of this. It is unlikely that these cilia are actively motile but again there is no certainty of this. They consist of a short, thick, proximal segment which contains nine pairs of sub-fibres plus two central ones. The distal segment is narrow and tapering, containing

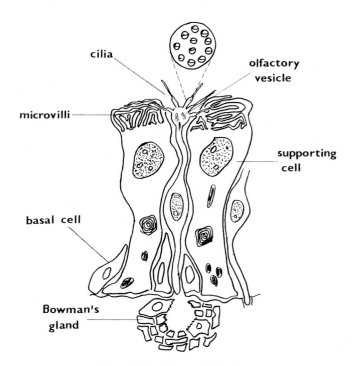

FIG. 1. The olfactory epithelium.

only half the number of sub-fibres. The proximal process of the receptor cell is invested by the basal cells until it pierces the basement membrane and is surrounded by Schwann cell cytoplasm. These axons form parallel fasciculi in the submucosa and pass through the openings in the cribriform plate to end in the bulb.

The supporting cell is thicker and its nucleus is at a more superficial level than that of the receptor cell. Its squat distal process ends in a surface of microvilli branching out in all directions and fusing with other branches. This network extends beyond the receptor cilia. The supporting cells are too complex to suggest a purely mechanical function, but exactly what their function is remains unclear.

The basal cell is a small polygonal cell which lies on the basement membrane and envelopes the axons of the receptor cells immediately beyond the supporting cells.

Bowman's glands lie beneath the basement membrane and consist of two types of cells; dark and light. Their secretions remain unrecognized and their function is thus unknown.

The yellowish-brown *olfactory pigment* is present as granules both in Bowman's glands and in the supporting

Regarding the olfactory mucosa itself, Ottoson's work from 1956 onwards has been the main contribution. Placing an electrode on the surface of the olfactory area of a frog, he directed a puff of odourized air at it. A slow, negative monophasic potential was developed (Fig. 3) and he termed this an *electro-olfactogram* (*e.o.g.*). Studies on other animals have shown this to be essentially the same response in all species. Cocaine studies have shown that the potential comes from the receptor cells and not the

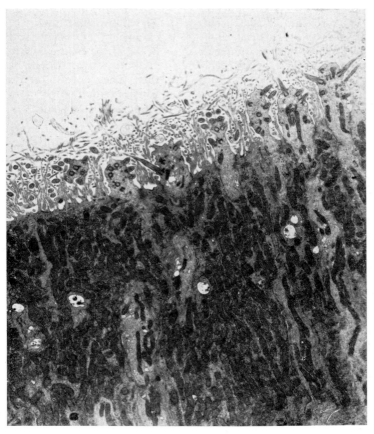

Fig. 2. Olfactory epithelium of the mouse. Electronmicrograph (× 5000), showing the surface structure drawn in Fig. 1. (Prepared by L. H. Bannister and H. Philipp, Guy's Hospital, London.)

cells. It consists mainly of lipids and the products of their auto-oxidation. There is little in the way of carotenoids in the human although these are present in the cow.

Normal human material is difficult to obtain in good enough condition and Fig. 2 has been prepared from the olfactory epithelium of the mouse by Dr. L. H. Bannister at Guy's Hospital.

Electrophysiology

The receptor cell detects minute quantities of odorous substances and the stimulus is transduced to a coded message that provides the brain with information about the quality and quantity of the chemical involved.

Over the last 20 years a great deal of information has been obtained and the impression is that of an important and continuous advance.

nerve fibres. The relationship between the e.o.g. and a generator potential for the transmitted nerve impulse is not clear, but it is possible that the e.o.g. is composite including perhaps the generator potential.

The e.o.g. responses to various substances presented at the same intensity has been studied. This has shown a considerable variation in duration and it is possible that this diversity represents the persistence of the olfactory sensation produced by some substances as compared with others. These potentials are altogether extremely slow (4–6 s) as compared with corresponding potentials in other sense organs. This may well be due to the fact that odorous particles have to pass through a layer of mucus in order to reach the membrane, and that excitation depends on the number of particles that reach the receptors per unit of time and is very gradual.

millivolts

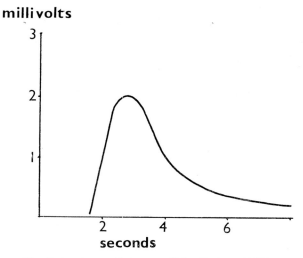

FIG. 3. An electro-olfactogram. (After Ottoson, 1956.)

Ottoson claimed that the increase in the amplitude of the e.o.g. had a logarithmic relationship with odour intensity. Adaptation tests on the frog preparation show very little, decline in the response with continuous stimulation. The olfactory organ is therefore among the slowly adapting sensors, which is difficult to explain in view of the well-known, rapid adaptation to smell. When the incoming impulses are measured at the bulb they can be seen to retain their strength at that level also, despite repetition. These facts suggest that the mechanism of adaptation is placed within the bulb itself.

Gasser (1956) using fish preparations was able to show that the action potential of the olfactory nerve was a single wave with a conduction velocity of 0.2 m.s^{-1}, which is slow and conforms with the axon diameter average of $0.2 \mu\text{m}$. Beidler and Tucker (1955) were able to record neural discharges from a bundle of fibres, responding to odorous stimuli, as they entered the bulb. They integrated the asynchronous responses into a running average.

The electrical activity of the olfactory bulb has been studied by many workers including Adrian (1956, 1959). He showed that there are large differences in the spatial patterning of excitation produced by different substances. It is possible that this pattern is due to differential distribution of the different odorous molecules in the nasal cavity. On the other hand the olfactory mucosa is very even and odours can be recognized just as well if inserted by the posterior choanae. If the excitation pattern in the bulb reflects the distribution of molecules on the olfactory mucosa, there are other likely factors such as the velocity of the air current and the composition of the surface film. There is also a temporal patterning in the bulb which is to some extent similar to the receptor response. Frequency component analysis of responses was carried out by Hughes and Hendrix (1967) on conscious rabbits with stainless steel macro-electrodes implanted into the olfactory bulb. The results were striking as the lowest frequency components represented respiration and sniffing rates. The highest frequency components appear in bursts at the beginning of a discharge and did not vary with different substances.

They may therefore represent a signal of odour presence only. Somewhat lower frequency components carried with the different chemicals and in particular high molecular weight substances, especially floral odours, show their main response between 37 and 75 Hz. Low molecular weight substances such as camphor respond between 75 and 125 Hz. There also appears to be both inhibitory and excitatory responses and variation according to the site of the electrode. The central regulative effects on the bulb are still unclear (Carreras *et al.*, 1967) but it is likely that the thalamus, as well as the reticular formation, influences it.

Theories of Smell

Although the first steps in the development of olfactory theory have been attempts at classifying the different smells, these are now of purely historical interest. Nevertheless since earliest times the theories of smell could be grouped into two main divisions: a *corpuscular theory* where the olfactory organ is stimulated by chemicals in particulate form, and a *wave theory*. In the latter case odorant substances are believed to emit waves by analogy with vision and hearing. The present representatives of the corpuscular concept have become dominated by the stereochemical theory. This idea was clearly stated by Moncrieff (1948) and developed to its present form by Amoore (1952).

The theory suggests that different shapes of molecules will fit into certain available molecular sites in the olfactory receptors and requires two pre-requisites from odorous substances: volatility and a molecular configuration that is complementary to certain sites on the receptor system. It implies that there must be primary odours of the sense of smell, and also that the sites which will receive them must have physical dimensions which correspond to the shape and size of the odorous molecules.

By surveying the chemical literature, Amoore made lists of pure compounds of known chemical structure which possessed the same smell. From the principle of probablity he accepted that rigid molecules, able to fit a given combination of two or more sites, are likely to be much less common than those fitting one site only. In that way the primary odours are likely to be the common ones.

The smell lists suggested that camphoraceous, floral, ethereal, minty, musky, putrid and pungent were the primary odours. Scale models of these molecules can be constructed from knowledge of similar compounds, X-ray crystallography, electron-diffraction etc. If receptor sites for molecules of these dimensions exist then their shapes can easily be worked out. Pungent compounds are usually highly reactive chemically with strongly electrophilic radicals while putrid compounds are usually nucleophilic. It may well be that the receptor site contains groupings giving them an opposite charge.

A vibrational theory is at present being widely discussed. It should be made clear, however, that it has no connection with the older wave theories which involved waves set in motion by a distant source. Modern vibrational theory refers to intra-molecular vibration and although by no means new, it is Dyson's (1937) theory and its development by Wright (1954) which interests us today. Molecules undergo many vibrations and it appears to be the low frequency range which contains the "osmic frequencies". According to Wright these had to be below 500 wave numbers to function in the conditions within the nose.

There are many difficulties in testing this theory and at present it is by no means entirely convincing.

More recently Davis (1953, 1957, 1962) offered a "Penetration and Puncturing Theory". He supposed that large, rigid, often awkwardly shaped, odorant molecules penetrate the membrane of the olfactory cell, leaving a slowly healing hole. The exchange of ions which would then take place would initiate excitation of nerves by short-circuiting the membrane resting potential. The quality of the odour will depend on the rate of diffusion of the odorant through the membrane relative to the subsequent rate of healing. As the membranes of different cells may also vary in their healing capacity, certain substances like musks would stimulate only cells with slowly healing membranes. Small molecules like ether which are weakly absorbed would not.

Despite great activity, smell theory today has still not reached a conclusion. Until such a time it will hold back clinical progress. The situation is, however, hopeful as research in this field is now experimental rather than speculative.

Tests of Smell

The lack of a theory of smell has contributed to the absence of widely accepted methods of testing smell. This has resulted in a profusion of tests so vast that it is not possible to review them here. We shall confine ourselves to a discussion of certain salient points and recent advances.

Objective tests such as those based on pupillary, cardiovascular, respiratory, psychogalvanic or electroencephalographic changes have not been of clinical value. Those based on haematogenous stimulation have also never attained practical application. We are left, therefore, with subjective tests of one type or another, and of a varying degree of sophistication.

Measurement of the olfactory threshold can be done in two ways: as a measure of the minimum perceptible odour (M.P.O.) and as a measure of the minimum recognizable odour (M.R.O.). The M.R.O. has not been found

as dependable as the M.P.O. because many other problems are involved in recognition. Recognition tests in general are of only limited use and Sumner (1962) suggested that only a few simple substances should be used when identification is required.

Measurement of the M.P.O. has been done in every conceivable way. Proetz's (1924) olfactometer has been an important contribution. It consisted of a rack containing 100 bottles of 10 different odorants at different dilutions. He coined the unit "olfact" to provide a quantitative element. It was the M.P.O. for a substance for many people expressed in grams per litre.

Another approach was that of Elsberg et al. (1936) who used a blast injection from a small bottle. This led to great interest in olfactory measurement particularly in Neurology.

It was modified by the author (Douek, 1967, 1970) so that it could be brought closer to modern theory. Seven blast olfactometers (Fig. 4) contained representatives of Amoore's primary odours and the results were expressed as the M.P.O. for each substance measured as volume units.

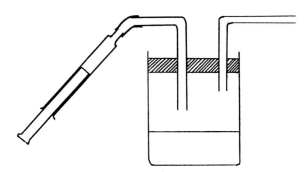

Fig. 4. A small blast olfactometer.

The whole was graphically represented as an *olfactory spectrogram* (O.S.G.)—(Fig. 5). Although there was a useful correlation between the O.S.G. and pathological conditions, it would be wrong to consider this to be a form of proof of the primary odour theory.

There have been many criticisms of these simple systems

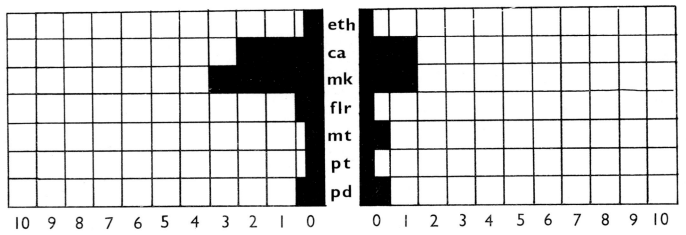

Fig. 5. An olfactory spectrogram—normal except for some reduction in musky and camphoraceous smell.

mostly based on the lack of regulation of the number of molecules entering the nose and on the variability of the stimulus pressure. Complex apparatus has been devised to overcome this (Stuiver, 1960; Bozza et al., 1960; Eyferth, 1969). The author believes that the use of these complex systems of stimulus delivery are misleading if the purity of the odorant is not ascertained. Chemical purity of a liquid can usually only be guaranteed to a certain degree; it is variable between the different compounds and decomposition products are an important source of impurities in odorant substances. An even greater reason for uncertainty is the probability that the percentage impurity alters and may be magnified in the vapour as opposed to the liquid. As odorants can be selectively absorbed onto the walls of the apparatus (Douek and Poynder, 1973), the stimulus itself may be grossly impure. Analysis by gas/liquid chromatography would be essential in a parallel apparatus or in series adding to the bulkiness of the whole. Although such systems may be essential for experimental work they have a less prominent place in clinical testing.

Abnormalities of Smell

Abnormalities of smell may be quantitative, such as anosmia or hyposmia if reduced in threshold, hyperosmia if there is a greater sensitivity to smells: or else they may be qualitative, causing distortions of smell known broadly as "parosmia".

These symptoms can be caused by simple local lesions in the nose such as vasomotor rhinitis or by serious intracranial disease. Any abnormality of smell warrants investigation. The olfactory investigation of intracranial lesions was considered of considerable importance at a time when other less subjective tests were not available. Elsberg and Stewart (1938), Spillane (1938) and Zilstorff-Pedersen (1955, 1964) produced a considerable body of observation which could be summarized in the following manner.

Pressure on the olfactory nerve or tract such as that exerted by an olfactory groove meningioma will raise the smell threshold. Supratentorial intracerebral neoplasms may give a normal threshold but, with olfactory stimuli, fatigue is more persistent. There is a tendency for an odorous stimulus applied to the side in which a tumour is present to be felt as if it came from the opposite side. Spillane (1938) has called this phenomenon "olfactory alloaesthesia".

Abnormalities due to local nasal lesions have been studied by the author for some years, using the O.S.G. technique of testing and a number of findings were made. (Douek, 1973). Patients with a deviated nasal septum are unlikely to lose their sense of smell. If they have lost it there is probably some other cause and it would be wrong to suggest that they can be treated by septal surgery. Patients with rhinitis of various types tend to give a similar O.S.G. with a loss variable both quantitatively and qualitatively. It was not possible to differentiate between the various types of rhinitis by their olfactory changes as demonstrated in this way, but some unexpected changes did have a clinical significance. Patients with mucosal changes of

rhinitis who complained of parosmia tended to have lost the ability to smell one or two modalities completely. This absence of perception was given the name "anosmic zone" and the presence of such zones did have an association with distortion of smell. Other patients with parosmia, who had an entirely normal O.S.G., probably belonged to a different group.

A further group of patients who claimed to have lost the sense of smell responded almost completely to stimulus by large quantities of odoriferous vapour. The response, however, was fleeting and the olfactory sensation was the same whatever the stimulus used. The term single non-discriminating (S.N.D.) response was given to this phenomenon and it bore a very poor prognosis.

Two patients were recently studied by O.S.G. and both had scrape biopsies of the olfactory mucosa taken by the author. The tissues were prepared for electron microscopy (L. H. Bannister and H. Philipp) and produced features of considerable interest.

The first patient suffered from a severe chronic rhinitis of infective origin and had lost the sense of smell almost completely. Electron microscopy (Fig. 6) showed that the olfactory epithelium was grossly altered. There seems to have been extensive replacement of sensory cells by abnormal respiratory epithelium, including goblet cells bearing motile cilia. Some cells were present which did not fit exactly into any category but their internal structure suggested that they were modified supporting cells.

The second patient had had an episode of influenza which she had caught from a sister who in turn had caught it from a neighbour. All three women had lost the sense of smell but only one came to be examined. Electron microscopy (Fig. 7) again showed a greatly modified epithelium, but this time the most dramatic changes were seen in the subepithelial layers. All neuronal elements had disappeared and the most characteristic structures were fibroblasts and the large quantities of collagen which surrounded them. In other words scar tissue had replaced the nerve fibres of the olfactory cells and probably also the autonomic nerve fibres which are present in the area.

Altogether there is still very little information on the changes which occur when the sense of smell is damaged.

Pheromones

Few aspects of olfaction have attracted more interest in recent years than the discovery of pheromones. Their existence in primates, much less in man, has not been demonstrated beyond doubt but the subject is of such potential importance that it should be recognized here.

The name pheromone was first used to describe sex-attractants in insects and they have also been known as ectohormones. They are chemical substances formed by glands and which affect the behaviour, development and reproduction of individuals. They differ from hormones as, while the latter are secreted within and by the individual that they will affect, pheromones are secreted by one individual and carry information to others. Hormones are not species specific and their use in medical treatment has been largely due to the fact that they can be extracted from

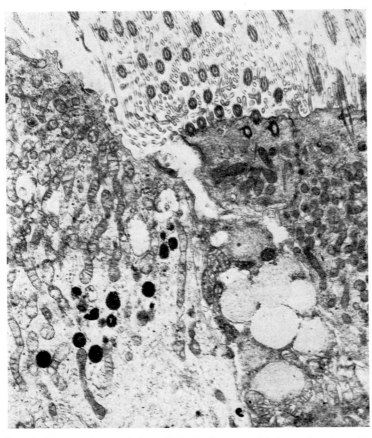

FIG. 6. Electronmicrograph (×10 000) of olfactory epithelium of patient with loss of smell from chronic rhinitis. (Prepared by L. H. Bannister and H. Philipp, Guy's Hospital, London.)

the secreting glands of other animals. Pheromones, however, appear to be species specific although there may be some overlap between related insect species.

The existence of chemical signals of this type given out by one individual and received by the olfactory organ of another, is found among insects and have been used commerically as pesticides.

In mammals, Whitten (1956) has shown the effect of anosmia in mice. He showed that if a number of females are kept together there occurs a suppression of oestrus, but if a male is introduced among them a new cycle is induced so that oestrus becomes synchronized in the group. Bruce (1959) showed the olfactory control which male mice exert on the female. If a mated female is put in the presence of a strange male even as late as four days after conception, the pregnancy will fail and she will return to oestrus. Bruce demonstrated that this blocking effect was due to olfactory impulses.

Michael and Keverne (1970) carried out a series of experiments using rhesus monkeys. It appeared from these that there is a component in the vaginal secretions of the female which provides an olfactory stimulus which induces sexual activity in the male.

No pheromone has been discovered in humans and one should be careful not to confuse a process of conditioning to a particular smell with a true pheromone. It is important,

however, not to overlook the possibility of such substances in these days of deodorants and contraceptive pills.

REFERENCES

Adrian, E. D. (1956), "The Action of the Mammalian Olfactory Organ," *J. Laryng.*, **70:** 1.

Adrian, E. D. (1959), "Des réactions éléctriques du système olfactif.," *Actualités Neurophysiol. (Paris)*, **1,** 1.

Amoore, J. E. (1952), "Smell and Molecular Shape," *Perfum. essent. Oil Rec.*, **43,** 321.

Beidler, L. M. and Tucker, D. (1955), "Response of Nasal Epithelium to Odor Stimulation," *Science*, **122,** 76.

Bozza, G., Calearo, C. and Teatini, P. (1960), "On the Making of a Rational Olfactometer," *Acta oto-laryng. (Stockh.)*, **52,** 189.

Bruce, H. M. (1959), "An Exteroceptive Block to Pregnancy in the Mouse," *Nature, Lon.*, **184,** 105.

Carreras, M., Mancia, D. and Mancia, M. (1967), "Centrifugal Control of the Olfactory Bulb as Revealed by Induced Slow Potential Changes," *Electroenceph. clin. Neurophysiol.*, **23,** 190.

Davis, J. T. (1953), "A Theory of Smell," *Int. Perfum.*, **3,** 17.

Davis, J. T. and Taylor, F. H. (1957), "Olfactory Thresholds and Molecular Size and Absorption Energies," *Proc. II Int. Congr. Surf. Activ.*, Vol. 4, p. 329. London: Butterworths.

Davis, J. T. (1962), "Penetration and Puncture Theory," *Symp. Soc. exp. Biol.*, **8,** 1.

Douek, E. (1967), "Smell: Recent Theories and Their Clinical Applications," *J. Laryng.*, **81,** 431.

Douek, E. (1970), "Some Abnormalities of Smell," *J. Laryng.*, **84,** 1185.

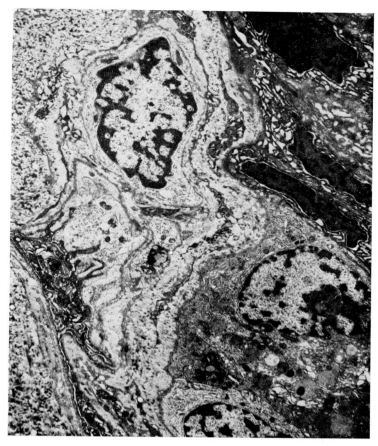

FIG. 7. Electronmicrograph (×5000) of olfactory epithelium of patient with anosmia following influenza. (Prepared by L. H. Bannister and H. Philipp, Guy's Hospital, London.)

Douek, E. (1973), *The Sense of Smell and its Abnormalities.* London and Edinburgh: Churchill-Livingstone.

Dyson, G. M. (1937), "Smell and Molecular Vibrations," *Perfum. essent. Oil Rec.*, **28**, 13.

Elsberg, C. A., Levy, I. and Brewer, E. D. (1936), "New Method for Testing the Sense of Smell," *Science*, **83**, 211.

Elsberg, C. A. and Stewart, J. (1938), "Quantitative Olfactory Tests," *Arch. Neurol. Psychiat.*, **40**, 471.

Eyferth, K. (1969), "Notiz über ein einfaches olfactometer," *H.N.O. (Berl.*, **17**, 14.

Gasser, H. (1956), "Olfactory Nerve Fibres," *J. gen. Physiol. (Baltimore)*, **39**, 473.

Michael, P. R. and Keverne, E. B. (1970), "Primate Sex Pheromones of Vaginal Origin," *Nature (Lond.)*, **225**, 84.

Moncrieff, R. W. (1949), "Odor and Molecular Shape," *Amer. Perfum.*, 453.

Ottoson, D. (1956), "Analysis of the Olfactory Epithelium," *Acta physiol. scand.*, suppl. 122.

Proetz, A. (1924), "A System of Exact Olfactometry," *Ann. Otol. (St. Louis)*, **33**, 746.

Spillane, J. D. (1938), "Olfactory Alloaesthesia," *Brain*, **61**, 393.

Stuiver, M. (1960), "An Olfactometer with a Wide Range of Possibilities," *Acta oto-laryng. (Stockh.)*, **51**, 135.

Sumner, D. (1962), "On Testing the Sense of Smell," *Lancet*, **2**, 895.

Whitten, W. K. (1956), "Effect of Removal of Olfactory Bulbs on Gonads of Mice," *J. Endocr.*, **14**, 160.

Wright, R. H. (1954), "Osmically Significant Vibrational Modes," *J. appl. Chem. (London)*, **4**, 611.

Zilstorff-Pedersen, K. (1955), "Further Studies on Blast-olfactometry," *Acta oto-laryng. (Stockh.)*, **45**, 268.

Zilstorff-Pedersen, K. (1964), "Determinations and Variations of Olfactory Thresholds," *Arch. Otolaryng. (Chicago)*, **79**, 412.

35. NASAL FILTRATION

A. C. HILDING

The function of nasal filtration has become a subject of increasing interest in the decades of the '60's and the '70's with the ever-widening scope of studies and publications concerning airborne occupational hazards and airborne pollutants affecting the entire population or certain regions (Corn and Burton, 1967; Fry, 1970; Hounam *et al.*, 1971, 1972; Acheson *et al.*, 1968; Brain, 1970; Buckley and Loosli, 1969; R. Frank, 1970; N. R. Frank *et al.*, 1969; Fry and Black, 1973; Morrow, 1970; Proctor and Swift, 1972; Speizer and Frank, 1966). The dramatic emphasis given to our surroundings in recent years by a new consciousness of the importance of preserving our various ecological systems has brought some of the natural defence systems of the body, such as nasal filtration, into a sharper focus of interest than they have probably ever enjoyed. Just being aware of the capabilities of these systems may help us in making judicious and well-balanced decisions allowing people, industry and ecological systems to exist together with the least amount of unnecessary restriction on any group and the greatest opportunity to enhance the future of all the groups.

It is satisfying, for those of us who would like to have decisions in this important field of our environment made with the greatest availability of scientific information, to know that entire symposiums are being devoted to such subjects as "Inhaled Particles" (Inhaled Particles and Vapours, 1961; Inhaled Particles and Vapours II, 1967; Inhaled Particles III, 1972), "Air Pollution Medical Research" (Annual Air Pollution Medical Research Conferences started in 1960, in recent years the papers have been published in *Archives of Environmental Health*) and "Inhalation Carcinogenesis" (Inhalation Carcinogenesis, 1970). Well-known workers from many disciplines and many parts of the world have contributed their knowledge and experience to these meetings, the proceedings of which are available to us in the literature.

The year 1970 saw the inception of publication in England of a journal, *Aerosol Science* (Pergamon Press, Great Britain), which is offering much of importance to those working in the field of respiratory tract physiology. The American publication, *Archives of Environmental Health* (American Medical Association, Chicago) devotes considerable space to environmental factors related to the respiratory tract and airborne foreign matter. Certainly these are but a few examples of this type of literature, but they serve to point out the emphasis we have been observing in recent years on the behaviour of the respiratory tract toward inhaled environmental substances.

The major purpose of the nose is to conduct and to prepare inspired air for safe reception into the lungs. In addition to adjusting temperature and humidity, this involves cleansing the air of polluting substances—particulate matter, micro-organisms and some gases. The nasal mucosa is perhaps more exposed to the environment than any other part of the body. Even the skin is not exposed to a blast of rapidly-flowing, raw air 18 or 20 times a minute.

Filtration not only requires the removal of pollutants from the air stream, but involves the disposal of this collected material.

Air Flow Through Tubes

A suspension of dust particles in a gas flowing smoothly (laminar flow) through a tube of uniform diameter does not deposit much of the suspended material. When such a tube is lined by wet blotting-paper and is warmed, in imitation of the nasal passages, gas (air) passing through it in laminar flow becomes neither warmed nor humidified to any great extent. If the tube through which the suspended dust flows contains constrictions, bends or dilatations, deposition of dust particles takes place just beyond the constrictions and bends and within the dilatations (Bernoulli's phenomenon) (Proetz, 1953; Williams, 1970). When the flow is turbulent and the tube is warmed and lined with wet blotting paper, air passing through becomes both warmed and humidified (Ingelstedt, 1970). Turbulence is necessary for effective deposition of particulate matter and for warming and humidifying.

Air Flow Through the Nose

The nose is anatomically irregular. At the anterior nares, inspired air divides into two jets, which are directed up and back. Upon entering the preturbinal areas, it expands in the larger space there. Then the middle and inferior conchae divide the flow into irregular, flat ribbons in the common, middle and inferior meatuses. Since all of these meatuses are irregular from front to back, the air streams must continually change shape to conform. The directions of flow also change. In the common meatus, the flow is in the form of an arc—up, back and down, in the inferior and middle meatuses, the direction is more nearly straight back. At the posterior choanae, the streams from the meatuses from both sides unite to make a single stream, which then makes a sharp turn downward to pass through the pharynx and then somewhat forward to enter the larynx. There are eddies about the posterior margin of the soft palate, in the pharyngeal recesses (Rosenmüller's fossae), about the base of the tongue, the pyriform fossae and the posterior part of the mouth and about the epiglottis. The flow within the nose is turbulent as the air passes through the narrow spaces, over irregularities, such as the conchae and septal ridges and as it makes the changes of direction (Proctor, 1965, 1966; Proctor and Swift, 1972; Bridger and Proctor, 1970).

The volume in the nasal cavities (excluding the sinuses) is about 7 or 8 ml on each side. Thus, during inspiration or expiration of 500 ml of air in quiet breathing, the volume of contained air must change more than 30 times. The volume and shape of the air passages are altered from time to time through changes in the volume of the blood flow in the erectile tissue over the conchae and septum (Takagi *et al.*, 1969; Drettner, 1961). The volume of the pharynx also varies, depending upon contraction of the palatine and pharyngeal muscles and the position of the tongue. Thus, the flow within the nose and pharynx is turbulent.

The degree of turbulence within the nose depends upon the velocity of air flow, increasing with increasing velocity (Fig. 1). During quiet respiration, the velocity changes

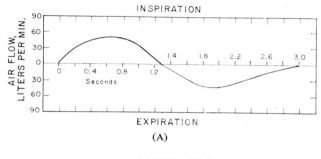

(A)

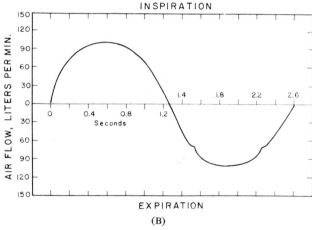

(B)

FIG. 1. (A) Mean respiratory air flow for subjects seated on a Krogh bicycle ergometer riding at 0 watts, breathing through minimal resistance. (B) Same with the subjects riding at 102 watts. (Redrawn from Silverman *et al.*, 1951.)

during each inspiration. The average flow rate is about 15 l.min⁻¹, but it begins at zero, then accelerates to a maximum velocity of 40 l.min⁻¹, then decelerates to zero again, all in 1 or 2 s. The maximum velocity is sustained for 55–60 per cent of the time of inspiration.

Bridger and Proctor (1970) found that there is a limit to the increase in nasal air flow from inspiratory effort. Up to a point, the volume of air-flow increases with increased inspiratory effort but, when a critical transnasal pressure is reached, there is no further increase in air flow with increased inspiratory effort. They placed the "flow-limiting segment" about where the upper nasal cartilages are attached to the pyriform margins of the maxilla. When the negative pressure within the nose reaches a critical point, the erectile tissue in this area becomes engorged with blood and reduces the cross-sectional area, thus preventing further increase in air flow.

Air Conditioning and Recycling

According to the second law of thermodynamics, the nasal lining loses heat to inspired air, if this is below body temperature, as is usually the case. Additional heat is lost through evaporation of the water necessary to humidify the air. The quantity of this heat loss is equal to the mass of water times the heat of vaporization. Thus, considerable heat and water are lost to inspired air. It is of importance that a portion of both be recycled and used again (Ingelstedt, 1970). This also has an effect on filtration. As the air flows out during expiration, it is warmer than the cooled nasal walls and, therefore, gives back part of its heat. In addition, the contained water vapour condenses on the cooled walls, restoring to them the heat of vaporization. This recycling of heat and moisture is of fundamental importance to the normal functioning of the nasal mucosa.

Deposition

The nasal deposition of particulate matter suspended in inspired air depends upon the nature of the particles and certain physical factors. The size, shape and density of the particles are pertinent. The forces involved in deposition include air resistance, velocity, inertia, gravity, diffusion and, under unusual circumstances, electric charge. These factors vary in magnitude with the velocity of air flow and the times for transit from place to place within the system and from moment to moment throughout the breathing cycle (Hatch and Gross, 1964). In general, the larger and heavier the particles, the sooner they deposit (Hatch, 1961; Hatch and Hemeon, 1948). Some particles form aggregations and some hygroscopic dusts take on water, becoming larger until they reach an equilibrium determined by vapor saturation at the ambient body temperature. Bacteria, although small, may form agglomerates (Laurenzi *et al.*, 1964) or may be included in droplets. Viruses can also be enclosed in droplets. All of these then behave as larger particles and are deposited in the nose (Lippmann, 1970b).

Effect of Inertia or Resistance

A large, heavy particle moving at a high velocity, will not follow the air flow in sharp turns and in eddies. Its inertia tends to keep it on a straight trajectory and it cuts across the lines of flow to impact against the bounding walls. Smaller particles and those of low density are more influenced by air resistance and tend to remain suspended longer in turns and eddies. In other words, the force, due to viscosity of the air which tends to keep the particles in the stream, is proportional to the surface area.

The shape of the particles also makes a difference. Air resistance acts more upon an irregularly shaped particle than upon a round one. At low velocities, when turbulence is small, relatively large particles may remain suspended. When velocity is high and turbulence great, even relatively small particles become deposited. Consequently, the rate of deposition and the size of particles deposited, vary greatly during each inspiration. At the low velocity of air flow during the beginning of inspiration, the efficiency of filtration—deposition—is relatively low and even large particles may pass through the nose. As the velocity of flow accelerates, so does that of the suspended particles and turbulence increases. As a consequence, filtration is more effective and smaller and smaller particles strike the walls to become deposited. During deceleration, the reverse is true.

Effect of Gravity

The effect of gravity upon the particles depends, obviously, upon their mass and density and upon the size of the airway and time and velocity of flow and the air resistance. The greater their mass and density, the more rapidly the particles will sediment. The larger the airway and the greater the air resistance, the slower they will settle. Obviously, the greater the time involved, the greater the sedimentation. Inertial deposition increases with the flow rate whereas sedimentation increases as the flow rate decreases. In neither instance are the effects upon particle deposition linear (Hatch and Gross, 1964). (*See below*—Physics.)

Effect of Diffusion

The overall effect of diffusion on particles within the nose is probably negligible. For particles 0·5 μm (micrometers) in diameter, the diffusion rate, according to Davies (1946) is several hundred thousand times slower than that for organic vapours. Deposition by diffusion of droplets or particles, even above 0·1 μm is negligible, at all flow rates.

Location of Deposition

After the inspired air has passed through the anterior nares, it expands, filters through the hairs in the vestibule, constricts again at the limen nasi, then expands into the preturbinal area, and then strikes the anterior ends of the inferior and middle conchae. Here, in the anterior third of the nose, a large portion of the suspended material is deposited. The exposure of the lining mucosa of this part of the nose to harsh environment from the incoming blast of raw air is so great that cilia cannot survive it. The epithelium here is squamous or transitional in character and this type extends over the anterior portions of the conchae. Further deposition takes place as the air stream changes direction to flow back instead of up. Turbulence and deposition take place about the conchae and any ridges which may be present upon the septum. Again, more deposition takes place in the pharynx as the air stream turns sharply downward and as it passes through the eddies about the palate, toruses, tongue and epiglottis.

Gases

Certain noxious gases contained in inspired air are removed by solution in the lining mucous blanket of the respiratory tract. The respiratory secretion is a buffer at about pH 7·0–7·2 and tends to neutralize both acid and basic gases. Diffusion undoubtedly is a factor in the deposition of gas molecules.

The Tract Beyond the Nose

Although the tracheobrachial tree is not part of the nose anatomically, the entire tract, from the tip of the nose to and including the terminal bronchioles, is a single physiologic unit as far as conduction, cleansing and conditioning of respired air is concerned. The nose furnishes from 50–70 per cent of the total gas flow resistance (Butler, 1960; Hugh-Jones *et al.*, 1962) necessary for the physiology of air flow in and out of the pulmonic portion of the lungs (distal to the terminal bronchioles). This resistance is probably also important in the proper perfusion of the lungs.

Nasal irritants have been found to cause bronchial constriction and also to change the depth and rate of breathing (Corn and Burton, 1967; Binger and Gaarde, 1931).

Ogura and his colleagues (1970, 1971) have made a number of research studies, which have revealed a relationship between nasal obstruction and increased lower airway resistance. Nasal obstruction undoubtedly, under these circumstances, would also have an effect on the filtration efficiency of the nose. Drettner (1970), in studying the nasobronchial reflex, found that it was principally homolateral and that it was transmitted from the nasal mucosa to the lungs, probably via the trigeminal and vagus nerves. It is supposed that these nasopulmonary and nasobronchial reflexes increase bronchial tone in cases of nasal obstruction (Sercer, 1930, 1952) and increase pulmonary resistance and decrease compliance (Corn and Burton, 1967; R. Frank, 1970). Physiologically, the nose acts as a factor in the control of respiration (Williams, 1969).

The velocity of flow in the trachea is relatively low (lower than in the nose) but even here the flow is turbulent (Drettner, 1970; Brody, 1966; Ingelstedt and Toremalm, 1960) and deposition continues—in fact, all through the larynx, trachea and bronchial tree. Beyond the bifurcation of the primary carina, for the first six or eight branchings, the surface area of the epithelium lining the tract increases but the combined cross-sectional area does not increase. However, after the first six or eight branchings (generations), both increase—the combined cross-sectional area of the tract sharply and surface area enormously. The flow rate decreases correspondingly as the total cross-sectional area increases. The terminal bronchi are only a fraction of a millimeter in diameter and suspended particles must pass very close to the lining mucous blanket and some deposit, even though the velocity is here very low. Finally, in the alveoli, the air movement is reduced to the point where it consists mainly of diffusion of molecules—Brownian movement. Remaining fine particles—one-tenth of a micrometer (micron) or less in diameter—that have not already been deposited through gravity may deposit by diffusion—impact with moving gas molecules. As previously stated, some of the fine particles (about 0·5 μm in diameter) may not be deposited at all, but may flow out again during expiration. This size does not actually enter the alveoli. It travels only as far as mass movement of the air continues and remains suspended there until expiration.

Physics of Nasal Deposition

A number of workers have studied in detail the physics of particle deposition; among them Morrow (1959, 1960, 1970) and Landahl (1950). Landahl divides the nose into four regions in calculating the deposition of particulate matter. The hairy region in the vestibule is the first. He divides the hairs into two groups and considers that the projection of the two groups combined covers half of the area of each of the external nares. In his calculations he takes the diameters of the hairs of the two groups to be 150 μm and 50 μm respectively. The probability of impaction of dust particles against the hairs he takes to be the sum of two similar terms, P_h' and P_h''—one for each group of hairs. He writes the equation for one group thus:

$$P_h' = f' \left[\frac{150 \left(\rho d^2 V/D'\right)^3}{3 \times 10^{-6} + \left(\rho d^2 V/D'\right)^2 + 150 \left(\rho d^2 V/D'\right)^3} + \frac{d}{D'} \right] \tag{35.1}$$

where f' = the fraction of projected area covered by one
group (150 μm) of hairs
V = average velocity of air flow (cm.s^{-1})
D' = diameter of the hairs (cm)
ρ = particle density
d = particle diameter (cm)

The equation for the 50 μm group would be similar. The sum of the two would be the total probability of impaction, P_h, if the hairs were evenly distributed. Since they are not, he makes a correction.

From his calculations he concludes that a substantial part of the particles removed from the air stream in the nose are removed by the hairs. He does not mention the additional factors of the expansion of the airways within the vestibule, or of the dryness of the hairs.

Within the nose proper, deposition takes place through: (1) inertia (impaction), (2) gravity sedimentation, and, to a minor degree, through (3) diffusion.

(1) Inertial Deposition

When a flowing air stream carrying a dust particle makes a change of direction, due to its inertia the particle tends to continue in a straight line but meets resistance as it moves across the line of flow. The direction it takes is determined by the balance between air resistance and inertial force. The "stopping distance" of the particle as it moves through the air is proportional to the balance of the two forces acting upon it. Hatch and Gross (1964) give this value as

$$h_s = \frac{U_t U \sin \theta}{g} \tag{35.2}$$

where h_s = the stopping distance
U = the velocity of the air stream
θ = the angle of the bend
U_t = terminal velocity of fall
g = acceleration due to gravity

The probability of inertial deposit is proportional to the ratio of stopping-distance to the diameter of the airway.

Landahl (1962) obtained two equations from the inertial parameter $U_t U \sin \theta / gW$, where W is the channel dimension (Landahl, 1950):

$$\text{Inertial deposition } I = 1 - \frac{1}{12} \left(\frac{gW}{U_t U \sin \theta} \right)^2$$
$$+ \frac{1}{108} \left(\frac{gW}{U_t U \sin \theta} \right)^3 \tag{35.3}$$

assuming that the velocity distribution across the stream is parabolic. Assuming air velocity to be uniform, the probability of deposit is expressed by the equation:

$$I = \frac{2U_t U \sin \theta}{gW} \tag{35.4}$$

Landahl used the averages of these two equations to express the value of inertial deposition.

(2) Gravity Sedimentation

Fine particles falling through air fall at a constant velocity such that air resistance balances the weight of the particle. Particles of low density or irregular shape offer more surface to air resistance than dense or round ones, hence settle more slowly. The following equation (Hatch and Gross, 1964) shows the relation of size and density to terminal velocity of fall:

$$U_t = \frac{\sigma g d^2}{18\gamma} \tag{35.5}$$

where U_t = terminal velocity of fall
σ = particle density
g = acceleration due to gravity
d = particle diameter
γ = air viscosity

To determine the rate, time, dimensions and shape of airways and flow rate, gravity must be taken into account. Landahl (1962) does this in the following expression for circular airways:

$$S = 1 - \exp \left[- (0 \cdot 8 U_t t \cos \psi)/R \right] \tag{35.6}$$

where S = sedimentation coefficient
t = time
ψ = angle
R = radius

For the nasal airways, which are far from round, he modifies the exponential parameter to read:

$$S = 1 - \exp \left[-(1 \cdot 3 U_t t \cos \psi)/W \right] \tag{35.7}$$

where W = the channel dimensions.

Assuming the angle $\psi = 45°$ and expressing time (t) and dimensions (W) in terms of area of the walls (A_t) and air flow F, the equation becomes:

$$S = 1 - \exp \left[-(0 \cdot 46 A_t U_t)/F \right] \tag{35.8}$$

(3) Diffusion

When the diameter of a particle approaches and becomes smaller than the mean free distance between air molecules, air resistance decreases and a correction must be made (Hatch and Gross, 1964). But, since deposition by diffusion (except for gases) (Brownian movement) is considered to be negligible in the nose, this is mainly of importance deeper in the respiratory tract (Fig. 2).

Because of all of the irregularities of channel shape and size and irregular and changing flow-rates (Fig. 3) and the variable turbulence during respiration—variable pyramiding upon variable (Dennis, 1972)—accurate values for nasal deposition cannot be expected through mathematics. To arrive at true values, experimental measurement is necessary. Yet, the theoretical and experimental results are surprisingly close to one another (Fig. 4).

CLINICAL AND EXPERIMENTAL DETERMINATIONS

The efficiency of nasal filtration has been studied by many workers using a number of different techniques (Lippmann, 1970a, b; Asset *et al.*, 1956; Asset, 1957;

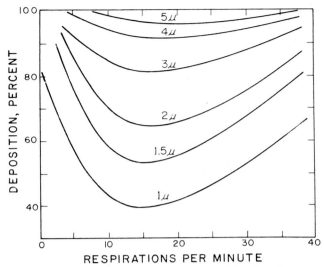

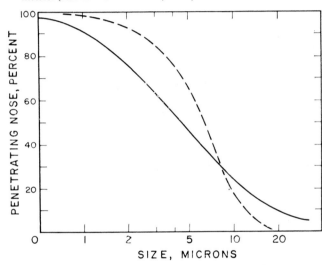

Fig. 3. Variations of total respiratory deposition in relation to breathing frequency for different sized particles. Size in micrometers. (Redrawn from Dennis, 1961.)

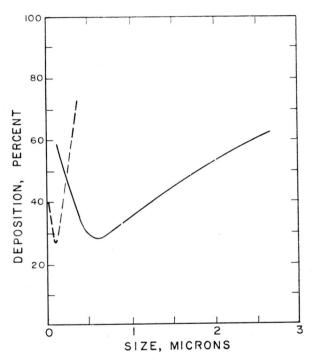

Fig. 2. Percentage of respiratory deposition in relation to particle size in micrometers (microns), showing increase in deposition of submicronic particles by diffusion as they grow smaller. (Reprinted with permission from Dautrebande and Walkenhorst (1961), in *Inhaled Particles and Vapours* (C. N. Davies, Ed.). Pergamon Press Ltd.)

Fig. 4. Percentage of inhaled particles passing through (penetrating) the nasal chamber in relation to particle size in micrometers (microns). Mean of a variety of particles. Air flow 18 l/min. Experimental findings (solid line) are compared with theory (calculated findings). (Redrawn from Landahl, 1950.)

Hilding *et al.*, 1967; Landahl and Black, 1947; Palm *et al.*, 1956; Lehmann, 1935; Brain, 1970; Tourangeau and Drinker, 1937; Meurman, 1948; Acheson 1968; Fry and Black, 1973; Davies, 1946; Boyland *et al.*, 1947; van Wijk and Patterson, 1940; Landahl and Hermann, 1950; Frank *et al.*, 1969; Frank, 1970; Speizer and Frank, 1966; Amdur, 1966; Dalhamn, 1961; Dalhamn and Sjöholm, 1963; Henry *et al.*, 1969; Anderson *et al.*, 1971; Bridger and Proctor, 1970; Bates *et al.*, 1965; Dennis, 1961, 1972; Dautrebande and Walkenhorst, 1961; Fry, 1973; Hatch, 1961; Hatch and Hemeon, 1948; Hatch and Gross, 1964; Hounam and Black, 1971, 1972; Landahl, 1950; Morrow, 1959, 1960, 1970; Proctor and Wagner, 1965; Proctor, 1966; Proctor and Swift, 1972; Proetz, 1953; Wolfsdorf *et al.*, 1969).

Asset and Gongwer (Asset, 1957; Asset *et al.*, 1956) tested the noses of freshly killed experimental animals by placing the decapitated heads in a 6·7 m (22 ft) wind-

tunnel in a stream of air flowing at 1·12 m.s⁻¹ (2·5 m.p.h.) and containing aerosols of triphenylphosphate. The particles were of low density, i.e. 1 200 Kg.m⁻³ (1·2 gm/cm³) and of a diameter averaging 1·3 μm. They recorded penetration of the nose (not deposited) of 92 per cent. Objection to these studies might be made on the grounds that the air flow was unidirectional for 10–20 min and that the animal was dead. During respiration, of course, the air flow is to and fro with inspiration, lasting (in man) 1–2 s only, and with warming and moistening of the mucous membrane during expiration. The authors found no appreciable difference in the size and shape of the nasal passages after death as compared with the ante-mortem state and apparently they assumed there would likewise be no change in filtration efficiency.

In some experiments that we did (Hilding *et al.*, 1967),

passing 20 ml of cigarette-smoke-laden air through the noses of anesthetized rabbits and guinea pigs, a definite difference was found between the filtration efficiency before death and that after death—the latter being less efficient. Also, during life, the efficiency varied with the depth of anesthesia, being greater under light than under very deep anesthesia. Under light anesthesia, 40 per cent of the smoke was filtered out, while under very deep anesthesia and after death, only 23 and 22 per cent respectively was filtered out.

Landahl and Black (1947) passed three types of particles (corn oil, sodium bicarbonate and tricalcium phosphate) through the noses of volunteers. They found that deposition was greater at higher velocities of flow than at lower. The oil droplets did not deposit as well as the sodium bicarbonate, probably because of the lower density. At flow rates of 10, 17, 29 and 60 l.min^{-1}, the particle diameters corresponding to 50 per cent penetration (and deposition) were found to be 8, 5, 5 and 2 μm respectively for corn oil droplets. For sodium bicarbonate particles, at 17 and 60 l.min^{-1}, the diameters for 50 per cent penetration were 2 and 1 μm. Average flow rate in man in quiet respiration is about 15 l.min^{-1}. At this flow rate, particles (sodium bicarbonate and calcium phosphate) <0·6 μm hardly deposited at all and above 10 μm. almost all did.

Palm and his colleagues (1956) tested dust retention in the noses of man, guinea pigs and monkeys. They used clay dust varying in size from 0·5–5 μm in man and in the guinea pig from 0·1–3 μm. At 3 μm, in the guinea pig, deposition in the nose was almost 100 per cent, becoming progressively less with decreasing particle size. This was more efficient than in man—probably because of the smaller air passages in the guinea pig. Efficiency in monkeys and man was found to be about the same. Up to 1 μm, there was almost no retention in the nose. At a diameter of 2 μm, about 60 per cent and from 3–5 μm, 70–80 per cent was retained in the nose.

The efficiency of nasal filtration in a group of 426 miners who, at work, were subjected to silica dust, was studied by Lehmann (1935). Of these, 185 were found to be healthy, but the other 241 suffered from some degree of silicosis. The method of examination consisted essentially of blowing dusty air into the nose while the subject held his breath, and of recovering it through the mouth. From 10–70 per cent of the dust was filtered out in the nose. Among the healthy subjects, 63 per cent had retention efficiencies of over 40 per cent (some up to 70 per cent). In 19 per cent, the efficiency lay between 30 and 40 per cent and in only 18 per cent, below 30. Among the 241 having silicosis, only 20 per cent showed retention of over 40 per cent of the dust. Seventeen per cent of the silicotics had retention figures between 30 and 40 per cent and well over half—62 per cent—had below 32 per cent nasal retention of dust. Lehmann concluded that silicosis tended to develop in those workers who had low nasal filtration. He recommended that these nasal tests be made upon the workers annually and that those with poor nasal filtration be placed in other work, where dust is not a problem.

In the experiments in which recovery of air is made through the mouth, it should be borne in mind that some of the retention (filtration) probably takes the place in the mouth. Brain (1970) made some measurements that indicated this.

Meurman (1948) reviewed the literature on the effects of industrial dusts in the respiratory tract and contributed an excellent clinical study of 529 workers in lime and cement industries, over a period of 9 years. He described very well the area of dust deposition in the nose—mostly on the inactive area in the anterior third (Fig. 5A)—and compared the deposition in the nose, pharynx, larynx and trachea. He found it to be much greater in the nose than elsewhere and that it decreased progressively through the pharynx, the larynx and the trachea. Among his interesting findings was the discovery that even under a crust of dust 2 mm thick in the anterior portion of the nose, the underlying mucous membrane usually appeared to be normal.

Meurman's studies led him to conclude that lime and cement dust were almost devoid of danger for the upper respiratory tract under the conditions of industrial hygiene of that era. However, in workers whose exposure was of long duration and whose mucous membranes possessed a "weak resistance", these dusts might cause chronic mucosal changes with harmful symptoms, as well as producing a marked impairment of smell.

Fry and Black (1973) have recently made studies in which they determined that 45 per cent of dust particles retained in the nose are collected in the anterior third. Clearance from this area required from 20 min to 3 h and it varied greatly between individuals. This would be expected, considering the non-ciliated character of the epithelium in the anterior third of the nose.

Acheson and his colleagues (1968) made an industrial, environmental and epidemiological study of cases of nasal cancer occurring in three counties in southern England. They concluded that this was an industrial disease caused by inhalation of particles of wood in woodworkers in the furniture industry. The rate was about 1000 times greater than that in the general population.

Tourangeau and Drinker (1937) did nasal filtration experiments with finely ground limestone dust on six randomly selected subjects. They prepared the dust by blowing it into a 45·3 m^3 cabinet and allowing it to settle for 20 min. After 20 min "only those particles comparable in size to silica particles found in silicotic lungs remain suspended". They do not state the diameters of the particles. Each subject then entered the cabinet and the filtration efficiency of the nose was tested. They concluded, from the tests on these six subjects, "We have found nothing to indicate that the nonobstructed human nose will prevent inhalation of fine dust. Anatomically we can see no reason at all why it should be a good filter—compared with dust filters in commercial use, the efficiency of the nose is trifling. In general, nasal efficiency of the normal nose is too low to be of importance in preventing fine dust from reaching the lungs." Yet these workers plotted Lehmann's data on probability paper and found that the median or geometric average of nasal efficiency is 27·5 per cent for silicotics and 56 per cent for normals—differences which are statistically significant. Obviously, the filtration in the nose *is* of importance.

The results of the study are really not at variance with those of the other studies cited. The other workers tested a variety of particles and gases with a profile of sizes varying from molecular up to 15 μm in diameter. All found that the very small, irregular particles, especially those of low density, penetrated the nose. Tourangeau and Drinker selected a single type and size of irregular particle, which is known to penetrate the nose: obviously—because it is found in the lungs of silicotics. It is rather surprising that as much as 30 per cent of this type and size was retained in the nose in some of their tests.

Davies (1946) studied droplet filtration in rabbits. Many other workers have studied nasal deposition of particles. Boyland and his colleagues (1947) compared filtration of droplets in man, goats and rabbits. He found that variations in breathing rate were important. The noses of man and goat were comparable in efficiency and the rabbit nose was somewhat more efficient than these two. Van Wijk and Patterson (1940) found that at 17 breaths/min the human nose filtered out 80 per cent of silica particles 2 μm in diameter but only 25 per cent of those 0·2 μm in diameter.

Gas Absorption

Not only particulate matter but noxious gases as well are present at times in inspired air. Can the nose remove any of these? The answer is in the affirmative. Turbulence and diffusion are both instrumental in bringing the gas molecules into close contact with the mucous blanket. Retention depends on the solubility and reactivity of the gases. Those of high solubility are rapidly taken up by the mucous blanket and the tissues of the nose. Those that are only slightly soluble are not effectively removed from the inspired air until they reach the depths of the lungs, where the air-tissue contact is very high (Hatch and Gross, 1964; Buckley and Loosli, 1969). The pH of the respiratory secretion is about neutral (7·0–7·2). It contains dissolved proteins which would act as buffers that would serve to neutralize acidic and basic gases.

Landahl and Herrmann (1950) studied the retention of selected vapors and gases as these passed through the nose; as they put it, "extending the investigation of particulate retention to particles of molecular size". Alcohol and acetone vapours and ammonia and hydrogen cyanide gases were tested. The experimental apparatus used consisted of a device which delivered a known constant concentration of the experimental gas mixed with air to a face mask covering the subject's nose and mouth. The mixture was delivered at a low positive pressure. Another tube extended from the mouth, through the mask, to a sampling device. As the subject held his breath, a sample of the air containing the experimental gas was passed through the nose and out of the mouth tube at a fixed rate of flow. At the same time, a control sample was drawn from within the mask. The difference between the test gas or vapor contained in the two samples indicated the amount retained in the nose, i.e. filtered out.

In the case of alcohol, between 43 and 70 per cent was retained at a flow rate of 18 l.min^{-1}. The time of sampling varied from 0·5–60 s. The highest rate of retention occurred with the shortest sampling time. Since the time for normal inspiration is only 1–2 s, it would be expected that filtration efficiency would be decreased by a sampling time as long as 50 s.

With concentrations ranging from 0·3–4 μmol.l^{-1}, the retention rate of hydrogen cyanide gas at 18 l.min^{-1} varied from 19–23 per cent. The retention figure for acetone varied from 26–40 per cent at 5·2 μmol.l^{-1} and ammonia at better than 80 per cent at 2·9 μmol.l^{-1}. When the subject inhaled the ammonia gas through the nose (and into the lungs) and exhaled through the mouth, up to 92 per cent was retained—only 12 per cent more than in the nose alone.

Frank and his associates (1969); Speizer and Frank (1966); Amdur (1966); Brain (1970) and Dalhamn (1961) studied the uptake of sulfur dioxide (SO_2) in the nose. Dalhamn used anesthetized rabbits for this purpose. His experiment was done in a moist, warm chamber, thus preventing cooling and drying of the mucosa. He drew the gas-air mixture through the nose and into the trachea for 45 min continuously. Samples for analysis were taken from the trachea each 15 min after exposure began. At 100 p.p.m. only 4–6 p.p.m. came through into the trachea; at 200 p.p.m., 6–8 p.p.m. came through. It was not until concentration reached 300 p.p.m. that appreciable amounts —25–30 p.p.m.—penetrated the nose. He concluded that, in rabbits, the concentrations of SO_2 which must be inhaled, before effect on ciliary beating in the trachea becomes discernible, must exceed by many-fold that found in smog. The filtration efficiency probably would be still greater in the to and fro flow of normal respiration as compared with the unidirectional flow for 45 min. The nose of man would probably be somewhat less efficient than that of the rabbit.

Nitrogen dioxide, being less soluble than sulfur dioxide, is not absorbed to a great extent in the nose, but penetrates deeper into the respiratory tract (Henry, 1969; Dalhamn, 1963).

When dissolved, sulfur dioxide forms sulfurous acid. The proteins in nasal secretion, even though this secretion is very small in volume, could buffer many parts per million for a considerable length of time—especially if ciliary activity were maintained allowing frequent replacement of nasal secretion.

Other experiments by Dalhamn showed that, in the tracheas of rats exposed directly to 10 p.p.m. SO_2 stopped ciliary action in 5 min and ammonia and formaldehyde in 1 min. This may explain why sulfur dioxide is so much more irritating when taken in through the mouth rather than through the nose. One would suppose that the much higher concentrations of sulfur dioxide for 45 min, as used in these experiments, would stop ciliary action in the nose. If so, the efficiency of nasal filtration of sulfur dioxide and ammonia found in these experiments and those of Landahl and Herrmann (1950) would not depend upon continuing ciliary action unless the neutralization of the gases takes place in the anterior portion of the nose, allowing ciliary function to continue farther posterior.

Dalhamn also observed that there did not seem to be an end—saturation point—to the absorption. At 45 min, sulfur dioxide was absorbed as fast as in the beginning. The same was true for nitrogen dioxide, but at a much lower level (Dalhamn and Sjöholm, 1963).

Desorption

Frank and his colleagues found that after sulfur dioxide had been inhaled through the nose and absorbed, it desorbed during expiration and that this continued as long as 25 min after the end of exposure (Frank *et al.*, 1969). Speizer and Frank (1966), making similar measurements, found that 15 per cent of the original concentration inspired was desorbed again.

Deposition of Deposited Material

The pollutants deposited upon the mucous blanket are entangled in it and eventually are carried with it into the stomach. Ciliary streaming in the nose has been the subject of many studies (Anderson *et al.*, 1971; Proctor, 1969; Proctor and Wagner, 1965; Hilding, 1932, 1935; Asmundsson and Kilburn, 1970; Proetz, 1953; Tremble, 1947, 1948, 1953; Negus, 1949) which have provided us with an understanding of the general functioning of the mucociliary mechanism. The lining secretion in the nose and bronchial tree is composed of two layers—a watery layer in which the cilia stand and beat and a mucinous layer which overlies the tips of the cilia and which they push along. The mucinous layer is dimensionally thin—a few micrometers (microns) normally—but it is viscid. It stretches readily but will sustain a certain degree of traction. Also it is elastic but incompletely so. It is strongly hysteretic. These physical properties make it possible for the mucociliary stream to flow cleanly over, past, and around obstructions, such as areas of squamous epithelium in the anterior third of the nose, the squamous islands on the epiglottis, and, in the lower tract, the squamous-covered vocal folds and around bronchial openings.

The rate of flow in the mucous blanket varies greatly throughout the tract (Hilding, 1932, 1935; Ewart, 1965). The anterior third of the nose drains largely through traction upon the mucous blanket by cilia located more posterior (Fig. 5A). Gravity probably plays a role here because the direction of flow is down and back. The rate of flow in these areas may be only a few millimeters per hour. Over the ciliated areas, the flow in general is about 10 mm.min⁻¹ and gravity is unimportant. Where cilia are active, the flow upward directly against gravity is as rapid as downward, for instance in the sinuses and trachea. But, the flow rate in the ciliated nasal areas varies in more or less inverse proportion to the exposure to inspired air. The rate is great in the middle and inferior meatuses than in the common meatus. The direction of flow is back and somewhat down, both upon the nasal septum and lateral nasal wall. The downward component is probably due to traction by the more active cilia in the protected meatuses (Fig. 5B and C). The pollutants are thus carried with the blanket to the soft palate and lateral pharyngeal wall, whence the swallowing mechanism takes charge and conducts them down the esophagus and into the stomach.

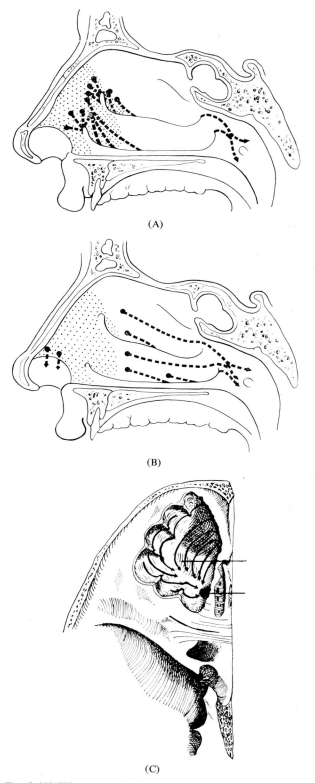

(A)

(B)

(C)

FIG. 5. (A) Ciliary streaming from the inactive areas (non-ciliated) in the anterior third of the nose. Drainage of these areas is accomplished mainly by traction upon the mucous blanket and movement is slow. (Hilding, 1932.) (B) Ciliary streaming on the lateral wall of the nose. These areas are ciliated and the flow is rapid (8–10 mm/min). (Hilding, 1932.) (C) Drainage within a frontal sinus as observed at a necropsy.

Sakakura and his colleagues (1973) found that experimentally induced rhinovirus infection in man compromised the effectiveness of the mucociliary mechanism in both those with normal nasal morphology and those with abnormal nasal morphology. This is consistent with a study of the pathology of the nasal epithelium in the common cold, which I made many years ago. The surface cells, together with their cilia, were exfoliated during these infections (Hilding, 1944).

The mucociliary stream in the lower tract forms an inverted river flowing vertically upward against gravity. The rate is slow in the tributaries—bronchioles—perhaps just 0.5–1.5 mm.min^{-1} (Iravani, 1971; Asmundsson and Kilburn, 1970). The velocity increases progressively toward the trachea and larynx, as the streambed (combined circumferences of the air passages) grows narrower. In the trachea, the flow may be 15 mm.min^{-1} or more. The pollutants that escaped deposition in the nose, and were deposited in the tracheobronchial tree, are carried up in this stream to the larynx, where they are conducted over the posterior margin and into the esophagus to be swallowed.

The pollutants that are deposited in the alveoli are removed in special ways. The alveolar walls are not ciliated. Ciliated epithelium, no matter how short the cells, is not a suitable membrane for the exchange of gases. The distribution of cilia ceases in the terminal and respiratory bronchioles. Phagocytic cells, both free and fixed, ingest particles, which have escaped deposition in the upper tract. The former make their way to terminal bronchioles where they and their ingested materials reach the ciliary escalator and are thereby removed. Some phagocytes (or naked particles) enter the alveolar walls and are carried to regional lymph nodes or are otherwise disposed of. Despite all of these elaborate filtration and defense mechanisms, some small amounts of polluting particles (carbon) remain more or less harmlessly in the tissues and lymph nodes of nearly all people. Under special circumstances, where dust, such as that from asbestos or silica, is inhaled over long periods of time, these retained particles may cause serious disease (Lehmann, 1937).

In addition to the mechanical removal of microorganisms with the mucous blanket, there are contained chemical compounds that destroy the organisms. For a great many years, muramidase (lysozyme) has been known to kill and fragment most airborne bacteria. In addition, the respiratory secretion contains a number of secretory immunoglobulins, IgA being the most abundant (Hughes and Johnson, 1973).

Hughes and Johnson (1973) reported a study on nasal secretory immunoglobulin A which demonstrated a marked circadian rhythm, varying as much as four-fold during the day. The highest concentration occurred between midnight and 0800 h, with the low-value period during the afternoon (1400–1700 h). They found a marked individual as well as a seasonal difference. They believed that the low concentration during the afternoon might be instrumental in permitting viral infection.

Bates and his colleagues (1965) had an unusual opportunity to study an outbreak of tuberculosis at the Arkansas Negro Boys' Industrial School. The controlled living pattern of all of the boys and the tuberculosis-control program in effect at the outbreak provided an unusual opportunity to study the epidemiology. They concluded that the spread of the tubercle bacilli was by the airborne nuclei of dried droplets. One of the boys with cavity-formation sang in the school choir with 21 other boys, 20 of whom were initially tuberculin-negative, but 60 per cent shortly became positive reactors.

These authors (Bates et al., 1965) did experimental studies on rabbits and found that a single bacterium was much more effective in producing lung lesions than were large aggregates, which were filtered out by the nose. They quoted Ratcliff and Palladino (1953) as demonstrating in guinea pigs, mice and rats that almost all tubercle bacilli inhaled as single organisms reach the alveoli and produce lesions. These clinical and experimental experiences indicate the importance of particle size for penetrating the nose and conductive tract down to the alveoli. Similar experiences were reported by others who studied the transmission of airborne disease (Proctor, 1966; Yamashiroya et al., 1966; Couch et al., 1966). The concept of particle size must be kept in mind in developing and using therapeutic aerosols, including those used for immunization, which are intended to reach the lower tract (Wolfsdorf et al., 1969; Dautrebande, 1962).

The antiseptic chemical in the nasal secretion are so effective that, although the nasal vestibule is heavily contaminated, it is difficult to procure a positive bacterial culture from the posterior portion of the normal nose, under usual circumstances, unless special techniques are used. Additional immune bodies occur in the tissues, epithelium and submucosa. Any particulate or bacterial pollutants that might penetrate these defenses are met by phagocytes.

When considering the importance of the nose in preparing the respired air for use in the alveoli, the question naturally arises, "What would happen if the nose were bypassed?" In general, the body is well protected from deleterious effects from the loss of organs and tissues—even important ones. If necessary, the heart, in the case of aortic stenosis, can hypertrophy and produce several times the normal amount of work. If one kidney is lost, there is enough capacity in the remaining one, if normal, to avoid any renal failure. A considerable part of the trachea may be denuded of epithelium without any great deleterious effect upon ciliary streaming. The magin of safety there is wide. If the nasal function is lost, for instance, through laryngectomy, the trachea and bronchial tree will take over that function and compensate. After a period of time (perhaps a year or more), the inspired air will be properly moistened, warmed and cleansed with practically no resultant irritation or excess secretion to disturb the patient. Even the recycling of heat in the expired air after laryngectomy improves with time (Ingelstedt and Toremalm, 1960). As far as filtration is concerned, this function is reasonably well compensated following laryngectomy. The compensated state for all of the described functions is understood to occur at low levels of activity of the individual so afflicted.

SUMMARY

The nose is a highly efficient filtering mechanism. It removes particulate matter, gases and microorganisms from inspired air. All of these materials are not equally well removed under all circumstances. Deposition of particles varies with the size, shape and density. In general, particles of 5 μm in diameter (aerodynamic diameter) and above are removed almost completely by the nose. About 50 per cent of the particles of 2–3 μm in diameter are retained in the nose and, of those 1 μm in diameter, almost none is filtered out. Much of the particulate matter which penetrates the nose is removed from the inspired air lower down in the tract. The lowest efficiency of deposit, considering the entire tract, occurs at a dimension of about 0·5 μm. This size particle is too small to sediment or be removed by inertial effects and it is too large to deposit by diffusion, as particles less than 0·1 μm will do.

The physical forces involves in filtration are inertia (momentum), gravity, diffusion, and air resistance due to viscosity. These factors vary with the rate of respiration and from moment to moment within each respiratory cycle. Turbulence is characteristic of the air flow though the nose. The greater the velocity of flow, the greater the turbulence and the greater the particle deposition by inertia. The slower the velocity of flow, the slower the movement from place to place within the system, the greater the sedimentation due to gravity.

Microorganisms that have formed conglomerates or are enclosed within droplets are apt to deposit in the nose. Most airborne microorganisms are destroyed quickly in the mucous blanket by contained immune bodies. Single organisms, or those attached to the nuclei of dried droplets, are apt to penetrate the nose and enter the lower part of the tract, even as far as the alveoli, where they are deposited by diffusion (Brownian movement).

Filtration efficiency varies with the rate of breathing. It is least at 18 or 20 respirations per minute and increases both with slower and with more rapid breathing. The slower breathing rate allows more time for sedimentation and the increased velocity of flow, with rates above 20 per minute, promotes deposition by inertia.

Some gases, such as sulfur dioxide, alcohol and ammonia, are well absorbed in the nose, while others, such as nitrogen dioxide and hydrogen cyanide, are less well absorbed. Some gases which are absorbed during inspiration are partially desorbed during expiration. Diffusion plays a large role in the absorption of gases.

Materials (pollutants) removed from the inspired air are taken into the mucous secretion which covers the epithelial surfaces within the nose. If these materials remain there, they are carried with this secretion by ciliary action into the pharynx and esophagus to be swallowed. What transpires after that, depends upon the nature of the pollutants.

The mucous secretion within the nose is produced by goblet cells within the epithelium or glands lying deep to it. Proper functioning of the mucociliary mechanism within the nose depends in part upon the recycling of the heat and moisture carried by the expiratory air and returned to the mucous blanket and mucous membrane.

Those wishing to pursue any of the many facets of nasal filtration will be amply rewarded in their search for informative studies not only in the individual articles which are being published with ever-increasing frequency in our major medical journals, but in the reports of symposia held on this and closely related subjects (*Inhalation Carcinogenesis*, 1970; *Inhaled Particles and Vapours*, 1961, **II**, 67; *Inhaled Particles*, 1972). Outstanding research workers, both clinical and laboratory, have contributed papers and participated in the discussions for these symposia. We have mentioned by name only a few such gatherings; the medical indices will yield an additional goodly supply.

REFERENCES

Acheson, E. D., Cowdell, R. H., Hadfield, E. and Macbeth, R. G. (1968), *Brit. med. J.*, **2**, 587.

Anderson, Ib., Lundquist, G. B. and Proctor, D. F. (1971), *Arch. Environ. Health*, **23**, 408.

Amdur, M. O. (1966), *Arch. Environ. Health*, **12**, 729.

Asmundsson, T. and Kilburn, K. H. (1970), *Amer. Rev. Resp. Div.*, **102**, 388.

Asset, G. (1957), *AMA Arch. Ind. Health*, **15**, 119.

Asset, G., Gongwer, L. E. and Ryan, S. (1956), *AMA Arch. Ind. Health*, **13**, 597.

Bates, J. H., Potts, W. E. and Lewis, M. (1965), *New End. J. Med.*, **272**, 714.

Binger, M. W., Gaarde, M. W. and Markowitz, J. (1931), *Amer. J. Physiol.*, **96**, 647.

Boyland, E., Gaddum, J. H. and McDonald, F. F. (1947), *J. Hyg.*, **45**, 290.

Brain, J. D. (1970), *Ann. Otol., Rhinol., Lar.*, **79**, 529.

Bridger, G. P. and Proctor, D. F. (1970), *Ann. Otol., Rhinol., Lar.*, **79**, 481.

Brody, A. W., Stoughton, R. R., Connolly, T. L., Shehan, J. J., Navin, J. J. and Kobald, E. E. (1966), *J. Lab. clin. Med.*, **67**, 43.

Buckley, R. D. and Loosli, C. G. (1969), *Arch. Environ. Health*, **18**, 588.

Butler, J. (1960), *Clin. Sci.*, **19**, 55.

Corn, M. and Burton, G. (1967), *Arch. Environ. Health*, **14**, 54.

Couch, R. B., Cate, T. R., Douglas, R., Gordon, R., Jr., Gerone, P. J. and Knight, V. (1966), *Bact. Rev.*, **30**, 517.

Dalhamn, T. (1961), *Amer. Rev. Resp. Dis.*, **83**, 566.

Dalhamn, T. and Sjöholm, J. (1963), *Acta physiol. scand.*, **58**, 287.

Dautrebande, L. and Walkenhorst, W. (1961), *Inhaled Particles and Vapours*, p. 110 (C. N. Davies, Ed.). London: Pergamon Press.

Dautrebande, L. (1962), *Microaerosols*, p. 37. New York: Academic Press.

Davies, C. N. (1946), *Proc. roy. Soc. B*, **133**, 282.

Dennis, W. L. (1961), *Inhaled Particles and Vapours*, p. 88 (C. N. Davies, Ed.). London: Pergamon Press.

Dennis, W. L. (1972), *Inhaled Particles III*, Vol. 1, p. 91 (W. H. Walton, Ed.). Unwin Brothers Ltd., The Gresham Press, Old Woking, Surrey, England.

Drettner, B. (1961), *Acta oto-laryng., suppl.* 166.

Drettner, B. (1970), *Ann. Otol., Rhinol., Lar.*, **79**, 499.

Ewert, G. (1965), *Acta oto-laryng., suppl.* 200.

Frank, N. R., Yoder, E., Brain, J. D. and Yokoyama, E. (1969), *Arch. Environ. Health*, **18**, 315.

Frank, R. (1970), *Ann. Otol., Rhinol., Lar.*, **79**, 540.

Fry, F. A. (1970), *J. Aerosol Sci.*, **1**, 135.

Fry, F. A. and Black, A. (1973), *J. Aerosol Sci.*, **4**, 113.

Hatch, T. and Hemeon, W. C. L. (1948), *J. industr. Hyg.*, **30**, 175.

Hatch, T. (1961), *Bact. Rev.*, **25**, 238.

Hatch, T. F. and Gross, P. (1964), *Pulmonary Deposition and Retention of Inhaled Aerosols*. New York: Academic Press, Inc.

Henry, M. C., Erhlich, R. and Blair, W. H. (1969), *Arch. Environ. Health*, **18**, 580.

Hilding, A. C. (1932), *Arch. Otolaryng.*, **15**, 92.

Hilding, A. C. (1935), *Practitioner's Library of Medicine and Surgery*, Vol. II, p. 661. New York: Appleton Century Co.

Hilding, A. C. (1944), *Trans. Amer. laryng. Ass.*, **66**, 137.

Hilding, A. C., Filipi, A. N. and Elstrom, J. H. (1967), *Arch. Environ. Health*, **15**, 584.

Hounam, R. F., Black, A. and Walsh, M. (1971), *J. Aersol. Sci.*, **2**, 47.

Hounam, R. F., Black, A. and Walsh, M. (1972), *Inhaled Particles III*, Vol. 1, p. 71 (W. H. Walton, Ed.). Unwin Brothers Ltd., The Gresham Press, Old Woking, Surrey, England.

Hugh-Jones, P., McGrath, M. W. and West, J. B. (1962), *Pulmonary Structure and Function*, p. 77 (A. V. S. deRueck and Maeve O'Connor, Eds.), Ciba Foundation Symposium. Boston: Little, Brown & Co.

Hughes, E. C. and Johnson, R. L. (1973), *Ann. Otol., Rhinol., Lar.*, **82**, 216.

Ingelstedt, S. and Toremalm, N. G. (1960), *Acta oto-larnyg.*, suppl. 158, p. 81.

Ingelstedt, S. (1970), *Ann. Otol., Rhinol., Lar.*, **79**, 475.

Iravani, J. (1971), *Pneumologie*, **144**, 93.

Landahl. H. D. and Black, S. (1947), *J. industr. Hyg.*, **29**, 269.

Landahl, H. D. (1950), *Bull. math. Biophys.*, **12**, 43, 161.

Landahl, H. D. (1962), Quoted by Hatch and Gross, 1964.

Landahl, H. D. and Herrmann, R. G. (1950), *Arch. industr. Hyg.*, **1**, 36.

Laurenzi, G. A., Berman, L., First, M. and Kass, E. H. (1964), *J. clin. Invest.*, **43**, 759.

Lehmann, G. (1935), *J. indistr. Hyg.*, **17**, 37.

Lehmann, G. (1937), *Arbeitsphysiologie*, **9**, 572.

Lippmann, M. (1970a), *Ann. Otol., Rhinol., Lar.*, **79**, 519.

Lippmann, M. (1970b), *Inhalation Carcinogenesis*, p. 55 (M. G. Hanna, Jr., P. Nettesheim and J. R. Gilbert, Eds.). U.S. Atomic Energy Commission, Division of Technical Information, Oak Ridge, Tenn.

Meurman, O. H. (1948), *Acta oto-Laryng.*, suppl. 73.

Morrow, P. E. (1959), U.S. Atom. Energy Comm., Wash. 1023: 113 (9–15–59).

Morrow, P. E. (1960), *Health Physics*, **2**, 366.

Morrow, P. E. (1970), *Inhalation Carcinogenesis*, p. 103 (M.G. Hanna, Jr., P. Nettesheim and J. R. Gilbert Eds.). U.S. Atomic Energy Commission, Division of Technical Information, Oak Ridge, Tenn.

Negus, V. E. (1949), *Thorax*, **4**, 57.

Ogura, J. H. (1970), *Ann. Otol., Rhinol., Lar.*, **79**, 496.

Ogura, J. H. and Harvey, J. E. (1971), *Acta oto-laryng.*, **71**, 123.

Palm, P. E., McNerney, J. M. and Hatch, T. (1956), *AMA Arch. Ind. Health*, **13**, 355.

Proctor, D. V. and Wagner, H. N., Jr. (1965), *Arch. Environ. Health*, **11**, 363.

Proctor, D. F. (1965), *Clin. Anesthesia*, **1**, 13.

Proctor, D. F. (1966), *Bact. Rev.*, **30**, 498.

Proctor, D. F. (1969), *Ann. Otol., Rhinol., Lar.*, **78**, 518.

Proctor, D. F. and Swift, D. L. (1972), *Inhaled Particles III*, p. 59 (W. H. Walton, Ed.). Unwin Brothers Ltd., The Gresham Press, Old Woking, Surrey, England.

Proetz, A. W. (1953), *Applied Physiology of the Nose*, 2nd edition, p. 138. St. Louis: Annals Publ. Co.

Ratcliffe, H. L. and Pailadino, V. S. (1953), *J. exp. Med.*, **97**, 61.

Sakakura, Y., Sasaki, Y., Togo, Y., Wagner, H. N., Jr., Hornick, R. B., Schwartz, A. R. and Proctor, D. F. (1973), *Ann. Otol., Rhinol., Lar.*, **82**, 203.

Sercer, A. (1930), *Acta oto-laryng.*, **14**, 82.

Sercer, A. (1952), *Arch. Ohr.-, Nas.- u. Kehlk Heilk.*, **161**, 264.

Silverman, I., Lee, G., Plotkin, T., Sawyers, L. A. and Yancey, A. R. (1951), *AMA Arch. Ind. Hyg. Occup. Med.*, **3**, 461.

Speizer, F. E. and Frank, N. R. (1966), *Arch. Environ. Health*, **12**, 725.

Takagi, Y., Proctor, D. F., Salman, S. and Evering, S. (1969), *Ann. Otol., Rhinol., Lar.*, **78**, 40.

Tourangeau, F. J. and Drinker, P. (1937), *J. industr. Hyg.*, **19**, 53.

Tremble, G. E. (1947), *Canad. med. Ass. J.*, **56**, 255.

Tremble, G. E. (1948), *Laryngoscope*, **58**, 206.

Tremble, G. E. (1953), *Laryngoscope*, **63**, 619.

van Wijk, A. M. and Patterson, E. S. (1940), *J. industr. Hyg.*, **22**, 41.

Williams, H. L. (1969), *Ann. Otol., Rhinol., Lar.*, **78**, 725.

Williams, H. L. (1970), *Ann. Otol., Rhinol. Lar.*, **79**, 513.

Wolfsdorf, J., Swift, D. L. and Avery, M. E. (1969), *Pediatrics*, **43**, 799.

Yamashiroya, H. M., Ehrlich, R. and Magis, J. M. (1966), *Bact. Rev.*, **30**, 624.

36. AIR CONDITIONING FUNCTION

POUL STOKSTED AND MUNIR A. KHAN

The nose is the most important organ and the most prominent feature of the human face. It has been assigned many important functions. In order to have an understanding of this complex organ it is necessary to start with the development of the nose.

Embryology

The face and nose have a very complex phylogenetic and ontogenetic history. There are three phylogenetic stages in the embryology of the human nose: (a) the piscine; (b) the amphibian; (c) the mammalian. This results in the development of the nose as first a predominantly olfactory organ and later a predominantly respiratory organ. The differentiation of the central face starts at the third week of intra-uterine life from five primordia situated around the stomodaeum (primitive oro-nasal cavity): (a) superior to it is the fronto-nasal process; (b) lateral to it is the right and left maxillary process; and (c) inferior to it the paired mandibular processes.

As mentioned above, the nose begins to form at the third week of the embryonal life—thickened epithelial areas appear on both sides above the stomodaeum, these are convex ectodermal masses and are termed the "olfactory placodes".

The areas invaginate in the fourth week and form the shallow "olfactory pits" by proliferations of surrounding mesoderm. These open ventro-caudally and are separated from each other by the broad fronto-nasal process. The fronto-nasal process subdivides into secondary processes at the end of this stage, i.e. into (a) a single, median, large nasal field; (b) right and left medial nasal processes (processi globulares); and (c) right and left lateral nasal processes, forming the early medial and lateral boundaries respectively of the primitive nasal pits (Fig. 1).

Growth and fusion of the maxillary processes with the medial and lateral nasal processes form the inferior boundary of the nasal pits, separating them from the early oral cavity. Blind sacs or "primary nasal fossae" result. These communicate with the exterior by the nostrils ("anterior nares") and are occluded by epithelial plugs which disappear by resorption at the end of the fifth week. Communication with the oral cavity is established by dorsal growth of these primary nasal fossae and rupture of he oronasal membrane. Thus the posterior apertures, (choanae) of the nose ("posterior nares") are formed during the seventh week of fetal life.

Laterally, the obliteration of the nasolacrimal sulcus ("naso-optic furrow") takes place by fusion of the lateral processes with the maxillary processes, while medially, the lateral portions of the upper lip are formed by conjunction of the medial nasal processes with the maxillary processes. The central portion of the upper lip and the philtrum are formed by fusion of the medial nasal processes with each other and with the lower part of the fronto-nasal process.

Limitation from below occurs at the end of the sixth week following growth of the "primary palate". Ridges (palatine processes) appear on the medial sides of the maxillary processes. The palate is formed from the anterior portion. The ridges fuse anteriorly with the premaxillary process, and posteriorly with each other. General broadening of the head shifts the widely separated primitive nasal

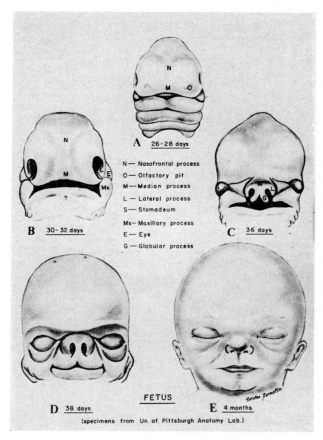

N — Nasofrontal process
O — Olfactory pit
M — Median process
L — Lateral process
S — Stomadeum
Mx — Maxillary process
E — Eye
G — Globular process

A 26-28 days
B 30-32 days
C 36 days
D 38 days
FETUS
E 4 months
(specimens from Un. of Pittsburgh Anatomy Lab.)

FIG. 1. The progressive development of the formation of the nose and surrounding structures. (From *Fundamentals of Anatomy and Surgery of the Nose*, by Kenneth H. Hinderer, M.D.)

fossa to the midline of the face, narrowing and modifying the broad mass of the single median fronto-nasal process and ultimately forming the primary nasal septum. Fusion of the septum and the palatine processes divides the nasal cavity into the left and right nasal fossae. The nasal conchae (turbinates) develop on the lateral walls of the nasal fossae and the paranasal sinuses expand and pneumatize into their relative bones from the corresponding nasal meatuses. The external nose is fairly well defined by the end of the eighth week.

The nasal capsule and septum are initially cartilaginous. Later, certain parts persist and form the cartilaginous part of the skeleton of the nose; other areas become ossified as individual bones, and certain parts remain rudimentary. The nasal bones develop in membrane overlying the cartilage which they replace following resorption. The ossification of the septum starts from an important centre at the junction of the anterior end of the vomer, the maxilla, premaxilla and the cartilaginous septum.

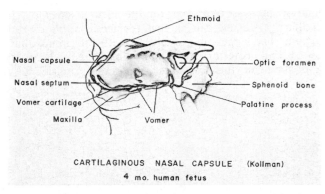

CARTILAGINOUS NASAL CAPSULE (Kollman)
4 mo. human fetus

FIG. 2(a). (From *Fundamentals of Anatomy and Surgery of the Nose*, by Kenneth H. Hinderer, M.D.)

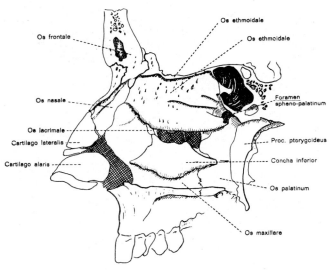

FIG. 2(b). Bony construction of the lateral wall of the nasal cavity. (*Grant's Atlas of Anatomy*, 1962.)

Anatomy, Vascularization and Innervation of the Nose

The nasal framework consists partially of bony and cartilaginous vaults, which are covered by a mucous membrane. The nose is divided into two completely separated cavities by a partition, the nasal septum. The two nasal cavities have openings to the exterior at the nostrils, via the posterior choanae into the nasal part of the pharynx and via various openings into the so-called paranasal sinuses (Fig. 2a and b).

Not less than eight bones contribute to the composition of the lateral wall of the nasal cavity: the nasal, frontal ethmoid, lacrimal, maxillary, palatine, sphenoid and the inferior nasal concha. Openings in this bony wall are

found: in the inferior meatus for the nasolacrimal duct in the middle meatus to the frontal sinus, the maxillary sinus and the anterior ethmoidal cells, in the superior meatus to the posterior ethmoidal cells and also the spheno-palatine foramen, in the spheno-ethmoidal recess to the sphenoid sinus. Excepting the spheno-palatine foramen, these foramina, are not closed by mucous membrane. The bony connection with the maxillary sinus is much larger than the opening in the mucous membrane. A large part of the hiatus semilunaris (maxillaris) is closed by means of a membrane, formed from the mucous membranes of the nasal cavity and the maxillary sinus. The bony sphenopalatine foramen, situated between the sphenoid and palatine bones in the upper posterior part of the lateral nasal wall forming a connection between the bony nasal cavity and the spheno-palatine fossa, is completely covered by mucous membrane (Fig. 3).

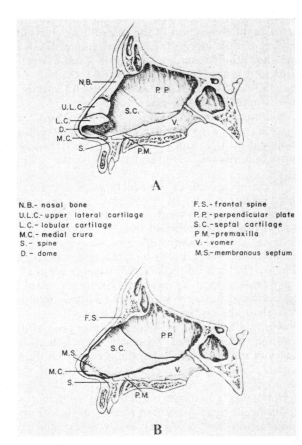

N.B.- nasal bone
U.L.C.- upper lateral cartilage
L.C.- lobular cartilage
M.C.- medial crura
S.- spine
D.- dome

F.S.- frontal spine
P.P.- perpendicular plate
S.C.- septal cartilage
P.M.- premaxilla
V.- vomer
M.S.- membranous septum

FIG. 3. Anatomy of the septum and associated structures. (From *Fundamentals of Anatomy and Surgery of the Nose*, by Kenneth H. Hinderer, M.D.)

The front part of the lateral nasal wall is made of cartilage. It consists mainly of two cartilages, the lateral cartilage and the lateral part of the greater alar cartilage. There is no reinforcement between these cartilages and the maxillary bone. The lower part of the external nose is rather flexible in relation to the bony wall owing to this.

The nasal septum consists of a bony and a cartilaginous part. The bony part is made up mainly by the perpendicular plate of the ethmoid bone and by the vomer bone. These two bony plates are joined at the upper and lower wall of the nasal cavity, to the cristae septales of the frontal, sphenoid, palatine and maxillary bones. The septal cartilage separates the medial crus of the greater alar cartilage from its fellow.

Vascularization

The most important supply of blood occurs through the spheno-palatine artery, which arises from the maxillary

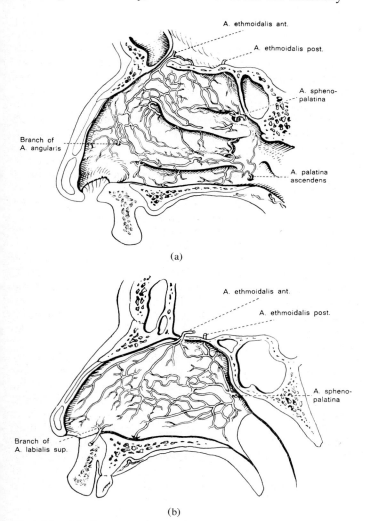

(a)

(b)

FIG. 4. (a) and (b) The septal vascular system. (*Grant's Atlas of Anatomy*, 1962.)

artery. The artery traverses the spheno-palatine foramen into the nose and then lies under the mucous membrane of the lateral wall, in a position corresponding to the bottom of the sphenoid sinus. Several branches, posterior nasal arteries, spread out over the lateral nasal wall and nasal septum, some of them extending for a short distance into the bony wall (Fig. 4a and b).

The anterior and posterior ethmoidal arteries, which run through the lamina cribrosa, bring blood to the top part of the nose, both the septum and the lateral wall, including the olfactory region.

Venous drainage takes place by means of veins which follow the arteries. It is important to note that the anterior and posterior ethmoidal veins run towards the orbit and join together to form the superior ophthalmic vein, which enters the cavernous sinus. Thus there is a connection between the vascular areas of the nose and the dural sinus.

Electron-microscopic studies of nasal mucosa obtained from the concha have shown a pronounced fenestration of the endothelial layer of the capillaries and a corresponding porosity of the surrounding basal membrane which is adjacent to the ciliated mucous membrane. Cauna (1970) is of the opinion that the moisture of the nose is provided mainly by the vast network of fenestrated capillaries found immediately underneath the respiratory epithelium and has observed that damage to the fenestrated capillaries causes dryness of the nose and crust formation.

The venules have, in contrast to the capillaries, continous endothelium but a pronounced porosity of the basal membrane with direct contact between the endothelial cells and the surrounding smooth muscle cells.

All the arterioles were found to be contracted with the preparation technique used, even so thinner parts of the walls were also seen suggesting that the vessels in a dilated condition have a porous area and that there is direct connection between the epithelial cells and myoepithelial elements.

The arterial segments of the arterio-venous anastomoses were found to be thick walled. The endothelial tube consists of several layers of complex lacework surrounded by a thick layer of smooth muscle cells. The transitional erectile cavernous tissue in the conchae, allows several combinations of changes in the mucosal temperature and its volume.

Innervation

The innervation of the mucous membrane, with regard to sensation, takes place through the trigeminal nerve. The ophthalmic nerve as well as the maxillary nerve furnish this area with branches. The anterior ethmoidal nerve arises from the former, which together with the similarly named artery, pass through the cribriform plate (lamina cribrosa) of the ethmoid and branch out along the septum. The external nasal nerve branches off to the epidermis of the outer nose.

The second branch of the trigeminal nerve, the maxillary, penetrates the foramen rotundum on its way to the spheno-palatine fossa and there it ramifies into a number of branches of which the spheno-palatine nerves penetrate the spheno-palatine foramen into the mucous membrane of the nose and extend along the lateral wall and the septum.

Autonomic Nervous System

The vasomotor nerve supply is derived from the autonomic nervous system. The sympathetic pre-ganglionic branches are derived from the first and second thoracic segments of the spinal cord. The postganglionic fibres pass from the superior cervical ganglion to the plexus around the internal carotid artery and then via the deep petrosal nerve and nerve of the pterygoid canal (Vidian nerve) to the sphenopalatine ganglion from where they continue without synapsing to the conchae (turbinates).

Resection or procaine-block of the cervical sympathetic ganglion is followed by hyperaemia, swelling and hyper-secretion of the nasal mucosa. Resection of the para-sympathetic innervation results in a shrunken, pale mucous membrane and excessive drying followed by crusting.

Resection of the nerve of the pterygoid canal, containing both sympathetic and parasympathetic fibres, is able to relieve the dysfunction of the conchae in patients suffering from vasomotor rhinitis (Golding-Wood, 1962).

The response to stimulation of the cervical sympathetic is an immediate and intense vaso-constriction. The threshold of stimulation for this response is remarkably low and mere handling of the sympathetic chain elicits a response. Stimulation of the parasympathetic nerve supply in the facial nerve, central to the genicular ganglion or of the greater petrosal nerve, causes dilatation of the nasal blood vessels.

How the autonomic outflow is regulated is not known with certainty, though it is probable that the hypothalmus may act as an integrating centre receiving numerous afferent impulses including emotional stimuli from higher centres. Normally the vasomotor balance may be temp-orarily disturbed by such factors as: circulating catechola-mines, emotion, posture, exercise and change of external temperature or humidity but as a rule without any feeling of discomfort. However, it is probable that, in those sub-jects suffering from vasomotor rhinitis, this balance is constantly disturbed, most commonly in favour of para-sympathetic hyperactivity. In these individuals, the mechanism of control is not only unbalanced but hypersen-sitive. Psychogenic, endocrine drugs may influence it in doses which only induce subliminal changes in unaffected subjects.

The exact termination of the nerve fibres is uncertain. The erectile vessels have a very rich innervation, to such a degree that it seems that each smooth muscle fibre receives its own innervation. There is a very rich sympathetic innervation of the wide veins of the erectile tissue, in contrast to the sparse adrenergic innervation in most other tissues. This unusually highly developed innervation apparatus must be of great importance in regulating the blood flow. So the nose, and especially the turbinate apparatus, appears as an organ having an abundant and intricate blood supply as well as nervous supply.

The conchae and the nasal mucous membrane are in-fluenced by a variety of reflex responses affecting in particu-lar the cardiovascular and respiratory system. The conchae also respond to thermal stimuli applied to the skin as shown by Ralston and Kerr and by Drettner. A more direct response is seen by compressing the jugular veins, which causes swelling of the conchae, as shown by van Dishoeck. The reaction fails to appear in cases of thrombosis of the jugular vein.

The Glands

In man, as in the monkey, the glands of the lamina propria of the respiratory region can be divided into two groups; larger ones, which open into crypts in the region of the internal ostium, i.e. anterior nasal glands, and the smaller ones, which are scattered throughout the entire region. The former can be divided into a medial or septal group and a lateral group, called anterior medial nasal glands and the lateral nasal glands respectively.

In addition to the anterior nasal glands, there are smaller glands scattered throughout the entire respiratory region. Their acini are placed in groups in the superficial part of the lamina propria and a small excretory duct proceeds straight up to the surface from each group, where they penetrate the epithelium.

Numerous duct openings are visible even to the naked eye in the region of the internal ostium, both on the septum and along the limen nasi by anterior rhinoscopy. Each duct opening is covered by a droplet of clear serous fluid. After applying a mechanical stimulus to the vestibule, one can observe the droplets increase in size prior to the sneez-ing reflex. Furthermore, in a few cases the droplets can be observed to increase during inspiration and decrease during expiration; this is probably caused by the changes in pressure.

The glands of the nose have been studied in particular by Zuckerkandl and by Brunner, who have demonstrated the presence of both serous and mucous of alveolar-tubular type, as well as a smaller number of glands of mixed type. The glands open into small crypts on the surface of the mucous membrane and are provided with long secretory ducts, round which Zuckerkandl has demonstrated a close-meshed capillary network that strangulates the glands during the dilating phase of the conchae, so that secretion can be evacuated only during the relaxing phase of the pseudo-erectile tissue. With such an arrangement the serous secretion will always be evacuated in the nasal cavity which has the largest respiratory lumen and at the place where the possibility of evaporation is greatest.

The innervation of the nasal glands appears to be differ-ent from that of the salivary glands. The human sub-mandibular and parotid glands and the submandibular gland of the mouse possess dual autonomic nerve supply, the adrenergic innervation being dominant in man.

The secretion of the glands is dependent upon their blood supply. Blood vessels of the nasal glands are richly innervated by adrenergic and cholinergic axons. Therefore, the nasal glands are affected by the adrenergic element of the autonomic nervous system through the innervation of their blood vessels.

Histology and Histopathology of the Nasal Mucosa

The respiratory membrane of the nose is similar in structure to that of the trachea and bronchial tree and shows a pseudostratified columnar epithelium, generally ciliated. But the cilia are often lacking, and the epithelium becomes stratified. Under normal conditions the anterior ends of the lower and middle conchae may represent areas of hyperplastic columnar epithelium or even of squamous metaplasia. These can be considered physiological rather than actual pathological changes. There is considerable individuable variation to the exact position of the transition from the stratified squamous epithelium of the vestibule to that of the respiratory epithelium of the nose. The term "pseudo-stratified ciliated epithelium" is generally applied to the nasal epithelium of the lower respiratory tract. This is due to the variation in depth of their nuclei in the columnar cells, which gives a false appearance of stratification.

The nasal mucosa varies in thickness in different parts of the nasal cavity. The thickness of the mucous membrane has to do with the amount of tunica propria and the character of the contained blood spaces and vessels. Under pathological conditions the character of the surface epithelium may undergo considerable alteration or metaplasia. The respiratory epithelium rests upon a cribriform connective tissue membrane, the membrana propria or basement membrane.

There are cells filled with mucin between the columnar cells, and these are greatly increased under irritating stimuli. They assume the shape of a goblet and are therefore called goblet cells. This is one source of the protective mucous coating of the nasal epithelium. Mucus is likewise secreted by the seromucinous glands of the entire nasal cavity. The goblet cells are probably identical to the ciliated columnar cells but when irritated by chemical or bacterial toxins are greatly increased in number, actually due to mutation of the ciliated columnar cells. After the goblet cell had disgorged itself, it collapses and the nucleus migrates to the central zone of the cell cytoplasm. The cytoplasm retracts towards the nucleus after the cell has disgorged itself and again becomes granular in character.

Valves and Baffles of the Nose

The lobule is the caudal component of the external nose. It consists of the tip, the alae, columella and the membranous septum. Each half of the lobule encircles the beginning of its corresponding nasal passage, the vestibule. Each vestibule is bounded laterally by the ala, medially by the mobile septum and columella, proximally by the cul-de-sac, limen nasi, and the ostium internum vestibuli, and distally by the nostrils.

The cul-de-sac is the space between the lateral cartilage above and the lateral crus of the greater alar cartilage and is lined by non-hair-bearing skin lying on the aponeurotic attachment between the two cartilages.

The cul-de-sac serves as a resistance (baffle) during inspiration, while the recess on the inside of the nasal tip, called the ventricle, presents a baffle during expiration. The free ends of the medial and lateral crura, the free ends of the conchae and the soft palate are other baffles and valves that may be mentioned.

The terminal (interior) part of each lateral cartilage is so thin that it is able to follow the respiration movement. This part of the lateral cartilage makes a 10° angle with the septum and is not attached to the septum for a considerable distance. This is the nasal valve of the nose (Mink) enclosing the narrowest part of the nasal passage, the internal ostium. The alar cartilage overrides the caudal part of the lateral cartilage in the valve area. The alae are attached to the alar portion of the nasalis muscle, which contract during inspiration and open the vestibule and the internal ostium during this phase of respiration. At the same time

a pull possibly occurs on the inferior conchae with a flattening of these during inspiration.

Some investigators have expressed the opinion that the nasal valve, in combination with the anterior ends of the conchae, is the main regulator of the airstream, just like a waterfall, where the bed of the fall determines the flow and main resistance to the water, while rocks at the bottom create a resistance which can be compared to the resistance of the nasal cavities.

If we look into the nose, we will find an anterior part consisting of the nasal atrium and the agger nasi, which corresponds to the outer nose, a structure unique for the human race. This part of the nose may well be an isolating device together with the paranasal sinuses, the purpose of which is to protect the nose against the changes in temperature and humidity of the surrounding atmosphere.

The conchae are situated on the sidewalls. The large inferior concha runs smoothly into the nasal atrium in the front and has a free end at the back, while the middle concha is just the opposite. At the back of the nose the posterior choanae form the connection to the nasal part of the pharynx, where the airstream is influenced by the movements and contractions of the uvula and the soft palate. Why the nose structures have this construction, and its relationship to the sinuses, is not fully understood. Tomography of the nose at various levels shows, however, that the cavity is divided into a number of shallow compartments between the conchae and the septum and between the conchae themselves, indicating the very close contact between the airstream and mucous membrane.

Air Conditioning

Many hundreds of years ago it was believed that the function of respiration was to cool the blood. Even as late as the beginning of the nineteenth century, the conducting airways were usually regarded as a passive tubular system simply conducting air to and from the lungs. In 1829, Magendie was the first to suggest that the nose had an active respiratory function: to warm and moisten the air inspired.

The primary function of the nasal cavities can be classified as: olfaction, air conditioning by heating and humidification of the inspired air, protective filtration and the cleansing action by the cilia.

In man, the nose is part of the natural respiratory route. It warms and moistens the inspired air and is thereby supposed to protect the tracheo-bronchial tree and the delicate alveolar epithelium. But, in addition, the mucous membrane of the nasal cavities recovers part of the heat and moisture from the expired air.

It is generally assumed that the inspired air is warmed to body temperature after having passed through the upper respiratory airways, and that this air, when in the alveoli, is saturated with moisture. According to several investigators, the inspired air is almost completely conditioned after passing the nasal cavities.

Despite fundamental differences in the structure of the nasal and oral cavities as yet no convincing evidence has been produced that the inspired air is conditioned less well during oral breathing than during nasal breathing. Clinical experience, however, suggests that the inspired air is not so well prepared by mouth breathing, dryness and catarrhal conditions of the throat and larynx being more common among mouth breathers. In various works, Ingelstedt and Toremalm have discussed the measurements done with their thermo-electric psychrometer and have pointed out, that, from the functional point of view, the subglottic space is the ideal place for measuring the air conditioning (Fig. 5).

conditioning and body heat regulation, it has been repeatedly demonstrated that heating and moistening of air by the nose is adequate to prepare inspired air for the vital process of pulmonary gas exchange.

Some physiological studies indicate that the nasal mucosa alone can adequately condition inspired air under moderate conditions of temperature and humidity. Other studies have lead to the conclusion that the human nose cannot prepare air adequately under extremely low

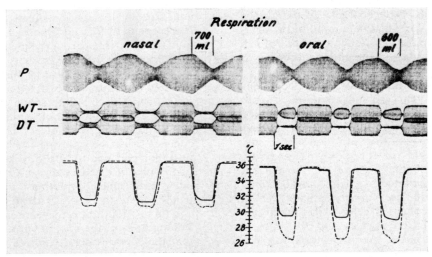

Fig. 5. Simultaneous recordings of the pneumograms from the same subject during nasal or oral breathing at room temperature.
P   = Pneumograph.
WT = Wet thermoelement.
DT = Dry thermoelement.

Adequate moisture is essential for the maintenance of the integrity and normal functional activity of the respiratory mucosa, and especially for the function of its cilia.

The secretion produced by the glands and goblet cells is of great importance, not only because it filters off airborne irritants and thereby prevents them from penetrating the mucosa, but also because it gives up moisture to the inspiratory air. Any dehydration of the mucous blanket covering and protecting the cilia increases the viscosity of the secretion and slows down the motion of the cilia, on which drying has a severe or even fatal effect. Impairment of ciliary function renders the mucosa more susceptible to injury by air-borne irritants.

Most investigators have focused their interest on changes in the temperature and moisture content of the respiratory air, mainly to elucidate the extent to which the upper airways contribute to air conditioning. The results thereby obtained should reasonably reflect the function of the respiratory mucosa with its vessels, glands and goblet cells and of the nervous mechanism governing this function.

Heat and Moisture Exchanges in Respiratory Mucous Membrane

The nose is a simple organ with a subsidiary function of smell but it has a unique heat controlling mechanism, independent of the respiratory system. Despite the loss of intranasal complexity necessary for keen olfaction, air

temperatures and moisture content. Nonetheless, the nasal mucosa being first in line to receive the raw material is at the mercy of the physical laws governing heat and moisture exchange of gases.

Air entering the human nose is usually below saturation and also cooler than the temperature of the body core. When it reaches the lung, it is either completely saturated with moisture or very nearly so, and is warmed to body temperature. Heat transfer, in general, occurs by the physical processes of convection, conduction and radiation. Of the three physical processes radiation seems to be the most important, followed by conduction and convection respectively.

The rate of vaporization of water molecules (while leaving the surface of the mucosa and mixing with the air passing over) depends upon temperature, surface area, vapour pressures and ventilation (movement of gas above the mucosal surface). In the confined areas of the nose, these factors favour rapid uptake of moisture from the mucosal surface toward the lamellae of inspired air. During expiration, the highly saturated and heated air looses water and heat to the cooler and drier surface.

Sources of Respiratory Moisture

(1) Transudation

The large amount of water released by the nasal mucosa cannot be derived from secretory glands. The mucous disappears almost completely from the mucous glands of the trachea under atropinization although the amount of water given off is not reduced. Therefore it can be concluded that moisture in the respiratory tract is due to transudation rather than secretion. The racemose secretory glands in the mucosa have serous elements and there is evidence that one type of secretory cell can change into another or that the mucous cell can secrete a non-mucous material. The goblet cells continue to secrete when the respiratory membrane is atropinized.

Negus believed that, although the hydrostatic pressure of lamina propria is low, it is sufficient for water to pass to the epithelial surface because of the osmotic pressure of mucous surface.

(2) Secretion

The respiratory mucous membrane of the nose, as described previously, has an abundant supply of various glands. Goblet cells also appear in abundance in the respiratory lining membrane and produce the glycoprotein mucin. The relative number of glands in the respiratory tract secreting a serous material is not known. Cells which are histologically serous are characteristically found in gland structures which secrete enzymes. In the respiratory mucous membrane, however, no enzymatic activity has been demonstrated. It is probably that these cells serve to supply water to the surface membrane to keep the viscosity of mucus at a low level.

When inspired air reaches the lung alveoli it is completely saturated with moisture. Here oxygen and carbon dioxide freely diffuse between the air sacs and capillaries, obeying the physical laws governing the passage of dissolved gases through membranes. The hydrostatic pressure of the moisture in alveolar air appears to balance the osmotic pressure of plasma so that no fluid exchange occurs in the lung alveoli.

Biochemical Considerations

The biochemical processes involved in heat and moisture exchange through respiratory mucous membrane in general and nasal mucosa in particular have received little attention *per se*. However, cellular metabolism, involving proteins and carbohydrates with its many complicated chemical transformations through the mediation of oxidative and reductive enzymes, occurs in nasal tissue as in tissue elsewhere in the body. Heat and moisture exchange involves chiefly physical processes; chemical reactions, in the main, are concerned with maintaining the integrity of the tissues.

Changes in the normal cellular and intercellular chemistry occurring with nasal infections, allergy, glandular abnormalities, emotional disturbances and imbalances in the autonomic nervous system can, however, produce changes in the respiratory mucosa.

Hyaluronic acid is capable of holding water in the colloid suspension as a gel. There is evidence that abnormalities in the chemistry of this substance result in mucosal swelling and nasal obstruction. Corticosteroids and ACTH play an important role in maintaining the integrity

of collagen and ground substance, as also do the sex hormones.

Calcium ions play an important role in the permeability of membranes, affecting the passage of water through the respiratory epithelium and endothelium. Hydrogen ion concentration also affects the health of the mucosal tissue. Congested nasal mucosa in disease states is often on the alkaline side of pH 7. Normal nasal tissue and fluids are on the acidic side.

Nasal Cycle
Definition and Historical Background

In order to understand nasal respiratory physiology one should familiarize oneself with the effect produced by the nasal cycle.

The term nasal cycle was first noticed and described by Kayser in 1895. "If a patient has one sided obstruction of the nose, which in the course of a few hours will shift to the other side while the previously obstructed side opens up, his ability to breathe through his nose remains normal and he does not have to resort to mouth breathing." In other words, the alternating changes in patency of the two nasal cavities were called nasal cycles. Kayser, however, suggests that this alternating congestion and decongestion in the erectile tissues of the nasal mucosa of the lateral wall and septum, which he though might be caused by a central autonomic influence, did not influence the total nasal patency. In 1923, Lillie took up this problem and observed that, as one nasal chamber is opening up and its mucosal glands are throwing off their secretions, the erectile tissues of the opposite nasal chamber are filling with blood and the secretions of the mucosal glands diminishing.

Later, in 1936, in a clinically more comprehensive and careful study, Heetderks confirmed Lillie's observations. An individually characteristic nasal cycle, occupying from about 30 min to about 5 h from one corresponding phase to another, is present in about 80 per cent of normal individuals while in an upright position. The effect of posture on the changes in the swellings of the erectile tissues of the nasal chambers is produced by the effect of gravity. About 80 per cent of people have a definite cycle of reaction. In general, damp and cold atmosphere brings about the greatest swelling of the conchae, and dry warm air a little less, while optimal atmospheric conditions (humidity 50–60 per cent, temperature 13–18°C) cause cycles of least degree. The cycle seems to be most active during the adolescent age (explained on hormonal activity). The physiological activity is decreased with increasing age (often with the simultaneous appearance of demonstrable atrophic changes in the nasal mucosa). The same nose responds differently at various times under apparently the same conditions. These cycles, including both the phase of filling as well as the phase of emptying on the same side, occur over a period, ranging from 50 min to 4 h. In general, more time is required under favourable conditions, when the cycle is of less degree. These reactions of the conchae can be explained by the great amount of air conditioning the nose has to perform and also as a reflex mechanism preventing free entrance of air. The average time, however, under all atmospheric conditions for a complete cycle is approximately $2\frac{1}{2}$ h.

Stoksted (1952) was the first to study the nasal cycle rhinomanometrically. In a series of papers he and his associates confirmed the observations of Kayser (1895), Lillie (1923) and Heetderks (1927). He calculated total nasal resistance by adding the conductances of the separate nasal chambers (conductance being the reciprocal of resistance) and found that the combined resistance remained practically constant, despite the constantly changing volumes of the erectile tissues in the two nasal chambers. The rhythmicity of the cycle is maintained through the peripheral autonomic centres, the sphenopalatine and stellate ganglia—so connected that an increase in tonus in one set of centers may give a decrease in tonus in the other two. The peripheral centres are regulated by a central sympathetic centre, possibly located in the hypothalamus, which by altering tonus could increase or decrease the cross section of a nasal chamber and in this way make it possible for the nasal airway to act in the cybernetic control of respiration.

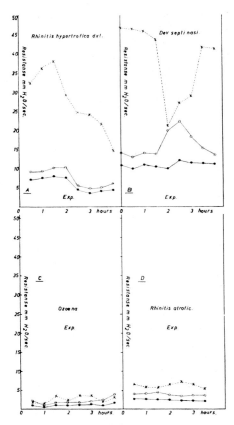

FIG. 7. (A) Rhinomanometric curves of a patient with hypertrophic rhinitis. (B) Deviation of the septum. (C) Ozaena. (D) Atrophic rhinitis.

Nasal Cycle in Pathologically Distorted Noses

When one nasal chamber is abnormally narrow and the other abnormally wide, very little respiratory air passes through the narrow side. Almost the entire volume of respired air is carried through the wider side and, unless bilateral obstruction of sufficient degree to force mouth-breathing is present, this volume will be adequate for the required alveolar oxygenation without increased work. If the conchal congestion on the wide side, owing to cyclic change, is severe, the recurring episodes of symptomatic nasal respiratory obstruction, with dyspnea and forced mouth breathing, may take place. It may be feared that the complaint of dyspnea might seem to be on a psychic basis to a poorly informed and/or inexperienced examiner who looks into the wide side of the nose during the shrunken phase of the erectile tissues. In atrophic rhinitis, the congestion-decongestion of the nasal cycle is very much reduced and a very low nasal resistance is present. Both in atrophic and non-atrophic vasomotor rhinitis, both nasal cavities react to stimulation synchronously and to an exaggerated degree so that the cyclic pattern is disturbed and a morbidly increased nasal resistance is present, It is desirable to compare instantaneous determinations in a given individual to those made some hours or days previously. It is necessary to make a graph of measurements of a nasal cycle taken at 10 min intervals over a period of

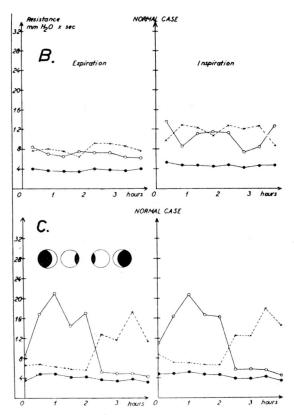

FIG. 6. Rhinomanometric curves during inspiration and expiration from two normal persons. (B) From a person with high and small nose with equally small conchae, it gives only small amplitudes during the nasal cycle. (C) From a person with a broad and low nose, large prominent conchae which showed large alternating conchae movements and the nasal cycle was $2\frac{1}{2}$ h.

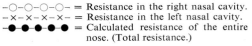

−○−○−○−○− = Resistance in the right nasal cavity.
−×−×−×−×− = Resistance in the left nasal cavity.
−●−●−●−●− = Calculated resistance of the entire nose. (Total resistance.)

at least 3 hr on each occasion, so that the data can be super-imposed at a coinciding phase of the nasal cycle. Generally, the duration of a cycle can be between 2 and 5 h and in some of the cases the duration of a cycle can go up to 8 h. The duration of a cycle is usually constant in a given person during repeated examination. In individuals having

warming of the nasal mucosa by infra-red rays with long wavelengths causes a swelling of the mucosa, while shorter wavelengths cause an initial widening of the nasal passage.

Local skin warming causes an initial widening of the nasal passage followed by mucosal swelling. General warming causes mucosal swelling.

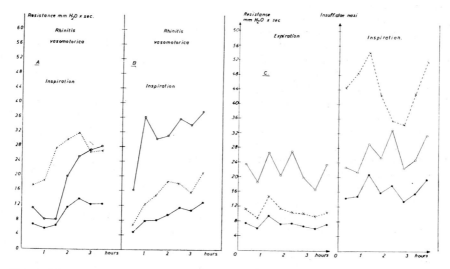

FIG. 8. (A) and (B) Rhinomanometric curves from patients with vasomotor rhinitis. (C) Curves during expiration and inspiration from a patient with alar insufficiency.

acute or chronic sinusitis or significant deflection of the nasal septum, the nasal cycle is irregular, while amplitudes differ on the two sides and maximal amplitudes exceed those of cycles in normal noses.

Influencing Factors

Factors influencing the nasal cycle by their action on the nasal mucosa as a whole are manifold and diverse, e.g. the influence of posture. There is the influence of increased hydrostatic pressure of the blood in the head when lying down, in a head-high position (15° angle to the floor) and a head-low position (also in a 15° angle to the floor). In normal persons, there is no change in the total nasal patency but, in patients with atrophic vasomotor rhinitis, there is a considerable decrease in total nasal patency in the head-low position which rapidly increases again in the head-high position. The rapidity with which this happens points to vasodilatation and not to extravascular escape of fluid as the cause of the decreased nasal patency. The vascular hypotonicity may be due to parasympathetic preponderance. The same mechanism may be responsible for the well known side-effect of sympatholytic and ganglion blocking agents, e.g. nasal obstruction especially on lying down. In these cases a parasympathetic predominance exists, as is also the case in Horner's syndrome. Vasoconstriction or sympathetic reaction occurs in sudden fright situations (emotional influences), and vasodilatation of parasympathetic reaction in anxiety situations.

Cooling of the back and of the inspiratory air, and of the skin with or without cooling of the inspiratory air, may all be followed by a narrowing of the nasal passage. Local

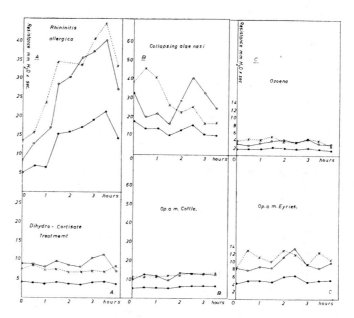

FIG. 9. Some rhinomanometric examinations before and after treatment. (A) Typical curves from a patient with vasomotor rhinitis after treatment with hydrocortisone 21-acetate. (B) Inspiratory curves from a patient with alar insufficiency. (C) Ozaena patient.

Hyperventilation causes swelling of the nasal mucous membranes, and dyspnoea a widening of the nasal airway.

The important function of the nose besides air conditioning is to offer a resistance to breathing in connection with the function of the lungs. This rheostatic effect influences the exchange of air in the alveoli and contributes to building up a sufficiently great oxygen partial pressure in the alveoli as well as to encourage the diffusion of oxygen into the blood, and the venous reflux to the right chamber of the heart. An increased respiratory resistance gives rise to an increase in the carbon dioxide content of the blood which, by its action on the respiratory centre, produces a deeper and slower breathing rate; at this level the patient can breathe without difficulty. Beyond a certain resistance this compensation fails. Consequently, oral breathing will supervene when lung compensation of nasal stenosis fails. The ability of the individual patient to compensate for a nasal stenosis varies. In some patients, the type of respiration changes, while others completely or partially lack this ability, and quickly resort to mouth breathing even in the presence of a very moderate stenosis.

A patient may have to resort to mouth breathing while having a normal nose, when, because of bad pulmonary function, the normal nasal resistance cannot be overcome by the lungs. Normal rhinometric values in a patient with mouth breathing may therefore suggest an underlying pulmonary or cardiac deficiency, or also a nasal neurosis.

Compression of the jugular vein normally causes swelling of the homolateral conchae. This does not occur in sigmoid sinus thrombosis.

There may be vasoconstriction in the nasal mucous membranes after the ingestion of either cold or warm food, even with tube-feeding.

The nasal cycle may stop after application of vaso-constrictor drops, to resume its activity when the drug activity is over. The so-called rebound effect of nose drops, a period of nasal stuffiness after the vasoconstriction phase, is nothing but the resumption of cyclic activity.

What actually goes on in the conchae during the cycle has not yet received much attention. A swelling of the mucous membranes may be due to arterial hyperaemia, venous engorgement, oedema, or to combinations of these. The temperature of the mucosa of the swollen side is usually higher than that on the shrunken side, but this does not necessarily mean that the swelling is caused by arterial hyperaemia. The nasal mucosa is cooled by the inspiratory air, and the cooling is less on the swollen side. That the conchal volume changes are due to changes in blood volume, at least at the moment of reversal, seems to be beyond doubt because of the rapidity with which this occurs (Figs. 6, 7, 8 and 9).

REFERENCES AND FURTHER READING

Arey, L. B. (1954), *Developmental Anatomy*, 6th edition. Philadelphia: W. B. Saunders Co.
Ash, J. E. and Raum, M. (1956) *Atlas of Otolaryngic Pathology*. American Registry of Pathology, Roskin Photo ofsett Corp., N.Y.
Boyd, J. D. (1933), *J. Anat.* (*Lond.*) **67**, 409.
Broman, J. (1918), *Year-book of the University of Lund*, **14**, 1.
Bojsen-Møller, F. (1965), *Int. Rhin.*, **3**, 117.
Cauna, N. and Hinderer, K. H. (1969), *Ann. Otol., Rhinol., Lar.*, **78**, 865.
Cauna, N., Hinderer, K. H. and Wentges, R. T. (1969), *Amer. J. Anat.*, **124**, 187.
Cauna, N., Cauna, D. and Hinderer, K. H. (1972), *J. Neurocytology*, **1**, 49.
Cottle, M. H. (1960), *Amer. Rhin. Soc.* Illinois: Chicago.

Cottle, M. H. (1968), *Int. Rhin.*, **6**, 7.
Dalström, A. and Fuxe, K. (1965), *Acta oto-laryng.*, **59**, 65.
Dankmeijer, J. (1964), *Int. Rhin.*, **2**, 37.
Dishoeck, H. A. E. van (1935), *J. Hyg.*, (*Lond.*) **35**, 185.
Dishoeck, H. A. E. van (1957), Lecture read for the American Rhinol. Soc., Yale University, New Haven (University Press, Leyden), 23 pp.
Dishoeck, H. A. E. van and Majer, E. H. (1964), *Allergische Erkran-kungen und neurovasculäre Störungen der Nase und ihrer Neben-höhlen*. Berendes-Link-Zöllner; HNO Bd. 1, G. Thieme, Stuttgart.
Drettner, B. (1960), *Acta oto-laryng.*, suppl., **158**, 111.
Drettner, B. (1961), *Acta oto-laryng.*, suppl., **166**, 109.
Eggston, A. A. and Wolff, D. (1947), *Histopathology of the Ear, Nose and Throat*. Baltimore: Williams Wilkins Comp.
Ewert, G. (1966), *Int. Rhin.*, **4**, 25.
Golding-Wood, P. H. (1962), *J. Laryng.*, **76**, 969.
Gregory, W. K. (1929), *Our Face from Fish to Man: a Portrait Gallery of Our Ancient Ancestors and Kinsfolk Together with a Concise History of Our Best Features*, N.Y.: p. 122. G. P. Putnam's Sons.
Grillo, M. A. (1966), *Pharmacol. Rev.*, **18**, 387.
Heetderks, D. R. (1927), *Amer. J. med. Sci.*, **174**, 231.
Hinderer, K. H. (1971), *Fundamentals of Anatomy and Surgery of the Nose*. Birmingham, Alabama, U.S.A.: Aesculapius Publishing Co.
Hlaväcek, V. and Loyda, Z. (1963), *Acta oto-laryng.* (*Stockh.*), 56.
Ingelstedt, S. (1956), *Acta oto-laryng.*, suppl. 131.
Ingelstedt, S. and Toremalm, N. G. (1960), *Acta oto-laryng.*, suppl., **158**, 1.
Ingelstedt, S. and Toremalm, N. G. (1961), *Acta physiol. scand.*, **51**, 1.
Ingelstedt, S. (1970), *Ann. Otol., Rhinol., Lar.*, **79**, 475.
Kayser, R. (1895), *Arch. Laryng. Rhin.*, **3**, 101.
Kern, E. B., Personal communication.
Keuning, J. (1963), *Int. Rhin.*, **1**, 57.
Keuning, J. (1968), *Int. Rhin.*, **6**, 99.
Lillie, H. (1923), *J. Iowa St. med. Soc.*, **13**, 403.
Majer, E. H. (1964), *Int. Rhin.*, **2**, 71.
Masing, H. (1967), *Int. Rhin.*, **5**, 63.
Masing, H. (1970), *Int. Rhin.*, **8**, 17.
McKillick, E. (1935), *J. Physiol.*, **84**, 162.
Mink, P. J. (1920), *Physiologie der obern Luftwege*, 150 pp. Leipzig: Vogel.
Mitchell, G. A. G. (1954), *J. Laryng.*, **68**, 495.
Naumann, H. H. (1961), *Die Mikrozirkulation in der Nasen-schleim-haut*. Zwangl. Abhandl. aus dem Gebiet der Hals-Nasen-Ohren-Heilkunde, Heft 7, 96 pp. Stuttgart: Thieme-Verlag.
Negus, V. (1958), *The Comparative Anatomy and Physiology of the Nose and Paranasal Sinuses*, 402 pp. Edinburgh/London: Living-stone.
Negus, V. (1964), *Int. Rhin.*, **2**, 3.
Ogura, J. H. and Stoksted, P. (1958), *Laryngoscope*, **68**, 2001.
Ogura, J. H. (1964), *Ann. Otol., Rhinol., Lar.* (*St. Louis*), **73**, 381.
Rosen, Z. (1963), *Int. Rhin.*, **1**, 10.
Rundcrantz, H. (1964), *Acta oto-laryng.*, **58**, 283.
Schaeffer, J. P. (1956), *The Genesis, Development and Anatomy of the Nose*. Hagerstown, M. D.: Coates, Prior Comp., Inc.
Semenov, H. *Personal Communications Concerning the Nasal Valves.*
Spoor, A. (1965), *Int. Rhin.*, **3**, 27.
Stockinger, L. and Burian, K. (1963), *Acta oto-laryng.* (*Stockh.*), **56**, 376.
Stockinger, L. (1963), *Z. Zellforsch.*, **59**, 443.
Stoksted, P. (1952), *Acta oto-laryng.*, **42**, 175.
Stoksted, P. (1953), *Acta oto-laryng.*, suppl., **109**, 159.
Stoksted, P. (1953), *Acta oto-laryng.*, suppl., **109**, 176.
Stoksted, P. (1954), *Acta oto-laryng.*, **44**, 259.
Stoksted, P. (1956), *Rhinomanometriske Naesefunktionsundersøgel-ser.* København: Aug. Christensens Bogtrykkeri.
Stoksted, P. and Nielsen, J. Z. (1957), *Ann. Otol., Rhinol., Lar.* (*St. Louis*), **66**, 187.
Stoksted, P. (1960), *Acta oto-laryng.*, suppl., **158**, 110.
Swindle, P. F. (1935), *Ann. Otol., Rhinol., Lar.*, **44**, 913.
Tatum, A. L. (1923), *Amer. J. Physiol.*, **65**, 229
Töndury, G. (1950), *Acta anat.*, **11**, 300.
Toremalm, N. G. (1960), *Acta oto-laryng.*, **52**, 461.

Uddströmer, M. (1940), *Acta oto-laryng.*, suppl., **42**, 146.

Williams, H. L. (Ed.) (1970), *Report of Committee on Standardiz-ation of Definitions, Terms, Symbols in Rhinometry of the American Academy of Ophthalmology and Otolaryngology*. Rochester, Minnesota, U.S.A.: American Academy of Ophthalmology and Otolaryngology.

Winslow, C. E. A., Greenburg, L. and Herrington, L. D. (1934), *Amer. J. Hyg.*, **20**, 195.

Wustrow, F. (1951), *Z. Anat. EntwGesch.*, **116**, 139.

Zuckerkandl, E. (1885), *Ohrenheilk.*, **19**, 86; also in (1884), *Denkschr. der Math.-Naturwiss. Classe der K. Acad. Wiss., Wien*, **49**.

Zwaardemaker, H. (1894), *Arch. Laryng. Rhin.*, **1**, 174.

37. ACOUSTIC ASPECTS OF NASAL FUNCTION

JYRKI KYTTÄ

The nose has—in addition to the functions mentioned in previous chapters——a phonetic function, to which we "automatically" resort in communication.

The three cavities important in speech, the oral, pharyngeal and nasal cavities, modify the "glottal tone" that is transmitted from the vocal folds by an air stream. The pharyngeal cavity participates in producing all the ingressive and egressive sounds that use lung air; whereas we can regulate whether the air escapes through the oral and/or the nasal cavity. There are three different possibilities: through the oral cavity, e.g. *i* and *s*; through the nasal cavity, e.g. *n*; and through both the nasal and the oral cavities, e.g. *ã* and *s̃*.

Sounds that have the nose as a resonator (the "nose-sounds" can be divided into three groups: nasals, nasal vowels and nasalized vowels.

When a nasal (i.e. nasalized consonant) is produced, the tongue occludes the oral cavity just as with the plosives, but the velum is lowered. Articulatorily, only the position of the velum palatinum distinguishes a nasal from a plosive. When producing a nasal vowel and a nasalized vowel, both the oral and the nasal cavities act as resonators; the velum is lowered, and air has access both to the mouth and to the nose. Articulatorily and acoustically there need not be any difference between a nasal vowel and a nasalized vowel. In some languages, nasal vowels presuppose a phonemic opposition between oral and nasal vowels.

There are nasal vowels in, for example, French, Polish and Portugese. The English and the Finns, on the other hand, use their noses for phonation considerably less often than people speaking the above-mentioned tongues, as there are no nasal vowels in either language, only nasalized vowels and the three nasal consonants proper, *m*, *n* and *ng*.

In speech, the velum is lowered and raised without special attention being paid to it. The function of the velum is linguistically binary in regard to the nose passages. When oral sounds are uttered, the velum prevents nasal resonance from being produced; when nasal sounds are uttered the velum is lowered and nasal resonance produced. Physiologically, the function of the velum, however, is not so categorical. On the contrary, there are countless different positions the velum can assume while being lowered and raised.

Björk (1961), when investigating the velopharyngeal function with a cineradiograph and a synchronized sound spectrograph, found that the velum was lowered in the middle of the expression in 12 ms, and raised in 15 ms, on the average. On the same occasion he also investigated what effect the speed of speech has on the speed of the velopharyngeal movement. Three speaking tempos were used, the duration ratios of which equalled those of 100:200:300; the corresponding duration ratios of the velopharyngeal movement equalled those of 100:130:160. In other words, the experiment proved that the speed at which the velum was lowered and raised increased statistically significantly when the speed of speech was changed.

"On the average, the velum is lowered and raised, when a certain period of time after the nasal has passed. The length of this period depends on e.g. the speaking tempo, the vowel quality, and the position of the vowel in regard to the nasal. When the speed of speech increases, the speed at which the velum is lowered and raised does not increase infinitely, but at a certain point the 'ceiling' is reached. After that, the nasalized portion of the vowel increases with the speed of speech, because the movement of the velum does not become any faster after the ceiling has been reached. Rapid and reduced speech is thus according to the above-mentioned hypothesis more nasalized than slow and accurately articulated speech" (Hurme, 1968). The analysis by Björk supports this hypothesis.

ACOUSTIC STRUCTURE OF NASAL CONSONANTS

According to the pronouncing place, *m* can be characterized as a labial, *n* as a dental and *ng* as a palatal nasal. The *m*-sound resembles the plosive *b* (in that closure between the upper and lower lips is loose) as well as the plosive *p*, in which the closure is tighter than in *b*. The adjoining vowels colour the *m*-sound as well as the other labials very clearly. In *m*, as well as in the other nose-sounds, the velum is slightly lowered. The tongue tends to maintain the position of the preceding vowel, but without touching the velum.

In the *n*-sound, the point of contact for the tongue-tip is usually medioalveolar, but it can also be prealveolar. The position of the lips depends mainly on the preceding vowel. The plosives that correspond to *n* are *d* and *t*.

The pronouncing place of the *ng*-sound is post-palatal, but it becomes mediopalatal in connection with a front vowel, as the back of the tongue touches the velum. Compared with other nasals, the distance between the lips as well as the interdental distance is here the longest. *K* and *g* are the corresponding plosives.

When nasals or nasal consonants are produced, the nasal and pharyngeal cavities together act as a resonator; the oral cavity which is coupled to the primary resonator acts as a secondary resonator, the size of which varies in different nasals. In addition to the formant pattern produced by the primary resonator, the nasals have additional distinctive features, i.e. the anti-resonances produced by the oral cavity, and the oral formant transitions. In the sonagram, vowel formants seem to extend into the nasal segment, especially if nasals are between two vowels.

In the nasal spectrum, the formant that occurs low, at 200–300 Hz, obviously predominates. This formant is generally understood to occur when the nasal and pharyngeal cavities together act as a resonator. Because of the damping effect of the nasal cavity, the formant area is rather broad; also the other nasal formants are generally broader than the oral formants. According to several investigators, the nasal formants occur at approximately the following frequencies: 250, 1 000 and 2 000 Hz (Nakata, 1959; Fant, 1960; Kaspranskij, 1965).

According to Fant (1968), a voiced occlusive nasal (nasal murmur) is characterized by a spectrum in which F2 is absent. A formant at approximately 250 Hz, generally extending into the adjacent vocalic segment, dominates the spectrum, but several weaker high-frequency formants (not always seen in spectrograms) occur, one typically at 2 200 Hz. These higher formants are generally weaker than for laterals. The bandwidths of nasal formants are generally larger than in vowel-like sounds.

The vowel formants proper are of secondary importance in the nasals. F1 is found to be 300–430 Hz, F2 500–1 900 Hz, and F3 1 800–2 600 Hz. The nasal *m* lacks a third formant because of the bilabiality of this sound. Different nasals are, however, comparatively similar as regards their acoustic structure. We therefore identify them mainly by means of the glide in the adjoining vowels (Malecot, 1956).

Being vowel formants proper, F1 and F2 are of secondary importance in the nasals themselves, but perform a definite transition, decisively influencing the acoustic pattern of the preceding and following vowels. Thus, the initial *m*, during the transition to the following vowel, causes an upward glide of F1 and F2, whereas the intermediate *m* causes the opposite phenomenon in the preceding vowel. The initial *n* causes shifting of F1 upwards, and of F2 downwards, if the F2 of the vowel that follows *n* permits this. When *n* is in intermediate position the F1 of the preceding vowel falls and F2 rises subject to the above condition as regards F2.

In the case of *ng*, approximately the same phenomenon occurs as in the medial *n*, but it is often less distinct because the F1 area is broader than above. Thus if one covers the nasal sound in the sonagram, it is possible, in the transition phase of the F1 and F2 of the preceding or following vowel, to say which of the nasals is concerned in each case. F3 is not affected by the proximity of a nasal (Fig. 1).

According to Nakata, the identification of separate nasals

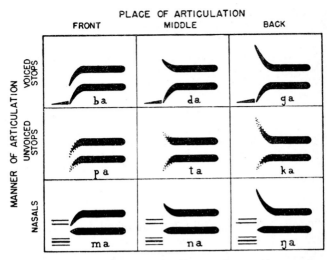

Fig. 1. Spectrographic patterns that illustrate the transition cues for the stop and nasal consonants in initial position with the vowel *a*. The dotted portions in the second row indicate the presence of noise (aspiration) in the place of harmonics. (After Liberman, 1957.)

depends on the frequency of the second nasal formant (FN2). *M* was the most common estimation, when the frequency of the formant in question was 1 100 Hz; *n* when FN2 was 1 700 Hz and *ng* when FN2 was 2 300 Hz and *ng* when FN2 was 2300 Hz. These results were obtained by listening tests made with synthetic speech; with real speech it is not as unambiguous as this.

In addition to formant transition and formant resonances playing an essential part in the acoustic identifiability of the nasals, there is also another phenomenon which is characteristic of the nasals alone and directly contrasted with the formant resonances. This is the anti-resonance produced by the oral cavity. Fant (1960) stated: "The effect of the mouth cavity as a side chamber, shunting the sound transmission through the pharynx-nose system, is to cause a shift of resonance frequencies and to introduce anti-resonances. It has been vertified by supplementary analog experiments that an increase of the coupling area to the mouth cavity, as in the case of an incomplete lowering of the velum or a lowered tongue position, shifting the mouth cavity anti-resonance up to 100 Hz, causes a neutralization of the 1 000 Hz nasal formant." Anti-resonance can be observed as "gaps" which become very prominent, especially in sections (Fig. 2).

NASALIZATION OF VOWELS

Additional information about the factors affecting the nasalization of vowels is obtained by investigating the impedance of the nasal and oral cavities. If the impedance of the nasal cavity is higher than that of the oral cavity, the effect of the nasal resonator on the acoustic quality of the sound is small. However, if the impedance of the oral cavity is higher than that of the nasal cavity, the nasal cavity, the nasal resonator has considerable effect on the acoustic outcome. The effect is strongest for those ranges of frequency where the difference between the impedances is largest, especially in the proximity of the first formant.

The impedance of the oral cavity is highest for the nasal consonants proper (in these cases the oral cavity is completely occluded), as in them the effect of the nasal resonator on the acoustic outcome is distinctly clearer than that of the oral resonator.

Voiced vowel-like nasal sounds (nasalized vowels) possess the nasal characteristics as a distortion superimposed on the vowel spectrum. Typical nasalization cues are the addition of the first nasal resonance in the region below the first formant of the vowel-like (open) sound and a simultaneous weakening and shift up in frequency of the first formant F1. A relative reduction of F3 or F2 (palatal articulation) is often seen (Fant, 1968).

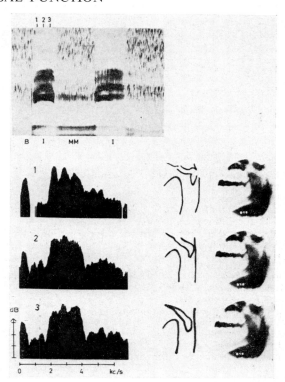

Fig. 3. Spectrographic analysis of the vowel *i*. The following three factors could be mentioned as the characteristic features of nasalized vowel: intensity growing in the area of 50 Hz; intensity weakening in the area of about 500 Hz; appearance of comparatively weak and diffuse components between the vowel formants in the area of 1 000–2 500 Hz. (After Björk, 1961.)

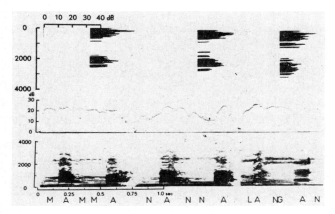

Fig. 2. Spectrographic analysis of the anti-resonance found in nasals and appearing in the sections as "gaps". It is seen that the gap is broadest in the labial *m*, narrower in the apicodental *n*, and narrowest in the dorso-velar *ng*. (After Kyttä, 1964.)

In brief, the following three factors are characteristic of a more or less nasalized vowel:

(1) Intensity growing in the area of 250 Hz.
(2) Intensity weakening in the area of about 500 Hz.
(3) Appearance of comparatively weak and diffuse components between the vowel formants in the area of 1 000–2 500 Hz (Fig. 3).

The nasalization of vowels is rather similar in Finnish and in British English, i.e. more regressive than progressive. In American English the vowels are, practically speaking, completely nasalized on both sides of the nasal (Hurme).

According to several studies, vowels are more nasalized in an unstressed than in a stressed position (e.g. Wiik, 1965), In British English, the duration of the nasalized portion of the vowel is a little longer after a nasal than in front of it, while in Finnish, the nasalized portion of the vowel is about twice as long after the nasal than in front of it. Apparently the velopharyngeal function is slower when speaking American English than when speaking the other mentioned languages. This is in line with assertions that American English is a "carelessly articulated tongue", with nasal features, in which the duration of the nasalized portion of the vowel does not seem to depend on the degree of "openness" of the vowel. Nasality has, obviously, a better chance to act as a distinctive feature in American than in British English. For example, in the word *bent* the vowel is com-

pletely nasalized in American English; in British English perhaps about one-half of the vowel is nasalized. "In the series vowel + nasal consonant + oral consonant, like *bent* (bɛnt), . . ., *bank* (bæŋk), nasality has clearly a distinctive part to play. The nasality of a vowel helps in the identification of words *bent/bet* and *bank/back* possibly as much as the nasal consonant; in fact, the nasality of the vowel may be even more important" (Delattre, 1965).

Many phoneticians have studied the acoustic aspects in the nasalization of vowels. Plenty of these "acoustic" correlates of nasalization have been found. Hurme has collected the opinions of various investigators (Table 1). In it the acoustic correlates are divided into four groups:

(I) The total intensity of the vowels is weakening. The weakening of separate formants and the broadening of their bandwidths all have a weakening effect on the total intensity.

(II) The first formant of a nasalized vowel is weakening in regard to the other formants, the width of F1 is increasing and the mean frequency is rising. Or both groups together: The first formant of the nasalized vowel is weakening in comparison to the other formants, and the intensity of the vowel is weakening.

(III) Nasal formants at certain frequencies, anti-resonances at certain frequencies and shifting of the oral formants on the frequency scale. All these changes can be understood by explaining the nasal resonance as an

Table 1

THE ACOUSTIC ASPECTS IN THE NASALIZATION OF VOWELS AFTER VARIOUS INVESTIGATORS
(After Hurme, 1968)

	Joos, 1948	Smith, 1951	Durand, 1953	Delattre, 1954	Hockett, 1955	House, 1956	Hattori, 1958	Truby, 1959	Fant, 1960	Björk, 1961	Plich, 1964	Wiik, 1965
I The total intensity of the vowel weakening						○	○	○	○		○	
F2 weakening		○										
F3 weakening		○										
"widening of all formants"									○	○		
"weak and diffuse components"							○					
II F1 bandwidth increasing					○	○						
F1 weakening in comparison with the other formants		○		○		○			○	○		
F1 mean frequency rising						○		○	○			
III 250 Hz formant				○				○			○	○
Extra formant (low)									○		○	
F2 unchanged (frequency and intensity)				○								
F2 frequency rising			○					○				
F3 frequency falling			○	○								
F3 frequency rising					○							
No changes in the vowel formant frequencies									○	○		
1 000 Hz formant	○	○							○			○
2 000 Hz formant		○		○		○			○			○
Extra formants	○											
Anti-formant 500 Hz							○					
Anti-resonance 500–900 Hz												○
Anti-resonances vary 500–1800 Hz						○			○			
Anti-resonance 900 Hz	○											
Anti-resonance between 200–1 200 Hz											○	
Anti-formants 300, 1 500 and 4 000 Hz										○		
F3 disappearing						○						
IV F4 intensity growing			○									
F4 intensity falling				○								
Formants above the F4 weakening			○									
Irregularities above F4						○						
7 500 Hz formant					○							

alternation between maximal and minimal intensities (between pole and zero). According to investigators, the intensity maxima (for nasal formants) are found to be at about 250, 1 000 and 2 000 Hz, the intensity minima (the anti-resonances) are found between the nasal formants.

(IV) It is typical of the lat five acoustic correlates that they are concerned with factors which are in the frequency range above 3000 Hz. Most of these can be explained by means of the alternation between intensity maxima and minima. The effect of frequencies that are as high as this on auditory perception is rather small. Delattre *et al.* (1954) have convincingly refuted the appearance of the 7 500 Hz nasal formant with, for example, synthetic speech.

On these grounds, all the acoustic correlates of vowel nasalization that various investigators have listed can be included in the acoustic theory by means of the concepts of resonance and anti-resonance. Because of anti-resonance and the 250 Hz nasal formant, the mean frequency of the

first oral formant may rise, the total intensity may fall and the bandwidth of the formant may increase. When a vowel is nasalized, its total intensity weakens due to the anti-resonance. The effect of nasalization on the second and third formants of the vowel depends on the quality of the vowel as well as the degree of nasalization.

EFFECT OF NASAL CAVITY CHANGES

Complete closure on one side of the nose (e.g. with a piece of cotton wool dipped in saline) does not produce an audible change. In the sonagram, one observes a general weakening of energy in the higher frequencies (Fig. 4b). Thus, marked septal deviations, hypertrophic conchae or polypi on one side have no appreciable influence upon the acoustic pattern of the nasal.

If, after this, changes are produced in the nasal passage of the other side—one side being completely closed—it is is observed that the glotto-pharyngeal-nose cavity formant remains at 250 Hz as long as the lowest nasal passage is free, and become even stronger if there is an obstacle in the middle or upper passage of the nose. The resonance of the upper nasal passages is either missing or becomes weaker, more diffuse and similar to noise in the sonagram (Fig. 4c). The converse effect obtains if the lowest passage of the nose is closed (Fig. 4b). If one continues the experiments with closure of the nose, so that the nasal passages are otherwise free but the nostrils are closed, it is observed that FN1 formant rises to 350 Hz. If the obstacle is pushed deeper

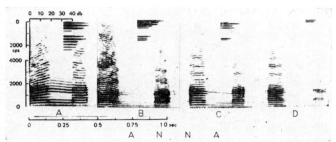

Fig. 4. Spectrographic analysis of the nasal sound *n*. (A) the nose is completely open; (B) one side ot the nose is closed; (C) one side of the nose and the upper passages of the other side are closed; (D) one side of the nose and the lowest passage of the other side are closed. (After Kyttä, 1970.)

into the nose, it is observed that this formant rises further, and when a point approximately 4 cm from the nostrils has been reached, the formant rises to 500–1 000 Hz, which is the same frequency for the anti-resonance. The nasalization stops, and the nasal consonant in question changes into some other sound. In some cases, it may start to resemble the preceding, or subsequent, vowel or—which is most common—*m* gets the acoustic structure of *b* or *p*, *n* that of *d* or *t*, and *ng* that of *g* or *k*, as it was somehow to be expected, and as was discussed in the beginning of this presentation when listing the corresponding plosives.

When the converse situation (increased nasal patency, as in rhinitis atrophicans or ozaena) is examined, sonographic methods do not reveal anything noteworthy. The widening of the nasal passage, as well as the increase in the cavity volume, apparently cause falling of the formant frequency, but because individual variations are great, it has not been possible to prove calculated frequency changes.

Attempts have also been made to ascertain the influence of the side cavities of the nose, especially the most accessible of these, the cheek cavities, on nasality (Kyttä, 1970). After

filling first one of the cheek cavities and then the other with radio-opaque material (Dianosil ᴿ), the consistency of which is comparatively thick, sonagrams were recorded in the usual manner, making use also of a nose microphone. No appreciable changes were observed. It is apparent, therefore, that the oral and nasal stress needed for normal speech is so small that hardly any side cavity resonance appears; the situation is obviously different in singing or perhaps in reciting, because the performer needs then a larger soundboard, and co-operation of the side cavities is necessary, perhaps even decisive.

CONCLUSION

We need and utilize the nose comparatively frequently for phonation, because nasalization is a common rather than an exceptional phenomenon, even for vowels. The nasals proper demand rapid velopharyngeal function, satisfactory straightness of the septum and one or other side of the conchae to be free from obstructions for the glotto-pharyngeal-nose cavity formant to be generated so that our ears can accept the countless individual nuances in the way that we use nasals.

REFERENCES

Björk, L. (1961), *Acta radiol.*, suppl. **202**, 82.
Delattre, P. (1965), *Comparing the Phonetic Features of English, German, Spanish and French.* Weinheim.
Delattre, P., Liberman, A. and Cooper, F. (1954), *J. acoust. Soc. Amer.*, **27**, 769.
Durand, M. (1953), *Studia Linguistica*, **7**, 33.
Fant, G. (1960), *Acoustic Theory of Speech Production.* The Hague.
Fant, G. (1968), *Manual of Phonetics.* Amsterdam.
Hattori, S., Yamamoto, K. and Fujimura, O. (1958), *J. acoust. Soc. Amer.*, **30**, 267.
Hockett, C., Quoted by Hurme, 1968.
House, A., quoted by Hurme, 1968.
Hurme, P. (1968), *Suomenkielen laudatur-työt.* Turun Ylioposto.
Joos, M. (1948), *Language*, **24**, 136.
Kaspranskij, R. (1965), *Phonetica*, **12**, 165.
Kyttä, J. (1964), *Acta oto-laryng. (Stockh.)*, suppl. **195**.
Kyttä, J. (1970), *Acta oto-laryng. (Stockh.)*, suppl. **263**.
Liberman, A. (1957), *J. acoust. Soc. Amer.*, **29**, 117.
Malecot, A. (1956), *Language*, **32**, 274.
Nakata, K. (1959), *J. acoust. Soc. Amer.*, **31**, 661.
Pilch, H. (1964), *Phonemtheorie I.* Birsfelden.
Smith, S. (1951), *Folia phoniatr.*, **3**, 165.
Truby, H. (1959), *Acta radiol.*, suppl. **182**.
Wiik, K. (1965), *Finnish and English Vowels.* Turku.

SECTION IX

THROAT

PAGE

38. DEVELOPMENTAL ANATOMY OF LARYNX   529

39. COMPARATIVE MORPHOLOGY OF LARYNX   536

40. NEUROLOGY OF THE LARYNX   546

41. LARYNX—MEASUREMENT OF FUNCTION   574

42. DEGLUTITION   591

38. DEVELOPMENTAL ANATOMY OF THE LARYNX

M. H. HAST

In the broad concept of developmental anatomy, the ontogeny of the larynx can be viewed from the fertilization of the ovum to the death of the individual organism. The morphogenesis of the larynx extends from its first visualization in the fourth week of embryonic life to the ossification of its cartilaginous structure in senescence. From its period of development in the embryo to the last stages of growth in puberty, the larynx is constantly changing. In

layer of the pouch and ectoderm of each groove then join, with each arch separated from its fellow arch, cranially or caudally, by an epithelial plate. Each arch contains a cartilaginous or bony core, a main blood vessel, muscles and nerves. From the five (or six) pharyngeal (branchial) arches and pouches arise the derivatives of the face, nose, palate, ear, tongue, pharynx, larynx, trachea, bronchi, lungs, tonsils, thyroid, parathyroids and thymus glands.

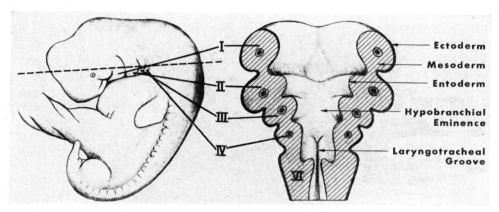

FIG. 1. Drawing of human embryo in the fifth week (CR 6·5 mm) to illustrate (1) external configuration of branchial region and (2) coronal section through the wall of the pharynx, dramatically enlarged, to demonstrate topography of the branchial arches and pouches.

this chapter, our attention will focus on that period of development in the human embryo in which the morphology of the larynx is established. Although this division of time occupies only some five weeks in the total life of the individual, it is during these stages of embryonal development that particular structures are laid down, a knowledge of which is essential for an understanding of both normal and abnormal form and function in the postnatal larynx.

THE BRANCHIAL REGION OF THE EMBRYO

Since the morphogenesis of the larynx is inseparable from that of the branchial arches a discussion of these structures and their derivatives is of singular importance to the topic of this chapter.

The branchial arches (Fig. 1) parallel the gill-arches of fish and some amphibians. In the human embryo, five arches are developed which are separated by four ectodermal grooves. On the same plane as the ectodermal groove, the pharyngeal entoderm presses aside the middle germ-layer (mesenchyme) and swells laterally to form the pharyngeal pouches (fourth gestational week). The entodermal

In this chapter, the discussion will be confined to the derivatives of branchial arches III, IV, V (?)* and VI.

In the branchial arches, the entodermal (inner) layers of arches (and pouches) III, IV and VI differentiate into the epithelium of the root of the tongue, pharynx, larynx, trachea, parathyroid and thyroid glands, thymus, epiglottis, tonsils, oesophagus and lungs.

Some entodermal anomalies would include a diverticulum of the pyriform fossa (arch III), hyperplasia of the epiglottis and vestibular folds (IV), congenital web of the vocal folds (IV), cysts of the laryngeal part of pharynx, larynx and thyroid gland (IV), laryngocoele (IV) and anomalies of the trachea (VI).

The mesodermal (middle) layer gives origin to the connective tissue of the tongue and neck region, the blood vascular and lymphatic systems, the muscles of the neck and larynx and the skeletal elements which include the hyoid bone and cartilages of the larynx. Mesodermal anomalies would include thyroid deformities (arch III), laryngeal stenosis and asymmetry (IV), chondromalacia (IV),

* A rudimentary inconstant arch which does not form typically on the human embryo. The ultimobranchial body is either a derivative of the disputed pouch V or of the pharyngeal entoderm in that region.

malformation of the laryngeal cartilages (IV and VI) and
an aneurysm of the internal carotid artery (III).

The ectodermal germ-layer (outer) of arches III, IV and
VI gives rise to the epidermis of the middle and lower neck,
and to the ninth (glossopharyngeal), tenth (*vagus*) and
eleventh (*accessory*) cranial nerves, respectively. The
superior laryngeal nerve, a branch of the vagus, is a nerve
of the fourth arch whereas the inferior (recurrent) laryngeal
is primarily a sixth arch nerve (cranial root of accessory).
In the post-embryonic period, the left recurrent laryngeal
nerve remains with the sixth arch artery (*ductus arteriosus*),
while the right nerve migrates cranially and laterally to the
fourth arch artery (subclavian), as a result of the disappearance of the right homologue of the sixth arch artery.

comes to lie between branchial arches IV and VI. The
caudal end of the laryngotracheal tube eventually develops
into the lung bud. As development continues, the margins
of the laryngotracheal groove fuse in a caudo-cranial
direction; a tracheoesophageal septum eventually is
formed which separates the laryngotracheal tube from the
oesophagus (seventh week).

During the fifth and sixth weeks, CR 5–10 mm, the
laryngeal aditus is modified by the growth of three masses of
tissue (comprising the furcula of His, 1885). The anterior
mass is the future epiglottis, a probable derivation of
the hypobranchial eminence (and arch IV); the two
lateral masses or swellings of mesenchymal tissue found
on the floor of the pharynx are the anlage of the arytenoids

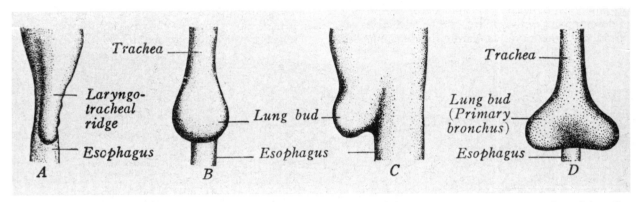

FIG. 2. Early stages of the human respiratory primordium: (*A*) at 2·5 mm, ventrally; (*B*) and (*C*) at 3 mm, ventrally and laterally; (*D* at 4 mm, ventrally. ×75. (From Arey, 1965.)

A frequent anomaly of ectodermal origin is the branchial
cyst. Ganglia of the seventh (*facial*), ninth and tenth
cranial nerves receive contributions from overlying patches
of ectoderm designated as epibranchial placodes. Cranial
nerves are dependent on the epibranchial placode for their
full development. Usually, placodal vesicles undergo
complete regression and disappear. If these placodes
persist, they could give rise to branchial (cervical) cysts.
The cysts, lined with stratified squamous epithelium, will
be found along the surface of the carotid sheath deep to
the sternocleidomastoid muscle.

EMBRYOLOGY OF THE LARYNX

The respiratory primordium, consisting of the larynx,
trachea and lungs, arises from a ventromedian diverticulum
of the foregut (groove of the furcula) caudal to the fourth
pharyngeal pouch. This depression, called the laryngotracheal groove or ridge, appears during the fourth week
in embryos of fourteen somites (crown rump 2·5 mm). As
development continues lateral furrows develop on each
side of the diverticulum along a line of union of the groove
and oesophagus. These furrows become progressively
deeper, eventually join, and form the laryngotracheal tube
(Fig. 2). The cranial end of this tube, which is posterior to
and proximal to the hypobranchial eminence, develops
into the primitive laryngeal aditus or slit. This aditus,
which appears at the crown rump (CR) 4 mm stage,

(vertical ridges of arch VI). These masses of tissue approximate each other medially and move cranially to the base of
the tongue (Fig. 3). The result is the addition of a transverse component to the top of the sagittal slit forming a
"T" shaped aditus (Fig. 4). The epithelial masses of the
aditus then join, closing the laryngeal slit until the end
of the second month.

The vocal folds and thyroarytenoid muscle are not
differentiated until the mesenchymal mass of cells that
forms the future glottis has split and the ventrodorsal depth
of the thyroid cartilage has increased. With the development of the thyroid cartilage during the second month,
the vocal folds are drawn out between the intrathyroid
lamina and the arytenoid cartilages. The normal formation
of the vocal folds, however, is intimately related to the
development of the sinus of the larynx and the vestibular
folds. During this period, there is an outpouching of the
lateral and inferior portion of the laryngeal cavity, extending from the eminence of the arytenoid anteriorly to the
floor of the primitive vestibule. The apex of this evagin-
ation forms the saccule of the larynx and the proximal and
wider portion of the sinus of the larynx. The fibrous basis
of the vestibular fold is produced by a condensation of
mesenchyme. With the development of the sinuses (between the fourth and fifth arches), the vocal and vestibular
folds are separated, the mass splitting during the third
month. The aryepiglottic folds are formed by an elongation
of the lateral fourth arch mass, which runs from the hypo-

branchial eminence (epiglottis) to the upper prominence of the sixth arch (arytenoid eminence).

It is interesting to note that if there is a failure of the epithelial primordium of the vocal folds to split (reopen) in the sagittal plane in the eighth week, a congenital atresia of the larynx would probably result. A congenital web between the folds is another anomaly seen in neonates. Although laryngeal webs are commonly found at

cuneiform cartilages probably develop from the blastema of the aryepiglottic folds, with the cuneiform tubercle forming earlier than the corniculate tubercle (Rudan, 1965).

The thyroid cartilage develops as two lateral plates (derived from the ventral cartilaginous portions of arch IV) (Fig. 5) which fuse in the mid-ventral line united by a membrane. Development of the thyroid cartilage is almost complete by the ninth week (Fig. 6); its superior cornu,

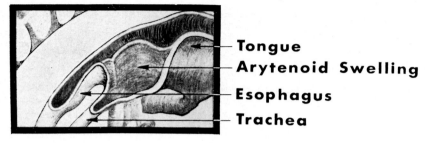

FIG. 3. View of the laryngeal region in a 5½-week-old embryo (CR 10 mm) showing the relationship, at this early stage, of the tongue, arytenoid eminences, oesophagus and trachea. (After Blechschmidt, 1961.)

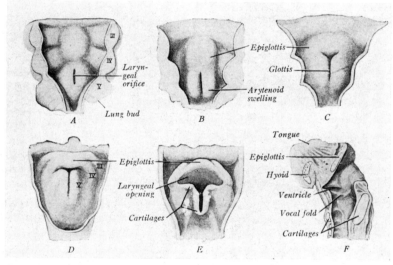

FIG. 4. Development of the embryonic larynx and at birth: (A) 4 weeks (5 mm); (B) 5 weeks (9 mm); (C) 6 weeks (12 mm); (D) 7 weeks (16 mm); (E) 10 weeks (40 mm); (F) at birth. (From Arey, 1965.)

the level of the glottis anteriorly, webs also can occur in the infraglottic area and supraglotically between the vestibular folds or (rarely) in the intercartilaginous part of the rima glottidis (posterior commissure).

The Cartilages

Skeletal elements of the hyoid bone and larynx are mesodermal derivatives of the branchial arches. The lesser cornu and upper part of the body of the hyoid develop from arch II, while the greater cornu and lower part or remainder of the body of the hyoid bone develop from the ventral portion of arch III.

The epiglottis is probably developed from fusion of the caudal portion of the hypobranchial eminence (copula of His) and ventral ends of the third and fourth arches. The

however, remains fused to the greater cornu of the hyoid until the twelfth or thirteenth week.

The arytenoid cartilages and the corniculate cartilages are derivatives of arch VI and develop from the arytenoid swellings (Fig. 3). In the early period of their development, the arytenoids are fused to the cricoid cartilage; they will separate with the appearance of the cricoarytenoid joint, achieving almost full development and their future shape by the end of the embryonic period. The vocal processes are formed later, in conjunction with development of the vocal (thyroarytenoid) ligament and thyroid cartilage; development occurs during the end of the second and beginning of the third month.

The cricoid cartilage also develops as two cartilaginous centres of the sixth arch. The centres unite ventrally in the

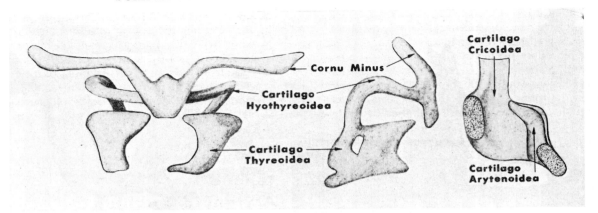

FIG. 5. Three figures to illustrate the hyoid bone and laryngeal cartilages in an embryo of approximately 7 weeks of age (CR 21 mm). (After Kallius, 1897.)

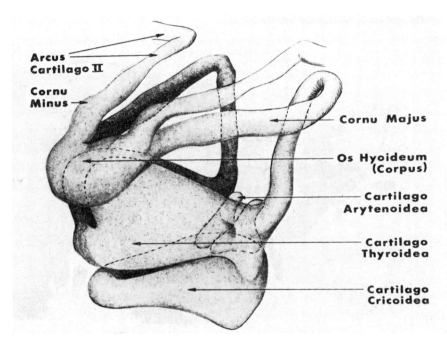

FIG. 6. Skeletal structure of the larynx and hyoid bone in the early fetal period of 9 weeks (CR 47 mm). (After Wind, 1970.)

early developmental period of the larynx. Fusion of the dorsal lamina occurs during the seventh week of embryonic life. It is also during this period that the tracheo-oesophageal septum has developed to at least the first tracheal ring and future fusion of the cricoid. If the rostral advancement of the tracheo-oesophageal septum is arrested, preventing the dorsal fusion of the cricoid cartilage, a laryngotracheo-oesophageal cleft will result. The cleft should not be confused with the large interarytenoid notch that persists even into the fetal period (Fig. 4).

The laryngeal cartilages chondrify at varying developmental stages. Chondrification of the thyroid and cricoid cartilages begins at the end of the seventh gestational week. The arytenoids develop more slowly, chondrifying at the beginning of the third month; the corniculates do not start to chondrify until the end of the third month. The

epiglottis, unlike the hyoid bone and other cartilages of the larynx, contains little cartilaginous tissue until the beginning of the fifth month of fetal life.

The Epithelium

The anlage of the epithelium of the larynx is found in the epithelial lamina, a ventromedially disposed fold in the foregut (Walander, 1950). The laryngeal epithelium, like that of the base of the tongue and pharynx, is of entodermal origin and is derived from arches (or pouches) IV and VI. Significant changes in the epithelial lining of the larynx become apparent in the later embryonal and early fetal stages between 8 and 12 weeks (CR 40–90 mm). The primitive mesenchymal tissue of the glottis develops into cuboidal and eventually stratified squamous. The anterior surface of the epiglottis, the aryepiglottic folds and piriform fossa are also lined with stratified squamous epithelium. The balance of the interior lining of the larynx changes from an embryonic polyhedral variety of cell to ciliated pseudostratified columnar epithelium.

The Extrinsic Muscles

The anlage of the extrinsic laryngeal muscles derives from the epicardial ridge as part of the primitive infrahyoid muscle mass. This mass divides into superficial and deep layers, with each layer further separating into two. The omohyoid and sternohyoid muscles result from a split of the superficial layer longitudinally into a medial and

slit and epiglottic sphincter (transverse arytenoid, aryepiglottic and lateral cricoarytenoid muscles) and that pair which opens the glottic sphincter (posterior cricoarytenoid).

It is at the 7 mm stage (Fig. 7) where the anlage of the cricoid and arytenoid cartilages can be recognized, that one can first differentiate both an "inner" and "external" constrictor (Frazer, 1910).

As the inner constrictor is the primordium for all of the intrinsic laryngeal muscles of the larynx discussed above, the cricothyroid is probably formed from the external constrictor muscle of the pharynx, a derivative of the fourth arch. These inner and external planes of cells are more

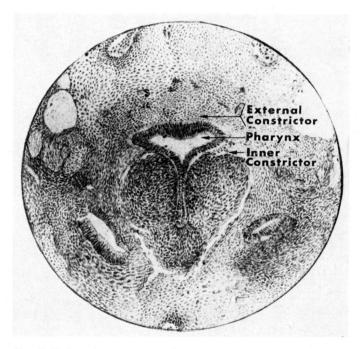

FIG. 7. Embryonic larynx of CR 7 mm (32 days); microscopic drawing. ×56.

lateral part; the thyroid and sternothyroid muscles are formed as a consequence of the deep layer becoming attached to the oblique line of the thyroid cartilage, ultimately separating into an upper and lower part. In regard to the pharyngeal constrictors, the stylopharyngeus is derived from the third arch and the cricopharyngeus from the fourth arch.

The Intrinsic Muscles

In the early stages (4–6 mm), the primitive glottic slit is observed surrounded by condensation of undifferentiated mesenchyme; the cells are denser at the glottis and appear to be migrating peripherally. The primordium of the laryngeal muscles appears first as an intrinsic sphincter, lying within the anlage of the thyroid cartilage and at the level of the cricoid. From this author's studies, it appears that the laryngeal myoblasts are strung in the form of a ring or sphincter in the the 7–10 mm embryo. As development continues, this sphincter of muscle fibres separates into individual masses of muscle, those that constrict the glottic

clearly defined in the CR 10–12 mm embryo. Until we reach the CR 13 mm stage of development, however, judgments as to the recognition of individual muscles are more speculative than reliable (Fig. 8). It is during the seventh gestational week (CR 13–17 mm), when the development of the cartilages has advanced to a more easily recognizable form, that the intrinsic muscles can be definitely differentiated.

The most developed muscles in the 13 mm embryo are the transverse arytenoid and the posterior cricoarytenoid. The primordium of aryepiglottic musculature can also be distinguished at this stage. The cricothyroid, like the thyroarytenoid muscle is still difficult to differentiate until the CR 15 mm embryo, although the cricothyroid probably separates from the pharyngeal constrictor as a separate mass by the 10–12 mm embryo. The thyroarytenoid is, however, well differentiated from the lateral cricoarytenoid in the CR 18 mm embryo (Fig. 9).

Finally, it is in the CR 19–23 mm embryo that we observe the laryngeal muscles passing through their last stages

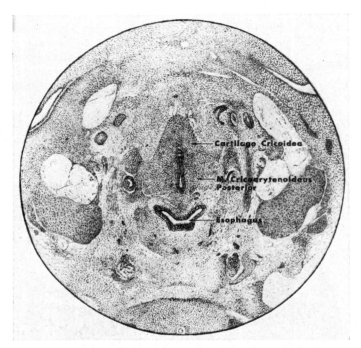

FIG. 8. Embryonic larynx of CR 13 mm (42 days); microscopic drawing.
×32.

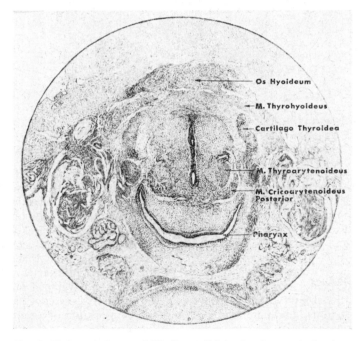

FIG. 9. Embryonic larynx of CR 18 mm (45 days); microscopic drawing.
×30.

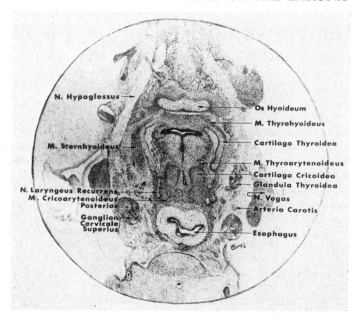

Fig. 10. Embryonic larynx of 21 mm (48 days); microscopic drawing. × 18.

of embryonic development and differentiation (Fig. 10). All intrinsic muscles are now clearly visualized, with the transverse arytenoid, posterior cricoarytenoid and cricothyroid muscles still dominant. The next stage (24–30 mm) marks the end of the embryonic period and the beginning of the fetal stage of laryngeal growth, with the larynx taking on much of its future postnatal form during the eighth and eleventh week of prenatal life (Fig. 6).

REFERENCES AND FURTHER READING

Arey, L. B. (1965), *Developmental Anatomy*, 7th edition. Philadelphia: Saunders.

Bardeen, C. R. (1910), *Manual of Human Embryology*, Vol. 1 (F. Keibel and F. P. Mall, Eds.). Philadelphia: Lippincott.

Blechschmidt, E. (1961), *The Stages of Development Before Birth*. Philadelphia: Saunders.

Blumberg, J. B., Stevenson, J. K., Lemire, R. J. and Boyden, E. A. (1965), *Surgery*, **57**, 559.

Davies, D. V. (Ed.) (1967), *Gray's Anatomy*, 34th edition. London: Longmans Green.

Frazer, J. E. (1910), *J. Anat. Physiol.*, **44**, 156.

Hamilton, W. J., Boyd, J. D. and Mossman, H. W. (1972), *Human Embryology*, 4th edition. Baltimore: Williams and Wilkins.

Hast, M. H. (1970), *Otolaryng. Clin. Amer.*, **3**, 413.

Hast, M. H. (1972), *Ann. Otol., Rhinol., Lar.*, **81**, 524.

His, W. (1885), *Anatomie Menschlicher Embryonen*, Heft 3. Leipzig.

Holinger, P. H. and Brown, W. T. (1967), *Ann. Otol., Rhinol., Lar.*, **76**, 744.

Iffy, L., Shepard, T. H., Jakobovits, A., Lemire, R. J. and Kerner, P. (1967), *Acta anat.*, **66**, 178.

Kallius, E. (1897), *Anat. Hefte*, **9**, 302.

Lewis, W. H. (1910), *Manual of Human Embryology*, Vol. 1 (F. Keibel and F. P. Mall, Eds.). Philadelphia: Lippincott.

Lisser, H. (1911), *Amer. J. Anat.*, **12**, 27.

Negus, V. (1949), *The Comparative Anatomy and Physiology of the Larynx*. New York: Hafner.

Pattern, B. M. (1968), *Human Embryology*, 3rd edition. New York: McGraw-Hill.

Rudan, A. S. (1965), *Dokl. Akad. Nauk. S.S.S.R.*, **160**, 1444.

Soulié, A. and Bardier, E. (1907), *J. Anat. Physiol.*, **43**, 137.

Strazza, G. (1888), *Med. Jahrb.*, ser. 3, **2**, 105.

Streeter, G. L. (1945), *Contr. Embryol.* Carneg. Instn., **31**, 27.

Streeter, G. L. (1948), *Contr. Embryol.* Carneg. Instn., **32**, 133.

Walander, A. (1950), *Acta anat.*, **10**, suppl. 13.

Willis, R. A. (1962), *The Borderland of Embryology and Pathology*, 2nd edition. London: Butterworth.

Wind, J. (1970), *On the Phylogeny and the Ontogeny of the Human Larynx*. Groningen: Wolters-Noordoff.

39. COMPARATIVE MORPHOLOGY OF THE LARYNX

SUSAN P. DENNY

"What a piece of work is man! How noble in reason! How infinite in faculty! In form and moving how express and admirable! In action how like an angel! In apprehension how like a god! The beauty of the world! The paragon of animals!"

(*Hamlet*, Act II, Sc. 2)

The significance of the combination of human brain and body is perhaps best shown by man's most important innovation: language. Only humans use sounds for speech, although all animals communicate with their fellows, many by the use of less refined sounds. Bees dance to direct the swarm to food, wolves warn-off intruders by marking their territories with scent, one bird call announces danger, another invites love-making. Besides employing all these methods of communication (odours, bodily movements and simple sounds), humans use language, a huge repertory of sounds that can be combined as units to express very complex facts and ideas. The prairie dog's quick high-pitched barks can send up a vague alarm but they cannot be specific. However, they have developed a type of society which consisted of millions of animals on the Great Plains before man came, and a major element in their success was the vocabulary of barks and calls, "a language" that is one of the most precise systems of communication in non-human societies. Such communication obviously depends on the brain, for some animals equal man in vocal performance without mastering language. Myna birds and parrots mimic a man's voice perfectly; they can even be taught to repeat sentences of several words, but they cannot combine elements from different sentences, learned by rote, and use them to construct a third sentence. Language is so clearly dependent on brainpower that its dependence on the body is often overlooked. Chimpanzees appear to have a brain capable of abstract thought. They can, for example, stack several boxes on top of one another to reach a bunch of bananas. They can also produce a wide range of sounds. They ought to be able to talk. They have been taught to use the American sign-language, originally designed for the deaf. But the best results for speech have been to get them to say "mama" or "papa" and a few other infant words. Only recently has the reason for this failure been traced. A chimpanzee lacks the pharynx that enables humans to articulate vowel sounds. It is the structure of the larynx in animals which limits their sound production and it is this same structure in humans which has allowed man to be the only animal to have acquired speech. Learning to talk was the last of man's major evolutionary achievements and, with the discovery of speech, man acquired an immensely powerful tool for speeding-up his cultural evolution. The members of man's hunting and gathering bands made good use of their ability to communicate verbally with one another: to plan a hunt, pass on information or agree upon a rendezvous. But the greatest ability was to learn from the accumulated experience of others, other people, other groups. Before the birth of language, man's experiences were brief and transitory; when a man died, his experiences died with him. By means of language, the shared experiences of mankind could be preserved and kept accessible over the course of many generations, first through folklore and legend and then through the written word.

Having looked at man, let us compare the use of sounds for communication in a variety of other animals. Sounds can be divided broadly into those designed for the survival of the individual and those designed for the survival of the species. Animals cries can be used for *defence* by frightening away an aggressor, for example, the barking of dogs, the hissing of birds, snakes and cats, the screaming of monkeys, the screeching of geese, and the snorting of bulls. Cries are also emitted to obtain help, but this is uncommon in animals other than Primates. However, kangaroos yell in fear, as do cattle, deer and horses. The cry for food is common among young birds and mammals, even though it has the danger of attracting enemies. *Offence* by intimidation is by development of the defensive cry. Dogs are vocal when on the track of their prey; an elephant trumpets and a bull bellows. When prey is sought most animals are silent.

Though every animal has a keen instinct to preserve itself, it has an even greater urge to preserve the species. The initial stage of this is *finding a mate*. It is usual for the male to call to the female. Insects, crickets and grasshoppers stridulate with their wingcases, and, amongst the Amphibians, frogs and toads, for example, are very vocal in the pairing season. Amongst the Reptiles, alligators, crocodiles and tortoises are also vocal. Birds sing to proclaim their territory and to find a partner. It is to be noted that songbirds have often a dull plumage, whereas brightly coloured birds are often silent and usually have a complex display which compensates for their lack of vocalization. Parrots, however, are brightly coloured and noisy, though not endowed with song. Nocturnal birds such as nightjars and owls are vocal, to retain communication with their mates. Not only is sound used to find a mate but it is also used to keep her (or him) by repulsing intruders.

Sounds are also used in *communication* between parents and young, a function of obvious importance. The slight differences between the calls of parents in a penguin colony, for example, enable a bewildered youngster to find his own parents among thousands of birds. Sound is of great value for communication in species which live in trees or amongst grass and bushland, and in creatures who are constantly on the move such as chimpanzees. It is less important in less mobile animals such as gorillas, koala bears and sloths. Nocturnal animals also tend to be very vocal since the dark inhibits the use of visual communication. Individual communication is not the ultimate to which phonation is directed, but communication within the group or society is important, especially when danger is imminent.

The nature of sound production in the various species is

correlated with the nature of their hearing. There is little purpose in an animal producing a complex series of sounds if other species and members of his own species are unable to perceive these via their ears or similar organs. Thus sound production is correlated with hearing, and, similarly, deafness is a good reason for the absence of voice. Deafness is a physiological defect in some animals, such as snakes, and it is a pathological inheritance in some human infants, who require special speech training if they are to learn to speak. The structure of the larynx thus shows considerable variation, depending on whether noise or tone shall be the result of this activity, whether pitch shall be low or high, and whether the range shall be wide or limited, as well as what quality of tones shall be produced. In some animals, phonation is unnecessary or little used because other senses, such as olfaction, touch or vision are better developed. The total use of other senses usually occurs in animals other than mammals, such as insects, fish and reptiles. All mammals use their ears, eyes, larynx and nose to some degree. However, depending on the species, they tend to rely on one or more of the senses which are better developed. Man's sense of smell is less developed than his vocal powers.

Let us review some of the modifications of the larynx associated with olfaction, respiration and deglutition.

Olfaction is of great importance to many animals and, when the pulmonary apparatus was evolved, a system was necessary in which air would circulate through the nose, which communicates with the mouth in all animals organized on such a pattern. In some cases, the opening of the nasal tract into the food tract is not in direct relationship with the opening of the larynx, as in the dog, gorillas, muntjac and tiger. Other animals, however, have an opposite arrangement. For example, the crocodile has evolved a mouth flap. In mammals, the necessity of separation has resulted in the evolution of a flap, the epiglottis, arising at the cranial end of the larynx and lying in contact with the palate to close the gap between the nasal part of the pharynx (nasopharynx) and the laryngeal aperture. The degree of development of the epiglottis depends on the habit of the animal concerned. Thus a well developed epiglottis is found in echidnas (spiny anteaters) and in all Australian marsupials with a keen sense of smell, in rodents, such as the jerboas and cavies, and in lagomorphs (hares and rabbits), as well as in antelopes, deer and goats. There is an additional modification in man relating to the position of the larynx, since the palate in man is proportionately shorter than it is in other animals. The shape of the palate is also altered, there being a central uvula, which is absent in most animals. This is a relic of a longer and more complete palate. The epiglottis would be sufficiently large to close the gap, provided the larynx were in the position it occupies in other animals, that is, opposite the base of the skull. But in man the larynx lies low in the neck opposite the lower border of the 4th cervical vertebra. Descent to this position occurs in the fetus and in childhood. Partly responsible for this is the erect posture and the recession of the jaws.

Certain modifications involving, but not confining themselves to, the larynx are concerned with *respiration*. These modifications involve expansion of the larynx, variations in the arytenoid cartilages and in the relative lengths of the arytenoid vocal processes, there being many interesting relationships between the latter and the activity of the species. Thus antelopes and horses have vocal processes closely approximating the optimum length, whereas those of man are relatively short, because he has no need for a wide glottal opening and also because he requires long membranous margins to the glottis for purposes of both phonation and fixation of the thorax.

A specialized mechanism of respiration is the presence of *air-sacs*. These are found in a variety of animals and have a variable structure and usage. Buccal air-sacs are found in the mouth of many frogs. Nasal air-sacs are found in monitor lizards and in the bladder-nosed seal. There are tracheal air-sacs in as diverse a group as chameleons, female emus, and a species of spider monkey. Syringeal air-sacs are important in many birds such as ducks and swans. Unlike the other types of sacs, where rebreathing of air is the primary function, the syringeal air-sacs of birds are part of the specialized vocal organ—the syrinx. In birds, there is also a system of air-sacs (cervical, thoracic and abdominal) in connection with the lungs, thus maintaining a method of internal respiration. Finally, there are the laryngeal air-sacs, which are found in a wide variety of animals, including bats. The nature of these will be discussed in detail later.

The larynx was evolved by an increase in size, by tilting of its aperture and by the addition of an epiglottis. Together with the close relationship of the latter to the soft palate, these developments have introduced complications when *swallowing* is necessary, and certain modifications have consequently occurred. In microsomatic animals, such as the Californian "sea lion", the dingo and the walrus, there is a small or absent epiglottis and no trouble with swallowing. The larynx is easily closed when dealing with liquid or solid food. However, in animals that live on a herbivorous diet, a large amount of semi-liquid food is ingested over a prolonged period. A mechanism must therefore be developed whereby liquids or semi-solids can pass from the mouth into the oesophagus without inundating the larynx. This mechanism is the lateral food channel which is present on either side of the larynx. Fish-eating mammals, such as dolphins, porpoises and toothed whales, all swallow along the very efficient lateral food channel. The high spout-like larynx, its margins supported by epiglottic and cuneiform (Wrisberg) cartilages, extends into the nasal part of the pharynx wherein it remains permanently. The nasal passage opens on the top of the head by a single aperture protected by a muscular valve and so placed as to allow these cetaceans to inspire and exhale, with no interruption to swallowing. Whalebone whales, however, have a poorly-protected larynx. This is associated with their habit of taking plankton and water into the mouth and expelling the latter through their sieve of baleen or whalebone, swallowing only the separate mass of plankton.

PARTICULAR ASPECTS: THE CHIROPTERA

Space does not allow for a comprehensive account of all known variations in the structure of the larynx. The author therefore considers it would be more profitable to concentrate on one group of animals only, the order Chiroptera (bats). These have been the subject of special study by the author and an attempt will be made to relate structural modifications to functional differences. The importance of the larynx to bats cannot be over-emphasized, for most of this group of mammals rely solely on echolocation to find food, and to find their way around generally.

The Chiroptera are divided into two suborders, the Megachiroptera and the Microchiroptera. Of the former, only *Rousettus* can orientate acoustically. *Rousettus* uses pulses of sound which are audible and which are produced

"Rotring" ink pens flow easily on this surface. The sheets were attached by sellotape to the projection face of a Zeiss "Ultraphot" microscope and the main structures were traced on the sheet. These were then coloured so that similar structures could easily be recognized (Fig. 1). The plastic sheets were displayed in a specially-designed and constructed aluminium box, to which a temporary light source was added. By removing the appropriate lid, the sheets were placed in numerical order and, from the front, a three-dimensional effect was obtained. Two species have been

TABLE 1

GENERAL INFORMATION ON THE BATS STUDIED

Superfamily	Family	Species	Location	Distribution of Species	Roosting Habitat of Species
Emballonuroidea	Emballonuridae	Saccopteryx biliniata	Panama	Central and South America	Trees and caves
	Rhinopomatidae	Rhinopoma hardwickei	Egypt	Africa, Asia	Caves
	Noctilionidae	Noctilio leporinus	Panama	South America	Sea caves, hollow trees (characteristically *Ceiba pentandra*)
Rhinolophoidea	Rhinolophidae	Rhinolophus ferrumcquinium	East Africa	Old World only	Caves or buildings
		Rhinolophus fumigatus	East Africa	Old World only	Caves or buildings
	Hipposideridae	Hipposideros caffer	East Africa	Old World only	Caves or buildings
	Nycteridae	Nycterio macrotis	East Africa	Africa, Malaya	Caves or under rocks
	Megadermatidae	Lavia frons	West Africa	Africa	Trees
		Cardioderma cor	East Africa	Africa, Asia	Caves and trees
Phyllostomatoidea	Phyllostomatidae	Phyllostomus hastatus	Panama	Central and South America	Caves
		Pteronotus parnellii	Panama	Central and South America	Caves
		Glossophaga soricina	Panama	Central and South America	Caves, trees
	Desmodontidae	Desmodus rotundus	Panama	Central and South America	Caves, trees

by tongue-clicking. Other Megachiroptera find their way by olfaction and vision. The Microchiroptera have evolved a system independently of *Rousettus*. They use echolocation not only to avoid obstacles but also to locate and to catch their prey. Those that feed on fruit or other animals no doubt use olfactory information as well. They send out loud ultrasonic pulses of high frequency sound which are reflected by objects in their path. Depending upon the species, the sounds are emitted through the mouth or the nostrils. In bats which emit their sonar pulses nasally, the larynx often fits into the nasal part of the pharynx, mechanically separating the trachea from the mouth. Most bats which emit their orientation pulses nasally have a nose-leaf, the structure of which varies considerably throughout the group.

Table 1 shows a list of the species which have been studied and these are arranged according to Simpson's (1945) classification.

Methods of Study

In addition to the use of serial sections, the structure of the larynx was studied in a few representative species of bats by the use of a three-dimensional model. This method is based upon the work of Bart (1969), Graham (1952), Griffiths (1970) and Morris (1972). A plastic sheet was cut into 15 × 20 cm sections, which proved ideal, since black

studied by this method, *Rhinolophus ferrumequinum* and *Lavia frons*, chosen for their different laryngeal structure.

As in man, the larynx of bats consists of a scaffolding and a series of muscles covered by an epithelial membrane provided with numerous mucous glands for purposes of lubrication. However, the larynx is very large in comparison with other species. Certainly, the muscles of the bat larynx are large and in many species, a system of air-saccules has been found and, though this has been attributed to the mixing and rebreathing of air (Negus, 1949), it seems more likely to be related to the emission of the echolocation pulses.

Cartilages

As in man, the framework of the bat larynx consists primarily of the thyroid, cricoid and arytenoid cartilages.

The thyroid cartilages shield the intrinsic part of the larynx. The thyroid notch is above and in front. On either side, below the notch and flaring outwards, are the thyroid laminae (alae). Extending upwards from each lamina to the hyoid bone is the superior cornu and, downwards to the cricoid, the less prominent inferior cornu. The thyroid cartilage articulates only with the cricoid and for this purpose there are two articular facets on each inferior cornu. These facets meet with the corresponding facets on the cricoid. The cricothyroid joint permits the cricoid to tilt

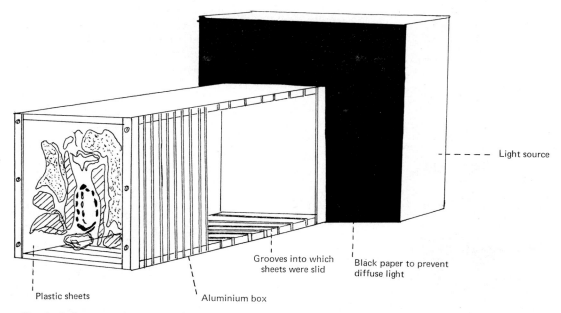

Light source

Grooves into which
sheets were slid

Black paper to prevent
diffuse light

Plastic sheets

Aluminium box

FIG. 1. A diagram to show the aluminium box and temporary light source constructed to exhibit the plastic sheets.

slightly on the thyroid. In all species of bat studied the thyroid cartilage was very thin. As in man, the cartilage is of the hyaline type.

The cricoid cartilage is a complete ring of cartilage in the human larynx. However, this ring structure was observed in only three of the bat species studied, namely, *Lavia frons* and *Cardioderma cor* (of the family Megadermatidae), and *Desmodus rotundus* (of the family Desmodontidae). It was uncertain whether or not the cricoid cartilage was a complete ring in *Phyllostomus hastatus* and in *Glossophaga soricina*. The fact that other species did not show this structure is probably due to a modification of the larynx in these species to form air-saccules. An interesting feature of these cartilages in bats is that they are subject to ossification, which presumably makes them more rigid structures although there is variability amongst species as to the degree of ossification. Suffice to say that the thyroid and cricoid cartilages in both the Rhinolophoidea and the Emballonuroidea showed the greatest degree of ossification, but that members of phyllostomatoidea also showed some degree of ossification. Besides the thyroid, cricoid and arytenoid laryngeal cartilages, there are two corniculate cartilages, one on top of each arytenoid cartilage, and two cuneiform cartilages, one in each aryepiglottic fold. These were not easily identified since they appear small and relatively insignificant in bats.

Air-sacs

One of the most interesting aspects of the anatomy of the bat larynx is the absence or presence of air-saccules and their variable structure.

Both species of the Rhinolophidae (the Horseshoe Bats) studied, *Rhinolophus ferrumequinum* and *Rhinolophus fumigatus*, possess air-sacs (Fig. 2). These have previously been reported both by Wassif and Madkour (1968–9) in Egyptian bats, and by Roberts (1972). It appears that, in *Rhinolophus sp.*, the 1st and 2nd tracheal rings are expanded to form a pair of small lateral pouches. The tracheal rings from the third to the fifth are fused dorsally to form a broad dorsal pouch which fails to ossify mid-dorsally. The rings fuse with the body of the pouches laterally and dorsally (Fig. 2) Histologically, the lining of both the sacs and the laryngeal lumen is seen to be columnar epithelium and pseudostratified, with ciliated epithelium present posteriorly towards the oesophagus. In the closely related species, *Hipposideros caffer*, an obvious similarity can be seen in the pattern of the air-sacs (Fig. 3). There are, again, two pairs of pouches supported by a cartilaginous ring.

In *Nycteris macrotis* there are a pair of large laryngeal pouches just caudal to the cricoid cartilage (Fig. 4a, b). They are large and extend caudally to the level of the 10th tracheal ring. The pouches join the trachea between the cricoid cartilage and the 1st tracheal ring. In *Lavia frons* and *Cardioderma cor*, both members of the family Megadermatidae (false vampire bats), pouches were absent (Figs. 5 and 6a, b). However, the larynges of these animals showed a complete cricoid ring, an unusual feature in bats (Fig. 6b).

Pteronotus parnellii (the moustache bat) has one dorsal air-sac strengthened, as seen previously in other bats, by a ring of cartilage (Fig. 7a, b). However, the internal structure is noticeably different from that found in the pouches of the Rhinolophoidea, and one is immediately aware of invaginations whose epithelial lining is still columnar or pseudostratified, with ciliated cells dorsally. This type of structure seems more suited to the mixing and rebreathing of air than are the pouches of Rhinolophoidea. However, even in those species of bats which do not possess saccules, the laryngeal lumen is often bulbous and invaginated at its posterior end. This leads one to believe that the larynx of bats generally is very flexible and can be expanded or contracted at will, when the need arises, to force a larger amount

Key to Illustrations

Salivary Tissue	
Muscle	
Thyroid Gland	
Cartilage	

Key to Abbreviations

AC	Arytenoid Cartilage
CC	Cricoid Cartilage
TC	Thyroid Cartilage
CR	Cricoid Ring
TA	Thyroarytenoideus Muscle
LL	Laryngeal Lumen
LP	Laryngeal Pouch
MC	Mucous Cells
VC	Vocal folds
OESO	Oesophagus

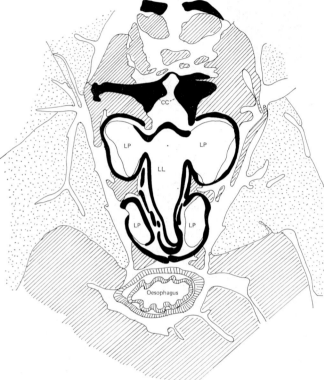

FIG. 2. A drawing of a section through the larynx of *Rhinolophus ferrumequinum*.

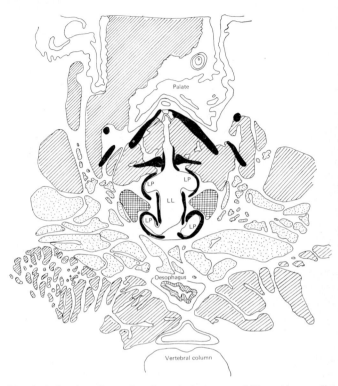

FIG. 3. A drawing of a section through the larynx of *Hipposideros caffer*. (*See* Fig. 2, for Keys to Illustrations and Abbreviations.)

a species with piscivorus teeth which feeds by flying low over water and catching fish with its feet, such a function is a possibility, for it must echolocate and breath while feeding. Possible explanations for the presence of air-sacs will be discussed later.

of air through the larynx to modify the acoustic character of sound pulses.

Returning to the other members of the phyllostomatoidea, neither *Desmodus*, the vampire bat, nor *Phyllostomus* possess air-saccules. Laryngeal sections of *Desmodus* show a complete cricoid ring, but noticeable is the small, simple oesophagus modified for a liquid diet. (*Desmodus* lives on the blood of mammals.)

Noctilio leporinus (the fisherman bat), *Rhinopoma hardwickei* (one of the mouse-tailed bats), and *Saccopteryx biliniata* (the white-lined bat) all possess similar larynges. Figure 8 shows the ventricle-like air-sacs exemplified by the genus *Noctilio*. These are lined by cubical or simple epithelium in *Noctilio* and *Saccopteryx*, but by ciliated epithelium in *Rhinopoma*. Initially, these sacs seemed to be similar to the ventricles of the larynx in man. However, the sacs are below the vocal folds and are fused to them in part. It is difficult to ascertain whether or not these sacs are used for the mixing and rebreathing of air. In *Noctilio leporinus*,

Vocal folds

Another interesting anatomical detail, possibly connected with the air-sacs and ultimately with echolocation, is the structure of the vocal folds (cords). In the species of bats which possess air-sacs (*Rhinolophus ferrumequinum*, *Rhinoluphus fumigatus*, *Hipposideros caffer*, *Nycteris macrotis*, *Pteronotus parnellii*, *Noctilio leporinus*, *Rhinopoma hardwickei* and *Saccopteryx biliniata*), the vocal folds are shorter and thicker than those in the species without air-sacs (*Phyllostomus hastatus*, *Desmodus rotundus*, *Glossophaga soricina*, *Cardioderma cor* and *Lavia frons*), where the folds are longer and thinner (Fig. 8). Theoretical considerations will be discussed later.

Salivary tissue

In all sections of the bat larynx, one of the most noticeable structures is the abundance of salivary tissue surrounding the larynx proper. Internally, the laryngeal lumen is well supplied with mucous cells all functional for lubrication.

Epiglottis

The cartilage of the epiglottis is yellow fibro-cartilage and consists of a central flat broad plate with a superior notch but no lateral or median processes. In section it resembles a horseshoe, united to the top of the thyroid

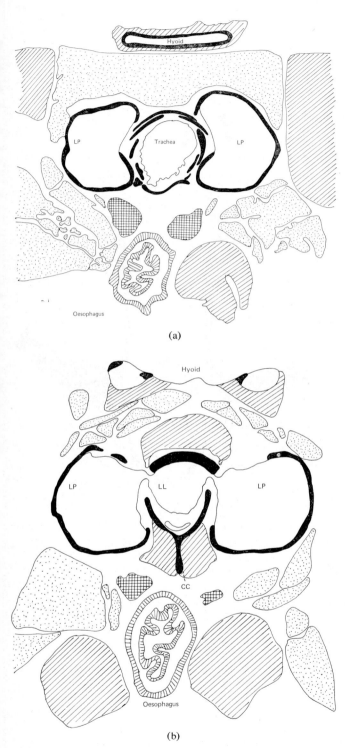

(a)

(b)

FIG. 4(a) and (b). A drawing of a section through the larynx of *Nycteris macrotis*. (*See* Fig. 2, p. 540, for Keys to Illustrations and Abbreviations.)

cartilage by a ligament. Soft coverings of connective tissue and mucosa extend the size of the epiglottis, which stands above the laryngeal aperture as a broad, flap-like process Unlike in man, but as in most other mammals, the epiglottis of bats is in contact with the soft palate, thus not losing its original olfactory function.

Musculature

The extrinsic and intrinsic muscles of the larynx are similar in all the bats studied and bear close resemblance to those present in man, though in comparison they are well developed in size.

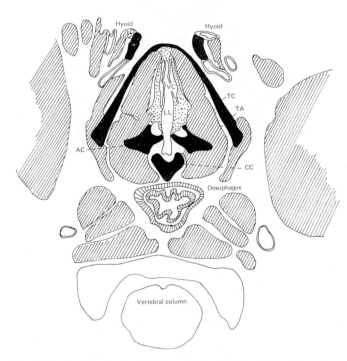

FIG. 5. A drawing ot a section throu h the larynx of *Lavia frons*. (*See* Fig. 2, p. 540, for Keys to Illustrations and Abbreviations.)

Intrinsic muscles—External adductors—the cricothyroideus muscles originate from the cricoid cartilage, each muscle spreading out fanwise to gain attachment to the inner surface and inferior border of the lamina of the thyroid cartilage and to its inferior cornu. Contraction of these muscles causes the approximation of the anterior parts of the cricoid and the thyroid cartilages. This causes an increase in the distance between the anterior parts of the laminae of the thyroid and the arytenoid cartilages. The result of this is elongation of the vocal fold and lengthening of the glottis, as in man.

Internal adductors—The functions of this group, which in bats corresponds to the cricoarytenoideus and thyroarytenoideus of man, are to close the aperture of the larynx during swallowing and brings the vocal folds together.

Abductors—These are represented by the posterior cricoarytenoidei, which have the function of opening the glottis.

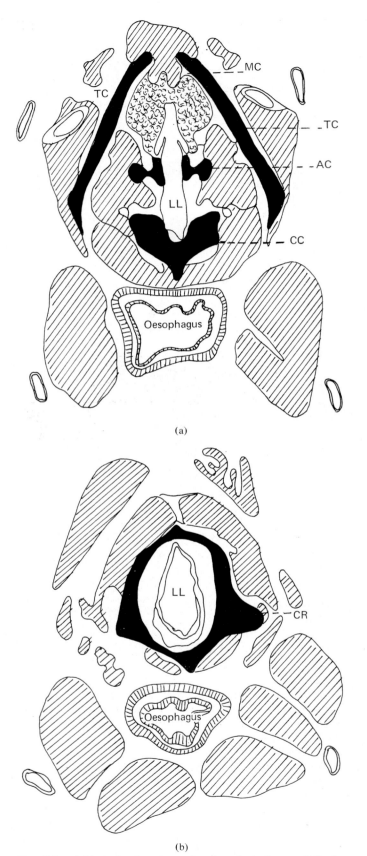

(a)

(b)

FIG. 6(a) and (b). A drawing of a section through the larynx of *Cardioderma cor*. (*See* Fig. 2, p. 540, for Keys to Illustrations and Abbreviations.)

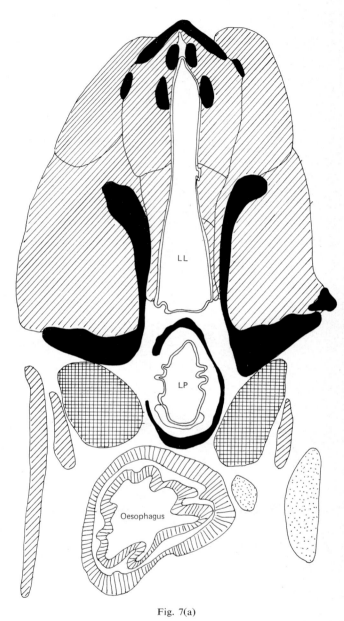

Fig. 7(a)

FIG. 7(a) and (b). A drawing of a section through the larynx of *Pteronotus parnellii*. (*See* Fig. 2, p. 540, for Keys to Illustrations and Abbreviations.)

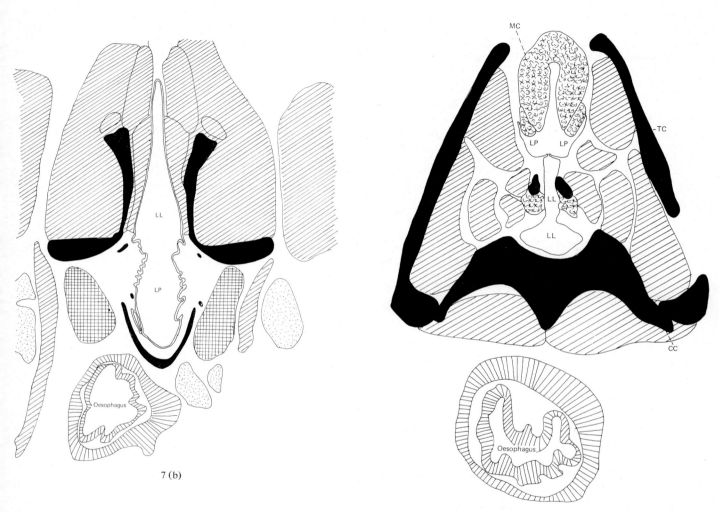

7 (b)

Fig. 8. A drawing of a section through the larynx of *Noctilio leporinus*.
(*See* Fig. 2, p. 540, for Keys to Illustrations and Abbreviations.)

FUNCTIONAL CORRELATIONS

As so little research has been conducted on the anatomy of the bat larynx, it would be both difficult and unwise to attempt to make positive conclusions from the results obtained to date. However, many interesting correlations and deductions may be made from information at present available.

As previously mentioned, Negus (1949) believed air-sacs to be concerned with the mixing and rebreathing of air, but recent work by Roberts (1972) indicated that Rhinolophidae and Hipposideridae may vary vocal tract resonance to produce changes in the frequency of emitted sounds. The laryngeal, pharyngeal and nasal cavities of Rhinolophidae and Hipposideridae are rigid bony structures and, if a variable resonance is used, it must be tuned. A change in resonance from 70–80 kHz. corresponding to observed changes in the peak frequency in *Rhinolophus ferrumequinum*, would require an increase in length of 14 per cent for a small pipe, whether "open" or "closed". Such a

TABLE 2

SIZE RELATIONSHIPS OF AIR-SACS (VARYING MAGNIFICATIONS)

Species	Left Ventral Sac (in mm)		Right Ventral Sac (in mm)		Left Dorsal Sac (in mm)		Right Dorsal Sac (in mm)		Single "Dorsal" Sac (in mm)	
	Width	Length	Width	Length	Width	Length	Width	Length	Width	Length
Rhinolophus ferrumequinum ×37·5	25	37	29	39	11·5	28	11·5	30	—	—
Actual size	0·65	1·0	0·8	1·1	0·3	0·75	0·3	0·8	—	—
Hipposideros caffer ×25	9	10	10	10	7	17	8	17	—	—
Actual size	0·36	0·4	0·4	0·4	0·2	0·2	0·32	0·6	—	—
Nycteris macrotis ×35	32	50	38	56	—	—	—	—	—	—
Actual size	0·9	1·4	1·1	1·6	—	—	—	—	—	—
Pteronotus parnellii ×32·5	—	—	—	—	—	—	—	—	32	38
Actual size	—	—	—	—	—	—	—	—	1·0	1·1
Noctilio leporinus ×35	4	21	4	22	—	—	—	—	—	—
Actual size	0·1	0·6	0·1	0·6	—	—	—	—	—	—

TABLE 3

SIZE RELATIONSHIPS OF AIR SACS (×32·5 MAGNIFICATION)

Species	Left Ventral Sac (in mm)		Right Ventral Sac (in mm)		Left Dorsal Sac (in mm)		Right Dorsal Sac (in mm)		Single "Dorsal" Sac (in mm)	
	Width	Length	Width	Length	Width	Length	Width	Length	Width	Length
Rhinolophus ferrumequinum	22	33	25	36	10	25	10	25	—	—
Hipposideros caffer	12	15	12	15	10	22	10	22	—	—
Nycteris macrotis	42	53	45	55	—	—	—	—	—	—
Pteronotus parnellii	—	—	—	—	—	—	—	—	36	50
Noctilio leporinus	4	25	4	27	—	—	—	—	—	—

relatively large change is hardly compatible with bony cavities. Cavities can, however, be tuned by other means. Helmholtz resonators, for example, are tuned by their neck length, area of cross-section of the neck or cavity volume. Cavities which could act as Helmholtz resonators are the lateral, dorsal and caudal pouches or air-sacs that are found in Rhinolophidae, Nycteridae Hipposideridae, Emballonuroidea and in *Pteronotus parnelli* (of the superfamily Phyllostomatoidea). Thus, tuning could occur by muscle action at several points in the vocal tractor even at the external nares. *Pteronotus parnelli* may differ from other species since it emits pulses through the mouth instead of the nose, forming its lips into a megaphone shape.

To collect more information concerning the relationship between air-sacs and emitted pulses, the sizes of the air-sacs were determined. Table 2 shows the results at varying magnifications. These relate to the accompanying diagrams although the actual size was easily determined and is also shown on the table. Table 3 shows a better relationship since all results are for the same magnification. Table 4 shows the average size of the animals by two criteria, body

TABLE 4

SIZE RELATIONSHIPS BETWEEN THE SPECIES POSSESSING AIR-SACS

Species Studied	Average Body Size	Length of Forearm
Rhinolophus ferrumequinum	35–110 mm	30–75 mm
Hipposideros caffer	35–110 mm	33–105 mm
Nycteris macrotis	45–75 mm	36–60 mm
Pternotus parnellii	40–67 mm	35–63 mm
Noctilio leporinus	70–132 mm	54–92 mm

size and the length of the forearm. The size of the animal may be important, though a small animal need not necessarily have a small larynx, and similarly a large animal, a large larynx. Initially, the results show that *Noctilio leporinus* has the smallest pouches or air-sacs and larynx, yet it is the largest of the five bats studied. *Rhinolophus ferrumequinum* and *Hipposideros caffer*, two closely related species, are similar in both body size and in forearm size, and in the size of the dorsal pouches, though it appears that

the ventral air-sacs of the former are larger. *Nycteris macrotis* and *Pteronotus parnelli* are similar in both body size and air-sac size, though it must be remembered that the latter species possesses a posterior sac whereas the former possesses a pair of tracheal sacs. However, the larynx size as a whole is similar in both species. Members of both species are larger than those of other species of bats studied.

REFERENCES AND FURTHER READING

Bart, J. L. (1969), "A Sectionalized Model of a Human Embryo," *Med. biol. Ill.*, **19**, 52–53.

Fischer, H. and Gerken, H. (1961), "Le Larynx de la Chauvesouris (*Myotis myotis*) et le Larynx Humain," *Ann. Oto-laryng. (Paris)*, **78**, 577–585.

Graham, A. (1952), "Histological Drawings in Pen and Ink," *Med. biol. Ill.*, **2**, 99–103.

Griffin, D. R. (1958), *Listening in the Dark*. Yale University Press.

Griffin, D. R., Dunning, D. C. and Cahlander, D. A. and Webster, F. A. (1962), "Correlated Orientation Sounds and Ear Movements of Horseshoe Bats," *Nature (Lond.)*, **196**, 1185.

Griffiths, D. A. (1970), "A Working Paper Model of the Human Larynx," *Med. biol. Ill.*, **20**, 41–47.

Hinde, R. A. (1966), *Animal Behaviour*. New York: McGraw Hill.

Matthews, L. H. and Knight, M. (1963), *The Senses of Animals*. London: Museum Press.

Milne, L. J. and Milne, M. J. (1963), *The Senses of Animals and Men*. Deutsch.

Morris, E. W. T. (1972), "A Method of Reconstruction from Serial Sections," *Med. biol. Ill.*, **22**, 103–105.

Negus, V. (1949), *Comparative Anatomy and Physiology of the Larynx*. London: Heinemann.

Novick, A. and Leen, N. (1969), *The World of Bats*. Lausanne: Edita.

Pye, Ade (1972), "Variations in the Structure of the Ear in the Different Mammalian Species," *Sound*, **6**, 14–18.

Pye, J. D. (1968), "Hearing in Bats," in *Hearings Mechanisms in Vertebrates* (A. V. S. De Reuck and J. Knight, Eds.), Ciba Foundation Symposium. London: Churchill.

Pye, J. D., Flinn, M. and Pye, A. (1962), "Correlated Orientation Sounds and Ear Movements of Horseshoe Bats," *Nature (Lond.)*, **196**, 1186.

Roberts, L. H. (1972), "Variable Resonance in Constant Frequency Bats," *J. Zool. (Lond.)*, **166**, 337–348.

Simpson, G. G. (1945), "The Principles of Classification and a Classification of Mammals," *Bull. Amer. Mus. nat. Hist.*, **85**, New York.

Stevens, S. S. and Warshofsky, F. (1966), *Sound and Hearing*. Time-Life.

Tinbergen, N. (1966), *Animal Behaviour*. Time-Life.

Wassif, K. and Madkour, G. (1968–9), "The Structure of the Hyoid Bone, Larynx and Upper Part of the Trachea in some Egyptian Bats," *Bull. zool. soc. Egypt*, **22**, 15–26.

Wood, P. and Leonard, J. N. (1973), *The Emergence of Man: Life before Man*. Time-Life.

40. NEUROLOGY OF THE LARYNX

B. D. WYKE AND J. A. KIRCHNER

"As to the motor acts of phonating and articulating, we seem not aware usually of thinking about them at all! . . .
How is it the mind can seem to do these things and yet not know how they are done?"

Sir Charles Sherrington [*Man on his Nature*, 1942]

This Chapter summarizes the current status of understanding of the neurological systems controlling the activity of the intrinsic and extrinsic musculature of the larynx related to respiration, swallowing and phonation, concerning which there have been (at long last) major experimental and clinical advances in the last decade.[1] To this end, some relevant neuro-anatomical and neurophysiological data bearing on the efferent and afferent innervation of the laryngeal tissues are first reviewed, after which consideration is given to the rôle of these neurological systems in regulating the activity of the laryngeal muscles in spontaneous breathing, in swallowing, and in speaking and singing—for understanding of the mode of operation of these neurological mechanisms is fundamental to the needs of laryngologists, neurologists, linguistic scientists, phoneticians and speech therapists dealing with disorders of laryngeal function.

LARYNGEAL MOTOR SYSTEMS

Laryngeal Motor Units

In no normal human striated muscle (including the laryngeal muscles) does a single motoneurone innervate a single muscle fibre: instead, through its terminal axonal branches each alpha motoneurone controls the activity of a population of muscle fibres whose number varies from muscle to muscle, from a minimum of 3 to a maximum of over 3000.[2] Each alpha motoneurone and its related population of muscle fibres constitutes a *motor unit*; and neurologically engendered changes of tension in striated muscle are therefore effected in stepwise fashion by increases or decreases in the number and frequency of firing of active motor units therein, small (and brief) changes being effected by recruitment or derecruitment of small motor units (containing few muscle fibres) and large (and more prolonged) changes by variations in the number of active large motor units (containing many muscle fibres per unit).[2] Such changes in motor unit activity (whose individual maximal discharge frequency does not anywhere exceed 50 Hz) may be monitored experimentally and clinically by the procedure of electromyography (*q.v.*)—although it must be remembered that the recordings of motor unit potentials thereby obtained are not necessarily a direct measure of the tension being generated by

the muscle producing them.[3] Consideration of the sizes and functional properties of motor units in the laryngeal muscles is therefore essential in any analysis of their motor control mechanisms.

In the light of the above data, most workers have assumed that the *intrinsic laryngeal muscles* would contain small motor units—although estimates of their average sizes in man have varied widely (for technical reasons implicit in the various methods employed for the determinations) from a minimum of 2–3 muscle fibres per unit[4] to 250 fibres per unit.[5] Modern anatomical, histochemical and physiological studies of the intrinsic laryngeal muscles indicate, however, that the sizes and functional characteristics of their contained motor units are not uniform throughout the laryngeal musculature—or indeed, even within the individual muscles.[6] Furthermore, investigation of this matter is complicated by the fact that some individual fibres in these muscles (including those in man) are innervated through more than one neuromuscular junction—the proportion being greatest (up to 80 per cent of fibres) in the thyro-arytenoid muscles and least (about 5 per cent or less of fibres) in the posterior crico-arytenoid muscles, with intermediate values (about 30 per cent of fibres) in the cricothyroid and lateral crico-arytenoid muscles.[7]

In view of the continued absence of precise data on this matter, the best that can be said at present is that the intrinsic muscles with the fastest contraction times[8] (such as the vocalis and lateral crico-arytenoid muscles—contraction times 12–18 ms in the monkey, 14–19 ms in the dog and 11–22 ms in the cat) probably consist mainly of small motor units containing less than 20 fibres per unit, whereas muscles with slower contraction times[8] (such as the cricothyroid and posterior crico-arytenoid muscles—contraction times 28–48 ms in the monkey and 30–50 ms in the dog and cat) probably consist of a high proportion of larger motor units containing perhaps up to 200–250 diffusely distributed fibres per unit. This is not to say, however, that these latter muscles do not contain some small, fast-contracting motor units in addition—for neurophysiological experiments suggest

---

[1] For more detailed reviews covering this period, *see* Brewer (1964); Wyke (1967b); Bouhuys (1968); Wyke (1969a); Kirchner (1970); Greene (1972); Wyke (1973b).
[2] Fulton (1943); Feinstein *et al.* (1955); Buchthal (1961); Andrew (1966); Basmajian (1967); Wyke (1969b).

[3] Weddell *et al.* (1944); Lippold (1952); Bigland and Lippold (1954); Basmajian (1967); Lenman (1969).
[4] Ruëdi (1959); Piquet and Barets (1960).
[5] Faaborg-Andersen (1957); English and Blevins (1969).
[6] *See* Hast (1966, 1967a, b); Knutsson *et al.* (1969); Ohyama *et al.* (1972a, b) and Wyke (1973b) for reviews and discussions of this matter.
[7] Piquet *et al.* (1957); Rudolph (1960); Zenker (1964a); Rossi and Cortesina (1965); Abo-El-Enein (1967); Bowden (1973).
[8] Mårtensson and Skoglund (1964); Hast (1966a, b, 1967a, b, 1969); Hall-Craggs (1967); Hirose *et al.* (1969); Hast and Golbus (1971); Edström *et al.* (1973).

that they do (at least, in experimental animals), although their proportion remains as yet undetermined.[9]

As far as the *extrinsic laryngeal muscles* are concerned—which, for the purposes of this account, are taken arbitrarily to include the muscles attached to the external surfaces of the thyroid and cricoid cartilages other than the cricothyroid muscle[10]—no reliable data are available to indicate their motor unit sizes or related functional properties.[11] This hiatus in knowledge is particularly regrettable in view of the relevance of such data for the interpretation of the electromyographic studies of the activity of these muscles in relation to respiration, phonation and swallowing[12] that are described later in this Chapter.

Laryngeal Motor Nerves

The alpha motor nerve fibres innervating the motor units in the *intrinsic laryngeal muscles* reach them from their parent nerve cell bodies in the nucleus ambiguus in the medulla oblongata through branches of the ipsilateral recurrent laryngeal nerve—except for the cricothyroid muscle (which is innervated through the external branch of the superior laryngeal nerve and sometimes (additionally) by motor nerve filaments that traverse the pharyngeal plexus from the vagus nerve) and the interarytenoid muscle (which is innervated from both recurrent laryngeal nerves, and not at all from the internal laryngeal nerve).[13] For the neurolaryngologist, the crude accounts of these nerves given in conventional text-books of anatomy need to be supplemented by the more precise details of their topographical distribution that are available elsewhere.[13]

In human nerves generally, alpha motor fibres are large myelinated axons whose diameter lies in the Group I range (up to 25 μm);[14] and as the electrophysiological (excitability, conduction velocity and action potential dimensions) and biochemical parameters of nerve fibre function are related to fibre diameter,[14] this aspect of laryngeal motor nerves is of practical importance. Early studies of the fibre diameter spectra of the recurrent and external laryngeal nerves were confused by species differences and by a variety of technical neurohistological problems:[15] however, more recent anatomical and physiological studies in the cat, dog, monkey and man[16] reveal that the laryngeal motor nerve fibres vary widely in diameter, but in general are somewhat smaller than those innervating striated muscles elsewhere, most of them being between 6 μm and 10 μm in diameter (but with a few as large as 20 μm). This correlates with the fact that the conduction velocity of most laryngeal motor nerve fibres is slower (about 50–65 m.s^{-1}), and that their refractory periods are longer, than is the case with the majority of nerve fibres supplying motor units in the limb muscles—particularly as the branches of these motor fibres decrease in diameters of 4–6 μm (with conduction velocities of 30–40 m.s^{-1}) as they traverse the terminal muscular branches of the laryngeal nerves. Each recurrent laryngeal nerve contains between 500 and 1000 myelinated nerve fibres (but with more larger—and hence faster-conducting—fibres in the left nerve), and each external laryngeal nerve between 100 and 250 such fibres—but the proportion of these that are efferent in function remains undetermined at present, for each nerve also contains an unknown proportion of myelinated afferent fibres from a variety of sources, as well as many more that are unmyelinated.

Semon's[17] suggestion (almost a century old now) that motor fibres innervating the vocal fold adductor and abductor muscles might lie in separate bundles within the recurrent laryngeal nerve trunk has been shown to be untenable by neurohistological study:[18] in fact, the motor fibres destined for these two groups of muscles do not separate from one another until they enter the terminal intralaryngeal branches of the nerve.[19] Likewise, later proposals that the motor fibres innervating these two groups of muscles might differ in their respective diameters and thus be differentially susceptible to conduction blockade by compression, cooling or local anaesthesia of the recurrent laryngeal nerve have been shown to be invalid by specific neurohistological and neurophysiological studies of the matter.[20] Such purported explanations of the so-called "Semon's Law," which is one of the historic myths of laryngology, are thus completely unfounded in the light of modern studies of laryngeal neurology[21] and therefore should be abandoned once and for all by laryngologists.

Although small motor units are generally innervated by finer diameter nerve fibres than are large motor units,[22] the marked differences in the contraction characteristics of the individual intrinsic laryngeal muscles in response to stimulation of their motor fibres in the laryngeal nerves probably reflect differences in the functional properties

---

[9] Murakami and Kirchner (1972); Edström *et al.* (1973) and Discussion in Wyke (1973b).

[10] In this account, the cricothyroid muscle is arbitrarily included with the intrinsic laryngeal muscles—although it is external to the laryngeal cartilages, and although some of its motor units operate "extrinsically" whilst others operate "intrinsically" from a functional point of view [*see* Discussion in Wyke (1973b)].

[11] Other than a study by Hast (1968) in the dog of the contraction characteristics of the sternohyoid and thyrohyoid muscles—both of which have contraction times (50–52 ms) that are longer than those of the intrinsic laryngeal muscles.

[12] Fink *et al.* (1956); Doty and Bosma (1956); Bosma (1957); Faaborg-Andersen and Sonninen (1959, 1960); Zenker and Zenker (1960); Zenker (1964b); Faaborg-Andersen and Vennard (1964); Kawasaki *et al.* (1964); Levitt *et al.* (1965); Faaborg-Andersen (1965); Murakami and Kirchner (1971a, 1973).

[13] Ónodi (1902); Lemere (1932a, b); Mayet (1956); Bowden and Scheuer (1961); Van Harreveld and Tachibana (1961); Kirchner (1966); Abo-El-Enein (1967); English and Blevins (1969); Murakami and Kirchner (1971b); Rueger (1972); Bowden (1973).

[14] Wyke (1969b).

[15] *See* Abo-El-Enein (1967) and Bowden (1973) for discussion.

[16] Tomasch and Britton (1953); Ogura and Lam (1953); Murray (1957); Krmpotić (1958); Scheuer (1964); Peytz *et al.* (1965); Eyzaguirre *et al.* (1966); Abo-El-Enein (1967); Shin and Rabuzzi (1971); Bowden (1973).

[17] Semon (1881).

[18] Sunderland and Swaney (1952).

[19] Williams (1951, 1954); Pichler and Gisel (1957); Keros and Nemanic (1967); English and Blevins (1969); Murakami and Kirchner (1971b); Rueger (1972).

[20] Pollis (1969); Ohyama *et al.* (1972a); Fukuda and Kirchner (1972).

[21] *See also* Faaborg-Andersen (1964); Kirchner (1970); Kotby and Haugen (1970c); Terracol and Greiner (1971); Fukuda and Kirchner (1972).

[22] *See* Granit (1970).

of their contained muscle fibres (or of their neuromuscular junctions) rather than major differences in the diameters of their related motor nerve fibres.[23] This is illustrated by the fact that the fatiguability of the intrinsic laryngeal muscles in response to protracted stimulation of their motor nerves is much less than that of limb muscles in the same species;[24] and by the fact that maximal motor unit activity is attained in the posterior crico-arytenoid muscle at lower frequencies (20–40 Hz) of stimulation of motor fibres in the recurrent laryngeal nerve than are necessary to generate maximal activity in the vocal fold adductors (which requires stimulus frequencies of 30–70 Hz), whereas variations in stimulus voltage (at constant frequency) have no such marked differential effect.[25]

The motor units in the *extrinsic laryngeal muscles* are innervated by nerve fibres that traverse the pharyngeal and cervical plexuses.[26] Thus, the thyropharyngeal and cricopharyngeal muscle components are supplied by motor fibres derived from cells in the nucleus ambiguus[27] that reach the muscles from the vagus nerve through its filamentous contributions to the pharyngeal plexus; whilst the thyrohyoid and sternohyoid and sternothyroid muscles are supplied through the cervical plexus by motor fibres whose parent nerve cells are located in the anterior horns of the first, second and third segments of the cervical spinal cord (the thyrohyoid muscle is innervated from the C1 and C2 segments by fibres which run part of their course in the hypoglossal nerve trunk: the sternothyroid muscle is innervated mainly from the C3 segment by way of the descending cervical nerve and the ansa hypoglossi). Nothing is known, however, of the diameter ranges or correlated functional properties of these motor nerve fibres.

The presence of fusimotor as well as alpha motor fibres in the laryngeal nerves has not yet been demonstrated directly. However, the intrinsic (as well as the extrinsic) laryngeal muscles in the cat and man certainly contain muscle spindles in which intrafusal muscle fibres are identifiable; and the fibre diameter spectra of the recurrent and external laryngeal nerves in these species[28] embrace fibre sizes of the same order (1–6 μm) as those of the fusimotor nerve fibres found in muscle nerves in other parts of the body.[29] It seems highly likely, therefore, that some at least of the smaller diameter fibres in the laryngeal nerves will turn out to be fusimotor efferents when this technically difficult matter is specifically examined by modern neuro-anatomical and neurophysiological techniques.

Finally, it should be noted that the laryngeal nerves also contain small diameter vasomotor and secretomotor fibres of sympathetic (superior and middle cervical ganglion) and parasympathetic (dorsal nucleus of vagus) origin.[30] The vasomotor fibres regulate the calibre of the laryngeal blood vessels and the vascular glomeruli in the laryngeal mucosa (sympathetic vasoconstrictor fibres traversing the superior laryngeal nerve whilst parasympathetic vasodilator fibres reach the larynx through the the recurrent branch of the vagus nerve):[31] the secretomotor fibres control the activity of the laryngeal glands that secrete lubricant mucus.[32]

Laryngeal Motoneurone Pools

As previously indicated, the nerve cells controlling the motor units in the intrinsic laryngeal muscles and in the extrinsic thyropharyngeal and cricopharyngeal musculature are located in the *nucleus ambiguus*, which extends as a longitudinal column (about 16 mm in length) of large, multipolar neurones (lying medial to the spinal nucleus of the fifth nerve) within the ventrolateral part of the medulla oblongata.[33] The motor axons leave the nucleus on its dorsal aspect, and then curve laterally and ventrally to exit from the medulla in the rootlets of the ipsilateral (mainly) vagus and cranial accessory nerves: most of the fibres (in fact, all except those destined for the cricothyroid muscle) actually leave the medulla by the latter route and subsequently (in the jugular foramen) transfer to the vagal nerve trunk, whilst the fibres innervating the cricothyroid muscle enter the vagal rootlets directly.[34] In view of the bilateral synchrony and symmetry of laryngeal muscle function, it should be noted that some fibres from each nucleus ambiguus cross the midline within the medulla oblongata to enter the contralateral vagus or cranial accessory nerves.[35]

Cyto-architectural and degeneration studies[36] have shown that the laryngeal motoneurones are located at the lower (caudal) pole of the nucleus ambiguus (in the so-called nucleus retro-ambigualis) and that, within this region of the nucleus, the motoneurone pools of the individual laryngeal muscles have a specific rostro-caudal topographical distribution in relation to one another rather than being randomly intermingled. Most rostrally located are the cricothyroid motoneurones, followed in order caudally by the motoneurone pools of the posterior crico-arytenoid, thyro-arytenoid, lateral crico-arytenoid and interarytenoid muscles: the thyropharyngeal and cricopharyngeal motoneurones are, however, located rostral to the cricothyroid motoneurone pool along with those innervating the rest of the pharyngeal and aryepiglottic musculature. Correlated with these observations is the fact that patients with bulbar poliomyelitis may sometimes show selective loss of function in individual laryngeal

[23] Mårtensson (1963); Mårtensson and Skoglund (1964); Nakamura (1964); Ohyama *et al.* (1972a, b); Edström *et al.* (1973).

[24] Edström *et al.* (1973).

[25] Capps (1958); Brewer and Dana (1963); Nakamura (1964); Hast (1966a, b); Takenouchi *et al.* (1968); Kotby and Haugen (1970c); Murakami and Kirchner (1972).

[26] Lemere (1932a); Hwang *et al.* (1948); von Lanz (1955); Levitt *et al.* (1965); Murakami and Kirchner (1971a, 1973).

[27] Earlier assumptions [see Kirchner (1958) and Levitt *et al.* (1965) for discussion] that the striated fibres of the cricopharyngeus muscle might be innervated by sympathetic and/or parasympathetic efferent fibres have been shown (Lund and Ardran, 1964; Levitt *et al.* 1965; Murakami and Kirchner, 1973) to be unfounded.

[28] Zenker (1964a); Scheuer (1964); Abo-El-Enein (1967); Bowden (1973).

[29] *See* Leksell (1945); Matthews (1972).

[30] Porta (1950); Mitchell (1954).

[31] Scevola (1950); Koizumi (1953); Ardouin and Maillet (1965); Shin *et al.* (1970); Terracol and Greiner (1971).

[32] Johnson (1935); Ardouin and Maillet (1965).

[33] Brodal (1969).

[34] DuBois and Foley (1936); Réthi (1951).

[35] Obersteiner (1912).

[36] Szentágothai (1943); Hofer (1944, 1947); Getz and Sirnes (1949); Réthi (1951); Szabo and Dussardier (1964); Lawn (1966).

muscles[37]—indicating that the virus may selectively invade cells in particular motoneurone pools within the nucleus ambiguus.

In relation to what has been said concerning the possibility of a fusimotor system related to the laryngeal muscles, it should be noted here that none of the cytological investigations of the nucleus ambiguus just mentioned have identified small motoneurones therein that might qualify as laryngeal fusimotor neurones. This does not exclude the possibility of their presence, however, for such neurones were not sought by any of the workers quoted: clearly, then, this important matter urgently requires specific neuro-histological investigation. There is likewise no information as to whether or not the laryngeal motoneurones in the nucleus ambiguus are provided with a Renshaw cell system—although in view of the rôle of this system in modulating and limiting the frequency of motoneurone discharge elsewhere[38] (except in the phrenic nucleus[39]), this matter is highly relevant to the problem of regulation of the discharge frequency of laryngeal motoneurones, especially in relation to phonation.[40]

Finally, it should be noted that antidromic activation of cells in the nucleus ambiguus in response to stimulation of motor fibres in the laryngeal nerves and in the vagal nerve trunk has been demonstrated,[41] and that micro-electrode recordings of the "spontaneous" discharges of neurones located in this nucleus have been reported.[42]

Suprabulbar Influences on Laryngeal Motoneurones

The activity of the laryngeal motoneurones located in the nucleus ambiguus is influenced by projections that reach them from the cerebral cortex and from the mesencephalic tectum and cerebellum, as well as by reflexogenic inputs entering the lower brain stem from various receptor systems located within the larynx itself and within the lungs (*see* page 555).

Direct Cortical Projection Systems

Fibres from cells located in the inferior paracentral and postero-inferior frontal regions of each cerebral cortex (*vide infra*) descend (with the corticospinal fibres) through the anterior part of the posterior limb of the internal capsule and the central region of the cerebral peduncle (where they lie dorso-medially) to the medulla oblongata in the *corticobulbar tract*.[43] There they project to the laryngeal motoneurone pools located in the nucleus ambiguus, the few larger diameter fibres (derived from cells in Layer V of the inferior precentral gyrus) relaying directly onto the laryngeal motoneurones whilst the many smaller diameter fibres (derived from smaller neurones in the inferior precentral and postcentral cortex) relay indirectly through interneurones scattered throughout the laryngeal motoneurone pools. Most of these cortical projection fibres cross the midline within the pons and upper medulla oblongata (traversing the medial lemnisci on the way) to enter the contralateral motoneurone pools, but some remain ipsilateral—so that each cerebral cortex projects to laryngeal motoneurones on both sides of the brain stem.

Animal experiments[44] (some of them quite old, but unjustifiably forgotten) likewise demonstrate that bilateral responses may be evoked in the intrinsic laryngeal muscles, or in the motoneurones innervating them, by stimulation of the inferior frontal region of the cerebral cortex in either cerebral hemisphere (although the contralateral cortical projection system has a higher threshold and a longer transmission time than the ipsilateral projection system), and that the responsible cortical projection fibres leave the mainstream of the direct corticofugal pathway proximal to the medullary pyramids. Electrical stimulation of the cerebral cortex in unanaesthetized human subjects has likewise shown[45] that activity of the laryngeal muscles (associated with vocalization) may be effected from the inferior precentral region of each cerebral hemisphere, and also from a region on the supero-medial aspect of each hemisphere lying anterior to the precentral gyrus (the so-called "supplementary motor area"); whilst similar vocalizations sometimes occur as part of a focal motor seizure sequence associated with the presence of irritative lesions in the same regions of cortex[46] or in the anterior portion of the temporal lobe in the non-dominant hemisphere.[47] On the other hand, unilateral excision of the inferior precentral cortical region (or of the supplementary motor area) from either hemisphere (or the performance of unilateral hemispherectomy) does not permanently abolish control of the laryngeal muscles during speech—although there is temporary dysphonia (and dysarthria) after such operations. However, bilateral destructive lesions of the inferior paracentral cortical regions or of the central portions of the internal capsule—such as may occur in cerebrovascular disease, to produce the syndrome of suprabulbar (or "pseudobulbar") palsy—certainly produce persisting phonatory paresis of the vocal fold musculature (with bowing of the vocal folds), whereas unilateral lesions in these same regions (as in postapoplectic hemiplegia) do not.[48]

Taken together, then, these anatomical, physiological and clinical data indicate that voluntary bilateral control of laryngeal motoneurones may be effected through the corticobulbar projections from either cerebral hemisphere, but particularly through those derived from the inferior precentral and postero-inferior frontal sections of the cerebral cortex of the dominant hemisphere.

Indirect Projection Systems

Clinical neurologists have long been familiar with the fact that phonatory disturbances of laryngeal muscle

---

[37] *See also* Faaborg-Andersen and Jensen (1964); Luchsinger (1965).
[38] *See* Wilson (1966); Wyke (1969b); Granit (1970).
[39] Gill and Kuno (1963a, b).
[40] *See* Discussion in Wyke (1973b).
[41] Porter (1963); Merrill (1970); Bianchi (1971).
[42] Cohen (1973).
[43] Déjerine (1914); Furstenberg (1937); Szentágothai and Rajkovits (1958); Kuypers (1958a, b, c); Ranson and Clark (1959); Brodal (1969).
[44] Krause (1884); Semon and Horsley (1890); Katzenstein (1905, 1908); Furstenberg and Magulski (1955); Kirikae *et al.* (1962); Rudomín (1964, 1966); Hast and Milojevic (1966).
[45] Penfield and Rasmussen (1949); Penfield and Roberts (1959).
[46] Penfield and Jasper (1953); Wyke (1959).
[47] Wyke (1958).
[48] Furstenberg (1937); Penfield and Roberts (1959); Konorski (1961).

function (in addition to articulatory disorders) are associated with the dyskinetic diseases (such as Parkinson's disease, athetosis and Sydenham's chorea, for example) and with the presence of traumatic, neoplastic, vascular and degenerative lesions in the cerebellum.[49]

As far as the dyskinetic diseases are concerned, it seems that the disturbances of laryngeal motoneurone function result from interruption of activity that is normally propagated to them indirectly (and unconsciously) from the cerebral cortex by way of relays through the *basal ganglia* and *brain stem reticular system* during phonation,[50] in addition to that delivered through the direct corticobulbar pathways mentioned above.

As for the *cerebellum*, a combination of anatomical, physiological and neuropathological studies[51] indicates that it is the relay systems traversing its anterior lobe (some of which may be driven reflexly by projections from the laryngeal afferent systems)[52] that are particularly concerned with co-ordination of laryngeal motoneurone activity during phonation—although the precise details of the complex relevant pathways have not yet been delineated.[53]

Projections also reach the nucleus ambiguus from the *tectal nuclei* of the midbrain through the lateral part of the tectobulbar tract. As some of these fibres arise in the nuclei of the inferior colliculi to which the cochlear nuclei project[54] via the lateral lemniscus, they may provide a pathway mediating some of the reflex effects on the laryngeal muscles of acoustic stimulation mentioned later (at page 564).

LARYNGEAL AFFERENT SYSTEMS

The larynx is provided with three principal sets of intrinsic afferent systems[55]—operated respectively from receptors located in the laryngeal mucosa, in the capsules of the intercartilaginous joints of the larynx and in the laryngeal muscles themselves—that exert co-ordinated reflex influences on the activity of the laryngeal motoneurones.

Laryngeal Mucosal Afferent Systems

Everyday experience clearly testifies to the exquisite tactile and pain sensitivity of the mucous membrane lining the larynx. This sensitivity is subserved by two related types of receptor nerve ending embedded in the laryngeal mucosa, the afferent fibres from which traverse the laryngeal nerves to reach the lower brain stem. In addition, recent neurophysiological studies[56] suggest that the laryngeal mucosa may also be provided with chemosensitive nerve endings.

Neurohistological examination of the laryngeal mucosa[57] reveals that it contains glomerular corpuscular nerve endings embedded in the submucosa, together with a plexus of unmyelinated nerve fibres from which free nerve endings extend into the epidermal layers of the mucous membrane (this latter system being more dense in the supraglottic mucosa (especially posteriorly) than in its infraglottic regions). These receptor systems are innervated by medium and small diameter myelinated afferent fibres, and by unmyelinated afferent fibres, that enter the laryngeal nerves and have their parent cell bodies in the ganglion nodosum—those from each half of the supraglottic mucosa traversing the ipsilateral internal branch of the superior laryngeal nerve, whilst those from the infraglottic mucosa enter the ipsilateral and contralateral recurrent nerves through their terminal mucosal branches (derived mainly from the posterior division of each recurrent nerve):[58] in addition, afferent fibres from the mucosa lining the cricothyroid membrane enter the external branch of the superior laryngeal nerve.[59] It is probable (though not yet directly proven) that the glomerular corpuscles function as low-threshold mechanoreceptors and that the plexiform system is the pain-receptor system of the laryngeal mucosa: the morphological nature of the chemosensitive nerve endings is entirely undetermined at present—although they appear to lie mainly in the subglottic mucosa and to be innervated by fine, unmyelinated nerve fibres that traverse the recurrent laryngeal nerves.[60]

Supraglottic Mucosa

It has long been known[61] that stimulation of receptors located in the supraglottic mucosa provokes mass reflex contraction of the occlusal (sphincteric) musculature of the larynx, and gives rise to changes in the activity of the respiratory musculature generally (including coughing)[62]—as when foreign bodies (such as food particles) enter the upper orifice of the larynx. Similar reflex effects are also elicitable by direct electrical stimulation of mucosal afferent fibres in the superior laryngeal nerve[63]—as well as reflex activation of middle-ear (stapedius and tensor tympani) muscles[64] and of vagal parasympathetic efferent neurones, the latter effect being manifest (*inter alia*) by

[49] See Zentay (1937); Ottonello (1941); Wyke (1947); Luchsinger and Arnold (1965); Canter (1965); Greene (1972).
[50] Kappers *et al.* (1936); Rudomín (1965a); Hassler (1956); Crosby (1964); Dunker (1968).
[51] Katzenstein and Rothmann (1911, 1912); Bender (1928); Hassler (1956); Dunker (1968).
[52] Lam and Ogura (1952).
[53] See Wyke (1947); Dow and Moruzzi (1958) and Brodal (1969) for discussion of the available data.
[54] Rose *et al.* (1963); Brodal (1969).
[55] See Wyke (1967, 1969a, 1971, 1973b) for reviews.
[56] See Widdicombe (1973b) and p. 554.
[57] Matsumoto (1953); Koizumi (1953); Roberto (1957); Rudolph (1960); König and von Leden (1961a); Van Michel (1963); Ardouin and Maillet (1965); Wyke (1973b).
[58] DuBois and Foley (1936); Brocklehurst and Edgeworth (1940); Andrew and Oliver (1951); Ogura and Lam (1953); Sampson and Eyzaguirre (1964); Eyzaguirre *et al.* (1966); Wyke (1967, 1969a, 1973a); Kirchner and Suzuki (1968); Suzuki and Kirchner (1969); Rueger (1972).
[59] Lemere (1932a); Andrew (1956); Suzuki and Kirchner (1968).
[60] Boushey *et al.* (1972); Widdicombe (1973b); Widdicombe and Richardson (personal communication).
[61] See Negus (1929, 1949); Ardran and Kemp (1967); Kirchner (1970); Murakami and Kirchner (1972a).
[62] Gracheva (1950); Murtagh and Campbell (1954); Mündnich (1956); Yamashita and Urabe (1959, 1960); Bianconi and Molinari (1962); Campbell *et al.* (1963); von Leden and Isshiki (1965); Korpáš and Gajdoš (1971); Korpáš (1972).
[63] Aldaya (1936a); Ogura and Lam (1953); Seymour and Henry (1954); Doty and Bosma (1956); Mündnich (1956); Yamashita and Urabe (1959); Mårtensson (1963); Eyzaguirre *et al.* (1966); Kirchner and Suzuki (1968); Suzuki and Kirchner (1969b); Kotby and Haugen (1970c); Murakami and Kirchner (1971, 1972a).
[64] McCall and Rabuzzi (1973).

increased motility of the small intestine[65] and by brady-cardia.[66] The sphincteric mucosal reflex response is abolished by topical anaesthesia of the laryngeal mucosa,[67] by bilateral (but not by unilateral) division of the internal or superior laryngeal nerves[68] and by sufficiently advanced degrees of general anaesthesia.[69]

The electrical stimulation studies mentioned above[63] also show that it is the larger diameter afferent fibres in the superior laryngeal nerve (that is, those derived from the corpuscular mucosal mechanoreceptors) that principally transmit the impulses evoking reflex laryngeal occlusion,[70] and that excitation of such fibres in one superior laryngeal nerve reflexly activates (through polysynaptic relays) laryngeal motoneurones in the nucleus ambiguus on both sides of the medulla oblongata—leading to synchronous bilateral activation of the sphincteric musculature. More intense stimulation of the same nerve (producing additional excitation of the small diameter fibres located therein) leads to bodily responses consistent with activation of a pain afferent system—which supports the view that the plexiform and free nerve endings embedded in the mucosa (which are innervated by the small diameter afferent fibres) constitute a mucosal pain receptor system.

Finally, recordings of the afferent nerve impulse traffic in the superior laryngeal nerve[71] show that much (but not all) of it is abolished by topical anaesthesia of the laryngeal mucosa, that the conduction velocities of the fibres located therein display two peaks (at 50 and 15 m.s^{-1}), and that increased afferent activity in the faster-conducting fibres is provoked by gentle direct mechanical stimulation of the supraglottic mucosa—facts again consistent with the view that this nerve contains two populations of afferent fibres, the larger diameter (lower-threshold, faster-conducting) fibres being mucosal mechanoreceptor afferents whilst the smaller diameter (higher-threshold, slower-conducting) fibres are mucosal pain afferents. Most of the supraglottic mucosal mechanoreceptors appear to have relatively slowly-adapting behavioural characteristics, and their responses are sensitive to changes in mucosal surface temperature within a range from 27·4–32°C.[72] The rôle of the supraglottic mucosal mechanoreceptors in influencing laryngeal muscular activity during swallowing is considered at page 560.

Subglottic Mucosa

The infraglottic region of the laryngeal mucosa contains the same morphological variety of receptor nerve endings (but with fewer corpuscles) as does the supraglottic mucosa, but their related afferent nerve fibres reach the brain by different routes. Most of the subglottic mucosa receives its afferent innervation from fibres that traverse the recurrent laryngeal nerve;[73] but a diamond-shaped area of the anterior subglottic mucosa (namely, that lining the cricothyroid membrane) is innervated by afferent fibres in the external laryngeal nerve[74]—which, therefore, is certainly not a pure motor nerve in spite of what many anatomical and surgical text-books still say.

Direct stimulation of this latter region of mucosa has shown[75] that it contains low-threshold (mainly slowly-adapting) mechanoreceptors whose discharges can be recorded in afferent fibres in the external laryngeal nerve, and whose activity is totally abolished by topical anaesthesia of this region of mucous membrane. Furthermore, stimulation of afferent fibres in one external laryngeal nerve evokes reflex efferent discharges in both recurrent laryngeal nerves—but with a shorter latency (15 ms) in the ipsilateral than in the contralateral (latency 30 ms) recurrent nerve: these reflex responses are abolished by proximal local anaesthetic or compression blockade of the stimulated external laryngeal nerve. Afferent fibres from this region of the laryngeal mucosa do not enter the internal or recurrent laryngeal nerves in significant numbers.[76]

The afferent fibres from each half of the remainder of the subglottic mucosa (including that covering the vocal folds) mainly enter the ipsilateral recurrent laryngeal nerve, although some enter the contralateral nerve (especially from the posterior mucosa). Direct, gentle mechanical stimulation of any part of this region of the mucosa (with probes or puffs of air) reveals that it contains both slowly-adapting and rapidly-adapting mechanoreceptors of low threshold whose discharges can be recorded from afferent fibres in the recurrent laryngeal nerves, and that these receptors are most densely aggregated in the mucosa covering the anterior and posterior portions of the vocal folds.[77] Afferent discharges from these receptors evoke bilateral reflex changes in the activity of the vocal fold musculature, produced by polysynaptic activation of laryngeal motoneurones in both nuclei ambigui; and such discharges (and their reflex effects) are abolished by topical anaesthesia of the infraglottic mucosa[78] and by sufficiently advanced degrees of general anaesthesia.[79] As with the mucosal afferents in the external laryngeal nerve (vide supra), the reflex latency[80] of recurrent nerve mucosal afferents in respect of their activation of ipsilateral recurrent laryngeal motoneurones is less (being about 25 ms) than that obtaining in respect of contralateral recurrent motoneurones (which is about 40 ms). The possible significance of these subglottic mucosal mechanoreceptors in the control

[65] Andersson *et al.* (1950).
[66] Suzuki and Kirchner (1967).
[67] Wyke (1968); Kirchner and Suzuki (1968).
[68] Wyke (1968).
[69] Wyke (1968, 1973b).
[70] Stimulation of mechanoreceptors in the pharyngeal mucosa (innervated from the glossopharyngeal and pharyngeal nerves) may also evoke reflex laryngeal occlusion (Murakami and Kirchner, 1971), which may be further modified by trigeminal inputs from orofacial (including periodontal) mechanoreceptors (Sessle and Storey, 1972).
[71] Aldaya (1936b); Andrew and Oliver (1951); Ogura and Lam (1953); Sampson and Eyzaguirre (1964); Eyzaguirre *et al* (1966); Mei and Nourigat (1967); Kirchner and Suzuki (1968).
[72] Sampson and Eyzaguirre (1964); Eyzaguirre *et al.* (1966).

[73] Sampson and Eyzaguirre (1964); Eyzaguirre *et al.* (1966); Wyke (1967, 1969a, 1971, 1973a); Kirchner and Suzuki (1968); Suzuki and Kirchner (1969); Rueger (1972).
[74] Lemere (1932a); Andrew (1956); Suzuki and Kirchner (1968).
[75] Suzuki and Kirchner (1968).
[76] Mårtensson (1964); Suzuki and Kirchner (1968).
[77] Bianconi and Molinari (1960, 1962a); Sampson and Eyzaguirre (1964); Eyzaguirre *et al.* (1966); Wyke (1967, 1969a, 1971, 1973a); Kirchner and Suzuki (1968); Suzuki and Kirchner (1969).
[78] Bianconi and Molinari (1962a); Wyke (1968, 1969a, 1971, 1973a, b); Suzuki and Kirchner (1969).
[79] Wyke (1968, 1973b).
[80] Suzuki and Kirchner (1969).

of the activity of the laryngeal muscles in respiration and phonation is considered later.

Laryngeal Articular Afferent Systems

The fibrous capsules of the synovial intercartilaginous joints of the larynx (that is, the cricothyroid, crico-arytenoid, thyro-epiglottic and thyrohyoid joints) are provided with receptor nerve endings[81] that are basically similar in morphology, distribution and behaviour to those found in the fibrous capsules of all the other synovial joints in the body.[82] As far as the cricothroid and crico-arytenoid joints are concerned, both are liberally provided with low-threshold, rapidly-adapting corpuscular (Type II) mechanoreceptors and with a pain-sensitive (Type IV) plexus of unmyelinated nerve fibres, whilst the capsule of the crico-arytenoid joint additionally contains a small number of low-threshold, slowly-adapting corpuscular (Type I) mechanoreceptors.[83]

The corpuscular mechanoreceptors embedded in the capsules of these two joints are innervated by medium-sized (5–10 μm) myelinated afferent fibres that enter specific articular branches of the related laryngeal nerves, whilst the pain-sensitive (Type IV) plexus system in each joint is supplied mainly by unmyelinated afferent fibres (2 μm or less in diameter) that enter the same articular nerves. Each crico-arytenoid joint is innervated by articular branches derived from the ipsilateral internal laryngeal nerve (or sometimes from the ramus communicans that links the superior with the recurrent laryngeal nerve): the cricothyroid joint is innervated partly by articular branches of the ipsilateral recurrent laryngeal nerve (or the ramus communicans) and, to a greater extent, by articular afferent fibres that enter the ipsilateral external laryngeal nerve.[84] The cell bodies of all these articular afferent fibres are probably located in the ganglion nodosum of the vagus nerve.[81]

Neurophysiological studies[85]—involving direct electrical stimulation of the individual laryngeal articular nerves or graduated passive movements of the individual laryngeal joints combined with oscilloscopic recordings of the afferent impulse traffic evoked thereby in the articular afferent nerve fibres and simultaneous, multichannel electromyographic recording of the activity of the intrinsic and extrinsic laryngeal muscles—have shown that rapid movements of the individual joints in appropriate directions stimulate the mechanoreceptors contained therein. The afferent discharges thus evoked are transmitted polysynaptically to nucleus ambiguus motoneurones on both sides of the brain stem through the superior and recurrent laryngeal nerves to evoke co-ordinated reflex changes in the activity of the mucles on both sides of the larynx. It is now clearly established, therefore, that the laryngeal

joints are equipped with a powerful, highly sensitive and rapidly-acting arthrokinetic reflex system, the significance of which for the co-ordinated control of the laryngeal musculature in respiration and phonation is considered further at pages 558 and 564.

Laryngeal Myotatic Afferent Systems

Whilst there is no doubt that the extrinsic laryngeal muscles (including the thyropharyngeal and cricopharyngeal musculature) contain stretch-sensitive mechanoreceptors in the form of muscle spindles,[86] there is no more contentious subject in the whole field of laryngeal neurology than the presence or absence of stretch-sensitive mechanoreceptors in the intrinsic laryngeal muscles.[87] This latter matter will therefore be considered first and in some detail in this section of this Chapter, in an attempt finally to resolve this critical problem.

Myotatic Mechanoreceptor Systems in the Intrinsic Laryngeal Musculature

Although the presence of *muscle spindles* has long been (and by some continues to be) denied in the intrinsic laryngeal muscles, reports of their histological identification in small numbers in these muscles in the cat, dog, monkey and man have appeared irregularly for over 50 years;[88] and more recent studies with modern neurohistological techniques have clearly established that each of the intrinsic laryngeal muscles (in the cat and man) certainly contains a few small muscle spindles.[89] Equally clear from these same studies, however, is the fact that the spindles are very few in number in each muscle (although more numerous in man than in other species)—so much so, that in most circumstances they are unlikely to exert significant reflexogenic influences on the activity of the intrinsic laryngeal muscles[90] (as is also the case in the diaphragm.[91]). Their small number may also account for the fact that fusimotor neurones have not yet been identified in the nucleus ambiguus or in the laryngeal nerves (*see* p. 548): for the fact that attempts to record spindle afferent discharges in laryngeal nerve fibres after administration of decamethonium bromide or suxamethonium (succinylcholine) (which stimulates muscle spindles)[92] have thus far been unsuccessful;[93] and for the observation[94] that myotatic stretch reflexes in the intrinsic laryngeal muscles are suppressed at stages of general (barbiturate) anaesthesia that are less advanced than those required to abolish monosynaptic reflex effects elicited from muscle spindles in other muscles of the body.

[81] Andrew and Oliver (1951); Jankovskaya (1959); Gracheva (1963); Kirchner and Wyke (1964a, b, 1965b); Abo-El-Enein (1967); Wyke (1967a, b, 1969a, 1973a).

[82] *See* Wyke (1967a, 1972).

[83] Kirchner and Wyke (1964a, b, 1965a, b); Abo-El-Enein (1967); Wyke (1967b, 1969a, 1973a).

[84] Gracheva (1963); Kirchner and Wyke (1964a, b, c, 1965a, b); Kirchner and Suzuki (1968); Suzuki and Kirchner (1968).

[85] Andrew (1954b); Kirchner and Wyke (1964c, d, 1965a, b); Wyke (1967b, 1968, 1969a, 1971, 1973a); Suzuki and Kirchner (1968); Kirchner and Suzuki (1968).

[86] Winckler (1957a); Fernand (1970); Matthews (1972).

[87] *See* Hosokawa (1961); Abo-El-Enein (1967); Bowden (1973) and Wyke (1973b) for comprehensive reviews of this subject.

[88] Nakamura (1915); Sugano (1929); Sunder-Plassmann (1933a, b); Brocklehurst and Edgeworth (1940); Goerttler (1950); Winckler (1957b); Paulsen (1958a, b, c); Withington (1959); Bowden *et al.* (1960); König and von Leden (1961b); Lucas Keene (1961); Bowden (1963); Rossi and Cortesina (1965); Voss (1966).

[89] Lucas Keene (1961); Bowden (1963, 1973); Rossi and Cortesina (1965); Voss (1966); Abo-El-Enein and Wyke (1966b); Abo-El-Enein (1967); Grim (1967); Wyke (1967b, 1971, 1973b, c); Baken (1971).

[90] Paulsen (1958c); Wyke (1967, 1973b).

[91] *See* von Euler (1968, 1973); Campbell *et al.* (1970).

[92] *See* Granit *et al.* (1953); Matthews (1972).

[93] Hirose (1961); Mårtensson (1973).

[94] Abo-El-Enein and Wyke (1966); Wyke (1968).

More relevant to the problem of a stretch-sensitive mechanoreceptor system in the intrinsic muscles of the larynx is the large number of *spiral nerve endings* that are coiled around individual laryngeal muscle fibres[95]—as is the case also with stretch-sensitive receptors in the external ocular, suboccipital and other small muscles.[96] Each such spiral is innervated by a medium-sized, myelinated afferent fibre and consists of a varying number of coils (from 2 to 8) that are tightly wrapped around individual muscle fibres over a distance of 100–250 μm, usually near the efferent neuromuscular junctional region. Not all the fibres in an intrinsic laryngeal muscle possess such receptor endings: instead, they are found on small bundles of relatively thin contiguous muscle fibres that are separated from other similarly innervated bundles by larger muscle fibre bundles that lack these nerve endings. There is only one spiral ending on each muscle fibre—even on those fibres that possess multiple neuromuscular junctions.

There can no longer be any doubt, then, that the intrinsic laryngeal muscles of man and the cat (as well as of some other species) are provided with a system of receptor nerve endings (spindles and spiral endings) whose morphology and disposition (being respectively in parallel with and coiled around the laryngeal muscle fibres) would qualify them as stretch-sensitive mechanoreceptors. In this regard, the intrinsic laryngeal muscles more particularly resemble the external ocular muscles—with which they also share the functional characteristics of delicate gradation of tension and invariable bilaterally co-ordinated synchrony of operation. It should be noted further that at their tendinous attachments to the laryngeal cartilages the intrinsic laryngeal muscles are additionally furnished with miniature tendon organs, whose behaviour and reflexogenic effects[97] resemble the larger tendon organs that are related to muscles elsewhere.[98]

In spite of these neurohistological data, however, morphology is not enough in such a highly contentious matter as this. But fortunately, two sets of neurophysiological observations are available that should serve to settle this issue once and for all, when taken in conjunction with the results of the histological studies that have just been described.

Afferent Discharges from Myotatic Mechanoreceptors in the Intrinsic Laryngeal Muscles

Although denied by earlier workers, the modern studies of the fibre calibre spectra of the laryngeal nerves referred to at p. 548 show (in man and the cat) that they contain afferent fibres whose diameters embrace those of the fibres innervating the muscle spindles, spiral endings and tendon organs described above. It has therefore been possible (in animal experiments) to record the afferent discharges

evoked in such fibres within the laryngeal nerves by the application of graduated stretch to individually isolated intrinsic laryngeal muscles.[99]

These studies indicate that most of the myotatic mechanoreceptor afferents from the intrinsic laryngeal muscles (including the cricothyroid muscle) traverse the ipsilateral recurrent laryngeal nerve, whilst some enter the ipsilateral internal nerve and a few enter the contralateral recurrent nerve from certain of the muscles. None, however, traverse the external laryngeal nerve—which explains why previous attempts[300] to record afferent discharges in this nerve in response to stretching of the cricothyroid muscle have been uniformly unsuccessful. The threshold of the myotatic mechanoreceptors (in the cat) to an applied stretch load is about 30–50 mN (3–5 g), and their afferent discharge frequency increases progressively up to a peak stretch load of about 150–200 mN (15–20 g): furthermore, these receptors adapt only very slowly in the presence of sustained stretches.

As these afferent discharges in response to applied muscle stretches persist after topical anaesthesia of the laryngeal mucosa and after local anaesthetic infiltration, electrocoagulation, disarticulation or denervation of the laryngeal joints,[101] and as they may be aborted during active contraction of the stretched muscles provoked by stimulation of the related motor nerve fibres,[102] they can only be derived from stretch-sensitive mechanoreceptors distributed in the intrinsic laryngeal muscles in parallel with or wrapped around the muscle fibres.[103] It is not possible at present to decide what the relative contribution of the muscle spindles and spiral nerve endings to this afferent discharge may be although, in view of the relative paucity of the former, it would seem likely that most of the afferent activity provoked by moderate degrees of stretch is derived from the latter receptor system.[103] With more intense stretch (or with sufficiently powerful active contraction of the muscles) a contribution from the tendon organs is added to (or constitutes all of) the afferent activity derived from muscle receptors.[104]

Myotatic Reflexes in the Intrinsic Laryngeal Muscles

The final (and functionally the most relevant) evidence for the existence of a myotatic reflexogenic system in the intrinsic laryngeal muscles is provided by direct electromyographic demonstration of stretch reflex responses in the muscles themselves.[105] Thus, if one end of an intrinsic laryngeal muscle be freed from its cartilaginous attachment its motor unit activity (both tonic and respiratory phasic) is immediately and continuously thereafter reduced substantially in comparison with the still attached, contralateral homologous muscle: but application of gradually

---

[95] Sunder-Plassmann (1933a, b); Rudolph (1961); Lucas Keene (1961); König and von Leden (1961b); Van Michel and Gerebtzoff (1962); Gracheva (1963); Abo-El-Enein and Wyke (1966b); Abo-El-Enein (1967); Wyke (1967, 1969a, 1971, 1973a, b, c).

[96] Cooper and Daniel (1949); Cooper et al. (1955); Cooper and Fillenz (1955); Bowden (1963, 1973).

[97] Abo-El-Enein and Wyke (1966b); Abo-El-Enein (1967); Wyke (1973c).

[98] See Bridgman (1968, 1970) and Matthews (1972).

[99] Abo-El-Enein and Wyke (1966a, b); Abo-El-Enein (1967); Wyke (1967b, 1969a, 1970, 1971, 1973a, b, c).

[100] Andrew (1956); Paulsen (1958c); Mårtensson (1963, 1964).

[101] Abo-El-Enein and Wyke (1966b); Abo-El-Enein (1967); Wyke (1973a, b).

[102] Bianconi and Molinari (1961, 1962b); Mårtensson (1964).

[103] See Wyke (1973b, c).

[104] See Mårtensson (1964); Abo-El-Enein and Wyke (1966b); Rudomín (1966b).

[105] Abo-El-Enein and Wyke (1966a, b); Abo-El-Enein (1967); Wyke (1967, 1968, 1969a, 1971, 1973a, b, c).

increasing stretch to its detached end progressively restores its tonic and phasic-respiratory activity. Such myotatic reflex facilitation of motor unit activity is evident immediately a stretch-stimulus load in excess of 30 mN (3 g) is applied, persists throughout the whole period of applied stretch and disappears immediately the stretch stimulus is removed. Furthermore, stretching of one intrinsic laryngeal muscle not only facilitates its own motor unit activity but also augments that in its contralateral homologue and in its ipsilateral synergists, at the same time inhibiting activity in its antagonists (for example, stretching the isolated left cricothyroid muscle not only facilitates its own motor unit activity but also augments that in the right cricothyroid, left thyro-arytenoid and left lateral crico-arytenoid muscles while reducing the activity of the posterior crico-arytenoid muscle). The fact that these reflex responses to stretch arise from low-threshold, slowly-adapting mechanoreceptors (that is, from the spiral endings and spindles) located in the stretched muscle is confirmed by the fact that they are still elicitable after topical anaesthesia of the laryngeal mucosa, and after local anaesthetic infiltration, electrocoagulation, disarticulation or denervation of the laryngeal joints.[101]

Several features of these intrinsic laryngeal myotatic reflexes—and in particular, their considerable sensitivity to depression by barbiturates[106]—suggest that they are polysynaptic and not monosynaptic. This would accord with the observation,[107] based on simultaneous stimulation of and recording from the laryngeal nerves, that monosynaptic reflex responses are not elicitable therein—an earlier claim to the contrary[108] having been shown to be unfounded—and reinforces the suggestion that the spiral endings, rather than the muscle spindles, are the principal source of this reflexogenic activity.

Finally in this connexion, it should be noted that if stretch-stimulus loads in excess of 150–200 mN (15–20 g) be applied to the individual intrinsic laryngeal muscles, their on-going motor unit activity (both tonic and phasic-respiratory) is progressively inhibited as the degree of applied stretch increases; and this inhibition persists throughout the whole period of application of the stretch, disappearing abruptly when it is removed.[109] Furthermore, this inhibitory reflex effect is intensified if active contraction of the muscle is occurring at the time the stretch stimulus is applied to it. These observations suggest that the inhibitory myotatic reflexes are provoked from relatively high-threshold mechanoreceptors lying in series with the muscle fibres—represented probably by the tendon organs mentioned at p. 553.

Consideration of the foregoing observations should finally dispel any lingering doubts as to whether or not the intrinsic laryngeal muscles are invested with myotatic reflexogenic systems—for clearly they are. Hopefully, then, this long argument can be regarded as at an end, and consideration can now be given to the possible rôle of these systems in influencing the respiratory and phonatory activity of the intrinsic laryngeal musculature.

Myotatic Reflexes in the Extrinsic Laryngeal Muscles

As already indicated, the extrinsic laryngeal muscles (in contrast to the intrinsic muscles) are liberally provided with muscle spindles: and tendon organs are also related to their tendinous attachments. As might be expected, then, these muscles display phasic and tonic facilitatory myotatic reflexes of characteristic muscle spindle origin, together with higher-threshold inhibitory reflexes derived from their tendon organs.[110] The operations of these reflexes with changes in head posture, with vertical movements of the larynx in swallowing, and in respiration and phonation, are considered later.

Laryngeal Chemoreceptor Afferent Systems

A recent discovery of considerable importance is the identification of a chemoreceptor system in the laryngeal mucosa,[111] stimulation of which exerts potent reflex effects on the brain stem mechanisms that control breathing (apart from the production of coughing). Thus, it has been found that exposure of the laryngeal mucosa to low concentrations of ammonia gas, cigarette smoke and riot control (CS) gas gives rise reflexly to slow, deep breathing. Even more important, however, is the demonstration that exposure of the laryngeal mucosa to low (5–6 per cent) concentrations of carbon dioxide (which are similar to the carbon dioxide concentrations to which the laryngeal mucosa is normally exposed as the expired air sweeps over it) produces similar reflex changes in the pattern of breathing.

The structural nature of these chemosensitive nerve endings has not yet been determined, but they appear[112] to be innervated by unmyelinated afferent nerve fibres that traverse the recurrent laryngeal nerves. However, in view of the fact that the subepithelial cells of Langhans in the laryngeal mucosa have been shown[113] to be innervated by rosettes of unmyelinated nerve terminals whose structural arrangement is similar to that of the chemoreceptors in the carotid and aortic bodies, it may be that these cells and their nerve supply represent the laryngeal chemoreceptor system.

Extralaryngeal Afferents in Laryngeal Nerves

Before concluding this section on laryngeal afferent systems, it must be pointed out (because of its experimental and clinical relevance) that the laryngeal nerves contain afferent fibres innervating receptor systems located in extralaryngeal tissues—in addition to those related to the receptor systems in the laryngeal tissues themselves that have already been described.

A combination of degeneration and electrophysiological recording studies has shown that such extralaryngeal

---

[106] Abo-El-Enein and Wyke (1966b); Wyke (1968).
[107] Mårtensson (1963).
[108] Esslen and Schlosshauer (1960).
[109] Abo-El-Enein and Wyke (1966a, b); Abo-El-Enein (1967).

[110] See Abo-El-Enein and Wyke (1966b); Murakami and Kirchner (1973); Wyke (1973b).
[111] Boushey et al. (1972); Boushey and Richardson (1973); Widdicombe (1973b).
[112] Widdicombe (1973b); Widdicombe and Richardson (personal communication).
[113] Ardouin and Maillet (1965).

afferent fibres are derived from baroreceptor and chemoreceptor endings located in the arch of the aorta[114] and from pulmonary mechanoreceptors.[115] These fibres ascend from the chest along the wall of the trachea to enter the (mainly left) recurrent laryngeal nerve at the level of the upper tracheal rings (where they are readily irritated by the tracheal distension produced by intubation or bronchoscopy): they then pass rostrally from the recurrent nerve to the superior laryngeal nerve by way of the ramus communicans, finally to enter the proximal part of the vagus nerve (their cell bodies being located in the vagal nodose ganglion).

Pulmonary Afferent Systems Influencing Laryngeal Activity

It is now established[116] that the lungs are provided with three principal types of afferent system; and recent experimental studies have shown that each of these pulmonary afferent systems may exert differential reflex influences on the activity of the nucleus ambiguus motoneurones controlling the activity of individual laryngeal muscles (*see* Table 1)—in addition to their effects on primary respiratory neurones.

TABLE 1

LARYNGEAL REFLEX EFFECTS OF PULMONARY
AFFERENT SYSTEMS*

Muscles	Pulmonary Stretch Receptors	J-receptors	Lung Irritant Receptors
Inspiratory muscles	Inhibition	Inhibition	Stimulation
Expiratory muscles	?	Inhibition	Inhibition
Laryngeal abductors (inspiratory)	Inhibition (? stimulation)	Stimulation	Stimulation
Laryngeal adductors (expiratory)	Inhibition	Stimulation	Stimulation
Laryngeal resistance	Decreased	Increased (may be sustained)	Increased (never sustained)

* From Widdicombe (1973c).

Stretch-sensitive Pulmonary Mechanoreceptors

Stimulation of activity in the myelinated vagal afferent fibres innervating these slowly-adapting receptors by passive inflation of the lung reflexly alters the activity of recurrent and external laryngeal motoneurones, and thereby modifies the reciprocally-related patterns of activity that occur in the vocal fold adductors and ab-

ductors.[117] The overall effect seems to be reflex inhibition of both adductor and abductor activity (Table 1), with the more powerful effect being on the vocal fold adductor motoneurones—although sometimes the abductor (posterior crico-arytenoid) motoneurones may instead be facilitated.[118] In addition, while the inspiratory motor units in the cricothyroid muscle are inhibited by lung inflation, expiratory motor units in the same muscle are facilitated by this manoeuvre[119]—as is also the case with inspiratory and expiratory motoneurone activity in the recurrent laryngeal nerve.[120] On the other hand, interruption of these pulmonary afferent fibres on one side inactivates the ipsilateral cricothyroid muscle so that the vocal fold assumes a partially abducted (so-called "intermediate") position—such as is observed in patients with carcinoma of the upper oesophagus or lung apex, or immediately after cardiothoracic operations.[121]

Lung Irritant Receptors

These rapidly-adapting receptors, distributed as unmyelinated nerve terminals in the epithelial lining of the walls of the bronchi and bronchioles, are stimulated by inhalation of chemical irritants and by distortion of the caudal airway walls (as with bronchospasm, and large deflations and inflations of the lung).[122] Such stimuli evoke episodic discharges in the small myelinated vagal afferent fibres that innervate the receptor nerve terminals; and this afferent activity reflexly facilitates the activity of laryngeal motoneurones innervating both the vocal fold adductors and the vocal fold abductors[123] (Table 1), thereby increasing laryngeal resistance in expiration and decreasing it during inspiration.

J (Juxta-capillary) Receptors

Although their histological structure has not yet been fully determined, these receptors appear to be unmyelinated nerve terminals distributed in the alveolar-capillary membrane: their afferent fibres are mainly unmyelinated, and traverse the vagus nerves.[122] They are stimulated in the presence of lung damage (as with pulmonary congestion, oedema and micro-embolism, and with inhalation of strongly irritant gases),[124] and the afferent discharges thereby evoked reflexly excite the motoneurones innervating the vocal fold adductors and abductors (Table 1). However, this effect is more sustained and is more powerful in respect of the adductor motoneurones, so that there is a persisting increase in laryngeal resistance throughout the respiratory cycle[123]—unlike the phasic variations in

[114] Andrew (1954a); Jewett (1964); Suzuki and Kirchner (1967); Strauss *et al.* (1973).
[115] Agostoni *et al.* (1957); Molinari and Pivotti (1962); Jewett (1964).
[116] *See* Widdicombe (1964, 1973a, c); von Euler (1973) and Wyke (1973b) for reviews and discussion.
[117] Green and Neil (1955); Joels and Samueloff (1956); Bianconi and Raschi (1959); Molinari and Pivotti (1962); Bianconi *et al.* (1963, 1967); Eyzaguirre and Taylor (1963); Rudomín (1966a); Suzuki and Kirchner (1969); Suzuki *et al.* (1970); Barillot and Bianchi (1971); Fukuda *et al.* (1973).
[118] Bianconi *et al.* (1967); Suzuki and Kirchner (1969); Widdicombe (1973c).
[119] Rudomín (1966a).
[120] Bianconi and Raschi (1959); Eyzaguirre *et al.* (1966).
[121] Fukuda and Kirchner (1972).
[122] Fillenz and Woods (1970); Widdicombe (1973a); Stransky *et al.* (1973).
[123] Widdicombe (1973a, c); Stransky *et al.* (1973).
[124] Paintal (1970); Widdicombe (1973a).

glottal resistance produced by activation of the rapidly-adapting irritant receptors (*vide supra*).

Lingual Afferent Systems Influencing Laryngeal Activity

It should also be noted that afferent impulses derived from stretch-sensitive mechanoreceptors (including muscle spindles) in the intrinsic and extrinsic tongue musculature are capable of affecting reflexly the activity of the intrinsic muscles of the larynx. Thus, it has been shown[125] that activation of the appropriate afferent fibres in one hypoglossal nerve reflexly excites polysynaptic efferent discharges in the (mainly) ipsilateral recurrent (but not external) laryngeal nerve, the relevant afferent fibres leaving the hypoglossal nerve extracranially to join the vagus nerve at the level of the ganglion nodosum. Such a hypoglosso-laryngeal reflex system[125] is clearly relevant to co-ordination of laryngeal activity with tongue activity in the processes of swallowing and phonation, and its operations in regard thereto should be specifically investigated.

BEHAVIOURAL ASPECTS OF LARYNGEAL NEUROLOGICAL SYSTEMS

Respiratory Activity

From a functional viewpoint, the intrinsic and extrinsic muscles of the larynx constitute an integral part of the striated respiratory musculature,[126] so the behaviour of the neurological mechanisms controlling this fundamental aspect of their activity will be considered here in the light of the foregoing morphological and physiological data.

Intrinsic Laryngeal Musculature

Although the activity of the intrinsic muscles of the larynx has long been known to vary in concert with that of the rest of the respiratory musculature, there has been considerable uncertainty regarding the temporal relations of this oscillatory activity to the phasic events of the respiratory cycle—and even more regarding the neurological mechanisms responsible for its production and control.[127] However, recent clinical and neurophysiological investigations[128] have thrown some light on this important matter.

In lightly anaesthetized animals or patients (whether breathing through the larynx or through a tracheostomy tube[129]), and in unanaesthetized human subjects (whether breathing or holding the breath),[130] continuous (*tonic*) background motor unit activity is apparent electromyographically to varying degrees in each of the intrinsic muscles of the larynx (as well as in direct recordings from their related motoneurones). In view of previous arguments on this point,[131] it should be noted that this tonic activity is progressively reduced by increasing general anaesthesia—but to differing degrees and at different rates in the individual laryngeal muscles,[132] so that the distribution of tonic activity within the intrinsic laryngeal musculature depends on the presence or absence of anaesthesia and (critically) on the degree of the latter. Other experiments[133] have shown that this tonic activity is generated primarily (but not exclusively) from the reflexogenic input that is delivered continuously to the laryngeal motoneurones from the low-threshold myotatic mechanoreceptors located in the intrinsic laryngeal muscles, in response to the stimulation provided by the normal slight stretch that prevails in each muscle between its cartilaginous attachments (and which is affected by head posture).[134] This myotatic reflexogenic influence appears to be operative on laryngeal motoneurones against a background of excitation thereof from neurones located in the caudal brain stem reticular system.

Electromyographic recordings in man[135] and animals[136] have revealed that, during quiet breathing, phasic motor unit discharges are superimposed on the tonic activity in the laryngeal muscles in synchrony with the respiratory cycle, but that the time relations of this activity differ in the individual muscles. In anaesthetized preparations, these time relations (as well as the distribution of the phasic respiratory activity within the laryngeal musculature) are also affected by the degree of anaesthesia obtaining at the time.[137]

In quiet natural breathing, the *cricothyroid muscle* displays[138] low-grade, biphasic changes of motor unit activity in relation to the spontaneous respiratory cycle that appear as grouped motor unit potentials, one burst occurring at the beginning of each inspiration and another (sometimes shorter) burst at each expiration. Different motor unit populations within the muscle appear to be involved in these two events[139]—particularly in view of the facts that when breathing occurs through a tracheostomy, when the laryngeal mucosa is topically anaesthetized or denervated, or when the degree of general anaesthesia is increased slightly, the expiratory burst is abolished although a reduced inspiratory burst still persists;[140] whereas the

[125] Sauerland and Mizuno (1968).

[126] Negus (1929, 1949, 1965), Campbell *et al.* (1970); Kirchner (1970); Wyke (1973b).

[127] *See* Pressman (1942); Faaborg-Andersen (1957, 1965); Buchthal (1959); Murakami and Kirchner (1972b) and Wyke (1973a) for reviews.

[128] *See* Eyzaguirre *et al.* (1966); Wyke (1968, 1973a); Murakami and Kirchner (1972b).

[129] Bianconi and Raschi (1959, 1964); Abo-El-Enein and Wyke (1966b); Kotby and Haugen (1970b); Wyke (1973a); Cohen (1973).

[130] Faaborg-Andersen (1957, 1964, 1965); Buchthal (1959); Zenker and Zenker (1960); Knutsson *et al.* (1969); Kotby and Haugen (1970a, b); Sutton *et al.* (1972).

[131] Semon (1890); Weddell *et al.* (1944); Fink *et al.* (1956); Faaborg-Andersen (1957, 1964a, 1965); Fabre *et al.* (1962); Mårtensson (1964); Kotby and Haugen (1970a, b); Wyke (1973b).

[132] *See* Brewer and Dana (1963) and Wyke (1968, 1973a, b) for details.

[133] Abo-El-Enein and Wyke (1966b); Wyke (1973a).

[134] Sutton *et al.* (1972).

[135] Weddell *et al.* (1944); Feinstein (1946); Fink *et al.* (1956); Faaborg-Andersen (1957, 1964, 1965); Buchthal (1959); Buchthal and Faaborg-Andersen (1964); Hiroto *et al.* (1964); Yagi (1964a); Knutsson *et al.* (1969); Kotby and Haugen (1970a, b); Haglund (1973).

[136] Green and Neil (1955); Nakamura *et al.* (1958); Rattenborg *et al.* (1963); Rudomín (1966a, b); Murakami and Kirchner (1972b); Wyke (1973a).

[137] Bosma and Koivisto (1962); Brewer and Dana (1963); Eyzaguirre *et al.* (1966); Wyke (1968, 1973a, b); Suzuki and Kirchner (1969b).

[138] Fink *et al.* (1956); Nakamura *et al.* (1958); Faaborg-Andersen (1957, 1965); Buchthal and Faaborg-Andersen (1964); Hiroto *et al.* (1964); Rudomín (1966a, b); Konrad and Rattenborg (1969); Suzuki *et al.* (1970); Murakami and Kirchner; (1972b); Wyke (1973a).

[139] Rudomín (1966a, b); Suzuki *et al.* (1970); Wyke (1973a, b); Haglund (1973).

[140] Rudomín (1966b); Wyke (1968, 1973a).

inspiratory burst is selectively depressed by detaching one end of the muscle from its cartilaginous attachment[141] or by passive lung inflation[142] and selectively facilitated by respiratory obstruction.[143]

The *thyro-arytenoid* and *lateral crico-arytenoid* musculature displays a more prolonged monophasic alteration in its respiratory-linked activity, which is augmented at the onset of expiration and (in the case of the thyro-arytenoid) continues to increment as expiration develops until it terminates abruptly at, or shortly after, the onset of inspiration.[144] In lightly anaesthetized animals,[145] and in unanaesthetized human subjects,[146] the thyro-arytenoid muscle may also show a separate, brief increment in its motor unit activity at the onset of inspiration that is almost synchronous with that occurring in the cricothyroid muscle[147] or (in its vocalis portion) follows slightly after the cricothyroid inspiratory burst.[148] These respiratory oscillations of motor unit activity are substantially reduced (although not abolished) by breathing through a tracheostomy instead of through the larynx, and by detaching the muscles at one end from their cartilaginous attachments:[149] they are also critically affected by small variations in the degree of general anaesthesia obtaining in anaesthetized preparations[150]—which facts may explain why a recent experimental study[151] failed to detect respiratory-linked activity in these muscles in tracheostomized, anaesthetized animals.

The *posterior crico-arytenoid* muscle displays[152] a sinusoidal pattern of fluctuation in its motor unit activity during the respiratory cycle, which activity begins to increase at the end of each expiration and thereafter continues to increment until the ensuing inspiration reaches its peak, decreasing rapidly before the next expiration begins. This inspiratory activity commences, therefore, just prior to the inspiratory increase in phrenic nerve discharge and in diaphragmatic and intercostal muscle activity:[153] it is relatively resistant (compared with the respiratory activity in the other laryngeal muscles) to depression by increasing general anaesthesia.[154] The motor units in this muscle do not all behave uniformly during the respiratory cycle however—for some are active throughout inspiration whilst others discharge only for limited periods, and yet others (which can be recruited by respiratory obstruction or development of hypercarbia) normally remain inactive.[155]

Activity in this muscle is inhibited by moderate passive inflation of the lungs, but facilitated by forced inflation and by passive lung deflation[156]—presumably due respectively to reflex effects on its motoneurones from the pulmonary stretch receptors and lung irritant receptors (Table 1).

Having described the respiratory-linked behaviour of the intrinsic laryngeal muscles, it is now necessary to consider how this co-ordinated activity is neurologically generated and controlled. As might be expected, many workers over the years[157] have held that the activity of the laryngeal musculature responsible for the movements of the vocal folds during the respiratory cycle is directed exclusively (via projections to the nucleus ambiguus) from the respiratory nuclei in the lower brain stem, in concert with that of the primary respiratory musculature. However, the activities of these two groups of muscles are actually not synchronous, for the vocal folds abduct just prior to the inspiratory inflow of air produced by contraction of the diaphragm and intercostal muscles,[158] largely (although not entirely) due to bilateral contraction of the posterior crico-arytenoid muscles; and (as noted at p. 556) recordings of the electrical activity of these (and of the other) intrinsic laryngeal muscles and of their motor fibres in the recurrent laryngeal nerve reveal[159] that their inspiratory motor units are activated (in quiet breathing) some 20–100 ms before the inspiratory discharge of phrenic motoneurones commences, and become inactive just before the expiratory air flow commences. That the basic (albeit not exclusive) modulation of the respiratory activity of the intrinsic laryngeal muscles is provided through relays from the respiratory nuclei in the lower brain stem to the nucleus ambiguus is evidenced by demonstration that rhythmical waxing and waning of laryngeal motoneurone discharge persists to varying degrees (even in decerebrate animals) after production of total muscular paralysis by administration of neuromuscular blocking agents,[160] after diversion of the respiratory air stream out of the larynx,[161] after topical anaesthesia of the laryngeal mucosa,[162] after interruption of pulmonary afferents by bilateral division of the vagus nerves distal to the origin of the recurrent laryngeal nerves,[163] and after complete de-afferentation of the larynx.[164] It has also been shown[165] that direct electrical stimulation of the inspiratory region of the medullary reticular system on one side leads to bilateral activation of the vocal fold abductors, whilst stimulation of the expiratory region provokes bilateral

[141] Abo-El-Enein and Wyke (1966b); Wyke (1973a).
[142] Rudomín (1966a).
[143] Suzuki *et al.* (1970).
[144] Green and Neil (1955); Nakamura *et al.* (1958); Sawashima *et al.* (1958); Yagi (1964a); Wyke (1973a).
[145] Abo-El-Enien (1967); Wyke (1973a).
[146] Weddell *et al.* (1944); Feinstein (1946); Fink *et al.* (1956); Faaborg-Andersen (1964); Buchthal and Faaborg-Andersen (1964); Kotby and Haugen (1970).
[147] Buchthal (1959); Wyke (1973b).
[148] Faaborg-Andersen (1957); Buchthal (1959).
[149] Abo-El-Enein (1967); Wyke (1973a).
[150] Brewer and Dana (1963); Wyke (1968, 1973a, b).
[151] Murakami and Kirchner (1972b).
[152] Green and Neil (1955); Sawashima *et al.* (1958); Buchthal (1959); Rattenborg *et al.* (1963); Kotby and Haugen (1970a, b); Murakami and Kirchner (1972b); Wyke (1973a).
[153] Green and Neil (1955); Nakamura *et al.* (1958).
[154] Brewer and Dana (1963); Wyke (1968, 1973a, b); Suzuki and Kirchner (1969).
[155] Suzuki and Kirchner (1969); Murakami and Kirchner (1972b).

[156] Murakami and Kirchner (1972b); Fukuda *et al.* (1973).
[157] Semon (1890); Semon and Horsley (1890); Negus (1929); Green and Neil (1955); Andrew (1955); Rudomín (1966b); Kirchner (1970).
[158] Green and Neil (1955); Nakamura *et al.* (1958); Murakami and Kirchner (1972b)
[159] Green and Neil (1955); Nakamura *et al.* (1958); Bianconi and Raschi (1959, 1964); Bianconi *et al.* (1963); Eyzaguirre and Taylor (1963); Eyzaguirre *et al.* (1966); Wyke (1973a); Cohen (1973).
[160] Nakamura *et al.* (1958); Suzuki and Kirchner (1969b); Stransky *et al.* (1973); Cohen (1973).
[161] Nakamura *et al.* (1958); Sampson and Eyzaguirre (1964); Murakami and Kirchner (1972b); Wyke (1973a).
[162] Wyke (1968, 1973a).
[163] Green and Neil (1955); Wyke (1973a); Stransky *et al.* (1973); Fukuda *et al.* (1973).
[164] Suzuki and Kirchner (1969b); Stransky *et al.* (1973).
[165] Kurozumi *et al.* (1971).

adductor muscle activity (with latencies of 15–25 ms depending on the phase of respiration obtaining at the moment of stimulation). Thus, whilst it is clear that the basic respiratory modulation of the activity of the intrinsic laryngeal motoneurones located in the nucleus ambiguus is effected from neurones in the nearby respiratory nuclei of the caudal brain stem reticular system, it seems that the reticular respiratory neurones controlling the laryngeal motor units are not the same cells that project to the phrenic and intercostal motoneurone pools – especially as the different time relations of the activity of laryngeal and primary respiratory (that is, phrenic and intercostal) motoneurones are not explicable solely in terms of differences in conduction time from the reticular respiratory nuclei to the respective motoneurone pools.[166]

Although the primary control of the phasic respiratory activity of the intrinsic laryngeal motoneurones is effected from reticular neurones in the lower brain stem (on a background of tonic activity maintained in the laryngeal motoneurone pools), there is substantial evidence that this influence may be secondarily modulated to different degrees by a number of the peripherally-operated reflexogenic systems that have already been described and whose respiratory influences will now be considered *seriatim*.

Evidence has already been presented to show that a variety of *pulmonary afferent systems*, including the stretch-sensitive mechanoreceptor system, may modify reflexly the activity of laryngeal motoneurones. Furthermore, there is evidence that the reflex effects of afferent discharges from pulmonary mechanoreceptors upon laryngeal motoneurones are not secondary to (or even coincident with) their effects upon primary respiratory neurones,[167] and that phasic driving of laryngeal motoneurones from pulmonary mechanoreceptors can be effected in animals paralyzed with gallamine triethiodide (*Flaxedil*) by artificial ventilation.[168] Nevertheless, all the available data indicate[169] that although pulmonary reflexogenic mechanisms may modify the activity of laryngeal motoneurones in a variety of circumstances of altered ventilation, they do not play a major part in engendering the rhythmical oscillations of motor unit activity that occur in the intrinsic laryngeal muscles in normal quiet breathing.

Other observations[170] have been interpreted as indicating that the respiratory activity of the intrinsic laryngeal muscles may depend to some degree upon *laryngeal mucosal reflexogenic influences*, operated from the mucosal mechanoreceptors in response to the fluctuations in intralaryngeal (and especially subglottic) air pressure that occur with the respiratory ebb-and-flow of air through the larynx.[171] Further weight appears to be lent to this view by the fact that respiratory-linked discharges can be recorded in afferent fibres in the superior laryngeal nerve,[172] by the fact that

electrical stimulation of this nerve (or of its internal branch) modifies laryngeal motor unit activity,[63] and by the fact that direct mechanical stimulation of various parts of the supraglottic and subglottic laryngeal mucosa (including with gentle puffs of air) evokes afferent discharges in the related laryngeal nerves[77] that reflexly excite laryngeal motoneurones.[75,78] However, although such mucosal afferent activity is suppressed by topical anaesthesia of the mucosa,[71,75,78] this procedure makes only a slight difference to the respiratory oscillations in motor unit activity of the intrinsic laryngeal muscles that occur in quiet breathing:[173] furthermore, phasic respiratory discharges can still be detected in some recurrent laryngeal motoneurones after complete de-afferentation of the larynx[174] and after general anaesthesia has been advanced to the point where laryngeal reflex responses to direct mucosal stimulation have been abolished.[175] It should also be noted that the respiratory-linked phasic discharges mentioned above as occurring in the superior laryngeal nerve are only markedly apparent in the presence of obstructed breathing (when the extrinsic laryngeal muscles are powerfully involved and thus produce mechanical distortions of the supraglottic mucosa), and that the lesser activity seen in unobstructed breathing is abolished when the intrinsic muscles are paralyzed by recurrent nerve section.[176] Finally it should be added that, although direct opening of the larynx to the atmosphere[177] or the performance of tracheostomy[178] both markedly reduce the respiratory oscillations of laryngeal motor unit activity in quiet breathing, they do not always abolish them immediately—and the significant reduction in laryngeal muscular activity that does then occur (and which may eventually become complete in the vocal fold abductors) is not simply the result of diversion of the respiratory air stream away from the laryngeal mucosa.[179] In the light of present knowledge, then, it seems that although laryngeal mucosal reflexogenic systems make a significant contribution to the control of the intrinsic laryngeal musculature in swallowing and in phonation (*vide infra*), they are not critically involved in influencing the phasic oscillations of motor unit activity that occur in this musculature in quiet breathing—probably because of the lower range of subglottic pressure variation that then obtains (and which therefore recruits only a small proportion of the mucosal mechanoreceptor population), in contrast to the higher pressures that are associated with speaking and singing.

In view of the fact that the intercartilaginous joints of the larynx are liberally provided with low-threshold (mainly rapidly-adapting) mechanoreceptors whose afferent discharges exert significant phasic reflex effects on intrinsic laryngeal motoneurones, it is pertinent to enquire whether such *laryngeal arthrokinetic reflexogenic systems*

[166] *See* Cohen (1973).
[167] Fukuda and Kirchner (1972); Cohen (1973).
[168] Suzuki and Kirchner (1969b); Stransky *et al.* (1973).
[169] *See* Green and Neil (1955); Bianconi *et al.* (1967); Wyke (1973a); Fukuda *et al.* (1973).
[170] Aldaya (1936a, b); Petitpierre (1943); Campbell and Murtagh (1956); Sampson and Eyzaguirre (1964); Kirchner and Suzuki (1968).
[171] Van den Berg (1956, 1964).
[172] Aldaya (1936b); Petitpierre (1943); Sampson and Eyzaguirre (1964); Eyzaguirre *et al.* (1966).

[173] Wyke (1968, 1973a); Suzuki and Kirchner (1969b).
[174] Suzuki and Kirchner (1969b).
[175] Wyke (1968).
[176] Petitpierre (1943); Sampson and Eyzaguirre (1964); Eyzaguirre *et al.* (1966).
[177] Sampson and Eyzaguirre (1964).
[178] Wyke (1968), 1973a); Sasaki *et al.* (1973).
[179] Wyke (1973a); Sasaki *et al.* (1973).

might be implicated in the production of the respiratory oscillations in the activity of these motoneurones. Laryngologists have long been familiar with the fact that the laryngeal joints move during quiet breathing,[180] and their patterns of movement in this (and other) circumstances have been analyzed radiographically in some detail:[181] but these joint movements are the *result* of the respiratory activity of the muscles acting upon the articulated laryngeal cartilages, and such activity persists in laryngeal motoneurones to some degree after complete de-afferentation of the larynx.[174] Laryngeal arthrokinetic reflex effects cannot therefore be fundamentally involved in the production of the phasic oscillations of laryngeal motoneurone activity that are associated with the respiratory cycle: nevertheless, such reflexes may be secondarily involved in eliciting some of the respiratory-linked motor unit activity observed in the intrinsic muscles once their primary inspiratory and expiratory activity is set in train by discharges delivered from the reticular respiratory nuclei to the nucleus ambiguus, in much the same way as the respiratory activity of the intercostal muscles is modulated by arthrokinetic reflex influences from mechanoreceptors located in the capsules of the costovertebral and costotransverse joints.[182] Consistent with this view is the fact that the respiratory oscillations of motor unit activity in the intrinsic laryngeal muscles are substantially reduced (and their pattern modified) when ventilation occurs through a tracheostomy (in which circumstance, movements of the laryngeal joints are markedly reduced), and the observation that bilateral local anaesthetic infiltration of the cricothyroid joints or destruction of the receptors located in the capsules thereof by electrocoagulation significantly reduces (although does not abolish) the initial inspiratory burst of motor unit activity that normally occurs in the cricothyroid muscles as tracheal traction rotates the cricothyroid joints.[183]

The remaining reflexogenic system that requires consideration in the present context is that related to the low-threshold mechanoreceptors located in the intrinsic laryngeal muscles (evidence for whose existence has already been presented): for a series of experimental observations[184] suggests that *laryngeal myotatic reflexogenic systems* do have a significant modulating influence on the respiratory activity of the intrinsic laryngeal musculature. Thus, as mentioned previously at p. 553, detaching one end of an intrinsic laryngeal muscle from its cartilaginous attachment (thereby freeing it from the slight stretch to which it is normally subject between its attachments) not only reduces its tonic motor unit activity but also markedly attenuates (in amplitude and frequency) its respiratory-linked phasic motor unit discharges. Furthermore, re-imposition of graduated passive stretch to the detached muscle progressively restores its phasic respiratory activity at the same time (and to the same degree) as it restores its

tonic activity. As these modulating effects of varied muscle stretching on the oscillating respiratory activity of the intrinsic laryngeal muscles (as well as on their tonic motor unit activity) are still elicitable after topical anaesthesia of the entire laryngeal mucosa and after local anaesthetic infiltration, electrocoagulation or denervation of the laryngeal joint capsules, they are clearly effected by the reflex effects of afferent discharges from the stretch-sensitive mechanoreceptors located in the intrinsic laryngeal muscles themselves on related laryngeal motoneurones.[185] It therefore seems that the effectiveness of the discharges from the primary inspiratory and expiratory neurones in the brain stem reticular system upon the laryngeal motoneurones located in the nucleus ambiguus is conditioned, throughout the respiratory cycle, by the prevailing background reflex input to these latter motoneurones from the myotatic receptors in the intrinsic laryngeal muscles.[185] This influence appears to be particularly important in maintaining vocal fold adductor activity during expiration, after its initiation (just prior to the commencement of the expiratory flow of air) from reticular respiratory neurones: for the elevation of subglottic pressure that ensues as the expiratory air flow commences imparts an upward stretching force to the already adducted vocal folds and the muscles attached thereto, thereby augmenting the afferent discharge from the low-threshold myotatic receptors located therein. The removal of this influence by the performance of tracheostomy also helps to explain why this procedure considerably attenuates the respiratory oscillations of motor unit activity that occur normally in the intrinsic laryngeal muscles when breathing *per vias naturales*.[185]

Extrinsic Laryngeal Musculature[186]

The oscillating movements of the glottis that are associated with the respiratory cycle are not due solely to the phasic variations in the activity of the intrinsic laryngeal muscles that have been described, for they are also affected by changes in the activity of the extrinsic laryngeal muscles (and of the suprahyoid musculature) that are associated with the slight vertical displacements of the larynx (downwards during inspiration, upwards during expiration) that occur during the normal respiratory cycle, and which are considerably enhanced during augmented breathing.[187]

Electromyographic studies of various of these muscles in quietly breathing subjects[188] have shown that low-grade, phasic changes in motor unit activity occur in most (but not all) of them during the respiratory cycle—although there is uncertainty regarding the precise temporal relations of this activity to the sequence of events in the cycle, particularly as its pattern is critically affected by changes in head posture. In augmented breathing, however, activity in the

[180] Negus (1929, 1949); Fink *et al.* (1956); von Leden and Moore (1961); Bosma and Koivisto (1962).
[181] Ardran and Kemp (1966, 1967).
[182] Yamamoto *et al.* (1956, 1960); Godwin-Austen (1969); Vrettos and Wyke (1973).
[183] Kirchner and Wyke (1965b); Wyke (1973a).
[184] Abo-El-Enein and Wyke (1966b); Abo-El-Enein (1967); Wyke (1968, 1973a, c).

[185] Wyke (1973a, b, c): Sasaki *et al.* (1973).
[186] *See* p. 547 for definition.
[187] Petitpierre (1943); Mitchinson and Yoffey (1947); Andrew (1955); Armstrong and Smith (1955); Fink *et al.* (1956); Zenker and Zenker (1960); Rattenborg *et al.* (1962); Faaborg-Andersen (1964a, 1965); Zenker (1964b); Kotby and Haugen (1970a).
[188] Fink *et al.* (1956); Zenker and Zenker (1960); Faaborg-Andersen (1965); Kotby and Haugen (1970a, b).

extrinsic laryngeal muscles is greatly increased—particularly in the sternothyroid and thyrohyoid muscles—as it is also during swallowing and phonation.

Fortunately, however, a recent detailed experimental study[189] of the respiratory activity of the extrinsic laryngeal muscles has somewhat clarified this problem. Thus the *sternothyroid muscle* was found to display more-or-less continuous, low-grade motor unit activity (perhaps because the animal was placed in a supine, head-extended posture) that is phasically augmented during the inspiratory phase of quiet breathing,[190] during which there is slight descent of the thyroid cartilage. Similar tonic activity is present in the *thyrohyoid muscle* (and in its motor nerve fibres),[191] but this is biphasically reduced in mid-inspiration and late in expiration. The *thyropharyngeus muscle* likewise shows continuous tonic activity, on which phasic motor unit discharges are superimposed during expiration;[192] but the related *cricopharyngeus muscle* generally shows only continuous tonic activity that displays no phasic modulations related to the respiratory cycle[189]—even with augmented breathing (although passive inflations and deflations of the lung evoke phasic activity in this muscle). Further experiments in this study suggest that the respiratory-linked phasic activity just described is generated from respiratory neurones in the brain stem reticular system through projections therefrom to the motoneurone pools of the individual extrinsic muscles, and that this activity can be modified through pulmonary mechanoreceptor and arterial chemoreceptor inputs to the respiratory nuclei. It also appears that such respiratory displacement of the laryngeal cartilages as does occur in quiet breathing is generated passively by episodic inspiratory traction from the trachea and oesophagus,[192] and that this secondarily affects motor unit activity in the extrinsic laryngeal muscles by altering reflexogenic afferent discharges to their motoneurones from the stretch-sensitive muscle spindles embedded therein and from the mechanoreceptors in the laryngeal joints.

Swallowing Activity

During swallowing, the larynx is pulled upwards in the neck into the pharynx and its pharyngeal orifice is occluded (thereby sealing off the airway from the alimentary tract) while respiration is inhibited and the pharyngo-oesophageal orifice opens, all as the result of a highly complex series of reflexes. As this account is concerned only with the mechanisms controlling the contributions of the intrinsic and extrinsic laryngeal muscles to total swallowing behaviour, the reader is referred elsewhere[193] for integrated accounts of the whole elaborate process.

Intrinsic Laryngeal Muscles

In terms of their rôle in swallowing, the vocal folds and their related intrinsic muscles represent the most caudal in a triple-tiered system of occlusive sphincters surrounding the rostral portion of the airway,[194] and when in apposition can resist pressures from above to more than 13 kPa (100 mm Hg).[195]

When ingested material (solid or liquid) enters the inferior pharynx and stimulates the low-threshold mechanoreceptors embedded in its mucosa, the impulses evoked thereby are transmitted (via afferent fibres traversing the pharyngeal plexus and the glossopharyngeal and vagus nerves) to the nucleus of the tractus solitarius in the medulla oblongata,[196] whence they are relayed bilaterally to the nucleus ambiguus and the caudal brain stem reticular system. In the former location they facilitate the motoneurones innervating the vocal fold adductors on both sides of the larynx and inhibit those supplying some of the motor units in the posterior crico-arytenoid muscles whilst facilitating others,[197] thereby forcefully occluding the glottis and tensing the vocal folds: in the latter location, they inhibit the discharge of the inspiratory neurones. These reflex effects are further reinforced should any of the ingested material enter the pharyngeal aditus of the larynx (as it often does in young babies) and stimulate the mechnoreceptors located in the supraglottic mucosa.

Contraction commences first in the thyro-arytenoid and interarytenoid musculature, whilst the cricothyroid muscle contracts later (after the pharyngeal constrictors); but all this activity is preceded by decreased motor unit activity in the posterior crico-arytenoid muscles that allows initial downward and medial movement of the arytenoid cartilages.[198] Adduction of the vocal folds commences anteriorly and develops progressively in a posterior direction until they are in the apposition throughout their length—at which moment, supplementary closure of the more rostral vestibular (false vocal) folds commences as a result of contraction of the aryepiglottic musculature.[199] On completion of the swallow, both the vocal and the vestibular folds fly apart at high velocity (the adductor musculature related to the former relaxing completely for a brief moment) and the respiratory cycle is resumed (often with an initial expiration). Finally, it should be emphasized that all this activity is reflexly initiated and controlled from the pharyngeal and laryngeal mucosal mechanoreceptor system and is not voluntarily produced—thus, it occurs unaltered in decorticate and decerebrate mammals, in patients with upper brain stem lesions producing a state of akinetic mutism, in sleep, and before recovery of consciousness in patients emerging from general anaesthesia.

Extrinsic Laryngeal Muscles

Laryngologists and neurologists know that closure of the glottis during swallowing is not the exclusive prerogative of the reflexly co-ordinated changes in motor unit activity in the intrinsic laryngeal muscles that have just been described,

---

[189] Murakami and Kirchner (1973).
[190] This has also been observed in unanaesthetized human subjects (Fink *et al.*, 1956; Kotby and Haugen, 1970a).
[191] *See also* Murakami and Kirchner (1971a).
[192] *See also* Mitchinson and Yoffey (1947); Zenker (1964).
[193] Negus (1929, 1949); Pressman (1941, 1953, 1954); Doty and Bosma (1956); Bosma (1957); Shedd *et al.* (1961); Kawasaki *et al.* (1961); Ardran and Kemp (1967); Doty (1968); Kirchner (1970).

[194] *See* Luchsinger and Arnold (1965); Kirchner (1970).
[195] Brunton and Cash (1883).
[196] Brodal (1969); Sessle and Storey (1972).
[197] Mündnich (1956); Doty and Bosma (1956); Bosma (1957); Faaborg-Andersen (1957, 1965); Mårtensson (1963); Kawasaki *et al.* (1964); Murakami and Kirchner (1971b, 1972a).
[198] Doty and Bosma (1956); Faaborg-Andersen (1957, 1965); Ardran and Kemp (1967).
[199] Pressman (1941, 1953); Kirchner (1970).

for it can still be effected to some degree (without voluntary effort) in patients with bilateral loss of function of the recurrent laryngeal nerves (as a result of lesions of the nerve trunks, or of bulbar poliomyelitis involving the nucleus ambiguus) by reflex activity of the extrinsic laryngeal musculature. The reflex involvement of these muscles in the normal swallowing process has been clearly demonstrated in electromyographic and radiographic studies,[200] and has been the subject of a recent experimental investigation.[201]

In normal swallowing, the larynx is elevated in the neck by approximation of the thyroid cartilage to the hyoid bone,[202] effected by contraction of the thyrohyoid (and longitudinal pharyngeal) musculature accompanied by relaxation of the cricopharyngeus musculature.[203] Both of these effects are produced reflexly by stimulation of the inferior pharyngeal and supraglottic mucosal mechanoreceptors and can be reproduced experimentally by stimulation of afferent fibres in the superior laryngeal nerve.[204] The upward excursion of the thyroid cartilage is limited by a simultaneous increase in the activity of the cricothyroid muscles that also contributes to vocal fold adduction, and which is produced reflexly partly by afferent discharges from the mucosal mechanoreceptors,[204] partly by myotatic reflexes generated by stretch stimulation of the mechanoreceptors located within these muscles, and partly by arthrokinetic reflex effects from the mechanoreceptors in the capsules of the moving cricothyroid joints. This cricothyroid muscle activity also contributes to the small ascent of the cricoid cartilage that occurs in normal swallowing,[205] but which is substantially less than that of the thyroid cartilage. Limitation of thyroid cartilage ascent is also sometimes assisted by an increase in sternothyroid muscle activity that is engendered by similar reflex mechanisms. Finally, it should be noted (not least, by laryngeal, thyroid and other neck surgeons) that the occlusal pressure generated reflexly in the glottis is substantially less in the absence of extrinsic muscular activity than it is when these muscles are operating normally.[206]

Phonatory Activity

Phonation is not the prerogative of the human species, for many animals utilize the larynx (as well as other mechanisms) to produce sounds of varying degrees of complexity and expressiveness[207]—but none approaches man in respect of the range and precision of control of the laryngeal musculature that is displayed during phonatory activity. Furthermore, although human beings may learn to phonate after extirpation of the larynx (by using oesophageal speech, for example), after excision of the vocal folds, or after complete denervation of the laryngeal muscles, their phonatory range is then grossly restricted and their speech is manifestly abnormal.[208] The phonatory behaviour of the neuromuscular apparatus of the larynx therefore clearly merits detailed study as the essential physiological substratum of human verbal communication: for whilst human speech is not merely a modified form of breathing,[209] most workers in this field would agree with the late Wallace O. Fenn[210] that "vocalization has evolved as an ingenious exploitation of the breathing mechanism for the purpose of meaningful communication"—and nowhere has this evolutionary exploitation been more remarkable than in the neurological mechanisms that control the laryngeal musculature.

Although some animals (for example, the horse and the ass) normally phonate during inspiration, this is almost impossible for human beings as a means of sustained speech (although a few such examples have been recorded),[211] and normal human phonation (both in speaking and singing) is accomplished by controlled expiration through adducted and tensed vocal folds after an initial inspiration. In general terms, intensity of the voice is determined by the degree of subglottic pressure maintained against the glottic resistance by the expiratory mechanisms,[212] whilst the pitch of the sounds uttered (which may embrace a range of as many as 2100 changes)[213] is primarily a function of the length, tension, mass and posture of the vibrating vocal folds.[214]

Many muscles (at least 40) are involved in the determination of these (and other) parameters of vocalization,[125] but the present account deals only with the mechanisms controlling the phonatory activity of the intrinsic and extrinsic laryngeal musculature—and in order to avoid a needless waste of space, it should at once be said that the so-called "neurochronaxic" theory of phonation propounded some twenty years ago by Husson[216] is completely untenable on both neurophysiological and physical grounds[217] and that all contemporary workers in this field agree that phonation is governed (as far as the larynx is concerned) by the interaction of aerodynamic forces in the respiratory tract with the myo-elastic properties of the vocal folds.[218] This interaction involves (*inter alia*) the

[200] Fink (1956); Doty and Bosma (1956); Kawasaki *et al.* (1964); Levitt *et al.* (1965); Ardran and Kemp (1967).

[201] Murakami and Kirchner (1971a).

[202] Fink (1956); Ardran and Kemp (1967).

[203] Doty and Bosma (1956); Kirchner (1958); Kawasaki *et al.* (1964); Doty (1968); Murakami and Kirchner (1971a).

[204] Murakami and Kirchner (1971a).

[205] Ardran and Kemp (1967); Murakami and Kirchner (1971a).

[206] Murakami and Kirchner (1971a, 1972a).

[207] *See* Negus (1929, 1949); du Brul (1958); Lanyon and Tavolga (1960); Napier and Barnicot (1963); Luchsinger and Arnold (1965); Lieberman (1968); Wyke (1973b); Peters and Ploog (1973).

[208] *See* Luchsinger and Arnold (1965); Diedrich (1968); Brodnitz (1971); Greene (1972).

[209] Mead and Bunn (1973); Wyke (1973b).

[210] Fenn (1968).

[211] Moses (1958); Brodnitz (1973); Kollár (1973).

[212] Van den Berg (1956); Draper *et al.* (1960); Ladefoged (1960, 1968, 1973); Ladefoged and McKinney (1963); Isshiki (1964, 1965); Yanagihara and Koike (1967); Mead *et al.* (1968); Koyama *et al.* (1969); Ueda *et al.* (1971); Stevens and Klatt (1973); Wyke (1973b).

[213] Cohen (1879).

[214] Van den Berg (1958); Isshiki (1959); Hollien (1960); Hollien and Curtis (1960); von Leden (1961); Rubin (1963); Luchsinger and Arnold (1965); Bouhuys (1968); Damsté *et al.* (1968); Hirano *et al.* (1970); Koyama *et al.* (1971); Stevens and Klatt (1973).

[215] *See* Luchsinger and Arnold (1965); Wyke (1967b); Greene (1972).

[216] Husson (1950, 1962); Portmann *et al.* (1955, 1956).

[217] Floyd *et al.* (1957); Negus *et al.* (1957); Van den Berg (1958); Weiss (1959); Rubin (1960); von Leden (1961); Dedo and Dunker (1967); Kirchner (1970); Greene (1972).

[218] *See* Brewer (1964); Bouhuys (1968); Kirchner (1970); Greene (1972) and Wyke (1973b) for comprehensive reviews of this matter.

co-ordinated activity of the intrinsic and extrinsic laryngeal muscles, each of which groups will now be considered in the light of the foregoing general comments.

Intrinsic Laryngeal Muscles

The earlier electromyographic studies of the phonatory activity of individual human intrinsic laryngeal muscles[219] disclosed that the utterance of single phonemes is associated with a specific sequence of changes in motor unit activity in these muscles that consists basically of an increase in adductor (cricothyroid, thyro-arytenoid, lateral crico-arytenoid, interarytenoid) activity and a decrease in abductor (posterior crico-arytenoid) activity. Furthermore, correlation of the electromyographic recordings with microphonic recordings of the vocal output[220] showed that the adductor facilitation and abductor inhibition both commence some 350–550 ms before the audible utterance (the precise prephonatory interval sometimes varying with the intensity and frequency of the tone uttered) and continue throughout (and sometimes for slightly longer than) the utterance: the duration of the prephonatory interval is similar in all of the intrinsic muscles of a particular subject for a given utterance.

This phonatory activity represents a modification imposed on the tonic activity obtaining in the intrinsic muscles in the absence of phonation, and involves a change in the number and firing frequency of the active motor units therein. Thus, single motor unit recordings from the cricothyroid muscle[221] have shown a prephonatory increase in discharge frequency of up to 25 s^{-1}, followed (as the audible utterance commences) by a lower discharge frequency of 15–20 s^{-1} that declines to 10–15 s^{-1} as the utterance comes to an end. Slightly higher motor unit frequencies (up to 40 s^{-1})—but with a similar temporal variation—have been recorded[221] from the vocalis muscle; whereas in the posterior crico-arytenoid muscle[221] the tonic frequency falls by about 60–70 per cent in the prephonatory period, after which motor unit activity ceases momentarily as the audible utterance commences and then returns irregularly and continues until it comes to an end. In most circumstances of phonation of single phonemes the maximal motor unit frequency in the adductor muscles is about 25–30 s^{-1}, and in no circumstance does it ever exceed 50 s^{-1}.[222]

More recent analyses of the phonatory activity of the intrinsic laryngeal muscles[223] have provided further details, including the relations of their activity to repetitive and sustained utterances, and to variations in the pitch, loudness and phonetic nature of the sounds uttered.[224] Thus the rapid repetition of phonemes leads to a reduction in the duration of the prephonatory interval to values of between 50 and 350 ms in different subjects—but now there is no direct correlation between the activity of the intrinsic laryngeal muscles during the utterance and the loudness of the emitted sound, although there are significant relationships with variations in its pitch and phonetic nature. Thus, as the pitch of a (voiced) sound being uttered is increased (within a particular register), there is a correlated increase in the motor unit activity in all the vocal fold adductor musculature that is greatest in the cricothyroid and vocalis muscles;[225] but there is no correlated decrease in abductor (posterior crico-arytenoid) muscle activity, for this in fact increases during the utterance as vocal pitch rises.[226] It therefore seems that whilst the activity of the posterior crico-arytenoid muscles is briefly inhibited during the prephonatory phase, their activity is augmented to an increasing degree during utterances of increasing pitch so that they contribute to the associated increasing tension of the vocal folds: these muscles (or, at least, some of their contained motor units) can therefore function during phonation of voiced sounds (especially vowels) as a tensing mechanism of the vocal folds in the presence of synchronous adductor muscle activity, as well as operating as an abduction mechanism in the presence of adductor muscle relaxation (as in quiet respiration and in the production of voiceless consonants). Finally, it should be noted that the prephonatory activity in the intrinsic laryngeal muscles described at p. 563 is initiated some 50–100 ms prior to the rise in subglottic pressure that is associated with commencing phonation, and that it occurs even when phonation is attempted in the presence of a tracheostomy by non-laryngectomized patients.[227]

Consideration of these observations of the phonatory behaviour of the intrinsic muscles of the larynx in the light of the experimental studies of their neurological control mechanisms that have been described in the earlier parts of this Chapter has led to the following proposals[228] regarding the neurological mechanisms involved in engendering and regulating such behaviour—proposals that suggest that the laryngeal activity involved in the utterance of each phoneme during speaking and singing involves a temporal sequence of three sets of neuromuscular events, comprising (in order) prephonatory tuning of the laryngeal musculature, phonatory reflex modulation of its activity, and further adjustments in response to acoustic monitoring of the vocal output.

Prephonatory Tuning

The occurrence of the brief (but large) changes in motor unit activity that occur in the intrinsic laryngeal muscles immediately prior to each audible utterance (and also in advance of the arrival of the expiratory air stream in the larynx) indicates that, in order to utter an intended sound, the length, tension, mass and mutual posture of the vocal folds must be *preset* in advance of each utterance.[229] As

[219] Katsuki (1950); Faaborg-Andersen (1957, 1964a, 1965); Spoor and van Dishoeck (1958); Buchthal (1959); Greiner *et al.* (1960); Zenker and Zenker (1960); Buchthal and Faaborg-Andersen (1964).

[220] *See also* Faaborg-Andersen (1957, 1965); Buchthal and Faaborg-Andersen (1964); Hirose (1971); Sutton *et al.* (1972).

[221] Faaborg-Andersen (1957, 1965); Sutton *et al.* (1972).

[222] Katsuki (1950); Faaborg-Andersen (1957, 1965); Sawashima *et al.* (1958).

[223] Faaborg-Andersen (1965); Hiroto (1966); Hiroto *et al.* (1967); Wyke (1967b, 1969a); Kotby and Haugen (1970a, b); Terracol and Greiner (1971); Hirose (1971); Gay *et al.* (1972); Sutton *et al.* (1972).

[224] Faaborg-Andersen (1965); Sutton *et al.* (1972).

[225] Katsuki (1950); Faaborg-Andersen (1957, 1965); Sawashima *et al.* (1958); Hiroto (1966); Hiroto *et al.* (1967); Gay *et al.* (1972).

[226] Hiroto *et al.* (1967); Kotby and Haugen (1970a, b); Dedo (1970); Gay *et al.* (1972).

[227] Terracol and Greiner (1971).

[228] Wyke (1967b, 1969a, 1970, 1971, 1973d).

[229] *See also* Wyke (1973b, d).

this initial process involves (in the case of voiced sounds) synchronously an increase in adductor and a decrease in abductor muscle activity, the vocal folds are approximated towards one another before vocal fold vibration (and thus audible phonation) commences—a fact also apparent in high-speed cinématographic pictures of the phonating larynx[230]—whereas they are abducted prior to the utterance of voiceless consonants.

It is suggested[228] that this process of prephonatory tuning —which is carried out repeatedly during continuous speech and singing—represents the principal *voluntary* contribution to control of the laryngeal musculature during phonation, being effected through the corticobulbar projections to the laryngeal motoneurones. Clinical neurological and neuro-psychological studies indicate[231] that this control is norm-ally effected on laryngeal motoneurones on both sides of the brain stem primarily (but not exclusively) by the bilateral projections thereto from the inferior paracentral region of the cerebral cortex in the dominant cerebral hemisphere. In other words, it is suggested that a subject—having decided upon the sequence of sounds that he wishes to make[232]—voluntarily presets the posture of his vocal folds and the tension pattern of his intrinsic laryngeal muscula-ture into a state that his past experience (acquired mainly during the period of infantile speech maturation) leads him to believe will produce the desired sound, just prior to each utterance. Disturbances of function in this corticobulbar system—due either to structural lesions somewhere along its course, or to abnormalities of functional maturation (such as may result from infantile deafness)—may therefore be expected to produce distortions of this prephonatory tuning process that result in a variety of abnormalities of speech that may include some types of stammering.[233]

Phonatory Reflex Modulation

But once the expiratory column of air is voluntarily set into motion and the subglottic pressure begins to rise— which events also begin prior to the utterance of audible sounds, but after prephonatory tuning of the vocal fold musculature[234]—it will be apparent that the adducted vocal folds (and the laryngeal cartilages to which they are at-tached) will be deflected from their preset phonatory pos-ture. That such deflections (in an upwards and outwards direction) do occur to a limited degree during phonation of voiced sounds has been shown in radiological and cinémato-graphic studies of the larynx, the deflection of the vocal folds commencing anteriorly and progressing posteriorly as the subglottic pressure continues to rise.[235]

In view of the fact[236] that during the utterances of normal conversational and declaratory speech the subglottic pres-sure rises to values of 490–980 Pa (5–10 cm H_2O), in singing with moderate loudness (*mezzo forte*—about 70 dB(A)) to between 980 and 1960 Pa (10 and 20 cm H_2O), and to peak values of about 4·9–6·9 k Pa (50–70 cm H_2O) when singing *fortissimo* (about 100–110 dB(A)), it is clear that the required laryngeal resistance and vocal fold tension can only be maintained against these pressures by enhanced activity in the laryngeal musculature—whose occurrence is clearly evidenced in electromyograms recorded from the intrinsic laryngeal muscles throughout the utterance of voiced sounds.[219,223] It is this activity that limits the up-wards and outwards deflection of the vocal folds and con-tinuously maintains their tension, length and mass near to or at the repeatedly preset desired values during running speech and song; and consideration of the time relations involved in such adjustments[237] makes it clear that they can only be effected by sensitive and rapidly-acting reflex mechanisms operated mainly from receptor systems located within the laryngeal tissues themselves. It has therefore been suggested[238] that this corrective or stabilizing process is largely controlled by the combined effects of the varying afferent discharges delivered reflexly to the laryngeal motoneurones from the low-threshold mechanoreceptors located in the subglottic laryngeal mucosa, in the intrinsic laryngeal muscles themselves and in the capsules of the laryngeal joints such that the fluctuating Bernouilli forces created by the pulsatile flow of air through the glottis generate[239] vibrations of appropriate amplitude and fre-quency in the vocal folds throughout each utterance.

Although the *subglottic mucosal mechanoreceptors* des-cribed at p. 551 are probably not stimulated to a significant degree by the air pressure fluctuations associated with quiet breathing, their threshold is such that they are certainly capable of stimulation by the subglottal pressure surges that occur during speaking and even more during singing, so that their afferent discharges then exert co-ordinated reflex effects on the activity of the intrinsic laryngeal muscu-lature.[240] Direct evidence of their contribution to the reflex control of the intrinsic laryngeal muscles during phonation is now in fact available from studies of the changes that occur in the voice during speaking and singing as a result of topical anaesthesia of the subglottic mucosa[241]—in spite of the fact that the occurrence of such changes following mucosal anaesthesia has sometimes been denied by earlier workers,[242] usually because they anaesthetized the supra-glottic rather than the infraglottic mucosa. There can be no doubt, then, that once the expiratory air flow is set in train during phonation, the fluctuating discharges from the subglottic mucosal mechanoreceptors (some of which are

---

[230] *See* Farnsworth (1940); von Leden (1961); Moore *et al.* (1962); Fink (1962); Dunker and Schlosshauer (1964); Sonninen (1968); Cooper *et al.* (1971); Sovak *et al.* (1971); Cavagna and Camporesi (1973).

[231] Penfield and Rasmussen (1949); Penfield and Roberts (1959); Luchsinger and Arnold (1965); Maria Wyke (1971).

[232] *See also* Wyke (1973b, d).

[233] Penfield and Roberts (1959); Lennenberg (1962); Jones (1966); Wyke (1970, 1971).

[234] Lieberman (1968); Klatt *et al.* (1968); Proctor (1973); Ladefoged (1973).

[235] *See* von Leden (1961); Moore *et al.* (1962); Ardran and Kemp (1967); Bouhuys (1968); Kirchner (1970); Sovak *et al.* (1971); Cavagna and Camporesi (1973).

[236] Rubin *et al.* (1967); Lieberman (1968); Klatt *et al.* (1968); Lade foged (1973); Proctor (1973); Wyke (1973b).

[237] Hast and Milojevic (1966); Lieberman (1968); Klatt *et al.* (1968); Wyke (1973b).

[238] Wyke (1967b, 1969a, 1970, 1971, 1973b, d).

[239] Luchsinger and Arnold (1965); Flanagan (1968); Lieberman (1968); Cavagna and Margaria (1968); Cavagna and Camporesi (1973); Stevens and Klatt (1973); Wyke (1973b).

[240] Wyke (1969a, 1970, 1971, 1973b).

[241] Proctor (1973); Gould and Okamura (1973); Wyke (1973b).

[242] *See* Zemlin (1969).

rapidly-adapting whilst others are slowly-adapting) that mirror the changes in subglottic pressure exert co-ordinated reflex modulating effects on motor unit activity in the intrinsic laryngeal muscles that contribute to maintenance of the preset phonatory posture throughout each utterance. Because of the higher subglottic pressures that obtain in declamatory speech and singing, however, this mechanism is probably more important to the phonation of actors and singers than it is in everyday conversational speech.[243]

Added to the effect of this modulating mucosal reflex mechanism is that of the *myotatic mechanoreceptor reflex systems*,[244] whose morphological basis and functional characteristics have been described at p. 552. The mechanoreceptors in the intrinsic laryngeal muscles behave as low-threshold, slowly-adapting stretch receptors, and are therefore stimulated during phonation as soon as the subglottic pressure rises and begins to stretch the tissues of the vocal folds: likewise, their afferent discharge is maintained throughout each utterance at frequencies that vary with the magnitude of this stretching force. In view of the tonic reflex effects that this afferent discharge exerts on the intrinsic muscles of the larynx, it will be clear that these myotatic reflex mechanisms must make a substantial contribution to maintenance of the phonatory posture and tension of the vocal folds that is initially established during the voluntary prephonatory tuning process.[244] Their excitation in the posterior crico-arytenoid muscles during phonation may also contribute to the motor unit activity that often develops in these muscles during audible utterances, in place of the inhibition of their activity that is associated with the initial phase of prephonatory tuning.

The third of the triad of phonatory modulatory reflex systems is that operated by the low-threshold *articular mechanoreceptors*[245] embedded in the fibrous capsules of the intercartilaginous joints of the larynx. As most of these receptors are rapidly-adapting, they intermittently emit brief bursts of impulses in response to the rapid movements of the laryngeal joints that occur during phonation[246] which are delivered to the laryngeal motoneurones, and thereby effect phasic reflex alterations in the activity of the intrinsic laryngeal muscles throughout each utterance.

It will be clear from this account that the laryngeal tissues (mucosa, muscles and joint capsules) are equipped with an array of mechanoreceptor reflexogenic systems that exert a combination of tonic and phasic modulating effects on motor unit activity in the intrinsic laryngeal muscles during phonation. *Tonic* reflex effects are exerted from some of the subglottic mucosal receptors (those that are slowly-adapting), together with the intramuscular myotatic mechanoreceptors; whilst superimposed *phasic* reflex adjustments are effected from the rapidly-adapting subglottic mucosal mechanoreceptors and the articular mechanoreceptors. It is therefore suggested[247] that the co-ordinated activity of this triad of laryngeal reflexogenic systems during phonation, operating on laryngeal motoneurones against the background influence of the corticobulbar pro-

jections thereto, is responsible for the fluctuating motor unit activity that is apparent electromyographically[219,233] in the intrinsic laryngeal muscles throughout each utterance.

Acoustic Automonitoring

Once a sound has begun to be uttered, the subject's acoustic monitoring of his own on-going vocal output—either directly, or indirectly from reverberations in a room, concert hall or theatre—may lead to further fine readjustments of the motor unit activity obtaining in the intrinsic laryngeal muscles during the utterance (as well as in the activity of the respiratory and oropharyngeal musculature).[248] Empirical evidence of this automonitoring relation between acoustic input and laryngeal muscle activity during phonation is readily apparent in the abnormal voice quality of congenitally deaf children and of adults with long-standing hearing defects, in the phonatory disorders that occur in patients with intracerebral lesions that interrupt the cortico-cortical projections from the temporal acoustic cortex to the inferior paracentral cortex, and in the disturbing effects of delayed or distorted auditory feedback upon the phonatory processes of normal speakers and singers[249] —but it has not yet been specifically investigated by students of laryngeal function (although the relation with control of the respiratory muscles during phonation has been studied).[250]

In untrained speakers this acoustic automonitoring process is largely unconscious (that is to say, it is reflex): but in trained speakers, actors and singers deliberate voluntary control of phonation of a high order of precision in response to acoustic automonitoring may be acquired by practice. Likewise, speech therapists can train patients with various speech disorders (including stammerers) to control their phonatory processes by listening carefully to their own speech or to supplementary acoustic signals provided by the therapist.[251] These latter facts would (at first sight) imply that the changes in laryngeal muscle activity thus engendered are effected *voluntarily* through the corticobulbar tract system, the discharges in which are modified in response to perception of the on-going acoustic input reaching the auditory sectors of the temporal cerebral cortex.[252] However, consideration of the probable time relations that would be involved in such a mechanism in relation to the time relations of the phonatory activity of the laryngeal muscles[253] suggests that more rapidly acting *acoustico-laryngeal reflexes* might also be implicated—operating, perhaps, through the brain stem projections of the cochlear nuclei to the caudal reticular system, the inferior collicular

[243] *See* Gould and Okamura (1973); Wyke (1973b).

[244] Wyke (1967b, 1969a, 1971, 1973b, d).

[245] Wyke (1967b, 1969a, 1970, 1971).

[246] *See* Ardran and Kemp (1966).

[247] Wyke (1967b, 1969a, 1970, 1971, 1973b, d).

[248] *See* Luchsinger and Arnold (1965); Mysak (1966); Wyke (1967b, 1973a).

[249] Lee (1950, 1951); Winckel (1952); Black (1955); Meyer-Eppler and Luchsinger (1955); Fairbanks (1955); Stanton (1958); Konorski (1961); Yates (1963); Grémy and Guérin (1963); Timmons and Boudreau (1972).

[250] Woldring (1968).

[251] *See* Luchsinger and Arnold (1965); Van Riper (1971); Greene (1972).

[252] But it should be noted in this regard that prephonatory tuning of the middle-ear (stapedius and tensor tympani) muscles also occurs along with (but slightly later than) prephonatory tuning of the laryngeal muscles (Salomon and Starr, 1963; Shearer and Sommons, 1965)—and this appears to be effected reflexly partly by afferent impulses from laryngeal receptors (McCall and Rabuzzi, 1973).

[253] Marslen-Wilson (1973).

nuclei, the olive or the cerebellum.[254] Further speculation in this area is profitless in the absence of specific data—but a neurophysiological investigation of the possible existence of an acoustico-laryngeal reflex system in the brain stem clearly needs to be undertaken.

Finally, it should be added that previous ideas of the relative importance of acoustic automonitoring in the processes controlling phonation[255] need modification, in view of the fact that deafness acquired in adult life does not lead to deterioration of speech quality until the deafness has been present for some time;[256] that a well-trained singer can immediately emit a note of designated pitch and loudness without "searching" for it;[257] and that some such singers can continue to phonate accurately even when they cannot hear their own voices[258] (as in certain sections of some Wagnerian operas, or in the presence of acoustic masking). On the other hand, however, untrained "pop" singers in recording studios have to be provided with headphones so that they may hear their own voices (which would otherwise be drowned in the deafening noise made by their accompanists) in order to perform.

Extrinsic Laryngeal Muscles[259]

The extrinsic (as well as the intrinsic) laryngeal muscles make a significant contribution to the adjustments of the status of the vocal folds that occur in speaking and singing—a fact that is of considerable practical importance to head-and-neck and thyroid surgeons as well as to laryngologists, speech therapists and teachers of speaking and singing. The nature of this contribution has been examined during speaking and singing in radiological and electromyographic studies,[260] the essential findings of which are summarized here.

During phonation—and particularly during singing—vertical displacements of the larynx in the neck occur, especially with variations of vowel utterance and at extremes of pitch and vocal intensity;[261] and these vertical displacements, which are associated with changes in the length, tension and posture of the vocal folds,[262] involve alterations in the activity of the extrinsic (and cricothyroid) laryngeal muscles that commence (like those in the intrinsic muscles) some 300–500 ms prior to each audible utterance. Utterance of low-pitched sounds (e.g. at 175 Hz), or of sounds at high intensity, involves a caudal displacement of the larynx that is associated with increased motor unit activity in the sternothyroid and thyrohyoid muscles (more in the former than the latter), whereas high-pitched (e.g. at 490 or 517 Hz) or low-intensity utterances involve

laryngeal ascent that is produced by increased activity in the thyrohyoid muscles combined with sternothyroid inhibition.[263] Still higher-pitched uttrances (e.g. at 715 Hz), however, are associated with increased sternothyroid (as well as thyrohyoid and cricothyroid) activity that results in descent of the larynx to a position similar to that seen during the utterance of low-pitched sounds.[263] It is also relevant to note that mutual approximation of the vocal folds can be achieved in patients with bilateral lesions of the recurrent laryngeal nerves by contraction of the muscles that elevate the thyroid cartilage to the hyoid bone —an action that supplements that of the cricothyroid muscles.[264]

In young people with still flexible thyroid cartilages, mutual approximation and tensing of the vocal folds at higher pitches of phonation is further aided by activity in the thyropharyngeus muscle,[265] bilateral contraction of which produces medial displacement of the thyroid laminae towards one another and an anterior shift of the thyroid attachment of the vocal folds. On the other hand, the shortening of the vocal folds that occurs with low-pitched utterances is associated with increased activity in the cricopharyngeus muscle.[265] Finally, it should be emphasized that these phonatory changes in extrinsic laryngeal muscle activity are accompanied by, and are co-ordinated with, changes in the activity of the longitudinal pharyngeal musculature (mainly the stylopharyngeus and palatopharyngeus components) and of the muscles linking the hyoid bone to the mandible and to the thoracic cage[266]— all of which mechanisms combine to produce (inter alia) the changes in voice quality associated with alterations in the posture of the head on the neck that are well known to professional speakers and singers.[267]

In addition to these observations on human subjects, some recent experimental studies of extrinsic laryngeal muscular activity[268] are pertinent in the present context. Thus, it has been shown that reflex activation or direct electrical stimulation of the extrinsic laryngeal muscles is capable of producing significant changes in vocal fold position and tension, and that increased activity in these muscles (probably the result of myotatic reflex afferent discharges from their contained muscle spindles) provides a significant counterforce to the action of the thyro-arytenoid musculature in tensing the vocal folds.. During artificially induced phonation in the dog,[269] selective bilateral activation of the sternothyroid muscles results in a decrease in vocal pitch and intensity as the larynx moves caudally in the neck and vocal fold tension (and subglottic pressure) is reduced; and other changes in vocal quality are associated with activation of the inferior pharyngeal (thyropharyngeus

[254] See Kappers et al. (1936); Garde (1965); Whitfield (1967); Brodal (1969).

[255] Winckel (1952); Luchsinger and Arnold (1965); Mysak (1966).

[256] Kirchner and Suzuki (1968); Winckel (1973); Wyke (1973b, d).

[257] Kirchner and Suzuki (1968); Winckel (1973); Wyke (1973b, d).

[258] See Dunker and Schlosshauer (1964); Wyke (1973b, d).

[259] See p. 547 for definition.

[260] Sonninen (1956, 1968); Zenker and Zenker (1960); Faaborg-Andersen and Sonninen (1960); Zenker (1964b); Faaborg-Andersen and Vennard (1964); Faaborg-Andersen (1965); Ardran and Kemp (1966, 1967); Damsté et al. (1968).

[261] Sonninen (1956, 1968); Faaborg-Andersen and Sonninen (1960); Faaborg-Andersen and Vennard (1964); Luchsinger and Arnold (1965).

[262] Zenker and Zenker (1960); Zenker (1964b); Sonninen (1968); Damsté et al. (1968).

[263] Faaborg-Andersen and Sonninen (1960); Arnold (1961); Zenker (1964b); Ardran and Kemp (1966).

[264] Luchsinger and Arnold (1965); Ardran and Kemp (1967).

[265] Zenker (1964b); Hiroto (1966).

[266] Fink (1956); Faaborg-Andersen and Sonninen (1960); Ardran and Kemp (1960); Réthi (1962); Zenker (1964b); Faaborg-Andersen and Vennard (1964); Luchsinger and Arnold (1965); Sonninen (1968); Wyke (1973b).

[267] See Ardran and Kemp (1960); Zenker (1964b); Sonninen (1956, 1968); Jones (1972); Sutton et al. (1972); Wyke (1973b).

[268] Evoy (1968); Murakami and Kirchner (1971); Ueda et al. (1972).

[269] Ueda et al. (1972).

and cricopharyngeus) musculature and of the suprahyoid muscles.

Aryepiglottic Musculature

Before leaving this subject, reference must be made to the changes that occur in the aryepiglottic folds during phonation at the same time as the other laryngeal muscular phenomena that have been described—for these may affect the degree of supraglottal damping applied to the vibrating air stream after it has traversed the glottis, and thus influence the quality of the voice.[270]

The protective sphincteric reflex contraction of the aryepiglottic musculature that occurs in response to mechanical stimulation of supraglottic mucosal receptors and during swallowing has already been noted: but laryngoscopic, cinématographic and radiological studies of the phonating larynx have revealed[271] changes in the morphology of the vestibular folds and laryngeal ventricles indicative of contraction of this musculature (as well as of the extrinsic muscles) during phonation also. These changes involve tightening and rostral displacement of the vestibular folds and expansion of the ventricles, and occur in a manner indicative of reflex contraction of the aryepiglottic musculature—although electromyographic confirmation of such activity has not yet been provided. It seems significant in relation to phonation, however, that only in man (amongst the primates) is the aryepiglottic musculature well developed[272]—even though the anthropoid apes also have prominent vestibular folds.[273]

It would thus appear that the tightening and elevation of the vestibular folds that occurs during normal phonation diminishes their intrusion into the vibrating supraglottic air stream, and thereby reduces their damping effect thereon; whilst the associated changes in volume and shape of the ventricles alter their resonance characteristics (which are especially important in the enunciation of vowels).[274] Furthermore, this contraction mechanism is particularly active in bass singers singing in low chest register, so that the supraglottic larynx becomes an acoustic filter that amplifies the lower tones at the expense of the higher partials;[275] and it may also be used for voice production by patients with bilateral paralysis of the vocal fold musculature, or in whom the vocal folds have been surgically removed.[276]

Consideration of all the data reviewed in this section of the Chapter makes it clear that the normal phonatory processes of speaking and singing require precise temporal co-ordination of a highly complex series of neuromuscular events which—as far as the larynx is concerned—involves a combination of voluntary and reflex control systems that together regulate the activity of the intrinsic and extrinsic laryngeal musculature. It is of especial importance

for the clinician to appreciate that these events are organized (in respect both of the intrinsic and extrinsic laryngeal musculature, as well as of the respiratory musculature generally) in a temporal sequence of prephonatory tuning, phonatory reflex modulation and acoustic automonitoring processes. Disturbance of the activity of any of these components will result in disordered phonation.

REFERENCES

Abo-El-Enein, M. A. (1967), *Functional Anatomy of the Larynx*. Ph.D. Thesis, University of London.

Abo-El-Enein, M.A. and Wyke, B. D. (1966a), "Myotatic Reflex Systems in the Intrinsic Muscles of the Larynx," *J. Anat. (Lond.)*, **100**, 926–927.

Abo-El-Enein, M. A. and Wyke, B. D. (1966b), "Laryngeal Myotatic Reflexes," *Nature, (Lond.)*, **209**, 682–686.

Agostoni, E., Chinnock, J. E., de Burgh Daly, M. and Murray, J. G. (1957), "Functional and Histological Studies of the Vagus Nerve and its Branches to the Heart, Lungs and Abdominal Viscera in the Cat," *J. Physiol. (Lond.)*, **135**, 182–205.

Aldaya, F. (1936a), "Les modifications réflexes de a respiration par l'excitation du nerf laryngé supérieur," *C. R. Soc. Biol. (Paris)*, **123**, 104–105.

Aldaya, F. (1936b), "Le contrôle réflexe de la respiration par la sensibilité du larynx," *C. R. Soc. Biol. (Paris)*, **123**, 1001–1002.

Andersson, B., Landgren, S., Neil, E. and Zotterman, Y. (1950), "Reflex Augmentation of Intestinal Motility Caused by Stimulation of the Superior Laryngeal Nerve," *Acta physiol. scand.*, **20**, 253–257.

Andrew, B. L. (1954a), "A Laryngeal Pathway for Aortic Baroreceptor Impulses," *J. Physiol. (Lond.)*, **125**, 352–360.

Andrew, B. L. (1954b), "Proprioception at the Joint of the Epiglottis of the Rat," *J. Physiol. (Lond.)*, **126**, 507–523.

Andrew, B. L. (1955), "The Respiratory Displacement of the Larynx: A Study of the Innervation of Accessory Respiratory Muscles," *J. Physiol. (Lond)*, **130**, 474–487.

Andrew, B. L. (1956), "A Functional Analysis of the Myelinated Fibres of the Superior Laryngeal Nerve of the Rat," *J. Physiol. (Lond.)*, **133**, 420–432.

Andrew, B. L. (Ed.) (1966), *Control and Innervation of Skeletal Muscle*. Dundee: Thompson.

Andrew, B. L. and Oliver, J. (1951), "Nerve Endings at the Joint of the Epiglottis," *J. Physiol. (Lond.)*, **112**, 33–35.

Andrew, B. L. and Oliver, J. (1951), "The Epiglottal Taste Buds of the Rat," *J. Physiol. (Lond.)*, **114**, 48P.

Ardouin, P. and Maillet, M. (1965), "Etude des fibres nerveuses amyéliniques de la corde vocale," *Acta oto-laryng.*, **59**, 225–233.

Ardran, G. M. and Kemp, F. H. (1960), "Movements of the Hyoid Bone Relative to the Thyroid Cartilage on Neck Flexion," *J. Anat. (Lond.)*, **94**, 285.

Ardran, G. M. and Kemp, F. H. (1966), "The Mechanism of the Larynx. I. The Movements of the Arytenoid and Cricoid Cartilages," *Brit. J. Radiol.*, **39**, 641–654.

Ardran, G. M. and Kemp, F. H. (1967), "The Mechanism of the Larynx. II. The Epiglottis and Closure of the Larynx," *Brit. J. Radiol.*, **40**, 372–389

Armstrong, B. W. and Smith, D. J. (1955), "Function of Certain Neck Muscles During the Respiratory Cycle," *Amer. J. Physiol.*, **182**, 599–600.

Arnold, G. E. (1961), "Physiology and Pathology of the Cricothyroid Muscle," *Laryngoscope*, **71**, 687–753.

Baken, R. J. (1971), "Neuromuscular Spindles in the Intrinsic Muscles of a Human Larynx," *Folia phoniat.*, **23**, 204–210.

Barillot, J.-C. and Bianchi, A.-L. (1971), "Activité des motoneurones laryngés pendant les réflexes de Hering-Breuer," *J. Physiol. (Paris)*, **63**, 783–792.

Basmajian, J. V. (1967), *Muscles Alive. Their Functions Revealed by Electromyography*, 2nd edition. Baltimore: Williams and Wilkins.

Beckmann, G. (1956), "Experimentelle Untersuchungen über den akustischen Einfluss der Kehlkopfventrikel auf die Stimmproduktion", *Arch. Ohr.-, Nas.- u. Kehlkheilk.*, **169**, 485–491.

---

[270] Van den Berg (1955); Fink (1962b); Luchsinger and Arnold (1965); Ardran and Kemp (1967); Moore (1971); Brodnitz (1971); Greene (1972).

[271] Fink (1962b); Réthi (1962); Ardran and Kemp (1967).

[272] Negus (1929, 1949).

[273] Negus (1929, 1949); Fink (1956).

[274] Van den Berg (1955); Luchsinger and Arnold (1965).

[275] *See* Beckmann (1956); Greene (1972).

[276] Luchsinger and Arnold (1965).

Bender, L. (1928), "The Cerebellar Control of the Vocal Organs," *Arch. Neurol. Psychiat. (Chicago)*, **19**, 796–833.

Bianchi, A.-L. (1971), "Localization et étude des neurones respiratoires bulbaires: mise en jeu antidromique par stimulation spinale ou vagale," *J. Physiol. (Paris)*, **63**, 5–40.

Bianconi, R., Cangiano, A. and Raschi, F. (1967), "Influenze di afferenze vagali polmonari sui motoneuroni laringei nel respiro spontaneo e nell' iperventilazione. II. Insufflazione polmonare," *Acta med. Rom.*, **5**, 215–223.

Bianconi, R., Corazza, R. and Raschi, F. (1963), "Attività elettrica dei muscoli intrinseci della laringe e posizione delle corde vocali nella iperventilazione con aria e nell' apnea ipocapnica," *Arch. Sci biol. (Bologna)*, **47**, 376–389.

Bianconi, R. and Molinari, G. (1960), "Impulsi afferenti nel nervo laringeo ricorrente, nel gatto," *Boll. Soc. ital. Biol. sper.*, **36**, 1750–1752.

Bianconi, R. and Molinari, G. (1961), "Studio elettroneurografico della terminazione propriocettivi del nervo ricorrente nei muscoli intrinseci della laringe, nel gatto," *Boll. Soc. ital. Biol. sper.*, **37**, 657–658.

Bianconi, R. and Molinari, G. (1962a), "Fibri afferenti a distribuzione laringea nel nervo ricorrente, nel gatto," *Arch. Sci. biol. (Bologna)*, **46**, 112–120.

Bianconi, R. and Molinari, G. (1962b), "Electroneurographic Evidence of Muscle Spindles and Other Sensory Endings in the Intrinsic Laryngeal Muscles of the Cat," *Acta oto-laryng.*, **55**, 253–259.

Bianconi, R. and Raschi, F. (1959), "Osservazioni sull'attività elettrica dei nervi ricorrenti nel gatto," *Boll. Soc. ital. Biol. sper.*, **35**, 1917–1918.

Bianconi, R. and Raschi, F. (1964), "Respiratory Control of Motoneurones of the Recurrent Laryngeal Nerve and Hypocapnic Apnoea," *Arch. ital. Biol.*, **102**, 56–73.

Bigland, B. and Lippold, O. C. J. (1954), "The Relation Between Force, Velocity and Integrated Electrical Activity in Human Muscles," *J. Physiol. (Lond.)*, **123**, 214–224.

Black, J. W. (1955), "The Persistence of the Effects of Delayed Sidetone," *J. Speech and Hear. Dis.*, **20**, 65–68.

Bosma, J. F. (1957), "Deglutition: Pharyngeal Stage," *Physiol. Rev.*, **37**, 275–300.

Bosma, J. F. and Koivisto, E. (1962), "Laryngeal and Pharyngeal Respiratory Motions in the Rabbit: Cinematographic Observations," *Ann. Otol., Rhinol., Lar.*, **71**, 341–355.

Bouhuys, A. (Ed.) (1968), *Sound Production in Man*. New York: New York Academy of Sciences.

Boushey, H. A. and Richardson, P. S. (1973), "The Reflex Effects of Intralaryngeal Carbon Dioxide on the Pattern of Breathing," *J. Physiol. (Lond.)*, **228**, 181–191.

Boushey, H. A., Richardson, P. S. and Widdicombe, J. G. (1972), "Reflex Effects of Laryngeal Irritation on the Pattern of Breathing and Total Lung Resistance," *J. Physiol. (Lond.)*, **224**, 501–513.

Bowden, Ruth E. M. (1963), "Muscle Spindles in the Human Foetus," *Acta biol.*, **9**, 35–39.

Bowden, Ruth E. M. (1973), "Innervation of Intrinsic Laryngeal Muscles," in *Ventilatory and Phonatory Control Systems: An International Symposium*, pp. 370–378 (B. D. Wyke, Ed.). London: Oxford University Press.

Bowden, Ruth E. M., Lucas Keene, M. F., Gooding, M., Mahran, Z.Y. and Withington, J. L. (1960), "The Afferent Innervation of Facial and Laryngeal Muscles," *Anat. Rec.*, **136**, 168.

Bowden, Ruth E. M. and Scheuer, J. L. (1961), "Comparative Study of the Nerve Supply of the Larynx in Eutherian Mammals." *Proc. zool. Soc. Lond.*, **136**, 325–330.

Brewer, D. W. (Ed.) (1964), *Research Potentials in Voice Physiology*. New York: State University of New York.

Brewer, D. W. and Dana, S. T. (1963), "Investigations in Laryngeal Physiology: the Canine Larynx," *Ann. Otol., Rhinol., Lar.*, **72**, 1060–1075.

Bridgman, C. F. (1968), "The Structure of Tendon Organs in the Cat: a Proposed Mechanism for Responding to Muscle Tension," *Anat. Rec.*, **162**, 209–220.

Bridgman, C. F. (1970), "Comparisons in Structure of Tendon Organs in the Rat, Cat and Man," *J. comp. Neurol.*, **138**, 369–372.

Brocklehurst, R. J. and Edgeworth, F. H. (1940), "The Fibre Components of the Laryngeal Nerves of *Macaca Mulatta*," *J. Anat. (Lond.)*, **74**, 386–389.

Brodal, A. (1969), *Neurological Anatomy in Relation to Clinical Medicine*, 2nd edition. London: Oxford University Press.

Brodnitz, F. S. (1971), *Vocal Rehabilitation*. Rochester, Minnesota: American Academy of Ophthalmology and Otolaryngology.

Brodnitz, F. S. (1973), "Discussion," in *Ventilatory and Phonatory Control Systems: An International Symposium*, p. 360 (B. D. Wyke, Ed.). London: Oxford University Press.

du Brul, E. L. (1958), *Evolution of the Speech Apparatus*. Springfield, Illinois: Thomas.

Brunton, T. L. and Cash, T. (1883), "The Valvular Action of the Larynx," *J. Anat. Physiol.*, **17**, 363–378.

Buchthal, F. (1959), "Electromyography of Intrinsic Laryngeal Muscles," *Quart. J. exp. Physiol.*, **44**, 137–148.

Buchthal, F. (1961), "The General Concept of the Motor Unit," *Res. Pub. Assoc. nerv. ment. Dis.*, **38**, 3–30.

Buchthal, F. and Faaborg-Andersen, K. L. (1964), "Electromyography of Laryngeal and Respiratory Muscles: Correlation with Phonation and Respiration," *Ann. Otol., Rhinol., Lar.*, **73**, 118–123.

Campbell, C. J. and Murtagh, J. A. (1956), "Electrical Manifestations of Recurrent Nerve Function," *Ann. Otol., Rhinol., Lar.*, **65**, 747–765.

Campbell, C. J., Murtagh, J. A. and Raber, C. F. (1963), "Laryngeal Resistance to Air Flow," *Ann. Otol., Rhinol., Lar.*, **72**, 5–31.

Campbell, E. J. M., Agostoni, E. and Newsom Davis, J. (1970), *The Respiratory Muscles: Mechanics and Neural Control*, 2nd edition. London: Lloyd-Luke.

Canter, G. J. (1965), "Speech Characteristics of Patients with Parkinson's Disease. II. Physiological Support for Speech," *J. Speech and Hear. Dis.*, **30**, 44–49.

Capps, F. C. W. (1958), "Abductor Paralysis in Theory and Practice Since Semon," *J. Laryng.*, **72**, 1–31.

Caraceni, T. and Zibordi, F. (1964), "Studio elettromiografico dei muscoli intrinseci laringei dell'uomo in condizioni fisiologichi," *Arch. ital. Otol.*, **75**, 478–499.

Cavagna, G. A. and Camporesi, E. M. (1973), "Glottic Aerodynamics and Phonation," in *Ventilatory and Phonatory Control Systems: An International Symposium*, pp. 76–88 (B. D. Wyke, Ed.). London: Oxford University Press.

Cavagna, G. A. and Magaria, K. (1968), "Airflow Rates and Efficiency Changes During Phonation," *Ann. N.Y. Acad. Sci.*, **155**, 152–164.

Cohen, J. da Silva Solis. (1879), *The Throat and Voice*. Philadelphia: Lindson and Blakiston.

Cohen, M. I. (1973), "Discussion and Supplementary Statement III," in *Ventilatory and Phonatory Control Systems: An International Symposium*. pp. 468–471 (B. D. Wyke, Ed.). London: Oxford University Press.

Cooper, F. S., Sawashima, M., Abramson, A. S. and Lisker, L. (1971), Looking at the Larynx During Running Speech," *Ann. Otol., Rhinol., Lar.*, **80**, 678–682.

Cooper, S. and Daniel, P. M. (1949), "Muscle Spindles in Human Extrinsic Eye Muscles," *Brain*, **72**, 1–24.

Cooper, S., Daniel, P. M. and Whitteridge, D. (1955), "Muscle Spindles and Other Sensory Endings in the Extrinsic Eye Muscles: the Physiology and Anatomy of These Receptors and of Their Connections with the Brainstem," *Brain*, **78**, 564–583.

Cooper, S. and Fillenz, M. (1955), "Afferent Discharges in Response to Stretch from the Extraocular Muscles of the Cat and Monkey and the Innervation of These Muscles," *J. Physiol. (Lond.)*, **127**, 400–413.

Crosby, E. (1964), "Anatomical Considerations," in *Research Potentials in Voice Physiology*, pp. 43–46 (D. W. Brewer, Ed.). New York: State University of New York.

Damsté, P. H., Hollien, H., Moore, P. and Murry, T. (1968), "An X-ray Study of Vocal Fold Length," *Folia phoniat.*, **20**, 349–359.

Dedo, H. H. (1970), "The Paralyzed Larynx: An Electromyographic Study in Dogs and Humans," *Laryngoscope*, **80**, 1455–1517.

Dedo, H. H. and Dunker, E. (1967), "Husson's Theory: An Experimental Analysis of His Research Data and Conclusions," *Arch. Otolaryng.*, **85**, 303–313.

Déjerine, J. (1914), *Sémiologie des affections du système nerveux.* Paris: Masson.

Diedrich, W. M. (1968), "The Mechanism of Esophageal Speech," *Ann. N.Y. Acad. Sci.*, **155**, 303–317.

Doty, R. W. (1968), "Neural Organization of Deglutition," in *Handbook of Physiology*, Sec. 6, Vol. IV, pp. 1861–1902 (C. F. Code, Ed,). Washington: American Physiological Society.

Doty, R. W. and Bosma, J. F. (1956), "An Electromyographic Analysis of Reflex Deglutition," *J. Neurophysiol.*, **19**, 44–60.

Dow, R. S. and Moruzzi, G. (1958), *The Physiology and Pathology of the Cerebellum.* Minneapolis: University of Minnesota Press.

Draper, M. H., Ladefoged, P. and Whitteridge, D. (1960), "Expiratory Pressure and Air Flow During Speech," *Brit. med. J.*, **1**, 1837–1843.

DuBois, F. S. and Foley, J. O. (1936), "Experimental Studies on the Vagus and Spinal Accessory Nerves in the Cat," *Anat. Rec.*, **64**, 285–307.

Dunker, E. (1968), "The Central Control of Laryngeal Function," *Ann. N.Y. Acad. Sci.*, **155**, 112–121.

Dunker, E. and Schlosshauer, B. (1964), "Irregularities of the Laryngeal Vibratory Patterns in Healthy and Hoarse Persons," in *Research Potentials in Voice Physiology*, pp. 151–184 (D. W. Brewer, Ed.). New York: State University of New York.

Edström, L., Lindquist, C. and Mårtensson, A. (1973), "Correlation Between Functional and Histochemical Properties of the Intrinsic Laryngeal Muscles in the Cat," in *Ventilatory and Phonatory Control Systems: An International Symposium*, pp. 392–404 (B. D. Wyke, Ed.). London: Oxford University Press.

English, D. T. and Blevins, C. E. (1969), "Motor Units of Laryngeal Muscles," *Arch. Otolaryng.*, **89**, 778–784.

Esslen, E. and Schlosshauer, B. (1960), "Zur Reflexinnervation der inneren Kehlkopfmuskeln," *Folia phoniat.*, **12**, 161–169.

von Euler, C. (1968), "The Proprioceptive Control of the Diaphragm," *Ann. N.Y. Acad. Sci.*, **155**, 204–205.

von Euler, C. (1973), "Control of Depth and Rate of Respiratory Movements," in *Ventilatory and Phonatory Control Systems: An International Symposium*, pp. 95–101 (B. D. Wyke, Ed.). London: Oxford University Press.

Evoy, M. H. (1968), "Experimental Activation of Paralyzed Vocal Cords," *Arch. Otolaryng.*, **87**, 155–161.

Eyzaguirre, C., Sampson, S. and Taylor, J. R. (1966), "The Motor Control of Intrinsic Laryngeal Muscles in the Cat," in *Muscular Afferents and Motor Control* (Nobel Symposium), pp. 209–225 (R. Granit, Ed.). Stockholm: Almquist and Wiksell.

Eyzaguirre, C. and Taylor, J. R. (1963), "Respiratory Discharges of Some Vagal Motoneurones," *J. Neurophysiol.*, **26**, 61–78.

Faaborg-Andersen, K. L. (1957), "Electromyographic Investigation of Intrinsic Laryngeal Muscles in Humans: An Investigation of Subjects with Normally Movable Vocal Cords and Patients with Vocal Cord Paresis," *Acta physiol. scand.*, **41**, suppl. 140, 1–149.

Faaborg-Andersen, K.L. (1964a), "Electromyography of the Laryngeal Muscles in Man," in *Research Potentials in Voice Physiology*, pp. 105–129 (D. W. Brewer, Ed.). New York: State University of New York.

Faaborg-Andersen, K. L. (1964b), "The Position of Paretic Vocal Cords," *Acta oto-laryng.*, **57**, 50–54.

Faaborg-Andersen, K. L. (1965), "Electromyography of Laryngeal Muscles in Humans: Technics and Results," in *Aktuelle Probleme der Phoniatrie und Logopädie*, Vol. 3, pp. 1–72 (F. Trojan, Ed.). Basel: Karger.

Faaborg-Andersen, K. L. and Jensen, A. M. (1964), "Unilateral Paralysis of the Superior Laryngeal Nerve," *Acta oto-laryng.*, **57**, 155–159.

Faaborg-Andersen, K. L. and Sonninen, A. (1960), "The Function of the Extrinsic Laryngeal Muscles at Different Pitch: An Electromyographic and Roentgenologic Investigation," *Acta oto-laryng.*, **51**, 89–93.

Faaborg-Andersen, K. L. and Vennard, W. (1964), "Electromyography of Extrinsic Laryngeal Muscles During Phonation of Different Vowels," *Ann. Otol., Rhinol., Lar.*, **73**, 248–254.

Fabre, P., Husson, R. and Roëlens, R. (1962), "Physiologie phonatoire laryngée: séparation expérimentale des fonctions cloniques et toniques de la musculature laryngée par la glottographie électrique dite 'respiratoire'," *C. R. Acad. Sci. (Paris)*, **255**, 1526–1528.

Fairbanks, G. (1955), "Selective Vocal Effects of Delayed Auditory Feedback," *J. Speech and Hear. Dis.*, **20**, 333–346.

Farnsworth, D. W. (1940), "High Speed Motion Pictures of the Human Vocal Cords," *Bell Lab. Rec.*, **18**, 203–208.

Feinstein, B. (1946), "The Application of Electromyography to Affections of the Facial and Intrinsic Laryngeal Muscles," *Proc. roy. Soc. Med.*, **39**, 817–819.

Feinstein, B., Lindegård, B., Nyman, E. and Wohlfart, G. (1955), "Morphologic Studies of Motor Units in Normal Human Muscles," *Acta anat. (Basel)*, **23**, 127–142.

Fenn, W. O. (1968), "Perspectives in Phonation," *Ann. N.Y. Acad. Sci.*, **155**, 4–8.

Fernand, V. S. V. (1970), "The Afferent Innervation of Two Infrahyoid Muscles of the Cat," *J. Physiol. (Lond.)*, **208**, 757–771.

Fillenz, M. and Woods, R. I. (1970), "Sensory Innervation of the Airways," in *Breathing: Hering-Breuer Centenary Symposium*, pp. 101–107 (R. Porter, Ed.). London: Churchill.

Fink, B. R. (1956), "The Mechanism of Closure of the Human Larynx," *Trans. Amer. Acad. Ophthal. Otolaryng.*, **60**, 117–127.

Fink, B. R. (1962a), "Adaptations for Phonatory Efficiency in the Human Vocal Folds," *Ann. Otol., Rhinol., Lar.*, **71**, 79–85.

Fink, B. R. (1962b), "Phonatory Adaptations in the Upper Larynx of Man," *Ann. Otol., Rhinol., Lar.*, **71**, 356–362.

Fink, B. R. (1962c), "Tensor Mechanism of the Vocal Folds," *Ann. Otol., Rhinol., Lar.*, **71**, 591–599.

Fink, B. R., Basek, M. and Epanchin, V. (1956), "The Mechanism of Opening of the Human Larynx," *Laryngoscope*, **66**, 410–425.

Flanagan, J. L. (1968), "Source-system Interaction in the Vocal Tract," *Ann. N.Y. Acad. Sci.*, **155**, 9–15.

Floyd, W. F., Negus, V. E. and Neil, E. (1957), "Observations on the Mechanism of Phonation," *Acta oto-laryng.*, **48**, 16–25.

Fukuda, H. and Kirchner, J. A. (1972), "Changes in the Respiratory Activity of the Cricothyroid Muscle with Intrathoracic Interruption of the Vagus Nerve," *Ann. Otol., Rhinol., Lar.*, **81**, 532–537.

Fukuda, H., Sasaki, C. T. and Kirchner, J. A. (1973), "Vagal Afferent Influences on the Phasic Activity of the Posterior Crico-arytenoid Muscle," *Acta oto-laryng.*, **75**, 112–118.

Fulton, J. F. (1943), *Physiology of the Nervous System*, 2nd edition (revised). London: Oxford University Press.

Furstenberg, A. C. (1937), "Anatomical and Clinical Study of Central Lesions Producing Paralysis of the Larynx," *Ann. Otol., Rhinol., Lar.*, **46**, 39–54.

Furstenberg, A. C. and Magielski, J. E. (1955), "A Motor Pattern in the Nucleus Ambiguus: its Clinical Significance," *Ann. Otol., Rhinol., Lar.*, **64**, 788–793.

Garde, E. J. (1965), "Le réflexe cochléo-phonatoire: état actuel de la question," *Rev. Laryng.*, **85**, 632–638.

Gay, T., Hirose, H., Strome, M. and Sawashima, M. (1972), "Electromyography of the Intrinsic Laryngeal Muscles During Phonation," *Ann. Otol., Rhinol., Lar.*, **81**, 401–409.

Getz, B. and Sirnes, T. (1949), "The Localization Within the Dorsal Motor Vagal Nucleus: An Experimental Investigation," *J. comp. Neurol.*, **90**, 95–110.

Gill, P. K. and Kuno, M. (1963a), "Properties of Phrenic Motoneurones," *J. Physiol. (Lond.)*, **168**, 258–273.

Gill, P. K. and Kuno, M. (1963b), "Excitatory and Inhibitory Actions on Phrenic Motoneurones," *J. Physiol. (Lond.)*, **168**, 274–289.

Godwin-Austen, R. B. (1969), "The Mechanoreceptors of the Costovertebral Joints," *J. Physiol. (Lond.)*, **202**, 737–753.

Goerttler, K. (1950), "Die Anordnung, Histologie und Histogenese der quergestreiften Muskulatur im menschlichen Stimmband," *Zeit. Anat. Entw. Gesch.*, **115**, 352–401.

Gould, W. J. and Okamura, H. (1973), "Inter-relationships Between Voice and Laryngeal Mucosal Reflexes," in *Ventilatory and Phonatory Control Systems: An International Symposium*, pp. 347–360. (B. D. Wyke, Ed.). Oxford University Press.

Gracheva, M. S. (1950), "Reflexogenic Zones of the Larynx (Russian Text)," *Vestn. oto-rino-laring.*, **12**, 12–17.

Gracheva, M. S. (1963), "On the Sensory Innervation of the Loco-motor Apparatus of the Larynx (Russian text)," *Arkh. Anat. Gist. Embr.*, **44**, 77–83.

Granit, R. (1970), *The Basis of Motor Control.* New York: Academic Press.

Granit, R., Skoglund, S. and Thesleff, S. (1953), "Activation of Muscle Spindles By Succinylcholine and Decamethonium: the Effects of Curare," *Acta physiol. scand.*, **28**, 134–151.

Green, J. G. and Neil, E. (1955), "The Respiratory Function of the Laryngeal Muscles," *J. Physiol.* (*Lond.*), **129**, 134–141.

Greene, Margaret C. L. (1972), *The Voice and Its Disorders.* 3rd edition. London: Pitman.

Greiner, G. F., Isch, F., Isch-Treussard, C., Ebtinger-Jouffroy, J., Klotz, G. and Champy, M. (1960), "L'électromyographie appliquée à la pathologie du larynx," *Acta otolaryng.*, **51**, 319–331.

Grémy, F. and Guérin, C. (1963), "Etude du glottogramme chez l'enfant sourd en cours de rééducation vocale," *Ann. d'otolaryng.* (*Paris*), **80**, 803–815.

Grim, M. (1967), "Muscle Spindles in the Posterior Crico-arytenoid Muscles of the Human Larynx," *Folia morphol.*, Prague, **15**, 124–131.

Haglund, S. (1973), "The Normal Electromyogram in Human Cricothyroid Muscle," *Acta oto-laryng.*, **75**, 448–458.

Hall-Craggs, E. C. B. (1967), "Contraction Times and Metabolism in Rabbit Laryngeal Muscles," *J. Anat.* (*Lond.*), **101**, 181–182.

Hassler, R. (1956), "Die extrapyramidalen Rindensysteme und die zentrale Regelung der Motorik," *Dtsch. Z. Nervenheilk.*, **175**, 233–258.

Hast, M. H. (1966a), "Physiological Mechanisms of Phonation: Tension of the Vocal Fold Muscle," *Acta oto-laryng.*, **62**, 309–318.

Hast, M. H. (1966b), "Mechanical Properties of the Cricothyroid Muscle," *Laryngoscope*, **76**, 537–548.

Hast, M. H. (1967a), "Mechanical Properties of the Vocal Fold Muscle," *Pract. oto-rhino-laryng.* (*Basel*), **29**, 53–56.

Hast, M. H. (1967b), "The Respiratory Muscle of the Larynx," *Ann. Otol., Rhinol., Lar.*, **76**, 489–497.

Hast, M. H. (1968), "Studies on the Extrinsic Laryngeal Muscles," *Arch. Otolaryng.*, **88**, 273–278.

Hast, M. H. (1969), "The Primate Larynx: a Comparative Physiological Study of Intrinsic Muscles," *Acta oto-laryng.*, **67**, 84–92.

Hast, M. H. and Golbus, S. (1971), "Physiology of the Lateral Crico-arytenoid Muscle," *Pract. oto-rhino-laryng.* (*Basel*), **33**, 209–214.

Hast, M. H. and Milojevic, B. (1966), "The Response of the Vocal Folds to Electrical Stimulation of the Interior Frontal Cortex of the Squirrel Monkey," *Acta oto-laryng.*, **61**, 196–204.

Hirano, M., Vennard, W. and Ohala, J. (1970), "Regulation of Register, Pitch and Intensity of Voice: an Electromyographic Investigation of Intrinsic Laryngeal Muscles," *Folia phoniat.*, **22**, 1–20.

Hirose, H. (1961), "Afferent Impulses in the Recurrent Laryngeal Nerve in the Cat," *Laryngoscope*, **71**, 1196–1206.

Hirose, H. (1971), "An Electromyographic Study of Laryngeal Adjustments During Speech Articulation: a Preliminary Report," *Haskins Lab. Status Rept. on Speech Res.*, Jan.-June, pp. 107–116.

Hirose, H., Ushijima, T., Kobayshi, T. and Sawashima, M. (1969), "An Experimental Study of the Contraction Properties of the Laryngeal Muscles in the Cat," *Ann. Otol., Rhinol., Lar.*, **78**, 297–306.

Hiroto, I. (1966), "The Mechanism of Phonation: its Pathological Aspects," *Pract. otolaryngol.*, Kyoto, **59**, suppl., 1–229.

Hiroto, I., Hirano, M., Toyozumi, Y. and Shin, T. (1964), "Function of Laryngeal Muscles," *Oto-rhino- and laryng. Clin.*, **57**, 1–9.

Hiroto, I., Hirano, M., Toyozumi, Y. and Shin, T. (1967), "Electromyographic Investigation of the Intrinsic Laryngeal Muscles Related to Speech Sounds," *Ann. Otol., Rhinol., Lar.*, **76**, 861–872.

Hofer, G. (1944), "Zur motorischen Innervation des menschlichen Kehlkopfes," *Z. ges. Neurol. Psychiat.*, **177**, 783–796.

Hofer, G. (1947), "Zur motorischen Innervation des menschlichen Kehlkopfes," *Mschr. Ohrenheilk.*, **81**, 57–69.

Hollien, H. (1960), "Vocal Pitch Variation Related to Change in Vocal Fold Length," *J. Speech and Hear. Res.*, **3**, 150–156.

Hollien, H. and Curtis, J. F. (1960), "A Laminagraphic Study of Vocal Pitch," *J. Speech and Hear. Res.*, **3**, 361–371.

Hosokawa, H. (1961), "Proprioceptive Innervation of Striated Muscles in the Territory of Cranial Nerves," *Tex. Rep. Biol. Med.*, **19**, 405–464.

Husson, R. (1950), *Etude des phenomènes physiologiques et acoustiques fondamentaux de la voix chantée.* Thèse de la Faculté des Sciences, Université de Paris.

Husson, R. (1962), *Physiologie de la phonation.* Paris: Masson.

Hwang, G., Grossman, M. I. and Ivy, A. C. (1948), "Nervous Control of the Cervical Portion of the Esophagus," *Amer. J. Physiol.*, **154**, 343–357.

Isshiki, N. (1959), "Regulatory Mechanism of the Pitch and Volume of Voice," *Oto-rhino-laryng. Clin.*, **52**, 1065–1094.

Isshiki, N. (1964), "Regulatory Mechanism of Voice Intensity Variation," *J. Speech and Hear. Res.*, **7**, 17–29.

Isshiki, N. (1965), "Vocal Intensity and Airflow Rate," *Folia phoniat.*, **17**, 92–104.

Jankovskaya, N. F. (1959), "The Receptor Innervation of the Perichondrium of the Laryngeal Cartilages" [Ukranian text], *Arkh. Anat. Gist. Embr.*, **37**(8), 70–75.

Jewett, D. L. (1964), "Direct Nervous Pathways Between the Cervical Vagus and the Aortic or Superior Laryngeal Nerves Traversed by Baroreceptor, 'Pulmonary Stretch' and Other Fibres in the Cat," *J. Physiol.* (*Lond.*), **175**, 358–371.

Joels, N. and Samueloff, M. (1956), "The Activity of the Medullary Centres in Diffusion Respiration," *J. Physiol.* (*Lond.*), **133**, 360–372.

Johnson, J. (1935), "Effect of Superior Laryngeal Nerves on Tracheal Mucus," *Ann. Surg.*, **101**, 494–499.

Jones, F. P. (1972), "Voice Production as a Function of Head Balance in Singers," *J. Psychol.*, **82**, 209–215.

Jones, R. K. (1966), "Observations on Stammering After Localized Cerebral Injury," *J. Neurol. Neurosurg. Psychiat.*, **29**, 192–195.

Kappers, C. U. Ariëns, Huber, G. C. and Crosby, E. C. (1936), *The Comparative Anatomy of the Nervous System of Vertebrates, Including Man*, 2 vols. New York: Macmillan.

Katsuki, Y. (1950), "The Function of the Phonatory Muscles," *Jap. J. Physiol.*, **1**, 29–35.

Katzenstein, J. (1905), "Ueber ein neues Rindenfeld und einen neuen Reflex des Kehlkopfes," *Arch. ges. Physiol.*, **29**, 396–400.

Katzenstein, J. (1908), "Über die Lautgebungsstelle in der Hinrinde des Hundes," *Arch. Laryng. Rhin.* (*Berl.*), **20**, 501–524.

Katzenstein, J. and Rothmann, M. (1911), "Zur Lokalization der Kehlkopfinnervation in der Kleinhirnrinde," *Neurol. Zbl.*, **30**, 1146–1147.

Katzenstein, J. and Rothmann, M. (1912), "Zur Lokalisation der Kehlkopfinnervation in der Kleinhirnrinde," *Beit. Anat. Physiol. Pathol. Therap. Ohres.*, **5**, 380–389.

Kawasaki, M., Ogura, J. H. and Takenouchi, S. (1964), "Neurophysiologic Observations of Normal Deglutition," *Laryngoscope*, **74**, 1747–1780.

Keros, P. and Nemanic, D. (1967), "The Terminal Branching of the Recurrent Laryngeal Nerve," *Pract. oto-rhino-laryng.* (*Basel*), **29**, 5–10.

Kirchner, J. A. (1958), "The Motor Activity of the Cricopharyngeus Muscle," *Laryngoscope*, **68**, 1119–1159.

Kirchner, J. A. (1966), "Atrophy of Laryngeal Muscles in Vagal Paralysis," *Laryngoscope*, **76**, 1753–1765.

Kirchner, J. A. (Ed.) (1970), *Pressman and Kelemen's Physiology of the Larynx.* Rochester, Minnesota: American Academy of Ophthalmology and Otolaryngology.

Kirchner, J. A. and Suzuki, M. (1968), "Laryngeal Reflexes and Voice Production," *Ann. N.Y. Acad. Sci.*, **155**, 98–109.

Kirchner, J. A. and Wyke, B. D. (1964a), "Innervation of Laryngeal Joints, and Laryngeal Reflexes," *Nature* (*Lond.*), **201**, 506.

Kirchner, J. A. and Wyke, B. D. (1964b), "The Innervation of the Laryngeal Joints in the Cat," *J. Anat.* (*Lond.*), **98**, 684.

Kirchner, J. A. and Wyke, B. D. (1964c), "Laryngeal Articular Reflexes," *Nature* (*Lond.*), **202**, 600.

Kirchner, J. A. and Wyke, B. D. (1964d), "Electromyographic Analysis of Laryngeal Articular Reflexes," *Nature* (*Lond.*), **203**, 1243–1245.

Kirchner, J. A. and Wyke, B. D. (1965a), "Afferent Discharges from Laryngeal Articular Mechanoreceptors," *Nature (Lond.)*, **205**, 86–87.

Kirchner, J. A. and Wyke, B. D. (1965b), "Articular Reflex Mechanisms in the Larynx," *Ann. Otol., Rhinol., Lar.*, **74**, 749–768.

Kirikae, H., Hirose, H., Kawamura, S., Sawashima, M. and Kobayashi, T. (1962), "An Experimental Study of Central Motor Innervation of the Laryngeal Muscles in the Cat," *Ann. Otol., Rhinol., Lar.*, **71**, 222–241.

Klatt, D. H., Stevens, K. N. and Mead, J. (1968), "Studies of Articulatory Activity and Airflow During Speech," *Ann. N.Y. Acad. Sci.*, **155**, 42–54.

Knutsson, E., Mårtensson, A. and Mårtensson, B. (1969), "The Normal Electromyogram in Human Vocal Muscles. *Acta otolaryng.*, **68**, 526–536.

Koizumi, H. (1953), "On the Sensory Innervation of the Larynx in the Dog," *Tohoku J. exp. Med.*, **58**, 199–210.

Kollár, A. (1973), "Inspiratorische Phonation bei der Behandlung von Stimmstörungen," *Folia phoniat.*, **25**, 221–224.

König, W. F. and von Leden, H. (1961a), "The Peripheral Nervous System of the Human Larynx. I. The Mucous Membrane," *Arch. Otolaryng.*, **73**, 1–14.

König, W. F. and von Leden, H. (1961b), "The Peripheral Nervous System of the Human Larynx. II. The Thyroarytenoid (Vocalis) Muscle," *Arch. Otolaryng.*, **74**, 153–163.

Konorski, J. (1961), "Pathophysiological Analysis of Various Forms of Speech Disorders and an Attempt at Their Classification," in *Pathophysiological Mechanisms of Disorders of Higher Nervous Activity After Brain Lesions in Man*, pp. 1–10. Warsaw; Polish Academy of Science.

Konrad, H. R. and Rattenborg, C. C. (1969), "Combined Action of Laryngeal Muscles," *Acta oto-laryng.*, **67**, 646–649.

Korpáš, J. (1972), "Expiration Reflex From the Vocal Folds," *Physiol. bohemoslov.*, **21**, 671–675.

Korpáš, J. and Gajdoš, E. (1971), "Mechanoreception of the Respiratory Tract in Guinea-pigs," *Physiol. bohemoslov.*, **20**, 623–630.

Kotby, M. N. and Haugen, L. K. (1970a), "The Mechanics of Laryngeal Function," *Acta oto-laryng.*, **70**, 203–211.

Kotby, M. N. and Haugen, L. K. (1970b), "Critical Evaluation of the Action of the Posterior Crico-arytenoid Muscle, Utilizing Direct EMG-study," *Acta oto-laryng.*, **70**, 260–268.

Kotby, M. N. and Haugen, L. K. (1970c), "Attempts at Evaluation of the Function of the Various Laryngeal Muscles in the Light of Muscle and Nerve Stimulation Experiments in Man," *Acta oto-laryng.*, **70**, 419–427.

Koyama, T., Harvey, J. E. and Ogura, J. H. (1971), "Mechanics of Voice Production. II. Regulation of Pitch," *Laryngoscope*, **81**, 47–65.

Koyama, T., Kawasaki, M. and Ogura, J. H. (1969), "Mechanics of Voice Production. I. Regulation of Vocal Intensity," *Laryngoscope*, **79**, 337–354.

Krause, H. (1884), "Ueber die Beziehungen der Grosshirnrinde zu Kehlkopf und Rachen," *Arch. ges. Physiol.*, **8**, 203–210.

Krmpotić, J. (1958), "Anatomisch-histologische und funktionelle Verhältnisse des rechten und des linken Nervus recurrens mit Rücksicht auf die Geschwindigkeit der Impulsleitung bei einer Ursprungsanomalie der rechten Schlüsselbeinarterie," *Arch. Ohr.-, Nas.-u. Kehlheilk.*, **173**, 490–496.

Kurozumi, S., Tashiro, T. and Harada, Y. (1971), "Laryngeal Responses to Electrical Stimulation of the Medullary Respiratory Centers in the Dog," *Laryngoscope*, **81**, 1960–1967.

Kuypers, H. G. J. M. (1958a), "An Anatomical Analysis of Cortico-bulbar Connexions to the Pons and Lower Brain Stem in the Cat," *J. Anat. (Lond.)*, **92**, 198–218.

Kuypers, H. G. J. M. (1958b), "Some Projections From the Pericentral Cortex to the Pons and Lower Brain Stem in Monkey and Chimpanzee," *J. comp. Neurol.*, **110**, 221–255.

Kuypers, H. G. J. M. (1958c), "Cortico-bulbar Connexions to the Pons and Lower Brain Stem in Man: an Anatomical Study," *Brain*, **81**, 364–388.

Ladefoged, P. (1960), "The Regulation of Sub-glottal Pressure," *Folia phoniat.*, **12**, 169–175.

Ladefoged, P. (1968), "Linguistic Aspects of Respiratory Phenomena," *Ann. N.Y. Acad. Sci.*, **155**, 141–151.

Ladefoged, P. (1973), "Respiration, Laryngeal Activity and Linguistics," in *Ventilatory and Phonatory Control Systems: An International Symposium*, pp. 299–307 (B. D. Wyke, Ed.). London: Oxford University Press.

Ladefoged, P. and McKinney, N. (1963), "Loudness, Sound Pressure and Subglottal Pressure in Speech," *J. acoust. Soc. Amer.*, **35**, 454–460.

Lam, R. L. and Ogura, J. H. (1952), "An Afferent Representation of the Larynx in the Cerebellum," *Laryngoscope*, **62**, 486–495.

Lanyon, W. E. and Tavolga, W. N. (Eds.) (1960), *Animal Sounds and Communication*. Washington: American Institute of Biological Sciences.

von Lanz, T. (1955), *Praktische Anatomie*. Berlin: Springer.

Lawn, A. M. (1966), "The Localisation, in the Nucleus Ambiguus of the Rabbit, of the Cells of Origin of Motor Nerve Fibres in the Glossopharyngeal Nerve and Various Branches of the Vagus Nerve by Means of Retrograde Degeneration," *J. comp. Neurol.*, **127**, 293–305.

von Leden, H. (1961), "The Mechanism of Phonation," *Arch. Otolaryng.*, **74**, 660–676.

von Leden, H. and Isshiki, N. (1965), "An Analysis of Cough at the Level of the Larynx," *Arch. Otolaryng.*, **81**, 616–625.

von Leden, H. and Moore, G. P. (1961), "The Mechanics of the Crico-arytenoid Joint," *Arch. Otolaryng.*, **73**, 541–550.

Lee, B. S. (1950), "Effects of Delayed Speech Feedback," *J. acoust. Soc. Amer.*, **22**, 824–826.

Lee, B. S. (1951), "Artificial Stutter," *J. Speech and Hear. Dis.*, **16**, 53–55.

Leksell, L. (1945), "The Action Potentials and Excitatory Effects of the Small Ventral Root Fibres to Skeletal Muscle," *Acta physiol. scand.*, **10**, suppl. 31, 1–84.

Lemere, F. (1932a), "Innervation of the Larynx. I. Innervation of Laryngeal Muscles," *Amer. J. Anat.*, **51**, 417–432.

Lemere, F. (1932b), "Innervation of the Larynx. II. Ramus Anastomoticus and Ganglion Cells of the Superior Laryngeal Nerve," *Anat. Rec.*, **54**, 389–407.

Lenman, J. A. R. (1969), "Integration and Analysis of the Electromyogram and Related Techniques," in *Disorders of Voluntary Muscle*, pp. 843–876. (J. N. Walton, Ed.). London: Churchill.

Lennenberg, E. H. (1962), "A Laboratory for Speech Research at the Children's Hospital Medical Center," *New Engl. J. Med.*, **266**, 385–392.

Levitt, M. N., Dedo, H. H. and Ogura, J. H. (1965), "The Cricopharyngeus Muscle: an Electromyographic Study in the Dog," *Laryngoscope*, **75**, 122–136.

Lieberman, P. (1968a), "Primate Vocalisations and Human Linguistic Ability," *J. acoust. Soc. Amer.*, **44**, 1574–1584.

Lieberman, P. (1968b), "Vocal Cord Motion in Man," *Ann. N.Y. Acad. Sci.*, **155**, 28–38.

Lippold, O. C. J. (1952), "The Relation Between Integrated Action Potentials in a Human Muscle and its Isometric Tension," *J. Physiol. (Lond.)*, **117**, 492–499.

Lucas Keene, M. F. (1961), "Muscle Spindles in Human Laryngeal Muscles," *J. Anat. (Lond.)*, **95**, 25–29.

Luchsinger, R. (1965), "Beitrag zur Diagnostik (Elektromyographie) isolierter peripherer Lähmungen des N. laryngeus cranialis," *Folia phoniat.*, **17**, 105–114.

Luchsinger, R. and Arnold, G. E. (1965), *Voice, Speech, Language*. Belmont, California: Wadsworth.

Lund, W. S. and Ardran, G. M. (1964), "The Motor Nerve Supply of the Cricopharyngeal Sphincter," *Ann. Otol., Rhinol., Lar.*, **73**, 599–617.

McGall, G. N. and Rabuzzi, D. D. (1973), "Reflex Contraction of Middle-ear Muscles Secondary to Stimulation of Laryngeal Nerves," *J. Speech and Hear. Res.*, **16**, 56–61.

Mårtensson, A. (1963), "Reflex Responses and Recurrent Discharges Evoked by Stimulation of Laryngeal Nerves," *Acta physiol. scand.*, **57**, 248–269.

Mårtensson, A. (1964), "Proprioceptive Impulse Patterns During Contraction of Intrinsic Laryngeal Muscles," *Acta physiol. scand.*, **62**, 176–194.

Mårtensson, A. (1973), "Discussion," in *Ventilatory and Phonatory Control Systems: An International Symposium,* pp. 389–390 (B. D. Wyke, Ed.). London: Oxford University Press.

Mårtensson, A. and Skoglund, C. R. (1964), "Contraction Properties of Intrinsic Laryngeal Muscles," *Acta physiol. scand.,* **60,** 318–336.

Matsumoto, T. (1950), "Innervation, Especially Sensory Innervation, of the Laryngeal Mucosa Except the Epiglottis," *Tohoku med. J.,* **45,** 11–18.

Matthews, P. B. C. (1972), *Mammalian Muscle Receptors and Their Central Actions.* London: Arnold.

Mayet, A. (1956), "Zur Innervation des M. cricothyroideus," *Anat. Anz.,* **103,** 340–343.

Mead, J., Bouhuys, A. and Proctor, D. F. (1968), "Mechanisms Generating Subglottic Pressure," *Ann. N.Y. Acad. Sci.,* **155,** 177–181.

Mead, J. and Bunn, F. C. (1973), "Speech as Breathing," in *Ventilatory and Phonatory Control Systems: An International Symposium,* pp. 33–38 (B. D. Wyke, Ed.). London: Oxford University Press.

Mei, N. and Nourigat, B. (1967), "Etude électrophysiologique des neurons sensitifs du nerf laryngé supérieur," *C. R. Soc. Biol.* (*Paris*), **162,** 149–153.

Merrill, E. G. (1970), "The Lateral Respiratory Neurones of the Medulla: Their Associations with Nucleus Ambiguus, Nucleus Retro-ambigualis, the Spinal Accessory Nucleus and the Spinal Cord," *Brain Res.,* **24,** 11–28.

Meyer-Eppler, W. and Luchsinger, R. (1955), "Beobachtungen bei der versögerten Ruckkopplung der Sprache," *Folia phoniat.,* **7,** 87–99.

Mitchell, G. A. G. (1954), "The Autonomic Nerve Supply of the Throat, Nose and Ear," *J.. Laryng.,* **68,** 495–516.

Mitchinson, A. G. and Yoffey, J. M. (1947), "Respiratory Displacement of the Larynx, Hyoid Bone and Tongue," *J. Anat. (Lond.),* **81,** 118–120.

Molinari, G. A. and Pivotti, G. S. (1962), "Sul reperto di fibre tensocettrici polmonari nel nerve laringeo ricorrente," *II Valsalva,* **38,** 207–214.

Moore, G. P. (1971), *Organic Voice Disorders.* Englewood Cliffs, New Jersey: Prentice-Hall.

Moore, G. P., White, F. D. and von Leden, H. (1962), "Ultra-high Speed Photography in Laryngeal Physiology," *J. Speech and Hear. Dis.,* **27,** 165–171.

Moses, P. J. (1958), "Psychosomatic Aspects of Inspiratory Voice," *Arch. Otolaryng.,* **67,** 390–393.

Mündnich, K. (1956), "Anatomische und histologische Untersuchungen und Experimente zur Physiologie und Pathologie des menschlichen Kehlkopfes," *Arch. Ohr.-, Nas.-u. Kehlkheilk.,* **169,** 190–196.

Murakami, Y. and Kirchner, J. A. (1971a), "Reflex Tensor Mechanism of the Larynx by External Laryngeal Muscles," *Ann. Otol., Rhinol., Lar.,* **80,** 46–60.

Murakami, Y. and Kirchner, J. A. (1971b), "Electrophysiological Properties of Laryngeal Reflex Closure," *Acta oto-laryng.,* **71,** 416–425.

Murakami, Y. and Kirchner, J. A. (1972a), "Mechanical and Physiological Properties of Reflex Laryngeal Closure," *Ann. Otol., Rhinol., Lar.,* **81,** 59–71.

Murakami, Y. and Kirchner, J. A. (1972b), "Respiratory Movements of the Vocal Cords: an Electromyographic Study in the Cat," *Laryngoscope,* **82,** 454–467.

Murakami, Y. and Kirchner, J. A. (1973), "Respiratory Activity of External Laryngeal Muscles: an Electromyographic Study in the Cat," in *Ventilatory and Phonatory Control Systems: An International Symposium,* pp. 430–448 (B. D. Wyke, Ed.). London: Oxford University Press.

Murray, J. G. (1957), "Innervation of the Intrinsic Muscles of the Cat's Larynx by the Recurrent Laryngeal Nerve: a Unimodal Nerve," *J. Physiol. (Lond.),* **135,** 206–212.

Murtagh, J. A. and Campbell C. J. (1954), "Laryngeal Spasm," *Laryngoscope,* **64,** 154–171.

Mysak, E. D. (1966), *Speech Pathology and Feedback Theory.* Springfield, Illinois: Thomas.

Nakamura, F. (1964), "Movement of the Larynx Induced by Electrical Stimulation of the Laryngeal Nerves," in *Research Potentials in Voice Physiology,* pp. 129–135. (D. W. Brewer, Ed.). New York: State University of New York.

Nakamura, F., Uyeda, Y. and Sonoda, Y. (1958), "Electromyographic Study on Respiratory Movements of the Intrinsic Laryngeal Muscles," *Laryngoscope,* **68,** 109–119.

Nakamura, N. (1915), Cited by Hosokawa (1961).

Napier, J. and Barnicot, N. A. (Eds.) (1963), *The Primates. Zool. Soc. Lond. Symp.,* **10,** 1–285.

Negus, V. E. (1929), *The Mechanism of the Larynx.* London: Heinemann.

Negus, V. E. (1949), *The Comparative Anatomy and Physiology of the Larynx.* London: Heinemann.

Negus, V. E. (1965), *The Biology of Respiration.* Edinburgh: Livingstone.

Negus, V. E., Neil, E. and Floyd, W. F. (1957), "The Mechanisms of Phonation," *Ann. Otol., Rhinol., Lar.,* **66,** 817–829.

Obersteiner, H. (1912), *Anleitung beim Studium des Baues der nervösen Zentralorgane im gesunden und kranken Zustande.* Leipzig: Deuticke.

Ogura, J. H. and Lam, R. L. (1953), "Anatomical and Physiological Correlations on Stimulating the Human Superior Laryngeal Nerve," *Laryngoscope,* **63,** 947–959.

Ohyama, M., Ueda, N., Harvey, J. E. Mogi, G. and Ogura, J. H. (1972a), "Electrophysiologic Study of Reinnervated Laryngeal Motor Units," *Laryngoscope,* **82,** 237–251.

Ohyama, M., Ueda, N., Harvey, J. E., Mogi, G. and Ogura, J. H. (1972b), "The Action of Certain Neuromuscular Blocking Agents on the Laryngeal Muscles in the Dog," *Laryngoscope,* **82,** 483–489.

Ónodi, A. (1902), *Die Anatomie und Physiologie der Kehlkopfnerven.* Berlin: Coblentz.

Ottonello, P. (1941), "Singolari alterazioni della loquela (incoordinazione verbo-mimico-emotiva) rilevate nel de corso dei processi morbosi endocranici con interessamento dell' apparato cerebellare," *Riv. Patol. nerv. ment.,* **57,** 131–161.

Paintal, A. S. (1970), "The Mechanism of Excitation of Type-J Receptors and the J-reflex," in *Breathing: Hering-Breuer Centenary Symposium,* pp. 59–70 (R. Porter, Ed.). London: Churchill.

Paulsen, K. (1958a), "Untersuchungen über das Verkommen und die Zahl von Muskelspindeln im M. vocalis des Menschen," *Z. Zellforsch. mikr. Anat.,* **47,** 363–366.

Paulsen, K. (1958b), "Über Vorkommen und Zahl von Muskelspindeln in inneren Kehlkopfmuskeln des Menschen (M. cricoarytenoideus dorsalis, M. cricothyroideus)," *Z. Zellforsch., mikr. Anat.,* **48,** 349–355.

Paulsen, K. (1958c), "Über die Bedeutung von Muskelspindeln und Schleimhautreceptoren bei der Phonation," *Arch. Ohr.-, Nas.-u. Kehlkheilk.,* **173,** 500–503.

Penfield, W. and Jasper, H. (1954), *Epilepsy and the Functional Anatomy of the Human Brain.* London: Churchill.

Penfield, W. and Rasmussen, T. (1949), "Vocalization and Arrest of Speech," *Arch. Neurol. Psychiat. (Chicago),* **61,** 21–27.

Penfield, W. and Roberts, L. (1959), *Speech and Brain-Mechanisms.* Princeton: Princeton University Press.

Peters, M. and Ploog, D. (1973), "Communication Among Primates," *Ann. Rev. Physiol.,* **35,** 221–242.

Petitpierre, C. (1943), "L'activité respiratoire du nerf laryngé supérieur," *Helv. physiol. pharmacol. Acta,* **1,** 325–328.

Peytz, F., Rasmussen, H. and Buchthal, F. (1965), "Conduction Time and Velocity in Human Recurrent Laryngeal Nerve," *Danish med. Bull.,* **12,** 125–127.

Pichler, H. and Gisel, A. (1957), "The Clinical Significance of the Ramification of the Recurrent Laryngeal Nerves," *Laryngoscope,* **67,** 105–117.

Piquet, J. and Barets, A. (1960), "Observations sur l'innervation motrice du muscle vocal," *Acta oto-laryng.,* **51,** 203–206.

Piquet, J., Hoffmann, K. and Husson, R. (1957), "Recherches histologiques sur le nerf récurrent et sur les plaques motrices de la musculature laryngée intrinsique de l'homme," *Montpellier méd.,* **51,** 367–380.

Pollis, R. (1969), *Diameters of Nerve Fibers Supplying the Abductor and Adductor Muscles of the Larynx,* M. D. Thesis, Yale University.

Porter, R. (1963), "Unit Responses Evoked in the Medulla Oblongata by Vagus Nerve Stimulation," *J. Physiol (Lond.),* **168,** 717–735.

Portmann, G., Humbert, R,, Robin, J.-L., Laget, P. and Husson, R. (1955), "Etude électromyographique des cordes vocales chez l'homme," *C. R. Soc. Biol. Biol. (Paris)*, **149**, 296–300.

Portmann, G. Robin, J.-L., Laget, P. and Husson, R. (1956), "La myographie des cordes vocales," *Acta oto-laryng.*, **46**, 250–263.

Pressman, J. (1941), "Sphincter Action of the Larynx," *Arch. otolaryng.*, **33**, 351–377.

Pressman, J. (1942), "Physiology of the Vocal Cords in Phonation and Respiration," *Arch. Otolaryng.*, **35**, 355–398.

Pressman, J. (1953), "The Sphincters of the Larynx," *Trans. Amer. Acad. Ophthal. Otolaryng.*, **57**, 724–737.

Pressman, J. (1954), "Sphincters of the Larynx," *Arch. Otolaryng.*, **59**, 221–236.

Proctor, D. F. (1973a), "Breathing Mechanics During Phonation and Singing," in *Ventilatory and Phonatory Control Systems: An International Symposium*, pp. 39–57 (B. D. Wyke, Ed.). London: Oxford University Press.

Proctor, D. F. (1973b), "Discussion," in *Ventilatory and Phonatory Control Systems: An International Symposium*, pp. 293–295 (B. D. Wyke, Ed.). London: Oxford University Press.

Ranson, S. W. and Clark, S. L. (1959), *The Anatomy of the Nervous System*, 10th edition. Philadelphia: Saunders.

Rattenborg, C. C., Barton, M. D., Kain, M. L., Logan, W. J., Konrad, H. R. and Holaday, D. A. (1963), "Reflex Activity of the Larynx During Breathing," *Anesthesiology*, **24**, 139–140.

Rattenborg, C. C., Kain, M. L., Logan, W. J. and Holaday, D. A. (1962), "Laryngeal Opening During Inspiration," *Fed. Proc.*, **21**, 446.

Réthi, A. (1951), "Histological Analysis of the Experimentally Degenerated Vagus Nerve," *Acta morph. Acad. Sci. Hung.*, **1**, 221–234.

Réthi, A. (1962), "L'innervation du larynx," *Acta otorinolaryngol. ibero-amer.*, **13**, 585–595.

Roberto, V. (1957), "La distribution et les aspects morphologiques du contingent nerveux dans la muqueuse du larynx de l'homme," *Montpellier méd.*, **51**, 322–366.

Rose, J. E., Greenwood, D. D., Goldberg, J. M. and Hind, J. E. (1963), "Some Discharge Characteristics of Single Neurons in the Inferior Colliculus of the Cat," *J. Neurophysiol.*, **26**, 294–320.

Rossi, G. and Cortesina, G. (1965), "Morphological Study of the Laryngeal Muscles in Man," *Acta oto-laryng.*, **59**, 575–592.

Rubin, H. J. (1960), "The Neurochronaxic Theory of Voice Production – a Refutation," *Arch. Otolaryng.*, **71**, 913–920.

Rubin, H. J. (1963), "Experimental Studies on Vocal Pitch and Intensity in Phonation," *Laryngoscope*, **73**, 973–1015.

Rubin, H.J., LeCover, M. and Vennard, W. (1967), "Vocal Intensity, Subglottic Pressure and Air Flow in Relationship to Singers," *Folia phoniat.*, **19**, 393–413.

Rudolph, G. (1960a), "Recherches neurohistologiques sur l'innervation de la corde vocale," in *Activités neurophysiologiques*, 2ème ser., pp. 321–345. Paris: Masson.

Rudolph, G. (1960b), "Multiple Innervation von Muskelfasern im *M. vocalis* des Menschen," *Experientia*, **16**, 551–553.

Rudolph, G. (1961), "Spiral Nerve Endings (Proprioceptors) in the Human Vocal Muscle," *Nature (Lond.)*, **190**, 726–727.

Rudomín, P. (1964), "Some Aspects of the Reflex Activation of the Recurrent Laryngeal Motoneurones of the Cat," *Bol. Inst. Estud. med. biol. (Méx.)*, **22**, 341–353.

Rudomín, P. (1965a), "The Influence of the Motor Cortex Upon the Vagal Motoneurones of the Cat," *Acta physiol. latino-amer.*, **15**, 171–179.

Rudomín, P. (1965b), "Recurrent Laryngeal Nerve Discharges Produced Upon Stimulation of the Bulbar Pyramidal Tract and Nearby Structures," *Acta physiol. latino-amer.*, **15**, 180–190.

Rudomín, P. (1966a), "The Electrical Activity of the Cricothyroid Muscles of the Cat," *Arch. int. Physiol.*, **74**, 135–153.

Rudomín, P. (1966b), "Some Aspects of the Control of Cricothyroid Muscle Activity," *Arch. int. Physiol.*, **74**, 154–168.

Ruëdi, L. (1959), "Some Observations on the Histology and Function of the Larynx," *J. Laryng.*, **73**, 1–20.

Rueger, R. S. (1972), "The Superior Laryngeal Nerve and the Interarytenoid Muscle in Humans: an Anatomical Study," *Laryngoscope*, **82**, 2008–2031.

Salomon, G. and Starr, A. (1963), "Electromyography of Middle Ear Muscles in Man During Motor Activities," *Acta neurol. scand.*, **39**, 161–168.

Sampson, S. and Eyzaguirre, C. (1964), "Some Functional Characteristics of Mechanoreceptors in the Larynx of the Cat," *J. Neurophysiol.*, **27**, 464–480.

Sasaki, C. T., Fukuda, H. and Kirchner, J. A. (1973), "Laryngeal Abductor Activity in Response to Varying Ventilatory Resistance." In press.

Sauerland, E. K. and Mizuno, M. (1968), "Hypoglossal Nerve Afferents: Elicitation of a Polysynaptic Hypoglosso-laryngeal Reflex," *Brain Res.*, **10**, 256–258.

Sawashima, M., Sato, M. Funasaka, S. and Totsuka, G. (1958), "Electromyographic Study of the Human Larynx and its Clinical Application," *Jap. J. Otol.*, **61**, 1357–1364.

Scevola, P. (1950), "A proposito dei dispositivi di blocco a livello dei vasi arteriosi e venosi del labbro vocale," *Arch. ital. Otol.*, **61**, 234–242.

Scheuer, J. Louise (1964), "Fibre Size Frequency Distribution in Normal Human Laryngeal Nerves," *J. Anat. (Lond.)*, **98**, 99–104.

Semon, F. (1881), "Clinical Remarks on the Proclivity of the Abductor Fibres of the Recurrent Laryngeal Nerves to Become Affected Sooner Than the Adductor Fibres, or Even Exclusively, in Cases of Undoubted Central or Peripheral Injury or Disease of the Roots or Trunks of the Pneumogastric, Spinal Accessory, or Recurrent Nerves," *Arch. Laryng.*, **2**, 197–222.

Semon, F. (1890), "On the Position of the Vocal Cords in Quiet Respiration of Man, and the Reflex Tonus of Their Abductor Muscles," *Proc. roy. Soc. Lond.*, **48B**, 156–159; 403–405.

Semon, F. and Horsley, V. (1890), "Experimental Investigation of the Central Motor Innervation of the Larynx," *Philos. Trans. roy. Soc. Lond.*, **181B**, 187–211.

Serra, C. (1964), "Neuromuscular Studies on Various Oto-laryngological Problems," *Electromyography*, **4**, 254–294.

Sessle, B. J. and Storey, A. T. (1972), "Periodontal and Facial Influences on the Laryngeal Input to the Brain Stem of the Cat," *Arch. oral Biol.*, **17**, 1583–1595.

Seymour, J. C. and Henry, H. S. (1954), "Some Experimental Observations on the Innervation of the Larynx in Cats," *J. Laryng.*, **68**, 225–228.

Shearer, W. M. and Sommons, F. B. (1965), "Middle Ear Activity During Speech in Normal Speakers and Stutterers," *J. Speech and Hear. Res.*, **8**, 203–207.

Shedd, D. P., Kirchner, J. A. and Scatliff, J. H. (1961), "Oral and Pharyngeal Components of Deglutition," *Arch. Surg.*, **82**, 373–380.

Shin, T. and Rabuzzi, D. D. (1971), "Conduction Studies of the Canine Recurrent Laryngeal Nerve," *Laryngoscope*, **81**, 586–596.

Shin, T., Rabuzzi, D. D. and Reed, G. F. (1970), "Vasomotor Responses to Laryngeal Nerve Stimulation," *Arch. Otolaryng.*, **91**, 257–261.

Sonninen, A. A. (1956), "The Role of the External Laryngeal Muscles in Length-adjustment of the Vocal Cords in Singing," *Acta oto-laryng.*, suppl. 130, 1–102.

Sonninen, A. A. (1968), "The External Frame Function in the Control of Pitch in the Human Voice," *Ann. N.Y. Acad. Sci.*, **155**, 68–89.

Sovak, M., Courtois, J., Haas, C. and Smith, S. (1971), "Observations on the Mechanism of Phonation Investigated by Ultraspeed Cinefluorography," *Folia phoniat.*, **23**, 277–287.

Spoor, A. and van Dishoeck, H. A. E. (1958), "Electromyography of the Human Vocal Cords and the Theory of Husson," *Pract. oto-rhino-laryng. (Basel)*, **20**, 353–360.

Stanton, J. B. (1958), "The Effects of Delayed Auditory Feedback on the Speech of Aphasic Patients," *Scot. med. J.*, **3**, 378–384.

Stevens, K. N. and Klatt, D. H. (1973), "Current Models of Sound Sources for Speech," in *Ventilatory and Phonatory Control Systems: An International Symposium*, pp. 279–292. (B. D. Wyke, Ed.). London: Oxford University Press.

Stransky, A., Szereda-Przestaszewska, M. and Widdicombe, J. G. (1973), "The Effects of Lung Reflexes on Laryngeal Resistance and Motoneurone Discharge," *J. Physiol. (Lond.)*, **231**, 417–438.

Strauss, S. G., Fukuda, H. and Kirchner, J. A. (1973), "Arterial Baroreceptor Fibers in the Recurrent Laryngeal Nerve," *Ann. Otol., Rhinol., Lar.*, **82**, 228–234.

Sugano, M. (1929), "On the Laryngeal Nerves" (Japanese text), *J. oto-rhino-laryng. Soc. Japan*, **35**, 1338–1361, 1362–1375, 1369–1400.

Sunderland, S. and Swaney, W. E. (1952), "The Intraneural Topography of the Recurrent Laryngeal Nerve in Man," *Anat. Rec.*, **114**, 411–426.

Sunder-Plassmann, P. (1933a), "Über den Nervenapparät des Musculus vocalis," *Zeit. Hals.-, Nas.-, Ohrenheilk.*, **32**, 493–499.

Sunder-Plassmann, P. (1933b), Über den Nervenapparät des menschlichen Glottisöffners, Musculus crico-arytenoideus positicus," *Z. Hals-, Nas.- u. Ohrenheilk.*, **32**, 586–598.

Sutton, D., Larson, C. R. and Farrell, D. M. (1972), "Cricothyroid Motor Units," *Acta oto-laryng.*, **74**, 145–151.

Suzuki, M. and Kirchner, J. A. (1967), "Laryngeal Reflex Pathways Related to Rate and Rhythm of the Heart," *Ann. Otol., Rhinol., Lar.*, **76**, 774–780.

Suzuki, M. and Kirchner, J. A. (1968), "Afferent Nerve Fibers in the External Branch of the Superior Laryngeal Nerve in the Cat," *Ann. Otol., Rhinol., Lar.*, **77**, 1059–1070.

Suzuki, M. and Kirchner, J. A. (1969a), "Sensory Fibers in the Recurrent Laryngeal Nerve: an Electrophysiological Study of Some Laryngeal Afferent Fibers in the Recurrent Laryngeal Nerve of the Cat," *Ann. Otol., Rhinol., Lar.*, **78**, 21–32.

Suzuki, M. and Kirchner, J. A. (1969b), "The Posterior Crico-arytenoid as an Inspiratory Muscle," *Ann. Otol., Rhinol., Lar.*, **78**, 849–865.

Suzuki, M., Kirchner, J. A. and Murakami Y. (1970), "The Cricothyroid as a Respiratory Muscle: its Characteristics in Bilateral Recurrent Laryngeal Nerve Paralysis," *Ann. Otol., Rhinol., Lar.*, **79**, 976–984.

Szabo, T. and Dussardier, M. (1964), "Les noyaux d'origine du nerf vague chez le mouton," *Z. Zellforsch. mikr. Anat.*, **63**, 247–276.

Szentágothai, J. (1943), "Die Lokalisation der Kehlkopfmuskulatur in den Vaguskernen," *Z. Anat. Entw. Gesch.*, **112**, 704–710.

Szentágothai, J. and Rajkovits, K. (1958), "Der Hirnnervenanteil der Pyramidenbahn und der prämotorische Apparat motorischer Hirnnervenkerne," *Arch. Psychiat. Nervenkr.*, **197**, 335–354.

Takenouchi, S., Koyama, T., Kawasaki, M. and Ogura, J. H. (1968), "Movements of the Vocal Cords," *Acta oto-laryng.*, **65**, 33–50.

Terracol, J. and Greiner, G. F. (1971), *Le larynx: bases anatomiques et fonctionelles*. Paris: Doin.

Timmons, B. A. and Boudreau, J. P. (1972), "Auditory Feedback as a Major Factor in Stuttering," *J. Speech and Hear. Dis.*, **37**, 476–484.

Tomasch, J. and Britton, W. A. (1953), "A Fibre Analysis of the Laryngeal Nerve Supply in Man," *Acta anat. (Basel)*, **23**, 386–398.

Ueda, N., Ohyama, M., Harvey, J. E., Mogi, G. and Ogura, J. H. (1971), "Subglottic Pressure and Induced Live Voices of Dogs with Normal, Reinnervated and Paralyzed Larynges. I. On Voice Function of the Dog with a Normal Larynx," *Laryngoscope*, **81**, 1948–1959.

Ueda, N., Ohyama, M., Harvey, J. E. and Ogura, J. H. (1972), "Influence of Certain Extrinsic Laryngeal Muscles on Artificial Voice Production," *Laryngoscope*, **82**, 468–482.

Van den Berg, J. (1955), "On the Role of the Laryngeal Ventricle in Voice Production," *Folia phoniat.*, **7**, 57–69.

Van den Berg, J. (1956), "Direct and Indirect Determination of the Mean Subglottic Pressure," *Folia phoniat.*, **8**, 1–24.

Van den Berg, J. (1958), "Myoelastic-aerodynamic Theory of Voice Production," *J. Speech and Hear. Res.*, **1**, 227–244.

Van den Berg, J. (1964), "Some Physical Aspects of Voice Production," in *Research Potentials in Voice Physiology*, pp. 63–101. (D. W. Brewer, Ed.). New York: State University of New York.

Van Harreveld, A. and Tachibana, S. (1961), "Innervation and Reinnervation of Cricothyroid Muscle in the Rabbit," *Amer. J. Physiol.*, **201**, 1199–1202.

Van Michel, C. (1963), "Considérations morphologiques sur les appareils sensoriels de la muqueuse vocale humaine," *Acta anat. (Basel)*, **52**, 188–192.

Van Michel, C. and Gerebtzoff, M. A. (1962), "Aspects particuliers de l'innervation motrice dans les muscles striés de type squelettique chez les mammifères," *Verhandl. I. Europ. Anatomen-Kongr., Strasburg* (1960), pp. 408–427 (M. Watzka and H. Voss, Eds.). Jena: Fischer.

Van Riper, C. (1971), *The Nature of Stuttering*. Englewood Cliffs, New Jersey: Prentice-Hall.

Voss, H. (1966) "Untersuchungen über Vorkommen, Zahl und individuelle Variation der Muskelspindeln in den Muskeln des menschlichen Kehlkopfes," *Anat. Anz.*, **118**, 305–309.

Vrettos, X. C. and Wyke, B. D. (1973), "Articular Reflex Systems in the Costovertebral Joints," *Proc. Brit. Orthopaed. Res. Soc.*, Oct., pp. 16–17.

Weddell, G., Feinstein, B. and Pattle, R. E. (1944), "The Electrical Activity of Voluntary Muscle in Man Under Normal and Pathological Conditions," *Brain*, **67**, 178–257.

Weiss, D. A. (1959), "Discussion of the Neurochronaxic Theory (Husson), *Arch. Oto-laryng.*, **70**, 607–618.

Whitfield, E. C. (1967), *The Auditory Pathway*. London: Arnold.

Widdicombe, J. (1964), "Respiratory Reflexes," in *Handbook of Physiology*, Sec. 3, Vol. I, pp. 585–630 (W. O. Fenn and H. Rahn, Eds.). Washington: American Physiological Society.

Widdicombe, J. (1973a), "Pulmonary Reflex Mechanisms in Ventilatory Regulation," in *Ventilatory and Phonatory Control Systems: An International Symposium*, pp. 131–143 (B. D. Wyke, Ed.). London: Oxford University Press.

Widdicombe, J. (1973b), "Supplementary Statement II," in *Ventilatory and Phonatory Control Systems: An International Symposium*, pp. 465–468 (B. D. Wyke, Ed.). London: Oxford University Press.

Widdicombe, J. (1973c), "Discussion," in *Ventilatory and Phonatory Control Systems: An International Symposium*, pp. 144–153 (B. D. Wyke, Ed.). London: Oxford University Press.

Williams, A. F. (1951), "The Nerve Supply of the Laryngeal Muscles," *J. Laryng.*, **65**, 343–348.

Williams, A. F. (1954), "The Recurrent Laryngeal Nerve and the Thyroid Gland," *J. Laryng.*, **68**, 719–725.

Wilson, V. J. (1966), "Regulation and Function of Renshaw Cell Discharge," in *Muscular Afferents and Motor Control* (Nobel Symposium), pp. 317–329 (R. Granit, Ed.). Stockholm: Almqvist and Wiksell.

Winckel, F. (1952), "Elektroakustische Untersuchungen an der menschlichen Stimme," *Folia phoniat.*, **4**, 93–113.

Winckel, F. (1973), "Acoustical Cues in the Voice for Detecting Laryngeal Diseases and Individual Behaviour," in *Ventilatory and Phonatory Control Systems: An International Symposium*, pp. 248–260 (B. D. Wyke, Ed.). London: Oxford University Press.

Winckler, G. (1957a), "L'innervation proprioceptive des muscles soushyoïdiens et genio-hyoïdien chez l'homme," *Arch. Anat. (Strasbourg)*, **40**, 171–178.

Winckler, G. (1957b), "Les différents critères de l'innervation proprioceptive des muscles du larynx chez l'homme," *Arch. Anat. Pathol., Paris*, **33**, 141–143.

Withington, J. Louise (1959), *Comparative Studies of the Nerve Supply of the Larynx with Special Reference to the Afferent Innervation of the Musculature*, Ph.D. Thesis, University of London.

Woldring, S. (1968), "Breathing Patterns During Speech in Deaf Children," *Ann. N.Y. Acad. Sci.*, **155**, 206–207.

Wyke, B. D. (1947), "Clinical Physiology of the Cerebellum," *Med. J. Aust.*, **2**, 533–540.

Wyke, B. D. (1958), "Surgical Considerations of the Temporal Lobes," *Ann. roy. Coll. Surg. Engl.*, **22**, 3–24.

Wyke, B. D. (1959), "The Cortical Control of Movement: A Contribution to the Surgical Physiology of Seizures," *Epilepsia*, **1**, 4–35.

Wyke, B. D. (1967a), "The Neurology of Joints" (Arris and Gale Lecture), *Ann. roy. Coll. Surg. Wngl.*, **41**, 25–50.

Wyke, B. D. (1967b), "Recent Advances in the Neurology of Phonation: Phonatory Reflex Mechanisms in the Larynx," *Brit. J. Dis. Communic.*, **2**, 2–14.

Wyke, B. D. (1968), "Effects of Anaesthesia Upon Intrinsic Laryngeal Reflexes," *J. Laryng.*, **82**, 603–612.

Wyke, B. D. (1969a), "Deus ex machina vocis: Analysis of the Laryngeal Reflex Mechanisms of Speech" (Jansson Memorial Lecture), *Brit. J. Dis. Communic.*, **4**, 3–25.

Wyke, B. D. (1969b), *Principles of General Neurology. An Introduction to the Basic Principles of Medical and Surgical Neurology.* London and Amsterdam: Elsevier.

Wyke, B. D. (1970), "Neurological Mechanisms in Stammering: an Hypothesis," *Brit. J. Dis. Communic.*, **5**, 6–15.

Wyke, B. D. (1971), "The Neurology of Stammering," *J. psychosomat. Res.*, **15**, 423–432.

Wyke, B. D. (1972), "Articular Neurology: a Review," *Physiotherapy*, **58**, 94–99.

Wyke, B. D. (1973a), "Respiratory Activity of Intrinsic Laryngeal Muscles: an Experimental Study," in *Ventilatory and Phonatory Control Systems: An International Symposium*, pp. 408–429 (B. D. Wyke, Ed.). London: Oxford University Press.

Wyke, B. D. (Ed.) (1973b), *Ventilatory and Phonatory Control Systems. An International Symposium.* London: Oxford University Press.

Wyke, B. D. (1973c), "Myotatic Reflexogenic Systems in the Intrinsic Muscles of the Larynx," *Folia morphol.*, *Prague*, **21**, 113–118.

Wyke, B. D. (1973d), "Laryngeal Neuromuscular Control Systems in Singing: a Review of Current Concepts," *Folia phoniat.* In press.

Wyke, Maria A. (1971), "Dysphasia: a Review of Recent Progress," *Brit. med. Bull.*, **27**, 211–217.

Yagi, M. (1964), "Electromyographic Study on Respiratory Movement of the Intrinsic Laryngeal Muscles," *Clinica otorhinol. Jap.*, **56**, 389–397.

Yamamoto, S., Miyajima, M. and Urabe, M. (1960), "Respiratory Neuronal Activities in Spinal Afferents of Cat," *Jap. J. Physiol.*, **10**, 509–517.

Yamamoto, S., Sugihara, S. and Kuru, M. (1956), "Microelectrode Studies on Sensory Afferents in Posterior Funiculus of Cat," *Jap. J. Physiol.*, **6**, 68–85.

Yamashita, T. and Urabe, K. (1959), "Über den Stimmbandtensorreflex," *Z. Laryng. Rhinol. Otol.*, **38**, 759–766.

Yamashita, T. and Urabe, K. (1960), "Glottisschlussreflex und M. cricoarytaenoideus posterior," *Arch. Ohr.-, Nas.-u. Kehlkheilk.*, **177**, 39–44.

Yanagihara, N. and Koike, Y. (1967), "The Regulation of Sustained Phonation," *Folia phoniat.*, **19**, 1–18.

Yates, A. J. (1963), "Delayed Auditory Feedback," *Psychol. Bull.*, **60**, 213–232.

Zemlin, W. R. (1969), "The Effect of Topical Anaesthesia on Internal Laryngeal Behaviour," *Acta oto-laryng.*, **68**, 169–176.

Zenker, W. (1964a), "Vocal Muscle Fibers and Their Motor Endplates," in *Research Potentials in Voice Physiology*, pp. 1–17 (D. W. Brewer, Ed.). New York: State University of New York.

Zenker, W. (1964b), "Questions Regarding the Function of External Laryngeal Muscles," in *Research Potentials in Voice Physiology*, pp. 20–29 (D. W. Brewer, Ed.). New York: State University of New York.

Zenker, W. and Zenker, A. (1960), "Über die Regelung der Stimmlippenspannung durch von aussen eingreifende Mechanismen," *Folia phoniat.*, **12**, 1–36.

Zentay, P. J. (1937), "Motor Disorders of the Central Nervous System and Their Significance for Speech. I. Cerebral and Cerebellar Dysarthrias," *Laryngoscope*, **47**, 147–156.

41. LARYNX—MEASUREMENT OF FUNCTION

HANS VON LEDEN

INTRODUCTION

The past decades have witnessed increasing interest in the maintenance and restoration of the normal physiological processes in all branches of medicine. This concentration on the function of various human organs or systems has resulted in the development of objective examinations for their measurement. In the field of laryngology, the importance of mass communications and the evolution of surgical procedures for the improvement of voice have created new interest in the improvement of function studies for the accurate diagnosis of laryngeal diseases and voice disorders. These modern diagnostic studies do not replace the traditional examination of the larynx and voice. Current adaptations of electronic facilities complement the eyes and ears of the examiner and furnish precise measurements for prognostic and therapeutic purposes.

Measurements of laryngeal function may be classified into four main categories: vibratory studies, laryngeal dynamics, vocal acoustics and neuromuscular tests. Abnormalities in the vibratory pattern of the vocal folds can be determined by various examinations, e.g. stroboscopy, glottography or cinematography. Aerodynamic investigations of the sound producing system present valuable information about the efficiency of the larynx in translating air pressure into acoustic signals. Several acoustic tests afford an accurate assessment of the acoustic parameters of the sound produced. Ancillary facilities include the utilization of electromyography for the evaluation of different laryngeal muscles, neurosensory studies for the determination of the neurologic component, and computers for an analysis of mathematical models and complex measurements.

The resulting data present a kaleidoscopic picture of the larynx in action and an accurate assessment of the end product—the human voice. This multidimensional approach permits a comprehensive image of the vocal function for diagnostic and prognostic studies, medicolegal evaluations, therapeutic determinations, and for applied research in laryngology and phoniatry. The medical application of these scientific measurements offers substantial clinical benefits for both physician and patient, for their sensitivity often permits the discovery of early changes in the larynx before the eyes and ears of the examiner detect the underlying physiologic or pathologic aberrations.

VIBRATORY MEASUREMENTS

The complex vibratory pattern of the vocal folds during phonation represents one of the best indicators of laryngeal function. The intricate movements of the vocal folds depend on several interrelated factors: the substance and tension of the vocal folds, the texture of the mucous membrane and the subglottic pressure. Virtually all diseases (inflammations, neoplasms, fibroses, paralyses) of the sound producing system affect one or more of these elements. Special techniques are necessary for the study of vibratory phenomena, because the unaided human eye is limited to the perception of 5 distinct images per second. By contrast, during normal phonation the vocal folds oscillate at speeds of 100–250 vibrations per second and a singer may attain 1 000 or even 2 000 excursions per second during the production of a high note.

In recent years, various methods have been employed for an evaluation of the vibratory pattern, but only three of these techniques have stood the test of scientific experience. The most accurate measurements are obtained from ultra-high speed motion pictures of the vibrating vocal folds, but the expense of this technique limits its application. For routine determinations of the vibratory pattern, stroboscopy and/or glottography contribute adequate measurements with a much lower investment of time and expense.

LARYNGO-STROBOSCOPY

Stroboscopy produces an optical illusion in which an object moving rapidly and periodically appears to stand still or move very slowly. This illusion is attained by the intermittent but regular presentation of the object to the viewer. The phenomenon is based on Talbot's law which relates to the persistence of vision in the human eye. Each image lingers on the retina for 0·2 s after the exposure.

If this principle is applied to the vibrating vocal folds, the rapid oscillations appear to be arrested or greatly slowed. Synchronization of the changes in illumination with the frequency of vibration results in an apparent standstill of the vocal folds in any desired position, thus permitting a sharp image of the phonating structures (Fig. 1). A slight variation in the rate of illumination

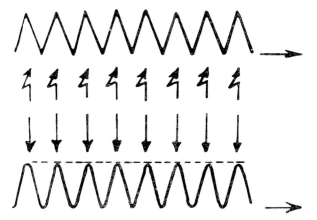

FIG. 1. Laryngostroboscopy (schematic drawing). Synchronization of stroboscopic pulses (upper graph) with frequency of laryngeal vibrations (lower graph) results in apparent arrest of motion.

changes in relation to the frequency of vibration results in a slow motion effect, because each successive light impulse strikes a different phase of the vibratory cycle (Fig. 2).

A modern electronic synchronstroboscope, such as the model Timcke KS-3, permits an evaluation of the vibratory

pattern during phonation via indirect laryngoscopy (Fig. 3). The voice of the subject or patient is picked up by a contact microphone below the larynx and directed to the electronic control unit where the sound waves are filtered

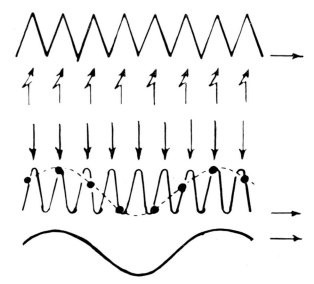

FIG. 2. Laryngostroboscopy (schematic drawing). Variation in relative frequencies of stroboscopic pulses (upper graph) and laryngeal vibrations (middle graph) produces slow motion effect (lower graph).

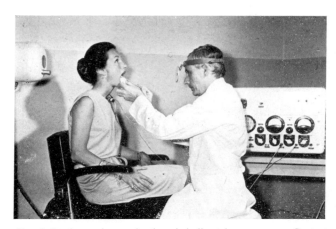

FIG. 3. Stroboscopic examination via indirect laryngoscopy. Contact microphone below larynx delivers vocal frequency to electronic control unit (right) and to stroboscopic lamp (left).

and amplified. The fundamental frequency of the voice is transmitted via electronic pulses to a xenon lamp which emits an intermittent beam of light at the same rate. Thus the repetition rate of the light flashes always corresponds to the frequency of the vocal fold vibrations, regardless of any change in pitch.

The light beam is directed by an ordinary head mirror to the laryngeal mirror and thence to the larynx as in any indirect laryngoscopy. A semi-automatic auxiliary light system provides illumination of the larynx before voice production, while the examiner prepares for the examination. Meters on the instrument panel indicate the fundamental frequency from 65–1 000 Hz as well as the intensity

of the phonation. In an aphonic subject the frequency of
the flashes of light can be controlled directly with the aid
of an audio-frequency generator. A foot pedal permits a
change in the phase angle of the light flashes in relation to
the sound impulses so as to obtain a stationary image of
the vocal folds at any instant of their vibration, or the more
typical slow motion effect. Additional attachments permit
automatic registration of frequency and intensity variations
for comparative studies or as a permanent repository.

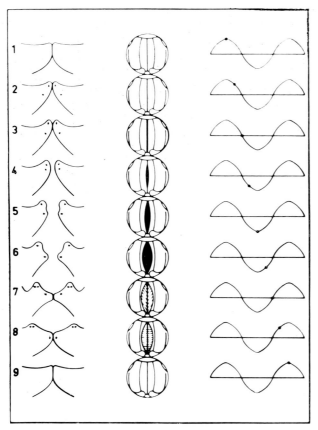

Fig. 4. Laryngostroboscopy—clinical application. Schematic
drawings of events during one vibratory cycle at low pitch: (left)
vertical section through centre of vocal folds; (centre) laryngoscopic image; (right) slow motion effect of stroboscopy. (From
Schönhärl, 1960.)

A typical stroboscopic evaluation of the larynx utilizes
both the still and slow motion effects of this technique. The
moving picture presents a general orientation regarding the
functional adjustments of the vocal folds and the ability of
the patient to maintain a constant tone. It also affords
information regarding the relative excursions of the two
vocal folds and phase variations in the vibratory cycle at
different levels of pitch and intensity (Fig. 4).

The still picture presents a sharp and clear image of the
vocal fold margins during the different phases of the
vibratory cycle, in contrast to the diffuse blur visible to the
naked eye. Deliberate phase variations of the still picture
through the full cycle of 360° demonstrating fine details of
laryngeal behaviour are of clinical significance because

they may be associated with qualitative changes in the
human voice.

A stroboscopic examination, therefore, offers a simple
and effective screening technique for differentiating
physiologic and pathologic abnormalities of the larynx.
Important applications of this diagnostic tool include the
diagnosis of functional disorders of the larynx, the extent
of organic disease, the differentiation between benign and
malignant neoplasms, the degree of laryngeal paralyses,
and the evaluation of traumatic and fibrotic changes in the
vocal folds.

GLOTTOGRAPHY

Electro-glottography is a simple technique for the
registration of vocal fold vibrations without impeding the
normal process of phonation and articulation. In this
procedure the vocal folds act as the plates of a capacitor
which is introduced into an ac cicuit. The larynx
represents a capacitative reactance for the alternating
current which remains always at the same frequency. The
movements of the vocal folds produce a change in this
reactance which is amplified and registered electronically.

The accuracy of the measurements has been improved in
recent models, such as Loebell's glottograph (manufactured by Martin Gruber, K.G.). For the operation of
this equipment one round electrode is applied to the neck
on each side of the larynx. These electrodes connect with
a small electronic unit which includes the generator as well
as the amplifier and measuring device. The results of the
examination may be registered on an oscilloscope or
polybeam recorder (Fig. 5).

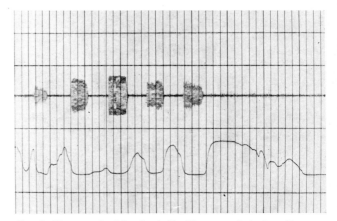

Fig. 5. Glottography (after Loebell). Upper graph depicts vibratory
movements during vowels a, e, i, o, u; lower graph demonstrates
respiratory movements within larynx during identical time
interval.

The advantages of this technique include the small size
of the portable electronic unit which is powered by a
flashlight battery, the relative simplicity of its construction,
and its adaptability to different methods of registration.
The same unit can be utilized for simultaneous measurements of the respiratory and phonatory movements
within the larynx. A careful analysis of the resulting
glottogram presents valuable information about hyper- or
hypo-kinetic disturbances of the laryngeal muscles,

paralytic or paretic weaknesses, or structural changes in the vibrating vocal folds as a result of oedema, inflammation or neoplasms.

ULTRA-HIGH SPEED PHOTOGRAPHY

A more detailed study of the vibrating vocal folds calls for the use of ultra-high speed cinematography. Ultra-high speed pictures afford a unique opportunity to study the complex vibratory oscillations of the vocal folds at different frequencies and intensities. Presentation of the moving film in ultra-slow motion displays the rapid movements of each vibratory cycle with a tremendous magnification of the time factor. Frame by frame projection of the same sequence discloses the minute details of motion at each instant and permits accurate measurements for graphic representation. The high speed of the photography also captures the short but significant transient phenomena which may affect voice production.

This technique also permits the study of laryngeal function during non-linguistic phenomena, such as a cough, laughter, or clearing of the throat, which occur too rapidly and too irregularly for the demonstration of the data by any other method. In addition, ultra-high speed photography facilitates comparative studies with artificial and cadaver larynges which can be modified to reproduce selected vibratory patterns. An analysis of these movements often affords valuable information regarding puzzling physiologic adjustments in the human larynx; in other cases, the study of comparative motion pictures provides confirmation of presumptive evidence.

Since ultra-high speed photography is both costly and time consuming, the design of this equipment requires special consideration. The examination of the patient should simulate an indirect laryngoscopy in the clinical setting of a physician's office, and the position and mounting of the camera should assure maximum flexibility in following the movements of the mirror in the patient's throat. A modern apparatus for laryngeal cinematography, such as the unit constructed by the author and his associates (Fig. 6), combines the following advantages:

The central feature of this equipment is a standard laryngeal mirror which is mounted on a sound probe leading to a tape recorder. This mirror is manually inserted by the examiner into the patient's throat, and the larynx is visualized as in any indirect laryngoscopy. A large concave mirror directs the light beam to the laryngeal mirror and thence to the vocal folds. The image of the larynx returns via the laryngeal mirror and through an opening in the concave mirror to a beam splitter which divides the image in two directions—10 per cent to the examiner and 90 per cent to the camera. The beam splitter in turn is mounted on a swivel so that the photographer can keep the camera centred on the larynx, irrespective of movements of the patient or of the examiner.

The requirements of colour photography at speeds of several thousand frames per second require the employment of a Xenon light or of a powerful incandescent lamp. In the United States, the Wollensack FASTAX camera (Model W.F. -4S) has proved its adaptability for laryngeal photography. The capacity of this equipment ranges from 30–120 m of 16 mm film. Special resistors control the speed from 1 000–5 000 frames (pictures) per second; this speed can be increased by the use of a special accelerator to more than 8 000 frames per second.

An effective method of sound proofing is essential to minimize the screeching noise of the Fastax camera, and to permit satisfactory simultaneous recordings of the patient's voice. A tracing of the acoustic signal can also be

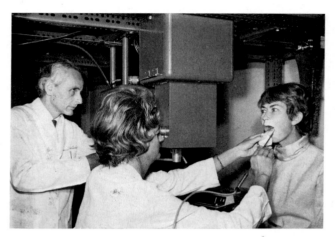

FIG. 6. Ultra-high Speed Photography. Examiner (centre) views larynx via peep hole and manipulates laryngeal mirror in patient's throat (right). Photographer (left background) centres camera with aid of swivel stick.

recorded on the film to facilitate a comparison between the visual image of the vocal fold vibrations and the resulting sound. The camera can be controlled either by the examiner with a foot switch or by the photographer with a hand button.

A photographic record presents a valuable repository of larnygeal function and appearance on a specific date. An analysis of the laryngeal adjustments conveys important information regarding the movements within the larynx: colour, texture and the motility of the different structures are clearly captured and identified (Fig. 7). Frame by frame analysis with graphic representation permits accurate measurements of laryngeal function, even during brief transient manoeuvres (Fig. 8).

There is often a perplexing disproportion between the subjective vocal symptoms of a patient and the objective laryngeal findings during a routine laryngoscopic examination. Many patients with moderate or severe voice changes present but little visible evidence in the larynx to explain these vocal abnormalities. In such cases, ultra-high speed photography of the larynx often discloses physiologic variations in the vibratory pattern which account for the acoustic manifestations. This type of examination has also proved of paramount importance for basic research in laryngeal physiology and patho-physiology.

AERODYNAMICS

After extensive investigations, my associates and I have reached the conclusion that aerodynamic investigations

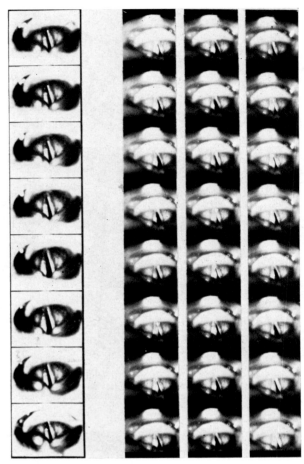

FIG. 7. Laryngeal Cinematography. Sequence from motion picture of unilateral vocal fold (cord) paralysis during phonation: (left) at normal speed, right vocal fold moves freely while left fold remains in intermediate position; (right) at ultra-high speed, excursions of paralyzed vocal fold can be observed during successive vibratory cycles.

present the most accurate objective measures for quantitative and qualitative determinations of laryngeal function. This evaluation agrees with our present understanding of phonation as an aerodynamic phenomenon. Basic investigations at different research institutions support the observation that laryngeal function depends primarily on the delicate balance between the subglottic pressure and the glottal resistance. Measurements of these aerodynamic factors should, therefore, denote the efficiency of the larynx in transforming air pressure into acoustic signals.

This concept substantiates the importance of the subglottic pressure for laryngeal function studies; for any significant variation in the air pressure affects the process of phonation at the level of the larynx. Respiratory function studies form an essential component in any aerodynamic evaluation of phonation. Such a determination requires one of the basic pulmonary examinations, because an impairment of pulmonary function requires an appropriate adjustment in the laryngeal evaluations.

PNEUMOTACHOGRAPHY

The central feature of the aerodynamic equipment is a pneumotachograph which is designed for measurements of the air flow rate and the air volume (Fig. 9). This apparatus consists of a respiratory mask, a laminar flow register (composed of a 400 mesh monel wire screen having an area of 20.5 cm^2), a highly sensitive bi-directional differential gas pressure transducer (e.g. Sanborn No. 270), and a carrier pre-amplifier (e.g. Sanborn No. 350–1000B). An integrating pre-amplifier (e.g. Sanborn No. 350–3700) records the air volume by integrating the flow rate. The gradient of the integrated curve at any given point indicates the mean flow rate. Air volume and air flow rate are displayed on two channels of a polybeam recorder (e.g. Sanborn Model 568–100).

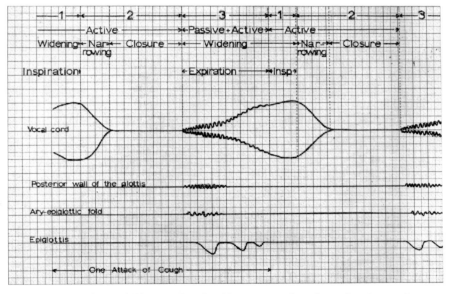

FIG. 8. Ultra-high Speed Photography. Graphic representation of transient laryngeal movements during a cough.

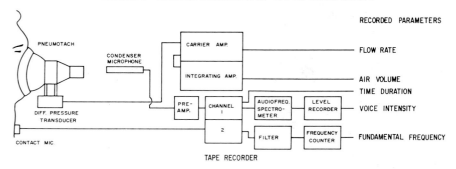

FIG. 9. Pneumotachography. Schematic view of electronic components.

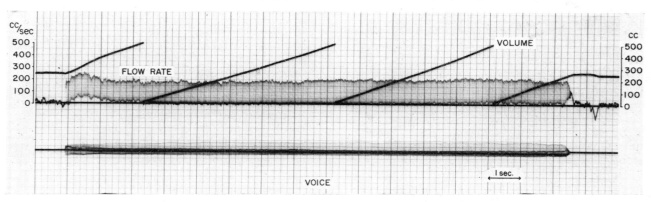

FIG. 10. Pneumotachography. Simultaneous registration of the flow rate, volume of air and voice signal during sustained phonation in subject with normal voice. Total volume 3460 ml (cc), mean flow rate 150 ml. s^{-1} phonation time 23·1 s.

The voice signal is picked up by a capacitative microphone (Bruel and Kjaer No. 4134) which is located near the outlet of the pneumotachograph. The sound is amplified by a pre-amplifier and recorded on a tape recorder at a constant recording level. The amplified sound waves are registered on the third channel of the polybeam recorder (Fig. 10). The sound pressure level of the voice signal is measured with a level recorder (Bruel and Kjaer No. 2305) and an audio-frequency spectrometer. If a visual display of the voice intensity is desired, the amplified sound waves are rectified with a linear converter and transmitted to a fourth channel of the polybeam recorder.

Several techniques may be used to determine accurately the fundamental frequency of the voice:

(a) The short term fundamental frequency can be measured by tracing the sound wave peaks on an oscillographic picture. A contact microphone is placed against the skin over the trachea to obtain the fundamental frequency.

(b) The average fundamental frequency can be calculated automatically by an electronic counter (e.g. Hewlett-Packard No. 5223-L); again the sound waves are picked up by a contact microphone.

(c) The overall fundamental frequency is readily obtained with the aid of a sound spectrograph (Kay Sonagraph Model 6061-A). The close agreement between these three methods assures an accurate objective determination of the fundamental frequency of the voice.

Additional components may be added to this system for special studies as indicated. For measurements of the subglottic pressure, for instance, a guarded 16 gauge needle may be introduced into the tracheal lumen above

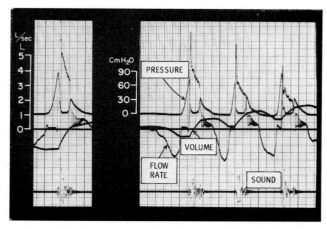

FIG. 11. Pneumotachography. Simultaneous registration of subglottic pressure flow rate, air volume, and sound during single cough (left), and triple cough (right).

or below the third tracheal ring. The subglottic pressure is transmitted to a pressure transducer (e.g. Sanborn No. 286-B), delivered into a carrier amplifier and registered on an additional channel of the polybeam recorder (Fig. 11).

Air pressure signals can also be picked up by an ultra-miniature pressure transducer (e.g. Whittaker No. 1015-S),

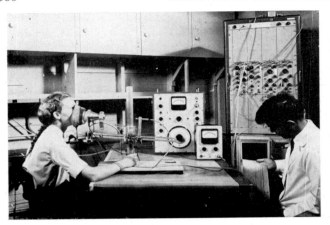

FIG. 12. Aerodynamic Function Studies: (left) patient at pneumo-tachograph; (right) examiner at polybeam recorder.

disorders or psychosomatic problems. With the aid of pulmonary function studies, these data may be related to the balance of power and resistance at the level of the larynx.

Accurate measurements of the air flow rate during phonation provide valuable information regarding laryngeal function. In normal men the air flow rate ranges from 90–175 ml.s^{-1} (c.c./sec.), while normal women register 80–160 ml.s^{-1} (c.c./sec.). By comparison, the air flow rate in pathologic subjects may extend from 50–1 150 ml.s^{-1} (c.c./sec.). Extremely high readings are usually obtained in patients with a paralysis of the recurrent laryngeal nerve. An increase in the air flow rate is also observed in other patients with poor closure of the glottis during phonation, as occurs with tumours or myasthenia laryngis. By contrast, low readings are often found in patients with contact ulcers and other diseases associated with excessive tension in the laryngeal muscles.

The total volume of air consumed during maximally sustained phonation (at given pitch and intensity levels) appears to have a definite physiologic significance. There is an important correlation between this phonation volume (*PV*) and the vital capacity (*VC*). At medium pitch and intensity between 3 l and 6 l of vital capacity,

placed at any desired point in the vocal system. The air pressure signals converted by the transducer are directed into a high-gain pre-amplifier (e.g. Sanborn 350-2700C), and registered on the polybeam recorder. However, accurate examinations of the pressure in the lower respiratory passages are uncomfortable for the subject.

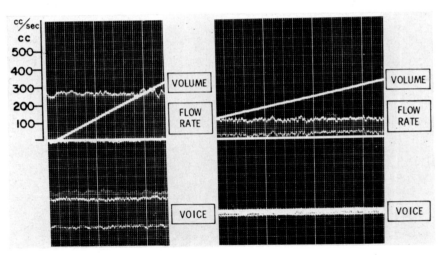

FIG. 13. Aerodynamic Recordings: (left) normal subject; (right) low air flow rate suggests increased glottic resistance (hypertension of vocal muscles).

They are usually not required for clinical evaluations, because respiratory function tests provide a satisfactory substitute for this purpose.

Aerodynamic studies of laryngeal function require no special preparation and are readily performed with the average subject or patient (Fig. 12). The simplicity of instructions and the lack of discomfort assure the co-operation even of highly emotional singers or fearful children. A decrease in the mean air flow rate and the air volume suggests an abnormal tension of the laryngeal structures (Fig. 13). By contrast, an increase in the mean air flow rate indicates a weakness of the neuromuscular component with an abnormal escape of air (Fig. 14). Fluctuations of the air flow rate give valuable information regarding specific laryngeal diseases, functional voice

the relation between these two factors is represented by the equation

$$PV = 0.86 \times VC - 891 \qquad (41.1)$$

The phonation volume is also related to the mean flow rate (*MFR*) and the maximum duration of phonation (*MPT*), as expressed by the equation

$$PV = MFR \times MPT \qquad (41.2)$$

This equation permits the calculation of the maximum phonation time for any subject. A comparison of this predicted maximum phonation time and the actual phonation time of the patient leads to the establishment of the phonation time ratio (*PT*), which may be expressed as a percentage of the normal value:

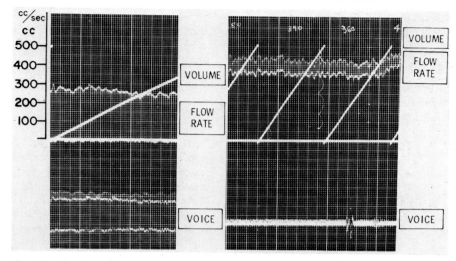

FIG. 14. Aerodynamic Recordings: (left) normal subject; (right) high air flow rate and high air volume suggest lowered glottic resistance (hypotension of vocal muscles).

$$PT = \frac{Actual\ MPT}{Predicted\ MPT} \qquad (41.3)$$

One of the most accurate indicators of laryngeal function appears to be the vocal velocity index (VVI), which refers to the ratio of the mean flow rate to the vital capacity:

$$VVI = \frac{MFR}{VC} \qquad (41.4)$$

The 95 per cent confidence limit in normal subjects ranges from 2·26 per cent to 2·76 per cent, with a mean value of 2·51 per cent. In a large series of cases, a statistical comparison using F-ratio tests between the vocal velocity index of normal subjects and of patients with organic laryngeal diseases showed a significant difference. A smaller difference in the statistical variation was observed between the normal subjects and the patients with functional voice disorders (Iwata and von Leden, 1970).

The simplest clinical indicator of the aerodynamic parameters is the phonation quotient (PQ), which represents the ratio of vital capacity to maximum phonation time:

$$PQ = \frac{VC}{MPT} \qquad (41.5)$$

This determination requires only a respirometer and a stop watch, while all other measurements necessitate the use of a pneumotachograph and other electronic equipment. Although the phonation quotient provides useful clinical information of laryngeal dysfunction, it is not specific for different laryngeal diseases. A comparison has demonstrated that the phonation quotient is a less sensitive indicator for the determination of laryngeal function than the mean air flow rate or the vocal velocity index.

Measurements of these factors provide important data on the overall vocal function. This information is of special value for the determination of faulty vocal habits and the evaluation of surgical procedures or protracted voice therapy. With the current development of operative techniques for the improvement of voice, the utilization of an objective test has been imperative to measure the pre-operative impairment and the post-operative improvement. The application of these tests in numerous patients with laryngeal diseases and voice disorders has demonstrated their validity and their value for the assessment of laryngeal function. During radiotherapy of malignant lesions or during prolonged therapy, these objective function studies have proved so sensitive that they usually signal convalescence of the patient before the clinical examination confirms the improvement.

RESPIRATORY FUNCTION TESTS

Current facilities for pulmonary function studies vary from an inexpensive respirometer to a complex body plethysmograph. A simple water sealed spirometer of the Benedict Roth type (like the Collins 9-litre respirometer) permits recording of the vital capacity and multiple oxygen uptake determinations (Fig. 15). The component ventilograph records basal minute ventilations as well as maximum breathing capacity. With appropriate attachments, the same equipment can be employed for timed vital capacity measurements and for the recording of respiratory excursions on a multiple channel electronic galvanometer. For a complete range of pulmonary function studies, the body plethysmograph represents the most accurate apparatus.

For the evaluation of a patient with voice difficulties, the mechanical function of the lung and thorax can be estimated from vital capacity studies. The tidal volume, expiratory reserve volume, inspiratory capacity and one-stage vital capacity are calculated. These indicators present valuable data regarding the function of the lungs during normal and forced respiration. The resulting measurements are compared with the predicted vital capacity (*VC*) in normal subjects of the same age and height derived from Baldwin's formulae:

$$VC \text{ (male)} = (27 \cdot 63 - 0 \cdot 112 \times \text{age}) \times \text{height} \quad (41.6)$$
$$VC \text{ (female)} = (21 \cdot 78 - 0 \cdot 101 \times \text{age}) \times \text{height} \quad (41.7)$$

Significant abnormalities in the vital capacity require an appropriate adjustment in the interpretation of aerodynamic tests of laryngeal function, for it is apparent that major changes in the function of the bellows (lungs) affect the air pressure and air flow phenomena at the level of the larynx.

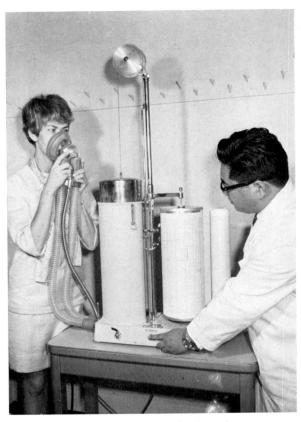

Fig. 15. Spirometer.

ACOUSTICAL STUDIES

A thorough acoustical evaluation of the voice provides paramount information about the organ of voice production. Current investigations suggest that an acoustical analysis of the voice may provide the earliest accurate information about faulty vocal habits or pathologic changes in the larynx. Even minor variations in the vibratory pattern are accompanied by transient pressure changes across the glottis which are reflected acoustically in disturbances of the vocal signal.

The voice of the subject must be recorded in a sound proof room in order to assure an accurate acoustic analysis. The examination should include a sample of the patient's spontaneous speech for an evaluation of his vocal habits. Since the vowels reflect the performance of the larynx, special attention must be devoted to the recording of the five cardinal vowels, sustaining each vowel for several seconds at moderate loudness and medium pitch. A determination of the lowest and highest frequencies is required for an evaluation of the pitch range. The singing of a scale is helpful for an impression of the subject's musical aptitude. Finally the patient should read aloud a carefully selected transcript, like the rainbow passage in the English language, which includes all major components of speech sounds.

High fidelity equipment, such as the Ampex Model 350 tape recorder and an Electrovoice No. 666 supercardioid microphone, are essential for an accurate acoustic analysis. *Frequency* determinations indicate the patient's habitual pitch and the extent of his vocal range. An abnormally high pitch often reflects a psychosomatic factor; an abnormally low pitch may indicate an increase in the vocal mass from an inflammation, a neoplasm or from other organic changes; it may also reflect a studied imitation of a social or cultural trend. The *intensity* of the voice is directly related to vocal habits and voice disorders. Abnormal loudness characterizes a certain personality type and suggests an important aetiological factor. A weak voice may be the result of protracted abuse, misuse or overuse; it may also be related to pathological changes in the larynx or in the lungs. A spectrographic analysis permits an accurate determination of the voice *quality* and an objective measurement of hoarseness.

SONAGRAPHY

For sound spectrography, the recorded vowels are reproduced at controlled intensity levels, particular frequency characteristics, with the aid of a sonagraph, (Kay Model 6061-A). This apparatus permits visual presentation of the three parameters of the acoustical structure of voice—frequency, intensity and time (Fig. 16). With the use of a narrow band filter setting, the sound spectrograms of normal subjects phonating sustained vowels appear to have centain basic characteristics, regardless of the difference in vowel sounds. Within the range of the formant frequencies, the transverse striations corresponding to the fundamental harmonic frequencies are regularly spaced (Fig. 17). By contrast, the sound spectrograms of hoarse voices demonstrate abnormal harmonic changes and noise components.

On the basis of extensive spectrographic experiments, Yanagihara has introduced an acoustical classification of the hoarse voice which is based on (1) noise components in the main formants of vowel sounds, (2) loss of acoustical energy in the harmonic components, and (3) cycle-to-cycle variations in the fundamental frequencies of the major vowels (Fig. 18). Based mainly on Yanagihara's observations, the following classification of hoarseness is suggested:

Type 1: Regular harmonic components are mixed with noise components chiefly in second and third formants of vowels /e/ and /i/.

Type 2: Noise components in second formants of vowels /e/ and /i/ predominate over harmonic components, and extend to vowel /a/. Slight additional noise components in high frequency region above 3 kHz.

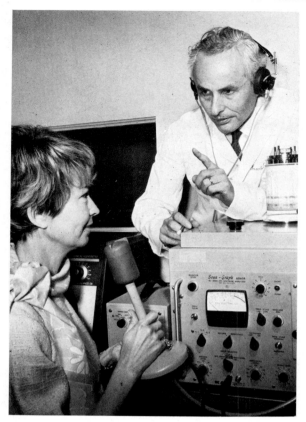

FIG. 16. Spectrographic analysis of voice with the aid of a Kay Sonagraph

A comparison of these objective acoustical studies with the subjective perception of the same voice by experienced observers stresses the clinical importance of this approach. Incipient hoarseness is associated with acoustical changes in the higher formants of the vowels /e/ and /i/ where the human ear is least sensitive. Thus, in some cases, early disorders of the voice may be discovered by sound spectrograms before the human ear perceives these changes as hoarseness. This early detection of laryngeal problems is of special importance for singers, actors and professional voice users whose vocal organs can be placed at rest and treated before further damage occurs.

Refinements of the sound spectrographic analysis have permitted a more direct visualization of the vocal spectrum in terms of the frequency and time factors. This modification, the contour display spectrogram, is more popularly known as a "voice print", and is obtained with the aid of a contour display unit (Kay Model 6070-A) mounted on a sound spectrograph (Kay Model 6061-A). The reproduction is carried out at controlled intensity levels using particular frequency characteristics. For an accurate analysis of the acoustical pattern, two different contour spectrograms should be obtained for each patient:

(1) a voice print with a normal scale up to 8 kHz to demonstrate the acoustical energy distribution for the entire frequency range, and

(2) a voice print with an expanded scale up to 2 kHz to show the details of energy distribution in the critical first formant.

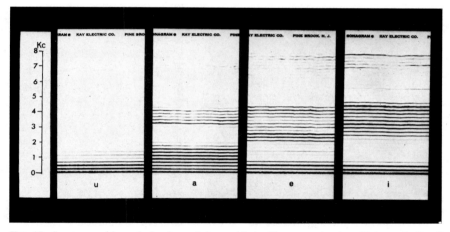

FIG. 17. Spectrographic analysis of vowels in a subject with a normal voice. Note regularity of fundamental frequency and formant structure.

Type 3: Second formants of vowels /e/ and /i/ totally replaced by noise components. Noise components in second formant of vowel /a/ predominate over harmonic components. Additional noise components above 3 kHz intensified and expanded.

Type 4: Second formants of all vowels replaced by noise components. First formant shows loss of normal periodicity. High frequency noise components intensified and expanded.

This three-dimensional acoustical examination provides additional information about the type and the extent of the laryngeal involvement. The clearly defined contour lines of the voice print provide accurate amplitude discrimination in 6 dB steps, and the gradations in shading offer a convincing image of the acoustical energy distribution. The acoustical energy distribution in the first formant appears to be of special significance for recognition of pathological conditions of the larynx. There appears to be

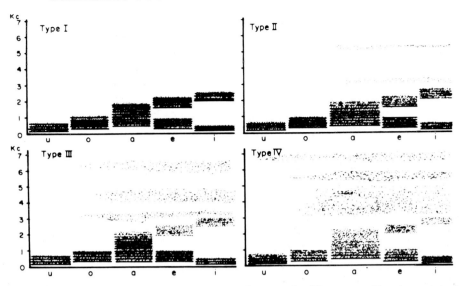

FIG. 18. Schematic presentation of sonagrams at different levels of hoarseness. Note increment of noise components and loss of high frequency harmonic components as hoarseness increases. (From Yanagihara, 1967b.)

a fundamental relationship between the degree of hoarseness and the distribution of acoustic energy. In slight hoarseness the energy is distributed mainly above 4 kHz (Fig. 19), while in moderate degrees of hoarseness the energy appears most pronounced in the middle frequency range (Fig. 20). As the hoarseness increases, the distribution of energy extends throughout the harmonic range and the fundamental frequency demonstrates marked irregularities.

Although various laryngeal diseases with slight hoarseness produce similar sonagrams according to Yanagihara's classification, the comparative voice prints permit comprehensive studies of the acoustic energy distribution in different formant bars, especially in the first formant. As the degree of hoarseness increases, the formant bars widen and become irregular in both frequency and time. These changes may be related to the increment of noise components and to the fluctuations of the fundamental frequency. In patients with laryngeal neoplasms and severe hoarseness, for instance, the voice prints are characterized by marked irregularity in the acoustic energy for the entire frequency range, as indicated by irregular islands of energy distribution of varying intensities. These findings are most conspicuous in the lower frequencies: extensions of high energy distribution from the first formant bar coalesce with the adjoining fundamental and second formant bars at many points, with a disintegration of the formant pattern (Fig. 21). By contrast, patients with unilateral laryngeal paralysis and severe hoarseness present entirely different voice prints. The first formant bar indicates a much lower energy distribution, there is less communication between adjoining formants, and the contrasts are less pronounced (Fig. 22). These findings differ sharply from regular sonagrams which suggest the same classification for all patients with severe hoarseness. The clinical application of contour spectrography provides important information

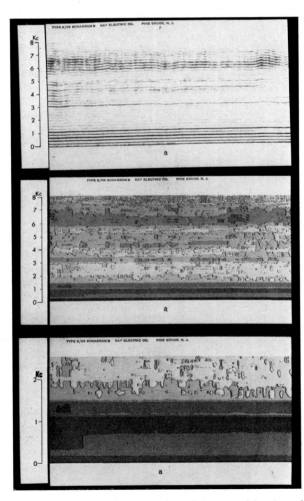

FIG. 19. Acoustic Spectrography: Sonagram (above) and voice prints of slight hoarseness (mild laryngitis).

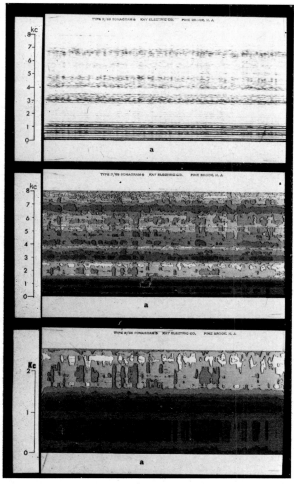

FIG. 20. Acoustic Spectrography: Sonagram (above) and voice prints of moderate hoarseness (moderate laryngitis).

about the acoustical correlates of the hoarse voice and the underlying laryngeal pathology.

USE OF COMPUTERS

In recent years, computer science has affected every other branch of science. The medical applications of this new technique have resulted in multiphasic screening programs which emphasize the early detection and prevention of disease. Current investigations suggest a simple and inexpensive method of discovering disease of the vocal system from an acoustical evaluation of the voice with the aid of computers. This approach is based on the observation that transient pressure changes across the glottis are reflected acoustically in disturbances of the fundamental frequency and amplitude patterns.

For this evaluation, the acoustic signal is picked up by a contact microphone (e.g. Sony F-96) which is placed over the pre-tracheal skin directly above the manubrium sterni. A special foam rubber adapter assures air-tight coupling and prevents artificial distortions of the signal. This technique provides a high signal-to-noise ratio which is important for the extraction of the fundamental period in patients with hoarse voices. The acoustic signal is recorded on one channel of a high fidelity tape recorder (e.g. Ampex Model 350). A reference signal from an oscillator (e.g. Bruel and Kjaer No. 1024) is recorded on the second channel of the tape recorder in order to assure an accurate time display for the entire system. The recording signals are played back into a Visicorder (Honeywell Model 1108) and registered on the photo-sensitive recording paper (Fig. 23). A magnification system is employed to assist in the actual measurements of pitch perturbations or amplitude modulations.

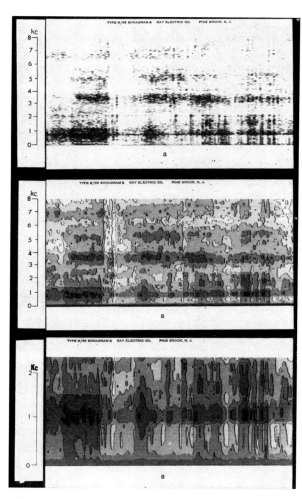

FIG. 21. Acoustic Spectrography: Sonagram (above) and voice prints of severe hoarseness (carcinoma of vocal folds).

The measured values of the recorded signals are subjected to data processing with a digital computer, such as a PDP-8. The digital data may be presented as a series of correlation coefficients in the form of correlograms. These correlograms show the serial correlation coefficient as the ordinate and the fundamental periods as the abscissa. The serial correlation coefficient is shown for each lag between 1 and 15 fundamental periods because pathologic changes in the larynx manifest themselves primarily as short term modulations. A positive peak at any given point indicates a positive correlation at the fundamental period, whereas a negative peak suggests a negative correlation.

For example, a typical correlogram of the amplitude modulations in a normal subject demonstrates a smooth

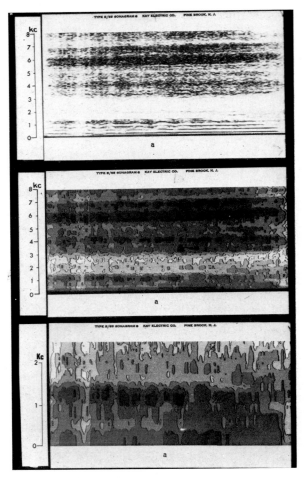

FIG. 22. Acoustic Spectrography: Sonagram (above) and voice prints of severe hoarseness (vocal fold paralysis).

lag of one period. This type of correlogram is commonly observed in patients with benign organic changes affecting the vibratory margin of the membranous vocal folds (Fig. 25).

The correlogram of a patient with unilateral paralysis shows no evidence of significant periodicities except for a frequent elevation at the lag of one period, which indicates a correlation between consecutive periods. The graph shows variable irregularities throughout the entire range of 15 fundamental periods. This type of correlogram is commonly associated with the clinical condition of incomplete approximation during phonation (Fig. 26). Malignant lesions and other large neoplasms of the vocal folds result in correlograms with marked positive and negative peaks representing an apparent periodic modulation throughout the 15 fundamental periods calculated. Extreme acoustical patterns of this type of amplitude modulation are found in patients with advanced malignancies of the larynx (Fig. 27).

Similarly, correlograms of pitch perturbations demonstrate significant differences between normal subjects and patients with laryngeal disease. Further refinements in the equipment and in the techniques of data processing should lead to even greater specificity in the results, as well as to an effective, inexpensive, time saving process for the examination of large populations and for the early discovery of laryngeal diseases and voice disorders.

SUPPLEMENTARY FUNCTION STUDIES

The supplementary examination of laryngeal function includes techniques which have been perfected at various research institutions. The most effective studies have utilized radiologic principles or electromyographic techniques. Radiology in particular has proved valuable not only for an analysis of the structural changes of the vocal folds within the larynx, but also for an evaluation of the thoracic cavity and of the resonance chambers in the head and neck. Electromyography remains the only tool for an

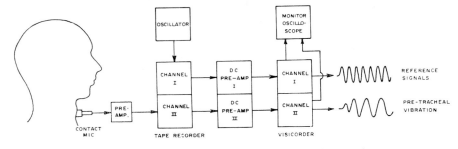

FIG. 23. Acoustical Evaluation of voice. Schematic drawing of electronic components.

outline without significant irregularities at successive fundamental points (Fig. 24). By contrast, a patient with a small vocal nodule demonstrates irregularities of the graph between 2 and 10 lags, suggesting irregular short term perturbations of the amplitude in the acoustical signal. Again there is a high correlation between successive fundamental periods, as indicated by a positive value at a

effective determination of the electric changes in the neuromuscular component.

RADIOLOGY

The radiologic examination of the chest and resonance chambers in the head and neck is widely practised through-

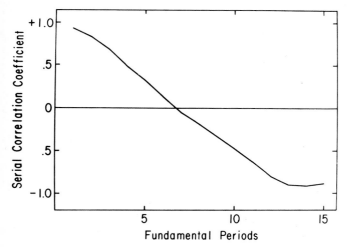

FIG. 24. Acoustical Evaluation of voice. Correlogram of normal voice.

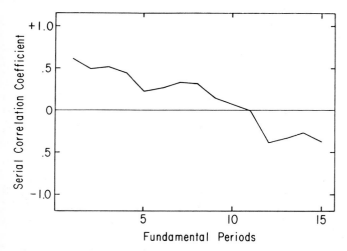

FIG. 25. Acoustical Evaluation of voice Correlogram of patient with benign vocal nodule.

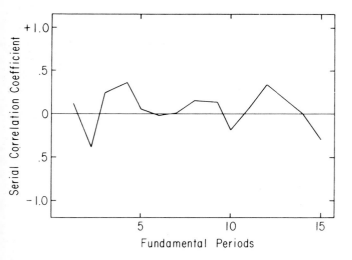

FIG. 26. Acoustical Evaluation of voice. Correlogram of patient with unilateral vocal paralysis (intermediate position).

out the world and requires no further elucidation. By contrast, radiologic techniques for an evaluation of the laryngeal function represent certain inherent difficulties, such as the speed of the vibrating vocal folds and their rapid changes in position and mass during phonation. A number of different approaches have been utilized to overcome these difficulties.

Postero-anterior and lateral films of the larynx provide useful information about the position of the laryngeal skeleton at different frequencies and intensities; they provide no useful data for the analysis of endolaryngeal events. Laryngology with the aid of radio-opaque materials outlines the contour of the tissues within the larynx and provides helpful information about the location and mass

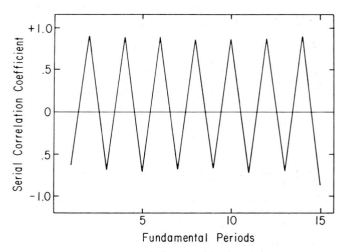

FIG. 27. Acoustical Evaluation of voice. Correlogram of patient with advanced carcinoma of vocal folds.

of the phonating structures. However, the superimposition of successive segments detracts from the usefulness of this technique.

The development of laminagraphic techniques represents a great advance for the radiologic study of laryngeal phenomena. This method permits measurements of the cross sectional area and thickness of the vocal folds at specific intervals along their length. Tomographic studies of laryngeal function have proved especially effective when the radiologic image is captured on a moving picture film. Various techniques have been employed to synchronize this motion picture with the sound produced at the time of photography.

The development of a stroboscopic unit for laminagraphy carries these investigations an additional step further. This technique avoids the composite effect of successive vibratory cycles which result in a blurred image of the rapidly vibrating vocal folds. The stroboscopic laminagraph (Strol) presents a series of laminagraphic photographs which display coronal cross sections of the vocal folds at ten different phases of the vibratory cycle (Fig. 28). For measurements of the cross sectional area and thickness, the examiner evaluates one or more pictures of the folds in their closed phase; for studies of the vibratory action, the entire series is utilized. This system

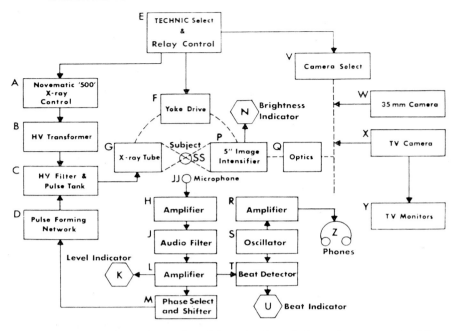

FIG. 28. Stroboscopic Laminagraphy: Schematic view of electronic components. (From Hollien, Coleman and Moore, 1968.)

has the advantage of eliminating any modification of phonation, such as the introduction of a laryngeal mirror or the protrusion of the tongue. Unfortunately, the cost of construction and utilization limits the application of this promising technique.

ELECTROMYOGRAPHY

Electromyographic investigations of the laryngeal muscles and neurosensory studies of the laryngeal nervous system have added significant contributions both to fundamental research and to our knowledge of laryngeal physiology. However, the technical difficulties of these procedures and the associated discomfort limit their routine use for the clinical evaluation of laryngeal function.

While an electromyographic examination of the extrinsic laryngeal muscles is relatively simple and can be conducted readily with concentric needle electrodes and routine electromyographic equipment, this type of investigation provides limited information about the physiology of phonation. The clinician is interested primarily in the function of the vocalis muscle and the other tiny intrinsic muscles of the larynx which change the configuration of the glottis and participate directly in the regulation of vocal pitch, intensity and quality. The small size of these structures and their location within the cartilaginous framework of the larynx necessitates special equipment, a skilful technician and a co-operative subject.

The best technique for the insertion of the electrodes into the intrinsic laryngeal muscles is the transcutaneous approach developed by Hiroto, Hirano and their associates. Two-hooked wire electrodes of special design are adapted for insertion into each of the different intrinsic laryngeal muscles, and introduced through hollow curved needles by a skilled operator. High-gain pre-amplifiers intensify the

electric impulses which are registered on a multi-hecannl tape recorder (Fig. 29). For immediate visual demonstration they may also be recorded on a polybeam recorder (e.g. Sanborn Model 568) or on a cathode ray oscilloscope

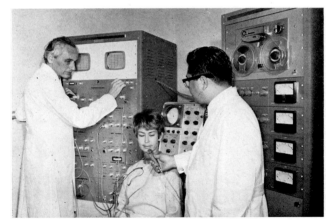

FIG. 29. Electromyography of the Vocal Folds. Electrical potentials are picked up by hooked needle electrodes and directed to multi-channel electromyograph (left) and multi-channel tape recorder (right).

(e.g. Tektronics Model 565). Simultaneously, with the electromyographic recording, the voice signal is picked up from the skin in the pre-tracheal area and registered on another channel of the polybeam recorder or oscilloscope for the purpose of visual analysis.

MATHEMATICAL MODELS

The idea of modelling the human vocal folds in an attempt to produce synthetic speech is not new, but digital computer simulation of vocal fold motions is a very recent development. Flanagan (1972) at the Bell Telephone Laboratories has pioneered this line of investigation, in an effort to produce more natural speech with vocal tract synthesizers.

Simulated vocal fold motions with various adjustments of register, pitch, intensity and quality should be of value

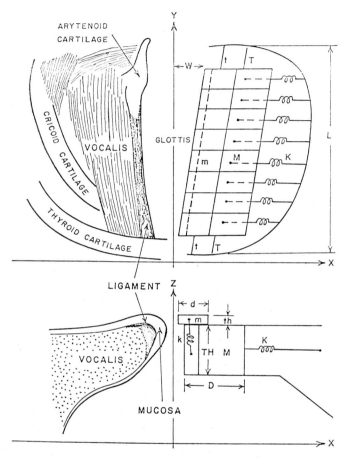

Fig. 30. Mathematical Model of Vocal Folds. T and t represent tensions in the vocalis and ligament, respectively. K represents the coupling of the vocalis to the thyroarytenoid muscle. k is the coupling between the mucous membrane and the ligament. M is the mass of each ligament-vocalis section, whereas m is the mass of a mucosal section. L is the overall length, W is the position of the arytenoids, and the thickness and depths th, Th, d, and D are self-evident. (From Titze and Strong, 1975.)

in determining the fundamental physical and physiologic principles of phonation. The computer simulation may prove of even greater value in the identification of abnormal voice patterns and pathological changes. However, such investigations presume a sophisticated synthesizer which permits adjustments for different sections and constituents of the vocal folds.

Until recently, the most complex model consisted of two coupled masses for each cord. Each mass had one degree of freedom perpendicular to the direction of the flow, which limits its adaptation for applied research in laryngeal physiology. Titze has developed a mathematical model for digital simulation of phonation which obviates

many of these objections. Titze's system consists of a periodic structure of 16 coupled masses for each of the vocal folds, an 18 section cylindrical tube approximation of the pharynx and mouth, and a similar 12 section approximation of the nasal tract. Special care was taken to model separately the functions of the vocal ligament, the vocalis muscle, and the covering mucous membrane (Fig. 30).

With this model it is possible to simulate phonation in the different frequencies, intensities and qualities of phonation and to measure the response with a high degree of accuracy. Transient responses, such as coughs or voice breaks, can also be simulated. The parameters which control the nature of this phonation are the subglottic pressure, the external tension applied to the vocal ligament, the vocalis muscle, the mucous membrane and the internal tension of the vocalis muscle.

Titze has proved that the simulated motions of the vocal folds, the output pressure, and the glottal waveshape closely resemble those of human voice. Vertical and horizontal phase difference have been observed in segments of the vocal fold. It is apparent that this ingenious new development provides an entirely new dimension for fundamental research on phonation, with opportunities for clinical measurements of abnormal or pathologic voice production.

FURTHER READING AND REFERENCES

Beckett, R. L. (1969), "Pitch Perturbation as a Function of Subjective Vocal Constriction," *Folia phoniat.*, **21**, 416–425.

Böhme, G., Aust, S. and Heinemann, M. (1969), "Spirographische Untersuchungen bei Glottisstenosen," *Folia phoniat.*, **21**, 112–120.

Cooper, F. S., Sawashima, M., Abramson, S. and Lisker, L. (1971), "Looking at the Larynx During Running Speech," *Ann. Otol., Rhinol., Lar.*, **80**, 678–682.

Cornut, G. (1971), "Vibrations normales et pathologiques des cordes vocales etudiees a l'aide du Sonagraph," *Folia phoniat.*, **23**, 234–238.

Damste, P. H. (1968), "Study of Phonation; Applications," *Folia phoniat.*, **20**, 65–88.

Dedo, H. H. and Hall, W. N. (1969), "Electrodes in Laryngeal Electromyography," *Ann. Otol., Rhinol., Lar.*, **78**, 172–180.

Dudgeon, D. E. (1970), "Two-Mass Model of the Vocal Cords," *J. Acoust. Soc. Amer.*, **48**, 118.

Dunker, E. and Schlosshauer, B. (1958), "Klinische und experimentelle Studien über Stimmlippenschwingungen," *Arch. Ohr.-, Nas.-, u. KehlkHeilk.*, **172**, 363–380.

Dunker, E. and Schlosshauer, B. (1961), "Unregelmässige Stimmlippenschwingungen bei funktionellen Stimmstörungen," *Z. Laryng. Rhinol. Otol.*, **40**, 919–934.

Faaborg-Andersen, K. (1957), "Electromyographic Investigation of Intrinsic Laryngeal Muscles in Humans," *Acta physiol. scand.*, **41**, suppl. 140.

Faaborg-Andersen, K. and Vennard, W. (1964), "Electromyography of Extrinsic Laryngeal Muscles During Phonation of Different Vowels," *Ann. Otol., Rhinol., Lar.*, **75**, 1248.

Fabre, Ph. (1957), "Un procédé électrique percutane d'inscription de l'accolement glottique au cours de la phonation: glottographie de haute fréquence: premiers résultats," *Bull. Acad. nat. Méd.*, **141**, 66–69.

Fabre, P. (1958), "Etude comparée des glottogrammes et des phonogrammes de la voix humaine," *Ann. Oto-laryng. (Paris)*, **75**, 767–775.

Flanagan, J. L. (1972), *Speech Analysis, Synthesis, and Perception.* Berlin: Springer.

Gay, T., Hirose, H., Strome, M. and Sawashima, M. (1972), "Electromyography of the Intrinsic Laryngeal Muscles During Phonation," *Ann. Otol., Rhinol., Lar.*, **81**, 401–409.

Hirano, M., Koike, Y. and Joyner, J. (1969), "Style of Phonation, an Electromyographic Investigation of Some Laryngeal Muscles," *Arch. Otolaryng.*, **89**, 902–907.

Hirano, M., Koike, Y. and von Leden, H. (1968), "Maximum Phonation Time and Air Usage During Phonation, Clinical Study," *Folia Phoniat.*, **20**, 185–201.

Hirano, M. and Ohala, J. (1969), "Use of Hooked-wire Electrodes for Electromyography of the Intrinsic Laryngeal Muscles," *J. Speech and Hear. Res.*, **12**, 362–373.

Hirano, M., Ohala, J. and Vennard, W. (1969), "The Function of Laryngeal Muscles in Regulating Fundamental Frequency and Intensity of Phonation," *J. Speech and Hear. Res.*, **12**, 616–628.

Hirano, M., Vennard, W. and Ohala, J. (1970), "Regulation of Register, Pitch and Intensity of Voice," *Folia phoniat.*, **22**, 1–20.

Hirose, H. and Gay, T. (1973), "Laryngeal Control in Vocal Attack: An Electromyographic Study," *Folia phoniat.*, **25**, 203–213.

Hirose, H., Gay, T. and Strome, M. (1971), "Electrode Insertion Techniques for Laryngeal Electromyography," *J. acoust. Soc. Amer.*, **50**, 1449–1450.

Hiroto, I., Hirano, M., Toyozumi, Y. and Shin, T. (1967), "Electromyographic Investigation of the Intrinsic Laryngeal Muscles Related to Speech Sounds," *Ann. Otol., Rhinol., Lar.*, **76**, 861–872.

Hollien, H., Coleman, R. and Moore, P. (1968), "Stroboscopic Laminagraphy of the Larynx During Phonation," *Acta oto-laryng.*, **65**, 209–215.

Hollien, H. and Colton, R. H. (1969), "Four Laminagraphic Studies of Vocal Fold Thickness," *Folia phoniat.*, **21**, 179–198.

Hollien, H., Curtis, J. and Coleman, R. F. (1968), "Investigation of Laryngeal Phenomena by Stroboscopic Laminagraphy," *Med. Res. Engineer.*, **7**, 24–27.

Hollinger, P. H., Lutterbeck, E. F. and Bulger, R. (1970), "Xeroradiography of the Larynx," *Ann. Otol., Rhinol., Lar.*, **81**, 806–808.

Ishizaka, K. and Flanagan, J. L. (1972), "Acoustic Properties of a Two-Mass Model of the Vocal Cords," *J. acoust. Soc. Amer.*, **51**, 91.

Isshiki, N. (1964), "Regulatory Mechanism of Voice Intensity Variation," *J. Speech and Hear. Res.*, **7**, 17–29.

Isshiki, N. (1965), "Vocal Intensity and Air Flow Rate," *Folia phoniat.*, **17**, 92–104.

Isshiki, N. and von Leden, H. (1964), "Hoarseness—Aerodynamic Studies," *Arch. Otolaryng.*, **80**, 206–213.

Isshiki, N., Yanagihara, N. and Morimoto, M. (1966), "Approach to the Objective Diagnosis of Hoarseness," *Folia phoniat.*, **18**, 393–400.

Iwata, S. (1972), "Periodicities of Pitch Perturbations in Normal and Pathologic Larynges," *Laryngoscope*, **82**, 87–96.

Iwata, S. and von Leden, H. (1970), "Clinical Evaluation of Vocal Velocity Index in Laryngeal Diseases," *Ann. Otol., Rhinol., Lar.*, **79**, 259–268.

Iwata, S. and von Leden, H. (1970), "Phonation Quotient in Patients with Laryngeal Diseases," *Folia phoniat.*, **22**, 117–128.

Iwata, S. and von Leden, H. (1970), "Pitch Perturbations in Normal and Pathologic Voices," *Folia phoniat.*, **22**, 413–424.

Iwata, S. and von Leden, H. (1970), "Voice Prints in Laryngeal Diseases," *Arch. Otolaryng.*, **91**, 346–351.

Iwata, S., von Leden, H. and Williams, D. (1972), "Air Flow Measurement During Phonation," *J. Communic. Disorders*, **5**, 67–79.

Johnson, T. H., Jr. (1970), "Spray Aerosol Laryngography," *Arch. Otolaryng.*, **92**, 511–513.

Koike, Y. (1969), "Amplitude Modulations in Patients with Laryngeal Disease," *J. acoust. Soc. Amer.*, **45**, 839–844.

Koike, Y. and Hirano, M. (1968), "Significance of Vocal Velocity Index," *Folia phoniat.*, **20**, 185–201.

Koike, Y., Hirano, M. and von Leden, H. (1967), "Vocal Initiation: Acoustic and Aerodynamic Investigations of Normal Subjects," *Folia phoniat.* **19**, 173–182.

Koike, Y. and Perkins, W. H. (1968), "Application of a Miniaturized Pressure Transducer for Experimental Speech Research," *Folia phoniat.*, **20**, 360–368.

Koike, Y. and von Leden, H. (1969), "Pathologic Vocal Initiation," *Ann. Otol., Rhinol., Lar.*, **78**, 138–147.

Köster, J. P. and Smith, S. (1970), "Zur Interpretation elektrischer und photoelektrischer Glottogramme," *Folia phoniat.*, **22**, 92–99.

Large, J. W. (1971), "Observations on the Vital Capacity of Singers," *The NATS Bulletin*, **28**, 34–52.

Lieberman, P. (1963), "Some Acoustic Measures of the Fundamental Periodicity of Normal and Pathologic Larynges," *J. acoust. Soc. Amer.*, **35**, 344–353.

Lieberman, P. (1967), *Intonation, Perception, and Language*. Cambridge, Mass.: M.I.T. Press.

Lieberman, P. (1968), "Vocal Cord Motion in Man," *Ann. N.Y. Acad. Sci.*, **155**, 28–38.

Loebell, E. (1968), "Über den klinischen Wert der Elektroglottographie," *Arch. Ohr.-, Nas.-, u. Kehlk Heilk.*, **191**, 760–764.

Luchsinger, R. and Arnold, G. E. (1965), *Voice-Speech-Language*, Belmont, Calif.: Wadsworth Co.

Luchsinger, R. and Pfister, K. (1959), "Ergebnisse von Kehlkopfaufnahmen mit einer Zeitdehnerapparatur," *Bull. schweiz. Akad. med. Wiss.*, **15**, 164–177.

Michel, Cl. van (1967), "Les artéfacts en glottographie," *Rev. électro. Diag. Ther.*, **4**, 3.

Michel, Cl. van, Pfister, K. and Luchsinger, R. (1970), "Electroglottographie et cinématographie laryngée ultrarapide; Comparaison des resultats," *Folia phoniat.*, **22**, 81–91.

Michel, Cl. van and von Leden, H. (1969), "L'Electroglottométre Mark 4, son principe, ses possibilités," *Folia phoniat.*, **21**, 145–157.

Nessel, E. (1960), "Über das Tonfrequenzspektrum der pathologisch veränderten Stimme," *Acta oto-laryng.*, **157**, 1–45.

Ohala, J. (1966), "A New Photo-electric Glottograph," *Working Papers in Phonetics*, **4**, 40–52. University of California, Los Angeles.

Perkins, H. and Koike, Y. (1969), "Patterns of Subglottal Pressure Variations during Phonation: A Preliminary Report," *Folia phoniat.*, **21**, 1–8.

Ringel, R. and Isshiki, N. (1964), "Intra-Oral Voice Recordings: An Aid to Laryngeal Photography," *Folia phoniat.*, **16**, 19–28.

Rubin, H., LeCover, M. and Vennard, W. (1967), "Vocal Intensity, Subglottic Pressure, and Air Flow Relationships in Singers," *Folia phoniat.*, **19**, 393–413.

Sawashima, M., Abramson, A. S., Lisker, L. *et al.* (1970), "Observing Laryngeal Adjustments During Running Speech By Use of a Fiberoptics System," *Phonetica*, **22**, 193–201.

Sawashima, M., Sato, M., Funasaka, S. and Totsuka, G. (1958), "Electromyographic Study of the Human Larynx and its Clinical Application," *Jap. J. Otol.*, **61**, 1357–1364.

Schönhärl, E. (1960), *Die Stroboskopie in der praktischen Laryngologie*. Stuttgart: Geo. Thieme.

Schönhärl, E. (1962), "Zur klinischen Bedeutung der Stroboskopie," *Z. Laryng. Rhinol.*, **41**, 568–573.

Schönhärl, E. (1963), "Beitrag zur Qualitativen Stimmanalyse," *Z. Laryng. Rhinol. Otol.*, **42**, 130–139.

Seidner, W., Wendler, J. and Halbedl, G. (1972), "Mikrostroboskopie," *Folia phoniat.*, **24**, 81–84.

Smith, S. (1970), "Laryngographische Untersuchungen der Stimmlippen," *Folia phoniat.*, **22**, 169–170.

Sovak, M., Courtois, J., Haas, C. and Smith, S. (1971), "Observations on the Mechanism of Phonation Investigated By Ultraspeed Cinefluorography," *Folia phoniat.*, **20**, 277–287.

Steinhauer, R. E. (1969), "Voice Prints: A New Aid in Detecting Criminals," *Saturday Rev.*, **52**, 56–59.

Titze, I. (1973), *The Human Vocal Cords: A Mathematical Model, Dissertation*. Brigham Young University. Provo, Utah.

Titze, I. and Strong, W. J. (1972), "Vocal Cord Model for Singing," *J. acoust. Soc. Amer.*, **51**, 138.

Titze, I. and Strong, W. J., (1975), "Normal modes in vocal cord tissues," *J. acoust. Soc. Amer.*, **57**, 736–744.

Vallancien, B. (1955), "Analyse comparative des mouvements glottique des cordes vocales par la Stroboscopie et ultracinematographie," *J. franç. Oto-Rhino-Laryng.*, **4**, 3.

Vallancien, B. (1968), "Etude radiologique de la phonation: Aspect technique," *Folia phoniat.*, **20**, 156–181.

Vallancien, B., Gautheron, B., Pasternak, L., Guisez, D. and Paley, B. (1971), "Comparaison des signaux microphoniques, diaphanographiques et glottographiques, avec application au laryngographe," *Folia phoniat.*, **20**, 371–380.

Van Den Berg, J. W. (1962), "Modern Research in Experimental Phoniatrics," *Folia phoniat.*, **14**, 81–149.

Vennard, W. (1967), *Singing: The Mechanism and the Technic.* New York: Carl Fisher.

Vennard, W. and Irwin, J. W. (1966), "Speech and Song Compared in Sonagrams," *NATS Bulletin*, **23**, 18–23.

von Leden, H. (1965), "Research in Laryngeal Physiology. Clinical Applications," *Eye, Ear, Nose, Thr. Monthly*, **44**, 41–49.

von Leden, H. (1968), "Objective Measures of Laryngeal Function and Phonation," *Ann. N.Y. Acad. Sci.*, **155**, 56–67.

von Leden, H. (1971), "Datos Objectivos en el Diagnostico Laringeo," *Acta oto-rhino-laryng. Ibero-Amer.*, **22**, 258–274.

von Leden, H. (1971), "Neuere Funktionsteste des Larynx," *HNO*, **19**, 225–231.

von Leden, H. (1972), "New Horizons in Laryngology," *Acta oto-laryng.*, **74**, 332–338.

von Leden, H. and Isshiki, N. (1965), "An Analysis of Cough at the Level of the Larynx," *Arch. Otolaryng.*, **91**, 3–10.

von Leden, H. and Koike, Y. (1970), "The Detection of Laryngeal Disease by Computer Technics," *Arch. Otolaryng.*, **81**, 616–625.

von Leden, H., Le Cover, M., Ringel, R. L. and Isshiki, N. (1966), "Improvements in Laryngeal Cinematography," *Arch. Otolaryng.*, **83**, 482–487.

von Leden, H., Yanagihara, N. and Werner-Kukuk, E. (1967), "Teflon in Unilateral Vocal Cord Paralysis: Pre- and Post-operative Function Studies," *Arch. Otolaryng.*, **85**, 666–674.

Wendler, J., Seidner, W., Halbedl, G. and Schaaf, G. (1973), "Tele-Mikrostroboskopie," *Folia phoniat.*, **25**, 281–287.

Werner-Kukuk, E. and von Leden, H. (1969), "Laryngeal Trauma—Importance of Objective Laryngeal Function Tests," *Pract. oto-rhino-laryng.*, **31**, 166–173.

Werner-Kukuk, E. and von Leden, H. (1970), "Vocal Initiation: High Speed Cinematographic Studies of Normal Subjects," *Folia phoniat.*, **22**, 107–116.

Werner-Kukuk, E., von Leden, H. and Yanagihara, N. (1968), "The Effect of Radiation Therapy on Laryngeal Function," *J. Laryng.*, **82**, 1–15.

Winckel, F. (1957), "Technik und Anwendung der Laryngostroboskopie," *Z. Laryng. Rhinol.*, **36**, 574–585.

Yanagihara, N. (1967a), "Hoarseness: Investigations of the Physiological Mechanism," *Ann. Otol., Rhinol., Lar.*, **76**, 472–488.

Yanagihara, N. (1967b), "Significance of Harmonic Changes and Noise Components in Hoarseness," *J. Speech and Hear. Res.*, **10**, 531–541.

Yanagihara, N. and Koike, Y. (1967), "The Regulation of Sustained Phonation," *Folia phoniat.*, **19**, 1–18.

Yanagihara, N., Koike, Y. and von Leden, H. (1966), "Phonation and Respiration—Function Study in Normal Subjects," *Folia phoniat.*, **18**, 323–340.

Yanagihara, N. and von Leden, H. (1966), "The Cricothyroid Muscle During Phonation—Electromyographic, Aerodynamic, and Acoustic Studies," *Ann. Otol., Rhinol., Lar.*, **75**, 987–1006.

Yanagihara, N. and von Leden, H. (1967), "Respiration and Phonation: The Functional Examination of Laryngeal Disease," *Folia phoniat.*, **19**, 153–166.

Yanagihara, N., von Leden, H. and Werner-Kukuk, E. (1966), "The Physical Parameters of Cough," *Acta oto-laryng.*, **61**, 495–510.

42. DEGLUTITION

W. S. LUND

Deglutition is the transfer of solids and liquids from the buccal cavity to the stomach brought about by complex co-ordinated reflex action.

It is convenient for descriptive purposes, to divide the act into three stages:

(1) Oral.
(2) Pharyngeal.
(3) Oesophageal.

These three stages correspond to the three anatomical regions through which the bolus passes, but it must be emphasized that swallowing is a continuous and integrated manoeuvre, the initiation of the first phase inevitably leading to the automatic completion of the whole process.

Oral Stage

In this first stage, the tongue is involved in squeezing food out of the mouth and oropharynx. When swallowing begins, the tip of the tongue is raised to the back of the upper incisor teeth and is then applied to the palate from before backwards so squeezing the contents of the mouth into the pharynx. As the tongue rises in the fore part of the mouth the back of the tongue is lowered and brought forward so creating adequate space for the reception of the bolus in the pharynx. When the tail of the bolus has been expelled from the mouth, the back of the tongue arches backwards to meet the soft palate and pharyngeal wall. The bolus is squeezed downwards by the wave of contraction of the pharyngeal constrictors as it is applied to the soft palate and the tongue from above downwards. No account of the variations in the behaviour of the tongue in swallowing can be understood without following the movements of the hyoid bone, to which most of the extrinsic muscles of the tongue and the floor of the mouth are attached: the contraction of these muscles influence the volume and disposition of the tongue's substance relative to the mouth cavity.

Normal individuals swallow the contents of the mouth in the midline furrow in the tongue. When chewing, food may pass down the upper lateral food channels at the sides of the tongue to the valleculae as in the rabbit. Patients with a gap in the palate (congenital or acquired) may also divert food to the sides of the tongue, and may plug the gap by raising the tongue in the midline. Patients with holes in the cheek, e.g. a gunshot injury, learn to swallow down the opposite side as do patients with unilateral weakness of the tongue.

When the subject is at rest, breathing through the nose with the mouth closed, the volume of the tongue nearly fills the mouth cavity: the soft palate is applied to the back of the tongue and there is an adequate space between the back of the tongue and pharyngeal wall for the subject to breathe.

After food has been introduced into the mouth, the mandible is usually raised and the lips closed. Food must either be stored in the cheek pouches or contained in the mouth proper. In the first case, there need be no displacement of the tongue, but in the second, the tongue and floor of the mouth must be lowered to create space. The average content of the mouth which can be swallowed as a single bolus is about 15 ml of food and fluid. Space for this will normally be made by lowering the tongue and floor of the mouth and the hyoid bone: the teeth are normally not tightly apposed. If a large volume of food is held on the tongue, accommodation is provided by lowering the mandible.

During the act of swallowing, the jaws are brought together as the tongue fills the mouth cavity to displace the mouth contents, the hyoid bone is raised towards the lower border of the mandible. Maximum elevation of the hyoid bone is reached as the tail of the bolus is being expelled from the mouth and is maintained as the tongue arches backwards to displace the bolus downwards. These movements of the hyoid bone relate to the need to adjust the volume of the tongue: as the bolus is displaced from the mouth the tongue reoccupies its position of rest in the mouth cavity, but since the tongue must also arch backwards to displace the bolus downwards, the volume of the tongue necessary to occlude the mouth must be further reduced by raising of the floor of the mouth. In other words, maximum elevation of the hyoid bone is indicative of maximum contraction of the mylohyoid muscles, thus reducing the mouth proper to the smallest possible size. If a large bolus is swallowed, the tongue (and hyoid bone) must be pulled well forward to provide adequate accommodation for the bolus to be taken into and through the pharynx; thus, maximum displacement of the hyoid forwards relates to the degree of distention of the oropharynx.

Under certain circumstances the whole of a mouthful may not be swallowed as a single bolus. When a large mouthful is taken, the subject may elect to swallow it by a series of boluses. To do this, he releases a quantity of the content into the pharynx by parting the tongue and soft palate and then raising the tongue in the back of the mouth behind the junction of the hard and soft palates, so cutting-off the bolus in the pharynx from the rest of the contents of the mouth proper. The contents of the pharynx are then cleared by apposition of the constrictors to the back of the tongue and soft palate in the usual manner. In these circumstances, there is no oral phase of swallowing until the last mouthful is to be expelled.

Thus, it is possible to dissociate the fore part of the tongue from swallowing and to use it for some other purpose while swallowing is continuing. The fore part of the tongue may be lowered in the front of the mouth to create suction as when drinking or as part of the mechanism of suckling, or with the mouth open as in pint-swallowing, to create a large cavity into which food can be taken or poured. With the conclusion of all these acts it is necessary to clear the mouth either by dribbling with the head inclined forwards or by using the whole of the tongue to swallow the contents of the mouth.

The fore part of the tongue is also used for manipulation of food in preparation for mastication and in the formation of consonants in speech; manipulation of food may continue during pharyngeal swallowing.

The anterior third of the tongue which corresponds with the free portion in conjunction with the lips and jaws, is mainly responsible for procedures requiring manipulation in feeding and in speech. These include:

(1) Taking food from a spoon or fork, e.g. lapping, licking and pulling food such as grass.

(2) Manipulation of food in the fore part of the mouth, including cleaning the teeth and palate.

(3) Expressing the contents of a teat or nipple and the initial stage of swallowing.

(4) In speech to form consonants, and to whistle.

(5) To express emotion.

The middle third of the tongue which corresponds to the region opposite the molar teeth is concerned with:

(1) The expression of food onto the molars for chewing.

(2) The passage of food into the upper lateral food channels at the side of the tongue.

(3) When elevated it may be used to:

(a) Cut off the mouth cavity from the pharynx, e.g. when regulating the swallowing of a large mouthful by multiple boluses.

(b) Alter the shape of the oropharyngeal cavity to form vowel sounds.

(c) Plug a hole in the hard or soft palate, or cheek.

(d) Compensate for a paralysed soft palate by preventing or reducing nasopharyngeal reflux in the pharyngeal phase of swallowing.

The posterior third acts mainly:

(1) As a wadge of tissue in the pharyngeal phase of swallowing, which when apposed to the soft palate and pharyngeal constrictors displaces the bolus downwards and helps to turn down the epiglottis.

(2) When the mouth is closed, apposition between the posterior third of the tongue and the soft palate normally closes-off the mouth cavity at rest.

(3) The posterior third of the tongue can be apposed to the pharyngeal wall to close-off the airway to reinforce or substitute for laryngeal closure in certain circumstances, e.g. some normal subjects when bearing down or in patients who can use glossopharyngeal breathing, but who cannot close the larynx.

The whole of the tongue is normally concerned from before backwards in the co-ordinated peristaltic wave which squeezes food from the mouth into the lower pharynx and by the reverse response as it is lowered from before backwards it creates suction as seen in continuous swallowing associated with suckling or drinking.

Pharyngeal Stage

The Normal Mechanism of Swallowing

In the erect position, the first half of the bolus is passed through the pharynx into the oesophagus by means of thrust from the tongue, assisted by gravity. The peristaltic wave usually commences when the tongue expressor wave reaches the soft palate. With a moderate-sized fluid bolus, the head of the bolus has often entered the oesophagus before the pharyngeal peristaltic wave has commenced. This moves rapidly and smoothly downwards, clearing the pharynx of the hind part of the bolus and pushing it through into the oesophagus. Normally, no hold-up occurs at the cricopharyngeal sphincter as the wave of relaxation, preceding the contraction of the pharynx reduces the resting tone of the cricopharyngeal muscles. The peristaltic wave involves the sphincter as it descends, producing tight closure of it, the sphincter then relaxing and returning to its resting state after the peristaltic wave has passed.

Studies conducted by Ardran and Kemp (1961) show that swallowing in the lower half of the pharynx occurs down the lower lateral food channels which extend from the edge of the lateral pharyngo-epiglottic folds downwards and backwards around the laryngeal air passage to the level of the cricopharyngeal sphincter, where they fuse and become one channel continuous with the lumen of the oesophagus. These channels are functional entities and serve to transmit fluid or semi-fluid substances around the mouth of the larynx, thus preventing spill into the laryngeal airway. During swallowing the bulk of a bolus is usually deflected to either side of the mouth of the larynx and comparatively little passes directly over the edge of the tongue or the epiglottis down the midline: if the bolus is large the larynx is pulled further forwards to accommodate it and the two channels become one posteriorly.

In normal young persons during quiet breathing, the lower lateral food channels are either obliterated or reduced to narrow clefts. If the pharynx is distended with air, as in the Valsalva manoeuvre, the cavity is increased in depth and the lateral food channels are opened and partly taken into the lumen of the pharynx. The arytenoids and the body of the cricoid cartilage are moved forwards, permitting the two channels to communicate posteriorly; the piriform fossae lose their triangular or piriform shape and become two shallow depressions in the lateral aspects of the floor of the distended pharynx.

In old persons, the lower lateral food channels are frequently not obliterated at rest as in young people and may contain saliva or food residues.

When swallowing in the erect position, a bolus is usually directed down the midline of the tongue to the level of the median glosso-epiglottic fold when it is deflected into the vallecula on either side. The epiglottis is tilted backwards towards the posterior pharyngeal wall and serves to arrest the head of the bolus as it descends upon the back of the tongue. As the bolus accumulates upon the epiglottis it spills over the lateral pharyngo-epiglottic folds into the food channels on either side of the mouth of the larynx and passes forwards into the piriform fossae: at this stage a small quantity of fluid may spill directly over the edge of the epiglottis over the open entrance to the larynx. As the bulk of the bolus enters the upper pharynx, the larynx is raised towards the hyoid bone, the contents of the piriform fossae are expressed upwards and backwards, and the lower part of the lateral channels is open to allow the bolus to spill downwards and backwards towards the midline: the columns meet over the back of the cricoid cartilage at the

level of the upper border of the cricopharyngeus muscles. which then open to allow the bolus to enter the oesophagus. During the descent of the two streams below the epiglottis some fluid frequently passes behind the arytenoids joining the two columns: this path is used whenever one side is partly or completely obstructed below this level.

When the bulk of the bolus has entered the upper oropharynx, the tongue moves backwards towards the posterior pharyngeal wall and meets the contraction due to the pharyngeal constrictors. The tongue of the epiglottis is gradually displaced with the bolus and is bent downwards at the side so that it is arched like a monk's hood over the larynx. Each half of the epiglottis serves as a chute to deflect the bulk of the bolus to either side of the midline. A certain amount of the bolus is always displaced down the midline, but this proportion of the total bolus is small unless the amount swallowed is comparatively large, when room is made to accommodate it by taking the larynx further forwards. As the main mass of the bolus is expressed from the oropharynx, the soft palate is lowered and applied to the tongue and the posterior pillars of the fauces are also brought forwards. The tongue of the epiglottis is pressed forwards over the mouth of the larynx until its tip is over the back of the cricoid cartilage. As the tail of the bolus is expressed from the pharynx, the larynx is lowered; the lateral food channels are cleared from above downwards. Finally, the cricopharyngeus muscles contract and express the last of the bolus into the oesophagus. Only a small residue normally remains in the pharynx: this is situated over the base of the tongue upon the downturned epiglottis in what are now backward-turned valleculae. When the airway is re-established, as the larynx returns to the position of rest, the tongue of the epiglottis springs upwards and the small residue which remains upon the epiglottis is either retained in the valleculae or spilt into the lower lateral food channels and held in the piriform fossae.

If a person swallows with the head turned fully to one side, the bolus is deflected down the lower lateral food channel on the side opposite that to which the head is turned: the whole of an average-sized bolus may be swallowed down the one lateral channel. Old people with rigidity of the spine or other lesions may not be able to turn the head enough to obstruct totally the side to which the head is turned. Many instruments, such as a test-meal tube, the gastroscope and oesophagoscope, may be passed entirely down one side.

When a normal person swallows lying supine, the bulk of the bolus is still directed to the side of the larynx, but it takes a relatively postero-lateral course: the laryngeal opening, which is situated anteriorly, is not necessarily surrounded by the bolus unless the amount swallowed is large. The course of the bolus is likewise influenced by gravity when the patient swallows lying prone, or on one side. The effect of gravity is important in consideration of the problems of management of patients with pharyngeal palsy.

Epiglottis and Closure of the Larynx During Swallowing

Ardran and Kemp (1956) stated that there are several components associated with the above action. In the first component when the bolus of food begins to spill down the back of the tongue, the lumen of the laryngeal vestibule is invariably narrowed: this is due to the rocking movement of the arytenoids downwards, forwards and inwards with resulting narrowing of the glottis, bulging inward of the vestibular folds, forward movement of the cartilages of Wrisberg and obliteration of the interarytenoid space.

The second component produces backward tilting of the leaf of the epiglottis towards the posterior pharyngeal wall. The manner in which this is brought about depends upon the position of the larynx and hyoid relative to the cervical spine and lower jaw at the moment swallowing is initiated.

In normal individuals at rest in the erect position the leaf of the epiglottis is closely approximated to the tongue. With the passage of the bolus from the mouth into the pharynx the descent of the barium is checked by a ledge constituted by the backward-tilted epiglottis; this is the phase of vallecular arrest. At this stage the lumen of the laryngeal vestibule is usually reduced in size, but not closed.

As the mass of the bolus accumulates on the epiglottis, the larynx and hyoid are usually elevated towards the lower jaw, the hyoid rotates so that its greater cornuae become horizontal (rather than parallel with the lower border of the mandible) producing further backward tilting of the epiglottis towards the pharyngeal wall. This may result in complete closure of any remaining gap between the epiglottis and pharyngeal wall, thus completely checking any spill of the bolus.

With further displacement of the bolus from the mouth the hyoid and larynx are moved forwards and further upwards: contact between the epiglottis and posterior wall is not longer maintained and barium spills over the edge of the epiglottis into the lateral food channels on either side of the laryngeal entrance: the laryngeal lumen, though narrow, is usually not completely closed and a little barium may enter the vestibule at this time and pass down as far as the laryngeal ventricle. During this swallowing-stage the leaf of the epiglottis projects backwards above the entrance of the larynx into the stream of the descending bolus, the epiglottis is raised in the middle and bent down at the side and serves to deflect the bulk of the bolus to one or both sides of the larynx (*vide supra*).

With further descent of the bolus the whole of the hyoid bone is approximated more closely to the thyroid cartilage. The cricothyroid visor is opened which allows the arytenoid masses to be tilted bodily forward, the various components reducing the lumen of the vestibule to about a third of the antero-posterior diameter in quiet breathing.

At any stage during the bolus descent, but always when it has been expressed past the larynx, there is backward bulging of the lower part of the epiglottis into the vestibular lumen due to apposition of the thyroid cartilage to the hyoid; this in turn also results in further bulging of the vestibular folds and obliteration of the ventricles. The total effect of all these movements is to oppose the dorsal surface of the epiglottis to the cartilages of Wrisberg and obliterate the laryngeal lumen from the level of the vocal fold to the superior laryngeal aperture.

The final component of laryngeal closure is the sealing of the laryngeal aperture by the sudden downward turning of the leaf of the epiglottis within the column of the bolus. This action results from a number of factors, viz. the sustained approximation of the thyroid to the hyoid, both structures being elevated to the lower jaw, force is transmitted to the bolus as the tongue moves backward to the palate and posterior pharyngeal wall, the leaf of the epiglottis is pressed down by the descending peristaltic wave against the arytenoid masses and any residue of the bolus which lies beneath it is displaced from the entrance to the larynx.

In all normal individuals, the pharynx is not squeezed entirely clear of the bolus; there is always a small residue left upon the dorsal surface of the downturned leaf of the epiglottis, i.e. the ventral surface when the epiglottis was erect. If the leaf of the epiglottis was not present this residue would lie over the laryngeal entrance. When the airway is re-established the residue is swept upwards into the valleculae as the leaf of the epiglottis rises to the erect position.

There are, of course, modifications of the above sequence of events, for example when an individual swallows into a large, air-filled pharyngeal cavity, or when lying supine, etc.

Oesophageal Stage

Before discussing the final part of deglutition some mention should be made of the cricopharyngeal sphincter which forms the junctional zone between the pharynx above and oesophagus below.

Cricopharyngeal Sphincter

Lund (1965) states that the sphincter at rest is normally closed and remains so even when subjected to raised pressure from above or below. The cricopharyngeus muscles can relax, however, to allow air, etc., to pass either up or down. The sphincter provides a zone of elevated pressure which is approximately 1·6 kPa (12 mm Hg) above the pressure in the upper part of the oesophagus.

When swallowing occurs the sphincter initially relaxes but does not open, the bolus then passing through the relaxed sphincter by means of a thrust from the tongue assisted by gravity. The cricoid is displaced forwards by the bolus, the sphincter opening at this stage. At about the time the bolus enters the oesophagus the peristaltic wave commences at the top of the pharynx. This moves rapidly and smoothly downwards, clearing the pharynx of the hind part of the bolus and pushing it through into the oesophagus. The peristaltic wave involves the sphincter as it descends, producing the tight closure characteristic of the second stage of the sphincter changes. After the peristaltic wave has passed the sphincter relaxes, returning to its resting state.

Oesophagus

The oesophagus functions essentially as a conducting tube for conveying substances to and occasionally from the stomach. During discussion of deglutition, Slome (1971) writes that in the intra-thoracic oesophagus the intra-luminal pressure corresponds to the intra-pleural pressure. However, the pressure varies considerably with inspiration and expiration and particularly with the latter if the glottis is closed as in coughing, straining, etc. During swallowing, peristaltic waves pass down the oesophagus with waves of positive pressure reaching 6·67–13·3 kPa (50–100 mm mercury). The form of the wave varies somewhat with the nature of the swallowed substance, but with liquids and semi-solids there is an initial negative wave due to elevation of the larynx drawing on the cervical oesophagus. This is followed by an abrupt positive wave, coinciding with the entry of the bolus into the oesophagus. Next comes a slow rise of pressure, succeeded by a final, large positive pressure wave which rises and falls rapidly, this being the peristaltic stripping wave.

Secondary peristaltic waves arise locally in the oesophagus in response to distention and complete the transportation of bolus portions which have been left after the primary peristaltic wave. Tertiary oesophageal contractions are irregular, non-propulsive contractions involving long segments of the oesophagus frequently occurring during emotional stress. The velocity of oesophageal transport is more rapid in the upper oesophagus than in the distal half, due to the differences in muscle type and neural mechanism of the propagation of the peristalsis.

At the lower end of the oesophagus there is a zone of raised pressure about 3 cm in length, extending above and below the diaphragm, with a mean pressure of approximately 1 kPa higher (c. 8 mm Hg) than the intra-gastric pressure which can be regarded as the location of the "physiological sphincter" of the oesophago-gastric region. As with the cricopharyngeal sphincter, the oesophago-gastric sphincter which is normally in tonic contraction undergoes relaxation before the peristalsis reaches it, with a reflex preventing contraction occurring immediately the bolus has passed into the stomach.

The physical consistency of the swallowed material determines to some extent the mechanism involved in its passage through the oesophagus. When fluid is swallowed it may be projected from the pharynx to the oesophago-gastric junction in about 1 s (the subject standing) well ahead of the peristaltic wave. In consequence of this rapid passage the swallowing of corrosive fluids causes burns, often localized to the distal end of the oesophagus. When the bolus is solid or semi-solid it is passed down the oesophagus by a peristaltic contraction of the oesophageal musculature, gravity playing little part in the process.

In the upper part of the oesophagus peristalsis progresses rapidly. In the lower one-third the contraction wave is more sluggish, the differences in motor activity being related to the muscular coat being striated in the former situation and unstriated in the latter.

It is not in the context of this book to deal in any detail with the method of closure of the oesophago-gastric sphincter and prevention of reflux, but some reference to the numerous theories should be made. These vary from an anatomical sphincter composed of a thickening of the circular muscle, a pinch-cock action of the diaphragm, the gastric muscular loop of Willis, the oblique oesophago-gastric angle, a mechanical valve mechanism by mucosal folds or rosette, an external pressure gradient on the supra- to infra-diaphragmatic parts of the oesophagus with a flutter valve effect, to finally a physiological intrinsic muscle sphincter.

Undoubtedly the latter situation exists, producing a region of raised intra-luminal pressure extending above and below the diaphragm. This is believed to be due to several of the above factors, the chief component of the "sphincter" being a segment of intrinsic muscle of the oesophagus, close to the oesophago-gastric junction which is normally in tone and contracts and relaxes as a single functional unit.

Nervous Regulation of Deglutition (Fig. 1)

Swallowing is a brain stem reflex involving two components, bucco-pharyngeal and oesophago-gastric stages.

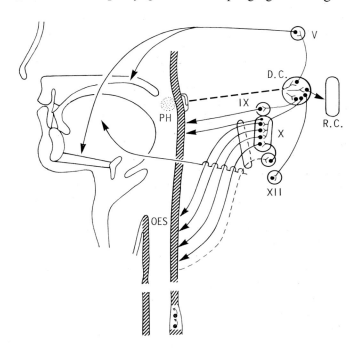

NEURAL MECHANISM OF THE DEGLUTITION REFLEX

Fig. 1.

The sensory receptors are concentrated mainly in the oro-pharyngeal area. The afferent pathways are derived from IX, the pharyngeal and internal laryngeal branches of X and V.

Afferent impulses pass to the solitary fasciculus of the brain stem, then being relayed to a specific neurone population of the reticular formation in the medulla constituting a "swallowing centre".

The efferent limb of the reflex arc comprises motor neurones supplying striated muscle located in the motor cranial nuclei of V, VII, IX and XII, together with the nucleus ambiguus of X. The neurones supplying the plain muscle of the distal oesophagus are in the dorsal nucleus of X.

There is no clinical or experimental evidence to suggest that the motor nerve supply to the cricopharyngeal sphincter is derived from either the recurrent laryngeal nerve or the autonomic nervous system. It is more likely that it is supplied by the pharyngeal branch of X.

A swallowing centre in the functional sense is located in the medulla in close relation to but distinct from the "respiratory centre" in the reticular formation. Medullary lesions may abolish the swallowing reflex without arresting respiration, but these centres are inter-connected and respiration is always inhibited during swallowing.

The centre is bilateral and consists of two half-centres. Destruction of the half-centre on one side eliminates the response of the ipsilateral swallowing muscles. The two half-centres are linked by inter-neurones, thus ensuring the normal integrated bilateral response of the muscles of the mouth, pharynx and larynx in swallowing.

The reflex stimulation of the deglutition centre results in a co-ordinated motor discharge producing contraction of the palatal muscles, the elevators of the larynx, adductors of the vocal cords, and the elevators of the pharynx. It also produces a co-ordinated peristaltic wave of contraction of the pharyngeal constrictors and the oesophageal musculature, the former being accompanied by inhibition of the cricopharyngeal sphincter.

There are experimental findings to imply that the sphincter changes are probably due to a reflex arc, stimulated by the peristaltic wave when it reaches a level just above the sphincter. It is likely that this "sphincter reflex" is merely part of a series of co-ordinated reflexes which give rise to the peristaltic wave itself. It is suggested that the nerve supply to the cricopharyngeus muscles (a definite entity in the dog) constitutes the efferent pathway of this reflex arc. The fibres passing in these nerves are either excitatory or inhibitory, producing contraction or relaxation of the sphincter respectively. The latter change is probably due to a reduction of the nerve impulses which normally pass continuously to the sphincter maintaining its resting tone. The arrangement of the afferent pathways is uncertain, but it may be formed by nerve fibres in the pharyngeal wall derived from the pharyngeal branch of X.

When a swallow is produced by stimulation of the upper pharynx an initial wave of relaxation passes downwards. When it reaches a point just above the sphincter, the reflex arc is stimulated and the sphincter relaxes. This is followed by a contraction wave which also passes down the pharynx, but in this case stimulates the reflex to produce contraction of the sphincter. Thus, the sphincter initially relaxes and then contracts, both changes being co-ordinated with the peristaltic wave.

When the pharynx is experimentally divided above the sphincter in the dog, the peristaltic wave is unable to pass downwards in the normal way. As a result the afferent pathway is not stimulated and the normal sphincter changes do not occur, even though the nerve supply to the cricopharyngeus muscles is intact. Similarly, the sphincter again fails to function normally if the nerve supply to the cricopharyngeus muscles is divided but the pharynx is continuous with the sphincter. In this case it is the efferent pathway which has been destroyed.

To *summarize*, sphincter actions depend on the integrity of the nerve supply to the cricopharyngeus muscles and also on continuity between the pharynx above and the sphincter below.

The peristaltic wave in the upper oesophagus is also part of the reflex response excited by the initial stimulation of the pharyngeal sensory receptors and is mediated through the extrinsic nerves dependent upon the integrity of the vagal oesophageal plexus.

This main reflex mechanism excited from the pharynx is supplemented by secondary reflex responses, which are initiated by the stimulation of sensory endings in the oesophageal mucosa by the bolus of food. Afferent impulses from these receptors evoke reflexly, via the vagi and the medullary deglutition centre a peristaltic contraction of the oesophageal muscle above the bolus, pushing it onward. Thus the bolus itself causes a series of reflex contractions, each one providing the stimulus for the reflex contraction of the succeeding segment of the oesophagus. If the propulsion of the bolus to the stomach is not effected by the initial peristaltic wave of the deglutition reflex, then this accessory reflex mechanism will complete the transportation through the upper oesophagus.

In the lower oesophagus in which the muscle coat is composed of smooth muscle, the propagation of the wave of peristalsis is independent of the extrinsic nerve supply. The co-ordination of peristaltic contraction is dependent here on the intra-mural myenteric plexus.

Clinical Applications

Pharyngeal Dysphagia

The cranial nuclei containing the cell bodies of the neurones supplying the muscles in swallowing lie close together in the medulla. Lesions in this region, such as those of bulbar poliomyelitis, motor neurone disease, or thrombosis of the posterior cerebellar artery may cause dysphagia. The palatal and pharyngeal muscles may be paralysed, but the cricopharyngeal sphincter is usually unaffected and will relax normally. Very rarely there may be a complete hold-up of the bolus at the level of the sphincter in a total pharyngeal palsy. On the one hand nasal regurgitation may occur and on the other laryngeal spill with coughing or swallowing. In these cases a cricopharyngeal myotomy may be indicated, but it should be remembered that there is a risk of oesophageal contents refluxing upwards through the divided sphincter, particularly if the oesophagus is also paralysed.

Peripheral lesions of IX and X, if unilateral, do not produce any serious disorder of swallowing.

Dysphagia is a common symptom in myasthenia gravis. Transmission of motor nerve impulses at the motor end plates at the neuro-muscular junction is defective. In this disorder the cricopharyngeal sphincter is also affected as well as the other muscles of the pharyngeal phase of swallowing. Difficulty in swallowing may also be a feature of the increased motor-neurone excitability in tetanus.

"Globus hystericus" describes the sensation of a lump in the throat, usually at supra-sternal notch or cricoid level, without apparent cause. In the absence of some unsuspected local condition, for e.g. inco-ordination between the cricopharyngeal sphincter and the pharynx, or a very small posterior pharyngeal diverticulum (as shown on cineradiography), the majority of these patients have some degree of reflux oesophagitis. The symptom is due to

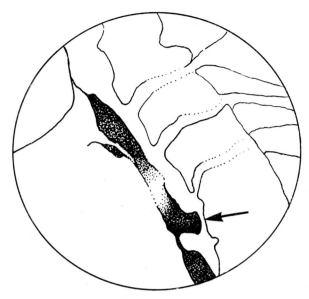

FIG. 2. Ciné swallow: 25 frames per second. Barium shown black (lateral projection of pharyngo-oesophageal region). Arrow shows a small pouch. Above it there is some pharyngeal residue indicating a weak expressor wave. Below can be seen the prematurely contracted crico-pharyngeal sphincter.

referred sensation from the lower oesophagus, antacids being an effective treatment.

The posterior pharyngeal or Zenker's diverticulum occurs at the level posteriorly between the upper and lower halves of the inferior constrictor muscles, i.e. the thyro- and crico-pharyngeal muscles respectively. This pouch arises as a result of a combination of early closure of the crico-pharyngeal sphincter and weakness or inco-ordination of the pharyngeal peristaltic wave.

If the peristaltic wave is likened in a normal swallow to the smooth, progressive squeezing of a toothpaste tube (held upside down) from the bottom to the top, then a similar analogy can be drawn to describe the formation of these early pouches (Fig. 2). If one starts to squeeze the toothpaste down from the bottom of the tube (the peristaltic wave sweeping down the pharynx) and then suddenly with the other hand squeeze the tube in front of it (the crico-pharyngeal muscles contracting) a bulge in the tube will appear between the two flattened parts (this is the equivalent of the pouch). Thus the pouch is formed when the sphincter is closing and not when it is relaxing, relaxation being usually adequate.

Achalasia of the oesophago-gastric junction is usually due to degeneration of the ganglion cells of Auerbach's plexus at this region. The oesophagus is dilated and its muscle hypotonic. Radiological studies show that in swallowing, the oesophageal peristalsis is weak or absent. Feeble, non-propagated contractions occur simultaneously in different parts of the oesophagus. The disorder is a true failure of relaxation and not a cardiospasm or hypertonus of the musculature of the lower oesophagus.

REFERENCES

Ardran, G. M. and Kemp, F. H. (1956), *Brit. J. Radiol.*, **29**, 205.
Ardran, G. M. and Kemp, F. H. (1961), *J. Laryng.*, **75**, 358.
Lund, W. S. (1965), *Ann. roy. Coll. Surg.*, **37**, 225.
Slome, D. (1971), *Diseases of the Ear, Nose and Throat*, 3rd edition, Vol. 1, p. 235.

SECTION X

VOICE, SPEECH AND LANGUAGE

PAGE

43. VOICE AND SPEECH   599

44. LANGUAGE AND SPECIFIC LANGUAGE DISORDERS IN CHILDREN   609

43. VOICE AND SPEECH

D. B. FRY

The one faculty which beyond any question marks off man from the rest of the animal kingdom is that of speech. Many scientists have tried through observation, experiment and speculation to arrive at a firm basis for this distinction and although it has been argued, for example, that in the chimpanzee and also in primitive man the anatomy of the vocal tract was such as to preclude the development of speech (Lieberman, 1968, 1972; Lieberman *et al.*, 1972) the great weight of evidence is in favour of the view that it is man's brain, by its structure and in particular by its enormous capacity for processing information, which makes speech possible. All communication by speech demands a high degree of brain activity, whether connected with the sending out of speech or with its reception, partly because such communication is based on language and all linguistic information is carried in the brain (Penfield and Roberts, 1959).

Speech is such an everyday process and is so over-learned in the individual that it is regarded as being a single, unified activity; all speech is thought of as being of the same character and as being the output of one mechanism. This is far from being the case. In every act of speaking a number of components need to be distinguished and the relation between these components, and hence the nature of speech, varies from one individual to another and from one occasion to another. One important distinction is that between social behaviour and individual behaviour. Speech serves as a means of communication between human beings only because it constitutes one form of social behaviour, because we can all recognize, when people are talking, repeated patterns of behaviour which are the coded form of the language patterns which lie behind our communication. At the same time, speech embodies individual behaviour, much of it highly idiosyncratic, which is not encoded or to be decoded in terms of the language system. This conveys information about the speaker's mood, his reactions to the situation and to his listeners, his state of health, his immediate past history and many other things. Much of this information is gleaned by listeners, whether the speaker means them to do so or not, because of their previous experience as human beings rather than as speakers of a particular language, but here again some weight is to be given to the social component since they are relying on a knowledge of the conventions of their society in evaluating individual behaviour. In much the same way speech may give information about the long-term history of the speaker, about his family, educational, social and regional background.

If we consider only the production of speech, as distinct from its reception, these two components can be characterized perhaps more clearly as a *communicative* and an *expressive* component. A speaker begins talking usually with the intention of "telling something" to his listeners and in order to achieve this object he has recourse to his memory stores which refer to the language he is using. He calls upon stored information about the vocabulary, the syntax, the grammar and the phonological system of the language in order to select words appropriate to his meaning, to construct sentences and grammatical forms and to build up sound sequences which will be readily decoded by his listeners. This last process includes selecting rhythmic patterns and intonations which fit what he intends to say and conform to the patterns of the language, so that, for example, a question shall appear as a question and not as a statement. The possible intonations for an English question are as much a part of the grammar of English speech as are the words and grammatical forms which may make up a question (Halliday, 1967).

All this constitutes the communicative component of the speech and communication by speech is possible and successful precisely because speaker and listeners share common information about the language. It is not possible, however, for a speaker to confine himself to the communicative component when speaking; whether he wishes it or not, an expressive element will be added to his communication. Often this will be quite overt; he may, for example, ask a question and at the same time express indignation that it should be necessary to ask the question, or he may make a statement and show that he is emotionally involved in contradicting something which has just been said. In other cases the effects are much less obvious, as frequently when the speaker expresses by his intonation or tone of voice that he is immensely flattered by what has been said. Even where the speaker uses a neutral tone, the expressive component is still there in the very absence of any marked emotional colour in the speech and it is present again, on a more physiological level, when speech conveys simply that the speaker has a cold or is feeling tired.

The effects of these two components, communication and expression, cannot of course always be clearly distinguished in the speech output since they interact to a considerable degree. It is worth noting, perhaps, that a much greater proportion of ordinary speech is predominantly expressive than we usually imagine and speakers are very often expressing their emotional reaction when both they and we, as listeners, believe them to be stating a fact or giving an intellectual judgment. The mechanisms by which the two components operate in speech form the subject of the rest of this chapter. The whole of speech activity is based on the use of mechanisms which serve other and more vital functions in the human body, those of breathing, swallowing and chewing. In speech, the working of these mechanisms is adapted to serve the three main purposes of respiration for speech, phonation and articulation and we can view the system as one in which highly developed and sophisticated functions are superimposed upon more vital and hence more primitive ones. The expressive component in speech is more closely connected with these primitive functions and, as we shall see, influences respiration and phonation particularly. The communicative component is a later development, both in the individual and in man himself, and depends very largely on the more sophisticated activity of articulation. The infant already has at his disposal the means of expressive utterance, which he in fact shares with many animals; he then learns to add to this the capacity for communication, which distinguishes him from the animals, but he does this without ever losing the capacity for expression.

RESPIRATION FOR SPEECH

Speaking is a form of physical work and as such requires a supply of energy. This is provided by the flow of air from the lungs during the expiratory phase of breathing. There are no normal circumstances in which speech takes place during the inspiratory phase though children will sometimes adopt this technique in play and there are isolated cases in which it may take place in adults for some very special reason (Wyke, 1973). Speaking on the inspired air is very inefficient and cannot be maintained for very long.

During quiet breathing the time taken for one breath cycle, i.e. inspiration plus expiration, varies from one individual to another and from one occasion to another, depending on the conditions. The range of variation among individuals is rather larger than is generally supposed; there are some in whom the rhythm of ordinary quiet breathing is as slow as 10 breaths min^{-1} and others in whom it is as high as 20 breaths min^{-1}. An average for a large sample of subjects is likely to be in the region of 15 breaths min^{-1} (Skarbek, 1967).

If 1 cycle takes 4 s, this time will be about equally divided between inspiration and expiration, each phase occupying about 2 s. Since speech makes use of the expiratory phase only, there must clearly be a breaking of this even rhythm during speech, for if it were maintained, a speaker would be compelled to spend just as much time in taking in breath as he did in uttering what he wants to say. In fact the rhythm is drastically altered in speech; breath is taken in much more rapidly than in quiet breathing and the expiratory phase is made to last very much longer than the inspiratory. The duration of the expiratory phase depends upon the particular utterance planned by the speaker but it may in rather extreme cases last up to about fifty times as long as the inspiratory phase (Peterson, 1957). This change in the breathing rhythm is brought about by a somewhat delicate balance between the action of the muscles of exhalation and inhalation, a balance which is continuously changed in the course of an utterance in such a way as to maintain almost constant air pressure below the glottis (Draper et al., 1959).

The moments at which the speaker breathes in are determined normally at the linguistic level of organization and according to syntactic considerations. The brain is continually occupied with the forward planning of what is to be said and, at one level, the plan provides for breath pauses which will coincide with the end of a phrase, clause or sentence (Goldman-Eisler, 1968). How often a breath is taken depends upon the style and the tempo of the speech sequences. While speaking in public, for example, a speaker will adopt a relatively slow tempo and tend to take more breaths at phrase and clause endings; the more rapid tempo of conversation, on the other hand, will entail fewer breaths. This is one level at which the influence of the expressive component is very marked, since a speaker who is feeling very emotional and is allowing free expression to his emotion will tend to take in breath more frequently during speech; if he is trying to inhibit the expression of emotion in speech, however, the effect is likely to be the opposite and the frequency of breathing may be decreased (Goldman-Eisler, 1968).

With regard to the amount of air taken in during speech, it can be said in general that this is little if any greater than that taken in during quiet breathing. In this respect there is considerable individual variation. Although subjects who take in relatively large amounts of air in quiet breathing tend to do the same during speech, it is nevertheless quite common to find subjects who regularly take in less air for purposes of speech (Gray and Wise, 1959; Idol, 1936). An equally interesting observation is that speakers do not by any means necessarily require more air in order to speak loudly than to speak at a conversational level, and in fact many speakers use rather less (Idol, 1936). This is to be accounted for by the fact that the acoustic intensity of the speech output is less dependent upon the amount of air available than upon the efficiency of the laryngeal mechanism and the associated vocal tract.

MECHANISM OF PHONATION

Since only the expiratory phase of breathing is used for speech, the power supplied by the lungs takes the form of air-flow in one direction. In order that this power may be transformed into an acoustic output, the first requirement is a mechanism for converting the uni-directional flow into fluctuations or oscillations within the range of frequencies which produce the sensation of sound in the human hearing mechanism. The larynx provides the basic means for this conversion.

Adduction of the vocal folds interposes a barrier in the path of air flowing to or from the lungs. If the vocal folds are adducted when air is flowing from the lungs, then air pressure builds up in the trachea against the under surface of the folds. As the pressure increases, a condition is reached in which the obstacle presented by the vocal folds to the flow of air can no longer withstand the pressure and consequently the folds open, allowing air to flow momentarily into the pharynx. This release of pressure results in the return of the vocal folds to the closed condition, owing in part to the elasticity of the folds and in part to the Bernoulli effect, which is the developing of a negative pressure in cases where air is flowing through a narrow opening into a wider tube. When the folds are again closed, the cycle of events begins to be repeated, air pressure builds up once more and the vocal folds open and close again as before. The opening and closing of the folds continues so long as air is flowing from the lungs and the folds are held in the adducted position (Van den Berg, 1968).

In this way the larynx mechanism converts uni-directional air-flow from the lungs into a series of puffs of air whose frequency is determined by the physical conditions obtaining in the larynx. The mass, length and tension of the adducted folds and the general level of subglottal pressure all influence the degree of pressure increase which the closure will withstand and also the rapidity with which the folds open and return to their closed position, hence determining the time taken for each cycle of opening and closing. The sound resulting from this glottal action is the sound of voice and the frequency of the glottal cycles is responsible for the voice pitch which is heard by a listener. An average value for the frequency of the vocal tone in the speech of male speakers is 120 hertz (cycles per second) and in female speakers is about one octave above this, 240 Hz (hertz).

A major difference between speaking and singing is that, during speech, the period of the vocal fold vibration changes continuously whereas in singing it remains relatively constant for appreciable lengths of time. The sliding pitch changes which are characteristic of speech result from the fact that successive cycles of opening and closing have different periods. The range of variation differs as between men, women and children. It differs among individuals and from utterance to utterance. At the low end of the range is found the phenomenon which is referred to as "creaky voice" by English authors and as "vocal fry" by Americans, which is characterized by alternating longer and shorter voice periods (Fourcin, 1972). This effect is heard very frequently in English speech where it regularly marks the end of a final falling intonation pattern. Measurements in this part of the range show frequencies as low as 50 Hz or even 30 Hz and these very low frequencies are to be found in the speech of women as well as men. At the other end of the scale, men's speech will not generally show voice frequencies above about 400 Hz and women's not above 500 Hz (Denes, 1962). The difference in the mean frequency for men and women, in the face of this considerable overlap in the ranges, is accounted for by the proportion of time during which women's speech uses higher frequencies.

The range of voice frequencies in a single utterance depends on both the communicative and the expressive elements. The intonation patterns in a given language form an important part of the linguistic system and they dictate the general outline of the frequency variations to be used in a particular utterance. The expressive component then determines the actual range which these variations will cover; if the speaker is very emotional and is expressing pleasure, excitement, indignation or anger, the range will be wide; if he is expressing awe or disgust or contempt, the range will be narrow, and if he is unemotional, the range will lie between the two.

The period of vibration is not the only dimension along which the vocal fold action varies. A number of factors affect also their mode of vibration. When the larynx is producing low frequencies, the vocal folds are relatively slack and during the closed phase of their vibration, the surfaces which are in contact have an appreciable vertical height. When the folds begin to open in response to increased pressure below, contact is broken first on the underside, the puff of air progresses upwards and a little later breaks the contact at the upper surface. By this time, the lower edges of the folds have begun to close again, so that there is a rolling motion of the surfaces which are in contact in the vertical plane and a consequent vertical phase difference in the flow of air (Sonesson, 1968). The production of higher frequencies requires a marked increase in the tension of the vocal folds, with a consequent thinning of the edges and a considerable reduction in the surfaces which are in contact during the closed phase, and there is now no vertical phase difference (Van den Berg, 1968). There are naturally many intermediate adjustments of the vocal folds and all such changes are important because they affect the waveform of the vocal fold vibration. As a result we hear not only variations in the pitch of the voice but also changes in the voice quality.

The relation between the open and the closed phase of the vocal fold vibration is one feature of the glottal waveform which shows a good deal of variation. At low frequencies of vibration the closed phase may occupy up to about half of the time for the complete cycle; at higher frequencies, the open phase takes up a larger proportion of the cycle than the closed phase and for very high tones, the vocal folds move towards each other but do not attain complete closure at any point in the cycle. The ratio of closed to open phase is also connected with variations in the loudness and the quality of the vocal tone and with the efficiency of the larynx as a sound generator. If the closed phase is relatively long and the open phase gives rise to a pulse of considerable amplitude, the glottal wave will produce a sound of great acoustic power for the expenditure of a small amount of exhaled air. This condition often obtains in the case of practised speakers and in singers who make the larynx work with a high degree of efficiency when producing high tones as well as low ones. An additional effect in these circumstances is brought about by the more rapid closing action of the vocal folds which provides a sharper wavefront at the rise of the glottal wave and hence a glottal tone which is richer in high harmonics. Tones of low intensity, whether spoken or sung, will generally have characteristics which are the converse of these; the open phase of vibration will be relatively long, the pulses of low amplitude and the wavefront not very sharp so that the resulting sound is richer in low than in high harmonics (Flanagan, 1958; 1972).

Again in the matter of voice quality the expressive element in speech plays its part. The speaker's emotions find their expression through larynx action not only by means of the pitch pattern but through the selection of the appropriate voice quality. Additional tension in the vocal folds and the associated structures gives rise to the loud, harsh quality appropriate to expressions of anger, indignation and aggression, or to the quieter but still hard-edged tones of disgust or contempt; a moderate degree of tension produces the rounder tones of pleasure or affection and a low degree of tension gives the long open phase and the breathy quality which expresses the emotions of awe or fear.

THE LARYNGOGRAPH

The problem of obtaining reliable information about the functioning of the larynx as a sound generator is one which is not easily solved. Much has been learned from the study of the behaviour of excised larynges and by the examination of the human larynx during speech, with the aid of the laryngoscope, by means of still or cinéphotography generally with stroboscopic devices (Van den Berg, 1968). X-ray tomography has also been used, as has a trans-glottal illumination technique in which a small light source is introduced by way of the nostril and the naso-pharynx and interruptions in the light effected by movements of the vocal folds are registered by means of a photo-cell applied to the external surface of the throat below the larynx (Lisker *et al.*, 1969; Sawashima, 1972). A major disadvantage of nearly all such methods is that it is difficult for a subject to continue normal speech production.

A great deal of valuable information about larynx functioning is now being gained through the use of the *laryngograph*, a device which has been perfected and described by Fourcin (1971), and which makes possible the reliable monitoring of larynx action without interference with normal speech. A pair of surface electrodes is placed in contact with the skin of the neck, one on each side at the level of the larynx. A high frequency signal, of the order of 1 MHz, passes from one electrode to the other and the amplitude of the signal picked up varies according to the state of affairs in the larynx. The major factor is the degree of contact between the vocal folds; when there is good contact, the impedance to the signal falls and there is consequently a high level of signal picked up by the second electrode. When the folds are not in contact, the impedance rises and the signal level falls. The waveform of the output is therefore a reliable indication of the degree of contact between the vocal folds and of the variation in this quantity with time.

The curves shown in Fig. 1 are typical of those obtained with the laryngograph. Since there is an increase in the signal when the vocal folds are in contact, a rise in the curve indicates closure of the folds. The output of the laryngograph has been correlated with the results of direct photography of the larynx and the correspondences between the laryngograph curve and the phases of vocal fold action are indicated in Fig. 1. With suitable electronic equipment it is possible to derive and to plot automatically from the curves the successive periods of vocal fold vibration. Such frequency curves taken together with the glottal waveforms afford a very valuable basis for the study of normal speech and also of pathological conditions (Fourcin, 1971).

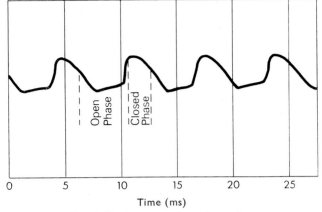

Time (ms)

FIG. 1. Laryngogram of a male speaker.

FUNCTIONS OF THE LARYNX IN SPEECH

Phonation is an important element in speech because the sound generated at the glottis is what makes speech generally audible to listeners; it acts as the carrier-wave for speech information (Dudley, 1939). Variations in vocal fold frequency are the major vehicle for intonation patterns which are a part of the language system and serve vital communicative and expressive functions. In addition, the larynx fulfils other functions in speech which are directly connected with the working of the language system. The chief of these is concerned with the switching on and off of vocal fold vibration. Although the vocal folds are in vibration for a considerable proportion of the time during which speech is actually being sent out (approximately 70 per cent of the time in English speech), there are a number of sounds which require that the larynx tone should be switched off. These are the voiceless consonants such as *p*, *t*, *k*, *s*, *f*, etc. in English. Whenever these sounds occur in the stream of speech the vocal folds are returned to the adducted position and remain there until the sound of voice is next required. The switching action, whether on or off, is accurately synchronized with movements of other articulators, such as the opening of the lips for *p* or *b*. It has been shown experimentally that, for example, a difference of some 30 ms in the moment of the onset of vocal fold vibration relative to the opening of the lips is enough to differentiate *p* from *b* for the majority of English listeners (Lisker and Abramson, 1970).

Larynx action is involved in some other forms of articulatory activity. In certain contexts, the vocal folds are adducted and separated again without the initiating of vibratory movement. This results in the sound known as the *glottal stop* which frequently accompanies the production of *p*, *t* and *k* in the dialects of London and the south of England and may replace the articulation of *t* and *k*. For the production of *h* sounds the vocal folds are brought and held sufficiently close together to produce marked turbulence as the air passes through the glottis either with or without simultaneous vibration of the folds. Similar action is required for whispering, in which there is no vibration of the vocal folds but the noise generated by turbulence at the glottis replaces the sound of voice as the carrier for speech information. In more intense whispering (as in a stage whisper) the anterior part of the vocal folds may be adducted and turbulence set up at the cartilaginous glottis. In all whispering, the overall intensity of the speech, and hence its carrying power, is very much reduced.

MECHANISMS OF ARTICULATION

The sound generated at the larynx carries a very restricted range of speech information. If it were transmitted direct to a listener, and with the aid of the laryngograph it is possible to do this experimentally, he would be able to recognize the intonation and rhythm of what was said, would pick up information about the mood of the speaker and, if the speaker were someone whom he knew well, would probably be able to identify the speaker. He would not, however, be in a position to take in the words, phrases and sentences and would be unable to decode the message from the linguistic and hence communicative point of view. Most of the information of this kind is transmitted through the modulation of the glottal tone brought about by the action of the muscles used in articulation.

The larynx mechanism is coupled to the *vocal tract*, that is the air tube which leads from the larynx through the pharynx and mouth, and also through the nasal part of the pharynx (nasopharynx) and nose, to the outer air. The effect of articulatory action is continually to modify the configuration of the vocal tract and so modulate the larynx tone. The syllabic structure of speech is one important result of this modulation. During a large proportion of any speech sequence, the air passage through the vocal tract is relatively wide open and a high level of sound energy is radiating from the speaker's lips. Each high amplitude stretch of speech is flanked by low amplitude stretches so that continuous speech forms a rough alternation of low and high amplitude sounds. The reduction in amplitude is brought about by introducing a constriction or a complete blockage of the air path at some point in the vocal tract and the articulations which effect this are those of the consonant sounds. Vowel articulations leave the tract relatively open and any sequence consists of syllables, each made up of a vowel with consonant articulations on either side. The principal articulator for vowel sounds, and for the majority of consonants as well, is the tongue; for vowels, the tongue forms a constriction at some place in the oral section of the vocal tract, thus modifying its resonances, as we shall see in the section on the acoustic aspects of speech. From the point of view of articulation, vowel sounds are classified according to the place and the degree of the constriction into categories such as front, back, open and close vowels (Gimson, 1970; Jones, 1956).

Consonant articulations call for rather more dimensions of classification which are summarized in Table 1. The majority of consonants depend on the setting up of turbulence at some point in the vocal tract, either by forming a very narrow constriction and increasing the air-flow through it, or by blocking the air passage completely and then allowing a sudden release of the air pent up behind the obstruction. The result in both cases is audible noise which can be generated at different points in the tract and one of the chief dimensions of classification is the place of maximum constriction or the *point of articulation*. In the case of *p*, for example, this is at the lips, for *s* it is at the alveolar ridge and for *k*, at the velum. The method by which the noise is generated gives another dimension; the fricative mode is that in which a narrow constriction produces turbulence which lasts for an appreciable time, the plosive mode is that in which a complete obstruction is followed by a sudden release of air and there is a third mode in which a complete closure is followed by a slower release involving friction noise; this gives rise to the affricates. There is a whole group of consonants, shown in the lower half of the table, in which no noise is generated so that the sounds are essentially vowel-like. The nasal sounds are made with a complete closure of the oral air passage but with the velum lowered and the passage through the nasal part of pharynx open; lateral sounds are made with a closure at the mid-line of the oral cavity but with an open passage at the sides of the tongue and semi-vowels are brief vowel articulations which are followed immediately by a true vowel articulation of longer duration (Gimson, 1970; Jones, 1956).

TABLE 1
THE CONSONANT PHONEMES OF ENGLISH

Manner of Articulation	*Place of Articulation*						
	Bi-labial	*Labio-dental*	*Dental*	*Alveolar*	*Palatal*	*Velar*	*Glot-tal*
Plosive	p b			t d		k g	
Affricate				tʃ dʒ tr dr			
Fricative		f v	θ ð	s z ʃ ʒ			h
Nasal	m			n		ŋ	
Lateral				l			
Semi-vowel				r	j	w	

Table 1 is Table III, p. 46, in Whetnall and Fry, *The Deaf Child.*

Finally there is the possibility that the consonant articulation may or may not be accompanied by vocal fold vibration. In cases where the symbols are shown in pairs in the table, the first of a pair refers to a consonant in which the larynx mechanism is switched off and no vocal fold vibration accompanies the articulation, the second to a consonant during which the folds are vibrating; thus *p*, *t*, *f*, *s*, for example, are *voiceless* consonants while *b*, *d*, *v* and *z* are *voiced*. The consonants in the lower part of the table, the nasals, laterals and semi-vowels, are all voiced in most contexts in English.

On the speech production side, the whole range of articulations, both vowel and consonant, form the vehicle for the distinctions necessary to the phonological system of the language and thus provide the basis for the communicative component. This component would almost disappear from, for example, English speech if the speaker did not have the means of implementing distinctions like those between *pick* and *lick*, *hid* and *had*, or *rim* and *rib*. The transposing of such distinctions on to the acoustic and perceptual planes will be dealt with in the following sections.

SPEECH MECHANISM AS AN ACOUSTIC SYSTEM

The main reason for treating the physiological speech mechanism as a system comprising two principal components, the larynx and the vocal tract, lies in the acoustic function of these two elements. As we have said, the vocal folds generate a carrier wave which is modulated by the vocal tract; the glottal wave is referred to as the *source function* and the resonance characteristics of the vocal tract as the *system function*. Each puff of air set up at the level of the vocal folds excites the resonances of the vocal tract, setting the air in the tract into forced vibrations. Both the source function and the system function change continuously during a speech sequence and hence the sound-waves which are radiating from the speaker's lips and nostrils, and which are the resultant of these two functions, present a waveform which is continuously changing (Fant, 1960; Flanagan, 1972).

THE SOURCE FUNCTION

A number of the ways in which the source function varies have already been noted. In speech, the frequency of the vocal fold vibration is likely to lie somewhere within the range of approximately 50–500 Hz but it changes continuously so that the period of successive cycles of opening and closure is different. The amplitude of the pulses generated at the glottis also varies and so too does the actual waveform of the laryngeal tone. Typical waveforms, as they are registered by the laryngograph, were shown in Fig. 1. Fig. 2 shows a further example obtained

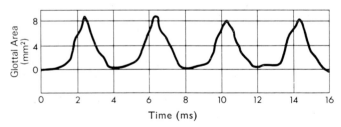

FIG. 2. Glottal area function obtained from high-speed photography of a male speaker. (After Gill, 1962.)

by direct photography of the vocal folds from above (Gill, 1962). Here the area of the opening between the edges of the vocal folds is plotted against time and therefore a rise in the curve indicates an increase in the degree of opening; the distinction between the open and the closed phase is more immediately visible than in the laryngograph curves.

The approximately triangular waveform in Fig. 2 is typical of the shape of the glottal wave. Like other periodic or quasi-periodic waves it can be regarded as being the summation of a number of sine waves whose frequencies are all terms in a harmonic series based on the fundamental frequency, which is itself determined by the period of the

complete cycle of opening and closing of the vocal folds. Such a pulse wave will have a spectrum like that shown in Fig. 3; the fundamental frequency is the component having the highest amplitude, all successive harmonics are represented in the spectrum and the amplitude of these harmonics falls off exponentially as their frequency rises. The spectrum shown here is that of a glottal tone transduced by the laryngograph and analysed by means of a spectrograph. It will be seen that there is still some considerable amplitude of harmonics above 3000 Hz. The possible variations in glottal wave-form mentioned earlier, such as the change in the relations of the open and closed phase of the vocal fold movement, the sharpness of the wave front and the amplitude of the wave will all produce changes in the spectrum of the resulting sound. Some of these effects will appear in the distribution of minor peaks of energy in the spectrum of the kind which are to be seen in Fig. 3 but more generally they will influence the proportion of higher to lower harmonics in the total spectrum. Since the source function drives the resonances of the vocal tract, such variations will in turn affect the quality of the sound which leaves the speaker's lips and will be heard by listeners as differences in the "brightness" or "roundness" and so on of the voice quality.

THE SYSTEM FUNCTION

The larynx is coupled to the vocal tract which is the column of air connecting the sound generating mechanism with the outer air. Like any other air column, that of the vocal tract will have normal modes of vibration and therefore will act as an acoustical resonating system, but it has peculiar properties in that not only the effective length but also the cross-sectional area of the column can be varied in a great variety of ways. The length can be changed by small vertical movements of the larynx structures and by lip movements which extend the column at its outer end and the shape of the tube can undergo a very large number of modifications through movements of the tongue, soft palate and lips. All such adjustments alter the resonances of the whole vocal tract.

We will consider first a simplification of the system in which the vocal tract is represented as a straight cylinder of uniform cross-section. In the adult male speaker the length of the tract is of the order of 17 cm and a realistic estimate of the cross-sectional area of such a cylinder would be about 6 cm^2. When the air in a cylinder of these dimensions is forced into vibration by a sound source which is closely coupled to it, the first three resonances are found to occur at 500, 1500 and 2500 Hz (Fant, 1960; Flanagan, 1972). This approximation to the human vocal tract is clearly not a very close one. In its simplest form, during the production of steady-state vowels, the tract consists of at least two tubes, of different lengths and cross-sections, connected together by a constriction. However it has been found that theoretical models of the acoustical behaviour of the vocal tract, based on the general principle of considering it as a series of tubes joined by constrictions, do give reasonable approximations to the acoustic output of the speech mechanism. For a full treatment of these theoretical models, *see* Flanagan (1972).

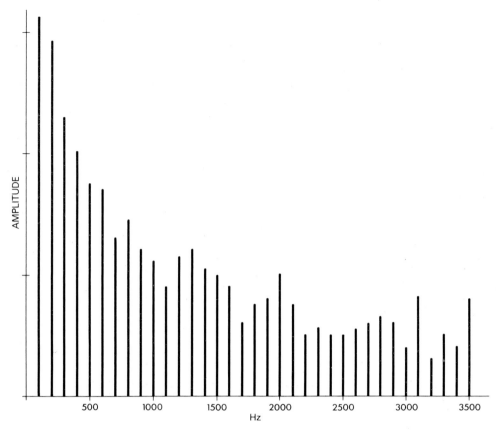

FIG. 3. Spectrum of a glottal wave obtained from a laryngogram. (After Fourcin, 1972.)

Acoustically then, the vocal tract presents a number of resonances which are excited by the glottal tone or by any other sound which is fed into the tract. The frequencies at which these resonances appear depend upon the configuration of the whole tract and each resonance is referred to as a *formant* of the resulting speech sound. It is usual to label formants by numbering them 1, 2, 3 and so on, beginning with the lowest resonance; thus the sound produced by a cylinder of the dimensions given above would have Formant 1 (F1) at 500 Hz, Formant 2 (F2) at 1500 Hz and Formant 3 (F3) at 2500 Hz.

The resonances of the vocal tract largely determine the spectrum of the sound which leaves the speaker's mouth, since each formant tends to introduce a peak of energy. The spectrum of the glottal tone is therefore transformed by its transmission to the outer air. Fig. 4 shows one example of the changes which may take place. On the right of the figure is reproduced the spectrum of the glottal tone; in the middle is an outline drawing of the vocal tract giving an indication of its configuration for a particular vowel and on the left is a typical spectrum for this vowel sound. It is quite possible for the human vocal tract to take on a shape which gives rise to formants at approximately 500, 1500 and 2500 Hz. The resulting sound is close to the vowel heard in a Southern English pronunciation of the word *bird* and it is the configuration and spectrum for this sound which are shown in the figure.

It will be seen that the constriction in the vocal tract for this vowel is somewhere about the middle of the oral space. If this constriction is moved further forward, the acoustic effect is to lower the frequency of F1 and to raise the frequency of F2 and of F3. Moving the constriction further back, raises the frequency of F1 and lowers the frequency of F2 but makes little change in F3 (Flanagan, 1972).

The first three formants fulfil the most important linguistic functions since variation in these resonances distinguishes many of the sounds used in languages. Variations in the higher formants generally serve to differentiate individual speakers and moods. From the listener's point of view, the frequencies of F1 and F2 go very far towards specifying a vowel sound and the sounds forming the vowel system of a given language are often described by giving the average values for these frequencies. It is necessary to collect samples from a reasonably sized group of representative speakers and the mean formant frequencies are then obtained through the use of a spectrum analyser. Such a mean value indicates the middle of a frequency band over which the formant frequency is likely to vary. Table 2 gives the means for a group of speakers of Southern English for 11 vowels which form a part of the English vowel system (Wells, 1962). This system also includes a number of diphthongs in which there is a marked change in the configuration of the vocal tract, and hence in the formants, during the production of the sound; such sounds cannot of course be specified by a single value of F1 and of F2.

The amplitude of the spectral peaks due to the formants

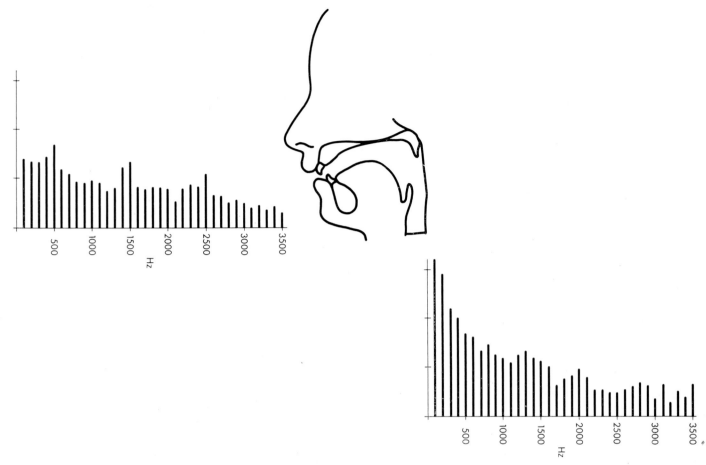

Fig. 4. Spectrum of the glottal wave, configuration of the vocal tract and spectrum at the lips for a vowel like that in the English word *bird*.

also varies from vowel to vowel and from one formant to another. On average, the intensity of F2 is some 12 dB lower than that of F1, and of F3, 28 db. lower than F1.

TABLE 2

MEAN FORMANT FREQUENCIES OF ENGLISH VOWELS
(After Wells)

	$F1$ (Hz)	$F2$ (Hz)
i:	300	2300
i	360	2100
e	570	1970
a	750	1750
a:	680	1100
o	600	900
o:	450	740
u	380	950
u:	300	940
ʌ	720	1240
ə:	580	1380

The formant values given in this table are based on data from a group of English subjects, reported by Wells (1962).
Table 2 is Table V, p. 56 in Whetnall and Fry, *The Deaf Child.*

Variation with different vowels is up to 5 dB in F1, up to 20 dB in F2 and can be as much as 23 dB in F3 (Peterson and Barney, 1952).

An important feature of the vocal tract is its high degree of damping which ensures that the resonances which it exhibits are not highly tuned. This is important from the language point of view since it is essential that vowel differences, for example, which are recognized on the basis of the location of the formants, should not be too much affected by changes in the fundamental frequency at which the vocal tract is driven by the glottal tone. Every shift in this fundamental frequency involves the generation of a different series of harmonics but owing to the damping of the tract and the relatively flat character of its resonance curves, there is always some energy in the glottal tone which will excite the resonances which constitute the formant regions. Because of this, vowel differences remain easily recognizable when vowels are uttered on fundamental frequencies which cover a wide range.

The band-width of these resonances can be derived from the spectra of vowels and these measurements give an average of 50 Hz for F1, 65 Hz for F2 and 100 Hz for F3 (Dunn, 1961).

Before leaving the subject of the resonances of the vocal tract it must be noted that the resonance pattern is somewhat modified if the effect of the air passage through the nose is added to that of the oral tract. For the majority of English sounds the velum is raised and obstructs the flow of air into the nose. In these conditions, sound transmission into the nasal part of the pharynx (nasopharynx) is very inefficient and there is little radiation of sound from the nostrils. In the production of the nasal consonants *m*, *n* and *ng*, however, the velum is low and the air passage through the nasal part of the pharynx and nostrils is open, while the passage through the oral tract is completely obstructed at some point. The nasal passage, in this arrangement, constitutes a side-branch to the main tract and the acoustic effect is to enhance the amplitude of the lowest formant, to introduce a spectral minimum, rather than a maximum, in the frequency region where F2 is to be found in oral vowels and to reduce the amplitude of higher frequencies generally (Flanagan, 1972; Fujimura, 1962).

NOISE COMPONENTS IN SPEECH

Up to the present we have considered only the case in which the resonances of the vocal tract are excited by the periodic glottal tone. The resonances will however be excited by any source which is coupled to the vocal tract. This is clear from the special case of whispered speech in which the vibration of the vocal folds is replaced by turbulence at the glottis, thus providing a broad spectrum noise as the source function. Whispered speech, so long as it is audible, is perfectly intelligible to a listener because the resonances of the vocal tract are being varied in exactly the same way as in voiced speech and the necessary distinctions between sounds are still possible.

Apart from this special case, however, during ordinary speech for some 30 per cent of the actual speaking time the vibratory mechanism of the larynx is switched off and the voice source function is replaced by some other source. This occurs during the production of all the voiceless consonants (*see* Table 1). In describing the articulation of these sounds, we noted that they depend on the setting up of turbulence at some point in the tract, in some cases by forming a narrow constriction and forcing air through it and in others, by closing the tract altogether and then releasing the air sharply in a short burst of noise. In both cases the noise generator is placed at different points in the tract for different consonants. For the fricative sounds, the noise generator is a constriction between upper teeth and lower lip for *f*, between upper teeth and tongue blade for *th*, tongue tip and upper alveolar ridge for *s*, tongue blade and the back of the alveolar ridge for *sh* and at the glottis for *h*. The acoustic picture for these sounds is even more complex than for vowels since the sound source is no longer sited constantly at one end of the tract, but may be placed at different distances from the glottis. Further, the noise actually generated at a given point of articulation depends upon the shape and size of the constriction and on the rate of air-flow through it. The variety of noises which occur in speech is the outcome of the complicated interaction between the noise source and the resonances of the vocal tract with which it is coupled, which of course means the whole vocal tract including both the length of it which happens to lie behind the constriction as well as that which lies forward of it. We shall confine ourselves here to some descriptive comments on the resulting sounds.

In the English fricative system we have two sounds, *f* and *th*, made at the extreme forward end of the tract, with a narrow slit-like constriction and low rate of air-flow. The resulting sounds are of low over-all intensity, with a marked rise in the level of spectral energy in the band from 6000–8000 Hz. The fricatives *s* and *sh* have the constriction considerably further back in the vocal tract, have a larger and rounder constriction but also a much higher rate of air-flow. The resulting sounds are both of much higher intensity than *f* and *th* (on the average about 12 dB). The spectra of *s* and *sh* are very different from each other; the further forward placing of the constriction in *s* introduces a spectral minimum at about 3000 Hz and there is a sharp rise in spectral energy in the region of 4000–6000 Hz. For *sh* the spectrum is considerably flatter and there is a high level of noise energy from about 2000 Hz upwards. The remaining member of the fricative group, *h*, has the noise source at the glottis and the resonances of the tract are therefore the same as for vowels and in fact *h* has marked formants which correspond to those of whatever vowel follows it in the phoneme sequence (Flanagan, 1972; Hughes and Halle, 1956).

Similar factors determine the acoustic character of the stop consonants, those in which there is a complete closure of the tract followed by a sudden release of air which generates a short burst of noise. For the sound *p*, the closure is made by the two lips and when the air is released the resulting pulse excites the resonance of the whole tract, giving a noise-burst with a peak of energy in the low frequencies between 300 Hz and 400 Hz. The closure for *t* is made at the upper alveolar ridge at just about the same place as the constriction for *s* is made, so that the release produces a short-lived noise with the frequency characteristic of *s*, that is a sharp peak of energy in the band from 4000–6000 Hz. In producing *k*, the closure at the velum divides the tract approximately into two equal sections and the noise-burst of *k* is intermediate between those of *p* and *t*, in the region of 1800 Hz (Halle *et al.*, 1957; Liberman *et al.*, 1952).

The one case that remains to be considered is that of the voiced consonants, which have already been referred to in the section on articulatory mechanisms. The voiceless stop and fricative consonants which have just been discussed all have their voiced counterparts during the production of which both glottal tone and noise generators are functioning. The noise components are similar to those of the corresponding voiceless sounds and to them is added the glottal tone, filtered by the particular configuration of the vocal tract. The resulting waveform at the lips is quasi-periodic, the periodicity being caused by the train of pulses from the larynx, with a random noise wave-form superimposed upon each period. From the point of view of the spectrum of the sounds, the general effect is the addition of low frequency energy to the spectrum of the corresponding voiceless sound with a marked diminution of the intensity level of the noise.

This last feature is of some importance with respect to the English system of stops, affricates and fricatives. The voiced version of all these sounds is made with vibration of the vocal folds when it occurs within a speech sequence, but whenever any of these sounds occurs at the very beginning or end of an utterance, the voice component is usually absent. Even the consonant *h*, which is generally regarded as being voiceless, has a voiced version used by many speakers in the middle of such words as *ahead*, *boyhood*, etc. Where "voiced" consonants occur without vocal fold vibration, the listener has to make use of other features in order to distinguish *b* from *p*, *z* from *s* and so on.

The importance of the various acoustic features of sounds that have been outlined above lies in the fact that they afford the basis for making the sound distinctions demanded by language systems. The use of such items of acoustic information, generally referred to as *acoustic cues*, by language users is a very complex matter and will not be dealt with in this chapter. There is an extensive literature on the subject and a summary of some of the evidence is to be found in Fry (1970). Original papers are listed in the references under Cooper *et al.* (1952), Delattre *et al.* (1952 and 1955), Fry *et al.* (1962), Harris (1958), Liberman *et al.* (1954 and 1957), Lisker and Abramson (1970), and O'Connor *et al.* (1957).

REFERENCES

Cooper, F. S., Delattre, P. C., Liberman, A. M., Borst, J. M. and Gerstman, L. J. (1952), *J. acoust. Soc. Amer.*, **24**, 597.

Delattre, P., Liberman, A. M., Cooper, F. S. and Gerstman, L. J. (1952), *Word*, **8**, 195.

Delattre, P. C., Liberman, A. M. and Cooper, F. S. (1955), *J. acoust. Soc. Amer.*, **27**, 769.

Denes, P. and Milton-Williams, J. (1962), *Language and Speech*, **5**, 1.

Draper, M. H., Ladefoged, P. and Whitteridge, D. (1959), *J. Speech Hear. Res.*, **2**, 16.

Dudley, H. (1939), *J. acoust. Soc. Amer.*, **11**, 139.

Dunn, H. K. (1961), *J. acoust. Soc. Amer.*, **33**, 1737.

Fant, G. (1960), *Acoustic Theory of Speech Production*.

Flanagan, J. (1958), *J. Speech Hear. Res.*, **1**, 99.

Flanagan, J. (1972), *Speech Analysis, Synthesis and Perception*, 2nd edition.

Fourcin, A. J. (1972), in *Proc. 7th Int. Congr. Phonetic Sciences*, p. 48.

Fourcin, A. J. and Abberton, E. (1971), *Med. biol. Instrum.*, **21**, 172.

Fry, D. B., Abramson, A. S., Eimas, P. and Liberman, A. M. (1962), *Language and Speech*, **5**, 171.

Fry, D. B. (1970), in *New Horizons in Linguistics*, p. 29 (J. Lyons, Ed.).

Fujimura, O. (1962), *J. acoust. Soc. Amer.*, **34**, 1865.

Gill, J. (1962), in *Proc. 4th Int. Congr. Phonetic Sciences*, p. 167.

Gimson, A. C. (1970), *An Introduction to the Pronunciation of English*.

Goldman-Eisler, F. (1968), *Experiments in Spontaneous Speech*.

Gray, G. W. and Wise, C. M. (1959), *The Bases of Speech*, 3rd edition. New York: Harper.

Halle, M., Hughes, G. W. and Radley, J-P.A. (1957), *J. acoust. Soc. Amer.*, **29**, 107.

Halliday, M. A. K. (1967), *Intonation and Grammar in British English*.

Harris, K. S. (1958), *Language and Speech*, **1**, 1.

Hughes, G. W. and Halle, M. (1956), *J. acoust. Soc. Amer.*, **28**, 303.

Idol, H. R. (1936), in "Studies in Experimental Phonetics," *Louisiana State University Studies*, **27**, 79.

Jones, D. (1956), *An Outline of English Phonetics*, (8th edition).

Liberman, A. M., Delattre, P. and Cooper, F. S. (1952), *Amer. J. Psychol.*, **65**, 497.

Liberman, A. M., Delattre, P. C., Cooper, F. S. and Gerstman, L. J. (1954), *Psychol. Monogr.*, No. 68.

Liberman, A. M., Harris, K. S., Hoffman, H. S. and Griffith, B. C. (1957), *J. exp. Psychol.*, **54**, 358.

Lieberman, P. (1968), *J. acoust. Soc. Amer.*, **44**, 1574.

Lieberman, P. (1972), in *Proc. 7th Int. Congr. Phonetic Sciences*, p. 258.

Lieberman, P., Crelin, E. S. and Klatt, D. S. (1972), *Amer. Anthrop.*, **74**, 3.

Lisker, L., Abramson, A. S., Cooper, F. S. and Schvey, M. H. (1969), *J. acoust. Soc. Amer.*, **45**, 1544.

Lisker, L. and Abramson, A. S. (1970), in *Proc. 6th Int. Congr. Phonetic Sciences*, p. 563.

O'Connor, J. D., Liberman, A. M., Delattre, P. and Cooper, F. S. (1957), *Word*, **13**, 25.

Penfield, W. and Roberts, L. (1959), *Speech and Brain Mechanisms*.

Peterson, G. E. (1957), in *Manual of Phonetics*, 1st edition p. 139 (L. Kaiser, Ed.).

Peterson, G. E. and Barney, H L. (1952), *J acoust. Soc. Amer.*, **24**, 175.

Sawashima, M. (1972), in *Trends in Linguistics*, **12**, 12.

Skarbek, A. (1967), "The Significance of Variations in Breathing Behaviour in Speech and at Rest," Ph.D. Thesis, University of London.

Sonesson, B. (1968), in *Manual of Phonetics* (2nd edition, p. 45) (B. Malmberg, Ed.).

Van den Berg, J. (1968), in *Manual of Phonetics*, 2nd edition, p. 278 (B. Malmberg, Ed.).

Wells, J. C. (1962), "A Study of Formants of the Pure Vowels of British English," M.A. Thesis, University of London.

Whetnall, Edith and Fry, D. B. (1971), *The Deaf Child*. London: Heinemann.

Wyke B. (Ed.) (1973), *Int. Symp. on Ventilatory and Phonatory Control Systems*.

44. LANGUAGE AND SPECIFIC LANGUAGE DISORDERS IN CHILDREN

MICHAEL RODDA*

Language and Language Theory

The major problem in discussing specific language disorder as a clinical condition is that the concept grew up in the post-war era under the umbrella of the emerging discipline of Audiology. Although psycho-acoustics was one of the parent disciplines of audiology, the discussion of specific language disorder failed to keep abreast of changes in the thinking of psycholinguists, sociologists and experimental psychologists—changes which had profound impact on our understanding of language development and perceptual processing. The resulting misconceptions have, even today, a continuing influence on clinical and remedial practice, and it is only recently that their harmful effects have begun to be realized. The art of clinical diagnosis of specific language disorder is made difficult because it is seen as a "disease" rather than a loose description of a variety of disabilities involving a number of different types of perceptual, linguistic or language problems. Description has concentrated on the auditory rather than the perceptual or cognitive systems, and the problem has been seen as one of abnormality rather than one of delayed or arrested development, equated with the adult conditions of aphasia rather than with language learning in normal children. Space does not permit me to write the treatise on developments in other disciplines which is really required, but reference must be made to the work of Shannon and Weaver, Chomsky and Bernstein, and a brief description of their influence is necessary if the reader is to follow the author's line of argument.

The late 1940's and 1950's saw the building of a systematic theory of information transmission in experimental psychology. The theory stemmed from the need to provide a means for making theoretical predictions in telecommunications and represents the contribution of Shannon and Weaver (1949) to this discussion. Their book on the *Mathematical Theory of Communication* concentrated not on the content or meaning of transmitted information, only on the probability of interaction between separate units of information measured in purely physical terms. Its importance to psychology was in providing a conceptual framework in which perception and language could be analysed as processes rather than events. Whilst earlier workers had attempted to do this, they lacked the analytical tools for making the transition, and without these tools the conceptual task was too complex to be handled by purely verbal analysis. In contrast, B. F. Skinner had a theory of learning based on a traditional stimulus response (S-R) theory. It fell to a linguist, Chomsky, to challenge the supremacy of Skinner's position and expose the fallacies of too rigid an application of S-R theories. His first major work

(Chomsky, 1957) began a new approach to linguistics and language learning, introducing to a wider audience the concept of transformational grammar and precipitating the decline if not the demise of the S-R theorists. Coincidently, Chomsky's thesis was published in the same year as Skinner's own treatise (Skinner, 1957) and only a year or two later Bernstein (1958, 1959) was also attacking, though less directly than Chomsky, the S-R position. Bernstein established language as a sociological as well as a cognitive variable and whilst he was easier to ignore than Chomsky the changing mood of psychology meant that his influence could not be ignored. His differentiation of public from formal language was particularly important and will be described later in more detail.

Skinner was never able to reconcile S-R theory with Chomsky's analysis. Judith Greene (1973) states: "Chomsky sees no problem here whilst Skinner thinks he has already solved it." She also suggests that the "vitriolic terms of Chomsky's original review" may have affected Skinner, but he has remained equally unresponsive to all critics and it is unlikely that Chomsky's tone has much to do with Skinner's reaction. It fell to Osgood (1963) to make some attempts to bring S-R and Chomskian theories closer together, but his failure to appreciate that they are concerned with different processing levels made his attempts rather futile. S-R theory has little of importance to say about the use of linguistic rules but it does help us to understand how linguistic or other stimuli activate the use of language. Chomsky helps us to explain the creativity of language—the way language independent in its form and structure from internal or external stimuli can be generated from within. The relationships between linguistics and information theory were seen more clearly, but only in the 1960's were the two approaches fully reconciled. Miller, in particular, through *Plans and the Structure of Behaviour*, written jointly with Galanter and Pribram, had much to do with the reconciliation. However, he only succeeded because "transformational grammar", the key concept in Chomsky's theory, was amenable to the introduction of rules based on probability—the concepts of information theory. Coupled with Bernstein's rather independent formulation of the sociological role of language, it was possible by the mid-1960's to clearly differentiate the five components of learning, linguistics, perception, cognition and language, but the literature on specific language disorder continued to be written as if language existed independently of and included all of these other attributes, as if language were a separate "faculty" independent of and not associated with its development in normal children. Given this, it is not surprising that "specific language disorder" is a concept mainly ignored by disciplines other than audiology and why it is exceedingly difficult to relate the literature on the topic to a suitable operational framework.

---

* The views expressed in this chapter are solely those of the author, and do not necessarily reflect the policy of the Department of Health and Social Security of Great Britain.

Definition of Language Disorder

Before carrying any discussion of specific language disorder further it is important to define it as an audiological concept as precisely as possible. Clinically it is characterized rather than defined as "a disability in understanding and/or expressing linguistic symbols, which is not remedied by traditional approaches to language instruction, and cannot be attributed to a defect in general intelligence, primary emotional disorder, a defect in sensitivity to sound, a defect in the peripheral speech mechanisms, or social or educational deprivation" (Farrant, 1971; by reference to the work of Barry 1961; Benton 1964; Calvert, Ceriotti and Ceile, 1966; Institute on Childhood Aphasia, 1962; and McGinnis, Kleffner and Goldstein, 1956). This process of definition by exclusion means that the classification and diagnosis of specific language disorder is confused. The term often degenerates into a catch phrase despite the existence of the recognizable clinical condition, and Eisenson (1968) has even gone as far as suggesting that as many as 90 per cent of children described as having "congenital aphasia" are misdiagnosed. Similarly, Di Carlo (1960) found of 67 children classified as "language disordered", only 4 met his diagnostic criteria—the majority of the others were either peripherally deaf or mentally retarded.

Despite the difficulties, there is a fair measure of agreement on a theoretical definition. Only a few suggestions, such as Orton's (1937) that the disorder may have a familial basis, sound slightly off-key, and in a survey of 18 residential schools for the deaf in the United States Mullins (1968) found full agreement by the staff of 11 schools with a theoretical definition—the staff of the other 7 schools qualifying rather than rejecting this definition. As with Mullins, the disability is generally seen to be associated with a defective ability to perceive the "temporal sequences" of sounds—the origin of this idea being found in classroom observation of the inability of language-disordered children to respond efficiently to rhythm or to properly sequence words (Monsees, 1957; Nicholas, 1962; Lea, 1965), but Farrant (1971) has pointed out that there is a possible confusion of cause and effect in these observations. It may be that experience with language provides the basic experience necessary for learning to process and code auditory stimuli briefly separated in time, rather than the reverse, as is assumed by most other writers on specific language disorder. Even if this suggestion is invalid, the literature frequently confuses the psychological and physiological aspects of the disability and is prone to apply physiological concepts as psychological explanations, a comment we shall now analyse in more detail.

Aetiology and Classification of Specific Language Disorder

The view that specific language disorder results from central nervous system damage has been expressed frequently (McGinnis, Kleffner and Goldstein, 1956; Monsees, 1957; Benton, 1964; Cole and Kraft, 1964; Taylor, 1964; Eisenson, 1968), but much of the theorizing borders on the fanciful. Less fanciful but equally unprofitable have been attempts, such as those of Myklebust (1954) and Hardy (1956) to describe specific aetiological classes of language disorders which associate with *differential* damage to the central nervous system. Most authorities now reject this approach (*see* Reichstein and Rosenstein, 1964), and, whilst accepting that there is a clinical entity of "specific language disorder", see this as a broadly based syndrome resulting from fairly diffuse damage, rather than seeing it as a highly localized neurological condition. Indeed Lenneberg (1964) goes even further and argues that the concept of intact but non-functional language mechanisms is meaningless in children. He suggests that the basic "language acquisition device" is impaired and different aspects of the disability are merely different reflections of the same basic aetiology. Certainly, whatever their value for adults, terms such as congenital word deafness, verbal auditory imperception, oligophasia, idiopathic language retardation, congenital verbal imperception and auditory symbolic disorder have little clinical significance when discussing specific language disorder in children.

Equally misleading have been attempts to divide specific language disorders into "receptive", "expressive" and "associative" conditions, analogous to Head's (1926) classical analysis of aphasia. McGinnis, Kleffner and Goldstein (1956); Lenneberg (1964) and Eisenson (1966) have all discussed the interdependence of language functions in children, and directly or by implication have concluded that purely expressive aphasia in young children is extremely rare. The major problem is a developmental impairment of language-learning skills which has some similarities to the receptive or associative condition, but is conceptually misunderstood if the analogy with the adult disorder is taken too far. Eisenson gives the clearest description, and feels the few children who understand but are unable to reproduce speech, more probably suffer from oral or verbal apraxia than aphasia. It cannot be emphasized too strongly that the differences between neurological damage to an established linguistic processing system in adults and damage to an unestablished and developing system in children are considerable. Whilst the classification has real meaning in the adult disorder, the plasticity of the neurological systems in the child means any attempt to divide language disorders into expressive, receptive or associative conditions imposes on the disorder a functional differentiation having little, if any, relevance to the language-learning processes which ought to form the focus of our attention in young children.

We have to turn to the work of Lotz (1970) to find a multiple classification system which is relevant to these language-learning characteristics. She has identified two main groups, each showing different learning problems in the classroom. The first group have attentional deficiencies and as a result randomly oscillate between distractability and perseveration. The second group have fundamental difficulties in integrating sensory input, in memory storage and in recall from memory. If they show attentional difficulties these are secondary to the major problem. Both types of children have limited ability to interpret environmental stimuli—one cannot attend to or cannot differentiate between competing stimuli, the other cannot interpret stimuli to which they have attended. For both groups, inability to perceive and organize objects, events and relationships in sensory stimuli leads to linguistic and cognitive deficiencies, particularly during the early years when cognitive and perceptual growth interact so crucially with each other. It is unfortunate that we have chosen to term the disability specific language disorder. Perhaps, the American term, specific learning disability, is a more appropriate one because specific language disorder is a developmental, perceptual and linguistic not a language impairment, and the characteristic retardation of emotional and social development which accompanies rather than results from the language impairment confirms this point of view.

Further confirmation is found in studies such as those of Wilson, Doehring and Hirsh (1960) and Farrant (1971) which have concentrated directly on diagnosis and have shown that the real problem is one of "diagnostic plurality". For example problems of auditory and visual association were identified by Wilson, Doehring and Hirsch for only 6 of the 14 children they studied. Their failure to identify uniform characteristics in groups of language disordered children is usually thought to result from either a failure in initial diagnosis or from a concentration on attributes which do not, from hindsight, reflect the major diagnostic criteria. In reality, the nature of specific language disorder is such that any group of children present differing profiles of impairment of learning and language skills, and diagnosis and remediation must be based on an understanding of language development, language learning and language functioning as part of a complex interactive perceptual, cognitive and linguistic processing system. Diagnosis and educational remediation must identify, directly or indirectly, the form of the processes, responses and outputs characteristic of the individual child. It must be more than mere "labelling". It must permit the clinician, the teacher and others to make suggestions about appropriate methods of developing *perceptual* and *cognitive* skills. It must not assign the child to an arbitrary class in a continuum of disability—the characteristic meaning of a clinical diagnosis of specific language disorders even when arrived at by many experienced practitioners.

Language Development

Language forms the base of a pyramid from which children develop and determines not only communication skill but social skill. It has been defined as a system of conventional symbols having reasonable uniformity in a given culture (Lewis, 1968), but such a definition ignores the universal nature of the deep structure of language and is only properly applied to the surface structure. The failure to appreciate this means that the processes underlying the development of linguistic skills in children with language and communication disorders has not been described adequately even though a number of texts describe various aspects of language development and ability in normal or other groups of handicapped children (e.g. McNeil, 1970; Harrison, 1958; Smith, 1962; Peins, 1962; Spradlin, 1963; McCarthy, 1964). Figure 1 attempts to do so with some assistance from Affolter (1968) and attempts to show how a developmental continuum can permit a range of conditions

to exist within the broad classification of specific language disorder.

The figure shows a *Condition*, a *Process* associated with that condition, a *Response* generated by the underlying process, and an *Output* determined by the appropriate process and response. The schemata described are developmental—*Reflex*, *Hearing*, *Listening* and *Communication* flow into one another as do the associated outputs of *Emotive Sound*, *Babbling*, *Imitation* and *Echolalia*, and *Speech, Reading and Writing*. The end-product is language in its various forms as achieved under optimum conditions by normal children and adults. Although hearing impairment and specific language disorder are properly regarded as separate clinical disabilities with different aetiologies, both disorders are characterized in Fig. 1 by a developmental failure in perceptual or linguistic skills. Their clinical differences arise because they represent organic or maturational retardation at different points on a normal to abnormal continuum.

On the normal to abnormal continuum severely hearing-impaired children develop emotive sounds and babbling, and it is reasonable to conclude that both the reflex and auditory processing levels are intact. The language problems of such children concern the need to develop listening and communication skills whether in an auditory or some other modality, and without these skills speech development will stop. It is more difficult to identify the level at which processing is malfunctional in the child with a specific language disorder, but the aetiology is probably at the more basic "hearing" or "reflex" level of Fig. 1. Again, without appropriate experiences, development will not take place, but in this case the retardation occurs at an earlier developmental age.

The apparent confusion arising from the suggestion that the hearing-impaired child cannot listen and the child with a specific language disorder cannot hear arise because characteristically we measure function by reference to the integrity of the organic systems. The figure does not describe these mechanisms, but rather the ability of a complex neuropsychological system to perceptually process incoming sensory stimuli. We are not concerned with the physical disability, *per se*, but with effect that this has on the the language learning process. Prescribing a hearing aid for a child does not restore auditory discrimination skills. Such skills can only develop through use, and the primary learning task for the child in the classroom is learning to listen. Similarly, the child with a specific language disorder may have an intact peripheral hearing system, but the inability to make acoustic sense of what he hears often results in inhibition of the response to sound. For him, the first learning task in the classroom is learning to hear not learning to discriminate which can only come after hearing has developed. However, it is important to remember that by drawing arbitrary lines on a continuum we run the risk of reinforcing the conceptual errors identified in the previous section. The real question is not what a hearing-impaired child or a child with a specific language disorder is like, but rather what are the prescriptive characteristics of this individual child—the profile rather than the labelling approach clearly conceptualized in Carroll's (1964) definition of word

DEVELOPMENTAL MODEL OF AUDITORY FUNCTION
(Adapted from Affolter, 1968)

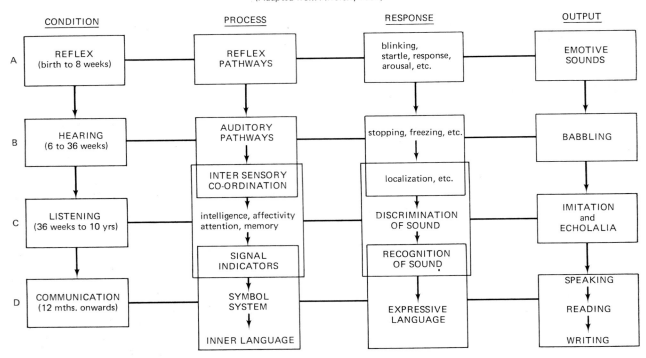

FIG. 1. Shows how auditory and language function develops from basic auditory reflex responses in normal children.

classes and Jenkins' (1958) illustration of the negative stereotypes characteristic of disability.

Specific Language Disorder and Hearing Loss

Despite the statements made in the previous section, it is possible to identify some differences between hearing-impaired and language disordered children, and as long ago as 1930 Ewing differentiated between peripheral hearing-impairment resulting from damage to the hearing system up to and including the brain stem nuclei and specific language disorder resulting from damage to the central nervous system. Most writers are vague about the supposed site of the damage in specific language disorder, but Benton (1966) suggests bilateral damage between the cochlea nuclei and the temporal cortices. Worster-Drought (1965) also suggests bilateral damage involving the auditory word area. The prevailing professional view is that hearing loss and specific language disorders in children are usually found together (see Rappaport, 1964), but caution is needed in accepting this as a definitive conclusion. Most of the studies cited (e.g. McGinnis, 1963 and Eisenson, 1966) have used children for whom a real or a presenting hearing loss is likely to be the main initial symptom, and there is a lack of information about the existence of specific language disorders in other groups of children. Without this information it is dangerous to assume that children with specific language disorders are significantly more prone to have organic hearing losses.

The association of specific language disorder and hearing loss not only lacks a sound statistical basis, but also raises other questions because inattention to sound is a characteristic of many children with language disorder (see Benton, 1964; Lenneberg, 1964; Purdie, 1966). Inattention is easily confused with hearing impairment and makes audiometric differentiation of language disorder and peripheral hearing loss difficult (Monsees, 1957; Barry, 1961; Ewing, 1962; Nicholas, 1962; Taylor, 1964; Purdie, 1966). Figure 2, reproduced from Farrant (1971), shows that the diagnostic criteria used in such testing are primarily based on inconsistency of response rather than on more objective criteria. Particularly important is the discrepancy between responses to meaningful and non-meaningful stimuli, difficulties in conditioning prior to conducting a performance test of hearing, unreliable responses during such a test and ease of distraction by visual stimuli. These negative factors are the main ones used in clinical diagnosis, although, when available, sleep or evoked response audiograms to provide important supplementary information—all of which adds to the process of definition by exclusion which is a primary and regrettable aspect of clinical practice.

Sporadic attempts have been made to improve on the situation described in the previous paragraph and to develop more positive methods for differentiating hearing-impaired and language disordered children. A baseline of theoretical knowledge exists for doing this in the field of experimental psychology involving work such as that of Conrad (1972). The author has also shown that a sequential test of auditory discrimination and a test using systematic cueing of auditory responses gives better results (Rodda, 1973). Despite these efforts, diagnosis is still based on an essentially pragmatic validation—the success or otherwise of the child is an educational programme designed for hearing-impaired children. It is generally assumed (e.g. Rappaport, 1964) that language disordered children gain only minimal benefit from the curriculum of such a school, but some workers

Peripherally Hearing-impaired Child	Language disordered Child	Reference
1. Hearing difficulties directly related to the pure-tone audiogram.	Auditory inefficiency over and above that which would be expected from audiometrically determined hearing loss.	McGinnis (1963); Taylor (1964).
2. Close relationship between results of pure tone and speech audiometry.	Considerable discrepancy between results of pure-tone audiometry and speech audiometry.	Nicholas (1962); Taylor (1966a).
3. Close correspondence between audiograms obtained in the waking state and by sleep ERA.	The sleep ERA indicated better hearing than suggested by results of conventional audiometric tests in the waking state.	Ewing (1962); Goldstein (in Rappaport, 1964); Gordon (1966); Monsees (1957); Taylor (1964); Worster-Drought (1965).
4. Consistent response to audiometric tests and environmental sounds.	Inconsistent response to audiometric tests and everyday sounds.	Douglas, Fowler and Ryan (1961); Hardy and Pauls (1959); International Conference on Audiology (1957); Monsees (1957); Myklebust (1954).
5. A performance test of hearing can be carried out from the age of about 3 years.	Cannot be conditioned to respond to a performance test of hearing, at an age when this would normally be expected	Douglas, Fowler, and Ryan (1961); International Conference on Audiology (1957); Purdie (1966); McGinnis (1963); Taylor (1964, 1966b).
6. Can respond to sound when visually or otherwise engaged.	Often fails to respond to sound when visually or otherwise engaged.	Myklebust (1954); Taylor (1964, 1966a); Benton (1964).

Fig. 2. This shows the criteria used to audiometrically differentiate peripherally hearing-impaired and specific language disordered children (reproduced from Farrant, 1971).

disagree and accept McConnell's (1964) contention that "although the non-peripheral group tended to show plateaux effects for longer periods, and were more inconsistent both in achievement, and from one to another, the study demonstrated that the results of intensive acoustic oral stimulation for such children are favourable". The explanation for these divergent points of view may be found

in the work of Farrant (1971) and the emphasis it places on motivation and learning in not only children with specific language disorders, but in children with peripheral impairment of hearing. The problem arises because we fail to question the effects of classroom instruction on different types of children and tend to assume that the same educational techniques have the same overall impact, irrespective of the wide range of individual differences children bring to and develop in the classroom.

Motivational Disturbance in Specific Language Disorder

The concept of perceptual defence is a well established psychological phenomenon (see Kleinman, 1957; Broadbent and Gregory, 1967), and the existence of "functional" hearing losses in children with specific language disorders is clearly established. Mark and Hardy (1958) suggest, unless the child has a secondary hearing impairment, responses to sound of language disordered children are usually normal up to about 4 years of age. If this is so, apparent hearing losses in children with specific language disorder must have psychologically based aetiology. Certainly the suggestion that these losses are an emotional reaction in language disordered children is a recurring theme in the literature (D'Asaro, 1962; Kleffner, 1959; Stark, 1966) further supported by the suggestion of Eisenson (1966) and McReynolds (1966)) that the closer auditory stimuli approximate to conventional language the more likely they are to be inhibited. Seemingly, inhibition of acoustic responses to sound is a secondary characteristic of the disorder resulting from the stress generated in trying to cope with visual or auditory stimuli which consistently fail to convey meaning.

Farrant (1971) has given a great deal of attention to this problem, and has produced a comprehensive summary of the theoretical basis of the motivational difficulties facing language disordered children and of the implications these have for education. Figure 3, reproduced from Farrant, shows how central nervous system dysfunction results in a failure of the auditory stimulus to convey information which in turn results in failure when specific language disordered children are taught by the traditional teaching methods of schools for deaf children. Failure generates anxiety, causing aversive responses to the stimulus and these aversive responses produce inhibition of sound. To overcome this problem, she used operant conditioning techniques and "stimulus shaping" to generate desired responses in an "errorless learning" situation. Such techniques replace failure by success, "desensitise" anxiety, and by removing the cause of inhibition remove a secondary cause of educational failure and lack of auditory response. Farrant, herself, points out that remedial language programmes, such as those of McGinnis (1963) and Lea (1966), intuitively utilize these principles, but differ in one crucial respect—the transfer from a simultaneous visual/auditory presentation to auditory presentation alone is abrupt, and prevention of errors in the final stages of learning is not possible.

In contrast to the prevailing opinion, Elliot and Armbruster (1967) found that the only significant differences between peripherally deaf and language disordered children at the Central Institute for the Deaf, St. Louis, were in age of diagnosis, age of prescription of hearing aids and age of school placement. They feel that if "speech pathology" children received the same early treatment as hearing-impaired children differences in the academic achievement of the two groups would at least be "smaller". Farrant also found, under carefully controlled conditions that the approximation to language of the auditory stimulus did not affect the degree of motivational disturbance. However, stress generated by a given stimulus; it does not change the essentially reactive nature of the process.

Specific Language Disorder and Primary Emotional Disturbance

The natural extension of problems of perceptual defence and language inhibition is into the field of primary emotional disturbance in children, but, as in hearing impairment,

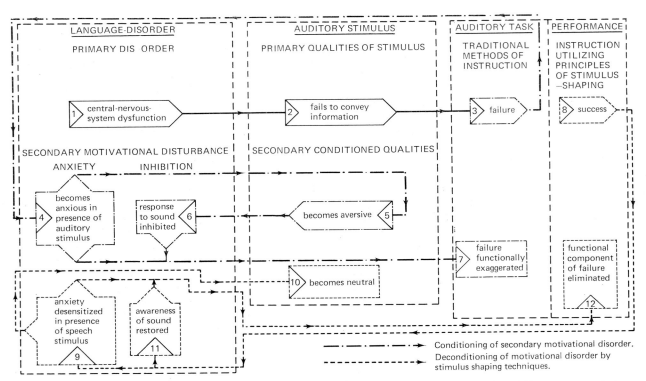

FIG. 3. Shows the hypothetical causes of motivational disturbance in children with specific language disorder and how operant techniques may reduce such problems. (Reproduced from Farrant, 1971.)

she suggests that such results complement rather than contradict those of other studies and provide an explanation of some of the discrepancies. Her explanation emphasizes that hearing-impairment as well as specific language disorder can sometimes be associated with inhibition of auditory or language responses because perceptual defence is determined by the stress produced by a stimulus not by its objective significance. One of the initial purposes of education of deaf children is the removal or prevention of inhibition of sound responses, but pre-school instruction of language disordered children is also specifically geared to dealing with their language problems. Although techniques differ for the two groups, the goal of the instruction is the same for each. It is not surprising that group differences are not statistically significant because inhibition of response to sound in children is a secondary reaction to, not a characteristic of specific language disorder. Whether or not it occurs will be determined by the social, educational and psychological history of the child not by his or her educational classification. It will be present in most severely impaired children who have not had early remedial training, but such training only reduces the amount of

diagnostic differentiation between childhood autism and specific language disorder is difficult. Despite the work of Creak (1961), O'Gorman (1967) and Wing (1973), part of the problem is the definition of the autistic condition is nearly as imprecise as the definition of specific language disorder, covering a wide range of malfunctional skills and concentrating on subjective rather than objective criteria. Even if this were not so research by Tubbs (1966) using the Illinois Test of Psycholinguistic Abilities has shown that as well as being linguistically retarded, autistic children have different profiles of linguistic skills from normal or mentally retarded children. These linguistic characteristics place autism in the same dimensional framework as specific language disorder. Moreover, the linguistic characteristics cannot be regarded as secondary effects. Although Lenneberg (1964) has suggested that there can be no situation in which the primary emotional condition in autism is remediated independently of the communication problem, more soundly based research by Rutter (1968) does not confirm Lenneberg's position and shows autistic children continue to be linguistically retarded even when their emotional problems show improvement. Whatever the effects of treatment, the linguistic aspects of the autistic condition makes diagnostic differentiation from specific language disorder difficult, but not impossible since in practice the two syndromes can be clearly distinguished (Benton, 1964; De Hirsh, 1967; Wakstein and Wakstein, 1962).

Autistic-type symptoms in language disorder are usually thought to be secondary, and in this assumption may lie the genesis of the conceptual problem of trying to differentiate two handicaps which apparently have a common aetiology in language impairment. The so called secondary symptoms may be simply less developed than those seen more clearly and pathologically in children whose major handicap is autism, although McGinnis (1963) and Lea (1966) would disagree with this idea and strongly express the view that aphasia and autism are distinct disabilities. If the two disabilities are not related, it is difficult to understand why secondary emotional problems decrease when a child with a specific language disorder begins to acquire language (see Barry, 1961; Kaftein, 1961; McGinnis, 1963; Wilson, 1964), but we need to be cautious in accepting this statement as proven fact. As previously suggested the expressed objectives of educational programmes may differ from their practical effects and, perhaps, language teaching does not remediate language but explicitly or implicitly remediates emotional problems. Fortunately, the insoluble dilemma posed by this question can be clarified if not fully resolved, by reference to more experimentally based research.

Kanner (1951) was first to postulate central nervous system damage as a cause of autism, but the work of Hutt and his associates (1964; 1970) postulates more specifically that the aetiology is to be found in chronic hyper-arousal of the lower brain structures. The repetitive mannerisms of rocking, tapping, finger twirling or wrist flicking could be displacement mechanisms which result from and reduce the amount of arousal. In confirmation of their hypothesis, Hutt and his associates found that the characteristic EEG pattern of autistic children is a predominantly low voltage, generalized activity, lacking any clearly established rhythm. In a complementary study Rodda (1973), basing his work on that of Ittleson and Kutash (1961), has postulated that anxiety as opposed to behavioural inhibition is the primary problem of the language disordered group, and that this also leads to a high level of arousal, but it is cortically, rather than subcortically mediated. Finally, Stratton and Connolly (1973) have undertaken one of the rare studies, investigating the ability of new-born infants to process auditory intensity, pitch and rhythm. They improved on earlier studies, such as those of Bartoshuk (1962) and of Eisenberg and associates (1966), by specifically controlling intensity and pitch, so enabling the three physical dimensions to be investigated independently. Their results showed that young infants clearly have ability to discriminate pitch and intensity but responses to the temporal characteristics of sound were found to be "rather more elusive". Stratton and Connolly point out that this finding tends to confirm Whitfield's (1967) suggestion that intensity and pitch discrimination are mediated subcortically, whereas discrimination of temporal patterns occurs at the cortical level.

If confirmed, the importance of the studies described in the previous paragraph is in showing the existence of similar but phylogenetically differentiated mechanisms in specific language disorder and childhood autism, consistent with the idea of a continuum of language disorder, ranging from autism at one extreme to hearing impairment at the other. At the moment this can only be regarded as a tempting and appealing hypothesis but, if true, the suggestion that many of the mannerisms of the autistic child are "displacement" activities could apply equally to children with a specific language disorder and to children with peripheral impairment of hearing. Displacement will be minimal in the hearing-impaired child because the need to discharge tension will also be minimal. It will be most frequently observed in the autistic child because of pathological damage to the structures of the lower central nervous system directly involved in attending to and processing sensory stimuli.

Language and Memory

To fully understand the nature of the problem, it is necessary to understand information processing in cognition and to appreciate that there are three different types of information storage system. Memory consists of a sensory information store, a short term memory and a long term memory. Information must be held in the sensory information store before it can be transferred to memory for use cognitively or linguistically (see Norman, 1968). Crowder and Morton (1969) have clearly demonstrated the existence of the "pre-categorical" level in the auditory modality, and Conrad (1964) had earlier demonstrated a visual equivalent. Both Conrad and Crowder and Morton show that integration of auditory and visual stimuli can and does take place in short term memory, and this offers a possible explanation of the intersensory aspects of specific language disorder.

Memory processing is also important because pre-categorical auditory as opposed to acoustic discrimination is a major and common factor to both perception and language. Again of the specialists in the field of specific language disorders, Eisenson (1966) has come closest to understanding this. In emphasizing that the problem is not the sequential material itself, he implicitly identifies the perceptual/linguistic/cognitive interaction so characteristically ignored by other workers even though research has not always seemed to support his position. Analysis shows such research has not only usually used non-verbal material, but has also used tasks which can be mediated by non-linguistic strategies (see Withrow, 1964; and Furth and Pufall, 1966 as examples). Therefore, it is not incompatible with the view that specific language disorder is a perceptual and linguistic handicap, not a language handicap. Impairment of information processing systems will affect both language and non-language tasks, but will not affect tasks which can be performed on the basis of direct stimulus-response associations. Negative results so far support and extend rather than contradict the analysis started by Eisenson and developed by the author here and elsewhere (Rodda, 1973). Rodda's (1973) research and that of Tallal and Piercy (1973) offer positive evidence for the hypothesis that impairment of perceptual and linguistic processing is the primary characteristic of specific language disorder. Rodda compared normally hearing, hearing impaired and language disordered children on a test of auditory/visual integration. Language disordered children showed a developmental lag best explained as a retardation of linguistic rather than acoustic, visual or language skills. Tallal and Piercy used sequential and discriminatory auditory tasks to test the performance of "aphasic" children. They similarly concluded that impairment of auditory perception of rapidly presented sequences resulted from a failure to discriminate auditory quality not from a specifically temporal effect. Effron (1963), Benton (1964), Lowe and Campbell (1965), Stark (1967) and Eisenson (1968) have all shown or hypothesized "temporal sequencing" problems as a symptom or cause of the handicap, but the work of Tallal and Piercy, in particular, offers significant qualification of these studies. Sequencing seems to be a secondary effect not a primary symptom or cause. It shows up as a result of the perceptual and linguistic difficulties not because the ability of the system to cope with auditory or other inputs separated in time is neurologically malfunctional. The neurological damage is associated with a much more general and diffuse effect than has been previously hypothesized.

Language and Behaviour

Earlier reference was made to Bernstein's influence on the sociological and behavioural analysis of language. His research and theory provides a link between language as a perceptual and as a communication process. The theory differentiates between two forms of language—*public language* and *formal language*, and between two coding systems—restrictive and elaborative codes. All except the pathologically impaired have a public language; the possession of a formal language depends upon educational, familial and social experience. Public language has relatively simple grammatical construction, uses statements and demands as questions, uses statements as reasons and conclusions, is personalized, makes simple and limited use of adjectives, adverbs and conjunctions, lacks generality and uses idiomatic expressions as tags. The converse is true of formal language (Bernstein, 1961). Restrictive codes are a primary characteristic of public language, and are used to a lesser degree in formal language. Such codes are particularistic in their meaning and social reference, whereas elaborative codes are more universal. Restrictive codes are learned informally and relatively quickly. Elaborative codes require much longer periods of formal and informal learning.

If we remember their different disciplinary associations, there is a striking similarity between Chomsky's description of deep structure and Bernstein's description of public language. The cardinal error Bernstein makes is in assuming that formal language is a "better" vehicle for thinking than public language. Deep and surface structure and public and formal languages are different aspects of the linguistic process, and the basic deep structure or public language is a far more fundamental aspect of cognition than the surface structure or formal language. The seriously impaired language disordered child may have difficulty in attaching linguistic names or sounds to objects but, even so,

much diagnosis and remediation is based on the surface structure and formal language. Consequently, diagnostic errors are made and even techniques which successfully teach the child to name or label objects build in language retardation by failing to expose him to appropriate linguistic experiences. Before the child can use formal language he has to develop inner language and a knowledge of the transformational rules which generate surface structure from deep structure. If he lacks this knowledge he will be unable to cope with even "simple" language because it has inbuilt assumptions about his ability to use transformational rules.

Language Acquisition

Accepting that fruitful discussion of specific language disorder requires a developmental approach, similar to that of Bernstein, the question of what kind of developmental approach is the most profitable has still to be resolved. Three major types of models are found in the literature. Mental faculties models of language acquisition postulate increasing capacity with age. Ethological models postulate specific age periods during which capacity to acquire language is maximum. Theories of an "inborn" and specific facility for language acquisition predict maximum capacity during the early years, declining thereafter until the learning of new language after puberty becomes extremely difficult (Lenneberg, 1967). Unfortunately most work with language disordered children has adopted the ethological approach, as befits its close association with education of the deaf, whereas it is the specific facility theory which has proved the most profitable in applied work with a whole variety of language handicaps, and the one to which the concepts discussed in the previous sections are most applicable (*see* McNeill, 1966; and Callaway, 1970). The consequence of adopting the ethological approach is the failure to appreciate that the perceptual and cognitive skills involved in language acquisition or processing are the same for auditory or visual stimuli, and in hearing or speaking are independent of the stimulus used to transmit the information. This in turn creates a situation in which most clinical and remedial work dealing with specific language disorders concentrates on the surface rather than the deep structure of language because speech as discussed and defined in most of the literature concerned with teaching deaf children is thought of only in terms of the product of the transformational rules which have generated it from the deep structure of language. The constraints imposed by these confusions will be difficult to overcome unless we can break away from the theoretical mould which closes the door to seeing language problems as merely facets of rather than the specific identifying features of the disorder.

To understand these conceptual errors it is necessary to understand the major distinctions made by Chomsky. In the final form of his theory Chomsky differentiates semantic, syntactic, and phonological components. Deep and surface structure are characteristics of the syntactic component but the surface structure of language is generated by the transformation of the basic rules of deep structure into complex *semantic and grammatical* rules. The sensory processes involved are second order to the perceptual, linguistic, cognitive processes and every sentence has both a deep and a surface structure, the latter being generated as a result of obligatory makers in the simple, active, affirmative and declarative sentences of the deep structure. When the sensory processes are impaired, as in peripheral deafness, they can possibly be replaced prosthetically, or another sensory system can take their place, without any *direct* effect on language acquisition skills. Pathologically or environmentally malfunctioning central processes present more of a problem. At present, there is no technical way to replace or repair them and alternative sensory systems simply input information into the same impaired process. Although it has never been suggested that technical prosthesis exists for specific language disorder, nevertheless, the approach has been prosthetically orientated. The effect has been to emphasize neurological damage as an explanation rather than a cause of the disability, with the added advantage that such an approach does not raise any questions about the ethological concepts so curiously ingrained in the application of audiology to children.

Despite the prevailing confusion, some teachers of deaf children (*see* Streng, 1972, or Simmons, 1968) have appreciated the difference between a technical prosthesis and cognitive development. They have emphasized exposing children as early as possible to linguistic as well as acoustic experience but the intuitive nature of these developments has led to inaccuracies in their application in the classroom. The oral versus manual controversy in the education of deaf children is, perhaps, the classic example and whilst not directly concerned with language disorders it does have considerable relevance for the wider problem. Current emphasis is on the use of manual communication with "non-oral" but not with "normal" deaf children. Many of the children described as "non-oral" are not hearing-impaired —they are children with linguistic and cognitive rather than perceptual handicaps. The reduced rate of input of information characteristic of manual communication as used in English classrooms will help these children, but only because the complexity of the task is reduced not because an auditory form is replaced by a visual one. If the child is deaf the problem is different. Deaf children can be classified as articulators or visualizers (Conrad, 1971), and whilst Conrad's experimental research does not provide a viable clinical technique, it does confirm that the differentiation between oral and manual is perceptual and not, as commonly supposed, linguistic. Much of the current thinking and writing on this topic in the U.K. adds to the existing confusion and will continue to do so as long as this crucial distinction is not clearly articulated.

Evaluating Language Performance

The principles rather than the type and level of the problem are clearly illustrated in current discussions of the language used in inner city areas of the U.S.A. The traditional view of such language was that it directly developed from the English used in the southern States (Williamson, 1971). More recently, it is regarded as originating from a number of West African languages such as Hausa, Wolof, Twi and Mende which have been modified by exposure to a number of European languages, particularly the original and North American forms of Portuguese, Dutch, French and English (Dillard 1972). Taylor (1973) has described the commonest feature of this "Black English". It lacks copula verbs, as in the statement "*He black*" rather than "*He is black*" or "*Who he?*" rather than "*Who is he?*". It does not distinguish between gender for third person plural pronouns. It does make a distinction between second person singular and second person plural, for example "*yu*" (singular) and "*una*" (plural). Prefixing or suffixing of third person plural objective case pronouns is used to generate plural nouns, as in "*dem boy*" rather than "*those boys*". Obligatory morphemes for plurals are not required, for example "50 cent", nor are obligatory markers for the third person singular of verbs or for possessives, as in "*he work here*' and in "*John cousin*". The language does use specified phrases to announce the beginnings of sentences such as "*dig*" or "*look here*", and also uses intonational ranges to mark meaning differences.

Clinical evaluation of speech and language in speech pathology takes little account of these differences because the methods of evaluation are based on the psychological concept of standard "norm". Consequently, tests such as the Illinois Test of Psycholinguistic Abilities (ITPA) and the Language Modalities Test of Aphasia can have seriously misleading implications when used with children using non-standard dialects or non-standard languages. Taylor (op. cit.) points out that classifying a pronunciation of "*toofbrush*" or a statement "He from Chicago" as abnormal often fails to consider their accuracy as a dialectical pronunciation or in applying linguistic rules different from those usually used in test construction. It can lead to a diagnosis of linguistic retardation or abnormality in children or adults whose performance is superior when judged by a more appropriate set of rules for pronunciation and grammar. The problem is not as serious in Great Britain as in the U.S.A., but there is an undoubted need for greater awareness, since it will grow as immigrant cultures become more widely established in our society and such children are already over-represented in schools for deaf children. Moreover, the described inadequacies seriously question the use, and if used, the interpretation, of such tests with pathologically impaired children, whether hearing handicapped or language disordered, and must be related to the need to develop diagnostic techniques providing more useful information to remedial specialists.

Conceptualization, Language and Environment

We noted, almost at the beginning of this chapter, the work of Eisenson (1968) and Di Carlo (1960) showing that mentally handicapped children are frequently classified as having a specific language disorder, particularly when retardation is combined with a peripheral hearing impairment. The difficulty arises because the interaction between intellectual development and environment is notoriously complex (*see* Helmuth, 1968, 1969 and 1971; Jones, 1970), and mental retardation has a social as well as a diagnostic concept. Diagnostic findings cannot be based simply on intelligence test performance when discussing the identification of multiply handicapped children or differential diagnosis (*see* Mercer, 1971). Reed (1970) has described the most appropriate tests to use with children with language and communication disorders, but would agree that the use of such tests to simply assign an "Intelligence Quotient" to a child is highly dangerous and misleading. Ives (1967) carries the argument further and shows how sensible diagnosis must concern itself with the nature of intelligence rather than regarding intelligence as a unitary concept. He shows that sensory motor skills, perception and memory are basically not affected by hearing impairment, but deficiencies in language development restrict the ability to operationally relate concepts, generalize from concepts, abstract

required for thinking but the deep structure of language is—indeed, it can be argued that it is thinking, and Furth's position can be misunderstood unless it is clearly understood that "thinking without language" really means thinking without depending on the ability to transform deep into surface structure.

To carry the discussion further, it is necessary to reintroduce the concept of memory processing and to remind the reader that memory consists of three stages—precategorical, short-term and long-term. Processing and the interaction between memory and cognition will be different at each of these levels, and a fair amount of research has

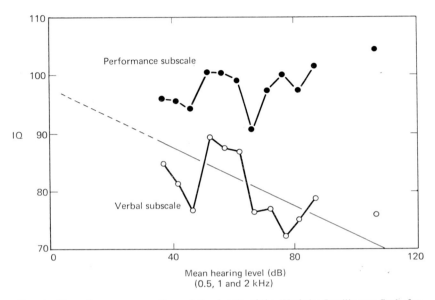

FIG. 4. Shows how scores on the verbal subscale of the Wechsler Intelligence Scale for Children are predicted by average hearing loss in the better ear, whereas scores on the performance subscale are not. (Reproduced from Hine, 1970.)

ideas from concepts and apply logical processes to concepts. The general principles uncovered by Ives would apply equally to both hearing impaired and language disordered children, differing only in detailed effect. Whilst it may be repetitive of earlier statements, it cannot be emphasized too strongly that a prescriptive approach is mandatory if reliable and useful diagnostic information is to be obtained.

Most of the research relevant to this discussion has been concerned with evaluating the effect of hearing impairment rather than language disorder on intelligence. It began with the classic work of Pinter and Reamer (1916) with over 2000 children in 26 schools for the deaf in the United States, but possibly the most useful work has been undertaken by Hine (1970). He analysed test scores on the Wechsler Intelligence Scale for Children (WISC) for 100 orally proficient partially hearing children, and figure 4 summarizes his results. A predictive relationship between intelligence and hearing exists only when verbal mediation is required. However, Furth (1966 and 1973) has cogently argued that this problem results from inadequate linguistic experience, not from a lack of speech or verbal language. Unfortunately, the correctness of his reasoning is obscured by his loose use of the term language. Surface language is not

been undertaken with both hearing-impaired and normal children and adults investigating the relationship between the different processing levels and thinking (for example, Pinter and Paterson, 1917; Blair, 1957; Olssen and Furth, 1966; Furth and Pufall, 1966; Winitz, 1969 and Rosenthal, 1970). Ling (1973) presented an extensive synopsis of the relevant studies to the 1973 International Conference on Auditory Techniques and four important conclusions can be drawn from the existing research: (i) It is the ability to undertake linguistic coding and not a special capacity for auditory analysis which leads to dominant hemisphere specialization in speech perception; (ii) The auditory qualities of speech are mediated in both hemispheres; (iii) Ordering deficiencies in hearing impaired children results from the use of tasks requiring verbal mediation for their effective performance and not from a basic defect in "sequencing" skills; and (iv) Deaf children can be sub-divided into "articulators" and "visualizers" (Conrad, 1970)—articulators function analogously to hearing children whereas visualizers use a linguistic system based on visual not auditory perception. Unfortunately, most of the work concentrates on the dimensions (*see* Murray, 1969 and Morton, 1970) or the stages of memory (*see* Waugh and Norman,

1965; Atkinson and Shriffin, 1968 and Norman, 1968) without providing the information necessary to distinguish children with different types or levels of language or communication disorder (Wallace, 1972). Despite the lack of this theoretical baseline, some attempts have been made to approach the problem from the practical end of the continuum, but they either failed to compare language disordered children with children having other kinds of communication disorders, or they have used such a wide definition of brain injury that statistically non-significant differences were a foregone conclusion (Bowling, Fish and Walters, 1963; Gray and D'Asaro, 1965; Williams, 1965). To obtain more useful information, we have to return to the work of experimental psychologists and consider the role of personality in language processing.

Language, Personality and Cortical Arousal

In the discussion of specific language disorder and primary emotional disturbance reference was made to cortical arousal in specific language disorder. Eysenck's (1967) classical text summarizes the basic thesis that extraversion and intraversion, cortical arousal and learning interact with each other—intraversion being characterized by a higher degree of cortical excitation and extraversion by a lower degree. Savage (1964) and Marton and Eurban (1966) have shown Eysenck's hypothesis to have a real basis in central nervous system physiology. Walker and Tarte (1963), Osbourne and Farnkiewicz (1972) and Osbourne (1973) have all gone on to show that words and language are the mediating mechanism between the psychological reactions of personality and physiological control through cortical arousal, but other work on the relationship between personality, attention and memory has tended to lose direction and concentrate mainly on the search for "plausible mechanisms" rather than on the dynamics of the selective process. Hamilton, Hockey and Quinn (1972), in discussing this problem refer to the need to investigate the stimulus modality, the characteristics of the stimulus itself and which aspects of the stimulus are selected for processing. There is, as they point out, evidence that different levels of cortical arousal produce different information selection strategies and they refer to the work of Hamilton (1969), Kanarick and Peterson (1969) and Hockey (1969). This work shows that increased complexity of the tasks results in increased and optimal dispersion of attention between different information sources. Similar, but more practical results, were obtained by Fountain and Lynn (1966) who found that children's sensitivity to complex stimuli is closely related to the level of arousal, and high arousal, whether of physiological or environmental aetiology, seems to result in increased long-term retention in memory at the cost of short-term performance (Hamilton, Hockey and Quinn, 1972).

Experiments using the "critical flicker fusion frequency" of visual stimuli have shown that anxiety affects the perceptual responses of children with specific language disorders. The effect increases cortical arousal, and in a similar but more pathological way than with non-impaired children results in difficulties in attending to and processing complex stimuli (Rodda, 1971, 1973). The basic problem is in the complexity of the processing task, not in the complexity of language itself and Farrant found little relation between response and language complexity because the processing difficulties remained constant even though the linguistic character of the stimulus changed. Language disordered children probably have such a high level of pathological cortical arousal that its effects are concentrated entirely on the short-term system, preventing increased long-term retention because short-term processing breaks down completely or nearly completely.

Certainly, whatever the explanation of the results of this work, it offers strong evidence for the main theme of this chapter. Language problems are a secondary aspect of specific language disorder which is an unusual but not unique aspect of perceptual processing difficulties with all the implications that this has for linguistic and cognitive functioning. Rather than resulting from specific damage to distinct neurological systems the aetiology of the disorder is to be found in a general disruption of the central nervous system when used to analyse incoming perceptual stimuli.

Conclusion

Current confusion about the diagnosis and remediation of specific language disorder has been well summarized by Farrant (1971). After reviewing the literature, she concludes:

> Although it is commonly assumed that children educationally classified as language disordered have a common underlying central nervous system disorder, no attempt is made to objectively verify this. Monsees (1961) and Nicholas (1962) believe that if a child fails to learn language by a whole-word method, but succeeds in learning by the McGinnis "Elemental approach involving special patterning", then he "has indicated that he has a central disorder involving the perception of temporal sequence". This "empirical approach" has been strongly criticized by Lenneberg (1968) and Birch (in *Institute on Childhood Aphasia*, 1962, pp. 30–31).

Clinical diagnosis of specific language disorder is difficult and prone to error. Its educational remediation is, at least in part, dependent on good luck rather than good management. This state of affairs will continue until specific language disorder is seen as a psychological rather than a neurological handicap. Language function is not a specific neurological entity and, therefore, whilst neurology can help, it can only add to our understanding. It cannot provide an explanation of specific language disorder, and it certainly cannot provide the diagnostic information which is required to prescribe for these patients if clinical practice is to become more scientific. Such a change can result only from seeing specific language disorder for what it is—a psychological problem dealing with sensory processing skills and linguistic rather than language development. It lies somewhere on a continuum between autistic children at one extreme and inner city black children at the other, but we have yet to decide exactly where.

ACKNOWLEDGEMENTS

I am indebted to Dr. Wendy Farrant, and Mr. W. D. Hine, for permission to reproduce Figs. 2 and 3 and Fig. 4 respectively. I am also indebted to Dr. Farrant for the stimulus she has given to my thinking in past years through her willingness to discuss and critically appraise our own work and that of others. Finally, I have to thank Mr. C. F. Knocker for all his help in the preparation of the manuscript and in proof-reading—crucial tasks in which his ability far exceeds mine.

REFERENCES

Affolter, F. (1968), "Thinking and Language," in *Vocational Rehabilitation of Deaf Persons* (G. T. Lloyd, Ed.). Washington, D.C.: Department of Health, Education and Welfare.

Atkinson, R. C. and Shriffin, R. M. (1968), "Human Memory," in *Psychology of Learning and Motivation* (K. W. Spence, Ed.). New York: Academic Press.

Barry, H. (1961), *The Young Aphasic Child.* Washington, D.C.: Alexander Graham Bell Association for the Deaf.

Bartoshuk, A. K. (1962), "Human Neonatal Cardiac Acceleration to to Sound: Habituation and Dishabituation," *Perceptual and Motor Skills*, **15**, 15–27.

Benton, A. L. (1964), "Developmental Aphasia (D.A.) and Hearing Damage," *Cortex*, **1**, 40–52.

Benton, A. L. (1966), "Language Disorders in Children," *Canadian Psychologist*, **7**, 298–300.

Bernstein, B. (1958), "Some Sociological Determinants of Perception," *Brit. J. Sociology*, **9**, 159–174.

Bernstein, B. (1959), "A Public Language: Some Sociological Implications of a Linguistic Form," *Brit. J. Sociology*, **10**, 311–326.

Bernstein, B. (1961), "Social Class and Linguistic Development," in *Economy, Education and Society* (A. H. Halsey, J. Floud and A. Anderson, Eds.). New York: Harcourt, Brace and World.

Blair, F. X. (1957), "A Study of Visual Memory of Deaf and Hearing Children," *Amer. Ann. Deaf*, **102**, 254–263.

Bowling, E. B., Fish, C. H. and Walter, J. R. (1963), "A Comparison of Auditory Differentiation in Aphasoid and Non-aphasoid Children," *J. Amer. Speech and Hear. Ass.*, **5**, 775.

Broadbent, D. E. and Gregory, M. (1967), "Perception of Emotionally Toned Words," *Nature*, **215**, 581–584.

Callaway, E. R. (1970), "Modes of Biological Adaption and Their Role in Intellectual Development," *P.C.D. Monographs*, Vol. 1, No. 1.

Calvert, D. R., Ceriotti, M. A. and Geille, M. A. (1966), "A Program for Aphasic Children," *Volta Rev.*, **68**, 144–153.

Carroll, J. B. (1964), *Language and Thought.* New York: Prentice Hall.

Chomsky, N. (1957), *Syntactic Structures.* New York: Mouton.

Cole, M. and Kraft, M. B. (1964), "Specific Learning Disability," *Cortex*, **1**, 302–313.

Conrad, R. (1964), "Acoustic Confusions in Immediate Memory," *Brit. J. Psychol.*, **55**, 75–84.

Conrad, R. (1970), "Short-term Memory Processes in the Deaf," *Brit. J. Psychol.*, **61**, 179–195.

Conrad, R. (1971), "The Effect of Vocalizing on Comprehension in the Profoundly Deaf," *Brit. J. Psychology.*, **62**, 147–150.

Conrad, R. (1972), "Short-term Memory in the Deaf: a Test for Speech Coding," *Brit. J. Psychol.*, **63**, 173–180.

Creak, M. (1961), "The Schizophrenic Syndrome in Children," *Brit. med. J.*, **11**, 889–890.

Crowder, R. G. and Morton, J. (1969), "Precategorical Acoustic Storage (PAS)," *Perception and Psychophysics*, **5**, 365–373.

D'Asaro, N. J. (1962), "Language Disorders and Related Learning Problems," *J. Amer. Speech and Hear. Ass.*, **4**, 411.

De Hirsh, K. (1967), "Differential Diagnosis Between Aphasic and Schizophrenic Language in Children," *J. Speech Hear. Dis.*, **32**, 3–10.

Di Carlo, L. N. (1960), "Differential Diagnosis of Congenital Aphasics," *Volta Rev.*, **62**, 361–364.

Dillard, J. (1972), *Black English.* New York: Random House.

Douglas, F. M., Fowler, E. P. and Ryan, G. M. (1961), *A Differential Study of Communication Disorder.* New York: Columbia—Presbyterian Medical Centre.

Effron, R. (1963), "Temporal perception; aphasia and déjà vu," *Brain*, **86**, 403–424.

Eisenberg, R. B., Coursin, D. B. and Rupp, N. R. (1966), "Habituation to an Acoustic Pattern as an Index of Differences Among Human Neonates," *J. Aud. Res.*, **6**, 239–248.

Eisenson, J. (1966), "Perceptual Disturbance in Children with Central Nervous System Dysfunctions and Implications for Language Development," *Brit. J. Disorders of Communication*, **1**, 21–32.

Eisenson, J. (1968), "Developmental Aphasia: A Speculative View with Therapeutic Implications," *J. Speech Hear. Dis.*, **33**, 3–13.

Elliot, L. L. and Armbruster, V. B. (1967), "Some Possible Effects of the Delay of Early Treatment of Deafness," *J. Speech Hear. Res.*, **10**, 209–224.

Ewing, A. W. G. (1930), *Aphasia in Children.* Oxford: Oxford University Press.

Ewing, A. W. G. (1962), "Central Deafness Pedagogy," *International Audiology*, **1**, 106–111.

Eysenck, H. J. (Ed.) (1967), *Biological Basis of Behaviour.* Springfield: Thomas.

Farrant, W. (1971), *An Experimental Investigation of Cognitive and Behavioural Disorders Associated with a Variety of Auditory Deficiencies.* Unpublished Ph.D. Thesis, University of Manchester.

Fountain, W. and Lynn, R. (1966), "Change in Level of Arousal During Childhood," *Behav. Res. and Therapy*, **4**, 213–217.

Furth, H. G. (1966), *Thinking Without Language: Psychological Implications of Deafness.* New York: The Free Press.

Furth, H. G. (1968), "Propositional Thinking in Deaf Underachieving Boys," in *Vocational Rehabilitation of Deaf Persons* (G. T. Lloyd, Ed.). Washington, U.S.A.: Department of Health, Education and Welfare.

Furth, H. G. (1973), *Deafness and Learning.* Belmont: Wadsworth.

Furth, H. G. and Pufall, F. B. (1966), "Visual and Auditory Sequences Learning in Hearing-impaired Children." *J. Speech Hear. Res.*, **9**, 441–449.

Gray and D'Asaro (1965), "Auditory Perceptual Thresholds in Brain-injured Children," *J. Amer. Speech and Hear. Ass.*, **8**, 49–56.

Greene, J. (1973), *Psycholinguistics.* London: Penguin.

Gordon, N. (1966), "The Child Who Does Not Talk. "Problems of Diagnosis with Special Reference to Children with Severe Auditory Agnosia," *Brit. J. Disorders of Communication*, **1**, 78–84.

Hamilton, P. (1969), "Selective Attention in Multi-source Monitoring Tasks," *J. exp. Psychol.*, **82**, 32–37.

Hamilton, P., Hockey, G. R. J. and Quinn, J. C. (1972), "Information Selection, Arousal and Memory," *Brit. J. Psychol.*, **63**, 181–189.

Hardy, W. G. (1956), "Problems of Audition, Perception and Understanding," *Volta Rev.*, **58**, 289–300.

Hardy, W. G. and Pauls, M. D. (1959), "Significance of Problems of Conditioning in G. S. R. Audiometry," *J. Speech Hear. Dis.*, **24**, 123–126.

Harrison, S. (1958), "A Review of Research in Speech and Language Development of the mentally Retarded Child," *Amer. J. men. Defic.*, **63**, 236–240.

Head, H. (1926), *Aphasia and Kindred Disorders of Speech.* London: Cambridge University Press.

Helmuth, J. (1968/69/71), *The Disadvantaged Child, Volumes 1, 2 and 3.* New York: Bruner/Mazel.

Hine, W. D. (1970), "Verbal Ability and Partial Hearing Loss," *Teach. Deaf*, **68**, 450–459.

Hockey, G. R. J. (1969), *Environmental Stress and Attention to Complex Visual Displays.* Unpublished Ph.D. Thesis, University of Cambridge.

Hutt, C., Hutt, S., Lee, D. and Ounsted, C. (1964), "Arousal and Childhood Autism," *Nature*, **204**, 908–909.

Hutt, S. J. and Hutt, C. (Eds.) (1970), *Behaviour Studies in Psychiatry.* Oxford: Pergamon Press.

Institute on Childhood Aphasia (1962), *Childhood Aphasia.* San Francisco, U.S.A.: California Society for Crippled Children and Adults.

Ittleson, H. W. and Kutash, J. (1961), *Perceptual Changes in Psychopathology*. Springfield: Thomas.

Ives, L. A. (1967), "Deafness and the Development of Intelligence," *British J. Disorders of Communication*, **2**, 96–111.

Jenkins, J. J. (1958), "An Atlas of Semantic Profiles for 360 Words," *Amer. J. Psychol.*, **71**, 688–699.

Jones, R. L. (1970), *New Directions in Special Education*. Boston: Allyn and Bacon.

Kaftein, O. (1961), *A Differential Study of Communication Disorder* (F. M. Douglas, E. P. Fowler and G. M. Ryan, Eds.). New York: Presbyterian Medical Centre.

Kanarick, A. F. and Peterson, R. C. (1969), "Effects of Value on the Monitoring of Multi-channel Displays," *Hum. Factors*, **11**, 313–320.

Kanner, L. (1951), "A Discussion of Early Infantile Autism," *Dig. Neurol. Psychiat.*, **19**, 158–159.

Kleffner, F. R. (1959), "Teaching Aphasic Children," *Education*, **79**, 413–418.

Kleinman, M. L. (1957), "Psychogenic Deafness and Perceptual Deafness," *J. abnorm. soc. Psychol.*, **54**, 335–338.

Lea, J. (1965), "A Language Scheme for Children Suffering from Receptive Aphasia," *Speech Pathology and Therapy*, **8**, 58–68.

Lea, J. (1966), "The Education of Children Suffering from Receptive Aphasia," *The Slow Learning Child*, **13**.

Lenneberg, E. H. (1964), "Language Disorders in Children," *Harvard Educational Review*, **34**, 152–177.

Lenneberg, E. H. (1967), *Biological Foundations of Language*. New York: Wiley.

Lewis, M. M. (1968), *The Education of Deaf Children: The Place of Fingerspelling and Signing*. London: H.M.S.O.

Ling, A. H. (1973), "Sequential Processing in Hearing Impaired Children," Paper presented to *International Conference on Auditory Techniques*, Pasadena, California.

Lotz, B. M. (1970), "Differential Diagnosis: Childhood Autism and Learning Disabilities." Personal communication.

Lowe, A. D. and Campbell, R. (1965), "Temporal Discrimination in Aphasoid and Normal Children," *J. Speech Hear. Res.*, **8**, 313–314.

McCarthy, J. J. (1964), "Research on Linguistic Problems of the Mentally Retarded," *Mental Retardation Abstracts*, **1**, 3–27.

McConnell, F. (1964), "Response of Two Groups of Non-language Children to Training," *Folia phoniat*, **16**, 172–182.

McGinnis, M. A., Kleffner, A. and Goldstein, R. (1956), "Teaching Aphasic Children," *Volta Rev.*, **58**, 239–244.

McGinnis, M. A. (1963), *Aphasic Children: Identification and Education by the Association Method*. Washington D.C.: Alexander Graham Bell Association for the Deaf.

McNeill, D. (1966), "Developmental Psycholinguistics," in *The Genesis of Language* (F. Smith and G. A. Miller, Eds.). Cambridge, Mass.: M.I.T. Press.

McNeill, D. (1970), *The Acquisition of Language: The Study of Developmental Psycholinguistics*. New York: Harper and Row.

McReynolds, L. V. (1966), "Operant Conditioning for Investigating Speech Sound Discrimination in Aphasic Children," *J. Speech Hear. Res.*, **9**, 519–528.

Mark, H. G. and Hardy, W. G. (1958), "Orientating Reflex Disturbance in Central Auditory or Language Handicapped Children," *J. Speech Hear. Dis.*, **23**, 237–242.

Marton, M. and Urban, I. (1966), "An Electroencephalographic Investigation of Individual Differences in the Process of Conditioning," *Proceedings of 18th International Congress on Experimental Psychology*, pp. 106–109.

Mercer, J. R. (1971), "The Meaning of Mental Retardation," in *The Mentally Retarded Child and his Family* (R. Koch and J. C. Dobson, Eds.). New York: Bruner, Mazel, Butterworths.

Miller, G. A., Galanter, E. and Pribram, K. H. (1960), *Plans and the Structure of Behaviour*. New York: Holt, Rinehart and Winston.

Monsees, E. K. (1957), "Aphasia in Children, Diagnosis and Education," *Volta Rev.*, **59**, 392.

Morton, J. (1970), "A Functional Model for Memory," in *Models for Human Memory* (D. A. Norman, Ed.). New York: Academic Press.

Mullins, J. B. (1968), "Provisions for the Education of Aphasic Children in Public Residential Schools for the Deaf in the United States," *Dissertation Abstracts*, **29**(4–A), 1134–1135.

Murray, D. J. (1969), "Modality-Specific Cues as Factors Determining Short-term Memory Performance," Paper presented at *AAAS Symposium*, Boston.

Myklebust, H. R. (1954), *Auditory Disorders in Children*: A Manual for Differential Diagnosis. New York: Grune and Stratton.

Nicholas, M. (1962), "The Asphasic Child," *J. Irish med. Ass.*, **50**, 42–46.

Norman, D. A. (1968), *Memory and Attention*. New York: Wiley.

O'Gorman, G. (1967), *The Nature of Childhood Autism*. London: Butterworth Press.

Olsen, J. E. and Furth, H. G. (1966), "Visual Memory Span in the Deaf," *Amer. J. Psychol.*, **109**, 480–484.

Orton, S. (1937), *Reading, Writing, and Speech Problems in Children*. New York: Grune and Stratton.

Osbourne, J. W. and Farnkiewicz, R. G. (1972), "Arousal as a Word Attribute," Unpublished study cited in Osbourne (1973).

Osbourne, J. W. (1973), "Extraversion, Neuroticism and Word Arousal," *Brit. J. Psychol.*, **64**, 559–562.

Osgood, C. E. (1963), "On Understanding and Creating Sentences," *Amer. Psychologist*, **18**, 735–751.

Peins, M. (1962), "Mental Retardation: a Selected Bibliography on Speech, Hearing and Language Problems," *J. Amer. Speech Hear. Ass.*, **4**, 38–40.

Pinter, R. and Reamer, J. F. (1916), "Learning Tests with Deaf Children," *Psychological Monographs*, No. 20.

Pinter, R. and Patterson, D. G. (1917), "A Comparison of Deaf and Hearing Children in Visual Memory for Digits," *J. exp. Psychol.*, **2**, 76–88.

Purdie, A. C. (1966), "Experimental Methods of Training Young Aphasic Children," *Teach. Deaf*, **64**, 218–225.

Rappaport, S. R. (Ed.) (1964), *Childhood Aphasia and Brain Damage: Differential Diagnosis*. Narbeth, Pa.: Livingston.

Reed, M. (1970), "Deaf and Partially-hearing Children", in *Psychological Assessment of Mental and Physical Handicaps* (P. Mittler, Ed.). London: Methuen.

Reichstein, J. and Rosenstein, J. (1964), "Differential Diagnosis of Auditory Deficits—a Review of the Literature," *Exceptional Children*, **31**, 73–82.

Rodda, M. and Sutton, G. (1971), "Intersensory Facilitation and the Diagnosis of Functional Hearing Loss," *Acta oto-laryng.*, **69**, 107–111.

Rodda, M. (1973), "Experimental Tests for Use in Diagnosing Language Disorder," *Brit. J. Audiology*, **7**, 9–15.

Rosenthal, W. S. (1970), *Perception of Auditory Temporal Order as a Function of Selected Stimulus in a Group of Aphasic Children*. Unpublished Ph.D. Thesis, Stanford University.

Rutter, M. (1968), "Concepts of Autism. A Review of Research," *J. Child Psychology and Psychiatry*, **9**, 1–25.

Savage, R. D. (1964), "Electro-cerebral Activity, Extraversion and Neuroticism," *Brit. J. Psychiatry*, **110**, 98–100.

Shannon, C. E. and Weaver, W. (1949), *The Mathematical Theory of Communication*. Urbana: University of Illinois Press.

Simmons, A. A. (1968), "Content Subjects Through Language," in *Curriculum: Cognition and Content* (H. G. Kopp, Ed.). Washington: A. G. Bell Association.

Skinner, B. F. (1957), *Verbal Behaviour*. New York: Appleton, Century, Crofts.

Smith, J. O. (1962), "Speech and Language of the Retarded," *Training School Bulletin*, No. 58.

Spradlin, J. E. (1963), "Language and Communication of Mental Defectives," in *Handbook of Mental Deficiency* (N. R. Ellis, Ed.). New York: McGraw-Hill.

Stark, J. (1966), "Performance of Aphasic Children on the I.T.P.A.," *Exceptional Children*, **33**, 153–158.

Stark, J. (1967), "Atypical Development and Behaviour in Some Non-verbal Children," *Brit. J. Disorders of Communication*, **2**, 146–151.

Stratton, P. M. and Connolly, K. (1973), "Discrimination by Newborns of the Intensity, Frequency and Temporal Characteristics of Auditory Stimuli," *Brit. J. Psychol.*, **64**, 219–232.

Streng, A. H. (Ed.) (1972), *Syntax, Speech and Hearing: Applied Linguistics for Teachers of Children with Language and Hearing Disabilities*. New York: Grune and Stratton.

Tallal, P. and Piercy, M. (1973), "Defects of Non-verbal Auditory Perception in Children with Developmental Aphasia," *Nature*, **241**, 468–469.

Taylor, I. G. (1964), *Neurological Mechanisms in Speech and Hearing in Children*. Manchester: Manchester University Press.

Taylor, I. G. (1966a), "Disorders of Communication in Deaf and Hearing-impaired Children," in *Proceedings of a Symposium on the Psychological Study of Deafness and Hearing Impairment*. London: British Psychological Society.

Taylor, I. G. (1966b), "Hearing in Relation to Language Disorders in Children," *Brit. J. Disorders of Communication*, **1**, 11–20.

Taylor, O. L. (1973), "Sociolinguistics and the Practice of Speech Pathology," *Rehabilitation Record*, May/June, 14–17.

Tubbs, V. K. (1966), "Types of Linguistic Ability in Psychotic Children," *J. Mental Deficiency Research*, **10**, 230–240.

Wakstein, M. P. and Wakstein, D. J. (1962), "The Syndrome of Childhood Psychosis Versus the Syndrome of Receptive Aphasia," *J. Amer. Speech and Hear. Ass.*, **4**, 410–411.

Walker, E. L. and Tarte, R. D. (1963), "Memory Storage as a Function of Arousal and Time with Homogeneous and Heterogeneous Lists," *J. Verbal Learning and Verbal Behaviour*, **3**, 112–129.

Wallace, G. (1972), *Short-term Memory and Coding Strategies of the Deaf*. Unpublished Ph.D. Thesis, McGill University.

Waugh, N. C. and Norman, D. A. (1965), "Primary Memory," *Psychol. Rev.*, **72**, 89–104.

Whitfield, I. C. (1967), *The Auditory Pathways*. London: Arnold.

Williams, J. B. (1965), "Auditory Figure—Ground Discrimination in Dysphasic Children," *J. Amer. Speech and Hear. Ass.*, **7**, 407.

Williams, C. E. (1969), "Early Diagnosis of Deafness and its Relation to Speech in Deaf, Maladjusted Children," *Developmental Medicine and Child Neurology*, **11**, 777–782.

Williamson, J. A. (1971), *A Varied Language*. New York: Holt, Rinehart and Winston.

Wilson, L. F., Dochring, D. G. and Hirsch, J. (1960), "Auditory Discrimination Learning by Aphasic and Non-aphasic Children," *J. Speech Hear. Res.*, **3**, 130–137.

Wing, L. (1973), "Psychotic Children," in *Stresses in Children* (V. P. Varma, Ed.). London: University of London Press.

Winitz, H. L. (1969), *Articulatory Acquisition and Behaviour*. New York: Appleton Century Crofts.

Withrow, F. B. (1964), "Paired Associate Learning of Moving Sequences by Deaf Children," *Volta Rev.*, **66**, 555–557.

Withrow, F. B. (1966), "Acquisition of Language by Deaf Children with Other Disabilities," *Volta Rev.*, **66**, 555–557.

Worster-Drought, C. (1965), "Observations on Congenital Auditory Imperception," *Teach. Deaf*, **63**, 4–11.

GROUPS	SUBGROUPS	SEROTYPES	CLINICAL CONDITION MOST OFTEN ASSOCIATED WITH INFECTION
Myxoviruses	Influenza	A B C	Influenza Influenza, "colds" "colds"
Paramyxoviruses	Parainfluenza	1 2 3 4	Croup; "colds"; influenza Croup; pharyngitis Pneumonia; "colds" Mild "colds"
	Respiratory syncytial	Only 1	Bronchiolitis; pneumonia; "colds"
Picornavirus	Enterovirus	Coxsackie virus A 21 Coxsackie virus B3 Echo 19	Pharyngitis; "colds"; pneumonia "Colds"; laryngotracheitis; pneumonia "Colds"
	Rhinovirus	More than 90	"Colds"; bronchitis
Adenovirus		1,2,5,6 3,4,7,14,21	Pharyngitis; conjunctivitis; pneumonia Epidemics in schools and military camps
Coronavirus		At least 3	"Colds"

This process was first described with bacterial viruses, or bacteriophages as they are usually called, and the process called lysogeny. The bacterial cells carrying the viral genome are lysogenic and under certain stimuli produce virus particles and are lysed, releasing the bacterial virus (phage particles). The presence of the integrated phage genome may alter the antigenic make up of the bacterial cell or cause it to become toxigenic as in the case of *Corynebacterium diphtheriae*. It is now clear that a similar process can occur in animal cells, the cells being altered in their growth pattern and becoming neoplastic (*see* review by Sambrook, 1972). Some viruses are defective, their nucleic acid not containing all the information necessary for the production of new virus particles. With these viruses a double infection is necessary. In addition to the defective virus, there has to be a helper virus which provides the information lacking in the defective virus. This is, in some cases, the information for the coat protein and in these viruses the antigenic structure and host range of the defective virus will depend on which helper virus is used. The range of helper viruses varies from one defective virus to another. In some there may be only one, while in others, a number of

to the host will vary from one to the other. Often, the host in which the least damage is caused will be the most important from the point of view of assuring the survival of the virus. For all classification purposes it is necessary to choose criteria. Previous classifications of viruses were based on the major host or type of disease produced, but, as more was learned about the biology of viruses and their structure, these classifications were not found to group together viruses of similar type. For example, the viruses which can cause respiratory disease (*see* Table 2) are a very mixed group. Viruses are currently classified as shown in Table 3. Thus they are first divided into RNA or DNA containing viruses and then on the basis of the symmetry of the arrangement of the protein units (capsomers) forming the capsid or shell of the virus particle. A further subdivision depends on the presence or absence of a lipid-containing envelope which is determined by sensitivity to inactivation by lipid solvents such as ether or chloroform. A scheme of viral taxonomy based on this classification, but using latin binomials, has been proposed by the International Committee on Nomenclature of Viruses (Wildy, 1971). However, the problem of establishing meaningful families and

OTOLARYNGOLOGICAL BIOLOGY AND PATHOLOGY

	PAGE
45. VIROLOGY	625
46. BACTERIOLOGY	638
47. MYCOLOGY	645
48. PARASITOLOGY	661
49. HISTOPATHOLOGY OF NOSE AND THROAT	667

45. VIROLOGY

K. E. K. ROWSON

Definition

It is impossible to define a virus satisfactorily in a few simple sentences and it is equally difficult to define a virologist because the people who work with viruses come from almost every scientific discipline. There are morphologists interested in the geometry of the arrangement of the protein subunits or capsomers from which the outer shell of the virus is constructed, taxonomists interested in the classification of viruses in relation to other microorganisms, geneticists who find in viruses a useful model system, cancer researchers, biochemists and, of course, molecular biologists, as well as a host of different workers interested in the diseases produced by viruses in plants, insects and other animals.

Lwoff (1957) defined viruses as strictly intracellular and potentially pathogenic entities with an infectious phase and (1) possessing only one type of nucleic acid, (2) multiplying in the form of their genetic material, (3) unable to grow and to undergo binary fission, and (4) devoid of an enzyme system for energy production. This definition stresses the non-cellular nature of viruses, their dependence on host cell metabolism, and that, at some stage in their reproductive cycle, the virus is reduced to an element of genetic material, the nucleic acid. Luria (1959) defined viruses as units of genetic material, capable of replicating in a host cell and, in the process of replication, able to produce any mechanism necessary for their transmission to other host cells. This definition emphasizes the role of viruses as units of genetic material capable of organizing their transfer to other host cells rather than their lack of metabolic self-sufficiency. More recently, Luria and Darnell (1968) have defined viruses as entities whose genetic constitution or genome is an element of nucleic acid, either deoxyribonucleic (DNA) or ribonucleic acid (RNA), which is replicated inside living cells and then uses the synthetic machinery of the cell to synthesise the viral proteins for the formation of virus particles which contain the viral genome and transfer it to other cells. The above definitions attempt to convey the two qualities of viruses, namely their possession of specific genetic material which, in a host cell, behaves as part of the cell, and their ability to package this genetic information in a specialized particle, the virus or virion (a name given to a whole virus particle), for transmission to a new host cell.

None of the viruses is much more than 200 nm in diameter and the majority are much smaller, but size would not appear to be one of their important biological properties as it is conceivable that virus particles several micrometres in diameter could be made in plant or animal cells. However, the small size of viruses has played an important role in determining the technical features of virology. It was by filtration that bacteria and viruses were first separated and filter-passing viruses discovered. Similarly, pathogenicity is not an important biological characteristic and the fact that the first viruses to be identified were those causing disease in plants and animals was merely because they were recognized by this property. Now that viruses can be detected in other ways many non-pathogenic viruses have been discovered. Intracellular parasitism is a property viruses share with other classes of microorganisms, but parasites such as the leprosy bacillus and the rickettsiae have a highly organized structure with ribosomal and mitochondrial systems or their equivalents. Their need to parasitize cells probably reflects a requirement for certain complex substances and not a lack of cellular organization as with the viruses. The psittacosis-lymphogranuloma venereum group of organisms which were originally classified with the viruses are now not regarded as viruses because they contain two types of nucleic acid and also appear to retain their organized form in their intracellular phase, in which they grow in size and divide by binary fission.

Table 1 shows some of the important differences between viruses and other microorganisms.

TABLE 1
SOME OF THE IMPORTANT DIFFERENCES BETWEEN VARIOUS GROUPS OF MICROORGANISMS

Organisms	Replication by Binary Fission	Contain RNA and DNA	Contain Ribosomes	Grow in Artificial Media	Sensitive to Interferon
Bacteria	+	+	+	+	−
Rickettsia	+	+	+	−	−
Psittacosis group	+	+	+	−	+
Viruses	−	−	−	−	+

A complete virus particle consists of (a) internal proteins and nucleic acid (either RNA or DNA), (b) protein molecules or capsomers arranged with either cubical or helical symmetry around the nucleic acid to form the capsid or shell of the virus particle and (c) an outer lipid-containing envelope which is present only in some viruses such as the myxoviruses. When a virus particle enters a cell it is uncoated and the nucleic acid which contains all the information necessary to produce new virus particles is released and replicated. New virus proteins are formed by the cell under the direction of the viral nucleic acid, and new virus particles are formed. They are released from the cell surface by budding over a long period without the

cell being killed. The viral nucleic acid also codes for a number of proteins which are not part of the viral particle but have functions related to viral replication and the control of host cell activity. These viral proteins can be demonstrated in virus infected cells by biochemical and immunological techniques.

Some viruses do not at once replicate when they enter a cell. In such cases, the viral nucleic acid is integrated into the cellular nucleic acid where it is replicated with the cell genome and functions as though it were a part of the normal cell but imparting to the cell certain new characteristics.

antigenically different, but related, viruses can act as helpers (*see* review by Rapp, 1969).

Classification of Viruses

Viruses are often subdivided, according to the nature of their hosts, into plant viruses, animal viruses and bacterial viruses or bacteriophages, but some plant viruses can multiply in their insect vectors. There is therefore no sharp division into these three subgroups. Each virus has a range of hosts in which it can replicate and the damage it does

TABLE 2

VIRUSES ASSOCIATED WITH ACUTE RESPIRATORY INFECTIONS

GROUPS	SUBGROUPS	SEROTYPES	CLINICAL CONDITION MOST OFTEN ASSOCIATED WITH INFECTION
Myxoviruses	Influenza	A B C	Influenza Influenza, "colds" "colds"
Paramyxoviruses	Parainfluenza Respiratory syncytial	1 2 3 4 Only 1	Croup; "colds"; influenza Croup; pharyngitis Pneumonia; "colds" Mild "colds" Bronchiolitis; pneumonia; "colds"
Picornavirus	Enterovirus Rhinovirus	Coxsackie virus A 21 Coxsackie virus B3 Echo 19 More than 90	Pharyngitis; "colds"; pneumonia "Colds"; laryngotracheitis; pneumonia "Colds" "Colds"; bronchitis
Adenovirus		1,2,5,6 3,4,7,14,21	Pharyngitis; conjunctivitis; pneumonia Epidemics in schools and military camps
Coronavirus		At least 3	"Colds"

This process was first described with bacterial viruses, or bacteriophages as they are usually called, and the process called lysogeny. The bacterial cells carrying the viral genome are lysogenic and under certain stimuli produce virus particles and are lysed, releasing the bacterial virus (phage particles). The presence of the integrated phage genome may alter the antigenic make up of the bacterial cell or cause it to become toxigenic as in the case of *Corynebacterium diphtheriae*. It is now clear that a similar process can occur in animal cells, the cells being altered in their growth pattern and becoming neoplastic (*see* review by Sambrook, 1972). Some viruses are defective, their nucleic acid not containing all the information necessary for the production of new virus particles. With these viruses a double infection is necessary. In addition to the defective virus, there has to be a helper virus which provides the information lacking in the defective virus. This is, in some cases, the information for the coat protein and in these viruses the antigenic structure and host range of the defective virus will depend on which helper virus is used. The range of helper viruses varies from one defective virus to another. In some there may be only one, while in others, a number of

to the host will vary from one to the other. Often, the host in which the least damage is caused will be the most important from the point of view of assuring the survival of the virus. For all classification purposes it is necessary to choose criteria. Previous classifications of viruses were based on the major host or type of disease produced, but, as more was learned about the biology of viruses and their structure, these classifications were not found to group together viruses of similar type. For example, the viruses which can cause respiratory disease (*see* Table 2) are a very mixed group. Viruses are currently classified as shown in Table 3. Thus they are first divided into RNA or DNA containing viruses and then on the basis of the symmetry of the arrangement of the protein units (capsomers) forming the capsid or shell of the virus particle. A further subdivision depends on the presence or absence of a lipid-containing envelope which is determined by sensitivity to inactivation by lipid solvents such as ether or chloroform. A scheme of viral taxonomy based on this classification, but using latin binomials, has been proposed by the International Committee on Nomenclature of Viruses (Wildy, 1971). However, the problem of establishing meaningful families and

SECTION XI

OTOLARYNGOLOGICAL BIOLOGY AND PATHOLOGY

PAGE

45. VIROLOGY   625

46. BACTERIOLOGY   638

47. MYCOLOGY   645

48. PARASITOLOGY   661

49. HISTOPATHOLOGY OF NOSE AND THROAT   667

TABLE 3

Classification of DNA Viruses

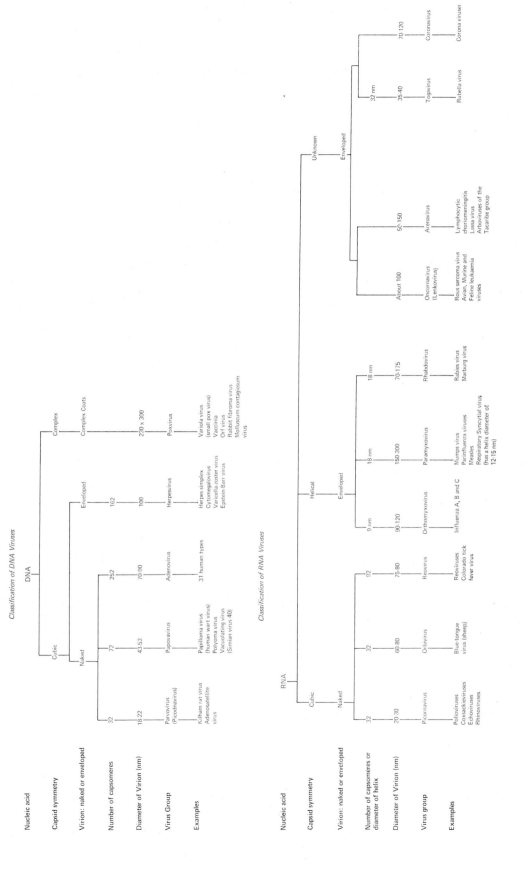

Nucleic acid	DNA				
Capsid symmetry	Cubic				Complex
Virion: naked or enveloped	Naked			Enveloped	Complex Coats
Number of capsomeres	32	72	252	162	
Diameter of Virion (nm)	18-22	43-53	70-90	100	230 × 300
Virus Group	Parvovirus (Picodnavirus)	Papovavirus	Adenovirus	Herpesvirus	Poxvirus
Examples	Kilham rat virus Adenosatellite virus	Papilloma virus (human wart virus) Polyoma virus Vacuolating virus (Simian virus 40)	31 human types	Herpes simplex Cytomegalovirus Varicella-zoster virus Epstein-Barr virus	Variola virus (small pox virus) Vaccinia Orf virus Rabbit fibroma virus Molluscum contagiosum virus

Classification of RNA Viruses

Nucleic acid	RNA								
Capsid symmetry	Cubic			Helical			Unknown		
Virion: naked or enveloped	Naked			Enveloped			Enveloped		
Number of capsomeres or diameter of helix	32	32	92	9 nm	18 nm	18 nm	About 100	50-150	32 nm
Diameter of Virion (nm)	20-30	60-80	75-80	90-120	150-300	70-175			35-40
Virus group	Picornavirus	Orbivirus	Reovirus	Orthomyxovirus	Paramyxovirus	Rhabdovirus	Oncornavirus (Leukovirus)	Arenavirus	Togavirus
Examples	Polioviruses Coxsackieviruses Echoviruses Rhinoviruses	Blue tongue virus (sheep)	Reoviruses Colorado tick fever virus	Influenza A, B and C	Mumps virus Parinfluenza viruses Measles Respiratory Syncytial virus (has a helix diameter of 12-15 nm)	Rabies virus Marburg virus	Rous sarcoma virus Avian, Murine and Feline leukaemia viruses	Lymphocytic choriomeningitis Lassa virus Arboviruses of the Tacaribe group	Rubella virus

genera has not been solved and the use of latin binomials is still controversial.

Structure of Viruses

Virus particles show a remarkable uniformity of size and shape. This, and the fact that some of the small viruses have only enough nucleic acid to code for some six to ten different proteins, leads to the view that the virion must have a regular geometric form (Crick and Watson, 1956). Electron microscopy has confirmed this prediction, and all viral capsids appear to be assembled from protein structural units (capsomers) arranged with either helical or cubical symmetry, as shown in Fig. 1. The virions of many

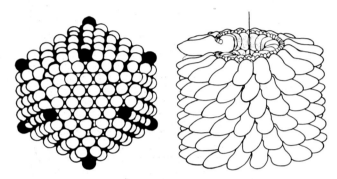

FIG. 1. Diagram showing the two types of capsid symmetry: helical on the right and cubical on the left, the solid black capsomers are at the 12 vertices of the icosahedron.

plant viruses consist of helical capsids with no outer envelope. The best known example of such a virus is the rod-shaped tobacco mosaic virus. In a number of animal viruses, the rod-shaped structure is wound inside a complex envelope giving the complete virion a spherical appearance. Examples of such viruses are the myxoviruses and poxviruses. Many viruses have nearly spherical capsids which, under the electron microscope, reveal regular features showing them to be icosahedra with 12 vertices, 20 faces and 30 edges. Only those viruses with a large number of capsomers appear at first sight to be icosahedral. Adenoviruses with 252 capsomers look icosahedral but herpesviruses with 162 capsomers do not. Icosahedral viruses, however, often have a hexagonal outline but some, such as wart virus with 72 capsomers, appear spherical (see Fig. 2 and also Madeley, 1972). Some bacteriophages have a very complex structure with a tail and specialized attachment organs on the tail down which the nucleic acid is injected into the bacterium.

Infection with Viruses

Viruses can replicate only within cells and they enter the body via the skin or mucous membranes. Probably they cannot penetrate the intact skin but enter via wounds, small abrasions, insect bites or inoculations. Most commonly viruses gain entry via the upper respiratory and alimentary tracts. Entry via the respiratory tract is not confined to viruses which cause disease of the respiratory tract. Generalized virus infections such as chicken pox and infectious mononucleosis may use this route. Having gained entry

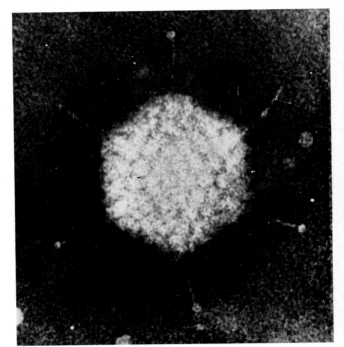

FIG. 2a

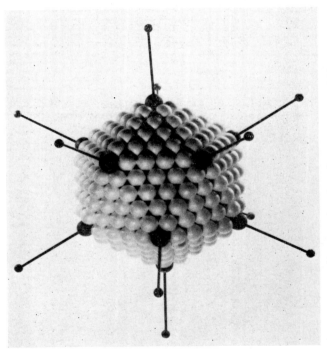

FIG. 2b

to the body, the virus particle must attach to a suitable cell, penetrate this cell and be uncoated to release the viral nucleic acid.

The intial attachment of the virus particle to the cell is probably mediated by electrostatic forces. The site of this attachment is specific and it is the specificity of this initial phase of viral infection which determines the host range of the virus. If the cells of a particular species or tissue are unable to provide the virus with an attachment site, then these cells will clearly be safe from infection by that virus. A number of viruses can attach to red cell membranes by specific receptors on the cell surface. As one virus can attach to two cells, a lattice of cells and virus can build up and become sufficiently large to be visible by the naked eye.

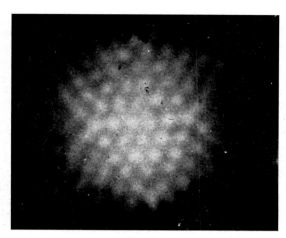

FIG. 2c

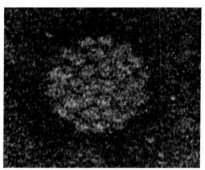

FIG. 2d

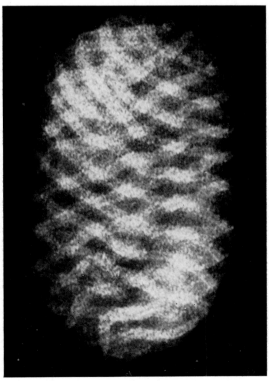

FIG. 2e

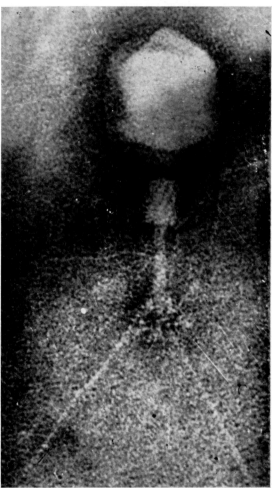

FIG. 2f

This process of haemagglutination can be used to help in the identification of viruses and in the titration of virus preparations. Serial dilutions of a virus preparation of, say, influenza virus, are prepared and, to each dilution, red cells are added. At a certain point in the dilution series, visible agglutination of the red blood cells will cease to occur and this is the titre of the virus.

The nucleic acid from certain viruses can infect cells but the nucleic acid is much less efficient than the complete virus and not all viruses yield an infectious nucleic acid (Sanders, 1964).

Bacteriophages attach by their tails to specific receptors on the bacterial cell wall and the viral nucleic acid is injected down the tail, through the cell wall which has been weakened at the attachment site. The bacteriophage protein

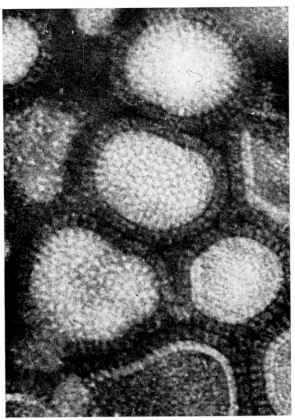

FIG. 2g

FIG. 2. Negatively stained virus particles. (a) Adenovirus particle showing the structures attached to the 12 vertices. (×600 000.) (b) Model of
adenovirus particle. (c) Adenovirus particle showing icosahedral array
of capsomeres. (×550 000.) (d) Human wart virus. (×650 000.)
(e) Orf virus particle showing the complex spiral surface structure.
(×320 000.) (f) T_2 phage particle showing the tail. (×470 000.)
(g) Influenza virus particles showing the surface spikes which at the
periphery form a fringe. (×33 750.) (Photographs kindly supplied
by Dr. H. G. Pereira (a and b) and Professor R. W. Horne (c, e, f and g).)

coat remains at the cell surface and plays no further part
in the process of infection. In contrast to the bacterial
cell wall, the animal cell membrane is very much less rigid
and virus particles attached to the cell surface are taken into
the host cell by a process of active ingestion similar to
pinocytosis by which fluid droplets gain entry. The virus
particle is engulfed by the cell membrane and it is in this
vesicle that the virus coat is removed and nucleic acid released. After penetration and uncoating, an infectious virus
cannot be demonstrated in the cell. This is the so-called
eclipse phase and lasts until new viral nucleic acid and
protein have been produced and new mature virus particles
assembled.

Growing Viruses in the Laboratory

For virus replication it is necessary to use living plant
or animal cells. The easiest method is to inoculate a suspension of virus particles into a suitable plant or animal
and then, after an appropriate interval, to remove certain
tissues and extract the newly formed virus. However,

laboratory animals have a number of disadvantages. The
most difficult of these to overcome is that they frequently
carry viruses and so virus preparations made from animal
and plant tissues may be contaminated with unwanted
agents. There are a few viruses which cannot be satisfactorily grown in any other way and, for these, animals must
be used but most viruses can be grown in embryonated
eggs or tissue cultures.

The developing chick embryo provides a ready made
tissue culture free of known contaminants except the fowl
leukaemia virus which is probably present in all eggs but
for most purposes, this virus causes no complications. The
eggs must be incubated for 9–12 days before inoculation
and the virus can then be inoculated onto the chorioallantoic membrane or into the allantoic cavity, the amniotic
cavity, the yolk sack or the embryo. The choice of site
depends on the virus being used. For example, to isolate
influenza virus from a throat swab the material must be
injected into the amniotic cavity but subsequent passages
can be made in the allantoic cavity.

For many years it has been known that viruses could be
grown in tissue cultures. Vaccinia virus was first grown in
1913 in small pieces of tissue in drops of plasma (Steinhart
et al., 1913) but the use of tissue cultures was not a practical
proposition until the advent of antibiotics made it easy
to prevent bacterial contamination.

The discovery, in 1949, that poliovirus would grow in
human embryonic and monkey tissue cultures gave a great
stimulus to the use of tissue cultures in virology (Enders
et al., 1949). The susceptibility of the intact animal to infection with a particular virus is of little help in predicting
whether or not the virus will grow in the cells in culture.
Some viruses will grow in cultures of cells from resistant
animals while others will not grow in cultures of cells from
susceptible animals. There are basically two types of
tissue cultures: primary cultures and continuous cell lines.
Primary cultures consist of cells freshly removed from the
animal and placed in culture either as small organized
pieces of tissue or broken up with trypsin to form a single
cell suspension. In either case, the cells are usually grown
on a glass or plastic surface in a tube or in a bottle. The
cells grow and for a time the cultures can be divided into two
or more subcultures at weekly intervals but, with most
cultures, growth gradually slows and eventually the culture
dies out. Occasional cultures, however, take on a new lease
of life, the morphology of the cells changes and they can
be subcultured indefinitely. This change in cultural behaviour is called *transformation* and the cells are described
as transformed. Transformed cells are very useful in the
laboratory as they can be kept growing, obviating the need
for fresh animal tissues. However, they are not suitable for
growing all viruses and they have a very abnormal chromosome pattern. They have in fact probably undergone a
neoplastic change and are therefore not used to make virus
vaccines for human use. In the last few years, lines of
human cells have been grown which retain their normal
morphology and diploid chromosomal configuration but
can be grown in the same way as transformed cells except
that after about 50 subcultures they die out. A stock of
these cells is usually kept frozen in liquid nitrogen so that,

when the line in use dies out a fresh line can be started from the frozen cells.

There are many formulae for tissue culture media but they all consist basically of a balanced salt solution, which provides the correct osmotic pressure, pH and essential inorganic ions, glucose as a source of energy and antibiotics to prevent the growth of bacterial contaminants. To this must be added essential amino-acids, vitamins and animal serum. The role of the serum is not fully understood but it is very difficult to grow cells without it. In place of, or in addition to, the amino-acids and vitamins, various protein hydrolysates, yeast extracts and embryo extracts can be used. Sera may contain viral antibodies and other inhibitory substances and these must be tested for before the sera are used otherwise viral replication in the culture may be prevented. The rate of growth of a culture can be slowed down by reducing the concentration of serum in the medium and it is usual to do this before inoculating the virus. Tissue cultures are not always free from contaminating viruses which were present in the cells before culture. Monkey kidney cell cultures often produce simian viruses and human tonsil cultures adenoviruses (*see* Paul, 1970, for techniques of tissue culture).

Some viruses growing in cultures give no indication of their presence and the cells or supernatant fluid have to be removed and tested by animal inoculation or some other means to demonstrate their presence. Fortunately, however, many viruses cause degeneration or necrosis of the cells. They are described as having a cytopathogenic effect (CPE) (*see* Fig. 3c). Other viruses, such as the one causing measles, induce the formation of syncytia or multinucleate giant cells. The myxoviruses do not produce a CPE but, if red blood cells are added to the culture medium, they stick to the infected cells which can be seen as clumps by light microscopy (*see* Fig 3d). Infected cells can also be visualized if the culture is exposed to appropriate viral antibody labelled with a dye which fluoresces in ultra-violet light. A more complicated method of demonstrating that a culture is infected is to add a cytopathogenic virus, the growth of which is prevented by the presence of the other virus. This is one method used to detect the presence of rubella virus in cultures used to isolate this virus from clinical material. A very useful technique used with cytopathogenic viruses is to cover the cell monolayers with soft agar after the virus has been given time to adsorb. This prevents spreading widely and from each focus of infection only a small area or plaque of cell degeneration is produced. The cell sheet can be stained and the number of infective doses in a virus preparation can be determined (*see* Fig. 3e and f). Plaques produced by different viruses, or even strains of the same virus, vary in size and appearance, and this technique can be of help in virus identification, or in genetic studies.

Diagnosis of Virus Diseases

The diseases caused by different viruses are often clinically indistinguishable, and, if an accurate diagnosis is to be made, laboratory investigations are necessary. However, if these investigations are not to be a waste of the laboratories' time, the specimens must be properly taken at the correct

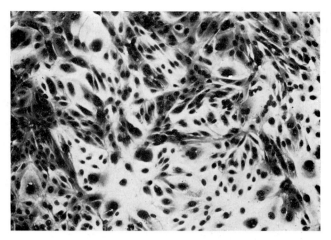

Fig. 3a

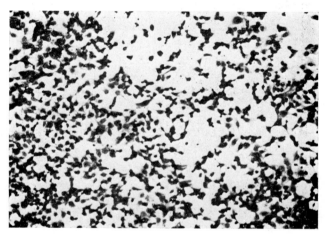

Fig. 3b

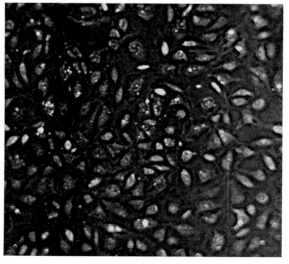

Fig. 3c

time in the course of the disease and transported to the laboratory under satisfactory conditions. If there is any doubt, the clinician should seek advice from the laboratory. The laboratory diagnosis of viral infection depends on demonstrating either the presence of the virus or a rising titre of antibodies. A virus may be demonstrated by direct microscopy of clinical material or by isolation of the virus

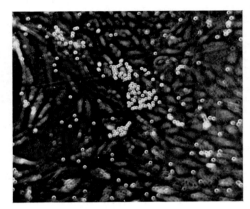

FIG. 3d

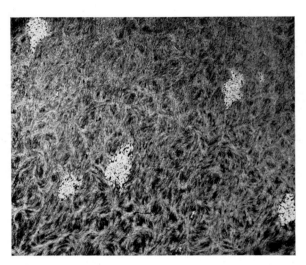

FIG. 3e

in animals, eggs or tissue cultures. Direct microscopy is rapid, giving a result in a few hours but can be used only in a very limited number of diseases. Two methods are available: electron microscopy and immunofluorescence. The viruses causing smallpox and chickenpox are morphologically quite different and adequate amounts of virus for electron microscopy can be obtained from the skin lesions. Electron microscopy is therefore the method of choice in making this important differential diagnosis. The presence of viral antigens in cells removed from the upper respiratory tract with a throat swab, or in the cerebrospinal fluid, can be demonstrated by the direct or indirect fluorescent antibody technique (see Nairn, 1969). In the direct method, the cells on a glass microscope slide are covered with antibody which has been conjugated with a fluorescent dye. After incubation at 37°C, the unabsorbed antibody is washed off and

the slide is examined under an ordinary microscope but with an ultraviolet light source. Cells which have viral antigen against which the antiserum has been prepared fluoresce. In the indirect method, the cells are first exposed to unlabelled antiserum against the appropriate viral antigen, and, after incubation, washed to remove uncombined antibody. The cells are then exposed to a fluorescent

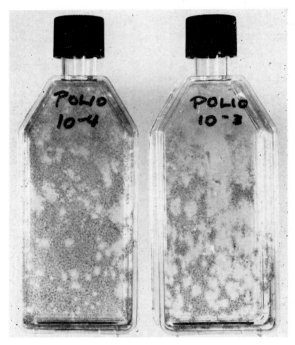

FIG. 3f

FIG. 3. Tissue culture cells. (a) Normal HeLa cells. (b) Primary monkey kidney cells. (c) Cytopathic effect produced in HeLa cell culture by poliovirus. (d) Monkey kidney cell culture infected with influenza virus and showing haemadsorption. (e) HeLa cell monolayer showing herpes simplex virus plaque. (f) Monkey kidney cell monolayer showing poliovirus plaques.

labelled anti-gamma globulin which combines with the serum used in the first stage. The slide is examined as in the direct method. The indirect method has the advantage of being slightly more sensitive and requiring only one labelled serum which can be used with different unlabelled sera. Obviously it is possible to look for only one virus in each test, so the method is most useful in confirming a fairly likely diagnosis such as herpes simplex encephalitis or respiratory syncytial virus infection in a young child.

Many viruses, including those which infect the respiratory tract, are readily inactivated outside the body, whereas the enteroviruses which multiply in the cells lining the intestinal tract and depend for their survival on transmission by the faecal-oral route can survive for a day or more at room temperature. The survival of all viruses can be improved by keeping the specimen just above 0°C. Because certain viruses, such as respiratory syncytial virus and the parainfluenza viruses, are inactivated by freezing, the former practice of transporting specimens for virus isolation in solid carbon dioxide is no longer recommended. It is now of a condition, such as sudden hearing loss, on isolated cases.

Pathogenesis of Virus Diseases

The invasion of a tissue by a virus can result in damage to the cells by a direct action of the virus on the cells, or as a result of the immune reaction mounted against the virus. Many viruses kill the cells in which they replicate and the effect of this on the animal will depend on the tissue involved. In the respiratory tract, the results may be slight or severe, but repairable, while in the central nervous system the damage may well be permanent. The changes produced by certain viruses in cells are very characteristic, as for ex-ample, the production of inclusion bodies. These are often seen in poxvirus infections and rabies, where the presence of Negri bodies are useful in making a post-mortem diagnosis, especially in animals. Some viruses, such as herpes simplex and cytomegalovirus, produce polykary-ocytes or syncytia, presumably because of some change in the cell membrane. The immune response is in most cases protective, but, in respiratory syncytial virus infection in infants and lymphocytic choriomeningitis virus infection in mice, the reaction between virus infected cells and anti-body leads to a much more damaging pathological change than when the infection occurs in the absence of antibodies. Viruses enter the body via the skin, respiratory or gastro-intestinal mucous membranes. In the case of the respiratory disease producing viruses, the primary site of infection is where the important pathological changes take place and the virus remains localized, but, in generalized virus in-fections such as measles or poliomyelitis, the virus, after replication in the primary site, spreads via the lymphatic system or blood stream to the secondary sites of virus replication where the characteristic lesions are produced. With most generalized virus infections, the viraemic phase is so short lived that it is difficult to demonstrate.

Virus infections are often silent. If the antibody levels in a group of individuals are followed, a number will produce antibodies to viruses such as mumps, rubella or Epstein-Barr virus, showing that they have been infected without developing any disease. The human fetus can be damaged by a maternal rubella virus infection without the mother suffering any clinical disease. Viruses may also become latent in infected animals. The best known latent infection in man is herpes simplex. After a primary infection, usually in childhood, the virus may remain in the tissues and pro-duce recurrent herpetic lesions, usually round the mouth, when stimulated by nonspecific factors such as ultra-violet light, fever or emotional disturbances. How the herpes simplex virus is maintained in the tissues is not known, but in another form of latency, seen in tumour-producing viruses, the viral nucleic acid is integrated with the cell genome in some way similar to the integration of bacterio-phage nucleic acid into the bacterial genome. The so-called slow viruses, which are better called persistent viruses, have a very prolonged incubation period of several months to a few years during which time they remain latent in the body (see Royal College of Pathologists Symposium, 1972; Hotchin, 1971). The tumour-inducing viruses differ from others only in their ability to produce tumours. Tumour

viruses are found in four groups of DNA viruses and one group of RNA viruses (Epstein, 1971). As well as producing tumours on injection into suitable animals, most tumour viruses transform normal cells in culture into neoplastic cells. This is similar to the change which primary cell cultures undergo spontaneously at times and involves a change in morphology and in growth habit. Normal cells are inhibited from further growth by contact with each other and, when growing on a surface, they form a mono-layer. Transformed cells do not show contact inhibition and grow over each other resulting in the piling up of the cells. Figure 4 shows two colonies of BHK cells (continuous

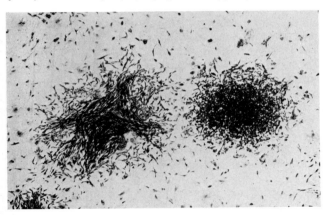

Fig. 4. Colonies of hamster cells developing from a suspension of cells plated out after exposure to polyoma virus. The colony on the left has grown from a transformed cell and the one on the right from an untransformed cell. (Photograph kindly supplied by Professor M. Stoker.)

line of baby hamster kidney cells) one of which has grown from a cell transformed by polyoma virus and the other from a normal cell. Work on the induction of tumours at the cellular level has been made possible by the study of virus-induced transformation of cells in culture. The DNA tumour viruses, on entering a cell, either replicate and produce new virus or transform the cell, the viral nucleic acid being integrated with the cell genome. The information carried by the viral nucleic acid codes for a number of new proteins which can be demonstrated as new antigens in the transformed cells. However, the property which gives the transformed cells their ability to escape the normal control systems and produce tumours in animals has not yet been determined. Cells transformed by DNA viruses do not produce new infective virus particles but the virus may be rescuable by hybridization of the transformed cells with another type of cell (Watkins and Dulbecco, 1967). The RNA tumour viruses produce infectious virus in the cells which have been transformed, the virus budding from the surface of the transformed cells. In order for the inform-ation in the viral RNA to be integrated into the cellular DNA, a DNA copy of the viral RNA is made by a reverse transcriptase present in all RNA tumour viruses (Temin, 1971). These viruses are responsible for naturally occur-ring tumours in fowls and for leukaemia in a number of species, but some of the most potent tumour producing DNA viruses such as polyoma and simian virus 40 produce suggested that specimens be packed in an expanded polystyrene box which also contains a plastic bag full of water ice. Specimens for virus isolation should be taken when the patient is first seen, since the chances of successful virus isolation are usually very much less late in the course of the disease. Enteroviruses may be isolated from faeces quite late in cases of encephalitis or meningitis. It is, nevertheless, very much better to isolate the virus from the CSF in the early stages, since enteroviruses are often found in the faeces of normal humans; their isolation from the faeces is not very convincing proof that they are the cause of a central nervous system disease. Respiratory viruses become difficult to isolate within a day or two of the onset of symptoms and they are easily inactivated on a throat swab. A swab should therefore be rubbed vigorously over the throat so that as much mucus and cellular material as possible are obtained. It should then be shaken in 2 ml of virus transport medium (obtained from the laboratory) and sent to the laboratory as rapidly as possible, preferably packed with water ice. Transport medium consists of a balanced buffered salt solution and some protein such as $0\cdot2$ per cent bovine plasma albumin. Viruses survive much better in protein solutions than in plain salt solutions. Table 4 gives some indication of the specimens best suited for the isolation of some common viruses, together with the methods used in the laboratory (see Sixth Annual A.S.C.P. Research Symposium., 1972).

A single serological test is seldom of any value in making a virological diagnosis. Antibodies to many viruses are so commonly present in the serum of healthy individuals that only a rising antibody titre can give an indication of recent infection. For this reason, it is important, if there is any likelihood that serological tests will be required, to take a sample of blood and store the serum the first time the patient is seen. Many serological tests are used for measuring antibody levels (Melnick, 1969), but the one most commonly used is the complement fixation test (Taylor, 1967) which can be used for most of the respiratory viruses. It is difficult to prepare complement fixing antigens from the enteroviruses so that the more time-consuming neutralization test in animals or tissue cultures is often used. The complement fixation test has the advantage of using a group antigen in the case of influenza virus and adenovirus so that it is not necessary to use each individual type, which would make the test impractical. Viruses which haemagglutinate are prevented from doing so by the presence of antibodies. Consequently antibodies to these viruses can be titrated by haemagglutination-inhibition tests. Although this test appears simple, non-specific inhibitors of haemagglutination are present in some sera and have to be destroyed. The test is nevertheless useful in typing influenza strains since, unlike the complement fixation test, it is type-specific. Antibodies to viruses which do not haemagglutinate can be measured by the indirect haemagglutination test. In this test the virus is adsorbed onto the surface of tanned red blood cells and these are agglutinated in the presence of antibodies. Fluorescent antibody tests are used to detect some virus antibodies, notably those to the Epstein-Barr (infective mononucleosis) virus, but the end point in this test is not

very sharp. Precipitation in agar gels is used to detect some antibodies such as those to Australia antigen, but this test is most useful in showing up a number of different antibodies in a serum. Radio-immunoassay has not yet been used much, but seems to be a method with considerable potential (Sönksen, 1974).

The interpretation of laboratory tests requires care. Virus infections are extremely common and many are asymptomatic, so that the isolation of a virus or detection of a rising titre of antibodies does not necessarily mean that the infection is responsible for the patient's disease. This applies especially to enteroviruses isolated from faeces. A virus isolated from a fluid such as CSF which is normally sterile has obviously much more significance. Respiratory virus infections are common and must from time to time occur at the same time as other unrelated diseases. Cases of, for example, sudden hearing loss occur sporadically through the year, and if such a patient presents during an influenza epidemic, paired sera may well show a rise in titre. It is always unwise to base any views on the causation

Table 4

SPECIMENS SUITABLE FOR ISOLATION OF SOME COMMON VIRUSES
AND THE LABORATORY METHODS USED

Viruses	Specimen	Method of Examination
Picornavirus Group		
1. Poliomyelitis	CSF, Faeces	1. Hela or MK cells.
2. Coxsackie A	Throat swabs, PM material	2. Inoculation of new born mice.
3. Coxsackie B	Throat swabs, PM material	3. Hela or MK cells, Inoculation of new born mice.
4. Echo viruses	Throat swabs	4. MK cells.
5. Rhinoviruses	Throat swabs	5. HEK, WI38, MK cells.
Adenoviruses	Throat swabs, Conjunctival swabs, Faeces, PM material	Hela cells.
Myxovirus group		
1. Influenza	Throat swabs	1. Amniotic cavity of embryonated eggs or MK cells.
2. Para-influenza	Throat swabs, Nose swabs	2. MK cells.
3. Mumps	CSF (in patients with aseptic meningitis) PM material	3. Amniotic cavity of embryonated eggs or MK cells.
4. Respiratory syncytial		4. Hela cells.
5. Measles	Throat swabs, conjunctival swabs, blood, urine	5. HEK, HA or MK cells.
Herpes virus group		
1. Herpes simplex	Vesicle fluid, swabs from lesions, CSF.	1. Inoculation onto chorio-allantoic membrane of embryonated eggs or HA or Hela cells.
2. Varicella-zoster	Vesicle fluid	2. HA or WI38 cells.
3. Cytomegalovirus	Saliva, Urine, Liver bopsy, PM material	3. HEK cells.
Poxvirus group Variola	Vesicle fluid, scrapings from lesions, Scabs, PM material	Electron microscopy, Inoculation onto chorio-allantoic membrane of embryonated eggs. Immunological tests—precipitation or complement fixation.
Lymphocytic choriomeningitis	CSF	Intracerebral inoculation of mice.
Rubella virus	Throat swabs, Nasal swabs, Serum	Green MK cells.

MK   monkey kidney
HEK human embryo kidney
WI38 human diploid cell line from human lung
HA   human amnion

46. BACTERIOLOGY

T. A. REES

INTRODUCTION

On October 10th, 1676, Anton van Leeuwenhoek initiated the science of bacteriology with his observations of bacteria in "pepper water". Seven years later he recorded the existence of oral bacteria in tartar taken from his own teeth and from those of an eight-year-old child. But the scientific treatment of disease had to wait another two centuries for the work of Louis Pasteur and Robert Koch. The relatively sudden realization that bacteria were the aetiological agents of disease produced an enormous amount of descriptive work, in the course of which much was learned of the structure and behaviour of pathogens and, incidentally, of non-pathogens as well, because there was initially no means of distinguishing between them. It was to meet this need that Robert Koch formulated his now famous postulates in which he set out a simple set of conditions that he hoped would make the distinction clear:

(1) The organism should be found in all cases of disease.
(2) The organism should be grown for several generations outside the body of the host.
(3) The organism so grown should be able to reproduce the disease in susceptible animals.

Unfortunately, Koch based his postulates on an "all or none" concept of pathogenicity, and no account is taken of the carrier state, in which pathogens can be isolated from susceptible humans or animals in apparent good health. Neither is there allowance for the role of the so-called "opportunist" bacteria, nor indeed of the physiological state of the host which can permit such organisms to assume the role of pathogens. Koch has nevertheless provided a useful set of working rules which have been applied successfully to most of the common diseases of bacterial origin. Leprosy remains problematic however, because nobody has yet succeeded in culturing *Mycobacterium leprae*.

MORPHOLOGY

There are three principal forms or shapes of the bacterial cell:

(1) Spheroidal, i.e. the coccus. These may occur in chains (streptococcus), in clusters like grapes (staphylococcus), in pairs (diplococcus) and other groupings.
(2) Cylindrical or rod-shaped, i.e. the bacillus. Bacilli may occur singly as in coliforms, or in chains as in species of proteus and the anthracoids.
(3) Helical, i.e. the spirillum and the spirochaete. Typical of this form are *Borrelia Vincenti* of Vincent's angina, and *Treponema pallidum* of syphilis.

The comma-shaped vibrio can be regarded as a special instance where the organism is curved through only one part of one turn of the helix, e.g. *Vibrio cholerae*.

The standard unit of measurement used in the description of bacteria is the micrometre, μm. (*micron* or μ), which is 10^{-6} of a metre or one thousandth of a millimetre.

All bacteria are enclosed by a semi-rigid wall within which lies the cytoplasmic membrane, a selectively permeable structure intimately involved with the osmotic behaviour of the cell. External to the cell wall may be found a capsule. This is not present in all bacteria, but can be characteristic of a particular group. It is not vital to the organism, and there are various techniques by which it can be removed experimentally. Where a bacterium is potentially virulent, the possession of a capsule is essential for the manifestation of this; though the mere possession of a capsule is no guarantee of virulence since they are also known to occur in commensals. Most capsules are composed of polysaccharides. For example, many strains of *Streptococcus* form a capsule of hyaluronic acid. Virulent pneumococci form acidic polysaccharide capsules that vary in composition from one type to another. However, *Bacillus anthracis* and other species of the same genus are exceptions to this and have capsules formed by a polypeptide made from units of glutamic acid. A capsule adds considerably to the bulk of an individual organism, and a colony will acquire a moist appearance and sometimes an extremely mucoid and viscid consistency. Species of the genus *Klebsiella* exhibit this property beautifully.

Some bacteria are able to move about in a lively manner where the consistency of the surrounding medium permits. This motion is effected through the use of one or more fine appendages which are often longer than the bacillary body in which they originate. Each of these structures is a *flagellum*, arising from its own basal body situated just below the cytoplasmic membrane. The wavelength of flagellar undulations and the number and siting of flagella on the bacterium are characteristic of the species. They can be removed by mechanical means without harm to the bacterium and are soon regenerated. There is some considerable variation in the antigenic constitution of flagella, even within a species, and this has allowed the preparation of specific antisera of great diagnostic value, particularly in the case of a pathogen such as *Salmonella* with its large number of different species.

Electron microscope studies of gram-negative bacilli have brought to light the existence of yet another kind of fine appendage to the bacillary body. These are the *fimbriae*, or *pili* as they are now commonly known. They apparently arise from basal bodies as do the flagella, but are shorter and straighter. A special function has been assigned to certain pili: this is discussed below.

BACTERIAL MULTIPLICATION

This is normally by the process referred to as binary fission, wherein the parent cell simply divides into two equal-sized daughter cells. There is inward growth of the success has been achieved in the treatment of keratitis due to herpes simplex virus with idoxuridine (Patterson and Jones, 1967) and the use of this substance in the treatment of herpes simplex encephalitis is life-saving (Nolan et al., 1970). Unfortunately idoxuridine is toxic and suitable only for parenteral use in serious disease such as encephalitis, though it can be applied topically, with some success, in treating hepetic skin lesions. Idoxuridine is very insoluble in water and most ordinary solvents but it is remarkably soluble in dimethyl sulphoxide. A 5 per cent solution in this solvent can be applied to skin lesions with a brush three times a day. This treatment is reported to increase the rate of healing and to reduce the pain in cases of herpes simplex (MacCallum and Juel-Jensen, 1966) and in cases of herpes zoster (Juel-Jensen et al., 1970). The treatment does not eliminate the virus from the body and fresh lesions at new sites must be treated in the same way. Cytarabine is another drug active against herpes simplex virus. It is water soluble and can be given parenterally but is toxic to the bone marrow. It has however been used in the treatment of generalized herpes (Juel-Jensen, 1970). Metisazone is used in the treatment of smallpox and vaccinia gangrenosa (Connolly, 1966) and amantadine is reported to reduce the duration of fever and symptoms in influenza (Galbraith et al., 1973).

There have been hopes for many years that interferon would be a useful chemotherapeutic substance. It is active against a wide range of viruses but it is specific for the species of cells in which it is produced and it has proved difficult to produce in quantity and to purify (Kleinschmidt, 1972). Also, to be effective, it must be given very early on in the infection, preferably even before infection. There are now a number of substances which stimulate interferon production and one of these may prove to be of clinical use. These also stimulate cell mediated immunity and may be of use in the treatment of neoplastic disease (Gresser, 1972).

REFERENCES

Bauer, D. J., St. Vincent, L., Kempe, C. H., Young, P. A. and Downie, A. W. (1969), Amer. J. Epidem., 90, 130.

Bellussi, G., Filippi, P. and Scalfi, L. (1959), Acta oto-laryng. (Stockh.), suppl. 147, 1.

Berglund, B. (1967), Acta paediat. scand., suppl. 176, 9.

Berglund B. and Halonen, P. (1970), E.E.N.T. Digest, 32, 37.

Connolly, J. H. (1966), Practitioner, 197, 373.

Crick, F. H. C. and Watson, J. D. (1956), Nature, 177, 473.

Durocher, J. (1972), Arch. intern. Med., 129, 143.

Enders, J. F., Weller, T. H. and Robbins, F. C. (1949), Science, 109, 85.

Epstein, M. A. (1971), Lancet, 1, 1344.

Galbraith, A. W., Oxford, J. S., Schild, G. C. and Watson, G. I. (1969), Lancet, 2, 1026.

Galbraith, A. W., Schild, G. C., Potter, C. W. and Watson, G. I. (1973), J. Roy. Coll. gen. pract., 23, 34.

Gresser, I. (1972), Adv. in Cancer Res., 16, 97.

Grönroos, J. A., Kortekangas, A. E., Ojala, L. and Vuori, M. (1964), Acta oto-laryng. (Stockh.), 58, 149.

Halsted, C., Lapow, M. L., Balassanian, N., Emmerick, J. and Wolinsky, E. (1968), Amer. J. Dis. Child., 115, 542.

Hotchin, J. (1971), Monographs in Virology, vol. 3. Basel: Karger.

Juel-Jensen, B. E. (1970), Brit. med. J., 2, 154.

Juel-Jensen, B. E., MacCallum, F. O., Mackenzie, A. M. R. and Pike, M. C. (1970), Brit. med. J., 4, 776.

Kleinschmidt, W. J. (1972), Ann. Rev. Biochem., 41, 517.

Luria, S. E. (1959), Immunity and Virus Infections, p. 188. (V. Najjar, Ed.). New York: Wiley.

Luria, S. E. and Darnell, J. E. (1968), General Virology, 2nd edition. New York: Wiley.

Lwoff, A. (1957), J. gen. Microbiol., 17, 239.

MacCallum, F. O. and Juel-Jensen, B. E. (1966), Brit. med. J., 2, 805.

Madeley, C. R. (1972), Virus Morphology, London. Churchill Livingstone.

Melnick, J. L. (1969), An Analytical Serology of Microorganisms, vol. 1, p. 411 (J. B. Kwapinski, Ed.). New York: Wiley.

Nairn, R. C. (1969), Fluorescent Protein Tracing. Edinburgh: Livingstone.

Nolan, D. C., Carruthers, M. M. and Lerner, A. M. (1970), New Engl. J. Med., 282, 10.

Patterson, A. and Jones, B. R. (1967), Trans. ophthal. Soc. U.K., 87, 59.

Paul, J. (1970), Cell and Tissue Cultures. Edinburgh: Livingstone.

Rapp, F. (1969), Ann. Rev. Microbiol., 23, 293.

Report of the Public Health Laboratory Service Working Party on Rubella (1970), Brit. med. J., 2, 497.

Royal College of Pathologists Symposium (1972), "Host-Virus Reactions with Special Reference to Persistant Agents," in J. clin. Path. (G. Dick, Ed.).

Sambrook, J. (1972), Adv. in Cancer Res., 16, 141.

Sanders, F. K. (1964), Techniques in Experimental Virology, p. 277 (R. J. C. Harris, Ed.). New York: Academic Press.

Schiff, G. M. (1969), Symp. Series in Immunobiol, Standard vol. 11, p. 83. Basel: Karger.

Sixth Annual A.S.C.P. Research Symp. on Laboratory Diagnosis of Viral Infections (1972), Amer. J. clin. Path., 57, 731.

Sönksen, P. H. (Ed.) (1974), Brit. med. Bull., Vol. 30, No. 1.

Steinhart, E., Israeli, C. and Lambert, R. A. (1913), J. infect. Dis., 13, 294.

Taylor, C. E. D. (1967), Progress in Microbiological Techniques, p. 1 (C. H. Collins, Ed.). London: Butterworths.

Temin, H. T. (1971), Ann. Rev. Microbiol., 25, 609.

Tilles, J. G., Klein, J. O., Jao, R. L., Haslem, J. E., Feingold, M., Gellis, S. S. and Finland, M. (1967), New Endl. J. Med., 277, 613.

Tóth, M., Barna, M. and Valtay, B. (1965), Acta Paediat. Hung., 6, 367.

Watkins, J. F. and Dulbecco, R. (1967), Proc. nat. Acad. Sci., 58, 1396.

Wildy, P. (1971), "Classifications and Nomenclature of Viruses" in Monographs in Virology, vol. 5 (J. L. Melnick, Ed.). Basel: Karger.

Yoshie, C. (1955), Jap. J. med. Sci. Biol., 8, 373.

only active against the extracellular virus. They can nevertheless prevent the spread of infection from cell to cell in most cases. However, some viruses, such as herpes simplex, may spread from cell to cell directly without being exposed to antibody while others, such as the lactic dehydrogenase virus of mice, form infective virus antibody complexes. Most viruses, however, on combination with antibody become unable to attach to cells because of blockade of their receptor sites. Phagocytosis of virus particles by macrophages, and cell mediated immunity may play a part in containing virus infections and in recovery, but they may also be damaging in certain infections.

Prevention of Virus Diseases

The control of virus diseases by isolation and quarantine measures is usually impractical because of the number of silent or mild infections which are not diagnosed and so maintain the virus in the population. However, there are a few notable exceptions, such as rabies and foot and mouth disease, but it is only possible to exclude these diseases from relatively small and sea-girt areas such as Britain. To eliminate a virus from the world population is only feasible when there is no animal reservoir and the disease is easily identified with a few mild cases and with no silent carriers. Smallpox is an example of such a disease and it seems likely that if the present progress is maintained it should be eliminated within a few years.

Virus infections leave behind them a very considerable degree of resistance to further infection with the same virus, or a virus with very similar antigenic composition. The immunity depends on the presence of immunoglobulins in the plasma and mucous membranes. The history of artificial immunization goes back to Jenner's use of cowpox virus to prevent smallpox. He discovered the important principle that resistance to a virulent virus could follow infection with a less virulent related virus. The viruses used today in live virus vaccines have mostly been attenuated in the laboratory by passage in tissue cultures or laboratory animals. A good antibody response can be obtained by the injection of inactivated virus vaccines, but the immunity is not usually as long lasting as that following the use of live vaccine. Live vaccines also have the advantage that they can be given by mouth in the case of poliomyelitis vaccine or by throat spray for influenza vaccine. This makes them cheaper and easier to administer, and a relatively small dose of virus is required to initiate infection, which reduces production problems. However, they have certain disadvantages. The virus replicates in the vaccinated person and he may infect his contacts. This is not a bad thing if the virus maintains its attenuated condition, but theoretically, on repeated passage in man by the natural route it could regain virulence. Nevertheless, live poliomyelitis vaccine has been in wide use for some years and no untoward incidents have occurred. Live vaccines may contain adventitious viruses from the animals, eggs or tissue culture cells in which they are made. This danger, however, is not confined to live vaccines since some of the early batches of poliomyelitis inactivated vaccine contained live simian virus 40, which is more resistant to inactivation than poliomyelitis virus. All vaccines have to be carefully

checked, batch by batch, for contaminants and antigenic potency, which adds considerably to their cost. The use of continuous cell lines for virus vaccine production would have the advantage of freedom from viruses such as simian virus 40 which are often present in primary cultures, but the similarity of spontaneously transformed cells to tumour cells makes them unacceptable at present for vaccine production.

Inactivated virus vaccines give a better antigen response if they are given with an adjuvant, but in a small number of cases adjuvants give rise to the formation of inflammatory cysts which may require surgical intervention. Adjuvants are therefore not used in humans for routine immunization. Virus particles contain several antigens, not all of which are required for the production of protective antibodies, and some of the viral antigens cause undesirable reactions such as fever, especially in young children. It is possible to break up influenza virus and remove from the vaccine much of the protein which causes side effects, while retaining the antigen which is important in producing resistance. Passive immunity occurs naturally in infants due to the passage of maternal antibodies across the placenta and it is an important factor in protecting infants against virus infections in the first six months of life. It can be produced by the injection of antiviral serum (usually, pooled human gamma globulin). It has the advantage of giving immediate protection but the resistance conferred lasts for three weeks at the most. The gamma globulin must be given within a few days of exposure and is useless once symptoms have appeared. It can be used to protect against, or attenuate, hepatitis, measles or smallpox, or in pregnant women exposed to rubella. Under experimental conditions, immunoglobulin can prevent rubella virus viraemia (Schiff, 1969) and presumably infection of the foetus, but, in clinical practice, its administration to pregnant women after exposure to infection appears to be of very little if any value in preventing the development of rubella (Report of the P.H.L.S., 1970). This is no doubt because of the inevitable time lapse between infection and the injection of immunoglobulin. Hyperimmune animal sera can be used to give passive immunity but there is a danger of serum sickness and antibodies are produced against the foreign gamma globulin. Consequently a second dose of serum from the same species will be eliminated very rapidly and be of no therapeutic use.

Antiviral drugs can be used to prevent certain virus diseases. They have the advantage of providing immediate protection but the number of occasions on which they can be used usefully is limited. Metisazone (methisazone) has been given to smallpox contacts and has proved effective (Bauer et al., 1969). Amantadine has been used successfully in a family environment to prevent secondary cases of A2 influenza (Galbraith et al., 1969).

Treatment of Virus Diseases

In most virus infections there is no specific therapy, and, even if it were possible to prevent virus replication by chemotherapy, it would be of limited value in many virus diseases because most of the damage to the tissues has taken place by the time symptoms appear. However, some tumours only in the laboratory and not in the wild state. Polyoma virus, a common infection of adult wild mice, has to be injected into newborn mice or hamsters and simian virus 40 into hamsters. On injection into animals, the tumour viruses probably transform cells within a few hours but tumours do not usually appear for a month or two. The long latent period is almost certainly occupied in a struggle between the tumour cells and the immune system which recognizes the transformed cells with their new antigens as abnormal (Durocher, 1972).

Virus infections, particularly those localized to the respiratory tract (Table 2), and also some generalized infections, such as measles, predispose to secondary bacterial infection. With the exception of a proportion of cases of acute tonsillitis due to *Streptococci*, viruses are the cause of virtually all acute primary infections of the upper respiratory tract. It is a common clinical observation that infection of the middle ear often follows either measles or a virus infection of the respiratory tract (Toth *et al.*, 1965). The ear is open to invasion by viruses in the throat and it is a widely accepted assumption that a bacterial otitis is often preceded by a viral otitis. However, although on occasion a number of respiratory viruses have been isolated from the middle ear (*see* Table 5), there is no evidence that any,

TABLE 5

VIRUSES ISOLATED FROM THE MIDDLE EAR CAVITY

Virus	Clinical Disease	Reference
Influenza A	1. From 4 of 10 children with acute otitis media during an influenza epedemic.	Yoshie (1955)
	2. From patients with influenza and otitis media.	Bellussi *et al.* (1959)
Coxsackie B4	From 8-year-old child with perforated drum and acute otitis media.	Tilles *et al.* (1967)
Adenovirus type 3	From 8-year-old child with bullous myringitis.	Tilles *et al.* (1967)
Respiratory syncytial	From 22 children age 1–38 months during 2 outbreaks of respiratory syncytial virus infection.	Berglund and Halonen (1970)
Parainfluenza 2	From 1 child of 106 with acute otitis media.	Halsted *et al.* (1968)

except respiratory syncytial virus, can invade the middle ear and cause a purely viral otitis media, and this virus produces only a very mild disease in infants (Berglund, 1967; Berglund and Halonen, 1970). The role of viruses in otitis media thus appears to be to predispose to bacterial invasion. If fluid is taken from the ear early in the disease, bacteria, usually in pure culture, can be grown in most cases (Grönroos *et al.*, 1964). Body cavities such as the middle ear which are open to the surface of the body yet remain sterile must have some active mechanism for maintaining this condition. It is perhaps not surprising that a viral disease can upset this mechanism, perhaps by impairing ciliary movement or altering the pH.

Resistance to Virus Infection

This may be specific or non-specific. Specific resistance results from past infection or therapeutic immunization and is mainly due to the presence of immunoglobulins in

the blood and in the secretions of the upper respiratory tract. Non-specific resistance depends on many factors. There is the mechanical barrier of the skin and the mucus of the respiratory tract which is swept outwards by the cilia. Viruses trapped in the mucus may be removed before they can attach to a suitable cell. These secretions also contain substances which can inhibit adsorption of viruses to host cells. The level of certain hormones may affect resistance. Cortisone, for example, increases the susceptibility of experimental animals to infection. The mechanism of action is not clear but cortisone inhibits the production of interferon and depresses the immune response. All viruses have a limited range of susceptible species and the resistance of the uninfectable species probably depends on their cells not having receptors for the virus. The susceptibility of cells for infection depends on their capacity for virus attachment and penetration. Non-primate cells which are insusceptible to infection by poliovirus fail to absorb the intact virus but are able to replicate the virus if the viral nucleic acid is introduced into the interior of the cell. The tissues of a susceptible animal are not all equally infectable, and tissue tropism was a criterion used in virus classifaction at one time. Individuals vary in their susceptibility to infection and it is possible, by selective breeding to obtain mice which are much more resistant than the average to a selected virus. This increased resistance is genetic but it may well depend on many other factors. Myxomatosis has become a much less lethal disease in rabbits due not only to the natural selection of more resistant animals but also to the selection of less virulent strains of virus. It is obviously a disadvantage to the virus to kill its host and there is a tendency for the less virulent strains to prosper providing they can still remain as infective and transmissable. Age is another factor in non-specific resistance. The young are usually more susceptible than the adult, and not always because of their lack of antibodies. New born mice are susceptible to coxsackie viruses and arbovirus infections to which adults are completely resistant.

Interferon is a protein produced by cells infected with live or inactivated virus or with certain foreign nucleic acids. It is able to protect normal cells against the dangers of viral infection and to prevent virus replication in these cells. It is active against a wide range of viruses, but not all, and it is specific for the species producing it. Interferon probably plays an important role in controlling virus infection and in the recovery from virus diseases. In experimental animal infections, the appearance of interferon in the plasma coincides with a reduction in the production of virus and the beginning of the end of the infection. The normal recovery from virus infections, but not from bacterial infections, of agammaglobulinaemic patients who produce little or no antibody is probably due to interferon.

The specific immunity which follows recovery from virus infections is dependent mainly on the presence of immunoglobulins in the plasma and in the secretions of the respiratory tract. The duration of immunity following a single infection is difficult to assess, since subclinical infections in immune individuals with viruses such as measles and mumps are probably frequent and give a boost to the antibody level. Antibodies do not penetrate cells and are therefore cross-resistance to framycetin, streptomycin and neomycin (Rees, 1971).

How are drug-resistant strains produced? This can happen through any of the following processes:

Selection. This is an essentially Darwinian process in which a small number of initially resistant bacteria are favoured by the widespread use of a drug active against the majority of strains of that organism. Proliferation of the "hospital staph" is probably attributable to this process. So too is the dramatic rise in the incidence of strains of beta-haemolytic streptococci resistant to tetracycline (*see* Fig. 2). In Britain in 1958, less than 1 per cent of strains

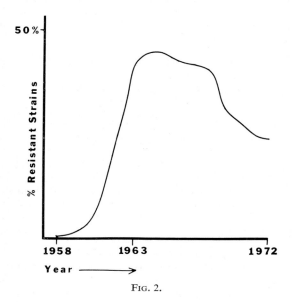

FIG. 2.

showed any resistance, but there followed a dramatic increase in this figure until, by 1963, it was well in excess of 40 per cent (Dadswell, 1967). Realization that this and related antibiotics were rapidly decreasing in usefulness, and also that it had unfortunate cosmetic effects on the teeth of growing children (Zegarelli *et al.*, 1960, Frankel and Hawes, 1964) brought about a considerable reduction in the quantities prescribed, with a consequent fall in the incidence of resistant strains (Rees, 1971a).

Induction. Though large populations of bacteria will throw off very small numbers of antibiotic resistant mutants, it is a fact that sensitive strains can sometimes be made resistant by exposure to a particular drug. This often appears in a step-wise manner as if a series of mutations were taking place. In the case of streptomycin, resistance, when it appears, does so in a single step so that the organism becomes highly resistant in the space of one subculture. But it is a pleasure to record that in all the years of its availability, no beta haemolytic streptococci or pneumococci have yet become resistant to the penicillins.

Transduction. We have seen how this process is involved in bacterial genetic exchange. It now appears that this mechanism can be the means of transmission of phage-like particles or plasmids which mediate drug resistance, and resistance to tetracycline, streptomycin, erythromycin and

chloramphenicol has been readily transmitted in this way *in vitro*.

Conjugation. Transmission of resistance by this route again involves plasmids, i.e. particles of extra-chromosomal genetic material. First described among species of Shigella in Japan in 1959 (*see* review by Watanabe, 1963), it was soon found to have a world-wide distribution, the first European report coming from England in 1962. The plasmid determining resistance does not move from one cell to another on its own account, but requires the presence of a second particle known as a "resistance transfer factor". Resistance transferred in this manner to uninfected cells is inherited by the daughter cells after division, so that all subsequent cells of a particular line will remain resistant once the line has become infected. Known as "infective drug resistance", this process occurs widely in both Gram-negative and Gram-positive organisms. The fact that it can take place between organisms in the human gut, and the ease with which it can be propagated *in vitro* have been viewed with a certain amount of alarm, but against this it can be argued that the process occurs much less easily *in vivo*, and that infected strains have a much lower rate of reproduction.

BACTERIAL TOXINS

The normal bacterial flora survives in the crevices and cavities of the body without harm to the host. Other bacteria are unable to survive without inducing in the host damage which may or may not be reversible. These are the pathogens, and the extent to which they are able to survive the host's defence mechanisms is a measure of their virulence. They mediate their pathological effects in a number of ways.

Exotoxins. Some of the more classical diseases are produced by the release from the invading organism of extremely toxic diffusible proteins which are easily distributed to distant parts of the body. Such are diphtheria, tetanus, gas gangrene; and these diffusible substances are called *exotoxins* because they are mostly extracellular substances which can be removed from a broth culture by simple bacterial filtration, purified and characterized as discrete chemical entities. Some are neurotoxins, some necrotoxins, leucocidins and so on, but all are susceptible to heat and are easily destroyed at 60°C. They will also undergo a slow loss of their toxic activity if left on the bench at room temperature, but without alteration of antigenic specificity. In either case, the resulting "toxoid" is then usable for prophylactic purposes. On occasion, the exotoxins are able to facilitate the spread of disease about the body, i.e. they act as "spreading factors". When this is so, the exotoxins are actually enzymes, such as hyaluronidase (released by streptococci, clostridia, staphylococci and strains of *C. diphtheriae*) or collagenase and lecithinase (released by *Cl. Welchii*). Exotoxins are for the most part produced by Gram-positive bacteria, but a few are secreted by Gram-negative bacteria, and a good example of this would be the neurotoxin of *Shigella shigae* which is one of the most toxic substances known to science.

Endotoxins are produced exclusively by Gram-negative bacteria of whose cells they seem to be a part, and differ from exotoxins in many respects. They are more resistant to heat and cannot be toxoided. Antigenically they appear to be identical with the somatic antigen of the smooth form of the cell. Neutralization with antibody is possible, but this process never goes to completion as it can with exotoxins. They are much less toxic than exotoxins, and have a common pharmacological action irrespective of the bacteria from which they were produced. Lipopolysaccharide in composition, endotoxins are regularly pyrogenic, can induce leucopenia and hyperglycaemia, and bring about endothelial damage leading to haemorrhage. Endotoxins derived from Gram-negative organisms in the gut may also pass into the circulation and become involved in haemorrhagic or ischaemic shock.

IMMUNITY AND RESISTANCE TO DISEASE

The term "immunity" implies complete or almost complete protection, and when it comes to be applied to the ability of the normal subject to avoid infection by microbes in the environment, it can be misleading. Indeed, resistance is a far better term, since the ability to resist infection can vary widely from one subject to another, and also within a particular individual from time to time. Mechanisms of resistance are usually discussed under two headings. These are:

(1) Non-specific or innate.
(2) Specific or acquired. This in turn can be divided into *active* and *passive* resistance.

Non-specific

The first barrier encountered by a potentially infective organism is the skin, and this is a mechanical barrier to further progress. In the skin live many harmless bacteria, the normal or resident flora, occupying the superficial layers, hair follicles, ducts of sebaceous glands and so on, from which it is impossible to dislodge them by scrubbing with soap or antiseptic and water. Other "transient" bacteria dwell in or on the skin but do not long survive because of the apparent effect of perspiration and sebaceous secretions. Further mechanical barriers are encountered at the mucous membranes and moist surfaces which are equipped to trap and expel the tiny particles which find their way on to them.

There are also chemical barriers, in the form of secretions. Lysozyme was first described by Fleming (1922). It is found in leucocytes, nasal fluids, saliva, tears and intestinal mucus. It is able to cause lysis by virtue of its action on certain amino-polysaccharides found in the walls of cells of some Gram-positive bacteria (unfortunately this action does not extend to the usual pathogens). But it can sometimes kill without the need for lysis, as happens in the case of coagulase-negative staphylococci which are exposed to lysozyme at an acid pH.

Perspiration and sebaceous secretions also come into the category of chemical barriers. Colebrook (1930, 1941) showed that *Streptococcus pyogenes* has a lower survival rate when smeared on human skin than when merely spread on a glass surface. This and similar effects are due to the presence of saturated fatty acids ranging from caprylic (C8) to undecylinic (C11) acid. Oleic acid can also be recovered from human skin, and lactic acid from perspiration.

A further barrier to invasion is the presence of the normal flora, not only in the skin, but the mucous membranes and the intestine as well. The mere presence of such a normal flora is usually sufficient to prevent the establishment of potential pathogens, but if the resident organisms are reduced or eliminated as a side-effect of treatment by antibiotics, the way is left open for invasion by less well-disposed bacteria. This has been known to occur after treatment with tetracyclines, with replacement of the normal gut flora by:

(a) Resistant strains of *Pseudomonas* and *Proteus*, giving rise to diarrhoea.
(b) *Candida albicans* which can invade:

(1) the mouth causing soreness or thrush,
(2) lower in the gut causing diarrhoea, or
(3) at the far end, causing pruritis ani.

(c) *Staphylococcus pyogenes* which can invade the small intestine producing superficial necrosis of the mucosa and giving rise to a copious diarrhoea full of staphylococci. This form of infection has also been known after treatment with concurrent penicillin and streptomycin.

Apart from its physical presence, the normal flora also plays a part in chemical defence by virtue of antagonistic substances which it produces. For example, the meningococcus and diphtheria bacillus can be killed by hydrogen peroxide formed by salivary streptococci. Tissue cells too can effectively resist invasion. Experiments in the guinea-pig have shown that the lesions of military TB are found in almost all organs but the kidney. Extracts of this tissue have been shown to contain spermine, a tetra-amine which has a pronounced inhibitory effect on *M. tuberculosis in vitro* when allowed to act in the presence of the enzyme spermine oxidase. The production of interferon by cells in response to infection by virus is discussed in the chapter on Virology.

Infection of normal tissues usually leads to a fall in pH due to the production of lactic acid by intense local activity, and this is sometimes sufficient to kill bacteria. In the event of a tissue being devitalized by injury, subsequent fall in oxygen tension may leave the way open for infection by obligate anaerobes such as *Clostridia sp.* in the form of spores. The presence of an exudate may serve to dilute toxins released by an infecting organism, while the formation of a fibrin network may assist by restricting the movement of organisms from the lesion. It may also facilitate the phagocytosis of capsulated bacteria which would normally escape in an entirely fluid medium (Wood, 1953).

When an organism succeeds in penetrating the skin or crossing into the tissues by other means, it is confronted by the cellular and humoral defence mechanisms of the body, and is shortly phagocytosed by cells which at other times are involved in scavenging the debris of worn out body cells. These phagocytes are of two types. Macrophages can be found lining the sinuses of lymph nodes, spleen, liver and bone marrow, or moving about as histiocytes through the tissues. Some leucocytes are also phagocytic, particularly the neutrophils, and it is these which first assemble in any large numbers at the focus of infection, migrating by chemotaxis through the capillary walls and in the direction of the invading bacteria. The wandering macrophages or histiocytes are slower to arrive, taking up not only the invading bacteria but also those leucocytes that have succumbed to them. The system is remarkably efficient even against some pathogens, though when presented with a choice of bacteria, leucocytes tend to prefer the avirulent ones to the virulent, and bacteria such as *Strep. pneumoniae* possessed of thick polysaccharide capsules are able to resist phagocytosis in the tissues of the normal subject. However, phagocytosis is made much easier in the presence of a fraction of the serum proteins. This particular fraction, the gamma globulin will be discussed in more detail below when dealing with the specific response to infection. Here it is sufficient to say that they can also have an apparently non-specific action wherein they are able to form a protein coat over the outsides of the bacteria. In this way the bacterial surface is greatly modified and the organism made much more susceptible to phagocytosis. Serum proteins endowed with this ability were originally called "opsonins", and the process of making the bacterium more vulnerable to phagocytosis "opsonization".

Once phagocytosis has taken place it does not necessarily mean that it is followed by bacterial death. Indeed, some bacteria are able to multiply within the phagocyte which may then serve to carry them to another site in the body before it dies, thus spreading the infection, and *Staph. pyogenes, Haem. influenzae* and *M. tuberculosis* can, for example, be disseminated in this manner.

Specific Resistance

Every minor cut introduces numbers of bacteria into the peripheral circulation and lymphatics where they are soon dealt with. But there are some occasions where the number of organisms so introduced, or gaining access elsewhere, are not rapidly removed, and the ensuing infective process offers a challenge to the host which results in a state of altered resistance. This state of resistance is an *increased* ability to resist further invasion by the same bacterium; that is to say, the resistance is specific, and the onset of this new state is commonly associated with alteration in the serum and lymph proteins.

There are several classes of protein present, all in colloidal solution, and they are easily separated and identified by the technique of electrophoresis. This depends on the fact that the protein molecules in solution carry a small electric charge, and when these are subject to a *direct* current (in a conducting medium), the molecules will migrate at a speed which is proportional to the charge they bear. As this charge is more or less constant for a particular class of molecule, there will be gradual separation of the protein mixture into its constituents as the "fast" proteins out-

strip the "slow" ones. If electrophoretic separation is made by Tiselius' method, a series of peaks is obtained which not only permits identification of the protein components but also allows a quantitative estimation of each, since the size of the peak is proportional to the amount present (*see* Fig. 3).

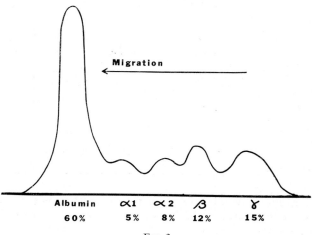

FIG. 3.

The fastest moving fraction is albumin, followed by the globulins. First of all, the α fraction with two peaks α_1, and α_2. These are followed by the β fraction and last of all, the slowest, γ fraction. It is with this γ globulin that specific resistance is associated and this can be demonstrated in the following manner: type-specific pneumococcal polysaccharide is used as antigen to immunize rabbits. When serum from these animals is treated with more pneumococcal polysaccharide, serum antibody is removed in the ensuing antigen-antibody reaction. This is matched by a reduction only in the γ region of the electrophoretic profile. Subsequent research has shown that the γ globulin fraction is a heterogeneous mixture of what are now called *immunoglobulins* (or Ig) on account of their antibody activity (*see* Table 3) and each is distinguished from the others by the addition of a single Roman letter after the prefix Ig.

Because it is the most abundant of the immunoglobulins, IgG is probably responsible for most of the work involved in the neutralization of bacterial toxins, and also in the promotion of phagocytosis which it does by forming complexes with bacteria which then adhere to the phagocytic cells. It passes more readily than any other immunoglobulin into extravascular tissue spaces and this property permits its passage across the placenta when it presumably comes to be of some use to the neonate in the first week or so of life.

IgA is found in secretions such as nasal fluids, saliva, tears, colostrum and in the lungs and gastro-intestinal tract. It is secreted by local plasma cells, the individual IgA molecules forming pairs or *dimers* which enter into a stabilizing chemical combination with a further secretory component (protein) formed by local epithelial cells. The presence of IgA in these secretions points to its role in the defence of the more vulnerable body surfaces.

TABLE 3

HUMAN IMMUNOGLOBULINS. THE MAJOR CLASSES AND THEIR PROPERTIES

	Molecular Weight	Normal Serum Levels	% Total Immunoglobulins	Crosses Placenta	Fixes C'	Fixes to Mast Cells (if in Homologous Skin)	Fixes to Macrophages
IgG	150 000	8–16 g. l.$^{-1}$ (53–107 μmol. l.$^{-1}$)	80	Yes	Yes	No	Yes
IgA	160 000+ polymers	1·4–4 (9–25 μmol. l.$^{-1}$)	13	No	No	No	Not known
IgM	900 000	0·5–2 (0·6–2·2 μmol. l.$^{-1}$)	6	No	Yes	No	No
IgD	185 000	0–0·4 (0–2·2 μmol. l.$^{-1}$)	1	No	Not known	No	Not known
IgE	200 000	17–450 μg. l.$^{-1}$ (85–2250 μmol. l.$^{-1}$)	0·002	No	No	Yes	Not known

IgM molecules also link up with one another, but in this case there are five in each group or *pentamer*, and for this reason they are sometimes called *macroglobulins*. With several reactive sites bound into one large molecule, the macroglobulins act as very efficient agglutinins, and, since they are for the most part found in the blood stream, their activity would appear to be especially significant in the event of bacteraemia.

IgD has been identified as a class of immunoglobulin, but so far no firm evidence has been put forward to demonstrate its activity as antibody.

IgE is present in serum only at very low levels, though there is an appreciable rise in the event of certain parasitic infections. It is synthesized by a very small percentage of plasma cells and readily becomes bound to mast cells. The antigen/antibody reaction which follows challenge with the appropriate antigen causes mast cell degranulation with its associated release of histamine and other vasoactive amines, a reaction which is at the basis of the symptoms of hay-fever and like diseases.

Primary and Secondary Response

In most instances, antibody production can be induced at will by means of vaccination or "immunization". This can be done in respect of all proteins because they are all antigenic, and since bacteria and many of their toxic by-products contain protein, use is made of this for prophylactic purposes. Dead bacteria or denatured toxin (toxoid) are usually injected in a series of doses spread over a period of time in order to induce a high level or titre of antibodies. Unfortunately, not all antibodies confer protection, e.g. syphilis, and even when they do, there are antigens which induce only a transient response for reasons that are not properly understood, e.g. *Vibrio cholerae*, and this is why there is no regular system of vaccination against certain diseases.

In those instances where an antibody response is known to occur, it follows the injections in an episodic manner. After the first dose of antigen has been given, there is a pause or latent period before the appearance of antibody in the circulation and this initial appearance of antibody is the primary response. If the antigen has been in solution, e.g. diphtheria toxoid, no primary response may be detected.

A second dose of antigen given after a suitable interval, will induce a further response which begins more quickly, rising faster and higher than the first. This is the secondary response, and it varies in magnitude according to the interval since the primary response, falling off if this has been too long and not rising high enough if too short. The second dose of antigen is therefore given at the optimum interval, a period which has long been established for the more general forms of vaccination. "Booster" doses may thereafter be given from time to time.

Passive Resistance

Members of the public are widely vaccinated against diseases such as diphtheria and tetanus, obtaining high and persistent degrees of protection. But there remains that section of the populace who receive no vaccination and therefore remain at greater risk. In the event of one of them falling sick with one of these infections, there is no time for the active induction of high antibody titres and recourse is had to the transference to the patient of antibodies in the form of high titre serum. Such prophylactic sera are prepared in animals which are bled at regular intervals once they have achieved a satisfactory antibody level, and the protection that it confers is described as "passive" because it has not been produced actively in the patient's own body.

Accounts of persisting sensitivity of streptococci to the penicillins (*see* p. 703) have not proceeded without challenge. For example, strains of pneumococcus showing significantly increased resistance to penicillin have been isolated from an aboriginal child in Australia and from fifteen New Guineans. These pneumococci were also partially resistant to the cephalosporin antibiotics.

Evidence for the virulence of these organisms is incomplete, however, since most were isolated from healthy persons (Hansman *et al.*, 1971).

REFERENCES

Colebrook, L. (1930), Ministry Health, Dept. Comm. on Maternal Morbidity and Mortality, Interim Report, Appendix D.

Colebrook, L. (1941), *Bull. War Med.*, **2**, 73.

Dadswell, J. V. (1967), *J. clin. Path.*, **20**, 641.

Fleming, A. (1922), *Proc. roy. Soc. B*, **93**, 306.

Frankel, M. A. and Hawes, R. R. (1964), *J. oral Therap. Pharmacol.*, **1**, 147.

Griffith, F. (1928), *J. Hyg. (Camb.)*, **27**, 113.

Hansman, D., Glasgow, H., Sturt, J., Devitt, L. and Douglas, R. (1971), *New Engl. J. Med.*, **284**, 175.

Lederberg, J. (1947), *Genetics*, **32**, 505.

Lederberg, J., Lederberg, E., Zinder, N. D. and Lively, E. R. (1951), *Cold Spr. Harb. Symp. quant. Biol.*, **16**, 413.

Rees, T. A. (1971), *Pract. oto-rhino-laryng.*, **33**, 388.

Rees, T. A. (1971a), *Lancet*, **1**, 938.

Watanabe, T. (1963), *Bact. Rev.*, **27**, 87.

Wood, W. B., Jr. (1953), *Harvey Lectures* 1951–52, *Series* 47, N.Y.: Academic Press.

Zegarelli, E. V., Denning, C. R., Kutscher, A. H., Tuoti, F. and DiSant'Agnese, P. A., (1960), *Pediatrics*, **26**, 1050.

Zinder, N. D. and Lederberg, J. (1952), *J. Bact.*, **64**, 679.

FURTHER READING

Cruickshank, R., Duguid, J. P., Marmion, B. P. and Swain, R. H. A. (1973), *Medical Microbiology*, Vol. 1. Edinburgh and London: Churchill Livingstone.

Elek, S. D. (1959), *Staphylococcus Pyogenes and Its Relation to Diseases*. Edinburgh: E. & S. Livingstone.

Garrod, L. P., Lambert, H. P. and O'Grady, F. (1973), *Antibiotic and Chemotherapy*. London: Churchill Livingstone.

Gell, P. G. H. and Combs, R. R. A. (1973). *Clinical Aspects of Immunology*. Oxford: Blackwell Scientific Publications.

Turk, D. C. and May, J. R. (1967), *Haemophilus Influenzae. Its Clinical Importance*. London: English Universities Press.

Williams, R. E. O., Blowers, R., Garrod, L. P. and Shooter, R. A. (1966), *Hospital Infection. Causes and Prevention*. London: Lloyd-Luke.

Wilson, G. S. and Miles, A. A. (1964), *Topley and Wilson's Principles of Bacteriology and Immunity*. London: Edward Arnold.

47. MYCOLOGY

MYRA McKELVIE

INTRODUCTION

The notion that fungi are frequent causes of disease is foreign to most otorhinolaryngologists. They recognize that a number of these organisms prove to be a nuisance, especially in the patient whose immune mechanisms are depressed by steroids or other agents; also in those patients whose usual bacterial flora has been disrupted by a range of wide spectrum antibiotics. Many fungi are found in the upper air and food passages, as well as in the external ears of patients without overt disease. It is often debatable whether or not these organisms are the cause of the condition under investigation. Microbiologists look for them secondarily, their immediate attention being directed to a relatively narrow range of bacteria. Moreover, therapy directed towards fungi yields, to the otolaryngologist, a far from dramatic response, accustomed as he is to the immediately rewarding results of antibiotics. The sluggishness of the resolution of fungal lesions is frequently less than persuasive. It is, with some justification, hard to persuade him that here is a range of conditions warranting more than perfunctory attention. His pathological colleague, in the face of this, together with the infrequent requests for culture, and other characteristics, of these organisms, tends to report only the most gross and impressive swabs and smears.

One should, however, hasten to point out that fungi have been of considerable value to the human race. Fungi may provide food or be used in food processing or in the production of drugs. The use of fungi as food is almost certainly older than the human species itself. Some tropical ants feed principally on a fungus which they cultivate for this purpose. There are possibly as many edible fungi known to the *mycophagist* (collector and eater of wild mushrooms) as there are pathogenic fungi known to the *mycologist*. The field mushroom (*Agaricus campestris*), common cultivated mushroom (*Agaricus bisporus*) and the truffle (*Tuber melanosporum*) are well known in Europe. The ear fungus (*Auricularia polytricha*) plays a probably greater role in the Oriental, especially Chinese, cuisine. Selected strains of *Saccharomyces cerevisiae* are used for baking bread or brewing, *Penicillium roqueforti* is used for the preparation of Gorgonzola, Roquefort and Stilton cheeses, *Aspergillus oryzae* is used to prepare soy sauce from soy bean (*Glycine max*) and, in the Orient also, *Monascus purpureus* is used to prepare *ang-khak* (a colouring agent for Chinese red rice and red wine). Indeed, *Monascus* is as much a food as a food-colouring material since, for centuries, the Chinese have deliberately cultivated it on rice kernels to use as such. Finally, there is the use of fungi to provide medicine with an increasing range of antibiotics (*see* Chapter 50). This listing of the uses of fungi is not provided solely in mitigation in the case of "*Homo* v. *Fungi*". It is, contrariwise, to provide a basis for conceptions regarding a greater role that fungi may play in the pathogenesis of disease. This will be discussed later.

Martin (1955) and subsequent mycologists have challenged the view that fungi are primitive plants. They are therefore now classified as a separate kingdom of organisms

(Whittaker, 1969). Over 70 000 species have been described. Although having some structural similarities to the algae (a primitive type of plant), the fungi characteristically contain no photodynamic pigment. Thus, like animals and bacteria, they are *heterotrophic*, i.e. they require organic materials as a source of energy. The great majority of fungi are *saprobic*,* i.e. they subsist on dead organic matter. The rest of the fungi are *parasitic*, i.e. they live on other living organisms without rendering a service in return.

Fungi may also be broadly classified as *moulds* (filamentous fungi), *yeasts* (unicellular fungi) or *dimorphic* fungi (having both mould and yeast forms). The moulds

is afforted either by pre-existing disease (metabolic disorders, chronic anaemias, leukaemias or lympho-reticular disorders), or by administration of certain drugs (corticosteroids; cytotoxic agents). Unfortunately, the term "opportunistic", whilst not having gained universal acceptance, is here to stay. The term "obligate pathogen" is, however, open to considerable criticism. All fungi are essentially *facultative pathogens*, i.e. they are saprobic but become pathogenic only in unusual circumstances. Even *Histoplasma capsulatum* (the causative organism of histoplasmosis), which is frequently cited as a non-opportunistic fungus, infects many people who show no clinical signs of infection. It would appear that the

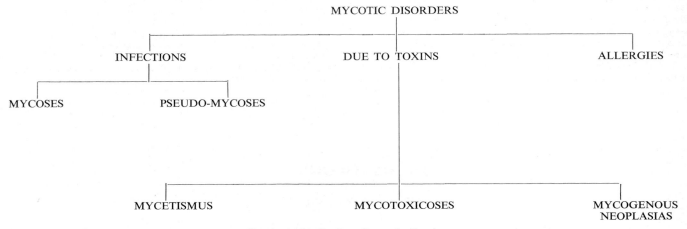

Fig. 1. A classification of mycotic disorders.

grow as branching filaments, *hyphae*. The mass of interlacing fungi that makes up a fungus colony is known as a *mycelium*.

A more formal classification of the fungi depends on a consideration of the nature of their sexual processes. In this respect, fungi are classified as *phycomycetes*, *ascomycetes*, *basidiomycetes* or *fungi imperfecti*. Phycomycetes characteristically form non-septate hyphae at the aerial ends of which are *sporangia* (spore cases). These sporangia contain *sporangiospores* (asexual spores). Sexual spores (zygospores) are produced in the phycomycetes by the fusion of the tips of two hyphae. Ascomycetes characteristically form septate hyphae, whose asexual spores are termed *conidia* and sexual spores, *ascospores*. Conidia are formed on special hyphae termed *conidiophores*, by the process of hyphal constriction. Ascospores are formed in an *ascus* which contains 2, 4 or 8 spores. Basidiomycetes also have septate hyphae. Sexual fusion of these produces a club-shaped *basidium*, the surface of which carries four (sexual) *basidiospores*. The *fungi imperfecti* includes all those fungi (the majority) in which a sexual stage has not yet been observed. Morphologically, however, the majority of this group resemble the ascomycetes.

Fungi which cause disease in man have also been classified into *opportunistic* (infecting when the opportunity presents itself) and *obligate* pathogens. The "opportunity"

"unusual circumstances" for fungal infection are primarily provided by variations in the *host response* and not by variations in fungus infectivity. This would appear to apply both to fungal allergies and to the mycoses. It should be noted that fungal infections, with the notable exception of the tineas, differ from virus and bacterial infections in being contracted from the external environment and not from other people or animals.

Figure 1 classifies human disorders where fungi play an important aetiopathological role. It will be convenient to use this classification as a basis for discussion.

MYCOSES

Figure 2 shows a classification of the *mycoses*, i.e. the fungal infections, which are of otolaryngological interest. They are usually subdivided into the *superficial* (*surface*) mycoses and the *deep* (*systemic*) mycoses. In superficial mycoses, the fungi are present only in the epidermis and its surface appendages (hairs and nails) or on the epithelial surfaces of mucous membranes. The deep mycoses comprise the fungal infections of the dermis and deeper tissues. This classification is not a hard and fast one; some organisms which are generally associated with superficial infections may, on occasion, give rise to a deep mycosis. This applies to *Candida* (nearly a quarter of all mycotic deaths in the U.S.A. are attributed to this organism) and, in Algeria at least, to *Trichophyton* (Hadida and Schousboe, 1959).

---

* This term is preferred to saprophytic since the latter implies a plant relationship.

Superficial Mycoses

Dermatophytoses

These are a group of superficial fungus infections of keratinized tissues, i.e. the epidermis, hair and nails. The causative organisms belong to one of the three genera, *Trichophyton*, *Microsporum* or *Epidermophyton*. Two of these dermatophytoses are of otolaryngological interest, i.e. *tinea capitis* (ringworm of the scalp) and *tinea barbae*. *Kerion* is a complication of ringworm of the scalp and is probably due to secondary infection. It is characterized

wherever possible. Scrapings from the edge of suspect skin lesions, after cleaning with 70 per cent ethanol, provide suitable material for study. For microscopic examination the material should be mounted in 10 per cent potassium hydroxide. The purpose of the alkali is to clear the specimen. Young hyphae appear as long, undulating branching threads. Older hyphae have many septa, at which points they eventually break to produce the barrel-shaped, or rounded, arthrospores. The media most commonly used for the isolation of these dermatophyte fungi are the modern equivalents of Sabouraud's maltose peptone agar.

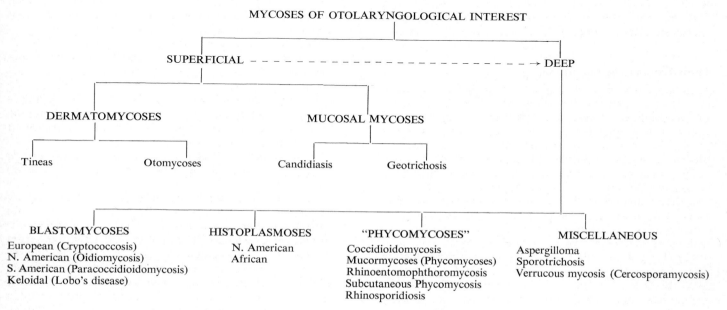

FIG. 2 A classification of the mycoses of otolaryngological interest.

by the formation of nodular, exudative pustules which may lead to scarring. *Favus* is a protracted disease of the scalp which affects children under fourteen years of age in countries surrounding the Mediterranean Sea or of Southern Asia. It is due to *Trichophyton schoenleinii*. Characteristically, there are patches of sulphur-yellow scabs, the healing of which may lead to permanent hairless scars.

About 50 per cent of dermatophyte species are *anthropophilic* (transferred from man to man), such as *Microsporum audouinii* which is the principal cause of *tinea capitis* in Canada, Nigeria and the U.S.A. (Ajello, 1960), and *Trichophyton violaceum* which is the principal cause of the condition in southern Europe, the U.S.S.R. and China; others are *zoophilic* (transferred from animals to man), such as *M. canis*, which is the commonest cause of tinea capitis in Australasia, Britain and India, and *T. verrucosum* which is a common cause of tinea barbae. Other organisms, such as *T. mentagrophytes*, are equally prevalent as a parasite of man and of other animals; this dermatophyte is also a common cause of tinea barbae.

The diagnosis of these infections by purely clinical means is not always possible. Direct microscopy and cultural examination of selected material should therefore be made

Contamination with bacteria may be troublesome so that the addition of an antibiotic is advisable. Most of these fungi will yield a growth in two to three weeks, when the particular dermatophyte can be identified. The three genera of dermatophytes can be distinguished by the appearances of their *macroconidia*, large, elongated conidia, the compartments of which are divided by transverse septa. *Epidermophyton* produces medium-sized, pear-shaped, relatively thick-walled structures; *Microsporum* produces large, fusiform structures with thick walls and many septa; *Trichophyton* produces small, irregular cylindrical structures with thin walls.

Topical treatment is sometimes effective and should always be used even if its action is only that of killing spores and the removal of infected debris. Compound benzoic acid, i.e. Whitfield's ointment (BPC) is a well-established preparation. A more recently introduced compound, clotrimazole, in the form of a cream, has been found to be an effective antifungal agent (Clayton and Connor, 1973; Polemann, 1973). Oral griseofulvin provided the first (and up to the present time the only) systemic treatment for ringworm. This is an antifungal antibiotic derived from several species of *Penicillium* and first isolated by

Oxford and his associates in 1939. Successful results were reported with the drug in experimentally induced ringworm infections in guinea pigs by Gentles (1958). Immediately afterwards, the drug was reported to be successful in man (Williams *et al.*, 1958). The mode of action of griseofulvin is by preventing invasion of the epidermal keratin by the ringworm fungi; the old susceptible keratin is shed and replaced by resistant griseofulvin-containing new keratin. The time required for cure therefore depends on the rate of replacement of keratin. The drug is carried to all parts of the body, including the epidermis and enters the living keratin precursor cells. The precise way in which griseofulvin acts *in vivo* has not yet been fully elucidated although it is clear that its beneficial action in ringworm infection results from its presence in keratin (Gentles *et al.*, 1959).

Otitis Externa and Otomycosis

Otitis externa is a term used to describe inflammatory disease of the external acoustic meatus. The development of the condition is associated with local itching, and is followed by progression to varying degrees of pain, and a clinical picture of mild to severe local inflammation associated with serous or purulent discharge. The disease is a common one and much has been written with regard to the aetiology. Multiple pathology appears to be common (McKelvie and McKelvie, 1966). The majority of fungi isolated from lesions of otitis externa are generally considered to be saprobic in nature and can commonly be isolated from normal healthy skin (Haley, 1950; Lea *et al.*, 1958). The part that these organisms play in the production and maintenance of otitis externa and the factors which allow them to grow in profusion under certain environmental conditions remain obscure. However, in the presence of such underlying conditions as seborrhoeic or atopic eczema, psoriasis, contact dermatitis and bacterial infections, especially with *Staphylococcus*, *Streptococcus*, *Proteus* and *Pseudomonas*, proliferation of the fungi will take place. *Aspergillus niger* (Fig. 3) is probably the commonest pathogenic organism isolated and is also considered to be of importance by Sharp and his colleagues (1946) and by Gregson and La Touche (1961). However, other fungi have also been isolated, e.g. *Candida albicans* (Smyth, 1961), dermatophytes (English, 1957; Smart and Blank, 1955), *Mucor* and *Penicillium* (McBurney and Gulledge, 1955).

In evaluating *treatment* for acute diffuse external otitis, Senturia (1973) gave little attention to fungi as aetiological agents. Since otitis externa is associated with the accumulation of débris, underlying dermatoses and both bacterial and fungal infections, effective therapy must take all these into account. Regular and effective aural toilet is necessary in order to clean the external meatus of débris. Local corticosteroids will assist in the reduction of inflammation and, where bacteria are present, these should be treated with the appropriate local antibiotic. In view of their action against both bacteria and fungi, quinoline compound preparations are of considerable value. In cases associated with infection with *Candida*, treatment with nystatin or amphotericin B is recommended (Pyman, 1959).

Candidiasis

Candidiasis is an acute, or subacute, infection of the mouth, pharynx or oesophagus caused by a yeast-like fungus, *Candida albicans* (monilia).

Candida albicans is the most frequent aetiological agent of candidiasis and is capable of causing any of the clinical types of this mycosis. *Candida albicans* belongs to the group of budding yeasts which, under certain conditions, are characterized by elongation of buds to form cylindrical pseudohyphae. This is the form in which the organism is encountered in pathological lesions. The consistent association between clinical candidiasis and some deeper-seated potentiating cause has long been recognized. *Candida albicans* is a weak pathogen and its establishment often depends on the presence of some underlying pathological condition, or other predisposing factor. Some of these are well known, e.g. as a sequel to the therapeutic use of wide-spectrum antibiotics. Other conditions known, or suspected, to be associated with candidiasis are infancy, old age, pregnancy, endocrine imbalance, including diabetes mellitus, blood dyscrasias, malnutrition, obesity, antibiotic or steroid therapy, drug addiction, abnormal laceration of the skin and postoperative states.

Shaheen (1965) has called attention to the role of *Candida sps.* in the Paterson Brown-Kelly (Plummer Vinson) syndrome.

Normal human serum possesses anticandidal activity (Roth *et al.*, 1959; Louria and Brayton, 1964). It would appear that there are at least two factors, one of which is specific for *C. albicans*. The anticandidal activity of serum is reduced in mucocutaneous and systemic candidiasis, Hodgkin's disease and leukaemias. Infants do not attain adult levels of anticandidal serum activity until about the age of seven months. This is therefore presumably a factor governing the age incidence of thrush. Taschdjian and Kozinn (1957) also observed that unless *C. albicans* grows in ordinary cultures taken from the neonate in the first three days of life, thrush rarely develops.

In addition to the reduction of serum anticandidal activity in patients suffering from neoplasias of the leukaemia-lymphoma group, there is also a decrease in the mobility of the diseased lymphocytes (Schrek, 1963). This is undoubtedly responsible for the high incidence of candidal infections in this group of patients.

Laboratory diagnosis is made by microscopic examination of material from mucosal or dermal lesions to demonstrate the budding cells and hyphae of *Candida*. Material is also cultured on Sabouraud's modified agar at 303 K (30°C) or at room temperature. The typical yeast-smelling colonies appear within three days.

In oral candidiasis (thrush), the tongue, soft palate, buccal mucosa and other oral surfaces are characteristically covered with discrete, or confluent, patches of a creamy white pseudomembrane. Removal of this leaves a red oozing surface. While neither so firm nor extensive as a diphtheritic membrane, that of oral candidiasis may be deep or extensive enough to be painful and to interfere with swallowing or, in the case of oral thrush in infants, with breathing. Oral candidiasis often extends to the angles of the mouth, causing fissuring. The role of the yeast in chronic glossitis is equivocal although it can usually be isolated in culture.

Candidiasis may be restricted to the larynx (Yonkers, 1973), where it may give rise to laryngeal hyperkeratosis (Tedeschi and Cheren, 1968).

or lozenges, it effectively controls *Candida* infections of the mouth. Owing to the toxicity of the drug when administered parenterally, its use in this way should be limited to the treatment of more severe infections (Bindschadler and Bennett, 1969).

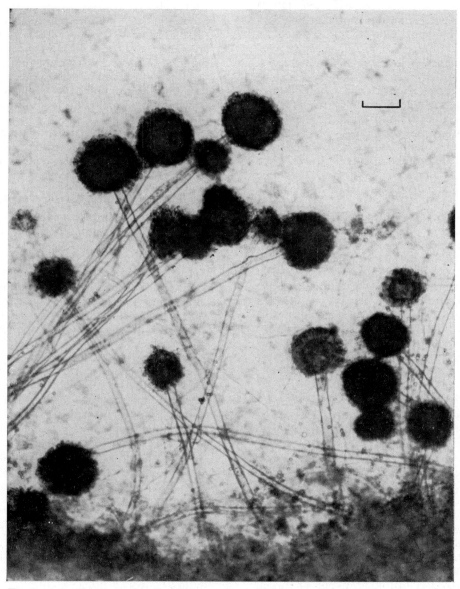

FIG. 3. *Aspergillus niger* cultured on Sabouraud's medium from a case of otitis externa. Scale = 50μm (By courtesy of Professor L. Michaels.)

Candidiasis can be a severe and fatal complication in a patient whose resistance has been reduced because of chronic disease or its treatment. In certain cases, the lesions caused by *Candida* are widespread, extending over the mucous surface of the upper respiratory and alimentary tract.

Nystatin (an antibiotic derived from *Str. noursie*) has a specific action against *C. albicans*. The drug is not absorbed from the gastrointestinal tract and therefore must be applied to the site of infection. Amphotericin B is also used in the treatment of candidiasis. In the form of tablets

Geotrichosis

Geotrichum candidum is responsible for white growths appearing in the cracks in the skin of over-ripe tomatoes. Rarely, it causes infection of the oral cavity, gastrointestinal tract and lower respiratory tract. This mycosis is usually secondary to some other disorder or is associated with a mixed infection. Because *G. candidum* is so commonly found on, in or around man, its mere isolation does not, of course, establish it as an aetiological factor. Nevertheless, when infection occurs, it is similar to that of *C.*

albicans (white growth on mucosal surfaces) and it is also similarly responsive to nystatin and amphotericin B.

Deep Mycoses

Deep mycoses of the head and neck can pose a difficult diagnostic problem. As Hoffarth and his colleagues (1973) point out, they may present a clinical picture indistinguishable from that of carcinoma. One doctor suffered an amputation owing to the mistaken histological interpretation of a biopsy specimen. The histological picture of a deep mycosis is that of a chronic inflammatory reaction; the causative fungi are of low virulence and do not produce exotoxins. Although different degrees and forms of inflammatory reaction are produced, no histological reaction is peculiar to infection by any particular fungus. As Symmers (1968) says, the thing that distinguishes a mycotic lesion from similar lesions of other inflammatory diseases is the presence of the causative fungus in the tissues. The three keys to the diagnosis of any deep mycosis are in the hands of the clinician, the microbiologist and the histopathologist. The clinician must be knowledgeable about the existence and the characteristics of particular fungal infections; the microbiologist must refuse to regard any fungus cultured from potentially infected material as a contaminant or a saprobe unless it has been exonerated from aetiological involvement by a full investigation; the histopathologist must be able to recognize fungi in sections of infected tissue. But, as Symmers points out, the demonstrable presence of a fungus in a histological preparation does not preclude the possibility of another co-existent disease. This is in addition to the pre-existing disease which has permitted the "opportunistic" fungal infection.

Cryptococcosis (European Blastomycosis: Torulosis)

This is defined as a chronic, granulomatous infection of worldwide distribution caused by *Cryptococcus neoformans* and contracted through inhalation of infected dust, with a predilection for spreading to the central nervous system (meningoencephalitis) although other tissues may also become involved (Btesh, 1973).

C. neoformans is a true yeast, reproducing by budding. It forms neither hyphae nor pseudohyphae. These cells are about 5–15 μm in diameter and surrounded by a thick mucinous capsule which is well defined in Indian ink preparations. This capsule is unique amongst those of the pathogenic fungi in being stained with mucicarmine. This stain is consequently the only histological stain of special diagnostic significance in mycopathology.

Normal human serum can inhibit the growth of *C. neoformans* (Baum and Artis, 1961).

Thirty per cent of cases of cryptococcosis are associated with Hodgkin's disease or disease of the reticulo-endothelial system (Zimmerman and Rappaport, 1954).

Virulent strains of this fungus are commonly found in abundance in pigeon nests and droppings (Emmons, 1955). It is generally considered that the organism is inhaled and initially involves the lungs. However, Briggs and his colleagues (1974) have reported the occurrence of *nasal cryptococcosis* where it was suspected that this was the initial lesion. Norris and Armstrong (1954) have also reported the occurrence of membranous cryptococcal nasopharyngitis. Meningoencephalitic cryptococcosis may present neuro-otologically. The condition may be confused with vestibulocochlear schwannoma (Rose *et al.*, 1958). Although neurocryptococcosis usually presents insidiously with a chronic course, it may present with *vertigo*, severe headache and vomiting of sudden onset. In these cases, there is associated evidence of a rapidly spreading intracranial lesion for which frequent lumbar puncture is required to prevent irreversible optic nerve damage.

Although one can gain assistance from serological testing (Kaufman and Blumer, 1968), diagnosis still depends upon clinical recognition of the disorder together with isolation of the organism.

Briggs and his colleagues treated their case successfully with amphotericin B and flucytosine. The course of the disease under treatment was monitored using specific slide latex agglutination tests.

North American Blastomycosis (Oidiomycosis)

North American blastomycosis is defined as a chronic, suppurative and granulomatous infection caused by *Blastomyces dermatitidis* and which is transmitted by inhalation of conidia. The initial, pulmonary infection characteristically spreads to other organs (Btesh, 1973).

B. dermatitidis is a dimorphic fungus which occurs as small, thick-walled budding spheres in infected tissues. When grown on special glucose agar, brown colonies develop which show branching septate hyphae with round or pear-shaped spores.

The organism has been isolated from the soil (Denton *et al.*, 1961) and recovered from both the dog (Robbins, 1954) and the horse (Benbrook *et al.*, 1948). Judging by blastomycin skin tests, less than 3 per cent of infected subjects show signs of the disease (Smith *et al.*, 1958).

The condition is likely to confront the otolaryngologist as a facial lesion characterized as a verrucous granuloma with central scarring. Alternatively, it may occur as chronic laryngitis with pulmonary involvement (Bennett, 1964). The condition is treated with a course of intravenous amphotericin B.

South American Blastomycosis (Paracoccidioidomycosis)

This is defined as a chronic, systemic infection occurring in Central and South America, most frequently in males, particularly manual labourers and farmers, which is caused by *Blastomyces brasiliensis* (Btesh, 1973).

The condition occurs predominantly in Argentina and Brazil. It is fatal in about 40 per cent of untreated cases. The first granulomatous ulcerating lesions are usually in the oral mucosa from which peripheral and lymphatic spread occurs. Thus the disease may be primarily mucocutaneous with lesions of the mouth, nose and face, or it may extend as far as the ileocaecal region. It must be distinguished from other chronic granulomatous lesions of the mouth and from oral carcinoma (Furtado *et al.*, 1954; Hildick-Smith *et al.*, 1964). The condition is treated with amphotericin B. Cures are obtained in cases receiving maximally tolerated intravenous doses of amphotericin B for a sufficient period of time (Gonçalves, 1962).

Keloidal Blastomycosis

Keloidal blastomycosis, formerly termed Lobo's disease, is defined as a keloidal infection due to *Paracoccidiodes loboi*, similar to cutaneous paracoccidioidomycosis (South American blastomycosis), but milder and without lymphadenopathy (Btesh, 1973).

This condition is rarer than the other blastomycoses. Probably less than 100 cases have been reported. Surinam appears to be a particularly endemic focus (Wiersema and Niemel, 1965).

Clinically, keloidal blastomycosis resembles the milder type of South American blastomycosis except that visceral

strated that bats in Central America are frequent hosts for the fungus and are capable of contaminating bat guano from intestinal lesions. It has been suggested that some of the puzzling epidemiological aspects of urban histoplasmosis in the U.S.A. might be explained by an association with *Eptesicus fuscus*, a bat which lives in old buildings (Emmons *et al.*, 1966). As a corollary of this association, histoplasmosis should always be suspect in any undiagnosed illness in subjects who handle bats.

As Moore and Jorstad (1943) have pointed out, histoplasmosis is important to otolaryngologists because it can simulate carcinoma, rhinoscleroma, laryngeal tuberculosis,

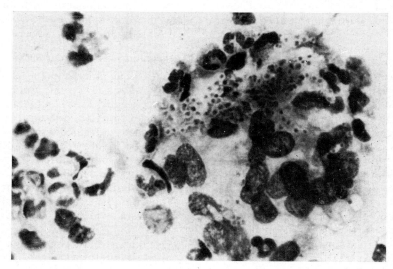

FIG. 4. Oral histoplasmosis. Smear from tongue showing a dense conglomerate of macrophages containing phagocytosed *Histoplasma capsulatum*. Leishman stain. ×1000. (By courtesy of Professors O. P. and R. M. Gupta.)

dissemination does not occur and the patient may remain in good general health for forty years. Contrary to what is implied by its name, the lesions are not always keloidal. Consequently, Emmons and his colleagues (1970) prefer the original name, Lobo's disease. The lesions, which appear as elevated, crusted, fungating plaques, may be localized to the face. Histological sections show the dermis to be replaced by exuberant giant-cell granulomas containing the fungi. Fungus cells, which are about 8 μm in diameter, are best demonstrated with the Grocott-Gomori methenamine silver nitrate stain. Chains of three to four cells are observed; these fungal cells often have two or three daughter cells.

Treatment is wide surgical excision where feasible.

Histoplasmosis

This is usually a systemic infection originating in the lungs by inhalation and spreading to other organs via the pulmonary lymphatics. It is due to *Histoplasma capsulatum*, an endoparasite of the reticuloendothelial cells. It is thus a reticuloendothelial cytomycosis. The fungus grows freely in soil which is contaminated by the faecal droppings of chickens, starlings, blackbirds and other avian species (Chin *et al.*, 1970). Klite and Diercks (1965) have demon-

leishmaniasis and otitis media. Conversely, leishmaniasis has been repeatedly mistaken for histoplasmosis (Woo and Reimann, 1957; Zinneman *et al.*, 1961). Histoplasmosis may also cause nasal septal ulceration. Laryngeal and tracheal lesions may be associated with generalized histoplasmosis or they may be primary, showing as a superficial ulceration of the vocal folds (Withers *et al.*, 1963). Acute tracheal obstruction secondary to a *Histoplasma* mediastinal granuloma has also been described (*see* Chapter 68).

The histopathological picture of, for example, oral histoplasmosis, is shown in Fig. 4. Here, a dense conglomerate of macrophages containing oval bodies (*H. capsulatum*) about 1–3 μm in size is seen surrounded by what appears to be a capsule.

Histoplasmosis is world-wide but particularly prevalent in the Mississippi-Ohio River Valleys. A related disorder, *African Histoplasmosis*, due to *H. duboisii*, occurs in West Central Africa and affects particularly the skin and cranial bones.

As with a number of other fungi, *H. capsulatum* is best demonstrated histopathologically by means of the Grocott-Gomori silver methenamine (hexamine) stain. Immunofluorescence microscopy also serves to differentiate *H. capsulatum* from *Leishmania donovani*, from which it might be indistinguishable with routine (hematoxylin-eosin) stains. Immunodiagnostic techniques comprise a skin hypersensitivity test (*histoplasmin* skin test) and use of a micro-Ouchterlony *immuno-diffusion* technique. Several arcs may develop in such antigen-antibody systems with sera from patients with histoplasmosis. One, the "M", precipitin band occurs as a result of the reaction of the antibody and the histoplasmin skin test antigen; another, the "H", is not related to the skin hypersensitivity test but usually appears during current infections. The "H" antibodies always accompany "M" antibodies but may not be adequately developed in some infected subjects. The histoplasmin skin test has also been reported to have been negative in at least one case of oral ulcerative histoplasmosis until one year after cure by amphotericin B (Drouhet, 1968).

Coccidioidomycosis

This fungal disorder, due to *Coccidioides immitis*, the most important of the pathogenic phycomycetes, is endemic in the semi-arid areas of the south-west U.S.A., northern Mexico and the Gran Chaco (northern Argentina and Paraguay). These areas correspond to an ecological zone termed the lower sonoran life zone (Emmons *et al.*, 1970). This is characterized not only by the low rainfall and high summer temperature, but also by a particular fauna, i.e. rodents such as those of species of *Perognathus*, *Dipodomys* and *Citellus*. Many of these rodents have naturally acquired pulmonary coccidioidomycosis (Emmons, 1942). It has been estimated that ten million people in the U.S.A. have been infected with *C. immitis* (Chick, 1962). Clinically, this mycosis may take the form of a primary infection (perhaps as an influenzal-like illness), disseminated infection or residual pulmonary disease following the primary infection. Mumma (1953) has recorded coccidioidomycosis of the epiglottis. An immunodiffusion technique is now used for the immunodiagnosis of this disease (Bailey *et al.*, 1965).

Hildick-Smith (1963) has pointed out that, in contrast to most systemic mycotic diseases, coccidioidomycosis is not predisposed to by diabetes, the leukaemias or the lymphomas.

Mucormycoses

Mucormycosis is defined as an acute, usually fatal if untreated, systemic fungal disease, caused by species of *Absidia*, *Mucor* and *Rhizopus*, originating usually in the nose and paranasal sinuses and spreading to other organs. It causes an acute inflammatory process with abscess formation in the affected organs (Btesh, 1973). The organisms penetrate the walls of arteries supplying nasal and paranasal structures and initiate thromboses and infarcts of the cheek and brain (Baker, 1960).

Almost invariably the organisms that have been isolated have belonged to one of two species of *Rhizopus* (*R. arrhizus* or *R. oryzae*). Moreover, *Absidia* and *Mucor* have never been recorded as having produced a cerebral infection. The term *rhinocerebral mucormycosis* is thus perhaps a little misleading, although the order to which these genera belong is the Mucorales. A more appropriate term might be the one used by Abramson and his colleagues (1967) and

by Battock and his colleagues (1968), i.e. *rhinocerebral phycomycosis*.

As Clark (1968) points out, the phycomycoses, i.e. the mucormycoses, are usually associated with immunological incompetence or metabolic disorders, especially ketosis. Indeed, a third of what become fatal neuromycotic infections present as paranasal sinus infections in diabetics (Burns, 1959).

Amphotericin B inhibits hyphal transformation of the spores of *R. oryzae* in rats and protects infected rabbits from otherwise lethal doses of this organism (Chick *et al.*, 1958). Thus this drug, given intravenously, and, if appropriate, in conjunction with antidiabetic therapy, can cure what would otherwise be a fatal condition (Burrow *et al.*, 1963).

Subcutaneous Phycomycosis

In 1956, Lie-Kian-Joe and his colleagues described *subcutaneous phycomycosis* in Indonesia and Burkitt and his colleagues (1964) subsequently described the condition in Uganda. The disease is characterized by extensive subcutaneous indurated lesions. Deeper structures may, however, be involved and the causative organism has been isolated from the posterior wall of the pharynx at the level of the cricoid cartilage (Clark, 1968). The causative organism is *Basidiobolus haptosporus*. It is now considered that *B. meristosporus*, which has also been cited as a causative organism, is identical with *B. haptosporus* (Emmons *et al.*, 1970).

Williams and his colleagues (1969) have described the ultrastructure of *B. haptosporus*. The eosinophilic sleeve (Splendore-Hoeppli phenomenon) which surrounds hyphae consists of collagen, lysosomes and degenerating mitochondria.

Rhinoentomophthoromycosis

The fungus *Entomophthora coronata* was isolated from nasal polyps of horses in Texas in 1962. The first human case was diagnosed in a man from Grand Cayman Island (Bras *et al.*, 1965); this island in the Caribbean is about 300 km north-west of Jamaica. Subsequently, a series of cases was reported from Nigeria and initially described under the term "rhinophycomycosis" (Martinson, 1963; Martinson and Clark, 1967).

The histopathology of the lesions resembles that of subcutaneous phycomycosis, i.e. subcutaneous eosinophilic granulomas. In the tissues, the organism resembles *B. haptosporus*, i.e. exhibiting broad hyphae with few septa. The two conditions are, however, clinically distinct. Rhinoentomophthoromycosis originates in the inferior nasal concha and spreads to the paranasal sinuses and subcutaneous tissues of the upper lip and the upper face (Figs. 5–7).

Rhinosporidiosis

This is a chronic granulomatous disease of the mucous membranes, especially of the nose, pharynx or conjunctivae, which is caused by *Rhinosporidium seeberi*. It is endemic in Southern India (Satyanarayana, 1960) and in Ceylon (Karunaratne, 1964). Ninety per cent of all

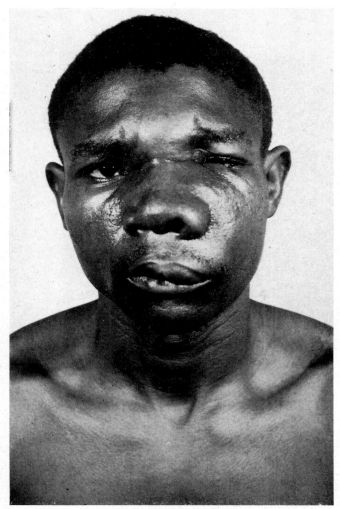

FIG. 5. Rhinoentomophthoromycosis involving glabella, dorsum of nose, left cheek, left ala nasi and left half of upper lip. (Reproduced by courtesy of Professor F. D. Martinson.)

spores in the mature sporangium (Fig. 10) are released through a pore in the chitinous shell. In many specimens, however, few trophocytes or sporangia are seen, only collapsed, empty and partly-destroyed chitinous shells (Fig. 11).

Rhinosporidiosis would still appear to be a surgical problem in that removal of the granulations from the upper air passages is the usual treatment required. To date it would appear to have resisted the newest chemotherapeutic agents, but it is possible that they will be applied successfully in the near future.

Aspergilloma and Aspergillosis

While the main literature (e.g. more recently, Crompton and Milne, 1974) on systemic aspergillosis concerns broncho-pulmonary manifestations, the problems associated with paranasal sinus infections caused by *Aspergillus sp.* are now attracting attention (Veress *et al.*, 1973).

Although *A. niger* is usually associated with otomycosis, *A. fumigatus* is the usual aetiological agent of pulmonary aspergillosis. A pansinusitis may also be due to *A. fumigatus* infection (Adams, 1933). The *primary paranasal aspergillus granuloma* (PAG) is, however, apparently due to the *A. flavus-oryzae* group of organisms. This paranasal granuloma, although rare in the rest of the world, is common in northern Sudan (Miloshev *et al.*, 1966; Milošev *et al.*, 1969). Unlike the other nasal mycoses, PAG is rarely visible rhinoscopically. The condition usually presents as a unilateral painless proptosis. PAG is, in fact, the most common cause of unilateral proptosis in the Sudan (Aal and Milošev, 1969). There may be radiological evidence for destruction of the ethmoid cells and the maxilla.

With conventional (e.g. hematoxylin-eosin) staining, the histological picture of PAG is that of non-specific giant cell granulomata. Indeed, this was the original designation of the tumour before its true condition was recognized. Staining with PAS (periodic acid Schiff reagent) or silver methenamine reveals the true fungal nature. Septate hyphae are seen surrounded by giant cells with a fibrous tissue background. Culture studies show the organism to be *A. flavus*. This organism is a common soil fungus in the Sudan (Tarr, 1955). It also frequently inhabits the nasal cavity of normal subjects (Sandison *et al.*, 1967). Milošev and his colleagues (1969) consider that this organism then becomes pathogenic when conditions in the paranasal sinuses become relatively anaerobic following mucosal thickening or polyp formation secondary to repeated inflammation.

The *larynx* may also be infected by *Aspergillus*. However, as with other laryngeal mycoses, this is almost always secondary to more extensive involvement of the tracheo-bronchial tree. Nevertheless, *primary laryngeal aspergillosis* has been described (Rao, 1969; Ferlito, 1974). Laryngoscopy shows ulceration of the vocal fold. Histological examination of biopsied specimens shows an ulcerated area covered with granulocytic and cellular débris intermixed with broad hyphae exhibiting dichotomous branchings and transverse septation (Fig. 12).

reported cases occur in this area. Sporadic cases occur in other parts of the world, particularly in Uganda (Engzell and Jones, 1973). Clinically, the condition usually shows as friable, polypoid lesions of the nasal cavity and, where the condition is not endemic, is commonly misdiagnosed as "nasal papilloma".

The disease is not contagious but is believed to arise from traumatic inoculation. Although a fungus has not yet been isolated from the soil, it is believed that there is a saprobic phase in the soil, as well as the parasitic phase in the tissues (Karunaratme, 1964). Karunaratme refers to the earliest stage of the organism which can be identified in tissues as *trophocyte* (Fig. 8). This is a spherical cell with a diameter ranging from 6 to 60 μm. It has a chitinous shell with a small, centrally placed nucleus surrounded by vacuolated cytoplasm which frequently shows shrinkage artefact. Nuclear division occurs when the diameter attains about 50 μm. This immature sporangium (Fig. 9) contains many small naked nuclei embedded in cytoplasm. The

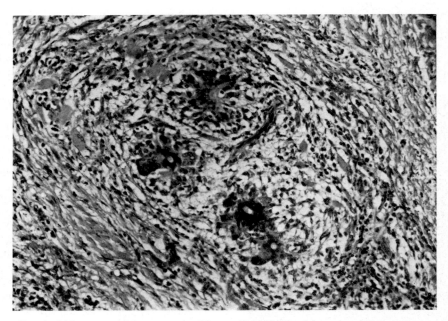

Fig. 6. Rhinoentomophthoromycosis. Biopsy. Epithelioid cells are arranged in palisades around necrotic eosinophilic granular substance with hyphae in centre. H. & E. stain. ×160. (Reproduced by courtesy of Professor F. D. Martinson.)

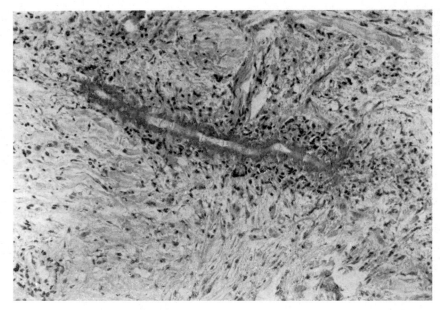

Fig. 7. Rhinoentomophthoromycosis. Section showing hypha surrounded by necrotic substance with diffuse chronic inflammation in the surrounding tissues. H. & E ×180 (Reproduced by courtesy of Professor F. D. Martinson.)

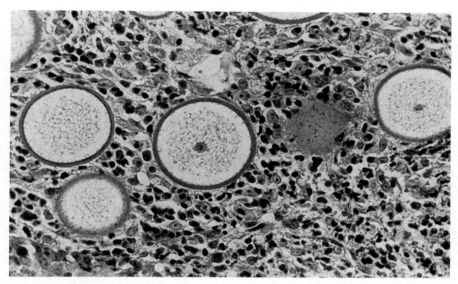

FIG. 8. Rhinosporidiosis. Four trophocytes surrounded by a chronic inflammatory reaction; two show a central nucleus surrounded by cytoplasm. The cytoplasm has contracted away from the chitinous shell. H. & E. ×400. (Reproduced by courtesy of Drs. U. C. G. Engzell and A. W Jones.)

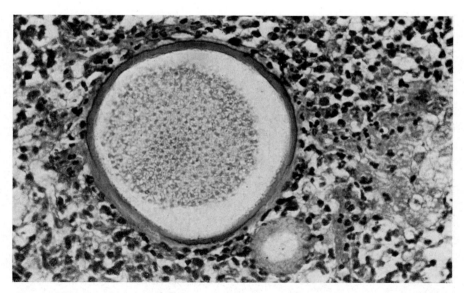

FIG. 9. Rhinosporidiosis. An immature sporangium containing small naked nuclei embedded in cytoplasm. H. & E. stain. ×400. (Reproduced by courtesy of Drs. U. C. G. Engzell and A. W. Jones.)

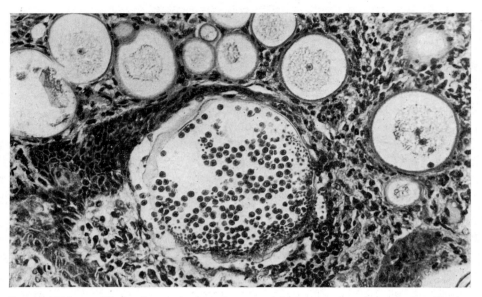

FIG. 10. Rhinosporidiosis. A mature sporangium containing spores of varying maturity. The immature spores are situated adjacent to the chitinous shell. Numerous trophocytes are seen. H. & E. stain. ×400. (Reproduced by courtesy of Drs. U. C. G. Engzell and A. W. Jones.)

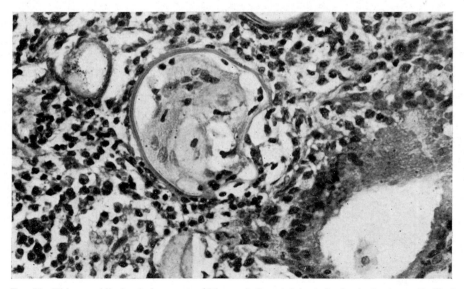

FIG. 11. Rhinosporidiosis. A degenerate chitinous shell containing a foreign body giant cell. H. & E. stain. ×400. (Reproduced by courtesy of Drs. U. C. G. Engzell and A. W. Jones.)

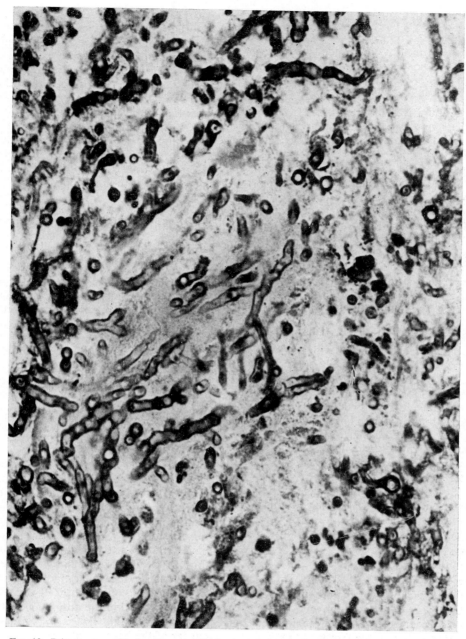

FIG. 12. Primary aspergillosis of larynx. The hyphae are broad and exhibit dichotomous branching and transverse septation. These features are characteristic of aspergilli. H. & E. stain. ×160 (Reproduced by courtesy of Dr. A. Ferlito.)

Sporotrichosis

This chronic subcutaneous lymphatic disorder is due to *Sporothrix schenckii**. The lesions may be granulomatous or they may suppurate, ulcerate and drain.

Sporotrichosis was frequently diagnosed in France at the beginning of this century and then became common in South African gold mines. This epidemic was eradicated by treating timber used in the mines with fungicides. The condition is of otolaryngological interest since it may involve the face and from there spread to the oropharyngeal mucous membranes.

Verrucous Mycosis (Cercosporamycosis)

A single case of infection by *Cercospora apii* was reported from Indonesia (Lie-Kian-Joe *et al.*, 1957). The condition was characterized by ulcerative lesions of the face. These lesions extended and had a fatal outcome.

* Emmons and his colleagues (1970) point out that this fungus is so unlike the type and related species of *Sporotrichum* that mycologists are now accepting Carmichael's recommendation of this term.

PSEUDOMYCOSES

For the sake of completeness, reference will be made to two conditions which are clinically confounded with the mycoses, i.e. *actinomycosis* and *mycosis fungoides*.

Actinomycosis

This is a chronic suppurative disease caused by an anaerobic organism, *Actinomyces israelii*. It is now agreed that the *Actinomyces* are not fungi but filamentous bacteria. *A. israelii* is normally found as a harmless commensal of the oral cavity and digestive tract. In the pathogenesis of actinomycosis, Holm (1950) attributes a synergistic activity to *associated bacteria*. *Cervicofacial actinomycosis* ("*lumpy jaw*") is the most common clinical type of the disease. It is characterized by induration and localized granulomatous areas which suppurate and drain to the skin surface through sinus tracts. The organism is usually organized into firm yellowish colonies in the pus coming from the sinuses. This is the basis of the so-called "*sulphur granules*". Bone involvement usually precedes the appearance of the sinus tracts. The infection may arise from dental or parodontal disease.

As Tamoney and Sammartino (1967) pointed out, one should always bear actinomycosis in mind when one is dealing with a painless, non-tender, possibly fluctuant, indolent facial lump.

Actinomycosis may also involve the middle-ear cleft (Leek, 1974). Nasal actinomycosis has occurred following the implantation of xenologous processed bone for atrophic rhinitis (Thomas *et al.*, 1974). A headache, initially thought to be psychogenic, was subsequently shown to be due to actinomycosis of the sphenoid sinus (Per Lee *et al.*, 1974).

Since the introduction of penicillin for the treatment of actinomycosis by Herrell in 1944, the prognosis has been appreciably altered. However, this antibiotic must be administered for not less than three months and used in conjunction with surgery to drain abscesses and to extensively excise diseased tissue.

Mycosis Fungoides

"*Mycosis fungoides*" is perhaps the greatest misnomer in the whole of medicine; it is a neoplasm and not a mycosis. It may, however, bear some clinical resemblance to a mycosis. This is attested for by the fact that the first case of coccidioidomycosis to be finally recognized as such at the end of the nineteenth century was initially diagnosed as mycosis fungoides.

Although denied a separate existence by Symmers (1932), this rare condition is accepted as a distinct entity by others, e.g. Block and his colleagues (1963). The condition almost always begins as a chronic benign dermatitis. This non-specific cutaneous eruption may be present for years. Subsequently, skin tumours with the characteristic histopathology of the condition develop. This histopathology is that of a polymorphic intradermal infiltrate containing atypical reticular cells together with the characteristic intra-epidermal Pautrier's abscesses. Concurrently in the development, there is progression from an associated benign lymphadenopathy to a malignant lymphomatous adeno-

pathy. The evolution of the disease may represent a primary failure of host resistance in limiting the disease to the skin or a development of new, more virulent cell types which metastasize readily. Early in the disease, it is distinguishable from other malignant lymphomas solely on the basis of the characteristic cutaneous histopathology. The relationship of this disease to other diseases, such as the so-called "*mid-line granuloma*", is mentioned in Chapter 49.

Mycosis fungoides may present otolaryngologically, beginning as an otitis externa (Strahan and Calcaterra, 1971), or with involvement of the oral mucosa and adjacent respiratory tract (Cohn *et al.*, 1971). Treatment (palliative) is by means of radiotherapy.

MYCOTOXINS

Mycetismus

Tyler (1963) has reviewed *mycetismus* (mushroom poisoning). He recognizes four basic types of mushroom poisons. Clinically, there may be gastro-intestinal, including hepatic, neurological and psychological effects.

Mycotoxicoses

This refers to the group of conditions resulting from the ingestion of foods which have been contaminated by toxin-producing fungi. *Stachybotryotoxicosis*, which occurs in the Ukraine, is due to exposure to hay contaminated with *Stachybotrys alternans*. Affected subjects have pharyngitis, an axillary skin rash and mild leucopenia (Gajdusek, 1957).

Mycogenous Neoplasias

Fungi of the *A. flavus-oryzae* series produce a group of hepato-carcinogens, i.e. the *aflatoxins*, of which aflatoxin B is the most potent. Indeed, it is a thousand times more potent than any known hepatocarcinogen. *A. flavus* contaminates foodstuffs in many parts of the world. Epidemiological studies by Van Rensburg and his colleagues (1974) have shown that the incidence of primary liver cancer is a function of aflatoxin intake. Are there any possible parallels for this in the otolaryngological area? We have already mentioned the observation of the occurrence of *A. flavus* as a commensal in the nose. Clifford (1970) has alluded to this as a possible factor in discussing the aetiology of cancer of the nasal part of pharynx.

The possibility of contamination of food by carcinogenic mycotoxins must be taken seriously when considering the aetiology of cancers other than those of the liver. It may not matter that the affected organ is not along the route of ingestion. Phenomena of selective concentration and/or synergism may account for cancer development at remote anatomical sites. One should therefore consider whether or not the high incidence of cancer of the nasal part of pharynx or of the oesophagus in parts of China is, for example, related to the use of soy sauce (this is prepared by fermenting soya beans by *A. oryzae*). As was pointed out previously, the Chinese deliberately cultivate some fungi, e.g. *Monascus purpurea*, for use not only as a food-colouring agent but also as a food itself. "Yellowed" rice is heavily contaminated with *Penicillium islandicum*. This fungus produces *islanditoxin* which has been shown to be carcinogenic (Uraguchi *et al.*, 1961). Another fungus, *Alternaria padwickii*, is the cause of stackburn disease. This disease affects rice crops in South China, Malaysia, the Philippines and Thailand, but not those in North China, Japan or Korea. This correlates with the geographical incidence of carcinoma of the nasal part of pharynx in that region of the world. Is this coincidental? Moreover, this disease also affects rice in North Africa, where there is also a relatively greater incidence of carcinoma of the nasal part of pharynx.

ALLERGIES

Over a hundred years ago, Blackley recognized that fungi have a role in the causation of allergies. He said that spores of *Pencillium glaucum* and *Chaetomium sps.* caused "bronchial catarrh". However, it was not until Feinberg's (1935) report that fungi were accepted as causes of *asthma*, and of *hay fever*. Other fungi have now been shown to be potently allergenic, especially *Aspergillus fumigatus*.

The proportion of allergies due to fungi appears to be *geographically dependent*. Over half of allergic individuals may react to fungal allergens in Britain, but only 15 per cent in Germany (Fraenkel, 1938). As Maunsell points out, the relatively low concentration of fungal spores at sea, in the Arctic regions, in the deserts and in the high mountainous regions of the world may explain the freedom from attacks in these areas of fungus allergic patients. In Britain, subjects with a *Cladosporium* sensitivity come predominantly from the higher and drier parts of the country. This corresponds with the geographical distribution of this fungus (Maunsell, 1954).

The atmospheric concentration of fungal spores may show *temporal*, as well as spatial, variations. Thus the spores of *Cladosporium sp.*, the commonest fungus in many parts of the world, reach a seasonal peak between July and September. Year to year variations in the fungal spore content of the atmosphere also occur (Adams, 1964).

The incidence of fungal allergies also appears to be inversely related to *age*.

Although there may be specific sensitization to fungal spores, especially in children (Sellers and McKenzie, 1947), it is usual for affected subjects to show multiple allergy to inhaled spores and other allergens, such as pollen and house dust. Although a mite *Dermatophagoides sps.* is considered to provide the principal allergenic factor in house dust, the spores of a number of fungi are also present (Schaffer *et al.*, 1953). Blankets, furniture stuffing, mattresses and pillowcases may be the source of these fungi (Conant *et al.*, 1936). The most common fungus found in damp houses is *Merulius lacrymans* which is the cause of dry rot. A number of allergic subjects react to this (Frankland and Hay, 1951).

Pepys (1969) has described a condition termed *allergic bronchopulmonary aspergillosis*. This is a hypersensitivity lung disease due to colonization of the respiratory tract with *A. fumigatus*. Species of *Aspergillus* are also responsible for *Malt workers* lung. This is an occupational disease due to the inhalation of spores of fungi of this genus (Riddle and Grant, 1967). *Suberosis* is another occupational respiratory fungal allergy. It is an extrinsic allergic alveolitis which affects workers in the cork industry and is due to inhaling the dust of mouldy cork. The source of the antigens in this disorder is *Penicillium frequentans* (Ávila and Villar, 1968; Ávila and Lacey, 1974).

Farmer's lung might be termed a pseudo-fungal respiratory allergy. The aetiological agent is a thermophilic actinomycete, especially *Micropolyspora faeni*. The antigens that are responsible for this allergic disorder are derived from inhaled spores of these organisms which grow in mouldy hay (Pepys *et al.*, 1963). The condition is not an uncommon disorder in some parts of the world. In some parts of Scotland about 9 per cent of farmers are affected (Grant *et al.*, 1972).

The field of fungal allergies has been recently extended by Wilson (1974). He reported a series of 30 subjects with *episodic vertigo* who also gave a history of hypersensitivity to fungal derivatives. This was verified by obtaining positive provocative intracutaneous or challenge feeding tests for hypersensitivity to yeasts. More than a half of the group gave a history of hypersensitivity to penicillin. Wilson suggested an antigenic cross-reactivity between penicillin, yeast and other fungi.

It is frequently impossible for subjects who are allergic to fungi to avoid the environments which contain the responsible fungi, so that hyposensitization remains the principle method of treatment. In homes where fungal allergens are a problem, *paraformaldehyde* (trioxymethylene) has been recommended as a fungicide (Criep *et al.*, 1958).

CONCLUSIONS

It is clear that fungi play an important role in disorders which concern, or should concern, the otolaryngologist. Moreover, for the various reasons given, this role is an expanding one, with suggestions that it may be much greater than we had hitherto assumed.

REFERENCES

Aal, A. O. A. and Milošev, B. (1969), *Sudan med. J.*, **7**, 5.
Abramson, E., Wilson, D. and Arky, R. C. (1967), *Ann. intern. Med.*, **66**, 735.
Adams, K. F. (1964), *Acta Allerg.*, **19**, 11.
Adams, N. F. (1933), *Arch. Surg.*, **26**, 999.
Ajello, L. (1960), *Ann. N.Y. Acad. Sci.*, **89**, 30.
Ávila, R. and Lacey, J. (1974), *Clin. Allergy*, **4**, 109.
Ávila, R. and Villar, T. G. (1968), *Lancet*, **1**, 620.
Bailey, J. W., Huppert, M. and Chitjian, P. (1965), *Bact. Proc.*, M19.
Baker, R. D. (1960), in *Pathology*, Vol. I (W. A. D. Anderson, Ed.). St. Louis: Mosby.
Battock, D. J., Grausz, H., Bobrovsky, M. and Littman, M. L. (1968), *Ann. intern. Med.*, **68**, 122.
Baum, G. L. and Artis, D. (1961), *Amer. J. med. Sci.*, **241**, 613.
Benbrook, E. A., Bryant, J. B. and Saunders, L. Z. (1948), *J. Amer. vet. med. Ass.*, **112**, 475.
Bennett, M. (1964), *Lasyngoscope*, **74**, 498.
Bindschadler, D. D. and Bennett, J. E. (1969), *Infect. Dis.*, **120**, 427.
Block, J. B., Edgcomb, J., Eisen, A. and van Scott, E. J. (1963), *Amer. J. Med.*, **34**, 228.
Bras, G., Gordon, C. C., Emmons, C. W., Prendegast, K. M. and Sugar, M. (1965), *Amer. J. trop. Med. Hyg.*, **14**, 141.

Briggs, D. R., Barney, P. L. and Bahu, R. M. (1974), *Arch. Otolaryng.*, **100**, 390.

Btesh, S. (1973), "Communicable Diseases," Provisional International Nomenclature. Geneva: C.I.O.M.S., W.H.O.

Burkitt, D. P., Wilson, A. M. M. and Jelliffe, D. B. (1964), *Brit. med. J.*, **1**, 1669.

Burns, R. P. (1959), *Trans. Pacif. Cst. oto-ophthal. Soc.*, **40**, 83.

Burrow, G. N., Salmon, R. B. and Nolan, J. P. (1963), *J. Amer. med. Ass.*, **183**, 370.

Chick, E. (1962), *Amer. Rev. Resp. Dis.*, **85**, 702.

Chick, E. W., Evans, J. and Baker, R. D. (1958), *Antibiotics and Chemother.*, **8**, 506.

Chin, T. D. Y., Tosh, F. E. and Weeks, R. J. (1970), *Mycopathologia (Amst.)*, **41**, 35.

Clark, Betty M. (1968), 'The Epidemiology of Phycomycosis,' in *Systemic Mycoses* (G. E. W. Wolstenholme and Ruth Porter, Eds.). Ciba Foundation Symposium. London: Churchill.

Clayton, Y. M. and Connor, B. S. (1973), *Brit. J. Derm.*, **89**, 297.

Clifford, P. (1970), *Int. J. Cancer*, **5**, 287.

Cohn, A. M., Park, J. K. and Rappaport, H. (1971), *Arch. Otolaryng.*, **93**, 330.

Conant, N. F., Wagner, H. C. and Rackemann, F. M. (1936), *J. Allergy*, **7**, 234.

Criep, L. H., Teufel, R. A. and Miller, C. S. (1958), *J. Allergy*, **29**, 258.

Crompton, G. K. and Milne, L. J. R. (1974), *Brit. J. Dis. Chest*, **67**, 301.

Denton, J. F., McDonough, E. S., Ajello, L. and Ausherman, R. J. (1961), *Science*, **133**, 1126.

Drouhet, E. (1968), *Systemic Mycoses* (G. E. W. Wolstenholme and Ruth Porter, Eds.). Ciba Foundation Symposium. London: Churchill.

Emmons, C. W. (1942), *Publ. Hlth Rep. (Wash.)*, **57**, 109.

Emmons, C. W. (1955), *Amer. J. Hyg.*, **62**, 227.

Emmons, C. W., Klite, P. D., Baer, G. M. and Hill, W. B. (1966), *Amer. J. Epidemiol.*, **84**, 103.

Emmons, C. W., Binford, C. H. and Utz, J. P. (1970), *Medical Mycology*. Philadelphia: Lea and Febiger.

English, M. P. (1957), *J. Laryng.*, **71**, 207.

Engzell, U. and Jones, A. W. (1973), *J. Laryng.*, **87**, 1217.

Feinberg, S. W. (1935), *Wis. med. J.*, **34**, 254.

Ferlito, A. (1974), *J. Laryng.*, **88**, 1257.

Fraenkel, E. M. (1938), *Brit. med. J.*, **2**, 68.

Frankland, A. W. and Hay, M. J. (1951), *Acta allerg.*, **4**, 186.

Furtado, T. A., Wilson, J. W. and Plunkett, O. A. (1954), *Arch. Derm.*, **70**, 166.

Gajdusek, D. C. (1953), "Acute Infectious Hemorrhagic Fevers and Mycotoxicosis in the Union of Soviet Socialist Republics," in *Med. Sci. Publ. No. 2*. Washington D.C.: Army Med. Ser. Grad. School.

Gentles, J. C. (1958), *Nature*, **182**, 476.

Gentles, J. C., Barnes, M. J. and Fantes, K. H. (1959), *Nature*, **183**, 256.

Gonçalves, A. P. (1962), *Bol. Acad. nac. Med.*, **134**, 81.

Grant, I. W. B., Blyth, W. and Wardrop, V. F. (1972), *Brit. med. J.*, **1**, 530.

Gregson, A. E. W. and La Touche, C. J. (1961), *J. Laryng.*, **75**, 45.

Gupta, R. M. and Gupta, O. P. (1970), *Laryngoscope*, **80**, 472.

Hadida, E. and Schousboe, A. (1959), *Algérie méd.*, **63**, 303.

Haley, L. D. (1950), *Arch. Otolaryng.*, **52**, 202.

Herrell, W. E. (1944), *J. Amer. med. Assoc.*, **124**, 622.

Hildick-Smith, G. (1963), *Arch. Derm.*, **87**, 8.

Hildick-Smith, G., Blank, H. and Sarkany, I. (1964), *Fungus Diseases and their Treatment*. London: Churchill.

Hoffarth, G. A., Joseph, D. L. and Shumrick, D. A. (1973), *Arch. Otolaryng.*, **97**, 475.

Holm, P. (1950), *Acta Path.*, **27**, 736.

Karunaratne, W. A. E. (1964), *Rhinosporidiosis in Man*. London: Athlone Press.

Kaufman, L. and Blumer, L. (1968), *Appl. Microbiol.*, **16**, 1907.

Klite, P. D. and Diercks, F. H. (1965), *Amer. J. trop. Med. Hyg.*, **14**, 433.

Lea, W. A., Schusten, D. S. and Hanell, E. R. (1958), *J. invest. Derm.*, **31**, 137.

Leek, J. H. (1974), *Laryngoscope*, **84**, 290.

Lie-Kian-Joe, Eng, N-I. T., Kertopati, S. and Emmons, C. W. (1957), *Arch. Derm.*, **75**, 864.

Lie-Kian-Joe, Njo-Injo, T. E., Pohan, A., Van der Muelen, H. and Emmons, C. W. (1956), *Arch. Derm.*, **74**, 378.

Louria, D. B. and Brayton, R. G. (1964), *Nature*, **201**, 309.

McBurney, R. and Gulledge, M. A. (1955), *Ann. Otol.*, **64**, 1009.

McKelvie, M. and McKelvie, P. (1966), *Brit. J. Derm.*, **78**, 227.

Martin, G. W. (1955), *Mycologia*, **47**, 779.

Martinson, F. D. (1963), *J. Laryng.*, **77**, 691.

Martinson, F. D. and Clark, Betty M. (1967), *Amer. J. trop. Med. Hyg.*, **16**, 40.

Maunsell, Kate (1954), *J. Laryng.*, **68**, 765.

Milošev, B., Mahgoub, El S., Aal, A. O. A. and El Hassan, M. A. (1969), *Brit. J. Surg.*, **56**, 132.

Miloshev, B., Davidson, C. M., Gentles, J. C. and Sandison, A. T. (1966), *Lancet*, **i**, 746.

Moore, M. and Jorstad, L. H. (1943), *Ann. Otol.*, **52**, 779.

Mumma, C. S. (1953), *Arch. Otolaryng.*, **58**, 306.

Norris, J. C. and Armstrong, W. B. (1954), *Arch. Otolaryng.*, **60**, 720.

Oxford, A. E., Raistrick, K. H. and Simonart, P. (1939), *Biochem. J.*, **33**, 240.

Pepys, J. (1969), *Hypersensitivity Diseases of the Lung due to Fungi and Organic Dusts*. Basel: Karger.

Pepys, J., Jenkins, P. A., Feinstein, G. N., Lacey, M. E., Gregory, P. H. and Skinner, F. A. (1963), *Lancet*, **ii**, 607.

Per-Lee, J. H., Clairmont, A. A., Hofman, J. C., McKinney, A. S. and Schwarzmann, S. W. (1974), *Laryngoscope*, **84**, 1149.

Polemann, G. (1973), *Clinical Excerpts*, **35**, 57.

Pyman, C. (1959), *Med. J. Aust.*, **2**, 534.

Rao, P. B. (1969), *J. Laryng.*, **83**, 377.

Riddle, H. F. V. and Grant, I. W. B. (1967), *Thorax*, **22**, 478.

Robbins, E. S. (1954), *J. Amer. vet. med. Ass.*, **125**, 391.

Rose, F. C., Grant, H. C. and Jeanes, A. L. (1958), *Brain*, **81**, 542.

Roth, F. J., Jr., Boyd, C. C., Sagami, S. and Blank, H. (1959), *J. invest. Derm.*, **32**, 549.

Sandison, A. T., Gentles, J. C., Davidson, C. M. and Branco, M. (1967), *Sabouraudia*, **6**, 57.

Satyanarayana, C. (1960), *Acta oto-laryng. (Stockh.)*, **51**, 348.

Schaffer, N., Seidmon, E. E. and Bruskin, S. (1953), *J. Allergy*, **24**, 348.

Schrek, R. (1963), *J. Lab. clin. Med.*, **61**, 34.

Sellers, E. D. and McKenzie, Evelyn (1947), *Ann. Allergy*, **5**, 455.

Senturia, B. H. (1973), *Ann. Otol.*, suppl. 8.

Shaheen, O. H. (1965), *J. Laryng.*, **79**, 442.

Sharp, W. P., John, M. B. and Robison, J. M. (1946), *Tex. St. J. Med.*, **42**, 380.

Smith, J. G., Jr., Humbert, W. C. and Olansky, S. (1958), *Publ. Hlth Rep.*, **73**, 610.

Smyth, G. D. L. (1961), *J. Laryng.*, **75**, 703.

Strahan, R. W. and Calcaterra, T. C. (1971), *Laryngoscope*, **81**, 1917.

Symmers, D. (1932), *Arch. Derm.*, **25**, 1.

Symmers, D. (1968), *Systemic Mycoses* (G. E. W. Wolstenholme and Ruth Porter, Eds.), Ciba Foundation Symposium. London: Churchill.

Tamoney, H. J., Jr. and Sammartino, C. A. (1967), *J. Amer. med. Ass.*, **199**, 1002.

Taschdjian, C. L. and Kozinn, P. J. (1957), *J. Pediat.*, **50**, 425.

Tedeschi, L. G. and Cheren, R. V. (1968), *Arch. Otolaryng.*, **87**, 82.

Thomas, G. G., Toohill, R. J. and Lehman, R. H. (1974), *Arch. Otolaryng.*, **100**, 377.

Tyler, V. E. (1963), *Progr. Chem. Toxicol.*, **1**, 339.

Uraguchi, K., Sakai, F., Tsukioka, M., Noguchi, Y., Tatsuno, T., Saito, M., Enomoto, M., Ishiko, T., Shikaka, T. and Miyake, M. (1961), *J. exp. Med.*, **31**, 435.

Van Rensburg, S. J., Van der Watt, J. J., Purchase, I. F. H., Coutinho, L. P. and Markham, R. (1974), *S. Afr. med. J.*, **48**, 2508a.

Veress, B., Malik, O. A., El Tayeb, A. A., El Daoud, S., Mahgoub, E. S. and El Hassan, A. M. (1973), *Amer. J. trop. Med. Hyg.*, **22**, 765.

Whittaker, R. H. (1969), *Science*, **163**, 150.

Wiersema, J. P. and Niemel, P. L. A. (1965), *Trop. Geog. Med.*, **17**, 89

Williams, A. O., Lichtenberg, F. von, Smith, J. H. and Martinson, F. D. (1969), *Arch. Path.*, **87**, 459.

Williams, D. I., Martin, R. H. and Sarkany, I. (1958), *Lancet*, ii, 1212.
Wilson, W. H. (1974), *Laryngoscope*, **84**, 1585.
Withers, B. T., Pappas, J. J. and Erickson, Ethel E. (1963), *Arch. Otolaryng.*, **77**, 25.
Woo, Z. and Reimann, H. A. (1957), *J. Amer. med. Ass.*, **164**, 1092.

Yonkers, A. J. (1973), *Ann. Otol.*, **82**, 812.
Zimmerman, L. E. and Rappaport, H. (1954), *Amer. J. clin. Path.*, **24**, 1050.
Zinneman, H. H., Hall, W. H. and Wallace, F. G. (1961), *Amer. J. Med.*, **31**, 654.

48. PARASITOLOGY: OTOLARYNGOLOGICAL ASPECTS

F. E. G. COX

INTRODUCTION

No animal parasite is specific to the human ear, nose or throat. Those that occur in these sites are either there by accident or are likely to be found elsewhere in or on the body. To a parasite, the ear is not a delicate and complex organ, it is a source of food and somewhere to live. The skin and blood vessels provide nourishment for parasites while the external and middle ears provide suitable cavities in which parasites can survive. Cartilage, bone and nerves are seldom parasitized but can be seriously damaged by multiplying or migrating parasites and this kind of damage is usually irreversible. Otolaryngological disease caused directly by parasites therefore ranges from temporary hearing impairment, due to the blockage of the external acoustic meatus or the auditory tube by a growing parasite, to the complete destruction of the internal ear by a parasite that has migrated outwards from the nasal part of pharynx. In addition, the auricle of the ear may be slightly or seriously affected by insect bites or by parasites living in the skin. Indirect effects of parasites result from damage to the nerves supplying the ear and the actual effects vary according to the nerve affected and the degree of damage caused. The symptoms of parasitic diseases are seldom sufficient to indicate the presence of specific parasites and resemble the symptoms due to tumours and accidental lesions in particular nerves and parts of the brain. Diagnosis is usually best made by a parasitologist. Otolaryngological diseases due to parasites are mostly, but not wholly, tropical.

The parasites that cause otolaryngological disease belong to four separate phyla. These are the Protozoa, Aschelminthes, Platyhelminthes and Arthropoda. The Aschelminthes include the class Nematoda. The actual parasites which have been associated with diseases of the ear, together with their classification, are listed in Table 1. The classification of parasites is not at all satisfactory at the present time and several alternative, and equally good, classifications exist. The protozoa are single celled organisms which multiply by repeated divisions inside their vertebrate host. The other parasites are multicellular. The nematodes are the roundworms, platyhelminths include the flukes and tapeworms, and arthropods include insects and mites. The multicellular parasites do not usually multiply within their vertebrate hosts. Whereas protozoa cause damage while they are multiplying, multi-cellular animals cause damage while they are growing or migrating around their hosts.

Excellent general accounts of parasitic infections are given by Faust and his associates (1968, 1970) and by

TABLE 1

AN OUTLINE CLASSIFICATION TO GENUS OF THE ANIMAL PARASITES ASSOCIATED WITH OTOLARYNGOLOGICAL DISORDERS

Phylum PROTOZOA	
Class Zoomastigophora	*Leishmania, Trypanosoma*
Class Telosporea	*Toxoplasma*
Class Rhizopodea	*Entamoeba, Naegleria*
Phylum ASCHELMINTHES	
Class Nematoda	
Superfamily Ascaroidea	*Ascaris, Toxocara*
Superfamily Strongyloidea	*Ancylostoma, Uncinaria, Bunostomum, Angiostrongylus*
Superfamily Spiruroidea	*Gnathostoma, Gongylonema*
Superfamily Filaroidea	*Onchocerca*
Phylum PLATY-HELMINTHES	
Class Cestoda	*Taenia, Echinococcus*
Class Digenea	*Poikilorchis, Paragonimus*
Phylum ARTHROPODA	
Class Insecta	*Chrysomyia, Callitroga, Cordylobia, Wohlfahrtia, Sarcophaga, Phaenica, Phormia, Calliphora, Musca, Fannia, Oestrus, Dermatobia, Cutebria, Gastrophilus*
Class Arachnida	*Sarcoptes*
Class Pentastomida	*Linguatula*

Marcial-Rojas (1971). The neurological manifestations of parasitic infections are described in a variety of papers edited by van Bogaert, Käfer and Poche (1963) and by Spillane (1973).

PROTOZOA

Six species, or subspecies, of protozoa are associated with serious diseases of the ear and all cause forms of cutaneous leishmaniasis. Only one almost invariably occurs on the ear and this is *Leishmania mexicana mexicana* which causes the condition known as chiclero's ear or bay sore. The parasites multiply in the gut of a sandfly and are injected into the skin when the insect feeds. They multiply at the site of the bite which is usually on the auricle of the ear, but is sometimes elsewhere on the head, and a small cutaneous nodule forms. In about half the cases the infection is mild and the lesion heals spontaneously. In other cases, however, the nodule grows and may ulcerate. The growing ulcer eventually destroys the outline of the helix (the characteristic sign of chiclero's ear) and the infection persists in a chronic state until spontaneous recovery occurs, possibly several years later. By this time the auricle is permanently damaged.

Chiclero's ear is a disease of Central America. It occurs in the Yucatan area of Mexico, Guatemala, Honduras and probably extends into adjacent areas. It is a disease of rain forests and is contracted by chicleros, or chicle collectors, when they enter the forests.

The second form of New World leishmaniasis is mucocutaneous leishmaniasis or espundia. It is caused by *Leishmania braziliensis braziliensis* and is the most destructive form of cutaneous leishmaniasis. The initial lesion forms at the site of the sandfly bite but develops into a large ulcer which may heal spontaneously or may become an open weeping sore. Secondary infections are often initiated from the primary one and these are frequently in the oronasal and ear regions, and sometimes involve the larynx. This disease is also one of forests. Its geographical distribution, however, is further south than that of chiclero's ulcer and it occurs in Colombia, Venezuela, Brazil, Peru, Ecuador, Bolivia and Paraguay. Two other subspecies of *Leishmania braziliensis* may also cause damage to the ears. *L. braziliensis guyanensis* and *L. braziliensis panamensis* cause crater-like ulcers all over the body. Nasopharyngeal and otolaryngological involvement are rare and result directly from sandfly bites in these regions.

In the Old World, cutaneous leishmaniasis caused by *Leishmania tropica* normally results in the formation of a single self-healing lesion. Occasionally, and usually in immunological deprived cases, the initial lesion does not heal but spreads to produce large fleshy swellings. This condition is known as leishmaniasis cutanea diffusa. In Ethiopia this kind of leishmaniasis is relatively common. It is characterized by non-ulcerating nodules which spread over the extremities, including the ears, and the general appearance is that of lepromatous leprosy. Bray and his associates (1973) have named the causative organism of this condition in Ethiopia *Leishmania aethiopica*.

The diagnosis of leishmaniasis is based on the recognition of the clinical symptoms, the isolation of parasites from the lesion and immunodiagnostic techniques. The incidence of leishmaniasis is well known so clinical diagnosis is relatively simple. Most lesions heal spontaneously and life-long immunity to re-infection usually follows. The chemotherapy of leishmaniasis varies according to local strains and no single drug is effective everywhere. The diagnosis and cure of leishmaniasis, therefore, should be based on local knowledge of the disease. An excellent collection of papers on leishmaniasis has been published by the World Health Organization (1971).

Protozoa other than the leishmanias are only rarely encountered in otolaryngological disease. The trypanosomes that cause sleeping sickness in Africa, *Trypanosoma gambiense* and *T. rhodesiense*, and Chagas' disease in America may be seen in blood films taken from the ear, in sectioned material and occasionally in discharges. They are widely distributed in the body, particularly the African species, and cause no specific disease in the ear. The same is true of the malaria parasites which also occur in the blood. African sleeping sickness and malignant tertian malaria often cause cerebral damage and nerves may be destroyed during Chagas' disease. Meningoencephalitis sometimes occurs in the acute stage of Chagas' disease and this and other neurological conditions are described by Kafer and his associates (1963) and by Romana (1963). A general account of this disease is given by Koberle (1968). Toxoplasmosis, caused by *Toxoplasma gondii*, a natural parasite of cats, also causes damage to the central and peripheral nervous systems and this may, in time, affect the hearing. In all these situations the advanced state of the disease makes diagnosis and treatment necessary long before the ear becomes involved.

Entamoeba histolytica, the causative organisms of amoebic dysentery, has been known to affect the ear. The amoebae live in the gut but may invade the gut wall. From there they enter the bloodstream and are carried to the liver and occasionally elsewhere, setting up secondary sites of multiplication. Cutaneous involvement is rare but the lesion may give rise to an ulcer anywhere on the skin including the ear. By the time the ulcer has burst the patient is usually on the way to recovery. For practical purposes, cutaneous amoebiasis is only likely to occur in the tropics or in those recently returned from the tropics. The immunodiagnosis of amoebiasis is quick and reliable and a variety of good, but not excellent, drugs are available. A summary of our knowledge of amoebiasis is given by the World Health Organization (1969).

A recently discovered form of amoebiasis is due to accidental infection with a free-living soil amoeba *Naegleria fowleri*. Over 70 fatal cases are now known. In all cases, the amoebae were inhaled and entered the brain through the nose, rapidly causing acute meningoencephalitis. The progress of the disease is so rapid that otolaryngological investigations are unlikely to be called for but this condition must be likely to affect the ear. An account of the disease is given by Carter (1972).

NEMATODES

Most nematodes have the same basic form and the same basic life-cycle consisting of an egg, four immature larval stages and a sexually mature male or female adult. Many nematodes live in the lumen of the gut and some live in other tissues. The actual details of the life-cycle are many and varied. Man is a regular host for over ten species of nematodes and the occasional or accidental host of many more. Infections may begin with the ingestion of an egg, the ingestion of a larval form, usually in another animal, the active boring of a larva through the skin or the injection of a larva through the bite of an insect. Once inside the body, the young nematode may migrate around the organs before reaching its final site. It is this migration that causes most damage. In abnormal hosts the nematodes never reach the correct final site and continue to migrate all over the body. Such migrations cause considerable damage and worms that behave in this way are those most likely to affect the ear.

Ascaris lumbricoides is the most common nematode to infest man. The adults, which measure up to 35 cm, live in the small intestine and eggs pass out with the faeces of the host. When the egg is ingested a larval stage emerges and immediately burrows through the gut wall until it reaches a blood vessel. It is carried in the blood to the liver and lungs from which it passes to the bronchi and trachea and is then swallowed and grows to maturity in the small intestine. Sometimes the worm abandons the normal habitat in the small intestine and goes to the stomach or large intestine. Occasionally, adult worms pass from the stomach to the oesophagus, larynx and trachea. There are several records of worms leaving the trachea, entering the auditory tube and either causing suppuration of the middle ear or perforating the ear drum and emerging through the external acoustic meatus. Worms also migrate to the trachea after treatment with vermifuges or during anaesthesia. The large worms passing through the ear usually damage it beyond repair. Worms lodged in the middle ear have to be removed surgically. Cases of *Ascaris* in the middle ear are relatively uncommon and the best documented accounts are those by Kurma, Nakagawa and Suzuki (1961), who record a number of cases in Japan, and by Shah and Desai (1969) who describe a case in India. There is no easy method of diagnosis and suspicion of aural ascariasis must be based on the parasitological case history. In most cases diagnosis must be retrospective.

The ascarid nematodes of cats and dogs, *Toxocara cati* and *Toxocara canis*, occasionally cause serious diseases in children. The larvae emerge from swallowed eggs, burrow through the gut wall and are carried in the blood to the liver and lungs. If they reach the left side of the heart they may be distributed all over the body including the nervous system. The presence of these larvae in the brain and in the nerves of the eye or ear may cause partial blindness or deafness. Diagnosis is almost impossible but eosinophilia is a common sign of this condition.

The condition of harbouring aberrant migratory larval nematodes in the viscera or other deep tissues is called visceral larval migrans. Cutaneous larval migrans is caused by the larvae of quite different nematodes, cat and dog hookworms, burrowing under the skin. Hookworm infection ensues when the larvae penetrate the skin of the host. In the correct host the larvae are carried to the lungs in the blood or lymph, pass into the mouth, are swallowed and complete their development in the intestine. In the wrong host, the larvae migrate under the skin causing a condition known as creeping eruption. The paths of the larvae are marked by visible tracks in which the advancing end is red, swollen and itchy. *Ancylostoma braziliense*, a hookworm of dogs, cats and other carnivores is the most important species, but *A. caninum* and *Uncinaria steno-cephala* of carnivores and *Bunostomum phlebotomum* of

cattle also cause cutaneous larval migrans. Cutaneous larval migrans can occur anywhere in the skin and is most common on the limbs but the ears can be infected. The progressive tunnelling (20–50 mm each day) and intense itching are characteristic. Cutaneous larval migrans might be encountered during the examination of the external ear but apart from the cutaneous lesions, these larvae cause no otolaryngological disorder.

Angiostrongylosis is a condition caused by a nematode parasite of rats, *Angiostrongylus cantonensis*. The eggs of the nematode are passed out in the faeces of the rat and the larvae develop in a snail. The snail may be eaten by a rat or by another animal which is later eaten by a rat. In the rat, the worm passes from the stomach to the blood and eventually to the brain. Man becomes infected by eating snails or animals such as crabs, which have themselves fed on infected snails. The larvae emerge, penetrate to the bloodstream and are carried all over the body. The parasites induce granulomatous lesions in various parts of the body, including the spinal cord and brain, and cause parasitic eosinophilic meningoencephalitis, facial paralysis and vertigo. The symptoms are those of intracranial disease and eosinophilia of the spinal fluid without intense peripheral eosinophilia (which occurs in gnathostomiasis). Angiostrongylosis is essentially Pacific in distribution but the distribution of the parasite is much wider than this and includes Africa. An excellent general account of the disease and biology of the parasite is given by Alicata (1965) and specific cases are quoted by the South Pacific Commission (1967).

A number of spirurid nematodes infect man as an accidental host and the most important of these is *Gnathostoma spinigerum*. The condition of harbouring this worm is called gnathostomiasis. *Gnathostoma spinigerum* is normally a parasite in the stomach of carnivores including cats and dogs. The life cycle involves two other hosts, a copepod crustacean and a fish, frog or snake. The carnivore becomes infected when it eats one of the latter hosts. The larvae emerge and migrate through the liver and skeletal and connective tissues before returning to the stomach. Man becomes infected after eating uncooked, infected fish. The migrating larvae have been recovered from subcutaneous tissues, which is the most commonly infected site, and practically every other site including the mastoid and adnexa. In the central nervous system and brain, the larvae causes haemorrhagic tracts and the disease may result in eosinophilic myelo-encephalitis. In the soft tissues related to the mastoid, the worms may produce swellings and the discharge of blood from the ear. Human gnathostomiasis occurs all over South-East Asia, China, Japan, India, Australia, and has been recorded from Israel. It is so prevalent in Thailand that it is regarded as being endemic there. Over 500 cases were recorded in one hospital in Thailand over a 5-year period (Chitanondh, 1963). Cases of aural gnatho-stomiasis are rare but a fully documented account is given by Prasansuk and Hinchcliffe (1975). In this case, after a variety of symptoms including difficulty in hearing, earache, tinnitus and facial palsy, a 5 mm worm emerged through the tympanic membrane following which the hearing returned to normal. Another case resembling mastoiditis was recorded by Datta and Maplestone (1930). The subject of human gnathostomiasis has been reviewed by Chitanondh (1963) and accounts of eosinophilic myelenocephalitis due to this worm are given by Punyagupta and his associates (1968) and by Bunnag and his associates (1970).

Other spirurids that may infect man include *Gongylonema pulchrum* which normally occurs in the upper respiratory tract of ruminants. The larvae occur in cockroaches and beetles and man becomes infected by accidentally eating these insects or by drinking water contaminated with their remains. The worm burrows into the stomach and may reach a variety of sites including the oesophagus, mouth, tongue, palate and tonsils. The parasite is rare in man but about 30 cases have been recorded in various parts of the world.

The final group of nematodes to be considered are the filarial worms. Infection begins when the larvae are injected into the skin through the bite of an insect. The adults live in various tissues and produce larvae which enter the bloodstream to be taken up by insects once again.

Onchocerciasis is caused by *Onchocerca volvulus*. The larvae are injected into the skin by blackflies (Simuliidae) and a nodule develops at the site of the bite. Within the nodule the adults grow and eventually produce larvae which escape to the surrounding tissues. The nodules range from 1–80 mm in diameter and may cover much of the skin of an infected person. Onchocerciasis occurs in Central America and Equatorial Africa. In Africa, nodules on the head are relatively rare. In America, 92–98 per cent of the nodules are found on the head, mainly in the occipito-parietal region and involving the external acoustic meatus. The escaping larvae may also cause inflammatory reactions characterized by a rash and scaly appearance. Dermal papillae may appear after the death of larvae in the skin. Like the nodules, the rash and papillae are frequently found in the external acoustic meatus in the American form of the disease.

During the acute stage of the disease, the ears appear larger than usual and oedematous. There is occasional neuralgia involving the trigeminal nerve, tinnitus and intermittent or persistent impairment of hearing. During the chronic stage of the disease the skin is pigmented and the ears are deformed and become about twice as thick as normal.

The most serious consequence of onchocerciasis is the invasion of the cornea, conjunctiva and retina of the eye with occasional involvement of the optic nerve over a period of years. Diagnosis is usually based on the isolation of the larvae from skin scrapings. Nodules are best treated by surgery which removes the primary cause of the infection. Chemotherapy is effective but drugs have to be administered carefully in order to reduce the chances of allergic reactions following the release of antigen into the circulation. A full account of onchocerciasis is given by Nelson (1970).

PLATYHELMINTHES

Platyhelminthes are the flatworms. The most important parasitic forms are the Cestoda or tapeworms and the Digenea or flukes. Most tapeworms and flukes are intestinal parasites but a few may affect the ear.

Adult tapeworms in the intestines of their hosts usually cause little harm but the larval or developmental stages in intermediate hosts can cause serious diseases. Man may act as intermediate host to three important tapeworms, *Taenia solium* of pigs, *T. saginata* of cattle, and *Echinococcus granulosus* of carnivores. *Taenia solium* infects man as an adult worm and man becomes infected by eating uncooked pork. If a human ingests the eggs of the tapeworm he may become an intermediate host. The larvae hatch from the eggs, penetrate the gut wall and are carried by the blood to various sites including the central nervous system and brain. There they develop into bladder filled cysts with the head of the tapeworm on the inside. These cysts are called cystercerci. Cerebral cysticercosis frequently manifests itself as seizures but among other symptoms are violent headaches, vertigo and tinnitus. There are no eosinophils in the cerebrospinal fluid. Cysticercosis can usually be diagnosed by the recognition of calcified cysts in X-ray photographs. Accounts of neurocysticercosis are given by Proctor (1963) and by Canelas (1963). The beef tapeworm *Taenia saginata* does not cause cysticercosis in man (Pawlowski and Schultz, 1972).

Echinococcus granulosus is a small tapeworm of dogs and other carnivores. The intermediate host is usually a ruminant in which a large cyst containing many scolices develops in a variety of tissues. Man is occasionally infected by ingesting eggs passed out in the faeces of dogs. The young larva passes through the gut wall and is carried around the body in the blood. Eventually it comes to rest and grows into massive fluid filled cysts which may reach 15–20cm in diameter and may contain 2 1 of fluid and over 2 000 000 scolices. The cyst is called a hydatid and may be lodged in the brain causing serious neurological symptoms. Otological symptoms may occur and these depend on the position of the cyst. Diagnosis can be made using immunological techniques and treatment is by surgery and chemotherapy. Echinococcosis in the nervous system is discussed by Iniguez and Gurri (1963).

The parasitic flukes have complex life-cycles involving a mollusc and a vertebrate host. A number are parasitic in man but do not cause otolaryngological disease. One species however, *Poikilorchis congolensis*, has been found in subcutaneous abscesses behind the auricles of inhabitants of Zaire (Fain and Vandepitte, 1957). This parasite has eggs resembling those of *Paragonimus westermani*, the lung fluke of man. *Paragonimus westermani* itself, may cause neurological disorders. The adult worms are able to develop in a variety of sites outside the lungs. In 45 per cent of extrapulmonary cases there is a cerebral or spinal involvement resulting in epileptic seizures, paralysis and meningitis. Eosinophilic meningitis resembles that resulting from angiostrongylosis but occurs in Japan and other places where *Angiostrongylus cantonensis* is absent. The diagnosis of paragonimiasis is based on the recovery of eggs of the worm from the sputum. The parasite and the diseases it causes are described fully by Yokogawa (1965).

ARTHROPODS

The most important arthropod parasites of the ear are the dipterous insects belonging to two groups, the blowflies and the the warble flies. The eggs of these insects hatch to produce white elongate legless larvae or maggots which live in decaying or living flesh. Human ears are sometimes infected with these maggots. They live in the subcutaneous tissue for about two weeks before emerging to pupate on the ground. The condition of harbouring the larval stages of these flies is known as myiasis. General accounts of myiasis are given by van der Hoeden (1964) and Zumpt (1965).

Many flies, including such common flies as houseflies and bluebottles, are known to lay their eggs in unclean wounds. The species described below are those known to infect the ear although they are also found elsewhere. The larvae can be identified from the appearance of their spiracular plates diagrams of which are given in James (1947) and most entomology text books.

Chrysomyia bezziana, the Old World screw worm fly occurs in Africa, Southern Asia and the Far East. The female fly lays her eggs near wounds and bruises on sheep, man and other animals. The larvae burrow into unbroken skin and grow to over one centimetre in length causing swellings of considerable size. The female fly also lays eggs in body orifices including the ear which may be blocked by the developing larvae. Cases of infection of the pierced lobule of the auricle in women have been recorded.

Callitroga hominivorax is the American screw worm fly. The female sticks her eggs on to damaged or undamaged skin close to wounds on cattle, pigs, man and other animals. The larvae tunnel deeply into the tissues particularly the nasal and frontal sinuses and ears. The lesions are painful and may become secondarily infected and infections may terminate fatally.

Cordylobia anthrophaga is the African tumbu fly. The eggs are laid in bedding and the larvae burrow into the skin causing shallow burrows and swelling in man and dogs.

Wohlfahrtia magnifica, the Old World flesh fly, occurs in the Mediterranean region, Middle East and the U.S.S.R. Eggs are laid on the skin or in body orifices, usually the ear, of man and sheep. The larvae burrow into tender skin and babies are particularly prone to infection. Other species of *Wohlfahrtia* occur in other parts of the world.

Sarcophaga spp. are cosmopolitan and lay their eggs in wounds and body orifices of man and other animals.

Other blowflies that may cause aural myiasis include *Phaenica sericata*, the greenbottle fly, *Callitroga macellaria*, the secondary screw worm fly, *Phormia regina*, the black blowfly and *Calliphora vicina*, a bluebottle fly. Two muscid flies, *Musca domestica* and *Fannia canicularis*, are also known to have caused aural myiasis.

Three genera of warble flies infect man. *Oestrus ovis* is a cosmopolitan species in sheep, goats and man. The female fly deposits larvae around and in the nostril and nasal passages and they grow there for 3–12 months to reach lengths of 3 cm or more. Occasionally, the larvae are found in human ears.

Dermatobia hominis occurs in Central and South America. The female fly catches a mosquito or another blood sucking fly and cements her eggs to it. When the mosquito feeds the larvae emerge and enter the skin through the lesion made by the insect. The larva makes a perpendicular burrow and a very painful cyst is produced. The larva usually has to be removed surgically.

Cutebria spp. are also warble flies causing painful cysts requiring surgical removal. They lay their eggs at the openings of burrows of small mammals. The larvae enter the skin of practically any animal and cats, dogs and man are sometimes infected.

One other fly must be mentioned here. This is the widely distributed horse bot, *Gastrophilus intestinalis*. In man, the larvae cause swellings at the site of entry and also superficial serpiginous tunnels resembling those of cutaneous larval migrans. The larva normally occurs in the alimentary canal of horses but the life-cycle does not proceed to completion in man.

Although aural myiasis is relatively common in conditions of poor hygiene it is not at all common in Europe and the United States. In the United States, for example, only 5 cases of aural myiasis were recorded over the 10-year period 1952–62 (Scott, 1964) and only 1 additional case between 1962 and 1965 (Waldren, 1965). Harrison and Pearson (1968) list 11 species of flies known to have caused aural myiasis in North America. These are *Cochliomyia (Callitroga) hominovorax*, *C. macellaria*, *Oestrus ovis*, *Phaenicia sericata*, *Calliphora vicina*, *Phormia regina*, *Fannia canicularis*, *Hydrotea meteorica*, *Musca domestica*, *Sarcophaga citellivora* and *S. cooleyi*. It is interesting to note that a large number of species of flies are responsible for very few cases of aural myiasis so every fly that has ever caused any kind of myiasis is a possible cause of aural myiasis.

The diagnosis of aural myiasis is complicated by the fact that flies may be attracted to the discharge from an ear and thus a worsening of symptoms may be immediately related to the new infection. The larvae can usually be removed easily from the external acoustic meatus and, after cleaning, any inflammation quickly disappears.

Mites and ticks differ from insects in that the adults possess eight legs whereas insects possess six. Several mites occur on human skin and two kinds may be found in or on the ears as well as elsewhere on the body. *Sarcoptes scabei* spends its whole life on its host. The mite burrows in the skin and forms tunnels within the epidermis. The skin becomes sensitized and an allergic reaction occurs leading to scratching and secondary infections. Chiggers are the larval forms of mites that spend most of their lives free living. The larvae, which have six legs, bury their mouthparts into the skin and feed for several days or weeks causing intense itching. Occasionally other mites invade the skin. It is unlikely that only the ear would be infected with any mite and no aural complications other than superficial damage to the skin are known. Ticks also feed from the ear without causing any other damage.

The last category of conditions caused by insects and mites relates to the accidental entry of adults or larvae into the ear. Most insects are deterred from entering the external acoustic meatus by the waxy layer but some beetle larvae get into the ear and grow causing blockage. This condition is known as canthariasis.

PENTASTOMIDS

Members of the Pentastomida are best considered separately from the rest of the arthropods. They are worm-like creatures which possess hooks near the head but no limbs. The group is not well understood but all species are parasitic, the adults in carnivores and the larvae in herbivores. They are found mainly in reptiles but also in amphibians, mammals and, occasionally, birds. When the herbivore is eaten, the larvae emerge and cling to the mucosa of the pharynx, including its nasal part. Man is occasionally infected with *Linguatula rhinaria*, a parasite of domesticated animals, and with other species. These worms are usually 10 cm in length or larger, ringed and flattened and easily seen. The infection is acquired through eating uncooked meat. A full account of the pentastomids of man is given by Cannon (1942) and a more recent and general account is given by Nicoli and Nicoli (1966).

ANNELIDS

The only other animals likely to have an effect on the ear or nasal part of pharynx are leeches. These sometimes enter the latter cavity in a starved condition and attach themselves to feed on blood. The growing leeches may cause blockages. The condition is normally painless and harmless.

REFERENCES

Alicata, J. E. (1965), *Adv. Parasit.*, **3**, 223.

van Bogaert, L., Käfer, J. P. and Poch, G. F. (Eds.) (1963), "Tropical Neurology," *Proceedings of the First International Symposium*, Lopez Liberos Editores S.R.L. Argentina, Buenos Aires.

Bray, R. S., Ashford, R. W. and Bray, M. A. (1973), *Trans. roy. Soc. trop. Med. Hyg.*, **67**, 345.

Bunnag, T., Comer, D. S. and Punyagupta, S. (1970), *J. Neurolog. Sci.*, **10**, 419

Canelas, H. M. (1963), *Tropical Neurology* (van Bogaert, *et al.*, Eds.), p. 149.

Cannon, D. A. (1942), *Ann. trop. Med. Parasit.*, **36**, 60.

Carter, R. F. (1972), *Trans. roy. Soc. trop. Med. Hyg.*, **66**, 193.

Chitanondh, H. (1963), *Tropical Neurology* (van Bogaert, *et al.*, Eds.), p. 260.

Datta, S. and Maplestone, P. A. (1930), *Indian. med. Gaz.*, **65**, 314.

Fain, A. and Vandepitte, J. (1957), *Nature (Lond.)*, **179**, 740.

Faust, E. C., Beaver, P. C. and Jung, R. C. (1968), *Animal Agents and Vectors of Human Disease*," London: Henry Kimpton.

Faust, E. C., Russell, P. R. and Jung, P. C. (1970), *Clinical Parasitology*, 8th edition. Philadelphia: Lea and Febiger.

Harrison, B. A. and Pearson, W. G. (1968), *Milit. Med.*, **133**, 484.

van der Hoeden, J. (Ed.) (1964), *Zoonoses*. Amsterdam: Elsevier.

Iniguez, R. A. and Gurri, J. (1963), *Tropical Neurology* (van Bogaert, *et al.* Eds.), p. 91.

James, M. T. (1947), The Flies that Cause Myiasis in Man. Department of Agriculture Miscellaneous Publications No. 631. Washington.

Kafer, J. P., Poche, G. F., Monteverde, D. A., Blanco, D. F. and Tarsia, O. (1963), *Tropical Neurology* (van Bogaert, *et al.*, Eds.), p. 273.

Koberle, F. (1968), *Adv. Parasit.*, **6**, 63.

Kurma, K., Nakagawa, T. and Suzuki, J. (1961), *Otolaryngology (Tokyo)*, **33**, 1035.

Nelson, G. S. (1970), "Onchocerciasis," *Adv. Parasit.*, **8**, 173.

Nicoli, R. M. and Nicoli, J. (1966), *Ann. Parasit. hum. comp.*, **41**, 255.

Marcial-Rojas, P. A. (1971), *Pathology of Protozoal and Helminthic Diseases*. Baltimore: Williams and Wilkins.

Pawlowski, Z. and Schultz, M. G. (1972), *Adv. Parasit.*, **10**, 269.

Prasansuk, S. and Hinchcliffe, R. (1975), *Arch. Otolaryng.*, **101**, 254.

Proctor, N. S. F. (1963), *Tropical Neurology* (van Bogaert *et al.*, Ed.), p. 140.

Punyagupta, S., Juttijudata, P., Bunnag, T. and Comer, D. S. (1968), *Trans. roy Soc. trop. Med. Hyg.*, **62**, 801.

Romana, C. (1963), *Tropical Neurology* (van Bogaert *et al.*, Ed.), p. 273.

Scott, H. G. (1964), *Florida Ent.*, **47**, 255.

Shah, K. N. and Desai, M. P. (1969), *Indian J. pediat.*, **6**, 92.

South Pacific Commission (1967), Seminar on Helminthiasis and Eosinophilic Meningitis, Noumea, New Caledonia.

Spillane, J. D. (Ed.) (1973), *Tropical Neurology*. Oxford: Oxford Medical Publications.

Waldren, W. G. (1965), *Calif. Vector. Views.*, **12**, 73.

World Health Organization (1969), "Amoebiasis," Technical Report Series No 421.

World Health Organization (1971), *Bull. Wld. Hlth. Org.*, Part 4.

Yokogawa, M. (1965), *Adv. Parasit.*, **3**, 99.

Zumpt, F. (1965), *Myiasis in Man and Animals in the Old World*. London: Butterworth.

49. HISTOPATHOLOGY OF NOSE AND THROAT

LESLIE MICHAELS

TECHNIQUES IN HISTOPATHOLOGY

The Small Biopsy

Knowledge of the histological changes in disease of the ear, nose and throat has largely come about through the examination of biopsy material. Biopsies taken during oto-laryngological work are usually small, sometimes minute; it is important that surgeons and laboratory workers are trained in the taking and handling of these specimens. The skill and experience of the surgeon in selecting suitable tissue for biopsy is as important as the skill and experience of the pathologist in interpreting the biopsy. The patholo-gist is greedy in his requirements for plentiful quantities of tissue to make a certain diagnosis. He should try to temper this need with the knowledge that diseased tissue is very limited in the narrow passages of the ear, nose and throat.

There are precautions required in the taking of the biopsy that, although well-known, are so important that they can bear repeating. There must be the minimum of stretch-ing and pulling in removing the tissue. Working at a distance with a long thin instrument, often observing the area indirectly through a microscopic lens or mirror and with insufficient illumination, the otolaryngologist is at a particular disadvantage in this respect and biopsies often show this by the marks of mechanical trauma. The speci-men must not be allowed to dry as this will also ruin the histological appearances. Immediate hydration should be ensured by washing off the specimen from the biopsy forceps into the fixative, not by wiping it off, which can be a traumatizing procedure. Small biopsies are often taken from a number of different areas; to build up a detailed histological picture of the disease process these should be placed into separate labelled containers. A description of the symptoms of the patient, the site of the biopsies and the appearances of the lesion should accompany the specimens when they are sent to the histopathology laboratory; this information is essential to the pathologist in his interpretation of the findings.

In the processing of the small biopsy histopathology technicians must take care in embedding the specimen so that the correct orientation of the tissue fragment in the paraffin wax is obtained. Most small biopsies in oto-laryngology are taken from mucous membranes; it is imperative that the histological section be cut at right-angles to the mucosal surface. A section taken tangentially to the surface will be difficult or impossible to assess for such conditions as invasion by tumour or extent of an inflammatory process (Fig. 1). If wrongly embedded the paraffin block may be remelted and the tissue then reset at right-angles to the former level. Histology technicians become skilled with practice at identifying the mucosal and deep surfaces of these small biopsy fragments but in the early stages of their training they should be encouraged

to use a hand lens or magnifying glass to assist in this procedure. (Fig. 2).

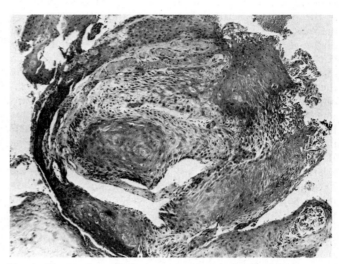

FIG. 1. Biopsy of vocal fold sectioned tangentially to epithelial surface. The epithelial cells are dysplastic, but it is impossible to determine whether invasion of lamina propria is present. Haematoxylin and eosin. (×120.)

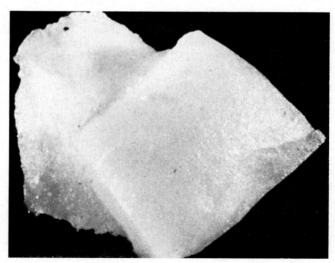

FIG. 2. Biopsy specimen of vocal fold photographed under dissecting microscope. The mucosal surface can be easily identified as a shiny pale layer.

The Frozen (Quick) Section in Otolaryngology

Otolaryngologists are often in doubt as to whether to request a frozen section for diagnosis in the course of an operation. They would enjoy the advantage of operating with histological insight, but are worried by the lack of accuracy which this procedure is reputed to have   What the surgeon can expect from a frozen section examination performed by an experienced histopathologist can be stated quite clearly. The average hospital laboratory can prepare a frozen section stained with haematoxylin and eosin in slightly less than ten minutes from the time of receiving the fresh specimen. The use in recent years of liquid nitrogen to quench the tissue and a cryostat to prepare the sections has led to the production of sections which are frequently almost equivalent to paraffin sections in their appearance. They are sometimes not quite as satisfactory to the pathologist trained mainly in the interpretation of high quality paraffin sections. In most cases an accurate diagnosis will be given which will be corroborated by the paraffin sections subsequently taken. In a few cases a mistaken diagnosis will be rendered. In cases of neoplasia these will almost always be situations in which the pathologist has given a benign diagnosis instead of a malignant one (false negative). The reverse is rare (false positive); this is because the pathologist takes care to report a section as indicating malignancy only if he is certain of the diagnosis. If he is in doubt he will render a benign or equivocal diagnosis so as to minimize any surgical procedure until the paraffin sections are available, which not only have a technical superiority over frozen sections, but also the possibilities of further and multiple sections, special stains, opportunities for consultation with colleagues and time for peaceful cogitation and reference to the literature on the subject. Thus if the pathologist reports a frozen section as showing malignancy the surgeon may confidently take the necessary action and it is by this service that frozen sections may be used to best advantage. If a major excision could be carried out under the same anaesthetic if malignancy were reported e.g. parotid or thyroid tumour, the surgeon should request a frozen section. The lines of resection during a major excision e.g. laryngectomy or glossectomy may be usefully examined by frozen section for the presence of malignancy. If present further excision is carried out until a negative report is obtained. Lymph nodes may be usefully subjected to frozen section in the course of laryngectomy or other major excisions. If positive, block dissection of the lymph node group may be performed. Table 1 gives a list of the main otolaryngological operations in neoplastic conditions together with the ways in which frozen sections may be of assistance and possible pitfalls.

I do not believe that frozen sections should be used in the diagnosis of the small mucosal biopsy as described above. The amount of material available is usually so limited that it should all be used for the paraffin section to obtain the maximum accuracy. A report on the paraffin section can usually be given within twenty-four hours. Some large institutions do carry out frozen sections on all specimens including small mucosal biopsies; it is held that the slightly diminished accuracy in using this material is more than compensated for by the immediate report given to the surgeon. The facilities required, particularly the large staff of pathologists who must be available for this purpose in the operating theatre, would seem to render this concept impracticable for most hospitals in the British Isles.

Laboratory Processing of the Specimen of Larynx and Block Dissection of Cervical Lymph Nodes

The usual extent of the laryngectomy specimen is the hyoid bone, thyroid and cricoid cartilages and a variable number of tracheal rings sometimes including the thyroid gland. In the histopathology laboratory the specimen is dissected by first making a longitudinal posterior incision through the interarytenoid tissue, the posterior lamina of the cricoid and the posterior wall of the trachea, so exposing the lumen of the larynx. A 2–3 cm length of glass rod jammed transversely between the cut sides of the tracheal rings will ensure that the specimen is fixed so that mucosal lesions are visible. This is useful for subsequent photography or if the specimen is to be wholly or partly used for display and teaching. Laryngectomy specimens whether to be partially sectioned for diagnostic purposes or to be serially sectioned *in toto* usually require decalcification because of ossification of the thyroid, cricoid and arytenoid cartilages. This is carried out after fixation. Decalcification of whole or sectioned larynges is carried out in the author's laboratory with RDO*. This proprietary preparation produces rapid decalcification while maintaining excellent staining properties (Wu and Michaels, 1969). The manufacturers of RDO have still not divulged its chemical composition. It does, unfortunately, contain some hydrochloric acid which has recently been shown to react with formaldehyde even in air to produce bischloromethyl ether (Keene, 1973). This substance has been shown to induce tumour formation in rats exposed to an inhaled air concentration of 0·1 ppm making it one of the most powerful carcinogens known. If RDO or any other hydrochloric acid containing decalcifying fluid is used, the larynx specimen should, therefore, be given an overnight wash in water to remove the formaldehyde prior to decalcification.

Serial sectioning of the whole larynx is a useful research method for the study of the spread of carcinoma of the larynx (Kirchner, 1969; Harrison, 1971). The larynx as a whole is processed, embedded in celloidin or in paraffin wax after opening up and removing the hyoid bone, the upper cornua of the thyroid cartilage and tracheal rings. Paraffin wax embedding has the advantage of speed (several weeks for the paraffin method as compared with about 6 months for the celloidin method) and of thinner sections (10–15 micrometres for the paraffin method as against 20–30 micrometres for the celloidin). Specimens may be embedded so that the larynx is cut coronally, sagittally or horizontally.

When block dissection of cervical lymph nodes is carried out at the same time as laryngectomy it is important to subject the specimen to a detailed examination of the maximum number of lymph nodes by a clearing method. In use in my laboratory is a method involving removal of the sternocleidomastoid muscle, dehydration in alcohols at 333 K (60°C) followed by clearing in methyl salicylate. The block dissection specimen is ready for selection of lymph nodes within about 1 week after operation. The nodes are identified by their position on a copy of Rouvière's

* RDO is obtained from Bethelem Instrument Ltd., Paradise House, Hemel Hempstead, Herts., England.

TABLE 1
FROZEN SECTIONS IN OTOLARYNGOLOGICAL SURGERY

Operation	Decisions Assisted by Frozen Section Report	Sources of False Negative Reports	Sources of False Positive Reports
Ear Radical removal of malignant tumour from temporal bone	Resection of facial nerve area Destruction of internal ear	Insufficient sampling	Cholesteatoma Middle ear glandular hyperplasia
Nose Lateral rhinotomy Partial maxillectomy Total maxillectomy Extended total maxillectomy	Extent of operation Orbital exenteration Removal of facial tissues and skin Removal of nasal septum	Insufficient sampling Plasmacytoma	Irradiated atypical seromucinous glands Organizing haematoma
Parotid Primary excision biopsy of superficial lobe	Proceed to type of parotidectomy	Well differentiated muco-epidermoid carcinoma	Cellular benign tumours especially mixed tumours and basal cell adenoma
Superficial lobectomy Total conservative parotidectomy Radical parotidectomy with sacrifice of facial nerve Extended radical parotidectomy	Extent of parotidectomy	—	—
Thyroid Lobectomy	Proceed to total thyroidectomy	Insufficient sampling Papillary adenocarcinoma Follicular adenocarcinoma	Adenoma
Tongue Hemiglossectomy Extended total glossectomy	Extent of glossectomy based on submucosal spread and muscle invasion	Insufficient sampling	Pseudo-epitheliomatous hyperplasia Irradiated atypical seromucinous glands
Larynx Partial laryngectomy Total laryngectomy Total pharyngolaryngectomy	Extent of laryngectomy	Insufficient sampling	—
Biopsy in a stridulous patient	Tracheostomy or emergency laryngectomy	Insufficient sampling	—
Laryngectomy if a pre-operative tracheostomy has been done	Excision of margin around stoma	Insufficient sampling	—
Pharynx and Cervical Oesophagus Partial pharyngectomy Laryngopharyngectomy	Extent of operation	Insufficient sampling	Pseudoepitheliomatous hyperplasia
Cervical Lymph Nodes Biopsy	Proceed to block dissection	—	Thymus Salivary gland inclusions

diagram and the pathological report indicates on this diagram which of the nodes shows metastatic carcinoma. (Hyams, 1974a)

HISTOPATHOLOGY OF THE NOSE AND PARANASAL SINUSES

The nose is subject to a wide variety of pathological conditions and problems arising in interpretation of biopsies taken from the nasal passages are the most frequent of those in otolaryngological histopathology. Table 2 gives a classification of the various conditions which may be encountered by histopathologists in biopsies of the nose. There follows a description of the histological features of the more important and difficult of the lesions listed in the Table.

Nasal Polyposis

A condition of swelling and polyposis of the nasal mucosa is produced in many different pathological conditions of the nose both benign and malignant. Although in many of these on gross inspection histological investigation is clearly required some of them appear similar to common nasal polyps. It, therefore, follows that all polypoid swellings of the nose that are removed must be subjected to histological examination.

The commonest type of nasal polyp is that due to allergy. In this condition the swelling is caused by marked oedema

TABLE 2

PATHOLOGICAL CONDITIONS OF THE NOSE AND PARANASAL SINUSES THAT
MAY BE ENCOUNTERED ON BIOPSY

Inflammatory Diseases
Infections:

    (a) bacterial—diphtheria, mycobacterial including leprosy, rhino-
        scleroma, syphilis
    (b) virus—measles
    (c) fungal—aspergillosis, North American blastomycosis, crypto-
        coccosis, coccidioidomycosis, histoplasmosis, rhinosporidiosis,
        mucormycosis
    (d) protozoal—leishmaniasis
Allergic and auto-immune conditions—nasal polyposis, relapsing
    polychondritis, amyloidosis
Unknown cause—Wegener's granuloma, "lethal midline granuloma",
    atrophic rhinitis, sarcoidosis, tuberculoid granuloma
Miscellaneous—mucocoele of paranasal sinuses, cholesterol granu-
    loma, organizing haematoma, pyogenic granuloma, xanthomatous
    degeneration

Neoplasms
Schneiderian mucosa—papillary adenoma, papillary adenocarcinoma
Seromucinous glands—mixed tumour (pleomorphic adenoma),
    muco-epidermoid tumour, adenocystic carcinoma, adenoma,
    adenocarcinoma
Squamous epithelium—everted squamous papilloma, inverted
    papilloma, squamous carcinoma
Melanocytes—malignant melanoma
Blood vessels—haemangioma, haemangiopericytoma, angiosarcoma
Muscle—rhabdomyosarcoma, leiomyoma, leiomyosarcoma
Lymphoid tissue—lymphosarcoma, plasmacytoma and histiocytic
    lymphoma
Connective tissue—fibroma, fibrosarcoma, fibromyxoma
Nervous system—neurilemmoma, neurofibroma, glioma, ectopic
    meningioma
Olfactory neurocytes—olfactory neuroaesthesiocytoma and olfactory
    neuroaesthesioblastoma
Cartilage and bone—chondrosarcoma, osteoma, ossifying fibroma,
    fibrous dysplasia, osteosarcoma, giant cell tumour
Tumours extending to nose and sinuses from other parts of the skull—
    ameloblastoma, meningioma, chordoma, paraganglioma
Metastatic neoplasms

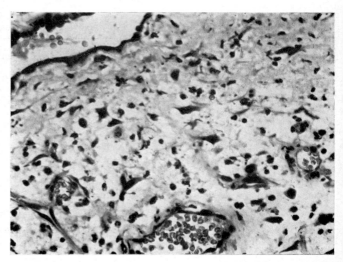

FIG. 3. Atypical stromal cells in nasal polyp obtained from a girl of 14
years. Note that some of atypical cells appear to be lining lymphatic
spaces.

of connective tissue and lymphatic vessels are severely
dilated. The respiratory epithelium shows intense goblet
cell hyperplasia and mucinous glands are similarly active.
The epithelial basement membrane is markedly thickened.
The most striking and specific feature of the allergic polyp
is the vast number of eosinophils that infiltrate the subepithelial tissue. The eosinophil infiltrate may give way to
a plasmacytic one presumably as the polyps become
secondarily infected. Antrochoanal polyps usually show
chronic inflammation, not an allergic type of inflammatory
change.

    The stromal mesenchymal cells of nasal polyps may
sometimes appear markedly atypical (Fig. 3). This is
occasionally seen in nasal polyps of children or teenagers
and may arouse anxiety as to the possibility of malignancy.
The nuclei of the atypical cells are swollen hyperchromatic
and irregular in shape, but mitotic figures are not seen.
The cytoplasm is abundant and contains numerous
minute vesicles or granules. These cells may sometimes be
identified as endothelial cells lining lymphatic vessels in
the stroma of the polyp. They probably arise as the result
of a degenerative process. Distinction from a malignant

tumour may be made from the fact that these lesions always
are less cellular than malignant neoplasms, other cytological
features of malignancy such as abnormal nuclear membranes and abnormal chromatin distribution are not
present and features of differentiation of particular neoplasms of this area such as the cross striations of rhabdomyosarcoma cannot be found.

Wegener's Granuloma

    This condition is one of a granulomatous vasculitis
which affects the upper respiratory tract and kidneys.
The lungs and other sites such as intestine are also frequently affected. The nose and/or the paranasal sinuses
are frequently the first or the main site to be affected by the
lesion of Wegener's granuloma which gradually appears
ulcerated, necrotic or crusted. Widespread and relentlessly progressive necrosis and ulceration in the nose as
are typical of lethal midline granuloma are not features of
Wegener's. The histological changes seen on nasal biopsy
of cases of Wegener's granuloma, are not specific for the
condition since similar changes may be seen in polyarteritis
nodosa and the relationship of the two conditions is
uncertain; moreover it is still uncertain whether patients
presenting with these histological features will always progress to renal and other lesions if left untreated. Nevertheless the histopathologist can recognize features which may
be described as "compatible with Wegener's granuloma"
on biopsy; without such histological changes the clinical
diagnosis, although it may be suspected, cannot be substantiated. These features are:

    (a) The presence of vasculitis. This may be acute or
chronic and often is accompanied by fibrin exudation in
the walls of blood vessels (Fig. 4). The internal elastic
lamina of arteries may be ruptured by the inflammatory
process.

    (b) A granulomatous infiltration of histiocytes,
lymphocytes, plasma cells and notably multinucleate

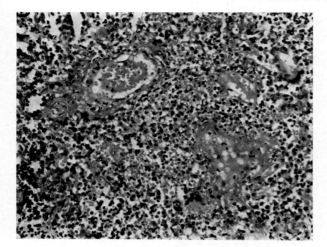

FIG. 4. Acute inflammation of walls of blood vessels in biopsy of nose in a case of Wegener's granuloma. (H. & E. ×166.)

giant cells, which may be of Langhans or foreign body type (Fig. 5).

Non-healing Granuloma

A condition which has been stated to be related to Wegener's granuloma is variously referred to as non-healing granuloma, midline granuloma, malignant granuloma, granuloma gangrenescens or Stewart's granuloma.

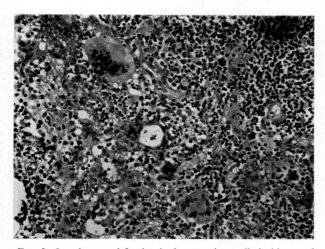

FIG. 5. Langhans and foreign body type giant cells in biopsy of nose in a case of Wegener's granuloma. Note small thickened blood vessel near the centre of the field. (H. & E. ×166.)

In "non-healing" granuloma the patient undergoes a relentlessly progressive ulceration of the nose without systemic involvement. Stewart (1933) described ten such cases and because various pathologists reporting on biopsy material in these cases could only find chronic inflammatory changes with certainty he suggested that the condition was basically granulomatous, i.e. inflammatory in origin. Friedmann (1964) was impressed by the similarity of this condition to Wegener's granuloma and stated that midline granuloma had two forms, (1) Stewart's type and (2) Wegener's type; intermediate forms existed between these two types. This concept and indeed the whole existence of

"midline granuloma" as a specific entity has not been universally accepted. Burston (1959) showed that more specific entities could often be diagnosed by persistent investigation in cases initially given the designation of midline granuloma. Eichel and Mabery (1968) felt that this condition did not actually exist as an isolated entity. Harrison (1974) found that by consideration only of the clinical aspects of the case he was able to decide on a mode of therapy which produced satisfactory results. Harrison treated patients with progressive local ulceration as neoplasms by irradiation; those cases showing less local but more systemic manifestations were more likely to be in the Wegener's group and were successfully managed with corticosteroids and azathioprine. The histological findings were not considered helpful.

Such a failure of histopathology to identify a cancerous type of ulceration has rarely been found in any other part of the body. Mycosis fungoides of the skin is an example of a similar situation, but such lack of correlation is rare. In fact, in spite of predictions to the contrary, identification of pathological processes by histological and cytological methods have become of the highest importance in the management of patients with suspected neoplasms. Because of this discrepancy between the cancerous behaviour of the lesions and the apparently inflammatory histological appearance of biopsies from them the author investigated material from 29 bases designated clinically as non-healing granuloma, most of them described by Harrison in his clinical study of 1974. Biopsy material was studied from these cases and, at first, without recourse to the clinical history. In seven cases, post-mortem histological material was available in addition to the surgical biopsies. In 18 of the 29 cases chronic inflammatory changes only were found. Some of these showed giant cells and vasculitis of the appearances found in Wegener's granuloma; correlation with the clinical findings to differentiate any specific type of inflammatory condition was not attempted. Three cases showed tumour tissue in the biopsy material; these were classified as histiocytic lymphoma (reticulum cell sarcoma), plasmacytoma and lymphocytic lymphosarcoma respectively. These patients had clinical appearances suggestive of neoplasm. The remaining eight cases all showed a peculiar and similar histological appearance in both biopsy and autopsy material from the nasal area. This took the form of widespread necrosis together with some areas of an atypical cell exudate (Necrosis with Atypical Cellular Exudate, NACE).

The atypical cells in cases showing NACE were a little larger than inflammatory cells with nuclei that varied from round to horseshoe-shaped with irregular protuberances. The chromatic material was irregularly distributed. Binucleate forms were present and mitotic figures were seen in each case. The cytoplasmic membrane was indefinite. Phagocytosed basophilic debris was frequently seen in the cytoplasm of the cells. Zones composed of such cells varied from very small areas to large parts of the available biopsy material (Figs. 6 and 7). Necrosis was always prominent and was usually of the coagulative type. It was seen between the tumour cells and also forming large eosinophilic cellular areas which frequently formed a

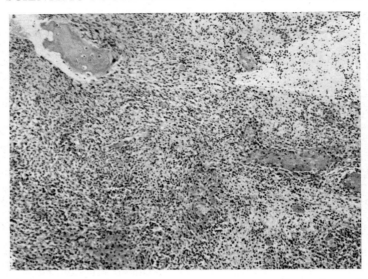

FIG. 6. Biopsy from ulcerating lesion of nose in 50-year-old man diagnosed as malignant granuloma. Photomicrograph shows an area of atypical cellular exudate with a residual fragment of bone (upper left), fibrin thrombi in capillaries (upper and centre right) and small areas of necrosis (lower centre). (H. & E. ×100.)

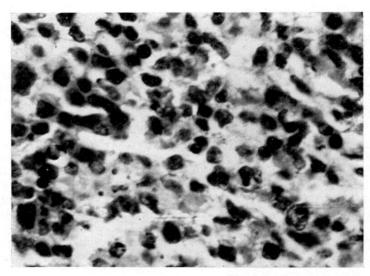

FIG. 7. High power view of part of preceding figure showing atypical cells with round to elongated nuclear shape and phagocytized intracytoplasmic particles. The cellular appearances are compatible with a diagnosis of histiocytic lymphoma (reticulum cell sarcoma). (H. & E. ×1 000.)

prominent feature of the biopsy material. The atypical cells possessed a fine reticulin pattern which surrounded each cell. Large areas of the necrotic zones showed a similar reticulin framework (Figs. 8A and B). In four cases, NACE tissue was seen to be invading nerve sheaths. In two cases there was invasion of skeletal muscle and in two cases histological evidence of invasion of facial bone by NACE was present. A number of vascular changes were evident. Some of these (subintiminal fibrous thickening and intimal foam cell infiltration of arteries) were found only in previously irradiated cases and the changes could be

explained on that basis. In two cases there was involvement of the walls of small vessels by atypical cellular exudate and, in five cases (two of them not irradiated), fibrin thrombi were found in small vessels within the areas of NACE.

The clinical findings in all cases showing NACE was that of a progressively ulcerating lesion involving the nose or nasal sinuses. In three cases NACE tissue was found at post-mortem examination in cervical lymph nodes and in one case as a discrete deposit in a kidney.

The author therefore believes, on the basis of the findings given above, that NACE represents a *malignant neoplasm*

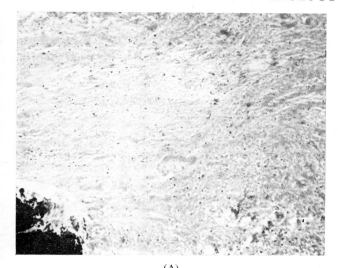

(A)

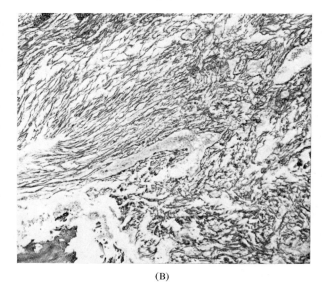

(B)

Fig. 8. (A) Biopsy from ethmoidal area from male of 24 with clinical diagnosis of malignant granuloma. Large areas of coagulative necrosis were found such as is seen here. A fragment of eroded bone is seen at the bottom left. (H. & E. ×100.) (B) Section taken from adjacent part of the same paraffin block as A. Note fine reticulin framework is what appeared to be necrotic tissue. The same bony fragment is, for reference, at bottom left. Gordon and Sweet's reticulin stain. (×100.)

which, although slowly growing, invades locally and eventually metastasizes to lymph nodes and further afield. The histological appearances of the NACE areas would suggest the designation *histiocytic lymphoma* for this neoplasm.

The question following remains: "Are there cases of progressive midline ulceration which after careful biopsy do not show NACE or any specific neoplastic condition?" This question cannot be answered with certainty, but, because of the impressive correlation of progressive midline ulceration with NACE in this series, the term "midline granuloma" should be abandoned. The use of this term may mislead clinicians into giving up the search for definite neoplasias and resorting to milder forms of therapy than are required for a malignant neoplasm.

Thus, the author is in agreement with Burston (1959) and with Eichel and Mabery (1968), i.e. that midline granuloma probably does not exist as a pathological entity; many of the cases which have been designated as midline granuloma are in fact lymphomas of histiocytic type. This group of neoplasms has provided much difficulty in diagnosis for a variety of reasons. Adequate biopsies of the nasal region are difficult to obtain, particularly in the ethmoidal area. When these small biopsies are examined they are found to be particularly prone to a process of necrosis; whether this is due to unusually active immunological processes as has been suggested by Harrison (1974) or whether it is the involvement of blood vessels within the tumour by tumour tissue, or other pathological processes as described above is difficult to say. As a consequence of the extensive necrosis, areas of atypical (i.e. neoplastic) cells are usually small and their identification is made even more difficult by the fact that they resemble inflammatory cells of histiocytic type in size and structure. The involvement of blood vessels by the neoplastic process and also by the small doses of irradiation with which this lesion has often been treated has created further difficulties by leading to its confusion with Wegener's granuloma, the nosology of which is already confused enough.

Tuberculoid Granulomas and Sarcoidosis

Foci of epithelioid cell and lymphocytic infiltration accompanied by Langhans and foreign body giant cells are frequently found in the nasal mucosa. The patients may be symptom free (the lesions being detected following examination of material removed during an unrelated minor operation such as submucous resection) or the condition may lead to the development of a polypoidal nasal mucosa. Biopsy material should be carefully examined for the presence of an aetiological agent by (at least) an acid fast stain and staining by the periodic acid Schiff method to detect the presence of mycobacteria and fungi, respectively. The presence of vasculitis in addition to the giant cell granulomata would suggest Wegener's granuloma. In the majority of cases of tuberculoid granuloma involving the nasal mucosa, however, no aetiological agent can be found. Some of these cases have manifestations of Boeck's sarcoidosis such as lung parenchyma changes and hilar lymph node enlargement on chest X-ray, skin lesions and changes in the small finger bones. It is questionable whether discrete tuberculoid granulomas of the nose without caseation or any detectable causative agent can be considered as manifestations of sarcoidosis in the absence of lung or other specific lesions. A positive Kveim test might be of help in these circumstances, but while the whole question of sarcoidosis remains *sub judice* the granulomatous nasal lesions must remain equally so.

Cholesterol Granuloma

Foci of haemorrhage and secondary change are common in the mucosae of the maxillary and frontal sinuses. Their cause in unknown and they are of quite benign import but they are significant clinically because they may be mistaken for a tumour or cyst. In the maxillary sinus this

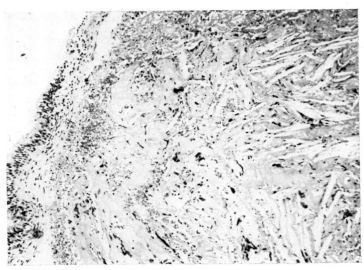

FIG. 9. Cholesterol granuloma of maxillary sinus. Cholesterol clefts are scattered among red cells and inflammatory cells and are surrounded by apposed foreign body type giant cells. (H. & E. ×120.)

lesion may appear as a large cystic bluish structure. Histologically haemorrhage is prominent and frequently has degenerated to haemosiderin containing histiocytes. Large clefts characteristically shaped like the crystals of cholesterol esters are scattered among the red cells and are surrounded by apposed foreign body type giant cells (Fig. 9). A turbid yellow fluid may be obtained from the affected sinus. Small foci with this type of histological change may also be seen in the vicinity of malignant tumours of the nose and a form of rhinitis has been described (rhinitis caseosa-pseudo-cholesteatoma) in which the characteristic histological change is cholesterol clefts and the foreign body giant cell reaction to them (Eggston and Wolf, 1947).

Papillary Adenoma

A papillomatous lesion reproducing the respiratory mucosa of the nose in papillary folds has variously been known as Schneiderian papilloma, papillary adenoma and cylindric cell papilloma. This benign tumour grows principally in the maxillary sinus and lateral wall of the nose. The principal feature is an everted frond-like series of folds of mucosa covered by respiratory epithelium. The cilia of the lining cells are often atrophic. Varying numbers of small mucus containing cystic structures are present among the epithelial cells which may be mistaken for rhinosporidiosis (Hyams, 1971) (Fig. 10).

Papillary Adenocarcinoma

A malignant counterpart of the papillary adenoma is the papillary adenocarcinoma. This condition usually presents with nasal obstruction and the nose contains polypoid masses of tumour. Radiological examination may show bone destruction. Microscopical examination reveals a neoplasm characterized by papillary outgrowths covered by columnar cells showing malignant characteristics

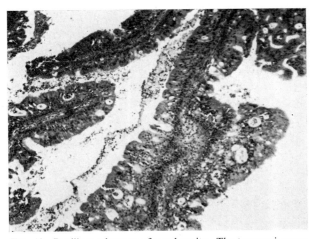

FIG. 10. Papillary adenoma of nasal cavity. The tumour is composed of frond-like folds of mucosa covered by respiratory epithelium with atrophic cilia. Small cystic structures are present among the epithelial cells. (H. & E. ×66·5.)

together with invading malignant glandular formations in which mucus productions is active (Fig. 11).

Adenocarcinomas of this histological type are particularly associated with the occupation of wood working (Acheson et al., 1968; Cowdell, 1968). Other occupational malignant lesions of the nasal passages are squamous carcinoma associated with the industrial refining of nickel (Morgan, 1958) and undifferentiated carcinoma of the nasal part of pharynx in Canadian bush pilots (Andrews and Michaels, 1967).

Tumours of Salivary Type Arising from Sero-mucinous Glands

The sero-mucinous glands of the nose and paranasal sinuses resemble salivary glands such as the submandibular gland not only in histological appearance, but also in the varieties of tumour which may arise from them. Three

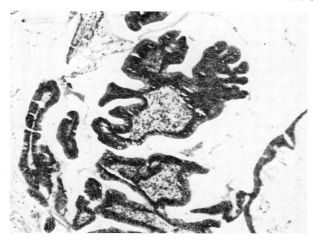

FIG. 11. Papillary adenocarcinoma of nasal cavity. Folds of hyperplastic columnar epithelium are embedded in pools of mucus. The patient was a seventy-two-year-old teacher of carpentry and had been a woodworker all his life. (H. & E. ×100.)

types of neoplasm in particular reflect the salivary structure of the nasal glands:

(a) Mixed tumour (pleomorphic adenoma).
(b) Muco-epidermoid tumour.
(c) Adenocystic carcinoma.

Mixed Tumour (Pleomorphic Adenoma)

These tumours usually arise on the lateral wall of the nose with a rather mucoid, translucent gross appearance associated with the development of the characteristic ground substance. The histological appearances of the nasal tumours are identical to those of salivary glands and enable them to be identified with no difficulty in the majority of cases. The cells adopt a "biphasic pattern" in all cases; there are glandular structures often with central eosinophilic secretion and there are cells, probably myoepithelial in origin which appear to have "dropped off" from the glands and are found lying singly in the stroma or ground substance (Fig. 12). The excess of the latter which may

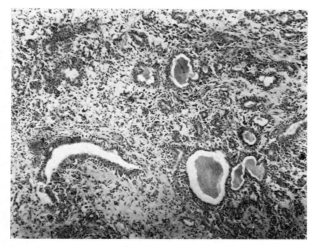

FIG. 12. Mixed tumour (pleomorphic adenoma) of nasal cavity. There is a biphasic pattern of glands and loose stromal cells lying in a mucoid ground substance. (H. & E. ×66·5.)

appear cartilaginous, mucoid or simply hyaline is the other histological characteristic of mixed tumours and it is by this combination of epithelial cellular structure and apparently mesenchymal ground substance (probably a secretion of epithelial cells) that this tumour derives its terminology as mixed or pleomorphic. Squamous metaplasia is common in these nasal mixed tumours, but is of no significance as regards malignancy (Fig. 13).

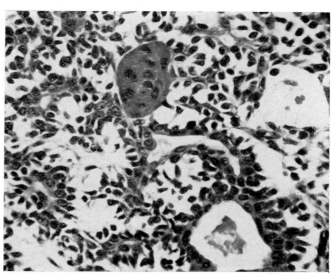

FIG. 13. Mixed tumour (pleomorphic adenoma) of nasal cavity. There is a biphasic pattern and an oval area of squamous metaplasia. (H. & E. ×380.)

The majority of these tumours, even those of considerable cellularity, are locally aggressive only and should be amenable to active surgical therapy, but not irradiation. Malignancy should be diagnosed in these tumours only in the presence of severe anaplasia and atypicism.

Mucoepidermoid Tumour

This tumour which is sometimes seen in the nasal passages is characterized by both mucus secreting and epidermoid elements. It usually arises in the nose itself where it forms a polypoid mass. Histologically both tall columnar mucus secreting cells and squamous cells with prickle and some keratin formation are interspersed (Fig. 14). The neoplasm is probably of duct cell origin and collections of squamous cells may be seen in relation to the lumina of neoplastic duct-like structures recapitulating the squamous metaplasia that may arise in the ducts of seromucinous or salivary glands (Fig. 15). Degrees of differentiation of both the secretory and the epidermoid elements may be seen and the malignant potential of the lesion increases in the poorly differentiated forms (Healey, 1970). We have found electron microscopy useful in detecting the presence of both secretory and squamous elements in tumours that by light microscopy would be regarded as undifferentiated carcinomas.

Adenocystic Carcinoma

The most malignant of the neoplasms of seromucinous gland origin, this lesion is frequent in the nose and maxillary sinus where it may present as nasal polyps or may be infiltrating into the surrounding bony tissues. The histological pattern is characteristic with cribriform collections of epithelial cells of a rather uniform appearance showing regular dark nuclei and little cytoplasm. The glandular spaces that appear in many cell masses are not lined by a discrete row of cells but appear as if "pushed

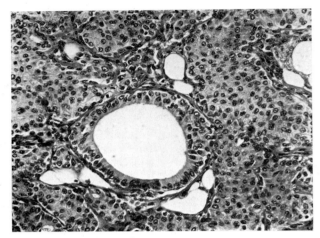

FIG. 14. Mucoepidermoid tumour of nasal cavity, well differentiated type. A mucous gland is surrounded by epidermoid cells. (H. & E. ×166.)

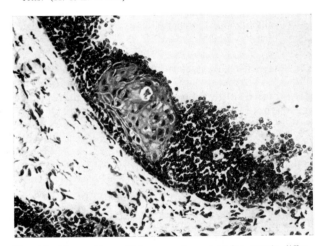

FIG. 15. Mucoepidermoid tumour of nasal cavity, poorly differentiated type. Columnar epithelial cells are represented by dark, apparently undifferentiated cells which, on electron microscopy, show secretory globules in their cytoplasm. A group of cells with squamous differentiation is present in a duct-like structure. (H. & E. ×166.)

into" the cell groups (Fig. 16). Large cylinders of mucus secretion that frequently are seen in these tumours give rise to the alternative, older designation of the lesion as "cylindroma". A solid variant of adenocystic carcinoma presents with minute glands in the tumour masses or completely solid clusters of tumour cells. The suggestion that this may be a more malignant form (Eby *et al.*, 1972) is unlikely since metastases of adenocystic carcinoma are usually composed of the more open form.

Local recurrence is common in adenocystic carcinoma after a variable period which may be many years. Lymph

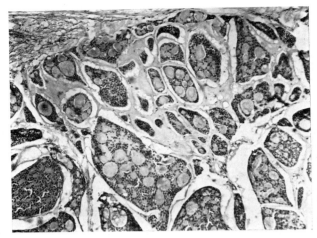

FIG. 16. Adenocystic carcinoma of nasal cavity. Cribriform collections of epithelial cells with numerous "cylinders" of secretion. (H. & E. ×88.)

node metastases are unusual in the nasal tumours. Distant metastases frequently develop after a long interval and the lungs represent the commonest site.

Adenoma and Adenocarcinoma

Tumours composed of glands lined by columnar cells of varying degrees of malignancy are sometimes seen in the nose. If there are no traces of one or other of the specific histological types of glandular tumour described above the possibility should be considered that the neoplasm is metastatic to the nose from a primary adenocarcinoma elsewhere in the body. Primary adenomas and adenocarcinomas are undoubtedly seen arising in the nose. They are usually locally invasive and they may be satisfactorily treated by wide local excision; they are probably not sensitive to irradiation.

Everted or Fungiform Squamous Papilloma

These lesions which are identical to those frequently seen on the uvula or tonsil, when arising in the nose are always found in the nasal septum (Hyams, 1971). They are exophytic growths with connective tissue cores in the fronds covered by squamous epithelium. Mucous cysts are commonly found among the epithelial cells of the neoplasm. There is no tendency to malignancy in this type of growth.

Inverted Papilloma

This lesion is often called Ringertz tumour or transitional cell papilloma, the latter from the supposed nature of the heaped-up cells lining the inverted sinuses of the tumour. This tumour arises from the lateral wall of the nose and paranasal sinuses, but never from the nasal septum (Hyams, 1971). The neoplasm presents as polypoid masses in the nasal cavity and sinuses. It may have a similar gross appearance to allergic nasal polyps, but usually is more opaque and never shows an elongated stalk. The microscopical appearance is striking and unlike that seen in any other tumour of the upper respiratory tract. The stroma of the polyp is interspersed by sinus-like tracts which are lined by thick layers of epidermoid cells which in places give way to pseudostratified columnar ciliated or secretory epithelium (Fig. 17). In some places the ciliated cells appear to form a row lining the inner surface of an epidermoid area. Serial sections suggest that this appearance may be due to abrupt

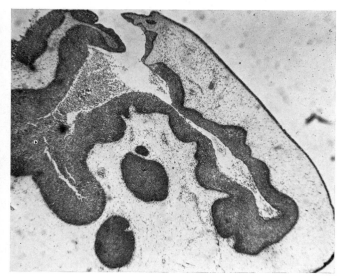

FIG. 17. The basic structure of an inverted papilloma. Sinus-like inversions of the surface epithelium are lined by metaplastic squamous epithelium with an occasional residual focus of respiratory epithelium. (H. & E. ×20.)

transitions between stratified squamous and pseudostratified columnar epithelium, the cells of the latter sending their long threads of cytoplasm down to the basement membrane at the sides of the former areas. The surface of the neoplasm is covered by similar alternating areas of squamous and columnar epithelium (Fig. 18). The stroma of the tumour commonly shows acute and chronic inflammation and neutrophils are frequently seen in considerable numbers infiltrating the squamous epithelial cells (Fig. 19). Eosinophils are common also in the stroma. The lesion may,

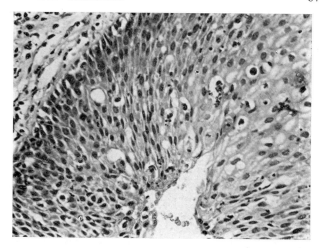

FIG. 19. Neutrophils in squamous epithelium in an inverted papilloma. (H & E. ×265.)

therefore, be summarized as a widespread and patchy process of squamous metaplasia affecting the surface and inverted sinuses of nasal mucosa with concomitant acute, chronic and allergic type of inflammation. The origin of the inverted sinuses would be crucial to an understanding of the histogenesis of this common and remarkable lesion. Are they derived from the ducts of seromucinous glands? This is unlikely because the acini of the glands are never seen in the lesion. More likely, perhaps is that surface epithelium pushes in the newly formed metaplastic areas as it develops rather than everting them as happens in the fungiform papilloma.

There is a strong tendency to recurrence of this tumour. A small but definite relationship to malignancy exists in this neoplasm and ranges from about 5 per cent (Osborn, 1970) to 13 per cent (Hyams, 1971). A figure as low as 2 per cent is obtained when those cases presenting with simultaneous inverted papilloma and squamous carcinoma are discounted (Osborn, 1970). The malignancy is always of the squamous carcinomatous variety, but may be poorly differentiated.

Malignant Melanoma

Malignant melanoma of the nose in the majority of cases is found in the nasal cavity and may involve the maxillary and ethmoid sinuses and the nasal part of pharynx. The tumour may be polypoid, but it usually presents infiltrating features with evidence of destruction of the bony maxillary sinus wall. A brownish coloration of the tumour is apparent in approximately two-thirds of the cases at operation (Gallagher, 1970). As elsewhere malignant melanomas of the nose can present as tumours composed of cuboidal cells, spindle cells or a mixture of both. The cellular type does not appear to be related to the degree of malignancy. Melanin pigment is always present and can be seen in moderate or large amounts by special staining. Its identity as melanin should always be confirmed by special staining procedures such as Fontana's silver stain followed by bleaching by "20 vols" hydrogen peroxide solution. The pigment should also be shown to be negative to staining

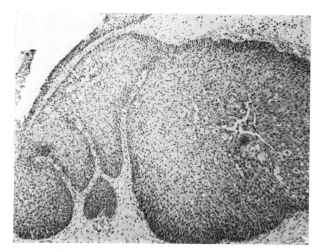

FIG. 18. Squamous metaplastic foci in inverted papilloma. (H. & E. ×66·5.)

for haemosiderin. The presence of pigment constitutes the most important diagnostic feature of malignant melanoma of the nose. Without melanin the diagnosis of malignant melanoma must remain unsure in a nasal tumour. The cuboidal type of cell may be associated with the grouping of tumour cells into small clumps each surrounded by a thin reticulin membrane. This alveolar pattern may mimic such tumours as alveolar soft part sarcoma or paraganglioma, but the presence of melanin pigment excludes these tumours. Mitotic figures are usually frequent in nasal melanoma, indeed these tumours are among the most active of neoplasms in mitotic rate. The presence of large eosinophilic nuclei has been stressed as a diagnostic feature of malignant melanoma of the nose, but this feature was prominent in only one-half of a series of 14 cases of this disease which I recently examined. Junctional activity is an important feature of dermal melanomas, but this change is unusual in malignant melanoma of the nose, perhaps because unlike the skin tumour only small amounts of normal nasal mucosa are removed with the nasal tumour (Fig. 20). Invading tumour cells are sometimes seen in the

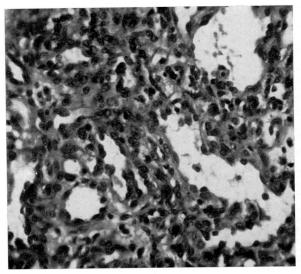

FIG. 21. Angiosarcoma of nasal cavity. Note vascular spaces lined by atypical cells. (H. & E. ×480.)

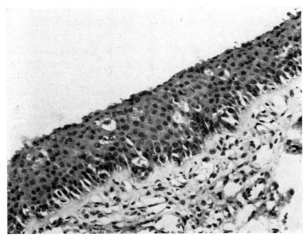

FIG. 20. Metaplastic stratified lining of nasal mucosa adjacent to malignant melanoma showing junctional activity among the basal layers. (H. & E. ×265.)

deeper layers of metaplastic squamous epithelium covering the tumour; this should not be confused with the junctional change that is found in the respiratory epithelium adjacent to the tumour.

The local origin of malignant melanoma in the nose is sometimes doubted on the grounds that melanocytes are not normally found there. Using special staining methods they may indeed be found there normally, particularly on the septum and it seems likely that such cells are capable of giving rise occasionally to these malignant tumours. Naevuses of the nasal mucosa are, however, exceedingly rare.

Haemangioma, Haemangiosarcoma and Organizing Haematoma

There is little histological difficulty usually associated with biopsy material from these tumours. Haemangiomas

are common particularly on the septum and they may be particularly exuberant in pregnancy. The normal nasal erectile tissue may be mistaken for haemangioma. Tumours composed of blood vessels lined by endothelial cells of active appearance may merit the term haemangioendothelioma and as an endothelial cell of still more active appearance is encountered the term haemangiosarcoma will be used implying a vascular lesion of aggressive activity. Metastasis is unusual in even the more malignant variants of this lesion (Fig. 21).

The histopathologist should be aware that organizing haematoma is commonly found in the nose and biopsies may be submitted by clinicians suspecting that this material is a neoplasm. Such material may be mistaken for haemangiosarcoma, since the endothelial cells of the penetrating capillaries are often very bizarre and mitotic figures are abundant among them. Careful examination will show

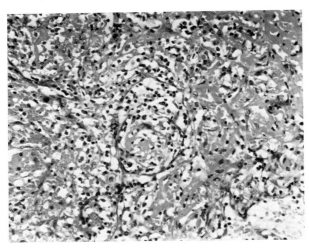

FIG. 22. Organizing haematoma of nasal cavity. Fibrin and blood clot are undergoing invasion by capillaries. Some of the accompanying fibroblastic cells are very bizarre. Note the large cell in mitosis on the upper left. (H. & E. ×265.)

differentiation to fibrous tissue away from the growing edge of the granulation tissue (Fig. 22).

Haemangiopericytoma

Stout and Murray in 1942 described a mesenchymal vascular tumour in which the component cells were present around the numerous capillary blood vessels of the neoplasm, but were definitely outside the endothelium of the vessels. On the basis of tissue culture findings these cells were felt to be derived from pericytes and so the term haemangiopericytoma was coined. Neoplasms with similar histological characteristics have since then been described in many sites. This is not surprising for if the explanation of Stout and Murray for the origin of this tumour is correct, capillaries and their pericytes, being ubiquitous, the tumours derived from them would be expected to be correspondingly so.

A small number of cases of haemangiopericytoma only has been described as originating in the nasal passages (Eneroth et al., 1969; Walike and Balley, 1971). This is unexpected in view of the abundant blood supply of the nasal mucosa. My experience does not support the idea that this is a particularly rare tumour of the nose. Many cases are probably put into another histological category, particularly fibrosarcoma, by histopathologists and, although this makes little difference to behaviour and treatment of the neoplasm it does seem that haemangiopericytomas warrant a separate histological grouping.

Haemangiopericytomas are found as polypoid, often vascular tumours of the nasal cavity. The sinuses are not involved. The tumour, which is situated beneath the epithelium of the nasal mucosa, presents an irregular shape with outgrowths of cells into the surrounding connective tissue. It has a marked intrinsic vascularity largely by small blood vessels many of which show somewhat thickened or hyalinized walls. Surrounding these blood vessels and definitely distinct from their endothelial cells are the usually somewhat elongated mesenchymal cells comprising the tumour. The nuclei are usually rather homogeneous with few or no mitotic figures. Cytoplasm is scanty (Fig. 23). Reticulin staining reveals not only the distinctness of the tumour cells from capillary endothelium, but also that each cell is surrounded by a layer of reticulin (Fig. 24). The tumour has about the same malignant potential as a fibrosarcoma. Local recurrence is a strong possibility particularly if surgical exision has not been complete. Distant metastases particularly to the lungs occasionally develop.

Rhabdomyosarcoma

Rhabdomyosarcoma has a significantly high incidence among nasal tumours. Unlike most other nasal tumours it affects the young predominantly, being found in children from birth to 15 years with a fairly uniform distribution through these age groups. Occasional cases are met with above the age of 50 years. The site of origin is about equally common in the nasal cavity, the maxillary sinus and the nasal part of pharynx. The lesion presents a polypoid and an infiltrating component with bone involvement to the base of the skull frequently complicating the latter.

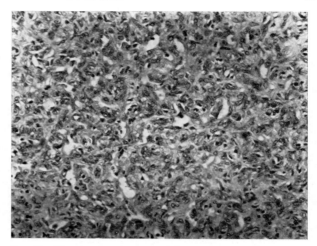

FIG. 23. Haemangiopericytoma of the nasal cavity. The tumour is composed of numerous blood vessels surrounded by mesenchymal cells, the "pericytes". (H. & E. ×265.)

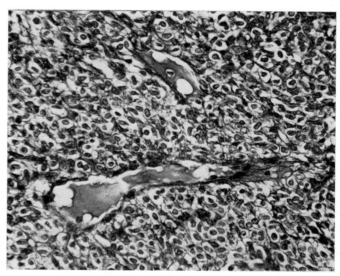

FIG. 24. Haemangiopericytoma of the nasal cavity. Note the fine thread of reticulin surrounding each tumour cell. The blood vessels and their lining endothelial cells are separated from the tumour cells by a layer of reticulin. Reticulin stain. (×390.)

Most cases of rhabdomyosarcoma are composed largely of embryonal cells. Sometimes the alveolar form of the tumour is seen in the nose, but this histological variation has no known significance in the natural history of the disease. All cases of embryonal rhabdomyosarcoma show largely undifferentiated cells (Fig. 25). Near the covering epithelium of the nose a loose arrangement of the tumour cells is often seen. The tumour cells are either rounded or elongated with little cytoplasm. Nuclear hyperchromatism is a common feature. In many cases no cross-striated fibres can be identified even after the use of a special staining method to demonstrate them such as phosphotungstic-acid haematoxylin. Although a rhabdomyoblast origin of these undifferentiated cells seems likely by comparison with cases showing some differentiation, the tumour may be only termed with accuracy a malignant mesenchymoma.

In other cases areas of definite skeletal muscle formation may be seen. These are usually elongated cells (sometimes strikingly thin cells) and possess cross-striations (Fig. 26). In one case that I have seen, a maxillary sinus lesion in a 48-year-old woman, adult muscle fibres were formed amid the sarcomatous areas and it is probably significant that

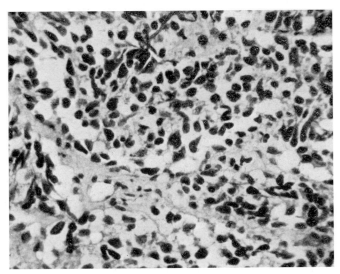

Fig. 25. Embryonic rhabdomyosarcoma of the nasal cavity. The tumour is composed of loosely arranged mesenchymal cells. Cross striations were not detected. (H. & E. ×480.)

such formations are known in the development of normal striped muscle (Fig. 27).

Rhabdomyosarcoma of the nasal passages is an extremely aggressive type of malignancy with a poor outlook for survival.

Extramedullary Plasmacytoma

The commonest site for plasmacytoma to present is in the bone marrow where it is almost always associated with changes in the serum proteins and often with the presence of Bence Jones protein in serum and urine. The next most common site for plasma cell tumours is in the upper respiratory tract. Here the majority of cases are seen as tumours of the nasal cavity and nasal part of pharynx, but primary involvement of the tongue, nasal cavity, sinuses and larynx is also found. The upper respiratory plasmacytoma is largely a disease of males, less than one-fifth of the patients being females. Most cases are over 50 years of age at presentation.

In the nose the tumour is a smooth sub-epithelial mucosal swelling which may be polypoid. It often shows evidence of soft tissue infiltration and sometimes infiltration of the bone. The histological appearance is that of solid sheets of plasma cells with various degrees of nuclear atypicism. The plasma cells may be on the one hand quite similar to the non-neoplastic cells seen in chronic inflammatory exudates (Fig. 28). On the other hand double or multiple nuclei may be frequent and mitotic figures and bizarre

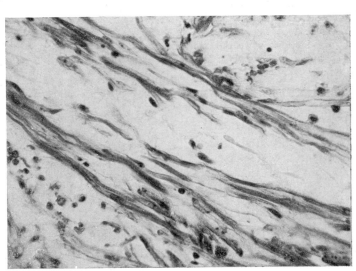

Fig. 26. Differentiated area of rhabdomyosarcoma of nasal part of pharynx. Note cross striations in some of the elongated tumour cells. Phosphotungstic acid haematoxylin. (×270.)

this patient has so far survived more than 3 years without recurrence. In some cases evidence of skeletal muscle origin is given by the presence of rounded areas of acidophilic material deposited in swollen or elongated tumour cells. Vacuoles in the cytoplasm of the tumour cells which on special staining with the periodic acid Schiff method, with and without diastase, can be demonstrated to be glycogen are visible in some tumours and enhance the impression of a skeletal muscle origin in these cases since

nuclei may also be present (Fig. 29). The nuclei frequently present large eosinophilic nucleoli. Unlike chronic inflammatory plasmacytic exudates, plasmacytomas often show a capillary stroma on which the tumour cells rest. The cells of extramedullary plasmacytoma sometimes adopt an alveolar arrangement somewhat resembling the acini of glandular tumours (Fig. 28).

Biochemical changes affecting proteins in the blood and urine are much less frequent in upper respiratory plasmacy-

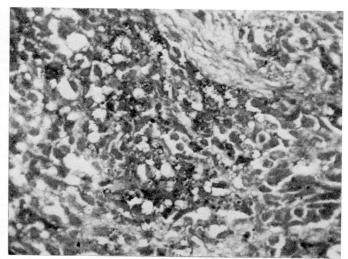

FIG. 27. Glycogenic deposits in vacuoles of tumour cells in embryonic rhabdomyosarcoma. Periodic acid Schiff. (× 380.)

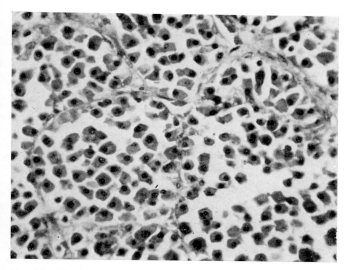

FIG. 28. Plasmacytoma of nasal cavity. The tumour is composed of differentiated plasma cells with a notable organoid pattern resembling a glandular tumour. (H. & E. × 380.)

toma than in the bone marrow variety of this tumour, presumably due to the much greater volume of tumour that the latter attains. There is no information available as to whether the extramedullary plasmacytoma usually produces a single immunologically specific immunoglobulin, like the medullary variety. Amyloid is produced in about 10 per cent of upper respiratory plasmacytomas; it is found within the tumour, sometimes in large amounts.

Plasmacytomas may spread widely from the site of origin. Multiple metastases to bones (like myeloma) and other organs such as lungs sometimes takes place. Plasmacytomas respond well to irradiation therapy.

Myxoma

This lesion is well known in the lower jaw where it is usually found in relation to an unerupted tooth, but it is also found in the upper jaw where only very occasionally

is it related to an unerupted tooth (Ghosh *et al.*, 1973). About one-half of the maxillary cases present in children. The tumour may be found involving any part of the maxillary bone, including the palate or nasal area. It presents grossly as a soft translucent mucoid tumour. Histologically the neoplasm resembles Wharton's jelly with loose myxoid

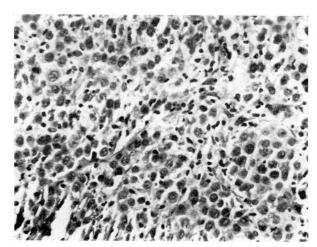

FIG. 29. Plasmacytoma of nasal cavity. A less differentiated plasmacytic lesion with an occasional mitotic figure. (H. & E. × 265.)

cells embedded in a ground substance containing variable quantities of collagenous stroma (Fig. 30). Sometimes blood vessels may be abundant and such cases may present with nose bleeds.

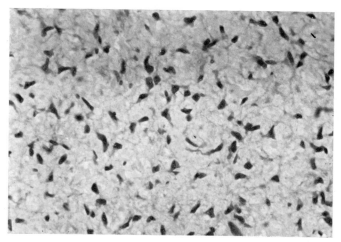

FIG. 30. Myxoma of the maxillary bone. The tumour is composed of loose myxoid cells embedded in a loose ground substance containing fibrils of collagen. (H. & E. × 320.)

This tumour does not metastasize but has a distinct tendency to recur unless aggressively excised.

Neurogenic Tumours

Neurogenic tumours are important in otorhinolaryngology. These neoplasms are not infrequent in the upper respiratory tract and tongue and a form of neurogenic tumour, the neurilemmoma, is the commonest tumour of the eight cranial nerve.

There are two distinct varieties of neurogenic tumour. Both are composed of Schwann cells and collagenous fibres. In the neurilemmoma (Schwannoma) the Schwann cells are patterned into organoid formations, particularly palisading, sometimes with whorled arrangements of the palisaded Schwann cells. These areas of the neurilemmal tumour are collectively known as Antoni A areas. Within the same tumour Antoni B areas are usually found; they are composed of loose connective tissue with scattered histiocytes and foam cells (Fig. 31). The other variety of

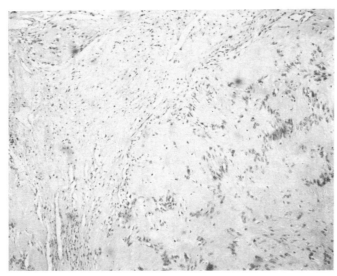

FIG. 31. Neurilemomma (Schwannoma) of nasal cavity. Note palisaded Antoni A areas on the right and looser Antoni B areas on the left. (H. & E. ×80.)

neurogenic tumour, the neurofibroma, shows a non-specific arrangement of Schwann cells and collagen. Nerve fibres usually traverse the tumour sometimes in considerable numbers (Fig. 32). Neurofibromas have a small, but distinct, tendency to undergo malignant change. Malignant change in Schwannomas is very rare. Von Recklinghausen's disease of the skin, in which neurogenic tumours present as multiple subcutaneous lesions together with *café au lait* patches shows both neurofibromas and neurilemmomas. It is the neurofibromas usually that undergo malignant degeneration in von Recklinghausen's disease. Neurogenic tumours of the head and neck may accompany von Recklinghausen's disease or may be found alone without the skin lesions.

Glioma

This term is applied to a mass in the nose composed of cerebral tissue. It is a misnomer because both the cellular elements of brain tissue may be found, viz. neurocytes and glial cells constituting what is sometimes referred to as "ganglioglioma"; moreover it is not necessarily a neoplasm. There are three forms of this condition:

(a) Congenital herniation of brain tissue, often into the root of the nose in infants. Histologically glial tissue

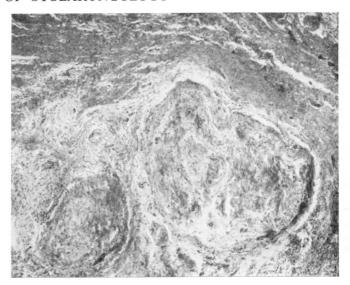

FIG. 32. Neurofibroma of nasal septum. The two demarcated areas at bottom centre are nerve bundles. Most of the tumour is composed of spindle cells and loosely arranged collagen. Haematoxylin and van Gieson. (×80.)

only is seen, the component astrocytes often showing swollen cytoplasm (gemistiocytic astrocytes).

(b) Traumatic herniation of brain tissue. This is seen occasionally after a particularly extensive nasal operation. Neurocytes are seen as well as glial tissue.

(c) Tumour-like formations of ectopic brain tissues sometimes present in the nose on areas such as the turbinates which are remote from the cribriform plate. These lesions usually show glial tissue only, but nerve cells may rarely be present (Fig. 33).

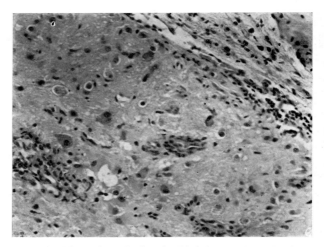

FIG. 33. Glioma (ganglioglioma) of inferior nasal concha (turbinate). The lesion is composed of astrocytes, glial fibres and occasional nerve cells. Note lymphocytic exudation around lobule of tumour. (H. & E. ×265.)

Olfactory Neuroblastoma

A tumour of the olfactory neurocytes has been more clearly categorized in recent years. It is also termed olfactory esthesioneuroblastoma and there has been a tendency to separate a more differentiated form, the olfactory esthesion-eurocytoma. The neoplasm originates high up in the nasal cavity; sometimes the ethmoid sinuses are involved. Occasionally the tumour is found in the nasal part of pharynx. Grossly the lesion is smooth, covered by mucosa and frequently polypoid. The neoplasm forms a characteristic pattern which can be recognized under the low power

Chondrosarcoma

This tumour, as would be expected, may arise from the nasal septum to fill the lumen of one or both sides of the nose. It may also present exteriorly from the cartilaginous superstructure or may appear to arise from the middle or inferior turbinates. Involvement of sinuses is not expected,

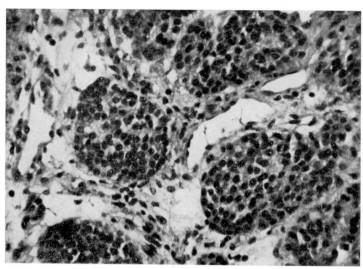

Fig. 34. Olfactory neuroblastoma. The photomicrograph is of the edge of the tumour where small lobules of tumour cells are present in a vascular stroma. (H. & E. ×380).

of the microscope. The tumour cells, composed of uniform round hyperchromatic nuclei with little cytoplasm, form rounded, lobular, well-defined masses.

The groups of cells at the edge of the tumour may be large or small, but are almost always rounded off into discrete collections and rarely appear to trail off as individual cells (Fig. 34). Rounded spaces often are seen between the tumour cells representing rosettes of the "pseudo" variety. When more glandular in appearance the rosettes are known as Flexner-Wintersteiner rosettes and if enclosing fibrillary material as Homer Wright rosettes, but these forms are rare in olfactory neuroblastoma. An axon stain such as the Bodian stain shows occasional fine axis cylinders between tumour cells (Fig. 35). Between the tumour cell masses there is a marked vascularity in most olfactory neuroblastomas, a feature which is again easily recognizable under the low power of the microscope.

The olfactory neuroblastoma is often mistaken for an anaplastic carcinoma, but the above light microscopical features help to separate it out quite distinctly as a separate entity when the histopathologist has some familiarity with it. Electron microscopical examination reveals membrane-bound neurosecretory granules in the cytoplasm of the tumour cells and neurites with neurofilaments and neuro-tubules, in confirmation of the neural nature of the tumour (Kahn, 1974). The tumour is locally aggressive and a small number of cases develop cervical lymph node and distant metastasis (Skolnick et al., 1966). Extensive surgical resection. irradiation or both measures have been recommended as therapy for this condition.

but in one case that I have seen the tumour invaded from the middle cranial fossa to involve the sphenoid sinus and nasal part of pharynx. Extensive involvement of the temporal bone with presentation in the nasal part of pharynx and middle ear has also been described (Leedham and Swash, 1972). The other site where the otolaryn-gological surgeon may expect to see chondrosarcoma from time to time is lamina of the cricoid cartilage.

Radiological evidence of invasion of nasal bones is to be expected. Histologically the features indicated by Lichten-stein and Jaffe (1943) as suggestive of malignancy in a cartilaginous lesion are useful in the recognition of these tumours. On this basis a cartilaginous lesion of the nose, ear or larynx showing any of the following features should be regarded as malignant: hypercellularity, enlargement, hyperchromatism or irregularity of nuclei; double or multiple nuclei; areas of dedifferentiation with appearance compatible with non specific sarcoma; marked enlargement of cartilage cells; mitotic figures among the cartilage cells (Fig. 36).

Difficulty may be experienced in distinguishing this lesion from pleomorphic adenoma. The presence of glandular acini is important in recognizing the latter. It may sometimes be useful to determine whether the alcian blue staining of the ground substance is diminished by hyaluronidase. The ground substance staining of cartilage is not eradicated by this enzyme in contradistinction to that of the epithelial mucin of mixed tumours. Difficulty may be further experienced in the differential diagnosis of a nasopharyngeal *chordoma* from chondrosarcoma. The

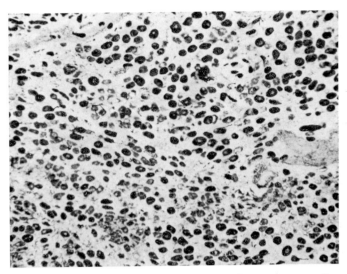

FIG. 35. Occasional very fine nerve fibres are seen between tumour cells. Bodian's nerve fibre stain. (×380.)

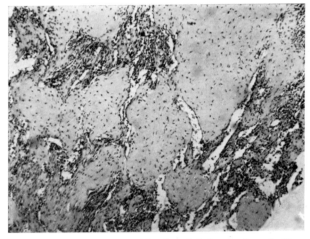

FIG. 36. Chondrosarcoma arising from inferior nasal concha (turbinate). Lobules of atypical cartilage are accompanied by groups of malignant mesenchymal cells. (H. & E. ×66.)

presence of physalliferous cells with the characteristic "soap bubble" cytoplasm is the accepted feature of chordoma but it must be admitted that the two conditions possess similarities in histological appearance and also in behaviour and may not always be distinguishable (Heffelfinger *et al.*, 1973).

Ossifying Fibroma

This lesion of the nose and sinuses has not been a well-defined entity in the literature. At times the terms osteoblastoma and osteoid osteoma have been applied to it, probably not accurately. It is stated to be synonymous with localized fibrous dyplasia and osteoma of the jawbones (Jaffe, 1958) but supposed histological differences from the former are sometimes invoked. Ossifying fibroma of the nose and sinuses has an approximately 2:1 ratio of incidence in females to males, a similar sex incidence to that of fibrous dysplasia in general. The tumour is found in the frontal or maxillary sinuses, within the bony walls of the sinuses and growing into the lumen where it may sometimes be covered by a layer of normal mucosa. In the nose it may arise from the turbinate bones particularly the middle turbinate and extend to fill the whole nasal cavity, sometimes growing into the nasal part of pharynx. The radiological appearances are those of a space occupying lesion involving the sinuses or facial bones and varying from radiolucent to dense depending upon the amount of bone present. Some lesions present a "ground glass" appearance produced by the fine bony deposits. Grossly the tumour is bony or gritty.

Three patterns of histological appearance may be recognized:

(1) This is found particularly in young people and shows oval, somewhat irregular, but not apparently anastomosing masses of primitive bone with central areas of calcification. These bony masses usually display flattened peripheral cells, probably the osteoblasts that have contributed to their formation. In the stroma between the calcified foci are spindle shaped cells of regular appearance (Fig. 37). These cells may display sometimes a somewhat whorled pattern resembling meningioma and the calcified bony foci characteristic of this form of ossifying fibroma may enhance the suspicion of psammoma bodies of meningioma, a lesion which may indeed be found sometimes in the nasal region.

(2) The feature of this variety of ossifying fibroma is the presence of anastomosing trabeculae of woven bone, confirmed as such by the lack of lamellar pattern of its constituent birefringent fibres. Again regular spindle cells and sometimes collagen are found between the trabeculae of woven bone. In all cases rows of osteoblasts are found on the surfaces of the trabeculae (Fig. 38).

(3) In this third pattern an anastomosing network of dense lamellar bony trabeculae is present. A poorly cellular intertrabecular stroma is present which may be quite vascular; in the latter case the possibility of the lesion representing a haemangioma of bone with the concomitant lamellar bony overgrowth that often accompanies such lesions should be considered. The borderline between this type of ossifying fibroma and osteoma, a well recognized entity in the region of the facial bones is impossible to define with certainty.

Osteosarcoma

This malignant tumour of bone is uncommon in the jawbones in comparison to the long bones. Aetiological factors that may be present are similar to those relating to osteosarcomas in other situations. In elderly patients presenting with this tumour the question of associated Paget's disease of the skeleton must be considered as an aetiological factor and clinical, radiological and biochemical studies should be carried out to elucidate this possibility. I have seen this tumour arising in the maxilla in a patient 23 years following irradiation of the nose for an unrelated tumour and also following ^{131}I treatment of papillary

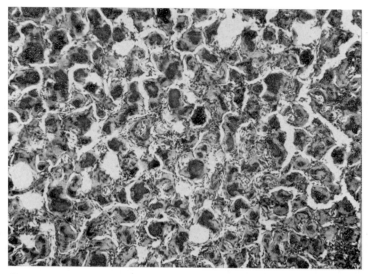

FIG. 37. Juvenile ossifying fibroma of concha. Rounded masses of bony tissue are separated by spindle cells. (H. & E. ×80.)

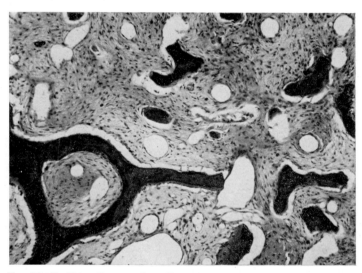

FIG. 38. Ossifying fibroma of maxilla. The lesion consists of anastomosing trabeculae of woven bone separated by fibroblastic cells. (H. & E. ×100.)

carcinoma of the thyroid; these examples of osteosarcoma in the upper jaw following irradiation recall the well-known radium watch-dial occupational osteosarcoma where, however, the long bones were the major sites of the lesions.

Osteosarcoma of the nose and sinuses usually involves the maxillary sinus and is found filling variable portions of the lumen as a fleshy, often haemorrhagic and frequently invading bony tumour. The ethmoid and sphenoid may also be involved as primary sites. The tumour spreads to invade the base of the skull and if the patient survives this, distant metastases particularly to the lungs are to be expected. Most patients are below the age of 30 except in the presence of concomitant Paget's disease.

The histological appearances are basically those of a sarcoma with superadded manifestations of bony tissue as osteoid, woven or lamellar bone. Cartilage is often quite prominent (Fig. 39). In the Paget's disease-associated osteosarcoma the features of that condition may also be seen in the biopsy if non-neoplastic bone is also available for examination, notably a mosaic appearance of cement lines indicating active bone deposition.

Giant Cell Tumour

A lesion of the nose and sinuses, under this category, is composed of multi-nucleated giant cells in a stroma of spindle cells. Such a lesion may fall into one of three separate groups:

(1) Benign giant cell tumour. It is questionable whether this condition is indeed a neoplasm and it is probable that it is identical to the epulis in the mouth sometimes termed giant cell reparative granuloma.

(2) The giant cell lesion associated with hyperparathyroidism often referred to as brown tumour from its frequently haemorrhagic nature (Fig. 40).

(3) An active neoplasm with a locally aggressive and sometimes metastatic activity equivalent to the giant cell tumour of long bones.

reparative granuloma and brown tumour of hyperparathyroidism on the one hand from the malignant giant cell tumour on the other hand. The benign lesions show cytoplasmic preponderance of their spindle cells and their giant cells are unevenly distributed and contain abundant cytoplasm. The malignant giant cell tumours show closely

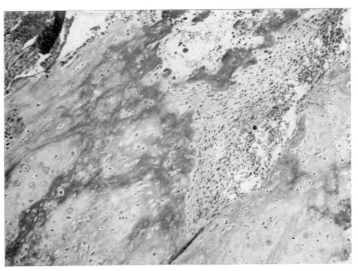

Fig. 39. Osteogenic sarcoma of nasal cavity. Tumour bone and cartilage are accompanied by malignant mesenchymal cells. (H. & E. ×100.)

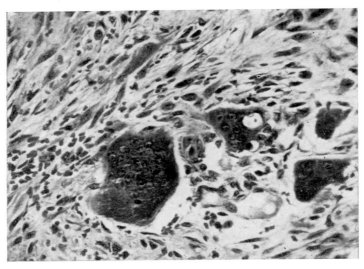

Fig. 40. "Brown tumour" of maxilla from a case of hyperparathyroidism secondary to renal failure. The infiltrate of giant cells and spindle cells could be indistinguishable from giant cell reparative granuloma. (H. & E ×480.)

These three conditions may be quite difficult to distinguish from each other histologically. The lesions in each group may be found in the nose, maxillary bone, filling the cavity of the sinus or invading the floor of the orbit. The sphenoid and ethmoid sinuses are sometimes also involved. The benign lesion of category (1) is usually seen below the age of 40. The malignant one presents at a later age group.

Friedberg and his colleagues (1969) give the histological criteria for distinguishing the benign entities of giant cell

packed spindle cells with large nuclei and giant cells which are uniformly distributed among the spindle cells and contain little cytoplasm. It must be admitted that while useful as a guide these criteria do not help in all cases. It is therefore essential in all cases of nasal tumours showing uniformly distributed giant cells in a cellular fibroblastic stroma that hyperparathyroidism be considered and excluded by clinical examination and serum calcium estimation. Secondary hyperparathyroidism (usually caused by renal failure) as well as the primary variety may lead to osseous maxillary giant cell lesions (Friedman *et al.*, 1974).

Nasopharyngeal Angiofibroma

The nasal part of pharynx shares many of the pathological processes described above in common with the nose and sinuses. It is exposed to, because of its content of lymphoid tissue and in keeping with the whole area of Waldeyer's ring, a much higher incidence of lymphoma, notably lymphosarcoma and also Hodgkin's disease. Amyloid deposits, which may recur after surgical removal, but rarely are associated with disseminated amyloidosis, are also more frequent in the nasal part of pharynx. Squamous carcinoma particularly the poorly differentiated and anaplastic varieties are more frequent in the nasal part of pharynx than in the nose and sinuses particularly in parts of Africa and in the Far East.

The nasopharyngeal angiofibroma, however, is a specific neoplasm confined to the nasal part of pharynx in young males. Considerable confusion has existed among clinicians and pathologists about this neoplasm; the problem is enhanced by the fact that choanal polyps are not uncommon in young people and may have a fibrous and/or vascular appearance. Following its origin in the nasal part of pharynx the nasopharyngeal angiofibromas may spread and become locally invasive. Fifteen per cent of these tumours show clinical evidence of extension to the maxillary sinus on the one or other side and the sphenoid sinus and sphenoid bone occasionally show evidence of invasion. Anterior extension into the nasal cavity is common.

The disorder is confined to males between 9 and 21 years of age. In an 18-year-old boy presenting with proptosis and X-ray evidence of erosion of the greater wing of the sphenoid, both his brother and his father had also been treated for nasopharyngeal angiofibroma. Such a family history is unusual, but indicates a possible genetic basis for the condition.

The neoplasm often presents a lobulated surface. Its deeper aspect frequently invades into the surrounding tissues. The vascularity of the surface and cut surface is marked, but the major feature of the neoplasm is its firm texture and the fibrous appearance of its cut surface.

The epithelium covering the lesion is often ulcerated. When present it may be normal mucosal squamous epithelium or respiratory columnar epithelium, as indeed may the normal nasopharyngeal lining be in this area. The tumour is composed of abnormal blood vessels and a fibrous stroma. The blood vessels may show a number of abnormalities. In many cases they are extremely long and thin with little branching and are arranged in rows parallel to the surface of the tumour. Often a thick medial layer is present in which there arises a sudden gap so that the vessel becomes only the thickness of the endothelium at this point. In some angiofibromas numerous smaller vessels are seen in addition to the larger ones. The vessels in this tumour frequently show a surrounding zone of pale staining very loose connective tissue. I have not been able to relate the cellularity of the stroma to previous treatment or to the age of the patient. The characteristic cell is a fibrocyte. Sometimes the nuclei of these cells may become very bizarre,

but the presence of numerous blood vessels characteristic of nasopharyngeal angiofibroma enables a diagnosis of this benign lesion to be made (Figs. 41, 42 and 43).

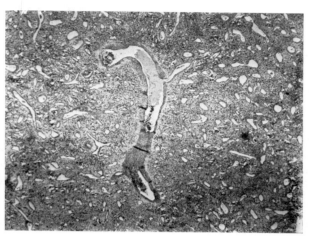

FIG. 41. Juvenile nasopharyngeal angiofibroma. Note abnormal blood vessels and stroma. (H. & E. ×20.)

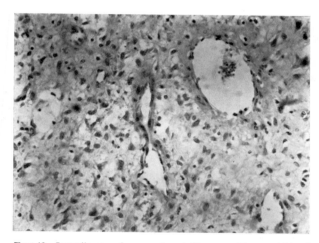

FIG. 42. Juvenile nasopharyngeal angiofibroma. Abnormal blood vessels and spindle cell stroma. (H. & E. ×265.)

HISTOPATHOLOGY OF THE TONSIL

In otolaryngological practice, biopsy material is submitted less frequently from the tonsil than from the nose, larynx or ear. Table 3 gives a list of diseases of the tonsil which may be encountered on biopsy.

Enlarged Tonsils

The removal of these structures for inflammatory disease is the commonest surgical procedure in otolaryngology. It is, perhaps, fortunate that they are submitted to the histopathologist more usually as a means of disposal of the specimen than with any problem as to the nature of the pathological change, for changes are difficult to interpret and usually non-specific. Nevertheless the tonsils (and accompanying adenoids) should be submitted to histological examination if only as a screening procedure to exclude early changes of a specific inflammatory or neoplastic

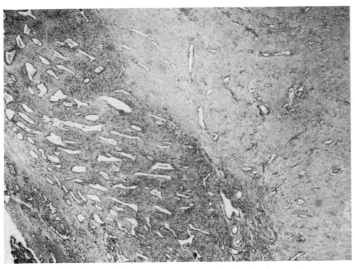

FIG. 43. Juvenile nasopharyngeal angiofibroma. This appearance of alternating layers of tumour with varying vascularity and stromal fibrosis is sometimes encountered but cannot be related to previous treatment. (H. & E. ×30.)

condition. Changes seen in the majority of tonsils removed for inflammation include lymphoid hyperplasia, foci of acute inflammation usually in the crypts and plasma cell infiltration, usually under the squamous epithelium, areas of fibrosis and small retention cysts of squamous epithelium (Porcelli, 1950). The relationship of these changes to the patient's clinical state is indistinct. It is likely that immunological and virological studies will yield more useful information in this regard than histopathology alone.

TABLE 3

PATHOLOGICAL CONDITIONS OF THE PALATINE TONSIL THAT MAY BE ENCOUNTERED ON BIOPSY

Inflammatory Diseases
Infections:

   (a) bacterial—acute follicular tonsillitis, diphtheria, syphilis, tuberculosis
   (b) virus—measles (Warthin-Finkeldy giant cells)
   (c) fungal—actinomycosis, North American blastomycosis
   (d) parasitic—trichiniasis

Unknown cause—hyperkeratosis pharyngis, lymphoid hyperplasia, fibrosis, tonsillolith, sarcoidosis
Degenerative—cholesterol granuloma, cartilage and/or bone deposition squamous retention cyst
Storage disease—Tangier disease

Neoplasms
Squamous epithelium—squamous papilloma, squamous carcinoma
Melanocytes—malignant melanoma
Seromucinous glands—mixed tumour (pleomorphic adenoma), muco-epidermoid tumour, adenocystic carcinoma, cystadenoma lymphomatosum (Warthin's tumour)
Blood vessels—haemangioma, Kaposi's sarcoma
Lymphatic vessels—lymphangioma
Muscle—rhabdomyosarcoma
Lymphoid tissue—pedunculated lymphoid tumour, lymphosarcoma, reticulum cell sarcoma, Hodgkin's disease, plasmacytoma

Hodgkin's Disease

It is commonly stated that Hodgkin's disease of the tonsil and nasal part of pharynx is very rare. Todd and Michaels (1974) saw 16 cases in Waldeyer's ring comprising 7 in the tonsil, 1 in the posterior pharyngeal wall and 8 in the nasal part of pharynx. The course of the disease process did not differ in these patients from that of the general pattern of Hodgkin's disease. The histopathological pattern however was of considerable interest. Using the Rye classification of Hodgkin's disease histology (Lukes *et al.*, 1966) most of the nasopharyngeal cases of Hodgkin's disease were of mixed cellularity type of the usual pattern. The majority of the cases of Hodgkin's disease involving the palatine tonsil were also classified as of mixed cellularity appearance, but in 4 of these cases a distinctly granulomatous appearance of the Hodgkin's neoplastic tissue was adopted (Figs. 44 and 45). This had been described by Lennert and Mestdagh (1968) as being a distinct feature of Hodgkin's disease in the tonsil. We, too, found it only in tonsillar cases, but where cervical lymph nodes were also available in these cases a granulomatous form of Hodgkin's infiltrate was present in the latter. The significance of this change is unknown and further study of these tonsillar Hodgkin's changes is indicated. Pathologists should endeavour to carry out histological examination of Waldeyer's ring in cases of Hodgkin's disease coming to post-mortem.

Tangier Disease and Other Lipidoses

In the tonsils as in the paranasal sinuses and middle ear, cholesterol ester crystals with foreign body giant cell reaction may result from a focal haemorrhage. Macrophages laden with cholesterol ester may accumulate also in the tonsil in a rare form of inherited lipoprotein disturbance which was first described among a group of families living on Tangier Island in Chesapeake Bay, Virginia. In patients with this condition, known as Tangier

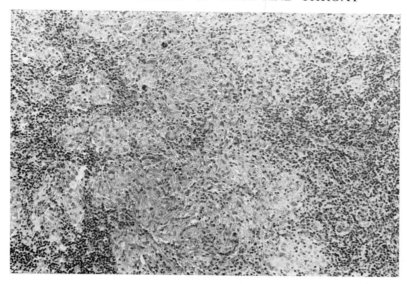

FIG. 44. Granulomatous Hodgkin's disease of tonsil. The neoplastic infiltrate is composed of epitheloid cells with occasional giant cells. (H. & E. ×175.)

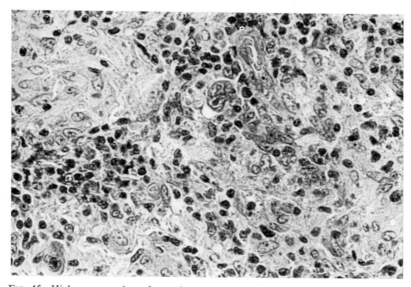

FIG. 45. Higher power view of granulomatous Hodgkin's disease of tonsil shows Reed Sternberg cell just above centre in a field of epithelioid cells. (H. & E. ×300.)

disease, plasma cholesterol levels are low while α_1-lipoproteins in plasma are absent (Fredrickson, 1964). The tonsils are enlarged by bright yellow streaks which are composed of collections of finely granular macrophages present mainly between the lymphoid follicles (Fig. 46). These cells are not accompanied by an inflammatory exudate of neutrophils and plasma cells. In Gaucher's disease the cytoplasmic granules stain green with Masson's trichrome and most other reticuloendothelial storage diseases contain granules which stain red by the P.A.S. method. In Tangier disease the cytoplasmic granules do not stain by this method. The affected cells may also be found in Tangier disease in the nasopharyngeal adenoidal tissue and in lymph nodes, thymus, colon, pyelonephritic scars of the kidney and in the ureter (Bale *et al.*, 1971).

HISTOPATHOLOGY OF THE LARYNX

Histological examination of biopsy material removed from the larynx at direct laryngoscopy plays an important part in the diagnosis of laryngeal disease. The use of the dissecting microscope in the observation of the larynx and the identification of areas to be selected for biopsy has enhanced the accuracy of diagnosis and treatment in this area. Table 4 shows the main lesions which may be encountered at biopsy.

Laryngeal Nodule

The commonest lesion encountered by the histopathologist in endoscopically removed biopsies is the laryngeal nodule. This lesion is often referred to as the vocal fold

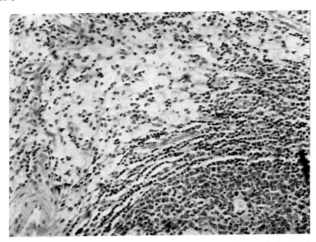

Fig. 46. Tangier disease involving adenoidal tissue. Pale lipid containing cells are present at the edge of a lymphoid follicle. (H. & E. × 300.)

(cord) polyp but, while the latter is an accurate designation of the advanced form of this condition, which appears as a polypoid protuberance from the vocal fold, the early stages may appear as a diffuse swelling of the fold (cord) or a localized thickening. These lesions are the result of the overuse of the vocal fold with resulting exudation of blood and blood products. Reinke's space of the vocal fold,

TABLE 4

PATHOLOGICAL CONDITIONS OF THE LARYNX THAT MAY BE ENCOUNTERED
ON BIOPSY

Inflammatory Diseases
Infections:

(a) bacterial—diphtheria, tuberculosis, scleroma, syphilis, lepromatous leprosy
(b) fungal—North American blastomycosis, coccidioidomycosis, histoplasmosis, moniliasis, actinomycosis, rhinosporidiosis
(c) parasitic—leishmaniasis, trichinosis

Auto-immune conditions—pemphigus, relapsing polychondritis
Unknown cause—Wegener's granuloma, sarcoidosis
Trauma—contact ulcer, intubation granuloma, laryngeal nodule (vocal fold polyp)
Endocrine deficiency—myxoedema
Lipidosis—lipoidosis cutis et mucosae

Neoplasms
Respiratory epithelium and seromucinous glands—adenocarcinoma, adenocystic carcinoma and carcinoid tumour
Squamous epithelium—squamous papilloma, pachyderma laryngis, dysplasia with or without hyperkeratosis, carcinoma *in situ*, invasive squamous carcinoma
Blood vessels—haemangioma
Muscle—rhabdomyosarcoma, granular cell myoblastoma
Lymphoid tissue—lymphoid hyperplasia, lymphosarcoma, plasmacytoma
Connective tissue—pedunculated fibroma, lipoma
Nervous system—neurilemmoma, neurofibroma
Cartilage—chondrosarcoma
Connective tissue—fibroma, fibrosarcoma
Nervous system—neurilemmoma, neurofibroma
Paraganglionic tissue—paraganglioma
Cartilage and bone—tracheopathia osteoblastica, chondroma, chondrosarcoma
Metastatic neoplasms

limited superficially by the squamous epithelium of the vocal fold and on the deep aspect by a thick elastic layer—the conus elasticus—does not possess the lymph drainage that is necessary to remove the exuded blood products. These then accumulate within that space and give rise to a variety of histological alterations. Almost all biopsies of laryngeal nodules show fibrin lying in the connective tissue and within dilated vessels. These amorphous eosinophilic deposits give an amyloid type of appearance to the biopsy but special stains for fibrin such as phosphotungstic acid haematoxylin and the Gram stain are usually positive while stains for amyloid are negative. Oedema, often of a basophilic type, frank haemorrhage and haemosiderin-containing macrophages are frequent. Fibroblasts may appear to have proliferated in the oedematous ground substance and some newly formed blood vessels may be present (Fig. 47). Patients with myxoedema may sometimes become hoarse and the vocal folds will be seen to be swollen. Biopsy examination shows histological appearances indisguishable from the basophilic oedematous form of the laryngeal nodule but in this case it is due to the deposition of the characteristic mucoid ground substance of myxoedema in the vocal fold.

Intubation Granuloma

Biopsies taken from this condition sometimes present a problem in diagnosis to the histopathologist. The histological appearances of this post-intubation lesion, which is always seen in the posterior part of the vocal fold are quite specific. The whole lesion has a spherical shape and projects somewhat above the level of the squamous epithelial surface of the vocal fold which it has replaced focally. The granuloma is composed mainly of vascular granulation tissue with a surface layer of fibrin. Usually there is a history of anaesthetic intubation. Recurrence of the lesion after attempts at local removal is quite common.

Laryngeal Cyst

Small cysts of the larynx are commonly removed at endoscopic biopsy. Most of these are situated in the vestibular fold (false cord) where they are the result of distension of the obstructed duct of a seromucinous gland. In these cases the adjacent seromucinous glands have undergone an oncocytic change—an eosinophilic granular transformation of cytoplasm (associated electron microscopically with an increase in mitochondria). It is likely that the "eosinophilic granular cell cyst" (Pinkerton and Beck, 1961) is mainly a mucous retention cyst of the larynx with oncocytic change of the adjacent seromucinous glands (Fig. 48). Small squamous epithelial lined retention cysts of the larynx are also encountered on endoscopic biopsy.

Haemangioma

Small cavernous or capillary haemangiomas are seen sometimes at biopsy mainly of the vocal folds. A lesion of particular urgency is the infantile subglottic haemangioma. This is easily recognized histologically as a tumour composed of closely packed blood vessels lined by swollen endothelial cells, identical to the cutaneous "haemangioendotheliomas" typically found in infants and likely to

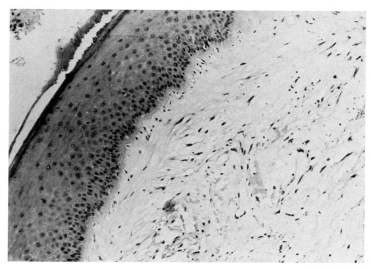

FIG. 47. Laryngeal nodule. Note fibrin deposition and increased vascularity of corium of vocal fold. The squamous epithelium shows hyperkeratosis with slight dysplasia and thickening of its basement membrane. (H. & E. ×300.)

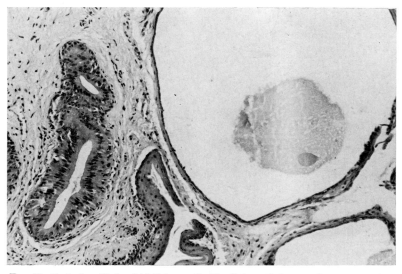

FIG. 48. Cyst of vestibular fold (false cord). The lining cells have undergone atrophy. Adjacent seromucinous glands show oncocytic change. (H. & E ×300.)

disappear spontaneously if left alone. The particular problem of these lesions in the subglottic position is that they are liable to produce stridor by obstruction of the narrow infantile tracheal lumen and even sudden death (Ferguson and Flake, 1961).

Squamous Papillomas

Squamous papillomas are common in the larynx and are usually seen on the vocal folds. The majority of case are single and in patients above the age of 20. They are usually cured by simple excision. The multiple recurrent lesions are usually in children and young adults. They may spread all over the larynx and into the trachea and bronchi. The histological appearance in both varieties of squamous papilloma is that of papillomatosis, multiple upward growths of squamous epithelium towards the lumen, with

their own cores of connective tissue. The squamous epithelium usually shows hyperkeratosis and parakeratosis. Dysplasia is present to a mild degree but is never serious enough to give concern about a possible malignant potential of the lesion (Fig. 49). We have sought virus particles electron microscopically in 10 biopsy specimens of the juvenile form of squamous papilloma of the larynx using both the tissue sectioning and negative staining methods, but have not found such particles.

Neurogenic Tumours

Neurilemmomas and neurofibromas are seen in the larynx from time to time and in the majority of cases the tumour is situated in the aryepiglottic fold bulging into the supraglottic space; it seems likely that a branch of the superior laryngeal nerve is involved in these cases. A few

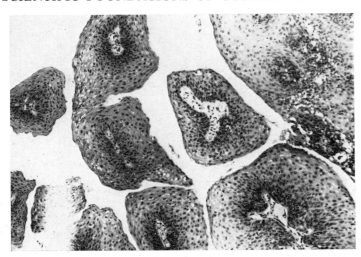

Fig. 49   Squamous papilloma of vocal fold. Frond-like projections with a central core of connective tissue and an outer covering of squamous epithelium. (H. & E. ×175)

cases have involved the vocal folds. Association with multiple neurofibromatosis (von Recklinghausen's disease) is encountered only rarely, there being 13 cases showing such an association in the world literature (Cummings *et al.*, 1969). The histological features of these growths are similar to those of neurogenic tumours elsewhere (*see above*). Ash *et al.* (1964) in a review of neurogenic tumours of the upper respiratory tract state that laryngeal neurogenic tumours are mostly of the neurofibromatous variety; more proximately in the mouth and pharynx neurilemmomas will predominate. Malignant transformation of only one case in each of these histological groups has been described in the larynx (Cummings *et al.*, 1969).

Granular Cell Tumour or "Myoblastoma"

The lesion which is commonly seen in surgical histology practice in such sites as subcutaneous tissue, tongue and other mucosal surfaces is well known also in the larynx. As its name implies it is composed of granular cells but its origin from primitive muscle cells has by no means been proven and indeed even its neoplastic nature is not certain. Most cases of granular cell tumour of the larynx present in the fourth decade. Males outnumber females in the ratio of 2:1. The laryngeal lesion usually arises on the vocal fold and without a predilection for any particular zone of that structure. The tumour is a sessile, raised swelling with a smooth mucosal covering. The histological characteristic of the lesion is the presence of rows and masses of cells with granular, eosinophilic cytoplasm. The nuclei are usually small and inconspicuous. Interstitial fibrous tissue is commonly found and the base of the lesion often gives an impression of deep invasion which belies the benign course of the disease (Fig. 50). The cytoplasmic granules are eosinophilic by ordinary staining and strongly positive by the periodic acid Schiff method. Their appearance by electron microscopy is quite specific and this may be a useful adjunct to histological diagnosis. The granules are irregular and up to 1 micrometre in diameter with a

specifically complex appearance of granular, vesicular tubular and amorphous components.

In the larynx, as in other mucosal surfaces, pseudo-epitheliomatous hyperplasia of the overlying squamous epithelium commonly, but not invariably, takes place. The proliferated squamous cells do not have significant dysplastic features. The differential diagnosis is from a histiocytic inflammatory lesion and paraganglioma. In the former pleocytosis is present while in granular cell tumour the cells are uniform. In paraganglioma, a much rarer layngeal neoplasm, the nuclear size of the tumour cells is greater, the granularity of the cells is less obvious and there is a considerable vascularity. Periodic acid Schiff staining does not show red cytoplasmic granularity in a paraganglioma, and in the latter electron microscopy reveals small membrane bound uniform granules. Malacoplakia is a lesion which has recently been identified in several cases in the upper respiratory tract (Hyams, 1974) where it might be confused with a granular cell tumour. The diagnosis would be made by the presence of Michaelis-Guttmann bodies; sometimes these structures are inconspicuous, the lesion consisting largely of histiocytic cells rather similar to the cells of granular cell myoblastoma. Squamous carcinoma may be erroneously diagnosed if a superficial biopsy shows the acanthotic squamous epithelium and the granular cells are not seen.

SQUAMOUS CARCINOMA OF THE UPPER RESPIRATORY TRACT

The frequency and importance of squamous carcinoma in the otolaryngological area suggest a need here for a separate discussion of the histopathology of this condition. Pathologists should be familiar with the patterns of growth of this tumour and otolaryngologists should also possess a good understanding of this field because their method of treatment will be dependent on the pathological findings. Some confusion of terminology and interpretation has crept into this subject and it would now seem desirable for histopathologists to review the matter objectively.

Histogenesis of Squamous Carcinoma

Squamous carcinoma arises from stratified squamous epithelium. This is a multi-layered covering in which mitotic activity is confined to the basal layers, and, as a

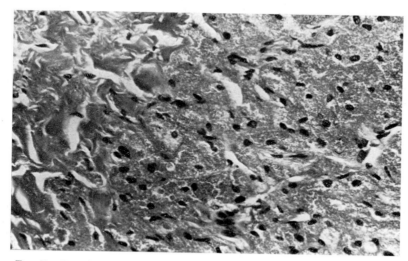

FIG. 50. Granular cell myoblastoma of vocal fold. Large cells with finely granular cytoplasm and small pyknotic nuclei. The amorphous material on the left is collagen. (H. & E. ×300).

result of this proliferation cells are pushed upwards and towards the surface where they undergo increasing differentiation. The latter is observed in the light microscope as the development of multiple "prickles" or fine inter-cellular bridges and an increase of keratinization culminating in the appearance on the surface of flattened dead cells composed largely of keratin. Electron microscopically the increased numbers of "prickles" are seen as an increase of intercellular processes each with a desmosome separating the cytoplasm of one cell from that of the other. Deeper cells possess tonofibrils which are related to the process of keratinization, and these structures increase in numbers towards the differentiated surface of the squamous epithelium. Squamous carcinoma may arise from an epithelium which has been of stratified squamous type *ab initio* or it may arise from squamous epithelium which is metaplastic in an area where the normal covering is columnar (usually of the pseudostratified, respiratory type in the upper respiratory tract). Such squamous metaplasia is frequent in the upper respiratory tract and because both the metaplastic epithelium and the squamous carcinoma derived from it are usually scanty producers of keratin the concept of "transitional" epithelium and "transitional" carcinoma has arisen. I do not feel that such a distinction is justified and believe that the concept of transitional carcinoma confuses the scientific appraisal of the tumour (*see below*).

The process of malignancy commences in the deepest aspects of the squamous epithelium. Cells produced there show nuclear atypia with irregularities of the nuclear membrane, an increase in nuclear chromatin content and

an irregularity of its distribution and an increase of nuclear size relative to the cytoplasm. These changes, which would be recognized as malignant in cytological preparations of individual cells, are collectively referred to as dysplastic or atypical. This process spreads from the basal layers to involve increasing amounts of the epithelium. It may be accompanied by hyperkeratosis (an increase of fully keratinized cells at the surface) but the latter has no ominous significance in itself (Fig. 51). The term leukoplakia, commonly representing a combination of hyperkeratosis and dysplasia should be abandoned in favour

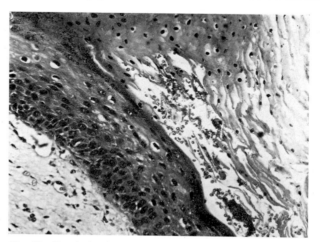

FIG. 51. Dysplasia of vocal fold with hyperkeratosis. The deeper four or five layers of cells are atypical. Note the presence of a granular layer. There is haemorrhage in the hyperkeratotic zone induced by the trauma of the biopsy operation. (H. & E. ×265.)

of a statement that there is hyperkeratosis together with an assessment of the degree of the dysplasia. It is only the latter that is important in the classification of the malignant potential of the lesion. When the whole thickness of the squamous epithelium has become involved by the dysplastic process the condition is now one of carcinoma *in situ* or intraepithelial carcinoma (Fig. 52). It is not known for how long the epithelium remains in this condition before the commencement of invasion, that is the penetration of tongues of malignant epithelium into the underlying

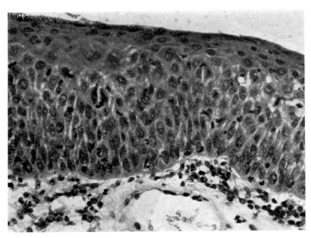

Fig. 52. Carcinoma *in situ* of vocal fold. All layers of squamous epithelial cells show atypical change and there is complete loss of cell polarity. (H. & E. ×265.)

connective tissue. It is likely that this takes a variable time and in some cases invasion may take place as soon as malignant cells have occupied the full thickness of the epithelium or even when only a small proportion of the epithelial thickness has become dysplastic. It is important to realize that these processes often involve a wide area of squamous epithelium. Dysplasia, carcinoma *in situ* and invasive carcinoma may be present simultaneously and if either of the former two lesions is present in a biopsy invasive carcinoma may be present in an unbiopsied area of mucosa. Thus these lesions should be regarded as serious ones, the patient kept under close observation and the biopsies repeated if any area shows the slightest suspicion of invasiveness.

Differentiation of Squamous Carcinoma

The method commonly used by histopathologists to assess the degree of differentiation of squamous carcinoma is that of the overall impression. The assessment is based on the least differentiated parts of the tumour and, depending on the degree of prickle formation and features of keratinization together with the overall degree of resemblance of the carcinoma to normal squamous epithelium the lesion is classified as well, moderately or poorly differentiated. The more differentiated the growth the less likely it is to recur locally after treatment and to metastasize to lymph nodes and by the blood stream; such is the assumption based on the idea that the speed of growth of the tumour and hence its likelihood to metastasize is inversely related to its differentiation. That there is some accuracy in this prediction is shown by the work of McGavran and his colleagues (1961) who studied the relationship between the degree of differentiation of the primary growth in 96 cases of squamous carcinoma of the larynx to the incidence of

lymph node metastasis. The cases of well differentiated squamous carcinoma showed 11 per cent metastasis, the moderately differentiated ones 22 per cent and of the poorly differentiated ones 49 per cent metastasized to cervical lymph nodes. This method is open to the serious criticism that the degree of differentiation presented by a small biopsy may be quite different from the overall differentiation of the main tumour mass. McGavran and his colleagues (1961) however found a fairly good correlation between the biopsy and the tumour as seen in the laryngectomy specimen. Nevertheless, although widely used because of its simplicity most pathologists are aware of the limitations of the method: the subjectivity of some of the criteria of differentiation used, the doubts about consistency between different observers of the same material and the same observer viewing the material at different times and the lack of adequate quantitation. The method of Broders in which the squamous carcinoma is classified as Grade I, II, III or IV on the basis of the enumeration of differentiated cells (Grade IV having the least number of differentiated cells) would seem to answer the last criticism. It has been admitted by proponents of the Broders method, however, that actual counting of the cells is impracticable and that other histological criteria, such as mitotic figures, should be taken into consideration in grading by the Broders method (Edmundson, 1948). This method, then, in the way that it is practised would seem to offer little or no improvement over the overall impression method. A satisfactorily objective method of prognosticating the growth potential of the cancer on the basis of its histological appearance has yet to be devised. It is likely that measurement of a number of cellular criteria including nuclear size and the use of a computer to analyse the data will replace the above methods as determinants of prognosis, but the new methods will require histopathologists to utilize more technical expertise and will be very time consuming.

Growth Patterns of Squamous Carcinoma

Squamous carcinoma may present a variety of patterns in addition to the variations of differentiation described above.

(a) Squamous Carcinoma with Infiltrating and Pushing Margins

Actively growing squamous carcinomas show an irregular jagged margin (Fig. 53) while tumours of slower growth have a more rounded lobular type of growing edge (Fig. 54). It has been shown that this change parallels squamous differentiation. Non-keratinizing carcinomas are associated with infiltrating margins to a significant degree, but well-differentiated tumours tend to have blunt margins. The tumours with infiltrating margins have a much higher incidence of lymph node metastasis (McGavran *et al.*, 1961). The degree of tumour alteration towards the infiltrating or blunt type has not been placed on a numerical basis; a useful approach towards such an investigation might be to assess the ratio of tumour area to the length of

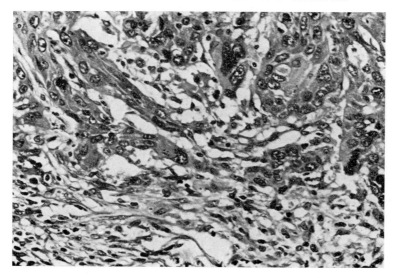

FIG. 43. Squamous carcinoma of larynx with infiltrating type of edge. Thin tongues of tumour cells penetrate the connective tissue. (H. & E. ×285.)

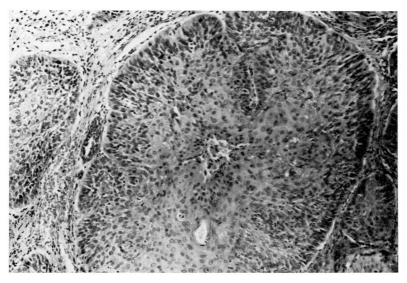

FIG. 54. Squamous carcinoma with "pushing" type edge. Rounded lobules of tumour cells constitute the margin. (H. &. E. ×285.)

growing edge by a standard method of histological quantitation. A higher ratio by this method might be expected to be associated with a lower yield of lymph node metastasis.

(b) Verrucous Squamous Carcinoma

Verrucous squamous carcinoma is a highly differentiated variant of squamous carcinoma which may develop in any mucosal surface of the nose and throat. It is a slowly growing neoplasm and rarely metastasizes to lymph nodes, but it may burrow deeply. Histologically it presents as a highly differentiated squamous neoplasm usually with a papillary structure over a wide base (Fig. 55). An important feature is said to be the presence of deep clefts visible to the naked eye within the tumour and microscopically lined by squamous epithelium. These clefts burrow from the surface deeply into the substance of the growth (Dockerty *et al.*,

1968). Two matters of practical importance arise in connection with this tumour. Firstly, on account of its great differentiation, the tumour may be mistaken by the histopathologist as a benign lesion, usually squamous papilloma and recurrence after several attempts at strictly local resection may take place before it is realized that it is in fact a well-differentiated malignant one. Secondly evidence exists that treatment of verrucous squamous carcinomas by radiotherapy may convert this neoplasm into a rapidly growing, metastasizing one with loss of histological differentiation (Proffitt *et al.*, 1970). When all has been said it must be admitted that doubt still exists as to the separation of verrucous squamous carcinoma as a clear cut entity from other squamous carcinomas. The study of many more cases is necessary particularly as regards its distinction from well-differentiated squamous carcinoma.

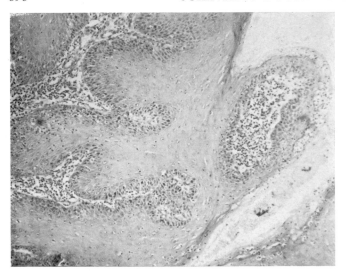

FIG. 55. Verrucous [squamous carcinoma of the mouth. Note large irregular rete pegs. (H. & E. ×80.)

(c) Spindle Cell Carcinoma

In association with or following treatment of squamous carcinoma of the head and neck there has been observed on many occasions the development of a tissue process composed of elongated cells resembling connective tissue.

concomitant undoubted squamous cell carcinoma which is often in the base or stalk of the polypoid masses. The carcinoma is often observed to be streaming off its cells into the spindle cell element (Fig. 56). The morphology of the latter is variable and there may be a close resemblance to fibrosarcoma, but at the junction of the squamous carcinoma and the spindle cell growth the cells are clearly of the same type. There is little doubt that this spindle cell lesion represents neither a reactive process nor a carcinosarcoma, but a variant of squamous carcinoma in which the carcinoma cells have developed a peculiar propensity for growing as spindle cells (Hyams, 1974b). This histological variation may be seen in lymph node metastasis of primary tumours exhibiting the spindle cell pattern. An analysis of 20 cases of spindle cell carcinoma of the larynx by Hyams (1974b) refuted the contention that this entity is of low-grade malignancy. It should be treated by radical, surgical and radiotherapeutic procedures similar to those which would be employed were the growth of the usual squamous histological appearance.

Squamous Carcinoma in the Nasal Part of Pharynx

In addition to squamous carcinoma of various degrees of differentiation and the special forms of squamous carcinoma described above, carcinomatous tumours are commonly seen in the upper respiratory tract which, although clearly of epithelial origin, show no differentiation

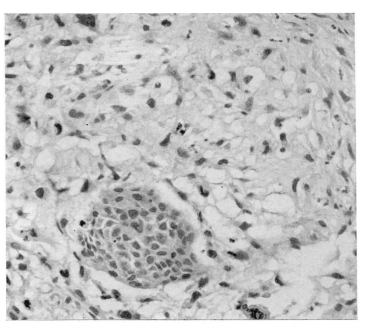

FIG. 56. Spindle cell carcinoma of vocal fold. The spindle cells are merging with cells of a downgrowth of invasive squamous carcinoma. (H. & E. ×250.)

This new formation, which is usually polypoid, has often been stated to represent a benign reactive process or pseudosarcoma (Lane, 1957) but the malignant course undoubtedly found in some cases has led to suggestions that this lesion represents a dual growth of sarcoma and carcinoma (Minckler *et al.*, 1970). Careful histological examination of these lesions leads to the discovery of

either in the squamous direction or towards a glandular structure. Such tumours are particularly common in the nasopharynx. Problems of terminology have arisen around these tumours which have appeared in many classifications and have haunted the pathology, surgery and radiotherapy of this field for at least 55 years. These problems would seem to arise from three main sources.

(1) The epithelium of the nasal part of pharynx, and also of other parts of Waldeyer's ring, has a close morphological relationship to the underlying lymphoid tissue and indeed recent immunological work has shown there is a shared function between lymphoid cells and epithelial cells in the production of secretory IgA. Perhaps largely because of the local presence of large amounts of lymphoid tissue, and also through a continuance of the same relationship in the process of epithelial neoplasia, carcinomas of the nasal part of pharynx are associated with large numbers of lymphocytes. This has given rise to the term "lympho-epithelioma" indicating a special form of tumour in which both types of cells share in the neoplastic process. Historically lympho-epitheliomas have been subdivided into the Regaud type (Jovin, 1926) in which columns of carcinoma cells are surrounded by lymphocytes and the Schminke-type (Schminke, 1921) in which the carcinoma cells are infiltrated by lymphocytes and may become individually scattered in a sea of lymphocytes (Fig. 57).

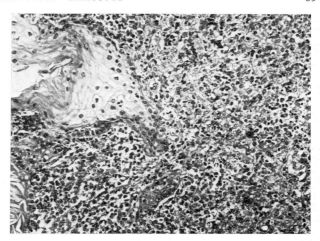

FIG. 58. Anaplastic carcinoma of nasal part of pharynx. Most of the tumour area show undifferentiated tumour cells prominently associated with lymphocytes. Necrosis is prominent. On the left is a squamous epithelial covering, the deeper cells of which are conspicuously giving rise to tumour. (H. & E. ×165.)

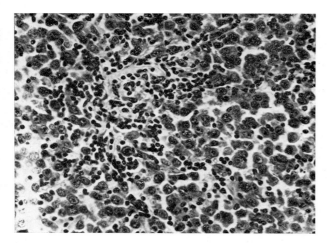

FIG. 57. "Lymphoepithelioma" of the nasal part of pharynx. Anaplastic squamous carcinoma cells are in close association with lymphocytes. (H. & E. ×265.)

A careful study of sections from cases of nasopharyngeal carcinoma has convinced me that these tumours in their undifferentiated form have a similar cellular constitution to more differentiated squamous carcinomas. The latter in some areas have a tendency to lose their "prickles" and keratinization and the cells in these areas may appear to fuse giving rise to the syncytial effect commonly associated with "lympho-epithelioma". The dropping off of tumour cells to form a sarcoma-like structure is well known in squamous carcinoma, as described above, and should such a process take place into lymphoid stroma the Schminke form of lympho-epithelioma will be accounted for. In about one-third of biopsies of undifferentiated nasopharyngeal carcinoma, careful examination will reveal squamous carcinoma *in situ* of the surface lining of the nasal part of pharynx or clear evidence of origin of carcinoma cells from the overlying squamous epithelium (Fig. 58). Electron microscopical examination of these undifferentiated neoplasms reveals the abundant tonofibrils and frequent desmosome-bearing intercellular pro-

cesses characteristic of squamous cells. When these tumours metastasize to a non-lymphoid organ such as the liver they are revealed as strictly epithelial tumours, free of lymphocytes. Lympho-epitheliomas are thus poorly differentiated squamous carcinomas with a close relationship to lymphocytes (with perhaps undiscovered tissue relationships additional to mere topographical proximity or immunological T-cell reaction) but nonetheless essentially epithelial tumours.

(2) An additional term that has given rise to confusion in this field, but which has been widely adopted, is transitional cell carcinoma. This has come about, as described above through the apparent existence of a form of epithelium in the upper respiratory tract "transitional" between the squamous and columnar. Thus tumours of rather regular, but undifferentiated, epithelial cells without the lymphoid stroma of lympho-epithelioma have been called transitional cell carcinomas particularly when seen to be arising from a transitional type of surface epithelium (Ewing, 1929). These tumours are also said to have a better outlook for the patient than squamous carcinomas or anaplastic carcinomas (Osborn, 1970). A study of tumours labelled as transitional carcinomas by other pathologists has convinced me of the essential squamous nature of these neoplasms; indeed it is difficult to support the separation of these tumours as a group at all since they merge with squamous carcinomas on the other hand and undifferentiated carcinoma on the other. It is not unreasonable to expect that squamous tumours in the upper respiratory tract will lack the keratinizing properties of squamous carcinoma of the skin, as the normal mucous membrane squamous epithelium is lacking in this respect. Because separation of these neoplasms as a histological entity is difficult, the assertion that transitional cell carcinomas have a better prognosis than other carcinomas is open to criticism. It seems likely that in putting these tumours into a group the proponents of the transitional cell concept have tended to select out two features: (a) those neoplasms

which are less keratinized and therefore more radiosensitive than more obviously squamous tumours and (b) neoplasms which have fewer features of dedifferentiation than anaplastic cancers and, therefore, are biologically less aggressive. A combination of these two features will give rise to a group with better prognosis, but the same results could probably be attained by typing on the basis of differentiation as discussed above.

(3) A third source of difficulty in the classification of nasopharyngeal carcinomas lies in the badly traumatized

have been described, but it is not generally realized that both irradiation and cytotoxic drugs can have a histologically differentiating effect on squamous carcinoma when effective. This phenomenon may prove to be of practical importance in future attempts to make therapy more specifically effective.

Glücksmann (1941) selected young areas of squamous carcinoma in biopsy represented by the buds of the growing edges of the tumour. In such areas he counted the entire cell population, determining the numbers of cells in each

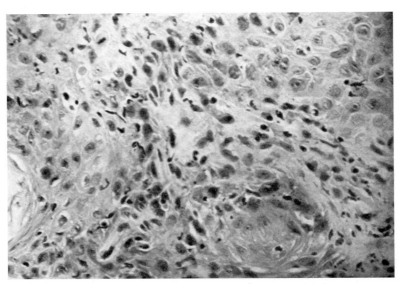

FIG. 59. Squamous carcinoma of the floor of the mouth. Biopsy before bleomycin treatment. (H. & E. ×300.)

appearance that many of the biopsies obtained from this situation show. This is because of the difficulty that is usually experienced by the surgeon in taking a satisfactory sample of tissue. Working without adequate visualization of the area to be biopsied usually from the front of the mouth with the necessity of obtaining tissue from behind and above the soft palate it is difficult to avoid the traumatizing action warned against in the first section of this chapter. As a consequence, and without criticism of the surgeon in this most difficult procedure, biopsy material from the nasopharynx often shows large areas of artefactual cell damage (Fig. 58). Frequently it is only just possible to recognize that there is a malignant tumour; the biopsy is too damaged for exact classification. Moreover since the standard treatment of nasopharyngeal carcinoma is irradiation a larger, more satisfactory surgical specimen will not be forthcoming to remedy the defects in histological identification. It must be admitted that nasopharyngeal tumours are among the most poorly studied malignant lesions for this reason and it is not, therefore, surprising that confusion exists in the literature on this subject.

Histological Effects of Treatment on Squamous Carcinoma

Non-specific effects of irradiation on squamous carcinoma such as necrosis, histiocytic and giant cell reaction

of four categories: dividing, degenerate, resting and differentiating. A similar study of a further biopsy taken from the patient was made after irradiation. It was found that in those tumours in which the subsequent appearance of the lesion indicated a favourable response to irradiation the numbers of differentiated cells increased after irradiation while the mitotic cells decreased. No such change was found in cases in which the response was poor. These observations, which have not passed into routine use account for the frequency of highly keratinizing squamous carcinoma seen in primary tumour sites and in lymph nodes of the head and neck after treatment by irradiation (Sclare, 1974).

Few cytotoxic drugs are effective against squamous carcinoma. Bleomycin, an antibiotic isolated in Japan in 1965 from the fungus *Streptomyces verticillus* has, however, been found to be particularly active against this tumour and the absence of toxic effects on the haemopoietic system enhances its value as a cytotoxic drug in head and neck squamous carcinoma (Grey and Michaels, 1972). We have found in serial biopsies taken of otolaryngeal squamous carcinoma that, in general, in those cases in which clinical shrinkage of the tumour was subsequently observed, keratinization became more pronounced in individual tumour cells and keratin pearls became larger and more numerous (Figs. 59, 60 and 61). Using the ultrastructural

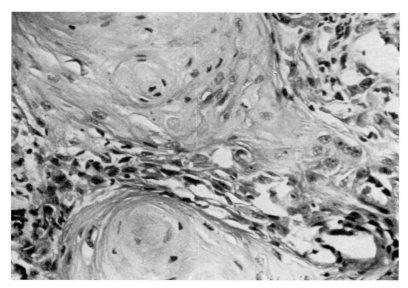

Fig. 60. Biopsy of tumour shown in Fig. 11 seven days after commencing therapy with bleomycin. Note increased keratinization. (H. & E. ×300.)

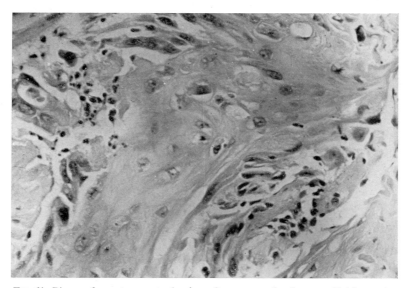

Fig. 61. Biopsy of same tumour twelve days after commencing therapy with bleomycin. Keratinization has advanced still further. (H. & E. ×300.)

criteria of tonofibrils and desmosome increase we noted a similar effect of bleomycin *in vivo* using a transplanted, poorly differentiated squamous carcinoma in mice and *in vitro* using the cells in monolayer tissue culture of a human, laryngeal squamous carcinoma (Michaels *et al.*, 1973).

A likely explanation for the increased squamous differentiation seen after treatment by both irradiation and cytotoxic drugs is that the actively dividing cells in the tumour are killed by these forms of therapy; the cells that survive will be the more differentiated ones, since they are resistant to both radiation and cytotoxic drugs. When a section of tissue is examined microscopically after treatment, a sample of approximately the same size is examined as in the pre-treatment biopsy. It, therefore, appears that there has been an increase in differentiated cells, although what has really happened is that undifferentiated cells have been eliminated.

There has been very little attempt to apply such observations to help in the all-too-frequently unsuccessful attempts at non-surgical therapy of squamous carcinoma. It is possible that quantitation of this phenomenon may be of value as a control of such therapy.

Descriptions given in the above survey of nose and throat histopathology represent the experience gained in a study of material in both the Institute of Laryngology and Otology, London and the E.N.T. Section of the Armed Forces Institute of Pathology, Washington, D.C. I am indebted to Dr. V. J.

Hyams, Director of the latter for allowing me to work in his Department and for the benefit of many discussions on otoaryngological histopathology.

Many conditions in which histopathologists contribute to the diagnosis and treatment of patients with nose and throat disorders are not described in detail. Consideration is given particularly to the pathology of the nose because of the frequency with which nasal conditions present problems in diagnostic histopathology and because of the absence of detailed work in this field. For diseases of the ear reference may be made to the recently published work by Friedmann (1974). Evans and Cruickshank (1970) have produced a useful study of salivary gland tumours.

REFERENCES

Acheson, E. D., Cowdell, R. H., Hadfield, Esme and Macbeth, R. G. (1968), *Brit. med. J.*, **1**, 587.

Andrews, P. and Michaels, L. (1967), *Lancet*, **ii**, 85.

Ash, J. E., Beck, M. R. and Wilkes, J. D. (1968), "Tumors of the Upper Respiratory Tract and Ear," in *Atlas of Tumor Pathology*, Section IV, Facsimiles 12 and 13, p. 77. Washington, D.C.: Armed Forces Institute of Pathology.

Bale, Patricia, M., Clifton-Bligh, P., Benjamin, B. N. P. and Whyte, H. M. (1971), *J. clin. Path.*, **24**, 609.

Burston, H. H. (1959), *Laryngoscope*, **69**, 1.

Cowdell, R. H. (1968), Personal communication.

Cummings, C. W., Montgomery, W. W. and Balogh, K., Jr. (1969), *Ann. Otol.*, **78**, 76.

Dockerty, M. B., Parkhill, E. M., Dahlin, D. C., Woolner, L. B., Soule, E. H. and Harrison, E. G. (1968), "Tumors of the Oral Cavity and Pharynx," in *Atlas of Tumor Pathology*, Section IV, Fascicle 10b. Washington, D.C.: Armed Forces Institute of Pathology.

Eby, L. S., Johnson, D. S. and Baker, H. W. (1972), *Cancer*, **29**, 1160.

Edmundson, W. F. (1948), *Arch. Derm. Syph.*, **57**, 141.

Eggston, A. A. and Wolff, Dorothy (1947), *Histopathology of the Nose and Throat*, p. 640. Baltimore: Williams and Wilkins Co.

Eichel, B. S. and Mabery, J. E. (1968), *Laryngoscope*, **78**, 1367.

Eneroth, A. A., Fluur, E., Söderburg, G. and Anggard, A. (1970), *Laryngoscope*, **80**, 17.

Evans, R. W. and Cruikshank, A. H. (1970), *Epithelial Tumours of the Salivary Glands*. London: W. B. Saunders Co.

Ewing, J. (1929), *Amer. J. Path.*, **5**, 99.

Ferguson, C. F. and Flake, C. (1961), *Ann. Otol.*, **70**, 1095.

Fredrickson, D. S. (1964), *J. clin. Invest.*, **43**, 228.

Friedberg, S. A., Eisenstein, R. and Wallner, L. J. (1969), *Laryngoscope*, **79**, 763.

Friedman, W. H. Perves, N. and Schwartz, A. E. (1974), *Arch. Otolaryng.*, **100**, 157.

Friedmann, I. (1964), *Proc. roy. Soc. Med.*, **57**, 289.

Friedmann, I. (1974), *Pathology of the Ear*. Oxford: Blackwell Scientific Publications.

Gallagher, J. C. (1970), *Ann. Otol.*, **79**, 551.

Ghosh, B. C., Huvos, A. G., Gerold, F. P. and Miller, T. R. (1970), *Cancer*, **31**, 237.

Glücksmann, A. (1941), *Brit. J. Radiol.*, **14**, 187.

Grey, P. and Michaels, L. (1972), *Med. J. Aust.*, **2**, 246.

Harrison, D. F. N. (1971), *Ann. Otol.*, **80**, 6.

Harrison, D. F. N. (1974), *Brit. med. J.*, **4**, 205.

Healey, W. V., Persin, K. H. and Smith, L. (1970), *Calwer*, **26**, 368.

Heffelfinger, M. J., Dahlin, D. C., McCarty, C. S. and Beabout, J. W. (1973), *Cancer*, **32**, 410.

Hyams, V. J. (1971), *Ann. Otol.*, **80**, 192.

Hyams, V. J. (1974a). Personal communication.

Hyams, V. J. (1974b), *Canad. J. Otolaryng.* In press.

Jaffe, H. L. (1958), *Tumors and Tumorous Conditions of the Bones and Joints*, p. 426. Philadelphia: Lea and Febiger.

Jovin, L. B. (1926), *Ann. Mal. Oreil. Larynx*, **45**, 729.

Kahn, L. B. (1974), *Hum. Path.*, **5**, 364.

Keene, B. R. T. (1973), *Chem. Brit.*, **9**, 424

Kessel, S. H., Echevarria, R. A. and Guzzo, F. P. (1969), *Cancer*, **23**, 920.

Kirchner, J. A. (1969), *Ann. Otol.*, **78**, 689.

Lane, N. (1957), *Cancer*, **10**, 19.

Leedham, P. W. and Swash, M. (1972), *J. Path.*, **107**, 59.

Lennert, K. and Mestdagh, J. (1968), *Virchows Arch. path. Anat.*, **344**, 1.

Lichtenstein, L. and Jaffe, H. L. (1943), *Am. J. Path.*, **19**, 553.

Lukes, R. J., Craver, L. F., Hall, T. C., Rappaport, H. and Rubin, P. (1966), *Cancer Res.*, **26**, 1311.

McGavran, M. H., Bauer, W. C. and Ogura, J. H. (1961), *Cancer*, **14**, 55.

Michaels, L., Grey, P. A. and Rowson, K. E. K. (1973), *J. Path.*, **109**, 315.

Minckler, D. S., Meligro, C. H. and Norris, H. T. (1970), *Cancer*, **26**, 195.

Morgan, J. C. (1958), *Brit. J. industr. Med.*, **15**, 224.

Osborn, D. A. (1970), *Cancer*, **25**, 385.

Pinkerton, P. H. and Beck, J. S. (1961), *J. Path. Bact.*, **81**, 532.

Porcelli, T. (1950), *Minerva paediat.*, **2**, 593.

Proffitt, S. O., Spooner, T. R. and Kosek, J. C. (1970), *Cancer*, **26**, 389.

Schmincke, (1921), *Beitr. path. Anat.*, **48**, 161.

Sclare, G. (1974), "The Histological Effects of Radiotherapy on Squamous Carcinoma," Paper presented to the Pathological Society of Great Britain and Ireland, July 1974.

Skolnick, E. M., Massari, F. S. and Tenta, L. T. (1966), *Arch. Otolaryng.*, **84**, 644.

Stewart, J. P. (1933), *J. Laryng.*, **48**, 657.

Stout, A. P. and Murray, M. R. (1942), *Ann. Surg.*, **116**, 26.

Todd, G. B. and Michaels, L. (1974), *Cancer*. **34**, 1769.

Walike, J. W. and Bailey, B. J. (1971), *Arch. Otolaryng.*, **93**, 345.

Wu, A. and Michaels, L. (1969), *Canad. J. med. Technol.*, **31**, 224.

SECTION XII

MATERIA OTOLARYNGOLOGICA

		PAGE
50.	GENERAL ASPECTS	703
51.	CYTOTOXIC DRUGS	725
52.	RADIOTHERAPY	733
53.	BLOOD TRANSFUSION	749
54.	SURGICAL IMPLANTS	762
55.	TRACHEOSTOMY TUBES	766
56.	AUDIOMETERS	772
57.	AUDIOMETRY	788
58.	CONDITIONS FOR HEARING TESTS	800
59.	AUDITORY PROSTHESES	805
60.	SELECTION OF HEARING AIDS	824
61.	ELECTROACOUSTIC REHABILITATION EQUIPMENT OTHER THAN HEARING AIDS	830
62.	AUDITORY REHABILITATION	839

50. MATERIA OTOLARYNGOLOGICA
GENERAL ASPECTS

R. HINCHCLIFFE

There is now a vast range of equipment and preparations which is available to the otolaryngologist. For purposes of discussion, these are classified into four groups (Table 1). Some of these the otolaryngologist shares equally with

TABLE 1
MATERIA OTORHINOLARYNGOLOGICA

I. Drugs
   A. Diagnostic
   B. Therapeutic
II. Ionizing Radiations
   A. Diagnostic
   B. Therapeutic
III. Structural Materials
   A. Animal tissues, i.e. transplants (grafts)
   B. Non-living Material
      (a) Implants
      (b) Other connecting, protecting and supporting materials
IV. Equipment, Instruments and Prostheses
   A. Mechanical
   B. Thermal
   C. Optical
   D. Electro-acoustic

other physicians and surgeons; others have been specially developed for otolaryngology. Consequently, a number of chapters, or parts of chapters, of this book are devoted to some aspect of what is termed *materia otolaryngologica*, by analogy to *materia medica*. This chapter merely seeks to give an overview of the topic and refer the reader to appropriate other chapters in this book. Section I (the greater part of this chapter) will deal with materials and instruments; Section II will deal with questions relating to the effectiveness, and economic use, of *materia otolaryngologica*. The latter section could equally well have been included in Chapter 2 (Statistics). However, since this subject represents a logical extension of *materia otolaryngologica*, it is included here.

I. MATERIALS AND INSTRUMENTS
Drugs

Chemical compounds may be employed in otolaryngology for either a diagnostic or a therapeutic purpose. An example of a drug employed for diagnostic purposes is the use of glycerol in the diagnosis of endolymphatic hydrops (Klockhoff and Lindblom, 1966). Temporary improvement of the hearing level in hydrops occurs about two hours after oral administration of glycerol in a dosage of 16 mmol. kg^{-1} body weight.

Perhaps the most important chemical compounds used therapeutically by the otolaryngologist are those which are most important to medical practitioners in general, i.e. the *antibiotics*. These are compounds which are produced by micro-organisms and which are deleterious to the reproduction, growth or survival of the cells of other organisms, including, in the case of some antibiotics, neoplastic cells. Together with other anti-neoplastic drugs, these anti-neoplastic antibiotics form the subject of the next chapter. The antibiotics which have a particular application in otolaryngology are predominantly derived from species belonging to two genera of organisms, i.e. the genus *Penicillium*, a fungal genus, and the genus *Streptomyces*, which is an actinomycete. Actinomycetes are now regarded as filamentous bacteria and so classified with these organisms instead of with the fungi. The penicillins and the cephalosporins, e.g. cefaloridine, inhibit mucopeptide synthesis. Mucopeptide is an important component of bacterial cell walls. The tetracyclines interfere with protein synthesis by blocking either the attachment of the transfer ribonucleic acid (*t*-RNA) amino acid complex to the ribosomes (15 nm diameter intra-cytoplasmic structures which are the sites of protein synthesis) or the transfer of the activated amino acid to the growing peptide chain. Streptomycin also interferes with protein synthesis by bacterial cells, probably by binding to that part of a ribosome whose function is to adsorb the *t*-RNA. Thus, as a consequence, it is hypothesized, messenger ribonucleic acids (*m*-RNA) are "misread" and incorrect proteins are synthesized.

Amphotericin B and nystatin belong to a group of what are termed polyenic antibiotics. These are characterized chemically by a macrocyclic lactone ring. These polyenic antibiotics inhibit the growth of a wide range of fungi, some algae and protozoa; they are, however, ineffective against bacteria, including actinomycetes, and animal cells. Their activity is related to the binding of the polyenes on the sterols in the cell membranes. Griseofulvin also interferes with cell wall formation and may inhibit nucleic acid synthesis.

New antibacterial compounds are now being produced by chemical treatments of naturally occurring antibiotics. Thus penicillin G (benzylpenicillin) can be hydrolysed to give 6-amino-penicillanic acid (Fig. 1). This can then be used as the basis for a whole new range of semi-synthetic penicillins, e.g. ampicillin, carbenicillin, cloxacillin, meticillin and oxacillin. Ampicillin is 6-(2 amino-2-phenyl-acetamido) penicillanic acid. This particular structure enables ampicillin to reach the site of mucopeptide synthesis in Gram-negative bacteria so it has a wider spectrum of activity than penicillin G itself. Cloxacillin, meticillin and oxacillin are not affected by staphylococcal penicillinase.

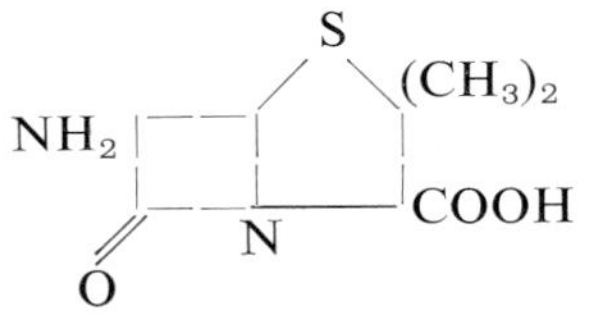

FIG. 1. 6-aminopenicillanic acid.

Pharmacokinetics deals with the time-course of drug concentrations in various parts of the body. As Thron (1974) points out, a pharmacokinetic system therefore consists of a set of anatomical points together with the drug concentrations at those points. If, within a certain anatomical region, the drug concentration is everywhere the same, the points in that region can be lumped together as a "compartment". In that case, one can speak of the quantity of drug in the compartment as well as the concentration. In pharmacokinetic analysis, a compartment can be treated as equivalent to a single anatomical point. The considerable mathematical complexities of multi-compartmental systems are best treated by using a completely general analysis based upon matrix algebra. Pharmacokinetic systems may be classified as either *linear* or *nonlinear* (so-called "dose-dependent") systems. Thron defines a linear system as one which obeys the principle of *superposition*. Thus, linearity can be tested by plotting the data for different doses and ascertaining whether or not there is superimposition (superposition) of the curves. However, one must plot plasma concentrations of the drug per unit dose of the drug as a function of time and not solely plasma concentrations as a function of time. As Westlake (1971) pointed out, the knowledge that a pharmacokinetic system is linear allows one to make important practical predictions about its behaviour. For example, the asymptotic drug levels on continuous infusion or repetitive dosage in a linear, time-invariant system can be predicted from the response to a single dose. Moreover, if one has measured the plasma concentrations after intravenous and intramuscular administration in a linear system, then one can predict the responses to various combinations of intravenous and intramuscular doses by simply adding the responses to be expected from the two injections given separately after multiplying each by an appropriate dosage factor. Similarly, if sustained release preparations exhibit the properties of linear systems, and part of the drug is released immediately, then the total response is the sum of the response to the rapidly-released and the slowly-released parts given separately.

It should be emphasized, however, that antibiotic drug concentrations in plasma or blood are not of primary importance except in septicaemias. What really matters is the concentration of an antibiotic (or other chemotherapeutic compound) in the infected tissues. Nearly thirty years ago, Florey and his associates (1946) showed that, after intramuscular administration, penicillin persisted

in the pus of a lesion for as long as twelve hours, whereas an effective blood concentration persisted for less than four hours. Antibiotic concentrations have been studied in lymph but these do not necessarily correspond to those in the interstitial fluid of the affected area. Attempts have therefore been made by Tan and his colleagues (1972), Chisholm and his colleagues (1973) and others to measure antibiotic concentrations in interstitial tissue fluid. Tan and his colleagues found, *inter alia*, that the concentrations of antibiotics in the tissue fluid were inversely related to the protein-binding property of the antibiotic. Thus flucloxacillin, which is more than 95 per cent protein-bound, attained barely detectable concentrations at any time. Chisholm and his colleagues studied interstitial tissue fluids using so-called "tissue cages". These cages consisted of closed but perforated 5 cm long silicone rubber tubes implanted beneath the skin of the abdomen and thigh of dogs. Following intramuscular (i.m.) injections, tissue fluid concentrations were always lower than the initial peak concentration of the drug in the serum. For drugs that were relatively slowly excreted, concentrations in the tissue fluid were similar to those in the serum after a period of six hours following administration. By contrast, the concentrations in the tissue fluid of those drugs that were excreted rapidly was unpredictable, being either negligible or maintained at concentrations significantly better than in serum. Although Chisholm and his colleagues did not analyse the time courses in serum and in tissue fluid of the various drugs they used, inspection of their results indicates that these will be compatible with the hypothesis that the growth of the drug concentrations in tissue fluids conforms to a Gompertz function and that the fall-off of concentration conforms to an exponential decay process (these particular functions are discussed in Chapter 1). The growth of drug concentrations in serum was so rapid compared to the sampling rate that insufficient data were available to indicate whether or not this function also exhibited a Gompertz curve. Figure 2 shows Chisholm's measurements for benzathine ampicillin concentrations in the tissue fluid as a function of time. In this figure, the concentrations are expressed in millimoles per cubic metre of tissue fluid per kilogram of animal (dog) per unit intramuscular dose in moles. The ascending curve (a) has been fitted to a Gompertz function, the equation of which is

$$C = 228 \, (0.003)^{0.986^t} \tag{50.1}$$

where C = concentration of benzathine ampicillin in mmol. m^{-3} of tissue fluid per mole of injected drug and per kg of animal (dog) at time t min after the i.m. injection.

The descending curve (b) has been fitted with an exponential equation where the concentration is given as

$$C = 524e^{-0.0024t} \tag{50.2}$$

where C has the same meaning as in equation (50.1) and e is the base of Napierian (natural) logarithms.

The point of intersection of the curves described by these two functions corresponds to the predicted peak concentration of the drug.

Figure 3 shows the fall in concentration of gentamicin in both blood (a) and in tissue fluid (b) following intra-

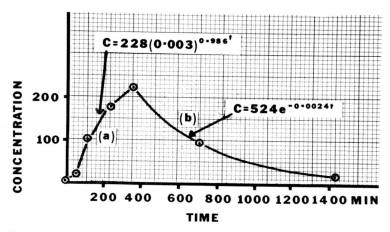

FIG. 2. Benzathine ampicillin concentration in tissue fluid as a function of time. Concentrations are expressed in millimoles per cubic metre of tissue fluid per kilogram of animal (dog) per unit intramuscular dose in moles. The ascending curve (a) has been fitted to a Gompertz function and the descending curve (b) has been fitted with an exponential function.

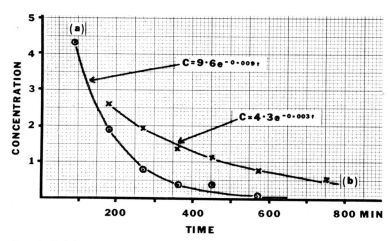

FIG. 3. Fall in concentration of gentamicin in both blood (a) and in tissue fluid (b) following intramuscular injection of the drug. The rising concentration is not shown but each curve starts from the measured peak concentration. Concentrations are expressed in moles per cubic metre of tissue fluid per kilogram of animal (dog) per unit intramuscular dose in moles. Exponential equations have been fitted to each curve.

muscular injection of the drug. The rising concentration is not shown but each curve starts from the measured peak concentration. The equation for the curve that has been fitted to the measured blood concentration is

$$C = 9.6e^{-0.009t} \qquad (50.3)$$

where C = concentration of gentamicin in mol. m^{-3} of serum per mole of injected drug per kg of animal (dog) at time t min after the i.m. injection.

The equation for the curve that has been fitted to the measured tissue fluid concentration is

$$C = 4.3e^{-0.003t} \qquad (50.4)$$

where C = concentration of gentamicin in mol. m^{-3} of the tissue fluid per mole of injected drug and per kg of animal (dog) at time t min after the i.m. injection.

Figure 3 shows that these exponential curves provide a good fit to the actual measurements. The values 0·009 and 0·003 in equations (50.3) and (50.4) are inverses of the time constants for the "decay" process for each of these curves. This indicates that the rate of disappearance of gentamicin from the blood serum is three times as fast as it is from tissue fluid. Thus, as the equations indicate, the time taken to halve the concentration of gentamicin in blood serum is 77 min, and, in tissue fluid, 231 min. Similarly, inspection of equation (50.2) indicates that the time taken for the concentration of benzathine ampicillin in tissue fluid to fall to a half is 289 min. In fact the time constants for the falling concentration of gentamicin and benzathine ampicillin in tissue fluid are little different. One therefore wonders to what extent the difference is due not to differences in drugs but to inter- or intra-animal variability. In the immediate future one would hope to see an answer to this question. Thus what one might term the basic pharmacokinetic constants of a drug should be listed along with its other characteristics. These basic constants would be the two parameters in the Gompertz growth function, i.e. constants g and h in equation (1.24), and the constant in the exponential decay function, i.e. k in equation (1.13) (see Chapter 1).

In respect of guidelines for the use of antibiotics in clinical practice, "seven deadly sins" of antibiotic administration have been listed, i.e.

(1) In pyrexia of unknown origin, antibiotic administration is not only futile but it delays appropriate diagnostic studies and exposes the patient to dangers of untoward reactions to the drug.

(2) Overdosage with certain antibiotics cause harm. The otolaryngologist is particularly aware of the ototoxic aminoglycosides. These are of such importance to him that a separate section of this book (Chapter 63) has been devoted to them.

(3) Combinations of antibiotics are generally bad since they encourage the use of ineffective doses of the individual agents.

(4) Failure to discontinue antibiotic treatment in the presence of reactions, or giving an antibiotic which has once caused potential serious untoward reactions constitutes a most dangerous misuse.

(5) Diseases due to viruses, which include about 90 per cent of upper respiratory tract infections, are untreatable with antibiotics.

(6) Reliance on chemotherapy without surgical intervention may hamper the chance of full recovery, e.g. cholesteatoma with infection.

(7) Chemoprophylaxis for surgery in a clean field is both futile and dangerous since infections which may then occur are frequently totally resistant to many or all antibiotics. A hospital in the U.S.A. reported the results of over 6 000 operations conducted over a nine-year period. The operations were classified as: (i) infected, (ii) contaminated, or (iii) clean elective; each of these three groups was subdivided according to whether or not antibiotics were given. In each of these three categories, the infection rate was higher in the patients receiving post-operative antibiotics than in those receiving none. This study was, however, a retrospective one and was not planned as a clinical trial. One therefore wonders whether or not a bias in the selection of patients to receive antibiotics could have accounted, partially or wholly, for the observations.

Ionizing Radiations

Diagnostic

(The therapeutic aspects of ionizing radiations are dealt with in Chapter 52.)

Nuclear Otolaryngology. Becquerel's discovery of *radioactivity* in 1896 was to be the precursor of a long series of studies by other Nobel Prizewinners, the Curies, Fermi and Hevesy, which culminated in the diagnostic use of *radioactive nuclides* (radionuclides) in medicine some 40 years later.

The term nuclide must be distinguished from the term *isotope*. Strictly, as Barnes and Rees (1972) point out, the word "isotope" should only be used when referring, in a comparative sense, to at least two types of atoms of one element. Thus ^{131}I, ^{132}I and ^{127}I are isotopes of iodine, and ^{60}Co and ^{57}Co are isotopes of cobalt. ^{60}Co and ^{131}I are not isotopes because they are different elements. The term "nuclide" refers to an individual type of atom, e.g. ^{60}Co, ^{131}I. Although common usage has resulted in the word isotope being used in the wider sense to cover the term nuclide, there is now a growing tendency to be rather more precise.

It will be noted that, in referring to a particular nuclide, the symbol for the element is prefixed by a number. This number is the *mass number* of the nuclide. The mass number is the whole number nearest in value to the atomic mass when that quantity is expressed in atomic mass units. The reference standard on this scale is the atomic mass of the carbon nuclide whose nucleus contains six *protons* and six *neutrons*, i.e. a mass number of 12.

The reader will recall that an atom is the smallest particle that exhibits the characteristic chemical properties of an element. Atoms consist of a *nucleus* surrounded by a ring, or rings, of *electrons*. The nucleus is composed of one (for the element hydrogen) or more *protons* (positively charged elementary particles of mass number 1) and, for all elements with an atomic number greater than 1, one or more *neutrons* (neutral elementary particles of mass number 1). The *atomic number* of an element defines the number of protons in the nucleus of an atom of that element. The *mass number* corresponds to the total number of protons and neutrons within the nucleus. Over 100 different elements are known and these are usually grouped in an ascending series according to the nuclear charge, which corresponds to the atomic number of the element. It is this that determines the chemical properties of the element. Atoms of the same atomic number may not all have the same mass number, i.e. there exist atoms with the same number of protons, but different numbers of neutrons in their nuclei. These individual types of atoms are termed *nuclides* and they may or may not be radioactive (*radionuclides*). Radionuclides disintegrate spontaneously with the emission of rays and particles of various types. They may be naturally occurring or artificially produced. Nuclides having the same number of protons in the nucleus but differing in other properties are referred to as being *isotopes* of one another; nuclides having the same number of neutrons in the nuclei, but differing in other ways, are referred to as *isotones*. Nuclides having the same atomic number and the same mass number but existing for measurable time-intervals in different states are referred to as being *nuclear isomers*. One state, that of lowest energy, is termed the *ground state*; all other states (of higher energy) are termed *metastable* states. The chemist uses one- or two-letter symbols to represent chemical elements, e.g. C for carbon, Na for sodium. This system has been extended by the atomic scientist to indicate, when dealing with nuclides, the atomic and mass number of these nuclides as well as whether or not the particular nuclide is a nuclear isomer. With this convention, the atomic number is given as a prescripted subscript and the mass number as a pre-scripted superscript to the symbol for the appropriate chemical element. Thus $^{127}_{53}I$ would indicate the naturally occurring iodine nuclide, which has a mass number of 127, and $^{131}_{53}I$ would indicate one of its isotopes (a radioactive one). A metastable isomer is indicated by the postscripted superscript m, e.g. $^{99}_{43}Tc^m$ (the metastable technetium nuclide of mass number 99). A postscripted n indicates a naturally occurring radionuclide. Thus $^{226}_{88}Ra^n$ indicates the naturally occurring radionuclide of radium.

Since the atomic number is implied by the chemical element, this number is redundant. It is thus usually omitted except in some equations describing nuclear reactions, when it is useful for describing the *disintegration* which occurs in radioactive nuclei. Disintegration refers to the change from one nucleus (parent) to another nucleus (daughter).

Nuclei containing 20, 50 or 82 protons, or 20, 50, 82 or 126 neutrons (the so-called *magic numbers*) are particularly stable. The *odd-even rule* of nuclear stability states that nuclides containing even numbers of neutrons and of protons are most stable; those with an even number of neutrons but an odd number of protons, or vice versa, are less stable; those with odd numbers of both neutrons and protons are least stable. Radioactive nuclei tend to decay towards stable arrangements (there is an appropriate ratio of neutrons to protons for each element); a disproportionately large number of neutrons is associated with processes which increase the number of protons and vice versa.

The rate of nuclear disintegration conforms to a particular pattern, i.e. the fraction of atoms present at any time which decay in each second is constant for a particular nuclide. This is therefore an exponential function (*see* Chapter 1). That is,

$$N = N_0 e^{-\lambda t} \qquad (50.5)$$

where N_0 = number of radioactive nuclei present initially, N = number of radioactive nuclei after time t, and λ = a time constant, which, in this expression, is referred to as the *transformation constant*.

In practice, it is more usual to refer to the *physical half-life*, or *half-value period* ($T_{0.5}$) of a nuclide, instead of the transformation constant. When we consider the physical half-life of a nuclide, then, in equation (50.5),

$$t = T_{0.5}$$
$$\text{and} \quad N = 0 \cdot 5 N_0$$
$$\therefore \ 0 \cdot 5 N_0 = N_0 e^{-\lambda T_{0.5}}$$
$$\therefore \ 0 \cdot 5 = e^{-\lambda T_{0.5}}$$
$$\therefore \ \ln 0 \cdot 5 = -\lambda T_{0.5}$$
$$\therefore \ T_{0.5} = 0 \cdot 693 / \lambda \qquad (50.6)$$

Physical half-lives for radionuclides range from less than a microsecond for polonium 217 to more than 10^{17} years for tin 124. Physical half-lives of radionuclides used in the otolaryngological area range from just over 2 h for iodine 132 to 57 days for iodine 125. Both of these radionuclides have been used in thyroid function tests but have not found a general application because of, on the one hand, too short a half-life, and on the other hand, too long a half-life. The physical half-life of 8 days for iodine 131

is more suitable and this iodine isotope has been more universally adopted.

The *biological half-life* of a substance is the time during which the process of elimination reduces the body content of that substance by one-half. The *effective half-life* of a radionuclide is the time during which the processes of elimination and radioactive decay together reduce the body content by one-half. The effective half-life is related to the biological half-life and the physical half-life by the expression

$$1/Te_{0.5} = 1/Tp_{0.5} + 1/Tb_{0.5}$$
$$\text{where } Te_{0.5} = \text{effective half-life}$$
$$Tp_{0.5} = \text{physical half-life}$$
$$\text{and} \quad Tb_{0.5} = \text{biological half-life.} \qquad (50.7)$$

A special unit is employed in nuclear physics to express activity of radionuclides. This is the *curie* (Ci). Although not an SI unit (*see* Chapter 1), it has been sanctioned for use with the International System for a limited time (12th CGPM, 1964, Resolution 7). The curie is now redefined in accordance with the recommendation of the International Commission on Radiological Units (1953), i.e. "The curie is a unit of radioactivity defined as the quantity of any radioactive nuclide in which the number of disintegrations per second is $3 \cdot 7 \times 10^{10}$".

The particular changes that the nuclei of radionuclides undergo on degeneration are several:

(1) Emission of alpha (α) particles (helium nuclei), e.g. the disintegration of the naturally occurring, but radioactive, radium nuclide to radon, which itself is radioactive, with the emission of alpha particles:

$$^{226}_{88}Ra^n \longrightarrow \ ^{222}_{86}Rn^n + \ ^{4}_{+2}He$$

This type of disintegration occurs only with nuclides whose atomic number is greater than 80.

(2) Emission of beta (β) particles (high-energy electrons):

$$^{1}_{0}n \longrightarrow \ ^{1}_{1}p + \ ^{0}_{-1}e$$

Since the nucleus of the nuclide gives a proton, the atomic number increases by 1. Thus, the disintegration of the phosphorus (atomic number 15) nuclide of mass number 32 is accompanied by the emission of β particles and the formation of sulphur (atomic number 16).

$$^{32}_{15}P \longrightarrow \ ^{32}_{16}S + \ ^{0}_{-1}e$$

(3) Emission of *positrons* (positive electrons), e.g. the disintegration of a particular radionuclide of phosphorus to produce a stable silicon atom and a positron:

$$^{30}_{15}P \longrightarrow \ ^{30}_{14}Si + \ ^{0}_{+1}e$$

A positron immediately combines with an electron to form two *photons* of electromagnetic radiation. A photon is a *quantum* (package) of electromagnetic energy.

(4) Emission of gamma (γ) rays.

In many cases, as Meredith and Massey (1972) point out, the ejection of the β particle or the positron from the nucleus completes the radioactive decay process. In other cases, the daughter nucleus, when formed, has too much energy for stability (the nucleus is said to be in an *excited state*). The excess energy is then emitted with the formation of electromagnetic radiation termed gamma (γ) radiation. Thus, in the disintegration of cobalt 60, an *excited* nickel nucleus is produced which immediately emits γ radiation, along with the electrons produced as the more immediate result of the cobalt decay.

$$^{60}_{27}Co \longrightarrow {}^{60}_{28}Ni + {}^{0}_{-1}e + \gamma$$

In some cases, the excited nuclear state following the emission of a β particle may be a nearly stable (metastable) one, remaining so for periods of up to days. The nuclear isomers of these metastable states also decay exponentially with emission of γ rays only. Thus, technetium 99m, which is produced when molybdenum 99 emits a β particle, also decays, with the emission of γ rays, to form technetium 99.

These various possible nuclear changes which we have just described are summarized by the *Soddy-Fajans Radioactive Displacement Law*, which in its contemporary, more inclusive, version states: "When a nucleus emits an alpha particle, the new nucleus formed has an atomic number of two less than the parent and a mass number of four less than the parent nucleus. When a nucleus emits a negative beta particle, the atomic number of the new nucleus formed is one greater than the parent nucleus but the mass number remains the same. The emission of a positron or the capture of an orbital electron decreases the atomic number by one without changing the mass number. Isomeric transition and gamma emission lead to no change in atomic number or mass number."

The particular interest of the otolaryngologist in nuclides is, of course, in respect of the radioactive nuclides (radionuclides), since he exploits them as a source of radiation. The therapeutic uses of radionuclides are discussed in Chapter 52. The diagnostic use depends also on the fact that radionuclides behave chemically exactly like their naturally occurring stable isotopes. Thus radionuclides can be used as *tracers* to *label* (*tag*) preparations containing the appropriate element, either in a chemical compound or otherwise.

The diagnostic radionuclides with which the otolaryngologist will be acquainted are tritium, xenon 133, gallium 67, the metastable nuclide of technetium 99 and the various radionuclides (predominantly those of the element iodine) used in the investigation of thyroid disorders.

The three isotopes of hydrogen are hydrogen, deuterium and tritium. *Tritium*, which has a mass number of 3, is the only one which is radioactive (half-life 12·3 years). Tritium, which decays by emitting electrons, is commonly used to label compounds for biochemical and pharmacological studies. Ishii and his colleagues (1967) have used tritiated (tritium-labelled) salicylate to study the uptake of this compound by the cochlea of the guinea pig. The use of tritiated thymidine in studying aural organogenesis is mentioned in Chapter 12.

Xenon 133 is a radioactive gas with a half-life of 5·3 days. Like tritium, it is a β-emitter (decays by emitting electrons).

It has been used to study the ventilation of the middle ear and paranasal sinuses by Kirchner (1974).

Gallium 67, which has a half-life of 78 h, decays by emitting γ rays and by electron capture. It has been used by Kashima and his colleagues (1974) to identify and localize *neoplasms* in the head and neck region. These authors performed 83 scans on 78 subjects who were all known, or suspected, to have malignant disease of the nose, throat or cervical region. Two days prior to the scanning, each subject was given 3 mCi ^{67}Ga citrate intravenously. This test was unable to detect *primary lesions* which were less than 20 mm in diameter. Of the 36 scans in subjects who were otherwise known to have *metastases* in the cervical lymph nodes, 33 were detected by this test. Of the 47 scans in subjects who were otherwise judged not to have cervical metastases, 10 were positive. Six of these 10 cases were due to inflammatory cervical masses.

Kornblut and his colleagues (1974) found gallium uptake of limited usefulness in the detection of squamous cell carcinoma and Vaidya and his colleagues (1970) have noticed failure of uptake in thyroid carcinoma which had previously been irradiated. It would appear that gallium concentrates mainly in viable than in necrotic tumour cells, and in the cytoplasm rather than in the nucleus (Hayes *et al.*, 1970).

Technetium 99m, in the form of sodium pertechnetate ($NaTcO_4$), is the radionuclide of choice for the diagnosis and localization of *brain tumours*. As Rowan (1972) says, it is presumed that selective concentration of this and other plasma-carried substances is the result of a selective focal breakdown of the blood-brain barrier. The metastable technetium is very suitable for this purpose for the following reasons. First, it produces negligible β particles. Owing to their absorption within the body, these radiations contribute to the hazard to the patient without contributing to the externally detectable radiation, i.e. that which is being used for diagnostic purposes. Secondly, it produces γ rays with energies of 140 keV (kilo-electron volts). Gamma rays with energies less than 50 keV are largely absorbed in the skull; those with energies higher than 500 keV present measuring problems. Thirdly, because of the short physical half-life (6 h), the radiation hazard to the patient is not a problem yet the time is sufficiently long to enable the test to be performed. Fourthly, since technetium is not protein-bound, it is readily eliminated from the body. Finally, it is relatively cheap and readily available. Normally, measurements of technetium uptake are made about 30 min to 120 min following a 5–10 mCi dose of the nuclide. When studies of organs other than the thyroid gland are being done, it is advisable to block uptake by this gland. For this purpose, 1·8 mmol potassium perchlorate is given by mouth 30 min before administration of the radionuclide. The perchlorate also blocks the choroid plexus which would otherwise selectively concentrate technetium and produce false positive scans.

As mentioned in Chapter 32, technetium 99m can also provide valuable information in the investigation of patients with disorders of *taste and smell*.

Radiosialography (*salivary gland scanning*) using technetium 99m, has been used routinely for the investigation of salivary gland *tumours* at the University of Michigan Medical Center since 1967. It is, however, suitable only for tumours greater than 10 mm diameter. The technique is similar to that used for investigating thyroid function (*see later*). A dose of 4 mCi of the nuclide is used and scanning is commenced a little earlier (15–20 min after i.v. injection of the nuclide). Moreover, atropine is given in a dose of 3 μmol 38 min prior to the injection of the pertechnetate. The prior administration of this drug eliminates, or, at least, minimizes, the secretion of radioactive saliva into the oral cavity. The presence of radioactive sources within the oral cavity would, of course, interfere with the results of scanning of the salivary glands. The technetium is avidly taken up by salivary gland tissue. Radionegative ("cold") nodules with a smooth outline are rarely malignant. Those with an irregular outline are generally malignant. Discrete radiopositive ("hot") nodules occur only in cases of Warthin's tumour (cystadenoma lymphomatosum). However, about half of Warthin's tumours show up as "cold" nodules, especially the more cystic ones (McCabe, 1975).

The use of technetium in studying *thyroid disorders* hinges on the fact that this element shows chemical similarities to iodine. When administered in the form of the pertechnetate ion, TcO_4, it behaves physiologically therefore very much the same as does iodine; it is concentrated in the salivary and thyroid glands. However, technetium differs from iodine in that it cannot be incorporated into tyrosine (the thyroid hormones precursor). It therefore diffuses out of the gland as the blood concentration falls. Nevertheless, this radionuclide can effectively separate hyperthyroid from euthyroid patients (Van't Hoff *et al.*, 1972). The usual dose of technetium 99m for a thyroid investigation is 1 mCi. This gives a total body dose of radiation of 10 mrad (Silver, 1968).

An *iodine* radionuclide was first used in the study of thyroid function by Hertz and Evans in 1938. Iodine plays a dominant role in thyroid physiology as a constituent of both thyroid hormones, i.e. thyroxine, tetraiodothyronine or T4 (Kendall, 1915), and triiodothyronine or T3 (MacLagan *et al.*, 1957). Although the concentration in the blood of the latter is only one-sixtieth of that of thyroxine, it is now considered to account for as much metabolic effect as does thyroxine. This is partly because the proportion of free serum triiodothyronine is about ten times that of free thyroxine, and partly because triiodothyronine is four times more potent than thyroxine. Moreover, triiodothyronine is the only thyroid hormone (apart from calcitonin) secreted by some subjects (Mack *et al.*, 1961).

The most common iodine nuclide in use for thyroid function studies is *iodine 131*, which is administered in the form of sodium iodide. Thompson (1974) states that, with present-day measuring apparatus, one need only use 5 μCi in thyroid uptake studies. This gives a total body dose of radiation of less than 10 mrad. Because of the differing forms of the percentage uptake curves, differentiation between euthyroid and hyperthyroid states is best made with an elapsed time of 4 h; that between euthyroid and hypothyroid states, with a time of 48 h. Unfortunately,

iodine uptake measures are very sensitive to the influence of many drugs, of which a comprehensive list has been given by Davis (1966), and changes in dietary iodine. Sachs and his colleagues (1972) reported two populations who consumed bread with differing iodine content. The bread of one population contained twenty-eight times as much iodine as that of the second. This population had normal radioactive iodine uptake of 5–15 per cent, compared with the second population of 15–40 per cent. Similarly, in iodine-poor areas of the world, where endemic goitre is common, high iodine uptakes are normally recorded. Thus, both in Mendoza Province, Argentina, (Stanbury *et al.*, 1954) and in West Irian* (Choufoer *et al.*, 1963), where inadequate dietary iodine is the rule, tracer uptakes of the order of 80 per cent are generally found.

Iodine-132 has also been used for clinical investigations (Hanbury *et al.*, 1954; Goolden and Mallard, 1958). Although this nuclide has higher β- and γ-energies which give greater dose rates to the tissues, this is more than offset by the shorter physical half-life (2·3 h). This radionuclide is therefore particularly recommended for studies that have to be conducted on children or on women during pregnancy. Morgans and Trotter (1958) used this nuclide in investigating the nature of the thyroid defect in Pendred's syndrome (*see* Chapter 9). The tracer is immediately discharged from the thyroid gland in this and similar peroxidase-iodinase defect disorders when potassium perchlorate is administered.

The distribution of radionuclide which is taken up by a thyroid gland is also helpful in deciding whether nodules that may be present are benign or malignant. The terms "hot", "warm", "cool" and "cold" have been applied to thyroid nodules to indicate the relative concentrating power of the nodule compared to adjacent or contralateral thyroid tissue (Silver, 1968). "Hot" (radiopositive) nodules are invariably benign (Perlmutter and Slater, 1956; Groesbeck, 1959) but about a quarter of "cold" (radionegative) nodules are malignant (Perlmutter and Slater, 1956). Horst (1959) and others have suggested that benign "cold" nodules can be differentiated from malignant "cold" nodules by the use of *phosphorus-32*. The study of Ackerman and his colleagues (1960) confirmed this but showed that false positive and false negative results may occur. After injecting 200–500 μCi phosphorus-32 intravenously, the scan becomes "hot" over malignant tissues owing to the incorporation of this particular radionuclide into active tumour tissue.

This brief description of the role of radionuclides in the investigation of thyroid disorders should not mislead the reader into assuming that uptake studies using these tracers form the principal, let alone sole, procedure for investigating thyroid dysfunction. As Havard (1974) points out in his excellent review, tests measuring the levels of thyroid hormones in the bloodstream are now being used increasingly in the diagnosis of thyroid disorders. Correspondingly, less emphasis is placed on *in vivo* tests of thyroid uptake of radionuclides.

The therapeutic use of radionuclides is discussed in Chapter 52.

* Formerly Netherlands New Guinea.

Measurement of Radionuclide Activity. The activity of radionuclides is measured by counting ionizing events. There are two principal types of counters for such a purpose, i.e. the *Geiger-Müller* type and the *scintillation counter.* The Geiger-Müller counter is based upon what is termed *gas amplification.* A thin wire anode is surrounded by a cylindrical metal cathode and the two are enclosed in a glass envelope containing gas at reduced pressure. The electrodes are maintained at a potential difference just too small to ionize the intervening gas. An ionizing particle entering the counter provides the necessary impetus to ionize the gas and so a current will momentarily pass.

The scintillation counter depends on the property exhibited by a number of compounds (anthracene, calcium tungstate, zinc sulphide) when exposed to ionizing radiations. Under these conditions, these compounds (termed *phosphors*) give out flashes of visible light, i.e. they *scintillate.* These compounds, when used in conjunction with a *photomultiplier tube,* form the basis for the scintillation counter. At one end of the photomultiplier tube is what is termed a *photocathode.* This is an electrode covered with light-sensitive material which emits electrons when light falls upon it. A series of special electrodes (*dynodes*) along the tube successively increase the number of electrons passing each stage to give a resultant amplification of more than one million.

Radiography. Perhaps no single discovery has contributed more to the improvement of diagnostic capabilities in the whole of medicine than has Roentgen's discovery of X-rays in 1895. Otolaryngology was, however, not to reap the benefits fully until the invention of *tomography* by Bocage in 1922 and the development of *non-linear (multi-directional)* tomography, using a special apparatus termed a *polytome,* by Sans and Porcher (1950).

In conventional radiography, the pattern on the X-ray film formed by the anatomical structures in which one is interested may be partially or wholly obscured by shadows cast by overlying and/or underlying structures. Although appropriate orientations of the patient to give particular views, e.g. that of Stenvers in the examination of the ear, frequently helps, tomography (*body-section radiography*) gives a clearer anatomical picture. Overlying and underlying structures are blurred out by a special technique which involves a controlled relative movement of the X-ray tube and the film during the exposure (Berrett *et al.,* 1973).

The general aspects of diagnostic radiography in otolaryngology have been discussed by Samuel (1952) and by Mittermaier (1969). A well documented report on the application of tomography to otolaryngology was produced by André and his associates (1968).

Linear (unidirectional) tomography of the nasal and paranasal structures is of particular value in detecting fractures as well as bone destruction due to malignant neoplasms. Antero-posterior (AP) linear tomograms are of value in the examination of the larynx, especially when the subject is phonating.

Non-linear (multidirectional) tomography (polytomography or polycyclic tomography) has been of particular value in respect of the examination of the ear and of the vestibulocochlear nerve. This is because they are encased within the temporal bone which offers as much radio-opacity as any anatomical structure. The application of non-linear tomography to the examination of the temporal bone is described by Lloyd (1973), as well as in Chapter 15 of this book. Wastie (1972) has reported the value of multidirectional (specifically, hypocycloidal) tomography in the examination of the nasal part of pharynx when carcinoma is suspect.

Chapter 15 also discusses the value of *zonography.* Zonography was first introduced by Ziedses des Plantes (1931). Zonography is narrow angle ($<12°$) tomography. The technical aspects of this subject have been studied by Westra (1966). The extent of blurring (S) for any structure outside the focal plane is given by

$$S = 2H \tan (\alpha/2) \qquad (50.8)$$

where H = distance of structure from focal plane and α = exposure angle in degrees.

Thus where the exposure angle (α) is small, as in zonography, the blurring of structures close to the plane of interest will be incomplete. Consequently, to achieve good results in zonography, it is necessary to have a radio-translucent zone (the *free zone*) before and behind the structure under investigation. For example, 10 mm sections of the petrous portion of the temporal bone can be conveniently studied by zonography if the position is such that the middle and posterior cranial fossa are aligned to constitute free zones. As Lloyd and Wylie (1971) point out, linear movements are particularly unfavourable in zonography where the aim is to produce maximal blurring with limited exposure angles. Circular movements are therefore more suitable.

Attenuation of X-rays. The radiodiagnostic properties of X-rays depend not only on the fact that these electromagnetic radiations pass through body tissues but that they pass through to varying degrees, i.e. they are variably attenuated. In Chapter 1, it was pointed out that the attenuation of X-rays is governed by an exponential law. This means that there is a *constant fractional reduction* in the intensity of an X-ray beam by equal added thicknesses of a given material. The *linear attenuation* coefficient, μ, in equation (1.14) is a measure of the fractional reduction of the X-ray beam per unit thickness of material as determined by considering a thin layer of material. For a given wavelength of the X-rays, μ will depend upon the density and the atomic number of the material under consideration. Bone (specific gravity of compact bone about 1·8 compared with a value of about unity for soft tissues) is not only denser than soft tissue but its average atomic number (about 13) is nearly twice as great; air has a specific gravity of the order of 10^{-3}. Thus, air containing cavities, bone and soft tissues, will attenuate X-rays to different degrees and so permit different amounts of the X-rays to reach the X-ray film.

The penetrating power of an X-ray beam is frequently defined in terms of the thickness of a given material which will reduce a narrow beam to one-half of its original value. This thickness is termed the half-value layer (HVL). If we denote HVL as D, it follows from equation (1.14) that

when $x = D$
and $I = 0\cdot 5I_0$
then $0\cdot 5I_0 = I_0 e^{-\mu D}$
$\therefore \ln 0\cdot 5 = -\mu D$
$\therefore D = 0\cdot 693/\mu$ (50.9)

i.e., the HVL is an inverse measure of the linear attenuation coefficient.

X-ray Films. The degree of blackening of X-ray films by the individual rays is expressed by a measure known as the (*photographic*) *optical density*. This is defined by the equation

$$Z = \log_{10}(I_0/I) \qquad (50.10)$$

where Z = optical density of the film, I_0 = intensity of light incident upon a small area of film, I = intensity of light transmitted by that area.

Thus optical density being a logarithmic ratio of two intensity measures is a similar mathematical function to the decibel. Optical density values encountered in radio-diagnosis usually range from about $0\cdot 3$ to $2\cdot 3$. This corresponds to fractions of light transmitted varying from a half down to a one two-hundredth. An X-ray film is characterized by the curve (hence, *characteristic curve*) relating optical density as a function of *Exposure* to X-rays (Fig. 4). In this context, Exposure (X) has a special meaning and it is therefore frequently written with a capital

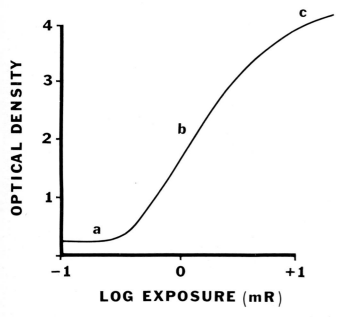

FIG. 4. Characteristic curve relating optical density to logarithm of Exposure (milliroentgens) to X-rays. The horizontal part ot the curve (a) is termed the fog level; the maximum slope of the curve, in the region (b), is termed the film gamma (Hurter and Driffield's development factor).

letter. The 1962 ICRU (International Commission on Radiological Units) defined Exposure as the quotient ΔQ by Δm where ΔQ is the sum of all the electrical charges on all the ions of one sign produced by air, when all the electrons (negative electrons and positrons) liberated by

photons in a volume element of air, whose mass is Δm are completely stopped in air. That is,

$$X = \frac{\Delta Q}{\Delta m} \qquad (50.11)$$

where X = Exposure in roentgens

The special unit of *Exposure* is the *roentgen* (R), one unit of which is equivalent to $2\cdot 58 \times 10^{-4}$ coulombs per kilogram of air. Thus the roentgen is not an SI unit (*see* Chapter 1), but the 1969 C.I.P.M. sanctioned its use for a limited time. The roentgen should be distinguished from the rad which is a special unit employed to express *absorbed dose* of ionizing radiations (*see* Chapter 52).

When *characteristic curves* of films are presented radiation exposure is expressed in terms of the logarithm of this measure in milliroentgens (Fig. 4). The maximum slope of this curve (in the region b in Fig. 4) is referred to as the film *gamma* (γ). The gamma (Hurter and Driffield's *development factor*) provides a convenient simple number to express the properties of the film. These properties are dependent on the method of manufacture of the film. The horizontal part (a) of the curve in Fig. 4 is termed the *fog level*. This background density is due, amongst other things, to the absorption of light by the film.

The difference in optical density between the various regions of a film is termed *contrast*. The contrast between two points on a film is measured as the difference in the optical densities of these two points.

The three principal components in *blurring*, or what Meredith and Massey (1972) term *unsharpness*, of the image are: geometric unsharpness (U_g), movement unsharpness (U_m) and screen unsharpness (U_s). Geometric unsharpness arises from the fact that X-rays originate from a finite-sized area on the target. Movement unsharpness arises from relative movements during the exposure time of the X-ray tube, film or object being X-rayed. Deliberate movement is, however, introduced in tomography to blur out structures in which the radiologist is not interested. Total unsharpness (U) is related to these three unsharpness components by the expression

$$U = \sqrt[3]{(U_g{}^3 + U_m{}^3 + U_s{}^3)} \qquad (50.12)$$

The interpretation of chest films has been shown to be influenced by the technical quality of the film (Fletcher and Oldham, 1949). However, a study of the interpretation of X-ray films of the paranasal sinuses indicated that the greater the experience, the less are observers' criteria disturbed by technical faults in the film (Hinchcliffe, 1961). For experienced observers, the technical quality may have no appreciable influence on interpretation.

Contrast Radiography. Information afforded by both ordinary and tomographic radiographic methods is improved by the use of *artificial contrast media*. As the name implies, these are preparations which produce contrast to enable one to delineate a particular anatomical structure; this structure (or structures) might otherwise produce an image whose optical density differs little from that of associated structures. Contrast media are classified as either negative or positive. Negative contrast media offer relatively less obstruction to X-rays and so produce an image on the X-ray film of greater optical density than would otherwise be the case; positive contrast media, by virtue of their high attenuation coefficients, produce an image of relatively less optical density. The commonest negative contrast medium is air, as in pneumoencephalography. The properties of positive contrast media are due to their containing elements of high atomic number, such as barium (atomic number 56) or iodine (atomic number 53). Thus barium sulphate is used for oesophagography, ethiodized oil (ethyl esters of iodinated fatty acids) for lymphangiography, iofendylate (ethyl 10-(p-iodophenyl)-undecanoate) for cisternomeatography (Scanlan, 1964) and sialography (Rubin *et al.*, 1955), and propyliodone (propyl ester of 3,5-diiodo-4-oxo-1-piperidine acetic acid) for bronchography, nasopharyngography (Walike, 1967) and laryngography (Harrison, 1969). Harrison advocates a procedure whereby the cocainized larynx is coated with propyliodone to enable the larynx to be viewed under conditions of quiet respiration and phonation. When the patient performs a Valsalva manoeuvre, the contrast medium is forced against the undersurface of the closed vocal folds outlining the subglottic space.

More recently, powdered tantalum (atomic number 73) has been used as a contrast agent in laryngography (Zamel *et al.*, 1970) and in tracheography (Hinchcliffe, 1970). As Nadel and his colleagues (1970) point out, tantalum adheres to airway mucosa, provides excellent detail of airways without filling them, does not interfere with respiratory function and has given no evidence for either local or systemic toxicity.

Structural Materials

Transplants

It has been long the surgeon's hope, as Billingham (1970) pointed out, that transplantation of tissues and organs from one human being to another and, perhaps even more ambitiously, from lower animals to man, would ultimately become a standard component of his art.

A *transplant* is a piece of *animal* tissue or whole organ which has been removed from an animal either immediately before, or some time previously, and transferred to the same, or another, animal and placed in the same, or a different, site. As Woodruff (1960) says, some authorities extend the term to cover not only living, but also non-living, tissues. Since *implantation* is defined as the introduction of portions of *non-living* material into an animal, the term *implant* would, in any case, cover a dead tissue transplant. *Explantation* is the process of removing living tissue from an animal and setting up cultures *in vitro*. *Explants* are the tissue pieces used for this. The terms "grafting" and "graft" are now held to be synonymous with "transplanting" and "transplant". However, some authorities restrict the word *graft* to denote transplants of living tissue (but not organs) which do not remain permanently attached to the original site by vascular connections.

Transplants may be classified in four ways. First, according to the relationship between donor and recipient.

Autograft is the term used where the donor and recipient are one and the same organism. If the donor and recipient are different organisms, but the donor has the same genetic constitution (genotype) as the recipient, e.g. identical twins, then the transplant is termed an *isograft*. Transplants from organisms of different genotypes but of the same species are known as *allografts*. Transplants from organisms of different species are termed *xenografts*. The term "homograft" or "homologous" transplant was formerly applied to an allograft but, as both Gorer (1961) and Snell (1964) have pointed out, this use of the term "homologous" was precisely opposite to the sense in which it is used by the biologist. The term heterologous transplant (or heterograft) was formerly used in describing xenografts.

Secondly, transplants may be classified according to the *recipient site*. *Heterotopic* transplants are surrounded by a different kind of tissue than before, e.g. a fat graft to the fenestra vestibuli. *Orthotopic* transplants are surrounded by the same kind of tissue as before, e.g. skin to skin defect. *Autotopic* transplants are those where the graft is replaced in its original site, i.e. it is a special case of orthotopic.

Thirdly, transplants may be classified according to the method of grafting, i.e. free or pedicle. Fourthly, a transplant may be classified according to its order, i.e. first, second . . . graft.

It is to be noted that blood transfusions are, in effect, graft, of a particular (fluid) tissue. Because of its importance, a special section (Chapter 53) has been devoted to this topic.

Metastases can be considered as spontaneous, pathological, heterotopic autotransplants. The developing fetus is a special, physiological allotransplant. In pregnancy, a condition of what is termed *temporary immunological inertia* occurs. During the pregnancy, the mother makes no attempt to reject the fetus. However, within a few months of the end of pregnancy, the mother's body will unequivocably reject tissue or organs transplanted from the offspring. Thus studies of the immunological mechanisms associated with viviparity should provide valuable information in regard to both GVH (graft versus host) and HVG (host versus graft) reactions. The principal HVG reaction—graft rejection—is well known; less well known are the GVH reactions which, experimentally at least, can lead to serious disease (runt disease) in animals (Billingham and Brent, 1957). Increasing knowledge of the mechanisms of the GVH and HVG reactions should provide a better understanding of the *immunobiology* of cancer. This topic is discussed by Morton (1974) in our companion volume *Scientific Foundations of Surgery*. Morton concludes that it is likely that immunotherapy will play an increasing role in the treatment of cancer. Unfortunately, at the present time, the patients most likely to respond to this form of treatment are those who are early cases. These patients have minimal residual tumour burden following treatment with other therapeutic modalities.

As Mackey (1970) and others have pointed out, the difficulties associated with transplantation of tissues and organs are not predominantly technical, but biological. This is because each organism possesses a mechanism for swiftly recognizing and rejecting any non-self living matter.

This mechanism, as initially demonstrated by Gorer (1937) on tumour transplants, is genetically determined. The terms originally used to denote the antibodies formed as a result of the transplantation of allogeneic cells (including erythrocytes) and the antigens which evoke them were *iso-antibody* and *iso-antigen* respectively. Unfortunately, as both Woodruff (1960) and Snell (1964) have pointed out, there are serious objections to the use of these two terms. Iso-antibodies are antibodies formed as a result of transplantation between individuals who are *not* isogenic, i.e. of the same genetic constitution (genotype). Following a similar use of the term *allotypic* by Dray and his colleagues (1962), Snell proposed that this term be used also to refer to what were formerly known as iso-antibodies and iso-antigens.

Gorer (1961) formulated (in immunological terms) the genetic theory of transplantation. This can be stated as follows: Normal and neoplastic tissues contain allotypic antigenic factors which are genetically determined. Allotypic antigenic factors present in transplanted tissue and absent in the host are capable of eliciting a response which results in destruction of the transplant. Under special circumstances, the response may not be elicited or the transplant may not be destroyed thereby.

The existence of Landsteiner's ABO allotypic antigen (blood group) system and its importance in connection with the compatibility of blood transfusions has been known since the beginning of this century. Although this allotypic antigenic system is a factor in transplant rejection it is not as important as what is termed the *HL-A (human leucocyte antigen)* system. The HL-A genetic system, which is one of the most complex so far described in man, is the principal histocompatibility system. The clinical status of transplant patients is correlated with the degree of tissue incompatibility in respect of the HL-A system (Batchelor and Joysey, 1969).

The HL-A system is inherited independently of the ABO and all other blood group systems apart from P_1. There is a negative association between the antigen P_1 and one of the HL-A antigens (Hronkova-Zoulkova et al., 1968).

The HL-A system is governed by a locus located on an autosomal chromosome. This locus is itself divided into several sub-loci. Each of these sub-loci is itself multi-allelic (*see* Chapter 9). The first sub-locus alternatively governs antigens HL-A1, HL-A2 (Mac), HL-A3, Dal5, Dal6 and Dal7. The second sub-locus alternatively governs antigens HL-A5, HL-A7, HL-A8, Da4, Da6 and Dag(6^B) (Dausset et al., 1968). Other antigens are probably governed by a third sub-locus. The symbol "Da" refers to Dausset's antigens.

There are ethnic differences in the prevalence of HL-A antigens. The HL-A1 antigen occurs in more than 20 per cent of Caucasians (Kissmeyer-Nielsen et al., 1968) but has not yet been detected in Asians.

Just as individuals can be "blood-typed", so they can be "tissue-typed". HL-A antigens are protein molecules situated on cell membranes. Fortunately, not only are they ubiquitous, being present throughout the body, but they are particularly represented in lymphocytes. Thus lymphocytes are generally used for "tissue-typing". The particular technique employed is usually a modified version of Ter-

asaki's microcytoxic technique (Mittal et al., 1968). With this technique, a comparison is made of the lymphocytotoxic activity of a standard serum of known HL-A characteristics against donor and recipient lymphocytes. Although there are several thousand possible combinations of HL-A antigens, some combinations are much more prevalent than others. Consequently, Dausset has calculated that there would be a 95 per cent chance of finding the correct donor from a potential donor population of 2 300. However, where allotransplants are concerned, correct tissue-matching of donor and recipient is not always possible. Recourse must therefore be made to the procedures for modifying the allograft reaction, by reducing, if not eliminating it.

There are three principal methods for *suppressing* the *allograft reaction*, i.e. use of cytotoxic sera, drugs or ionizing radiations.

Before the end of the last century, Metchnikoff studied antilymphocytic serum (ALS) but its potentialities in modifying the allograft reaction were not realized until Woodruff and Anderson's (1963) more recent work. The serum is usually prepared by injecting human lymphocytes into horses. ALS can promote not only the survival of allografts (Anderson et al., 1967) but also that of xenografts (Lance and Medawar, 1968).

A γ-globulin fraction of serum also has the property of prolonging the life of skin allografts in rats (Kamrin, 1959). This property of the γ-globulin has been shown to be due to the enzyme ribonuclease (Mowbray, 1967). As Billingham (1970) points out, this may be a normal homeostatic regulator of immunological reactivity.

The prelude to the clinical use of immunosuppressant drugs was Schwartz and Dameshek's (1959) observation that a thiopurine, mercaptopurine, prolonged the life of skin allografts in rabbits. Azathioprine, an imidazole derivative of mercaptopurine, was subsequently shown to be as effective as the latter drug in prolonging allograft survival but with less bone-marrow toxicity.

Both hydrocortisone (Krohn, 1954) and prednisone (Woodruff and Llaurado, 1956) are also effective in prolonging the survival of skin allografts in rabbits.

Whole-body irradiation by X-rays prolongs the survival of skin allografts in rabbits (Dempster et al., 1950). However, as regards clinical use, irradio-immunosuppression is still in the experimental stage. Current developments are following the lines of using compact external sources of ionizing radiation, e.g. a strontium radionuclide.

As Herbertson (1971) and others have pointed out, despite fundamental discoveries in general immunology and related sciences, practical methods of preventing the rejection of human allografts are often entirely inadequate or dangerously non-specific. Fortunately, as is mentioned in Chapter 65, the middle ear, at least, appears to be a "favoured site" for both allografts and xenografts. Thus the otologist is not so bedevilled by rejection mechanisms as are his colleagues dealing with other parts of the body. Reconstructive procedures in the rest of otolaryngology (*see* Chapters 66 to 68 inclusive) use principally autografts so again allograft and xenograft reactions are not of primary concern at the moment. The future may well, however, see a proliferation of the use of allografts and xenografts in otolaryngology. At present, transplants of the internal ear are considered to be not even remotely feasible. However, transplants of the adult eyes in the newt, *Triturus viridescens*, with return of vision have been reported (Stone and Zaur, 1940). Is the gap between the amphibian and the mammalian special sense organ too great to bridge?

Regeneration and Repair. The property to accept complicated organ transplants seems related to *regenerative* powers. After an intensive study, Needham (1964) concluded that regenerative power is primarily inversely related to evolutionary grade. The reason is probably that morphological, and especially histological, differentiation are directly related to the grade, so that, if de-differentiation is necessary as a precursor to regeneration, it becomes exceedingly difficult. Nevertheless, nearly 200 years ago, it was reported that a small, normally appearing eye with a transparent cornea, had regenerated in a salamander one year after incomplete removal of the original eye. Relevant to these neural regenerative properties is the work of Levi-Montalcini (1964) and others on the NGF (nerve growth factor). The preparation of an NGF antiserum raises questions of the possible medical control of schwannomas and other tumours of nervous tissue.

Non-Living Material

A variety of non-living materials find a use in otolaryngology either as surgical implants (*see* Chapter 54) or otherwise. The principal materials are metals, alloys and polymers. Their suitability for use is governed by certain physical, chemical and what might be termed, bioreactive, properties.

Types of Materials. A *metal* is one of the naturally occurring elements that are heavy, dense, fusible, malleable and opaque. There are about seventy of these but only a few (gold, plantinum, silver, tantalum and titanium) are used in the essentially pure state in surgery. Excluding the use of the noble metals for electrodes and in dental surgery, probably only titanium will be increasingly employed in the future. Titanium is more easily fabricated in useable form than other metals employed in surgery. It has a low position in the periodic table of elements (atomic number, 22; mass number, 48). This implies lightness and relative radio-translucency, permitting radiography after, for example, cranioplasty (Gordon and Blair, 1974).

Alloys are mixtures of metals. It is convenient to divide alloys into those based upon iron, i.e. *ferrous alloys*, and those not, i.e. *non-ferrous alloys*.

The *steels*, consisting of both iron and carbon, with or without other elements, are the most important of the ferrous alloys. The inclusion of carbon (between 0·15 per cent and 1·5 per cent by weight) increases the hardness of the iron. A *stainless steel* is a steel rendered corrosion-resistant by the addition of chromium (a minimum of 12 per cent by weight). Dependent on the microscopic structure, stainless steels are classified as *austenitic, ferritic* or *martensitic*. Both austenite (austenitic steels) and martensite (martensitic steels) contain nickel, but the former steel contains about twice as much (8–14 per cent by weight) as the latter. Increasing nickel contents above about 5 per cent are associated with decreased hardness and strength, but increased corrosion-resistance. Consequently, austenitic steels are preferred for use as implants, but martensitic steels for surgical instruments. Thus the British Standard (BS 5194: 1975) dealing with the requirements for stainless steel for such instruments specifies, *inter alia*, a maximum nickel content of 1 per cent. The addition of a few per cent of molybdenum to the austenitic steels further increases corrosion-resistance.

Amongst the non-ferrous alloys, those based on cobalt exhibit both high strength and corrosion resistance. Commercial preparations, e.g. Vitallium, are alloys of cobalt (about 75 per cent), chromium (about 20 per cent) and molybdenum (about 5 per cent).

Polymer-based materials comprise *elastomers, fibres* and *plastics*. Polymers consist of large molecules (*macromolecules*) built up from smaller units (*monomers*) to form a continuous chain of atoms joined together by *covalent* (non-ionic) chemical bonds. Thus the simplest organic polymer is polyethylene

$$\cdots \overset{\displaystyle H}{\underset{\displaystyle H}{C}} - \overset{\displaystyle H}{\underset{\displaystyle H}{C}} - \overset{\displaystyle H}{\underset{\displaystyle H}{C}} - \overset{\displaystyle H}{\underset{\displaystyle H}{C}} \cdots$$

whose monomer is ethylene

$$\overset{\displaystyle H}{\underset{\displaystyle H}{C}} = \overset{\displaystyle H}{\underset{\displaystyle H}{C}}$$

Elastomers (rubbers) are characterized by their ability to be deformed elastically to a considerable extent. This is because they are composed of long, coiled molecules. *Polyisoprene* (natural rubber)

$$\cdots CH_2 - \overset{CH_3}{\overset{|}{C}} = CH - CH_2 - CH_2 - \overset{CH_3}{\overset{|}{C}} = CH - CH_2 \cdots$$

is based upon the monomer, isoprene

$$CH_2 = \overset{CH_3}{\overset{|}{C}} - CH = CH_2$$

Polyisoprene molecules are cross-linked with sulphur atoms (vulcanized) to convert the compound from a fluid (latex) to the solid elastomer.

Silicone rubber (polydimethylsiloxane)

$$\cdots \overset{CH_3}{\underset{CH_3}{Si}} - O - \overset{CH_3}{\underset{CH_3}{Si}} - O - \overset{CH_3}{\underset{CH_3}{Si}} \cdots$$

is based upon the monomer dimethylsiloxane:

$$
\begin{array}{c}
CH_3 \\
\backslash \\
Si\!=\!O \\
\diagup \\
CH_3
\end{array}
$$

A whole range of polydimethylsiloxanes, i.e. the *dimeticones*, exist. This range includes not only elastomers but also fluids of variable viscosity. The actual physical form depends upon the length of the polymer chain and the degree of cross-linking. Particular molecular weights can be produced by varying the amount of what is termed a molecular chain terminator; in this case, chlorotrimethylsilane. The viscosity (resistance to flow) of dimeticone fluids is a function of their molecular weight. Fluids with viscosities ranging from less than $1 \times 10^{-6} m^2 . s^{-1}$ to more than $3 m^2 . s^{-1}$ are available. The viscosity grade of a dimeticone is frequently distinguished by a number which corresponds to the measure of viscosity (centistokes) in the CGS (centimetre-gram-second) system which preceded the SI system of units (*see* Chapter 1). The degree of cross-linking of the high molecular weight dimeticones governs the characteristics of the elastomer produced. As with the alcohols, industrial grades of the silicones may be toxic (Chaplin, 1969).

A *fibre* has been defined as a material whose length is at least a hundred times greater than its diameter. They are produced from bulk polymers by spinning processes. Collection of fibres are termed *yarns*, and these may be combined into planar structures termed *fabrics*. A fibre owes its characteristics to the longitudinal alignment of its molecular chains. This alignment is often reinforced by many interchain connections (usually electrovalent bonds). *Polyethylene terephthalate* fibres (Dacron; Teflon) are used for arterial prostheses.

Plastics are polymers in which various *additives* have been incorporated to improve the mechanical properties (*plasticizers*) or to stabilize the polymer chain against deleterious environmental agents (*stabilizers*).

Mechanical and Physical Properties. *Hardness* refers to the resistance of a material to surface abrasion. There are a variety of scales of hardness. The Mohs' scale is based upon a comparison of the ability of materials to scratch one another, so it is thus an ordinal scale (*see* Chapter 1). Other scales (Brinell, Rockwell, Vickers) depend on the amount of indentation produced in the material by a standard indentor. The higher the value of the measure on these scales, the harder the material. On the Vickers scale, high tensile steel has a hardness of about 500, and lead of about 5.

Metals may be *hardened* by alloying, and both metals and alloys may be hardened by certain procedures, which may or may not involve heating.

The application of a *tensile* (pulling) *force* to a piece of material, e.g. a rod, results in an overall extension of the material. Provided that this force does not exceed a certain value (the *elastic limit*), the specimen will return to its original length once the force has been removed. This property whereby a body, when deformed, automatically

recovers its normal configuration when the deforming force is removed, is known as *elasticity*. Figure 5 illustrates material which is undergoing elastic deformation in the region OW of the curve OZ. *Tensile stress* is expressed in terms of tensile force per unit area, the unit of which is the same as that for pressure, i.e. the pascal (*see* Chapter 1).

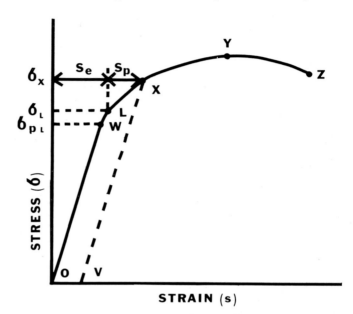

FIG. 5. A typical stress-strain curve. The curve is linear in the region OW. In this region any applied stress will be accompanied by a proportional amount of elastic strain. W indicates this proportional limit (σ_{PL}). When the applied stress is greater than a value σ_L (elastic limit, at L), e.g. a value σ_X, then plastic deformation occurs. When this stress is removed, the material follows the path XV to give a residual strain, i.e. a permanent deformation; this is the plastic component (S_p) in the total strain at X. The elastic component in the total strain at X is denoted by S_e. The stress at Y is termed the ultimate stress (tensile strength). The material breaks at point Z. Stress is measured in pascals; strain is dimensionless.

The measure of what might be termed "material response" is referred to as *strain*. Tensile strain is the ratio of elongation produced by the stress to the original length; it is therefore dimensionless. Since the part of the curve OW in Fig. 5 is linear, its equation is given by

$$\sigma = as + b$$

where σ = stress in pascals
s = strain
a = proportionality constant
and b = intercept in pascals

Since the intercept is zero,

then $\qquad\qquad\qquad \sigma = aS \qquad\qquad\qquad (50.13)$

This equation is the expression of *Hooke's Law*, i.e. the strain set up within an elastic body is proportional to the stress to which the body is subjected by the applied load.

The proportionality constant in the equation is usually referred to as *Young's modulus* and, in respect of tensile stress, is denoted by E

i.e. $\qquad\qquad\qquad E = \sigma/s \qquad\qquad\qquad (50.14)$

Young's modulus for metals is usually of the order of 200 GPa (gigapascals) (*see* Appendix 2). Polymers have values ranging from 0·5 GPa (politef) to 4·5 GPa (epoxy resins).

The *shear modulus* (of rigidity) is given by the ratio of shear stress to shear strain. The units for these measures are the same as for the corresponding measures in respect of tensile stress and strain. Shear moduli of elasticity for metals are usually in the range 20–100 GPa (stainless steel has a shear modulus of 84 GPa). Polymers have shear moduli ranging from 0·14 GPa (polyethylene) to 1·6 GPa (epoxy resins).

Lengthening of a rod subjected to tensile stress is associated with contraction in the transverse axis. The ratio of these two changes in dimensions is termed *Poisson's Ratio*,

i.e. $$P = c/s \qquad (50.15)$$

where P = Poisson ratio
c = transverse strain produced by longitudinal stress
and s = longitudinal strain produced by same longitudinal stress.

Stainless steel has a Poisson ratio of 0·28, politef, 0·4, and polyethylene, 0·45.

Torsion of a rod or a wire is a geometrical version of a shear stress.

The *bending* of a *beam* encompasses a combination of tensile, compression and shear stresses.

The *buckling* of *struts* is governed by the modulus of elasticity of the material. Struts, like columns (large perpendicular struts), are structural units working in compression (*compression structural members*), i.e. they are subject to a compressive stress. Thus cylindrical stapes prostheses are sometimes referred to as struts. However, these prostheses work as *tension structural members* as well, so that, in this respect, they are, by definition, *ties*. Euler was the first to derive a formula to calculate the maximum axial (longitudinal) load that a long, slender, ideal column could stand without collapsing. (At this point, however, the compression member, although stable, would no longer be straight but in the form of a sinusoid.) This maximum load (*critical load*) is given by

$$P = (K\pi^2 EI)/l^2 \qquad (50.16)$$

where P = critical load
E = Young's modulus of elasticity
I = moment of inertia of cross-sectional area
l = unsupported length of column
and K = a constant whose value depends upon the condition of end support of the column; it may have a value of 1 (both ends free to turn), 4 (both ends fixed) or 2 (one end fixed, other end free to turn).

It will be noted that elasticity and not the compressive strength of the material of the column determines the critical load. Moreover, the critical load is directly proportional to the moment of inertia of the cross-section. The moment of inertia of a surface is the product of its area (A) and the square of what is known as the *radius of gyration* (r). Thus for the case where both ends are free to turn, i.e. $K = 1$, we can substitute Ar^2 for I in equation (50.16), i.e.

$$P = \{(\pi^2 E)(Ar^2)\}/l^2 \qquad (50.17)$$

i.e. $P/A = (\pi^2 E)/(l/r)^2$

i.e. $s_{\text{crit}} = (\pi^2 E)/(l/r)^2 \qquad (50.18)$

where s_{crit} = critical stress
and (l/r) = slenderness ratio

Unfortunately, the Euler formula presupposes indefinite elasticity and also ignores the possible occurrence of a yield point (*see below*). Consequently, an extension of this formula (Perry-Robertson formula) has been derived to cater for these features. The Perry-Robertson formula is the basis, for example, of compressional structural member design covered in the British Standard BS 449: 1970.

A *yield point* is an abrupt inflexion in the curve relating strain to stress. If there is no yield point, the linear part of the curve may merge imperceptibly into the curvilinear part and definite points corresponding to the proportional limit or the elastic limit may not be detectable. In these cases, the elastic-plastic transition is defined by the *proof-stress*. This is a stress at which 0·2 per cent plastic strain is attained. It is determined by drawing a line parallel to the line OW in Fig. 5 and determining its point of interception with the curvilinear part of the graph.

The (*ultimate*) *tensile strength* is the maximum stress developed (Y in Fig. 5). Silicone rubber, politef, polymethyl methacrylate and high tensile steel have tensile strengths of 5 MPa, 23 MPa, 70 MPa and 2 GPa respectively.

The *tensile strength of healing wounds* has been studied by Howes and his colleagues (1929). For the first four days (*quiescent phase*), the tensile strength is negligible. After that, there is rapid growth of tensile strength (*phase of fibroplasia*) over the next ten days. The author has analysed Howes' data and fitted a Gompertz function (*see* Chapter 1) to the growth of the tensile strength of, for example, a skin wound:

$$T = 100 (1·14 \times 10^{-8})^{0·675^t} \qquad (50.19)$$

where T = percentage maximum tensile strength of wound and t = post-incisional time in days.

Thus, according to this equation, by the end of the fourth day, the tensile strength of the wound has reached only 2 per cent of the maximum which it will attain; on the fourteenth post-incisional day, it exceeds 90 per cent of the maximum tensile strength.

Repeated application of stress below the proportional limit can usually cause fracture. This phenomenon is termed *fatigue*. Curves showing the stress to produce fracture as a function of the number of cyclic stresses (usually plotted logarithmically) are termed S-N fatigue curves. With some materials there is a stress (*endurance* or *fatigue limit*) below which there is no fatigue failure. Such a condition occurs with ferrous alloys; here the endurance limit is about half the tensile strength. Other materials, principally plastics, exhibit no such limit; the curve approaches the N axis asymptotically.

The majority of metals and ceramics (clay-based

materials) are homogeneous and elastically *isotropic* (identical properties in whatever direction they are measured). Consequently, as Williams (1973) points out, they can be characterized by Young's modulus and the Poisson ratio. However, a number of polymer-based materials used are not so characterized. These materials are termed *visco-elastic*. With such materials, Young's modulus of elasticity changes with time. Therefore the modulus which is usually assigned to describe the tensile stress–strain characteristic of polymer-based materials is the *tensile creep modulus*. This is the ratio of stress to strain at a given time. If the modulus changes only with time and is not dependent upon the magnitude of the stress, the material is referred to as being *linear* visco-elastic; if the modulus is also a function of the magnitude of the stress, then the visco-elasticity is termed *non-linear*.

Photoelasticity is a badly chosen term that refers to certain changes in the optical properties of isotropic and transparent *dielectrics* (materials which offer relatively high resistance to the passage of an electric current but through which magnetic or electrostatic lines of force may pass) when subject to stresses. Since the end of the last century, the phenomenon has been used to study elastic stresses in glass or celluloid models of structures. Clark has used such models of the nose to study the role of the septum (*see* Chapter 66).

Physico-chemical Properties. *Corrosion* is the slow destruction of materials by chemical agents and electro-chemical reactions; *erosion* is the slow destruction of materials by mechanical agents. The biological environment into which implants are placed is hostile to both metallic and polymer-based materials. Normal physiological fluids are, in effect, highly oxygenated saline solutions (broadly equivalent to sea water) which present an environment conducive to corrosion. Moreover, enzymes which are present may attack the hydrocarbon bonds of polymers. This latter process is usually termed *biodegradation* (*see* Chapter 54).

Venable and Stuck (1938) showed that there was a correlation between the behaviour of a metal in biological fluids and its electro-chemical properties. These studies have since been extended (Hickman, 1953, and others) so that it is now possible to construct tables showing what is termed an electro-chemical potential series (galvanic series). The more successful implantable alloys and metals are shown in these tables to have electrode potentials in sea water of around $+200\,mV$ or more. The relationship between corrosion behaviour and the dual parameters of electrode potential and pH are displayed graphically in so-called Pourbaix (1966) diagrams.

Bioreactive Properties. A consideration of possible *tissue reactions* is important not only in respect of implants (*see* Chapter 54), but also in respect of other non-living surgical materials.

Granulomas in a number of otolaryngological sites have been attributed to glove powder. When the dangers of using the spores of fungi of the genus *Lycopodium* (club mosses) for glove powder became established (Antopol, 1933), powders containing talc came into use. However, it subsequently became clear that talc (magnesium silicate)

was itself hazardous, producing granulomas (Seelig *et al.*, 1943). Unfortunately, the corn starch which replaced talc as a basis for glove powders has itself been shown not to be free from this particular hazard. Pure starch will not produce a tissue reaction but corn starch for surgical glove powder is treated by a fairly extensive chemical process. This includes tanning with epichlorohydrin to make the granules resistant to autoclaving. Starch granulomatous reactions have followed operations on the sinuses (Ising, 1960) and on the stapes (Rock, 1967; Dawes *et al.*, 1973). In histological preparations and with examination using polaroid light, the starch granules are recognized as doubly refractile "Maltese cross" appearing particles of 10–$70\,\mu m$ diameter. Michaels and Shah (1973) have also drawn attention to granulomas arising in the middle ear cleft as a result of the use of insufflations containing corn starch powder as an "inert" base.

Possible *neoplastic* reactions to non-living structural material are discussed in Chapter 54.

Connecting, Protecting and Supporting Materials. A variety of non-living material is employed in otolaryngology as connecting, covering or supporting structural members. Thus, as examples of these three groups, we have sutures, dressings and stents. Many items in this group are of a basic cylindrical shape and can be considered as such when treated to a mechanical analysis. In reflecting on this theme, one can construct a classification of these various otolaryngological diagnostic and therapeutic cylindrical (or quasi-cylindrical) structures (Table 2).

Connecting materials may be classified as *adhesives*, *cements* or *sutures*. Adhesives have been defined as preparations which join two adjacent surfaces by chemical, or physico-chemical, interactions at the molecular level; cements are substances which act solely as a mechanical bond between adjacent surfaces which usually have relatively considerable irregularities (Charnley, 1970). Although a considerable amount of work has been done on tissue adhesives in surgery (Matsumoto, 1972), Houston's (1969) study showed that the strength of cyanoacrylate-bonded wounds fell progressively below that of sutured wounds after a post-operative period of three days. Further reference is made to adhesives in Chapter 54 and, in respect of the ear, in Chapter 65.

In assessing the strengths of sutures, Douglas (1949) pointed out that a more relevant and useful measure is the ultimate (breaking) stress of a knotted loop. Although it is important that a suture must retain sufficient tensile strength over the critical period of wound healing, it is equally important that the suture material does not provide any significant tissue reaction. Hitherto, suture materials have either been absorbable, i.e. the catguts (prepared from the submucous layer of the proximal third of the small intestine of sheep), or non-absorbable, i.e. natural or artificial fibres. The absorbable sutures were associated with appreciable tissue reaction and the non-absorbable ones with generally slight reaction. More recently, a synthetic absorbable suture material, polyglycolic acid, i.e. poly(oxy-carbonylmethylene), has been introduced. Not only is this material absorbable but it does not produce a tissue reaction (Echeverria and Jimenez, 1970).

TABLE 2

A. SOLID

USE / TYPE	DIAGNOSTIC	THERAPEUTIC	
		TEMPORARY	PERMANENT
FLEXIBLE	Bougies	← ———— Sutures ————→	
RIGID	Probes	Stents; Radioactive needles	Politef and stainless steel pistons

B. HOLLOW

USE / TYPE	DIAGNOSTIC	THERAPEUTIC	
		TEMPORARY	PERMANENT
FLEXIBLE	Auscultation tubes	Drainage tubes	Oesophageal, tracheal and vascular prostheses
RIGID	Needle and syringe; aural speculae; antral cannulae, endoscopes	Tracheostomy and tympano-stomy tubes	Endolymphatic shunt tubes

Cellulosics comprise those materials derived from the natural polymer, cellulose by chemical modification. Cellulose, a polysaccharide of glucose, is the compound of which the greater part of the cell walls of plants is composed. Cellulose is usually obtained from either cotton or wood pulp. Cotton, composed of 90 per cent cellulose, is derived from the seeds of plants belonging to the genus *Gossypium*. Cellulosic tapes with contact adhesives have a use for skin wound closure (Rothmie and Taylor, 1963) and facial neurorraphy (Freeman, 1965). More recently, Shah (1969) has used films of sodium carboxymethylcellulose with a polyethylene backing to cover tympanic membrane perforations. As well as using this procedure therapeutically, it can be used diagnostically to assess the degree to which a perforation accounts for a conductive hearing loss.

The term *stent* was originally applied to a mould made of Stent's (a nineteenth-century British dental surgeon) mass for the purpose of keeping a graft in position. Stent's mass is a plastic resinous material which sets into a hard substance. Nowadays the term "stent" has been extended to designate any material or object which is used to provide support, particularly for surgically repaired or reconstructed tubular structures. Thus, apart from the stents with which laryngologists are familiar, there are otologic stents. Akin and Tobin (1974) describe such a stent made from silicone rubber impression material. They point out how such a stent conforms to the criteria for an ideal ear pack. *Inter alia*, they emphasize that many of the failures

in tympanoplasty (e.g. blunting of the anterior sulcus, loss of ossicular continuity, retraction of the graft from the malleus) are attributable to improper packing. As well as these simple stents used in otolaryngology, composite stents also have a place. Thus Maran and Glover (1973) describe a modified McNaught (1950) keel (which is invaluable in the treatment of anterior glottic stenosis) for the treatment of posterior glottic stenosis. Their composite stent comprises a silicone rubber sheet moulded over the ends of a tantalum plate.

Hollow cylindrical structures, such as endoscopes and speculae, form the basic otolaryngological diagnostic instruments. Such structures also fill a number of therapeutic roles. The *tracheostomy tube* is of such singular importance in laryngological surgery that a special section of this book (Chapter 55) is devoted to this and its associated operations of tracheostomy and tracheotomy. The *tympanostomy tube* (so called "grommet" or "ventilating tube"), as Alberti (1974) has pointed out, was clearly described by Politzer and others in the nineteenth century. Its reintroduction by Armstrong (1954) in the middle of this century reaffirmed its effectiveness in the treatment of secretory otitis media, as demonstrated by Shah's (1971) study (*see* Fig. 3, Chapter 2). Moreover, the report by Hughes and his colleagues (1974) indicates that the use of the tympanostomy tube is essentially innocuous. Out of a total number of 838 introductions of tympanostomy tubes, a suppurative otitis media developed in less than

4 per cent of cases, closure of the membrane was delayed for more than six months in less than 2 per cent of cases and no case developed a sensorineural hearing loss. The use of tubing in other therapeutic roles is, however, not free from hazard, even when constructed of excellent biocompatible material such as silicone rubber. The Department of Health and Social Security, U.K., (1974) has warned against securing silicone rubber drainage tubes with retention sutures. Most silicone rubbers used in tubing manufacture have low tear resistance; thus, once cut or punctured, any hole extends easily to complete severance.

Instruments

The term *instrument* covers not only surgical tools (articles designed to help or enable the hands to apply force) but also objects for observing or measuring as well as objects for delivering some form of energy, or assisting in the delivery of some form of energy. Surgical instruments will be excluded from this discussion since they are properly the subject of articles on surgical techniques. Observing or measuring instruments are essentially diagnostic instruments; therapeutic instruments are usually associated with the delivery of a particular form of energy. A number of therapeutic instruments, e.g. hearing-aids, are by definition *prostheses* also. A prosthesis is defined as a fabricated substitute for a missing, or defective, bodily structure or function. However, internal prostheses, e.g. a stapes prosthesis, are not considered to be instruments, but may be classified as implants. It is convenient to classify instruments according to the physical principles employed, i.e. optical, radiological, thermal, electrical or electro-acoustic.

Optical Instruments. These include microscopes, endoscopes, fibroscopes, stroboscopes and more recently, lasers. All except the last are diagnostic instruments for either enhancing visual observation or permitting visual observation where it would not otherwise be possible.

Optical magnifying instruments are composed of lenses. A lens is an object made of transparent material and having two optical surfaces, one or both of which is curved. Its properties are dependent not only upon its shape but also upon it being a solid transparent object with an index of refraction which is appreciably greater ($>1\cdot5$) than that of air (unity). *Refraction* refers to the change of direction of light (or other radiation) which occurs when it passes from one medium to another in which its velocity of propagation is different. At the boundary of such medium, the angle of incidence and the angle of refraction of the light bear a particular relationship to one another. This relationship is expressed by Snell's Law which states that the ratio of the sine of the angle of incidence to the sine of the angle of refraction is a constant,

i.e. $$n = \sin i / \sin r \qquad (50.20)$$

where n = index of refraction, i = angle of incidence, and r = angle of refraction.

The power of a lens is the reciprocal of its focal length and is given by the equation

$$\phi = 1/f = (n - 1)\left(\frac{1}{r_1} - \frac{1}{r_2}\right) \qquad (50.21)$$

where ϕ = power of lens (m^{-1}), n = index of refraction, and r_1 and r_2 are the radii of curvature of the lens surfaces (m).

Microscopes. Nylén (1954) has discussed the development of the modern aural microscope. He himself was the first to use an operating microscope (monocular) for ear surgery (in 1921). Lundborg and Linzander (1970) have published a useful monograph, replete with colour photographs, dealing with the clinical applications of otomicroscopy. As Steffen and Urban (1969) point out, the operating microscope has now become a *sine qua non* for good otological surgery. These authors also report how adjustments can be made to compensate for refractive errors of the observer. Notwithstanding the value of these standmounted aural operating microscopes, there is a place for hand microscopes for diagnostic use. The Blackmore-Hallpike (1953) monocular ear microscope is particularly valuable in this respect. With a mass of under 400 g, it has a ×6 magnification and permits the use of instruments in the external acoustic meatus. Of the various otoscopes available, a binocular one with a ×3 magnification is available (Wilson, 1970).

Kleinsasser's (1968) modification of the ear microscope to provide for examination of the larynx has proved to be of particular value to surgery of the vocal folds.

Endoscopes. Endoscopes are basically very thin periscopes. Illumination may be by means of a small lamp at the distal end or at the proximal end. If the latter, then the light must be conducted down the tube by one means or another.

A technique of *sinoscopy* (endoscopy of the maxillary paranasal sinus) has been described by Illum and Jeppesen (1972), who also report the technique for photosinoscopy using a fibreoptic system. Illum and his colleagues (1972) also report the advantages of sinoscopy over radiographic examination of the maxillary sinus.

A number of *nasopharyngoscopes* are available for the examination of the nasal part of the pharynx. The smallest of these instruments is about 10 cm long and 2 mm in diameter, with the field of view about 30° at right-angles to the main axis. Larger instruments for the examination of the nasal part of pharynx are in the nature of pharyngeal periscopes. Clark (1967) has described a peroral instrument for the endoscopic examination and photography of the nasal part of pharynx. The endoscope proper fits inside an outer casing and can be rotated through 180° to view either the nasal part of pharynx or the larynx. Atropine is administered before the examination to decrease pharyngeal secretions and both the nasal cavities and the oral part of pharynx are sprayed with a lidocaine solution. When satisfactory anaesthesia is obtained, two rubber catheters are inserted through the nostrils and out through the mouth. Traction on the catheters draws the palate forward and the position is maintained by clamping.

The simplest *bronchoscope* is a rigid open tube up to 40 cm long and 9 mm diameter, with a small bulb for illumination at the distal end. Operating telescopes may be mounted through the tube. Some of the first ciné films taken through a bronchoscope were obtained using a quartz rod illuminating system to obtain the necessary illumination. Like the bronchoscope, the traditional *oesophagoscope* is a simple rigid rube with a length, for adults, of 48 cm and a diameter of 8 mm. The use of the *mediastinoscope* is reviewed by Palva (1963).

Fibreoptic Endoscopes. Because of their rigidity, the use of traditional endoscopes is limited. A system of glass fibres to carry images around corners was patented by Baird in 1927 and subsequently developed by Hopkins and Kapany (1954). Fibroscopes employ bundles of very fine glass fibres to do just this. Fibreoptic systems can be used either for viewing or as light guides for illumination.

With traditional (incandescent) sources of illumination, the illuminance of an object is inversely proportional to the square of the distance from the source. For fibreoptic illumination, this inverse square law does not hold for short working distances. The output end of a fibreoptic bundle, if round, can be considered as a circular disc of luminance B. An object on the central axis of the light beam from the bundle has an illuminance E, such that

$$E = \pi B(\sin u)^2 \qquad (50.22)$$

where u = angle subtended by the radius of the disc at the object.

Fibreoptic laryngoscopes and bronchoscopes of around 5 mm diameter facilitate and extend the scope of endoscopy in both the upper and the lower respiratory tract (Ikeda, 1970). Moreover, a fibreoptic endoscope may permit laryngoscopy when such a procedure using a traditional endoscope is impossible, e.g. in ankylosing spondylitis (Hains and Gibbin, 1973).

The modern flexible *fibreoptic bronchoscope* contains a fibreoptic viewing system, a light source and a multipurpose channel which can be used for anaesthesia, for guiding biopsy forceps or a bronchial brush, or for suction. Because of the small diameter, these instruments are usually introduced through the nose, although some bronchoscopists prefer to pass them through the mouth, through a conventional rigid bronchoscope or through an endotracheal tube. Because of their flexibility and small size, these instruments permit extension of the visible range to subsegmental bronchi with consequent improved detection of bronchial carcinoma. A review of nearly 25 000 fibreoptic bronchoscopic procedures by Credle and his colleagues (1974) indicated a fatality rate of the order of 1 : 10 000, with a complication (major) rate of the order of 1 : 1 000. The deaths (three) were due to excessive local anaesthesia or premedication (one case) or to the procedure itself. It would seem advisable to conduct the procedure transnasally which can usually be done with sedation alone. If a local anaesthetic is required, Credle and his colleagues recommend the use of 35 mol. m^{-3} lidocaine with a maximum dose of about 1 mmol. The studies of Karetzky and his colleagues (1974) show that the procedure is itself associated with a fall (up to 2·8 kPa) in arterial oxygen partial pressure (P_aO_2). Moreover, it appeared that the majority of subjects requiring bronchoscopy for a variety of respiratory disorders had an initial P_aO_2 of less than 10 kPa. A recent (1974b) Leading Article in the *British Medical Journal* therefore recommended careful assessment, including spirometry, of all patients before under-

going fibreoptic bronchoscopy. If the FEV (forced expiratory volume) is less than 1 litre, then the arterial or mixed venous $P\text{CO}_2$ must be measured. If the $P\text{CO}_2$ is raised, then the procedure should be conducted under general anaesthesia with adequate ventilation but no premedication.

With the latest *fibreoptic instruments* for *gastro-intestinal* investigations (Cotton and Williams, 1972; Salmon, 1974), an experienced observer can make a complete visual and biopsy survey of the oesophagus, stomach, duodenum and colon of conscious patients (Morissey, 1972; Cotton, 1973).

It is appropriate to conclude this section on fibreoptic endoscopy by quoting from a Leading Article (1974a) in the *British Medical Journal* which aptly referred to the "fibreoptic revolution": "The potential diagnostic and therapeutic applications of fibreoptic endoscopy are considerable but the feasibility of examination should not automatically assume its relevance or justify its expense."

Stroboscopes. A stroboscope is an instrument for viewing objects undergoing periodic, or quasi-periodic, motion, so that they appear stationary. Different stroboscopes use different methods to achieve this but those employed in otolaryngology use a flashing light to illuminate the moving object, e.g. the vocal folds (laryngostroboscopy). Since flashes can be made of extremely short duration using gaseous (e.g. xenon) discharge lamps, the object moves such a negligible distance that it appears sharply defined. The use of stroboscopy for the examination of the vocal folds is discussed in Chapter 41. McKelvie and his colleagues (1970) have reported the use of strobomicroscopy not only for the examination of the vocal folds but also for the examination of the eardrum.

Lasers. The theory of laser (light amplification by stimulated emission of radiation) and optical masers (microwave amplification by stimulated emission of radiation) has been set out by Schawlow and Townes (1958). Light from an ordinary source takes the form of small packets of light emitted by individual atoms. In a laser beam the light takes the form of a long train of waves, since emission from each atom is exactly in phase with all the others. This *coherence* is the essential characteristic of laser light energy. The coherence is both temporal and spatial. Thus laser beams can afford extremely high energy densities when focused on an area as small as a few micrometres diameter. A ruby crystal laser can produce a brief flash of light with a power of about a gigawatt (10^9 watts). The intensity at the focus of such a beam is sufficient to pierce a hole in a sheet of steel. Because of these properties, lasers can be used to destroy superficial tumours. The first successful results in eradicating malignancies were obtained with ruby crystal lasers by McGuff and his colleagues (1963). Lasers are now being applied in laryngology. Because of the existence of a critical minimum duration for painful stimulae and the brief duration of laser bursts, analgesia is not required.

Radiological Instruments. The use of ionizing radiations for diagnostic purposes is discussed earlier in this chapter and the use for therapeutic purposes is discussed in Chapter 52.

Thermal Instruments. Ideally, as Haas and Taylor (1948)

point out, a method of destroying functional biologic tissue should conform to the following criteria:

(1) Reversibility.
(2) Consistent reproducibility.
(3) Sharp delineation.
(4) Haemostasis.
(5) Flexibility.
(6) Safety.
(7) Simplicity.
(8) Rapidity.

Haas and Taylor studied experimental brain lesions on animals produced by a quantitative hypothermal method (cryogenic surgery, or just "cryosurgery"). They concluded that this method could meet the criteria that they had set out. Cryosurgical procedures can produce discrete circumscribed destruction of tissue with haemostasis and no danger of suppressive complications. The procedure has clear advantages over surgical excision which requires anatomical interruption and produces haemorrhage. Cryosurgery thus has a particular application in the treatment of neoplasms. Suitable equipment, such as that described by McKelvie and Shaheen (1967), utilizes the Joule-Thompson effect. This refers to the phenomenon of high-pressure gas flowing through a small orifice into a chamber rapidly changing temperature on expansion. At ordinary ambient temperatures and pressures, helium and hydrogen become warmer; all other gases become cooler. McKelvie and Shaheen's cryoprobes use nitrous oxide as a refrigerant; this gives a working "tip" temperature of 233 K. This temperature produces a 10 mm "ice ball" with a marginal temperature of 253 K. Holden and McKelvie (1972) have used this equipment to treat a series of patients with inoperable carcinoma of the floor of the mouth, oral and nasal cavities, pharynx (including the nasal part), paranasal sinuses and neck. A fifth of the cases failed to respond. In this context, a disadvantage of cryotherapy is that it is only local and not regional. There is also evidence that cryotherapy may render a tissue antigenic (Shulman *et al.*, 1967).

Cryotherapeutic procedures may also be used in hypophysectomy and in the treatment of epistaxis, nasal allergic and vasomotor conditions, and Ménière's disorder.

Electrical Instruments. A number of electrical instruments are available to the otolaryngologist for use in measuring the function of muscles and of nerves.

There have been two relatively recent developments of note in the application of electrical impedance techniques relevant to otolaryngology. First, Fourcin and Abberton (1971) have described an *electrolaryngograph*. This instrument depends on the fact that the output from a pair of electrodes on either side of the neck at the level of the vocal folds is a function of vocal fold contact (Fourcin, 1974). Secondly, Bäcklund and his colleagues (1969) have introduced a technique of electrical impedance *plethysmography* to measure vertebral artery function. By this method, the tissue impedance, which reflects volume changes caused especially by the pulse waves, is recorded. A reduced arterial blood flow results in smaller impedance variations with each pulse wave. Special electrodes for placing against

the posterior pharyngeal wall at the level of C2 have been constructed. Normally, rotation of the head when the subject is sitting or supine does not give rise to changes in the impedance compared to the initial position. However, with the head in the hanging position, with each pulse wave, a smaller impedance decrease than in the other positions is normally recorded, especially if the head is rotated in the direction opposite to the artery being studied. This indicates that some compression of the vertebral artery on one side is a normally occurring phenomenon in certain positions of the head. In patients with a clinical cervical syndrome, low pulse wave amplitudes simultaneous with nystagmus have been recorded. The latter can be regarded as an expression of brain stem ischaemia, caused by compression of the vertebral artery in association with a defective compensation via the circulus arteriosus (of Willis).

Electro-acoustic Instruments. Diagnostic electro-acoustic instruments, in the form of audiometers, are so important to the otolaryngologist that separate sections of this book have been allocated not only to audiometers (Chapter 56), but also to the techniques of using these instruments (Chapter 57) and the conditions required for their use (Chapter 58). Equally important are those rehabilitative/therapeutic electro-acoustic instruments (hearing aids and other sound amplifying equipment) which are so vital to those who are handicapped by virtue of a hearing loss. Three separate chapters (60–62) have therefore been allocated to this theme, including a final one on auditory rehabilitation.

In addition to the auditory prostheses, there are the vocal prostheses which provide a substitute voice after laryngectomy. Greene and his colleagues (1974) report a new laryngeal vibrator (so-called artificial larynx) where the sound is produced by a mechanical system driven by an electric motor. An unconventional flexible-drive system (spring-loaded plunger) causes a hammer to strike a diaphragm at a frequency of about 60 Hz. A compression spring between the plunger and the hammer produces a smoothing effect on the motion of the plunger and permits a certain degree of adjustment to the oscillation rate.

II. EFFICACY AND EFFICIENCY IN RESPECT OF USE OF MATERIA OTOLARYNGOLOGICA

Validation of Therapeutic Procedures (Clinical Trials)

Clinical trials are designed to test the *efficacy* of prospective (and sometimes not so prospective!) therapeutic procedures. The need to do this is now generally accepted. This applies as much to surgical procedures as to medical ones such as the administration of drugs.

The number of otolaryngological procedures whose efficacy has been established by *randomized comparative trials* (RCTs) is limited. Even those clinical trials which are published in medical journals have not been free from criticism. An analysis of over one hundred reports of clinical trials published in four British journals, showed that a third were unacceptable because of defects in methodology. However, in the otolaryngological area, Capel and McKelvie (1971), Holopainen and his colleagues (1971) and Somazzi and Wuthrich (1972) have all conducted double-bind trials of *disodium cromoglicate* insufflations in hay fever patients. The results of all three trials showed this treatment to be beneficial. The effect of the drug is to inhibit the release of histamine and other humoral mediators after the union of antigens with the reaginic antibodies on cell surfaces (Cox, 1967; Assem and Mongar, 1970). Also in hay fever patients, Harrison and Stanley (1972) conducted a double-blind crossover trial of *tetracosactide* (the compound formed of the first twenty-four of the thirty-nine amino acids of ACTH) in a dose of 170 nmol intramuscularly twice weekly. A significant improvement was demonstrated in 65 per cent of patients. Double-blind *hyposensitization* trials have also been conducted on asthmatics with or without perennial rhinitis who were allergic to house dust. Studies using extracts of both *Dermatophagoides farinae* (Maunsell et al., 1971) and *D. pteronyssinus* (Smith, 1971) have shown these extracts to be efficacious. Strong and his colleagues (1966) conducted a prospective study of the effects of *pre-operative radiation* (a total of 2 000 R spread over five successive days) to the entire neck as an adjunct to radical neck dissection for squamous carcinoma of the head and neck region. The two groups (radiation or no radiation) were matched by placing patients born on even-numbered days in one group and those born on odd-numbered days in the other. A statistically significant reduction in the incidence of recurrence was demonstrated, especially in respect of those subjects with histologically proven cervical node metastases. However, the similarity between different types of treatment for certain cancers underlines the need to take into account, in determining the treatment of choice, not only survival but also the quality of life of the survivors. When patients are permitted to express their feelings, evidence of social and psychological morbidity emerges.

Negative results from therapeutic trials are of as much importance as positive results since they can save us from applying useless procedures which may themselves not be without risk. Of note are Archard's (1967) demonstration that myringotomy alone is of no value in the management of secretory otitis media in children, Holborow's (1957) demonstration that, in children with sinusitis, maxillary sinus lavage is no more effective (perhaps less) when an antibiotic (penicillin) and/or a detergent (tyloxapol) is left in the sinus, and the various trials reported in Chapter 30 of the ineffectiveness of facial nerve decompression for Bell's palsy. The three therapeutic trials (McKee, 1963; Mawson et al., 1967; Roydhouse, 1969) in respect of adenotonsillectomy have still not satisfied clinical scientists. Cochrane (1971) concedes that "taken altogether the evidence, superficially, is in favour of the operation but, unfortunately, two major criticisms can be made against all three". The first criticism is that the comparison was made between "operation" and "no or inadequate medical treatment". The second criticism referred to the method of collecting data, basing it on parents' opinions.

As Wilson (1968) points out, therapeutic trials should include a report about any harmful or *undesirable effects* that may be caused by the new treatment. The mere statement "no toxic effects were noted" is generally inadequate since much depends upon how carefully they were sought. However, the use of a check list may actually interfere with the collection of side effects, including otological symptoms, when comparing the side effects of drugs (Huskisson and Wojtulewski, 1974). An accurate assessment of the incidence, nature and severity of side effects can come only from extensive clinical use of the drug or procedure. In the U.K., new drugs are released for general distribution by the Safety of Drugs (Dunlop) Committee if it accepts that the therapeutic efficacy, as demonstrated in clinical therapeutic trials, outweighs any toxic hazard that might so far have come to light. A drug may subsequently be withdrawn if information comes to hand that appreciable toxic effects exist. All those medical practitioners who note even suspected side effects should report these on the appropriate form to the Medical Assessor, Committee on Safety of Medicines, Finsbury Square House, London EC2B 2ZS.

Economics and Efficiency of Therapeutic Procedures

Cochrane (1971) has sought to distinguish between *efficacy* and *efficiency* in considering health care. (He does, however, because of a personal preference, use the term *effectiveness* in lieu of *efficacy*.) An *effective* (or efficacious) procedure, as we have just seen, is one which has been scientifically demonstrated to have a measurable effect in altering the natural history of a disorder for the better. *Efficiency* relates to the best use of materials and people in achieving the desired results in health care. Efficiency is of paramount importance for health services, where resources are limited so that priorities must be set. Thus *economic* considerations are basic to questions of efficiency.

In the late seventeenth century, Sir William Petty proposed to the British government that it undertake economic analyses of medical services. He argued that the government, by spending money, could, in the end, save money by saving lives and increasing productivity. Thus Petty was one of the first advocates of what came to be known as *cost-benefit analysis*. Techniques of cost-benefit analysis (Prest and Turvey, 1965) were subsequently devised to measure these problems relating to economics and to efficiency. Cost-benefit analysis is essentially similar to the method of financial appraisal used in private industry. However, unlike the decision-maker in private industry, public decision-makers must also take into account the benefits to society as a whole. The methods of cost-benefit analysis consist of estimating the financial returns (benefits) and outlays (costs) attributable to each of various competing projects (Glass, 1973). As defined by Roskill, a programme of cost-benefit analysis comprises three stages: first there is the identification of the relevant factors; secondly, there is quantitative measurement of their significance; thirdly, there is the expression in value terms of these quantities in order to permit aggregation of the costs and benefits due to different factors. Valuation means measurement in terms of money since the medium of money is the most convenient and easily understood general standard of comparison (Commission on the Third London Airport, 1970). As regards health care, the measurement of benefits is, as Pole (1968) has pointed out, a most intractable problem.

In discussing the cost of smoking, Atkinson and Meade

(1974) pointed to the number of different elements (factors) which are relevant:

(1) Medical treatment costs.
(2) Lost earnings as a result of sickness.
(3) Sickness benefit paid in case of sickness.
(4) Cost of premature death.
(5) Benefits not paid and taxes not received in the case of premature death.
(6) Resources employed in the production of tobacco.
(7) Tax revenue from tobacco duty.
(8) Pain and suffering to relatives.
(9) Nuisance to non-smokers and other externalities (including fire risk).

Even after a cost-benefit analysis, rules are required on which to base a decision. In their cost-benefit analysis of the treatment of varicose veins, Piachaud and Weddell (1972) said that the decision rule should be to choose the procedure that produces as good a clinical result as any other method and is the most economic in terms of man-power, money and resources.

Apart from a tentative incursion into this field by Ellis (1954), the approach to treatment which is outlined in this section has yet to be applied to otolaryngology. Ellis discussed the provision of a hearing aid *vis-à-vis* the fenestration operation for otosclerosis. The reader may find it an entertaining, yet profitable, exercise to attempt a cost-benefit analytical approach to the treatment of otosclerosis now that stapedectomy has superseded fenestration and the methods of cost-benefit analysis have been more fully elucidated.

CONCLUSIONS

The modern otolaryngologist clearly has an enormous range of materials and instruments placed at his disposal for both diagnostic and therapeutic purposes. Although there is an increasing number of sophisticated electrical diagnostic instruments, and an increasing number of nuclides and synthetic drugs for therapeutic purposes, the otolaryngologist is also making more and more use of natural materials, whether they be antibiotics or transplants. The future may also see an increasing use of sera. The production and use of all these things, it should not be forgotten, is subject to a number of administrative, legal and, possibly, economic restrictions (*see* Chapter 69). Even such instruments as aural and nasal forceps and items of equipment such as hospital bedside lockers must conform, at least in the U.K., to national standards (BS 3419: 1961 and BS 1765: 1951 respectively)!

REFERENCES

Ackerman, N. B., Shahon, D. B. and Marvin, J. F. (1960), *Surgery*, **47**, 615.
Akin, W. O. and Tobin, H. A. (1974), *Arch. Otolaryng.*, **99**, 462.
Alberti, P. (1974), *Laryngoscope*, **84**, 805.
Anderson, N. E., James, K. and Woodruff, M. F. A. (1967), *Lancet*, **i**, 1126.
André, P., Pialoux, P., Poncet, E., Dulac, G. L. and Francois, J. (1968), *La tomographie en oto-rhino-laryngologie*. Paris: Arnette.
Antopol, W. (1933), *Arch. Path.*, **16**, 326.
Archard, J. C. (1967), *J. Laryng.*, **81**, 309.
Armstrong, B. W. (1954), *Arch. Otolaryng.*, **59**, 653.
Assem, E. S. K. and Mongar, J. L. (1970), *Int. Arch. Allergy*, **38**, 68.
Atkinson, A. B. and Meade, T. W. (1974), *J. R. statist. Soc.*, **A137**, 297.
Bäcklund, L., Celestino, D., Eriksson, K., Johnson, L., Nylander, G. and Stahle, J. (1969), *Acta oto-laryng. (Stockh.)*, **68**, 303.
Baird, J. L. (1927), British Patent Specification, No. 285738.
Barnes, P. A. and Rees, D. J. (1972), *A Concise Textbook of Radiotherapy*. London: Faber and Faber.
Batchelor, J. R. and Joysey, V. C. (1969), *Lancet*, **i**, 390.
Berrett, A., Brünner, S. and Valvassori, G. E. (1973), *Modern Thin-section Tomography*. Springfield, Ill.: Chas. C. Thomas.
Billingham, R. E. (1970), *The Biology and Surgery of Tissue Transplantation*, Chap. 1. Oxford: Blackwell.
Billingham, R. E. and Brent, L. (1957), *Transpl. Bull.*, **4**, 67.
Blackmore, L. and Hallpike, C. S. (1953), *J. Laryng.*, **67**, 108.
Bocage, A. E. (1922), French Patent, No. 536464.
British Standard BS 1765 (1951), British Standards Institution, London.
British Standard BS 3419 (1961), British Standards Institution, London.
British Standard BS 449 (1970), British Standards Institution, London.
British Standard BS 5194 (1975), British Standards Institution, London.
Capel, L. H. and McKelvie, P. (1971), *Lancet*, **i**, 575.
Chaplin, C. H. (1969), *Plast. reconstr. Surg.*, **44**, 447.
Charnley, J. (1970), *Acrylic Cement in Orthopaedic Surgery*. Edinburgh: Livingstone.
Chisholm, G. D., Waterworth, Pamela M., Calnan, J. S. and Garrod, L. P. (1973), *Brit. med. J.*, **i**, 569.
Choufoer, J. C., Van Rhijn, M., Kassenaar, A. A. H. and Querido, A. (1963), *J. clin. Endocr.*, **23**, 1203.
Clark, G. (1967), *Arch. Otolaryng.*, **86**, 183.
Cochrane, A. L. (1971), *Effectiveness and Efficiency*. London: Nuffield Provincial Hospitals Trust.
Commission (Roskill's) on the Third London Airport (1970), *Papers and Proceedings*, Vol. VII. London: H.M.S.O.
Cotton, P. B. (1973), *Brit. med. J.*, **2**, 161.
Cotton, P. B. and Williams, C. B. (1972), *Brit. J. Hosp. Med.*, **8**, 35.
Cox, J. S. G. (1967), *Nature*, **216**, 1328.
Credle, W. F., Smiddy, J. F. and Elliott, R. C. (1974), *Amer. Rev. Resp. Dis.*, **109**, 67.
Dausset, J., Colombani, J., Legrand, L. and Feingold, N. (1968), *Nouv. Rev. Franç. Hémat.*, **6**, 841.
Davis, P. J. (1966), *Amer. J. Med.*, **40**, 918.
Dawes, J. D. K., Cameron, D. S., Curry, A. R. and Rannie, I. (1973), *J. Laryng.*, **87**, 365.
Dempster, W. J., Lennox, B. and Boag, J. W. (1950), *Brit. J. exp. Path.*, **31**, 670.
Department of Health and Social Security, U.K. (1974), Health Equipment Information No. 55, Nov. 54/74.
Douglas, D. M. (1949), *Lancet*, **ii**, 497.
Dray, S., Kelus, A., Dubiski, S. and Lennox, E. S. (1962), *Nature*, **198**, 785.
Echeverria, E. and Jimenez, J. (1970), *Surg. Gynec. Obstet.*, **131**, 1.
Ellis, M. (1954), *Brit. Encycl. Med. Practice*. London: Butterworths.
Fletcher, C. M. and Oldham, P. D. (1949), *Brit. J. industr. Med.*, **6**, 168.
Florey, M. E., Turton, E. C. and Duthie, E. S. (1946), *Lancet*, **ii**, 105.
Fourcin, A. J. (1974), *Ventilatory and Phonatory Control Systems*, Chap. 19 (B. Wyke, Ed.). Oxford University Press.
Fourcin, A. J. and Abberton, Evelyn (1971), *Med. biol. Ill.*, **21**, 172.
Freeman, B. S. (1965), *Plast. reconstr. Surg.*, **35**, 167.
Freeman, N. V. (1973), *J. Pediat. Surg.*, **8**, 213.
Glass, N. J. (1973), *Health Trends*, **5**, 51.
Goolden, A. W. G. and Mallard, J. R. (1958), *Brit. J. Radiol.*, **31**, 589.
Gordon, D. S. and Blair, G. A. S. (1974), *Brit. med. J.*, **2**, 478.
Gorer, P. A. (1937), *J. Path. Bact.*, **44**, 69.
Gorer, P. A. (1961), *Adv. Immunol.*, **1**, 345.
Greene, M. C. L., Atkinson, P. and Watson, B. W. (1974), *J. Laryng.*, **88**, 1105.

Groesbeck, H. P., (1959), *Cancer*, **12**, 1.
Haas, G. H. and Taylor, C. B. (1948), *Arch. Path.*, **45**, 563.
Hains, J. D. and Gibbin, K. P. (1973), *J. Laryng.*, **87**, 699.
Hanbury, E. M., Jr., Heslin, J., Stang, L. G., Jr., Tucker, U. D. and Rall, J. F. (1954), *J. clin. Endocr. Metab.*, **14**, 1530.
Harrison, D. F. and Stanley, I. M. (1972), *Practitioner*, **208**, 680.
Harrison, D. F. N. (1969), *Brit. med. J.*, **2**, 165.
Havard, C. W. H. (1974), *Brit. med. J.*, **1**, 553.
Hayes, R. L., Nelson, B., Swartzendruber, D. C., Carlton, J. E. and Byrd, D. L. (1970), *Science*, **167**, 289.
Hickman, J. (1953), *Proc. roy. Soc. Med.*, **8**, 644.
Hinchcliffe, R. (1961), *J. Laryng.*, **75**, 101.
Hinchcliffe, W. A., Zamel, N., Fishman, N. H., Dedo, H. H., Greenspan, R. H. and Nadel, J. (1970), *Radiology*, **97**, 327.
Holborow, C. A. (1957), *J. Laryng.*, **71**, 689.
Holden, H. B. and McKelvie, P. (1972), *Brit. J. Surg.*, **59**, 709.
Holopainen, E., Backman, A. and Salo, O. P. (1971), *Lancet*, **i**, 55.
Hopkins, H. H. and Kapany, N. S. (1954), *Nature*, **173**, 39.
Horst, W. (1959), in *Strahlenbiologie, Strahlentherapie, Nuklearmedicin u. Krebsforschung Ergebnisse*. Stuttgart: Thieme.
Houston, S., Hodge, J. W., Ousterhout, D. K. and Leonard, F. (1969), *J. Biomed. Materials Res.*, **3**, 286.
Howes, E. L., Sooy, J. W. and Harvey, S. C. (1929), *J. Amer. med. Ass.*, **92**, 42.
Hronkova-Zoulkova, J., Ivaskova, E. and Klouda, P. (1968), *Folia biol.*, **14**, 402.
Hughes, L. A., Warder, F. A. and Hudson, W. R. (1974), *Arch. Otolaryng.*, **100**, 151.
Huskisson, E. C. and Wojtulewski, J. A. (1974), *Brit. med. J.*, **2**, 698.
Ikeda, S. (1970), *Ann. Otol.*, **79**, 916.
Illum, P. and Jeppesen, F. (1972), *Acta oto-laryng. (Stockh.)*, **73**, 506.
Illum, P., Jeppesen, F. and Langebaek, E. (1972), *Acta oto-laryng. (Stockh.)*, **74**, 287.
Ishii, T., Bernstein, J. M. and Balogh, K. (1967), *Ann. Otol.*, **76**, 368.
Ising, U. (1960), *Acta chir. scand.*, **120**, 95.
Kamrin, B. B. (1959), *Proc. Soc. exp. Biol. (N.Y.)*, **100**, 58.
Karetzky, M. S., Garvey, J. W. and Brandstetter, R. D. (1974), *N.Y. St. J. Med.*, **74**, 62.
Kashima, H. K., McKusick, K. A., Malmud, L. S. and Wagner, H. N. (1974), *Laryngoscope*, **84**, 1078.
Kendall, E. C. (1915), *J. Amer. med. Ass.*, **64**, 2042.
Kirchner, F. R. (1974), *Laryngoscope*, **84**, 1894.
Kissmeyer-Nielsen, F., Svejgaard, A. and Hauge, M. (1968), *Nature*, **219**, 1116.
Kleinsasser, O. (1968), *Microlaryngoscopy and Endolaryngeal Microsurgery*. Philadelphia: Saunders.
Klockhoff, I. and Lindblom, U. (1966), *Acta oto-laryng. (Stockh.)*, **61**, 459.
Kornblut, A. D., Silberstein, E. B., Saenger, E. L. and Shumrick, D. A. (1974), *Arch. Otolaryng.*, **100**, 201.
Krohn, P. L. (1954), *J. Endocr.*, **11**, 78.
Lance, E. M. and Medawar, P. B. (1968), *Lancet*, **i**, 1174.
Leading Article (1974a), *Brit. med. J.*, **3**, 121.
Leading Article (1974b), *Brit. med. J.*, **3**, 542.
Levi-Montalcini, R. (1964), *Ann. N.Y. Acad. Sci.*, **118**, 199.
Lloyd, G. A. S. (1973), *Recent Advances in Otolaryngology*, Chap. 25 (Joselen Ransome, H. Holden and T. R. Bull, Eds.). Edinburgh: Churchill/Livingstone.
Lloyd, G. A. S. and Wylie, I. G. (1971), *Brit. J. Radiol.*, **44**, 940.
Lundborg, T. and Linzander, S. (1970), *Acta oto-laryng. (Stockh.)*, suppl. 266.
McCabe, B. F. (1975). Personal communication.
McGuff, P. E., Bushnell, D., Soroff, H. S. and Deterling, R. A. (1963), *Surg. Forum*, **14**, 143.
McKee, W. J. E. (1963), *Brit. J. Prev. Soc. Med.*, **17**, 49.
McKelvie, P., Grey, P. and North, C. (1970), *Lancet*, **ii**, 503.
McKelvie, P. and Shaheen, O. H. (1967), *Brit. med. J.*, **4**, 351.
McNaught, R. C. (1950), *Laryngoscope*, **60**, 264.
Mack, R. E., Hart, K. T., Druet, D. and Bauer, M. A. (1961), *Amer. J. Med.*, **30**, 323.
Mackey, W. A. (1970), *The Biology and Surgery of Tissue Transplantation* (J. M. Anderson, Ed.). Oxford: Blackwell.
Maclagan, N. F., Bowden, C. H. and Wilkinson, J. H. (1957), *Biochem. J.*, **67**, 5.

Maran, A. G. D. and Glover, G. W. (1973), *J. Laryng.*, **87**, 695.
Matsumoto, T. (1972), *Tissue Adhesives in Surgery*. London: H. K. Lewis.
Maunsell, K., Wraith, D. G. and Hughes, A. M. (1971), *Lancet*, **i**, 967.
Mawson, S. R., Adlington, P. and Evans, M. (1967), *J. Laryng.*, **81**, 777.
Meredith, W. J. and Massey, J. B. (1972), *Fundamental Physics of Radiology*. Bristol: John Wright & Sons.
Michaels, L. and Shah, N. S. (1973), *Brit. med. J.*, **2**, 714.
Mittal, K. K., Mickey, M. R., Springal, D. P. and Terasaki, P. T. (1968), *Transplantation*, **6**, 913.
Mittermaier, R. (1969), "Hals-Nasen-Ohren-Krankheiten in Röntgenbild," in *Ein Atlas für Klinik u. Praxis*. Stuttgart: Thieme.
Morgans, N. E. and Trotter, W. R. (1958), *Lancet*, **i**, 607.
Morissey, J. M. (1972), *Gastroenterology*, **62**, 1241.
Morton, D. L. (1974), *Scientific Foundations of Surgery* (C. Wells, J. Kyle and J. E. Dunphy, Eds.). London: Heinemann.
Mowbray, J. F. (1967), *J. clin. Path.*, **20**, 499.
Nadel, J. A., Wolfe, W. G., Graf, P. D., Youker, J. E., Zamel, N., Austin, J. H. M., Hinchcliffe, W. A., Greenspan, R. H. and Wright, R. R. (1970), *New Engl. J. Med.*, **283**, 281.
Needham, A. E. (1964), *The Growth Process in Animals*. London: Pitman.
Nylén, C. O. (1954), *Acta oto-laryng. (Stockh.)*, suppl. 116, p. 216.
Palva, T. (1963), *Arch. Otolaryng.*, **77**, 19.
Perlmutter, M. and Slater, S. L. (1956), *New Engl. J. Med.*, **255**, 65.
Piachaud, D. and Weddell, J. M. (1972), *Lancet*, **ii**, 1191.
Pole, J. D. (1968), *Screening in Medical Care*, Chap. 12. London: Nuffield Provincial Hospitals Trust; Oxford University Press.
Pourbaix, M. (1966), *Atlas of Electrochemical Equilibria in Aqueous Solutions*. Oxford: Pergamon.
Prest, A. R. and Turvey, R. (1965), *Econ. J.*, **75**, 683.
Rock, E. H. (1967), *Arch. Otolaryng.*, **86**, 8.
Rothmie, N. G. and Taylor, G. W. (1963), *Brit. med. J.*, **2**, 1027.
Rowan, J. O. (1972), *Scientific Foundations of Neurology* (M. Critchley, J. L. O'Leary and B. Jennett, Eds.). London: Heinemann.
Roydhouse, N. (1969), *Lancet*, **ii**, 931.
Rubin, P., Blatt, I. M., Holt, J. F. and Maxwell, J. H. (1955), *Ann. Otol.*, **64**, 667.
Sachs, B. A., Siegel, E. and Horwitt, B. N. (1972), *Brit. med. J.*, **1**, 79.
Salmon, P. R. (1974), *Fibre-optic Endoscopy*. London: Pitman Medical.
Samuel, E. (1952), *Clinical Radiology of the Ear, Nose and Throat*. London: Butterworths.
Sans, R. and Porcher, J. (1950), *J. Radiol.*, **31**, 300.
Scanlan, R. L. (1964), *Arch. Otolaryng.*, **80**, 698.
Schawlow, A. L. and Townes, C. H. (1958), *Phys. Rev.*, **112**, 194.
Schwartz, R. S. and Dameshek, W. (1959), *Nature*, **183**, 1682.
Seelig, M. G., Verde, D. J. and Kidd, F. H. (1943), *J. Amer. med. Ass.*, **123**, 950.
Shah, N. (1969), *Clin. Trials J.*, **6**, 207.
Shah, N. (1971), *J. Laryng.*, **81**, 283.
Shulman, S., Yantorno, C. and Bronson, P. (1967), *Proc. Soc. exp. Biol. (N.Y.)*, **124**, 658.
Silver, S. (1968), *Radioactive Nuclides in Medicine and Biology*. Philadelphia: Lea and Febiger.
Smith, A. P. (1971), *Brit. med. J.*, **4**, 204.
Snell, G. D. (1964), Transplantation, **2**, 655.
Somazzi, S. and Wuthrich, B. (1972), *Schweiz. med. Wschr.*, **102**, 776.
Stanbury, J. B., Brownell, G. L., Riggs, D. S., Preinette, H., Itoiz, J. and del Castillo, E. B. (1954), "Endemic Goitre," in *The Adaptation of Man to Iodine Deficiency*. Harvard University Press.
Steffen, T. N. and Urban, J. C. (1969), *Arch. Otolaryng.*, **90**, 380.
Stone, L. S. and Zaur, I. S. (1940), *J. exp. Zool.*, **85**, 243.
Strong, E. W., Henschke, U. K., Nickson, J. J., Frazell, E. L., Tollefsen, H. R. and Hilaris, B. S. (1966), *Cancer*, **19**, 1509.
Tan, J. S., Trott, A., Phair, J. P. and Watanakunakorn, C. (1972), *J. infect. Dis.*, **126**, 492.
Thompson, J. A. (1974), *Clinical Tests of Thyroid Function*. London: Crosby Lockwood Staples.
Thron, C. D. (1974), *Pharmacol. Rev.*, **26**, 3.
Vaidya, S. G., Chaudhri, M. A., Morrison, R. and Whait, D. (1970), *Lancet*, **ii**, 911.

Van't Hoff, W., Pover, G. G. and Eiser, N. M. (1972), *Brit. med. J.*, **4**, 203.
Venable, C. S. and Stuck, W. G. (1938), *J. Amer. med. Ass.*, **111**, 1349.
Walike, J. W. (1967), *Arch. Otolaryng.*, **86**, 676.
Wastie, M. L. (1972), *Brit. J. Radiol.*, **45**, 570.
Westlake, W. J. (1971), *J. Pharm. Sci.*, **60**, 882.
Westra, D. (1966), *Zonography, the Narrow-angle Tomography*. Amsterdam: Excerpta Medica. Foundation.
Williams, D. F. (1973), *Implants in Surgery*, Chap. 3 (D. F. Williams and R. Roaf, Eds.). London: Saunders.

Wilson, G. M. (1968), *Prescribers J.*, **8**, 95.
Wilson, T. D. H. (1970), *Arch. Otolaryng.*, **91**, 84.
Woodruff, M. F. A. (1960), *The Transplantation of Tissues and Organs*. Springfield, Ill.: Chas. C. Thomas.
Woodruff, M. F. A. and Anderson, N. F. (1963), *Nature*, **200**, 702.
Woodruff, M. F. A. and Llaurado, J. G. (1956), *Plast. reconstr. Surg.*, **18**, 251.
Zamel, N., Austin, J. H. M., Graf, P. D., Dedo, H. H., Jones, M. D. and Nadel, J. A. (1970), *Radiology*, **94**, 547.
Ziedes des Plantes, B. G. (1931), *Ned. Tijdschr. Geneesk.*, **75**, 5219.

51. CYTOTOXIC DRUGS

J. IAN BURN

INTRODUCTION

Practical cytotoxic chemotherapy has been in use now for 30 years, since the first patients were treated with nitrogen mustard in the autumn of 1942. However, there is nothing new in the concept of treating malignant disease by drugs and, indeed, it is the use of major ablative surgery and radiotherapy which are new in the field. Reference was made in the Ebers papyrus of Egypt to the use of plant remedies for what is thought to have been cancer as early as 1500 BC and throughout the ages malignant disease has been treated by the applications of chemicals, both locally and systemically. Substances as diverse as garlic and Coley's toxin have all been the subject of extravagant claims. The subject of plant remedies for cancer was reviewed by Hartwell (1960) and makes remarkable reading for the wide variety of substances recommended throughout the years. As emphasized by Hartwell, the empirical application of plants to the ailing human body, over thousands of years, has culminated in the development of many useful drugs for a number of diseases. "If there is any hope in a chemical treatment for cancer, it is reasonable to believe that such an agent is as likely to originate from a plant as from pure synthesis."

The first real impetus to the current concept of cancer chemotherapy, like so many other advances in medicine, was fortuitous. Extensive trials in the use of poison gases were carried out during World War II even though they were never used in conflict. A chance exposure of a group of workers to one of the nitrogen mustards resulted in a deficiency in their circulating blood cells. From this observation developed an extensive investigation into the use of the nitrogen mustards in the treatment of leukaemia and allied disorders. This in turn led to the recognition of the possible use of other alkylating agents in the treatment of cancer and the subsequent analysis of literally thousands of compounds. A few have proved suitable for clinical use.

Another observation in the 1940's that diets deficient in folic acid resulted in a blood picture resembling that caused by nitrogen mustard, provoked the eventual synthesis of antifolic compounds. Concomitantly, the fundamental observation that certain animal tumours regressed with the administration of yeast derivatives, led to the development of the group of anticancer agents known generically as antimetabolites. The resulting courageous use of a folic-acid antagonist, aminopterin (4-amino folic acid), in the treatment of acute leukaemia in children by Farber and his colleague (1948) heralded the real start of modern cancer chemotherapy.

Finally, among all the many antibiotics examined for their antibacterial potential, some were found also to have an anti-tumour effect, and notably the actinomycins. It is from these three basic groups, the alkylating agents, the antimetabolites and the antibiotics, that the majority of the anticancer cytotoxic agents at present in clinical use emanate. There are a few additional miscellaneous substances, but the majority of cytotoxic drugs fall into one or other of the three main categories,

In considering the historical aspects of cytotoxic cancer chemotherapy, it is impossible to acknowledge adequately the enormous role played by the basic biological sciences in the development of this mode of therapy. The unravelling of the genetic code and the elucidation of the chemistry of cell replication have enabled the synthesis of the modern anticancer cytotoxic agents, a subject dealt with in great detail by Sir Alexander Todd in the first Jephcott lecture at the Royal Society of Medicine (1959). Acknowledgement also must be made of the pioneering efforts of the U.S.A. in the development of rational cytotoxic cancer chemotherapy, initiated by the establishment of the Cancer Chemotherapy National Service Centre (CCNSC) in the mid-1950's. The history of the now world-renowned cancer chemotherapy screening programme undertaken at the National Cancer Institute, Bethesda (Zubrod *et al.*, 1966) is one of perseverance and massive endeavour. To date, approximately 150 000 compounds with known structures, and the same number of natural product extracts, have been screened (Wood, 1971). It is noticeable that the random selection of agents evident in the early years of the programme has now given way to a more rational selection of synthesized agents, specifically designed for the purpose of producing an anticipated anticancer effect.

Out of this gargantuan effort has come new hope for the realistic control of cancer by drug therapy. Although the massive American effort remains unparalleled, notable contributions have been made by many other countries. Much of our present knowledge of the action of the alkylating agents stems from 25 years of research at the Chester Beatty Cancer Research Institute in London.

The range of useful drugs has gradually increased and there are now about 30 that are in general use clinically. Despite the undoubted advances, however, cytotoxic cancer chemotherapy has as yet made only a limited impact upon the mortality figures from cancer. Lives have certainly been prolonged and a measure of control obtained, but total elimination of the cancer and cure has eluded all but a handful of malignant diseases. To date the most common cancers, including those of the head and neck region, have benefited minimally. The reasons for this disappointing result of 25 years' endeavour have been clearly detailed by Connors (1972), and relate essentially to the fact that the available agents have a selectivity for *all* dividing cells rather than human cancer cells as such. The vulnerability of normal tissues which are also proliferating rapidly, results in the relatively low therapeutic indices of the cytotoxics against cancer. In only a few instances are the cell kinetics of malignant tumours such that destruction of the cancer can be achieved before unacceptable toxicity occurs.

Tumours as a class are qualitatively similar to normal tissues and possess the same enzymes and consequently the same metabolic pathways (Griffin, 1961). There are certain quantitative differences among various tumours, however, and rapidly growing lesions in particular require increased amounts of nucleoproteins and the other components which are essential for the formation of new cells. As stated by Griffin, it is in this area of cellular replication that most of the effective cancer themotherapy occurs.

Continuing studies into the mechanism of action of the cytotoxic agents, some of which have now been shown to possess unique selectivity for cancer in experimental animals, are beginning to pay dividends in the treatment of human malignant disease. Much of the recent rationalization of cancer chemotherapy, such as the introduction of combination therapy, is due to detailed knowledge of the pharmacodynamics of the agents themselves and of the cytokinetics of tumour cell populations.

Excluding hormonal agents, which are not to be considered in the present context, the clinically effective cytotoxic-anticancer agents fall into the four broad categories referred to previously. These are: (a) alkylating agents, (b) antimetabolites, (c) antibiotics and (d) miscellaneous. The last named group includes a variety of agents of widely differing chemical structure and biochemical activity. A selection of the better known cytotoxic agents currently used clinically will be considered in detail to demonstrate the range of activity represented in cancer chemotherapy.

ALKYLATING AGENTS

The cytotoxic and hence the anti-tumour activity of these compounds in due to the possession of reactive alkyl groups in their structure. In many respects they appear to initiate the same biological effects as ionizing radiations, with markedly inhibitory effects on haemic, lymphatic and gonadal tissues. They also have carcinogenic and mutagenic effects. Their mechanism of action has been dealt with in great detail by Connors (1966). Connors gives, as typical of their effect, the replacement of the H atom of a molecule by an alkyl (RCH_2) group, according to the basic formula—

$$RCH_2X + HR^1 \rightarrow RCH_2R^1 + HX$$

Sites which are very reactive towards alkylating agents are termed nucleophilic centres. These include the ring nitrogens of nucleotides and nucleic acids. The anticancer cytotoxicity of alkylating agents is due to their direct reaction with deoxyribonucleic acids (DNA). According to Bodley Scott (1970), the point at which the reaction takes place is at the nitrogen atom in the 7-position on the imidazole ring of the purine base guanine. The two alkyl groups link together opposed guanine molecules on the two strands of DNA, where a twist in the helix approximates them. The result is that uncoiling of the helix is prevented and hence replication arrested. Bagshawe (1972) states that although repair *is* possible, many cells enter the mitotic processes before repair occurs and are thus likely to fail.

It is the cross-linkage effect on the DNA molecule, therefore, which essentially renders it useless to the cell. Although damage to other cellular components also occurs, it is the deactivation of the DNA and resulting interference with its replication which is mainly responsible for the cytotoxic action of the alkylating agents. Two or more of the reactive alkyl groups in the molecule are necessary for effective antineoplastic activity, and Bodley Scott (1970) has pointed out that agents with only one such group have less than 2 per cent of the potency of the bifunctional preparations.

As Connors (1966) has stated, the factors governing the effectiveness of the alkylating agents are the concentration of the agent at the site and the affinity of the site for alkylation. The latter will obviously depend upon the extent of DNA activity. Aliphatic mustards are especially dependent upon their concentrations at the site for the rate at which the reaction proceeds.

(a) The Nitrogen Mustards

Alkylating agents which can be used with relative safety in clinical practice are few in number. The nitrogen mustards, which are amine derivatives of mustard gas, are foremost among them. Their activity depends upon their reactive 2-chloroethyl radicals. The first of these agents to be used successfully clinically was chlormethine (*mustine hydrochloride*), methyl-bis (beta-chloroethyl)amine hydrochloride (Fig. 1). The solubility of this agent necessitates

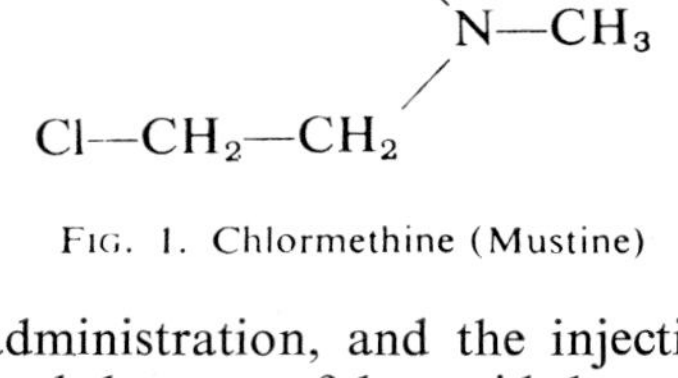

$$Cl—CH_2—CH_2$$
$$N—CH_3$$
$$Cl—CH_2—CH_2$$

Fig. 1. Chlormethine (Mustine)

intravenous administration, and the injection has to be made immediately because of the rapid changes which occur when the mustard is in solution.

Subsequently, a number of analogues were introduced in which the *N*-methyl group was replaced by other substitutes, thus affecting the solubility of the agent and its likely distribution within the body. Of these analogues, a popular one is *chlorambucil*, *p*-di-(2-chloroethylamino) phenylbutyric acid (Fig. 2). This agent was synthesized in the hope

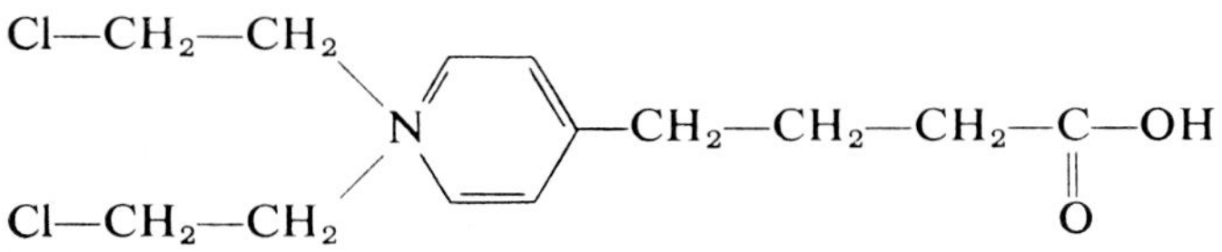

$$Cl—CH_2—CH_2$$
$$Cl—CH_2—CH_2$$
N
—CH_2—CH_2—CH_2—C—OH
O

FIG. 2. Chlorambucil

that its increased solubility would be advantageous. It has a marked destructive effect on the lymphoid series and a high "lymphoid/myeloid" ratio.

A third nitrogen mustard which has stood the test of time and has become one of the most popular of all cytotoxic agents is *cyclophosphamide* (Fig. 3), which is a cyclic phosphoramide mustard. It is inactive in its original form and is

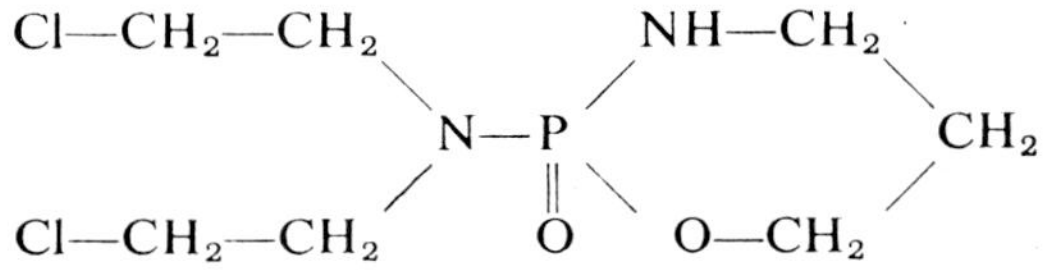

$$Cl—CH_2—CH_2$$
$$Cl—CH_2—CH_2$$
N—P
O
NH—CH_2
CH_2
O—CH_2

FIG. 3. Cyclophosphamide

activated primarily by hepatic microsomes. In the body, cyclophosphamide is converted in the liver into primary-activated metabolites of open-ring structure, which can be characterized chromatographically and tested for individual cytotoxicity. Much of the recent understanding of the activation of cyclophosphamide has been due to the use of mass spectrometry to study its metabolic products, and to observations made on the activation of the drug by hepatic microsomes in the rat after administration of ^{32}P labelled cyclophosphamide (Farmer, 1972). As a result of such studies, several of its metabolites have been shown to be more cytotoxic than the parent drug itself.

Enzymatic breakdown of cyclophosphamide occurs also to a limited extent in lung and kidney tissue. Tumour cells unfortunately cannot bring about this primary activation process, although it had been hoped that preferential activation would occur because of the high content of phosphoramidases in malignant tumours.

The primary activated metabolites of cyclophosphamide themselves are unstable. They are markedly hydrophilic and diffuse freely into malignant cells. Within the cell, the metabolites are converted into nor-*N*-mustard and *N*-2-chloroethyleneimine. These secondary metabolites tend to accumulate in the cell where they exert their powerful cytotoxic effect (Brock and Horhorst, 1967). Cyclophosphamide has the advantage that it tends to be less myelotoxic than many other alkylating agents.

(b) The Ethyleneimines

The only one of this group of alkylating agents which has remained popular is *thiotepa*, triethylene thiophosphoramide (Fig. 4). Ruddon and Mellett (1964) investigated the distribution of ^{14}C labelled thiotepa and its metabolites in

rats bearing Walker 256 tumours. No preferential uptake was observed in tumour tissue. Studies of the intracellular binding sites of the agent showed that much more of the ^{14}C activity was fixed in the *nuclear* fractions of both normal and tumour tissues than in the mitochondrial and microsomal fractions. Ruddon and Mellett were able to demonstrate association of the labelled alkylating agent with chromosomal material on autoradiography. They suggested that a single cross-link may prevent strand separation when thiotepa interacts with DNA, accounting for the extreme cellular damage caused by this drug.

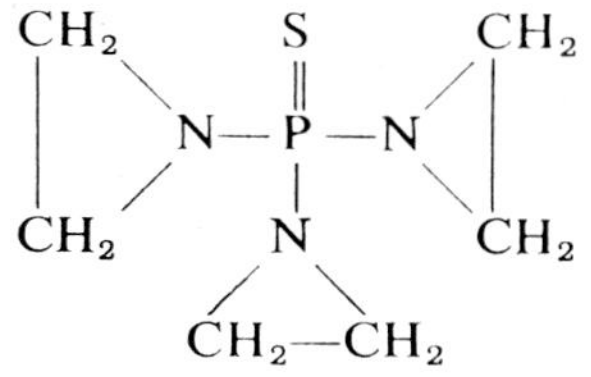

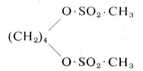

FIG. 4. Thiotepa

(c) The Methane Sulphonates

Members of this third group of biological alkylating agents have been shown to exhibit useful antineoplastic activity. The most popular agent *busulfan*, (1,4-dimethane sulfonyloxybutane) (Fig. 5) is of interest because of its

$$(CH_2)_4$$
O·SO_2·CH_3
O·SO_2·CH_3

FIG. 5. Busulfan

selective action upon the granular leucocytes, which makes it valuable in the treatment of chronic myeloid leukaemia. As observed by Bodley Scott (1970), in busulfan, the two alkylating radicals are separated by a distance critical for cross-linking of the opposed guanine bases in the DNA molecules. The higher and lower members in the series are less effective as cytotoxic agents.

ANTIMETABOLITES

Purists probably would not regard the antimetabolites as strictly "cytotoxic", but these important agents have certainly achieved a permanent role in the field of cancer chemotherapy.

The essential basis for their action is enzyme inhibition. Structurally they resemble certain vitamins, co-enzymes and normal intermediary metabolic products. They differ sufficiently from the normal substrates, however, to compete with them for binding to enzymes, either at the active site or elsewhere on the enzyme. They are thus able to inhibit essential metabolic processes. Bagshawe (1972) has explained that the competition either may be stoichiometric, that is on a proportionate "molecule-for-molecule" basis, or the antimetabolite may bind preferentially to the enzyme, as for example when methotrexate competes with folic acid.

Generally, the length of time for which antimetabolite action is maintained is more important than actual concentrations of the agent. When the concentration is such that the antimetabolite occupies most of the enzyme receptor sites, further increases in dose have little additional effect.

Antimetabolites have been widely used in cancer chemotherapy, primarily with the aim of interfering with the synthesis of nucleic acid by inhibiting the action of its precursors. To this end, much research has been directed towards developing effective folic acid antagonists and purine and pyrimidine analogues.

Methotrexate, 4-amino-N[10]-methyl-pteroyl-glutamic acid (Fig. 6), a folic acid antagonist, acts as an antimetabolite

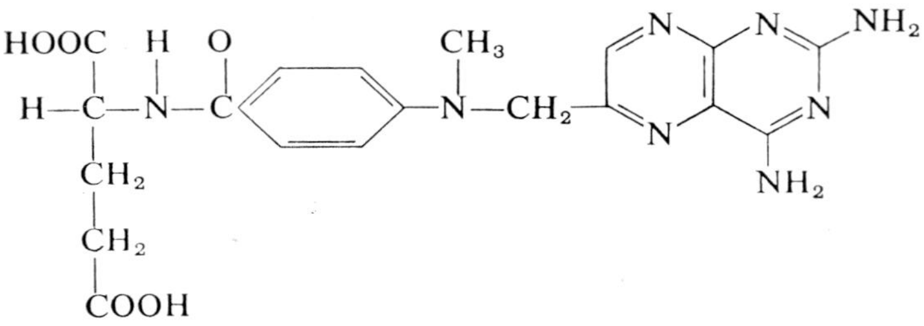

FIG. 6. Methotrexate

by preventing the reduction of folic acid to tetrahydrofolic acid by competing successfully for the enzyme which catalyses the process, dihydrofolic reductase. The affinity of methotrexate for the enzyme has been calculated to be 100 000 times greater than that of the normal substrate (*Brit. med. J.*, 1962). Hall and his colleagues (1966) stated that the binding of methotrexate with folic reductase is almost irreversible. The mere presence of target enzyme in tumour cells is not enough to ensure an effective anti-tumour effect, however.

Tetrahydrofolic acid is necessary for the conversion by methylation of deoxyuridilic acid to thymidylic acid, a key step in the eventual synthesis of DNA. Methotrexate binds the catalysing enzyme so that recycling of tetrahydrofolic acid stops. Inhibition of the synthesis of thymidine and of DNA interferes with cell proliferation. This inhibition can be prevented by the simultaneous administration of folinic acid (5-formyl tetrahydrofolic acid).

Clinically, methotrexate has been of considerable interest because of its apparent degree of specificity against squamous cell cancers. This as yet unexplained action is fortuitous in the context of head and neck malignancy. Methotrexate has been prominent in the treatment of such lesions, especially by regional techniques such as continuous intra-arterial infusion therapy.

Of all the pyrimidine antagonists synthesized and submitted to screening as potential anticancer agents, only a few have been found acceptable for clinical use. Of these, *fluorouracil* (Fig. 7) undoubtedly has become the most popular. A fluorinated pyrimidine it, or one of its metabolites, exerts its anti-neoplastic effect by blocking the methylation reaction of deoxyuridilic acid to thymidilic acid. It thus interferes with the synthesis of DNA and to some extent with that of ribonucleic acid (RNA).

Clinically, fluorouracil exhibits some apparent specificity of action against adenocarcinomas. The reason for this is undetermined. In a full and comprehensive account of the mechanism of action of purine and pyrimidine analogues,

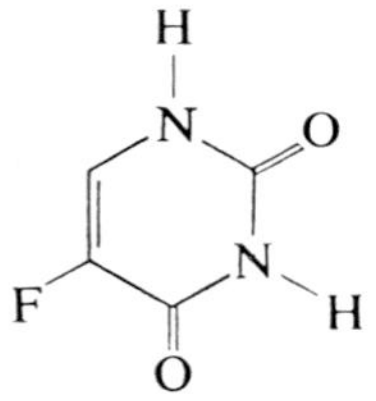

FIG. 7. Fluorouracil

Hutchings and Elion (1972) emphasized the potential scope for inhibiting biosynthesis of nucleotides and nucleic acid in future cancer chemotherapy. They made the valid point that, to date, the identification of loci of actions has been the main concern. Selectivity of action must be the next concept to pursue.

ANTIBIOTICS

The American National Cancer Chemotherapy Screening Programme examines a constant stream of moulds, emanating frequently from industrial laboratories, for antibiotic and anti-tumour agents. A number of antibiotics have been found to have anti-neoplastic activity, and a few have been accepted into clinical practice. There is increasing evidence that the mode of action of the different antibiotics is largely through enzyme inhibition. There is a marked resemblance structurally of many of the antibiotics to metabolites essential in the biosynthetic pathways of the cell. The pharmacodynamic action of the antibiotic group of anti-tumour agents has been reviewed in depth recently by Burchenal and Kreis (1972).

Azaserine, o-diazoacetyl-L-serine (Fig. 8), a naturally occurring diazo compound isolated from a *Streptomyces*,

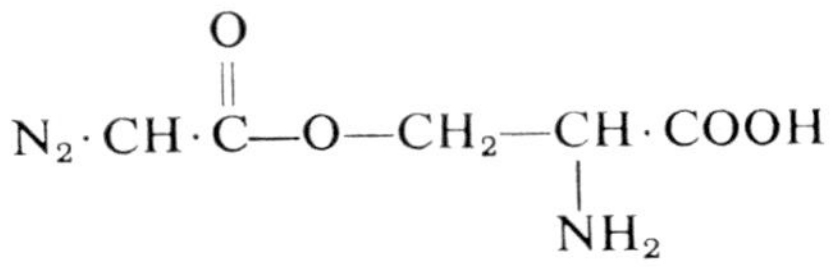

FIG. 8. Azaserine

is an antibiotic which acts as a glutamine antagonist. In the metabolic pathway for the synthesis of purines, azaserine blocks the conversion of formylglycineamide ribotide to formylglycineamidine ribotide. This agent has been used clinically mainly in the treatment of trophoblastic tumours.

Most of the actinomycins, which also are formed during the growth of various *Streptomyces* species, are too toxic for therapy, but *dactinomycin* (*actinomycin D*), a complex peptide (Fig. 9) is the exception. This agent causes a template defect by linking to the guanine groups of DNA. Dactinomycin has also been shown to inhibit RNA polymerase.

One of the most interesting of the newer antineoplastic

antibiotics is *bleomycin* (Fig. 10). This was first used clinically in the treatment of cancer in 1967. It consists of a group of sulphur-containing polypeptides and is produced from fermentation products of *Streptomyces verticillus*. It may be separated into its various fractions by column

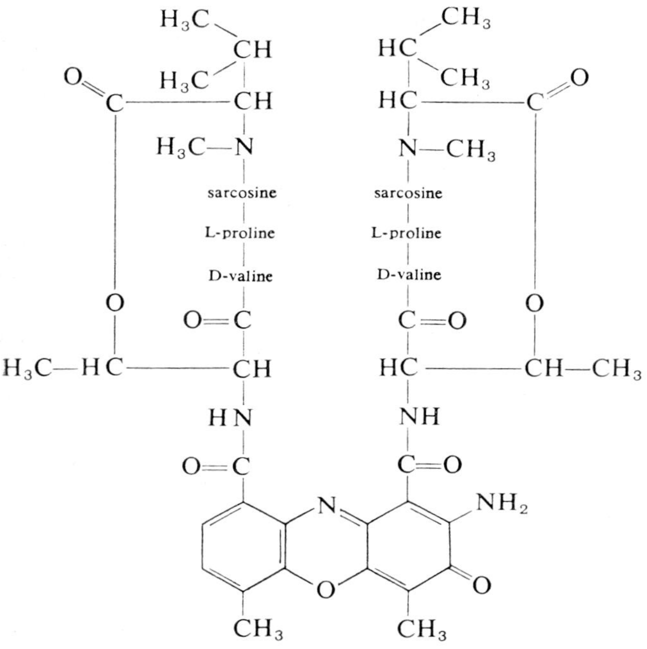

chromatography, and the main component in clinical use is the A2 fraction.

The antibiotic acts by inhibiting DNA synthesis and, to a lesser extent, RNA and protein synthesis. Terasima and Umezawa (1970) investigated the effect of bleomycin on mammalian S3 cells growing in culture. The types of dose-response curves obtained suggested to these writers the presence of fractions of varying sensitivity to the agent. Bleomycin is of particular interest in the context of head and neck cancer because of the reported successes in treating squamous cell carcinomas (Halnan *et al.*, 1972).

MISCELLANEOUS

There remain a group of miscellaneous cytotoxic agents which fit into none of the previous categories but which nevertheless are effective in clinical cancer chemotherapy.

Haddow and Sexton (1946) first reported the antineoplastic activity of urethane and, later, the closely related compound *hydroxycarbamide* (*hydroxyurea*) was introduced into clinical practice. With the simple empirical formula of $CH_4N_2O_2$, the agent's cytotoxic effect is due to inhibition of the reduction of cytidine diphosphate to deoxycytidine diphosphate (Bodley Scott, 1970), thus affecting the synthesis of DNA. Hydroxycarbamide does not appear to have an affect upon RNA activity (Ariel, 1970).

The plant *Catharanthus roseus* (*Vinca rosea*) of the family Apocynaceae, the West Indian periwinkle, is well-known now as the source of powerful cytotoxic agents, the vinca alkaloids (Johnson, 1968). They are quite unrelated to other

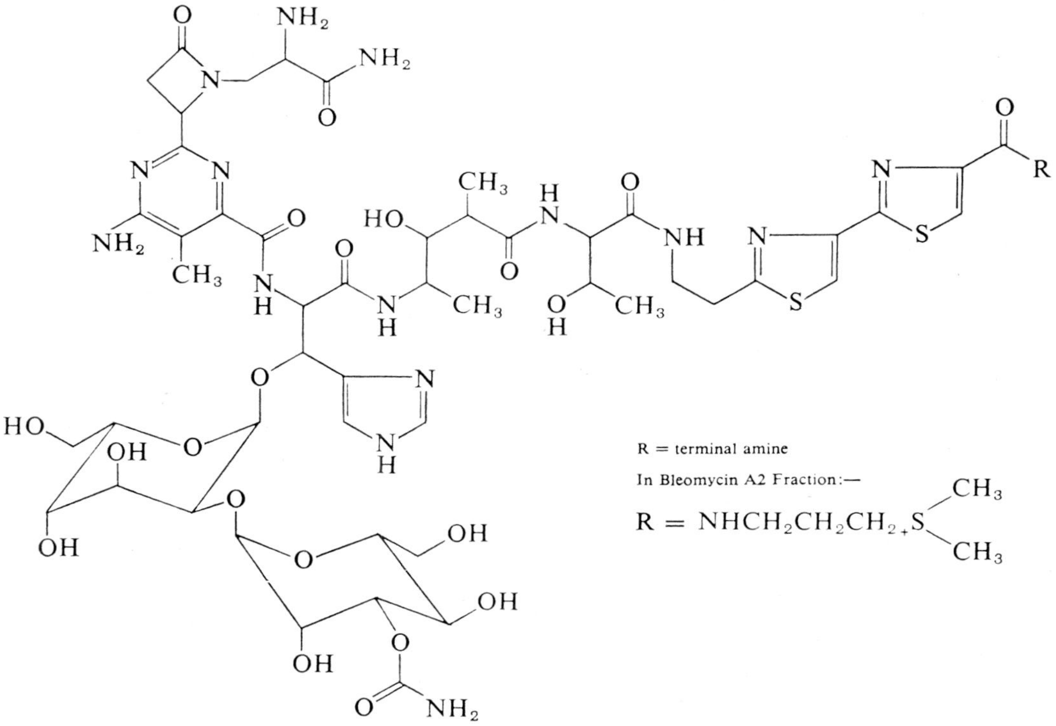

FIG. 9. Dactinomycin (Actinomycin D)

FIG. 10. Bleomycin

naturally occurring anti-neoplastic agents such as podo-phyllum and colchicine. Of the many alkaloids which can be isolated from the plant, two are suitable for clinical cancer chemotheraphy, *vinblastine* (vincaleukoblastine) and *vin-cristine* (leucocristine) (Fig. 11).

The two agents differ in minor respects, a methyl group of vinblastine being replaced by an aldehyde group in vin-cristine. The precise mechanisms by which these alkaloids inhibit tumour growth remains undetermined to a large extent, although it is clear that both cause arrest in meta-phase and that vinblastine interferes with transfer RNA.

rely upon exogenous sources of asparagine. L-aspara-ginase destroys plasma asparagine, thus depriving the leukaemic cells of an amino-acid essential for protein syn-thesis. DNA and RNA synthesis also are inhibited by asparaginase (Burchenall and Kreis, 1972).

In experimental systems, a high degree of correlation has been shown between sensitivity or resistance to L-asparaginase and the asparagine synthetase activity of the malignant neoplasm (Prager and Rothberg, 1972). This demonstration of a fundamental difference in metabolism between normal and certain malignant cells is of consider-

FIG. 11. Vinca Alkaloids

Studies in tissue culture suggest that vinblastine interferes with the metabolic pathways of amino-acids derived from glutamic acid. The mechanisms of action of the vinca alka-loids as far as they are known are discussed in detail by Marsden (1972). Certainly, the known arrest of mitosis caused by these agents does not explain the degree of tumour inhibition and toxicity which is experienced clinically.

All the aforementioned agents acts as cytotoxics by inter-fering with the reproductive capacity of the cells. The agent *L-asparaginase* is of particular interest because its mechan-ism of action is quite different. It can now be obtained from many different sources, including yeast, acid-fast bacilli, *Escherichia coli* bacteria and the plasma of certain mammals notably the guinea pig and related species. Not all of the forms of L-asparaginase isolated are active therapeutically, however, depending upon the rates of clearance from plasma and substrate specificity (Haskell *et al.*, 1972).

L-asparaginase is an enzyme which breaks down the amino-acid L-asparagine into aspartic acid and ammonia (Bodley Scott, 1970). All mammalian cells require aspara-gine for their continued survival. Most cells of the higher animals are capable of synthesizing the amino-acid, and are thus independent of an external supply. The observations by Neuman and McCoy (1956) that cells of the rat Walker 256 tumour would not grow in tissue culture without the addition of asparagine, led to the study of L-asparaginase as a possible anti-tumour agent and the eventual demon-stration of its anti-leukaemic effect in man. This anti-neoplastic activity occurs because certain leukaemic cells lack the enzyme asparagine synthetase and thus have to

able interest. Unfortunately, asparaginase-sensitive leu-kaemic cells rapidly develop resistance to L-asparaginase after exposure, presumably by the induction of asparagine synthetase in the resistant cells. This acquired resistance of leukaemic cells, together with the relative insensitivity of solid tumours, means that the earlier promise of L-asparaginase as an effective therapeutic anticancer agent has not been fulfilled. The interest of its theoretical impli-cations remains.

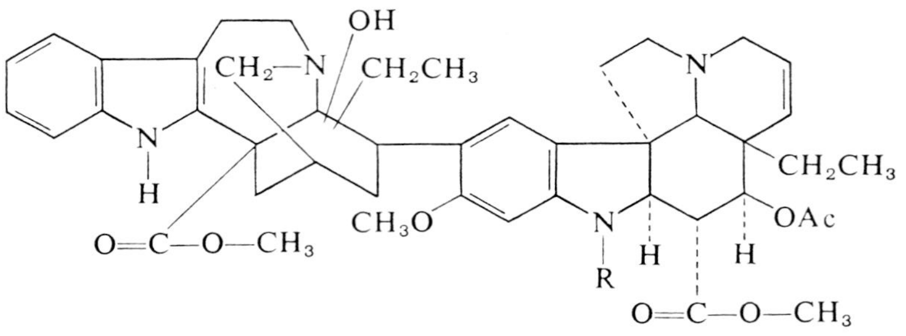

TUMOUR KINETICS

Cytotoxic drugs therefore act directly on malignant cells, damaging or destroying them by interfering with their ability to reproduce by mitosis. The rate at which cancer cells divide varies considerably from tumour to tumour. Many in fact divide at the same rate or even slower than cells of normal tissues. Unlike normal tissues, malignant tumours continue to increase in size because a proportion of their cells continue to multiply unchecked without ever develop-ing into normal mature tissue.

This abnormal behaviour of cancer cells has been described in detail by DeVita (1971) in an excellent account of the subject. At more complex levels of cellular organiz-ation, a cellular "brake" prevents overgrowth, this action being controlled by a feedback mechanism which is initi-ated probably by contact phenomena when the cells become crowded. In cancerous growth, the cells no longer cease to multiply when they reach this critical mass. Eventually, the continued uncontrolled growth will kill the host.

Studies of the mode of growth of a malignant tumour, given other stable conditions, suggest that this is exponential for the major part of its life (Breur, 1966). As the tumour becomes large, however, there is decay in the rate of growth which then becomes Gompertzian in nature (Simpson-Herren and Lloyd, 1970; Berenbaum, 1972). This progressive fall in the rate of growth has disadvantages in the context of cytotoxic chemotherapy, for, as a tumour responds to treatment and reduces in size, it may then adopt again the faster rate of growth of the smaller tumour.

The rate at which a tumour grows depends upon the mean cell reproductive cycle time; the size of the growth fraction, that is the proportion of cells participating in cell division; and the amount of spontaneous cell loss from death in situ, migration and exfoliation. These factors have a direct bearing on the effectiveness of cytotoxic chemotherapy.

The Cell Reproductive Cycle

Much is now known about the various phases of the cycle and there have been a number of excellent accounts of the subject in recent publications (Bagshawe, 1968; Andrews, 1969; Lamerton, 1969; Mendelsohn, 1969; Simpson-Herren and Loyd, 1970; De Vita, 1971). Autoradiographic studies after labelling cells that are synthesizing DNA with tritiated thymidine have identified precisely the various stages of the interphase period of the cycle; that is the period between two mitotic divisions.

At the completion of mitosis (M), the cell spends a variable period in a resting phase (G1–gap 1). During the resting phase, DNA synthesis for cell replication ceases although manufacture of repair DNA continues, as does synthesis of RNA and protein. Cells in this phase are still vulnerable to damage by cytotoxic chemotherapy agents to a variable extent. The G1 phase of the cycle varies from a few hours to many days in different tumours. This variability is one of the main causes of the markedly different doubling times among tumours.

Towards the end of the G1 phase, a critical period in the decision to divide occurs, known as the G1–S conversion period. An increased burst of RNA synthesis heralds entrance into a period of intense synthesis of replicating DNA (S phase). Entrance into this phase commits the cell either to divide or alternatively to remain polyploid. The cells are extremely vulnerable to certain of the cytoxic agents during this period. The length of the S phase is relatively short, 8–30 h, and is relatively constant for most cells in both normal and malignant tissues (DeVita, 1971).

The S phase is followed by another short period (2–8 h) before entry into mitosis, during which the cells cease to synthesize DNA although continuing with RNA and protein synthesis (G2–gap 2). When mitosis occurs, the rates of protein and RNA synthesis diminish abruptly while the genetic material re-arranges itself in the daughter cells. The time taken for mitosis is short and relatively constant among mammalian cells (30–90 min).

There is another phase in the cell cycle which is of considerable importance in cytotoxic therapy. This phase (G0) is an additional resting phase for cells which although viable are not contributing to tumour growth. Cells in this phase remain unlabelled with tritiated thymidine despite repeated attempts throughout the duration of the cell cycle. In other words, cells in G0 phase are not synthesizing DNA or RNA and are thus not vulnerable to the conventional cytotoxic agents. Cells presumably enter this inactive G0 phase in response to a variety of stimuli, or in the *absence* of the usual signal to divide, as a prolongation of the normal G1 phase. However, cells in G0 phase are fully capable of re-entering the active cell cycle at any time, upon receipt of the appropriate stimulus. It is this ability to revert to an actively dividing state that makes the cells in the dormant G0 phase a major, and as yet unsolved, problem in cancer chemotherapy.

As listed by Andrews (1969), the kinetic parameters of greatest important to cytotoxic chemotherapy include:

(1) The mean cell cycle times of the proliferative compartments of the cancer and of normal tissues in the host.
(2) The mean cell population doubling time of the cancer.
(3) The proportion of proliferating to total number of cancer cells, that is the growth fraction.

Studies of rates of regression of tumours treated by cytotoxic chemotherapy and sophisticated mathematical arguments, have been used to quantify the effects of various cytotoxic agents on malignant tumours. In experiments with hampster plasmacytomas treated with cyclophosphamide, Wilcox and his colleagues (1965) found that the treated tumours, decreased in a logarithmic fashion during the period of regression. He showed that, with the particular dose of cyclophosphamide used (about 80 per cent of the LD 10), the fraction of proliferating cells remaining viable was less than 1 per cent of the original total. Wilcox emphasized, however, that, due to the presence of non-proliferative cells, stroma and autolysis products, a good "proportionate" cell-kill may nevertheless be accompanied by only a small reduction in total tumour volume. In a subsequent publication, Wilcox (1966) dwelt on the chances of killing the "last surviving cell", which is the ultimate requirement of curative cytotoxic chemotherapy. He claimed that it is just as difficult to reduce 100 leukaemic cells to 1 with cytotoxic drugs as it is to reduce 1 000 000 cells to 10 000. A particular drug treatment eliminates the same *percentage* of proliferative cells present at the start, not the same *absolute* number of cells. This constant percentage reduction regardless of the original size is referred to as "first-order" kinetics. From his studies, Wilcox concluded that probably it was impossible to eradicate completely by the available cytotoxic agents any cancer that was palpable. He estimated that only micrometastases containing 10^3 cells or less could hope to be eliminated by present methods.

The arguments were extended by Berenbaum (1968). He showed mathematically that when the relation between the dose of the cytotoxic agent and the surviving fraction of the proliferating population was exponential, the elimination of the last survivor was more likely to be achieved by concentrating the total therapy into one or few massive doses than by using numerous small doses. However, not all these agents show exponential dose-response curves, notably the antimetabolites where the relationship is hyperbolic. Berenbaum showed that, with antimetabolites, logarithmic decreases in cell survival require logarithmic rather than linear increases in dose. These type of studies emphasize the naiveté of relying upon empiricism in deciding dose schedules.

There is no doubt that, as expressed by Andrews (1969), successful cytotoxic chemotherapy depends not only upon an understanding of the pharmacological actions of the various agents on the cancer and normal host tissues, but also upon the kinetic relationships involved. We are now in a much better position to decide appropriate dose schedules and to predict outcomes than in the earlier days of cancer chemotherapy. Unfortunately, we still do not possess cytotoxic agents which can be given safely in large enough doses and for sufficient time to make much impact upon human cancer. The need to ensure that all active and potential proliferating cells in the cancer are exposed at the appropriate time of the generation cycle is recognized but is as yet impracticable. The introduction of combination chemotherapy techniques and methods of protecting bone-marrow cells selectively should improve results to some degree.

The ultimate hope for successful cancer chemotherapy may lie in drugs which have a mechanism of action quite different from the current group of cytotoxic agents. Busch (1966) has developed the theory of cancer-specific messenger RNA's. He sees as a critical task for the future the identification and isolation from cells having as many as 30 000 messenger-RNA's, the few cancer-specific ones that govern the cancerous process. Success in this respect would pave the way for the development of a new class of cytotoxic agents designed specifically for the suppression of the activity of the cancer messenger ribonucleic acids.

REFERENCES

Andrews, J. R. (1969), *Cancer Chemother. Rep.*, **53**, 313.
Ariel, I. M. (1970), *Cancer*, **25**, 705.
Bagshawe, K. D. (1968) *Brit. J. Cancer* **22**, 698.
Bagshawe, K. D. (1972) *Brit. J. Hosp. Med.*, **8**, 677.
Berenbaum, M. C. (1968), *Cancer Chemother. Rep.*, **52**, 539.

Berenbaum, M. C. (1972), *Cancer Chemother. Rep.*, **56**, 563.
Bodley Scott, Sir Ronald (1970), *Brit. med. J.*, **3**, 259.
Brit. Med. J. (1962), in "To-day's Drugs," **2**, 1121.
Breur, K. (1966), *Europ. J. Cancer*, **2**, 157.
Brock, N. and Horhorst, H. J. (1967), *Cancer*, **20**, 900.
Burchenal, J. H. and Kreis, W. (1972), in *Cancer Chemotherapy II*, p. 41 (Brodsky and Kahn, Eds.). New York: Grune and Stratton.
Busch, H. (1966), in *Progress in Clinical Cancer*, p. 1 (Ariel, Ed.). New York: Grune and Stratton.
Connors, T. A. (1966), *Europ. J. Cancer*, **2**, 293.
Connors, T. A. (1972), in *Synopsis Report on Experimental Chemotherapy*. British Cancer Council.
DeVita, V. J. (1971), *Cancer Chemother. Rep.*, **2** (3), 23.
Farber, S., Diamond, L. K., Mercer, R. D., Sylvester, R. F., Jr. and and Wolff, J. A. (1948), *New Engl. J. Med.*, **238**, 787.
Farmer, P. B. (1972), "Abstracts," Meeting Brit. Ass. Cancer Research.
Griffin, A. C. (1961), in *Cancer Chemotherapy*, p. 49 (Lee Clark, Jr., Ed.). Springfield: Charles Thomas.
Haddow, A. and Sexton, W. A. (1946), *Nature*, **157**, 500.
Hall, T. C., Roberts, D. and Kessel, D. H. (1966), *Europ. J. Cancer*, **2**, 135.
Halnan, K. E., Bleehen, N. M., Brewin, T. D., Deeley, T. J., Harrison, D. F. N., Howland, C., Kunkler, P. B., Ritchie, G. L., Wiltshaw, E. and Todd, I. D. H. (1972), *Brit. med. J.*, **4**, 635.
Hartwell, J. L. (1960), *Cancer Chemother. Rep.*, **7**, 19.
Haskell, C. M., Canellos, G. P., Cooney, D. A. and Hardesty, C. J. (1972), *Cancer Chemother. Rep.*, **56**, 611.
Hutchings, G. H. and Elion, G. B. (1972), in *Cancer Chemotherapy II*, p. 23 (Brodsky and Kahn, Eds.). New York: Grune and Stratton.
Johnson, I. S. (1968), *Cancer Chemother. Rep.*, **52**, 455.
Lamerton, L. (1969), in *Normal and Malignant Cell Growth*, p. 1 (Fry, Griem and Kirsten, Eds.). London: Heinemann.
Marsden, J. H. (1972), in *Cancer Chemotherapy II*, p. 33 (Brodsky and Kahn, Eds.). New York: Grune and Stratton.
Mendelsohn, M. L. (1969), *Cancer Res.*, **29**, 2390.
Neuman, R. E. and McCoy, T. A. (1956), *Science*, **124**, 124.
Prager, M. D. and Rothberg, L. (1972), *Cancer Chemother. Rep.*, **56**, 339.
Ruddon, R. W. and Mellett, L. B. (1964), *Cancer Chemother. Rep.*, **39**, 7.
Simpson-Herren, L. and Lloyd, H. H. (1970), *Cancer Chemother. Rep.*, **54**, 143.
Terasima, T. and Umezawa, H. (1970), *J. Antibiot.*, **23**, 300.
Todd, Sir Alexander (1959), *Brit. med. J.*, **2**, 517.
Wilcox, W. S. (1966), *Cancer Chemother. Rep.*, **50**, 541.
Wilcox, W. S., Griswold, D. P., Laster, W. R., Jr., Schabel, F. M., Jr. and Skipper, H. E. (1965), *Cancer Chemother. Rep.*, **47**, 27.
Wood, H. B., Jr. (1971), *Cancer Chemother. Rep.*, **2**, (3), 9.
Zubrod, C. G., Schepartz, S., Leiter, J., Endicott, K. M., Carrese, L. M. and Baker, C. G. (1966), *Cancer Chemother. Rep.*, **50**, 349.

52. PHYSICAL AND BIOLOGICAL BASIS OF RADIOTHERAPY OF HEAD AND NECK CANCER

J. M. HENK AND J. F. FOWLER

INTRODUCTION

Radiotherapy is one of the many forms of medical treatment which were originally developed empirically without any rational scientific basis or knowledge of the biological mechanisms involved. Very soon after their discovery in 1895, X-rays were found to have effects on living tissues and were applied to a variety of inflammatory and neoplastic conditions for which there was no effective medical treatment available at that time Development of the use of radiation in medicine proceeded on a trial and error basis until the late 1920's when physical measurement of ionizing radiation became practicable, and a unit of radiation exposure, the röntgen, was defined. It was then possible to determine the dosages that could safely be given to various normal tissues, and which were effective in medical treatment. As more effective drug treatment became available for inflammatory conditions, and as the potential harmful effects of radiation, especially delayed carcinogenesis, became known, so the use of radiotherapy became more and more confined to the treatment of malignant neoplasms. Results steadily improved with increasing clinical experience, so that for example, in carcinoma of the lip and stage I glottic carcinoma, local control rates by radiotherapy have been greater than 90 per cent for over 30 years.

Experimental investigation of the biological effects of X-rays began soon after their discovery, but until the past 20 years laboratory studies made only small contributions to the understanding of the biological basis of radiotherapy Since the second world war the science of radiobiology has grown rapidly after receiving a considerable stimulus from the introduction of atomic weapons. A great deal is now known of the mechanisms whereby radiotherapy works; radiobiological studies are now able to suggest ways in which results of treatment may be improved. This chapter will endeavour to provide a resumé of the scientific basis of present-day radiotherapeutic practice and research.

NATURE OF IONIZING RADIATION

Radiations may be non-ionizing or ionizing. Ionizing radiations may be particulate, e.g. neutrons or pi-mesons (*see later*), or electromagnetic in type.

Ionizing radiation is so called because it knocks electrons out of atoms. Biological molecules can thereby be damaged. The important effect for cancer treatment is that living cells, both malignant and non-malignant, can be prevented from proliferating further.

Like radio waves, radar, infra-red rays, visible light, ultra-violet and diagnostic X-rays, the high energy X-rays and gamma-rays used in radiotherapy are types of electromagnetic radiation, which may be thought of as waves of both electrical and magnetic energy. The magnetic and electrical fields, at right angles to each other and to the forward motion of the beam, vary with time so that they move forward in much the same way as ripples move over the surface of a pond. Electromagnetic waves always move with the velocity of light, 3×10^8 m.s^{-1}. The distance between successive peaks of the wave is known as the wavelength. The number of waves passing a fixed point per second is the frequency. Electromagnetic rays may alternatively be thought of as a stream of "photons", or "quanta" i.e. packets of energy. Each energy "packet" contains an amount of energy proportional to the frequency. If a radiation has a *short wavelength* it will have a *high frequency* and so the energy per photon, the quantum energy, is large. The critical difference between non-ionizing and ionizing radiation is the size of these individual packets of energy. A radio wave may have a wavelength of 300 metres and has not sufficient quantum energy to knock electrons out of atoms. For visible light the wavelength is about one-tenth of a micrometre, and electrons are only ejected from specially light-sensitive substances such as photographic emulsion. The wavelength of X-rays is typically one million-millionth of a metre (10^{-12} m or 10^{-10} cm). The energy packets are large, so that electrons are knocked out of any atoms in materials through which the X- and gamma-rays pass including tissue, water and air. In the process chemical bonds are broken and the chain of events is initiated which ends in a biological change. It is not the total energy absorbed in tissue that causes the biological injury, but the highly localized effect of the large quantum packets of energy deposited within a few atoms' diameter of certain critical molecules in the cell, for example nuclear DNA or RNA. The amount of ionizing radiation required to sterilize all the cells in a block of human or animal tissue would only raise the temperature a few thousandths of one degree. Much greater amounts of heat delivered by the sun or by a cup of coffee have no such cell-sterilizing effects!

TYPES OF IONIZING RADIATION USED CLINICALLY

Although X-rays and gamma-rays do not differ in their main properties they are produced in different ways. X-rays are generated in an electrical machine which accelerates electrons to high energy and then stops them abruptly in a target usually made of tungsten. Linear accelerators of energy 4–20 million electronvolts* (Mev),

---

* One electronvolt (eV) is the kinetic energy acquired by an electron in passing through a potential difference of one volt in vacuum; 1 eV = $1\cdot602 \times 10^{-19}$ J.

betatrons of energy 15–45 MeV, and 60–300 kilovolt X-ray sets are the machines used.

Gamma-rays on the other hand are emitted from the nucleus of radioactive isotopes; their frequency depends on the isotope used. For example, both radium and cobalt-60 give penetrating gamma-rays of the same average energy as those produced by a 4 MeV linear accelerator, whereas gold-198 gives gamma-rays of similar energy to those from a 250 kV deep X-ray machine. X-rays and

Gamma-rays may also be used to treat cancer in accessible sites, by local application of small quantities of radioactive isotopes. The radioactive material may be contained in small tubes which can be packed into a cavity, e.g. the maxillary sinus after an antrostomy, known as intracavitary radiotherapy; the tubes may be applied to a surface in the form of a mould to treat a very superficial lesion, e.g. a basal-cell carcinoma of the scalp. Alternatively, needles, wires or seeds containing radioactive materials

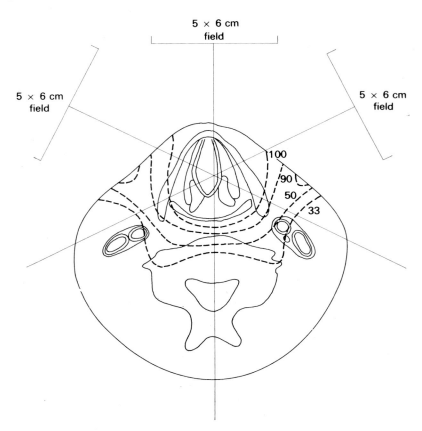

FIG 1. Transverse section through neck showing field arrangement for radiotherapy to the larynx. (Drawing by Mrs. S. King.) Isodose lines are expressed as percentages of the tumour dose.

gamma-rays at energies above 500 kV are known as supervoltage; their use has largely replaced that of the old-fashioned 250 kV "deep X-rays". Other types of radiation that are just coming into limited use at present will be mentioned in the final section.

Both X-rays and gamma-rays are used mainly for external radiation, i.e. as beams directed at the site of a tumour from outside the body. They can be "stopped down" by lead borders to give beams which are adjustable in cross-section from a few centimetres square or rectangular up to 20 × 20 cm. The radiation is attenuated as the beam passes through tissues (see below) so it is usual for nearly all cancers of the head and neck to use more than one beam portal, or "field" as each portal is called, in order to obtain as uniform a physical dose as possible over the whole tumour region while keeping the dose lower to the surrounding areas of normal tissue (Fig. 1).

may be inserted into the tissues; such techniques are known as "interstitial" and are discussed more fully later. Until the introduction of atomic reactors and cyclotrons, radium was the only radioactive substance available for medical use, but it has now been largely replaced by artificially produced radioactive isotopes such as cobalt-60, caesium-137 and iridium-192, which are safer and easier to handle.

DISTRIBUTION OF RADIATION IN TISSUES

Radiation of all types decreases in intensity as the distance from its source increases, according to the "inverse square law". This means that if the distance from the source is doubled the intensity falls to one-quarter; if the distance is halved, the intensity rises by a factor of four.

In addition, the radiation will also be attenuated by absorption and scattering in passing through matter, especially for low energy radiation. The decrease in intensity is usually rather greater from attenuation than from the inverse square law in external beams of radiation. For example, with supervoltage radiation from a standard cobalt-60 source, the intensity has fallen to one-half of the surface value at a depth of 10 cm. Twenty per cent of the total 50 per cent fall is due to the inverse square law, the other 30 per cent being due to attenuation.

By contrast 250 kV X-rays are attenuated to 50 per cent of the surface value at a depth of 6 cm. Supervoltage radiation is therefore able to deliver higher doses to deeper lesions, and is now used for most external beam therapy. Low-energy X-rays between 60–140 kV are absorbed over very short distances in tissue, falling to 50 per cent at between 4–20 mm depth; they are used to treat superficial skin tumours.

Certain types of supervoltage radiotherapy machines are designed to treat at such short distances, (about 10 cm) that the inverse square law fall-off is predominant. With such a machine the intensity has fallen to about 20 per cent of the surface value at 10 cm depth in tissue; a decrease of 50 per cent due to the inverse square law and of 30 per cent due to attenuation. Such short-distance treatment units are useful for the treatment of unilateral lesions in the head and neck.

At lower energies, absorption of X-rays varies considerably according to the density of the absorber, so that dosage to bone is much higher than soft tissue. This effect is not seen in the case of supervoltage X-rays. Irradiation of tumours close to bone, e.g. the lower alveolus, carried a high risk of bone necrosis in the days when 250 kV X-rays were the highest energy available. With the use of supervoltage bone necrosis is less of a problem.

High energy beams have a further advantage, illustrated in Fig. 2. The top few millimetres of skin and tissue absorb less dose from the beam than do tissues a few millimetres deep. This is because fewer electrons are "knocked on" from the air on to the skin surface than are knocked on from the uppermost layers of tissue into the subcutaneous tissues. The maximum dose in the beam therefore occurs at about 4 mm deep for cobalt-60 beams and up to a centimetre or two deep for linear accelerator beams. The skin dose may be only about one-third of that at the "dose maximum" just below the skin. The result is that severe skin reactions do not occur when supervoltage radiation is used. However, if cancer cells are suspected of being present in skin then no such sparing effect is wanted. It is easy to eliminate the skin-sparing by using a centimetre or more of wax or other tissue-equivalent "build-up material" placed in the beam close to the skin.

RADIATION DOSE: THE "RAD"*

The unit of radiation dose used in radiotherapy is the "rad" (from Radiation Absorbed Dose). This is useful because it measures simply the amount of radiation energy actually deposited in the tissues. Any radiation scattered outside the tissues cannot, of course, contribute to the biological effect and it is therefore not included in the meaning of absorbed dose in rads. One rad corresponds to the deposition of 100 ergs/g of tissue. In a submicroscopic scale this corresponds to an average of about one broken chemical bond per cubic micrometre of tissue, i.e. about 100 broken bonds per cell nucleus. Typical doses delivered in a course of radiotherapy may total several thousand rads, usually given over several weeks as doses of several hundred rads per daily session each lasting a few minutes.

EFFECTS OF IONIZING RADIATION ON THE CELL: CELLULAR AND ORGAN RADIOSENSITIVITY

The details of the physical deposition of radiation energy are quite well understood. Nevertheless, most details of the links between physical, chemical and biological effects have yet to be worked out.

Ionization (ejection of an electron) causes the majority of the immediate chemical changes in living material. *Excitation* (putting an electron into a different orbit in the same molecule) contributes less to radiation injury. Damage may be the *direct* result of an ionization somewhere within a critical molecule such as DNA (within 10^{-12} s) or it may be due to the *indirect* action of excited molecules which can diffuse for several microseconds before reacting chemically with a critical molecule. It is the indirect portion of radiation injury which can be altered by radiosensitizing drugs including oxygen or by large changes in dose rate (*see later*). Proteins and enzymes in the cell are less damaged by radiation than DNA, RNA or membranes. The result is that proliferation is the most radiosensitive function of the cell, and proliferative ability

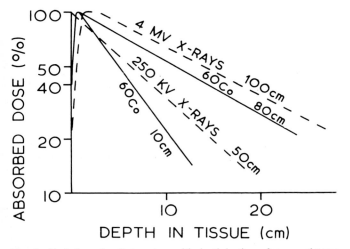

FIG. 2. Variation of radiation dose with depth in tissue for several types of commonly used treatment beam. A standard ^{60}Co beam has a treatment distance of 80 cm, but that at 10 cm distance is designed to treat unilateral lesions of the head and neck. Note that the absorbed dose for ^{60}Co and 4 MV X-rays is low at the skin surface and rises to its 100 per cent peak at depths of about 4 and 10 mm respectively.

* In 1969, the C.I.P.M. (Comité International des Poids et Mesures) sanctioned use of the rad with the International System for a limited time. 1 rad = 10^{-2} J. kg^{-1}.

is impaired by doses of radiation which are too small to affect the normal function of cells. A much higher dose of radiation is required to stop a differentiated cell from producing hormones, if that is its function, or keeping structural contact with its neighbour, than to stop proliferation. A cell which has been lethally damaged by irradiation does not break up and disappear at once. It usually does so at the next cell division, or even at the second or third attempt at division. Such a cell may remain present in the tissue for a cell cycle time or two as a "doomed" cell; it will appear intact, and can continue its vegetative function indefinitely provided it is not called upon to divide.

The final expression of biological damage may take hours, days, weeks, or even tens of years. This is because the gross effects, such as tumour regression or organ damage depend upon the death of cells. In the treatment of tumours the desired result is the killing, in the sense of prevention of proliferation, of all malignant cells. In normal tissues the main effects of radiation injury are also due, directly or indirectly, to the prevention of cell replacement.

No systematic differences in radiosensitivity have been found between malignant and normal cells proliferating at the same rate. Therefore the therapeutic advantages that have been found depend on quite small differences, especially on the relative ability of tumours and normal tissues to make good any radiation injury by the proliferation of more cells to replace those damaged or lost.

The relationship between dose of radiation absorbed and the proportion of cells which "survive" is described by a cell-survival curve. The term survival is used in the special sense of maintenance of "*reproductive integrity*", the ability to continue to proliferate indefinitely.

CELL SURVIVAL CURVES

A cell-survival curve describes the relationship between the dose of radiation absorbed and the proportion of cells which survive. The capability of a single cell to grow into a large colony or clone is proof that it has retained its reproductive integrity. Cells can be grown *in vitro* in culture dishes. Specimens of tissue can be cut into small pieces and the individual cells can be separated out by the use of trypsin, which dissolves and loosens the cell membrane. In this way a suspension of single cells can be made. After about 2 weeks of growing at 37°C (310 K) in sterile dishes, each surviving cell has doubled about 10 times to give rise to a colony of about 2^{10} (= 1000) daughter cells. This colony can easily be seen attached to the bottom of the culture dish (Fig. 3). The proportion of cells which survives a given dose of radiation can thus be counted and plotted against radiation dose. Cell survival curves are so basic to an understanding of the effects of radiation that a description of their main features is worth while.

Irradiation of a population of cells resembles a hail of bullets from a machine-gun aimed at a collection of targets, the bullets being the photons of energy and the targets the critical genetic apparatus of the cells. The thicker the hail of bullets, the larger the proportion of

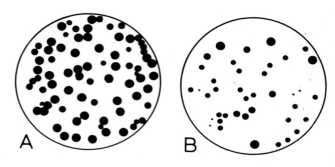

FIG. 3. Clones of cells, each originating from a single surviving cell, in culture dishes. Dish A is the unirradiated control. One hundred cells were seeded into it and allowed to grow for 10 days before being stained. There are 75 colonies. Dish B: 2000 cells were seeded into this dish before being exposed to 750 rads of X-rays. There are 40 colonies in the dish, corresponding to a surviving fraction of

$$\frac{40}{2000 \times 75/100} = 0.027.$$

targets hit. Therefore the higher the dose of radiation, the larger the *fraction* of cells killed.

Figure 4 shows a typical cell survival curve. The final part of it is straight if the proportion of surviving cells is plotted *logarithmically* on the vertical axis. This means that the surviving proportion falls by a factor of 10 for

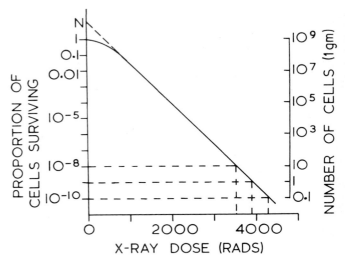

FIG. 4. A typical "cell survival curve" relating proportion of cells surviving (log scale on left) to radiation dose. N is the extrapolation number, from the straight (exponential) part of the cell survival curve. The right-hand scale gives the *number* of cells surviving per gram of tissue or tumour, assuming 10^9 viable cells per gram before irradiation (*see* text).

each additional radiation dose of 200–400 rads; this dose is denoted by D_{10}. At low doses however the cell killing process is less effective, so that a shallow initial slope or "shoulder" is seen on the survival curve. This shoulder represents that part of the radiation injury which can be repaired by the cell within a few minutes or hours. Where this shoulder is large, the cell is capable of considerable repair before the next dose is given. Often about two-thirds of the damage is repaired. Where the shoulder is small, as with some newer types of radiation such as neutrons, less repair will occur between successive dose fractions.

Nearly all the types of mammalian cell tested in the 20 years since cell survival curves have been measured have given survival curves which are very similar to that in Fig. 4. This is a much greater constancy than in the case of chemotherapeutic drugs. There are, however, differences within this range between cell lines and between different phases of the cell cycle.

For example, cell survival curves for lymphocytes seem to be somewhat steeper and have smaller shoulders than most other cells. Cells in the bone marrow are also intrinsically rather radiosensitive (D_{10} about 200 rads). Cells in skin and intestinal epithelium are slightly less radiosensitive, having D_{10} averaging about 300 rads and rather large shoulders. There are also differences, of about a factor or two in dose required to produce a given level of cell killing, depending on the phase of the cell in the proliferation cycle. Cells in mitosis are slightly more sensitive than cells in the late stage of DNA synthesis. No differences have been found, however, between cells from experimental tumours and cells from normal tissues. This is of course a most important point when we wish to eradicate a tumour but to leave normal tissues functioning, and is considered in more detail later.

In eradicating a tumour it is probably necessary to reduce the number of surviving cells to zero. It is sometimes alleged that immunological processes may finish the eradication if the number of viable cells is reduced to a few thousand, say, but the evidence for this in solid *human* tumours is questionable. In any case, even several hundred or a few thousand cells dealt with immunologically out of 10^{10} cells present would only save 20 or 30 per cent of the radiation dose and make no difference to the other considerations in this chapter.

As an example of the application of cell survival curves to illustrate what happens in radiotherapy, let us assume that a tumour of volume 10 cm³ contains 10^9 viable cells. Let us further assume that if just one of these cells remains viable after treatment the tumour has a 50 per cent chance of recurring. This will be the case if a dose of 3900 rads is given, from Fig. 4. If however a higher dose of 4300 rads is given, the cell survival becomes 10^{-10} so that "one-tenth of a cell" remains out of the original 10^9. This looks strange but simply means that, statistically, the chance of local recurrence is only one-tenth as great as before, i.e. it is 5 per cent now. Thus the change from a 50 per cent chance of non-recurrence, i.e. cure, to a 95 per cent chance of non-recurrence takes place over a narrow dose range, about 400 rads out of the total 4000. Similarly, a small decrease in total dose given would result in virtually nil chance of cure. Within this narrow band of radiation dose the radiotherapist exercises his skill. In practice, the single doses illustrated in Fig. 4 are not used; multiple daily doses are given instead; but the principle remains the same and the margin of error in order to avoid under-dosing is of the same proportional size.

REPAIR OF RADIATION INJURY: DOSE-TIME FRACTIONATION RELATIONSHIPS

If two radiation doses are given separated by an interval of several hours, they are less effective than the same total dose given at one session lasting only a few minutes. This is presumably because of the repair of intracellular damage, which can be regarded as corresponding to the restoration of the shoulder on the cell survival curve. Perhaps this is due to the replenishment of a pool of "repair enzymes" or of RNA; the details are not known. For example, in Fig. 5, the response to single doses of

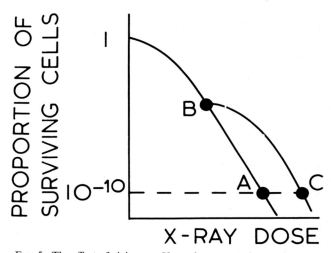

FIG. 5. The effect of giving two X-ray doses, spaced apart by about a day to permit full recovery of the "shoulder," is shown by the curve IBC. The response to a single dose of X-rays is curve IBA. An extra dose AC has to be given when the dose is given in two fractions instead of one.

radiation is shown by the usual survival curve BA. If however a smaller first dose is given, so that the surviving proportion is B, and further radiation doses are not given until 24 h later, the response will then follow BC instead of BA. The shoulder appearing after B is, to a first approximation, the same as the initial shoulder on the cell survival curve. This means that an extra dose, corresponding to AC has to be given when the dose is delivered in two sessions instead of one.

Similarly, when 20 or 30 sessions of irradiation are delivered at approximately daily intervals, as in external beam radiotherapy, each session is followed by repair. The total dose required, D_n, is considerably greater than if given as a single dose A. (Fig. 6a). Some examples are given in Table 1.

The total dose in radiotherapy is often about 3 times greater than the equivalent single dose, indicating that some two-thirds of the radiation injury seems to be repaired during X-ray treatment. Of course, if proliferation occurs in the irradiated tissues during the days or weeks of treatment, this too would require extra dose to be given in order to achieve a specified level of cell killing in the tissue. The effects of proliferation are not negligible but they are usually not as large as the effects of post-irradiation repair.

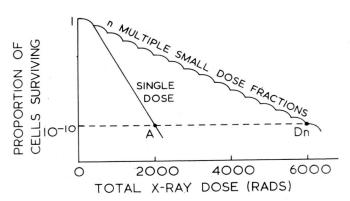

FIG. 6(a). The effect of giving many small fractions of X-rays, with intervals of at least a day to permit full recovery of the shoulder (upper curve). The single dose response is shown at A, as in Fig. 5. The total dose in n fractions, D_n, required to produce the same degree of biological effect as the single dose A, is much greater than the single dose.

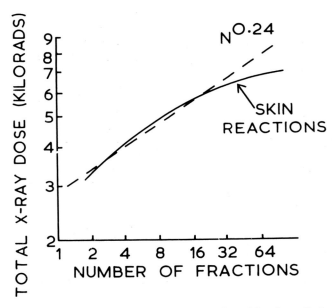

FIG. 6(b). Total tolerance dose versus number of fractions. Both scales of the graph are logarithmic and the resulting curve approximates to a straight line.

The way in which the total dose increases with the number of fractions and overall time is illustrated in Fig. 6b. A straight line relationship has been found to exist between the logarithm of total dose and the logarithm of overall time for "daily" treatments, i.e. 5 or 6 sessions each week. Strandquist (1944) found parallel lines for various degrees of radiation reaction in normal skin and for cure of superficial tumours. Fowler and Stern (1963) showed that, for skin damage, the effect of changing the number of dose fractions was greater than the effect of changing overall time. Ellis (1969) proposed a convenient rule of thumb for estimating these changes separately, so as to compare the effects of different fractionation schedules. He relates any schedule to a "Nominal Standard Dose" (theoretically the equivalent single dose,

TABLE 1

TYPICAL RADIOTHERAPY DOSES DELIVERED IN MULTIPLE FRACTIONS

10 fractions in 3 weeks	4500 rads
15 fractions in 3 weeks	5000 rads
20 fractions in 4 weeks	5500 rads
18 fractions in 6 weeks	5750 rads
30 fractions in 6 weeks	6500 rads

Note: These are the maximum tissue doses usually considered tolerable. They are often reduced depending on the size of the treated area and the type of normal tissue irradiated.

but in practice single doses are never used except for small superficial tumours) by means of the following expression:

$$\text{Total dose} = \text{NSD} \times N^{0.24} \times T^{0.11}$$

where NSD = nominal standard dose
N = number of dose fractions
T = treatment time in days

(NSD is expressed as "rets" (rad equivalent therapy); a radical tumour dose for head and neck cancer is between 1800 and 1950 rets)

Although this expression is an empirical approximation, it has been found to act as a reasonable guide to the total doses which normal tissues will tolerate over the range $N = 10–30$ and up to $T = 100$ (Fowler, 1971; Liversage, 1971).

Different schedules might cause more damage to the tumours than to normal tissues, as discussed later. It is however, usually the intention, in radical radiotherapy, to employ the highest dose that the normal tissues will tolerate in order to give the maximum possible radiation dose to the tumour.

THE OXYGEN EFFECT

Tumours tend to outgrow their own vasculature, so there are frequently areas in tumours with relatively poor blood supply. Even in very small tumours, tiny areas of necrosis can be seen histologically where capillary vessels have been pushed further apart than about 350 micrometres. This is because oxygen has a maximum diffusion range of about 150 micrometres before being metabolically used up. Other nutrients, such as glucose, diffuse further but oxygen is the critical one because it is used up in the shortest distance. Cells at the limit of the oxygen diffusion range will therefore be hypoxic, even in small tumours without overt central necrosis. In experimental animal tumours it has been found that between 1 and 50 per cent of the tumour cells are hypoxic but viable (Kallman, 1972). The histological and physiological features of human tumours are similar to those of experimental tumours in animals.

The importance of hypoxic cells is that they are intrinsically more resistant to X-ray killing than well-oxygenated cells. Figure 7 illustrates the difference. For a given level of cell killing in well-oxygenated cells A, a dose nearly three times greater is required to achieve the same level of cell killing in hypoxic cells E. Moreover, at a given X-ray dose, corresponding to A in Fig. 7, the degree of cell killing is much less in hypoxic cells, as shown at F: the

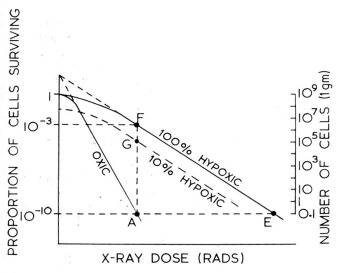

FIG. 7. The oxygen effect in radiotherapy. IA represents the single-dose cell survival curve for well oxygenated cells. IFE is the survival curve if all the cells are made hypoxic; X-ray doses some 2½ times greater are needed.

proportion of surviving hypoxic cells is one million times greater than the proportion of oxygenated cells. To be specific, if A represents a surviving proportion of 10^{-10} cells, the surviving fraction of hypoxic cells at F is 10^{-3}. Now if the tumour originally contained 10 per cent of hypoxic cells, the proportion of all cells left surviving is 10^{-4} as at G. If the tumour originally contained 10^9 cells, then 10^5 would survive and local recurrence would be certain.

It is clear that even a small proportion of hypoxic cells present in a tumour during X-ray treatment will dominate the response, making the tumour difficult or impossible to eliminate. The fact that radiotherapy is as successful as it is means either that the proportion of hypoxic cells is much smaller in human than animal tumours or that many hypoxic cells become better oxygenated as the tumour shrinks during the course of fractionated radiotherapy, as discussed later.

The main ways of dealing with the problem of hypoxic cells in tumours are:

(1) The use of multidose fractionation extending over several weeks, so as to permit reoxygenation of hypoxic cells to occur.

(2) Irradiation in high pressure oxygen.

(3) The use of new types of radiation beam which cause less difference in the response of hypoxic or oxygenated cells.

(4) The development of oxygen-mimicking radio-sensitizing drugs which will sensitize hypoxic cells, but not the well-oxygenated cells in normal tissue, to X-ray killing.

(5) The use of very low dose rates of X- or gamma-radiation.

These methods, which are still evolving, will be described below.

DOSE RATE: IMPLANTS

The cell survival curves shown above apply only if the individual doses of radiation are given in short spaces of time, at a rate of 50 rads/min or faster. Bedford and Hall (1963), working with Hela cells, demonstrated that, at rates below 45 rads/min, the cell-killing effect of a given number of rads depended upon dose rate. As the dose rate decreases so does the proportion of cells killed, presumably because at low dose rates a certain amount of intra-cellular repair of ionization damage is able to take place during the period of irradiation. Hall and his colleagues (1966) demonstrated that the dose-enhancing effect of oxygen was very much less at low dose rates; again working with Hela cells, they demonstrated oxygen enhancement ratios of 2·4 at 110 rads/min but 1·5 at 32 rads/h.

In external beam radiotherapy the times for each individual treatment are short; the tumour cells receive their radiation at well above 50 rads/min in most instances, so the dose rate is unimportant. Low dose rates however have been employed in clinical radiotherapy for many years in surface, intracavitary and interstitial techniques. The last named, in the form of an "implant", is commonly used to treat head and neck neoplasms. An implant aims to deliver a uniform dose of radiation by insertion of radioactive sources into the tumour and immediately adjacent normal tissues. It can be performed successfully only where the tumour is situated in accessible tissues into which the radioactive needles or wires can be inserted, e.g. the lateral border of the tongue and the buccal mucosa; large tumours and those immediately adjacent to bone are unsuitable for implant. Paterson and Parker (1934) devised geometrical rules for distribution of radium sources for both moulds and implants, in order to achieve a homogeneous dose of irradiation to the lesion treated. They also determined optimum time-dose factors from their clinical experience. They concluded that the best results were obtained if the radium needle implant remained in position for about 7 days and delivered a dose of around 6500 rads. The biological effect of such an implant is very similar to that of a course of external beam radiotherapy given in 30 daily treatments to a total dose of 6000 rads.

An implant has both physical and biological advantages over external beam therapy. The dose of radiation can be delivered to a more sharply defined volume of tissue immediately surrounding the tumour; the law of inverse squares ensures that dosage to surrounding tissues is low. The disadvantageous effect of tumour cell hypoxia is minimized by the low dose rate, usually between 30 and 40 rads/h, because the oxygen enhancement ratio is reduced, as mentioned above. Nevertheless, implants are not much favoured by radiotherapists because of the technical difficulty of inserting sources in exactly the correct positions, and also because of the radiation hazard to hospital staff. In the past few years the introduction of new techniques using flexible wires of radioactive iridium-192 inserted via fine polyethylene cannulae has partially overcome both these difficulties and led to a renewed interest in interstitial radiotherapy.

EFFECTS OF RADIATION ON NORMAL TISSUES

The anatomical and histological changes in various tissues following radiotherapy have been well described over the past 70 years. Details can be found in the comprehensive work of Rubin and Casarett (1968). Studies of radiation histopathology began almost as soon as ionizing radiation was first used clinically. At an early stage it was realized that radiation exerted the most profound effects on tissues where the cells were actively dividing. In 1906, Bergonnié and Tribondeau formulated a law stating that tissue radio-responsiveness depended on reproductive capacity, mitotic activity, and lack of differentiation of cells. These principles still generally apply although there are many exceptions, and it is now known that in the long term radiation can exert its most profound effects on more specialized tissues with low mitotic activity. New techniques involving the use of radio-active labelled DNA precursors have made it possible to estimate cell turnover times in most mammalian tissues. Knowledge of cell proliferation kinetics of tissues, and the phenomenon of mitotic death, can together explain the underlying mechanisms of radiation histopathology.

At the dose levels used in clinical radiotherapy an irradiated cell can usually survive and perform its normal function until such time as it is called upon to divide, when it may then die if there has been critical damage to the genetic apparatus in its nucleus. The first attempted mitosis of the cell may occur any time from a few hours to many years after irradiation, so the effect of the radiation in causing cell death can occur any time during the subsequent life of the individual. Cowdry (1950) has classified cells according to their mitotic activity.

(a) *Vegetative intermitotics*: those "stem" cells which have no function other than to perform cell division to replace cells rapidly lost in the body; for example, the basal cell layer of the epidermis and the stem cells of the bone marrow. Such cell populations are very sensitive to radiation and show evidence of radiation damage rapidly.

(b) *Differentiating intermitotics*: cells which have begun to differentiate but are still actively dividing to replenish a population of cells performing a specialized function, for example the prickle-cell layer of the epidermis and the myelocyte. This type of cell often has a higher mitotic rate than the vegetative intermitotic type. Radiation injury is therefore manifested rapidly; the time after radiation when pathological changes become manifest depends upon the cell population turnover rate, but is usually between a few days and a few weeks.

(c) *Reverting post-mitotics*: those cells which have differentiated to perform a specialized function and normally do not divide. They may however divide if part of the organ is destroyed by physical or chemical damage and attempted regeneration then occurs, as in liver cells or in osteoblasts. Such cells usually appear quite radio-resistant and may not show any evidence of histological changes despite high doses of radiation. If however there is injury to the tissue subsequent to radiation, so that the cells attempt to divide, they then express their latent radiation damage as mitotic death. In this way, trauma to an irradiated organ many years after radiation may cause necrosis, for example, a tooth extraction from an irradiated mandible.

(d) *Fixed post-mitotics*: those cells which have become so specialized that they have completely lost the power to divide, for example, the nerve cell and the granulocyte. This type of cell is very radio-resistant and normally only suffers after radiation if its blood supply is impaired.

Acute Effects

Pathological changes appear in actively-dividing tissues within a few days or weeks of beginning a course of radiotherapy. Such effects are known as "reactions", something of a euphemism for the inevitable damage to rapidly-dividing normal tissues which is the price that must be paid for destruction of a tumour by ionizing radiation. Such reactions may be unpleasant to the patient for a short period but are tolerable provided that careful attention is paid to radiation dosage and supportive care by the radiotherapist.

The *epidermis* is a typical example of a rapidly dividing tissue. The basal cell cycle time is about 5 days, and the epidermis is effectively 3 or 4 cells thick in the head and neck. The turnover time for the whole epidermis is therefore 3 or 4 times the cycle time of the basal layer, i.e. 15–20 days. Lethally irradiated cells undergo mitotic death within this period. Skin changes during radiotherapy therefore appear 2 or 3 weeks after the start of treatment, and do not reach their maximum for 5 or 6 weeks. Initially there is an erythema due to vaso-dilatation. As cell death proceeds there is loss of integrity of the prickle-cell layer leading to the flaking of the skin known as "dry desquamation". Very high doses of radiation produce a patchy ulceration with exudation known as "moist desquamation". Healing is fairly rapid, usually complete within about 3 weeks after completion of radiotherapy. The germinal epithelial cells of the *hair follicles* are particularly sensitive; epilation of any skin within a radiotherapy field is inevitable; the follicles can recover after small doses of radiation but if the dosage has been sufficient to produce a dry desquamative skin reaction, permanent epilation occurs.

The *mucosa* lining the upper respiratory and alimentary tract has a faster cell turnover time than the skin, so that radiation effects begin to appear within 10–14 days. Cell death leads to ulceration of the mucosa and an inflammatory response causing vaso-dilatation and a fibrinous exudate on the surface, which is almost inevitable in the course of radical radiotherapy of head and neck cancer. The time of appearance of this acute mucosal reaction varies with different parts of the mouth and pharynx as described by Coutard (1922); the areas of mucosa with the highest mitotic rates, e.g. the cheek, manifest their radiation damage before those areas, e.g. the dorsum of the tongue with a slower mitotic rate. Those epithelial cells which survive radiation are stimulated to divide more rapidly in response to the injury thereby re-populating the mucosa. Rapid healing is therefore the rule, and is usually complete within 2 or 3 weeks after completion of a course of radiotherapy; with the more prolonged fractionation schemes healing may in fact take place while the treatment is still in progress.

The *bone marrow* is one of the most mitotically active organs in the human body, being second only to the epithelium of the intestine in this respect. Irradiation of the marrow causes a rapid fall in production of blood cells. Changes in peripheral blood follow, depending on the life cycle of the different cell systems. White cells, being short-lived, disappear most rapidly, and the first change seen is a fall in total white count which may be followed a few days later by a fall in the platelet count. Red cell changes, if seen at all, occur several weeks later. Peripheral blood changes are only seen when a large proportion of the total body marrow is being irradiated. They are rarely a problem in the treatment of head and neck cancer.

Delayed Effects

Acute reactions, although unpleasant, heal rapidly and completely and are rarely the limiting factor in radiotherapy. Delayed effects occurring months or years after treatment are of much more consequence and limit the maximum doses which can safely be given. Late damage results from mitotic death of cells in slowly-dividing tissues, impairment of blood supply, and sometimes trauma acting as a mitotic stimulus to more specialized cells.

The *lens of the eye* is a good example of a slowly dividing tissue. Fibres are constantly being replaced throughout life by slow division of cells at the periphery of the lens. A dose of only a few hundred rads is sufficient to kill some of these cells, which undergo mitotic death several months or years after irradiation. The dead cells lead to the production of abnormal opaque fibres and consequently to a cataract, which develops gradually during a period between 1 and 10 years after the irradiation.

Small *blood vessels* are now generally believed to be the critical tissue responsible for most of the delayed histopathological effects of radiation. Proliferation kinetic studies of capillary endothelial cells in normal non-growing unstimulated mouse tissues by Tannock and Hayashi (1972) showed a turnover time of 2 months or more. Immediate vascular changes following irradiation are most likely to be physiological, as part of the inflammatory response to the rapid death of dividing cells. Pathological changes in the vessels themselves are not seen until mitotic death of endothelial cells begins several months after irradiation. The death of one endothelial cell will act as a mitotic stimulus to its neighbour which may then itself undergo mitotic death, so that a form of chain reaction of cell death may occur. Neighbouring intact endothelial cells are then over-stimulated and form localized hypertrophied areas which may partly or wholly occlude the vascular lumen. In this way, patchy areas of endarteritis obliterans occur. Dilatation of capillaries and venules distal to stenosed vessels results in the characteristic telangectasia sometimes seen in skin and mucosa after radiotherapy. Impairment of blood supply after radiotherapy is progressive, beginning within a few months after treatment and continuing for a number of years as more

and more endothelial lesions develop. It occurs in all patients to some extent but is not usually severe enough to impair the function of the irradiated organ. Progressive fibrosis is often associated with impairment of blood supply although the exact mechanism which stimulates fibroblastic activity is unknown; it may be related to changes in vascular permeability. Infection or trauma to irradiated organs may precipitate necrosis if the blood supply has been reduced and there is increased fibrous tissue.

Salivary glands present a special problem in radiotherapy. Salivary tissue is slowly-dividing; Glucksmann and Cherry (1971) consider the turnover time of the parotid serous acinar cells to be about 40 days. Nevertheless acute changes occur rapidly after irradiation, the mechanism of which is ill-understood. Swelling of salivary glands may occur within 24 h of the start of radiotherapy, followed by shrinkage a week or two later with production of a reduced volume of viscid saliva. After small doses, up to 2000 rads, recovery of full function occurs within about 8 months: higher doses result in atrophy and failure of secretion. Where a high dose is given to both parotid glands, e.g. in treating carcinoma of the nasal part of pharynx (nasopharynx), reduced salivary flow leads to unpleasant dryness of the mouth and predisposes to dental decay.

Mature *bone* and *cartilage* do not contain actively dividing cells. However, the osteoblast and the chondroblast may act as reverting post-mitotic cells if trauma acts as a stimulus to regeneration. This phenomenon may lead to mitotic death long after irradiation. A tooth extraction from an irradiated mandible may be just such a stimulus which together with impaired blood supply may lead to osteoradionecrosis. Attempted regeneration of irradiated bone may also occur if part of the bone has been eroded by tumour. Osteoradionecrosis may therefore follow successful treatment of a carcinoma of the alveolus if there was tumour invasion in bone initially, but not if there was no bone involvement. The same considerations apply to cartilage involvement in carcinoma of the larynx. For these reasons, invasion of bone or cartilage by tumour is generally regarded as an indication for treatment by surgery rather than radiotherapy.

The *neuron* is a fixed post-mitotic cell with no capacity for division and it is therefore highly radio-resistant. Nevertheless the cells of the central nervous system are critically dependent on their blood supply and any vascular endothelial damage here can easily lead to necrosis with catastrophic consequences. If injudiciously high doses of radiation are given to the brain or spinal cord symptoms and signs of damage characteristically begin between 9 and 18 months after the completion of radiotherapy. They then progress rapidly to become maximal after a few more months leading to a complete tetraplegia in the case of the cervical cord, or the death of the patient in the case of the brain stem.

Tolerance

The larger the dose of radiation given to an organ the greater the number of cells killed, and therefore the greater the chance of producing the late irreversible pathological effects described above. The concept of a tolerance dose has gradually developed in radiotherapy. This is defined as the maximum dose which can be given to an organ without producing serious pathological *sequelae*. It varies considerably between different tissues. At one extreme is the lens of the eye where a dose of as little as 400 rads may cause a cataract. At the other extreme 12 000 rads may be given to the uterine cervix without causing any serious *sequelae*. The radical tumour doses listed in Table 1 represent approximate tolerance for vasculo-connective tissue in the head and neck.

Tolerance doses in general depend inversely upon the volume of tissue irradiated. For example, a 6 × 4 cm area of skin may tolerate 5000 rads in 3 weeks, whereas a 20 × 15 cm area tolerates only 3000 rads in the same period.

EFFECTS OF RADIATION ON A SOLID TUMOUR

It was explained above that an irradiated cell may not die until it subsequently divides. A tumour will not shrink in volume unless dead cells are removed from it. If the dead (or strictly "doomed") cells are removed only slowly from a given tumour or tissue, then obvious clinical changes will occur only slowly. If however, the same proportion of "doomed" cells was created by a given dose of radiation in a tissue with a fast turnover rate, then shrinkage would be seen quickly. In this example the difference in "volume shrinkage rate" is due entirely to different cell population turnover rates, and not to any intrinsic difference in *cellular* radiosensitivity to the killing effect of radiation. In the past this distinction between "gross organ radiosensitivity" and "cell killing radiosensitivity" was not clearly made. The term "radiosensitive" has now been abandoned in favour of the two distinct terms "radioresponsive", referring to shrinking, and "radiocurable" referring to the chance of killing all tumour cells with tolerable radiation dosage.

In order to gain insight into the cellular and tissue changes occurring inside tumours, we can imagine the tumour to be made up of blood vessels, proliferating cells (P-cells), quiescent but potentially able to proliferate cells (Q-cells), differentiated cells (normally indistinguishable from Q-cells at any one time), and necrotic areas. The total number of viable cells in the tumour can be represented by P + Q and the proportion of those that are proliferating by P/(P + Q). This proportion is called the growth fraction (Steel, 1967). An indication of the growth fraction can be obtained by tritiated thymidine uptake studies, and less accurately but more simply from the mitotic index.

Many types of tumour grow until each capillary vessel is surrounded by a cylindrical annulus of "healthily" growing malignant cells of radius about 100 micrometres. This distance is the diffusion distance of oxygen, as described above. At the edge of this annulus lies a thin shell of cells, perhaps only one or two cells thick, which are starved of oxygen but not yet dead. Those are the most

dangerous cells; hypoxic and therefore resistant to X-ray killing, but still viable enough to regrow the tumour if left alive at the end of treatment. They are, of course, also difficult to reach with chemotherapeutic agents because these too have to diffuse outwards from the capillary vessels.

Studies in experimental tumours in animals have shown that the cell cycle time—the average time between successive mitoses—varies little as cells are pushed out along the 100 μm radius, but that the growth fraction decreases towards the edge. Cells that have been pushed beyond the hypoxic edge, out of reach of nutrients, will die. Whether they will be lysed or washed away, or whether they will remain in the tumour as necrotic masses, depends upon the type of tumour and its ability to clear away cellular debris.

If a tumour can get rid of cell debris, it is likely to shrink after treatment, at a rate depending on its clearance capacity and not just on the proportion of cells killed. This is why early clinical disappearance of a tumour mass is not a reliable guide to the ultimate probability of recurrence or cure, and should never be used as a signal to reduce the planned treatment dose or abandon radiotherapy in favour of surgery.

Referring to the cell survival curve in Fig. 4, it is obvious that two-ninths of a full treatment will reduce the number of viable cells in the tumour from 10^9 to 10^7, thereby killing 99 per cent of the malignant cells. The remaining 7/9 of the dose is necessary to bring the number of viable cells down from 10^7 to less than one. Any cell killing short of 10^{-8} is almost certain to lead to local recurrence. This means that a serious underdose would still kill 99 per cent of the cells, so that gross shrinkage could still occur, without any real chance of cure. This picture is commonly seen in present day chemotherapy where bone marrow depression limits the amount of drug that can be given. It can however be made use of clinically when radiotherapy is used palliatively (*see later*).

CLINICAL RADIOTHERAPY

Radiotherapy may be used as an adjuvant to the treatment of cancer by surgery, or it may be the sole method of treatment, either "radical", aimed at cure, or for palliation of symptoms. Cure of cancer can only be achieved if all reproductively viable malignant cells can be eliminated from the body. *Radical* radiotherapy aims to kill all such cells and is therefore applicable only to those cases where there are no detectable metastases present and where a high dose of radiation can safely be delivered to the entire tumour-bearing area. We have seen that the higher the dose given the greater the fraction of cells killed and therefore the greater the chance of eliminating all malignant cells. The radiotherapist therefore aims to administer the maximum doses which the normal tissues involved can tolerate so as to give the greatest chance of curing the tumour.

The *therapeutic ratio* of radiotherapy is defined as the tolerance dose of the relevant normal tissue divided by the tumour lethal dose. If this is greater than unity, radiotherapy may succeed; if it is less, the treatment must fail.

We have seen that the inherent radio-sensitivity of all mammalian cells, both normal and malignant, is very similar. Methods must be sought to enhance the relative effect of radiation on tumour cells compared with that on normal tissue, i.e. to obtain the best possible therapeutic ratio.

Tumour size is an important factor determining therapeutic ratio. The larger the tumour the greater the number of malignant cells, therefore the higher the chance that some cells will survive irradiation. At the same time, with larger tumours a larger volume of normal tissue must be irradiated, reducing the tolerance dose. An example of the influence of tumour size is seen in glottic carcinoma, where radiotherapy in most reported series cures over 90 per cent of T1 cases, but only about 65 per cent of T3 cases (*see* Chapter 1 for TNM classification of tumours).

Fractionation, i.e. dividing the dose of external beam radiotherapy into a number of treatments spread over a period of several weeks has long been known to improve therapeutic ratio. Regaud (1923), experimenting with the testes of rams and rabbits, found that fractionation increased the relative radiation damage to the testis compared with the scrotal skin. Although the testis is a doubtful model for tumours, similar principles were applied to clinical radiotherapy and it was indeed found that fractionation improved the therapeutic ratio. There are probably several factors which account for the beneficial effect of fractionation. Regaud's results are most likely explained by the fact that spermatic cells have a smaller shoulder to their cell-survival curve, i.e. less capacity for "recovery" than skin cells (Fig. 8). However,

determine experimentally. A more likely explanation of the benefit of fractionation may be in the differing reproductive capacity of normal and malignant tissues. Normal tissues possess a homeostatic mechanism whereby they

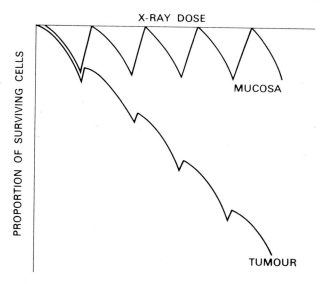

Fig. 9. Effect of fractionated radiotherapy on a tissue which replaces all the damaged cells by proliferation between successive fractions (upper curve); and on a tumour which proliferates little between fractions (lower curve).

attempt to keep the cell population constant; any form of injury, including radiation, which kills some cells, acts as a mitotic stimulus to the survivors which divide more rapidly to replace those lost. Tumours, being of their very nature disorders of growth mechanisms are less obedient to homeostatic laws, and less able to attempt to maintain a constant cell population. Tubiana (1970) and his colleagues have demonstrated increased growth rate of surviving tumour cells for a few days soon after radiation, but this is probably a non-specific stimulation by cell breakdown products or a transient improvement in relative availability of nutrition. If the mitotic response of the normal cell greatly exceeds that of the tumour cell, the effect shown in Fig. 9 will be seen. This effect can certainly be demonstrated in clinical radiotherapy. For example, Buschke and Vaeth (1963) showed that it was possible with very prolonged fractionation to cure carcinoma of the larynx without producing any visible mucosal changes during the treatment. However, prolongation will not necessarily avoid late radiation damage which depends on changes in more slowly dividing tissues.

The oxygen effect offers another explanation of the benefits of fractionation. Cater and Silver (1960) demonstrated a rising oxygen partial pressure ("tension") in tumours during a course of radiotherapy. Presumably as the well-oxygenated tumour cells die and are absorbed, there is a decrease in intercapillary distance with a relative increase in blood supply so that previously hypoxic cells become well oxygenated. Microangiographic studies by Rubin and Casarett (1966) have demonstrated an increase in the number of capillaries per unit volume in tumours

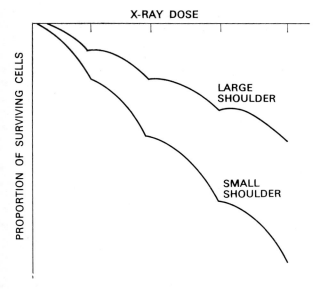

Fig. 8. Effect of fractionated radiotherapy on two cell populations. *Upper curve*: large shoulder, i.e. large capacity for repair between doses. *Lower curve*: small shoulder, i.e. small capacity for repair.

there is very little evidence available to suggest that this phenomenon explains the effect of fractionation on tumours. The sizes of shoulders for cells both in solid tumours and intact normal tissues are very difficult to during radiotherapy. Studies of the responses of animal tumours, e.g. those of van Putten and Kallman (1968), confirm this phenomenon of reoxygenation.

The ideal fractionation scheme for an individual tumour will depend on many factors, including the basic cell survival curve and the cell proliferation kinetic patterns of both the tumour and normal cells, the proportion of hypoxic cells in the tumour, and their rate of reoxygenation. It probably differs for every tumour. None of these parameters can be determined in the individual cancer patient, so the best that can be hoped for at present is to learn from clinical experience which fractionation scheme will give the best results in the largest proportion of patients with a particular type of tumour. This point remains controversial; the majority of radiotherapists favour about 30 fractions for treatment of head and neck cancer but some favour as few as 6 and others as many as 40. No radiotherapist's point of view can satisfactorily be refuted on either experimental or clinical grounds and there is an urgent need for more prospective controlled clinical trials to determine optimum fractionation schedules.

Apart from fractionation there are other methods under investigation to improve therapeutic ratios in radical radiotherapy. Nearly all these methods are aimed at overcoming the oxygen effect, this being the only known large difference in radiation response between normal and tumour cells which can readily be exploited. New techniques along these lines are discussed later.

Palliative radiotherapy aims to relieve symptoms in a patient with incurable cancer. A relatively small dose is given, sufficient to kill a significant proportion of the malignant cells thereby relieving a specific symptom such as bleeding, pain or obstruction, but insufficient to cause symptomatic normal tissue reactions.

Radiotherapy is sometimes given "*prophylactically*" after surgery to areas of potential spread, especially the lymph nodes draining the tumour site. The aim is to destroy microscopic foci of tumour. In these circumstances the number of malignant cells is smaller than in a clinically-apparent tumour, so that there is a good chance of eliminating all cells by a dose slightly lower than maximum tissue tolerance. Berger and colleagues (1971) showed that the incidence of subsequent lymph node metastases can be reduced significantly by giving 4500 rads over a period of 5 weeks, a dose which would have only a very small chance indeed of sterilizing a palpable carcinoma.

SURGERY AND RADIOTHERAPY

The outcome of a course of radical radiotherapy is always uncertain. Clinical evidence of a persistent mass at the end of a course of treatment does not necessarily indicate failure; for the reasons stated previously it often takes a further 1 or 2 months for all evidence of tumour to disappear. During this period biopsy is unreliable. Tumour cells which look intact histologically may have sustained lethal damage to their genetic apparatus but have not yet passed through mitosis. Such "doomed" cells, although visually apparently "viable", have lost their reproductive capacity and therefore are no threat to the patient; they will die when they attempt to divide. The only histological criteria of viability after radiotherapy which is at all reliable is the appearance of normal-looking mitoses in tumour cells. The vast majority of successfully treated squamous cell carcinomata will have disappeared by 2 months after the end of treatment; more slowly growing tumours such as adenoid cystic carcinoma may take very much longer. It is not unknown in the latter type of tumour for residual masses to persist unchanged for many years.

In some cases of squamous carcinoma after radiotherapy, viable tumour may persist. In other cases there may be complete regression but a recurrence may arise from microscopic remnants of viable cells which survive the radiotherapy. In either case "salvage" surgery may be feasible. The longer after radiotherapy that surgery is performed the greater the post-radiation vascular changes and therefore the higher the incidence of post-operative complications such as delayed healing, fistula formation, wound break-down, and most catastrophic of all, rupture of the carotid artery. In general, the optimum time to operate after the end of a course of radiotherapy is more than 3 weeks when all vasodilatation has subsided, and less than 3 months before any endarteritis obliterans appears. However, it must be stressed that modern radiotherapy does not increase the incidence of post-operative complication of head and neck surgery by more than about 20 per cent, even in the case of operations on recurrences several years after treatment.

Pre-operative radiotherapy has quite a different objective from radical radiotherapy. It is given to patients in whom a firm decision has been made to treat surgically, with the object of increasing the chance of cure. The concept of pre-operative radiotherapy is based on the hypothesis that cells disseminated at operation which may cause local recurrence or metastases are derived from the actively growing periphery of a tumour. Such cells have a good blood supply, are well-oxygenated and therefore radiosensitive. The hypoxic cells likely to survive radiotherapy are more centrally-placed and more certain to be removed at surgery.

The dose of pre-operative radiation should be large enough to kill the major proportion of the well-oxygenated cells but not large enough to cause significantly delayed wound healing or to increase the risk of post-operative complications. The maximum tissue tolerance doses used in radical radiotherapy should not be given pre-operatively; they are unnecessary and expose the patient to increased risk. Powers and Palmer (1968), working with a transplantable lymphosarcoma in mice, showed that a single dose of 500 rads would kill 99 per cent of the tumour cells but that 4 000 rads were required to cure the tumour. The former dose had no effect on wound healing but the latter caused a very marked delay. The same workers investigated the effect of a pre-operative dose of radiation on surgical cure rate in a variety of transplantable mouse tumours. In nearly all systems tested pre-operative radiotherapy significantly improved survival rates. For example, in the case of Gardener lymphosarcoma, no mice survived without treatment or after a dose of 500 rads alone; after excision without prior irradiation 53 per cent survived; but when 500 rads was given immediately before surgery, 85 per cent survived ($p = 0.001$). Similar results were obtained by Inch and McCredie (1963). In all the successful experiments the effective pre-operative dose was about one-third of that required to cure 50 per cent of tumours under test.

In clinical practice, there are two schools of thought on pre-operative radiotherapy, the low dose and the high dose. Low dose pre-operative radiotherapy consists of giving approximately 2000 rads in about 1 week's treatment and operating immediately, before any vasodilatation from acute radiation response occurs; this is less than half of a full radical treatment. The high dose method consists of giving 4000–5000 rads in 4 or 5 weeks and then waiting a further 4 weeks or so for the acute reaction to subside before operating; this is 75–85 per cent of a full radical treatment. Both methods have been found to give encouraging results in clinical practice but there is a need for more controlled clinical trials. Strong (1969) reported a controlled trial of radical neck dissection with and without low dose pre-operative radiotherapy. There was a significant decrease in local recurrence rate in the operation field in patients who had received radiotherapy. Hendrickson and Liebner (1968) compared high and low dose pre-operative radiotherapy for supraglottic cancer: they found no difference in results between the two. At the recommended dose levels neither high dose nor low dose pre-operative radiotherapy seriously increased post-operative morbidity. If there is, as seems likely, no difference between the two, then the low dose method should be preferred on the grounds of convenience.

An attractive-sounding policy sometimes employed for tumours where the relative merits of radiotherapy and surgery are in doubt, e.g. supraglottic carcinoma, is to give radiotherapy to a dose level similar to that used pre-operatively, and then to reassess the patient. If the tumour has regressed it is regarded as radio-responsive and additional treatment is given to make up a full radical course. If not, surgery is performed. Unfortunately, as explained previously, initial tumour shrinkage depends on many factors, apart from the proportion of cells killed. Suit and his colleagues (1965) found no correlation between regression rate and ultimate prognosis in mouth cancer. It is probably unwise, at the present state of our knowledge, to decide upon definitive treatment on the basis of early tumour shrinkage.

Post-operative radiotherapy is a possible alternative to pre-operative radiotherapy. On radiobiological grounds pre-operative radiotherapy should give more benefit. Post-operative radiotherapy cannot be expected to prevent the development of metastases due to cells disseminated by the blood at the time of surgery. It can only hope to prevent local recurrence arising from tumour cells left in the operation field. Such cells may well be poorly oxygenated in the post-operative period. In addition, the volume of the operative field which is potentially contaminated with malignant cells is always much larger than the original tumour, so that post-operative radiotherapy necessitates

irradiation of a large volume of normal tissues. These considerations have resulted in a paucity of animal experiments to test the possible value of post-operative radiotherapy. Perez and Olsen (1970) investigated the effects of single doses of radiotherapy given pre- and post-operatively on the surgical cure of transplanted mouse lymphosarcoma. A single dose of radiation improved the survival rates whether it was given before or after operation, but the survival rates were significantly higher in the pre-operatively treated compared with the post-operatively treated animals. This was true at all dose levels from 500 to 5000 rads, the greatest differences being seen at lower dose levels.

There are no results of controlled clinical trials of post-operative radiotherapy in head and neck cancer available. It is best reserved for those cases in whom surgery is thought to be incomplete because of either the operative findings or histological examination of the resected specimen. The clinical results of Fletcher and Evers (1970) suggest that in these circumstances post-operative radiotherapy given to maximum tolerance dosage may still control the disease in some cases. Low dose pre-operative therapy does not preclude subsequent post-operative radiotherapy.

FUTURE DEVELOPMENTS IN RADIOTHERAPY

Future developments in radiotherapy will include:

(a) Continuing developments in planned surgery with radiotherapy.
(b) Methods of delivering more exact dose distributions using new types of radiation machine.
(c) The use of radiation and cytotoxic drugs in combination.
(d) Methods of overcoming the problem of hypoxic cells.

Up to a few years ago, the main improvements in radiotherapy had occurred as a result of the first two approaches. The historical and logical precedent is therefore that these approaches might still lead to improvements. Nevertheless the room for such improvements now seems small.

The main developments from biological points of view arise in the various methods of overcoming the problem of hypoxic cells, and in the employment of very low dose rates. We shall describe three of the main methods at present under development for dealing with hypoxic cells: hyperbaric oxygen radiotherapy, fast neutron beams and chemical radiosensitizers. Combination treatments using cytotoxic drugs and radiotherapy will also be discussed.

(i) Radiotherapy in High Pressure Oxygen.

Hypoxia protects cells against radiation damage as explained previously, whereas raising oxygen partial pressure *above* physiological levels does not increase radiosensitivity. A significant proportion of tumour cells, but very few normal cells, are believed to be hypoxic. Consequently, provision of tumours and normal tissues with more oxygen should improve the therapeutic ratio of radiotherapy.

Breathing oxygen at atmospheric pressure makes only a small improvement in tumour oxygenation. The calculations of Thomlinson (1967) suggest a halving of the number of hypoxic cells in most tumours, probably insufficient to improve cure rates very much. Few clinical trials have so far been carried out using this method, and none has shown a benefit.

compression and decompression, bringing the total treatment time down to about 30 min. There is a small risk of oxygen-induced convulsions, about 1 per cent in most reported series. Stringent precautions must be taken to avoid fire and explosion. Consequently, the technique is time-consuming and is not in widespread use, although some 12 centres in the U.K. employ it. Fortunately, as can be seen from Fig. 7, the oxygen effect is greater the larger the X-ray dose given, so that a smaller number of larger

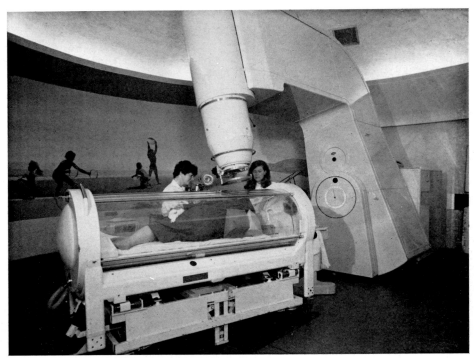

FIG. 10. Hyperbaric chamber for use in radiotherapy. (Photograph by Mr. R. Toogood.)

Inhalation of oxygen at raised pressure however increases the concentration of dissolved oxygen in plasma and extracellular fluid, so that diffusion distances from capillaries are greatly increased. At a pressure of about 300 kPa* (the maximum the human brain can tolerate without general anaesthesia) only about 0·1 per cent of tumour cells are calculated to remain hypoxic; a useful reduction from the 10–20 per cent found in most experimental animal tumours. However, this assumes normal blood flow rates in capillaries; if there is a reduced flow rate due to vasoconstriction, high pressure oxygenation may be ineffective (Milne *et al.*, 1973).

High pressure oxygen was introduced into clinical radiotherapy by Churchill-Davidson and his colleagues (1955). A one-man compression chamber is used (Fig. 10). For each treatment the patient must spend about 40 min in the chamber, allowing time for compression, saturation of tissues with oxygen, irradiation and decompression. Routine use of myringotomy and insertion of grommets avoids barotrauma and reduces the time necessary for

* About 3 standard atmospheres.

dose fractions are used with high pressure oxygen than in orthodox radiotherapy. Between 6 and 12 treatments are generally favoured over a period of 3 or 4 weeks.

Controlled trials by van den Brenk (1968) and Henk and his associates (1972) have provided convincing evidence of the existence of the oxygen effect in human head and neck cancer, and show that local tumour clearance can be improved significantly by the use of high pressure oxygen. The vulnerability of normal tissues is also increased to some extent, especially cartilage where the cells live at some distance from capillaries and therefore are presumably relatively hypoxic in normal circumstances. It is not yet clear whether the therapeutic ratio of radiotherapy is greater using a few large fractions in high pressure oxygen or many small fractions conventionally in air. Controlled trials to answer this question were reported by Chang and his associates (1973) in carcinoma of the oral part of pharynx (oropharynx) and Henk (1974) in carcinoma of the larynx. In both trials there appeared to be an advantage from high pressure oxygen, but the results did not reach statistical significance.

(ii) Fast Neutron Radiotherapy.

Fast neutron beams interact with tissue by knocking out protons, instead of electrons as X-rays do. These protons have a very high density of ionization along their short track, so that cells they damage are likely to be killed whether oxygen is present or not. The ratio of dose without oxygen present to the dose with oxygen present to produce the same biological effect is known as the oxygen enhancement ratio (OER). In Fig. 7 for example the OER is equal to the dose at E divided by that at A. The OER for X-rays is approximately 3, whereas for neutrons it is only about 1·7. Of course it would be ideal if the OER were as low as 1·0, but no particle which penetrates tissue sufficiently well for radiotherapy gives a value as low as that. The "therapeutic gain factor" for fast neutron beams can be estimated by dividing the OER for X-rays of 2·5 to 3 by the OER for neutrons, 1·7 (Alper, 1963). The quotient is about 1·6, representing the effective increase of dose to hypoxic cells in the tumour when neutrons are used instead of X-rays.

In general, types of radiation with densely ionizing particle tracks are called "high LET radiations". LET stands for "linear energy transfer" of energy from the particle to the medium it traverses. High LET radiations are associated with a reduced oxygen enhancement ratio.

Fast neutrons can be produced with good dose rates from cyclotrons and with rather lower dose rates from smaller deuterium-tritium (DT) machines. Their penetration in tissue is not quite as good as that of cobalt-60 gamma-rays; but with multiple-field treatments the dose distributions in tissue are comparable.

The main advantage of neutron beams is expected to be their ability to kill more hypoxic cells in tumours than X-rays do, for the same injury to normal tissues. Other advantages have been suggested but not proved. One is the fact that less repair takes place in cells after neutron irradiation than after X-irradiation, so that the total dose of neutrons increases much less steeply if the number of dose fractions is increased than in the case of X-rays (see Fig. 6). This should make the prescribing of neutron doses easier than with X-rays if changes in fractionation schedules are introduced. Another possible advantage is that not all tissues appear to have the same reduced repair after neutron irradiation, so that certain types of tumour might be more vulnerable to neutron treatment than others.

An early neutron trial in California in 1939–42 gave rise to very severe reactions in normal tissues (Stone, 1948) because the reduced repair in normal tissues, compared with that after X-rays, was not understood at the time. The patients were therefore overdosed when multiple dose fractions were given. Later, radiobiological experiments using the skin of pigs demonstrated this clearly (Fowler and Morgan, 1963), and showed that neutrons could safely be used in radiotherapy provided due attention was paid to dose-time fractionation relationships.

Clinical trials using neutrons have been in progress at Hammersmith Hospital since 1969 and favourable early tumour responses have been reported in advanced head and neck cases (Catterall, 1974). Clinical trials are just beginning in several other countries.

(iii) Pions.

Another type of high-LET radiation which may well be in clinical use shortly consists of negative pi-mesons, also called negative pions. Mesons are particles from atomic nuclei with mass intermediate between that of electrons and protons. They can only be produced from large particle accelerator installations working at 500 million electron volts or higher energies: Los Alamos, U.S.A.; Vancouver, Canada; Stanford University, U.S.A.; Zurich, Switzerland; and possibly the Rutherford Laboratory at Harwell are the only places capable of applying these beams clinically within the next few years.

Pion beams have two advantages. First, they give a strongly peaked physical dose distribution so that a designated thickness of tissue volume at depth receives about twice the radiation dose which is delivered to the overlying tissue (Fig. 11, Fowler and Perkins, 1961; Raju,

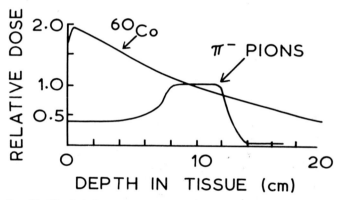

FIG. 11. Physical distribution of dose in tissue from negative pi mesons.

1973). This should, of course, be useful clinically. Second, when negative pions travel very slowly, at the end of their path in tissue, they are captured by positively charged nuclei of carbon, nitrogen or oxygen and cause these nuclei to "explode", giving several charged nuclear particles in the form of a tiny "star". These charged particles released in tissue in the dose peak have high LET, so they have a reduced oxygen enhancement ratio, as in the case of neutron beams. Negative pions therefore have the double advantage of excellent physical dose distributions and also the same biological advantage, of preferential killing of hypoxic cells, that neutron beams have (Raju, 1973). The OER values for pion beams so far measured have been about 1·7, i.e. quite similar to those of neutrons. Neither type of beam gives OER values as low as the 1·0 which would be desirable.

The value of improvements in physical dose distributions available with negative pions is controversial: some radiotherapists believe that adequate dose distributions can already be obtained using cobalt or linear accelerator beams, and that the outline of the tumour cannot be determined accurately enough to justify the precision obtainable with pions. Others do wish to use the sharper-edged treatment volumes. In due course clinical trials might tell which view is correct.

(iv) Chemical Radiosensitizers of Hypoxic Cells.

Recently drugs have been found which mimic the radiosensitizing action of oxygen and which are not too toxic for clinical use (Adams, 1973). These chemicals have been developed over a period of 10 years from basic research into the mechanism of the oxygen effect in radiobiology. Several compounds have been found to give 80 per cent of the full oxygen effect on cells in culture dishes, and also *in vivo* in experimental animals (Denekamp and Michael, 1972). The radiosensitizing effect on solid tumours in experimental animals have been found to be almost as great (Sheldon *et al.*, 1974). The drug has to be administered 1–2 h before each irradiation session. One such drug is metronidazole which is in common use to treat trichomoniasis at doses of less than 1g/day. For adequate radiosensitization however, some 10–20 g would have to be administered to the patient on each treatment day, and nausea prevents it. (Deutsch and Foster, 1975.) A somewhat more potent compound, a 2-nitroimidazole, is being investigated and improvements in this direction are expected to lead to clinical trials shortly. The dose enhancement ratios obtained in experimental tumours in mice have been just over 2·0, i.e. quite comparable with the gain factors of about 1·6 achieved with neutron or pion beams.

(v) Combination of Radiotherapy and Cytotoxic Drugs.

Most cytotoxic drugs are only effective against cells which are actively dividing. Unlike radiation, they do not affect the reproductive integrity of resting non-dividing cells, so the term "radio-mimetic" is now obsolete. Some drugs are "phase specific"; cells are only vulnerable if exposed to these drugs at a particular point in the mitotic cycle; fluorouracil for example only kills cells during the "S" phase, i.e. when they are actively synthesizing DNA. Other drugs are "cycle-specific" i.e. cells are vulnerable if exposed at any point in the mitotic cycle other than the resting phase: cyclophosphamide is an example.

Cytotoxic drugs alone rarely have more than a transient effect against most human solid tumours because of the large proportion of tumour cells that are in a resting phase at any one time, and it is impossible to obtain an adequate therapeutic ratio between the tumour and the vulnerable dividing normal tissue such as the bone marrow and gastro-intestinal epithelium.

When cytotoxic drugs are given in combination with radiotherapy the effect is usually merely additive on both dividing normal cells and tumour cells. The possible theoretical benefits of the cytotoxic drug are the chance of control of microscopic metastases, which seems very unlikely, or an improvement in therapeutic ratio between actively-dividing tumour and non-dividing vascular endothelium and other connective tissue cells. With some drugs, e.g. dactinomycin (actinomycin D), there is a true potentiation, i.e. the combined effect of the drug and the radiation is greater than the sum of the two effects when they are given singly; the possible benefits seem no greater than with an additive agent.

The drug which has been found to be most consistently effective in squamous carcinoma of the head and neck and most often combined with radiotherapy is the antimetabolite methotrexate, which inhibits DNA synthesis and is therefore "S" phase specific: Berry (1968) demonstrated that cells in tissue culture which survived exposure to methotrexate were more vulnerable to radiation and had a reduced oxygen enhancement ratio. He therefore proposed that a rational use of methotrexate would be a large dose of the drug followed soon after by radiation, to be repeated intermittently allowing rest periods for normal tissues to recover. The timing of such treatment is difficult, and in practice it is usual to give large doses of methotrexate by systemic or intra-arterial infusion to obtain some tumour regression before starting a course of radical radiotherapy. Several controlled clinical trials of combined radiotherapy and chemotherapy are in progress but none has yet shown any advantage over radiotherapy alone. The present position has been reviewed by Bleehen (1973).

REFERENCES

Adams, G. E. (1972), *Brit. med. Bull.*, **29**, No. 1 (Biological Basis of Radiotherapy), 48.
Alper, T. (1963), *Brit. J. Radiol.*, **36**, 97.
Bedford, J. S. and Hall, E. J. (1963), *Int. J. Radiat. Biol.*, **7**, 377.
Berger, D. S., Fletcher, G. H., Lindberg, R. D. and Jesse, R. H. (1971), *Amer. J. Roentgenol.*, **111**, 66.
Bergonnié, J. and Tribondeau, L. (1906), *C. R. Acad. Sci. (Paris)*, **143**, 938.
Berry, R. J. (1968), *Amer. J. Roentgenol.*, **102**, 509.
Bleehen, N. M. (1973), *Brit. med. Bull.*, **29**, 54.
Buschke, F. and Vaeth, J. M. (1963), *Amer. J. Roentgenol.*, **89**, 29.
Cater, D. B. and Silver, I. A. (1960), *Acta radiol.*, **53**, 233.
Catterall, Mary (1974), *Europ. J. Cancer*, **10**, 343.
Chang, C. H., Conley, J. J. and Herbert, C. (1973), *Amer. J. Roentgenol.*, **117**, 509.
Churchill-Davidson, I., Sanger, C. and Thomlinson, R. H. (1955), *Lancet*, **i**, 1091.
Coutard, H. (1922), *C. R. Soc. Biol.*, **86**, 1140.
Cowdry, E. V. (1950), *Textbook of Histology*, 4th edition. Philadelphia: Lea & Febiger.
Denekamp, J. and Michael, B. D. (1972), *Nature New Biol.*, **239**, 21.
Deutsch, G. and Foster, J. L. (1975), *Brit. J. Cancer*, **31**, 75.
Ellis, F. (1969), *Clin. Radiol.*, **20**, 1.
Fletcher, G. H. and Evers, W. T. (1970), *Radiology*, **95**, 185.
Fowler, J. F. (1971), *Brit. J. Radiol.*, **44**, 81.
Fowler, J. F. and Morgan, R. L. (1963), *Brit. J. Radiol.*, **36**, 115.
Fowler, J. F. and Stern, B. E. (1963), *Brit. J. Radiol.*, **36**, 163.
Fowler, P. H. and Perkins, D. M. (1961), *Nature*, **189**, 524.
Glucksmann, A. T. and Cherry, C. P. (1971), *Pathology of Irradiation*. Baltimore: Williams & Wilkins.
Hall, E. J., Bedford, J. S. and Oliver, R. (1966), *Brit. J. Radiol.*, **39**, 302.
Hendrickson, F. R. and Liebner, E. (1968), *Ann. Otol.*, **77**, 222.
Henk, J. M., Kunkler, P. B. and Smith, C. W. (1972), *Proc. of the 2nd Int. Congress of the Eur. Assn. of Radiol.*, p. 319, Amsterdam: Excerpta Medica.
Henk, J. M. (1974), *Laryngoscope*. In press.
Inch, W. R. and McCredie, J. A. (1963), *Cancer*, **16**, 595.
Kallmann, R. F. (1972), *Radiology*, **105**, 135.
Liversage, W. E. (1971), *Brit. J. Radiol.*, **44**, 91.
Milne, N., Hill, R. P. and Bush, R. S. (1973), *Radiology*, **106**, 663.
Paterson, R. D. and Parker, H. M. (1934), *Brit. J. Radiol.*, **7**, 592.
Perez, C. A. and Olsen, J. (1970), *Amer. J. Roentgenol.*, **108**, 396.

Powers, W. E. and Palmer, L. A. (1968), *Amer. J. Roentgenol.*, **102**, 176.

Raju, M. M. and Richman, C. (1973), *Current Topics in Radiation Research Quarterly*, **8**, 159.

Regaud, C. (1923), *Bull. Acad. nat. Med.*, **91**, 375.

Rubin, P. and Casarett, G. W. (1966), *Clin. Radiol.*, **17**, 220.

Rubin, P. and Casarett, G. W. (1968), *Clinical Radiation Pathology.* Philadelphia: W. B. Saunders Co.

Sheldon, P. W., Foster, J. L. and Fowler, J. F. (1974), *Brit. J. Cancer*, **30**, 560.

Steel, G. G. (1967), *Europ. J. Cancer*, **3**, 381.

Stone, R. S. (1948), *Amer. J. Roentgenol.*, **59**, 771.

Strandqvist, M. M. (1944), *Acta radiol.*, suppl. 55.

Strong, E. W. (1969), *Surg. Clin. N. Amer.*, **49**, 271.

Suit, H., Lindberg, R. and Fletcher, G. H. (1965), *Radiology*, **84**, 1100.

Tannock, I. F. and Hayashi, S. (1972), *Cancer Res.*, **32**, 77.

Thomlinson, R. H. (1967), *Modern Trends in Radiotherapy* (T. J. Deeley, Ed.). London: Butterworth.

Tubiana, M. (1971), *Brit. J. Radiol.*, **44**, 325.

Van den Brenk, H. A. S. (1968), *Amer. J. Roentgenol.*, **102**, 8.

Van Putten, L. M. and Kallman, R. F. (1968), *Frontiers of Radiation Therapy and Oncology*, Vol. 1, p. 162 (J. M. Vaeth, Ed.). Basle: Karger.

53. BLOOD TRANSFUSION

JOHN BOXALL

HISTORICAL

It is recorded that the transference of blood from the circulation of one living animal to another was made in the middle of the seventeenth century by Francesco Folli who was a Florentine physician. Within a few decades, blood from animal sources was transfused to a human being by Jean Denis of Montpellier. Considerable interest was shown in England by such persons as Sir Christopher Wren and Samuel Pepys but ignorance of the ABO groups alone resulted in at least a third of transfusion attempts between human subjects being incompatible. The use of a syringe by James Blundell (Lecturer at St. Thomas' and Guy's Hospitals) in 1824 made the transfusion of his patients with human blood possible. The avoidance of coagulation by removing fibrin (in 1835) overcame another prime difficulty. As late as the beginning of the twentieth century, Crile performed direct transfusion from the artery of a donor to the vein of a recipient. However, the volume of blood transfused could not be ascertained and the results were so hazardous that such work was regarded largely as experimentation. It seems that the simple necessity resulting from massive blood losses during the First World War led to the introduction, largely by American surgeons, of blood transfusion on a large scale. By that time, the discovery of three blood groups by Landsteiner (1900) and a fourth group by Decastello and Sturli (1902), as well as the independent work on blood-grouping carried out by Jansky (1907) and by Moss (1910), had laid a firm foundation for the understanding of hitherto unrecognized factors. Progress with anticoagulants (Agote, 1915) rendered direct transfusion unnecessary. The introduction of the improved technique met with opposition and anticoagulants were still in disfavour even as late as the 1920's. Another basic problem, i.e. that due to the rhesus factor, had to wait until the 1940's for elucidation. Medicine had been more concerned with blood letting than with blood transfusion.

NEED FOR TRANSFUSION

The *normal blood volume* is fairly constant when expressed in terms of unit body mass. For men, a value of 77 ml. kg^{-1} has been calculated from a method where circulating erythrocytes were labelled with a phosphorus radionuclide (Reeve and Veall, 1949); for women, the blood volume is 67 ml. kg^{-1} (Wadsworth, 1954) and for children, 75 ml. kg^{-1} (Russell, 1949).

Total blood loss in *microsurgical operations* on the ear, such as *stapedectomy*, is of the order of only 1 ml (Deacock, 1971) so that the question of blood replacement does not arise here.

Studies on children using a chromium 51 radionuclide method for labelling erythrocytes showed that the average blood loss in *adenoidectomy and tonsillectomy* was 11 8ml (Ruggles, 1960). Following his study of blood loss in adenoidectomy and tonsillectomy, Shalom (1964) concluded that, although the loss was greater the older the child, this was because the increasing age is associated with increasing body mass; the average blood loss per unit body mass (about 4 ml. kg^{-1}) was not a function of age. There was, however, considerable variation; blood loss per unit body mass for these children ranged from 1·4 to 19·1 ml. kg^{-1}. In 14 per cent of the cases, the loss was in excess of 6 ml. kg^{-1} (equivalent to 8 per cent of total blood volume). Shalom said that in two out of every five children undergoing adenoidectomy and tonsillectomy there was a loss sufficient to render an imminent need for fluid replacement. One child in the series of 50 cases required a whole blood transfusion. In adults, blood loss during tonsillectomy is about 3 ml. kg^{-1}. This last value and other values given in this paragraph so far refer to blood losses for operations under general anaesthesia. In respect of tonsillectomy on adults, the blood loss under local anaesthesia may be about one-tenth of that under general anaesthesia. In connection with re-anaesthetizing cases of adenoidectomy and tonsillectomy because of persisting postoperative haemorrhage, Davies (1964) has commented on the need to assess the haematological status of the patient. Anoxia occurring in a hypovolaemic patient can lead to cardiac arrest with extreme rapidity. Consequently, practically every one of these cases to be re-anaesthetized will require some replacement therapy; if the blood volume deficit is small, plasma may be given; if the deficit is large, whole blood must be used.

Shalom's (1964) data also showed that the blood loss in

major otolaryngological operations is of the order of 1 l (17 ml. kg^{-1}). However, there was an appreciable variation. Ninety per cent of the blood losses were in the range of ±10 ml. kg^{-1} around this central value. A number of factors are responsible for this variability. Clearly, the anatomical size of the operation is one factor. Block dissection of the cervical lymph nodes further increases blood loss; the use of hypotensive and hypothermic procedures reduces the loss (Loewy *et al.*, 1963). All the patients in Shalom's series received blood transfusions in an amount equal to, or a little above, the estimated blood loss. The haemoglobin concentrations in the blood on the first post-operative day differed little from the pre-operative values.

With the decreasing load of tedious laboratory investigations brought about by automation, more time is available to screen new patients as fully as possible; outpatients should have a full blood count and grouping performed as routine investigations. In addition to providing a useful lead to an expected clinical diagnosis, a resulting low haemoglobin concentration can often be treated in a simple manner, e.g. with iron preparations, long before admission to hospital. Failure to request these two simple tests may mean that an urgent request for a haemoglobin estimation, grouping and crossmatch arrives only following a haemorrhage during operation.

A haemoglobin level below 5 mmol. l^{-1} (8 gm per cent) will need to be carefully watched while levels below 4·35 mmol. l^{-1} (7 gm per cent) may well require blood transfusion unless operation can be delayed while iron therapy is given. There is a risk of cardiac complications when transfusing cases with a haemoglobin level of less than 6·2 mmol. l^{-1} (10 gm per cent). Consequently, transfusion taking place less than two days before operation is inadvisable in such cases. Patients with haemoglobin levels below 3 mmol. l^{-1} (5 gm per cent) are particularly at risk in this regard and should therefore be given *concentrated erythrocytes* ("*packed cells*") in small doses (250 ml) and transfused slowly (4–6 h) at two-day intervals. The prescription of a diuretic may help to reduce the cardiac burden. Exchange transfusions may also be considered in such cases. Where sickle cell anaemia is present, exchange transfusion may be considered prior to operation.

As an approximate guide, one unit (450 ml) of blood can be expected to increase the haemoglobin level by 0·6 mmol. l^{-1} (1·0 gm per cent) and, where no erythrocytes are being produced by the patient's own resources, one unit, administered each week, should maintain a normal haemoglobin level in an adult. Blood volume is usually readjusted within twenty-four hours of transfusion.

The effects of haemorrhage are similar to those of emotional shock but more sustained. The clinical signs include fainting, sweating, nausea and vomiting, and a cold clammy skin. Vaso-construction as a natural response will help to compensate for blood losses of up to 1 l. This loss is normally restored in a healthy individual in about 3 days. Where the systolic blood pressure falls below 13·3 kPa (about 100 mm mercury) and the pulse rate rises above 100 per minute, a volume less than 70 per cent of normal may be presumed; gross tissue haemorrhage will further

reduce such an estimate. During major operations, the loss of blood volume is usually 25 per cent more than is determined by careful estimation, e.g. by gauze weighing. A further reduction following operation is also not uncommon, especially in conjunction with infection; such losses may not become apparent from haemoglobin and packed cell volume (PCV) estimations.

The *packed cell volume* (haematocrit) estimation is of value in following the progress of haemorrhage. It is estimated with the use of Wintrobe or microhaematocrit tubes. The Wintrobe tube provides a useful dual role in that it first measures the erythrocyte sedimentation rate (ESR); secondly, the PCV is measured by centrifugation. The centrifugation is continued until the PCV remains constant; this may be achieved by a rate of, for example, 3000 r.p.m. for 30 min, depending upon the radius of the centrifuge arms. Edetic acid* is a suitable anticoagulant for this purpose. The author, however, prefers to use the Westergren technique for the ESR and the slightly less accurate microhaematocrit for PCV. The latter uses capillary tubing which is heparinized for capillary blood collection; alternatively, plain capillary tubing may be filled with venous blood containing edetic acid. The advantages of this capillary technique are simplicity and speed of operation; the tubes do not have to be filled with a predetermined volume of blood since readings can be performed on a sliding scale read out; centrifugation at 11 000 r.p.m. for five minutes usually suffices.

THE DONOR

Little use is at present made, in the U.K., of autologous blood, cadaver blood or the transfusion of autologous blood which has leaked into the peritoneal cavity, e.g. from a ruptured spleen.

An autologous transfusion is one in which the recipient has previously been the donor of the blood. It is thus formally equivalent to an *autogeneic* transplant. The method has been used to provide blood to replace that lost in elective surgical operations. The advantages of the method are that it avoids all risks of allotypic immune reactions and risks of transmitting infections such as serum hepatitis. The avoidance of allotypic immunization is, of course, particularly important in patients who are to receive tissue or organ transplants. The use of autologous transfusions could have a wider use than it has had hitherto. Milles and his colleagues (1971) described what they term a "leap-frog" technique of accumulating blood preoperatively. By restoring to the donor blood previously withdrawn, but immediately prior to this withdrawing a greater volume of blood, four units of blood which is less than two weeks old can be accumulated over the one-month period prior to operation. Sands and his colleagues (1968) have emphasized the value of autologous blood transfusions as a practical means for the replacement of blood loss in head and neck surgery. They also point out that an autogeneic

---

* An organic calcium chelator which removes the calcium ions which are essential for blood clotting. Chemically it is ethylenediaminetetra-acetic acid; sometimes abbreviated to EDTA.

transfusion is more economical than the conventional allo-geneic one, coming to only one-fifth of the cost of the latter. However, they advocate the need for supplemental iron medication with this type of transfusion.

The use of blood for transfusion from other human beings or from cadavers is formally equivalent to using *allogeneic* transplants.

The use of *cadaver blood* is not uncommon in the U.S.S.R. In such cases, the donors are individuals who have had a sudden cardiac arrest, e.g. due to electrical shock or myocardial infarction (Tarasov, 1960).

The British nationwide blood transfusion service provides a readily available source of human blood from *"normal"* subjects. This means that, in the main, donor blood has been carefully screened not only in respect of the safety of the recipient, but also of the donor. The criteria adopted in the selection of donors is that they should have normal haemoglobin levels, i.e. in excess of 8·4 mmol. 1^{-1} (13·5 gm per cent) for males and 7·8 mmol. 1^{-1} (12·5 gm per cent) for females, be free from hypertension, not pregnant, without isoantibodies following pregnancy or transfusion, and without a history of brucellosis, malaria, malignancy, serum hepatitis, sickle cell trait or syphilis. Donors are also excluded who harbour the hepatitis B (Australia) antigen, suffer from allergies or have had recent vaccinations or infections. The upper age limit for donors is sixty-five years. The author has noted a case of leukaemia in donor blood; even though the haemoglobin was normal, this became obvious macroscopically as a thick buffy coat after the stored blood had been allowed to settle. Donors are not bled more than twice yearly. This allows adequate time for renewal in women who lose about 50 ml of blood each month in menstruation. Apart from this temporary drop in haemoglobin concentration, the effect of the loss of one unit (equivalent to 180 ml erythrocytes) of blood on the donor is a diminution of tissue iron and an increase in the reticulocyte count. Donors are often advised to take ferrous sulfate for a period of one week following blood letting, this being the minimum time for the original haemoglobin level to be retained. Tetany is an occasional adverse effect of blood letting. This is due to alkalosis following emotional hyperventilation. Relief is afforded by breathing 5 per cent CO_2 or by breathing expelled air into a paper bag.

USE OF BLOOD

The sources of blood for transfusion are dependent upon the voluntary donor whose services, along with those of the transfusion collection service, are too valuable to be wasted. There are comparatively few otolaryngological disorders which call for an urgent, unforeseen, blood transfusion which cannot be postponed by the use of plasma or plasma substitutes until crossmatched blood is made available. The value of screening patients, e.g. by the mean corpuscular haemoglobin concentration (MCHC), blood film examination, ABO and Rh group determination and comprehensive erythrocyte antibody screen, at an early stage should never be underestimated. The practice of crossmatching and holding blood in reserve when its use

is not absolutely certain is wasteful; this wastage may amount to 30 per cent of stocks. The more recent practice of screening the patient's blood for antibodies and crossmatching only when the need is certain can drastically cut such losses without detrimental effects. Moreover, the efficient interchange of stocks of blood between hospital blood banks can effectively result in the use of more recent blood.

The actual rate of use of crossmatched transfusion blood is, however, often comparatively low because some units are crossmatched many times owing to excessive and unnecessary requests. Fortunately, many transfusion centres are able to prepare valuable fractions from expired plasma or fresh donations of blood and these will still be of value for general hospital use. Such units are usually labelled by blood transfusion centres for laboratory information. Thus packed cells may contain plasma replacement after cryoprecipitation (i.e. minus factors VIII and I) or may be platelet or leucocyte "free" when the latter have been removed for other use.

The *cost involvement* of transfusion blood (U.K.) from voluntary unpaid donors is now in excess of £30 per unit. Wastage must, therefore, be kept to a minimum by means of careful storage and using each unit as fresh as possible. Most laboratories naturally prefer to carry sufficient stock to cover any foreseen demand in addition to a small surplus for emergencies; unfortunately, small laboratories experience difficulty in using all their stock before expiry dates are reached unless frequent (weekly) exchange for fresher units can be arranged with larger hospital laboratories within their immediate vicinity.

Blood Fractions

With the aid of a separating machine, any blood layer can be removed by centrifugation and the remainder returned to the donor as thought necessary. Thus, various concentrates may be prepared in a concentrated and often stable form to be stored at temperatures which are too low for the preservation of whole blood.

Plasmapheresis is a useful technique for a transfusion centre to obtain large volumes of plasma. Plasma amounting to about one-half of the total blood volume removed may be obtained by centrifugation; erythrocytes are returned to the donor's circulation either following a saline drip or during a second visit when a further donation can be arranged. Where multiple donors are bled, stringent measures must be enforced to ensure that only their own erythrocytes are returned to them.

Erythrocytes

Transfused blood is destroyed within the patient's circulation at the rate of about 1 per cent each day. Agglutination and radioactive sodium chromate labelling techniques have confirmed that the normal life span of an erythrocyte is between 100 and 120 days (Berlin *et al.*, 1959). Destruction is, however, more rapid in conditions such as autoimmune haemolytic anaemia and in anaemia associated with the presence of cold agglutinins in pernicious anaemia and in rheumatoid arthritis. Other conditions where losses occur include chronic haemorrhage, fever, splenomegaly and even excessive venous sampling. Blood more than four weeks old should not be transfused because the life span of the erythrocytes will have become too short to make the transfusion worthwhile.

Concentrated erythrocytes (*packed red cells*) are valuable in conditions where blood volume should be minimized; they were first used extensively during the Second World War when vast quantities of plasma were under preparation and this fraction could then be provided. Units of whole blood are allowed to stand and sediment before plasma is drawn off or centrifuged. In view of the risk of infection by contaminating airborne bacteria, packed cells prepared from blood in glass bottles should be used immediately following their preparation. The introduction of the plastic bag as a transfusion blood container has eliminated this risk; plasma may be extruded through a tubing vent by applying gentle pressure to the outside of the sedimented bag. In addition, such containers have no dead space and present less risk of embolism occurring during transfusion.

Concentrated erythrocyte transfusions are of value where blood volume increase should be minimized. Thus otolaryngologists will find them useful in raising haemoglobin levels either prior to surgery in cases of chronic iron deficiency or in the transfusion of elderly patients with severe epistaxis.

The storage temperature should be as low as possible without actual freezing, i.e. 277–279 K (4–6°C). Should freezing occur, lysis and deterioration will be very rapid when the temperature is again raised. Depending upon the individual donor, probably only 75 per cent of the erythrocytes will survive the twenty-four hour period following transfusion if the blood has been stored for more than four weeks. The changes in electrolytes, rapid in the case of sodium but slow in the case of potassium, are reversible *in vivo* in the majority of surviving erythrocytes. Organic phosphate changes occur and oxygen capacity is lowered by the end of the first week.

Washed erythrocytes are prepared by centrifugation. This product may only be considered stable for a few hours after preparation; no antibodies are present.

Platelets

Studies using platelets labelled with chromium 51 radionuclide have shown that, within ten minutes of transfusion, only 65 per cent of the initially injected platelets are present in the circulation (Kotilainen, 1969). The percentage surviving, then falls off linearly by about 8 per cent per day, but with the final 5–10 per cent disappearing very slowly from the bloodstream. This tail extends to about 10–14 days and has been attributed to the presence of a type of platelet which is distinct from the shorter-lived, but more prevalent, variety (Aster and Jandl, 1964a).

The initial disappearance of platelets following transfusion is due to their being taken up by the spleen. Consequently, more platelets (about 90 per cent) are initially found to be present in the circulation of splenectomized patients, and less (of the order of 20 per cent) in patients with splenomegaly (Harker and Finch, 1969). A similar

smaller value is found in patients with idiopathic thrombocytopenic purpura.

In blood stored in the usual acid citrate dextrose solution at 277 K (4°C), there is a poor survival rate of platelets amounting to less than one-fifth after four days. This survival rate is improved by storage at room temperature, but the hazard of infection makes it unwise to use such blood.

Platelet rich plasma and *plasma concentrates* are prepared by centrifuging normal acid citrate dextrose platelet-rich plasma; additional acid citrate dextrose is added to bring the pH to 6·5 to ensure that the platelets do not aggregate. The concentrate is then stored at room temperature (storage is not improved at low temperatures). This fraction is used in platelet deficiency states, e.g. thrombocytopenia, epistaxis and haemorrhage associated with leukaemias. Repeat transfusions may, however, produce antibodies against platelet antigens unless the immune response has been impaired, e.g. by cytotoxic therapy. The maintenance of the platelet level is thrombocytopenia caused by drugs or irradiation is, however, difficult even with frequent transfusions; four units increase the adult count by about 70 000 mm^{-3}. This count is reduced to a half within a few days. The use of sibling donors may be the solution if the production of platelet antibodies is marked.

IgA and IgE immunoglobulins may cause pyrexial reactions in platelet rich plasma transfusions.

Other Fractions

Freeze-dried whole plasma is prepared from small pools of expired plasma from hepatitis antigen B-screened blood and is ABO antigen free. It does not contain factors VIII or V. It is a useful volume expander and a source of Factor I (fibrinogen) if reconstituted to triple strength.

The so-called *protein fraction* is mainly an albumin concentrate with a low globulin content; it is not isotonic. The total protein concentration is about 6 per cent. It is the preferred substitute for whole plasma (heat treatment lessens the risk of serum hepatitis by making this fraction Australia antigen free). It is used as an alternative to freeze-dried plasma.

Fibrinogen (freeze dried) is fractionated from freeze-dried plasma then freeze dried and reconstituted for use. It is used in hereditary afibrinogenaemia on its own and in conjunction with heparin in disseminated intravascular coagulation.

Albumin (freeze dried) is prepared as for the fibrinogen component. Salt poor albumin (SPA) in liquid form possesses low concentrations of sodium and potassium. These products are used in exchange transfusion in haemolytic disease of the newborn and in hypo-albuminaemia.

Immunoglobulins. This fraction is prepared by fractionation and used in the prophylaxis of viral and bacterial disease, suppression of Rh immunization and in the treatment of hypogamma-globulinaemia.

Cryofibrinogen precipitate is a source of factors I and VIII. It is prepared by snap freezing fresh plasma. After thawing at 293 K (20°C) the residual plasma is returned to the erythrocytes in the donation, the cryofibrinogen precipitate remaining is stored at 243 K (−30°C) for three months and thawed at 310 K (37°C) immediately before use. It is used in haemophilia.

Factor IX. Fresh frozen plasma (FFP) and Factor IX concentrate are used in the treatment of Christmas disease; FFP can be used for any coagulation protein deficiency.

Factors II, VII, IX and X. This fraction is prepared from acid citrate dextrose plasma and can be used whenever these factors are deficient.

Leukapheresis: This is a specialized production prepared by a mechanical centrifugal IBM separator. Using this apparatus, a large number of leucocytes may be prepared from a donor's blood (Judson *et al.*, 1968). The preparation is stable for a few hours only. It has been used in the treatment of gram-negative bacterial septicaemia in patients with acute leukaemia (Graw *et al.*, 1971).

Grouping sera are prepared from selected donors. Special procedures are used to make them specific. They are stable when stored at 253 K (−20°C). They are used in laboratory blood-grouping tests.

Plasma Substitutes

The beneficial effect of transfusion in the treatment of haemorrhage is primarily attributable to the sustained increase in blood volume that it produces. In this respect it is not therefore necessary to use blood for this purpose. The effect can just as well be achieved by using a fluid containing colloids with an osmotic pressure similar to that of plasma proteins (Bayliss, 1919).

The principal criteria for plasma substitutes are that they should: (1) be non-toxic, (2) not induce sensitization, (3) not be stored in the body for appreciable periods of time, and (4) not leave the circulation rapidly after infusion.

The two principal plasma substitutes in use are *dextran* and *povidone*.

Dextran is a polysaccharide formed by *Leuconostoc mesenteroides*, a species of bacteria belonging to the Lactobacillaceae. The dextran molecule consists of long chains of glucose units with a variable degree of branching. It is possible to make dextran compounds of a particular molecular weight by hydrolosis and subsequent fractionation. Preparations of dextran should have molecules with a molecular weight of about 70 000 since molecules with a molecular weight of less than this are rapidly excreted (Arturson and Wallenius, 1964), and those of a higher molecular weight promote rouleaux formation* *in vitro* and blood sludging *in vivo* (Thorsen and Hint, 1950). Rouleaux formation may be troublesome during subsequent laboratory crossmatching. Although the beneficial effects of the use of dextran are as good as those of plasma in the treatment of burns (Bull and Jackson, 1955), the use of dextran alone implies a failure to replace various plasma constituents such as coagulation factors. The infusion of dextran may therefore be associated with prolonged bleeding times. These prolonged bleeding times are not due solely to the failure to provide coagulation factors but also to the positive effect of interfering with platelet activity (Langdell *et al.*, 1958). Fortunately, clinical evidence of haemorrhagic

effects is infrequent in patients receiving dextran. Nevertheless, it is advisable to limit the amount of dextran given to any one patient to one litre.

Dextran may be purposely employed for its effect on blood coagulation. A randomized double-blind trial has shown that dextran 70, administered by intravenous drip during operation, significantly reduces the incidence of pulmonary embolism and mortality from this cause (Kline *et al.*, 1975).

Povidone is polyvinyl pyrrolidone. It is used as a plasma substitute much more extensively on the European continent than in Britain or in the U.S.A. A reluctance to use it stems from its not being metabolized by the body.

SELECTION OF BLOOD FOR TRANSFUSION

Introduction

Blood-grouping and crossmatching are a prerequisite to blood transfusion, which can be considered as an allotransplant of a particular fluid tissue.

Until a few decades ago, blood-grouping and crossmatching necessitated a fairly simple knowledge of the ABO and the Rh (rhesus) blood-group systems. Although a more thorough understanding of these systems, and some of the other 227 at present known to exist, has become necessary, errors still take place when procedures are overcomplicated or not properly understood. The intention, here, is primarily to present the methods for detecting offending substances and, at the same time, to draw attention to errors in technique. The ABO and rhesus bloodgroup systems are the ones of prime importance in blood transfusion; other systems are of secondary importance only.

At the present time, the selection of blood suitable for transfusion depends mainly on ascertaining the presence of certain antigens in the erythrocytes; these are genetically determined. However, platelets, immunoglobulins, soluble serum groups and other soluble blood group factors will doubtlessly prove to be very important in the future.

The A and B antigens attain their maximum effectiveness during puberty, whereas corresponding antibodies form during the first six months of life. Both erythrocyte antigen and serum antibody levels vary with age and between individuals.

Blood grouping sera are specially selected and standardized before use. Anti-A and anti-B sera are obtained from natural donors and anti-Rh sera is produced by natural immunization during pregnancy. The production of anti-Rh sera will eventually prove difficult unless artificial immunization is carried out.

Since it is necessary to remove unwanted antibodies from grouping sera and also to add additional substances, the production of these sera has become such a specialized procedure that it is customary to prepare these reagents in centralized laboratories. However, the careful testing of sera to ensure that they can detect weak subgroups must remain a routine procedure in any laboratory which undertakes blood transfusion work. Likewise, the patient's

---

* The tendency of erythrocytes to adhere to one another by their rims to form loose piles, which effect is due to differences in charges on cell surfaces.

serum must be tested against erythrocytes of known anti-genicity as a control for the erythrocyte grouping. The extent to which blood grouping can be undertaken will depend largely on the facilities available in the laboratory

TABLE 1

1900–10	Landsteiner groups (Decastello and Sturli; accepted for international nomenclature)	Jansky: AB, A, B, O → 4, 2, 3, 1	Moss: 1, 2, 3, 4
1911	Dungern and Hirszfeld	Subgroups of A (A₁ and A₂).	
1924	Bernstein	Inheritance of ABO system established as Mendelian in character, i.e. genotypes extended to AA, AO, etc.	
1927	Landsteiner and Levine	MN and P systems.	
1940–1	Landsteiner and Wiener	Rhesus (Rh) system.	
1946	Coombs, Mourant and Race	Kell (K) system (named after a patient).	
1946	Callender and Race	Lutheran (Lu) system.	
1946	Mourant et al.	Lewis (Le) system (named after a donor).	
1950	Cutbush, Mollison and Parkin	Duffy (Fy) system (named after a patient).	
1951	Allen, Diamond and Niedziela	Kidd (Jk) system (named after a patient).	
1950–70	Various authors described rare antigens often belonging to one family only.		
1956	Wiener et al.	"Cold" type of auto-immune haemolytic anaemia antibodies.	
1974	Two hundred and twenty-seven blood group systems identified. Further systems and platelet antigens being dealt with.		

and some cases may, depending upon the complexity of the problem, require further investigations to be undertaken elsewhere.

Blood group serologists must be given sufficient time and all pertinent clinical information. We are now passing into an era where O-negative blood is no longer considered to be that from a universal donor. Blood transfusion may be regarded as a transplant technique which we are only just beginning to understand.

Blood Group Systems

A brief historical summary is helpful in appreciating the relative importance of the various blood groups (see Table 1).

The earlier confusion in terminology (AB or Jansky group 4 or Moss group 1) was resolved by adopting Landsteiner's terminology. The names of later systems, e.g. Duffy, are those belonging to the patient and the system is denoted by a capital and small letter, e.g. Fy, and genes extended as Fy^a, Fy^b, etc. The Rh system is a notable exception. Here, three sets of alleles (alternative genes at one locus on a chromosome) occur. The principal blood group systems are shown in Table 2.

The ABO Blood Group System

Each parent donates one gene, either A, B or O, to their child which results in six possible genotypes AA, AO, BB, BO, AB and OO. The corresponding phenotypes, i.e. blood groups A, B, AB and O, may be determined with the use of anti-A serum (from a group B donor) and anti-B serum (from a group A donor). A drop of each of these sera is mixed with the unknown erythrocytes on a white tile at

TABLE 2
BLOOD GROUP SYSTEMS

(Numbered links) comprising:

System				Antibodies
ABO	(1) A₁ or A₂ or B or O / A₁ or A₂ or B or O			Naturally acquired or formed from immune response
Lewis	(1) L or 1 / L or 1	(2) Se or se / Se or se		
Lutheran	(1) Luᵃ or Luᵇ / Luᵃ or Luᵇ			From immune response
Rhesus	(1) C CᵂCˣ or c / C CᵂCˣ or c	(2) D or d / D or d	(3) E Eᵂ or e / E Eᵂ or e	
P	(1) P₁ or P₂ or p / P₁ or P₂ or p			
Kidd	(1) Jkᵃ or Jkᵇ or Jk / Jkᵃ or Jkᵇ or Jk			
Duffy	(1) Fyᵃ or Fyᵇ or Fy / Fyᵃ or Fyᵇ or Fy			
Kell	(1) K or K / K or k	(2) Kpᵃ or Kpᵇ / Kpᵃ or Kpᵇ		

Small laboratories are primarily concerned with ABO and rhesus systems but, when an antibody occurs, any of the many systems may be involved.

room temperature. The presence or absence of agglutination is observed after a few minutes gentle rocking of the samples. Genotypes AO and AA (phenotype A) are indistinguishable, as are genotypes BO and BB (phenotype B). The most common group resulting from this test in Britain is group O (46 per cent of the population); here no agglutination is seen. Agglutination with anti-A sera indicates group A (42 per cent); agglutination with anti-B indicates group B (9 per cent) and agglutination with both sera indicates group AB (3 per cent). The relative frequencies of the various blood groups differs widely outside Britain. As a result of genetic drift and natural selection, there may also be different distributions within a country.

The Rhesus System

The rhesus antigen system takes this name since the antigens are also present in the erythrocytes of the *Rhesus* monkey (Landsteiner and Wiener, 1940, 1941). According to Fisher's (1943) theory of rhesus interactions, a child receives one chromosome carrying three genes, which govern these antigens, from each parent; these genes are designated C, D or E (when dominant); with c, d and e (recessive) as alternatives (alleles) at the same loci. Second in importance only to the A and B antigens, they vary considerably in potency in the following order: D, C, c, E, e, whilst d has not been demonstrated as an antigen capable of producing a response. The Rh-positive fetus (D antigen present) may produce an immune response in a Rh-negative (D antigen absent) mother. The Rh-negative child will almost certainly form antibodies following transfusion with Rh-positive blood at any time during life. Certain hazards are therefore apparent and, although Rh immunization can be suppressed in the puerperium by passively administered antibody in the form of anti-D immunoglobulin (IgG), the transfusion of Rh-positive blood to a Rh-negative recipient must be avoided in spite of apparent compatability *in vitro*.

The primary immune response mechanisms are normally activated in about three weeks following immunization whilst the secondary response occurs in a shorter time (usually one week after the further stimulation).

The smaller laboratory dealing with routine blood group requests, with subsequent blood transfusion in mind, is primarily concerned with the D antigen. Standard techniques give good agglutination with either the heterozygote Dd or the homozygote DD form, whilst giving an even stronger reaction in the presence of E antigen, e.g. cDE.

A weak variant, "D^u *antigen*" (Stratton, 1946; Stratton and Renton, 1948; Race *et al.*, 1948), may react only with *incomplete** IgG. Incomplete anti-D is the commonest available form of this type of antiserum for routine grouping purposes. Procedures using such incomplete serum entail a fairly lengthy technique needing incubation and the provision of albumen or the use of the antiglobulin test before the cells will agglutinate. Improved antisera are currently available which are carefully selected to detect weak or low-grade D antigen strength; because of their

importance in donor selection and serological investigation, these are held by transfusion centres. Similarly, rarer typing sera for low-frequency antigens or weak expressions of antigen are also held by these centres Weak D variants are not always detected using complete I$_g$M (saline) anti-D. However, this antigen can absorb antibody and can subsequently produce a positive *indirect antiglobulin test**. The importance of the D^u antigen in blood transfusion is that donors possessing this antigen might incorrectly be designated as Rh negative; these donors would, nevertheless, stimulate antibodies in Rhesus-negative recipients

Blood Grouping

The use of so-called rapid sera allows for the *patient's provisional* blood group to be determined and a crossmatch to be started whilst confirmation of the patient's blood group using a tube technique can be run in parallel; this saves considerable time. In view of the fact that most transfusion discrepancies occur during the collection and labelling of samples, it is common practice to check the patient's group using a slide technique for confirmation of a previously-determined group. Antibodies to transfused blood may form within the space of a few days so that fresh serum should be obtained if requests are made for a repeat transfusion.

Grouping can be carried out on erythrocyte samples from clotted blood or blood which contains anticoagulant. The erythrocytes are normally washed in saline prior to grouping. Some agglutinogens, e.g. P, M, N, Lewis, are thermolabile. Erythrocytes are destroyed by freezing so that suspensions of them are stored at 277 K (4°C) to 279 K (6°C) and preferably tested not later than the day following collection. Serum to be used for crossmatch purposes is stored at deep-freeze temperatures in order that complement and unstable antibodies may be preserved.

Antibody Screen

In addition to considering the ABO and Rh (D) groupings, the patient's serum should be tested against a panel of erythrocytes containing known antigens. By such means the presence of an antibody against A, A$_1$, A$_2$, B; C, C^w, D, E, c, e; M, N, S, s; P$_1$; Le^a, Le^b; Lu^a, Lu^b; K, k, Kp^a, Kp^b; Js^a; Fy^a, Fy^b, Jk^a, Jk^b; Do^a; Xg^a; Co^a, Co^b; Sd^a; Vel; besides others, can be identified

The erythrocyte suspensions given below are an example of antigen combinations that might be used. This test is normally carried out using saline (room temperature), albumin with incubation at 310 K (37°C) and Coombs' method against two standard erythrocyte suspensions composed of mixed group O donors DCe or DcE who also possess the following antigens:

(1) DCe; c, e, f, k, Fy^a, Fy^b, Jk^a, Le^a, S, M, P, Lu^b, Xg^a;
(2) DcE; K, k, Fy^a, Jk^b, Le^b, S, s, M, N, P, Lu^b.

From the missing antigens, e.g. E, K, C^w, V, Jk^b, Le^b, s, N, Lu^a in cells of suspension (1) and C, C^w, V, Fy^b, Jk^a,

---

* When suspended in saline, an *incomplete antibody* will sensitize erythrocytes possessing the corresponding antigen, but will fail to agglutinate them.

* The production of agglutination by adding an anti-immunoglobulin serum (Coombs' reagent) to erythrocyte which have been sensitized by an incomplete antibody.

Le[a], Lu[a] and Xg[a], in suspension (2), the field can be narrowed and, with the aid of further, similar, suspensions, individual antigens can be recognized.

The purpose of the three methods (in saline, in albumin suspension or with anti-human globulin serum) helps to identify the type of antigen present:

Low temperature, 290 K (17°C), methods detect strong Rh and cold antibodies (anti Le[a], Le[b], M, P).

Incubation methods at 310 K (37°C) detect the weaker Rh antibodies.

Coombs' technique detects Kell, Duffy and Kidd antibodies.

A stronger reaction to the presence of an antibody in the patient's serum can be expected if the donor has a double dose of certain antigens, i.e. D, c, E, Fy[a], K, Jk[a], Le[a] and M.

The above examples are intended only as a general guide; some antigens may present themselves entirely outside this context, e.g. an anti-Kell antibody may react in saline and lead to the discovery of a new grouping system.

Besides the considerations given to antibodies which can affect erythrocytes, *other antibodies* exist with regard to leucocytes, platelets, proteins and serum allotypes. Usually, the clinical symptoms are manifest as rigor and pyrexia alone. The selection of suitable transfusion blood in these instances may require the services of a national panel and considerable delay in the "routine" pathology service must result.

HAEMOLYTIC DISEASE OF THE FETUS AND THE NEWBORN

This disorder is due to maternal antibody attacking the fetal and neonatal erythrocytes (Levine and Stetson, 1939; Levine *et al.*, 1941). In these cases of blood group incompatibility, e.g. a D-positive fetus with a D-negative mother, the fetal erythrocytes immunize the mother. The specific antibodies, e.g. anti-D, so produced, pass across the placental barrier into the fetal circulation. Haemolytic disease of the fetus and the newborn is of particular importance to the otolaryngologist since it may result in defects of hearing (Crabtree and Gerrard, 1950). In 95 per cent of cases, the antibody causing the disease is anti-D. In the remaining cases, the antibodies are usually either other Rh system antibodies or ABO antibodies (Halbrecht, 1944). If the haemolytic process is marked, then the neonate will exhibit severe jaundice (*icterus gravis neonatorum*). The jaundice is a result not only of the increased bilirubin production consequent on the haemoglobin breakdown but also of the inability of the newborn's liver to excrete bilirubin at a rate which is much more than about 1 per cent of the normal adult liver (Billing *et al.*, 1954). High plasma bilirubin concentrations (>200 mg. l^{-1}) produce staining and damage to the brain nuclei (Claireaux *et al.*, 1953). The latter condition is termed *kernicterus*. This is invariably a result of Rh group incompatibility but a case due to ABO group incompatibility has been recorded (Grumbach and Gasser, 1948). Data presented by Mollison and Cutbush (1954) indicate that the incidence of kernicterus increases linearly with an increase of plasma bilirubin concentration greater than 200 mg. l^{-1}. The increase is rapid so that a 100 per cent incidence would be expected from a plasma bilirubin concentration greater than 400 mg. l^{-1}. A high-frequency *hearing loss* may appear to be the only residual neurological deficit in kernicterus until the child is observed to be late in beginning to walk (Armitage and Mollison, 1953). Congenital sensorineural hearing losses observed with plasma bilirubin concentrations of <200 mg. l^{-1} may have been the result of the administration of high doses of menadiol sodium phosphate (Fisch and Norman, 1961).

In cases of haemolytic disease of the newborn, kernicterus can be almost entirely prevented by *exchange transfusion* within a few hours of birth. In the case of an Rh group incompatibility, the infant's Rh-positive erythrocytes are removed and replaced by Rh-negative erythrocytes (Allen *et al.*, 1950; Mollison and Walker, 1952). Finn (1960) pointed out that haemolytic disease of the fetus and newborn could be prevented by ensuring that an Rh-negative woman does not produce Rh antibodies. Subsequently, if any fetal erythrocytes are seen in the maternal circulation, the mother is now given *concentrated purified IgG anti-D* antibodies (Woodrow *et al.*, 1965; Clarke, 1968). The prevention of this antibody response is not antigen specific; the immunosuppressive mechanism involves the whole erythrocyte, probably through destruction within splenic macrophages (Woodrow *et al.*, 1975).

APPENDIX

Even very urgent calls for blood transfusion can usually be postponed by the provision of plasma or plasma substitutes, e.g. dextran, until grouping and some degree of crossmatching has been carried out. Where such services are not available, i.e. hospitals without a staffed laboratory in the immediate vicinity, group O Rhesus-negative blood may be stored and utilized. It is, however, most important that a blood sample for any subsequent laboratory investigation be taken prior to any such transfusion. Such samples are also invaluable if adverse reactions are found.

In any individual situation the clinician should know the minimum time required for blood to be crossmatched (Table 3). This is dependent upon transport, laboratory technique (including staffing arrangements) and donor availability. The approximate time-scale suggested here is independent of any such local variations which often account for most of the delay involved. Normally, blood will take about fifteen minutes to clot *in vitro* (glasstube) at body temperature and longer at room temperature. A sequestrenated, i.e. treated with trisodium edetate, or citrated sample (thrombin is anticomplementary) is therefore a useful addition to be used for grouping purposes where the matter is urgent.

Although group O Rh-negative blood would probably prove to be compatible where the group is unknown, antibody dangers increase with the amount administered and may severely restrict donor choice for subsequent transfusion. Where the ABO group is definitely known and a crossmatch cannot be done, uncrossmatched blood of the

TABLE 3

Time (min) After Receipt of Specimen in Laboratory	Clinician	Laboratory
0	Direct responsibility for transfusing plasma. Group O Rh negative blood to patient with unknown group where hospital does not have Laboratory Service to hand.	Specimen received; only uncrossmatched blood available.
5		Donor and patient's group checked as compatible
10	Useful advice from laboratory with regard to probable donor blood availability.	Crossmatch procedure starts.
45	Probable compatibility known.	(Coombs' washing.) Emergency testing: Group checked. Emergency testing: Crossmatch checked.
90–120	Decisive advice from laboratory as to compatibility.	Group and crossmatch fully checked after normal incubation time.

same ABO group should be given, and in the form of packed erythrocytes.

Let us consider an example where the patient's group is known to be group B Rh-negative with limited stocks of blood available and no crossmatching possible before transfusion. The choice of blood can only be group O Rh-negative or group B Rh-negative, followed by group B Rh-positive and group O Rh-positive as the stocks become exhausted.

The use of D-positive blood is an extreme measure in the case of a female patient of childbearing age. Any evidence for haemolytic disease of the newborn or a history of a previous transfusion (in either sex) would prohibit the use of the D-positive blood. It is, however, safe to give Rh-positive blood to Rh-negative elderly males who have no previous history of transfusion, especially when Rh-negative blood is in short supply.

Plasma protein fractions (PPF) are often employed in an emergency to treat any blood loss until compatible blood can be obtained.

It is essential for all branches of a hospital complex, i.e. clinicians, nursing staff, administration, transport, porters, pathologists and technologists, to be familiar with any aspect of blood transfusion which might at any given time become their concern. Not infrequently, the only contact between the clinician and the pathologist is the request form, yet hundreds of units of blood are expected to change hands without adverse reactions. Blood transfusion incompatibility is a far more likely occurrence through a fault

in comprehension rather than in laboratory technique. Unambiguous instructions by way of a request and subsequent report together with a carefully labelled specimen from the correct patient identified by a wrist band excludes many potential errors. All records of transfusion therapy must be included in the patient's notes and the following suggestions are intended as a helpful guide.

Specimen label: Patient's full name, Registered number, Ward, Date.

Request and report may be combined as a three-leaf no-carbon-required (NCR) form. One part is retained by the clinician and the second and third parts are sent to the laboratory. The second part is returned with completed report to the clinician and the third part is retained by the laboratory for record purposes. NCR duplicate or triplicate forms save a great deal of duplication as long as writing is legible using a ball-point pen. The labels used for labelling the donor's blood may be printed on adhesive paper coloured to match the colour code of various groups used by the transfusion centre; such additional aid can help in simple identification of the correct ABO and Rh group during primary identification, i.e. selecting units from a blood bank (see Table 4).

Grouping

Table 5 indicates a schema for routine ABO and Rh grouping. Agglutination is denoted by a plus sign and no agglutination by a negative sign. Items and results underlined are associated with the simple slide grouping technique. A complete test pattern may then be set up using a tube technique and left in parallel with the crossmatch—thus enabling both to be read concurrently. The four Roman numerals in the schema indicate some explanatory notes, viz.

(i) Optimal temperature for ABO testing is 278 K (5°C) but the test is carried out at 290 K (17°C) in order to avoid the action of cold agglutinins present in normal serum.

(ii) Test carried out at the optimum temperature of 310 K (37°C).

(iii) Both the presence of autoagglutinin (anti-I) and the occurrence of Rouleaux formation should be noted as they could mask the presence of antibodies other than anti-I. Rouleaux formation should disperse after the addition of an equal volume of saline.

(iv) These serum antibodies may not be present during infancy or in old age or in leukaemia or in agammaglobulinaemia.

Twenty per cent of group A subjects belong to a weaker subgroup, i.e. A_2; this can be ascertained by the use of specialized sera but it is not clinically significant.

Crossmatching

When deciding which techniques should be employed for routine *crossmatch* purposes, simplicity is a vital factor both in order to limit the time and to avoid possible confusion using multiple techniques. It is essential to carry out a *major crossmatch* to seek the presence of antibodies

TABLE 4
REQUEST FOR BLOOD TRANSFUSION AND/OR GROUPING

PATIENT'S SURNAME: FIRST NAMES:
SEX: DATE OF BIRTH: WARD: HOSP. REG. NO.:
BLOOD REQUESTED BY: TIME AND DATE DESPATCHED TO LAB:
☐: 10 ml CLOTTED BLOOD   (☐: ALSO EDETIC ACID SPECIMEN)
PATIENT IDENTIFIED AND BLOOD TAKEN BY:
CLINICAL DIAGNOSIS AND REASON FOR TRANSFUSION:

PATIENT'S ABO GROUP: RHESUS (D):
PREVIOUS TRANSFUSIONS: REACTIONS:
PREGNANCIES: HAEM. DISEASE NEWBORN: ERYTHROBLASTOSIS:
URGENCY: ☐—WITHOUT CROSSMATCH*; ☐—URGENT* (TELEPHONE DEPARTMENT)
☐: HOLD IN RESERVE FOR DATE: TIME:
NO. UNITS REQUIRED: ☐—UNITS WHOLE BLOOD; ☐—UNITS PACKED CELLS
☐: GROUP ONLY (SERUM WILL BE KEPT FOR 5 DAYS;
☐: DIRECT ANTIGLOBULIN (COOMBS') TEST

REPORT   (TO BE COMPLETED BY THE LABORATORY)
DATE AND TIME OF ARRIVAL: ☐: LABELLED CLOTTED SPEC
PATIENT IDENTIFIED AND BLOOD TAKEN BY: ☐: ALSO EDETIC ACID
DATE AND TIME OF REPORT: COMPATIBILITY TESTED BY:
PATIENT'S ABO GROUP: RHESUS:
NUMBER OF UNITS: ☐—AVAILABLE IN BLOOD BANK; ☐—SUPPLIED TO WARD

DONOR'S GROUP	UNIT REF. NO.	EXPIRY DATE	

LABEL FOR DONOR'S BLOOD (two part)

First part attached to Unit of blood.

ABO GROUP:	ABO GROUP:
RHESUS:	RHESUS:
	EXPIRES:
NAME:	NAME:
REG. NO.:	REG. NO.:
XM DATE:	XM DATE:
PATIENT'S SERUM DATE:	

Second part attached to Report by means of adhesive strip. Returned to Lab. in exchange for Units as and when required.

in the patient's serum which will react unfavourably with the donor's erythrocytes. Due consideration must be given as to the most favourable medium, i.e. saline or albumin, and as to whether direct agglutination or indirect agglutination (Coombs' test) is likely at varying optimal temperatures. Likewise, by means of a *minor crossmatch* and adequate donor grouping, the presence of antibodies in the donor's serum should be ascertained even though subsequent dilution within the patient's system may reduce their importance to that of a minor role.

Although agglutination is generally satisfactory at 310 K (37°C), the *optimal temperature* for different antibodies varies widely. In order to avoid non-specific agglutination (many healthy sera will agglutinate erythrocytes at 278 K), temperatures below 293 K (20°C) should be avoided:

$$< 303 \text{ K } (30°\text{C}) \text{ ABO}$$
$$> 308 \text{ K } (35°\text{C}) \text{ DEc K Fy}^a \text{ JK}^a \text{ S}$$

Le^a Le^b are temperature-independent).

Major Crossmatch

In order to detect antibodies present in the patient's serum where the corresponding antigen exists in the donor's erythrocytes, it is essential to include saline, albumin and indirect antiglobulin (Coombs') tests as separate techniques, e.g.

Saline* AB, P, M	Albumin† Rh	Indirect Antiglobulin Test K, Fy^a, Jk^a, S
A$_1$, Le^a, Le^b, I-H (K), (Rh), (S)	Le^a, Le^b, P, A, Ab, I-H (K)	Rh, Le, Le^{ba} (P$_1$), (M), (I-H)

Key: *Prevalent*, Likely, (Sometimes).
* For antibodies principally in IgM fraction.
† For antibodies principally in IgG fraction.

Minor Crossmatch (usually done by the Blood Transfusion Centre)

This procedure constitutes, together with donor screening, a search for antibodies within the donor's system. The minor crossmatch has limited application, i.e. it cannot be employed for any useful purpose where group O blood is transfused to A, B or AB recipients.

Donor Screening

Is designed to detect the presence of rare antibodies in the donor irrespective of the recipient. It has the additional advantage of illustrating incompatibility among multiple donors which would otherwise be inapparent from the major or minor crossmatch; these can detect immunization only in specified donor-patient relationships.

The Crossmatch Technique

Unlike antibodies in the IgM fraction, those in the IgG fraction possess insufficient molecular length for agglutination to occur in saline; a high protein medium such as 20 per cent bovine albumin is therefore necessary for their detection. Other antibodies, such as those of the Duffy and Kidd systems, can be detected only by the indirect anti-immunoglobulin test. Consequently, although individual laboratories vary, standard practice demands at least three basic conditions:

(a) A test at room temperature using a saline medium.
(b) A test at 310 K (37°C) using an albumin medium.
(c) An indirect anti-human globulin test.

A summary of the techniques involved during emergency and on routine occasions is illustrated:

(a) Saline Crossmatch. Room temperature and 310 K (37°C). Spin (or centrifuge) technique. Patient's serum (small volume, e.g. one drop) together with equal volume of donor's erythrocytes (N.B. Patient's serum must be fresh if transfusion has taken place previously. Donor's erythrocytes prepared as a 5 per cent suspension in saline after washing in saline by centrifugation.)

Emergency Crossmatch. Examine for agglutination after 15 min at room temperature following light centrifugation (e.g. 1000 r.p.m. for 1 min). For demonstrating: (i) direct incompatibility, e.g. ABO; (ii) cold agglutinins, anti-M, $-P_1$, $-A_1$.

Routine Crossmatch. As above, but with longer time (90 min) and no centrifugation. The test is carried out in duplicate at 290 K (17°C) and 310 K (37°C); check for agglutination.

(b) Albumin Crossmatch

Emergency Crossmatch. Equal volumes of the patient's serum and the donor's erythrocytes suspended in 20 per cent albumin are incubated at 310 K for 15 min. Examine for agglutination after light centrifugation.

TABLE 5

Serum	Unknown Erythrocytes — Possible resulting agglutination						Patient's Erythrocytes	Control Erythrocytes (Known Antigen)					
								A_1 cde/cde	A_2 cde/cde	B cde/cde	O cde/cde Kell +	O cde/cde Kell −	Rhesus + O CDe/cDE
	or	or	or	or	or								
(i) Anti-A	−	+	+	−	+	+		+	+	−	−		
Anti-A_1	−	+	−	−	+	−		+	−	−	−		
Anti-B	−	−	−	−	+	+		−	−	+	−		
Anti-A and B	−	+	+	+	+	+							
ABO group (phenotype)	O	A_1	A_2	B	A_1B	A_2B							
(ii) Anti-D *Rhesus*					+ Pos.	− Neg.						−	+
(iii) Patient's Serum / Autoagglutinin							+						

	Patient's Serum (iv) (Corresponding Agglutinins)	A_1	A_2	B	O	O
	O	+ and/or	+	+	−	
	A_1	−	−	+	−	
	A_2	+2%	−	+	−	
	B	+	+	−	−	
	A_1B	−	−	−	−	
	A_2B	+25%	−	−	−	

Possible genotypes   OO A_1A_1 A_2A_2 BB A_1B A_2B
A_1A_2 A_2O BO
A_1O

Routine Crossmatch. Patient's serum is incubated with an equal volume of donor's erythrocytes suspended in saline for 60 min. The supernatant fluid is replaced with 20 per cent albumin and read for agglutination after further incubation at 310 K for 30 min. If sufficient volumes are used, this part of the crossmatch may then be used for the indirect antiglobulin test.

(c) Indirect Antiglobulin Test (Coombs's Test). This test consists of adding antiglobulin serum to the donor's erythrocytes which have been washed three times in large volumes of saline following contact with the patient's serum under conditions where optimal sensitization takes place, i.e. those of the albumin crossmatch. Agglutination will denote the presence of a sensitizing antibody. The absence of agglutination will denote: (i) the absence of a sensitizing antibody; or (ii) inactive antiglobulin serum; or (iii) neutralization of the antiglobulin serum by residual (patient's) serum after inadequate washing. The inclusion of a separate carefully controlled sensitized erythrocyte suspension as a standard is necessary to exclude the last two possibilities.

Indirect antiglobulin test controls:

(i) Sensitized D-positive erythrocytes (i.e. using incomplete anti-D without albumin) are carried through with the test proper at 310 K; the addition of anti-human globulin produces agglutination.

(ii) Anti-human globulin to donor's cells, following triple saline wash.

(iii) Add anti-human globulin to donor's cells.

(iv) Add anti-human globulin to triple-washed donor's cells from the saline and albumin parts of the crossmatch proper after the examination for agglutination has proved negative; no agglutination should result.

The Incompatible Crossmatch

False reactions used to be common as a direct result of dust causing pseudoagglutination but with the advent of clean disposable plastic tubes such reactions are now rare. Rouleaux formation may usually be dispersed by adding equal volumes of saline to the test before reading. The action of cold agglutinins may be avoided by reading the test at 310 K (37°C).

An incompatible crossmatch requires a thorough investigation of the donor's antigens (*see previously*) and the patient's antibodies whether they be naturally occurring, such as anti-A_1 in a group A_2 patient who has been crossmatched with A_1 blood, or anti-P, -Le^a, -Le^b, or anti-Sd^a, or whether they be antibodies formed by an immune response, such as anti-D, -c, -E, -K, -Fy^a and -Jk^a; there is also the possibility of a false positive reaction. False negative reactions can usually be avoided if the laboratory is allowed adequate time to perform the necessary tests.

Incompatibility Reactions

In case a transfusion reaction should occur and need investigation, it is important for "used" blood containers to be returned unwashed to the laboratory and stored at 277 K (4°C). Such investigations are impossible without this simple precaution; all too often the hospital ward will (with the best of intentions) erroneously wash blood bottles or discard plastic containers. The serial number of any giving set involved should also be noted and reported to the appropriate laboratory.

The reactions caused by *incompatible transfusion* may not appear for 7–10 days. The clinical indications of incompatible transfusion are pyrexia, jaundice, burning sensations or back pains, apart from the more immediate signs of rigor or pyrexia. Both the donor's blood and the patient's blood must be investigated. A fresh sample and any previous specimen which the laboratory has filed should be collected from the patient and tested for antibodies. Group O blood which has been used during emergency in small amounts is unlikely to be the cause unless a one-in-four plasma dilution produces more than a trace of haemolysis with the patient's A_1 or B erythrocytes.

In incompatibility reactions, the laboratory should also test for haemoglobinaemia and mathaemalbuminaemia (Schumm's test), serum bilirubin (especially if the donor's blood is suspected of being in a poor state of preservation), carry out direct antiglobulin tests on the patient's erythrocytes and look for both spherocytes and erythrophagocytosis. Urine specimens should be examined for haemoglobin and urobilinogen. Blood should be taken with care in order to avoid haemolysis.

The donor's blood is also cultured for micro-organisms, including psychrophilic contaminants which thrive during cold storage. The donor's blood should also be examined for evidence of lysis, which may result from poor storage conditions or subsequent handling. The blood should also be retested for hepatitis virus, Australia antigen, malaria, syphilis and cytomegalovirus.

It is unwise to inject drugs into donor blood before transfusion because of the high risk of contamination involved. Fever and urticarial rashes are not uncommon after transfusion. Citrate toxicity or hypothermic reactions due to the very rapid transfusion of cold blood are sometimes seen following large transfusions.

Finally, as a additional measure to avoid infection, blood giving sets should be changed every twelve hours

REFERENCES

Agote, L. (1915), "Nuevo procidimiento para la transfusión de Sangre," *An. Inst. Clin. méd., Buenos Aires*, **1**, 1.

Allen, F. H., Jr., Diamond, L. K. and Niedziela, Bevely (1951), "A New Blood-group Antigen," *Nature*, **167**, 482.

Allen, F. H., Jr., Diamond, L. K. and Vaughan, V. C. III (1950), "Erythroblastosis Fetalis. VI: Prevention of Kernicterus," *Amer. J. Dis. Child.*, **80**, 779.

Armitage, P. and Mollison, P. L. (1953), "Further Analysis of Controlled Trials of Treatment of Haemolytic Disease of the Newborn," *J. Obstet. Gynaec.*, **60**, 605.

Arturson, G. and Wallenius, G. (1964), "The Renal Clearance of Dextran of Different Molecular Sizes in Normal Humans," *Scand. J. clin. Lab. Invest.*, **16**, 81.

Aster, R. H. and Jandl, J. H. (1964a), "Platelet Sequestration in Man. I: Methods," *J. clin. Invest.*, **43**, 843.

Aster, R. H. and Jandl, J. H. (1964b), "Platelet Sequestration in Man. II: Immunological and Clinical Studies," *J. clin. Invest.*, **43**, 856.

Bayliss, W. M. (1919), Spec. Rep. Ser. Med. Res. Coun. No. 25.

Berlin, N. I., Waldmann, T. A. and Weissman, S. M. (1959), "Life Span of Red Blood Cells," *Physiol. Rev.*, **39**, 577.

Bernstein, F. (1924), "Ergebnisse einer biostatischen zusammen-fassenden Betrachtung uber die erblichen Blutstrukturen des Menschen," *Klin. Wschr.*, **3**, 1495.

Billing, Barbara, Cole, P. G. and Lathe, G. H. (1954), "Increased Plasma Bilirubin in Newborn Infants in Relation to Birth Weight," *Brit. med. J.*, **2**, 1263.

Blundell, J. (1824), *Researches Physiological and Pathological.* London: Cox.

Bull, J. P. and Jackson, D. M. (1955), Quoted by Mollison, 1972.

Callender, Sheila T. E. and Race, R. R. (1946), "A Serological and Genetical Study of Multiple Antibodies Formed in Response to Blood Transfusion by a Patient with Lupus Erythematosus Diffuses," *Ann. Eugen.*, **13**, 102.

Claireaux, A. E., Cole, P. G. and Lathe, G. H. (1953), "Icterus of the Brain in the Newborn," *Lancet*, **ii**, 1226.

Clarke, C. A. (1968), Prevention of Rhesus Iso-immunisation," *Lancet*, **ii**, 1.

Clarke, R. and Fisher, Mary R. (1956), "Assessment of Blood Loss Following Injury," *Brit. J. clin. Pract.*, **10**, 746.

Coombs, R. R. A., Mourant, A. E. and Race, R. R. (1946), "*In Vivo* Iso-sensitisation of Red Cells in Babies with Haemolytic Disease," *Lancet*, **i**, 264.

Crabtree, N. and Gerrard, J. (1950), "Perceptive Deafness Associated with Severe Neonatal Jaundice," *J. Laryng.*, **64**, 482.

Cutbush, Marie, Mollison, P. L. and Parkin, Dorothy M. (1950), "A New Human Blood Group," *Nature*, **165**, 188.

Davies, D. D. (1964), "Re-anaesthetizing Case of Tonsillectomy and Adenoidectomy Because of Persistent Postoperative Haemorrhage," *Brit. J. Anaesth.*, **36**, 244.

Deacock, A. R. de C. (1971), "Aspects of Anaesthesia for Middle-ear Surgery and Blood Loss During Stapedectomy," *Proc. roy. Soc. Med.*, **64**, 1226.

Decastello, A. von and Sturli, A. (1902), "Uber die Isoagglutinine im Serum gesunder und kranker Menschen," *Münch. med. Wschr.*, p. 1090.

Dungern, E. von and Hirszfeld, L. (1911), "Uber gruppenspezifische Strukturen des Blutes III," *Z. ImmunForsch.*, **8**, 526.

Finn, R. (1960), "Erythroblastosis," *Lancet*, **i**, 526.

Fisch, L. and Norman, A. P. (1961), "Hyperbilirubinaemia and Perceptive Deafness," *Brit. med. J.*, **2**, 142.

Fisher, R. A. (1943), Cited by Race, 1944.

Graw, R. G., Jr., Herzig, G. P., Eyre, H., Goldstein, I., Henderson, E. S. and Perry, S. (1971), "Treatment of Gram Negative Septicaemia in Granulocytopenic Patients With Normal Granulocyte Transfusions," *Clin. Res.*, **19**, 491.

Grumbach, A. and Gasser, C. (1948), "ABO-inkompatibilitäten und Morbus haemolyticus neonatorum," *Helv. paediat. Acta*, **3**, 447.

Halbrecht, I. (1944), "Rôle of Hemagglutinins Anti-A and Anti-B in Pathogenesis of Jaundice of the Newborn (Icterus Neonatorum Precox)," *Amer. J. Dis. Child.*, **68**, 248.

Harker, L. A. and Finch, C. A. (1969), "Thrombokinetics in Man," *J. clin. Invest.*, **48**, 963.

Judson, G., Jones, A., Kellogg, R., Buckner, D., Eisel, R., Perry, S. and Greenough, W. (1968), "Closed Continuous-flow Centrifuge," *Nature*, **217**, 816.

Kline, A., Hughes, L. E., Campbell, H., Williams, A., Zlosnick, J. and Leach, K. G. (1975), *Brit. med. J.*, **2**, 109.

Kotilainen, M. (1969), "Platelet Kinetics in Normal Subjects and in Haematological Disorders," *Scand. J. Haemat.*, suppl. 5.

Landsteiner, K. (1900), "Zur Kenntnis der antifermentativen, Lytischen und agglutinierenden Wirkungen des Blutserums und des Lymphe," *Zbl. Bakt.*, **27**, 357.

Landsteiner, K. and Levine, P. (1926), "On the Cold Agglutinins in Human Serum," *J. Immunol.*, **12**, 441.

Landsteiner, K. and Levine, P. (1927), "Further Observations on Individual Differences of Human Blood," *Proc. Soc. exp. Biol. (N.Y.)*, **24**, 941.

Landsteiner, K. and Wiener, A. S. (1940), "An Agglutinable Factor in Human Blood Recognized by Immune Sera for Rhesus Blood," *Proc. Soc. exp. Biol. (N.Y.)*, **43**, 223.

Landsteiner, K. and Wiener, A. S. (1941), "Studies on an Agglutinogen (Rh) in Human Blood Reacting With Anti-rhesus Sera and With Human Isoantibodies," *J. exp. Med.*, **74**, 309.

Langdell, R. D., Adelson, E., Furth, F. W. and Crosby, W. H. (1958), "Dextran and Prolonged Bleeding Time: Results of a Sixty-gram, One-liter Infusion Given to One Hundred and Sixty-three Normal Human Subjects," *J. Amer. med. Ass.*, **162**, 346.

Levine, P., Burnham, L., Katzin, E. M. and Vogel, P. (1941), "The Role of Iso-immunization in the Pathogenesis of Erythroblastosis Fetalis," *Amer. J. Obstet. Gynec.*, **42**, 925.

Levine, P. and Stetson, R. (1939), "An Unusual Case of Intra-group Agglutination," *J. Amer. med. Ass.*, **113**, 126.

Loewy, A., Skolnik, E. M. and Sadove, M. S. (1963), "Hypothermia and Hypotension in Head and Neck Surgery," *Arch. Otolaryng.*, **77**, 277.

Milles, G., Langston, H. T. and Dalessandro, W. (1971), *Autologous Transfusions.* Springfield, Ill., U.S.A.: Chas. C. Thomas.

Mollison, P. L. (1972), *Blood Transfusion in Clinical Medicine*, 5th edition. Oxford and London: Blackwell.

Mollison, P. L. and Cutbush, Marie (1954), "Haemolytic Disease of the Newborn," *Recent Advances in Paediatrics* (D. Gairdner, Ed.). London: Churchill.

Mollison, P. L. and Walker, W. (1952), "Controlled Trials in the Treatment of Haemolytic Disease of the Newborn," *Lancet*, **i**, 429.

Moss, W. L. (1910), "Studies on Isoagglutinins and Isohemolysins," *Bull. Johns Hopk. Hosp.*, **21**, 63.

Mourant, A. E. (1946), "A 'New' Human Blood Group Antigen of Frequent Occurrence," *Nature*, **158**, 237.

Race, R. R. (1944), "An 'Incomplete' Antibody in Human Serum," *Nature*, **153**, 771.

Race, R. R. and Sanger, Ruth (1968), *Blood Groups in Man*, 5th edition. Oxford and London: Blackwell.

Race, R. R., Sanger, Ruth and Lawler, Sylvia D. (1948), "The Rh Antigen D^u," *Ann. Eugen.*, **14**, 171.

Reeve, E. B. and Veall, N. (1949), "A Simplified Method for the Determination of Circulating Red-cell Volume With Radioactive Phosphorus," *J. Physiol.*, **108**, 12.

Ruggles, R. L. (1960), "Blood Loss During Adenoidectomy and Tonsillectomy Measured With Radioisotopes," *Ann. Otol.*, **69**, 360.

Russell, Sheenah J. M. (1949), "Blood Volume Studies in Healthy Children," *Arch. Dis. Childh.*, **24**, 68.

Sands, C. J., Wood, R. P. II and Van Schoonhoven, P. V. (1968), "Autologous Blood Transfusions in Head and Neck Surgery," *Arch. Otolaryng.*, **88**, 423.

Shalom, A. S. (1964), "Blood Loss in Ear, Nose and Throat Operations," *J. Laryng.*, **78**, 734.

Stratton, F. (1946), "A New Rh Allelomorph," *Nature*, **158**, 25.

Stratton, F. and Renton, P. H. (1948), "Rh Genes Allelomorphic. to D," *Nature*, **162**, 293.

Tarasov, M. (1960), "Cadaveric Blood Transfusion," *Ann. N.Y. Acad. Sci.*, **87**, 512.

Thorsen, G. and Hint, H. (1950), "Aggregation, Sedimentation and Intravascular Sludging of Erythrocytes," *Acta chir. scand.*, suppl. 154.

Wadsworth, G. R. (1954), "The Blood Volume of Normal Women," *Blood*, **9**, 1205.

Wiener, A. S., Unger, L. J., Cohen, L. and Feldman, J. (1956), "Type-specific Cold Auto-antibodies as a Cause of Acquired Hemolytic Anemia and Hemolytic Transfusion Reactions: Biologic Test With Bovine Red Cells," *Ann. intern. Med.*, **44**, 221.

Woodrow, J. C., Clarke, C. A., Donohoe, W. T. A., Finn, R., McConnell, R. B., Sheppard, P. M., Lehane, D., Roberts, Freda M. and Gimlette, T. M. D. (1975), *Brit. med. J.*, **2**, 57.

Woodrow, J. C., Clarke, C. A., Donohoe, W. T. A., Finn, R., McConnell, R. B., Sheppard, P. M., Lehane, D., Russell, Shona H., Kulke, W. and Durkin, Catherine M. (1965), "Prevention of Rh. haemolytic Disease: A Third Report," *Brit. med. J.*, **1**, 279.

54. SURGICAL IMPLANTS

PETER McKELVIE

INTRODUCTION

Surgical implants are objects which are inserted into the body's tissues, and which become embedded, in order to give support or shape to, or add function to, an existing body structure, or which replace this. It is implied that implants will be present for a considerable time. For the purpose of this discussion, dental prostheses, suture materials, catheters and drains are excluded. The behaviour of the materials themselves is the major concern of this review. Mechanical, physical and chemical properties of these implanted objects are of great practical importance. Some may be metabolized, degraded or replaced by normal body constituents, being eventually resorbed, whilst others, the majority, are intended to be permanent, destined never to be incorporated as normal body constituents, remaining for ever a "foreign body".

The behaviour of these agents as materials, rather than as prostheses, is now a study much to the fore. Formerly, strength, malleability, ductility, elasticity and fatigue features, resistance to wear and ease of manufacture were the major considerations, whereas, now, aspects such as bio-compatibility and purity have gained ascendancy. The majority of these implants are fabricated from metals or plastics.

Progress in introducing new metals is necessarily slow, whereas the volume of polymer based materials (plastics) has been bewilderingly vast in volume and rapid in development. Since 1960 biomedical materials have been subject to more stringent quality control whereas, before that time, trial and error was much to the fore. Indeed, it is remarkable that trial and error has given rise to such success as it has.

GENERAL ASPECTS

The ideal implant material should resist fatigue, corrosion, degradation by electrolytes and enzymes, should yield neither diffusion nor degradation products and should elicit minimal tissue responses. These factors, each in themselves warranting detailed study, have been discussed in depth by Williams and Roaf (1973) and their timely book should be read by all wishing to pursue this subject further. They note the existence of a vast literature on implantables and rightly regret the extensive omission of the fine detail of the grades, purity and other physico-chemical properties of the implants discussed in so many communications. Without such information, workers have experienced difficulty in reproducing encouraging results reported by others. However, greater uniformity in implantable materials has recently become the rule. Many of the plastics used previously, and even currently, were devised for other than surgical purposes (silicone rubber excluded) and the work needed to render them non-toxic to tissue was relatively perfunctory.

A substance which is tolerated well and is encapsulated in a fine fibrous membrane when implanted in the form of a smooth mass, becomes much less innocuous than when rough surfaced or in a finely divided form. The cellular response (fibroblast, macrophage or giant cell) varies with the implant. In addition to the trauma of operation, implants, if finely divided, may enter the cytoplasm of macrophages. Larger particles elicit a foreign body giant cell reaction; massive implants of such materials later become encapsulated in fibrous tissue. Toxic agents leaching from the implant material result in very profuse fibrous tissue development.

The development of a neoplastic condition in response to those implant materials is undoubtedly rare in man, being virtually confined to some rodents (Winter, 1970; Oppenheimer et al., 1955). Calnan (1963) has pointed out that with the most successful materials (i.e. those eliciting minimal responses), the implant is encapsulated and wound healing proceeds as though the object were not present. Macrophage accumulations in this favourable situation do not proceed to giant cell formation, and a fibrous capsule, thin and avascular, surrounds the implant. This is in contrast to the granulomata which are regarded as acceptable by Charnley (1970).

The degradation of plastics is a chemical change occurring at the molecular level, in contrast to the electrochemical action in the case of metal corrosion. Plastics may degrade during storage (e.g. if exposed to heat or light) or during sterilization, or they may become toxic if immersed in sterilizing fluid. Some may become toxic due to additives used to counteract recognized forms of degradation to which a plastic might be liable.

The sterilizaton of these agents is subject to a comprehensive discussion by Williams and Roaf. The appropriate use of heat, irradiation and chemicals, including formaldehyde, ethylene oxide, ozone and propylene oxide are mentioned. It has been considered wise to avoid many of these agents in sterilizing prostheses coming in contact with the internal ear.

The reactions of the body tissues to these implants have been the subject of an immense series of communications, including the effects of the tissues on the implants and the effects of the breakdown products sometimes produced. Carcinogenicity is, of course, one feature which is examined. Neoplasia appearing in vulnerable experimental animals has been felt to warrant rejection of otherwise favourable materials. A search for immunological response to these implants, involving sensitization and rejection, indicates to date that these are not formidable, either as short or long term considerations. Finally, a most important feature is that surfaces to be in contact with blood must be ultra-smooth and have a compatible surface charge, otherwise haemolysis occurs. This is overcome in some very new materials by incorporating an adsorbed heparin layer.

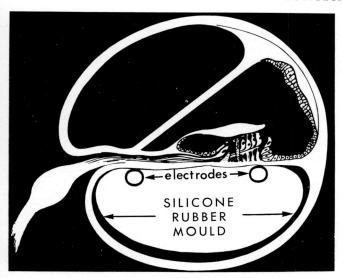

FIG. 1(a). Diagrammatic representation of a bipolar electrode experimentally implanted within the scala tympani of a cat. The intracochlear electrode consists of two 125 μm diameter gold wires with a coil diameter of 250 μm embedded in silicone rubber which has been moulded between etched steel plates to conform to the basal 9 mm of the cat scala tympani. (After Schindler and Merzenich, 1974.)

The features of otorhinological implants which differentiate them from some cardiothoracic or orthopaedic replacements are their small size, their proximity to vulnerable mucosal or epithelial surfaces, their performance in regions vulnerable to sepsis, and their applicability in heavily irradiated sites.

METAL IMPLANTS

The work which has gone into improving the tensile strength, malleability, corrosion resistance, quality control and design of metal orthopaedic implants has not been applied quite so rigorously to metal implants for the middle ear. However, structural failures there are rare and other types of failure are more difficult to lay at the door of a particular prosthesis.

Accounts of the relative merits of various metals are readily available in the orthopaedic literature, and excellently summarized by Williams and Roaf; indeed, the relative merits of substances of all types for these purposes are well laid out by them.

It is to be noted that, although metals are very heavy, their use either to give mechanical strength or to afford electrical conductivity (as in implanted electrodes) often cannot be avoided. Electrolytic effects can be minimized by using pure metals with suitable electronegativity, e.g. gold. However, purity and mechanical strength are at odds—strength relies on the inclusion of impurity to break up slip planes in the crystal lattice. For these reasons, when metals must be used, it is usual to employ one of three alloys:

(1) chromium-molybdenum,
(2) stainless steel, and
(3) cobalt-titanium.

To minimize electrolytic action, all metal implants should not only be made of the same alloy, but should also be of the same grade and from the same manufacturing batches. Of supreme importance is tight quality control during manufacture. Thus not only the use, but also the making of medical implant materials is a job for a specialist.

A special type of metal implant is that which serves as a substitute for the auditory receptor organ i.e. the cochlea. This refers to the so-called cochlear implant or intracochlear electrode (Simmons *et al.*, 1965; Michelson, 1971; House and Urban, 1973). This provides a means of by-passing the acoustic impedance matching mechanism of the middle ear and the acoustic analyzer mechanism of the cochlea to give direct electrical stimulation to the endings of the vestibulo-cochlear nerve (Fig. 1). As Simmons (1973) has pointed out, there are three possible goals for these auditory prosthetic devices. First, there is a device for giving sound sensations for a totally deaf individual without expecting much discrimination between various sounds. Information would be in regard to sound patterns and, as such, it should

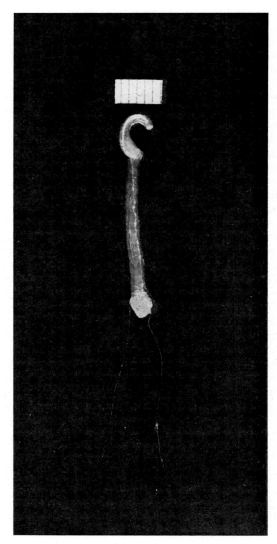

FIG 1(b). Photograph of one of the electrodes implanted in a cat. The electrode was inserted into the scala tympani via the round window. (After Schindler and Merzenich, 1974.)

serve as a supplement to lip reading. The second goal would be to improve the dynamic range of a severely hearing impaired individual without much improvement in speech discrimination. The third goal would be to improve speech discrimination. The latter would imply the encoding of intelligible speech and would require differential multi-channel stimulation. At the present time, the first goal can be met by a single wire electrode connected either to an induction coil implanted behind the ear or to a body surface button with which direct electrical contact can be made with the electrode. By this means, the acoustic speech signal which has been transduced to an electrical signal is delivered to the cochlea using a 90 per cent amplitude modulated 16 kHz carrier wave. Cadaver dissections had previously shown that an electrode would slip through the oval window and along the scala tympani for 20 mm without causing damage to the basilar membrane (House and Urban, 1973). Current discussion indicates that the metal parts of the implant which are not exposed as an electrode terminal may be embedded in any one of a wide range of inert polymers, while the noble metals are favoured for exposed parts. Gold or platinum is the metal of choice for making the electrodes. With these particular electrodes, ionization effects in perilymph or, worse still, gas formation, seem to be avoidable. A little of what has been learned from chronic implantation of electrodes in the brain, from cardiac pacemakers, or from electrical stimulation of perineal musculature to control incontinence may prove of value to this otological field. It is reported that there is no rising voltage requirement to overcome the insulation of the electrodes which is observed with the (much higher voltage) cardiac pacemakers.

Weinberg and Mahler (1964) have discussed the threats to neural tissue which are presented by the conditions at the electrode-electrolyte interface, and Parsonnet and his colleagues (1966) have discussed the electrical isolation of long term implanted electrodes in the tissues. Nevertheless, the implant surgeons appear to have escaped some of these difficulties. Indeed, it has been observed that the vestibulo-cochlear nerve can survive intracochlear electrode implantation for an appreciable time (Schindler and Merzenich, 1974).

In spite of the great effort that has already gone into this field, the technique of cochlear electrode implantation remains highly experimental, is an "unphysiological" method and, at the time of writing, is likely to offer limited advantages to the profoundly deaf. As Kiang (1973) has pointed out, while it is true that preconceived ideas can sometimes obstruct progress, it cannot be reasonable to ignore basic knowledge about how a system functions in trying to design replacement parts.

POLYMERS

Of the large range of medical polymers, only a few have found favour in otolaryngology. Some established, extremely well investigated agents in general use e.g. polymethyl methacrylate, have failed to become accepted in otolaryngology. Reference to the properties of the commonly used materials will be made.

Politef (polytetrafluoroethylene; Teflon) is extremely inert and highly tissue compatible. It is used both in the middle ear and in the vocal fold. Calnan (1963) has commented on the minimal tissue reaction it elicited, including the absence of giant cells so peculiarly a feature of more marked reactions. It is to be noted that finely divided politef particles do indeed elicit a greater degree of tissue reaction than smooth surfaced larger implants. The latter feature has been a boon in the middle ear where politef prostheses retain an excellent reputation for stability and biocompatibility. The permanently "wet" surface of the polymer prevents its fixation and immobilization to some degree (an asset in this situation). It should be added that, in the operation of stapedectomy, the perilymph in the internal ear is brought into contact with the prosthesis, which is an implant variously made of politef, stainless steel and a range of other materials. The internal ear survives this remarkably well, and surveys show only minor differences between the results obtained with the various prostheses. These differences are in connection with mechanical rather than with chemical features.

Using a long injection needle and an endoscope, both Arnold (1961) and Lewy (1966) have implanted finely divided politef paste in a unilateral, flaccid, paralyzed vocal fold. The procedure is used to splint and give bulk to the paralyzed fold, allowing the other (functioning) fold to occlude against it, so achieving phonation. The extremely ragged, shredded particles, 5–100 μm in size, suspended in glycerol, elicit a granuloma in the vocal fold. This resolves slowly over a period of about two years, the histiocytes and giant cells abating, to be replaced by a firm fibrous mass encapsulating the politef particles. Silicone (Rubin, 1965) and tantalum (Lewy, 1963) have also been inserted into the vocal fold for this purpose. Microlaryngoscopy now makes it easier to insert shaped masses into the vocal fold as an alternative to the injection of pastes.

Silicone rubber (Silastic), a silicon polymer, appears to have had more than the usual attention paid to its properties of biocompatibility, which indeed are remarkably good. Silicone rubber is such a good implant material because the body possesses no enzyme capable of degrading the Si-O bond. The excellence of silicone rubber, when used in sheet form in the middle ear to prevent adhesions in reconstructive surgery, is only slightly marred by the fact that ciliary function is impaired by contact with even the most inert substances.

Mention must be made of *polyhydroxylethylmethacrylate* (Hydron, PolyHEMA), not because of any effective application already in otolaryngology but rather because of its nature and possibilities. Polyhydroxylethylmethacrylate becomes ossified in the skin of the pig and is calcified in man. The spongy form of the implant allows exudate, erythrocytes and fibrin, followed by polymorphs and eosinophils to invade the pores. Fibroblasts and collagen follow within days, to be accompanied within a month by blood vessels and a little fibrous tissue. No outside fibrous capsule develops and so the sponge appears to be just such an agent as the implant surgeon seeks. As Calnan points out, one requires tissue cells to be freely mobile in such an implant, the correct tissue fluid environment to be present in and around the mass, the blood supply penetrating it, no degradation products, and chemical as well as physical stability. The agent can be prepared as a solid block (in dry gel form) which swells on implantation. It has been used for restoring bulk to the vocal fold.

ADHESIVES

Since fixation is commonly a difficulty, *surgical adhesives*, available for a decade, might be expected to have a use in the field of otolaryngology. Indeed, there have been hopes that the surgical suture might be supplanted by progress in chemical technology. A series of adhesives, mainly *cyano-acrylates*, has been produced. For the most part, they have fallen short of the ideal i.e. they should be stable, sterilizable, non-toxic, adhere in a moist field, be non-carcinogenic, not too endo- or exothermic when setting and minimally damaging to the surfaces to which they adhere. Naturally, any bonding can only be as good as the tissues involved.

The longer chain cyanoacrylates remain in limited use as adhesives, since methyl methacrylate is a "cement" (rather than a glue). They have been used for fixation in the middle ear (McKelvie, 1969).

It seems probable that, despite reservations over the toxicity of these polymers, better ones will be produced. Mecrilate (methyl 2-cyanoacrylate), the originally developed agent, has been well evaluated both by Sachs and his associates (1966), by Sewell (1966) and by Lehman and his associates (1967). Olsson and Rietz (1966) indicated possibilities in the fixation of bone grafts, Jesse (1966) the fixation of split skin grafts, and Thomas *et al.* (1963) the possibilities in the repair of bronchi. Mecrilate is completely eliminated in the course of time, although the longer chain derivatives, especially the more favoured isobutyl derivative (bucrilate), remains in situ indefinitely, being non-biodegradable. Smyth and Kerr (1974) have assessed the value of butyl cyanoacrylate (Histoacryl) as an ossicular adhesive in the middle ears of cats. The polymer was shown to be relatively non-toxic but functional results were poor. Slow progress in the development and availability of these glues probably stems from transatlantic anxieties about toxicity.

CONCLUSIONS

It is indeed unfortunate that no well ordered chart of the relative bioacceptabilities (and other qualities of implantability) of implantable materials can be made which could command universal approval. Each investigator, particularly those working with animal models and often also with variable polymers, is searching for different features. A lack of uniformity and agreement as to how suitability of materials, particularly the new plastics, should be assessed is also evident. Finally, it appears an inescapable conclusion that implantable materials, let alone the devices constructed from them, fall far short of "the real thing" on many occasions, but it seems that surgeons are going to fall back on them, *faute de mieux*, increasingly more frequently as they become more miniaturized and bio-acceptable.

REFERENCES

Arnold, G. (1961), "Vocal Rehabilitation of Paralytic Dysphonia: IV. Further Studies of Intracordal Injection Material," *Arch. Otolaryng.*, **73**, 290.

Arnold, G. (1964), "Further Experiences with Intracordal Teflon® Injection," *Laryngoscope*, **74**, 802.

Boedts, D., Roels, H. and Kluyskens, P. (1967), "Laryngeal Tissue Responses to Teflon," *Arch. Otolaryng.*, **86**, 110.

Charnley, J. (1970), "The Reaction of Bone to Self-curing Acrylic Cement," *J. Bone J. Surg.*, **52B**, 340, 358.

Dutton, J. (1959), "Acrylic Investment of Intracranial Aneurysms," *Brit. med. J.*, 597–602.

Goff, W. (1969), "Teflon® Injection for Vocal Cord Paralysis," *Arch. Otolaryng.*, **90**, 99.

House, W. F. and Urban, J. (1973), "Long Term Results of Electrode Implantation and Electronic Stimulation of the Cochlea in Man," *Ann. Otol.*, **82**, 504–510.

Jesse, R. H. (1966), "Clinical use of a Physiological Adhesive in the Fixation of Split Thickness Skin Grafts," *Proceedings of a Symposium on Physiological Adhesives.* Austin: University of Texas Press.

Kiang, N. Y. S. (1973), "Discussion," *Ann. Otol.*, **82**, 9.

Kirchner, F. R., Toledo, P. S. and Svoboda, D. J. (1966), "Studies of the Larynx after Teflon® Injection," *Arch. Otolaryng.*, **83**, 74.

Kliment, K., Stol, M., Fahoun, K. and Stockar, B. (1968), "Use of Spongy Hydron in Plastic Surgery," *J. Biomed. mat. Res.*, **2**, 237.

Lehman, R. A. W., Hayes, G. J. and Leonard, F. (1966), "Toxicity of Alkyl 2-cyanoacrylates. I. Peripheral Nerve," *Arch. Surg.*, **93**.

Lehman, R. A. W., West, R. L. and Leonard, F. (1966), "Toxicity of Alkyl 2-cyanoacrylates. II. Bacterial Growth," *Arch. Surg.*, **93**.

Lewy, R. (1963), "Glottic Reformation with Voice Rehabilitation in Vocal Cord Paralysis: The Injection of Teflon® and Tantalum," *Laryngoscope*, **73**, 547.

Lewy, R. (1964), "Glottic Rehabilitation with Teflon® Injection—The Return of Voice, Cough and Laughter," *Acta Oto-laryng.*, **58**.

Lewy, R. (1966), "Response of Laryngeal Tissue to Granular Teflon® in situ," *Arch. Otolaryng.*, **83**, 79.

McKelvie, P. (1969), "A Trial of Adhesives in Reconstructive Middle Ear Surgery," *J. Laryng.*, **83**, 2, 1105–1109.

Michelson, R. P. (1971), "Results of Electrical Stimulation of the Cochlea in Human Sensory Deafness," *Ann. Otol.*, **80**, 914–919.

Michelson, R. P. (1971), "Electrical Stimulation of the Cochlea," *Arch. Otolaryng.*, **93**, 317–323.

Olsson, S. E. and Rietz, K. A. (1966), "Polymer Osteosynthesis. II: An Experimental Study of Methyl 2-cyanoacrylate (Eastman 910 Adhesive) in Bone Grafting," *Acta chir. scand.*, Suppl. 367, p. 4.

Oppenheimer, B. S., Oppenheimer, Enid T., Stout, A. P., Willhite, Margaret and Danishefsky, I. (1958), "The Latent Period in Carcinogenesis by Plastics in Rats and its Relation to the Presarcomatous Stage," *Cancer*, **11**, 204.

Parsonnet, V., Zucker, I. R., Kannerstein, M. D., Gilbert, L. and Alvares, J. F. (1966), "The Fate of Permanent Intracardiac Electrodes," *J. surg. Res.*, **6**, 285.

Rubin, H. (1965), "Intracordal Injection of Silicone in Selected Dysphonias," *Arch. Otolaryng.*, **81**, 604.

Rubin, H. (1965), "Pitfalls in Treatment of Dysphonias by Intracordal Injection of Synthetics," *Laryngoscope*, **75**, 1381.

Rubin, H. (1965), "Dysphonia due to Unilateral Nerve Paralysis Treatment by Intracordal Injection of Synthetics: A Preliminary Report," *Calif. Med.*, **102**, 105.

Sachs, E. Jr., Erbengi, A., Margolis, G. and Wilson, D. H. (1966), "Fatality from Ruptured Intracranial Aneurysm after Coating with Methyl 2-cyanoacrylate (Eastman 910 Monomer, M2C-1)," *J. Neurosurg.*, **24**, 5.

Schindler, R. A. and Merzenich, M. M. (1974), "Chronic Intracochlear Electrode Implantation," *Ann. Otol.*, **83**, 202.

Sewell, I. A. (1966), "The Microvascular Responses Induced by Materials Used in Operative Surgery," *Brit. J. Surg.*, **53**, 8.

Simmons, F. B. (1973), "Discussion," *Ann. Otol.*, **82**, 9.

Simmons, F. B., Epley, J. M. and Lummis, R. C. (1965), "Auditory Nerve: Electrical Stimulation in Man," *Science*, **148**, 104.

Smyth, G. D. L. and Kerr, A. G. (1974), "Histoacryl (butyl cyno-acrylate) as an Ossicular Adhesive," *J. Laryng.*, **88**, 539–542.

Stone, J. W. and Arnold, G. E. (1970), "Intracordal Politef (Teflon®) Injection," *Arch. Otolaryng.*, **91**, 568.

Thomas, P. A. Jr., Nims, R. M., Hunt, R. D. and Aronstam, E. M. (1963), "Experimental Observations with a Plastic Adhesive, Methyl 2-cyanoacrylate as a Sealing Agent in Pulmonary and Bronchial Surgery," *Cohesive News*, **3**, 6.

Warren, A., Gould, F. E., Capulong, R., Glotfelty, E., Boley, S. J.,

Calem, W. S. and Levowitz, B. S. (1967), "Prosthetic Applications of a New Hydrophilic Plastic," *Surg. Forum*, **18**, 183.

Weinberg, J. and Mahler, J. (1964), "An Analysis of the Electrical Properties of Metal Electrodes," *Medical Electronics and Biological Engineering*, **2**, 299.

Wichterle, O. and Lim, D. (1960), "Hydrophilic Gels for Biological Use," *Nature* (*Lond.*), **185**, 117.

Williams, D. F. and Roaf, R. (1973), *Implants in Surgery*. London, Philadelphia, Toronto: W. B. Saunders & Co.

55. TRACHEOSTOMY TUBES

R. PRACY

INTRODUCTION

In common with circumcision, tracheostomy must be considered to be one of the oldest of surgical procedures. Authorities differ as to who carried out the first operation, but certainly it was described for the relief of airway obstruction in pre-Christian times. In spite of this, no perfectly satisfactory method of maintaining a patent airway and normal laryngo-tracheo-bronchial function by the use of a tube has yet been discovered. The purpose of this paper, therefore, is to describe the various tube designs currently available and to indicate the way in which they fulfil the requirements of an ideal tracheostomy tube. However, before this can be presented as a lucid account it is necessary to discuss the relevant structure and the function of the laryngo-tracheo-bronchial tree and to indicate what may be the effects of creating, deliberately, a temporary, semi-permanent or permanent fistula into the trachea. It will also be necessary to classify some of the conditions for which a tracheostomy may be required.

RELEVANT ANATOMY AND PHYSIOLOGY

For the purpose of this chapter, the laryngo-tracheo-bronchial tree must be considered as a surgical entity. It consists of a hollow rigid, or partially rigid, tube with a valved structure at its upper end. Both the wall and the lumen of the tube have a function. The lumen transports air and gross particulate matter during coughing and the wall is responsible for the transport of mucus and small particulate matter through the directional beat of the cilia. Throughout its length, the patency of the lumen is maintained and assured by the presence of varying amounts of rings of cartilage in the walls of the tube. The posterior wall of the trachea is deficient in cartilage and parts of the bronchi are unsupported by cartilage. The presence of rings, or parts of rings, in the trachea and bronchi is of considerable importance for if the tube were made up almost entirely of cartilage, flexibility of the airway would be lost and forced flexion of the neck could lead to kinking of the tube and consequent lower airway obstruction. Varying amounts of smooth muscle are found in the walls of the trachea and bronchi and the whole tube is lined by a ciliated mucosa, capable of sweeping mucus and debris upwards from the bronchi and out through the larynx. Mucus and debris discharged from the respiratory tract by this route may then be coughed up or swallowed. The sensory nerve supply to the larynx has a very low threshold and, particularly in children, very minor stimuli can produce severe laryngeal spasm. This function is purely protective as is the cough reflex and the importance of this must be borne in mind when a tracheostomy is established. Early operations were carried out solely for the relief of airway obstruction and probably the surgeon felt that once an efficient patent fistula had been established, the operation had achieved its objective.

EFFECTS OF MAKING A TRACHEOSTOMY

While it is certainly true that air access to the alveolar interface is of prime importance, one cannot overlook certain other aspects of laryngo-tracheal physiology, particularly when it is felt that the fistula may have to be maintained for any length of time.

Mucociliary transport, the ability to strain against a closed glottis, cough and speech are all important for normal life and all must be taken into account when planning for anything more than a very temporary situation. Recently, two other aspects of tracheostomy, relevant particularly to the child, have been brought to light, the importance of which were hitherto not appreciated. These are (a) in children, once a tracheostomy is established, the vocal folds cease to abduct and (b) the absence of a glottic expiratory tide of air removes what appears to be the all important stimulus to the growth of the larynx. These may have been responsible in the past for the considerable difficulties encountered in the removal of tracheostomy tube from the small child.

Once an artificial opening into the trachea is made, a "dead space" between that opening and the glottis will exist (Fig. 1). In that dead space there will be no tide of air in either phase of the respiratory cycle and since the transport of mucus appears to be dependent upon the expiratory tide of air, this will be affected with important consequences. Mucus will tend to stagnate and to fall

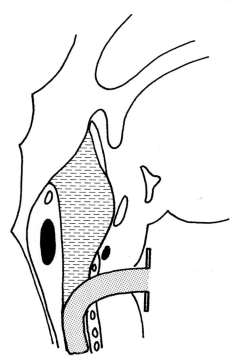

FIG. 1. Diagram showing "dead space" between tracheostomy and the glottis.

back into the bronchi and the lungs. In this stagnant fluid, pathogenic and saprophytic bacteria can multiply. At the best, therefore, there is a possibility of partial waterlogging of the lung, at the worst, blocking of the bronchi and pneumonic consolidation. In the special circumstances found in papillomatosis, pieces of tumour which necrose as the tumour outgrows its blood supply may be carried down into the lower respiratory tract in the stagnant mucus. This can lead to implantation of papilloma in the mucosa if it is traumatized, and to a fatal obstruction to the airway.

Obviously once the humidification supplied by the nasal mucosa is lost, the air inspired through the tracheostomy will have a drying effect upon respiratory mucosa. This drying concentrates the mucus and makes secretions more difficult to void. Furthermore, since the filtration effect of nasal vibrissae and mucosa is lost there will be a greater tendency to infection of the lower respiratory tract.

To summarize, therefore, the effects of creating a fistula into the trachea from the outside are:

(1) By-pass of all laryngeal functions. Cough is lost. Phonation is lost, and, in the child, development of the larynx ceases. The vocal folds cease abduction on inspiration.

(2) A dead space is created between the tracheal opening and the larynx from which mucus tends to fall back into the lower respiratory tract.

(3) The filtration and humidifying effect of the nasal mucosa is lost. Secretions will tend to be more viscid.

(4) There is a greater risk of infection.

(5) Any tube inserted through the fistula will act as a foreign body; since the tube will move against the

wall of the fistula during neck movements, swallowing and normal respiration, there is always a possibility of trauma to the track by abrasions unless the tube wall is very smooth.

THE PURPOSES FOR WHICH A TRACHEOSTOMY MAY BE REQUIRED

(1) Acute or chronic airway obstructions.

(2) For assisted ventilation in the medium-long or long-term—e.g. in central or peripheral respiratory or laryngeal paralysis or in chest injury.

(3) For drainage of the lower respiratory tract.

(4) As an essential preliminary for some surgical procedure on the larynx which may temporarily occlude the glottis.

DESIGNS OF TUBES (HISTORICAL)

Early tracheostomy tubes were made of bone, metal, gutta percha and rubber. The design varied but in general the tube was single and was expanded at its outer end in order to provide rings by which it could be secured in position by means of tape. Until relatively recent times (30 years ago) tracheostomies were carried out without an anaesthetic. An important feature of the design, therefore, was that the tube should be quickly and easily introduced. An interesting design of this type was Fuller's bi-valve tube (Fig. 2) which did in fact have an inner tube. By compressing the two halves of the outer tube a pointed cone

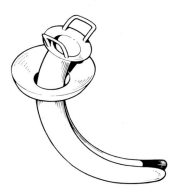

FIG. 2. Fuller's tracheostomy tube.

could be formed which could be introduced easily through a vertical incision through tracheal rings. For many years now, however, conventional tracheostomy tubes have been made of silver and have consisted of an inner tube which is marginally longer than the outer so that in the event of the lumen of the tube becoming blocked the airway could be cleared immediately by the removal of the inner tube. Tubes for adults were of two basic designs:

(a) A smooth curve in the arc of a circle, examples of which are Chevalier Jackson's, the King's College Hospital and the Edinburgh tracheostomy tube (Fig. 3).

(b) Tubes with a rounded angle and two straight segments, an example of which is Durham's (1869)

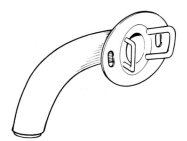

Fig. 3. Edinburgh tracheostomy tube.

"lobster-tail" tube (Fig. 4). This tube had the advantage that the guard could be moved to accommodate the vertical limb most satisfactorily in the lumen of the trachea. However, since the outer tube was rigid, both the introducer and the inner tube had to have a flexible curve in order to allow introduction and changing of the tube. The joints were complicated and potentially dangerous.

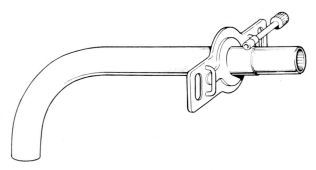

Fig. 4. Durham's "Lobster Tail" tracheostomy tube.

Tubes designed for children were either of adult designs reduced in size or special tubes designed by Parker (1879) and by Cubley.

Occasionally, situations arose in which the use of a metal tube were precluded as for example in a patient undergoing irradiation of the larynx, laryngeal part of pharynx or cervical oesophagus. A rubber tube designed by Morrant Baker was used for this purpose (Fig. 5). However, the

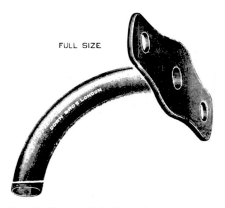

FULL SIZE

Fig. 5. Morrant Baker's tracheostomy tube. (By courtesy of Downs Surgical Ltd.)

tissues of the neck reacted violently to this tube and, because of the abrasive effect of the relatively rough wall, much granulations tissue was produced (Fig. 6 shows

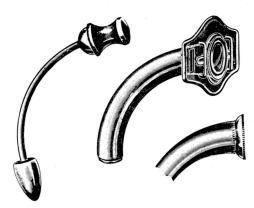

Fig. 6. Photograph of a Morrant Baker's tracheostomy tube under magnification.

Morrant Baker's tube under magnification). Trauma and tissue devitalization always favour the development of infections, and infection was a common accompaniment to the use of the tube.

With the discovery of flexible plastics (polyethylene, polyvinyl chloride and silicone rubber), a new generation of tracheostomy tubes was developed. As with the Morrant Baker tube an inner tube was not possible due to the reduction in the lumen size made necessary by the use of a sufficient thickness of plastic wall to keep the lumen patent. Certainly, they were an improvement on the Baker tube but again the surface was rough when compared with the metal tube. The position became complicated when certain polyvinyl chloride tubes were found to develop toxic impurities in the sterilization process.

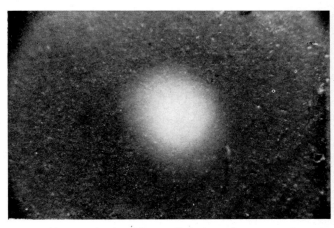

Fig. 7(a). Negus' tracheostomy tube. (By courtesy of Downs Surgical Ltd.)

A major advance in tracheostomy tube design had occurred twenty years or more before the introduction of plastic tubes. This was when Negus fitted the King's College Hospital Tube (Fig. 7a) with a de Santi's valve (Fig. 7b). This allowed the patient to breathe in through the tracheostomy tube and out through the glottis (Fig. 7c, d). Negus developed this type of tube to allow patients who had a bilateral abductor paralysis of the vocal folds to use the expiratory tide to phonate. It is not clear whether he appreciated the additional advantages of the use of a built-in expiratory valve. However, one disadvantage of

FIG. 7(b). de Santi's speaking aid valve for tracheostomy tube.

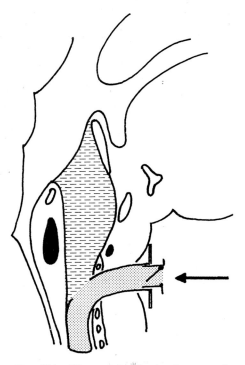

FIG. 7(c). Diagram showing inspiratory path through Negus type tracheostomy tube fitted with de Santi's valve.

the Negus modification was that, in general, in order to obtain an adequate peritubal space in the trachea, for the expiratory tide, a smaller bore tube than would be normally used was required if the patient was to have a strong enough voice.

Nearly twenty years ago, Wilson introduced a tube for children which showed two interesting developments. These were (1) the inner tube had a funnel shaped flange at its external end to which a respirator could be connected easily and (2) the outer tube had a fenestration on the shoulder which could be used during decannulation in association with a "blocker" to allow the child to breathe in and out through the glottis as a preliminary to decannulation. The two tubes were major advances in tracheostomy tube design though again it is not clear that Wilson fully appreciated what his instrument contributed to the patient's respiratory physiology.

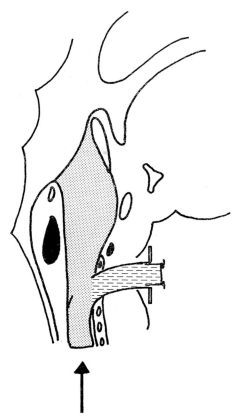

FIG. 7(d). Diagram showing expiratory path, i.e. through glottis, in patient fitted with Negus type tracheostomy tube with de Santi valve.

The Negus modification halved the humidification difficulty in adults and promoted physiological transport of mucus in the expiratory phase. The Wilson tube allowed normal respiratory exchange and near normal mucociliary transport when the blocker was in situ. At this point, the Swedes developed a most ingenious contribution to humidification. The "Swedish Nose" consisted of wire mesh metal discs housed in a plastic container. This could be inserted into the outer end of the inner tube. Water vapour in the expiratory tide was caught on the wire mesh and was returned to the tracheo-bronchial tree on inspiration. The discs were replaceable when they became blocked, but the apparent advantages were not realized in this country.

More recently, at Alder Hey Hospital in Liverpool, the Negus principle and the Wilson principle have been combined in the Alder Hey tube (Fig. 8) for children. In this tube, both the inner and outer tubes are fenestrated on the shoulder and a valve is inserted into the flange of the inner tube.

The guard of the tube is adjustable so that the holes in the shoulders of the tubes can be sited by a tracheoscope and brought into register with the tracheal lumen. Thus it is that the child is enabled to phonate, the stimulus to laryngeal growth is maintained and the stimulus to vocal fold abduction on inspiration is not lost.

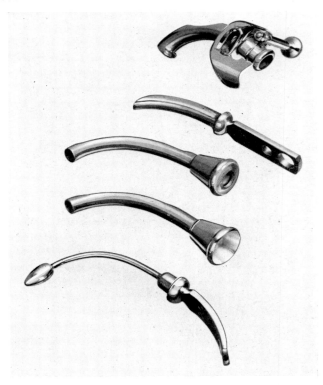

FIG. 8. Alder Hey type tracheostomy tube for children.

THE THEORETICAL IDEAL DESIGN OF TUBES

This will have to be considered under two headings, i.e. short-term and long-term, and long-term will have to be discussed according to whether it applies to the adult or to the child.

The modern *silver* tracheostomy tube usually consists of four parts—a *guard* attached to or connected to the *outer tube*, an *inner tube* and an *introducer*.

Plastic tubes are made on a mould in a single piece. It is therefore, relevant to examine why a mobile or semi-mobile guard was found to be necessary when tubes are made of metal. It will be appreciated that a shield is necessary to allow for the provision of lugs to which the retaining tape is attached. If, therefore, the head and neck are moved from side to side, or round a vertical axis, some play is available which leads to less movement of the outer/inner tubes complex. Obviously, this results in less trauma to the wall of the fistula and therefore to less likelihood of granuloma formation. This separate guard or shield is therefore seen to be an advantage. In the case of the plastic tube which is less rigid, it was felt that the separate shield could be dispensed with without increasing the risk of trauma. However, while this is certainly feasible, it is very important to use a smooth, shiny non-reacting plastic. Toxic reactions have been mentioned previously. There are further disadvantages. Tubes of this design with a single relatively thick plastic wall do not offer the patient the immediate relief in emergency which is offered by the possibility of removal of the inner tube. Moreover,

crusting due to drying of secretions can be very troublesome. Furthermore, it has proved difficult to fit these tubes with de Santi valves and to maintain the valve *in situ*. At the time of writing the future world position in regard to plastics is difficult to foretell. However, even if production of a cheap flexible tube remains possible, much will have to be done to improve the design before the metal tube can be discarded completely.

The *shape* and *bore* of tracheostomy tubes are important. A great deal of work has been done by the anaesthetists to study the flow patterns in both curved and angled airways. In general, flow of fluid (liquids or gases) in a tube may be *laminar* or *turbulent* (Fig. 9); in other words, the flow may be parallel to the walls of the tube or may be thrown into *eddies*, where one stream may turn on itself and push against another oncoming stream. Reynolds studied the behaviour of fluid flow experimentally. He found that the critical velocity range above which a fluid flow will be turbulent, below which it will be laminar and in which it will be either, depends on the velocity of flow, the size and shape of the conduit (tube) and the viscosity of the fluid. A ratio (*Reynolds' criterion* or *number*), encompassing the fluid velocity and viscosity, together with the length of the conduit, was found to be the same for all fluids at the critical velocity.

The rate of fluid flow through a tube is governed by *Poiseuille's Equation*, i.e.

$$V/t = (\pi r^4 \triangle p)/(8 \eta l) \qquad (55.1)$$

where
V = volume of fluid flowing in time t
r = radius of tube
l = length of tube
$\triangle p$ = pressure drop across ends of tube
and η = viscosity coefficient of fluid

The equation is valid only if the flow is laminar; this would not be true if the Reynolds' number is greater than 2000.

The central portion of the stream of fluid through the tube travels at a greater rate than the peripheral stream because the latter encounters the resistance from the wall. The head of a column of gas has therefore a convexity pointing in the direction of flow. If the curve of the tube is gradual and follows the arc of a circle of large radius, laminar flow may be preserved provided that the tube is o adequate bore. However, if the curve of the tube is of a relatively small radius and this curve connects two straight limbs, as in the sharply angled Durham's pattern, then turbulence is certain to occur. In the case of Durham's tube, the pockets created by the flexible joints on the inner tube tend only to increase the turbulence. Studies have been carried out on standard adult tubes of size 32 French gauge* (Fig. 10). The flow rates of 3 l. min^{-1}, 8 l. min^{-1} and 20 l. min^{-1} correspond to very low, low and average tidal volumes. It will be seen that there are wide variations in performance and in efficiency. The most linear flow appears to be achieved by a flow of 8 l. min^{-1}, which is equivalent to a tidal air of 500 ml and a respiratory rate of

* Calibres of tracheostomy tubes are now quoted in millimetres. For conversion of measures in French gauge (F.G.) to measures in millimetres (mm), divide the F.G. values by 3.

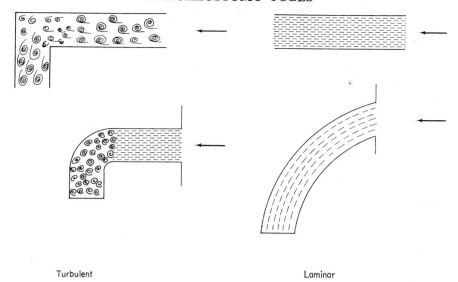

Turbulent   Laminar

FIG. 9. Diagram showing laminar and turbulent fluid flow and their dependence upon tube curvature.

0·27 Hz (16 respirations per minute). Although this would be normal for an adult resting in bed and in the ambulant patient, peak flow rates might otherwise reach as much as 60 l. min^{-1}. Figure 10 shows that with some tubes there is a significant reduction of efficiency as the flow rate increases.

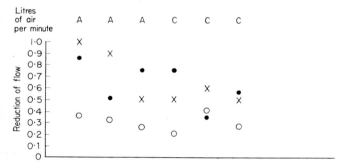

Reduction of flow through six tracheostomy tubes each of the same diameter (about 11 mm)

- ● ● = 3 litres input
- ○ ○ = 8 litres input
- X X = 20 litres input
- A = Angled tube
- C = Smooth curve

FIG. 10. Diagram showing reduction of air flow through six different tracheostomy tubes but each of the same diameter, i.e 32 F.G. (about 11 mm). Three of these tubes were angled (A), three showed a gradual, smooth curve (C). The dotted curve refers to a flow input of 3 l. min^{-1}; the interrupted line refers to a flow input of 8 l. min^{-1} and the continuous line refers to a flow input of 20 l. min^{-1}.

A smooth, gradual curve thus offers the best possibility of achieving a laminar flow. In the adult where a valve is not required in the short-term, it would appear that this requirement could be met most satisfactorily by a plastic tube of wide bore. In the long-term, where speech is an overriding consideration, a silver tube with a smooth, gradual curve and fitted with an expiratory valve appears to offer the most efficient system.

In the child, the position is somewhat different. The ratio of tube wall thickness to lumen size is higher than in the adult and therefore not as satisfactory. It is not possible to achieve the same comparative flow rates with silver and plastic tubes. Examination of the surface

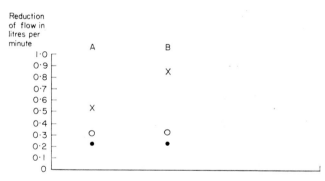

Comparison between child's pattern tubes in silver and polyvinyl chloride using similar flow rates showing higher frictional resistance of polyvinyl chloride

FIG. 11. A comparison of the flow resistance of two types of child's tracheostomy tubes, one a 7 mm silver tube (left hand side), the other an 8 mm polyvinyl chloride tube (right hand side)

structure of the plastic tube shows that it is as uneven as that of the silver tube. Moreover, the reduced bore makes crusting due to drying of the inspired air a problem. For these reasons, it seems that the valved silver tube still offers the most efficient type of tracheostomy tube for the child, because crusting is less likely to occur due to better provision in respect of humidity (Fig. 11). Abduction of the vocal folds will be maintained and the stimulus to laryngeal development will still present.

CONCLUSIONS

Much work yet remains to be done on the design of tubes for tracheostomy. The ideal material has yet to be found which will have to be as strong as metal so that the wall can be thin and the lumen large. The friction will need to be reduced, possibly by the use of materials such as politef or silicone rubber. Moreover, it will have to be possible to incorporate a speaking expiratory valve, which will not interfere with the ability of the nurse to aspirate secretions from the trachea and bronchi.

REFERENCES AND FURTHER READING

Crawley, B. and Cross, D. (1975), *Anaesthesia*, **30**, 4.
Durham, A. E. (1869), *Practitioner*, **2**, 212.
Lindholm, C. E. (1970), *Acta anaesth. scand.*, suppl. 33.
O'Dwyer, J. (1887), *Med. Rec.*, **32**, 557.
Parker, R. W. (1879), *Med. Chirurg. Trans.*, p. 42.
Salmon, L. F. W. (1975), *Proc. roy. Soc. Med.*, **68**, 347.
Toremalm, N. G. (1960), *Acta anaesth. scand.*, **4**, 105.
Toremalm, N. G. (1972), *Laryngoscope*, **82**, 265.

56. AUDIOMETERS

M. C. MARTIN

INTRODUCTION

At the time of writing (1974), the audiometer is almost 100 years old. Bunch (1943) gives credit to the Hartman "Acoumeter" as the first audiometer. This was produced in 1878. Bunch very adequately reviews the historical aspects of audiometers up to 1943; more recent historical surveys are those by Kranz (1963) and by Grason (1972).

An audiometer may be operationally defined as an electroacoustic instrument designed to measure hearing acuity. This chapter will deal only with audiometers that require the subject to give a response; other instruments such as the acoustic impedance bridge and the evoked response audiometer can be described as objective instruments because they rely on a physical measurement of behaviour to determine hearing acuity.

Developments in audiometers have been mainly confined to the use of more modern components and the incorporation of facilities for new tests that have become established. In practice, however, the use of new components and of new electronic techniques has been very slow, possibly due to the uncritical nature of the users and their lack of electronic knowledge. Audiometers in the form that we know them today became available in the 1930s, e.g. the Western Electric 6A in 1936 and the Maico D5 in 1937. Instruments of this type were in use in Great Britain in the 1930's. Room for technical development is not great and has been limited to the introduction of white noise, broad-and-narrow-band masking, the use of continuously variable inductance attenuators and the establishment of the self-recording audiometer described by Békésy.

Audiometers vary in complexity from simple portable instruments to large consoles. In practice, audiometers may be divided into the following four types, each having different facilities.

(1) Screening audiometer—limited frequency range and acoustic output, with air conduction only.

(2) Simple Diagnostic Audiometer—full frequency range but limited acoustic output; air and bone conduction with simple masking facilities.

(3) Diagnostic Audiometer—full frequency range and acoustic output; air and bone conduction; full masking facilities for speech and for pure tones; loudness balance facility; speech audiometry inputs.

(4) Advanced Diagnostic Audiometer—facilities as for the diagnostic audiometer but two independent channels, both frequency and amplitude modulation of test tones and ability to switch signals in a more flexible way. Normally this type of audiometer would be used for research purposes.

Recommended values for maximum outputs and frequency ranges are given in Table 1.

PURE TONE AUDIOMETERS

Design Features

Values for the various features of pure tone audiometers are standardized in International Electro Technical Commission Recommendations (IEC) 177 and 178 (1965).

The basic pure tone audiometer can be considered as being comprised of seven electronic parts (Fig. 1). The design features of these basic sections are as follows:

(1) *Pure Tone Generator*—The pure tones are generated electrically by an oscillator whose most important design feature ensures production of an accurate, stable frequency with low harmonic distortion. A further requirement is that if the oscillator is to be switched on and off by the interrupter switch none of the above parameters must alter during the on and off period. Catlin and Glackin (1964) describe a design meeting these criteria.

The easiest way of achieving the correct oscillator performance is to use an LC (inductance–capacitance) circuit as in Fig. 2. The LC circuit is easily tuned and frequencies can be changed by switching in capacitors of different values.

The greatest advantage, however, is that the resonant LC circuit does not change frequency or introduce distortion when the high voltage supply is switched on to the valve or transistor, thus allowing a simple form of tone interrupter switch to be used.

The other main type of oscillator used to generate pure tones is the RC (resistance–capacitance) oscillator (Fig. 3).

TABLE 1

MAXIMUM AIR AND BONE CONDUCTION OUTPUTS AT EACH FREQUENCY
FOR FOUR CATEGORIES OF AUDIOMETERS

(Where no figures appear, that frequency will not be required. Minimum hearing levels should be −10 dB at all frequencies. Where instruments are being used for hearing conservation programmes, it is advisable to have −20 dB as a minimum hearing level in order to cover all normally hearing persons.)

Frequency (Hz)	Screening		Simple Diagnostic		Diagnostic		Advanced Diagnostic	
	Air	Bone	Air	Bone	Air	Bone	Air	Bone
125					75		75	
250			80	35	90	40	90	40
500	60		100	50	110	60	120	60
1000	60		100	50	110	70	120	70
1500	60		100	50	110	70	120	70
2000	60		100	50	110	70	120	70
3000			100	50	100	70	120	70
4000	60		100	50	110	60	120	60
6000	60		90		110		110	
8000			80		90		90	

This type of oscillator suffers from the disadvantage that it cannot be switched on and off easily without causing both frequency change and distortion. Consequently, where RC oscillators are used they are normally left running and the tone switched on and off by a gating circuit at the output of the oscillator.

Both the LC and RC oscillators are of the fixed frequency type and are not easily made to be continuously variable over the 100 Hz to 8000 Hz range required for audiometric purposes. The beat frequency oscillator (BFO) is capable of meeting the requirements of continuously variable frequency audiometers. The signal from the BFO can be interrupted easily and modulated both in amplitude and in frequency.

A different form of continuous frequency audiometer is that described by van Dishoeck (1962). Here the test tone is swept at a fixed level and the subject indicates the frequency at which he no longer hears.

(2) *Interrupter Switch*. The interrupter switch on the manual audiometer is operated by the tester and allows the tone to be presented to the patient. The switch itself must be mechanically silent in operation and be capable of being operated without the patient seeing the operator's hand move. It must also not give any other indication to the patient that the tone has come on, e.g. lights flashing, clicks. Some audiometers have a facility for having the tone on and switching it off, as well as vice versa.

The interruption of the tone can be achieved by switching the supply voltage to the generator as in the LC oscillator (Fig. 2) or by the operation of a gate as in Fig. 3. Current practice is to use opto electronic switches which make use of light dependent elements (such as photo resistors and photo transistors) Automatic interruption of the signal at a constant rate is available on some audiometers but, owing to the regularity of pulsing, may give misleading results. Whichever system is used the characteristics of the rise and decay time of the pulse formed by operating the switch must conform to the following: "When the tone switch is moved to the "ON" position, the time taken for the sound pressure level produced by the earphone to attain −1 dB relative to its final steady value shall not exceed 0·2 s from the instant of operating the switch. The rate of increase of the sound pressure level produced by the earphone shall not exceed 500 dB s^{-1} in the region −20 dB to −1 dB relative to its final steady value. At no time during the build-up or decay of the tone shall the sound pressure level produced by the earphone attain a value exceeding +1 dB relative to its steady value in the "ON" position. When the tone switch is

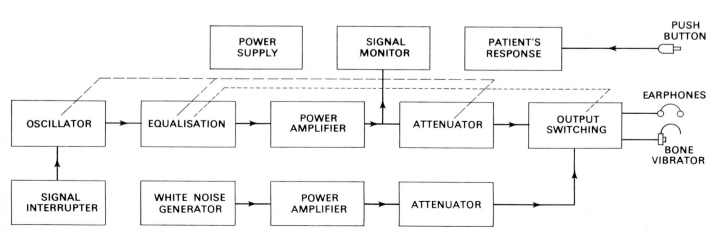

FIG. 1. Block diagram of a basic simple diagnostic audiometer. All parts joined by the interrupted lines have connections back to the frequency control switch. Thus altering the switch causes contacts connected to other parts of the circuit to be changed. The dotted lines joining equalization and output switching sections indicate that changes in equalization must be made where the output is changed from one headphone to another or when the bone vibrator is used.

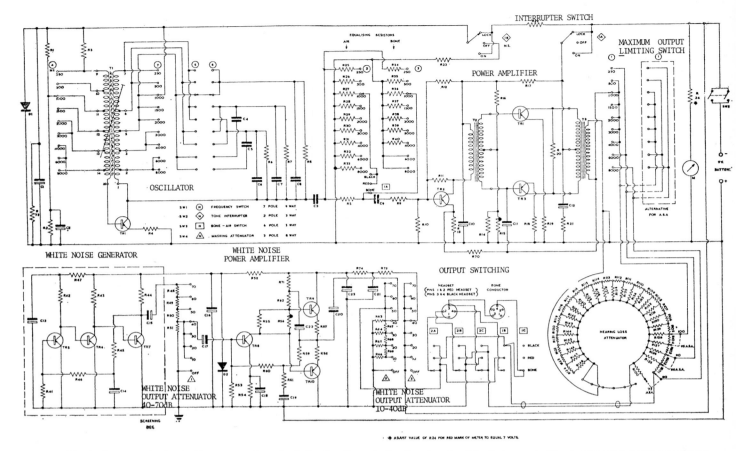

Fig. 2. Circuit diagram of a simple diagnostic audiometer indicating the main functional parts of the instrument. (By courtesy of Amplivox Limited.)

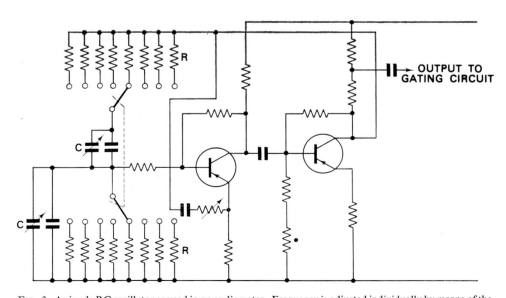

Fig. 3. A simple RC oscillator as used in an audiometer. Frequency is adjusted individually by means of the resistors marked R, while overall change to all frequencies is made by variable capacitors marked C.

moved to the "OFF" position the time taken for the sound pressure level produced by the earphone to decay from −1 dB to −60 dB relative to its steady value in the "ON" position shall not exceed 0·2 s from the instant of operating the switch. The rate of decay of the sound pressure level produced by the earphone shall not exceed 500 dB. s^{-1} in the region −1 dB to −20 dB relative to its steady value in the "ON" position." IEC 178 (1965).

(3) *Equalization.* The sound pressure level corresponding to the threshold of hearing varies with frequency and, if the zero on the hearing level dial of the audiometer is to be valid for each of the test frequencies, the output sound pressure must be varied for each frequency. The variation of sound pressure level is achieved by a set of equalizing attenuators situated between the oscillator and the power amplifier. A different set of equalizing resistors is used for each earphone and for the bone vibrator. The equalizing attenuators are switched by the action of the frequency selector switch. In older models of audiometers the setting up of the equalization was achieved by altering fixed resistors. Modern instruments tend to use preset potentiometers which allow precise adjustment. A typical equalizing circuit is shown in Fig. 2.

In continuously variable frequency audiometers an electromechanical cam system may be used to vary the output level with frequency.

(4) *Power Amplifier.* The output power available from the power amplifier determines the maximum sound pressure level available from the earphones and the bone vibrator, provided that the transducers are not overloaded. The amplifier must have low distortion and a good signal-to-noise ratio to meet standardized requirements, i.e. overall electrical noise should be 70 dB below the signal level and harmonics should be 30 dB below the fundamental at all frequencies.

The amplifier is often a Class B* push–pull output design. The advantages of this design are that, at low output levels, where the audiometer will be used most frequently, the current will be low and only at the higher levels will current become large, an important feature in battery operated instruments.

(5) *Hearing Level Control* (Output Attenuator): The hearing level control must be capable of adjusting the output sound pressure from below the threshold of hearing to some 110 dB above, and normally in 5 dB steps. This range of 120 dB is large and gives rise to design problems due to breakthrough of the signal and to electrical noise from the switch contacts.

Owing to the very small signals present at threshold (about 1 μV) any paths present due to stray capacitance or earth loops will cause the signal to by-pass the attenuator. Thus when attenuation is increasingly introduced the signal is reduced until a point at which break-through occurs is reached; beyond this point there is no further reduction of

signal level. Such faults give rise to a closing up of the attenuator steps. A range of 15 dB may, for instance, become 5 dB and threshold levels then appear to be very much better than they really are.

The movement of the attenuator control will cause a click to be heard as the switch moves from one position to another, particularly at high output levels. Consequently, attenuator switch contacts must be of a very high quality, and even then it will not be possible to remove the clicks at all levels. In manual audiometers the procedure should be to keep the tone off until the attenuator is turned to its position, thus avoiding the problem. In self recording audiometers the discrete steps of the switch are often replaced by a continuous wirewound tapped potentiometer, but these are prone to being noisy and are also liable to wear more quickly than stud switches. An alternative to the above methods is that used by one British manufacturer (Peters) who uses a continuously variable inductance coupled attenuator (Terman, 1943) (British Patent 1 146 261). This system has no switch contacts, but relies on a good mechanical system for ensuring the accuracy of the setting, giving an attenuator which is silent in operation.

Most attenuators, except this inductance coupled attenuator, are placed in the output of the audiometer and match the impedance of the earphone. The advantage of putting the attenuator in the output is that the signal and the inherent noise from the instrument are reduced together, thus ensuring that the required signal-to-noise ratio is achieved, particularly at the low output end of the scale. Owing to the limited power handling capabilities of the earphones and the bone vibrator it is necessary to limit the maximum output from the audiometer. This limiting is usually done by tappings on the attenuator which are selected by the frequency control switch. Limiting of output usually occurs at frequencies below 500 Hz and above 4 kHz (Table 1).

(6) *Power Supply.* The power supply for the audiometer may either be the main electricity or batteries. Design requirements for the power supply are that it should be able to supply sufficient current to the audiometer at high outputs without causing any undesired effect, e.g. excessive battery drain or overheating, and not induce any hum or other spurious signals at any setting. The supply must be stabilized against variations in the mains electricity and should be able to cope with a variation of ~10 per cent in supply voltage with a negligible change in performance. Battery audiometers must provide some indication of the state of the battery under load.

(7) *Switching Systems.* All audiometers, except single earphone types, must have a means of switching the signals from one earphone to another and also to the bone vibrator. The complexity of the switching will depend upon the type of audiometer. Table 2 lists the more favoured British switching combinations.

SIGNAL MONITORING

While not a main functional part of the audiometer an important addition is that of a signal monitor. It is reassuring to the tester to have some indication that a test tone is

---

* A Class B amplifier is a push–pull amplifier in which the transistors are biased approximately to cutoff. When operated in this manner, one of the transistors amplifies the positive half cycle of the signal voltage, while the other amplifies the negative half cycle. The output is then combined so that these half cycles give an amplified reproduction of the applied signal. The Class B amplifier is characterized by high efficiency, and large output power for a given transistor type.

TABLE 2

MORE FAVOURED SWITCHING COMBINATIONS
OF BRITISH AUDIOMETERS

Type of Audiometer	Switch Function
Screening	Select Headphone Left or Right
Simple Diagnostic	Above plus selecting bone vibrator and applying masking signal to opposite ear when using bone vibrator
Diagnostic	Above plus ability to put signal easily to left and right earphone one at a time though separate attenuators for loudness balance. Speech input–output as for loudness balance plus both left and right earphones together
Advanced Diagnostic	As above but with speech and masking to bone vibrator and ability to mix signals, or signal and noise in one earphone or bone vibrator

being presented to the patient. A visual indicator conveniently achieves this purpose. Many indicators, however, do not measure the test signal as recommended (Medical Research Council, 1947), but simply respond to a contact on the interrupter switch. Today, it is not difficult to fit circuitry that will detect the presence of the test signal prior to the attenuator and will indicate its presence. The indicator also allows levels to be set for speech audiometry.

SUBJECT'S INDICATOR BUTTON

While it is an easy matter to ask patients to acknowledge the presence of a signal by nodding their head, saying "yes" or raising a finger it is often better if a push button is available for the patient to press to indicate he has heard the signal. The push button simply lights a lamp on the front panel of the audiometer which gives the tester a clear indication of a response while allowing the patient more freedom in making a response. The push button should not introduce any click or other noise into the headphones.

SELF-RECORDING (AUTOMATIC) AUDIOMETERS

Von Békésy (1947) first described a method of audiometry where the patient controlled the setting of the hearing level control and adjusted it by means of a remotely controlled motor driven attenuator. Control is achieved by the patient pressing a hand held button when he hears the tone and keeping it pressed until he no longer hears it. He then releases the button until he again hears the tone, when he again presses the button. The patient continues to do this until told to stop. The effect of pressing the button is for the motor to drive the attenuator so as to reduce the output from the earphones and when the button is released

the motor is reversed and drives the attenuator in the opposite direction, thus increasing the output. The rotation of the attenuator is coupled mechanically or electrically to a writing system which records the movements; a continuous recording of the patient's reactions is thus made. With fixed frequency audiometers, the frequencies are changed automatically and when one ear has been tested the procedure is repeated on the other ear.

Self-recording audiometers have the advantage of providing a permanent record and of giving specialized diagnostic information but have the disadvantage of being more time consuming to use as well as making the test potentially more difficult for patients to undertake. The audiometers themselves are very much more expensive to purchase. Self-recording audiometers may be either of a fixed frequency or a continuously variable frequency type. The former are more frequently used for screening purposes, particularly in industrial hearing conservation programmes.

Variables on the audiometer are the rate of attenuation change and, in the case of variable frequency audiometers, the rate of frequency change. Proposed values for intensity change are 2.5 dB. s^{-1} as a preferred value with options of a half or double this figure. Values for frequency change are one octave per minute as a preferred value with half and double this value as options.

The effect of listening to a tone at a constant or slowly changing frequency is to cause adaptation and eventually fatigue. In order to overcome this effect which may have clinical significance, the tone is pulsed and a recommended value for pulse duration is 200 ms on and 200 ms off. Many audiometers have a choice of employing a continuous or a pulsed tone.

The widespread use of self-recording audiometry has led to an impression that the thresholds achieved with these instruments are identical with manual audiometry but, as Robinson and Whittle (1973) point out, this is not necessarily the case and the factors cited previously will all contribute to small changes.

Audiometers are also sometimes referred to as self-recording when they provide the operator with a system of guides for plotting conventional audiograms. These guides often take the form of an orthogonal pair of wires or scales which are moved with the movement of the frequency hearing loss controls and at their intersection a marker can be inserted to mark the audiogram chart. Some audiometers also have an audiogram drawn on the front of the instrument and bulbs light up at each setting of the controls thus enabling the operator to see and record the level without looking at each control.

SPEECH AUDIOMETERS

In order to be able to measure a patient's perception of speech one needs to deliver speech through earphones, or from a loudspeaker, at a known intensity and for the characteristics of the speech signal to be known. Fig. 4 shows a block diagram of a speech audiometer which may be a separate instrument or part of an audiometer. For loudspeaker outputs (free field or sound field being the

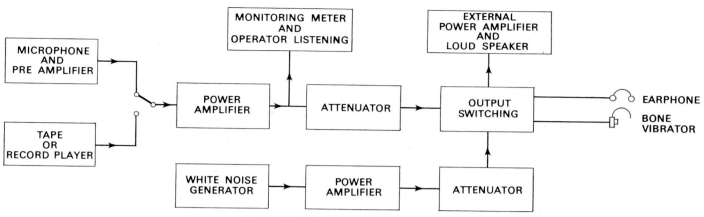

Fig. 4. Block diagram of a speech audiometer.

terms used to describe this method) an additional audio power amplifier is often required if an audiometer has speech facilities for earphone listening only. The simplest form of speech audiometer may be made by using an attenuator box with a built-in monitoring meter connected to a tape recorder and a pair of audiometric earphones. Knight and Littler (1953) described a simple speech audiometer and discussed the problems involved in speech audiometry. An essential feature of any speech audiometer is a monitoring earphone for the tester to hear the material being presented. At low levels, the tester may not be able to relate the patient's response to the score sheet without actually hearing the test words. The monitoring earphone may be of the inset type and should have loudness adjustment.

The reference zero for speech audiometry has not been standardized largely due to the present inability to measure speech signals in a way that will relate their content to a measured level. The information contained in speech is not easily related to the measurements made on the speech waveforms and different methods of measurement will indicate, apparently, different sound pressure levels for the same signal (Sjogren, 1973). The speech audiogram is often shown as an articulation curve the shape of this curve being determined by the speech forming the test material. Three reference points may be used on the articulation curve:

(1) The level at which 50 per cent of test words can be detected as being present (the threshold of detectability).
(2) The level at which some percentage of the speech material, usually 50 per cent, can be heard correctly (the threshold of discrimination).
(3) The level at which 100 per cent or a maximum of the material is heard correctly.

In spite of the problems involved in standardizing speech levels, those of around 20 dB SPL appear in the literature as the threshold of detectability (Carhart, 1966). In practice, users should take a group of normally hearing subjects and determine a normal speech audiometric curve from this group and for the particular form of presentation used. It is also essential that any speech audiogram should have written on it the sound pressure level that is used as a reference zero. As the sound pressure level for the 50 per cent score varies with material it is not a suitable point to standardize.

Scores achieved by a subject can easily be altered by the instructions given. It is therefore essential that the subject be given clear instructions as to how he should respond. If the subject is told to guess then scores will be higher than if he is told only to respond when he is certain that he is correct.

Recorded test material should have a calibration tone, normally 1 kHz, which may be used to set the monitoring meter on the audiometer to the same position at each test session. The level of the calibration tone on the recording relative to the speech material will determine the output range of the audiometer and also whether or not distortion will occur. Too low a level of calibration tone will cause the speech to be high and cause overloading of the audiometer's amplifier and subsequent distortion. Too high a level of calibration tone will cause the speech to be at a low level and consequently the audiometer will be incapable of delivering its maximum output. A suggested value is such that the value of the calibration tone is equal to the average speech level read off the same meter: the meter should preferably be of the peak reading type.

Speech audiometers do not lend themselves to be automatic or self-recording. Nevertheless, Stephenson (1973a and b) describes an experimental instrument based on a forced choice of two stimulus words. If a response is correct the output level is reduced and if incorrect the level is raised. Digital computer techniques are used to record correct responses and reaction times.

PAEDIATRIC AUDIOMETERS

When testing children between the ages of two and six, or older backward children, the tester conditions the child to respond correctly when the signal is presented. Conditioning may be achieved by means of games where a correct response results in a reward for the subject. Automated systems, such as the Peepshow audiometer (Dix and Hallpike, 1947), are available. The peepshow audiometer is a conventional audiometer which has a separate visual display system operated through the audiometer. When a test signal is presented and the child gives a correct response, the display lights up thus giving an automatic reward to the child. Many modifications of the peepshow have been used by workers all aimed at giving a more interesting reward for the child.

For very young children who cannot make a deliberate response such as by moving a toy or pressing a button, it is necessary to observe the child's response to an acoustic stimulus. The test often takes the form of a distracting signal presented through loudspeakers; pure tones or recorded real life sounds may be used. Crabtree (1972) describes a method of using filtered sounds to obtain a better indication of the threshold of hearing as a function of frequency.

The Stycar test (Sheridan, 1958) is the basis for most distraction tests and consists of making noises with common objects, such as tissue paper or a cup and spoon, and observing the reactions of the infant. The frequency spectra of these noises are often not what the tester assumes them to be and attention has been drawn to similarities in the spectra of different objects (Hodgson, 1972). The fundamental of the tone being sounded from wind instruments, such as pitch pipes, often does not appear (Delany, 1967; Martin and Barker, 1971).

A portable free field pure tone audiometer is now available commercially and is widely used for the testing of young children. (Crabbe and Denes, 1959; Denes and Reed, 1959.) The instrument consists of a battery operated oscillator driving a loudspeaker and covering the frequency range 250 Hz to 4 kHz at intensities up to 80 dB SPL at about 60 cm from the childs ear. The power output of this instrument is limited by the size of the loudspeaker that may be comfortably held and by the size of battery. The instrument is small enough to be held in the hand. Accurate audiometry with these instruments is restricted by the occurrence of diffraction and standing waves which make the sound pressure level at the patient's ear uncertain. To overcome these problems the RNID Technical Department has developed a simple hand held horn type loudspeaker system using filtered white noise in narrow bands which provides an output of 100 dB SPL at 90 cm. The white noise obviates most of the problems arising from standing waves.

Very small free field audiometers which are designed to be held almost entirely in the hand are available for testing infants (RNID, 1968). Generally, these very small audiometers have limited outputs and attenuator steps, and often only two or three test frequencies.

DELAYED AUDITORY FEEDBACK INSTRUMENTS

In the delayed auditory feedback test the patient speaks into a microphone whose output is fed to a system which delays the speech before replaying it to the patient through earphones. The effect of this procedure is to cause stuttering in most normal people and if the time delay and intensity are appropriate a complete blocking of the listener's ability to speak occurs. The test is of value in cases of malingering although there are people who are not affected by this technique. The delayed feedback is most easily produced with a modified tape recorder, where the signals are recorded by one tape head and replayed from a second head a variable distance away (Fairbanks and Jerger, 1951). The time delay between the two heads is, of course, dependent upon the distance between the heads and upon the tape speed; a third fixed head is useful for the tester to monitor the tape. It is of course a simple matter to have a recording of the patient's speech at the same time by means of a twin track recording. Fairbanks (1955) has shown that the maximum effect takes place with delays of around 0·2 seconds.

Delayed auditory feedback may also be used in a tapping task to alter tapping rates (Ruhm and Cooper, 1964). Price and Weaver (1964) describe electronic instrumentation which can be used with an audiometer to perform this task.

THE SISI TEST EQUIPMENT

Jerger and his associates (1959) described a test in which subjects are required to detect very small amplitude changes in a pure tone signal. The test procedure, Short Increment Sensitivity Index (SISI), involves producing an increase in amplitude of 1 to 5 dB on a continuous tone. The amplitude increase is contained in a 200 ms pulse every 5 seconds (Martin, 1972). Most ordinary diagnostic audiometers do not have the SISI facility built into them whereas some advanced diagnostic instruments do. For some audiometers, it is possible to obtain "add-on" units which provide the pulsing facility.

AUDIOMETRIC ZERO

While at first sight it might not be considered a difficult problem to arrive at an acceptable set of values of sound pressure level for the threshold of hearing for pure tones by earphone listening, it has proved to be a matter that has caused considerable difficulty over the years. To illustrate the problems involved the steps taken to achieve a standardized threshold for air and bone conduction will be described.

Subjects

A group of otologically normal subjects must be found who have no history of ear disease or of exposure to excessive noise. The age of the group must be limited and it is normally taken to be 18 to 25 years of age. Different age groups, however, will give rise to different threshold values. Even with children, thresholds have been shown to alter with age (Eagles et al., 1963; Delany et al., 1966; Lenihan et al., 1971) and with adults a large decline in hearing acuity occurs with advancing age (Hinchcliffe, 1959). A further effect that must be taken into account is the variation in individual thresholds with time; Delany (1970) has shown considerable individual variations with time and practice. A sufficiently large group, that is more than 20, should be used to ensure stable results.

Earphones

The measurement to be made is the threshold of hearing for earphone listening, and it is therefore essential that the earphone to be used is stable both in regard to its frequency response and in regard to its sensitivity. The method of coupling the earphone to the ear must also be specified, i.e. the type of earcap; different earcaps fitted to the same transducer can give rise to different threshold values. Moreover, the earphone must be applied to the ear by a known force which is sufficient to give a good acoustic seal. This is a factor which is often overlooked in routine audiometry where headbands may be allowed to become very slack, giving rise to spurious low frequency hearing losses. One of the most widely used earphones for audiometric testing is the Telephonics Type TDH 39 with MX 41/AR earcap. Figure 5 shows the frequency response of this and of other types of earphone.

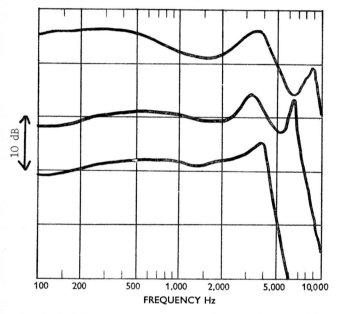

FIG. 5. Relative frequency response of three earphones used in audiometry. Constant voltage input with output measured on IEC wideband artificial ear. Upper curve is for S.T. & C. 4026. Middle curve is for Telephonics TDH39 with MX41/AR earcap. Lower curve is for Western Electric 705A.

Conditions for Testing

It is essential that threshold measurements on normally hearing subjects be undertaken in conditions of ambient noise that will ensure no masking of the test tones. Table 3 gives values of ambient noise in $\frac{1}{3}$rd octaves for measuring hearing levels down to the normal threshold of hearing. Fig. 6 shows a method of measuring background noise using a sound level meter (Berry, 1973). Subjects should spend some time in the quiet conditions before testing starts and should receive a practice session. The number of presentations of the tone should be limited, e.g. to four, at any level and by the method of limits the threshold found for a criteria of 50 per cent correct responses (Underwood, 1966). Instructions to the subject are most important since these can bias the results.

TABLE 3

THE MAXIMUM PERMISSIBLE SOUND PRESSURE LEVELS (dB RE 20 μPa) WHICH WILL PERMIT A LEAST HEARING LEVEL OF 0 dB TO BE MEASURED RE BS 2497: PART 3: 1972

(After Berry, 1973).

$\frac{1}{3}$-octave band centre frequency (Hz)	a For tests at 125 Hz, 250 Hz, 500 Hz and upwards	b For tests at 250 Hz, 500 Hz and upwards	c For tests at 500 Hz and upwards
31·5	68	68	78
40	63	63	73
50	58	58	68
63	54	54	64
80	48	49	59
100	44	44	54
125	39	40	50
160	34	32	46
200	29	29	42
250	26	26	38
315	30	30	33
400	24	24	24
500		19	
630		19	
800		20	
1000		21	
1250		23	
1600		26	
2000		34	
2500		37	
3150		41	
4000		43	
5000		40	
6300		37	
8000		37	

Acoustic Measurements

Acoustic measurements of the sound pressure level required to obtain the threshold of hearing can be made directly by inserting a probe tube microphone through the earcap to a point at the entrance of the meatus. These measurements, however, are extremely difficult to make and the more favoured method now is an indirect one. The ac voltage across the earphone is measured with a calibrated voltmeter and the rms reading that corresponds to the threshold for each test frequency for a given subject noted. The earphone used for the tests is then placed on an artificial ear or acoustic coupler and a voltage some 60 dB above that required for threshold applied to the earphone at each frequency used. 60 dB above threshold is used since the sound pressure levels at threshold are too small to measure easily in the coupler. The sound pressure level in the artificial ear is then measured and corrected for any differences between the voltage across the earphone for threshold and the voltage used for measurement on the artificial ear. The sound pressure level at threshold on an artificial ear for any subject is known as the Equivalent Threshold Sound Pressure Level (ETSPL) and when this sound pressure

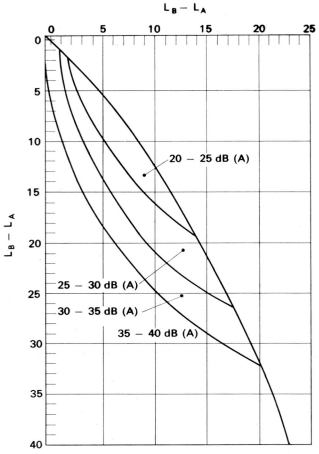

FIG. 6. Zones of maximum allowable sound level in dB(A) that ensure that an error of not more than 1 dB occurs at a hearing level of 0 dB (ISO, 1964). A sound level meter with A, B and C weighting networks is used in the following manner: (1) Measure the overall sound pressure levels in dB(A), dB(B) and dB(C); (2) Calculate the difference between dB(C) and dB(A), i.e. $L_C - L_A$; (3) Calculate the difference between dB(B) and dB(A), i.e. $L_B - L_A$; (4) From the figure locate the point whose co-ordinates correspond to $L_C - L_A$ and $L_B - L_A$. If the sound level in dB(A) is within the range of dB(A) values indicated for the zone in which the point lies then the room is suitable for testing for frequencies from 125 Hz upwards at hearing levels of 0 dB (ISO, 1964) and above.

level relates to a mean value for a group it is known as the Reference Equivalent Threshold Sound Pressure Level (RETSPL). The RETSPL is in fact the information presented in standards.

Standardization of Audiometric Zero

(Air Conduction)

From what has already been said, it may be difficult to see how very different values could be arrived at for audiometric zero but two areas have presented problems. These are in respect of subjects sampled, how they are tested and the artificial ear or acoustic coupler used for making comparisons.

In 1952, two laboratory investigations in Britain (Dadson and King, 1952; Wheeler and Dickson, 1952) provided threshold values for groups of known otologically normal

subjects which resulted in the production of a British Standard, BS 2497 (1954). Measurements were made on an artificial ear conforming to BS 2042 (1953) (Fig. 7) and using S T and C type 4026A earphones. In the U.S.A., the threshold of hearing was based on people sampled in a National Health Survey in 1937 and the results were

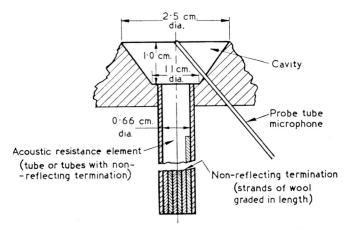

Principles of arrangement of artificial ear—microphone position A.

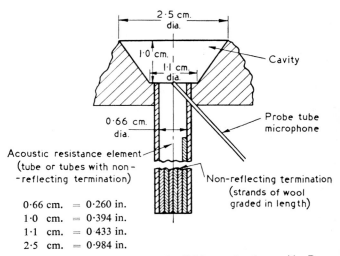

Principles of arrangement of artificial ear—microphone position B.

0·66 cm.	= 0·260 in.
1·0 cm.	= 0·394 in.
1·1 cm.	= 0·433 in.
2·5 cm.	= 0·984 in.

FIG. 7. Artificial Ear conforming to BS 2042:1953.

expressed in terms of a Western Electric Type 705A earphone using the American Standards Association's 9A acoustic coupler (Fig. 8). This is now also known as the IEC Provisional Reference Coupler IEC 303 (1970). The results from these two sets of measurements became known as the British and the American Standard for Audiometric Zero and differed by as much as 15 dB. Table 4 gives differences between the current ISO (International Standards Organization) standard and the American standard, the British standard being very close to the ISO at most frequencies. Naturally, a difficult situation arose with the American thresholds of hearing being some 10 dB less sensitive than those in the U.K. Other countries had also produced their own standards and only after a considerable amount of work was it possible for the International Standards Organization (ISO) to produce a standard ISO:R389:1970 which expresses the RETSPL not for one

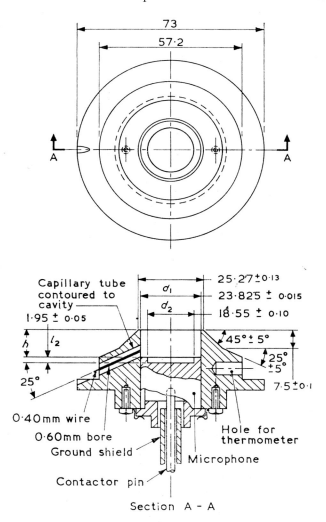

FIG. 8. IEC Interim Reference Coupler BS 4668:1971.

TABLE 4

REFERENCE EQUIVALENT THRESHOLD SOUND PRESSURE LEVELS FOR AMERICAN AND INTERNATIONAL STANDARDS

Frequency (Hz)	RETSPL dB relative to 20 μPa		Difference
	1951 ASA	1964 ISO	
125	54·5 dB	45·5 dB	9 dB
250	39·5	24·5	15
500	25	11	14
1000	16·5	6·5	10
2000	17	8·5	8·5
4000	15	9	6
8000	21	9·5	11·5

However, if earphones other than those specified are to be used then steps have to be taken to calibrate them either as outlined previously or by means of loudness balance procedures. It should be noted that each earphone has a different set of figures due to the interaction between the earphone and the acoustic coupler. If the acoustic coupler truly replicated the acoustic impedance of the ear as seen through an earcap then one set of figures should suffice for threshold. This indicates the difference between an acoustic coupler and an artificial ear. The latter attempts to duplicate the acoustic impedance of a typical real ear while the acoustic coupler is a simple device which does not attempt to do so. The development of such an artificial ear (Fig. 9a and b) has been undertaken (Delany et al., 1967), and has resulted in the introduction of a standard entitled The IEC Wideband Artificial Ear (IEC 318:1970; BS 4669: 1971). Further work by Delany (1969) has led to a single set of figures for threshold being standardized by the British Standards Institute (BS 2494 Part 3, B.S.I.:1972). These are tabulated in Table 6. Work is now being undertaken on an international basis to arrive at acceptable figures for an ISO Standard based on these figures.

Noise Excluding Enclosures for Earphones

Alternative earcaps are sometimes used on audiometric earphones, particularly those designed to exclude ambient noise. These noise excluding enclosures should reduce ambient noise, as its name implies, but not alter the calibration of the audiometer. In practice many enclosures not only do not alter the threshold but also do not attenuate the ambient noise, any more than the MX 41/AR earcap. (Coles, 1967; Martin et al., 1973.)

In evaluating noise excluding enclosures it is often felt by the listener that there is a large subjective effect in respect of the attenuation, but when this is measured and compared with the standard earcap little difference is found. It should also be noted that these enclosures are designed for adults and when used with children the attenuation is poorer by as much as 15 dB (Martin et al., 1973). Where the noise excluding enclosure alters the coupling of the transducer to the ear (often by introducing a large cavity), the characteristics of the earphone are altered and differences of up to 20 dB may be found, particularly at low frequencies. In testing the efficiency of noise excluding enclosures it is

earphone or one artificial ear but for five different combinations. While this was a step forward there were still inconsistencies (Delany and Whittle, 1967) and it did not permit manufacturers of audiometers to calibrate their instruments more accurately as the earphones used for standardization were not the ones used in practice. Considerable confusion reigned at this time and Rice and Coles (1967) found differences of up to 6·5 dB in the threshold values being used by different manufacturers of audiometers. While 6·5 dB may not be considered large in practical terms, if the maximum tolerances in output are added, i.e. ±5 dB., it is possible to achieve differences of 23 dB between audiometers that are within specification. An Addendum to R389 was produced in 1970 which expressed the RETSPL in terms of different earphones on the 9A acoustic coupler IEC (1970). Table 5 gives the values of RETSPL for a range of earphones in conjunction with the 9A coupler.

TABLE 5

RECOMMENDED REFERENCE EQUIVALENT THRESHOLD SOUND PRESSURE LEVELS IN THE 9-A COUPLER (AFTER BS 2497: PART 2: 1969)*
(For these data to be valid, the earphone is placed both on the ear and on the coupler with its earcushion, with one exception. When calibrating the Beyer DT 48 earphone on the 9-A Coupler, the cushion is removed and an adaptor, described by H. Mrass and H. G. Diestel, in *Acustica*, **9**, 61 (1959), is used. The values for the TDH-49 earphone are derived from a paper by M. E. Delany and L. S. Whittle in *Acustica*, **18**, 227 (1967).)

Frequency	Reference equivalent threshold sound pressure levels relative to 20μPa							
Hz	dB							
125	47·5	51·0	44·0	46·5	46·5	51·0	45·0	47·5
250	28·5	30·5	25·0	26·0	26·0	28·5	25·5	26·5
500	14·5	13·5	11·5	10·5	11·0	10·0	11·5	13·5
1000	8·0	6·5	6·5	5·0	7·0	6·0	7·0	7·5
1500	7·5	7·0	5·5	5·0	7·0	6·5	6·5	7·5
2000	8·0	7·5	7·5	7·5	9·0	6·5	9·0	11·0
3000	6·0	8·0	8·0	6·5	10·0	9·0	10·0	9·5
4000	5·5	10·5	9·0	13·0	13·5	9·0	9·5	10·5
6000	8·0	13·5	17·0	11·0	8·5	18·5	15·5	13·5
8000	14·5	20·5	13·0	13·0	11·0	14·0	13·0	13·0
Pattern of earphone*	Beyer DT 48 with flat cushion	S.T.C. 4026A	Permoflux PDR8 MX41/AR cushion	Permoflux PDR1 ADC case cushion	Permoflux PDR1 MX41/AR cushion	Permoflux PDR10 MX41/AR cushion	Telephonics TDH-39 MX41/AR cushion	Telephonics TDH-49 MX41/AR cushion

essential that the attenuation obtained be compared with a standard earcap and that the attenuations of the enclosure be measured with the transducer inside.

TABLE 6

REFERENCE EQUIVALENT THRESHOLD SOUND PRESSURE LEVELS IN A WIDE-BAND ARTIFICIAL EAR COMPLYING WITH BS 4669: 1971

Frequency	RETSPL relative to 20 μPa
Hz	dB
125	45·0
250	27·5
500	13·5
1000	8·0
1500	7·5
2000	10·5
3000	11·5
4000	13·5
6000	13·5
8000	16·0

Standardization of Audiometric Zero
(*Bone Conduction*)

The same steps taken for standardizing air conduction have to be undertaken with bone conduction. However greater difficulty exists in the production of an artificial mastoid with which to make measurements. The NPL (National Physical Laboratory) produced a design (Robinson and Whittle, 1967a), shown in Fig. 10, which was subsequently standardized by BSI (BS 4009 1966) for the U.K. In the U.S.A., Weiss (1960) produced an air damped artificial mastoid known as the Beltone Mastoid (Fig. 11a

and b) which does not contain rubber pads that are a feature of the NPL model.

Objections to the use of materials that might age have largely been overcome and experience (Whittle, 1970) has shown that, in practice, little ageing takes place. In order to produce an international standard it was decided that no specific design should be standardized and that only a set of mechanical impedances which all mastoids should present to a bone vibrator having a circular surface area of 1·75 cm² should be given. Owing to the problems involved, it was decided to term the measuring device a Mechanical Coupler, analogous to an Acoustic Coupler, to indicate that it only approximated a real mastoid. IEO 373 (1971) specifies the impedance requirements for such mechanical couplers.

In view of the difficulties in measuring the output from bone vibrators it is not surprising that threshold values have not been standardized and that considerable variations have occurred in the past. The importance of accurate bone conduction audiometry cannot be over emphasized since this constitutes a major diagnostic test; in practice the calibration of the bone vibrator is often totally ignored.

The testing of normal subjects for obtaining values for bone conduction thresholds requires not only very low ambient noise conditions, owing to the test ear being unoccluded, but a stated masking signal to mask out the non-tested ear and also a means of preventing airborne noise from the bone vibrator reaching the test ear. Whittle (1965) describes a method for overcoming these problems. A further factor at low frequencies is the harmonic distortion inherent in bone vibrators of the hearing aid type. Figure 12 shows the waveform for different output levels from a typical bone vibrator used on an audiometer.

In Britain, a standardized value for bone conduction thresholds in terms of acceleration measured on the British

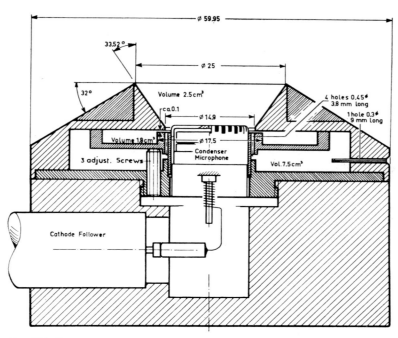

FIG. 9(a). Example of one specific design of IEC Wideband Artificial Ear (BS 4669: 1971).

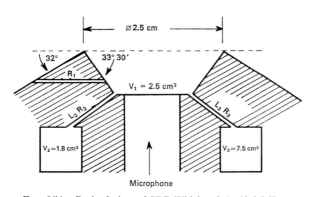

FIG. 9(b). Basic design of IEC Wideband Artificial Ear.

Standard artificial mastoid has been established. Lybarger (1966) has suggested values for the Weiss mastoid in the U.S.A. International comparisons of bone conduction threshold have shown considerable variations in thresholds measured in different countries and also a considerable variance in each set of results (Robinson and Whittle, 1966, 1967a). More recent work Flottorp (1973) has given further data very much in keeping with earlier results. In view of the problems involved in specifying bone conduction thresholds, BSI decided that a single value for acceleration was probably the most practical way of expressing the threshold; a figure of -30 dB relative to 1 m.s^{-2} is therefore recommended. It should be noted that this figure refers to an unoccluded test ear; some audiometer manufacturers calibrate their bone vibrators to cater for an occluded test ear. The effect of occlusion is to increase the sensitivity of the ear at frequencies below 1 kHz.

A small proportion of tests are made by placing the bone vibrator on the forehead and a correction has to be made for the reduced sensitivity which results. Table 7 gives suggested values for correcting from mastoid to forehead placement of the vibrator. Since the forehead is less sensitive, it reduces the degree of hearing loss by bone conduction that can be measured. This range is already limited in many audiometers.

TABLE 7

PROPOSED VALUES FOR CORRECTING FROM MASTOID TO FOREHEAD PLACEMENT OF A VIBRATOR

(After Whittle, 1965)

Frequency (Hz)	Forehead Sensitivity Relative to Mastoid Positions
500	-16 dB
1000	-11
2000	-7
4000	-5

AUDIOMETER CALIBRATION

In order to know that an audiometer is working correctly it is necessary to measure the following functions: frequency of test tone, purity of tone, output level through earphones and bone vibrator, effect of altering the attenuator (i.e. size of steps), rise and decay time of test tone and the level of background noise. It is possible to check an audiometer by measuring the hearing of subjects with known thresholds, but this does not give any indication of what is happening at other levels. However, it is essential that individuals using audiometers should listen to their instruments (and frequently) to ensure that there are no gross errors in the

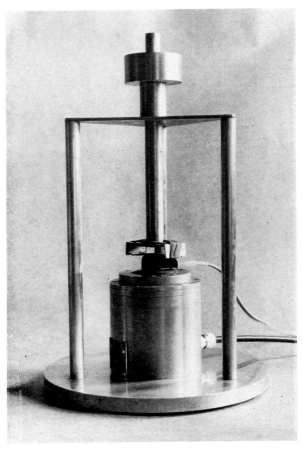

FIG. 10(a). Basic design of IEC Wideband Artificial Ear.

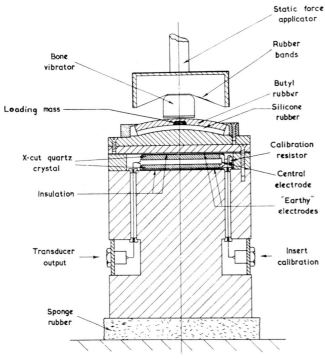

FIG. 10(b). National Physical Laboratory's artificial mastoid.

output or any spurious signals. Procedures for calibrating audiometers have been reported by Eagles and his associates (1963), Martens (1964), Harford (1965), Martin (1967) and Wilber (1972).

In order to fully calibrate an audiometer it is necessary to have an appropriate artificial ear or acoustic coupler together with selective amplifying equipment. A procedure that is often used is to measure the output from the audiometer at a level that is well above any noise, i.e. 60 dB HL (hearing level). At a 60 dB level there is sufficient sound pressure level developed in an artificial ear to enable a simple metering amplifier or valve voltmeter to measure the electrical output from the measuring microphone. Moreover, an electronic frequency counter can be connected to the amplifier to measure frequency simply and accurately. However the two measurements of frequency and output level at 60 dB are not sufficient in themselves and for a full calibration it is necessary to measure other parameters for which a selective amplifier is necessary. Harmonic distortion is best measured by means of a selective amplifier. By measuring the level of each harmonic the tester may then ensure that any degree of harmonic distortion is due to the test tones and not due to the presence of noise. With total harmonic distortion meters it is not always possible to separate noise from distortion. The selective amplifier is also necessary for measuring the accuracy of the attenuator steps. At high output levels there is no difficulty in measuring attenuator steps but at threshold levels there is considerable difficulty which can be overcome only by using a highly selective amplifier and a high test tone frequency, say 6 kHz, where the effect of ambient noise is negligible. In these calibration procedures, the measurements are all made acoustically. Experience with audiometer calibration services has shown that such acoustic measurements are feasible and do not require special conditions for the making of such measurements (Knox and Lenihan, 1958; Martin, 1967). Rise and decay times of test tones can be measured with the aid of a long persistence oscilloscope or a level recorder but for practical purposes a listening test will determine the presence of any abnormal times and also the presence of clicks and changes of tone. A listening test is also required to detect pure tones radiated acoustically from the audiometer.

Various surveys of audiometric equipment (Martin, 1968; Knox 1967) have shown that some users of audiometers pay insufficient attention to the state of their instruments which is somewhat surprising in view of the importance attached to audiometric tests.

MASKING

A wealth of literature exists on every aspect of masking. Here, it is intended to present only aspects of masking relevant to pure tone and speech audiometry.

Early audiometers (before 1950) provided masking in the form of low frequency sawtooth waveforms which were effective at low frequencies but much less so at higher frequencies. Difficulties also arose because of the harmonics "beating" with the test signal. The introduction of white noise generators using discharge tubes as the noise source

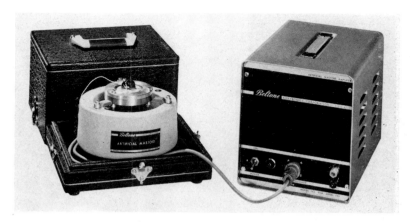

FIG. 11(a). An air-damped artificial mastoid.

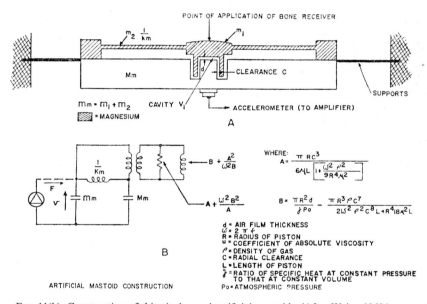

FIG. 11(b). Construction of this air-damped artificial mastoid. (After Weiss, 1960.)

provided a more efficient masking signal. Current audiometers usually use diodes as a noise source followed by a high gain amplifier. Later work showed that it was only necessary to have a narrow band (so-called critical bandwidth) of masking noise for each test frequency. This has the advantage of producing the same masking effect as a wide band noise but with a lower sound pressure level of the noise. In practice the critical bands (Table 8) suggested by Scharf (1970) can be approximated by one-third octaves and this conveniently allows existing specifications for filters to be used. IEC Recommendation 225 (1966) specifies performance figures for suitable filters.

Masking noise in audiometers falls into three categories:

(1) Broad band noise covering the full range of the earphones and giving a flat frequency spectrum, i.e. constant energy per cycle.

(2) Narrow band noise. This may be of constant bandwidth, approximate critical bands or be a constant percentage bandwidth.

TABLE 8

RECOMMENDED MINIMUM BANDWIDTHS FOR
NARROW-BAND MASKING

(The values tabulated are the critical band bandwidths
derived from Scharf's (1970) publication.)

Test Tone Frequency (Hz)	Critical Band Bandwidths (Hz)
125	100
250	100
500	115
750	145
1000	160
1500	225
2000	300
3000	470
4000	700
6000	1130
8000	1500

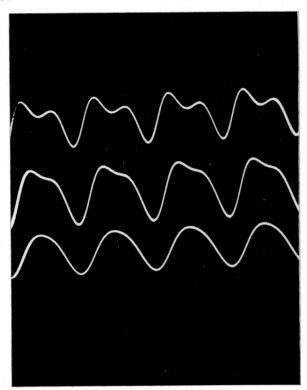

Fig. 12. Output from bone vibrator as measured on an artificial mastoid. Frequency 250 Hz. Upper trace is 45 dB above BSI threshold, middle curve 35 dB, lower curve 25 dB above threshold.

(3) A limited noise band. Simple high and low pass filters are chosen to reduce the noise at unwanted frequencies, i.e. for testing low frequencies, the high frequency energy is reduced. At mid frequencies, both filters are brought into play to give a simple band-pass effect.

For speech audiometry, broad band white (equal energy per cycle) or pink (equal energy per octave) noise is necessary as a masking signal. The use of competing speech signals as masking for speech has been shown to be even more effective than either white noise or white noise shaped to a speech spectrum (Olsen and Tillman, 1965). Studebaker (1964) has reviewed some of the practical problems found with audiometers using masking.

Standardization of the masking zero reference level for audiometers has not as yet been achieved owing to the difficulty in obtaining agreement on the bandwidth to be used for the noise and whether or not the level should refer to an effective masking level or simply the sound pressure level of the signal. The effective masking level can be considered as the threshold shift (in dB) produced by a stated amount of noise in the masked ear (Sanders, 1973). The manufacturer should state whether the masking noise and the test tone are fed through the same transducer or whether the two signals are fed separately to a bone vibrator and the earphone. The sound pressure levels of the masking signal are useful for calibration purposes and should be stated by the audiometer manufacturer. Where

there is a very large difference between the hearing levels of the two ears, the attenuation of some 50 dB which exists between the ears for air conducted sounds may not be sufficient to prevent cross-masking. The use of an insert (hearing aid) button receiver can increase the attenuation to 80 dB (Littler, 1967). Consequently, some audiometers have an insert receiver which provides the masking signal in place of, or in addition to, one earphone. Output levels from an insert receiver may be very much higher than from the main earphone. The disadvantages of this system lie in the variability of the masking signal owing to changes in positioning of the receiver in the ear.

A technique described by Peters and Littler and termed synchronous masking allows the masking and signal attenuators on an audiometer to be locked together so that any movement of the signal attenuator causes an equal change in intensity of the masking output.

THE FUTURE

The development of audiometers is dependent upon two factors. One of these is the evolution of new tests; the other is the advance of electronic technology. The latter has moved at such a rapid rate over recent years that a whole new generation of audiometers could be produced using recent electronic developments. The advantages to be gained from these new techniques would be mainly in the form of increased reliability. It is only recently that manufacturers have taken note of how audiometers are used in practice and ergonomic studies would probably reveal that considerable further improvements could be made. Earphones and bone vibrators present a limitation on performance at the present time and any improvements to these transducers would be reflected in more accurate audiometry. It must be remembered, however, that such developments need considerable sums of money. Consequently, developments may be limited for financial reasons; manufacturers of audiometers constitute small concerns and so are probably not able to provide the necessary financial backing.

At present audiology is firmly wedded to pure tone tests which, for clinical purposes, may be satisfactory. However where audiometry is undertaken for education or rehabilitation purposes, the pure tone is not an effective means of testing. New tests will therefore evolve using material which is not a pure tone but which resembles some form of sound heard in everday life. Speech is the most important form of sound in everday life and current work in the field of speech analysis and synthesis offer opportunities for a whole new range of tests and instruments.

ACKNOWLEDGEMENT

The considerable assistance of members of the Technical Department of the Royal National Institute for the Deaf, London, in the preparation of this chapter is gratefully acknowledged. Extracts from British Standards are reproduced by permission of the British Standards Institution, 2 Park Street, London W1A 2BS from whom copies of the complete standards may be obtained.

REFERENCES

Békésy, G. von (1947), "A new audiometer," *Acta Oto-laryng.*, **35**, 411–422.

Berry, B. F. (1973), "Ambient Noise Limits for Audiometry," *NPL Acoustics Report AC*60.

British Standard Institution
    BS 2042:1953. An Artificial Ear for the Calibration of Earphones of the External Type.
    BS 2497:1954. The Threshold of Hearing for Pure Tones by Earphone Listening.
    BS 4009:1966. Specification for an Artificial Mastoid for the Calibration of Bone Vibrators.
    BS 2497:Part 1, 1968. Specification for a Reference Zero for the Calibration of Pure-Tone Audiometers. Part 1. Data for Earphone Coupler Combinations Maintained at Certain Standardizing Laboratories. (Identical with ISO recommendation R389).
    BS 2497:Part 2, 1969. Data for Certain Earphones used in Commercial Practice (Technically identical with ISO recommendation R 389—Addendum 1).
    BS 2497:Part 3, 1972. Data for a Wide Band Artificial Ear Complying with BS 4669.
    BS. 2497:Part 4, 1972. Normal Threshold of Hearing for Pure Tones by Bone Conduction.
    B.S. 4668:1971. Specification for an Acoustic Coupler (IEC Reference Type) for Calibration of Earphones used in Audiometry. (Technically identical with IEC publication 303).
    B.S. 4669:1971. Specification for an Artificial Ear of the Wide Band Type for the Calibration of Earphones used in Audiometry. (Technically identical with IEC publication 318).

Bunch, C. C. (1943), *Clinical Audiometry.* St. Louis: C. V. Mosby.

Carhart, R. (1966), "Inconsistency Among Audiometric Zero Reference Levels," *ASHA*, **8**, 63–66.

Catlin, F. I. and Glackin, R. N. (1964), "Audiometer Design Principles for Long Term Stability," *ASHA*, **6**, 3.

Coles, R. R. A. (1967), "A Noise-attenuating Enclosure for Audiometer Earphones," *Brit. J. industr.*, **24**, 41–51.

Crabbe, H. and Denes, P. (1959), "Transistorized Audiometer," *Wireless World*, **65**, 563–565.

Crabtree, N. (1972), "Assessment and Treatment in Hearing Impaired Children," *Proc. roy. Soc. Med.*, **65**, 709–714.

Dadson, R. S. and King, J. H. (1952), 'A determination of the normal threshold of hearing and its relation to the standardization of audiometers," *J. Laryng.*, **66**, 366–378.

Delany, M. E. (1967), "A note on the acoustic output of several devices used in tests of hearing," *J. Laryng.*, **81**, 927–928.

Delany, M. E. (1969), "Proposed Values of RETSPL for the IEC Artificial Ear," *N.P.L. Aero Report AC*42.

Delany, M. E. (1970), "On the Stability of Auditory Threshold," *N.P.L. Aero Report AC*44.

Delany, M. E. and Whittle, L. S. (1967), "Reference Equivalent Threshold Sound Pressure Levels for Audiometry," *Acoustica*, **18**, 227–231.

Delany, M. E., Whittle, L. S., Cook, J. P. and Scott, V. (1967), "Performance Studies on a New Artifiical Ear," *Acoustica*, **18**, 231–237.

Delany, M. E., Whittle, L. S. and Knox, E. C. (1966), "A note on the use of self-recording audiometry with children," *J. Laryng.*, **80**, 1135–1143.

Denes, P. and Reed, M. (1959), "A Portable Free Field Audiometer," *Lancet*, **2**, 830.

Dishoeck, H. A. E. van (1962), *Technique of continuous audiometry,"* *Int. Audiol.*, **1**, 165–168.

Dix, M. R. and Hallpike, C. S. (1947), "The Peep Show," *Brit. med. J.*, **2**, 719.

Eagles, E. L., Wislik, S. M., Doerfler, L. G., Melrick, W. and Levine, H. S. (1963), "Hearing Sensitivity and Related Factors in Children," *Laryngoscope (St. Louis)*, U.S.A.

Fairbanks, G. (1955), "Selective Vocal Effects of Delayed Audiotory Feedback," *J. Speech Hear. Dis.*, **20**, 333–346.

Fairbanks, G. and Jerger, R. (1951), "A Device for Continuously Variable Time Delay of Headset Monitoring during Magnetic Recording of Speech," *J. Speech Hear. Dis.*, **16**, 162–164.

Flottorp, G. (1973), "Bone Conduction Threshold Data in Dahm, M.

(1973). Calibration Problems in Bone Vibration with Reference to IEC R 373 and ANSI 53. 13–1972," in *B & K Technical Review*, **2**, 31–37.

Grason, R. L. (1972), "Audiometric Measurement: 150 years of Applied Research," *Hearing Aid Dealer*, **23**, 13–15.

Harford, E. R. (1965), "Audiometric Calibration," in *Hearing Measurement* (I. M. Ventry, J. B. Chaiklin, R. F. Dixon, Eds.) New York: Appleton-Century-Crofts.

Hinchcliffe, R. (1959), "The Threshold of Hearing as a Function of Age," *Acoustica*, **9**, 303.

Hodgson, W. R. (1972), "Testing Infants and Young Children," chapter 26 in *Handbook of Clinical Audiology* (J. Katz, Ed.). Baltimore: Williams and Wilkins.

International Electrotechnical Commission (1965), IEC Publication 177, Pure Tone Audiometers for General Diagnostic Purposes.
    (1965) IEC Publication 178. Pure Tone Screening Audiometers.
    (1970) IEC Publication 303. IEC Provisional Reference Coupler for the Calibration of Earphones used in Audiometry.
    (1970) IEC Publication 318. The IEC Wideband Artificial Ear for the Calibration of Earphones used in Audiometry.
    (1971) IEC Publication 373. An IEC Mechanical Coupler for the Calibration of Bone Vibrators having a Specified Contact Area and being Applied with a Specified Static Force.

International Standard Organisation
    (1964) ISO Recommendation R 389 Standard Reference Zero for the Calibration of Pure Tone Audiometers.
    (1970) Addendum 1 to ISO Recommendation R 389—1964. Additional Data in Conjunction with the 9A Coupler.

Jerger, J., Shedd, J. L. and Harford, E. (1959), "On the Detection of Extremely Small Changes in Sound Intensity," *Arch. Otolaryng.*, **69**, 200–211.

Knight, J. J. and Littler, T. S. (1953), "The Technique of Speech Audiometry and a Simple Speech Audiometer with Masking Generator for Clinical Use," *J. Laryng.*, **67**, 248–265.

Knox, E. C. (1967), "An Audiometer Calibration Service—Is it Really Necessary?" *Sound*, **1**, 7–9.

Knox, E. C. and Lenihan, J. M. A. (1958), "The Scottish Audiometer Calibration Service," *Ann. occup. Hyg.*, **1**, 104–113.

Kranz, F. W. (1963), "Audiometer: Principles and History," *Sound* **2**, 20–38.

Lenihan, J. *et al.* (1971), "The Threshold of Hearing in School Children," *J. Laryng.*, **85**, 375–385.

Littler, T. S. (1967), "The Scientific and Clinical Aspects of Bone Conduction," *Sound*, **1**, 58.

Lybarger, S. F. (1966), "Interim Bone Conduction Thresholds for Audiometry," and *J. acoust. Soc. Amer.*, **40**, 1198.

Martens, A. E. (1964), "The Calibration of Audiometers," *J. acoust. Soc. Amer.*, **36**, 775.

Martin, F. N. (1972), "The Short Increment Sensitivity Index (SISI)," in *Handbook of Clinical Audiology* (J. Katz, Ed.). Baltimore: Williams and Wilkins.

Martin, M. C. (1967), "The RNID Audiometer Calibration Service," *J. Laryng.*, **81**, 833–847.

Martin, M. C. (1968), "The Routine Calibration of Audiometers," *Sound*, **2**, 106–109.

Martin, M. C., Barker, B. (1971), "Letter on Pitch Pipes," *Sound*, **5**, 106–107.

Martin, M. C., Lodge, J. J. and Williams, W. (1973), "Evaluation of Noise Excluding Enclosures for Audiometric Earphones," *Sound*, **5**, 90–93.

Medical Research Council (1947), "Hearing Aids and Audiometers" Special Report Series No. 261. London: H.M.S.O.

Olsen, W. O. and Tillman, T. W. (1965), "Re-evaluation of the Effects of Competing Speech on Aided Discrimination of Monosyllables," *J. acoust. Soc. Amer.*, **37**, 1205 (A).

Peters, J. E. and Littler, T. S. (undated), *The Synchronous Masking Technique.* Sheffield: Alfred Peters and Sons Ltd.

Price, L. L. and Weaver, O. R. (1964), "Modified Instrument for Pure Tone Delayed Auditory Feedback," *J. Speech Hear. Dis.*, **29**, 264–268.

Rice, C. G. and Coles, R. R. A. (1967), "Comments on the Lack of Standardization in Calibration of the Audiometer Earphones Most Commonly used in Great Britain," *J. Laryng.*, **81**, 829–832.

Robinson, D. W. and Whittle, L. (1966), "An International Ring Comparison of Bone Conduction Thresholds," *N.P.L. Report AP.* 23.

Robinson, D. W. and Whittle, L. S. (1967a), "Second Report on Standardization of the Bone Conduction Threshold," *N.P.L. Aero Report AC* 30.

Robinson, D. W. and Whittle, L. S. (1967b), "An Artificial Mastoid for the Calibration of Bone Vibrators," *Acustica*, **19**, 80–89.

Robinson, D. W. and Whittle, L. S. (1973), "A Comparison of Self-recording and Manual Audiometry," *J. sound. Vib.*, **26**, 41–62.

R.N.I.D. (1968), "Linco Paediatric Audiometer AU—1". Royal National Institute for the Deaf Test Report No. 6883.

Ruhm, H. B. and Cooper, W. A. (1964), "Delayed Feedback Audiometry," *J. Speech Hear. Dis.*, **29**, 4.

Sanders, J. W. (1972), "Masking," in *Handbook of Clinical Audiology* (J. Katz, Ed.). Baltimore: Williams and Wilkins.

Scharf, B. (1970), "Critical Bands," in *Foundations of Modern Auditory Theory*, Vol. 1. (J. W. Tobias Ed.). London: Academic Press.

Sheridan, M. (1958), *Manual for Stycar Hearing Tests*. Windsor: NFER Publishing Co.

Sjogren, H. (1973), "Objective Measurements of Speech Level," *Audiology*, **12**, 47–54.

Stephenson, P. W. (1973a), "An Automated Form of Speech Audiometry." Unpublished Ph.D. Thesis, University of Essex.

Stephenson, P. W. (1973b), "Reaction Time Measurements in Speech Discrimination Tasks—An Automated System with Closed Response Sets," *J. Phonetics*, **1**, 347–367.

Studebaker, G. A. (1964), "The Standardization of Bone Conduction Thresholds," *Laryngoscope*, **77**, 8.

Terman, F. E. (1943), *Radio Engineering*, p. 981 3rd Edition. McGraw-Hill.

Underwood, B. J. (1966), *Experimental Psychology*. New York: Appleton-Century-Crofts.

Weiss, E. J. (1960), "Air Damped Artificial Mastoid," *J. acoust. Soc. Amer.*, **32**, 1582.

Whittle, L. S. (1965), "A Determination of the Normal Threshold of Hearing by Bone Conduction," *J. sound Vib.*, **2**, 3.

Whittle, L. S. (1970), "Problems of Calibration in Bone Conduction," *Sound*, **4**, 33–41.

Wheeler, L. J. and Dickson, E. D. D. (1952), "The Determination of the Threshold of Hearing," *J. Laryng.*, **66**, 379.

Wilber, L. A. (1972), "Calibration: Pure Tone, Speech and Noise Signals," in *Handbook of Clinical Audiology* (J. Katz, Ed.). Baltimore: Williams and Wilkins.

57. AUDIOMETRY

J. J. KNIGHT

INTRODUCTION

Today hearing can be assessed with precision, providing that a number of important criteria are met. Some of these concern the design of the test instrument itself and the acoustic quality and calibration of its output with respect to agreed standards. Chapter 56 has dealt with these aspects and details are given there of some of the fundamental measures of hearing for which either national (British Standards) or International Recommendations and Standards have been produced. Human hearing is so very sensitive that its measurement is easily disturbed by adverse environmental conditions in the test room, particularly by too much background noise. Any distracting influence which will upset total concentration on the subject's listening task may affect the results of the test. However, the chief physical factor in the test room is the ambient noise level which ideally should be as low as possible, but in practice is recommended by the Department of Health and Social Security (1974) not to exceed 30 dB (A), in a room sound treated to give a reverberation time not exceeding 0·25 s (seconds). The environmental conditions required for audiometry are fully discussed in the chapter following, although the point needs stressing that there is a continual interaction between the subject whose hearing is to be tested, the room, the test and technique of the test, and the examiner. This chapter will deal with the fundamentals of hearing measurement using established techniques which involve a degree of co-operation on the part of the subject in some way acknowledging the presence of an acoustic stimulus.

Audiometry is practiced either to demonstrate that a person has hearing acuity within normal limits (as in school screening audiometry or in pre-employment audiometry) or to determine the extent of the departure from normality (as in assessment for possible medical or surgical alleviation of hearing loss, or for selection of a hearing aid). Furthermore, it is now used as a principal aid to diagnosis. The earliest, and the simplest, hearing tests were performed by measuring the response at threshold and often employed pure tones. The hearing level of a subject at a particular frequency is taken as the difference between the measured threshold and the accepted standard normal threshold. In psycho-acoustical usage, Fig. 1 illustrates the situation of a person with a hearing disorder affecting the high frequencies, compared with the average normal limits of hearing. In otolaryngological, and also in audiological practice, the corresponding pure-tone (threshold) audiogram is used as shown in Fig. 2.

Additional diagnostic information can be obtained from the results of pure-tone threshold tests with air-conducted sounds compared with the results from similar tests using a bone-conduction vibrator applied to the skull.

TUNING FORK TESTS

The foundations of many audiometric tests employed today were laid over two centuries ago when John Shore invented the tuning fork in 1711, a simple mechanical oscillator made of metal with a low damping factor to give a high degree of resonance. Thus, when struck in the correct way on a resilient pad, the fork oscillates at its natural frequency and radiates a pure tone. The basic tuning fork tests of hearing ascribed to Rinne, Weber,

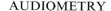

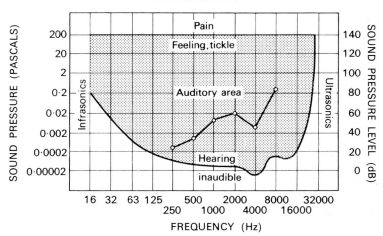

FIG. 1. Normal limits of hearing showing the thresholds of hearing and of pain, as plotted in psycho-acoustics. The raised threshold of a patient with impaired hearing is also shown. The threshold of hearing is for binaural listening in a free field. (Robinson and Dadson, 1957.)

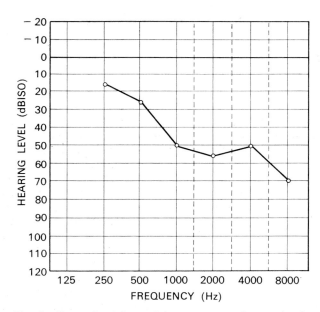

FIG. 2. Conventional form of the pure-tone audiogram for the patient of Fig. 1, plotted on the form agreed by the British Society of Audiology (B.S.A.) and the British Association of Otolaryngologists (B.A.O.).

Schwabach, Bing, Gelle and Pomeroy were reviewed some 40 years ago by a Committee appointed by the Section of Otology of the Royal Society of Medicine (1933) and were put on an excellent scientific basis.

At that time the National Physical Laboratory undertook the measurement of the decay time of otological tuning forks for air-conducted and for bone-conducted transmission and the Laboratory has continued to provide this service until recently. A 1000 Hz fork might have a decay of 1·6 dB. s^{-1} by air and 2·9 dB. s^{-1} by bone. Thus a subject for whom the fork became inaudible 20 s by air, and later 11 s. by bone, before the normally-hearing examiner's threshold was reached, would be deemed to have a hearing loss of 32 dB by air and 31 dB by bone. We would call this a sensorineural loss of approximately 30 dB at 1000 Hz. With large differences between the sensitivity of the two ears, the possibility of test sounds being heard by the better ear during tests of the poorer ear must be borne in mind. The procedure for masking is described in a later section. A noise source in the form of a Bárány box provides a means of masking the better ear for tuning fork tests. In the quiet test rooms we now use there is no reason why a tuning fork test should not be as accurate as one with the most sophisticated pure-tone audiometer. Once calibrated, the tuning fork's performance will not change, whereas the same cannot be said for all other electro-acoustic apparatus which needs re-calibration and service at frequent intervals. That pioneer of British scientific audiology, T. S. Littler was greatly impressed by the simplicity of the classical fork tests and advocated their widespread use e.g. Hinchcliffe and Littler (1961), and he detailed their application in his textbook (Littler, 1965). Johnson (1970) has lately reviewed the history of tuning fork tests in audiology.

Much of the fundamental scientific work on hearing measurement originated from the physicists and engineers in the national telephone laboratories. It was summarized in books by West (1932) in Britain, and by Fletcher (1930, 1953) in the U.S.A.

TESTS WITH PURE-TONE AUDIOMETERS

One disadvantage of the tuning fork in hearing tests lies in its uncontrolled intensity of radiated sound which decreases exponentially with time, or linearly with time when decibel units are employed. This no longer applies with a conventional pure-tone audiometer, where an electrically maintained oscillator supplies a controlled excitation to the earphones and bone-conduction vibrator. With a constant sound output available from the audiometer, the same basic tests to compare hearing for air conduction and for bone conduction with the standard values (zero decibels hearing level) are applicable as with tuning forks.

The basic tests have become routine procedures, but they need to be performed by trained audiological assistants who are constantly aware of the various pitfalls inherent in the procedures, understand the required performance and basis of calibration of the instruments, and are in sympathy with patients who are very young and those who are senile, and often ailing as well. Their task is to produce results of hearing tests for comparison with those standards obtained under the more ideal circumstances of testing young, healthy, normal subjects. Consequently, rigorous procedures must be applied in order to obtain repeatable results and ample time must be allowed the assistants in which to conduct the tests. There is sometimes a danger of otologists confusing the issue by requesting a whole series of different tests, where a single comparative test of air and bone-conduction thresholds at two or three central frequencies would confirm a tentative diagnosis. Sufficient time must always be allowed for application of the usual technical safeguards.

TEST PROCEDURE FOR CLINICAL AUDIOMETRY

In pure-tone threshold audiometry the psycho-acoustical procedure adopted is that of the method of limits described by Hirsh (1952), which was adopted by Dadson and King (1952) and by Wheeler and Dickson (1952) in collecting the normal threshold data on which the British and International Standards have been based. Slight variations exist in the detailed procedures for threshold determination described by Hinchcliffe and Littler (1958) and by Knight and Coles (1960) for use in audiometric surveys; both were based on the ascending method of tonal presentation of Hughson and Westlake (1944) and closely correspond to that endorsed by Carhart and Jerger (1959). For ordinary clinical purposes, a satisfactory procedure is as follows. The patient is told in simple language the aims of the test and the response required before the earphones are fitted by the assistant to obtain a good firm fit on the ears. The tones are presented first to the better ear in the order 1, 2, 4, 8, 0·5, 0·25 kHz and then 1 kHz again, the second determination at 1 kHz being the one finally noted.

The patient is first taught to respond by holding down the audiometer signal switch for the several seconds presentation of a pulse of 1 kHz tone at an estimated 40 dB above his threshold. The level is then reduced in 10 dB steps until the presentation is no longer acknowledged. At this stage it is worth asking the patient if he is sure that a faint sound cannot be detected, and to follow with a second short tone burst at this level. Next, an approach is, made from about 20 dB above this approximate threshold, reducing the tone in 5 dB steps and taking particular care to avoid a rhythm by altering the duration of both the tone burst and the silent interval within the approximate limits of one to three seconds. The threshold is crossed in a series of pulses of diminishing level and finally the "ascending" threshold is noted. Threshold is taken as the faintest level at which acknowledgement is given of at least

two out of four presentations of the tone with a duration between one and two seconds. Such a procedure applied to the ears at the six frequencies specified may take up to 15 min with each patient for air-conduction tests alone.

In bone-conduction tests, the better ear (for bone-conducted tones) is again tested first. This can usually be decided by an audiometric Weber test using a 500 Hz tone. If there is clearly a considerable difference in the bone-conduction thresholds between the ears, the better ear is tested without masking and with the vibrator on the mastoid process. The opposite ear is not fitted with an earphone unless masking is necessary, when due allowance must be made for a possible enhancement of the sensitivity to bone-conducted tones. Some workers have advocated forehead placement for the bone vibrator on account of a smaller intersubject variability, which is obtained at the expense of a 10–15 dB reduction in sensitivity.

CROSS HEARING

In air and bone-conduction audiometry where sound is applied to one ear, the contralateral cochlea is also stimulated by transmission through the bone of the skull. This is called cross hearing and is one of the pitfalls of audiometry to which reference has already been made. In the simplest case where there is a complete unilateral loss of hearing with normal hearing in the other ear, a "shadow" air-conduction audiogram will be obtained on the poorer ear showing an apparent average hearing loss of 40–65 dB according to frequency, if a suitable masking noise is not applied to the better ear when testing the worse. The detailed measurements are shown with Table 1 below.

If the tones are applied to a miniature hearing aid earphone the cross hearing is decreased in some cases to approximately 80 dB, according to Littler, Knight and Strange (1952). Other measurements have been given by Zwislocki (1953) and by Gyllencreutz and Lidén (1967). Subsequent re-examination of the 1952 data suggests that the early figures were unduly pessimistic for audiometer earphones and too optimistic for miniature earphones. It was later found that the degree of cross hearing with a miniature earphone is very variable among individuals. On average there is a slight improvement in the insulation across the head, but with some individuals there is greater attenuation with conventional earphones. Use of a different type of earphone for masking signals has additional disadvantages, not the least of which are a greater instability of sensitivity and placement uncertainties with the miniature earphone.

When testing by bone conduction, the average loss across the skull is approximately 5 dB. Thus in all bone-conduction tests, where the hearing level of each ear is required, a suitable masking procedure must be employed to eliminate response from the ear not being tested. In air-conduction tests, there is no need to mask if it has been already established that no element of conductive hearing loss exists, and there is no more than 40 dB apparent difference in sensitivity between the ears. In the presence of a conductive component, the situation is more complicated and masking must be introduced with less difference than 40 dB. In this case it is the difference

TABLE 1
CROSS HEARING WITH ONE NORMAL EAR AND COMPLETE UNILATERAL DEAFNESS.
TDH39 EARPHONE IN MX41AR EARCAP (N = 30)
(After Knight, 1960)

Frequency (Hz)	125	250	500	1000	2000	3000	4000	6000	8000
Mean (dB)	40·7	49·9	56·8	62·7	61·7	67·0	68·6	64·0	65·2
Stnd. Dev. (dB)	9·4	8·0	8·8	7·3	8·5	9·3	9·1	6·9	10·9

between the apparent (unmasked) air-conduction threshold of the test ear and the contralateral bone-conduction threshold which is of importance.

PRINCIPLES OF MASKING

Noise covering a wide or a narrow frequency band of the audible spectrum is generally used for masking in audiometry. In particular, in pure-tone audiometry, narrow bands of noise about one-third octave wide, centred on the test tone, are suitable. The concept of narrow band masking was first described by Denes and Naunton (1952). The masking effect on pure-tones becomes linear within a few decibels from threshold as shown in Fig. 3.

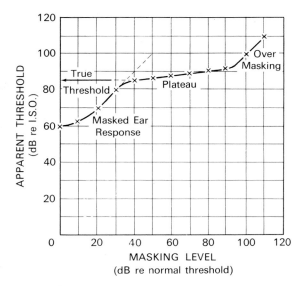

FIG. 3. Illustrating the graduated masking procedure applied to an air-conduction test. Patient has normal hearing in the masked ear, and an apparent threshold of 60 dB in the test ear which proves to be a true threshold of 85 dB with an appropriate degree of masking. The same principle applies to bone-conduction tests.

The principles of masking in clinical pure-tone audiometry were laid down by Littler (1950) and practised in the M.R.C. Wernher Research Unit on Deafness although they were not documented by him except in his book (Littler, 1965). In the case of air-conduction tests, with one ear within normal limits when the other gives an apparent (unmasked) hearing loss of more than 40 dB, the recognized procedure is to apply masking noise to the better ear at 10 dB above its threshold for the noise. If the measured threshold of the poorer ear is made worse, the masking noise must be increased by another 5 or 10 dB and the test repeated. When the threshold remains constant, despite successive increases in the level of noise to the better ear, the true threshold of the poorer ear has been attained. In this "graduated masking procedure", the aim is to determine the level of the plateau illustrated in Fig. 3.

These basic ideas must be carried out in the more complicated situations where the better ear is not normal and in all determinations of bone-conduction thresholds. There are no short cuts permitted in masking procedure, except in so far as it is often better to spend the available time with difficult cases in obtaining true (masked) thresholds at two or three important frequencies for air and bone, rather than pursue tests at all the octave frequencies from 125 to 8000 Hz.

Rainville (1955) proposed application of the masking noise by a bone-conduction vibrator to overcome difficulties in cases of conductive hearing loss. Jerger and Tillman (1960) modified the test and called it a test of sensorineural acuity level (SAL). The amount by which the noise transmitted by bone conduction shifts the impaired air-conduction threshold at a given frequency is compared to the shift produced in normal ears by the same noise. A shift of less than normal magnitude is taken to indicate a sensorineural loss equal to the difference between the normal shift and the observed shift. Lightfoot (1960) developed another variation of Rainville's test. Theoretically these tests have much to commend them but, in practice, there are difficulties and the tests have not been applied to any great extent in Britain.

OCCLUSION EFFECT

Whenever the ear canal is closed with the finger or is fitted with a plug, or even is covered by the earphone of an audiometer, the dynamics of the middle ear are affected under normal circumstances and the result is an increased sensitivity to bone-conduction stimulation, particularly for the lower audiometric frequencies. In conductive hearing loss, the occlusion is already present and no increase in loudness results from a bone-conducted tone on closing the ear canal. This is the basis of the Bing test for conductive hearing loss which is equally applicable to tests with a tuning fork or an audiometer.

It has often been stated in the past that the increased sensitivity on occluding the ear is an artefact produced by a reduction of the masking effect of ambient noise in the test room. That this is not the case is easily proved in any good audiometric room. Measurements of the occlusion effect with conventional audiometer earphones on uni-laterally hearing impaired subjects has shown that covering the impaired ear with an earphone improves the bone-conduction threshold and thereby reduces the cross hearing to the extent shown in Table 2.

TABLE 2
OCCLUSION EFFECT OF TDH39 EARPHONE IN MX41AR EARCAP (N = 6)

Frequency (Hz)	125	250	500	1000	2000	4000	8000
Occlusion (dB)	−12·5	−14·2	−4·2	−4·2	−3·3	+6·7	+12·5

Similar values have been measured in bone-conduction tests when an earphone is applied for masking purposes. Tables 1 and 2 together indicate that the cross hearing on unoccluded ears averages more than 60 dB at frequencies from 250 to 4000 Hz.

CARHART NOTCH

It was noticed during the era of fenestration surgery for otosclerosis that an apparent improvement often resulted in the post-operative bone-conduction hearing level, particularly around 2000 Hz. The notch in the pre-operative bone-conduction audiogram was first described by Carhart (1950). He showed that, with fixation of the stapes, the bone-conduction audiogram gave an unduly pessimistic indication of the so-called cochlear reserve to the extent given in Table 3 below.

TABLE 3
DEPRESSION OF BONE-CONDUCTION HEARING LEVEL
DUE TO STAPES FIXATION

Frequency (Hz)	250	500	1000	2000	4000
Depression (dB)	0	5	10	15	5

SELF-RECORDING AUDIOMETRY

It was Békésy (1947) who designed the first self-recording audiometer and, after this single publication to show its application, moved on to his many other researches. Soon the idea was taken up commercially and these audiometers began to appear in audiology research laboratories. The first in use in Britain was constructed at the Institute of Laryngology and Otology, London, and was demonstrated at the 1955 Physical Society Exhibition. McLay (1959) described a series of cases tested on this audiometer and later Hinchcliffe (1959) appraised some conflicting reports of the reliability and value of self-recording audiometers. Jerger (1960) described the characteristic four types of self-recorded audiogram obtained when traces are compared as a result of using pulsed (P) and then a continuous

(C) tone. These are reproduced in Fig. 4. Later Jerger and Herer (1961) described a fifth type of trace often obtained in non-organic hearing loss where, for no obvious reason, the continuous tone appears to be acknowledged at a quieter level than the pulsed tone and thus gives better indication of the true threshold.

A modification of the original Békésy audiometer principle was produced by McMurray and Rudmose (1956) for hearing tests in industry. Instead of using a continuous slow frequency sweep, the Rudmose self-recording audiometer selected six frequencies, usually 0·5, 1, 2, 3, 4 and 6 kHz, which were presented sequentially to the left and right ears for 30 s per frequency. Thus a complete hearing test could be performed in about 10 min including a short instruction and practice period for the subject. A typical chart is shown in Fig. 5.

At the present time, similar instruments are produced by several manufacturers and have many advantages in the clinical situation. While the older instruments had only an air-conduction output, the latest self-recording audiometers are comprehensive and include facilities for bone-conduction tests. One of the chief advantages of self-recording audiometers used in a busy clinic is that much of the tedium is removed from the assistant who performs the tests in having to decide whether the patient is really hearing, or not hearing, the presented tone. Precise instruction to the patient is essential in self-recording audiometry as well as a short practice period. Thereafter, every decision of the patient is recorded for later evaluation and the assistant need only supervise the conduct of the test. Less than 0·5 per cent of the adult patients from ear, nose and throat clinics are unable to perform the test satisfactorily, and those that have difficulty are often difficult to test by manual audiometry.

Self-recording audiometers are calibrated to the same standard normal thresholds as for conventional manual pure-tone audiometers. It is believed that this is a satisfactory first approximation pending acquisition of further data relating to the self-recorded threshold on which new standards can be based. Knight (1966) published results for 66 ears which indicated that there is slightly less than 1 dB difference between thresholds assessed in the two ways; self-recorded thresholds were the more sensitive. Robinson and Whittle (1973) have also reviewed this situation.

RECRUITMENT OF LOUDNESS

Recruitment of loudness refers to an abnormal growth of loudness with increasing intensity. It occurs predominantly in cochlear disorders and can be readily demonstrated in

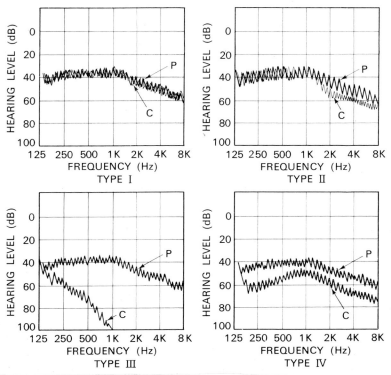

FIG. 4. Jerger's classification of self-recorded audiograms using pulsed (P) and continuous (C) tones.

Type I Predominates in middle ear lesions
Type II Predominates in cochlear lesions
Type III ⎫
Type IV ⎭ Predominate in VIIIth nerve lesions

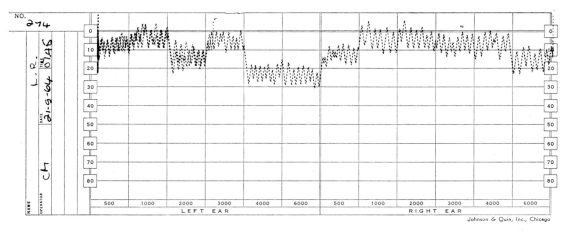

FIG. 5. Fixed frequency type of self-recorded audiogram introduced for hearing tests in industry. The tests at 500; 1000; and 2000 Hz for the left ear have been repeated finally, and show good agreement.

cases of Ménière's disease, which, characteristically, affects one ear. By matching the loudness of a tone applied alternately to the two ears, the phenomenon is revealed in the Alternate Binaural Loudness Balance test (ABLB). Some authors refer to recruitment as "regression".

It was first described by Pohlman and Krantz (1924), and Fowler (1936) devised the Loudness Balance Test. A classic summary of this and other so-called recruitment tests was published by de Bruine-Altes (1946). Since that time, the description and evaluation of numerous tests for recruitment have taken up a large section of the audiological publications. In Britain, the M.R.C. Unit at Queen Square has been particularly active in investigating the phenomenon by the Alternate Binaural Loudness Balance Test as it was held to be a means of distinguishing cochlear lesions (which recruit) from retrocochlear lesions (which generally do not recruit) (see Dix et al., 1948; Hallpike and Hood, 1959; Hood, 1969). Hood insists that loudness balance should be performed only when one ear is normal and that a fixed level of tone should always be presented to this better ear to be balanced by "bracketing" its loudness by altering the levels on the poorer ear. The tones should be presented alternately to the two ears in pulses of about 0·3 s duration with a changeover interval of twice this period. Several presentations of each pair of levels should be made before the patient says which ear heard the louder tone. With strict adherence to these rules, he claims a 90 per cent success rate in detecting nerve fibre lesions. However, there is not total agreement on Hood's method of fixing the level to the control ear nor on the necessity for the control ear to be normal, for the test only demonstrates a recruitment of one ear with respect to the other. If the better ear has a conductive hearing loss, or a non-recruiting sensorineural hearing loss, recruitment of the opposite ear will still be revealed. It is only when both ears recruit equally that recruitment of the test ear will be hidden on a loudness balance, and other means of detection must be used. Figure 6 shows the recommended form of presentation of the results of an ABLB test, with some of the results which may be obtained.

The alternate binaural loudness balance is accepted as the true method of measuring recruitment but, because of the requirement of one normal, or at least one non-recruiting ear against which the balance is performed, many other indirect methods have been proposed. One group of such methods has attempted to detect changes in the differential sensitivity to intensity as an indication of recruitment. This just noticeable change is called the difference limen for intensity. Békésy (1947) showed a threshold tracing of an ear with hearing loss having a reduced excursion at high frequencies and he considered this indication of a reduced difference limen to be a manifestation of recruitment. However, further investigations with self-recording audiometers (and a continuous test tone) have shown that the narrow excursions rarely occur below about 1500 Hz— even though the same ear may exhibit recruitment at 250 or 500 Hz on the alternate binaural loudness balance. It appears that both recruitment and the narrow high-frequency trace are related to cochlear lesions, which is

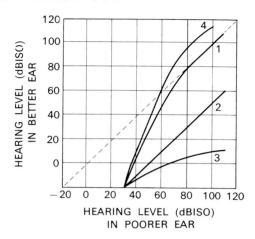

FIG. 6. Results of Alternate Binaural Loudness Balance Tests plotted in the form agreed by B.S.A. and B.A.O
(1) Complete Recruitment
(2) No Recruitment
(3) Loudness Reversal
(4) Over Recruitment

more important information than knowledge of whether the ear recruits.

In the normal ear, the difference limen for intensity near threshold is 3 or 4 dB at 1000 Hz; for tones 40 dB more intense, it is less than 1 dB. Lüscher and Zwislocki (1948, 1951) and Lüscher (1951) hence proposed a measurement of the difference limen at 40 dB above the threshold of the disordered ear as a recruitment test. A special circuit attached to the pure-tone audiometer enabled a steady tone to be modulated once or twice a second with an incremental intensity variable in the range 0·1–5 dB. By and large, normally-hearing persons and those with conductive hearing losses could detect variations of 1 dB or more, whereas some Ménière's disease patients with recruitment were sensitive to variations of 0·2 or 0·4 dB. However, the test was not found to be very reliable. Jerger (1952) proposed certain modifications to the original test and again this did not find great favour in Britain, although the original test has been used until recently in Europe.

Another variation of this type of test for cochlear involvement was proposed by Jerger, Shedd and Harford (1959) under the name of Short Increment Sensitivity Index (SISI). This requires the patient to report the number of 1 dB increments of 0·2 s duration heard at 5 s intervals on a steady tone 20 dB above his threshold; 20 presentations of the increment constitute the test. Normal hearing, conductive hearing loss and retrocochlear lesions tend to produce a poor score (0–15 per cent) while cochlear pathologies tend to give 80–100 per cent scores. As with the difference limen tests, this test is not used to any great extent in Britain, although it has a vogue in U.S.A.

Watson and Tolan (1949) describe the determination of a most comfortable loudness level (MCL) for pure tones. It can be traced most easily on self-recording audiometry and recruitment can be judged on inspection of its relation to the threshold curve. This procedure is used routinely in many clinical investigations by Hinchcliffe (1969).

Hood and Poole (1966) adopted a simpler test of the same character called the Loudness Discomfort Level test (LDL). In this, the patient is asked to indicate when a tone presented from a manually-operated pure-tone audiometer becomes uncomfortably loud as the intensity is increased from a hearing level of 80 dB. Ninety per cent of normally hearing subjects find 90–105 dB unpleasant, while the same figures apply to the disordered ears of patients with Ménière's disease, even though some may have losses of up to 80 dB. This finding is taken as a demonstration of the compression of loudness function that accompanies recruitment, together with a demonstration of the constancy of the upper limit of the loudness-intensity function.

In conductive and nerve-fibre hearing losses, where recruitment is not found, the LDL's are found to be raised. Hood and Poole conclude that if no discomfort is experienced in pure sensorineural losses with tones up to 120 dB hearing level there is a 90 per cent probability of the lesion being in the nerve fibre.

The test has great merit in its simplicity and the short time required for its performance. However, it has a disadvantage in that is operates near the maximum output of most audiometers, and all but the most experienced technicians might influence the result unconsciously by observing the hearing level control of the audiometer during performance of the test.

Finally, careful consideration needs to be given during all these tests to masking requirements for it is all too easy to obtain erroneous results in some cases by neglect of cross hearing.

ADAPTATION AND FATIGUE

Many different terms have been applied to the decline of threshold with time for a sustained tone. In certain disorders of hearing the decline is marked and it has therefore been studied extensively for diagnostic purposes both with self-recording audiometry—Hood (1950); Reger and Kos (1952), and with manual pure-tone audiometry—Hood (1955); Carhart (1957) and Stephens and Hinchcliffe (1968). Hood experimented with per-stimulatory and post-stimulatory fatigue. Carhart coined the term "tone decay" for per-stimulatory adaptation or fatigue at threshold. Slight variations of technique exist as applied to the conventional manual presentation of the test tone for measurement of tone decay.

A form of test currently used at the Royal National Throat, Nose and Ear Hospital, London, is as follows. A frequency is selected where an appreciable hearing loss exists. The patient is instructed to indicate as soon as the tone is no longer heard, and the tone is applied 5 dB above the measured threshold simultaneously with a stop watch being started. If the tone is heard for one minute, there is no tone decay. If the patient indicates that the tone has completely gone, the hearing level control is increased by 5 dB. The procedure is continued until one minute has elapsed since the onset of the first presentation. The decay is expressed as the difference between the final threshold level after one minute, and the original threshold level. The diagnostic value of the test is that cochlear disorders

seldom give a tone decay greater than 20 dB, while retrocochlear (nerve fibre) disorders often show more than 30 dB threshold decay in one minute. In normal hearing, and in conductive hearing loss, the tone can usually be heard for a full minute at 5 dB above threshold.

Workers investigating noise-induced hearing loss have often tried to relate temporary auditory fatigue, or temporary threshold shift (TTS), to the possible permanent threshold shift (PTS) which might result from more prolonged exposure to the noise. So far this approach has been unsuccessful; *see* Ward, Glorig and Sklar (1959) and Chapter 11.

EFFECT OF AGE ON HEARING

It has been shown that hearing sensitivity deteriorates systematically with time, at least from early adult life. Rosen and his colleagues (1964) indicated that exposure to noise in Western civilizations was responsible for much of this deterioration, but Bergman (1966) cast some doubt on this view. The differences between the hearing levels of the Mabaan tribe in the Sudan and, for example, the widely-accepted results of Hinchcliffe (1959) for random sample British rural communities are now largely attributed to nutritional differences among the populations in the two countries. Figure 7 shows the average effect of age on hearing according to Hinchcliffe.

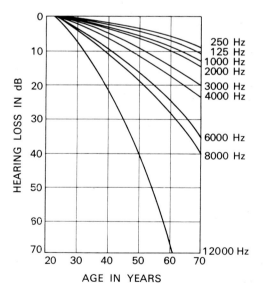

Fig. 7. Smoothed presbyacusis curves. The curve for 500 Hz is omitted to avoid overcrowding; it lies between the curves for 125 and 250 Hz. The curves are equally applicable to men and women up to the age of 54 years and for frequencies up to 2 kHz. Above this age and frequency the curves apply to women.

This average presbyacusis correction needs to be subtracted from any measured hearing level in order to establish the component due to aural pathology or exposure to noise etc.

EFFECT OF MECHANICS OF MIDDLE EAR ON THE AUDIOGRAM

The middle ear can be treated as a simple mechanical system comprising a mass, M; a stiffness, S; and a resistance, R. Then for a frequency, f, the mechanical impedance, Z of the system is given by

$$Z = \sqrt{R^2 + \left(2\pi f M - \frac{S}{2\pi f}\right)^2}$$

Thus, for the higher frequencies, the impedance will be largely controlled by the reactive term involving mass. Any increase in mass of the system will therefore increase the impedance at high frequencies giving a high frequency loss in the air-conduction audiogram, as occurs in advanced otosclerosis.

An increased stiffness, as in early otosclerosis, on the other hand, will result in a maximum effect at low frequencies, producing the so-called low-frequency "stiffness tilt" in the audiogram. Decreased stiffness, as in ossicular discontinuity, results in a high-frequency loss as does increased mass. Johansen (1950), among others, has reviewed the implications of the impedance formula given above.

Apart from these factors, transmission of sound through the middle ear is affected by the intra-aural reflexes (Reger, 1960). This is another example of an increased stiffness causing mainly a low-frequency insensitivity.

Sound transmission is also influenced by abnormal air-pressures (usually reduced pressure resulting from auditory tubal dysfunction) and by fluid in the middle ear. Great advances in the diagnosis of these conditions have been made in the last decade by application of techniques of measurement using the concept of acoustical impedance. These are considered fully in Chapter 19.

SPEECH AUDIOMETRY

The majority of the tests detailed above for use with pure-tone audiometers relied on threshold determinations. As we seldom listen to pure tones in ordinary life and only rarely are we concerned with threshold sounds, these tests are rather unrealistic. Those with disordered hearing are most handicapped by their difficulties in communication by speech, which is usually received at supra-threshold levels. Their problems are somewhat similar to those encountered by telephone engineers in communication problems over poor telephone links. Fletcher (1929) described the use of articulation curves relating to the percentage of speech sounds received correctly with various intensities. A similar method was adapted by Fry (1946) for testing the hearing of war-time aircrew and later was used for hearing aid evaluation and development by the Medical Research Council (1947). The British procedure has employed principally sentence lists and phonetically-balanced (PB) monosyllabic word lists (Fry and Kerridge 1939; Fry 1964), while workers in the U.S.A. have used the so-called spondee word lists (disyllabic

words of equal stress) and different monosyllabic phonetically-balanced lists (Egan, 1948).

Speech audiometry is used following pure-tone audiometry as a diagnostic aid (Coles, 1972), as a better means of assessing the social handicap, and in order to confirm the benefit of a particular hearing aid. An early form of free-field speech audiometer for clinical use was described by Knight and Littler (1953), but current practice generally employs the close-coupled earphone of the pure-tone audiometer, except for applications in hearing aid assessment. Some of the most reliable and well-used material for speech audiometry has been the 78 rpm discs produced for the M.R.C. Electro-Acoustics Committee which, unfortunately, were never transferred to long-play recordings. However, Fry (1964) has made available magnetic tape recordings of similar PB word lists.

The accepted form of the speech audiogram is shown in Fig. 8 which shows an average normal curve for a particular apparatus and a specified speech material; also the

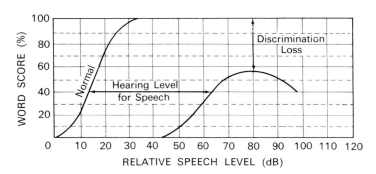

FIG. 8. Speech audiogram of a patient with a sensorineural hearing loss. Form is that agreed by B.S.A. and B.A.O.

curve of a patient with a moderately severe sensorineural hearing loss. The curve shows the hearing level for speech to be 50 dB (the displacement from normal at the 40–50 per cent articulation level) with a discrimination loss of 45 per cent. The hearing level for speech is sometimes referred to as the Speech Reception Threshold (SRT) in the U.S.A. While few national standards exist for speech audiometry, because of inherent difficulties in agreeing on the method of measurement of the sound pressure level of individual speech sounds, material for speech audiometry is available for most European languages including French, German, Spanish, Italian etc. Recently attention has been given to developing similar material in Arabic (Alusi et al., 1974), and a number of African languages (Muyunga, 1974).

Assessment of hearing loss by speech tests with a high-quality reproduction system takes us towards a real life situation but seldom are we able to listen under such ideal conditions without the intrusion of interfering sounds and background noises. These are sometimes deliberately introduced into speech audiometry for clinical purposes as was originally done during the war-time tests already referred to.

Independent of the use of these background noises it is of course imperative to mask appropriately the better ear during speech audiometry of the poorer ear when there is more than a 40 dB difference in hearing level. A wide frequency band of random noise is then required rather than the narrow-band noises used in pure-tone audiometry.

In U.S.A. attempts are being made to adapt to speech audiometry a modified rhyme test (MRT) for phonemic differentiation (Fairbanks, 1958; House et al., 1965) used for testing commercial and military communication equipment. As far as is known no use has been made of such material in Britain where most workers either employ the M.R.C. Word or Sentence lists, Fry's lists or, for children, various word lists developed at Manchester University (Watson, 1967).

DIAGNOSTIC AUDIOMETRY

Conductive Hearing Loss

This, the easiest form of hearing loss to alleviate medically, surgically or with a hearing aid, is diagnosed audiometrically when the bone-conduction threshold level is within normal limits (after due allowance for the Carhart notch) in the presence of a depressed air-conduction threshold level. Clinically, this would be detected initially by tuning fork tests and confirmed by pure-tone audiometry. However, the possibility of an ear being completely deaf must never be overlooked, particularly when it is presented during a busy out-patient clinic. The resulting false negative Rinne response can only be elucidated with strict adherence to the approved masking procedures already described.

The widespread introduction of acoustic impedance measurements (Chapter 19) has aided the diagnosis of some types of conductive hearing loss, particularly in young children, by an easy rapid measurement in which a minimum of co-operation is required from the patient.

Sensorineural Hearing Loss

When tuning fork tests and suitably-masked pure-tone audiometry indicate a bone-conduction threshold level depressed approximately to the extent of the air-conduction level, further tests are indicated to attempt to establish the site of the lesion. In unilateral cases, the first choice is the alternate binaural loudness balance (ABLB). It is generally agreed that the presence of recruitment indicates with a high probability that the disorder is seated in the cochlea, A self-recorded audiogram with pulsed tone, repeated with a continuous tone, should be used for additional evidence of a cochlear disorder. In a case of bilateral sensorineural hearing loss, where loudness balance is inappropriate, the self-recorded audiogram tests should be performed routinely. Here, if additional tests are required in order to exclude the possibility of a retrocochlear lesion, speech audiometry and a test for abnormal auditory adaptation should be used.

Cochlear disorders characteristically show recruitment and give a Type II self-recorded audiogram with con-tinuous-tone threshold appearing poorer than the corre-sponding pulsed-tone threshold at the higher frequencies.

Tests for abnormal auditory adaptation may show moderate "decay" and speech audiograms have a lower than normal slope with some discrimination loss.

During the 1950's, Langenbeck claimed to use masking noise to differentiate between cochlear and nerve fibre hearing losses. Nerve fibre lesions were found to give masking thresholds 10–15 dB higher than those found in cochlear disorders and in normal ears. An account of these findings is also given in his book (Langenbeck, 1962), but, after repeating this work, Palva and his associates (1953) concluded that the masked threshold was not a useful indicator for the differential diagnosis of these conditions.

Retrocochlear disorders may or may not show recruitment. They show abnormal degrees of "tone decay" which is also detected by a Type III or Type IV self-recorded audiogram. In addition they are distinguished from cochlear disorders by speech audiometry when the neural disorders almost invariably give poorer maximum discrimination scores than occur with cochlear disorders of similar average pure-tone loss (Coles, 1972).

Central Hearing Loss

This is discussed in Chapter 25.

Non-organic hearing loss

Until a few years ago non-organic hearing loss was considered to be extremely rare except in the Services, where it has often been reported in the extreme form of malingering. With the availability of objective forms of audiometry in clinical practice in Britain from 1965 (Beagley and Knight, 1966), many more cases have been found than had hitherto been suspected. Some of these have been in adults but, what is more surprising, is the prevalence of non-organic hearing loss in children (Beagley and Knight, 1967, 1968).

Frequently such cases can be detected by discrepancies between the results of pure-tone and speech audiometry; speech tests in non-organic hearing loss showing much better hearing levels than would be expected from the pure-tone audiogram. The Stenger test performed with tuning forks or audiometrically is also favoured. Self-recorded audiograms frequently show inconsistencies as well as overall a Type V result. Acoustic impedance measurements of the intra-aural reflex thresholds are of value, but the auditory evoked response threshold is crucial in such cases.

AUDIOMETRY IN INDUSTRY

It is more than two centuries since occupational hearing loss was recorded in coppersmiths and blacksmiths (Kylin, 1960), yet it is only in recent years that serious attempts have been made to prevent damage to hearing in noisy industrial processes. Following a series of investigations into noise-induced hearing loss in the Royal Navy by Coles and Knight (1965), a large-scale survey into hearing loss in British industry was sponsored by the Government (Knight, 1971). It has recently resulted in occupational noise-induced hearing loss being accepted on a limited scale for compensation purposes under the Industrial Injuries Act. Also there have been a number of successful common-law actions for damages in British courts for hearing loss, and this has produced a renewed interest in pre-employment, and periodic retest, audiometry in many industries where there is a potential noise hazard to hearing.

An account of the damaging effects of noise on hearing was given by Knight (1969) and a more complete analysis of the effects of noise on man by Burns (1974). In hearing tests in industry, there are three main problems. First, there is the difficulty of finding a suitably quiet situation in which to test hearing. This is sometimes overcome by employment of a mobile audiometric facility such as was described by Copeland and his colleagues (1964), which was used on the Government survey. The second problem often involves finding a suitably-trained nurse or technician to perform the audiometry, and to ensure that the audiometer remains in correct calibration. Finally, it is sometimes a difficult matter to decide how much of an individual's measured hearing loss is attributable to a particular noise when he has often had a multiplicity of noisy jobs in different firms—perhaps following service in the Armed Forces with its attendant gunfire exposure.

EVALUATION OF HEARING IN INFANTS AND YOUNG CHILDREN

It is just 50 years since Irene Ewing started her famous work at Manchester University on the ascertainment of hearing loss in infancy and early childhood. The endeavour was later formalized with the establishment of a Clinic for the Deaf in 1934 within the non-medical environment of the Department of Education of the Deaf where the Ewings led the world with their hearing test methods adapted for the younger age groups.

Their methods are well documented (Ewing, 1943); Ewing and Ewing, 1944; Ewing, 1957). Hearing loss in infants aged 1 week to 6 months is detected by means of a startle reflex in response to a loud sound. Normally this reflex is inhibited at an age of about 6 months. For children below the age of 5 years unable to respond to conventional audiometric tests, special sources of free-field test sounds in particular frequency bands were used at controlled intensities. Test situations were devised where, by behavioural observation, it could be decided whether the child under investigation had sufficient hearing to allow the development of speech. The range of sound sources covered voice, percussion toys (bell, drum, triangle etc.) and "meaningful sounds" (chink of feeding bottle, rustling paper etc.) Edith Whetnall, an otologist with special interest in children's hearing problems, introduced these basic tests with some modifications (Whetnall and Fry, 1964) to her Clinic at the Royal National Throat, Nose and Ear Hospital, London, in 1948. Taylor, who in 1965 succeeded Professor Sir Alexander Ewing in the chair created at the Department of Audiology and Education of

the Deaf, Manchester, gives a modern account of the Manchester techniques in his book (Taylor, 1964).

Briefly the free-field tests are of three types graded to suit developmental ages as follows:

(1) Distraction Tests (7 months to 18 months).
In order to pass these tests the infant is required to respond to low and high-pitched sounds at sound pressure levels not greater than 30 dB when presented out of sight at each side, and to turn towards the source.
(2) Co-operative Tests (18 months to 2½ years).
The child is required to discriminate very quiet speech (e.g. "show me your shoes") from both sides at 1 m; also to respond to high tones at sound pressure levels not greater than 30 dB, and to be able to locate the source.
(3) Performance Tests (from 2½ years).
The child is required to understand very quiet speech from both sides at 1 m; also to perform an activity test in response to a sound stimulus on one side at a time, to respond to high tones at sound pressure levels not greater than 30 dB, and to be able to locate the source.

When a child has carried out a free-field performance test satisfactorily he is then introduced to free-field audiometric tones (Denes and Reed, 1959) and thence transferred to the headset of a pure-tone audiometer for a more accurate test. Simple toys or coloured balls are employed to establish a conditioned response to the sounds. Here it needs to be mentioned, as in Chapter 56, that the basis of calibration for audiometers relies on the normal hearing level of young adults. An indication of the variation experienced in the hearing level of young children is given in the publications of Eagles and his colleagues (1963, 1967).

Another worker in this important, yet difficult, assessment field who has made many notable contributions is Fisch (1955, 1971) who has, among other developments, described the use of recorded sound stimuli (Fisch, 1965) for the children's free-field tests. Bench and his co-workers have recently undertaken a series of validation experiments to determine the most important factors involved in the detection of hearing loss in neonates with the startle reflex (Langford and Bench, 1973; Collyer and Bench, 1974).

Although forms of pure-tone audiometry can be practiced with children over the age of 2½ years, self-recording audiometry is not generally possible until the age of 6 or 7 is reached. Most children of 7 years are capable of tracing their thresholds very accurately, providing the usual precautions are taken of maintaining their interest and keeping the test duration reasonably short.

SCHOOL SCREENING AUDIOMETRY

Another important aspect of audiometry is that which relates to the checks which are routinely carried out on the hearing of 5–7-year-old children in schools. In school screening audiometry, pure-tone hearing tests are conducted by sweeping through the test frequencies at a fixed intensity of 20 dB hearing level to determine if each child hears all the tones presented. The tests are conducted in classrooms where, all too often, the ambient sound level is unduly high. The range of frequencies tested is normally from 250 to 8000 Hz, although 6000 and 8000 Hz are sometimes omitted.

Where the ambient noise is excessive, it will have the greatest masking effect on the lower frequencies, particularly on 250 Hz, and some screening audiometricians therefore raise the screening level to 25 dB at 250 and 500 Hz. Children who fail two successive tests are referred for more detailed hearing tests and examination under better conditions at an audiology clinic. Brooks (1970) suggested that a more suitable screening test is available using acoustic impedance measurements to exclude the possibility of a conductive hearing loss, together with a pure-tone screen at 4000 Hz to ensure the detection of a possible high-tone loss. The advantage to be gained with impedance tests of hearing is that they are relatively less sensitive to error from background noise, but there are the disadvantages of the more expensive and complex apparatus, and the longer time required for each test.

SUMMARY AND CONCLUSIONS

Some of the basic requirements for many of the so-called subjective tests of hearing have been reviewed which, together with the necessary medical examination, including, where required, radiography and blood tests, lead to a complete evaluation of most hearing disorders and hence to suitable treatment.

Fundamental to all the tests described is the necessity for adequately quiet and ventilated rooms, equipment of known performance and calibration and, what is equally important, a qualified audiological assistant to conduct the test according to an agreed procedure with sufficient time to apply an adequate masking routine.

The choice of the actual tests performed on a particular patient tends to vary widely from place to place as well as the procedure of test. In Britain, reliance is placed on accurate pure-tone audiometry, alternate binaural loudness balance, self-recording audiometry and tests of abnormal auditory adaptation, supplemented by speech tests as required. Objective tests of hearing also have an important part to play, but these are usually restricted to acoustic impedance measurements leaving evoked response audiometry and cochleography for solving problems of assessment incapable of solution by other means. Greater detail of some of the material described in this chapter is to be found in the works of Burns (1974); Davis and Silverman, (1970); Glorig (1965); Hirsh (1952); Littler (1965) and Watson and Tolan (1949).

REFERENCES

Alusi, H. A., Hinchcliffe, R., Ingham, B., Knight, J. J. and North, C. (1974), *Int. Audiol.*, **13**, 212.
Beagley, H. A. and Knight, J. J. (1966), *J. Laryng.*, **80**, 1127.
Beagley, H. A. and Knight, J. J. (1967), *J. Laryng.*, **81**, 347.
Beagley, H. A. and Knight, J. J. (1968), *J. Laryng.*, **82**, 693.
Békésy, von, G. (1947), *Acta otol-laryng.*, **35**, 411.
Bergman, M. (1966), *Arch. Otolaryng.*, **84**, 411.
Brooks, D. N. (1970), *J. Audiol.*, **9**, 22.
British Standards Institution. See Refs. Chapter 56.
Bruine-Altes, J. D. de (1946), "Symptoms of Regression in Different Kinds of Deafness," Thesis, Groningen: J. B. Walters.
Burns, W. (1974), *Noise and Man*, 2nd edition. London: Murray.
Carhart, R. (1950), *Arch. Otolaryng.*, **51**, 798.
Carhart, R. (1957), *Arch. Otolaryng.*, **65**, 32.
Carhart, R. and Jerger, J. F. (1959), *J. Speech Hear. Dis.*, **24**, 330.
Coles, R. R. A. (1972), *J. Laryng.*, **86**, 191.
Coles, R. R. A. and Knight, J. J. (1965), *J. Laryng.*, **74**, 131.
Collyer, Y. and Bench, J. (1974), *Brit. J. Audiol.*, **8**, 14.
Collyer, Y. and Bench, J. (1974), *Brit. J. Audiol.*, **8**, 37.
Copeland, W. C. T., Whittle, L. S. and Saunders, E. G. (1964), *J. Sound. Vibr.*, **1**, 388.
Dadson, R. S. and King, J. H. (1952), *J. Laryng.*, **66**, 366.
Davis, H. and Silverman, S. R. (1970), *Hearing and Deafness*, 3rd edition. New York: Holt, Rinehart, Winston.
Denes, P. and Naunton, R. F. (1952), *Proc. roy. Soc. Med.*, **45**, 790.
Denes, P. and Reed, M. M. (1959), *Lancet*, **ii**, 830.
Department of Health and Social Security (1974), *Hospital E.N.T. Services—A Design Guide*. London: D.H.S.S.
Dix, M. R. Hallpike, C. S. and Hood, J. D. (1948), *Proc. roy. Soc. Med.*, **41**, 516.
Eagles, E. L., Wishik, S. M. and Doerfler, L. G. (1963), "Hearing Sensitivity and Related Factors in Children," *Laryngoscope*. St. Louis.
Eagles, E. L., Wishik, S. M. and Doerfler, L. G. (1967), "Hearing Sensitivity and Ear Disease in Children: A Prospective Study," *Laryngoscope*. St. Louis.
Egan, J. P. (1948), *Laryngoscope*, **58**, 955.
Ewing, A. W. G. (1943), *J. Laryng.*, **58**, 143.
Ewing, I. R. (1943), *J. Laryng.*, **58**, 137.
Ewing, I. R. and Ewing, A. W. G. (1944), *J. Laryng.*, **59**, 309.
Ewing, I. R. and Ewing, A. W. G. (1957), *Educational Guidance and the Deaf Child*. Manchester: Manchester University Press.
Fairbanks, G. (1958), *J. acoust. Soc. Amer.*, **30**, 596.
Fisch, L. (1955), *J. Laryng.*, **69**, 479.
Fisch, L. (1965), *J. Laryng.*, **79**, 1077.
Fisch, L. (1971), *Sound*, **5**, 1.
Fletcher, H. (1929), *Speech and Hearing*. Princeton: Van Nostrand.
Fletcher, H. (1953), *Speech and Hearing in Communication*. Princeton: Van Nostrand.
Fowler, E. P. (1936), *Arch. Otolaryng.*, **24**, 731.
Fry, D. B. (1946), Unpublished Ph.D. Thesis, University of London.
Fry, D. B. (1964), *Lancet*, **ii**, 197.
Fry, D. B. and Kerridge, P. M. T. (1939), *Lancet* **i**, 106.
Glorig, A. (Ed.) (1965), *Audiometry: Principles and Practices*. Baltimore: Williams and Wilkins.
Gyllencreutz, T. and Lidén, G. (1967), *Acta oto-laryng.*, suppl. **224**, 229.
Hallpike, C. S. and Hood, J. D. (1959), *Acta oto-laryng.*, **50**, 472.
Hinchcliffe, R. (1958), *Acustica*, **9**, 304.
Hinchcliffe, R. (1959), *J. Laryng.*, **73**, 795.
Hinchcliffe, R. (1969). Personal communication.
Hinchcliffe, R. and Littler, T. S. (1958), *Ann. Occup. Hyg.*, **1**, 114.
Hinchcliffe, R. and Littler, T. S. (1961), *J. Laryng.*, **75**, 201.
Hirsh, I. J. (1952), *The Measurement of Hearing*. New York: McGraw Hill.
Hood, J. D. (1950), *Acta oto-laryng.*, suppl., 92.
Hood, J. D. (1955), *Ann. Otol.*, **64**, 506.
Hood, J. D. (1969), *J. Laryng.*, **83**, 695.
Hood, J. D. and Poole, J. (1966), *J. acoust. Soc. Amer.*, **40**, 47.
House, A. S., Williams, C. E., Hecker M. H. L. and Kryter, K. D. (1965), *J. acoust. Soc. Amer.*, **37**, 158.
Hughson, W. and Westlake, H. (1944) *Trans. Amer. Acad. Ophthal. Otolaryng.*, suppl., **48**, 1.
International Electrotechnical Commission. See Refs. Chapter 56.
International Organisation for Standardisation. See Refs. Chapter 56.
Jerger, J. (1952), *Laryngoscope* **62**, 1316.
Jerger, J. (1960), *Speech Hear. Res.*, **3**, 275.
Jerger, J. (Ed.) (1973), *Modern Developments in Audiology*, 2nd edition. New York: Academic Press.

Jerger, J. and Herer G. (1961) *J. Speech Hear. Dis.*, **26**, 390.

Jerger, J., Shedd, J. and Harford, E. (1959), *Arch. Otolaryng.*, **69**, 200.

Jerger, J. and Tillman, T. W. (1960), *Arch. Otolaryng.*, **71**, 948.

Johansen, H. (1948), *Acta oto-laryng.*, suppl., **74**, 65.

Johnson, E. W. (1970), *Laryngoscope*, **80**, 49.

Knight, J. J. (1960). Unpublished data.

Knight, J. J. (1966), *J. acoust. Soc. Amer.*, **39**, 1184.

Knight, J. J. (1969), *Chem. Engr.*, **47**, 108.

Knight, J. J. (1971), *Rivista de Acustica*, **2**, 172.

Knight, J. J. and Coles, R. R. A. (1960), *J. acoust. Soc. Amer.*, **32**, 800.

Knight, J. J. and Littler, T. S. (1953), *J. Laryng.*, **67**, 248.

Kylin, B. (1960), *Acta oto-laryng.*, suppl., 152.

Langenbeck, B. (1962), *Textbook of Practical Audiometry*. London: Arnold.

Langford, C. and Bench, J. (1973), *Brit. J. Audiol.*, **7**, 29.

Lightfoot, C. (1960), *Laryngoscope*, **70**, 1552.

Littler, T. S. (1950). Personal communication.

Littler, T. S. (1965), *The Physics of the Ear*. London: Pergamon.

Littler, T. S., Knight, J. J. and Strange, P. H. (1952), *Proc. roy. Soc. Med.*, **45**, 783.

Lüscher, E. (1951), *J. Laryng.*, **65**, 486.

Lüscher, E. and Zwislocki, J. (1948), *Acta oto-laryng.*, suppl., **78**, 156.

Lüscher, E. and Zwislocki, J. (1951), *J. Laryng.*, **65**, 187.

McLay, K. (1959), *J. Laryng.*, **73**, 460.

McMurray, R. F. and Rudmose, W. (1956), *Noise Control*, **2**, 33.

Medical Research Council (1947), Special Report Series No. 261. London: H.M.S.O.

Muyunga, C. (1974), Unpublished Ph.D. Thesis, University of London.

Palva, T., Goodman, A. and Hirsh, I. (1953), *Laryngoscope*, **63**, 842.

Pohlman, A. G. and Kranz, F. W. (1924), *Proc. Soc. exp. Biol. (N.Y.)*, **21**, 335.

Rainville, M. J. (1955), *J. Français d'oto-rhino-laryng.*, **4**, 851.

Reger, S. N. (1960), *Ann. Otol.*, **69**, 1179.

Reger, S. N. and Kos, C. M., (1952), *Ann. Otol.*, **61**, 810.

Robinson, D. W. and Dadson, R. S. (1956), *Brit. J. appl. Phys.*, **7**, 166.

Robinson, D. W. and Whittle, L. S. (1973), *J. Sound Vibr.*, **26**, 41.

Rosen, S., Bergman, M., Plester, D., El-Mofty, A. and Satti, M. H. (1962), *Ann. Otol.*, **71**, 727.

Royal Society of Medicine (1933), Report of Committee for the Consideration of Hearing Tests. Part 1, *J. Laryng.*, **48**, 22; Part 2, *J. Laryng.*, **48**, 77.

Stephens, S. D. G. and Hinchcliffe, R. (1968), *Int. Audiol.*, **7**, 267.

Taylor, I. G. (1964), *The Neurological Mechanisms of Hearing and Speech*. Manchester: Manchester University Press.

Ward, W. D., Glorig, A. and Sklar, D. L. (1959), *J. acoust. Soc. Amer.*, **31**, 791.

Watson, L. A. and Tolan, T. (1949), *Hearing Tests and Hearing Instruments*. Baltimore: Williams and Wilkins.

Watson, T. J. (1967), *The Education of Hearing Handicapped Children*. University of London Press.

West, W. (1932), *Acoustical Engineering*. London: Pitman.

Wheeler, L. J. and Dickson, E. D. D. (1952), *J. Laryng.*, **66**, 379.

Whetnall, E. and Fry, D. B. (1946), *The Deaf Child*. London: Heinemann.

Zwislocki, J. J. (1953), *J. acoust. Soc. Amer.*, **25**, 752.

58. CONDITIONS FOR HEARING TESTS

L. FISCH

INTRODUCTION

In all hearing tests it is essential to obtain a clear and unequivocal indication that the test sound was heard by the subject being examined. The nature of the signal from the subject depends on the type of test. There are three possible types of reaction to a test sound:

(1) A voluntary behavioural change.

(2) An involuntary behavioural change.

(3) A change in an autonomic function or a physiological reaction.

For example:

(1) The subject, to whom the procedure has been explained, is instructed to press a button activating a light signal, or to say "Yes", or to raise a hand when a test sound is heard (a voluntary signal).

(2) Hearing tests in free field with very young children (before they are able to co-operate) depend on behavioural observation; a sudden change in behaviour (a motor reaction, such as turning the head) constitutes the signal indicating that the test sound was heard. With children who are able to co-operate but cannot as yet understand verbal explanation of the procedure or when one cannot rely on themselves indicating that they heard the test sound, as is the case with adults, play audiometric techniques must be applied. The signal consists then of a movement that the child is taught to carry out, as a play, when the test sound is produced.

(3) In other tests, the signal consists of an involuntary reaction which is recorded by an electrophysiological method. The signal indicating that the test sound was perceived is then a change which occurs following production of the test sound, for instance, in the electro-encephalographic record, or in the electrical potential of the internal ear, as recorded in electrocochleography.

All the reactions following a test sound are subject to various influences and the responses are subject to modifications in a variety of ways. There is no absolute certainty of a reaction or a response occurring in any hearing test. A response may or may not occur even when the test sound is heard. In other words, a situation of probability exists. Some conditions favour a high probability of a response while other influences may reduce it considerably. This applies, not only to tests based on behavioural changes or voluntary signals, but also to electrophysiological tests based on involuntary changes of an autonomic function or a neurophysiological change.

AUDIOMETRY

The advantage of pure tone audiometry is that it is a, important single test which can be carried out easily quickly and economically, but only when certain conditions are fulfilled and strictly adhered to. The aim is to obtain a reliable response at threshold. The threshold of hearing is defined, for this purpose, as a consistent response which is obtained when the intensity is decreased in 10 dB steps until no response is obtained and then increased at 5 dB steps until a response is obtained, this response being obtained twice out of four trials.

There are many influences which will determine the probability of obtaining a threshold response. These are

EXTERNAL DETERMINANTS

ACOUSTIC CONDITIONS

VENTILATION

THE AUDIOMETER   CALIBRATION
                ERGOMETRICS

METHODS OF SIGNAL DELIVERY

DEGREE OF TRAINING OF   AUDIOMETRICIAN
                          STANDARD PROCEDURE

SIZE OF ROOM

OUTLAY AND APPEARANCE OF ROOM

TIME AVAILABLE FOR TEST

CONTACT AND COMMUNICATION WITH SUBJECT

Fig. 1.

INTERNAL DETERMINANTS

ABILITY TO GIVE SIGNAL

DEGREE OF COOPERATION

ANXIETY OF   SUBJECT
           EXAMINER

PHYSICAL TIREDNESS OF   SUBJECT
                       EXAMINER

MENTAL TIREDNESS OF   SUBJECT
                     EXAMINER

SPAN OF ATTENTION OF SUBJECT

GENERAL RELIABILITY OF   EXAMINER
                       MOTIVATION

Fig. 2.

external determinants (consisting principally of the physical conditions of the environment, of the methods of testing and of the machine) (Fig. 1) and internal determinants (Fig. 2) which exist within the tested subject and the examiner. The external ones are: acoustic conditions, ventilation, size, layout and appearance of the room, the audiometer, methods of delivery of the signal, communication with the subject, training of the audiometrician, and time available for the test. The internal ones are the human assets: degree of co-operation, ability to give a signal, anxiety, physical and mental tiredness, span of attention both of the subject and the examiner and general reliability of the examiner. These variables are interconnected and influence each other (Fig. 3). The external determinants influence the internal ones.

Acoustic conditions and ventilation are obviously closely related. The size of the room will determine its layout. The effort of the subject will be related to anxiety. Anxiety is related to ability to co-operate. The persistence of the audiometrician and her ability to persevere with the standard procedure is closely related to physical and mental tiredness and to span of attention. This is related to the time available for the test or the number of tests already carried out. External determinants will influence the internal ones. Ventilation will obviously influence comfort and degree of persistence or ability to maintain the effort. The size of the room may influence its layout and the method of the delivery of the signal. Many of these variables influence the ability to avoid the pitfalls inherent in these tests.

Even the simplified presentation of interconnexions, as illustrated in Fig. 3, indicates that we are dealing with a complex system. Viewing the situation in this manner enables us to gain insight into aspects of audiometry which would not otherwise be possible. Every part of a system is so related to its fellow parts that a change in one causes a change in all of them and in the total system. This is not a

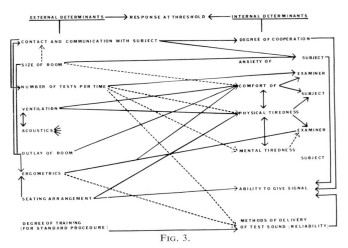

FIG. 3.

composite of independent elements, but an inseparable whole in which the elements are coherently interconnected. System thinking refers to the habit of concentrating on how these connections act and interact so as to produce quite unexpected behaviour resulting from the internal dynamics of the system. This concept enables us to analyse the complexity of the situation and to detect what influences can lead to the breakdown of the system. When planning audiometric rooms, they should be planned as a system. A close study of the inter-relations of the parts enables us to produce a model for an audiometric system and discover the processes which may interfere with its satisfactory functioning.

Of the many intricate relationships, one is the ability of the audiometrician to sustain the effort. The audiometrician herself is rarely considered with as much care as the machine or its calibration. Such properties as comfort, tiredness, span of attention and emotional aspects are almost dismissed as mere subjective aspects hardly worth considering. Strictly speaking the calibration or recalibration of the audiometrician, if this could be done, should be one of the most important aspects of audiometry. Ability to sustain the effort can be reduced when too many tests are required per session. There is good evidence to show that after a certain number of tests the results will become less reliable; this is often disregarded when a large number is requested. It is impossible to set absolute limits. On average, for a full threshold audiometric test in a co-operative adult, the audiometrician may need 15–30 min. When a few subjects are difficult, or when children are tested, the timetable is thrown out of gear.

Many variables can influence the ability or possibility of avoiding the pitfalls inherent in these tests, such as unintended visual signals associated with the delivery of the test sound by the examiner. Inability of detecting unreliable responses when the standard procedure is not strictly adhered to is another source of serious error. This may happen when the time is limited for a test, when the examiner is asked unreasonably to carry out a large number of tests, or when personnel are inadequately trained. Results may be presented as threshold responses when in fact they represent responses at much higher intensities.

The most important aspect of pure tone audiometry is

first of all that the response should be a reliable one and secondly that the final result should truly show a threshold response. The judgement whether a response was reliable rests entirely with the examiner. That the finally recorded result represents a threshold response depends not only on the examiner, but also to a great extent on the conditions in which the test is carried out. An examiner of the greatest reliability may not achieve good results in unfavourable conditions. Conditions for audiometry must be completely satisfactory. This is so because we are dealing with a complex system in which a fault in a single part can lead to the breakdown of the whole system.

PLAY AUDIOMETRY

Because of the high information value of pure tone audiometry it is desirable that with all children suspected of having a hearing impairment we should obtain a reliable threshold result as soon as it is feasible.

A physically and mentally normal child is able to co-operate in audiometry from the age of $2\frac{1}{2}$ years but he is not able to indicate reliably that he heard the test sound in a similar way as an older child or adult can. Moreover, many children who are presented for a hearing test are unable to communicate and verbal explanations of the procedure are impossible. It is, however, feasible or possible to train a child to perform a simple movement as part of a game when a test sound is produced and this performance serves then as a signal that it was heard. No verbal explanation is necessary—repetition of the performance will teach the child what is wanted.

The speed of learning to associate the required movement following the production of the test sound depends on a variety of factors. In addition to environmental influences, the most important aspect is the correct technique in training the child to carry out the performance required in play audiometry. This depends on the ability of the examiner to gain the child's confidence and reduce his anxiety. The examiner must be well trained in the correct techniques. Fundamentally this is a stage by stage procedure.

At the first stage of play audiometry the child is taught to carry out a movement (which later becomes the signal that the test sound was heard), when a sound is produced by a percussion instrument (a xylophone or a drum) so that the child can see and hear the source of sound. When he has learned the game and performed reliably, the second stage follows—that is performing when the source of the test sound is out of the child's field of vision.

When a reliable response is obtained, the third stage follows: practising to respond to pure tones from a small free field pure tone audiometer.

Again, when a reliable response is obtained the fourth important stage follows, that is introducing the child to the earphone. First a single earphone is used in conjunction with the same free field audiometer. Once a child accepts this and responds reliably, the fifth stage follows, that is transfer to the audiometry room for a full threshold test. The large earphones are presented gently, which is especially necessary with anxious children. Once a child accepts the large earphones freely and without anxiety, a skilful audiometrician should be able to complete a full test. But, with some children, even this stage is considered only as an introduction to a full audiometric test and an intermediate stage of practice audiometry is interposed. The essence of this procedure is that before a full threshold test is carried out, the child is gradually taken through various stages of preparation or practice in surroundings which allow us to reduce the child's anxiety, gain his confidence and achieve co-operation in the form of a play.

Conditions for stage by stage play audiometry must be satisfactory. Without them even the most skilful examiner cannot obtain satisfactory results. Suitable environment is a basic pre-condition for successful application of stage by stage play audiometry. For the initial stages it is essential to have a large friendly room specially structured for the initial hearing tests in free field. Such a room is essential in any case when children are to be tested who are restless and cannot be restrained. Even children who are on the move all the time can still be tested in such circumstances by observing their behaviour and reactions to test sounds in free field produced at an appropriate moment.

The size of such a room should be at least 4·5 by 6 m, acoustically treated and with the background noise level not exceeding 35 dB SPL. It should be ventilated by a silent ventilation system. The room should be carpeted. All the test materials and toys should be stored in cupboards mounted on the wall, off the floor and out of the reach of children. The room should be structured in such a way that it gives a pleasing and colourful appearance, without the impression of being a clinical examination room. It should be possible to eliminate sources of stimulation or distraction when this is required. One way observation facility is essential. The audiometry room for play audiometry should fulfil all of the physical specifications of an audiometric room in general, but additional special conditions are necessary. The size and appearance of the room is critical and above all it must not be a cubicle. An audiometric room for children should be not less than 3 by 4·5 m should give a pleasing and colourful appearance with close-carpeted floors, comfortable seats not only for the subject but also for the parent and for the examiner. The techniques of play audiometry require a close direct contact between the examiner and the child and special seating arrangements are necessary for this purpose.

TESTING INFANTS AND YOUNG CHILDREN IN FREE FIELD

It is essential to understand why and how a child reacts to a test sound and how such a reaction can be modified by various influences. Many influences can modify a reaction in such a way that even when the subject's hearing is normal a reaction may not occur. A child reacts to a test sound because it is a significant change in the environment. A reaction will occur in a similar fashion to any other type of change, such as light, movements of objects or people, vibration, or direct sensory stimulation (touch, puff of air on the skin, etc.). The probability that a child will respond to a test sound will increase directly when the

other changes in the environment decrease. The influences which modify reactions are:

(1) Environmental.
(2) Internal determinants (originating in the subject).

A sudden change becomes more significant when it occurs against an unchanging, still background. A distinct acoustic signal acquires greater significance when it occurs against an acoustically quiet environment. In order to increase the probability of response it is necessary to have not only a quiet room from the acoustic point of view but also to have complete stillness in every other respect. Any change in the environment, whether acoustical or visual (movement of any type), competes with the test sound and reduces the probability of response.

The environment (that is the room in which the tests are carried out), apart from the various transient changes, is determined by the size and quality of the room.

Exploration

When a child enters a room, the first reaction will be a desire to explore. Exploration of a new environment is a deep-seated urge, characteristic of all living creatures. When exploration is inhibited, it creates anxiety. Even infants unable to explore by moving about will explore by visual and auditory search. When the ability or possibility to explore is limited, anxiety will increase. Anxiety is one of the important internal determinants which greatly reduces the probability of response. The quality of the room can create anxiety of various degrees, depending on other influences as well. When the room is friendly, peaceful and structured in such a fashion that anxiety is reduced, the probability of response will increase.

The Size of the Room

Hearing tests in children must be carried out in a permissive setting. Children behave differently in rooms of different size, in the same way as an animal behaves differently in a cage as compared with its spacious natural environment. Cubicle-sized rooms, which are still used in many centres for testing children, are the equivalent to a cage. A child may not react at all in a cubicle-sized room, but the same child will behave differently in a room of large size and will react promptly. The size of the room also determines the possibility of the various modifications of the test procedures which are essential with various types of children. A room which is too small restricts these possibilities and thus reduces the probability of response.

Internal Determinants

These are distractibility, anxiety, arousal and habituation. The phenomenon of a subject's reaction to a test sound cannot be considered in isolation. It is not enough to consider it in relation to a few obvious variables. It is essential to realize that this phenomenon is part of a complex system in which it is related to many other parts. Moreover, it is not enough to study separately all the other variables. Even if we could measure all of them and express the results numerically (which is unlikely), it would not be sufficient. What is required is to see the interrelationships of the parts of the system. Figure 4 indicates some of the interrelationships which can be described as follows.

A child reacts to a test stimulus only when he is "ready to respond". Environmental influences and internal determinants interact and create the condition of "readiness to respond", a condition which can vary greatly according

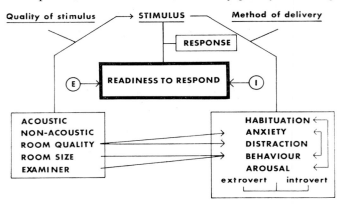

FIG. 4.

to these influences. The stimulus (test sound) combined with "readiness to respond" will result in a response. The stimulus is modified by the acoustic conditions of the environment. Its type and mode of application influences habituation.

All the environmental influences modify, in different ways, the internal determinants. The internal determinants also influence each other; habituation is related to arousal; anxiety is closely related to behaviour; behaviour is related to the size and quality of the room; room quality also influences distractibility; the size of the room influences the examiner, his behaviour, his method of testing and the behaviour of the subject.

It is essential in this context to emphasize the condition that we call "readiness to respond". It is the task of the examiner to recognize it in the child so that the test stimulus can be applied at the right moment and also that we should able to interpret the result in relation to this condition. It means that the examiner must be aware of all the influences which create and modify "readiness to respond". This indicates that the examiner, who is an important part of the environment, should be an experienced person with good fundamental knowledge of child behaviour, of child development and of various disabilities in children apart from a defect of hearing.

ELECTROPHYSIOLOGICAL TESTS

Tests based on recording physiological reactions by an electrophysiological method tend to be called "objective" as opposed to the "subjective" ones based on direct observation of a behavioural change, voluntary or involuntary. This distinction is incorrect. A consistent synchronous behavioural change is as "objective" as for example a change in the electro-encephalogram which still may have to be evaluated by the examiner in order to decide whether or not a change is acceptable as a reliable record of a reaction. It seems that, to some, the term "objective" is associated chiefly with the method of recording the results

of the test. If they are recorded automatically by a mechanical or electrophysiological device, this is considered "objective" because it seemingly eliminates the "subjective" interpretation of the reaction by an observer. However, provided the conditions are satisfactory, direct observations by a person can be more objective than some of the electrophysiological records when conditions for the latter are unsatisfactory. The term "objective" in this context is misleading because it may give the impression that an autonomic reaction occurs independently of any influences and that the probability of occurrence is as high as in any faultless electric or electronic input-output system. This is far from being true. If we take for example the heart rate as a reaction following the impact of a test sound (this could be used as part of a hearing test in a polygraphic method of testing including a variety of physiological changes), even the most "objective" method will not be valid if we do not pay attention to influences which may modify the reaction. The change of any function due to stimulation depends on the pre-stimulus level of that function, that is, the greater the excitation, the smaller the excitability. In this respect the most important single factor is the level of the particular physiological function during the immediate pre-stimulus period. For example, if the heart rate is already high, it will change little on stimulation. If the pre-stimulus level is low there will be a big change. And, most important, at a certain definite level, critical for each physiological function, there will be no change at all. Unless this is taken into account, the test results cannot be interpreted correctly. Unless one correlates the immediate pre-stimulus level of a function to the post-stimulus one, correct interpretation of the results is impossible. Concerning "objective" tests of hearing, many examiners think that because these tests are "objective" it is legitimate to disregard such "subjective" aspects as the "state" of the child, handling the child, the type of room and environment and the experience of examiners so far as child behaviour is concerned. Unfortunately, precisely because of the dismissal of these "subjective" influences, the "objectivity" of the test may be invalidated.

The state of the tested subject can be influenced to a significant degree by the conditions in which the test takes place and this applies not only to the physical conditions of the examination but also to the handling of the subject by the examiners. For instance, in Electric Response Audiometry (ERA), it will certainly depend on the environment and the handling of the subject, whether or not the test can be carried out with the subject fully awake, cooperative and quiet. The alternative is sedation which, however, changes the nature of the test and influences the results in an adverse manner. In electrocochleography which necessitates a general anaesthetic, much depends on pre-anaesthetic handling and undoubtedly the responses will also depend on a variety of external and internal determinants.

REFERENCES

Fisch, L. (1967), "The Physiology of Children's Reactions to Test Sounds in Free Field," *Int. Audiol.* **6**, 121.
Fisch, L. (1971), "The Probability of Response to Test Sounds in Young Children," *Sound,* **5**, 7.

59. AUDITORY PROSTHESES
(Technological Aspects)

M. C. MARTIN

INTRODUCTION

Prostheses are fabricated* objects which are placed in or on individuals to remedy or replace a defective function or structure. Otological prostheses are of particular importance and comprise both *auditory prostheses* (Fig. 1) to remedy defective auditory function and *aural prostheses* to

as in the conventional personal electronic hearing aid or it may employ an indirect *magnetic* or *radiation field,* as in hearing aids using audio-frequency inductive loops or radio-links respectively.

It is frequently forgotten that the conventional hearing aid represents only one of a number of types of auditory prostheses. Personal hearing aids constitute external

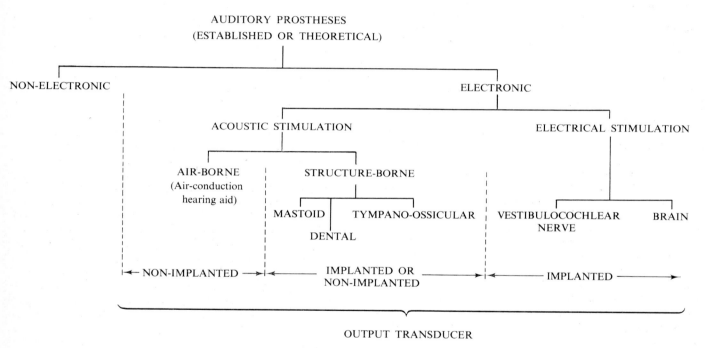

FIG. 1. Classification of auditory prostheses.

replace defective anatomical structures. This classification of otological prostheses is, as with many classifications, an artificial one; an aural prosthesis, e.g. a politef piston to replace a stapes, may, by restoring structure, also, as a consequence, restore function.

Auditory prostheses may be classified primarily in five ways, i.e. according to the physical nature (electronic or non-electronic) of the prosthesis, according to the physical modality of the signal, according to the anatomical route (or routes) used, according to whether or not the output transducer is implanted, and, finally, according to the nature of the link between the input and the output transducers. The first four types of classifications are encompassed in Fig. 1. The link between the input and output transducers may be by direct electrical connections

auditory prostheses. These are by far the commonest types of auditory prosthesis so that the greater part of this chapter will be devoted to them. Nevertheless, auditory prostheses in which at least some part is implanted in the body tissues (*internal* or *interno-external auditory prostheses*) are increasing in importance so that some mention will be made of these also.

PERSONAL HEARING AIDS

Historical

As Carver (1972) has pointed out, man devised the first hearing aid when he cupped his hand behind his ear. From very early times, a variety of *mechanical devices* (Anon, 1965) have been used to alleviate impairment of hearing; most of these have taken the form of the ear trumpet.

* *Fabrication* refers to the procedure of constructing or forming an assembled entity from a number of separate elements which must be joined together according to a definite predetermined plan.

The history of the *electronic hearing aid* is, however, naturally a short one. It began in 1900 with the introduction, in Austria, of a carbon microphone aid by Ferdinand Alt. In 1887, Alexander Graham Bell, who had a great interest in the problems of hearing loss, had tried his telephone on a partially hearing man who "held the telephone attached to the microphone to his ear and understood everything that was said, even when (Bell) went to the other end of the room, but when he took the telephone away, he was helpless" (Bruce, 1973). Bell did not, however, produce a wearable hearing aid.

During the period 1900–40 many forms of aids with carbon microphones were produced for use with both air and bone conduction outputs. By 1920, thermionic valve (*see* Chapter 5) aids were being produced. These used large triode valves and were powered by accumulators. These aids were extremely bulky but gave a considerably better performance than did the carbon aids. The introduction of very much smaller valves enabled manufacturers to produce aids in two parts capable of being carried on the body; these were called *Duopacks*. In 1943 the production of very small, low current consumption thermionic valves led British manufacturers to produce the first *Monopack* aids which contained batteries, microphone and amplifier in one small case. Further developments in battery and component design allowed body-worn aids to be reduced to a size comparable to that of the body-worn aids of today.

With the introduction in 1953 of transistors (*see* Chapter 5) in commercial quantities, body-worn hearing aids were made which required only a low voltage battery instead of the high and low voltage batteries previously required. Spectacle aids were first produced in 1954. Aids worn behind the ear appeared in 1956 and were followed in 1957 by aids worn completely within the external ear.

Goldstein (1933) has reviewed hearing aid developments up to 1930 and Watson and Tolan (1949) have continued this history up to 1943. Carver (1972) has described more recent developments.

Types

Non-electronic hearing aids comprise *auricles*,* *ear trumpets* and *speaking tubes* (Anon, 1965). These non-electronic hearing aids are sometimes referred to as acoustical aids and the method of amplification as mechanical. Although these devices may be considered something of an anachronism today, many elderly people with hearing losses prefer them to the modern electronic hearing aid. For some elderly patients, especially those with arthritic fingers, the controls of the electronic aid may be too difficult to manipulate. In many developing areas of the world, where the use of electronic aids is limited because of cost and lack of maintenance facilities, these non-electronic aids should find an application. The *speaking tube* is capable of delivering very high sound pressure levels to the ear if the mouthpiece of the tube is close-coupled to the speaker's mouth. Modern versions of these speaking tubes have been used in schools for the deaf

* The use of this term is, of course, unfortunate since the word 'auricle" also refers to the projecting part of the external ear.

in Europe. The frequency response of these close-coupled devices is good; the response suffers from small multiple resonances and a fall off of response (but only by about 5 dB per octave) only above 500 Hz. *Auricles* and *ear trumpets* supply only a small degree of amplification but this is sufficient for some slight to moderate hearing losses.

Over 400 models of *electronic hearing aids* are available on the British market at present (RNID, 1975). These models may be broken down into three basic categories, i.e. *body-worn aids*, *head-worn aids* and *special educational aids* such as auditory training units and group hearing aids. In addition, each of the above categories can be subdivided into *air-* and *bone-conduction* hearing aids.

Before describing any particular type of aid it must be appreciated that all the categories of hearing aids mentioned in the last paragraph work on the principle of amplifying sound by electronic means; they therefore have five basic parts. First, there is a microphone to receive sound and convert it to an electrical form; secondly, an amplifier to enhance the electrical signal; thirdly, an earphone to convert the electrical signal from the amplifier into an acoustic signal to be fed through the fourth part, i.e. an earmould,* into the ear canal. Finally, a source of power is required to operate the amplifier and this is usually some form of dry battery.

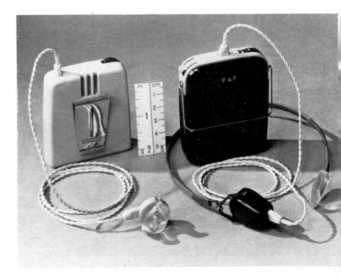

FIG. 2. Two British National Health Service MEDRESCO hearing aids. On the left, the OL56 air conduction aid with connecting cord, earphone and earmould. On the right, the OL58 bone conduction aid with connecting cord, transducer (vibrator) and headband. The OL57 is not shown but it looks exactly like the OL56 with an additional switch. The OL63 looks like the OL58 but it has a tone control and is used with an air conduction earphone. (RNID photograph.)

Body-worn Aids

A body-worn aid is one where the microphone, amplifier and battery are housed in a case which is worn on the body, usually the chest, and the earpiece is connected to a flexible pair of wires (*cord*) running from the ear to the case. Figure 2 shows two of the British National Health

* To avoid confusion with aural fungi, it is better to use one word instead of two when referring to this object.

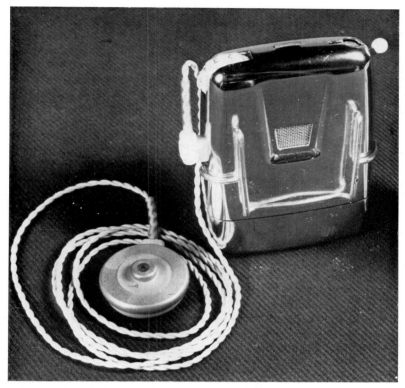

FIG. 3. A typical commercial body-worn hearing aid. (RNID photograph.)

ervice body-worn aids and Fig. 3 a typical commercial id.

Body-worn aids can be relatively large and, because of his, are capable of producing a very high level of sound ressure over the required range of frequencies.

Head-worn Aids

Head-worn aids may be divided into four types, i.e. *behind-the-ear*, *spectacle*, *in-the-ear*, or *headband* hearing ds. *Behind-the-ear* (*post-aural*) *aids* are worn behind the uricle; the sound from the aid is usually fed into the ear inal by means of a plastic tube.

The behind-the-ear aid is the most popular type of head-orn aid. This type accounts for 85 per cent or more of all ommercial sales in the U.K. (Board of Trade, 1970). It as considerable flexibility in its performance and is apable of giving high outputs which enables its use with earing losses of up to 80 dB or more. Figure 4 shows a pical behind-the-ear hearing aid.

Spectacle (Eyeglass) Aids have their components housed one or both arms of the spectacle frame (Fig. 5). The ectacle type of hearing aid provides a suitable structural amework for applying more recently developed systems ig. 6) of auditory prostheses. In cases of severe unilateral eafness where the patient cannot be helped with an aid, e suffers from an obvious difficulty in hearing on his deaf de. The "good" ear is capable of hearing sounds from e other side of the head but there is a marked area of shadow" in which sounds are greatly reduced in intensity. order to overcome this shadow effect, a microphone is

placed near to the deaf ear and the signals routed to the good ear. Harford and Barry (1965) refer to this system as contralateral routing of signals (CROS). If the good ear is normal, the sound is fed into that ear by means of an open

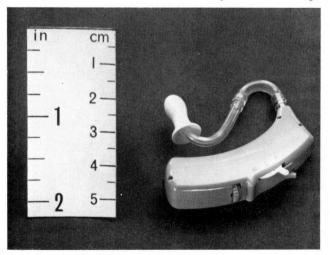

FIG. 4. A typical ear-level (postaural) hearing aid with switch for induc-tive pick-up coil (T), microphone (M) and off (O) positions. A tem-porary earpip is attached to the aid.

earmould. If the good ear suffers from some loss then a further microphone may be used and the sound fed in by a closed earmould (BICROS* system). Dunlavy (1968) has reviewed the use of CROS and has suggested (Dunlavy, 1974) a number of variations in the use of CROS. These

* Bilateral CROS system.

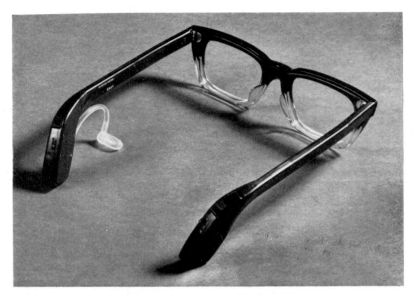

FIG. 5. A spectacle type hearing aid.

SPECTACLE HEARING AIDS

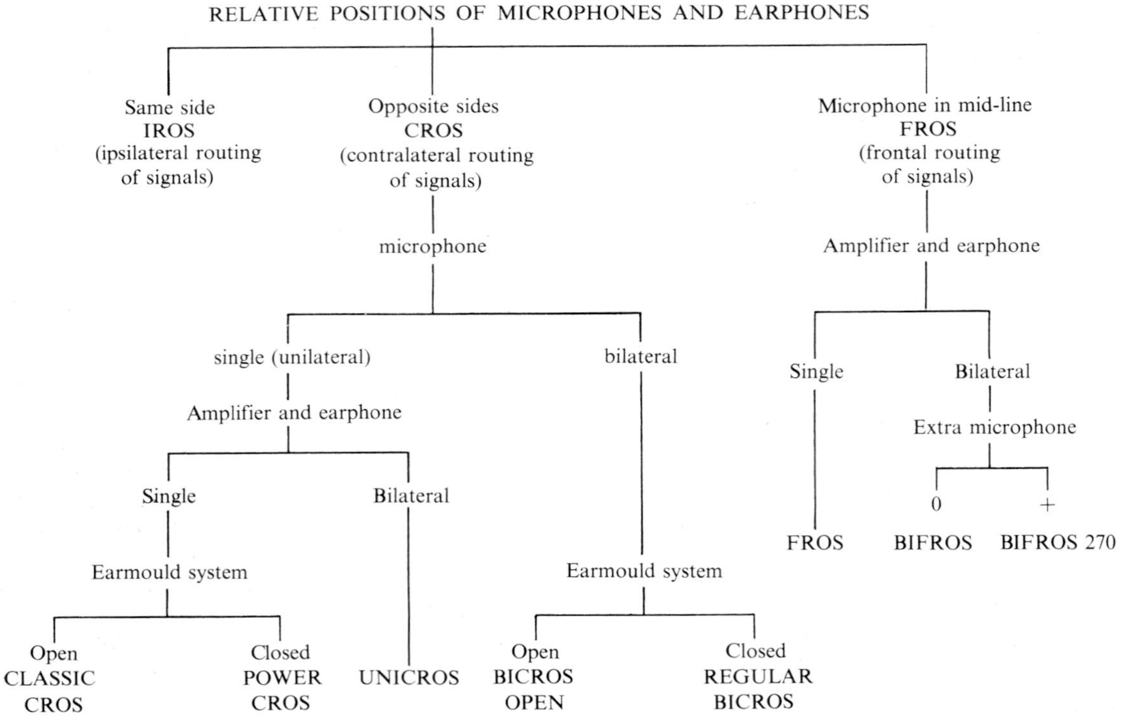

RELATIVE POSITIONS OF MICROPHONES AND EARPHONES

Same side
IROS
(ipsilateral routing
of signals)

Opposite sides
CROS
(contralateral routing
of signals)

Microphone in mid-line
FROS
(frontal routing
of signals)

microphone

Amplifier and earphone

single (unilateral)

bilateral

Single

Bilateral

Amplifier and earphone

Extra microphone

Single

Bilateral

0   +

FROS   BIFROS   BIFROS 270

Earmould system

Earmould system

Open
CLASSIC
CROS

Closed
POWER
CROS

UNICROS

Open
BICROS
OPEN

Closed
REGULAR
BICROS

FIG. 6. Classification of spectacle type hearing aids in respect of relevant positions on skull of microphones and earphones. Although the spectacle type hearing aid is eminently suitable for CROS systems, these can of course be used with other types of hearing aids.

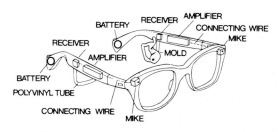

FIG. 7. A BIFROS hearing aid. One side has a closed earmould which is suitable for greater degrees of hearing loss; the other side has a tube inlet which is suitable for lesser degrees of hearing loss. The microphones are seen on the front of the spectacle frames. (Reproduced by courtesy of Dunlavy.)

...re listed in Table 1. One type (BIFROS, i.e. bilateral ...ontal routing of signals) is shown in Fig. 7.

TABLE 1

Classic CROS	Microphone on same side as that of deaf ear; earphone connected to good ear with open earmould.
Regular BICROS	Two microphones (one on each side) connected through single amplifier and earphone to closed earmould in better ear.
Open BICROS	Same as regular BICROS but with tube (open canal earmould system) in better ear.
UNICROS	One microphone feeding two amplifiers and two earphones. Closed mould fitted to poorer ear, tube (open canal earmould system) to better ear.
Power CROS	Same as classic CROS but with high gain and output amplifier and closed earmould. Minimizes feedback problems.
FROS	Frontal routing of signals. Microphone in front of spectacle frame feeding amplifier and earphone on same side.
BIFROS	A FROS system on each side (Fig. 7).
BIFROS 270	Same as BIFROS but with an extra microphone on each side set in side arms of spectacle aid.

"In-the-ear" (Intrameatal) Aids fit entirely within the ...oncha and external acoustic meatus.

Aids Worn on a Headband are used only in special cases ...here other methods of wearing an aid prove difficult, e.g. ...ith a malformed external ear.

...ducational Aids

Both body-worn and head-worn aids are limited in their ...erformance and it is only by the employment of large, ...gh-quality earphones that it is possible to improve on ...is performance. Large earphones, i.e. supra- and ...rcumaural headphone types are normally used in ...njunction with auditory training units and group hearing ...ds for educational purposes. These are discussed in ...hapter 61.

...one-conduction Aids

In cases of very severe conductive hearing loss and when ...a earmould cannot be used, e.g. in some discharging ears, ...one-conduction hearing aids may be fitted. A bone ...nduction transducer (bone vibrator) can be fitted on to a ...adband as in Fig. 2, or built into the arms of a pair of spectacles. Reinforced spectacle arms are available to hold a bone vibrator used with a body-worn aid. Bone vibrators are relatively inefficient devices and therefore require a more powerful amplifier to drive them than would be necessary for air conduction earphones. The frequency response of bone vibrators is poor below 500 Hz and does not usually extend above 4 kHz.

The performance of a bone vibrator is closely related to the contact pressure of the vibrator against the head. Consequently the relatively high pressure required for good performance may well cause discomfort in use.

Where a severe discharge from the ear prevents the use of an earmould, an alternative to bone conduction is the use of a lightweight external earphone on a headband similar to that used on a telephone. This type of earphone is provided in the British National Health Service range of aids. It is estimated that the proportion of cases requiring bone-conduction aids is only of the order of one or two per cent (Knight, 1970).

Performance

The performance of a hearing aid is usually specified in terms of its frequency response, maximum acoustic amplification and maximum acoustic output. Standardized methods of measuring the above parameters are detailed in British Standard 3171 (1968) and the International Electrotechnical Commission (I.E.C.) Publication 118 (1959). It is important to realize that the performance of an aid is measured in the absence of a user and in a very artificial, but reproducible, manner. The purpose of these measurements is to allow the collection of quantitative information on hearing aids for comparative purposes (I.E.C. Publication 126, 1961).

Measurement of Performance

To measure the performance of an aid it is placed in a non-reverberant acoustic enclosure (*anechoic chamber*) of known properties. For routine purposes, an *acoustic test box* is usually employed. A loudspeaker is driven from a pure tone oscillator and thus an acoustic signal at a known sound pressure level and frequency may be fed into the microphone of the hearing aid. This test signal is presented at frequencies within the range 100–10000 Hz, either at discrete frequencies or sweeping the entire range continuously. The output from the hearing aid is fed into a standardized acoustic coupler (I.E.C. Publication 126, 1961) which consists of a 2 cubic centimetres cavity in which the sound pressure level is measured (Fig. 8). The output from the measuring microphone in the acoustic coupler is amplified and fed to a pen recorder or display unit.

The acoustic coupler does not truly simulate the effect of a *real* ear. Sachs and Burchard (1973) have shown that considerable differences may arise between measurements on a real ear and on the I.E.C. coupler. A closer correspondence is found with Zwislocki's (1970) acoustic coupler (Richter and Diestel, 1973) (Fig. 9).

The standard method of measuring hearing aid performance does not take into account gross acoustic

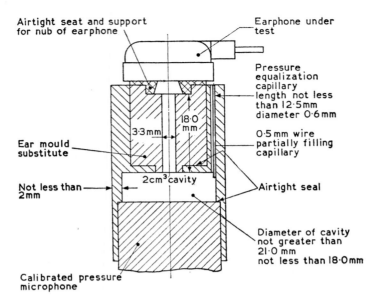

NOTE. This diagram is only intended as a schematic representation, illustrating the principle of construction.

1. Acoustic connection to the coupler

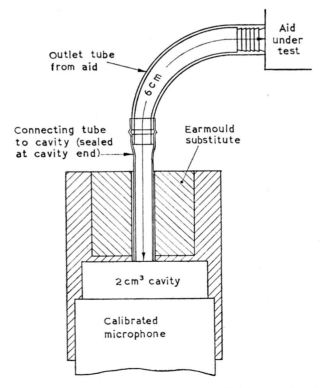

NOTE 1. When outlet tube from aid is not specified or supplied, the **connecting tube from** the cavity should be 6 cm long and connected directly onto the aid.

NOTE 2. The connecting tube should have an internal diameter of 2 ± 0.13 mm and external diameter of 3 ± 0.13 mm unless otherwise stated.

NOTE 3. All dimensions for cavity as for Fig. 1.

2. Form of coupling for hearing aids with acoustic connecting tubes

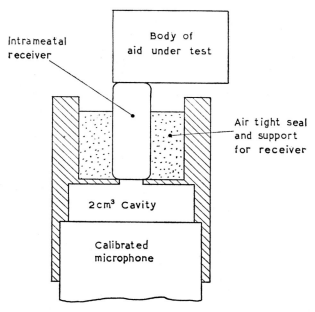

NOTE 1. Care should be taken that results are not influenced by mechanical coupling through the test apparatus, and it is recommended that the body of the aid be freely suspended.
NOTE 2. All dimensions for cavity as for Fig. 1.

3. Form of coupling hearing aids with intrameatal receivers

FIG. 8. Measurement of Hearing Aid Performance: a 2 cc acoustic coupler with three possible methods of connection (BS 3171:1968): (1) direct connection of insert earphone to the coupler, (2) a form of coupling for hearing aids with acoustic connecting tubes, and (3) a form of coupling for hearing aids with intrameatal earphones. For acoustic connecting tubes, a metal adaptor is now used and fitted on top of the earmould substitute. (Amendment No 1, 1973, to IEC Publication 118.)

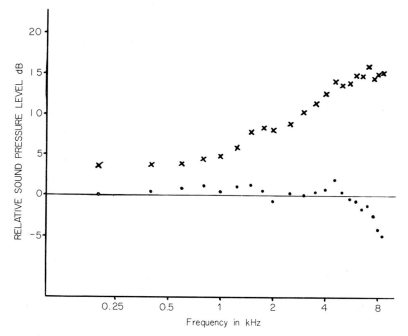

FIG. 9. Sound pressure levels in real ears compared with those developed in: IEC 126 2 cc coupler (x x x), and in Zwislocki coupler (. . .). (After Sachs and Burchard, 1973.)

effects due to the presence of the user. These are referred to as *body-baffle* and *head-baffle* effects (Fig. 10).

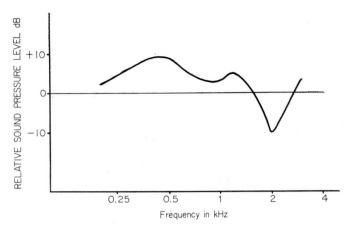

FIG. 10. Body baffle effect. Ratio of sound pressures when aid worn on chest to those delivered when aid suspended in free space. (Based on data obtained by D. Byrne.)

Frequency Response

The overall performance of a hearing aid is best described by a family of frequency response curves as in Fig. 11. From this it may be seen that the shape of the frequency response curve is dependent upon the input signal level at which it is measured. The true frequency response characteristic of the aid is that taken on a linear

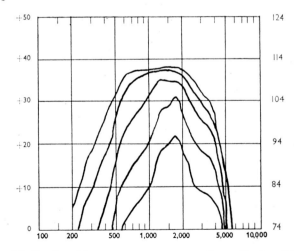

FIG. 11. Family of frequency response curves for an "in-the-ear" aid showing dependence of frequency response on input level. Horizontal axis gives frequency in hertz. Left hand vertical axis gives total output pressure in decibels re 0·1 pascals; right hand vertical axis in decibels SPL. Maximum gain. 1·3 V battery. Earphone coupled directly to 2 cc cavity. Acoustic input field: upper to lower curves in 10 dB steps; + 20 dB to − 20 dB re 0·1 Pa (94 dB to 54 dB SPL).

portion of the input-output characteristic; when limiting occurs the true frequency response is obscured. The acoustic amplification of the aid can be easily calculated at any frequency by subtracting the input signal level from the output level at a point on the linear portion of the input-output function, and when both of these quantities are expressed in decibels.

As the input signal level is increased, a proportional increase in output occurs up to a point (*saturation point*) where limiting commences. After this point is reached, any further increase in input results in no further significant increase in output and consequently the acoustic output represents the maximum obtainable. The value of the *maximum acoustic output* is of prime importance in selecting hearing aids. Aids should be chosen so that the maximum output has a value that is lower than the user's threshold of discomfort.

The frequency response characteristic of the hearing aid is largely determined by the individual responses of the microphone and the earphone. In general, the microphone influences the low frequency response of the aid while the earphone imposes limitations at the high frequency end of the response.

Microphones in valve hearing aids were almost always high output impedance devices employing piezo-electric crystals. These worked satisfactorily when coupled to the very high input impedance of a valve. With the introduction of germanium transistor amplifiers with low input impedances, crystal microphones were not satisfactory due to the resulting impedance mismatch. Consequently, low impedance magnetic microphones were introduced in transistor aids but, due to their small size, had a poor low frequency response. With the development of semi-conductor technology, high input impedances can now be obtained either by improved circuit designs or, better still by using field-effect transistors (FET) (*see* Chapter 5). The use of ceramic piezo-electric materials has therefore become possible.

A more recent development has been the introduction of the electret* microphone (*see* Chapter 7) which works in the same manner as a condenser microphone but with the polarizing charge held in an electret foil instead of being supplied from an external source. The electret microphone has the advantage that it has a very wide frequency response and is relatively insensitive to mechanical vibration, thus making it less prone to cause mechanical feedback in head-worn aids.

A recent development has been that of a *directional microphone* in which sounds coming from one direction, e.g. the rear, are attenuated with respect to sounds from another direction. This effect is achieved by means of two ports (holes) in the microphone which allows phase cancellation of the signal (Carlson and Killion, 1973).

Earphones for hearing aids are interchangeable on body worn aids and this provides a means of altering the performance of aids (Fig. 12). The low-frequency limitations of miniature (button) type earphones are largely due to acoustic leakage. With no leakage, usable response down to 20 Hz are easily obtained. At high frequencies the acoustic output is seriously limited as a result of the physical size of the transducer. Relatively wide-band frequency responses are possible, but not with high acoustic output. If high output is required then the bandwidth must be restricted. It is only possible to obtain wide bandwidth and high output with large external

* An electret is a permanently polarized piece of dielectric material it is therefore analogous to a magnet.

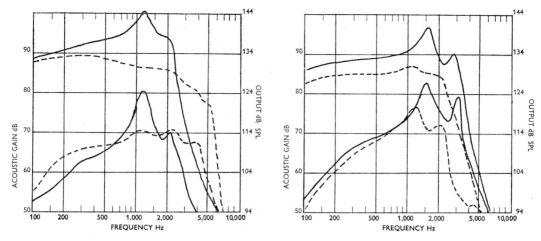

FIG. 12. Effect of four different earphones on gain, maximum acoustic output and frequency response of a hearing aid. In the left hand graph, the interrupted line refers to earphone of type A and the continuous line for earphone type B; in the right hand graph, the interrupted line refers to earphone type C and the continuous line to earphone type D. In each graph, the lower curves refer to the frequency response and acoustic gain for an input of 54 dB SPL with tone control set to N and gain control at maximum. The upper curves are for the maximum acoustic output (input 94 dB SPL). Output is measured in IEC 2 cc acoustic coupler.

earphones. Earphones are now available that are almost half the size of previous types, but retain comparable performances.

With body-worn aids, it is normal practice to connect a single earphone; however, in certain cases it may be desirable to stimulate both ears from the one aid. In this case it is possible to connect the earphones by means of a "Y" lead where the leg of the "Y" is connected to the aid and one earphone is connected to each of the two arms.

"Y" leads may be connected electrically in either a series or a parallel manner. In the latter case (sometimes referred to as a "V" lead), a pair of wires goes to each of the earphones and these pairs are connected together at the plug going into the aid. The series-connected "Y" lead however has two wires from the plug at the aid end of the lead, one wire going to each of the earphones. A common wire then connects the other side of each earphone. The manner of connection is important since, depending upon the impedance of the earphone and the output impedance of the aid, the effect of connecting two earphones instead of a single one might cause a severe drop in output, greater than the 3 dB due to sharing the output power between two equal loads.

The amplifier of a hearing aid imposes very few practical restrictions on the frequency response. The power output is limited only by battery current considerations and the efficiency of the microphone and the earphone.

Maximum Acoustic Output

The *maximum acoustic output (saturation sound pressure level)* of a hearing aid is defined as the greatest sound pressure level available from the hearing aid at a given frequency. It may be seen from Fig. 11 that, for low input levels, as the input sound pressure level increases, the output also increases in a linear fashion. However, a point is reached where the input-output characteristic becomes non-linear and a plateau is reached where no

further increase in output occurs with increase in input. This plateau defines the maximum acoustic output and *peak clipping* occurs here. Peak clipping, as its name indicates, is a clipping of the top and bottom of the signal thus providing instantaneous limitation, but with a large increase in distortion. At this maximum acoustic output the signal is particularly distorted at low frequencies. Owing to the low-pass filtering action of the earphone, the acoustic output at high frequencies exhibits non-linear distortion but does not suffer from harmonic distortion.* Consequently, the acoustic output waveform shows no distortion although no change in output occurs with increased input.

The *rated maximum sound pressure level* at a specified frequency is taken to be the lowest value of sound pressure level in the coupler at which the total harmonic distortion reaches 10 per cent.

Output Limitations

The maximum acoustic output can be varied in a number of ways but in only one of these does the action of the gain ("volume") control affect the maximum acoustic output. The point often overlooked in fitting hearing aids is that turning down the gain control reduces the gain but, if the input level is sufficiently intense, such as may easily occur unexpectedly, then the input sound will be high enough to drive the aid to its maximum output and possibly cause discomfort to the user. All hearing aids eventually limit the acoustic output by a peak-clipping action, but in some aids this peak clipping is made variable and an internal adjustment sets the output to a desired value. It should be noted, however, that this occurs only at the maximum

---

* *Harmonic distortion* refers to the production of *harmonic* frequencies at the output of the transducer when a sinusoidal voltage is applied to the input. A *harmonic (frequency)* refers to a frequency which is an integral multiple of the fundamental frequency; thus the *n*th harmonic is *n* times the fundamental frequency.

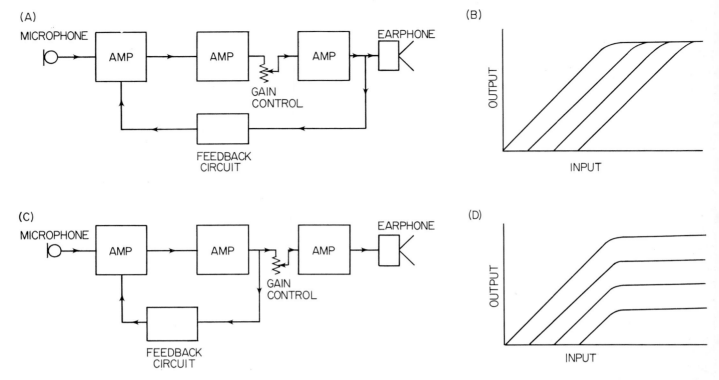

FIG 13. Two AGC systems: three stage amplifier with gain control inside AGC loop (A), and three stage amplifier with gain control outside AGC loop (C). (B) shows the input-output characteristics of the (A) system and the effect of reducing the gain control; maximum output remains constant when the gain is reduced. (D) shows the input–output characteristics of system (C) and the effect of reducing the gain control.

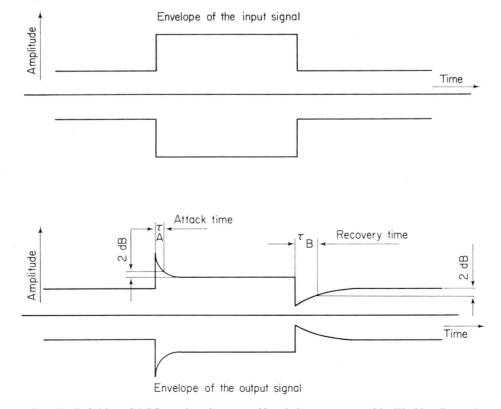

FIG. 14. Definition of AGC attack and recovery (decay) times as suggested by Working Group 6 (Hearing Aids) of IEC Technical Committee 29.

acoustic output of the aid and that the circuitry for this purpose is usually in the output stage.

An alternative method of controlling the output is by means of *automatic gain control* (AGC), which is also referred to as *automatic volume control* (AVC). This takes a finite time to operate and produces a reduced maximum output with little distortion. AGC in hearing aids usually

testing hearing aids with AGC and defines attack and decay times (Fig. 14). Values for AGC time constants vary and typical values have been a 20 ms attack time and a 200 ms decay time. Recently, very fast-acting AGC circuits have been produced with time constants of 5 and 50 ms; these are referred to as *instantaneous systems* by manufacturers. Trinder (1970, 1972) has described a

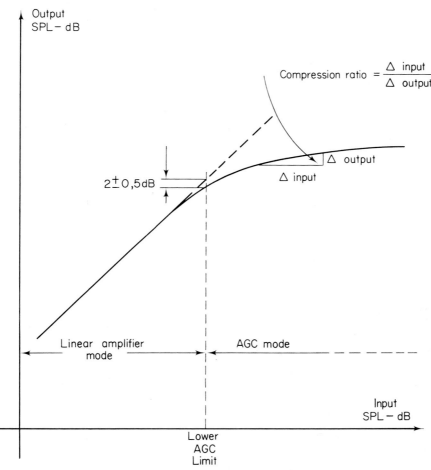

FIG. 15. Example of AGC steady state input–output graph as suggested by Working Group 6 (Hearing Aids) of IEC Technical Committee 29.

operates by taking a small part of the output signal and feeding it back to the first stage, where it is used to control the degree of amplification (Fig. 13). In most aids, the AGC is as above and the gain control of the aid is incorporated in the feedback loop. Recently, aids have been produced where the gain control is outside the AGC feedback loop and is situated before the output stage (Fig. 13). The effect of this is for the gain control to act as an output control and the full effect of the AGC is retained at all settings of the volume control. Figure 13 also shows the effect of the gain control on the input-output characteristics of the two forms of AGC.

Important features of AGC circuits are first, the time they take to operate (the *attack time*) and secondly, the time they take to return to normal (*decay* or "*release*" *time*). An I.E.C. draft Standard describes the method of

truly instantaneous system using *positive and negative logarithmic amplifiers*.

With some aids, the output limiting system is referred to as *compression amplification* or *linear dynamic compression* (LDC). However, it is difficult to separate the action of these systems from that of AGC, apart from different attack and decay times, and no agreement on standardization of these various terms has been reached. All such systems show an input-output characteristic as in Fig. 15.

Specification of Performance

The performance of a hearing aid depends upon a number of measures which are frequency dependent; this presents problems when single figures of overall performance are required. In the U.S.A., the Hearing Aid

Industry Conference (HAIC) (1961) produced a recommendation for calculating average gain and output figures. A method for determining the bandwidth was also described and is depicted in Fig. 16. American National Standard S3.3 (1960) describes the standardized method derived from the HAIC recommendation for use in the U.S.A. These

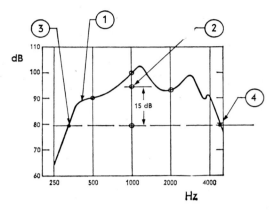

FIG. 16. HAIC method for calculating average gain and output, as well as bandwidths, of a hearing aid. The basic frequency response (1) is measured and the average of the 500, 1000 and 2000 Hz values is calculated (2). The lower frequency limit (3) and the higher frequency limit (4) are each taken as the point where the frequency response curve cuts a line 15 dB below the average value (2).

recommendations are, however, not universally accepted, although the method is widely used for expressing performance. The problem is in relating the measured performance to the effective performance of the aid in respect of the user. To date it is not known which part, or parts, of the frequency response characteristic determines the gain that a user will require and therefore an average of the values at three arbitrary frequencies may be misleading.

Jerger and Thelin (1968) have suggested a method of specifying the irregularity in frequency response by dividing up the amplitude into 2·5 dB sections and counting the number of times the frequency response curve crosses each 2·5 dB section.

The United States Veterans Administration (1970) have a method of measuring the uniformity of slope; this permits a decision as to which aid meets their requested criterion of a 5 dB per octave rise in frequency response. The method depends upon dividing the frequency range into 20 bands which give equal contribution to the intelligibility of speech (Kryter, 1950), and then taking gain values for the 20 points. A 5 dB per octave line is next drawn on the response curve 5 dB below the median value of these 20 points. The difference is then taken between the constructed line and the response of the aid. The mean difference then describes the degree to which the aid departs from the required response.

The now obsolete British Standard BS 3171:1959 described a method of rating the sensitivity of hearing aids by dividing the frequency range into three sections, i.e. 200–800, 800–2500 and 2500–4000 Hz. The average value of each of these frequency ranges was found by drawing a horizontal line so that the total area between the line and the frequency response curve above was equal to the area between the line and the frequency response curve below.

Although the HAIC and other indices provide a useful guide, they do not replace the full set of response curves and other data given by manufacturers.

Independent evaluations of the electro-acoustic performance of hearing aids are undertaken by Physikalisch-Technische Bundesanstalt (PTB) in Germany, (Brinkmann and Broksch, 1971, 1972), and by the Royal National Institute for the Deaf (RNID) in London (Denes and Fry, 1951). The RNID publish reports of hearing aid performance in their journal *Hearing*.

Performance of Current Aids

The four hundred or so models of hearing aids on the market at the present time (RNID, 1975) may be broken down into groups according to their gain, maximum acoustic output and frequency response. In terms of frequency response, it can be shown that the range and variation available is not very great (Martin, 1971). This is because the transducers used in most hearing aids are made by only one or two manufacturers. Thus, for the purposes of classification, frequency response can be ignored and only gain and output used as the criteria, as shown in Table 2.

TABLE 2

	Gain in dB at 1 kHz	Maximum Acoustic Output (dB SPL at 1 kHz)
Body-worn Aids		
Low	Under 40	Under 115
Medium	40–55	116–125
High	56–70	126–135
Very high	Over 70	Over 135
Head-worn Aids		
Low	Under 40	Under 110
Medium	40–55	111–120
High	55–60	120–125
Very high	Over 60	Over 125

The United States Veterans Administration (1970) have laid down three categories of gain and output for all aids purchased by them; these categories are given in Table 3. No aid may have a maximum gain of less than 29 dB or a maximum output of less than 97 dB SPL.

TABLE 3

Class	Average Maximum Gain in dB (1, 1·5, 2 kHz)	Average Maximum Power dB SPL (Random Noise Signal)
Mild	31–52	99–119
Moderate	41–62	120–129
Strong	58 or above	130–139

In a survey of 4975 aids issued in 1967, the Veterans Administration found that the aids which they provided were distributed as in Table 4.

TABLE 4

Strong power	13%	Body-worn aids	24%
Moderate power	44%	Post-aural aids	51%
Mild power	43%	Spectacle aids	24%

The frequency response, gain and output for some currently available aids are given in Fig. 17. These characteristics may be modified by the use of the controls

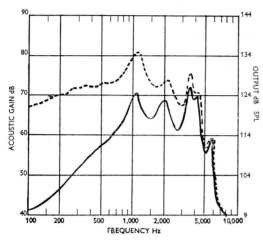

FIG. 17(A).

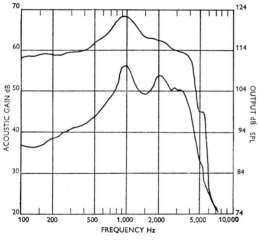

FIG. 17(B).

so that greater use can be made of the inductive loop system (*see* Chapter 61).

The degree of hearing loss that can be helped with any particular hearing aid is difficult to assess from theoretical considerations. However, as a general rule, losses of less than 70 dB can be assisted with body- or head-worn aids except, perhaps, "in-the-ear" aids. Losses of between 70 and 90 dB will require either a high, or very high, powered head-worn aid, or a body-worn aid. Losses of greater than 90 dB will normally only be effectively helped by a body-worn aid. It must be remembered, however, that the above figures are only rough guides and that many other factors such as intelligence, degree of determination, as well as the

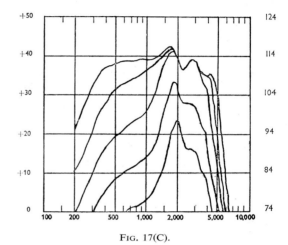

FIG. 17(C).

FIG. 17. Frequency response curves for three types of hearing aids: (A) high-powered spectacle aid (interrupted line is maximum acoustic output at maximum gain setting; acoustic input 94 dB SPL. Continuous line is frequency response at maximum gain setting with acoustic input of 54 dB SPL), (B) ear-level aid with ceramic microphone (upper curve is for maximum acoustic output with acoustic input of 94 dB SPL; lower curve is frequency response at maximum gain setting with acoustic input of 54 dB SPL), and (C) an "in-the-ear" type (horizontal axis is frequency in Hz, left hand vertical axis is sound output pressure in dB re 0·1 Pa; right hand vertical axis is output in dB SPL. Acoustic input field falls in 10 dB steps from +20 dB to −20 dB re 0·1 Pa, i.e. over range 94 dB to 54 dB SPL). All outputs are measured in IEC 2 cc acoustic coupler.

degree and the type of hearing loss will modify these criteria.

Circuit Design

Hearing aid amplifiers are basically simple audio-frequency amplifiers. Figure 18 shows a three-stage direct coupled hearing aid using discrete components. Integrated circuits (Fig. 19), where all three transistors and some resistors are formed on a semiconductor chip by diffusion processes, are used by some manufacturers (Dorendorf, 1966). The advantages of integrated circuits are disputed by some manufacturers who argue that the large number of external components required provide no saving over discrete components and that selection of circuits is needed to obtain the required electrical performance. It is necessary, however, to select transistors for discrete component amplifiers to ensure that a low-noise, high-gain amplifier is obtained. The amount of electrical gain

on the aid. Body-worn aids will often have a tone control switch as well as a switch for changing the input from the microphone to an inductive pick-up coil, or to a combined microphone and pick-up coil position. In this combined position, the microphone is often reduced in sensitivity because of the need to emphasize the signals coming from the pick-up coil, usually for educational purposes.

Head-worn hearing aids do not often have tone controls or pick-up coils. One would expect the introduction of a pick-up coil in the British National Health Service post-aural aid to be followed by its introduction into other aids

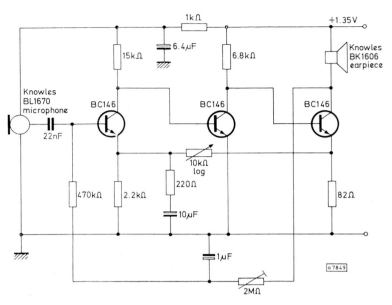

FIG. 18. Three-stage hearing aid circuit with 300 μW output

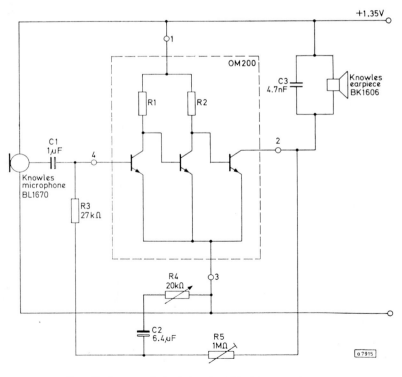

FIG. 19. Integrated circuit hearing aid with 200 μW output.

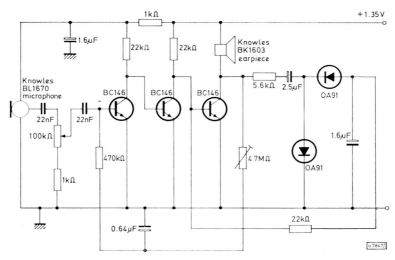

FIG. 20. Three stage circuit with AGC and 70 μW output. (Reproduced by courtesy of Mullard Limited.)

required is a function of the sensitivities of the transducers; their efficiency is low so that for an acoustic gain of, for example, 50 dB, an electrical gain of some 80 dB is required.

AGC circuits are usually of a simple nature as in Fig. 20 although, in more recent times, as already mentioned, more sophisticated circuits have been used which have fast attack and decay times. Integrated circuits with AGC incorporated are available to give up to 40 dB of compression. Veit (1973) has reviewed the design of AGC circuits.

An important design feature of the amplifier is the power consumption as, the higher the current drain, the shorter the battery life will be. Modern aids are made with current consumptions of between 0·5 and 2 mA, except for high-powered models where class B push-pull circuits (*see* Chapter 56) are used. In high-power aids, peak battery currents may be as high as 10–20 mA with quiescent currents of 0·5 mA.

Recoding Devices

In cases of profound hearing loss, where no useful high-frequency hearing exists, equipment has been produced which *transposes* the high frequencies down to the low frequencies that can be usefully used. Johannson (1959, 1966) has advocated a form of transposition that superimposes frequencies above 4 kHz on the linearly amplified low-frequency band. Figure 21 gives details of a wearable transposing type hearing aid.

An alternative to frequency transposition is analysis of the input sound and then *synthesis* in such a way that the output is contained within a narrow range of frequencies. Pimonow (1968) has described such a device.

Risberg (1969) has critically reviewed the use of recoding devices and Rowarth (1970) has reviewed the use of the synthesis techniques.

Earmoulds

The earmould is not a part of the hearing aid itself but is, of course, a vital part of the hearing aid system. The

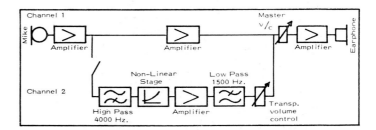

FIG. 21. Block diagram of a commercially available body-worn frequency transposing hearing aid. Channel 1 allows all signals to pass through while the lower channel (Channel 2) filters off all sounds below 4 kHz and then effectively distorts these high frequency signals. The distorted signal contains a large amount of low frequency energy which is then passed back to the normal channel through a low pass filter and superimposed on Channel 1. A switch allows the possibility of using the aid as a conventional body-worn instrument or as a transposing aid.

earmould performs the function of delivering the sound into the ear and holding the earphone, or even the aid itself, in position as well as preventing sound leakage back to the microphone; this sound leakage is termed *acoustic feedback* ("whistling").

Earmoulds are normally made from an impression taken from the user's ear. The impression material normally used today is silicone rubber. This is initially in the form of a soft pliable material into which is put a small portion of hardener just prior to insertion in the ear. The two materials are mixed together and then formed into a cone shape. The apex of the cone is placed into the external acoustic meatus and the material then pressed into the meatus and then into the rest of the external ear. It is most important to ensure that the *concha of the auricle*, including the *cymba conchae*, is filled with impression material since this part holds the earmould in position when fitted. The impression material is allowed to set (this takes a few minutes) and then removed from the ear and sent to an earmould manufacturer. It must be remembered that the manufacturer does not see the individual's ear and it is therefore important to ensure that as much detail as possible is contained in the impression. Some technicians cut the surplus material from earmoulds, often at the request of the manufacturer, but this, if not carried out carefully, can lead to earmoulds being produced with insufficient of the structure to obtain a purchase in the cymba.

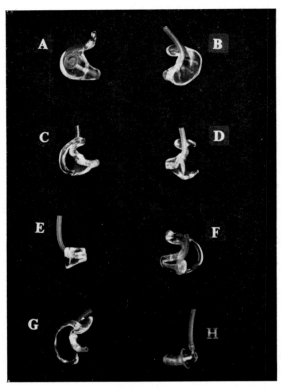

FIG. 22. Some current types of earmould: Type A is the familiar solid earmould supplied with body-worn hearing aids. It has a recess and snap-ring to accommodate the "button" receiver. Types B (shell) and C (skeleton) are the moulds most commonly used with earlevel aids. They are fitted with a length of plastic tubing which conducts the sound from the hearing aid receiver. Type D is a reduced form of skeleton earmould and is termed a three-quarter skeleton mould. Type E, the meatal tip mould, is reduced even further to the form of a plug which occludes the meatus. It is unsuitable when high degrees of amplification are required. Earmoulds A to E all effectively seal the ear canal, but in some situations a controlled "leak" past the ear-mould is desirable. This may be done either to reduce the "closed-in" feeling of pressure in the ear or to filter off excessive low frequency sound energy (for instance, if a person has a pronounced high-tone loss). Earmould Type F is equipped with a variable vent enabling the filter characteristics to be changed. The open earmould, Type G, carried the venting process to the extreme where the mould serves only to carry the sound conduction tubing into the ear canal. Finally, Type H is included to demonstrate a proprietary temporary ear pip which is available in a number of stock sizes. (After Grover, 1974.)

From a single aural impression it is possible to specify the type of mould required. Grover (1974) has suggested a basic terminology to cover the various types of mould available (Fig. 22), as has the National Association of Earmould Laboratories in the U.S.A. (Sachman *et al.*, 1973).

The fit of the earmould affects the low-frequency response of the aid as is shown in Fig. 23. In some cases, earmoulds are deliberately *vented* with an acoustic leak to

reduce low frequency levels for improved comfort and to use with CROS systems (*see previously*).

The earmould configuration affects the frequency response of the aid and Dalsgaard and his colleagues (1966) have shown the effect of varying the dimensions of various parts of the earmould. Where an acoustic tube is used, as in a post-aural aid, the length (Fig. 24) and bore (internal diameter) (Fig. 25) of the tube can affect the performance. The material used to form the final earmould is usually a hard, clear acrylic plastic. In cases where the user's skin is sensitive to this material, earmoulds can be made of vulcanite. Soft materials are also available which are claimed to be more comfortable for the user and yet allow a better acoustic seal in the ear, thus allowing a higher degree of amplification to be used without feedback problems.

Grover and Martin (1974) have shown that practical values of amplification of the order of 50 dB over the range 0·5–4 kHz can be obtained without difficulty when using conventional earmoulds. When it is not possible to have an earmould made by a manufacturer, or where speed is required, *cold-cure material* is available for making a mould direct from the aural impression. Self-curing materials of this type generate a considerable amount of heat so it is important to use the material in the correct manner and remove it from the ear in the prescribed time. A technique has been developed by one company* whereby, by placing a plastic tube in the meatus first and building up material around it, it is possible to make an earmould with a hole in it and thus eliminate the final drilling operation.

Selection of Aids

This is discussed in Chapter 60.

IMPLANTABLE AUDITORY PROSTHESES

The possibility of implanting a hearing aid would seem to offer considerable advantages to many deaf people. By implanting an aid it is hoped that all the psychological problems of wearing an aid would be removed and that a greater benefit in terms of speech perception would be obtained.

Four approaches to implanting auditory prostheses are possible; they differ radically in their methods.

Tympano-ossicular Auditory Implants

The simplest method is to use a conventional aid but with the microphone external to the head and the output transducer either fixed to the eardrum or built into the middle ear cavity. Goode (1970) has reviewed this area of work and points out that there are three primary drawbacks to the use of implants of this type:

(1) An operation is required for insertion and removal of the device.
(2) A potential source of infection is present.

* C.M.W. Laboratories Limited, Polymer Division, Preston New Road, Blackpool, Lancashire.

(3) Mediocre or poor acoustic performance may be substituted for improved cosmetic appearance.

In summing up, Goode makes the following appraisal: "Advances in medical technology not uncommonly precede their appreciation and proper application by physicians by an inordinate length of time. Such may be the case with implantable aids. However, the technical ability to implant a hearing aid and to make it work is much different than the necessity for doing so. It is the latter that is important. Advances from other fields that have the potential for being applied to the improvement of hearing certainly should be investigated in the laboratory."

Dental Auditory Implants

Under this heading mention should be made of *audiodontics* (hearing through the teeth). The main method of

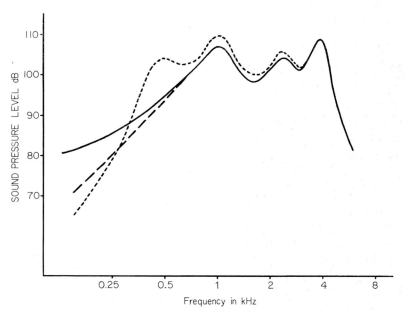

FIG. 23. Frequency response of a typical head-worn hearing aid modified by either acoustic leakage (interrupted line) or an earmould vent (dotted line). The unmodified response is shown by a continuous line.

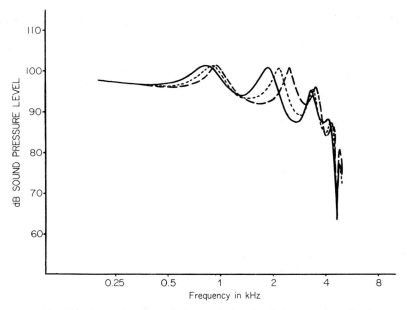

FIG. 24. This shows the effect of changes in length of the sound conduction tubing on the frequency response of an aid, as measured in a Zwislocki coupler. The continuous line indicates the response curve for a 50 mm length of tubing, the dotted line a 40 mm length and the interrupted line a 30 mm length.

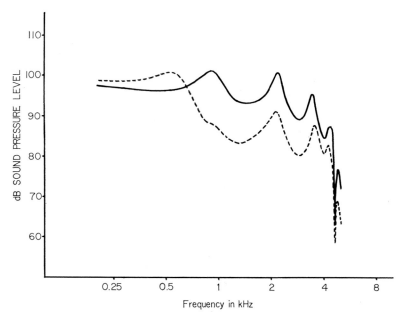

FIG. 25. Effect on frequency response curve of bore of sound conduction tubing attached to an earphone and as measured on a Zwislocki coupler. The continuous line indicates the response curve for tubing with a 2 mm bore; the interrupted line, the response curve for a 1 mm bore. Total tube length 40 mm.

stimulation is by means of vibrating the teeth. Dahlin (1972) has shown that the teeth are as sensitive as the mastoid process for bone conduction and that they are also less prone to change in sensitivity with change in position of the vibrator. Practical problems in fitting an aid of this type preclude its general use.

In a U.S. patent issued in 1961, Puharich has described a *dental radio receiver*. Radio frequency signals are received by a gold inlay, converted to electrical signals in the audio-frequency range by a subjacent rectifier crystal and "imparted to the nerve endings of the tooth for transmission to the brain". It was envisaged that the user would carry a small radio transmitter which would pick up sounds and transmit them to the tooth. Although the device would receive radio signals directly, it would, of course work best with an amplifier. In a subsequent patent, Puharich (1964) described circuitry for an amplifier to be mounted in another tooth. Although Puharich claims that this prosthesis works by electrical stimulation of the trigeminal nerve endings in the tooth, one wonders to what extent structure-borne acoustic signals are transmitted to the ear. Moreover we have yet to see practical applications of this technique.

Cochlear Implants

The third method is to implant an active electrode in the cochlea itself (*see* Chapter 54) and thus stimulate the vestibulocochlear nerve directly. A considerable amount of experimentation has shown that stimulation is possible but that it does not give rise to normal hearing (House and Urban, 1973; Merzenich *et al.*, 1973; Lawrence and Johnson, 1973). Most studies show that stimulation of the

basal turn of the cochlea appears to give rise to a sensation of hearing below 500 Hz.

Cortical Stimulation

The fourth method is to stimulate the auditory cortex of the brain. Dobelle and his colleagues (1973) have undertaken experiments on normally hearing patients during surgical exposure of the auditory cortex in the course of removing tumours. The extrapolation of the results to deaf patients is uncertain according to Dobelle, but he makes an analogy with stimulation of the visual cortex in blind people and concludes that this may give rise to reasons for optimism.

CONCLUSIONS

There are clearly a number of auditory prostheses other than the conventional hearing aid. The scope of these, particularly those with implanted transducers, may well expand appreciably in the future. Nevertheless, there is no doubt that, in the foreseeable future at least, the conventional hearing aid will remain the mainstay of auditory rehabilitation. Moreover, in view of research projects being conducted at the present, there are indications that, in contrast to the development of more sophisticated electronic prostheses, there will be an expansion in the use of non-electronic, i.e. acoustic, hearing aids, particularly for underprivileged rural communities in developing countries.

REFERENCES

Anon (1965), "Speaking Tubes. A Report from the RNID Technical Dept.," *Hearing*, **20**, 84.
Board of Trade (1970), *Business Monitor*, p. 77. London: H.M.S.O.

British Standard (1968) 3171, "Methods of Test of Air Conduction Hearing Aids," British Standards Institution, London.

Brinkmann, K. and Broksch, K. H. (1971), "Type Approved Testing of Hearing Aids by the Physikalisch-Technische Bundesanstalt," Part I, *J. Audiol. Tech.*, **10**, 6.

Brinkmann, K. and Broksch, K. H. (1972), "Type Approved Testing of Hearing Aids by the Physikalisch-Technische Bundesanstalt," Part 2, *J. Audiol. Tech.*, **11**, 32.

Bruce, R. V. (1973), *Alexander Graham Bell and the Conquest of Solitude*. Boston: Little Brown & Co.

Carlson, E. V. and Killion, M. (1973), "Subminiature Directional Microphones," Paper Presented at 4th Audio Engineering Society Convention.

Carver, W. F. (1972), "Hearing Aids. A Historical and Technical Review," in *Handbook of Clinical Audiology* (J. Katz, Ed.). Baltimore: Williams & Wilkins.

Dahlin, G. C., Collard, E. W. and Allen, F. G. (1972), "Audiodontics: Hearing Through the Teeth," Talk on 23rd March 1972 at 50th International Association for Dental Research. Las Vegas.

Dalsgaard, S. C., Johansen, P. A. and Chisnall, L. G. (1966), 'On the Frequency Response of Earmoulds," *J. Audiol. Tech.*, **4**, 126–139.

Denes, P. and Fry, D. B. (1951), *The Testing of Hearing Aids*, Booklet Number 490. London: National Institute for the Deaf.

Dobelle, W. H., Stensaas, S. S., Mladejovsky, M. G. and Smith, J. B. (1973), "A Prosthesis for the Deaf Based on Cortical Stimulation," *Ann. Otol.*, **82**, 445–463.

Dorendorf, H. (1966), "Integrated Semiconductor Circuits for Hearing Aid Amplifiers," *J. Audiol. Tech.*, **4**, 141–149.

Dunlavy, A. R. (1968), "CROS: A Review of Applications of Fittings Utilizing Contralateral Routing of Signals," *National Hearing Aid Journal*. July.

Dunlavy, A. R. (1974). Personal communication.

Goldstein, M. A. (1933), *Problems of the Deaf*. St. Louis, Mo., U.S.A.: Laryngoscope Press.

Goode, R. L. (1970), "An Implantable Hearing Aid," *Trans. Amer. Acad. Ophthal. Otolaryng.*, **74**, 128–139.

Grover, B. C. (1974), "The Shape of Earmoulds," *Hearing*, **29**, 232–233.

Grover, B. C. and Martin, M. C. (1974), "On the Practical Gain Limit for Post-aural Hearing Aids," *Brit. J. Audiol.*, **8**, 121–124.

HAIC (1961), "Standard Method of Expressing the Performance of Hearing Aids," Hearing Aid Industry Conference Inc., Washington D.C.

Harford, E. and Barry, J. (1965), "A Rehabilitative Approach to the Problems of Unilateral Hearing Impairment: The Contralateral Routing of Signals (CROS)," *J. Speech Hear. Dis.*, **30**, 121–138.

House, W. F. and Urban, J. (1973), "Long Term Results of Electrode Implantation and Electronic Stimulation of the Cochlea in Man," *Ann. Otol.*, **84**, 504–513.

I.E.C. Publication 118 (1959), *Recommended Methods for Measurements of the Electro-acoustical Characteristics of Hearing Aids*. Geneva: International Electrotechnical Commission.

I.E.C. Publication 126 (1961), *I.E.C. Reference Coupler for the Measurement of Hearing Aids Using Earphones Coupled to the Ear by Means of Ear Inserts*. Geneva: International Electrotechnical Commission.

Jerger, J. and Thelin, J. (1968), "Effects of Electroacoustic Characteristics of Hearing Aids on Speech Understanding," *Bulletin of Prosthetics Research*, pp. 159–197.

Johannson, B. (1959), "A New Coding Amplifier System for the Severely Hard of Hearing," *Proc. Third Int. Congress of Acoustics. Stuttgart*, **2**, 655–657.

Johannson, B. (1966), "The Use of the Transposer for the Management of the Deaf Child," *J. int. Audiol.*, **5**, 362–371.

Knight, J. J. (1970), "The Use of Bone Conduction Hearing Aids," *Sound*, **4**, 46–49.

Kryter, K. D. (1950), "Effects of Noise on Man," *J. Speech Hear. Dis. Monogr.*, supp. 1, 1–59.

Lawrence, M. and Johnson, L. (1973), 'The Role of the Organ of Corti in Auditory Nerve Stimulation,' *Ann. Otol.*, **82**, 464–472.

Martin, M. C. (1971), "Electroacoustic characteristics of hearing aids and sensorineural hearing loss". *Scand. Audiol Suppl.* 1.

Martin, M. C. (1973), "Hearing Aid Gain Requirements in Sensorineural Hearing Loss," *Brit. J. Audiol.*, **7**, 21.

Merzenich, M. M., Michelson, R. P., Petet, C. R., Schendler, R. A. and Reid, M. (1973), "Neural Encoding of Sound Sensation Evoked by Electrical Stimulation of the Acoustic Nerve," *Ann. Otol.*, **82**, 486–503.

Mullard (1969), *Mullard Hearing Aid Amplifier Circuits*. London: Consumer Electronics Division, Mullard Ltd.

Piminow, L. (1968), "Technical and Physiological Problems in the Application of Synthetic Speech to Aural Rehabilitation," *Amer. Ann. Deaf*, **113**, 275–282.

Puharich, A. H. (1961), U.S. Patent 2 995 637.

Puharich, A. H. (1964), U.S. Patent 3 156 787.

Risberg, A. (1969), "A Critical Review of Work on Speech Analysing Hearing Aids," in *I.E.E.E. Transactions on Audio and Electroacoustics*. AU-17, **4**, 290–297.

Richter, U. and Diestel, H. G. (1973), "The Frequency Response of an Insert Type Earphone at the Human Ear and Various Couplers," *J. Audiol. Tech.*, **12**, 146–167.

Rowarth, D. A. A. (1970), "The Re-Coding of Speech," *Sound*, **4**, 95–105.

RNID (1974), *Special Aids to Hearing*. London: Royal National Institute for the Deaf.

RNID (1975), "A List of Current Hearing Aids." Royal National Institute for the Deaf, London.

Sachs, R. M. and Burchard, M. D. (1972), "Insert Earphone Pressure Response in Real Ears and Couplers," *J. acoust. Soc. Amer.*, **52**, 183.

Trinder, E. (1970), "Experimental Hearing Aid Circuit with an Input-variable Transfer Function for the Correction of Cochlear Deafness," *Electronic Letters*, **7**, 1.

Trinder, E. (1972), "An Attempt to Correct Speech Discrimination Loss in Cochlear Deafness by Graded Instantaneous Compression," *Sound*, **6**, 62–67.

Veterans Administration (1970), "Hearing Aid Performance Measurement Data and Hearing Aid Selection Procedures," in *Contract Year* 1970. Washington: Veterans Administration.

Veit, I. (1973), "Practical Possibilities in the Design of Hearing Aids with Automatic Gain Control," *J. Audiol. Tech.*, **12**, 186–201.

Watson, L. A. and Tolan, T. (1949), *Hearing Tests and Hearing Instruments*. Baltimore: Williams and Wilkins Co.

Zachmann, T. A., Lankford, J. E. and Hahn, L. (1973), "Earmould Nomenclature," *J. Speech Hear. Dis.*, **38**, 456.

Zwislocki, J. J. (1970), "An Acoustic Coupler for Earphone Calibration," Report LSC-S-7. Laboratory of Sensory Communication, Syracuse University.

60. SELECTION OF HEARING AIDS

ANDREAS MARKIDES

Broadly speaking, a hearing aid can be described as any device that brings sound to the ear more effectively. Persons with a hearing impairment which cannot be remedied medically or surgically benefit to varying degrees from amplification through the use of hearing aids. In the last twenty-five years, mainly because of the increasing miniaturization of electronic components, hearing aids have tended to become both smaller and smaller (Lybarger, 1966) and more versatile in meeting individual needs. This has resulted in a plethora of hearing aids from tiny devices that can fit into the meatus, to group aids with multiple microphones and earphones and including, more recently, radio transmission aids. Every type of hearing aid has its advantages and disadvantages and some of these, together with the problems encountered in hearing aid selection, will be presented later in this chapter.

Modern developments in hearing aids have been influenced considerably by the recommendations embodied in two reports published just after World War II. One of these reports originated in the United Kingdom and it was produced by the Medical Research Council (M.R.C. Report); the other one came from the Psycho-Acoustic Laboratory of Harvard University (Harvard Report). Both reports were published in 1947 and although the two groups were working independently their conclusions were remarkably similar. Details regarding the recommendations of these two reports will be given in the course of this chapter.

Modern wearable hearing aids consist essentially of five parts—a microphone which transforms sound into electrical energy; a transistorized amplifying circuit; a battery that supplies energy; an earphone (receiver) that transduces the amplified electrical patterns back into sound; and a specially constructed earmould that channels sounds to the ear drum. A detailed description of each separate part of the hearing aid is given in the previous chapter.

Electroacoustic Characteristics of Hearing Aids

These have been discussed in the preceding chapter. Salient features of clinical importance will be mentioned here.

Frequency Response Curve

The frequency response curve, or frequency response characteristic of a hearing aid is a graph which shows how the gain (the amount of amplification which a hearing aid gives) changes with frequency.

According to the Hearing Aid Industries Conference (H.A.I.C.) in the U.S.A. the effective limits of the frequency range of an aid can be taken to be the points at the upper and lower ends of the curve intersected by a line drawn parallel to the base and 15 dB below the average gain at 500, 1000 and 2000 Hz (American Standard).

The M.R.C. Report recommended that the most useful frequency range of an aid was from 250 to 4000 Hz. Similarly, the Harvard report recommended a frequency range from 300 to 4000 Hz. Hudgins and his associates (1948), however, recommended a hearing aid with wider frequency response characteristics than those put forward in the above-mentioned reports. Work carried out at the University of Manchester (Watson, 1956) and recently

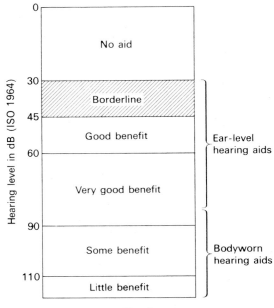

FIG. 1.

substantiated by Olsen and Carhart (1967), also showed that better patterns of speech were given back by severely deaf children when the response of the aid was relatively flat up to at least 6000, and, if possible, 8000 Hz.

The frequency response characteristics proposed by the M.R.C. and Harvard reports provided limited amplification in the low frequencies. Wedenberg (1954) and, later, Huizing (1959) pointed out that most hearing impaired children have better residual hearing in the frequency region below 750 Hz. This observation coupled with the fact that there exists sufficient information in these low frequencies to aid in the development of voice and language (Peterson and Barney, 1952; Watson, 1961) rendered some hearing aids unsuitable for such children.

It was with this view in mind that Ling (1964), Rice (1965) and Brinskey and Sinclair (1966) recommended the production of hearing aids with extended low-frequency amplification down to about 100 Hz. It may well be that the recommendations of both the M.R.C. and Harvard reports regarding the range of amplified frequencies are ideal for hearing impaired adults with mainly conductive hearing impairment. (It must be noted that the M.R.C.

report studied 228 adults, 61 per cent of whom had conductive hearing losses and the Harvard report dealt with 18 adult subjects with approximately half of them having conductive hearing impairments.) As has been shown, however, their applicability to children with severe hearing impairments is in question. Had hearing impaired children been included in these studies the recommendations might possibly have been appreciably different.

Working mainly within the frequency range of 250–4000 Hz, several studies attempted to identify patterns of amplification which would suit the majority of hearing aid users. The M.R.C. report recommended a 12 dB gain per octave from 250 to 750 Hz with either a flat curve extending to 4000 Hz or, for patients with high frequency losses, a rise of 6 dB per octave from 750–4000 Hz, with the gain at 750 Hz to be at least 40 dB. This became the design rule for the first "Medresco" hearing aids. The design rule for the later insert earphone "Medresco", however, is a gain of 7 dB per octave from 300 Hz to at least 3000 Hz with the gain at 750 Hz to be at least 52 dB. The Harvard report suggested that the gain should be a uniform one from 300 to 4000 Hz. As an alternative to this it suggested a moderate high tone emphasis of from 6 dB per octave throughout the range; with gain falling within the range of 40 dB as minimal to 80 dB as maximal.

Rice (1965), referring mainly to the needs of hearing impaired children, recommended a flat frequency response over the range of 250–4000 Hz with a maximum of 60 dB air to air gain. Two years later (Watson, 1967) put forward similar recommendations emphasizing the necessity for the aids to have a gain of not less than 65 dB if very deaf children were to hear their voices at the necessary levels.

The frequency response of most commercial bodyworn hearing aids can be altered through the use of a tone control (usually a three-position switch) which simply reduces the relative strength of the high frequency or the low frequency tones in the amplified signal. Another method of tone control is the use of alternative receivers with different frequency characteristics. Also for many years modifications of the earmould have been used with a view to changing the frequency response of hearing aids. Ewertsen and his associates (1957), for example, found that reproduction of high frequencies was better when an earmould with a short and wide canal was used instead of one with a long and narrow canal. Vented and open earmoulds were found to attenuate the amplified low frequencies and theoretically, such earmoulds are ideal for persons with high frequency sensorineural losses. This was partially verified experimentally by McClellan (1967) and by Hodgson and Murdock (1970). Lybarger (1958, 1967), however, warned against indiscriminate venting, since vents of different sizes were found to change the low frequency output differentially, and that certain sizes of vents may actually enhance the area around 500 Hz. It is also pointed out that venting creates a second acoustic leakage, thus increasing the possibility of acoustic feedback. Of course, the satisfactory performance of any hearing aid will depend on the efficiency with which the individual earmould fits the patient's ear. A bad seal at the meatus, for example, not only creates problems of acoustic feedback, poor retention and annoyance, but also has a detrimental effect on the low frequency response of the hearing aid (Boothroyd, 1965). This is very important, as most hearing impaired children are able to perceive only low frequency sounds.

Maximum Output

A hearing aid is expected to provide a sufficiently high level of output to enable hearing impaired people to hear speech at adequate levels above their thresholds. The usefulness of a hearing aid, therefore, depends not only on its frequency response characteristic of gain but also on its maximum output. The M.R.C. report concluded that the needs of most deaf people can be met with a hearing aid having undistorted maximum output of 120 dB (rms re 20 μPa). The Harvard report proposed 132 dB with variant maximum settings at 126, 120 and 114 dB. Rice (1965) was of the opinion that the maximum output level of a hearing aid should be restricted to 125 dB provided enough amplification was given in the 250–750 Hz frequency range. Watson (1967) preferred 130–135 dB as the maximum output level of a hearing aid.

It is difficult to be specific regarding clear-cut "desirable maximum output levels" of hearing aids. Indeed, such a question can only be answered on an individual basis. It is accepted, however, that the needs of the great majority of people suffering from sensorineural hearing losses can be met with wearable hearing aids having maximum acoustic outputs ranging from 110 to 130 dB SPL. For people suffering from mixed hearing losses, higher levels may be warranted. Similarly, children with severe hearing losses, 110–120 dB, may require outputs well in excess of 130 dB SPL.

The question arises, of course, as to whether powerful hearing aids cause further deterioration of hearing. Works by Kinney (1953, 1961), Møller and Rojskjaer (1960), Sataloff (1961), Ross and Truex (1965), Macrae and Farrant (1965), Ross and Lerman (1967), Macrae (1967, 1968) and Ballantyne (1970) uphold the idea that powerful hearing aids have a deleterious effect on the user's residual hearing. The opposite view was put forward by Holmgren (1940), Murray (1951), Naunton (1957), Brockman (1959), Whetnall (1964), Barr and Wedenberg (1965), World Health Organization (1967), Bellefleur and Van Dyke (1968) and Roberts (1970). Three years ago Markides (1971) evaluated all available literature on this topic and concluded that there was not as yet any conclusive scientific evidence that powerful hearing aids do or do not have an adverse effect on the user's residual hearing. In the absence of such evidence and in view of some evidence, though inconclusive, and theoretical predictions based on the energy concept of noise-induced hearing loss, a policy of caution is advisable when fitting hearing impaired persons, especially children, with powerful hearing aids.

Output Limitation

One of the fundamental principles in selecting a hearing aid is to choose an instrument with sufficient amplification and with a maximum acoustic output which is tolerable to the patient. This underlines the necessity of incorporating within a hearing aid a device for protecting the hearing aid user against high intensity sounds. Every electro-acoustic reproducing apparatus has, of course, a limited output. Two deliberate methods of limiting the output of a hearing aid have been devised, first, "peak clipping" (PC), and secondly, "compression amplification", also referred to as "automatic volume control" (AVC) or "automatic gain control" (AGC). The first method, which has been described by Licklider (1946) and recommended by the M.R.C. report, "clips" loud sounds at a predetermined level of amplification. According to the Harvard workers, however, "peak clipping" produces a great amount of harmonic and intermodulation distortion which can have severe effects on speech intelligibility in untrained listeners. They preferred the second method.

It was Littler (1944) who first recommended that protection from overamplification without distortion could be achieved through the use of compression amplification. The output of a hearing aid may be automatically limited when the intensity of the sound is greater than a predetermined level, or there may be systematic compression throughout the operating range. Hudgins and his colleagues (1948), in a follow-up study to the Harvard report, found distinct advantage in favour of compression amplification and there has been widespread preference for this method ever since, especially when dealing with hearing-impaired people suffering from an abnormally compressed dynamic range of hearing.

These studies used the first kind of compression amplification and it was mainly Caraway and Carhart (1967), followed by a small pilot study by Fleming and Rice (1969), which attempted a serious evaluation of the second kind of compression amplification, namely, the systematic compression of the speech signal throughout its dynamic range. The first writers used compression ratios of 1:1, 2:1 and 3:1 dB, while the second writers used compression ratios of 1:1, 2:1, 3:1 and 5:1. Trinder (1972) has improved on these compression systems. One problem associated with compression circuits is that amplification in noisy surroundings tends to become very unstable. In view of this, when recommending hearing aids with automatic volume control the audiologist must bear in mind the surroundings in which the hearing aid will be used most (Watson, 1970).

Main Types

Hearing aids may be conveniently classified into two major categories, i.e. those that can be worn and those that cannot. It should be noted, however, that "group hearing aids" are not considered as hearing aids by the International Electrotechnical Commission (I.E.C.).

Wearable (Personal) Hearing Aids

This category consists of bodyworn, post-aural, spectacle and in-the-ear aids.

The *bodyworn aids* are usually worn at chest level. There is a wide variety of such aids with differing electroacoustics properties. Generally speaking they are more powerful and they also provide amplification over a wider range of frequencies than the other types of wearable aids. In view

of this, they are particularly suitable for persons with severe hearing losses. Their conspicuousness and bulkiness, however, are definite drawbacks except for elderly people who cannot manage the smaller aids. The *post-aural aids* fit snugly behind the ear, thus satisfying strong aesthetic needs. They are less powerful than the high-powered bodyworn types but these days have a comparable frequency response. Because of this, they are of restricted value to persons with average hearing losses exceeding 80 dB. The *spectacle aids* which are housed in slightly enlarged spectacle frames have also been designed to meet obvious aesthetic needs. Their electro-acoustic performances are similar to those of the post-aural types but, owing to the possibility of separating the microphone and earphone, it is possible to produce higher gain and output than with post-aural aids.

The *in-the-ear aids* are tiny self-contained devices which can be accommodated wholly in the meatus. They exhibit limited performances in terms of amplification and frequency range and are of limited use. One problem that affects the efficiency of all ear-level types of aid is the high incidence of feed-back (or whistling) which occurs due to the close proximity of the microphone and the earphone.

Non-wearable Hearing Aids

This category, which includes auditory training units and group hearing aids is discussed in the next chapter.

Auditory training units are mostly found in schools and clinics for the hearing impaired and they are mainly used in the teaching of speech to hearing impaired children on an individual basis. They provide a high maximum output with a wide and flat frequency response characteristic. The group hearing aids have similar electro-acoustic properties as speech training units and are designed to cater for a group of three to ten hearing impaired children. These aids, however, limit freedom of movement by the pupils and as such they cannot be used for long periods.

Factors Affecting the Efficiency of Hearing Aids

Apart from the electro-acoustic limitations, environmental factors like the noise background, reverberation, and the distance of the speaker from the microphone impose further limitations on the final efficiency of a hearing aid.

In 1961, Sanders measured the noise levels in 47 classrooms in 15 different schools and he reported that the majority of classes exhibited noise levels well above 70 dBA while the levels of the voices of the teachers ranged from 64 to 70 dBA at 3 m. This, of course, is an unacceptable speech-to-noise ratio and one can well imagine the difficulties facing the hearing aid user. Extraneous noises can be avoided with careful siting of the school and unwanted sounds generated within the classroom can be dealt with through noise-reducing floor coverings and materials fixed to the base of movable objects.

Another important factor affecting the use of hearing aids is the reverberation of sound within the classroom. Most school classrooms have reverberation times ranging from 1·0 to over 3·0 s. John (1960) reported that even a reverberation time of 0·7 s gave a discrimination score of only 52 per cent in the case of hearing-impaired adults, whereas with a reduction in time to 0·5 s their scores increased to 70 per cent. He concluded that the reverberation time in classrooms should not exceed 0·5 s. The obvious way to reduce reverberation time is by careful sound-treatment of a room. John (1957) warned, however, that this needs to be achieved through skilful placement and choice of the absorbent materials. If such materials are concentrated in certain areas of the room, the desired effect may not be achieved. Moreover, some materials absorb high frequency sounds too effectively, thus removing from speech the very acoustic clues which are essential for intelligibility.

Another way of reducing the effects of reverberation is by speaking close to the microphone of the hearing aid, i.e. at a distance of about 0·6–0·9 m. Only a quiet conversational voice is needed at this distance, since a loud voice will cause overloading of the aid. Under such conditions, the hearing aid user receives the benefit of the direct sound and also reverberation is reduced. Dale (1962), working with partially-hearing children, reported that whereas their discrimination scores in a well treated room dropped by 6·8 per cent when the speaker moved from a distance of 1·2 m to one of 6·7 m from the microphone, in poor acoustic conditions the corresponding drop in score was 15·6 per cent.

In 1964, Watson conducted a study designed to take into consideration the overall effect of the frequency limitations of hearing aids, the poor acoustic conditions, the noise background and the distance of the speaker from the microphone. He observed a dramatic reduction in discrimination scores from 84·8 per cent in good acoustic conditions down to 35·2 per cent in an ordinary classroom with ambient noise between 55 and 60 dB. He concluded that the most effective use of hearing aids can be achieved only in acoustically well treated rooms.

Selection Procedures

There is universal agreement that the proper use of amplified sound is potentially a powerful tool in the education, habilitation and rehabilitation of the hearing impaired. Research in the University of Manchester over the last 30 years, described by Watson (1967), has shown that hearing impaired children can gain very great benefit from the early and systematic use of hearing aids. These benefits include greater facility in comprehension, greater skill in the use of language, more intelligible speech and improvement in psychological well-being.

Because of great individual differences both in pattern and degree of hearing loss, the question arises as to which hearing aid best meets individual needs.

Both the M.R.C. and the Harvard reports suggested that hearing aid selection was not necessary as the majority of cases could benefit from hearing aids which had moderate high frequency emphasis or uniform amplification. This generalization, however, has not been universally accepted.

Reddell and Calvert (1966) criticized the generalizations of the above two reports and, after carrying out an experiment with hearing aids having frequency-response characteristics custom-adjusted to the audiogram of each subject,

asserted that selective frequency amplification was the best technique for hearing aid selection.

Generally speaking, most workers in this field agree that the use of speech tests both in quiet and in noise is the most adequate approach to the *evaluation* of hearing aids. It is often argued, though, that differences in aided discrimination scores are brought about by the interaction of a number of variables and are clinically time-wasting and meaningless. This argument stems mainly from the study of Shore and his colleagues (1960). These authors studied the reliability of the measures obtained in hearing aid evaluations with 15 patients over a period of several days using the same four aids with each patient. They concluded that the discrimination scores obtained both in quiet and in noise varied from day to day and therefore their reliability was not good enough to warrant the investment of a large amount of clinical time. Soon after the publication of this study, however, McConnell and his colleagues (1960) and Jeffers (1960) reasserted the value of speech tests of hearing in selection of hearing aids. Nonetheless, Shore and Kramer (1963), followed by Resnick and Becker (1963), announced the discontinuation of hearing aid evaluations in their respective clinics, an action based mainly upon the recommendations of Shore and his colleagues. They adopted instead a new approach to hearing aid selection in which the time previously spent in comparative testing of hearing aids was now devoted to counselling the patient regarding his own hearing problems and then leaving him to make his own choice. Subsequent research showed that the views of Shore and his colleagues were not widely accepted. For instance, Jerger and his colleagues (1966) concluded that, with the use of sufficiently difficult speech material, one can show that certain hearing aids are superior to others.

This state of affairs did not satisfy Witter and Goldstein and in 1971 they reported a new method for hearing aid selection based on a quality judgement procedure. Here the potential hearing aid user is asked to try out several aids then rate them according to preference.

The above procedures relate solely to persons who can either co-operate in lengthy audiological investigations or are in a position to carry out complicated comparisons and evaluations. There remain, however, the whole population of very young hearing impaired children for whom complicated and lengthy audiological procedures are not feasible and yet their needs for amplification are crucial. Of course, the responses of these children to meaningful sound stimuli will give valuable information on the degree and pattern of their hearing impairment on which an intelligent guess regarding the selection of suitable hearing aids can be made. Once such selection has been made, however, it must not be considered final. The needs of these children can only be met through prolonged observation and experimentation with various types of hearing aids under audiological supervision.

Fitting of Hearing Aids

There are many audiological and psychological factors which affect the successful fitting of hearing aids. The most important ones are the degree and pattern of the hearing impairment of the patient, his speech discrimination ability both in quiet and in noise and his tolerance for loud sounds. Information on the above is essential before a decision is reached regarding the use of hearing aids. In most cases, however, the only audiological information available to the worker in the field, apart from a brief case history and personal observations, is a pure-tone audiogram. Therefore Fig. 1 is presented here with a view to providing a rough idea of the degree of benefit to be expected from amplification by means of hearing aids. These predictions, however, are based solely on the degree of hearing impairment for pure tones and as such they contain a considerable degree of unreliability.

It is also pertinent to note that there exists a marked relationship between degree of benefit from amplification and the pattern of hearing impairment. The most successful users of hearing aids are persons with relatively flat pure-tone audiograms.

Persons with steep high frequency losses, or with remnants of hearing at only a few frequencies, or with highly irregular patterns of hearing loss, are potentially poor users of hearing aids.

As a general rule persons with a bilateral moderate-to-severe hearing impairment (50–90 dB hearing levels averaged across 500, 1000 and 2000 Hz) should be fitted with binaural hearing aids. There are certain exceptions to this rule which will be presented later on. For these exceptions a single hearing aid should be fitted in the ear with the better speech discrimination ability. It is pointed out that the customary procedure of fitting patients with bilateral symmetrical hearing impairment with a single hearing aid with two earphones attached to a "Y" lead, thus stimulating both ears simultaneously, does not result in truly binaural listening; neither is it in general superior to the use of a single hearing aid. Rice has, however, shown that some children prefer a "Y" lead.

Binaural Hearing Aids

According to Hirsh (1950) interest in binaural hearing aids dates back to the beginning of this century, when Soret (1912) developed and patented a true stereophonic hearing aid system. It is only in the last two decades, however, with the introduction of the ear-level hearing aid, that substantial interest in binaural hearing aids was stimulated. It is pointed out that binaural hearing aids relate to true stereophonic or dichotic listening whereby each ear is stimulated separately through an independent channel consisting of microphone, amplifier and earphone. This must not be confused with the pseudobinaural, diotic or "Y"-lead system which employs one microphone and one amplifier to feed two earphones.

Markides (1974) reported that most of the experimental studies published were about equally divided as to whether two hearing aids were better than one with regard to speech facilitation in noise. The preponderance of subjective reports were undoubtedly in favour of binaural hearing aids but such reports can hardly be considered as conclusive. He stated that subjects with symmetrical conductive or symmetrical sensorineural hearing impairment and with average hearing levels of 50–90 dB (averaged across 500,

1000 and 2000 Hz) derived significant advantages in terms of speech discrimination and localization ability from binaural hearing aids as opposed to a single hearing aid. It was pointed out, however, that subjects with relatively flat hearing impairment in their better ear and with a steeply falling pure tone audiogram configuration in their worse ear were found to derive no advantage in terms of speech discrimination when wearing two hearing aids as opposed to one. These subjects, however, did benefit in localization ability from two hearing aids as opposed to one. Similarly those subjects who exhibited diplacusis derived no help or very little help from binaural hearing aids in terms of speech discrimination. Again, however, these subjects derived benefit in localization ability from two hearing aids as opposed to one.

Aids for Persons with Unilateral Hearing Loss

According to Bergman (1957), Malles (1963) and Harford and Musket (1964), persons with slight-to-moderate unilateral hearing impairment derive significant improvement in speech discrimination when fitted with a hearing aid in their affected ear. The same opinion results from the subjective experience and assertions of users of such hearing aids: while recognizing the potential bias of such "evidence", it cannot wholly be ignored.

The results of Markides' (1974) investigation did not bear out the findings of the above workers. He reported that the subjects in his investigation showed relatively little advantage in terms of speech discrimination enhancement when fitted with a single ear-level hearing aid in their affected ear. In fact, it was observed that in situations where they were required to listen to speech from the side of their good ear, a hearing aid in their bad ear had an adverse effect on their speech discrimination ability. This was true both for subjects with conductive and for subjects with sensorineural unilateral hearing impairment. Similar results were also observed with regard to localization. These conclusions, however, must be accepted with some reservation as it is generally agreed that it takes time to "acclimatize" to hearing aid(s) and the subjects tested here did not have such time.

It has also been suggested on many occasions that persons with severe or total unilateral hearing impairment receive substantial benefit in terms of speech discrimination and localization enhancement when fitted with the CROS (Contralateral Routing of Signals) hearing aid system. Markides (1974) reported that the CROS hearing aid, in situations where speech came from the side of the good ear and noise from the side of the bad ear, had a significantly adverse effect on speech discrimination. This is to be expected, as under such listening conditions the CROS hearing aid amplifies the background noise and then feeds it to the good ear, thus magnifying the masking potential of the background noise. The CROS hearing aid, however, was found to enhance speech discrimination to a significant level in listening situations where speech was coming from the side of the bad ear and with noise coming from the side of the good ear.

It is evident therefore that a CROS hearing aid when selectively used, e.g. by switching it on only when the wanted signal is at the deaf ear can benefit the user in terms of speech discrimination enhancement. Contrary to popular belief, however, the CROS hearing aid was not found to facilitate localization ability. In fact, it tended to interfere disastrously with localization. The potentiality of learning effects is considerable though, and it may well be that persons using the CROS hearing aid may find it useful with time.

REFERENCES

Ballantyne, J. (1970), "Iatrogenic Deafness," The 16th James Yearsley Memorial Lecture, *J. Laryng.*, October, 967–1000.

Barr, B. and Wedenberg, E. (1965), "Prognosis of Perceptive Hearing Loss in Children with Respect to Genesis and Use of Hearing Aid," *Acta oto-laryng.*, 59, 464–474.

Bellefluer, P. A. and Van Dyke, R. C. (1968), "The Effects of High Gain Amplification on Children in a Residential School for the Deaf," *J. Speech Hear. Res.*, 11, 343–347.

Bergman, N. (1957), "Binaural Hearing," *Arch. Otolaryng.*, 66, 572–578.

Boothroyd, A. (1965), "The Provision of Better Earmoulds for Deaf Children," *J. Laryng.*, 79, 320.

Brinskey, R. J. and Sinclair, J. (1966), "The Importance of Low Frequency Amplification in Deaf Children," *Audecibel*, 15, 7–20.

Brockman, S. J. (1959), "An Exploratory Investigation of Delayed Progressive Neural Hypacusis in Children," *Arch. Otolaryng. (Chicago)*, 70, 340.

Caraway, B. J. and Carhart, R. (1967), "Influence of Compressor Action on Speech Intelligibility," *J. acoust. Soc. Amer.*, 41, 1424–1433.

Dale, D. M. C. (1962), *Applied Audiology for Children.* Springfield: C. Thomas.

Davis, H., Stevens, S. S. and Nichols, R. H. (1947), *Hearing Aids: An Experimental Study of Design Objectives.* Cambridge: Harvard University Press.

Ewertsen, H. W., Ipsen, J. B. and Nielsen, S. C. (1957), "On Acoustical Characteristics of the Earmould," *Acta oto-laryng.*, 47, 312–317.

Fleming, D. B. and Rice, C. G. (1969), "New Circuit Development Concepts in Hearing Aids," *Int. Audiol.*, 8, 517–523.

Harford, E. and Musket, C. N. (1964), "Binaural Hearing with One Hearing Aid," *J. Speech Hear. Dis.*, 29, 133–146.

Hirsh, I. J. (1950), "Binaural Hearing Aids: A Review of Some Experiments," *J. acoust. Soc. Amer.*, 15, 114–122.

Hodgson, W. and Murdock, J. R. (1970), "Effect of the Earmould on Speech Intelligibility in Hearing Aid Use," *J. Speech Hear. Res.*, 13, 290–297.

Holmgren, L. (1940), "Can the Hearing be Damaged by a Hearing Aid?" *Acta oto-laryng.*, 28, 440.

Hudgins, C. V., Marquis, R. J., Nichols, R. H., Peterson, G. E. and Ross, D. A. (1948), "The Comparative Performance of an Experimental Hearing Aid and Two Commercial Instruments," *J. acoust. Soc. Amer.*, 20, 241–258.

Huizing, H. C. (1959), "Deaf Mutism: Modern Trends in Treatment and Prevention," *Ann. Otol. Rhin. Laryng.*, 5, 74–106.

I.S.O. R389 (1964), "Standard Reference Zero for the Calibration of Pure Tone Audiometers." International Organization for Standardization.

Jeffers, J. (1960), "Quality Judgement in Hearing Aid Selection," *J. Speech Hear. Dis.*, 25, 259–266.

Jerger, J., Speaks, C. and Malmquist, C. (1966), "Hearing Aid Performance and Hearing Aid Selection," *J. Speech Hear. Res.*, 9, 136–149.

John, J. E. J. (1957), *Educational Guidance and the Deaf Child* (Ewing, A. W. G., Ed.). Manchester University Press.

John, J. E. J. (1964), "Hearing Aids," in *Teaching Deaf Children to Talk*, by Ewing and Ewing. Manchester University Press.

Kinney, C. E. (1953), "Hearing Impairments in Children," *Laryngoscope*, 63, 220–226.

Kinney, C. E. (1961), "The Further Destruction of Partially Deafened Children's Hearing by the Use of Powerful Hearing Aids," *Ann. Otol.*, 70, 828–835.

Licklider, J. C. P. (1948), "The Influence of Interaural Phase Relations Upon the Masking of Speech by White Noise," *J. acoust. Soc. Amer.*, 20, 150–159.

Ling, D. (1964), "Implications of Hearing Aid Amplification Below 300 cps," *Volta Rev.*, 66, 723–729.

Littler, T. S. (1944), "Electrical Hearing Aids," *J. Inst. elect. Engrs.*, 91, 67–74.

Lybarger, S. F. (1958), "The Earmould as Part of the Receiver Acoustic System." Radioear Corp., n.d. Canousburg, Pa.

Lybarger, S. F. (1966), "A Discussion on Hearing Aid Trends," *Int. Audiol.*, 5, 376–383.

Lybarger, S. F. (1967), "Earmould Acoustics," *Audecibel*, 9, 19–22.

Malles, I. (1963), "Hearing Aid Effect in Unilateral Conductive Deafness," *Arch. Otolaryng.*, 77, 406–408.

Macrae, J. H. and Farrant, R. H. (1965), "The Effect of Hearing Aid Use on the Residual Hearing of Children with Sensorineural Deafness," *Ann. Otol.*, 74, 409–419.

Macrae, J. H. (1967), "TTS and Recovery from TTS After Use of Powerful Hearing Aids," *J. acoust. Soc. Amer.*, 43, 1445–1446.

Macrae, J. H. (1968), "Recovery from TTS in Children With Sensorineural Deafness," *J. acoust. Soc. Amer.*, 44, 1451.

Macrae, J. H. (1968), "Deterioration of the Residual Hearing of Children With Sensorineural Deafness," *Acta oto-laryng.*, 66, 33–39.

Markides, A. (1971), "Do Hearing Aids Damage the User's Residual Hearing?" *Sound* (now *Brit. J. Audiol.*), 5, 22–31.

Markides, A. (1974), "The Possibility of Restoring Binaural Hearing Advantages by Means of Wearable Hearing Aids," Ph.D. Thesis, Faculty of Engineering and Applied Science, Institute of Sound and Vibration Research, University of Southampton.

Medical Research Council (1947), "Hearing Aids and Audiometers," Special Report Series No. 261, H.M.S.O., London.

Møller, T. T. and Rojskjaer, C. (1960), "Injury to Hearing Through Hearing Aid Treatment (Acoustic Trauma)," Fifth Cong. of Internat. Soc. of Audiology, Bonn, Germany.

Murray, N. E. (1951), "Hearing Aids and Classification of Deaf Children," Report CAL-IR-2, Commonwealth Acoustic Laboratories, Sydney (Quoted by Macrae and Farrant).

McClellan, M. E. (1967), "Aided Speech Discrimination in Noise With Vented and Unvented Earmoulds," *J. Auditory Res.*, 7, 93–99.

McConnell, F., Silver, E. F. and McDonald, D. (1960), "Test-retest Consistency of Clinical Hearing Air Tests," *J. Speech Hear. Dis.*, 25, 273–280.

Naunton, R. F. (1957), "The Effect of Hearing Aid Use Upon the User's Residual Hearing," *Laryngoscope*, 67, 569–576.

Olsen, W. O. and Carhart, R. (1967), "Development of Test Procedures for Evaluation of Binaural Hearing Aids," *Bull. Prosthetic Res.*, 10, 22–49.

Redell, R. C. and Calvert, D. R. (1966), "Selecting a Hearing Aid by Interpreting Audiological Data," *J. Auditory Res.*, 6, 445–452.

Rice, C. G. (1965), "Hearing Aid Design Criteria," *Int. Audiol.*, 4, 130–134.

Roberts, C. (1970), "Can Hearing Aids Damage Hearing?" *Acta oto-laryng.*, 69, 123–125.

Ross, M. and Lerman, J. (1967), "Hearing Aid Usage and Its Effect on Residual Hearing: A Review of the Literature and an Investigation," *Arch. Otolaryng.*, 86, 639–644.

Sanders, D. A. (1961), "A Follow-up Study of Fifty Deaf Children Who Received Pre-school Training," Ph.D. Thesis, University of Manchester.

Sataloff, J. (1961), "Pitfalls in Routine Hearing Testing," *Arch. Otolaryng.*, 73, 717–726.

Shore, I., Bilger, R. C. and Hirsh, I. J. (1960), "Hearing Aid Evaluation: Reliability of Repeated Measurements," *J. Speech Hear. Dis.*, 25, 152–170.

Shore, I. and Kramer, J. C. (1963), "A Comparison of Two Procedures for Hearing Aid Selection," *J. Speech Hear. Dis.*, 28, 159–170.

Trinder, E. (1972), "An Attempt to Correct Speech Discrimination Loss in Cochlear Deafness by Graded Instantaneous Compression," *Sound*, 6, 62–67.

Watson, T. J. (1961), "The Use of Residual Hearing in the Education of the Deaf Children," *Volta Rev.*, 63, 487–492.

Watson, T. J. (1964), "The Use of Hearing Aids by Hearing-impaired Pupils in Ordinary Schools," *Volta Rev.*, **66**, 741–787.

Watson, T. J. (1967), "The Education of Hearing-handicapped Children. University of London Press.

Watson, T. J. (1970), "Hearing Aids," in *Scott-Brown's Diseases of the Ear, Nose and Throat*, Chap. 18 (Ballantyne and Groves, Eds.). London: Butterworth.

Wedenberg, E. (1954), "Auditory Training of Severely Hard of Hearing Pre-school Children," *Acta oto-laryng.*, supplement 110.

Whetnall, E. (1964), "Binaural Hearing," *J. Laryng.*, **78**, 1079–1089.

Witter, H. L. and Goldstein, D. P. (1971), "Quality Judgements of Hearing Aid Transduced Speech," *J. Speech Hear. Res.*, **14**, 312–322.

World Health Organization (1967), "The Early Detection and Treatment of Handicapping Defects in Young Children," Special Report Distributed by Regional Office for Europe, Copenhagen.

61. ELECTRO-ACOUSTIC REHABILITATION EQUIPMENT OTHER THAN HEARING AIDS

ELIZABETH C. KNOX

INTRODUCTION

With the continuing developments in hearing aid design and performance, it would appear to follow that there should be less need for additional electro-acoustic rehabilitation equipment for individuals with impaired hearing. There is still a demand, however, for equipment which will attempt to fulfil the following requirements:

(a) Provide amplification over all (or part of) the frequency range 50 Hz to 5 kHz, as deemed necessary, to make maximum use of residual hearing. (Until recently, hearing aids tended to have a restricted frequency response because of limitations in the microphone and in the earphone response.)

(b) Provide an amplifying device capable of large maximum output sound levels over all, or part, of a wide frequency range without presenting acoustic feedback problems. This is important for the education of those with severe impairment of hearing (the present coupling of an insert earphone/earmould combination to an ear poses feedback problems with high output levels).

(c) By having variable controls, will:

(i) Compensate for differences between the user's own voice and the teacher's voice. This is important when a hearing impaired child first uses an amplifying device for auditory training because, whereas the teacher's voice can be maintained at normal conversational level, the child's voice may be set at a very low or a very high level.

(ii) Allow for changes in the basic frequency response, gain and maximum available output of such an amplifying device. This facility is useful for selection of the most suitable amplification and is of particular importance when the hearing loss is not known.

(d) Enable a hearing-impaired person to hear a speaker who is at a distance and yet be independent of acoustic environment. This is necessary because a hearing aid is inefficient at a distance and its performance is dependent on the acoustic environment.

(e) Permit a hearing-impaired person to participate in a group situation, e.g. in a classroom where the pupil should hear his own voice, teacher's voice, fellow pupils' voices and any radio, television or similar equipment being used.

(f) Reinforce acoustic signals with visual and/or tactile signals.

(g) Transpose sound signals into the frequency range of residual hearing.

TYPES OF EQUIPMENT

The electro-acoustic rehabilitation equipment to be discussed here is as shown in Fig. 1.

Electro-acoustic rehabilitation equipment may be considered as falling into two main categories.

(A) *Equipment for communication purposes* and therefore basically *sound amplifiers*. This includes equipment used in the education of the auditory handicapped, such as individual auditory trainers, group hearing aids, loop systems (audio- and radio-frequency) and radio-frequency free-field systems.

Some of these systems are also of general use to the auditory handicapped, e.g. loop systems in public places, auditory trainers for communicating with hearing impaired adults. Other equipment, e.g. telephone amplifiers, are specifically designed for general use by hearing impaired individuals. (For descriptions of these devices, apart from educational equipment, see the R.N.I.D. publication *Special Aids to Hearing*.)

(B) *Equipment specifically designed for training* those with hearing impairments to make use of their residual hearing and to gain control of their articulatory movements. This equipment includes that in which the auditory stimulus is reinforced, or replaced, by visual and/or tactile information, i.e. it constitutes ancillary equipment.

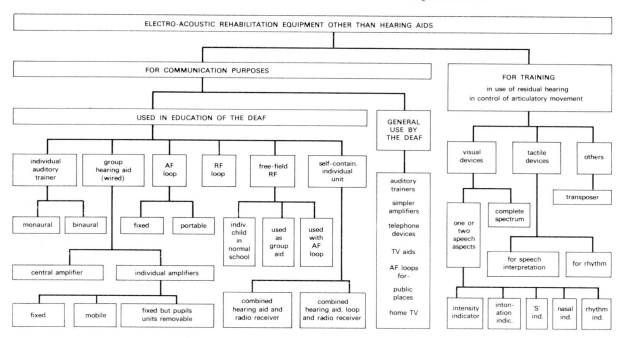

FIG. 1. Types of electro-acoustic rehabilitation equipment.

Sound Amplifying Equipment

Educational sound amplification systems have been in use for many years. According to Watts (1969), in his article on the historical development of auditory training, the first systematic attempt to use the hearing of children handicapped by a hearing loss was made by Itard at the beginning of the nineteenth century. Conversation tubes and other similar devices were being used in deaf education by 1892. The first electrical amplifying device for those with a hearing impairment was produced by Alt in 1900, and, by the late 1920's group hearing aids had been developed and were being successfully used in schools for the deaf. Developments in electronic technology, radio-communications and in the design of electro-acoustic transducers have led to an increase in the types of equipment now available for deaf education.

There are currently available six basic types of educational sound amplification systems:

(a) The individual auditory trainer.
(b) The group hearing aid system.
(c) The induction loop (audio-frequency).
(d) The induction loop (radio-frequency).
(e) The radio-frequency free-field system.
(f) The self-contained individually worn unit.

Individual Auditory Trainer

This unit basically consists of two microphones (one for the pupil; one for the teacher), an amplifier, an attenuator for each earphone and a pair of earphones (Fig. 2). The overall system is only as good as the weakest link in the system and therefore microphones, amplifier and earphones must be capable of handling the desired signal. The unit is normally battery operated. The complete system is port-

able and some of the recent models can be worn. The microphones may be handheld, lavalier (round the neck type), or desk type. The pupil's microphone may take the form of a boom microphone attached by a boom to the headset, the advantage being that the child speaks at a constant distance from the microphone. Acoustic feedback may be a limitation with the boom microphone. Moreover, when two different types of microphone are used, care must be taken that their characteristics are similar. It is desirable that each microphone has a separate gain control to compensate for possible differences in voice level between pupil and teacher. A meter, or other visual indicator, is incorporated to monitor voice level and can be used as a visual stimulus for the child.

The amplifier should have, as a basis, a wide, flat frequency response (preferably ± 3 dB in the range 50–8000 Hz) and should have facilities for altering this normal response. In some models, this is done by providing variable bass and treble attenuation controls. Some of these models have variable bass and treble boost and attenuation controls pivoting about 1000 Hz.

Darbyshire and Reeves (1969) studied the performance of 24 children on three different tone settings of an auditory trainer and their results indicate that the settings predicted to give the best discrimination score did in fact do so.

The amplifier may also incorporate peak clipping, automatic volume control or compression amplification (*see* Chapter 59).

The attenuators change in steps of 5 dB or are continuously variable. The range is usually about 50 dB.

The Telephonics TDH-39 moving coil earphone is often used in auditory trainers because of its extended and substantially flat response. The type of earphone cushion is also important. The circumaural earcap may reduce the

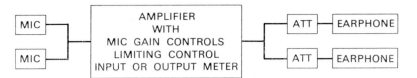

FIG. 2. The individual auditory trainer.

maximum acoustic output. Apart from the acoustic performance of the earphones and the cushion, consideration must also be given to the comfort and fitting of the instrument, as well as ensuring avoidance of acoustic feedback.

Kettlety (1973) outlines the principal characteristics of 14 auditory trainers currently available in Britain. The acoustic performance of current models of auditory trainers differs considerably. The maximum output may range from 125 to 140 dB SPL (HAIC) (*see* Chapter 59). The low end of the frequency range (HAIC) may range from 80 to 300 Hz, and the high end from 3000 to 8000 Hz. This variation is not unexpected since differing views are held regarding the desirable amplification for a profoundly deaf child.

Following three years of experimental work on the design of hearing aids, Littler and Rice (1964) concluded that the profoundly deaf child does not need an average SPL greater than 125 dB, or a frequency response higher than 4000 Hz. John (1957) has produced an auditory trainer with a response up to 8000 Hz; the experimental work of Watson and John (1960) indicated that deaf children could benefit from the use of this extended high-frequency range. Ewing and Ewing (1964) confirmed the conclusions of Watson and John. Dale (1962) advocates levels of up to 135 dB SPL. The work of Ling (1965) emphasizes the importance of amplification below 300 Hz for certain hearing-impaired children.

It is essential that an auditory trainer be chosen with the acoustic properties desired for the work in hand.

Apart from the basic parts described, an auditory trainer may have additional features:

(i) Input: for tape-recorder; for record player or radio; an induction pick-up coil.

(ii) Output: for vibrator or visual attachment.

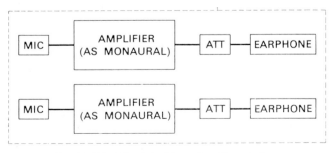

FIG. 3. Principle of the binaural auditory trainer.

Some auditory trainers have duplicate microphones and amplifiers to produce a true binaural effect (Fig. 3). Several researchers, including Poulos (1950), have shown an improvement in speech perception in certain circum-

stances when deaf children are listening binaurally instead of monaurally.

Auditory trainers are now widely used in schools for the deaf, in partially-hearing units, by peripatetic teachers of the deaf and by parents of deaf children in the home situation. The advantage of the auditory trainer is that it can amplify over a wide frequency range and up to high output levels *without distortion*; but, if it is to be effective, the listening level must be set as accurately as possible. Dale (1962) outlines several ways of setting listening level. Ewing and Ewing (1971) relate listening levels to the pure-tone audiogram.

An auditory trainer which has a selection of frequency responses can be used as a tool for assessing hearing loss. Auditory trainers can also be useful for communication with hearing-impaired adults in certain situations, e.g. interviews in social work departments, talking to the geriatric patient, group therapy in mental hospitals.

Group Hearing Aid (Wired System)

The group hearing aid was designed for use in the classroom situation where individual hearing aids are inefficient due to the distance between speaker and microphone and due to room acoustics (John, 1957).

The group hearing aid with its multiple microphones allows teacher and child to speak close to a microphone. It allows the children to receive the teacher's voice, other pupils' voices and their own voices. The use of high quality external earphones provides the children with high output levels of sound over an extended frequency range. Modern group hearing aids with their individual amplifiers allow the amplification of the speech delivered to each child to be individually selected. Mobile group hearing aids permit flexibility within the classroom.

The earlier models of group hearing aids often consisted of fixed desk microphones for pupils and neck-type (lavalier) microphone for teacher wired to a central amplifier in the classroom (Fig. 4). The output from the amplifier was fed to each child's desk where the plugged-in child's headset had controls for adjusting the level to each ear. Either external earphones on a headband or insert receivers comprised this headset. One disadvantage was that the settings of the central amplifier determined the frequency response presented to every child and also determined the limiting output level for every child. Thus this system did not allow for differences in the type of hearing loss.

More recent models of group hearing aid provide each child with his own independent amplifier (Fig. 5). This amplifier has controls (tone, gain, maximum output and earphone balance) which can be set with the aim of suiting the hearing loss of the individual child. These units, with

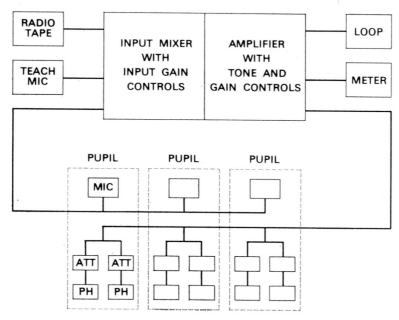

FIG. 4. Group hearing aid—common (central) amplifier.

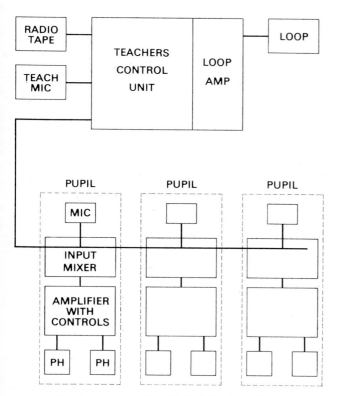

FIG. 5. Group hearing aid—individual amplifiers.

feeding tape-recorders, radio etc. into the system and an output for a loop. In some models, a meter is incorporated in the teacher's unit to monitor inputs. In other models, a separate output meter is supplied for plugging in to any of the children's units in order to measure output level.

Martin and Power (1965) have designed a group aid, using a plug-in modular system in which the children's unit, teacher's unit and loop amplifier unit were plugged into one main chassis on the teacher's desk. This provides ease in servicing. A further development was the mobile group hearing aid (Power, 1969). This complete system is contained within a cabinet on wheels. The unit may be either battery- or mains-operated. The children, who each have a combined microphone/earphone device (boom microphone or lavalier-type microphone suspended from headset lead) sit around the cabinet. This cabinet may have flaps acting as working surfaces. Thus the mobile unit provides group hearing aid facilities for younger children, with no restriction as to where the group is to be located. Provided that the combined headset microphones have long leads, older children can use the mobile unit by arranging their desks around it.

The more sophisticated group systems (fixed and mobile) allow for flexibility in their use, e.g. when necessary, a single pupil's unit can be used as an individual auditory trainer, or children can work in two independent groups, with different functions of the group hearing aid being used simultaneously.

The mobile group aid would appear to be more adapted than the fixed system to modern methods of education, where children tend to work individually or in groups, and where there are changes of activity within the classroom.

In one fixed-type group system, part of the child's desk unit (amplifier, microphone, headset) can be detached and worn in a harness by the child as an individual hearing aid.

microphone and headset, can be mounted on the children's desks with connecting leads between desks and linked to the teacher's control unit. The teacher has a lavalier-type microphone which can be plugged into the system at suitable points within the room. The teacher's control unit has a gain control for her own microphone, input facilities for

Induction Loop System (Audio-frequency)

The basic system as used in a classroom consists of a microphone, an amplifier, a loop of wire round the room and individual hearing aids which incorporate an induction pick-up coil (Fig. 6).

The microphone transduces the teacher's voice into an electrical signal which is amplified and fed into the loop.

in adjacent rooms. The aim therefore is to fit a loop configuration which will allow sufficient field within the room but as little as possible towards the walls of adjacent rooms (both horizontally and vertically) where it is desired to use loop systems. Bellefleur and McMenamin (1965), Bosman and Joosten (1965), Pearson (1968) and Heath and Lane (1969) have all described loop configurations designed to minimize overspill. Martin (1967) suggests that, in many

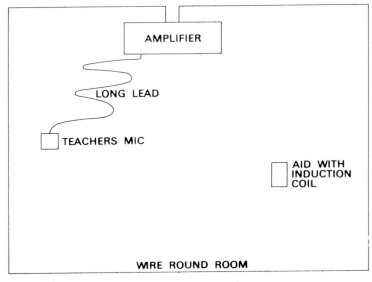

FIG. 6. Induction loop system (audio-frequency).

This electrical current flowing through the wire produces a *magnetic field* within the room, which induces an electrical signal in the coil of the hearing aid. This electrical signal is then amplified within the aid and transduced in the aid's earphone into sound in the usual way.

The teacher's microphone is normally designed for use at close range, so reducing the masking effect of background noise. A long lead is necessary to give the teacher some degree of mobility within the room. Heath and Lane (1969) also advocate the use of a fixed microphone in the room to give the child an appreciation of all sounds created within the room. The output of the amplifier should be the minimum required to produce sufficient magnetic field to saturate the aids when the gain (volume) control of the aid is set at maximum. Martin (1967) suggests that a power of 1 W is sufficient to operate a loop system in a classroom. Both the International Electrotechnical Commission (I.E.C.) and the British Standards Institution (B.S.I.) have publications in preparation which will recommend the intensity of the magnetic fields that should be used. Aids are currently designed for use in magnetic-field strengths of either 10 or 100 mA.m^{-1}.

The loop should be impedance-matched to the amplifier output and, ideally, should be around the walls of the room at the height at which the aids are used. Such a loop, however, would radiate a magnetic field outside the actual area of the loop for a considerable distance both horizontally and vertically, making use of loop systems impossible

cases, overspill problems are due to using excessive amplifier output power.

In most hearing aids, the induction coil is in a vertical position, i.e. designed for use in a horizontal magnetic field when the aid is being worn. If the aid is worn in any position other than the normal one, the performance may be impaired. Some recent aids are designed to allow the aid to be used efficiently in any orientation. The sensitivity of induction coils may vary according to the type of aid and this must be taken into account in classes where the children use various types of aid. A mode (function) switch on the aid allows selection of: (i) "microphone only" operating, (ii) "coil only" operating and, in many aids, (iii) "microphone and coil" operating. The choice as to whether the child uses the "coil only" or the "microphone and coil" position depends to a certain extent on the type of teaching being done and on the acoustic environment.

The main *advantages* of the loop system in a classroom are:

(i) The closeness of the teacher's voice to the microphone reduces the masking effect of background noise.

(ii) The effect of distance of the child from the teacher is eliminated.

(iii) Freedom of movement for children while still in acoustic contact with the teacher.

(iv) Any number of children can use the system.

(v) The output from tape-recorders, record player or television can be fed into the loop.

The main *disadvantages* of the loop system are:

(i) Overspill into adjacent rooms.

(ii) Microphone lead restricts movement of teacher (can be overcome by use of radio-microphone).

(iii) The child can monitor his own voice if he is on the "combined coil and microphone" position but he cannot efficiently pick up his fellow pupils who are at a distance.

Induction Loop System (Radio-frequency)

This system was developed to overcome the overspill problem of the magnetic induction loop system. It consists of a teacher's microphone, radio-frequency generator, combined mixer/amplifier, loop and special receiving device (Fig. 8). The electrical signal from the teacher's microphone modulates the RF (*radio-frequency*) carrier radiated by the loop. This modulated RF carrier is received

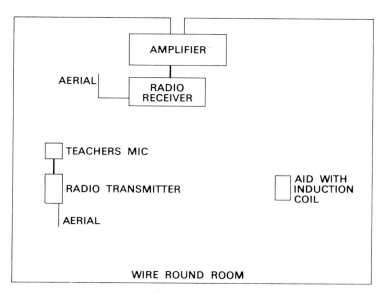

FIG. 7. Induction loop system (audio-frequency) combined with radio-microphone.

(iv) The performance of the system is limited by the performance of the individual aid. (This disadvantage is becoming less important with advances in hearing aid design but it is still important because of the enforced limitation of aid performances owing to acoustic feedback problems with earmoulds.)

The loop system is widely used in schools for the deaf, particularly with young children who must be able to move freely about the room and yet be in contact with the teacher's voice. It is also useful in assembly halls, domestic science and technical rooms and for participation in games, dancing and drama. The audio-frequency induction loop system combined with a radio-microphone (Fig. 7) has possibilities for the hearing-impaired child in the normal primary school where he is mainly in one room. It allows him to use his individual aid regardless of distance of the teacher. A portable amplifier and loop system is available for the pupil who has to change classrooms. This portable system can also be used for small groups of hearing-impaired children on visits outside their looped classroom.

Hearing-impaired adults can use the loop system for listening to television in the home (particularly useful in old people's homes). Aids designed for loop use only are commercially available. Some cinemas, churches and public places have loop systems installed for the benefit of those members of the public with impaired hearing.

A licence may be necessary to operate a loop system and information should be sought from the relevant authority.

by the children's special device. The children's devices which incorporate a microphone can be for desk use or worn on the body. External earphones, such as the TDH-39, rather than inserts, are often used. An additional special type of overhead microphone is sometimes incorporated to cover sounds from any part of the room.

The main *advantage* of this system is that closely situated classrooms can have systems operating on different carrier frequencies with the pupils' hearing devices tuned to the frequency operating in their own classroom.

The main *disadvantage* is that the sophisticated receiving devices are of use only when the child is within the radio-frequency loop.

Before considering the installation of any type of radio-microphone system, advice should be sought from the relevant authority as to whether or not the system is approved for use in the country concerned and what conditions are attached to the issuing of a licence.

Radio-frequency Free-Field System

Although the use of radio-communication in deaf education has been advocated for some time, e.g. by Schmael (1960) and by Bollid (1964), the size of both the transmitter and the receiver have limited the use of such equipment. Recent developments, however, have led to small radio transmitters and receivers which can be worn for lengthy periods by teachers and pupils respectively.

The teacher's unit consists of a combined microphone

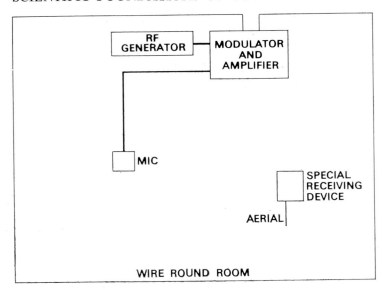

FIG. 8. Induction loop system (radio-frequency).

and radio-transmitter powered usually by a rechargeable battery. The pupil's unit consists of a radio-receiver, an amplifier and either an insert or external earphone (Fig. 9). This also is powered by a rechargeable battery. A microphone is usually incorporated in the pupil's unit in order that he may hear his own voice. A charger is provided for recharging both the pupil's and the teacher's units.

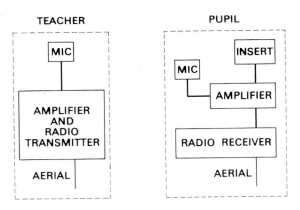

FIG. 9. Radio-frequency free-field system.

This system can be used for the hearing-impaired child in the normal school and in schools for the deaf, where each class has its allocated radio-frequency. The number of allocated frequencies depends on the total bandwidth allocated by the authorities and on the bandwidth used by the equipment. Narrow bandwidth radio systems have a poorer frequency response than wideband systems.

The *advantages* of the free-field RF system are:

(i) Freedom of movement for both teacher and pupils within the classroom.

(ii) Pupils' units can be adjusted as far as possible to suit each individual hearing loss.

(iii) Pupils receive teacher's voice at constant level.

(iv) Pupils can monitor their own voices.

(v) Adjacent classrooms can use systems without fear of interference from each other.

(vi) The class, together with the teacher, can operate the system outside the school, e.g. on educational visits.

One *disadvantage* is that the pupil will have to change to another form of aid when he is not in the class situation. Another is that the pupil can only pick up other classmates if they are within range of the microphone on his own unit or on the teacher's unit.

One important use of this system is the substitution of it for the conventional microphone and long lead used in the audio-loop system, thus giving freedom of movement to the teacher (Fig. 7).

Self-contained Individually Worn Unit

This may consist of a combination of radio-microphone receiver and individual aid which can be worn by the child (Fig. 10), or a combination of radio-microphone receiver,

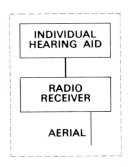

FIG. 10. Self-contained individually worn unit.

loop and individual aid which can be worn (Fig. 11). In both cases, the advantage is that the child always uses the same individual aid chosen to suit his hearing-loss and can add the additional facilities (radio-microphone, loop, high quality headset) as the situation requires.

These self-contained systems can be used in conjunction with either a radio-frequency loop system or a free-field radio-frequency system, or they can be separated from the radio-frequency section and used as a normal individual hearing aid.

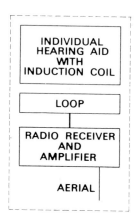

FIG. 11. Self-contained individually worn unit with loop system.

Transposing Equipment

In addition to individually worn transposing hearing aids, there are larger training units incorporating variable transposition facilities. One currently available model has five filters for total transposition of all the speech frequencies into a range below 400 Hz and only the pitch of the voice is normally amplified. The child can also simultaneously receive amplified speech which is not transposed.

Ancillary Equipment

For many years attempts have been made to produce equipment specifically designed for training the auditory handicapped and which aims to supplement or replace the sound signal with visual and/or tactile information. Watts (1965) and Good (1973) have traced the history and the technological development of these devices.

Visual Devices

A wide selection of *visual devices* are commercially available. They can be divided into those which visually display one specific aspect of speech and those which display a more complete speech pattern.

The first category includes:

The "S" indicator which can be helpful in cases of severe high frequency loss. A microphone picks up the sound produced, which is then analysed and the "S" content is visually displayed by a meter indication, a flashing lamp or the height of a vertical column. The work of Risberg (1968), of Martony (1969) and of Pickett (1971) attests the value of this equipment. To increase motivation when training young children, a relay allows operation of toys and slide projectors.

The *intonation indicator* for training of voice pitch register is useful for the deaf person where auditory feedback of the fundamental frequency is not possible. The vibration frequency of the vocal folds is picked up with a contact microphone that is held against the throat. The fundamental frequency may be displayed on a meter or on an oscilloscope.

The nasal indicator is intended to be used in training partially-hearing children in respect of nasalization or denasalization. In this case, the contact microphone is held against the alae nasi; vibrations are picked up, amplified and their intensity registered on a meter.

The rhythm indicator is important in the training of deaf children because incorrect rhythm can affect the intelligibility of the speech of the deaf child. The speech rhythm is displayed, via the microphone, on a long persistence cathode-ray tube arranged so that vertical spot deflection is independent of frequency and in direct proportion to voice amplitude.

One device described by Plant (1960) presents an immediate indication of pitch variation and, if desired, can also be used for indicating intensity. The pupil sees his voice as a light beam which is raised or lowered on the screen according to the voice pitch. It can be arranged for the width of the light beam to expand laterally, according to the intensity of the speech being received.

The work of Fourcin and Abberton (1971) on the electro-laryngograph could have applications to deaf education although not specifically designed for this.

The second category of visual speech equipment includes equipment which displays a more complete speech spectrum. In several devices, bandpass filters are used to analyse the frequency composition of speech and display this as varying vertical columns of light, or as different colours. The device described by Fant (1960) provides sixteen columns of light, the height of the column representing energy within that bandwidth. (In this model, ten bandwidths are also fed to tactile transmitters, one for each finger.) In currently available models the visual pattern can be frozen. A speech training programme using this type of apparatus is described by Searson (1965).

Other devices display a form of speech pattern on a cathode ray tube. The design work of Barton and Barton (1963) led to the production of the Calligraphone by Martin (1965) who states that the roulette figures displayed are suitable for showing differences in speech sounds that are not easily seen by other means. Montgomery (1967) describes a portable visual speech device which produces a running visual representation of speech sounds on the 7·5 cm screen of an oscilloscope. Still photographs of characteristic speech sounds are available for comparison and recently Montgomery has linked to the equipment teaching machines programmed to display the appropriate written word.

Gitlits (1972) describes recent experiments with an oscilloscope type of visible-speech apparatus which not only converts audible speech into symbols but also conveys its rhythmic structure.

Recent work has produced equipment which relates the visual speech waveform to the position and form of the tongue, as described by Pickett (1971), or to lip positions, as described by Boston (1973).

In most visual speech equipment, synchronized auditory amplification is included to utilize residual hearing.

Tactile Aids

As is indicated by Mulholland in her summary of developments up to 1963, early developments in using sophisticated equipment to interpret speech signals through the sense of touch does not appear to have proved of great benefit to the deaf child. Uden (1960), however, claims that it is frequently possible to awaken an awareness of the world of sound in deaf-mute children by exercising the sense of vibration in the body. One device used to encourage the child to exercise his sense of vibration is a specially designed wind instrument with notes selected on a keyboard and reproduced electronically at the required level through earphones or loudspeakers. Its early use is described by Vermeulen (1959) and by Nicholas and Maeliosa (1967) who give details of training programmes using the blow-organ and other musical instruments.

Several models of tactile vibrator are available commercially. These consist basically of a microphone, an amplifier and, sometimes, a transposer to transpose frequencies outside the sensitivity range of the skin into frequencies within the skin's limited sensitivity range, which Pickett (1971) gives as 100–800 Hz. Models intended for training in speech rhythm rather than in speech discrimination are simpler and have one vibrator which can be used on different parts of the body. The wrist, the sternum, the clavicle and the cervical vertebrae have proved to be favourable positions for the vibrator. In training for speech rhythm, amplified sound is simultaneously fed to the child through earphones. Neate (1972), in an interim report on her own findings, using simple tactile vibrators with a selected group of children, suggests that it is a worthwhile additional technique to use with very deaf children.

SUMMARY

No matter what type of system is chosen for communication purposes in the education of those with hearing impairments, the following points are important if full use is to be made of it:

(1) It is the *overall* performance of the complete system, i.e. amplification characteristics from input sound signal to output sound signal in the hearing impaired person's ear, which should be considered, and not the performance of any individual part of the system.

(2) Teacher and child (when old enough) should understand how the system works and the settings to be used to get maximum benefit in various situations.

(3) There should be some procedure for daily checking of the system.

(4) There should be facilities for quick maintenance and repair of the wiring and other components.

(5) There should be a programme for checking at regular intervals the acoustical, as well as the electrical, properties of the system.

REFERENCES

Barton, G. W. and Barton, S. H. (1963), *Science*, **142**, 1455.
Bellefleur, P. A. and McMenamin, S. B. (1965), *Volta Rev.*, **67**, 559.
Bollid, K. (1964), *North. Cong. for Spec. Educn.* (Stock.), June.
Bosman, P. A. and Joosten, J. M. (1965), *I.E.E. Transact. on Audio* AU13/3, **47**.
Boston, D. W. (1973), *Brit. J. Audiol.*, **7**, 95.
Dale, D. M. C. (1962), *Applied Audiology for Children*. Springfield: Chas. C. Thomas.
Darbyshire, J. and Reeves, V. (1969), *Sound*, **3**, 35.
Ewing, A. W. G. and Ewing, E. C. (1964), *Teaching Deaf Children to Talk*, Chap. II. Manchester University Press.
Ewing, A. W. G. and Ewing, E. C. (1971), *Hearing Impaired Children Under Five*. Manchester University Press.
Fant, G. C. M. (1960), *Modern Educational Treatment of Deafness* (A. W. G. Ewing and E. C. Ewing, Eds.). Manchester University Press.
Fourcin, A. J. and Abberton, E. (1971), *Med. biol. Ill.*, **21**, 172.
Gitlits, I. (1972), *T. of Deaf*, **70**, 420.
Good, J. W. (1973), *T. of Deaf*, **71**, 389.
Heath, L. E. and Lane, W. L. (1969), *T. of Deaf*, **67**, 285.
John, J. E. (1957), *Educational Guidance and the Deaf Child* (A. W. G. Ewing, Ed.). Manchester University Press.
Kettlety, A. (1973), *T. of Deaf*, **71**, 20.
Ling, D. (1965), *Volta Rev.*, **66**, 723.
Littler, T. S. and Rice, C. G. (1964). Unpublished data.
Martin, M. C. and Power, R. F. (1965), *Sound*, **1**, 33.
Martin, M. C. (1965), *Hearing*, **20**, 4.
Martin, M. C. (1967), *Sound*, **1**, 5.
Martony, J. (1969), *International Symposium on Speech Communication Ability and Profound Deafness* (Stock.), p. 345. Alexander Graham Bell Association.
Montgomery, G. W. G. (1967), *Scot. Educ. J.*, **25**, 808.
Mulholland, A. (1963), *Volta Rev.*, **65**, 513.
Neate, D. M. (1972), *T. of Deaf*, **70**, 137.
Nicholas, M. and Maeliosa, M. (1967), *T. of Deaf*, **65**, 161.
Pearson, F. J. (1968), *Sound*, **2**, 34.
Pickett, J. M. (1971), *Volta Rev.*, **73**, 147.
Plant, G. R. (1960), *T. of Deaf*, **58**, 132.
Poulos, T. H. (1950), *Volta Rev.*, **52**, 316.
Power, R. (1969), *Sound*, **3**, 14.
Risberg, A. (1968), *Amer. Ann. Deaf*, **113**, 253.
R.N.I.D. (1973), *Special Aids to Hearing*. R.N.I.D.
Schmaehl, O. (1960), *Modern Educational Treatment of Deafness* (A. W. G. Ewing, Ed.). Manchester University Press.
Searson, M. (1965), *T. of Deaf*, **63**, 370.
Uden, A. van (1960), *Modern Educational Treatment of Deafness* (A. W. G. Ewing, Ed.). Manchester University Press.
Vermeulen, R. (1959), *Silent World*, **14**, 61.
Watson, T. J. and John, J. E. J. (1960), *Modern Educational Treatment of Deafness*, p. 161 (A. W. G. Ewing and E. C. Ewing, Eds.). Manchester University Press.
Watts, W. J. (1965), *T. of Deaf*, **63**, 34.
Watts, W. J. (1969), *T. of Deaf*, **67**, 4.

62. AUDITORY REHABILITATION WITH SPECIAL REFERENCE TO CHILDREN

JOHN BENCH AND KEVIN MURPHY

INTRODUCTION

Even though the practice of preventive medicine is now widely accepted, there is still a natural concern for the acute condition. Hence the approach to chronicity, which tends to emphasize alleviation as much as cure, tends to be regarded with less urgency or indeed with less enthusiasm. In the case of impaired hearing one result of this imbalance has been the development of various kinds of pressure groups, usually established by parents or teachers, which aim to alert the public to the consequences of hearing loss. Although primarily aiming at helping children who have already been diagnosed, they also tend to publicize the fact of hearing loss and, as a result, put pressure upon community services for improved detection and diagnostic facilities as much as for further rehabilitative measures. Community medicine authorities in most developed countries now provide systems aimed at recognizing the possibility of hearing loss and encouraging referral to diagnosis, but the therapeutic aspects are often relatively weak. The results of the pioneer work in the field of risk registration (e.g. Sheridan, 1948) have spread rapidly throughout many parts of Europe, America, Australia and New Zealand, and improved detection procedures have led to a slow reduction in the age at which a child is brought to diagnosis and, hopefully, effective treatment.

Although it is not his main concern, it is clearly necessary that the auditory rehabilitator, or hearing therapist (as he or she is sometimes known) should not only have a sound grasp of the strengths and limitations of diagnostic methods for assessing hearing impairment, but should also understand the findings from clinical psychology, education and social work, and their interactions. Thus, no matter how early it begins, the likely success of a training programme is dependent not only on the treatment of the handicap, but on the degree of confidence which can be placed in the estimate of hearing deficit (an especially important point as regards young children and infants, for whom threshold measures are particularly difficult to achieve and which may tend to fluctuate); the extent to which it is possible to help the patient to understand the nature of his impairment and the effects which the impairment will have on his everyday life; and the success in conveying to parents, teachers and others with whom the patient comes into contact, the behavioural and intellectual concomitants of the hearing difficulties and therefore their own important role in his ameliorative programme.

Though we recognize that such factors are important we have decided that in the interests of selectivity we cannot do more than mention them. The same comments apply to the considerable controversies which exist throughout the area of diagnosis, remediation and rehabilitation. We would stress, however, that in nearly all cases of hearing impairment, the early stages of diagnosis and therapy are inextricably related, and we note that the term "diagnostic therapy" has been used to represent the complex processes involved in identifying hearing impairment, in experimenting with various forms of amplification, and in attempting to guide both parents and community in the first steps of rehabilitation (Matkin, 1973).

DEFINITION OF AUDITORY REHABILITATION

By auditory (or aural) rehabilitation we should, strictly speaking, refer to work which attempts to restore normality of auditory function to persons with impaired hearing or, if this is not possible, then to work which aims to make the most of the patient's residual hearing. Auditory rehabilitation has often been taken to include lipreading, sign language and speech conservation (Sanders, 1971; O'Neil and Oyer, 1973). We shall not concern ourselves with these, but propose to devote our review to the auditory aspects only.

We have chosen to deal with auditory rehabilitation and to omit mention of habilitation, because, in our opinion, the latter term involves a number of difficulties. As we have already remarked, the area of auditory rehabilitation is concerned with restoring normal hearing function or to optimizing the use of auditory residua. The expression "habilitation" is essentially prospective. It implies treatments to correct or alleviate a condition whose effects do not debilitate the patient now but which may become important at some future time. Although it is possible to conceive of problems which require habilitation of the individual with regard to future difficulties in certain fields (e.g. the U.S.A. "headstart programme", and the confounding effects of social class in attempts to promote educational attainments), there seems to be relatively little place for habilitation as regards auditory impairments. Even though such an impairment is likely to lead to educational and speech difficulties, the use of habilitation here has a reference to education and speech, and not to the auditory difficulty.

O'Neill and Oyer (1973) appear to have chosen to regard the development of such (specific) areas as speech and language as involving "habilitation", while they regard the development of "everyday communication" as the task of rehabilitation. This distinction also involves difficulties, for rehabilitation so described will subsume habilitation. Moreover, "everyday communication" involves such a plethora of different processes and their interactions that it defies analysis and treatment.

There is a conceptual distinction between the use of the term when applied to teaching an infant *de novo* compared to its use in describing attempts to restore function (Asp, 1973), especially in those cases where language structures have been developed before the impairment was incurred or at least where sufficient auditory experience of, e.g.

phonemic elements, has existed prior to the onset of impaired hearing. However, it is difficult to make practical use of this distinction since accurate audiometry is difficult to achieve with very young infants, especially as regards derivation of a tonal audiogram (Bench, 1974; Collyer *et al.*, 1974a, b). Even where it may be achieved, the relevance of a pure tone audiogram to hearing for speech is a continuing source of discussion.

AUDITORY REHABILITATION AND THE ACQUISITION OF SPEECH AND LANGUAGE

Auditory rehabilitation for children has received particular attention, especially in respect of younger children and infants. This is mainly because considerable evidence has accumulated to show that the normal acquisition of important elements of speech and language is largely contingent upon adequate hearing for speech over the age range of approximately 1–5 years (Renfrew and Murphy, 1964; Lenneberg, 1967; Rutter and Martin, 1972). Because of the importance of adequate speech hearing, we have chosen to give it special mention in what follows. Although it has been argued (Chomsky, 1968; Katz, 1966; McNeil, 1966; Slobin, 1966) that a child has an innate or fundamental capacity for language, even the more extreme nativists would accept that much of the shaping of language depends on experiential factors.

Although it is clearly recognized that hearing plays an essential role in the development of speech and language, it is extremely difficult, if not impossible, to describe such a role fully. Much has recently been written on the acquisition of language in infants and children with normal hearing, but we still do not know enough (Crystal, 1972; Friedlander, 1970), and much still remains to be discovered about the way in which speech and language are acquired by those children who suffer from various auditory disorders (Dale, 1972; Jones and Byers, 1971). We also need to know much more than we do at present about the auditory fluctuations which may occur in so-called normally hearing children, and the extent, if any, to which they are likely to constitute a threat to language growth in the first few years of life. We know next to nothing about such variations, and in particular we are unable to identify the extent to which they are stable or fluctuating, and/or attenuating, and/or distorting. Given such variables, the growth of signal processing (i.e. discrimination, decoding and encoding) prior to any expressive functions seems to be at risk. Add these phenomena to a sensorineural hearing loss and the problem is further complicated. Nonetheless, sufficient is already known to compel us to relate hearing problems in children within the wider field of what we have come to know as communication problems in order to achieve effective rehabilitation. This in turn leads on to yet wider issues because: "Children's personality adjustment as well as their development linguistically, socially and intellectually, now clearly have been found to be affected by problems in communication" (Ewing, 1973) and because: "any disturbance of either (the nervous system or the mind) in relation to communication must

have the most profound social effects because society is based upon communication" (Brain, 1965).

INTERVENING VARIABLES

We have felt it important to give this brief orientation before discussing in detail some recent work on auditory rehabilitation because there is a danger that, in a book devoted to the "Scientific Foundations of Otolaryngology", the wider issues involved would go unregarded, and that therefore the reader might be misled into regarding the problems as too closely associated with the impairment of the sensory end organ. While we recognize that our topic has its origin in disorders of the ear, the difficulties that ensue are the proper concern of disciplines other than otology, not least because the child is a developing being in many ways which involve complex interactions between a number of variables. Malfunction in one particular will have effects on many others, and, in the case of auditory impairment, it is not enough to restore auditory function, and then to assume that all will be well. For example, Critchley (1967) has remarked that aspects of hearing involve "brain stem startle reflexes, cortical representation of hearing, development of association areas and feedback mechanisms". Lloyd and Frisina (1965) have gone further to remark that hearing is important for "handling auditory symbols mechanically, chemically and electrically, as well as for the subsequent transmission of coded neural impulses to the areas of the brain important for speech and language. Important CNS processes include those such as perception, concept development and ideation". Adopting a rather different approach, Bench (1972) has referred to detection, discrimination, recognition, identification and interpretation of sound, examining the way in which the stimuli which impinge on the ear can be studied and related to past experience. Murphy (1972) on the other hand, has dealt with the feedback or self-monitoring proceesses whereby the child learns to check that his speech sounds conform to his linguistic intentions. Clearly the functions involved in what we refer to as "hearing" are so multifaceted that even a temporary failure of auditory input has far reaching effects on other areas. This is especially so for young children whose continuing development will cause higher order derangements to continue to accrue unless appropriate remedial action is taken (cf. Lewis, 1965).

THE CRITICAL PERIOD HYPOTHESIS

As we have remarked, considerable evidence has accumulated to show that normal hearing ability is particularly important for the development of language and speech in the first 5 years of life. It follows that the rehabilitation of impaired hearing is also of great importance at this time, perhaps more important than at any other age. Appreciation of this state of affairs has led to a proliferation of efforts towards the early identification of hearing impairment and also to attempts to alleviate such impairments from an early age, even in infancy. Unfortunately, however, the early identification of hearing loss is fraught with difficulties (Ling, 1970), and suitable therapy seems to be even more problematical. Despite this, a number of workers have gone so far as to implement diagnostic and therapeutic programmes for young infants, arguing from the critical period concept (Scott, 1962). They have reasoned that the experience of auditory and other stimuli during certain critical stages in infancy has profound, lasting and irreversible effects on subsequent development, and that deprivation of auditory experiences during such stages has long lasting deleterious effects on the acquisition of hearing skills and the development of speech and language. The result has been to create considerable confusion since, in their anxiety to emphasize the value of early diagnosis and therapy, too many workers have attempted to go beyond the notion of importance or value to the promulgation of scientific dogmas for which at present we lack convincing proof. Use of the word "critical" or "crucial" (Lenneberg, 1967; Pollack, 1967; Rubin, 1972) to describe the importance of a developmental period implies an irreversibility of the effects occurring during such a period as a result of normal stimulation. But if, after an infant or child has been impaired as a result of failure to receive adequate stimulation during a "critical period", a method can be found to change his condition back to normal, then it is clear that the so-called period is not critical after all. It seems impossible to be sure that the effects of some "critical period" are irreversible, and therefore "the usefulness of the critical period concept is belied by its own specificity. If a certain period in auditory development is postulated as . . . critical, this means that the effects of auditory stimulation in that period cannot be surpassed. It is difficult to see how this can be put to exhaustive empirical test. It seems more reasonable to forgo the critical part of the critical period hypothesis, and to adopt some such term as 'especially sensitive period', which allows us to recognize that certain periods in development may be important, perhaps very important, without necessarily being critical as regards irreversibility" (Bench, 1971). Moreover, it would seem that the use of the critical period concept implies a pessimistic outlook for work in rehabilitation. If the effects of "critical period" stimulation or its absence really were as specific and irreversible as the concept suggests, what point would there be in continuing the attempt to restore the affected individual to normal after the so-called "critical period" had run its course? At best, rehabilitation would have to be directed towards developing techniques to minimize the results of the damage, without any hope of obviating it.

AUDITORY TRAINING

In considering auditory rehabilitation, one of the first techniques which comes to mind is that of auditory training. This comprises a group of methods which attempt to stimulate or otherwise improve the effectiveness of the auditory mechanisms via controlled amplification. The concept of auditory training implies that the hearing handicapped either may not be using their residual hearing, or that they are making less than the maximum possible use of their residual hearing, or that they may be using their hearing inefficiently in the sense that they may tend to rely too much on non-auditory cues. Efficient use of residual hearing implies that the patient should be encouraged by means of frequency selective amplification to make fine discriminations (of a type not necessarily made by the normal hearer) between (speech) sounds which might otherwise seem very similar to one another. In this context it is noteworthy that Boothroyd (1967) has shown that certain hard-of-hearing children tend towards increased reliance on the low frequency components of speech.

One of the first fairly well described techniques for auditory training was recorded by Goldstein (1939) who taught the discrimination of musical tones. At about the same time, Ballenger (1936) and Goodfellow (1942) also published studies on similar work. These did not provide very conclusive evidence for the efficacy of auditory training, although Johnson (1939) claimed to have obtained some improvement when using verbal retention tests. It was not until 1948 that a reasonably comprehensive study was conducted (Di Carlo, 1948) on a sample of servicemen who had been issued with hearing aids. Di Carlo found some improvement for consonant recognition, and this work was soon followed by the studies of Larsen (1950), who reported that auditory training improved the recognition of phonetically balanced words. These studies provided some of the first reasonably valid empirical evidence to support the concept of auditory training. However, Clarke (1957), in a study of lipreading and auditory training in a group of hard-of-hearing schoolchildren, found that auditory training alone gave very little improvement for speech comprehension.

This early work may be summarized as showing that auditory training as a valid and reliable technique for assisting the communication of the hearing-impaired patient was not notably successful. The sum total of the studies quoted suggests that auditory training may be useful without implying that it is likely to be of more than minor utility. As O'Neil and Oyer have remarked (1973), there was a lack of standard tests necessary to evaluate the effectiveness of a training technique, and although much has been said by the practitioners of auditory training about its beneficial results, the practitioners themselves have in general omitted to research the effectiveness of their methods with anything like the degree of objectivity and rigour needed for a sound evaluation. Also, in too many cases they have failed to provide detailed and accurate records with which others might have made the evaluation. At this level, the effectiveness of auditory training remains an open question.

More recently, positive results for a programme of auditory training were reported briefly by Di Carlo (1958) and later by Lang and his associates (1962) for pre-school children. In the latter study, free field pure tone audiometry was followed by 1–1½ years of auditory training, with a finding that hearing-impaired children showed improvement for hearing level and speech development, whereas normal* (control) children showed no such changes.

---

* Normally hearing children do not seem to be a suitable form of control. It would have been more appropriate to use a hearing-impaired control group who were awaiting formal auditory training.

However, Lichtenberg (1966), comparing 3 groups of children who were normally hearing and speaking, normally hearing and speech defective, and hearing defective, reported that auditory training gave rise to a change in speech perception for both hearing impaired and normally hearing children. Bode and Oyer (1970) using Rhyme Tests found that concentrated auditory training for 32 adults suffering from sensorineural hearing loss produced significant changes for speech discrimination, and that speech discrimination increased with age, sensation level of stimuli and intelligence. Martony and colleagues (1972) also used a Rhyme test when studying 166 subjects aged between 10 and 22 years. They reported preliminary findings that, after classifying their children's audiograms by a method developed from that of Wedenberg (1954), discrimination for 4 kinds of rhythmical patterns differed for children with various kinds of residual low-frequency hearing.

VERBOTONAL PROCEDURE

This method, recently reviewed by Asp (1973), was developed by Guberina (1961, 1964) from experience with foreign language teaching for use with hard-of-hearing children. The method makes use of band-passed speech sounds, each comprising a consonant followed by a vowel (logatome) to estimate hearing and intelligibility thresholds, to give an octave by octave measure of the hearing pattern. The technique is thus a kind of compromise between pure tone and conventional speech audiometry. Once the hearing pattern has been assessed, the hearing-impaired child is trained to make use of his residual hearing for such aspects of speech as intonation, pauses, rhythm and phonemes at a setting of the training apparatus just greater than his threshold for intelligibility. Special apparatus (the SUVAG) has been designed for this method. Guberina (1970) later described the use of rhythmical body movements to "direct the student's listening". Although it has firm adherents (e.g. Perier, 1969), the verbotonal approach has generated some controversy, partly because Guberina himself appears not to have researched the effectiveness of this method very thoroughly. By contrast, Black (1968) has discussed the theoretical basis of the method and has concluded that the verbotonal auditory assessment was not to be regarded as an important aspect of the method and that patients who had some skills in speech recognition could improve their performance with training. Roberts (1969) compared the verbotonal method with a more conventional approach in a 13-month training study, finding that speech recognition improved more with lipreading and auditory training, than with auditory training alone. Tulasiewicz (1966) has given a theoretical description of the verbotonal method, a description of its accompanying SUVAG I and II machines and an account of a Cambridge experimental study with illustrative case histories on 4 children. It would appear that the verbotonal method may have been of some assistance in this study, but the patient numbers were small, and the controls were poor.

FREQUENCY TRANSPOSITION AND COMPRESSED SPEECH

The frequency transposer was developed by Johansson (1961). It consists of an amplifier, amplitude compression unit, and low and high pass filters. Its function is to transpose the higher audio-frequencies by heterodyning against a 4800 Hz reference tone into the low frequency area. Its especial application is to those severely hard-of-hearing patients who possess residual hearing for low frequencies, below 1500 Hz, say, but have no useful hearing for the higher frequencies. Frequency transposition thus presents the patient with a new frequency pattern for speech sounds, especially the fricatives. Wedenberg (1961) has suggested that training with the transposer leads to improved speech discrimination. However, the effectiveness of the frequency transposer has been further studied by Ling and Druz (1967) and by Ling (1968, 1969), who found only a marginal improvement with its use. More recently Biondi and Biondi (1968) have designed a transposer which makes use of a sample-and-hold process for the speech spectrum, with a sampling frequency variable from 1 to 4 Hz, and with variable degrees of transposition. The use of this instrument was also explored by Ling (1972) on a sample of 12 severely hard of hearing children. He found no advantage over more conventional amplification, but his results have been questioned by Biondi and Biondi (1972) who claim that Ling's data suggest that use of their apparatus does give an improvement in speech recognition.

Bandwith compression of vocoded (synthetic) speech has been described by Pimonow (1965, 1968) whose aim was to reduce the frequency bandwidth of speech without loss of important information. Pilot studies suggested that this approach has some beneficial effect on speech sound perception, but the results were not as great as anticipated. Guttman and van Bergijk (1958) used Bogert's (1956) VOBANC, which reduced the speech frequency range by a factor of 2. This was followed (Guttman and Nelson 1968) by further studies with coded speech, using an instrument which generated a low frequency pulse for every so-many zero crossings of high frequency sounds in speech. The method is currently being evaluated.

Amongst other work using frequency conversion may be noted that of Bennett and Byers (1967) who found that speech perception for a group of hard of hearing patients improved for material which was frequency-shifted by replaying tape recordings at 80 per cent of normal speed, but was worse for material slowed by 60 and 70 per cent. Raymond and Proud (1962) also used frequency shifting and claimed to find improved speech discrimination scores, which, however, did not approach the improvements found with conventionally (linearly) amplified speech. Ahlström and associates (1968) studied the effects of frequency transposition for consonant sounds in normally hearing subjects given a simulated hearing loss. They reported that the changes in consonant discrimination which occurred with training occurred rapidly (in contrast to many other reports, which, however, made use of more complex material). Discrimination was apparently based on voicing, duration and cluster consonants.

The studies outlined above present a rather common outcome insofar as the authors generally claim some improvement for the perception of speech material by the use of frequency transposition or compression, but in many cases this improvement was found to be less than that obtained from linear amplification, and rarely, if ever, approached the speech perception capabilities of the normal listener. In much of the work important controls were missing, e.g. for the Hawthorne effect, which Bench (1970) found to be considerable in a small scale study of 4 profoundly deaf children with only residual hearing for low frequencies. In this study, frequency and time compression were so combined as to lower the frequency of the speech material while maintaining the temporal characteristics close to those for the original material. An apparent improvement in the discrimination of word list material was found to be closely matched with a control improvement for acclimatization to the apparatus and experimental environment.

Work in this area has also been criticized by Risberg (1969). To develop Risberg's arguments, phoneme distortions with speech analysing hearing aids present the subject with new material, which is in some ways speech-like, but bears an unknown relation to speech as regards the speech analysing properties of the nervous system. Thus Liberman and associates (1967) have noted that perception of certain phonemes is related to relatively invariant acoustic loci associated mainly with second formant transitions. Transposition will shift the original acoustic locus, resulting in perception of a different sound, and breaking or distorting the speech perception code. Since this code is known to be highly efficient in conveying speech information, frequency transposition is likely to lead to a considerable diminution in efficiency and the implied recording will have to be learnt, not by any means an easy task. Even so, it is open to question that the new code will be accepted by the brain as a *speech* code, without loss of efficiency. On the other hand, the redundant nature of continuous speech may mitigate against problems arising from phonemic distortion. Work with an instrument designed by Thomas and Flavin (1970) for transposing only second formant speech information may shed some light on this problem. A discussion of processes associated with perception of the speech code is given by Roworth (1970) and by Velmans (1974). Areas for further research may include studies where speech material above, say, 4 kHz only is transposed—e.g. transposition of fricatives (Velmans, 1975), exploration of the interference effects between normal and frequency transposed/compressed speech, and more "basic" research into the speech coding processes and channel capacity of hard of hearing listeners, together with work of the type described by Pickett and his colleagues (Pickett and Martin, 1968; Pickett and Martony, 1970) on impaired discrimination for sound spectra.

HEARING AIDS AND AUDITORY REHABILITATION

Since the field of hearing aids and their uses is discussed at length elsewhere, we shall limit our remarks to certain brief comments followed by the consideration of some general aspects of national and international provision.

Developments in electroacoustics over the past 30 years have led to production of hearing aids which, besides being smaller in size, also consume less power. It has thus proved possible to take advantage of recent power cell technology to produce aids more acceptable for social reasons and more convenient generally, which have a greater range of gain, and which are amenable in many instances to tailoring of frequency characteristics. However, too few available aids have sufficient gain at the low frequencies to be potentially useful to certain profoundly deaf individuals. There is some controversy for patients of this type on whether one or two aids should be fitted. Obviously, much of the potential benefit will be derived from one aid alone, but there are a number of minor factors (e.g. binaural aids assist in the reception of a localized source (Carhart, 1966), which suggest that the fitting of two aids may maximize the chances of good reception so long as the loss is similar binaurally and that the aids are matched for performance as far as technically possible.

It is common clinical practice to prescribe a hearing aid on the basis of the patient's pure tone audiogram (Liden and Kankhunen, 1969). This will go some way towards alleviating the hearing handicap, but by no means far enough, because the goal is for the patient to receive speech rather than pure tones. Speech processing seems to be based not on an analysis of the frequency structure of phonemes or words alone, but on the perception of the frequency and intensity characteristics of phonemes or words as a function of time, and also as a function of a code of predictions, since "speech" very rarely occurs in single word systems. Conventional speech audiometry with word lists would seem to be of more relevance than pure tone data (but see Coles *et al.*, 1973), but the final test should ideally be based on the reception of running speech to approximate to a "real life" situation in a region which must be well above the pure tone hearing threshold.

Mazeas (1972), studying a group of hearing-impaired children, analysed the auditory capacity of his patients in information terms, and found that one group derived considerable benefit (ICA scores) from their aids, whereas another subgroup did not. Children with a relatively high auditory capacity of greater than 7000 bits per second showed great benefit from conventional aids, but such aids were of much less help to children whose auditory capacity was less than this quantity. These points have also been noted by Jerger (1968). Jerger found that the relation of the electroacoustic properties of his aids and speech discrimination depended on the nature of the speech task, and recommended that standard sentence identification tests with competing messages should be developed as test vehicles.

Fitting hearing aids to the adult patient is a relatively simple task, since some at least of Jerger's proposals may usually be attempted when a good speech intelligibility threshold can be identified and the patient has sufficient maturity, energy, insight and desire for help to co-operate in the process of aid selection. Schultz and Kraat (1970) have suggested a way of measuring aspects of this situation.

Having said this, we are compelled to note that with the exception of Denmark, the U.S.A. and Australia, very few countries provide hearing aid evaluation as part of their Health Services. Indeed as far as we can ascertain only one country (Denmark) controls the import of hearing aids for hospital prescription.

In the case of infants the selection of hearing aids tends to veer between the need for adequate amplification on the one hand and the fear of trauma on the other. Because formal speech tests are not possible with young pre-lingually deaf children, present practice has concentrated on the attempt to match frequency response curves in the hearing aid to the presumptive audiogram of the young child. Since the development of methods for measuring the acoustic impedance of the ear, there has been increased recognition of the phenomenon of recruitment in young children, and as a result some centres are concentrating on the use of amplitude compression or various forms of vented earmoulds.

The dilemma which still faces the clinician fitting a hearing aid to a young child is the need to distinguish between the various reasons for its early rejection. Various soft, semi-soft or hard plastics have been used for ear moulds, and various shapes and masses have been investigated, but there is little or no valid evidence to guide the hearing aid fitter faced with a child aged 9 months who obviously resents his ministration.

Descriptions of structural design and function of hearing aids, their mode of control by child, parent or teacher, the position in which they should be worn, the ease which they detect patient voice as well as that of the speaker at a distance (Gengel et al., 1971; Carhart, 1946; Resmick and Becker, 1963; Jeffers and Smith, 1964) fill the technical literature. In recent years, research has also concentrated upon the condition of the aid and the manner in which it is worn or used. Two depressing reports in this area were presented by Martin and Lodge (1969) and by Fisch (1973). One surveyed the condition of the aids worn by a selected population in schools or special classes for hearing impaired children; the other examined the manner in which the aid was worn by a selected clinical population of children. Martin found that over 60 per cent were so damaged as to be of little or no use. Fisch found that 60 per cent were so fitted as to be of equally dubious value.

Although shelves are filled with publications on the effects of listening conditions (e.g. Boothroyd, 1967), the acoustic control of the environment in which children will wear aids is often completely neglected. For instance 50 per cent of school age children wearing hearing aids in the U.K. attend schools for normally hearing children (estimated from recent issues of "Health of the School Child", D.E.S.). The provisions of special acoustic conditions, sound damping, induction loops, or radio microphones for such children is so rare as to be almost fortuitous. (The above comment does not, of course, apply to the partially hearing units which for statistical purposes fall within the other 50 per cent of children wearing aids who are in receipt of full-time special educational treatment.)

In the case of children suffering from unilateral loss, or who present with a unilateral atresia, the fitting of a hearing aid is often delayed. Such children are usually expected to develop spoken language without the aid of amplification. Decisions about fitting aids in such cases are often based on educational criteria.

The fitting of hearing aids as practised in Danish speech and hearing clinics cannot be too widely publicized (Ewertsen, 1971; Bentzen, 1965). In such centres the hospital patient is not only fitted with the aid but is also given a formal course of instruction in its use. The case is reviewed at regular intervals to ensure that progress is satisfactory, that the original prescription was reliable, and that the aids and earmoulds are presenting no problems. Other countries have excellent centres, but these tend to represent the skills and enthusiasm of their staffs rather than national policy. The supervision of hearing aids in the early stages of their use is often completely divorced from their selection, and in the case of group aids which are usually more powerful than the majority of individual aids there may well be no discernable pattern of selection let alone supervision. In Chapter 61, Miss Knox describes a fascinating choice of devices available to the teacher of hearing-impaired children. The reader might well be excused the uneasy suspicion that such a plethora of technical materials may well be beyond many teachers, particularly those who were trained before such devices were available and who find difficulty in attending specialized refresher courses in their use. Many European countries have only recently developed an interest in auditory training, and in many of them, were it not for private enterprise, no facilities for deaf education would be available for children under the age of 7 years.

At the time of writing, the use of peripatetic teachers who visit the hearing-impaired child in his home before he reaches the statutory age for formal education is confined, as a national practice, to no more than about 10 countries. Some of the wealthiest and most highly developed countries in the world do nothing at a national level for young hearing-impaired children in their homes. Visiting such countries one is often heartened by the few centres which do provide excellent facilities for pre-school age children, but some countries have not yet freed deaf education from the criteria originally developed for children with normal hearing. As a result, parent guidance, child supervision, and validation of the new aid may be in the hands of voluntary agencies with variable quality of contact with the clinician who originally recommended the aid.

CONCLUSIONS

Although studies are now being done which have both an experimental and a sound logical basis, and which might properly find their place in a book devoted to the scientific foundations of otolaryngology, this work is still in its infancy. It is clear from our review that whereas it is now recognized that a firm basis of expertise has to be built up concerning the interaction of the hearing ability of the patient with his prosthesis, and that work in this area is continuing, studies of sufficient rigour are lacking. There are a host of social, educational and psychological factors, which are difficult to measure and control, but which nonetheless are of great importance.

If the promise of therapeutic services for hearing impaired individuals is to develop satisfactorily, there is a pressing need for a pattern of audiological training which will relate current linguistic information and theories to current information on amplification systems. Such a training pattern, though obviously including a considerable amount of diagnostic theory and practice, would place great emphasis on rehabilitation and perhaps on certain aspects of education. Such additional criteria, as with sensory and multi-sensory training, visual perception, and visual-tactile reinforcement procedures, would need to be evaluated and, where relevant, include development of present research into aspects of cognition.

As linguistic sciences and psycholinguistics develop, present information on the development of language in children with normal hearing would need to be extended to include children with various types and degrees of hearing impairment. In the course of time, developmental language tests for hearing-impaired children should facilitate the compilation of speech audiometric material which relates more accurately to hearing-impaired child's maturity and known language skills. When such tests are available a more realistic evaluation of hearing aids should be possible.

Hearing aid evaluation has (with certain exceptions) often tended to be unreliable and excessively subjective. To some extent, this has come about because of the failure to create the right training schemes for audiologists and a tendency to relate the budget of any provisions to a modest standard of clinical competence. In other words, shortage of money, information and, to a certain extent, concern, has led to a quality of training which precludes the provision of comprehensive national services in most of the developed countries we have studied.

As we have already pointed out, few of the developed countries provide a comprehensive hearing aid evaluation service. There is insufficient research on patient usage, on patterns of wear, on validation of criteria beginning from the earmould and taking in every characteristic of the aid, particularly with reference to patterns of usage, acoustic conditions, auditory tasks involved, social or occupational criteria and the like. In the case of children, such studies could begin from present information on induction loop systems, group hearing aids, and classroom acoustics but, as has already been stated, they would need to be based on a considerably deeper knowledge of language development in hearing-impaired children than is currently applied to the problem.

In order to advise the otologist in his responsibility for recommending the aid, the audiologist needs access to information and skills based on vastly improved and extended research criteria.

REFERENCES

Asp, C. W. (1973), *An Appraisal of Speech Pathology and Audiology*, p. 134 (J. W. Wingo and G. F. Holloway, Eds.). Springfield, Illinois: Thomas.

Ahlstrom, K. G., Risberg, A. and Lindhe, V. (1968), Institute of Education, Uppsala University, Sweden, Report 36.

Ballenger, H. C. (1936), *Ann. Otol.*, **45**, 632.

Bench, J. (1970). Unpublished observations.

Bench, J. (1972), *Speech Communication Ability and Profound Deafness.* Stockholm (1970), p. 39 (G. Fant, Ed.). Washington: Alexander Graham Bell Association.

Bench, J. (1974). Unpublished observations.

Bench, R. J. (1971), *Sound*, **5**, 21.

Bennett, D. and Byers, V. W. (1967), *J. Aud. Res.*, **7**, 105.

Bentzen, O. (1965), *J. Aud. Technique*, **4**, 168.

Biondi, E. and Biondi, L. (1968), *Alta Frequenza*, **37**, 728.

Biondi, E. and Biondi, L. (1972), *Speech Communication Ability and Profound Deafness*, Stockholm, 1970, p. 334 (G. Fant, Ed.). Alexander Graham Bell Association, Washington, Paper 33.

Black, J. W. (1968), Final report, R. F. Project 1688, Ohio.

Bode, D. L. and Oyer, H. J. (1970), *J. Speech Hear. Res.*, **13**, 839.

Bogert, E. (1956), *J. acoust. Soc. Amer.*, **28**, 399.

Boothroyd, A. (1967), *Int. Audiol.*, **6**, 136.

Brain, Lord (1965), *Children with Communication Problems*, 6. London: Pitman Medical Publishing Co.

Carhart, R. (1946), *Arch. Otolaryng.*, **44**, 1.

Carhart, R. (1966), *Int. Audiol.*, **6**, 285.

Chomsky, N. (1968), *Language and Mind*. New York: Harcourt Brace Jovanovich.

Clarke, F. R. (1957), *Educational Guidance and the Deaf Child*, p. 128 (A. W. G. Ewing, Ed.). Manchester: Manchester University Press.

Coles, R. R. A., Markides, A. and Priede, V. M. (1973), "Uses and Abuses of Speech Audiometry," in *Disorders of Auditory Function* (W. Taylor, Ed.). London and New York: Academic Press.

Collyer, Y., Bench, J. and Wilson, I. (1974a), *Brit. J. Audiol.*, **8**, 14.

Collyer, Y., Bench, J. and Wilson, I. (1974b), *Brit. J. Audiol.* In press.

Critchley, E. (1967), *Speech Origins and Development*. Springfield, Illinois: Charles C. Thomas.

Crystal, D. (1972), *Brit. J. Comm. Disord.*, **7**, 3.

Dale, P. S. (1972), *Language Development*. Hinsdale, Illinois: Dryden Press.

Di Carlo, L. M. (1948), *Volta Rev.*, **50**, 490.

Di Carlo, L. M. (1958), *Element School J.*, **48**, 160.

Ewertsen, H. W. (1971), 3rd Danavox Symposium, Copenhagen, p. 135.

Ewing, A. (1973), *Disorders of Auditory Function*, 8 (W. Taylor, Ed.). London: Academic Press.

Fisch, L. (1973), "Paedoaudiology at the Crossroads," Contribution to Brit. Soc. Audiol. Meeting.

Friedlander, B. Z. (1970), *Merill-Palmer Quart.*, **16**, 7.

Gengel, R. W., Pascoe, D. and Shore, I. (1971), *J. Speech Hear. Res.*, **36**, 341.

Goldstein, M. A. (1939), *The Acoustic Method*. St. Louis, Ma., U.S.A.: Laryngoscope Press.

Goodfellow, L. D. (1942), *J. Psychol.*, **14**, 53.

Guberina, P. (1961), *Vox et images de France*. Paris: Didier.

Guberina, P. (1964), *Proc. Internat. Congr. Educ. Deaf*, p. 279.

Guberina, P. (1970), *Rev. Phonét. Appliq.*, No. 16.

Guttman, N. and van Bergeijk, W. A. (1958), *Proc. 4th Int. Cong. Audiol.* Padua.

Guttman, N. and Nelson, J. R. (1968), *Amer. Ann. Deaf*, **113**, 295.

Jeffers, J. and Smith, C. R. (1964), *A.S.H.A.*, **6**, 504.

Jerger, J. (1968), "Effects of Electro-acoustic Characteristics of Hearing Aids on Speech Understanding," Progress Report. Houston Speech and Hearing Center, Houston, Texas.

Johansson, B. (1961), *Proc. 3rd Internat. Congr. Acoustics*, p. 658.

Johnson, E. H. (1939), *Amer. Ann. Deaf*, **84**, 223.

Jones, M. C. and Byers, V. W. (1971), *J. Learn. Disabil.*, **4**, 46–49.

Katz, J. J. (1966), *The Philosophy of Language*. New York: Harper and Row.

Lang, J. Oban, L., Palatas, G., Merei, V. and Csangi, Y. (1962), *Int. Audiol.*, **2**, 198.

Larsen, L. L. (1950), *Consonant Sound Discrimination*. Bloomington: Indiana University Press.

Lenneberg, E. H. (1967), *Biological Foundations of Language*. New York and London: John Wiley.

Lewis, M. M. (1965), *Children with Communication Problems*, 7. London: Pitman Medical Publishing Co.

Liberman, A. M., Cooper, F. S., Harris, K. S., MacNeilage, P. F. and Studdert-Kennedy, M. (1967), *Models for the Perception of Speech and Visual Form*, p. 68 (W. Wathen-Dunn, Ed.). Cambridge, Mass.: M.I.T. Press.

Lichtenberg, F. S. (1966), *Volta Rev.*, **68**, 426.

Liden, G. and Kankhunen, A. (1969), *Int. Audiol.*, **8**, 99.

Ling, D. and Druz, W. S. (1967), *J. Aud. Res.*, **7**, 133.

Ling, D. (1968), *Amer. Ann. Deaf*, **113**, 283.

Ling, D. (1969), *I.E.E.E. Trans. Audio Electroacoustics*, p. 298.

Ling, D. (1970), Paper presented at International Congress of Audiology, Dallas, Texas.

Ling, D. (1972), *Speech Communication Ability and Profound Deafness. Stockholm (1970)*, p. 323 (G. Fant, Ed.). Washington: Alexander Graham Bell Association.

Lloyd, L. L. and Frisina, R. D. (1965), *Proc. Nat. Conf. Parsons, Kansas*, p. 265. Parsons State Hospital and Training Center.

Martin, M. C. and Lodge, J. J. (1969), *Sound (Brit. J. Audiol.)*, **3**, 2.

Martony, J., Risberg, A., Spens, K. E. and Agelfors, E. (1972), *Speech Communication Ability and Profound Deafness. Stockholm (1970)*, p. 75 (G. Fant, Ed.). Washington: Alexander Graham Bell Association.

Matkin, N. D. (1973), "Evaluation of Hearing Handicapped Children," in *Proc. V Danavox Symp.*, p. 93 (E. Kampp, Ed.). Ebeltoft, Denmark.

Mazeas, R. (1972), *Speech Communication Ability and Profound Deafness. Stockholm (1970)*, p. 99 (G. Fant, Ed). Alexander Graham Bell Association.

McNeil, D. (1966), Psycholinguistics Papers. Edinburgh University Press.

Murphy, K. P. (1972), *The Child with Delayed Speech* (M. Rutter and J. A. M. Martin, Eds.). London: Heinemann.

O'Neil, J. J. and Oyer, H. J. (1973), *Modern Developments in Audiology*, pp. 211, 216, 222 (J. Jerger, Ed.). New York: Academic Press.

Perier, O. (1969), *Proc. Int. Cong. Rehab. Disabl.* Dublin.

Pickett, J. M. and Martin, E. S. (1968), *Amer. Ann. Deaf*, **113**, 259.

Pickett, J. M. and Martony, J. (1970), *J. Speech Hear. Res.*, **13**, 347.

Pimonow, L. (1965), *Cahiers d'acoustique*, **133**, 151.

Pimonow, L. (1968), *Amer. Ann. Deaf*, **113**, 275.

Pollack, D. (1967), *Int. Audiol.*, **6**, 243.

Raymond, T. and Proud, G. (1962), *Arch. Otlaryng.*, **76**, 436.

Renfrew, C. and Murphy, K. (Eds.) (1964), *The Child Who Does Not Talk*. Heinemann, London: Spastics International Medical Publications.

Resmick, D. M. and Becker, M. (1963), *A.S.H.A.*, **5**, 695.

Risberg, A. (1969), *I.E.E.E. Trans Audio Electroacoust.*, AU-17.

Roberts, L. (1969), "The Verbotonal and Regular Programmes in the Metropolitan Toronto School for the Deaf: A Descriptive Study," Research Dept. Metropolitan Toronto School Board, Toronto.

Roworth, D. A. A. (1970), *Sound (Brit. J. Audiol.)*, **4**, 95.

Rubin, M. (1972), *J. Comm. Disord.*, **5**, 195.

Rutter, M. and Martin, J. A. M. (Eds.) (1972), *The Child with Delayed Speech*. London: Heinemann.

Sanders, D. A. (1971), *Aural Rehabilitation*. New Jersey: Prentice Hall.

Schultz, M. C. and Kraat, W. W. (1970), *J. Speech Hear. Dis.*, **35**, 37.

Scott, J. P. (1962), *Science*, **138**, 949.

Sheridan, M. (1948), *The Child's Hearing for Speech*. London: Methuen.

Slobin, D. I. (1966), *The Genesis of Language* (F. Smith and G. A. Miller, Eds.). Cambridge, Mass.: M.I.T. Press.

Thomas, I. B. and Flavin, F. E. (1970), *J. Audio Eng. Soc.*, **18**, 56.

Tulasiewicz, W. F. (1966), *Rev. Phonét. Appliq.*, p. 68.

Velmans, M. (1974), *Brit. J. Audiol.*, **8**, 1.

Velmans, M. (1975), *Language and Speech*. In press.

Wedenberg, E. (1954), *Acta Otolaryng.*, suppl. 110.

Wedenberg, E. (1961), *Proc. 3rd Internat. Congr. Acoustics*, p. 658.

SECTION XIII

TOXICOLOGY

PAGE

63. OTOTOXIC DRUGS   849

64. RHINOTOXIC DRUGS   862

63. OTOTOXIC DRUGS

JOHN BALLANTYNE

Aminoglycoside Antibiotics. By far the most important of the ototoxic drugs are the "unruly family of basic streptomyces antibiotics" (Hawkins, 1959), which are closely related to one another in their microbiology, pharmacology and toxicity.

For many years streptomycin, dihydrostreptomycin, neomycin, viomycin, framycetin, vancomycin and kanamycin have been "known or suspected to be toxic to the labyrinth to a greater or lesser degree when administered parenterally" (Leach, 1962). More recently, gentamicin, capreomycin and tobramycin have been added to this formidable list.

All the aminoglycoside antibiotics share a peculiar capacity to damage the internal ear, some of them affecting mainly the spiral organ of Corti, others the vestibular labyrinth.

Although in adults streptomycin is mainly vestibulotoxic, its cochleotoxic effect is much more pronounced in infants (Székely and Draskovich, 1965; Pražić and Salaj, 1972). Streptomycin (Robinson and Cambon, 1964) and dihydrostreptomycin (Kern, 1962) may also cross the placental barrier in concentrations sufficient to damage the fetal ear.

The most cochleotoxic of the basic streptomyces antibiotics are kanamycin and neomycin, and even small doses of these drugs may be toxic when administered parenterally (Šupáček, 1972). Sensorineural losses may also occur after oral administration (Ballantyne, 1970), or even after topical application. Hearing loss has been reported after injection of joint cavities (Campanelli *et al.*, 1966), irrigation of surgical wounds (Kelly *et al.*, 1969) and superficial dressing of burns. The aminohexoses are particularly well absorbed after intrabronchial (Lorian, 1962) and intrapleural (Leach, 1962) administration; and Fuller (1960) has described two cases of sensorineural hearing loss in children following the treatment of bronchiectasis with an aerosol containing neomycin. Hearing losses have also followed rectal and colonic irrigations with this drug (Fields, 1964).

The earliest symptom of the ototoxic patient is often one of high pitched tinnitus, which may be noticed some time before the subjective onset of hearing loss. Although vertigo may also be present, there is usually efficient compensation for a vestibular disturbance, and the most serious toxic effect of the basic antibiotics is a sensorineural hearing loss, usually irreversible and typically affecting mainly the high frequencies (Fig. 1). At a certain stage of gentamicin ototoxicity, a Z-shaped audiogram may be observed (Huizing, 1972) and recruitment may be demonstrated (Lidén, 1953).

The hearing loss caused by the streptomyces antibiotics will not uncommonly appear after a long latent period, and it usually becomes progressively worse as treatment is continued. It may not appear until some time after the drug has been discontinued, and thereafter it may progress even further (Šupáček, 1972).

Some families appear to have an unusual predisposition to the toxic effects of the aminohexoses (Podvineć and Stefanović, 1966; Miszke, 1972), and in elderly people dangerous concentrations may appear in the blood even with ordinary doses.

Diuretics. Maher and Schreiner (1965) were the first to describe sensorineural hearing losses due to etacrynic acid (Edecrin), a powerful diuretic which is given either by mouth or by intravenous injection. In many of their cases, hearing loss occurred either during or immediately after treatment with this drug, and it was characterized by a temporary hearing loss in patients with renal failure. Since that time, Schneider and Becker (1966), Schmidt and Friedman (1967), Ballantyne (1970) and others have reported instances of transient hearing loss after administration of etacrynic acid, but it was not until 1969 that Pillay and his colleagues (1969) reported permanent hearing losses.

Venkateswaran (1971) recorded a case of transient but severe hearing loss in a case of chronic renal failure treated with intravenous furosemide (Lasix) and Lloyd-Mostyn and Lord (1971) describe a case of permanent hearing loss following intravenous injection of this drug in large doses.

Anti-Protozoal Agents. Drugs used in the treatment of malaria include quinine and chloroquine and McKinna (1966) has reported two cases of congenital hearing loss in infants whose mothers had taken high pre-natal doses of quinine, in attempts to induce abortion.

Salicylates. Salicylates may cause a hearing loss when taken by mouth (Ghose and Joekes, 1964; McCabe and Dey, 1965; Gignoux *et al.*, 1966; Silverstein *et al.*, 1967) or very rarely when applied topically, as in a compound ointment (Perlman, 1966). Although the hearing loss is usually reversible, recovery of hearing may be delayed or incomplete and permanent hearing loss may result (Gignoux *et al.*, 1966); Jarvis, 1966).

Anti-Heparinizing Agents. Ransome *et al.* (1966) recorded several cases of sensorineural hearing loss due to an anti-heparinizing agent, hexadimethrine bromide (Polybrene). The drug had been given to patients who were being treated for renal failure by haemodialysis, during the course of which heparin was given as an anti-coagulant. No fewer than 6 of the 14 patients so treated developed varying degrees of sensorineural hearing loss, often severe.

Cytotoxic Agents. There have been several reports of sensorineural hearing loss after regional perfusions of nitro-

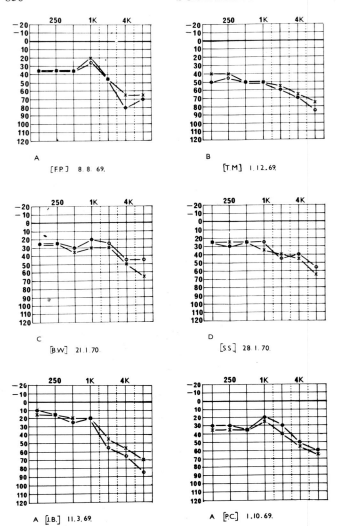

FIG. 1. Audiograms of six patients with neomycin ototoxicity. *Upper*: 4 patients with liver disease complicated by porto-systemic encephalopathy (PSE) and treated with neomycin only. *Lower*: 2 patients with liver disease complicated by PSE and ascites and treated with neomycin and diuretics. o = right ear; x = left ear.

gen mustard (Conrad and Crosby, 1960; Lawrence *et al.*, 1961; Young *et al.*, 1961; Schuknecht, 1964; Cummings, 1968).

Anti-convulsant Drugs. In recent years it has been recognized that overdosage with certain anti-convulsant drugs, especially phenytoin, may be associated with disorders of balance (Nozue *et al.*, 1973). These may be acute, when they resemble in every respect a "posterior fossa syndrome", the clinical features of which disappear rapidly as soon as the drug is withdrawn; or, much more commonly, chronic, when imbalance continues in the patient, often a young epileptic who has received repeated doses of anti-convulsants over a long period of time (Ajodhia and Dix, 1974). Detailed studies of the spontaneous, so-called "Rebound Nystagmus" which may occur in such cases have shown that it is associated with chronic cerebellar degeneration (Hood *et al.*, 1973), with loss of the Purkinje cells of the cerebellar cortex (Hoffman, 1958). Other drugs

used in the treatment of epilepsy, such as ethosuximide (Zarontin), may have similar vestibulotoxic effects; and chronic overdosage with phenobarbital may lead to imbalance and vertigo due to its depressant effects upon the vestibular connections within the brain-stem.

Topical Aural Preparations. There is growing concern about the potential ototoxicity of a variety of preparations applied topically to the ears, whether they be installed as drops or put in the middle ear during the course of stapedectomy, tympanoplasty or mastoidectomy. These include the ototoxic antibiotics.

Much has been written about the potentially harmful effects of absorbable gelatine sponge (Gelfoam, Sterispon) upon the internal ear, notably by Bellucci and Wolff (1960), but it is less well known that formaldehyde is used, in addition to gelatin, in the preparation of these products. In a retrospective study of 265 stapedectomies reported by Shenoi (1973), a severe cochlear hearing loss occurred in no less than 20 ears. The incidence of such hearing loss in those cases in which Sterispon was used as an oval window seal was twice as high as in those in which fat had been used.

Bicknell (1971) has recorded an incidence of sensorineural hearing loss in more than 14 per cent of 97 patients who had had simple myringoplasties; and the one factor that was common to all these cases was that the pre-operative sterilization of the ear had been done with chlorhexidine (Hibitane) in spirit.

Ototoxic Synergism. The combination of several ototoxic agents administered either serially or together, may cause potentiating damage to the cochlea.

Nilges and Northern (1971) have described a case of kanamycin ototoxicity in which synergism occurred in a cochlea which had been "primed" by anti-malarial drugs taken 3 weeks earlier. Previous treatment with one ototoxic antibiotic may also render the spiral organ more susceptible to subsequent treatment with another (Frost *et al.*, 1960).

Furthermore, there is experimental evidence that exposure to noise may predispose the inner ear more readily to antibiotic insult, and that acoustic and cochleotoxic damage may be additive (Darrouzet and de Lima Sobrinho, 1962).

ROUTES OF ACCESS TO THE INTERNAL EAR

When they are given systemically, or applied topically to areas other than the ears themselves, the ototoxic antibiotics presumably are carried to the labyrinthine fluids via the blood stream. This toxic effect is greatly enhanced if these drugs are given by the intrathecal route (Ranta, 1958), when they probably gain access to the internal ear by way of the cerebrospinal fluid and perilymph. Other possibilities include secretion into the perilymph from the vessels of the spiral ligament, or directly into the endolymph from the stria vascularis (Hawkins *et al.*, 1967). Yet another possible route is from the vas spirale of the cochlea into the cortilymph.

When the streptomyces antibiotics are applied topically to the middle ear (Spoendlin, 1966; Kohonen and Tarkkanen, 1969), they may reach the perilymph by permeating either the secondary tympanic (round window) membrane or the annular ligament; and thence they may reach the spiral organ by penetrating into the endolymphatic space from the scala vestibuli, through the vestibular membrane.

The aminoglycosides are probably eliminated from the internal ear by resorption in the stria vascularis (Osteyn and Tyberghein, 1968) and since this structure may itself be damaged by their toxic products, thus slowing still further the rate of resorption and hence the process of elimination, so these drugs are eliminated more slowly from the labyrinthine fluids than from the blood. Hence their level remains higher for a longer time in the internal ear, where the hair (sensory) cells are exposed to their noxious influence, than in the blood stream (Stupp and Rauch, 1965; Voldrich, 1965).

HISTOPATHOLOGY OF OTOTOXICITY

Aminoglycoside Antibiotics. Since Berg (1949) and Caussé (1949) first observed degenerative changes in the vestibular sensory epithelia and the spiral organ in animals treated with streptomycin, it has been widely supposed that the primary site of the toxic effects of the aminoglycoside antibiotics was in the sensory epithelia of the internal ear (Lindeman, 1969). For many years, the surface preparation technique of Engström (1951), a highly sophisticated development of that of Retzius (1881, 1884), has formed the basis of many studies on the histopathological changes in the sensory epithelia of animals treated with the aminoglycoside antibiotics. This is a quick and relatively simple method which is particularly well suited to the study of hair cell damage. The guinea pig is ideal for this purpose, because the hair cells of this animal form a remarkably constant pattern in such preparations (Fig. 2a).

COCHLEOTOXICITY

By focusing on to the hairs with the phase-contrast microscope, those on the outer hair cells of the normal cochlea are seen to be arranged in the form of the letter W. Amongst the earliest changes to be seen in guinea pigs treated with kanamycin (Hawkins and Engström, 1964) is a distortion of this normal W-pattern of the stereocilia on the outer hair cells. With increasing damage, the hairs of some cells are entirely lost and the whole cell may disappear, leaving a collapsed figure, or "phalangeal scar" (Fig. 2b).

After injecting guinea pigs with kanamycin, neomycin and framycetin, Engström and Kohonen (1965) found that degenerative changes in the sensory cells of the spiral organ followed the same general pattern with each of the three antibiotics, and that these changes advanced both with increasing dosage and with longer survival time.

Gonzalez et al. (1972) investigated the ototoxic effect of kanamycin in guinea pigs and, although every animal received the same amount of antibiotic, the time of sacrifice was varied between 1 and 12 weeks after treatment had been stopped. All animals which were sacrificed later than 8 weeks after cessation of treatment showed progressive damage to the hair cells and the cochlear nerve.

The outer hair cells of the basal turn of the cochlea are affected first, and the damage later progresses towards the apex. Degeneration of the inner hair cells, which are affected much later than the outer hair cells, also follows a clear-cut pattern, beginning at the apex and progressing towards the base. The extent of damage to the hair cells can be graphically recorded in the cochlear cytogram, or "cochleogram" (Fig. 3).

Friedmann et al. (1966) produced the first electron-microscopic study of changes produced in the cochlea by neomycin, and they confirmed that damage to the spiral organ in guinea pigs was most pronounced in the basal coil. Marked degeneration of the mitochondria was demonstrated in both outer and inner hair cells.

It is possible that those sensory cells which have the greatest metabolic activity are the first to be affected by the ototoxic antibiotics; and there is a considerable body of evidence that these are, in fact, the outer hair cells of the basal areas. For example, innervation of the outer hair cells in the basal coil of the cochlea is denser than in the apical coil (Smith, 1961; Engström and Kohonen, 1965) and this greater density of cells in the basal coil invites the supposition that the basal cells have a higher metabolic activity than those at the apex. Furthermore, oxygen consumption of the stria vascularis is higher in the basal than in the apical areas and Osteyn and Tyberghein (1968) found that the stria was always affected when the outer hair cells were damaged and the impairment in these two structures developed in parallel from base to apex.

The results of numerous animal experiments have been amply confirmed by several authors, in microscopic examinations of human temporal bones and with kanamycin, the findings in human ears have been identical with those of experimentally-induced lesions in animals (Benitez et al., 1962; Jørgensen and Schmidt, 1962; Matz et al., 1965).

The loss of hair cells after administration of ototoxic antibiotics first affects those which are provided with large granulated (Type 2) nerve-endings and, after the sensory cells have disappeared, the whole of the spiral organ may slowly collapse and the corresponding nerve fibres and ganglion cells degenerate.

The pattern of neural damage follows very closely upon that in the sensory cells and it is probably secondary to cochlear changes.

Although the hair cells and first-order neurones of the cochlear nerve have been generally regarded as the primary sites of ototoxic damage in the internal ear, Johnsson and Hawkins (1972) have emphasized that several forms of sensorineural deafness are associated with vascular changes in the cochlea and that these changes may often precede and may indeed be an important cause of, degenerative changes in the hair cells.

Experimental animals (cats and guinea pigs) were given large doses of neomycin and gentamicin, in order to study their effects upon the spiral organ and the stria vascularis. At autopsy all showed severe damage to the hair cells of the spiral organ and with the single exception of one cat which was sacrificed immediately after treatment, they all showed severe strial atrophy (Fig. 4). This was most severe in the basal turn, where only empty remnants of vessels and inter-vascular strands remained.

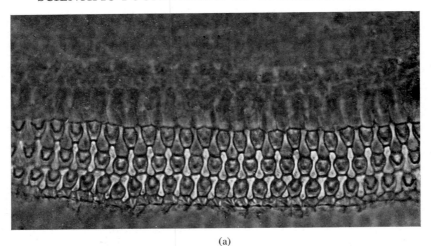

(a)

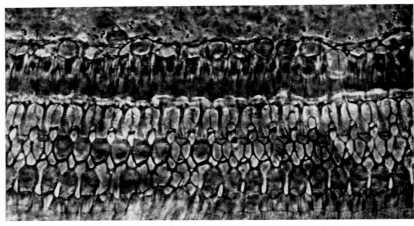

(b)

FIG. 2. Surface preparations of the spiral organ of Corti (guinea pigs). Phase-contrast photomicrographs. (a) Normal spiral organ, showing the regular pattern of the three rows of outer hair cells, each sensory cell being separated from its neighbours by narrow "phalangeal" cells. (b) Ototoxic damage to the spiral organ showing "phalangeal scars" in place of the degenerated cells. (By courtesy of Professor H. Engström.)

KANAMYCIN 400 MG/KG BODY WEIGHT FOR 8 DAYS (+ 14). 2 1/2 COILS F. BASE

●○○○●●○●●○○●●○●●○○●●○●●●○
●●●●●●●●●●●●●●●●●●●●●●●●●●
○○●○○●●○○●●○●●○○●●○○○○○○●●○●○
○●○○○○○○○●○○○●○○○○○○●○●●●●○

FIG. 3. "Cochleogram" of kanamycin-induced ototoxicity. All the cells in the first row of outer hair cells have degenerated. ○ = normal cells; ● = degenerated cells. (By courtesy of Professor H. Engström.)

Hawkins *et al.* (1972) have also studied other changes in the cochlear microvasculature of guinea pigs treated with gentamicin and they demonstrated destruction of the pericapillary spaces in the spiral ligament and external sulcus.

There are several named capillary networks in this region: *the supra-strial capillaries*, which are located in a specialized area of the spiral ligament, above the line of attachment of the vestibular membrane; the *ad-strial capillaries*, which are closely applied to the basal surface of the stria vascularis; the *post-strial capillaries*, which supply the tissues of the spiral ligament, and the *external sulcus capillaries*, which are continuous with the ad-strial and perhaps also with the post-strial vessels.

All these capillary networks are surrounded by a specialized pericapillary tissue (Fig. 5) and the presence of a pericapillary space appears to be characteristic of vessels which are actively engaged in filtration or reabsorption of fluid. This is readily destroyed by gentamicin and other aminohexose antibiotics.

VESTIBULOTOXICITY

In the earliest studies on the ototoxic side-effects of streptomycin and other related antibiotics, "the initial focus of attention was on the vestibular system" (Engström *et al.*, 1966).

Wersäll and Hawkins (1962), after parenteral injections

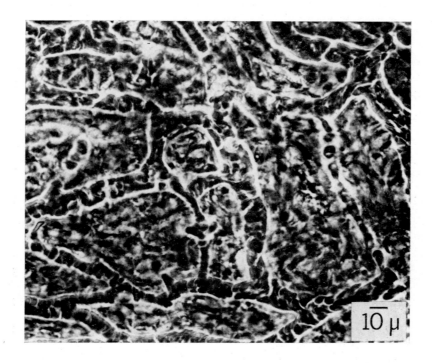

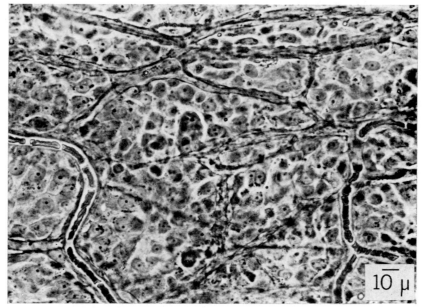

FIG. 4. Surface preparations of the stria vascularis. Phase-contrast photomicrographs. *Upper*: Normal stria vascularis from a 15-day-old beagle. *Lower*: Atrophic stria vascularis from a neomycin-treated cat, showing empty "ghosts" of capillaries and inter-vascular strands. (By courtesy of Professors L.-G. Johnsson and J. E. Hawkins, Jr. and *The Laryngoscope*.)

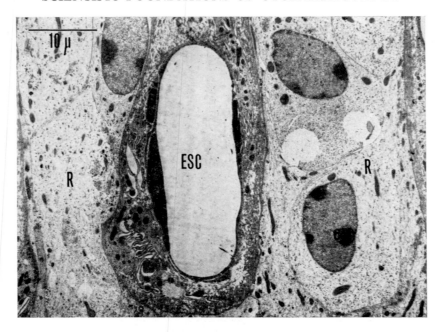

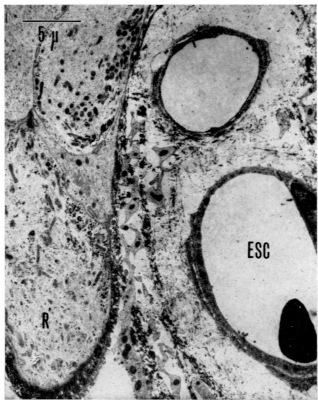

FIG. 5. Sections of external sulcus capillaries of the cochlea (guinea pig). Transmission electron microscopy. *Upper*: Part of a normal alternating pattern of root cells and external sulcus capillaries surrounded by pericapillary tissue (lower basal turn). *Lower*: Destruction of the pericapillary tissue surrounding an external sulcus capillary, in an animal treated with gentamicin (lower basal turn). R = roof cell; ESC = external sulcus capillary. (By courtesy of Professor J. E. Hawkins, Jr. and *The Laryngoscope*.)

of streptomycin in the cat, observed changes in the mitochondria, with swelling and vacuolization of the cytoplasm in the sensory cells, before there was any visible pycnosis of the nuclei and Duvall and Wersäll (1964), who studied the effect of parenteral injections of streptomycin in the guinea pig, postulated that the drug affected primarily the plasma membrane of the cells and the mitochondria.

In contrast with these earlier reports Spoendlin (1966) observed, by electron-microscopy, an agglomeration of chromatin in the nuclei of the more vulnerable Type I cells,

Damage to the stria vascularis has been demonstrated in guinea pigs by Quick and Duvall (1970) and it has been confirmed by Johnsson and Hawkins (1972) in cats. These latter authors have seen copious diureses in 5 cats which were given large doses of etacrynic acid and in all of them obvious strial lesions were seen *post-mortem*. These ranged from mild to severe, the extent of damage being apparently related to the total dosage of the drug. Although atrophic strial changes were found in the apical turn of the cochlea, they were most marked in the basal turn. There was an

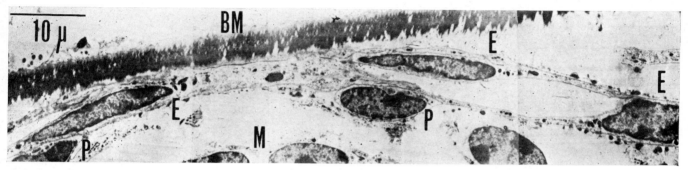

FIG. 6. Section of an external spiral vessel (guinea pig). Transmission electron microscopy. The section shows the constriction of an external spiral vessel produced by a single large dose of quinine hydrochloride (third turn). BM = basilar membrane; E = endothelial cells; P = pericytes; M = mesothelial cells. (By courtesy of Professor J. E. Hawkins, Jr. and *The Laryngoscope*.)

with later a loss of ribosomes and endoplasmic reticulum, as early as 12 h after intratympanic instillation of streptomycin in cats. The mitochondria and the membranes of nuclei and cells remained normal for some time thereafter.

Lindeman (1969a and b) investigated, in surface preparations, the effects of parenteral kanamycin and intratympanic streptomycin upon the vestibular sensory epithelia of guinea pigs. The degenerative changes which he observed followed a definite pattern which was the same in both groups of animals. These were more noticeable in the sensory epithelia of the ampullary cristae than in the macula utriculi and more in the latter situation than in the macula sacculi. They involved primarily the central areas of the cristae and the striolae of the maculae. Clear topographical differences in vulnerability could be seen within any sensory region and these probably represent differences in function.

These findings have been confirmed by Igarashi (1972), in his studies on the vestibulotoxicity of streptomycin, viomycin and gentamicin and by Watanuki *et al.* (1972) in their light-microscopic studies of surface preparations which show the toxic effects upon the peripheral vestibular sensory organs of intraperitoneal gentamicin.

In early studies with the scanning electron microscope, Wersäll *et al.* (1972) have demonstrated fusion of the stereocilia in the vestibular epithelia following the administration of gentamicin.

Diuretics. Matz, Beal and Krames (1969) reported severe destruction of the outer cells of the spiral organ, in a patient who had received only 50 mg of etacrynic acid and had died 10 days later. The inner hair cells were normal.

However, in animal experiments, hair cell damage has been conspicuous by its almost total absence and the main histopathological change has been one of strial atrophy.

unusual and apparently characteristic appearance in the stria (Fig. 6), with swollen osmiophilic cells clumped around the capillaries; further away from the capillaries there were areas of cellular atrophy which left numerous light and bare zones between the capillary loops. All these cats had numerous small vacuoles in the spiral ligament, and 3 of the 5 had large vesicles between the stria and spiral ligament, throughout the cochlea. Only the 2 cats which had the largest dosage showed any loss of outer hair cells, in the basal turn, the remainder having a normal population of sensory cells.

Anti-protozoal Agents. Two mechanisms have been postulated to account for capillary contractility in general; these are contraction of the pericytes (Rouget cells) and swelling of the endothelial cells. Both of these seem to be involved in vasoconstriction of the outer and inner spiral vessels in response to quinine; both of them appear to participate in bringing about a decrease in capillary diameter (Fig. 7) in the constricted outer spiral vessel of a guinea pig treated with a large single dose of quinine hydrochloride (Hawkins *et al.*, 1972).

A sort of precapillary sphincter seems to be present at the T-junctions of the outer spiral vessels and to become constricted in response to quinine.

In two cases of congenital hearing loss reported by McKinna (1966), in infants whose mothers had taken high pre-natal doses of quinine, degenerative changes were found in the spiral ganglion cells.

Salicylates. Vasoconstriction of the capillaries of the cochlear microvasculature may also be induced by salicylates (Hawkins, 1967).

Anti-heparinizing Agents. The histopathological changes found in the temporal bones of one patient who had been treated with hexadimethrine bromide (Polybrene) included:

gross degeneration of the spiral organ (Fig. 7a); degeneration of the stria vascularis (Fig. 7b); slight degeneration
of the spiral ganglion; thickening of the vestibular membrane; rupture and disorganization of the endolymphatic
sac and a fibrin-free exudate in the subepithelial connective
tissues of the otolithic maculae and the cupulae (Ransome
et al., 1966).

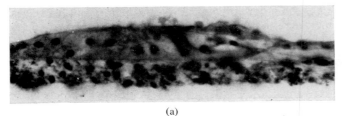

(a)

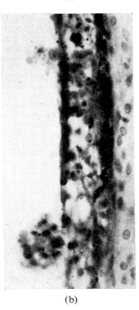

(b)

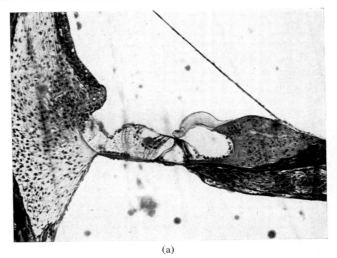

(a)

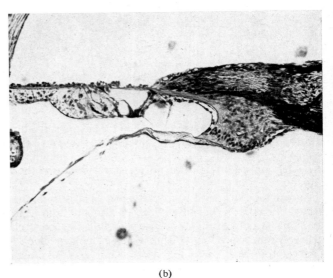

(b)

FIG. 7. Hexadimethrine toxicity (human). Section of cochlea. Light
microscopy. (a) Gross degeneration of the spiral organ. The shadowy
outline of the inner rod of Corti can be distinguished but otherwise no
other cellular elements are distinguishable, apart from a few scattered
nuclei (anterior middle half-turn). (b) Early degeneration of the stria
vascularis. There is breaking down of the superficial cell layer and
extrusion of degenerate elements of the middle cell layer (posterior
middle half-turn). (By courtesy of Miss Joselen Ransome, F.R.C.S.
and the *Journal of Laryngology and Otology*.)

FIG. 8. Sections of the spiral organ of the cat. Light microscopy.
(a) Normal spiral organ (middle coil). (b) Degeneration of the hair
cells, limbus cells and spiral ganglion cells, with collapse of the
vestibular membrane, in an animal in which 100 microgrammes of
formaldehyde had been put into the open fenestra vestibuli (middle
coil). (By courtesy of P. M. Shenoi, F.R.C.S.)

Cytotoxic Agents. Pathological changes have been
demonstrated in the spiral organs of patients treated with
regional perfusions of nitrogen mustard (Schuknecht, 1964;
Cummings, 1968).

Topical Aural Preparations. Bellucci and Wolff (1960)
suggested that damage caused to the membranous labyrinth
by absorbable gelatin sponge might be due to the release of
a chemical toxin. Shenoi (1973) has shown that absorbable
gelatin sponge BP (Sterispon) contains 0·367 per cent
formaldehyde and, in a series of experiments in cats, he has
demonstrated extensive degenerative changes in the cochlea,
after putting various known quantities of formaldehyde
into the open oval windows (Figs. 8a and b). These changes
did not occur when smaller quantities of formaldehyde

were used, nor when pure gelatin was placed in the oval
window.

OTOTOXIC ANTIBIOTIC CONCENTRATIONS
IN THE LABYRINTHINE FLUIDS

Stupp *et al.* (1967) have shown that the specific ototoxic
effects of the aminoglycoside antibiotics are related to the
high concentration and prolonged presence of these substances in the endolymph and perilymph of the internal ear.
In a series of experiments with 210 guinea pigs, varying
doses of kanamycin were given by subcutaneous injection
and subsequent estimations were made of the kanamycin
levels in the blood serum, heart muscle and perilymph.

After a single injection of 25 mg kanamycin sulphate
per kilogram body weight, the following levels of kanamycin

were obtained: in blood serum, 36 mg.l^{-1}; in heart muscle, less than 1 mg.kg^{-1}; in perilymph, 2·5 mg.l^{-1}. However, the kanamycin was almost totally eliminated from the blood serum 5 h later, whereas its concentration in the labyrinthine fluids showed only a slight tendency to decrease, exceeding the serum level tenfold. When the dosage of kanamycin was doubled (to a single injection of 50 mg.kg^{-1}), concentrations of the drug in blood serum and heart muscle were raised, but the kanamycin content of the perilymph rose much more, increasing by almost ten times. Rather surprisingly, when the dosage was increased still further (to a single injection of 250 mg.kg^{-1}) the kanamycin content of the labyrinthine fluids did not continue to rise, despite a higher concentration in the serum and a corresponding rise in tissue level (Fig. 9a). Nevertheless, after 5 h the kanamycin concentration in the perilymph began to exceed that in the serum and so it remained until the conclusion of the experiment 20 h later.

During long-term treatment with daily injections, there is a continuous accumulation of toxic substances in the internal ear (Fig. 9b). After a single injection (lower curve), the kanamycin level in the perilymph is the same as that in Fig. 9a. After 10 days of treatment (middle curve), there is a relatively slight but nevertheless significant rise in the kanamycin content of the labyrinthine fluids and after 20 days (upper curve), there is an even more pronounced increase.

It is important to realize that such long-term treatment has no influence on the kanamycin concentration either in the serum or in other tissues; therefore, one cannot blame a diminished excretory renal function for the high content of kanamycin in the internal ear.

Why, then, does the accumulation of toxic antibiotics take place only in the internal ear?

Kanamycin is eliminated only very slowly from the internal ear and even after 25 h this is not complete. When another injection is given on the following day, there is still about 10 per cent of the drug in the labyrinthine fluids from the previous day; therefore, this second injection must lead necessarily to an increase in the level of antibiotic in the internal ear. Hence its accumulation in the internal ear could possibly be explained by a constantly increasing residue of the drug in the perilymph and endolymph. Stupp *et al.* (1967) discovered that this residue in the internal ear fluids does not increase in relation to the rise in *concentration* in the internal ear. In fact, the higher its concentration, the quicker is kanamycin eliminated from the internal ear. This would prevent a progressive retention of toxic substances in the lymphatic fluids; yet the elimination of the streptomyces antibiotics from the internal ear is extraordinarily slow. There must therefore be some other explanation for their steady accumulation during long-term treatment.

These authors suggest that, during the initial steep ascent of concentration in the internal ear, when a toxic level is reached, an impairment of the cellular membranes in the internal ear and especially of their inter-cellular gaps, may take place. They postulate that enlargement of the cells and swelling of the nuclei, which have been described as the first morphological manifestations of intoxication (Müse-

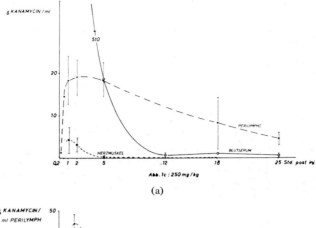

(a)

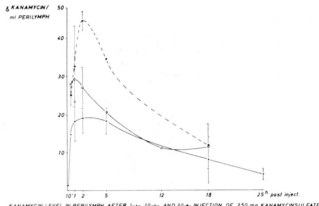

KANAMYCIN LEVEL IN PERILYMPH AFTER 1-·-, 10-○-, AND 20-•- INJECTION OF 250 mg KANAMYCINSULFATE /kg

(b)

FIG. 9. Kanamycin concentrations in the perilymph (guinea pig). (a) Variations in kanamycin concentrations in the perilymph, blood serum and heart muscle, from 0·2 and 25 h after injection, in a dosage of 250 mg per kilogram body weight. (b) Kanamycin levels in the perilymph after 1 injection (lower curve), 10 injections (middle curve) and 20 injections (upper curve), from 0·2–25 h later, during long-term treatment with daily injections of 250 mg per kilogram body weight. (By courtesy of Professor H. F. Stupp.)

beck, 1964; Kohonen, 1965), may lead to compression and occlusion of the inter-cellular gaps; that elimination of the toxic streptomyces substances, which depends entirely upon the existence of the extracellular spaces, may be blocked thereby. Kanamycin, by virtue of its toxic damage to these membranes, would block its own exit from the internal ear and, consequently, there would be a progressive accumulation of the antibiotic in the internal ear fluids. Hence, accumulation of the ototoxic antibiotics and also their delayed elimination may be accounted for by impaired diffusion.

In a more recent study, Stupp (1972) has evaluated both the antibiotic levels in the internal ear fluids and the extent of damage to the sensory hair cells caused by the aminoglycosides. He found that, the more toxic the substance, the higher was its concentration in the internal ear (Fig. 10), whether it was applied topically or given systemically by intramuscular injection.

On the other hand, when other antibiotics were applied, whether topically or systemically, basic differences became apparent. Thus, when applied intramuscularly the neurotoxic polymyxins and tetracyclines caused no damage,

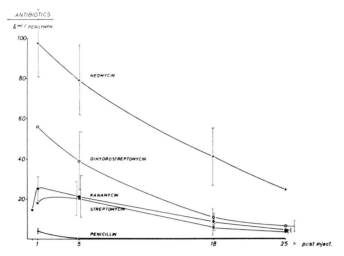

FIG. 10. Relationship of the ototoxicity of several antibiotics to their concentration in the perilymph, from 0·2 to 25 h after injection. (By courtesy of Professor H. F. Stupp.)

because of their inability to penetrate the internal ear through the blood-lymph barrier. However, when applied topically the polymyxins and to a lesser extent the tetracyclines also, caused damage to the sensory cells, as did chloramphenicol and (surprisingly) erythromycin. Only penicillin, independently of its mode of application, failed to produce any harmful effects upon the internal ear.

METABOLIC STUDIES IN OTOTOXICITY

Every living cell is a system of chemical reactions, most of which are controlled by enzymes. These intracellular enzymes (the catalysts of living cells) direct the processes of cellular metabolism. All metabolic processes utilize energy in the form of a common basic unit, which has its being in a substance called adenosine triphosphate (ATP).

Enzymes show a remarkable degree of specificity for the substance upon which they act and they are named after the reactions which they catalyze, by adding the suffix "ase" to the name of the substance upon which the enzyme acts; thus, for example, the enzyme adenosine triphosphatase (ATP ase) acts upon ATP.

Even after a drug has gained access to the labyrinthine fluids which bathe the sensory cells, there is still a cell membrane to cross before it can reach the cytoplasm, and substances acting upon nuclear material must also cross the nuclear membrane. Some pass also into such "organelles" as the ribosomes and mitochondria.

Enzyme action is responsible for maintaining the active transport of ions across cellular membranes, and ATPase, which is involved in sodium and potassium transport, has been found in the stria vascularis and spiral ligament of the guinea pig's ear (Iinuma, 1967). The ototoxic antibiotics can interfere with intracellular metabolic processes, and metabolic disturbances and specific inhibitors of the ATPase enzyme system will change the ionic content of the endolymph (Mendelsohn and Konishi, 1969; Konishi and Mendelsohn, 1970), leading to a fall in the potassium (normally high in the endolymph) and a rise in the sodium

ions. Kanamycin can damage the stria vascularis and can thus also lead to loss of membrane ATPase in the stria and the spiral ligament (Matz et al., 1965); Koide et al., 1966; Osteyn and Tyberghein, 1968).

Mendelsohn and Katzenberg (1972) have shown, in guinea pigs, that intraperitoneal injection of high doses of kanamycin sulphate can produce highly significant changes in the cation content of the endolymph, with a considerable fall in the potassium and a huge rise in the sodium content. They also found a fall in the endolymphatic (or endocochlear) potential (EP), corresponding to a reduction of the endolymphatic potassium level.

ELECTRICAL POTENTIAL CHANGES IN OTOTOXICITY

Wilson and Juhn (1970) and Cohn et al. (1971) have shown that etacrynic acid causes a decrease in potassium and an increase in sodium, concentration in the endolymph; there is also a marked increase in potassium in the perilymph. This would suggest that etacrynic acid inhibits active ion transport, with reversal of the potassium and sodium concentrations in the scala media and a consequent drop in the endocochlear potential (EP).

Mathog et al. (1970) have described depression of the cochlear microphonics (CM) and whole-nerve action potentials (AP), with almost complete recovery in 1 h.

More recently Prazma et al. (1972) have also studied the effects of etacrynic acid upon these various electrical indices of cochlear function (EP, CM and AP), in 27 guinea pigs. During their experiments, all these parameters were continuously recorded in response to auditory stimuli of 8000 Hz tone-bursts at 75 dB, at intervals of 20 ms. The drug produced reductions in EP, CM and AP, the strongest effect being observed in the cells, with a drop in CM which remained after 4 h, with no tendency to recover.

Bosher et al. (1973) found in rats that the normal endocochlear potential was rapidly replaced by a negative anoxic type of potential after the intravenous injection of etacrynic acid; recovery proceeded rapidly at first but became very much slower 30 min after the injection. The chemical composition of the endolymph remained unaltered until 35 min, at which time there occurred a progressive increase in sodium and a progressive decrease in potassium concentration, followed at 1 h by a gradual return towards normal. These authors believe that, initially, the drug probably causes a transient inhibition of the strial enzymes, followed by a more prolonged phase of altered membrane permeability, the latter giving rise to an accumulation of fluid in the intercellular spaces of the stria vascularis.

By recording averaged evoked responses (AER) from dural electrodes in 7 cats, Mathog and Matz (1972) were able to observe the changes produced immediately and after varying periods of time, by etacrynic acid. There was often a depression in cortical potential and an elevation of the auditory threshold, the onset and duration of these changes being apparently related to dosage. Similar effects were produced by furosemide. Even with dosages greatly in excess of those recommended for human patients, the changes in AER were transient and always reversible. In thus showing only transient effects upon the AER, it is probable that the permanent hearing loss recorded by some authors in patients with uraemia was due to the potentiating action of etacrynic acid upon a defective renal status.

OTOTOXICITY AND RENAL STATUS

There can be no reasonable doubt that the risk of ototoxicity is greatly enhanced by defective renal function.

Since the basic streptomyces antibiotics are excreted in the urine, it is to be expected that impairment of renal function may allow excessively high plasma levels to develop. Waisbren and Spink (1950), Goldner (1958), Körtge-Stöppler and Mittag (1958), Greenwood (1959), Ballantyne (1970) and Miszke (1972) have all emphasized that patients with renal dysfunction are particularly sensitive to the toxic effects of the aminoglycosides.

Many of the ototoxic antibiotics are themselves nephrotoxic, and the ability or inability of the kidneys to eliminate these drugs may determine, at least to some extent, the susceptibility of the individual to ototoxic damage.

The diuretics etacrynic acid and furosemide, both of which are in common use in cases of congestive heart failure, have been known to cause a hearing loss only in patients with renal failure. Hence other factors associated with renal failure, such as altered electrolyte balance, may also predispose to ototoxicity.

In this context there is particular interest in the cases of ototoxic damage caused by the anti-heparinizing agent, hexadimethrine (Ransome et al., 1966). There are certain resemblances between the structure of the stria vascularis and the glomerular tufts in the kidneys; and hexadimethrine is known to be nephrotoxic in high doses. Haller et al. (1962) have described a "constriction of the capillaries within the glomerular tufts", and it is possible that the drug may act in a similar way upon the microvasculature of the cochlea; and the anoxic degeneration of the stria vascularis so produced may lead to derangement of the electrolyte balance of the labyrinthine fluids.

The relationship of ototoxicity to renal status would suggest that damage to the stria vascularis probably plays a role of vital importance, in the ability of certain drugs to produce toxic effects upon the sensory cells of the internal ear.

MECHANISMS OF OTOTOXICITY

The precise mechanism by which some drugs exert their toxic effects upon the internal ear is not certain.

It has long been supposed that the ototoxic effect of the basic streptomyces antibiotics was due primarily to a direct assault of the toxic substances upon the sensory cells of the cochlear and vestibular neuroepithelia. Stupp et al. (1966) have demonstrated a gradual build-up of ototoxic antibiotic concentrations in the labyrinthine fluids, with a much slower clearance from them, measurable concentrations persisting for some time after the antibiotic has disappeared from the plasma.

Hawkins (1973) has suggested that, just as there is a highly effective blood-brain barrier against the aminoglycosides, so there may be a similar but less effective blood-ear, or haemato-labyrinthine, barrier which may be capable of impeding the entrance of undesirable blood-borne substances into the cochlear fluids. It must also play an essential part, he believes, in upholding the "micro-homeostasis" (environmental equilibrium) of the internal ear, which is expressed in the approximate constancy of the widely different concentrations of sodium and potassium ions in endolymph and perilymph.

This haemato-labyrinthine barrier must presumably depend upon the integrity of spiral ligament and stria vascularis, and their microvasculature, which is primarily responsible for the elaboration of the labyrinthine fluids. Evidence is presented by Hawkins (1973) that the basic streptomyces antibiotics can damage these "secretory" tissues, as well as those of the spiral prominence and outer sulcus which are thought to be "reabsorptive" in function.

In earlier work, Hawkins et al. (1950) found that streptomycin persisted in high concentrations in the kidney and continued to appear in the urine, after it had been eliminated from the blood serum. In the kidney, the antibiotic was bound to proteins of the renal tissues. The primary ototoxic action of the aminoglycosides may be compared with its nephrotoxic action, which affects membrane function and protein synthesis in tissues actively engaged in transporting water and ions on a considerable scale. Hence, injury to the hair cells is regarded as secondary to a disruption of the micro-homeostatic mechanisms which maintain the appropriate concentrations of sodium and potassium ions in endolymph and perilymph.

The haemato-labyrinthine barrier postulated by Hawkins (1973) may help to explain the relative slowness of the ototoxic processes when these drugs reach the internal ear in the blood stream. The process can be greatly accelerated by placing the ototoxic agent in the middle ear (Spoendlin, 1966; Wersäll et al., 1969), so that it may enter the cochlea via the secondary tympanic (round window) membrane, thus by-passing the blood-ear barrier and exerting a direct "explosive" toxic action upon the hair cells themselves.

The exact nature of the metabolic processes and enzyme systems which are affected by the ototoxic antibiotics is not yet known, but there is reason to believe that they may inhibit protein synthesis. For example, Spoendlin (1966), in electron-microscopic studies in cats, showed that whereas the nerve endings (which do not synthesize protein to any significant extent) were not damaged, the structures which were affected within the damaged cells were the nuclei and the ribosomes, both of which do synthesize protein.

Hence, somewhat paradoxically, the streptomyces antibiotics may act upon the sensory cells of the internal ear in much the the same way as they act upon invading bacteria.

PREVENTION OF OTOTOXICITY

Ototoxic drugs in general, and the aminoglycoside antibiotics in particular, should be avoided altogether unless they are essential to the survival or future well-being of the patient, especially in cases of renal or hepatic failure, in the very young and the very old, and in pregnant women. They should be used with great caution in those previously treated with potentially ototoxic agents, in those previously exposed to excessive noise, and in those with a known familial incidence of ototoxicity (Ballantyne, 1973).

When they *must* be used, the dosage and duration of their administration should be kept to the minimum consistent with the clinical control of the condition for which they have been prescribed; and even in the topical application of these drugs, one should limit the dosage to that which would be regarded as safe for systemic use, particularly in patients with open tympanic perforations and in those subjected to tympano-mastoid surgery, especially if the labyrinth has been exposed, either by surgery or by disease.

Many authors have recommended certain maximum doses of ototoxic drugs which should never be exceeded if their toxic effects are to be avoided (Erlanson and Lundgren, 1964; Sheffield and Turner, 1971; Ajodhia and Dix, 1974), and others have suggested the regular monitoring of serum levels (Geraci *et al.*, 1958; Meuwissen and Robinson, 1967; Line *et al.*, 1970); but it is only in recent times that serious attempts have been made to calculate a "safe" dosage of ototoxic drugs in accordance with the patient's renal status, although it has long been known that renal impairment exerts an adverse influence upon the development of ototoxicity (Waisbren and Spink, 1950; Goldner, 1958; Körtge-Stöppler and Mittag, 1958; Greenwood, 1959; Erlanson and Lundgren, 1964; Toma and Main, 1967).

The risk of administering kanamycin to patients with renal impairment cannot be over-estimated, and there is on record the case of one such patient who developed a sudden and severe deafness after receiving only 1 g of the drug (Toma and Main, 1967).

Mawer and his colleagues (Mawer *et al.*, 1972a) have developed a digital computer programme for calculating safe and effective doses of kanamycin for individual patients with renal insufficiency. The minimum input data consist of the patient's age, sex, body weight and serum creatinine, the estimated creatinine clearance providing the best basis for the estimation of renal clearance of the drug; the output includes a recommended regimen of kanamycin dosage, and the calculated serum concentrations of kanamycin expected to result.

In a later communication (Mawer *et al.*, 1972b), a simpler method has been described in which the computer programme described earlier has been used to construct a "nomogram" (Fig. 11a) from which a suitable dosage schedule may be obtained for any individual patient, provided that the serum creatinine concentration, the age, the body weight and sex are known. It is applicable to patients with all degrees of renal impairment, from normal function to severe oliguria and anuria; and it is used as follows:

(1) The serum creatinine concentrations appropriate to the patient's sex (Scale A) is joined to the patient's age (Scale B) with a straight line. Mark the point at which this straight line cuts line C.

(2) The mark thus produced on line C is joined with another straight line to the body weight (Scale D). Mark the points at which this line cuts the dosage lines L and M.

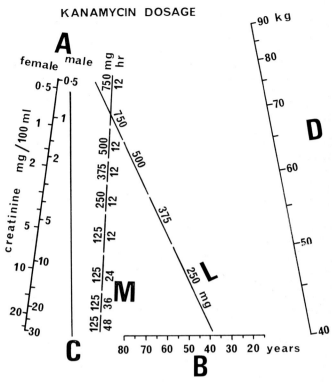

FIG. 11(a). Nomogram for kanamycin dosage. (After Mawer *et al.*, 1972b.)

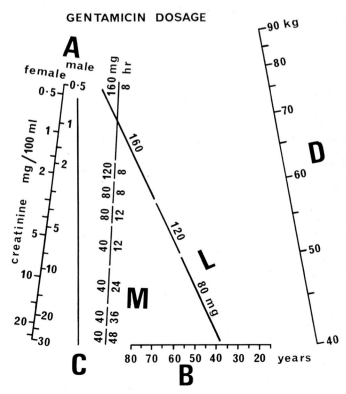

FIG. 11(b). Nomogram for gentamicin dosage. (After Ahmad *et al.*, 1974.)

(3) The loading dose is written against the marked part of Line L; the maintenance dose and the appropriate interval between doses are written against the marked part of line M.

(4) When the patient is severely oliguric or anuric, do not use the serum creatinine and age scales. To determine the dose schedule, join with a straight line the bottom of line C and the body weight on Scale D. Then proceed as in 2 and 3 above.

This nomogram is designed to produce serum concentrations of kanamycin within the accepted therapeutic range (10–30 mg.l^{-1}) 2 h after each dose; and a very similar one (Fig. 11b) has been developed for calculating gentamicin dosage (Mawer et al., 1974).

In patients with renal insufficiency it is still desirable to check the serum concentrations of these drugs by bio-assay once or twice during a course of treatment, and it is necessary to redetermine the dose schedule at intervals in patients in whom there are changing serum concentrations of creatinine due to alterations in renal function.

All patients receiving ototoxic drugs should be encouraged to report the onset of symptoms, however slight, of tinnitus, hearing loss, dizziness or ataxia; and regular audiometric checks should be made.

All new basic antibiotics should be submitted to laboratory tests of ototoxicity, preferably by the surface preparation technique of Engström (1951), which has the virtues of speed, simplicity and accuracy; and clinical trials should not be undertaken until it has become clear that such a new drug is at least as safe as streptomycin or gentamicin for the vestibular system, and significantly safer than kanamycin for the cochlea.

REFERENCES

Ajodhia, J. M. and Dix, M. R. (1975), Minerva otorinolaring, 25, 117.
Ballantyne, J. C. (1970), J. Laryng., 84, 967.
Ballantyne, J. C. (1973), Audiology, 12, 325.
Bellucci, R. J. and Wolff, Dorothy (1960), Ann. Otol., Rhinol., Lar., 69, 517.
Benitez, J. T., Schuknecht, H. F. and Brandenburg, J. H. (1962), Archaryng., 75, 192.
Berg, K. (1949), Ann. Otol., Rhinol., Lar., 58, 448.
Bicknell, P. G. (1971), J. Laryng., 85, 957.
Bosher, S. K., Smith, C. and Warren, R. L. (1973), Acta oto-laryng., 75, 184.
Campanelli, P. A., Grimes, E. and West, M. L. (1966), Med. Ann. Distr. Colombia., 35, 541.
Caussé, R. (1949), Ann. Oto-laryng. (Paris), 66, 518.
Cohn, E. S., Gordes, E. H. and Brusilow, S. W. (1971), Science, 171, 910.
Conrad, M. and Crosby, W. H. (1960), Blood, 16, 1089.
Cummings, C. W. (1968), Laryngoscope, 78, 530.
Darrouzet, J. and de Lima Sobrinho, E. (1962), Rev. Lar. Otol. Rhinol., 83, 781.
Duvall, A. J. and Wersäll, J. (1964), Acta oto-laryng., 57, 581.
Engström, H. (1951), Acta oto-laryng., 40, 5.
Engström, H., Ades, H. W. and Andersson, A. (1966), in Structural Pattern of the Organ of Corti, p. 120. Almqvist and Wiksell.
Engström, H. and Kohonen, A. (1965), Acta oto-laryng., 59, 171.
Erlanson, P. and Lundgren, A. (1964), Acta med. scand., 176, 147.
Fields, R. L. (1964), Arch. Otolaryng., 79, 67.

Friedmann, I., Dadswell, J. V. and Bird, E. S. (1966), J. Path. Bact., 92, 415.
Frost, J. O., Hawkins, J. E., Jr. and Daly, J. F. (1960), Amer. Rev. Resp. Dis., 82, 23.
Fuller, A. (1960), Lancet, i, 1026.
Geraci, J. E., Heilman, F. R., Nichols, D. R. and Wellman, P. M. (1958), Proc. Mayo Clin., 33, 172.
Ghose, R. R. and Joekes, A. M. (1964), Lancet, i, 1409.
Gignoux, M., Martin, H. and Cajgfinger, H. (1966), J. fr. Oto-rhinolar., 15, 631.
Goldner, A. I. (1958), N.Y. St. J. Med., 58, 2226.
Gonzalez, G., Miller, N. and Wasilewski, Valerie (1972), Ann. Otol., Rhinol., Lar., 81, 127.
Greenwood, G. J. (1959), Arch. Otolaryng., 69, 390.
Haller, J. A., Jr., Ransdell, H. J., Jr., Stowens, D. and Rubel, W. F. (1962), J. thorac. cardiovasc. Surg., 44, 486.
Hawkins, J. E., Jr. (1959), Ann. Otol., Rhinol., Lar., 68, 698.
Hawkins, J. E., Jr. (1967), in Deafness in Children, p. 156 (F. McConnell and P. H. Ward, (Eds.). Nashville: Vanderbilt University Press.
Hawkins, J. E., Jr. (1973), Audiology, 12, 383.
Hawkins, J. E., Jr., Beger, Valerie and Aran, J.-M. (1967), in Sensorineural Hearing Processes and Disorders, p. 411. (A. B. Graham, Ed.). Boston: Little, Brown and Co.
Hawkins, J. E., Jr., Boxer, G. E. and Jelinek, V. C. (1950), Proc. Soc. exp. Biol. N.Y.), 75, 759.
Hawkins, J. E., Jr. and Engström, H. (1964), Acta oto-laryng., suppl. 188.
Hawkins, J. E., Jr., Johnsson, L. S. and Preston, R. E. (1972), Laryngoscope, 82, 1091.
Hoffman, K. W. (1958), Neurology (Minneap.), 8, 210.
Hood, J. D., Kayan, A. and Leech, J. (1973), Brain, 96, 483.
Huizing, E. H. (1972), Audiology, 11, 30, suppl. Basel: Karger.
Igarashi, M. (1972), Audiology, 11, 16, suppl. Basel: Karger.
Iinuma, T. (1967), Laryngoscope, 77, 141.
Jarvis, J. F. (1966), J. Laryng., 80, 318.
Johnsson, L.-G. and Hawkins, J. E., Jr. (1972), Laryngoscope, 82, 1105.
Jørgensen, M. B. and Schmidt, M. R. (1962), Acta oto-laryng., 55, 537.
Kelly, D. R., Nilo, E. R. and Bergeren, R. B. (1969), New Engl. J. Med., 280, 1338.
Kern, G. (1962), Schweiz. med. Wschr., 92, 77.
Kohonen, A. (1965), Acta oto-laryng., suppl. 208.
Kohonen, A. and Tarkkanen, J. (1969), Acta oto-laryng., 68, 90.
Koide, Y., Stern, R., Röesler, H. K., and Daly, J. F. (1966), Laryngoscope, 76, 1769.
Konishi, T. and Mendelsohn, M. (1970), Acta oto-laryng., 69, 192.
Körtge-Stöppler, S. and Mittag, G. (1958), Münch. med. Wschr., 100, 1189.
Lawrence, W., Kuehn, P., Masle, E. T. and Miller, D. G. (1961), J. Surg. Res., 1, 142.
Leach, W. (1962), J. Laryng., 76, 774.
Lidén, G. (1953), Acta oto-laryng., 43, 551.
Lindeman, H. H. (1969a), J. Laryng., 83, 1.
Lindeman, H. H. (1969b), Acta oto-laryng., 67, 177.
Line, D. H., Poole, G. W. and Waterworth, P. M. (1970), Tubercle, 5, 76.
Lloyd-Mostyn, R. H. and Lord, I. J. (1971), Lancet, ii, 1156.
Lorian, V. (1962), Acta tuberc. scand., 42, 149.
McCabe, P. A. and Dey, F. L. (1965), Ann. Otol., Rhinol., Lar., 74, 312.
McKinna, A. J. (1966), Can. J. Ophthal., 1, 261.
Maher, J. F. and Schreiner, G. E. (1965), Ann. intern. Med., 62, 15.
Mathog, R. H. and Matz, G. J. (1972), Ann. Otol., Rhinol., Lar., 81, 871.
Mathog, R. H., Thomas, W. G. and Hudson, W. R. (1970), Arch. Otolaryng., 92, 7.
Matz, G. J., Beal, D. D. and Krames, L. (1969), Arch. Otolaryng., 90, 152.
Matz, G. J., Wallace, T. H. and Ward, P. H. (1965), Laryngoscope, 75, 1691.
Mawer, G. E., Ahmad, R., Dobbs, S. M., McGouch, J. G., Lucas, S. B. and Tooth, J. A. (1974), Brit. J. clin. Pharmacol., 1, 45.

Mawer, G. E., Knowles, B. R., Lucas, S. B., Stirland, R. M. and Tooth, J. A. (1972a), *Lancet*, **i**, 12.

Mawer, G. E., Lucas, S. B. and McGough, J. G. (1972b), *Lancet*, **ii**, 45.

Mendelsohn, M. and Katzenberg, I. (1972), *Laryngoscope*, **82**, 397.

Mendelsohn, M. and Konishi, T. (1969), *Ann. Otol. Rhinol. Lar.*, **78**, 65.

Meuwissen, H. J. and Robinson, G. C. (1967), *Clin. Pediat.*, **6**, 262.

Miszke, A. (1972), *Audiology*, **11**, 23, suppl. 1972. Basel: Karger.

Müsebeck, K. (1964), *Ann. Univ. Sarav.*, **11**, 159.

Nilges, T. C. and Northern, J. L. (1971), *Ann. Surg.*, **173**, 281.

Nozue, N., Mizuno, M. and Kaga, K. (1973), *Ann. Otol.*, **82**, 389.

Osteyn, F. and Tyberghein, J. (1968), *Acta oto-laryng.*, suppl. 234.

Perlman, V. L. (1966), *New Engl. J. Med.*, **274**, 164.

Pillay, V. K. G., Schwartz, F. D., Aimi, K. and Kark, R. M. (1969), *Lancet*, **i**, 77.

Podvinek. S. and Stefanovic P. (1966), *J. fr. Oto-rhino-lar.*, **15**, 61.

Pražić, M. and Salaj, R. (1972), *Audiology*, **11**, 25, suppl. 1972. Basel: Karger.

Prazma, J., Thomas, W. G., Fischer, D. and Preslar, M. J. (1972), *Arch. Otolaryng.*, **95**, 448.

Quick, C. A. and Duvall, A. J. (1970), *Laryngoscope*, **80**, 954.

Ransome, Joselen, Ballantyne, J. C., Shaldon, S., Bosher, S. K. and Hallpike, C. S. (1966), *J. Laryng.*, **80**, 651.

Ranta, L. T. (1958), *Acta oto-laryng.*, suppl. 136.

Retzius, G., in *Gehörorgane der Wirbeltieren*. Samson u. Wallin 1881 and 1884.

Robinson, G. C. and Cambon, K. G. (1964), *New Engl. J. Med.*, **271**, 949.

Schmidt, P. and Friedman, I. S. (1967), *N.Y. St. J. Med.*, **67**, 1438.

Schneider, W. J. and Becker, E. L. (1966), *Arch. intern. Med.*, **117**, 715.

Schuknecht, H. F. (1964), *Sth. med. J.*, **57**, 1161.

Sheffield, P. A. and Turner, J. S. (1971), *Sth. med. J. (Bgham. Ala.)*, **64**, 359.

Shenoi, P. (1973), *Proc. roy. Soc. Med.*, **66**, 193.

Silverstein, H., Bernstein, J. M. and Davies, D. Garfield (1967), *Ann. Otol., Rhinol., Lar.*, **76**, 118.

Smith, C. A. (1961), *Ann. Otol. Rhinol., Lar.*, **70**, 504.

Spoendlin, H. (1966), *Pract. oto-rhino-laryng. (Basel)*, **28**, 305.

Stupp, H. F. (1972), *Audiology*, **11**, 17, suppl. 1972. Basel: Karger.

Stupp, H. F. and Rauch, S. (1965), *Arch. Ohr., Nas.- u. KehlkHeilk.*, **185**, 500.

Stupp, H. F., Rauch, S., Sous, H. and Lagler, F. (1966), *Acta oto-laryng.*, **61**, 435.

Stupp, H. F., Rauch, S., Sous, H., Brun, J. P. and Lagler, F. (1967), *Arch. Otolryng.*, **86**, 515.

Šupáček, I. (1972), Audiology, **11**, 29, suppl. 1972. Basel: Karger.

Székely, T. and Draskovich, E. (1965), *Z. Laryng. Rhinol. Otol.*, **44**, 15.

Toma, G. A. and Main, B. J. (1967), *Postgrad. med. J.*, **43**, suppl. May, 46.

Venkateswaran, P. S. (1971), *Brit. med. J.*, **4**, 113.

Voldrich, L. (1965), *Acta oto-laryng.*, **60**, 243.

Waisbren, B. A. and Spink, W. W. (1950), *Ann. intern. Med.*, **33**, 1099.

Watanuki, K., Stupp, H. F. and Meyer zum Gottesberge, A. (1972), *Laryngoscope*, **82**, 363.

Wersäll, J., Björkroth, B., Flock, Å. and Lundquist, P.-G. (1971), *Arch. Klin. exp. Ohr.-, Nas.- KeklkHeilk.*, **200**, 1.

Wersäll, J. and Hawkins, J. E., Jr. (1962), *Acta oto-laryng.*, **54**, 1.

Wersäll, J., Lindquist, P.-G. and Björkroth, B. (1969), *J. infect. Dis.*, **119**, 410.

Wilson, K. S. and Juhn, S. K. (1970), *Pract. oto-rhino-laryng.*, **32**, 279.

Young, W. G., Jr., Lesage, A. M., Dillon, M. L., Lee, J. M., Collaway, H. A., Jr. and Reeves, J. W. (1961), *Ann. Surg.*, **154**, 372.

64. RHINOTOXIC DRUGS

L. H. CAPEL

The structure and function of the nose may be damaged by drugs applied topically for nasal disorder and by drugs taken by mouth for disorders elsewhere in the body. Because the dangers of prolonged topical administration are now widely recognized recent studies in man have been few, and such clinical studies as there are deal mainly with regimens prescribed by other clinicians or self administered.

Nasal symptoms due to drugs taken for disorders elsewhere in the body arise only from a few groups of drugs, and the symptoms may be missed because they are mild or misinterpreted: studies here too have been few. It is possible, however, to report what the author believes to be the consensus of critical opinion, noting that the toxic effects observed usually are what would be expected from the pharmacological properties of the drugs concerned.

It is probable that repeated topical administration of any drug eventually damages the nose, most important because most widely used are the topical vasoconstrictors. Other topically administered drugs include corticosteroids, antibacterial agents, antihistaminics, aromatic substances and astringents. Many commercial preparations contain a mixture of these. In the U.K. some may be bought without a prescription. Drugs applied to the nasal mucosa for their systemic effect, snuff and pituitary snuff are rare but interesting causes of local damage. Drugs taken orally also can adversely affect the nose; these include hypotensive agents, the contraceptive pill and anticonvulsants.

Topical Vasoconstrictors: "Decongestants"

Nasal vasoconstrictor drugs are commonly called decongestants. As most may also cause nasal congestion when applied topically this name is a bad one. Topically applied vasconstrictors constrict capillaries, arterioles and venous sinuses in the nasal mucosa, and it is probable that they all cause rebound vasodilatation involving mainly the deeper nasal sinuses, the superficial mucosa remaining blanched (Kully, 1945), so narrowing the nasal airway. The return of discomfort may result in the drug being applied again, perpetuating symptoms and eventually damaging nasal vasomotor structure and function. Perhaps the most widely reported offender is naphazoline, a potent sympathomimetic vasoconstrictor (Feinberg and Friedlander, 1945; Mentins, 1947; Walker, 1950; Goodman and Gilman, 1970).

Experiments on the nasal mucosa of rabbits have shown squamous metaplasia of the mucous membranes, fibrosis of subepithelial layers, chronic vascular dilatation and later sclerosis and constriction after topical naphazoline.

Possibly all topically administered sympathomimetic agents can cause after-congestion (Goodman and Gilman, 1970) and it is widely believed that prolonged use of them should be avoided.

Topical Antihistaminics, Antibacterial Agents and Antiseptics

Preparations containing antihistaminics, antibacterial agents and antiseptics, separately or combined, are widely available. Since each of these can cause skin hypersensitivity after repeated local application to the skin and to mucous membranes elsewhere, the same could happen in the nose. Such a development could be confused with the condition for which the application was used. There seem to be no important published studies of this.

Topical Corticosteroids

Corticosteroids are vasoconstrictor when applied to the skin and indeed the potency of topical corticosteroids can be assayed in this way. Corticosteroids applied to the skin regularly for very many months may cause atrophy of skin connective tissue.

There seem to be no reports of injury to the nasal mucosa from long use of topical corticosteroids, but in one study of their clinical use in perennial rhinitis nasal irritation was noted in a small proportion of patients taking hydrocortisone and dexamethasone snuff (McAllen and Langman, 1969).

Snuff

Medicinal properties are no longer claimed for snuff. Atrophy of the nasal mucosa can result from prolonged use (Harrison, 1964).

Pituitary Snuff

Allergic hypersensitivity to pituitary snuff may cause rhinorrhoea, apart from allergic reaction in the lungs (Pepys et al., 1966).

Antihypertensive Agents

Nasal stuffiness can result from antihypertensives such as guanethidine and bretylium tosylate acting as alpha-adrenergic blocking agents and from antihypertensives such as reserpine and methyldopa which deplete sympathetic nerve endings of their catecholamine stores (Ariens, 1967). Nasal stuffiness may, however, be a reasonable price for an effective antihypertensive. Failure to allow for the cause of the trouble may result in useless or troublesome medication. In such cases sympathomimetic agents such as ephedrine which act by releasing noradrenaline from sympathetic nerve endings will be even less effective than usual.

Anti-cholinergic Agents

Anti-cholinergic agents such as thiazinanium, oxyphenonium and certain drugs which act on mood may dry the nasal mucosa, but this is not necessarily rated as a toxic action. Indeed antidepressants such as imipramine have been recommended for rhinitis, possibly because of this action.

The Contraceptive Pill

Pregnancy may exacerbate rhinitis, and nasal stuffiness may similarly be a consequence of taking the contraceptive pill (Horan and Lederman, 1968).

Anticonvulsants

It is a personal impression that prolonged use of phenytoin may contribute to any nasal obstruction in epileptics. If this were confirmed it might be suggested that the drug causes proliferation of the tissues of the nasal conchae as it does in the case of the gums. In patients taking high doses because of epilepsy severe enough to require them to live in an institution thickening of the nose and lips was observed but no reference was made to symptoms of nasal obstructions (Lefebre, et al., 1972).

Catecholamine Depleting Agents

It is a common complaint of patients that drugs which at first appeared to help no longer do so. Some sympathomimetics which act by releasing noradrenaline from nerve endings, and so eventually depleting the store, characteristically behave in this way.

CONCLUSION

Prolonged use of topical vasoconstrictors, especially those containing naphazoline, are notorious perpetuators of nasal disorder. Antihypertensive agents may be overlooked as causes of stuffy nose, and so may the contraceptive pill; in both cases the usefulness of the drug may be thought to be a reasonable price to pay for any minor discomfort. Fortunately, apart from those due to naphazoline, nasal disorders due to drugs are rarely severe.

REFERENCES

Ariens, E. J. (1967), Internat. Rhinol., 5, 138.
Feinberg, S. M. and Friedlander, S. (1945), J. Amer. med. Ass., 128, 1095.
Harrison, D. F. N. (1964), Brit. med. J., 2, 1649.
Horan, J. D. and Lederman, J. J. (1968), Canad. med. Ass. J., 99, 130.
Kully, B. M. (1945), J. Amer. med. Ass., 127, 307.
Lefebre, E. B., Haining, R. G. and Labbé, R. F. (1972), New Engl. J. Med., 286, 1301.
McAllen, M. K. and Langman, M. J. S. (1969), Lancet, i, 968.
Mertins, P. S. (1947), J. Amer. med. Ass., 134, 1175.
Pepys, J., Jenkins, P. A., Lachmann, P. J. and Mahon, W. E. (1966), Clin. exp. Immunol., 1, 377.
Ryan, R. E., (1947), Ann. Otol., 56, 46.
Walker, J. S. (1952), J. Allergy, 23, 183.

SECTION XIV

RECONSTRUCTIVE SURGERY

PAGE

65. EAR 865

66. NOSE 882

67. LARYNX 894

68. TRACHEA 919

65. EXPERIMENTAL ASPECTS OF RECONSTRUCTIVE SURGERY: THE EAR

B. H. COLMAN

Although some functional studies have been carried out, most of the experimental work relating to the reconstruction of the ear is histological in nature and is concerned with grafting procedures and similar investigations in healthy animals with normal auditory tubes, healthy non-infected middle ears and, of course, non-otosclerotic ears.

It is a matter of regret that far too often insufficient experimental work is carried out before human operations are performed. Sometimes animal and human operations may be done in parallel, but too frequently the relevant animal investigations are done only as an afterthought.

In evaluating experimental work it is to be remembered that short-term animal results cannot always be extrapolated into human terms, either histologically or functionally and, although good results in animals may augur well for the equivalent human operation (e.g. the work relating to the grafting of ossicles), bad results do not necessarily exclude the possibility of success in the human patient (e.g. the work relating to stapes piston prostheses in animals usually gave poor results). These differences arise from various technical problems, the difficulties of operating on small unco-operative animals which have a high prevalence of spontaneous infections, and the different responses of the tissues and organs in different species of animals. Accordingly, although animal experiments are interesting and informative, the final test has to be with human patients. It is from these patients that clinical long-term information of the utmost value is obtainable, which with scientific examination of material obtained at operation and revision procedures, taken together with experimental results, helps final evaluation of disease processes and their correction by reconstructive methods.

If the hearing mechanism is to be successfully reconstructed it is essential that the surgeon should have some knowledge of the physical and acoustic properties of the external ear, tympanic membrane and middle ear mechanism. These have been discussed in earlier chapters. Moreover, if incoming sound energy is to produce an adequate disturbance of the cochlear partition, it seems reasonable to suppose that the surgeon should rebuild the damaged ear in such a way that it resembles the normal ear as closely as possible. On occasions when this cannot be achieved the surgeon can nevertheless provide a good level of hearing by building a system which, though differing greatly from the normal, provides good sound transmission to one cochlear window with, at the same time, effective sound protection at the other. The hearing mechanism in various types of disordered middle ear function and the mechanical principles involved in them in conditions such as total drum loss, round window baffle effect and columellar mechanism, have been well described by Groves (1971).

The reconstructive surgeon, in addition, must have a knowledge of the properties of the materials he is using for implantation, means of preservation when appropriate, and the behaviour of the implant and host tissues after reconstruction. The materials he uses may be xenograft, autograft, allograft or artificial, according to particular circumstances.

Xenografts are those in which the donor is of a completely different species from the recipient. They are seldom used in otology; problems of antigenicity are likely to be complex. Autografts are frequently employed, these grafts consist of tissue obtained from some part of the recipient himself. There may be problems relating to nutrition and revascularization, but immunological reactions are not to be expected. In the case of allografts, the tissue is obtained from a donor who belongs to the same species as the recipient, so that, unless the donor is an identical twin, the problem of immunological rejection is one that may have to be considered.

Tissue implants may be altered whilst awaiting use by drying, freeze-drying, refrigeration or preservation in various fluids, such as Cialit (sodium 2-ethylmercurithio-benzoxazole-5-carboxylate) or alcohol. They may be intentionally or accidentally modified by such treatment. Indeed, in the case of xenografts and allografts it is essential that their antigenicity should be reduced as much as possible by suitable treatment if rejection is to be avoided.

External Acoustic Meatus Reconstruction

For normal sound transmission across the middle ear, a prerequisite is normal delivery of sound energy to the tympanic membrane. Basic necessities for this are: (a) a patent meatus and (b) a normally shaped meatus with absence of any mastoid cavity.

Congenital meatal atresia remains a major problem in reconstructive ear surgery yet little experimental work is available relating to it. Reference may be made to the work of Wright and Colman (1973) who examined the behaviour of freeze-dried meatal allografts in dogs. Histological studies were made of the graft reaction at regular intervals up to two years and osteogenic activity was monitored by tetracycline fluoroscopy using techniques based on those described by Frost (1958, 1959) and by Woodruff and Norris (1955). Regional lymph nodes were examined for evidence of graft rejection. There was no allograft reaction and the implant acted as a scaffold for new bone formation followed by a continuous process of graft fusion with the host bone. In the longest term survivals the graft remained as a firm bony meatus of good thickness with scattered islands of dead bone still present in the body of the graft. As a result of their experiments, they felt justified in using a similar method as part of a staged treatment in selected human patients with congenital atresia of the ear. It may be noted that Smith (1973) has implanted posterior canal wall after experiments which led him to believe that with suitable methods of preservation an allograft could be implanted as a viable tissue.

Mastoid cavity obliteration has likewise received little attention experimentally, although Hohmann (1969) examined the fate of autogenous grafts and of processed xenogeneic bone in the mastoid cavity of primates and sought to investigate the long-and short-term fate of autogenous muscle and fat grafts in comparison with processed xenogeneic bone when implanted into the infected and non-infected mastoid cavity of monkeys. His observations were also concerned with the tissue response of the temporal bone, especially in the remaining deep pneumatic cell tracts. None of the grafts examined showed consistently good results, although the more radical the mastoidectomy the better were graft tissue fibrosis and cavity obliteration. He found that muscle became replaced by fibrous tissue which had a tendency to form a good seal between graft remnant and the bone. In long-term survivals, atrophy of the graft produced a few cystic spaces which could produce complications in an infected mastoid. Fat underwent absorption or liquefaction by fat necrosis and was not consistently replaced by fibrous tissue or by new bone formation. The survival of the fat graft was unpredictable and the end results so unrewarding that use of the fat appeared not to be justified in this context. He found that preserved xenogeneic bone became easily infected and consequently extruded from the cavity, the occurrence of foreign body and local allergic reactions suggested that the material may not be completely non-antigenic at least in primates. Merifield (1963) on the other hand, found that xenogeneic bone in the cat bulla behaved satisfactorily and became partially replaced by new bone and connective tissue. It would appear that further research is necessary in this field before a definite opinion can be formed.

As far as the response of the mastoid bowl and remaining air cells was concerned, Hohmann found that sometimes a collection of serous fluid, macrophages and occasional polymorphs was present, but this response was on a limited scale. No active or chronic bone disease could be identified in the invading bone surrounding the autogenous grafts. He was not able to produce cholesteatoma before grafting, neither was it found to have developed post-operatively in any animal in the series. The problem of persistence, or recurrence of disease, deep to an obliterative tissue of any kind is, however, one that will continue to be a source of anxiety to many otologists employing these methods.

Tympanic Membrane Replacement
(a) Experiments with Xenografts

The tympanic membrane has been repaired at various times using xenogeneic, autogeneic or allogeneic grafts and a certain amount of experimental work relates to each type of material. Earliest attempts at myringoplasty in fact were those with xenografts and include those reported by Stinson (1941) and by Ireland (1946). More recently, attention has again been directed towards xenografts by workers such as Jansen (1969, 1973) who used preserved serous membrane from calf intestine; no immunobiological graft reaction was found. The experimental basis for using tissues of this type is meagre, although the work of Patterson (1967) and of Cornish and Scott (1968) and of Hildmann and Steinbach (1971) is to be noted. Patterson pointed to the convenience of having preserved, stored, sterile tissues for use in drum repair and described the use of collagen film prepared from the deep flexor tendons of cattle. The grafting was carried out on cats which were killed up to 12 weeks later. He found that the chrome-tanned collagen incited an intense inflammatory reaction, but that untanned collagen was well tolerated by the host, attracted relatively few inflammatory cells, and was soon invaded by fibroblasts. By 6 weeks replacement of it was well advanced and by 12 weeks the collagen appeared to be completely replaced by fibrous connective tissue provided by the host.

Cornish and Scott (1968) described animal experiments with freeze-dried aortic valve cusps taken from humans, sheep and bullocks. The graft material was laid beneath the meatal and drum epithelium of recipient sheep. Other implants were placed as intra-tympanic grafts. The study was designed simply to assess the cellular reaction which might take place and was not an attempt to graft actual drum perforations. In no case did histological studies suggest any rejection reaction up to 3 months postoperatively. They subsequently felt justified in carrying out human myringoplasties using bullock aortic valve as drum replacement. Other animal experiments, however, in which bullock cusp had been placed in the rectus muscle of sheep, showed a strong antigenic response with disruption of the grafted valve and marked cellular infiltration with lymphocytes, macrophages and plasma cells representative of a rejection phenomenon. Potential antigenicity of the freeze-dried bullock valve material was further demonstrated in other experiments involving standard immunological techniques, although curiously it was not possible to detect relative immunoglobulin activity in the human patients. The authors suggested that although these graft materials are to some extent antigenic, the ear is for unknown reasons a "favoured site" for grafting without great risk of immunological problems. This point is one that is frequently made by a number of authors relating to various types of drum and ossicular grafts including Broek (1970) who observed that when an allograft ossicle is transplanted to a muscle site, rejection and resorption of the graft follow very rapidly. Although one can only speculate about the apparent tolerance of the middle ear towards grafts generally, it is suggested that one of the factors involved is the limited tissue contact between host and graft, especially in the case of ossicles which are suspended in an aerated space usually with extremely limited contact of the host tissues. Further studies, however, are clearly needed to clarify this matter.

Fascia was examined as a xenograft by Hildmann and

Steinbach (1971). They found that fresh xenogeneic fascia showed a strong inflammatory reaction. It was still present at 6 weeks and there were areas of tissue necrosis. No vital cells could be seen in the transplant and staining was poor in comparison with adjacent tissues. By contrast, the histological picture with xenogeneic fascia stored in Cialit was identical with that seen with Cialit-preserved allogeneic fascia. The inflammatory response was mild, fibrocyte cells could be seen between the fibres of the transplant and the texture of the fibrous tissue was especially satisfactory. From these experiments it might appear that suitably prepared xenogeneic tissues may have some part to play in myringoplasty, although most otologists to date have hesitated to use them clinically.

(b) Experiments with Autografts and Allografts

The most numerous studies concerning experimental myringoplasty have been concerned with various types of either fresh autogenous material or preserved allogeneic material. The renaissance in tympanoplasty arising from the pioneering work of Zöllner and of Wullstein resulted in many patients receiving fresh autogenous skin grafts of full or partial thickness, although problems of re-perforation, cyst formation and dermatitis soon became apparent. Skin, nevertheless, is again being used by certain otologists and basic studies reported by Tanaka (1970) are relevant and deserve attention by otologists using skin for drum repair. He examined the properties of skin taken from 14 different sites on the body and carried out histological and *in vivo* examinations of this material. He found that the structure and consequently the suitability of skin varied widely, depending upon the choice of the donor site. He concluded that transplants taken from the thigh, the back, the gluteal and retro-auricular regions were the most suitable grafting material if skin was the tissue selected for use, though thickness had to be carefully controlled if complications were to be avoided.

The major part of scientific research, however, has been concerned with either the experimental closure of artificially induced drum perforations in animals or with drum replacement in animals. These studies have usually been histological in nature though in assessing the results of experiments concerning grafted perforations in animals, especially in the cat, it has to be remembered that artificial perforations have a very pronounced tendency to spontaneous closure, even though the complete membrane may have been excised as far outwards as the fibrous annulus. Although this possibility must always be borne in mind, it does not necessarily invalidate those experiments designed to examine the way in which a tissue simply becomes incorporated into a healing eardrum.

Salén (1968) examined the histological behaviour of several types of fresh autogenous grafts in animals, but his report is made of greater importance by virtue of certain functional studies in which he investigated the acoustic properties of his tympanic membrane grafts by means of cochlear microphonic measurements. Although as many as 19 different types of tissues have been proposed since 1952 for drum grafts, comparatively few have been studied experimentally in any detail in this fashion. Using cats as his experimental animal, Salén investigated the behaviour of fresh unpreserved temporalis fascia, full-thickness skin, and cartilage with perichondrium. He found that full-thickness skin became fully integrated into the grafted eardrum and that grafts retained the histological character of skin. Glands, hair follicles and penetration by proliferating squamous epithelium caused the formation of intradermal epithelial cysts. In contrast to what is now known to occur in human patients, however, and which has caused most surgeons to abandon the use of full-thickness skin, no dermatitis was observed. Temporalis fascia grafts became reduced in bulk or replaced by a sparse amount of atypical connective tissue, except occasionally when the graft was grossly and microscopically unchanged. The cartilage component of his cartilage-perichondrial grafts usually persisted unchanged, but the perichondrium itself tended to behave like fascia. Functionally he found that each type of graft tended to impair slightly the transmission properties of the middle ear. This reduction was least pronounced at 1000 Hz, and most marked at 4000 and 8000 Hz. The impairment of transmission was less severe with temporalis fascia, but the differences were small.

Other experiments include those carried out by Withers and his team (1963, 1965) who examined fresh autogenous fascia, vein and canal skin in the cat when used for drum repair. They found vein became well revascularized and persisted as a viable graft whether used as an onlay or underlay. Temporalis fascia behaved similarly in their opinion, although sometimes foreign body giant cells were noted without any obvious cause. A composite graft consisting of temporalis fascia with hairless canal skin also took and thinned well. Their drum grafting experiments are of additional interest because they were combined with tympanoplasty procedures using politef* (polytetrafluoroethylene) and polyethylene ossicular prostheses. Although some of these plastic materials were extruded from some of the grafted ears others were retained satisfactorily and frequently became completely enclosed by middle ear mucosa. Survival times, however, were up to only 5 months maximum. Absorbable gelatin sponge (Gelfoam), which was used to support the implants, became completely absorbed.

Fresh oral mucosa, vein, temporalis fascia, mucosa and skin were examined in a major investigation by Paparella (1967). He examined the ability of these various types of graft to provide a functional and viable tympanic membrane in squirrel monkeys. In addition to myringoplasty, he used behaviourally conditioned animals to investigate various audiometric aspects of different kinds of tympanoplasty. In order to discourage spontaneous healing of the artificially induced perforations, he removed entire drum together with annulus and malleus. The implants all appeared to have the same ability to take satisfactorily. All healed properly to the edges of the ear canal, thinned well and provided a satisfactory new drum membrane. All types of graft underwent a certain amount of atrophy and all acquired an outer

* In this chapter, in all cases where reference is made to politef, polyethylene or silicone rubber, the particular proprietary preparations Teflon (Du Pont de Nemours Corporation), Polythene (Imperial Chemical Industries Limited) and Silastic (Dow Corning Corporation) respectively were employed.

layer of stratified squamous epithelium, which for obvious reasons in the case of skin grafts was much more pronounced than with other materials. The middle layer, i.e. the body of the graft, showed obvious fibroblastic activity with increased cellularity and with laying down of collagen, the tympanic surface of the grafts received an epithelial lining one or two cells thick. There seemed to be no significant difference in survival between the various grafting materials used. The primary vasculature of the grafts was observed to develop from the periphery, and occasionally a secondary blood supply came from adhesions from the promontory. Except for temporalis fascia, many small spaces developed in all the grafts with the appearance of lymphatic channels. Red blood cells were not identifiable within these spaces, suggesting that they were lymphatic rather than capillary, although of course there exists the possibility that blood cells may have been washed away by perfusion at the time of sacrifice. The observations concerning the vasculature are of special interest because most discussion has been speculative concerning the means by which grafts survive. Before the vasculature is established it is generally assumed that grafts are nourished from the adjacent fluids. Accordingly, it seems likely that if the graft is to persist as a vital structure it will have a better chance of survival if it has low metabolic needs.

Comparisons between autografts and allografts have been made by several investigators. Richards and McGee (1966) compared fresh autogenous vein with preserved allograft vein in the repair of newly created partial drum perforations in cats. Like Withers and his colleagues, they found that vein became an integral part of the healed drum and that although the smooth muscle fibres in vein degenerated and disappeared by 3 months, elastic fibres were intact and healthy even after a year. They noted that, by 7 days, invasion of the vein by blood vessels, polymorphs, macrophages and fibroblasts was already well advanced and that by 18 days well-defined bands of collagen fibres could be seen extending from one side of the tympanic defect to the other. Although some of these bands passed through the substance of the vein for the most part they extended along one or other surface of the graft. Growth of a stratified squamous epithelium across the superficial surface of the graft was complete by the 18th day, although growth of epithelium on the internal surface took about a week longer. They found no detectable difference in the fate of allografts as compared with fresh autografts. The response of surrounding tissues was identical in the two types of graft and they suggested that the eardrum, like the cornea for example, appeared to be a privileged site, exhibiting a high level of allograft acceptance.

As they carefully point out, however, this is an oversimplification of the facts because real allograft acceptance implies that living cells are transferred from a donor animal to the host and that these cells then proceed to live and function normally in harmony with the host's tissues. The fact would seem to be that in the case of preserved allografts clearly no living cells survive transfer, although within the graft there nevertheless may be plentiful amounts of antigenic materials.

The findings of Richards and McGee are in agreement with those of Williams and his co-workers (1965) who examined the behaviour of vein grafts in the ears of dogs. Using preserved vein, they, too, found that the graft became incorporated within the healed drum and that well stained elastic fibres persisted to give an appearance similar to that obtained with fresh autogenous vein.

Comparisons of fresh autologous fascia and Cialit stored allogeneic fascia were made by Hildmann and Steinbach (1971) in rabbits. As in previously quoted work, they found that fresh autogenous fascia appeared to be fully accepted, the graft became epithelialized on both sides, although the outer epithelium lacked normal regularity and the thickness of the graft tended to vary from one area to another. Cialit preserved allografts demonstrated no evidence of rejection, the epithelium on each side of the graft was remarkably similar to the normal and if anything the appearances were better than with fresh autografts.

Increasing clinical experience with temporalis fascia has repeatedly demonstrated its very high take-rate in human myringoplasty and has served to draw further attention to this material experimentally in its various forms and with various types of preservation. A number of investigations have been carried out in an attempt to demonstrate the inherent characteristics of this tissue which might account for its high survival rate. Patterson and his co-workers (1967) carried out tissue culture studies in combination with their animal experiments and found that specimens of human temporalis fascia and perichondrium showed no evidence of growth in tissue culture whereas vein and canal skin grew actively. They concluded that dry fascia as used for drum grafting was non-viable in any case and that this, together with its absence of metabolic requirements and high content of collagen and mucopolysaccharides would appear to account for the high take rate of dry fascia in human myringoplasty. In the repaired drums of their experimental animals, they found a clearly identifiable middle layer of connective tissue 2 weeks to 5 months after dry fascia grafting. By 3 months, the orderly arrangement of collagen fibres and numerous fibroblasts was a prominent feature. These appearances seem to be similar to those occurring with fresh autogenous fascia and would suggest a migration of cellular elements from surrounding tissue.

Smyth and his colleagues (1967, 1971) also carried out tissue-culture experiments using temporalis fascia and, like Patterson and his group, failed to observe fibroblast growth. They emphasized that although this does not necessarily indicate that fascial grafts are non-viable it does demonstrate that their metabolic demands are low and so they too concluded that this is an important factor in the high success rate with this material. Smyth and his colleagues pointed out that dried fascial grafts consist essentially of a sheet of collagen, possibly with some surviving fibroblasts, but of a very low level of antigenic activity. Autogenous and stored allogeneic fascial grafts, they believed, should not differ significantly in their behaviour. Indeed, this appears to be borne out in the histological part of their investigations in which they produced total drum perforations and repaired the defect with either fresh autogenous fascia or with allogeneic fascia which had been stored at 5°C in 5 per cent framycetin for a week prior to implant. They used an underlay technique with absorbable gelatin sponge as a support. The animals were sacrificed after 6 weeks and it was found that the graft had been satisfactorily accepted within the healed drum, as in the experiments of Hildmann and Steinbach. There was very little inflammatory reaction and the external surfaces had been epithelialized. Whilst recognizing the ability of perforations to close spontaneously in experimental animals, they nevertheless felt justified in using a similar technique for human patients and although healing with preserved allogeneic fascia was noticeably slower than with human autologous fascia, an extremely high success rate was obtained. They submit that, in human patients, any living fibroblasts which may by chance persist in an allograft are eliminated by the host's immune reaction and that the grafted tissue acts as a mere scaffold which may or may not be incorporated into the new drum.

The results of all these experiments with various types of tissues, various types of graft and with various methods of treatment enable certain general conclusions to be made which probably apply equally well to human drum repair, Although the clinical end results may be similar, regardless as to whether a particular tissue may be either fresh autograft or preserved allograft or even preserved xenograft in origin, it would appear that the recipient site deals with the implant in different ways. Fresh autogenous grafts probably survive as a living entity in the healed drum. Although it is not always easy to decide which living components of the healed drum belong to the graft and which have been provided by ingrowth, a complex structure such as skin is readily identifiable and obviously persists with little change. Accordingly, it seems reasonable to assume that other similar fresh autografts can behave in the same way. This is especially likely to be true in those materials that have been shown to have few metabolic requirements, even though it is not always easy to identify with certainty individual living cells which have survived transplant. Dried autografts may contain a few living components which have survived transfer, but probably behave more like suitably preserved allografts.

Suitable preservation of allografts demands treatment which is calculated to destroy the greater part of their antigenicity. Such grafts clearly do not contain living elements when preserved by the usual methods currently employed and act merely as scaffolds. Some non-viable components may persist, infiltration by host tissues slowly occurs, and epithelial coverings are supplied. Xenografts probably behave in essentially the same way as allografts, although clearly the destruction of their antigenicity is likely to be more complex and less complete with the methods of preservation currently employed.

At the present time, temporalis fascia appears to be the grafting material most commonly used clinically and there would appear to be good scientific reasons for selecting this tissue whether it be used fresh, dried or preserved.

Nevertheless, in spite of a very high take-rate often in excess of 97 per cent in human patients, many surgeons have at times expressed disappointment at the failure of all these materials to result in a tympanic membrane possessing a normal appearance. Thickening of the graft, blunting of the anterior sulcus and separation of graft from handle of malleus with consequent poor coupling are problems not yet satisfactorily solved and which sometimes are responsible for a poor hearing result.

It may be argued that the fibrous layer of the normal tympanic membrane should have metabolic characteristics similar to connective tissues elsewhere and that, if devitalized or preserved fascia can be successfully transplanted, it should be equally possible to transplant the middle fibrous layer of the drum itself, possibly even the whole area of the fibrous layer together with the annulus. Accordingly, various workers have been stimulated to examine the behaviour of preserved allogeneic tympanic membranes, initially in small drum defects and later as complete drum replacements. Drum allograft experiments will be discussed in a later section because the majority of such grafts when used clinically are employed in the form of composite grafts, i.e. drum with ossicles.

Ossicular Chain Reconstruction

Repair of the ossicular chain may be by means of plastic or metal struts, fresh autograft bone or cartilage, or preserved allograft bone or cartilage. Most experimental work relating to these three groups of materials has again been histological in nature and concerned with implants into healthy, non-infected middle ears.

A major study of the mechanical and acoustic properties of artificial ossicles, however, has been carried out by Gundersen (1971). Following a comprehensive study of the function and properties of the normal ossicular chain, he designed special prostheses of polythene and steel as incus replacements. As a result of his preliminary observations he concluded that if one is to make full use of the middle ear lever mechanism and of the normal drum oval window areal ratio then the malleus and stapes must be joined in the same way as in the intact chain. His investigations showed that the malleus and incus moved as one unit at sound pressures of up to 115 dB SPL and therefore he designed his prostheses so that the connection between them and the head of malleus was rigid. This he ensured by specially designed steel clips. Using the same apparatus as that used in his investigations of the normal mechanism, he proceeded to examine the sound transmission of the ear before and after inserting a prosthesis in fresh human temporal bones. Experiments were made with prostheses of various weights and shapes and the movements of prosthesis and stapes were measured by means of a stroboscope and film. Experiments on 94 temporal bone preparations showed an average of 4 dB poorer transmission with a prosthesis than with the natural chain. No alteration of the frequency characteristic of the chain could be demonstrated in either direction, and although the weight of the incus prosthesis was varied from 15–45 mgs this was not reflected in measurable changes of sound transmission. The occurrence of overtones was the same as with the intact ossicular chain. With the prosthesis in the ossicular chain he found linearity between input and output for pressures up to 115 dB as with the intact chain, and subsequently used prostheses of the same type in human patients undergoing tympanoplasty and requiring incus replacement.

Engineering studies have also been carried out by Longo and Byers (1971) who gave special attention to stapes replacement studies and developed a mechanical analogue system to help analyse the role of the acoustic transmission characteristics of prosthetic struts. The proposed model is to be regarded as a valuable tool in the analysis and design of present and future ossicular prostheses.

One of the few audiometric investigations is that of Benitez and Stein (1967) concerning incus allografts. Using healthy adult cats trained to respond audiometrically, hearing thresholds were established before and after incus transplantation. Complications of the type to be expected from attempts at functional reconstruction of the ossicular chain in small animals occurred in the majority of cats (and subsequently were demonstrated histologically) with consequent production of a conductive type hearing loss; but when good positioning and freedom from adhesions was obtained, audiograms taken 40 days post-operatively showed thresholds which were strikingly similar to those obtained pre-operatively.

Important sound transmission studies in human temporal bones have also been made by Andersen and his associates (1963) in Denmark in a comprehensive series of investigations. They observed changes in transmission properties with different connections to the oval window and found definite advantages with the use of ossicles. They accordingly concluded that in reconstructive operations ossicles should be replaced by ossicles.

Histological studies include those of Hohmann (1969) who in experiments with cats used a fresh incus autograft which was immediately re-implanted into the ear as in an incus interposition procedure. New callus had been laid down and a small amount of new bone showed up around the vascular channels. At 4 months it was found that some of the old bone was devitalized and that the osteocytes no longer stained. Later experiments were done with monkeys, as before it was found that with the passage of time old bone became replaced by new. Hohmann at the same time reported on the behaviour of fresh autograft bone taken from the mastoid cortex in monkeys. The graft osteocytes gradually disappeared and osteogenic reaction developed with consequent fusion of the graft to the malleus. The fibrous reaction in both sets of experiments was a notable feature, but probably no more than most investigators are accustomed to finding even in experiments in which no implants are used.

Autograft ossicle behaviour was examined further in monkeys by Taggart (1969). Each implanted ossicle became covered with mucous membrane and several of the autografts showed viable osteocytes from the original graft (his autografts were freshly taken in each case and re-introduced early). He also noted that many of the chondrocytes in the articular cartilage appeared to survive. New bone formation in the specimens was first noted along the surface and around the capillaries. Comparison was made with cancellous and with cortical xenografts taken from young calves. In the xenograft experiments there was, after the same period of time of 3–7 months, rather more extensive

bony replacement than with autograft material. He found no difference in the degree of epithelialization or scar tissue formed between the different types of material and felt that processed xenogeneic calf bone may well have a place in middle ear reconstruction, especially for those patients where suitable autogenous material was not available and in hospitals where facilities for taking allograft ossicles were absent.

As part of an experimental series of tympanoplasties in cats, Colman (1971, 1972) also examined the behaviour of autograft ossicles. He found that bone became replaced by a process of creeping substitution, during which the shape and size of the graft were in no way altered. The precise changes in the ossicles depended upon the survival time and the various replacement processes were invariably slow. At 18 weeks there existed a thin, outer shell of new bone on the surface of the ossicle. The interior of the ossicle showed extensive and irregularly shaped areas of devitalized bone without any surviving osteocytes indicating that the cells in these areas did not survive the ossicular transposition even though the ossicles were freshly taken, had not been kept in any preservative and were re-implanted after only a short period of time following removal from the ear. Numerous irregularly shaped islands of new bone deposition gradually occurred; the new bone was rich in osteocytes and appeared to be deposited in layers. Throughout the implanted ossicles, numerous spaces were present which characteristically were inside the regions of new bone formation; these spaces were loosely packed with vascular connective tissue. No osteoclasts could be identified in these areas, although there were very numerous osteoblasts closely packed together and lying in contact with the face of the newly formed bone. Even at 12 months, areas of devitalized bone which had not undergone replacement were still present in a number of animals.

The experience of many otologists is that autogenous grafts in human patients can produce good short-term results. On the other hand, there have been a substantial number of failures due to unsuspected areas of osteitis or cholesteatomatous disease in the transplanted ossicle as emphasized by Steinbach and Hildmann (1972) and it frequently happens that no suitable autograft ossicle is present in an ear which is being reconstructed. Accordingly, attention has been directed to the possibility of using preserved allografts and a number of investigators have designed experiments to compare the behaviour of autograft and allograft ossicles in animals. Wilson and his associates (1966), as well as other investigators, have shown that the histological changes were extremely similar with the two types of grafts, both types of graft appear to behave as non vital structures and both types are replaced by the same process of creeping substitution. The rate of substitution seems to vary from species to species though generally the rate of change is greater in the allograft than in an autograft. A possibly enhanced host response to the "foreign" graft has been suggested as an explanation of this in man.

The classical methods for examination of ossicles by conventional histological means can be criticized on the grounds that only inferential information on the status of bone metabolism can be obtained from the appearance number and site of osteoblasts, osteoclasts and osteocytes. Accordingly, various investigators have used tetracycline fluoroscopy techniques to examine the behaviour of transplanted ossicles. By this method Winter and Hohmann (1967) examined grafts which, as a result of the method of preservation, they regarded as definitely dead. They found that active calcium metabolism was occurring 3 months after implantation and concluded that the host tissues must be supplying the graft with cells by which to carry on osteogenesis. They suggested that the mineral components of the graft underwent very slow resorption and replacement. In the incus, activity was most marked near the body of the bone; less in the long process. In all cases, the lentiform process was the slowest to resume calcium metabolism. The transplanted ossicle apparently accepted ingrowth of a blood vessel from any nearby source and easily became fused to the wall of the tympanic cavity. The experiments suggested that bony fusion appeared likely if a protection barrier such as silicone rubber sheeting was not interposed. They emphasized that the validity of any animal study pertains only to that species being studied as it may not be a true reflection of what happens in the human; not only are there anatomical differences and species differences in response to grafting experiments, but, most important, it has to be remembered that the majority of experiments are conducted on healthy middle ears of animals (as mentioned in the introductory remarks to this chapter). Ossicular allografts in human patients, on the other hand, are usually done in ears which lack ossicles as a result of disease which may also have damaged or caused changes in the middle ear mucosa, the vascular supply of adjacent ossicles, and which may affect the vascular supply to the graft itself. Accordingly, caution has to be exercised when extrapolating animal experimental results to human patients in whom very long survival periods are expected and in whom recurrence of disease may occur at any time.

Benitez and McIntire (1968) used similar tetracycline labelling techniques to examine allograft incuses which had been preserved by refrigeration. Specimens were removed at periods ranging up to 12 months. Tetracycline activity was found as early as 28 days after implantation. The greatest bone remodelling seemed to take place from the 3rd to the 6th month. Remodelling was considerably diminished towards the 7th and 8th months and was negligible after 12 months in their animals. In two specimens, which provided a good display of osteoid seams, the period of time required to complete a Haversian lamella was 2–3 days. The maximum level of bone remodelling was observed at 3½ months after transplantation.

In the experiments of Touma and Maguda (1973), the complete ossicular chain was used as an allograft in the cat after preservation in 70 per cent alcohol. As in earlier experiments with individual ossicles, the ossicles in their experiment retained their normal overall shape and appearance macroscopically. The replacement process was again one of creeping substitution of bone which was first detected at the periphery of the ossicles and around blood vessels in the enlarged marrow spaces. Malleus, incus and stapes all remodelled in the same fashion. Bone replacement was again monitored using tetracycline labelling techniques and,

as in the animals investigated by Benitez and McIntire, it was found that greatest activity occurred between the 3rd and 7th month. The reaction of the internal ear to the stapes part of the implant, varied from inner hair (sensory) cell degeneration with hydrops, to total disorganization of the spiral organ and of the stria vascularis.

As previously indicated, there is evidence that the rate of creeping substitution may vary from one species to another and it is reasonable to suppose that the comparatively large ossicles of the human middle ear require much longer for replacement to reach completion. This is indeed borne out by the report of Kerr and Smyth (1972). They found that, in general, the formation of new bone in transplanted ossicles shows a fairly definite relationship to the time the ossicle has spent in the host middle ear, though in their experience

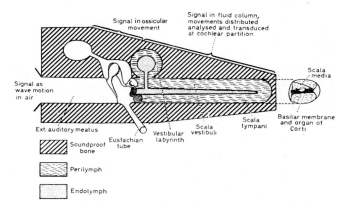

FIG. 1. *The normal sound-conducting mechanism.* Full advantage is taken of the drum-oval window areal ratio and of the lever mechanism in order to produce a satisfactory disturbance of the cochlear partition. (By courtesy of Mr. John Groves.)

the rate of creeping substitution was greater in autografts. This finding is at variance with the previously quoted findings of Wilson and his co-workers who found that allografts remodelled more quickly (in cats) and may be compared with the report quoted from Taggart who observed that xenografts (in monkeys) tended to be replaced more quickly. It is nevertheless generally agreed that the same sequence of events appears to be at work and it seems reasonable to assume that, given time, autograft and allograft ossicles will reach the same stage of replacement and finally become incorporated into the middle ear as totally vital and presumably stable sound conducting structures.

Cartilaginous struts are now not infrequently used by otologists to repair the ossicular chain and experiments concerning the behaviour of cartilage in the middle ear have been described by Smyth and Kerr (1970). They found that the behaviour of autogeneic and allogeneic cartilage grafts in the cat's middle ear showed remarkable similarities. Dead allo-cartilage remained dead. Four out of five living autografts remained alive despite the fact that in one case a chronic middle ear infection was present that persisted for the 18 months between surgery and sacrifice. On the other hand, the six dead allograft cartilage grafts remained as non-vital struts. In two of them small deposits of cellular osteoid were found on the surface, though even

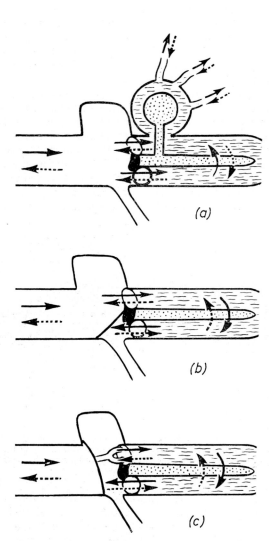

FIG. 2. *Common derangements of the sound-conducting mechanism.* In each illustration the direction of the displacement during the compression phase of an incident sound wave is represented by the continuous arrows, and during the rarefaction phase by the interrupted arrows. (a) *Total loss of drum and ossicular chain.* Displacement of the basilar membrane can occur only by virtue of the yielding of the vascular contents of the labyrinth, this yielding is mainly on the vestibular side so that the basilar membrane moves in that direction during compression. With absence of preferential sound transmission to the oval window combined with absence of sound protection at the round window a severe hearing loss is inevitable. (b) *Round window baffle effect.* The transformer mechanism of the middle ear is lost, but effective round window protection permits adequate disturbance of the cochlear fluids. The yielding of the basilar membrane during the compression phase is in the normal direction. (c) *Columellar mechanism.* There is loss of the normal lever ratio, but if adequate sound coupling and sound transfer to the oval window are provided, a good level of hearing can be restored. (By courtesy of Mr. John Groves.)

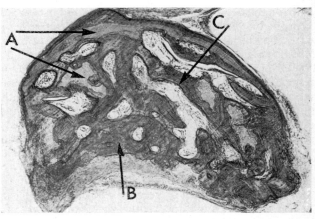

FIG. 3. *Incus transplant.* Fresh autografts and preserved allografts are dealt with by the same process of creeping substitution. Areas of devitalized bone are seen at "A", the new bone "B" stains more readily and is rich in osteocytes. The numerous irregularly shaped spaces "C" are filled with loose connective tissue and lined by osteoblasts. (Cat ear.)

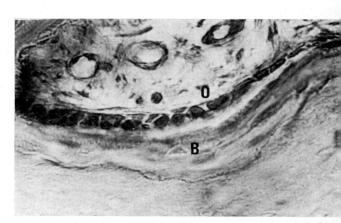

FIG. 4. *Transplant ossicle.* Closely packed osteoblasts "O" lying against new bone "B". (Cat ear.)

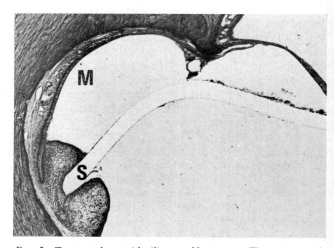

FIG. 5. *Tympanoplasty with silicone rubber insert.* The regenerated mucosa "M" is somewhat thicker than normal, but of good quality. It has become rather heaped up around the sharp edge of the implant "S".

after 15 months there was no suggestion that active substitution of the graft was occurring. There was no evidence of giant-cell resorption and the original overall shape of the cartilage graft was maintained in all but two of the implants, both of these being allogeneic. In one of these there was

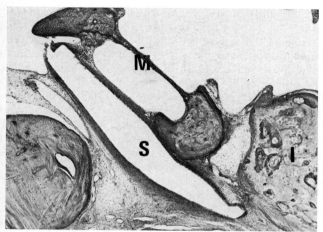

Fig. 6. *Experimental tympanoplasty*. The silicone rubber implant "S" has effectively prevented adhesions between attic wall and malleus "M". Note the remodelling incus "I".

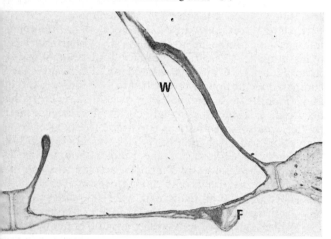

Fig. 7. *Oval window region with tantalum wire implant*. In the middle ear the wire was ensheathed by a thin layer of mucosa "W". No foreign body reaction was found. The wire was deliberately pushed through the footplate "F" and in the vestibule it had acquired a sheath of endosteum. (By courtesy of Professor Harold Schuknecht.)

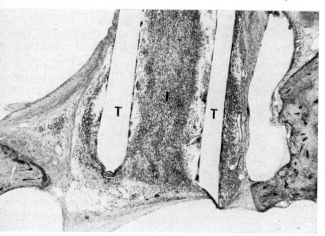

Fig. 8. *Stapedectomy with "polythene" tube implant*. An adipose tissue graft was used and at three months has been almost completely resorbed. The lumen of the tube "TT" contains loose fibrous tissue densely infiltrated with lymphocytes and polymorphs "I". Numerous foreign body giant cells surround the implant. (By courtesy of Professor Harold Schuknecht.)

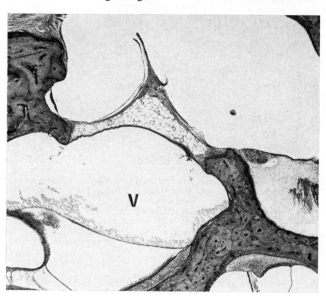

Fig. 9. *Stapedectomy with adipose tissue graft*. Adipose tissue is of fluid consistency at body temperature and accordingly moulds itself accurately to the size and shape of the oval window defect before acquiring a delicate connective tissue envelope with mucosal and endosteal coverings. Vestibule "V".

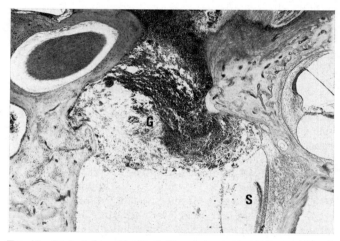

Fig. 10. *Oval window with absorbable gelatin sponge implant at 96 h*. A dense collection of polymorphs has invaded the "G". No membrane has formed on the vestibular surface. The saccule is implicated at "S". (By courtesy of Professor Harold Schuknecht.)

some bending of the strut, presumably due to excessive pressure, whilst in the other there had been some chronic infection in the middle ear for 18 months and some scalloping of the graft. Nevertheless, in both of these ears the authors felt there was little doubt that the cartilaginous grafts were able to act efficiently and effectively as sound-conductors. Fibrous tissue formed a capsule around every graft. Cracks in the cartilaginous struts were not a prominent feature and apart from those in one strut, were always

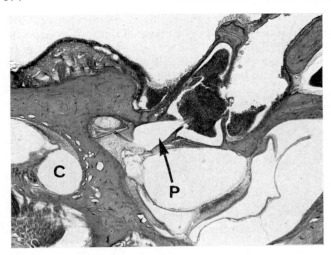

FIG. 11. *Stapes piston implant*. The site of the silicone rubber implant is indicated at "P". It is in satisfactory position between the stapes crura. There is a small collection of chronic inflammatory cells in the oval window niche, but otherwise the middle ear was healthy. At 13 weeks there is no evidence of a satisfactory layer of endosteum over the deep surface of the implant. There was severe internal ear damage with total sensory cell loss in the cochlea "C".

small and were always filled with fibrous tissue. The only exception was in the case of the one autograft which became devitalized and which cracked across its whole width; but, even in this case, fibrous tissue repair was occurring and functionally it appeared to be satisfactory.

The experimental evidence would accordingly seem to indicate that cartilage is well accepted in the ear and that there is every justification to use it in man provided its behaviour is not altered by the internal wiring that is usually necessary to give it extra strength in human ossiculoplasty.

Tympano-ossicular Allografts

For reasons that have already been described, there seemed to be good grounds for attempting to use complete eardrums as preserved allografts and, because plenty of experimental and clinical evidence is now available pointing to the success of techniques utilizing preserved ossicles, it seemed reasonable to attempt to transplant drum and ossicles as a single unit. It must be stated at once, however, that, in spite of very encouraging early results, many clinicians have now become somewhat disillusioned with the intermediate term results of such operations. The take-rate of the drum graft is often much less satisfactory than the rate routinely obtained with temporalis fascia, the functional results are no better and indeed often worse than those obtained with other less complicated and well tried methods as emphasized by Smyth (1973). Fellow contributors to the 1973 World Congress, however, including Austin, Smith and Lacha, were more optimistic, though it is clear that opinion is divided and that few otologists have been able to reduplicate the outstandingly good results of Marquet (1973) who in 1966 was first responsible for introducing the concept of tympanic, and later tympano-ossicular allografts.

There is very little literature relating to experimental work on allograft drums and composite grafts, but Dawkins (1970) succeeded in transplanting the whole tympanic membrane together with attached malleus and incus as a preserved allograft in Macaque monkeys as one anatomical unit. The grafts were stored at 4°C in Ciali for periods ranging up to 3 months and then washed for at least ½ h before use. Prior to implantation, the squamous epithelium was removed from the outer surface of the drum. The animals were sacrificed at various periods up to 1 year and their temporal bones sectioned to assess both the histological fate of the grafts and to review the accuracy of placement of the graft. Tetracycline studies were carried out to show mineralization and X-ray microscopy techniques were used to examine the ossicles before and after transplantation in order to discover if any change in shape or bone density occurred. The full details of the experiment will be awaited with interest although the author reported that, at the time of writing, no macroscopic evidence of rejection was occurring in any of the animals.

In a later paper, Dawkins (1971) reported the preliminary findings with composite grafts in the shorter-term survival of his animals. Micro-radiographic examination of ossicles removed up to 6 months showed no significant change compared to the appearances prior to their implant, though at 12 months, in an animal with otorrhoea, necrosis had occurred. His studies using tetracycline fluorescence methods showed some activity as early as 2 weeks after transplantation and, by 1 month, activity was obvious in both the handle of malleus and the head, although was less marked in the incus. By 3 months, activity was confined mainly to the distal ends of the long processes of the ossicles, the short process of incus and head of malleus. By months there was a sharp reduction in tetracycline activity.

Full histological sections of the temporal bones were only available for up to 3 months post-operatively at the time of his report and were only four in number. At 3 months the drum was intact, although thickened, the middle ear was well aerated. The heads of the ossicles were well covered by mucosa and only a few membranous adhesions were present. The tips of the malleus and incus, however, were eroded and there was no contact with the head of stapes. The ossicles were already fairly well vascularized and the enlarged marrow space, as seen in ordinary allograft ossicles, contained osteoblasts and osteoclasts with appearances of extensive bone remodelling. It would appear from his experiments that the weak part of the newly constructed ossicular chain is in the region of the incudo-stapedial joint. The longer-term report will be awaited with interest. It does appear that by acceptance of a drum malleus unit as an allograft the natural efficiency of the sound-collecting mechanism can be preserved; but as the author himself remarks it may be more satisfactory if a separate allograft incus is used in human patients to restore continuity between malleus and stapes in patients in whom composite grafts are utilized.

Further scientific information concerning drum and ossicular allografts is derived from human sources. Brandow (1969, 1973) found that in tympano-ossicular allografts the collagen fibres of the transplant are bio chemically and histologically similar to those in the original tympanic membrane which has been destroyed by disease and stated that they provide a new middle layer of the tympanic membrane which produced an almost perfect reconstruction of the original drumhead. He quoted Plester and Kahn as having carried out animal studies in guinea-pigs and cats which indicate that the collagen fibres of the graft are replaced by new collagen fibres from the host. He also quoted Marquet who examined histologically the appearance of a tympanic membrane 3 years following an allo-transplant operation. The graft was covered by normal epithelium and mucosa. The collagen network of fibres, both concentrically and radially, was almost indistinguishable from those of a normal eardrum as in his own case. There was no evidence that the graft had been absorbed and no evidence of any foreign body reaction. Whether the collagen fibres of the human drum transplant are replaced by the host is not yet known. It seems likely, however, considering what we know of other allografts, that these composite transplants are invaded by a slow process of creeping substitution so that eventually the donor tissue is almost completely replaced by new tissue from the host. It also has to be remembered that most allograft material regardless of its structure or preparation has some antigenic properties which may finally cause rejection and failure. The surgeon using these allografts does so in the hope that replacement is completed before rejection can occur. In discussing the qualities necessary, if tissue is to be used successfully as a composite graft, Marquet (1971, 1973) re-emphasized that immunologically competent structures in the tissue must be completely inactivated and expressed the view that this could only be achieved with either alcohol or Cialit as a preservative. Destruction of antigenic activity, he considered, could not be properly achieved by dry-freezing lyophylization or by autoclaving. His evidence suggested that the transplanted devitalized lamina propria of the drum simply acts as a scaffold over which epithelium grows and that the implanted meso-dermal elements of the drum preserve their structure, morphological shape and functional capacity even if they were not actually replaced by living cells.

The use of composite allografts will doubtless continue to attract the attention of surgeons both experimentally and clinically and it may be that with the passage of time and with improved knowledge relating to the reasons for failure our present good short-term human results will be followed by equally satisfactory permanent ones. It is already clear, however, that the transfer of a bulky drum-ossicular graft is far more complex than the transfer of either a small area of drum or a small, single ossicle.

Graft Preservation Techniques

Although various methods of graft preservation have been referred to in the previous sections, little has been said concerning the experimental aspects of the various techniques. Clearly, if a xenograft or allograft is to be used, and most especially if it has been taken from the donor post-mortem, then it is essential it must be bacteriologically sterile. Not all preservation methods are bactericidal in

nature, although the suitability of the actual method of preservation in this respect can be examined using conventional bacteriological techniques.

Although it has been suggested that the ear is a privileged site and that allogeneic tissues implanted in the ear are privileged tissues, the fact remains that allografts and xenografts are antigenic when taken and accordingly must be specially treated to reduce the level of antigenicity as far as possible. Graft rejection is otherwise inevitable. It will have already been noted that different investigators (like different surgeons) have utilized various methods of graft preservation. The method of preservation used is an important matter because it is closely related to the severity of immunological reaction which may or may not occur in response to an implanted drum and/or ossicular chain. This problem has been examined by Seiffert (1970). As a result of his experiments relating to the biological properties of various types of collagenous allografts, he concluded that deep-freezing hardly impaired the antigenicity of allografts whereas freeze-dried grafts provoked an antigenic response only in a few instances. Cialit stored grafts, on the other hand, apparently lost all their antigenicity. He raises the possibility that antigenicity depends upon enzyme content of the graft and that the inactivation of enzymes by Cialit could be an essential component of the modification produced by this chemical agent. His experiments suggested that antigenicity was greatest with freshly taken allografts, became progressively less with preservation by deep-freezing, and by freeze-drying and was least with Cialit preservation. Alcohol preservation was not examined, though most otologists, as a result of clinical experience, will equate alcohol with Cialit as producing a high degree of destruction of antigenic properties.

It is interesting to note that Smith (1973) as a result of experiments relating to different means of allografts storage, suggests that allografts which are maintained in tissue culture for sufficient time can lose their antigenic properties so that they can be successfully transferred as living grafts and become incorporated in the recipient's tissues as living implants. His experimental work included tetracycline studies. Clinically, by means of this technique he has been able to implant, apparently successfully, a complete block of tissue consisting of posterior wall of external meatus with drum, tympanic ring and ossicles.

Problems relating to the preservation of grafts, their sterilization, their antigenicity or non-antigenicity, as well as the host's immune response, continue of course to receive much attention in research fields generally. They will continue to be important to otologists whether or not the ear is in fact proven to be a "favoured site" immunologically.

Ossicular Adhesives and Sheet Implants

Reconstruction of the ossicular mechanism frequently presents the surgeon with problems of: (a) maintenance of ossicular implants in the desired position, (b) poor quality mucosa and/or adhesions.

Implanted ossicles are frequently supported by absorbable gelatin sponge as mentioned in earlier paragraphs.

Experimental evidence suggests that, when used in this way, it is readily liquified and evacuated without producing any harm. Provided the middle ear mucosa is of good quality and not traumatized in the course of the operation there is no evidence that absorbable gelatin sponge becomes organized or predisposes to formation of adhesions. On the other hand, if mucosa is deficient or traumatized and if apposing surfaces are not kept separated by suitable implants of plastic sheeting during healing, then adhesions may be encouraged. As an alternative to using absorbable gelatin sponge to support ossicular implants in good position, the surgeon may sometimes use special adhesives to maintain accurate contact between one ossicle and the next, but the experimental evidence relating to adhesives is somewhat disquieting.

Although adhesives are not widely used to maintain functional contact between implanted ossicles, they are nevertheless occasionally thought useful. That they can damage soft tissues and mucosa is recognized by most surgeons, but the possibility of bone damage is often overlooked. Kerr and Smyth (1970) reported on the use of methyl methacrylate in the course of experimental tympanoplasty carried out on cats. The most alarming positive finding in their series of experiments was the apparent ability of methyl methacrylate to destroy bone. This was not found in ears of animals killed less than 3 weeks after surgery, they therefore suggested that this is a slow process rather than an immediate reaction to the heat produced during polymerization. These workers also raised the possibility of internal ear damage resulting from the use of this preparation.

In a later paper, Kerr and Smyth (1971) examined bucrilate (isobutyl 2-cyanoacrylate) as an ossicular adhesive, but as in their experiment with methyl methacrylate they again obtained results on cats which led them to conclude that the substance was neither safe nor effective. A marked middle ear inflammatory reaction was found in all the cat ears examined, accompanied by damage to any bone with which the material had come into contact. Definite internal ear damage was present in most cases and, in addition, there was complete failure to achieve a functional result in the ears where ossicular continuity had been sought for. They felt that bucrilate could not be recommended in tympanoplastic surgery in man because of its potential damaging effect on the middle and internal ears and because of failure to enhance functional union between the ossicles. Indeed, they concluded that the future for better hearing results and tympanoplasty must lie to a large extent in improved operative technique rather than in a search for improved adhesives.

Plastic sheeting is frequently used in human tympanoplasty in order to discourage adhesion formation, promote middle ear ventilation and encourage a regeneration of mucous membrane. Politef is sometimes used for this purpose and its tolerance in the middle ear has been examined experimentally by Paparella (1967). He found it to be well tolerated and there was no foreign body reaction. In each animal the regenerated mucosa was of good quality, though its fibrous layer was much thicker than the normal. Sheeting manufactured from silicone rubber specifically for human implantation is now used extremely frequently in reconstructive middle ear surgery, especially in patients undergoing combined-approach tympanoplasty.

The behaviour of implants of this material, however, has received little attention experimentally. Colman (1971, 1972) examined the behaviour of silicone rubber film in the normal ears of cats and in the ears of cats subjected to experimental tympanoplasty procedures. He found that in the normal mesotympanum middle ear mucosa sometimes grew along the surface of the implant for a substantial distance. When the mesotympanum had been freshly stripped of mucosa, good regeneration occurred in comparison with controls and the regenerated mucosa generally was of good quality, though, as in Paparella's experiments, it was sometimes thickened. Suitably placed silicone rubber film discouraged adhesion formation, although this was less successful in the cramped spaces of the attic (epitympanic recess). A silicone rubber film implant over an atticotomy, however, helped minimize the prolapse inwards of soft tissues and consequent invasion of the attic by scar tissue. The inertness of the material when placed against bone in the region of the atticotomy was such that new bone would grow normally along the surface of the implant, and when silicone rubber film was implanted around a graft of malleus and/or incus remodelling occurred perfectly normally. It is reasonable to conclude that allograft ossicles in human patients remodel equally normally when silicone rubber film is implanted around them.

It was noted in some of Colman's animals, however, that, in certain implants located over the atticotomy defects and in close relation with the soft tissues, there was a patchy collection of lymphocytes and histiocytes, sometimes with giant cells. It is to be noted that these implants had been cleaned and sterilized in the same way as if intended for human implantation. Silicone rubber is generally regarded as being highly inert and it may be the cellular reaction was caused by tissue necrosis or possibly by inadequate preparation, cleaning and handling techniques. It was suggested that some of these reactions may not have been from the actual implant, but from contamination resulting from unsuspected fingerprints or dust particles and that the same kinds of reaction may occur in human patients although unsuspected by their surgeons.

In contrast, Paparella and Sugiura (1968) found a total absence of any foreign body reaction in their experiments with silicone rubber. They were examining, however, silicone sponge implants placed in the mesotympanum of the normal ear and were careful not to disturb or traumatize middle ear mucosa in any way. Their findings, accordingly, are not comparable.

The behaviour of films of silicone rubber has also been examined by Kerr and Smyth (1970) who, in their experiments, found satisfactory re-epithelialization of the middle ear without adhesions, inflammation or foreign body reaction. They found that regenerated mucosa was functionally satisfactory in appearance, although there was some deviation from normal. As in Colman's experiment, none of the specimens showed evidence of internal ear damage which might be attributed to the presence of silicone rubber film in the middle ear and it may reasonably be concluded that silicone rubber film, if properly cleaned and properly handled and sterilized, is a safe and valuable material for use in reconstructive ear surgery.

Experimental Aspects of Stapedectomy

Important early work relating to experimental surgical trauma in the region of the oval window was carried out by Bellucci and Wolf (1958) when interest in stapes mobilization was already causing otologists to think ahead to stapedectomy. They carried out various procedures in the oval window of monkeys and cats which demonstrated that the internal ear could be opened without being destroyed and drew conclusions which are still of significance to the stapes surgeon even though they are now frequently taken for granted or forgotten. They showed that, when the stapes was removed from the oval window, only a small quantity of perilymph escaped and that this could be safely done without damage to the internal ear. Trauma to the stapes and in the oval window area, they found, was followed by active repair processes which began promptly and apparently afforded a high degree of protection to the labyrinth. Vestibular and cochlear damage, however, could be caused readily, either by improper use of instruments or by displacement of bony fragments. They demonstrated that it was important to avoid trauma to the walls of the oval window niche if new bone formation was to be avoided, though fragments of bone which fell into the labyrinth did not themselves become osteogenic. They also demonstrated that, even when the stapes was mobilized to such an extent that it was actually removed and replaced, bony fixation would occur even in the normal ear. They thus forecast the forthcoming abandonment of the stapes mobilization operation. It is also interesting to note that, following stapedectomy in some of their animals, a membrane formed across the emptied oval window and was present as early as the 3rd day. In 4 of the 5 animals in this part of their investigation the spiral organ was in good, or in fairly good, condition.

Although stapedectomy is essentially an ossicular replacement, this type of reconstructive surgery is extremely different from that of other parts of the middle ear by virtue of the special oval window and internal ear relationships, as was demonstrated by these experiments. Even though the surgeon must have some knowledge of the materials which can be used to replace the stapes suprastructure and the experimental work relating to them, it is the closure of the oval window and the care of the internal ear itself that are of critical importance. A substantial amount of experimental knowledge is now available which relates to: (a) replacement of the stapes suprastructure, i.e. the head, neck and crura of the stapes, and (b) closure of the oval window and protection of the internal ear after removal of the stapes base (footplate).

In those human patients in whom the stapes suprastructure cannot be retained, a prosthesis of plastic, metal, bone or cartilage can be used. Sometimes these materials are used in combination with one another, or sometimes in association with a tissue graft to replace the stapes base as

well. Animal experiments concerned with the behaviour of foreign materials used as suprastructure replacements in the non-infected ear have been carried out in animals by a number of workers including Schuknecht and Oleksiuk (1960), Harris (1961), Lindsay (1961), Sooy and his co-workers (1961), Goldmann and his colleagues (1962) and Hohmann and his co-workers (1964).

The work of Schuknecht and Oleksiuk was concerned with the tolerance of the tissues of the middle and internal ear to the presence of tantalum wire in the cat. The lateral end of the wire was tightened around the long process of the incus, the opposite end was located either upon fractured pieces of stapes base or through a perforation of the base into the vestibule. The animals were killed 3–6 months later. Histological examination then showed that the wires were covered in the middle ear by a sheath of mucosa and in the vestibule by a sheath of endosteum. No connective tissue proliferation was evident around the wires at any point. In no case was any reaction observed in either middle ear or internal ear which could be attributed to the physical presence of the implant.

Harris was concerned with the properties of polyethylene when inserted as a stapes suprastructure replacement and likewise worked with cats. The polyethylene strut attracted some giant-cell reaction and usually became enveloped by a loose fibrous sheath. A substantial proportion of animals, however, developed excessive amounts of dense scar tissue in the ear and, although this was regarded as due to the atticotomy rather than the presence of the foreign body, this may be questioned in retrospect since it is now known that polyethylene in various body situations frequently elicits undesirable tissue responses, especially when implanted over a long term. Nevertheless, Lindsay, as well as Sooy and his colleagues, both found that polyethylene was well tolerated and was essentially non-reactive in the middle ear in their experiments.

The work of Goldmann and his team was likewise concerned with the search for a suitable material in place of the stapes suprastructure. They examined politef, steel and polyethylene tubing, the implants being each of similar diameter and length. The cats were sacrificed at intervals ranging from 1–4 months after operation. They found that politef tubing caused less reaction than polyethylene and merely became enclosed in a very thin envelope of mature fibrous tissue. There was complete lack of inflammatory reaction within the actual lumen of the politef tube, but polyethylene frequently produced a very significant cellular and foreign body reaction both in and around the tube whilst on a number of occasions the polyethylene itself became thickened and frayed.

Hohmann and his group also compared the behaviour of polyethylene and of politef and made a comparison with 316 SMo steel alloy in the middle ear cavity of healthy young rats. The animals were sacrificed at approximately their normal life span, i.e. between 1 and 2 years, although 5 elderly animals still surviving at the end of the experiment were killed at age 34 months. Suppurative otitis media developed in 27 per cent of the animals, the lowest instance was associated with a stainless steel implant and the highest occurred with polyethylene. The steel prosthesis never became enclosed in a fibrous tissue capsule, indeed there was practically no tissue reaction to it and no foreign body giant cells were found. In those animals with politef tube implants, tissue reaction was again very slight, although in the area of contact with the middle ear mucosa minimal fibrous reaction was observed. There was no encapsulation of the implant, the outside wall of the politef tube merely acquired a smooth sheath of acellular collagen. The polyethylene tubes in contrast, although of the same length and configuration as the politef, provoked much greater reaction. There was much more fibrous tissue at those points of contact with middle ear structures and usually fibrous tissue grew into the lumen of the tube. Infection had developed in 37 per cent of these ears (compared to only 16 per cent of the ears with a stainless steel implant) and foreign body giant-cell reaction was sometimes a marked feature. These authors also discussed the risk of sarcoma formation and noted that around 604 subcutaneous implants, 4 tumours occurred in relation to politef, one near a polyethylene insert.

The experimental evidence would thus suggest that the best suprastructure replacements are likely to be those fashioned from suitable alloys and/or politef. Nevertheless, the presence of a foreign material so near to the cochlea has persistently been the source of disquiet to some otologists carrying out stapedectomy and finding themselves unable to retain the patient's own suprastructure. Piccoli (1968) suggested that fresh autogenous cartilage could be used and examined the behaviour of a chondro-perichondral strut of autogenous origin in cats which were sacrificed between 15 and 180 days after insertion. The fragment of cartilage appeared to be constantly covered by middle ear mucosa and showed no evidence of degenerative phenomena or bony metaplasia, even in the longest survivals. As a result of his experiment, which was part of a stapedectomy procedure, he suggested that this material could provide a useful strut and offer the advantages of not provoking reactions which might result from a foreign body implant and which could be significant over the long term.

In a later investigation, Kerr and Smyth (1972) also used cats to examine the safety of allogeneic cartilage in the oval window area after preservation for several weeks in 70 per cent alcohol. The allogeneic cartilage was washed in saline for an hour before implantation and the results were compared with those obtained with fresh autogenous cartilage. The oval window in both groups of animals was closed by a sheet of autogenous fascia after the stapes base had been removed. Both autograft and allograft cartilage struts behaved in similar ways and appeared capable of providing permanent replacement for the stapes suprastructure. The general shape and appearance of the struts remained unaltered regardless of the duration of the experiment, there was no evidence of absorption of cartilage, nor of any foreign body reaction, nor of rejection phenomena in any ear. Evidence of cochlear damage due to the effect of alcohol preservative solution was searched for, but found absent. Few otologists, however, are likely to show enthusiasm for using chemically preserved struts in their human patients after total stapedectomy without far more experimental support for such a procedure.

Basic studies relating to experimental removal of the stapes base and reconstruction of the oval window were carried out by Colman (1960) working in Schuknecht's laboratory. His first report concerned the behaviour of fresh autogenous tissues when placed in the oval window of cats following total stapedectomy. Six types of graft were examined: skin, mucosa, vein, conjunctiva, connective tissue and adipose tissue and the animals were allowed to survive approximately 18 weeks. Of these 6 tissues, only skin was regarded as entirely unsuitable; even though very thin skin was used the graft proliferated in each case to produce a cholesteatoma-like cyst in the oval window recess. Mucoperiosteum from the auditory bulla was rather difficult to handle, but produced a very satisfactory membrane across the oval window, at the edges of which it maintained continuity with the mucosa of the mesotympanum. Its only disadvantage lay in the fact that it was possibly too delicate a membrane to consider for human use. Vein and conjunctiva persisted essentially unchanged, although the latter tended to contract to produce rather a thick graft. Subcutaneous connective tissue likewise persisted in an unchanged state; it simply acquired a covering of mucosa and endosteum on its lateral and medial surfaces respectively. The most satisfactory grafts were considered to be those consisting of adipose tissue. These persisted as a soft, pliable sheet of tissue which became enclosed on all sides by a thin connective tissue envelope with a cover as before of mucosa and endosteum on its two surfaces. The preference shown by Colman's experiments was for adipose tissue and this was subsequently employed in human patients reported by Schuknecht and his associates (1960). Rutledge and his co-workers (1965) later confirmed the highly satisfactory behaviour of autogenous fat when used as an oval window graft experimentally and also emphasized the absence of any serious internal ear complications with this tissue. There has been much debate since that time concerning the ultimate fate of fat cells in oval window grafts and it is interesting to note that Linthicum and Sheehy (1969) present a human temporal bone case report in which obviously viable fat cells were still very plentiful at 5 years.

In a further paper, Colman (1962) reported the internal ear changes in his same 18 animals. Certain of the complications can be attributed to faulty technique (e.g. electrocoagulation injury), to working on small animals, and to carrying out an operation which at that time was very new. The types of abnormality observed consisted of labyrinthitis with varying degrees of hydrops, saccule rupture and graft herniation. Blood contamination of the internal ear was found in 2 animals and small stapes base fragments were found in 5. Although the series of animals is probably too small for a valid relationship to be made between the internal ear changes and the type of graft used, it appeared that fatty tissue provided the best internal ear protection.

The abnormalities of the internal ear which are likely to be of most frequent interest to the otologist performing stapedectomy concern blood contamination, the behaviour of lost stapes base fragments, and damage to the spiral organ. Blood was found in the cochlea of 2 animals, but was absent from 6 others in which contamination was thought to have occurred. The red blood cells appeared to act as entirely inert foreign bodies, going wherever fluid currents and gravitational forces took them. These cells persisted in a good state of preservation and indeed appeared to survive longer in the cochlea than in the general circulation. It was found that removal of the red blood cells was undertaken by phagocytes and that these became active as early as the 10th day after operation. The scarcity of such scavenging cells indicated that blood clearance must be extremely slow when contamination is of any magnitude. There was no evidence from this experiment that blood or its breakdown products had any adverse effect on the internal ear structure. Hohmann (1960), in an animal study in which he injected blood deliberately into the labyrinth, reached similar conclusions. Reference may also be made at this point to the report from Linthicum and Sheehy (1969). They examined a human temporal bone which was removed 5 years after a stapedectomy in which gross blood contamination occurred. There was no clinical or histopathological evidence that the blood had been in any way harmful to the patient or to his hearing.

The behaviour of lost stapes base fragments is of direct practical importance. In several operations, Colman considered that several fragments of the base undoubtedly fell free into the vestibule and indeed sometimes they could be seen lying deeply in the vestibule with the saccular macula beneath. Other fragments of the stapes base edge appeared to fall free, but the histological appearances in these animals suggested that they merely hinged inwards on their endosteal attachments. It was clear that no harm resulted from the loss of fragments into the internal ear and, accordingly, there appears to be no justification for hazardous attempts at removing such fragments. The experimental evidence indicates that lost fragments float up and become adherent to the deep surface of the graft. They must do so while it is not endothelialized because they are usually incorporated beneath the intact endothelium and this is known to be completed about the 10th day.

Although a number of animals in the series showed changes in the spiral organ, there was in each case sufficient evidence, such as labyrinthitis, or electro-coagulation injury, to explain the damage. In some animals, stapes base removal was considered to be traumatic and, in these, special search was made histologically for evidence of stimulation injury, particularly in the regions corresponding to the lower middle and upper basal turns of the cochlea, which Tonndorf (1959) in his extensive studies on the hydrodynamics of the cochlea has shown to be the regions of maximal displacement of the cochlear partition during oval window manipulations. No damage was in fact found which could be attributed to stimulation in this region. The frequency of damage in the same region in experimental animals has been confirmed, however, by Singleton and Schuknecht (1959) in their investigation in which stapes trauma was deliberately caused. Cochlear injury was present in 4 of their 14 animals and was in the site predicted by Tonndorf.

That internal ear damage might sometimes be caused by improper handling of the graft has been emphasized by Hayden and McGee (1965) who also stressed the importance of careful techniques and the avoidance of crushing or drying grafts. They found a much higher rate of graft failure and internal ear damage with mishandled grafts. Not only did the graft itself tend to become altered to fibrous tissue when traumatized, but adhesions to the membranous labyrinth were encouraged.

Internal ear damage after experimental stapedectomy in cats and monkeys has also been described by Paparella and his co-workers (1966). The oval window was protected by allogeneic adipose tissue or silicone rubber sponge or gelatin sponge. In general, the internal ear changes were far more serious and far more extensive than those found in the animals in Colman's series. Severe cochlear damage was frequent as were labyrinthitis, fibrosis and osteogenesis in the oval window area. Complications of this severity, although known to occur in human patients, are fortunately extremely rare. These experiments, nevertheless, provide a useful reminder of what can sometimes happen, even though in these experiments the complications may be partly blamed on the difficulty of using cats for investigations of this kind, as well as on the type of materials used to repair the oval window.

Gelatin sponge has received the attention of a number of investigators in an endeavour to find a material which might prove more suitable than fresh autogenous tissue for oval window implantation and, although the material has now been used extensively in human stapes surgery, the results of work in experimental animals are rather variable and contradictory. In an investigation carried out by Bellucci and Wolf (1960) the behaviour of absorbable gelatin sponge implants in cats was compared with the results of vein grafting. Particles of lysed absorbable gelatin sponge were found showering into the vestibule and there was associated damage in the spiral organ. Fibrosis in the oval window area also tended to invade and destroy the cochlea though generally the fibrosis in the oval window area was less with absorbable gelatin sponge than with vein. A similar comparison was made by Sooy and his colleagues (1961) working with monkeys. They, too, found that fibrosis in the oval window region was more extensive with absorbable gelatin sponge than with vein and that in 4 of 10 such operations new bone formation was encouraged. More satisfactory results, however, were obtained by Harris (1961) in cats. He found that, in his animals, invasion of the interstices of absorbable gelatin sponge by fibroblasts, which occurred at 72 h, was usually followed by the formation of a satisfactory fibrous membrane with mucosal and endosteal coverings. Nevertheless, internal ear damage was present in 24 per cent of the animals and was often severe. A satisfactory membrane was generally obtained by Hohmann and his colleagues (1963) which consisted of endosteal and mucoperiosteal layers, and although a mild serous labyrinthitis occurred in some ears there was no evidence of serofibrinous, purulent or chemical labyrinthitis to be found.

The various stages by which absorbable gelatin sponge becomes replaced by a satisfactory membrane have been examined in detail by Kylander (1967). In monkeys, he found that absorbable gelatin sponge first became invaded by polymorphonuclear leucocytes and monocytes within 24 h and that the function of these cells is apparently to provide proteolytic enzymes which resorbed the absorbable gelatin sponge. As this invasion progressed, there was a dissolution of the absorbable gelatin sponge and formation of a fibrillary precipitate in the vestibule. Invasion by fibroblasts occurred within 48 h, but there was no intact membrane across the vestibular surface of the graft until after the 7th day. After 2 weeks, no absorbable gelatin sponge could be identified, but by this stage there was a good fibroblastic reaction present and many small blood vessels had developed. A month after operation there was a dense fibrous layer which later became thinned towards the 6th month. Severe labyrinthitis occurred in 20 per cent of the monkeys. It is difficult to decide from this report as from others to what extent internal ear damage can be blamed upon the nature of the actual implant utilized. Both good and poor results have been obtained experimentally with absorbable gelatin sponge implants as with tissue grafts and at the present time there is no satisfactory experimental evidence which would suggest cochlear damage from contained formalin in spite of recent warnings of this possible danger. Further investigation into this question would appear to be necessary.

The use of piston-type stapes prostheses of various kinds has gained widespread clinical popularity, although the related experimental work in animals has tended to emphasize the possible dangers which threaten when bad results are obtained. The behaviour of politef pistons has been examined by Hohmann and his co-workers (1963), by Rutledge and his colleagues (1965), and by Smyth and his colleagues (1967, 1968). Colman (1971, 1972) examined the behaviour of pistons made from silicone rubber in an experiment and also examined the performance of silicone rubber sponge in the oval window. These materials are regarded as being very highly inert if suitably prepared and handled according to the manufacturer's instructions. The unsatisfactory nature of some of the animal results may be attributed to poor preparation and handling techniques. It may be worth noting that similarly poor techniques are probably causing unnecessary and undesirable reactions in human patients after stapedectomy.

In the series of experiments carried out by Hohmann and his team, the politef piston was reinforced by connective tissue. In 4 of 5 animals they regarded the amount of fibrous tissue reaction and foreign body and inflammatory response as being minimal. The piston became surrounded by fibrous tissue in which some foreign body giant cells were present. In the remaining animal, which was the longest survivor, labyrinthitis and meningitis were present. These authors also noted that politef did not inhibit new bone formation and by special staining techniques they clearly demonstrated that new bone could form adjacent to the prosthesis.

The high incidence of serious internal ear reactions obtained by Rutledge and his colleagues (1965) with politef pistons in cats was attributed to several factors, including the use of too large a piston, ineffective sealing of the oval window by connective tissue, inadequate post-operative chemotherapy, and difficulties of technique. They emphasized the great importance of meticulous cleansing of the politef piston with detergent, autoclaving, proper con-

tainerization and handling only with proper instruments in order to avoid contamination of the implant.

Smyth and his co-workers (1968) assessed the internal ear defences against middle ear infection following stapedectomy with a politef piston reconstruction in cats. In certain animals in the series, the piston was reinforced by absorbable gelatin sponge. Microscopic evidence of some form of fibrous-tissue seal at the oval window was present in 16 out of 17 animals, although the thickness and integrity of the seal varied even in those animals in which absorbable gelatin sponge had been utilized. They found firm evidence to suggest that the presence of absorbable gelatin sponge promoted the formation of a more adequate and more protective oval window membrane although, nonetheless, there was evidence of some labyrinthine infection in each group of animals.

In the experiments carried out by Colman (1971, 1972), a small fenestra was made in the stapes base and a silicone rubber piston prosthesis inserted in cats which were allowed to survive up to 26 weeks. As in the experiment with politef pistons, absorbable gelatin sponge was used to reinforce the seal. Severe and diffuse labyrinthine damage was again an alarming feature. Although the piston in each case was in good position, there was never any attempt to produce either a layer of mucosa over it, nor a layer of endosteum beneath. Lymphocytes and histiocytes were sometimes present in the oval window area around the implant and were associated with a sero-fibrinous type of reaction in adjacent parts of the vestibule. Otitis media developed in one ear and was associated with total disruption of the cochlea. In a second group of experiments total stapedectomy was carried out on 8 ears, a piece of silicone rubber sponge fitted into the oval window in order to assess its suitability as a stapes base prosthesis and to make a comparison with soft tissue autografts. Maximum survival time for animals in this group was 56 weeks. He found that sponge implants easily became displaced, but that usually mucosa and endosteum covered the tympanic and vestibular surfaces satisfactorily. The overall results and the state of the internal ear was nevertheless inferior to those he obtained with tissue grafts and in one ear a lesion resembling reparative granuloma developed in the oval window. He regarded the results with silicone rubber as totally inferior in every way to the results previously obtained with various tissue autografts and concluded that, judging by the results of his animal experiments, the risks were totally unacceptable when translated into human terms.

In conclusion it would appear to be especially important in stapedectomy that experimental findings in animals should be correlated and considered in conjunction with human clinical and post-mortem material. A significant number of human temporal bones are now becoming available for scientific study from patients at various periods after stapedectomy, including those in the collection of Schuknecht (1971). With much experimental-animal material he also presents important human post-mortem findings in association with audiograms obtained at various times between operation and death. These human studies provide important information concerning the response of the human ear to otosclerosis, to surgical interference and of its tolerance to various prostheses that no animal investigations can clarify. Significant though animal investigations may be, it is only by the long term results in man that we can properly evaluate stapedectomy and other operations designed to reconstruct the middle ear mechanism.

REFERENCES

Andersen, H. L., Hansen, C. C. and Neergaard, E. B. (1963), *Acta oto-laryng. (Stockh.)*, **56**, 307.
Austin, D. F. (1973), Communication to Symposium on Tympanoplasty, X World Congress in Otorhinolaryngology, Venice.
Bellucci, R. J. and Wolff, D. (1958), *Ann. Otol.*, **67**, 400.
Bellucci, R. J. and Wolff, D. (1960), *Ann. Otol.*, **69**, 517.
Bellucci, R. J. (1963), *The Laryngoscope*, **78**, 580.
Benitez, J. T. and Stein, L. (1967), *Ann. Otol.*, **76**, 1026.
Benitez, J. T. and McIntire, C. L. (1968), *J. Laryng.*, **82**, 23.
Brandow, Jr., E. C. (1969), *Trans. Amer. Acad. Ophthal. Otolaryng.* **73**, 825.
Brandow, Jr., E. C. (1973), Communication to Symposium on Tympanoplasty, X World Congress in Otorhinolaryngology, Venice.
Broek, P. van den (1970), *Acta oto-rhino-laryng. belg.*, **24**, 79.
Colman, B. H. (1960), *J. Laryng.*, **74**, 858.
Colman, B. H. (1962), *J. Laryng.*, **76**, 411.
Colman, B. H. (1971), B.Sc. Thesis, University of Oxford.
Colman, B. H. (1972), *Acta oto-laryng. (Stockh.)*, **73**, 296.
Cornish, C. B. and Scott, P. J. (1968), *Arch. Otolaryng.*, **88**, 350.
Dawkins, R. S. (1970), *Acta oto-rhino-laryng. belg.*, **24**, 140.
Dawkins, R. S. (1971), *J. Laryng.*, **85**, 315.
Frost, H. (1958), *Stain Technol.* **33**, 273.
Frost, H. (1959), *Stain Technol.* **34**, 135.
Goldman, J. L., Nalebuff, D. J. and Druss, J. G. (1962), *The Laryngoscope*, **72**, 169.
Groves, J. (1971), *Scott-Brown's Diseases of the Ear, Nose and Throat*, 3rd edition, Vol. I, p. 82. Butterworth.
Guilford, F. R., Shortreed, R. and Halpert, B. (1966), *Arch. Otolaryng.*, **84**, 144.
Gundersen, T. (1971), *Prosthesis in the Ossicular Chain*. Universitetsforlaget Oslo/Bergen/Tromso.
Gundersen, T. (1972), *Arch. Otolaryng.*, **96**, 416.
Harris, A. J. (1961), *The Laryngoscope*, **71**, 131.
Hayden, R. C. and McGee, T. M. (1965), *Arch. Otolaryng.*, **81**, 243.
Hildmann, H. and Steinbach, S. (1971), *J. Laryng.*, **85**, 1173.
Hohmann, A. (1960), Quoted by Colman, B. H., in Ch.M. Thesis, University of Edinburgh, 1961.
Hohmann, A. (1962), *Otosclerosis*, p. 305. Henry Ford Hospital Symposium. Boston: Little, Brown & Co.
Hohmann, A. (1969), *Arch. Otolaryng.*, **89**, 229.
Hohmann, A. (1969), *The Laryngoscope*, **79**, 1618.
Hohmann, A., Stengl, T. A. and Long, V. (1963), *Arch. Otolaryng.* **78**, 578.
Hohmann, A., Hilger, J. A. and Carley, R. (1964), *Ann. Otol.*, **73**, 791.
Ireland, P. (1946), *Canadian Med. Soc. J.*, **54**, 256.
Jansen, K. (1969), *Z. Laryng. Rhinol.* **48**, 933.
Jansen, K. (1973), Communication to Symposium on Tympanoplasty, X World Congress in Otorhinolaryngology, Venice.
Kerr, A. G. and Smyth. G. D. L. (1970), *Arch. Otolaryng.*, **91**, 327.
Kerr, A. G. and Smyth, G. D. L. (1971), *Arch. Otolaryng.*, **94**, 129.
Kerr, A. G. and Smyth, G. D. L. (1972), *Oto. Cl. N. Amer.*, **5**, (1), 183.

Kylander, C. E. (1967), *Ann. Otol.*, **76**, 346.
Lacha, G. (1973), Communication to Symposium on Tympanoplasty, X World Congress in Otorhinolaryngology, Venice.
Lindsay, J. R. (1961), *Ann. Otol.*, **70**, 785.
Linthicum, F. H. and Sheehy, J. L. (1969), *Ann. Otol.*, **78**, 425.
Longo, S. E. and Byers, V. W. (1971), *Med. Res. Engng.*, **10**, 12.
Marquet, J. (1966), *Acta oro-laryng. (Stockh.)*, **62**, 459.
Marquet, J. (1970), *Acta oto-rhino-laryng. belg.*, **24**, 99.
Marquet, J. (1971), *J. Laryng.*, **85**, 523.
Marquet, J. (1973). Personal communication.
McIntire, C. and Benitez, J. T. (1970), *Ann. Otol.*, **79**, 1129.
Merifield, D. L. O. (1963), *Ann. Otol.*, **72**, 157.
Paparella, M. M. (1967), *The Laryngoscope*, **77**, 1755.
Paparella, M. M., Lim, J. J., Sugiura, S. and Bolz, A. (1966), *Arch. Otolaryng.*, **84**, 154.
Paparella, M. M. and Sugiura, S. (1968), *J. Laryng.*, **82**, 29.
Patterson, M. E. (1967), *Arch. Otolaryng.*, **86**, 486.
Patterson, M. E. Lockwood, R. W. and Sheehy, J. L. (1967), *Arch. Otolaryng.*, **85**, 287.
Richards, S. H. and McGee, T. M. (1965), *J. Laryng.*, **79**, 952.
Rutledge, L. J., Sanabria, F., Tabb, H. G. and Igarashi, M. (1965), *Arch. Otolaryng.*, **81**, 570.
Salén, B. (1968), *Acta. oto-laryng. (Stockh.)*, suppl. 244.
Schuknecht, H. F. (1964), *Arch. Otolaryng.*, **80**, 474.
Schuknecht, H. F. (1971), *Stapedectomy*. Boston: Little, Brown & Co.
Schuknecht, H. F., McGee, T. M. and Colman, B. H. (1960), *Ann. Otol.*, **69**, 597.
Schuknecht, H. F. and Oleksiuk, S. (1960), *Arch. Otolaryng.*, **71**, 287.
Seiffert, K. E. (1970), *Acta oto-rhino-laryng. belg.*, **24**, 27.
Singleton, G. T. and Schuknecht, H. F. (1959), *Ann. Otol.*, **68**, 1069.
Smith, M. F. W. (1973), Communication to Symposium on Tympanoplasty, X World Congress in Otorhinolaryngology, Venice.
Smyth, G. D. L. (1973), Communication to symposium on Tympanoplasty, X World Congress in Otorhinolaryngology, Venice.
Smyth, G. D. L. and Kerr, A. G. (1970), *Acta oto-rhino-laryng. belg.*, **24**, 53.
Smyth, G. D. L., Kerr, A. G. and Goodey, R. J. (1971), *J. Laryng.*, **85**, 891.
Smyth, G. D. L., Kerr, A. G. and Nevin, N. C. (1971), *J. Laryng.*, **85**, 1167.
Smyth, G. D. L., Kerr, A. G. and Jones, J. H. (1967), *The Laryngoscope*, **77**, 1684.
Smyth, G. D. L., Kerr, A. G. and Jones, J. H. (1968), *J. Laryng.*, **82**, 897.
Sooy, F. A., Barrios, X., Hambly, W. and Burn, H. (1961), *Ann. Otol.*, **70**, 808.
Steinbach, E. and Hildmann, H. (1972), *Z. Laryng. Rhinol.*, **51**, 659.
Stengl, T. A. and Hohmann, A. (1964), *Arch. Otolaryng.*, **80**, 72.
Stinson, J. (1941), *Ann. Otol.*, **50**, 178.
Taggart, J. P. (1969), *Arch. Otolaryng.*, **90**, 445.
Tanaka, J. (1970), *Nagoya J. med. Sci.*, **33**, 173.
Tonndorf, J. (1959), *The Laryngoscope*, **69**, 859.
Touma, J. B. and Maguda, T. A. (1973), *Ann. Otol.*, **82**, 62.
Williams, G. H., Guilford, F. R. and Halpert, B. (1965), *Arch. Otolaryng.*, **81**, 577.
Wilson, D. F., Pulec, J. L. and Van Vliet, P. D. (1966), *Arch. Otolaryng.*, **83**, 554.
Winter, L. E. and Hohmann, A., (1967), *Arch. Otolaryng.*, **86**, 44.
Withers, B. T., Hatfield, S. E. and Richmond, R. W. (1963), *The Laryngoscope*, **73**, 1022.
Withers, B. T., Mersol, V. and Hatfield, S. E. (1965), *The Laryngoscope*, **75**, 22.
Woodruff, L. A. and Norris, W. P. (1955), *Stain. Technol.*, **30**, 179.
Wright, J. L W. and Colman, B. H. (1973), *Acta oto-laryng. (Stockh.)* **75**, 159.

66. RHINOPLASTY

T. R. BULL

INTRODUCTION

Rhinoplasty surgery is now established and accepted by both the medical profession and the general public. Until fairly recently, however, cosmetic operations such as rhinoplasty, were viewed with some suspicion and disfavour by many doctors: this attitude was apparent to patients wanting advice about rhinoplasty and tended to encourage their furtive referral to a specialist surgeon without the advantage of advice from a general doctor, and this in turn, made rhinoplasty a fringe procedure. It is not surprising, therefore, that this operation with its difficult selection and technical problems has been delayed in acquiring a scientific basis and that the surgical development of good work has been relatively recent. Rhinoplasty is, nevertheless, rather a different form of surgery to that involving the excision of diseased tissue, and surgery for various forms of obstruction. Artistic judgement is involved. This is intangible and, by its very nature, rhinoplasty does not readily lend itself to scientific analysis: its place in surgery can be regarded as psychotherapeutic.

The number of papers on rhinoplasty, particularly from the United States, are increasing in the otolaryngology and plastic surgery journals, and good textbooks on the subject are now available (e.g. Rees and Wood-Smith, 1973). The emphasis in the literature is centred on surgical technique and its complications. Although there is a fairly uniform rhinoplasty procedure now adopted throughout the world, there is still much controversy over the surgery of the major alar cartilages.

Those surgeons having a large series of rhinoplasties and many years experience have contributed reflective papers on the general philosophy of this cosmetic surgery; the psychiatric aspects of the operation and the pitfalls of inexperienced selection of patients are well documented (Linn and Goldman, 1949). There are published reports on the results and follow up of most surgical operations: a good or bad result in cosmetic surgery, however, is obviously difficult to assess and papers describing results are a rarity. Rhinoplasty too has been the subject of limited scientific research, in that there has been little experimental work on either man or other animals. Nevertheless, anatomical details as they apply to this type of surgery, have been well described (Janeke and Wright, 1971) and the use of various implants in nasal reconstruction has been studied.

This chapter will discuss cosmetic or corrective rhinoplasty rather than the total or partial nasal reconstruction necessary following excision or destruction of the nose by trauma, surgery or disease.

SURGICAL TECHNIQUES

Most of the writing on rhinoplasty in the past decade has dealt with surgical technique. Surgeons who have used established methods and have been unhappy with the results have written to describe an alternative or improved technique aimed at displacing or discrediting previous methods. Earlier work centred on surgery to alter the nasal bones and septum, but recently attention has concentrated on the tip of the nose and the major alar (formerly, lower nasal, or lower lateral) cartilages. In so far as the basic steps are fairly universal, a standard technique for rhinoplasty could now be said to have been evolved. The fact that a personal preference for a certain appearance of the nose influences technique, will, of course account for some differences. The surgical result, whether good or indifferent, is not measurable quantitatively but is merely assessed by the surgeon and the patient, as well as by public reaction, and this does not lend a depth of science to its analysis.

Most patients seeking an alteration in the shape of their nose are not primarily concerned with their breathing or with their nasal airway; the air flow and nasal resistance may however, in some instances, be relevant to cosmetic rhinoplasty. The airway is often only relevant, in so far as the rhinoplasty technique runs a risk of impairing breathing. Clearly any operation to alter the shape of the nose must not compromise the airway or result in symptoms of nasal obstruction. External nasal deformity is not infrequently associated with a septal deviation limiting the size of one or other half of the nasal cavity, and septoplasty associated with the rhinoplasty should aim to improve nasal function.

THE SEPTUM

The submucous resection (SMR) has for decades formed a basic part of the rhinologists' technique to restore a normal airway in a case of a deviated nasal septum. When associated with rhinoplasty, however, it is a poor operation.

The submucous resection operation that is planned to be followed at a later stage by a rhinoplasty is unsatisfactory and constitutes poor operative staging. After the removal of septal cartilage, which the submucous resection entails, most rhinoplasty surgeons are reluctant to risk any degree of separation of the lateral (formerly, upper) nasal cartilages from the septum, for fear of causing saddling of the profile. Models of the nose have been made to assess the role of the septum in response to various stresses. These have shown that definite support is given by the septum. It is not simply retraction due to fibrosis after removal of excess septal cartilage in the submucous resection that causes saddling, but lack of support (Clark, 1971). The scope of the rhinoplasty is therefore limited by a submucous resection and the septum and lateral nasal cartilages, which may require reduction, are frequently inadequately corrected. If the caudal strut of the cartilaginous septum is removed during the SMR, either as a routine part of the surgical technique or because of dislocation anteriorly into the nasal vestibule, the subsequent rhinoplasty is again compromised.

A deviation of the septum frequently causes an external deformity with or without nasal obstruction. Septoplasty techniques have been introduced to obtain a good airway as well as correct the external deviation and, in most instances, the septoplasty is combined with the rhinoplasty. It is not possible, however, in every case to achieve a good result with one operation. It is probably better to aim to

cartilage is incised or excised in part, or "diced," and a pocket made in the columellar soft tissue into which the cartilage is replaced. Diagrammatically the techniques look attractive but in many cases they are unnecessary. The perverse nature of cartilage to twist and refuse to remain straight (regardless of surgical ingenuity) results in either a thick columella or a recurrence of the original deformity. The dislocated caudal portion of the columella in these cases is frequently redundant cartilage and excision of the projecting cartilage is the only treatment required. If the

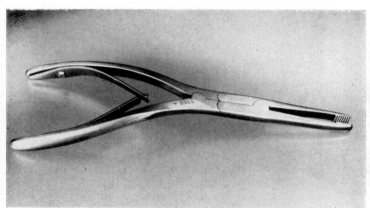
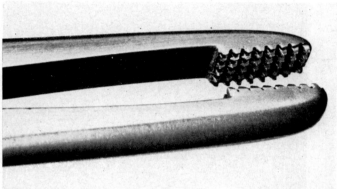

FIG. 1. The morcellizer for the cartilage of the nasal septum.

achieve the best rhinoplasty result possible but, if subsequently, despite septoplasty, the airway is imperfect, then to carry out a secondary operation to correct the septum.

Most septoplasty techniques involve incising the septal cartilage to break the "spring" with minimal excision of cartilage. Fracture of the maxillary crest and its displacement to the mid-line, as well as fracture of the vomer and the perpendicular plate of the ethmoid is also usually necessary. No one method is certain to induce deviated and dislocated cartilage to take up the desired mid-line position; the perverse tendency of the cartilage to return to its previous position is well known. This applies particularly to the externally apparent deviation of the septum. It is, therefore, unwise to promise a maintained straight nose following surgery for this deformity. "Dicing" of cartilage to reduce the spring has been practised for many years with such techniques as cross-hatching with a scalpel; more recently a surgical morcellizer (Rubin, 1967) has been used (Fig. 1). It has been demonstrated histologically that permanent changes in cartilage shape can be achieved in this way without necrosis or loss of support (Rubin, 1969). Mucous membrane overlying the cartilage is preserved with this morcellizing technique, which is also used for the lateral and alar cartilages. In all these cartilaginous incisions and morcellizing techniques, the mucous membrane overlying the cartilage requires elevation on one side of the septum only.

Dislocation of the caudal end of the cartilaginous septum frequently causes an ugly deformity and may also cause nasal obstruction by limiting the lumen of the vestibule (Fig. 2). Techniques to reposition this dislocated cartilage in the columella are described, in which the

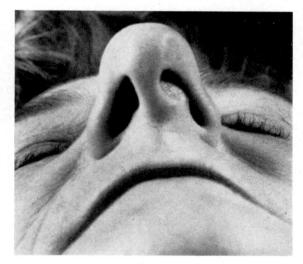

FIG. 2. Caudal dislocation of the cartilaginous septum into the left nasal vestibule, which causes nasal obstruction and an ugly deformity.

columella is *retracted*, however, efforts should then be made to reposition the cartilage or a graft used to add bulk to the columella.

The septum has a role in the normal development of the nose. Septal surgery is therefore generally deferred until after the age of 16 years. If gross nasal obstruction due to a congenital or traumatic septal deviation presents in a child, limited excision and reposition is the practice. Excision of the septal cartilage in growing rabbits alters the nasal growth considerably (although support of the rabbit snout is unaltered) (Sarnat and Wexler, 1967). Experimental surgery to the septum in rabbits also affects tooth eruption and occlusion, as well as the growth of the nose. It is therefore suggested that follow-up of nasal injuries in children to check nasal and dental development is advisable (Wexler and Sarnat, 1961). A septal haematoma in childhood, particularly if complicated by secondary

Methods of removing the hump with the chisel, saw or rasp, followed by infracture of the nasal bones, have changed little. A number of papers relate to preferences of technique for removing the bones and the lateral nasal cartilages (Skoog, 1966; Neuner, 1971) or to various methods of infracture with the saw or the osteotome. Basically, however, the technique is standard; interest in the nasal hump has diminished while attention to the

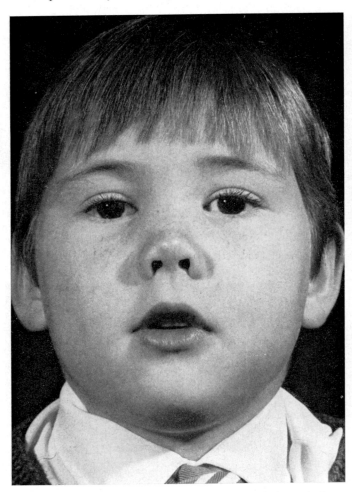 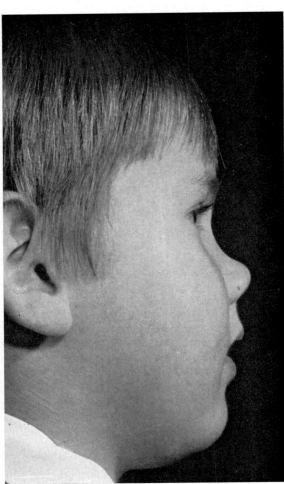

FIG. 3. This boy aged six received a nasal injury two years previously complicated by an infected septal haematoma. Collapse and shortening of the nose have already developed.

infection, invariably results in saddling and a small nose in later life. Implants to the nasal dorsum under the age of 10 years, to be replaced by a larger implant during adolescence, result in more normal development of the nasal soft tissues. Saddling with a small upturned nose occurring some years after a severe septal injury in childhood (Fig. 3) should not be ignored until late adolescence, when too little soft tissue limits the improvement possible with rhinoplasty (Heanley, 1973) (Fig. 4).

THE NASAL BONES

The prominent bony and cartilaginous nasal hump formed the main challenge in the early days of rhinoplasty.

minutiae of nasal tip surgery has increased. It is common practice, particularly in North America, to routinely deal with the nasal tip as the first step in rhinoplasty; hump removal and infracture—once the main part of the operation—is relegated to the closing stage. "As the tip is encountered first, it is corrected first," is Millard's (1965) uncompromising attitude. One generally agreed principle with hump removal has evolved: a much smaller bony and cartilaginous hump is now removed than hitherto. The saddling effect with a projecting tip deformity, when too large a nasal hump is removed, has been seen as a poor result of rhinoplasty all over the world (Fig. 3). Revision techniques are difficult and unsatisfactory, often requiring insertion of a plastic or bony graft. If excessive hump

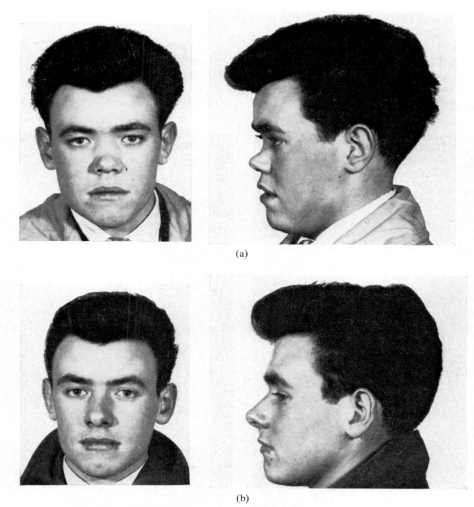

(a)

(b)

FIG. 4. What appear to be pre- and post-operative photographs demonstrating a graft for a saddle deformity of the nose are in fact photographs of identical twins. The brother in (a) shows the saddle short nose, with columellar retraction resulting from a childhood septal haematoma. His twin, (b), shows normal development of similar nasal structure with no past history of injury.

removal is associated with inadequate lowering of the lateral nasal cartilages and the septum, the postoperative deformity of saddling with a "polly beak" is even more complex to remedy (Fig. 5).

GRAFTS

Rhinoplasty commonly involves reduction of tissue, and nasal reduction is a synonym for rhinoplasty. Following trauma, with collapse of nasal support, or removal of extensive tissue surgically, there is a need for augmentation. Many substances have been used in the nose, but currently bone grafts or plastics are favoured. Marquit (1967) recorded 18 different types of nasal implants for saddle deformities which have been described. He estimated that a new material was advocated every 3 years.

Bone grafts have been in use for many years in the nose and both clinical and radiological follow-ups over a period of 20 years are available (Farina and Villano, 1971). About 90 per cent of these grafts have been satisfactory; infection and reabsorption accounts for the 10 per cent that fail. A plastic that is well accepted, can be easily fashioned to the shape required, and does not tend to migrate or extrude, is the ideal nasal graft. This makes a separate operation to obtain bone, with its attendant difficulties, unnecessary. Polyethylene and the early silicone rubber implants were well accepted but of a hard texture. The more recent silicone rubber sponge is more satisfactory for nasal reconstruction; grafts used for defects of the dorsum of the nose give good results with few complications. If the graft is placed by a separate mid-line columellar incision, rather than via the intranasal incision, displacement and extrusion is uncommon. Silicone rubber, along with other implants, is less effective when some tip support is required, for extrusion tends to occur. Silicone rubber, when used to deal with the difficult problem of lengthening a short nose, also gives complications (Davis, 1971). A polyamide mesh (Beekhuis, 1974) is also being used for saddle nose deformities and early reports suggested that displacement and extrusion are infrequent. Fat, which has also been used, resorbs and dermofat grafts, where the epithelium is removed from the skin, give bulk with little definition when used for the nose. Rib grafts, which have also enjoyed a

consider nasal tip surgery something best left to other surgeons.

Millard, one of the most prolific and readable of surgical writers, routinely removes a considerable part of the lateral nasal cartilages along with most of the lateral part (crus) of the major alar cartilages leaving about 1 mm of the caudal part of the alar rim. Complications are not

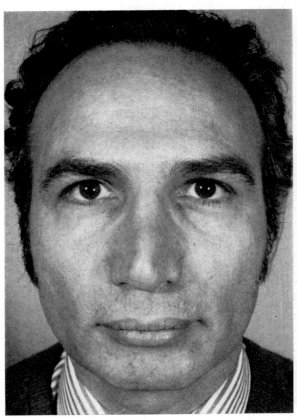 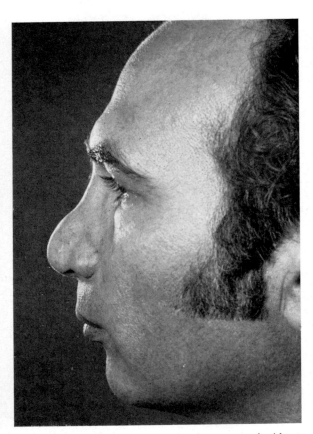

FIG. 5. The "Polly Beak" deformity following rhinoplasty. An excessively large bony nasal hump has been removed without reduction of the upper lateral cartilages and septum. In addition, there has been soft tissue hypertrophy over the dorsum of the septum. This deformity is difficult to correct.

vogue, tended to twist despite ingenious methods of introduction and of preparation to avoid this complication (Cinelli, 1966; Marquit, 1967).

When too much cartilage and mucous membrane, or vestibular skin, has been removed from the nose, revision rhinoplasty may require a composite graft. Cartilage from the nasal septum or skin and cartilage from the concha or helix of the ear are used to bridge gaps of vestibular lining when associated with loss from the lateral nasal and major alar (formerly, lower nasal) cartilage (Walter, 1969).

NASAL TIP

The lateral nasal cartilages and the major alar cartilages have been the subject of many papers and much controversy: opinions remain widely divergent on their importance for the shape of the nose. To those learning nasal surgery, dogma is so confusing and conflicting that one may almost

described by him and this technique has been employed for nearly 20 years in many hundreds of cases (Millard, 1965). In wide noses, the lateral parts of the major alar cartilages are removed. Collapse has not been a complication in his experience, providing mucosa and vestibular skin are preserved. That Millard's approach to rhinoplasty tends to be radical is suggested by the fact that 15 per cent of Millard's rhinoplasties have simultaneous mentoplasty and 90 per cent have a wedge resection of the alar base. Although a well established procedure, resection of the alar base to narrow a flared nostril or, on occasions, to assist in lowering a prominent nasal tip, is used by most surgeons infrequently and as a last resort rather than the method of first choice (Rees and Wood-Smith, 1973). Millard also advocates strip excision of a wedge of skin and soft tissue from the alar side-wall to thin the nasal tip. Tip techniques may, therefore, involve removal of considerable cartilage, skin and soft tissue.

Many advise extreme caution, however, when dealing with nasal tip cartilage. The alar cartilages have a definite physiological function and should never be radically resected, only modified (Safian, 1970). Not only however, are the views regarding either radical excision or preservation of the nasal cartilage conflicting, but there is a multiplicity of techniques described to either expose or to work on these cartilages.

septum. However, Anderson feels that the site of the intercartilaginous incision may cause cicatricial narrowing and this is one of the reasons for advocating the more caudal cartilage-splitting approach. Access to the major alar cartilage may also be achieved by a rim incision following the caudal margin of the cartilage, or via the intercartilaginous incision with retrograde dissection. There are many techniques for incising, excising, cross-

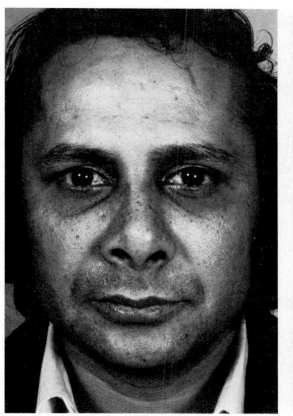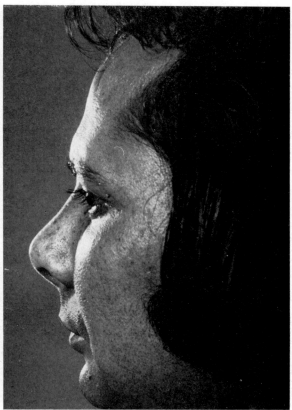

FIG. 6. Rhinoplasty with excessive removal of cartilage from the caudal aspect of the septum. This increases the naso-labial angle and results in a "pug nose" deformity.

The standard intercartilaginous incision between the lateral nasal cartilage and the major alar cartilage is the most widely used initial incision for exposure. The cartilage splitting incision described by Anderson (1971) is the basis of a new approach to rhinoplasty. The initial incision is made through the major alar cartilage close to the caudal margin. Elevation and exposure are through this approach. A similar technique is used by Millard. This approach gives ready access to the cephalic portion of the lateral part of the major alar cartilage which is excised routinely by those who advocate more radical tip surgery. An advantage of Anderson's approach is the reduction in the number of intranasal incisions. The commonly used inter-cartilaginous incision between the major alar and the lateral nasal cartilages may rarely cause narrowing at the "valve" of the nose, with distressing nasal obstruction, difficult or impossible to remedy by surgery. This complication is less likely to occur if mucosal continuity is preserved between the lateral nasal cartilages and the

hatching and suturing the major alar cartilages to give the desired alteration in shape; morcellizers are also used.

COMPLICATIONS

Techniques for correcting rhinoplasty errors are now well described and despite much teaching and writing on basic rhinoplasty aimed to avoid poor results, many cases need revision. Rhinoplasty leaves small margin for error and postoperative healing is not always predictable so, even in the best hands, poor results can occur. The first operation, as is so often the case in surgery, offers the best chance of a good result. Although revision rhinoplasty, if the surgical defect responsible for the deformity is carefully diagnosed and corrected, may be successful, third and fourth operations have a poor outlook.

Too much removal of tissue from one place with too little from another, results in the well recognized deformities with names such as *polly beak*, *parrot beak* and *pug nose* (Fig. 6) (Millard, 1969). The polly beak deformity after rhinoplasty is common. One unavoidable cause of this is the hypertrophy of connective tissue over the dorsal aspect of the septum and the lateral nasal cartilages. Rees, apart from paying attention to firm postoperative strapping, goes so far as to inject the supratip area of the nose postoperatively with triamcinolone to offset this complication.

produces some asymmetry of the tip and a "tent-pole" appearance (Fig. 7).

The "operated look" is descriptive of a nose that looks unnatural following rhinoplasty. Whistler was described as one who could hide the effort he put into his art. This attribute is necessary to those practising rhinoplasty. It is better to have a result that does not attract attention than a nose which has obviously had surgery. To do too little

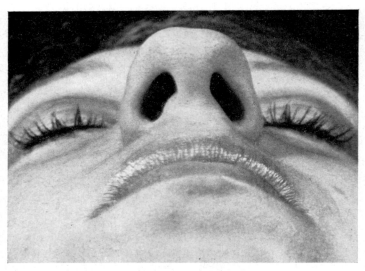

Fig. 7(a)

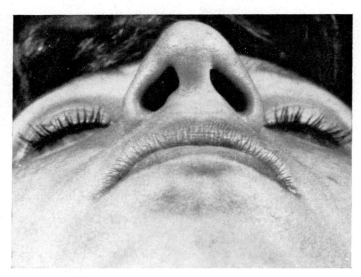

Fig. 7(b).

A more subtle post-operative problem of rhinoplasty is the production of a surgical or "operated" appearance. Techniques to the alae which involve removal of vestibular skin run the risk of postoperative "pinching" and this is the most obvious of these surgical appearances. Alar base resection also runs the risk of producing the postoperative appearance. The suturing of the septal processes (medial parts; formerly medial crura) of the major alar cartilages back-to-back, as advocated by Goldman, while it gives good tip projection may, particularly with thin skin,

rather than too much is the axiom, and the courageou surgeon who "operates his way out of trouble" leaves a result which makes revision surgery almost impossible. A good result should be the aim with rhinoplasty and although the attitude of perfection is advised by Smith (1973) in a reflective article on rhinoplasty, this attitude must be tempered with common sense. Parkes has said that perfection may be the enemy of good in rhinoplasty.

The patient with an unsatisfactory cosmetic result after rhinoplasty is dissatisfied, but if nasal obstruction also

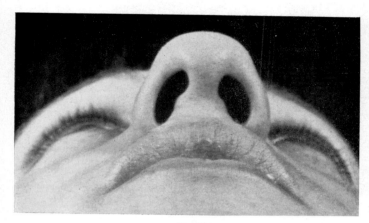

Fig. 7(c)

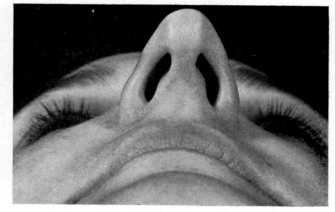
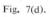

Fig. 7(d).

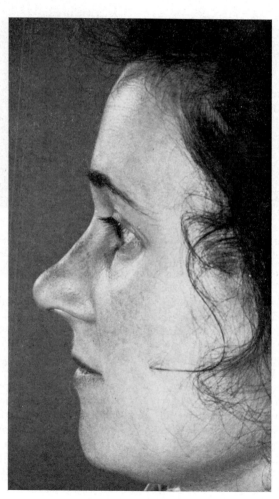

Fig. 7(e).

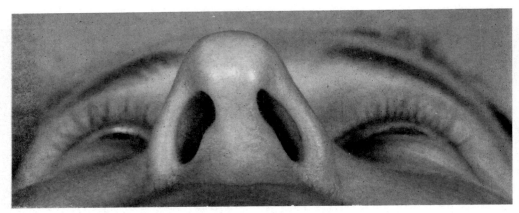

Fig. 7(f).

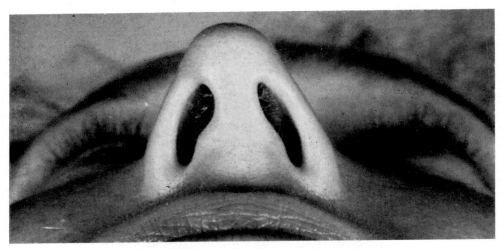

Fig. 7(g).

FIG. 7. A technique used for giving tip projection and dealing with square, or bifid, nasal tips is that advocated by Goldman. Division of the alar cartilages lateral to the dome, with the medial parts being sutured back-to-back, gives a good result as in 7(b) (Pre-op as 7(a)). This tip technique may, however, produce a projecting tip, described as a "tent-pole" deformity, as in 7(d) (Pre-op as 7(c)) and 7(e)(g) (Pre-op as 7(f)).

occurs the dissatisfaction is accentuated. Great care, therefore, is taken that techniques do not compromise the airway (Goldman, 1965). Removal of the hump and infracture of the nasal bones does not affect the airway, as the narrowing does not involve the part of the nose carrying the main airflow (Rees and Wood-Smith, 1973). Stenosis of the valve of the nose is one of the most common causes of nasal obstruction. It may follow a circular stenosis at the site of the intercartilaginous incision and transfixation incision. The lateral nasal cartilages are separated from the septum in a standard rhinoplasty technique but the preservation of the mucous membrane attachment is advised by Anderson to avoid narrowing the vestibule at this point. Too extensive alar base resection may also cause obstruction, and it is probable that radical removal of all of the lateral part of the major alar cartilage in some cases causes indrawing of the lateral wall of the nose on inspiration with nasal obstruction: the "knock-kneed" appearance of the alae is the characteristic appearance of this complication (Fig. 8). Surgical correction of these types of obstruction is difficult and unrewarding so the

primary technique should aim to avoid this complication. Occasionally splints are needed to support the lateral wall of the nose and ensure the integrity of the airway.

AGE IN RHINOPLASTY

Rhinoplasty is commonly requested in the late teenager or young adult. Surgery to the major alar cartilages under the age of 15 should be avoided for it may cause asymmetrical development of the tip. The development of a low cartilaginous hump several months after an initially good rhinoplasty, when the septum continues to grow, is a further problem when operating on the young (Fig. 9). With ageing, along with other facial changes, the nose droops. Surgery of the "mature" nose, as it is euphemistically described (Parkes and Kamer, 1973), is in line with society's emphasis on minimizing the ageing process. Consequently, this is becoming more common; rhinoplasty is not just for the young. The drooping tip is due to a relaxation of the tissue between the columella and the septal cartilage and between the lateral nasal and the

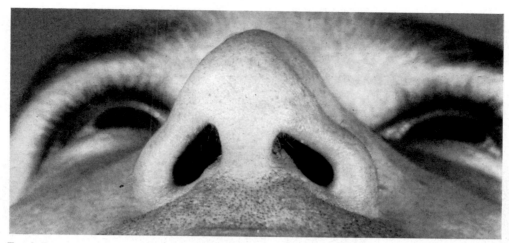

FIG. 8. Excessive removal of the lateral crus has led to alar collapse and the "knock-kneed" appearance. The airway is limited with this deformity.

major alar cartilages, so that the nose appears longer. This type of deformity can be corrected by excision of the cephalic part of the major alar cartilages with rotation of

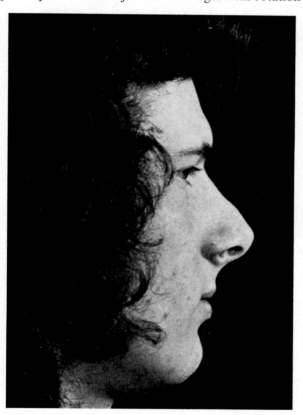

FIG. 9. A rhinoplasty was performed at the age of 16 giving a straight profile to this patient. One year later this cartilaginous hump has developed owing to continued growth of the septum.

the caudal portion. A high transfixation incision where a strut of cartilage remains in the columella is also necessary, along with a suspensory dressing maintained for 12 days postoperatively. These steps ensure that the tissue does not relax at the line of cartilage excision.

THE SELECTION AND PREPARATION OF PATIENTS

Patients unsuitable for rhinoplasty are not always readily detected. The relevant nasal factors, such as thick seborrhoeic skin, and soft frail major alar cartilages, which prejudice a good result, may be obvious, as may observation of associated facial faults such as a receding chin (Fig. 10), or a "crowded" or short upper lip (Fig. 11). The correct assessment, however, of the personality of the patient requesting rhinoplasty is of overall importance.

Most young women with a special complaint about a nasal hump or deviation, have a well adjusted attitude to rhinoplasty but men with an ill-defined non-specific concern about a relatively minor nasal deformity, can, if they are operated upon without psychiatric assessment, develop a major emotional problem. Specialists in rhinoplasty who simply examine the nose and do not think beyond the nasal correction, are certain to operate unwisely in some cases. Patients unsuitable for rhinoplasty do, however, for a variety of reasons, undergo surgery to their own detriment. Ideally, all rhinoplasty patients should have a preliminary psychiatric evaluation, but this is not a practical exercise in most centres and it remains up to the surgeons to learn to make this evaluation. In countries where litigation for malpractice is common the importance of this evaluation to the surgeon is very high.

Preoperative advice to the patient about operation is important, and in the United States of America, extensive handouts are used which, although they may confuse the patient with a surfeit of knowledge, serve to put beyond any medico-legal doubt that the patient has been well informed about the operation and its attendant hazards. Meticulous photographs are now a standard part of rhinoplasty and serve, preoperatively, to demonstrate to the patient the changes that will be made to the nose. The showing of a series of photographs of public figures of recognized good looks and a request for the patient to select their choice of nose is still practised: it is better to avoid this however as it tends to give the patient a misleading idea of what in fact it is possible to achieve with

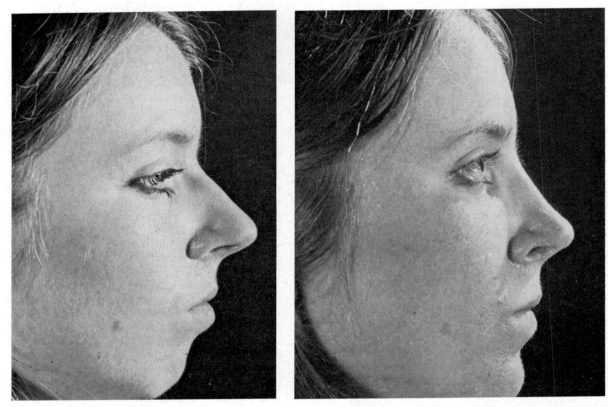

FIG. 10. This girl complains of a prominent nose. A receding chin, however, was also present, necessitating a mentoplasty with a rhinoplasty for a satisfactory result.

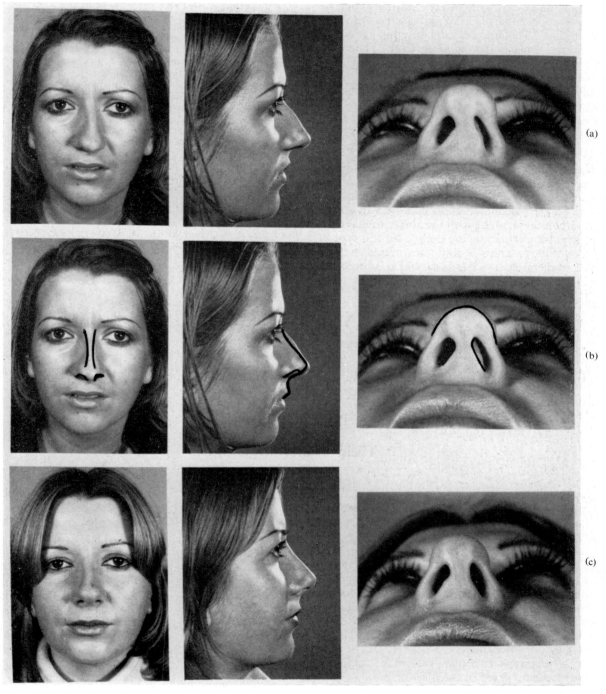

Fig. 11. Drawing (b) on the pre-operative photographs, (a) gives a realistic understanding of the results of rhinoplasty (c). These photographs demonstrate the correction of a nasal hump with deviation to the left of the nasal bones and septum. There is also alteration of the naso-labial angle, with correction of septum and "crowded" upper lip.

their particular nasal structure. Analysis of the face with measurements and grids to demonstrate the different facial proportions, is interesting but, in fact, most rhinoplasty surgeons do not find this analysis of practical benefit to the surgical procedure. The most realistic idea of what can be achieved with rhinoplasty can be given to the patient by reversing the preoperative photographs on an X-ray plate and sketching the changes that will be made (Fig. 11). Good photographs now form an essential part of rhinoplasty, and expert photographic assistance is necessary for preoperative analysis, and postoperative assessment of results.

CONCLUSIONS

Rhinoplasty which aims to improve the appearance of the nose depends on the diagnosis of the cause of the deformity and the application of the correct technique to remedy this. Surgical technique, experience with an artistic flair and common sense, along with the ability to make the relevant psychiatric evaluation, are needed for this type of surgery. Quantitative analysis and measurements have not, as yet, lent themselves to this work which is becoming an increasing part of ear, nose and throat surgery.

REFERENCES

Anderson, J. R. (1971), *Arch. Otolaryng.*, **93**, 284.
Beekhuis, G. J. (1974), *Laryngoscope*, **84**, 2.
Cinelli, J. A. (1966), *Arch. Otolaryng.*, **84**, 520.
Clark, G. M. (1971), *Arch. Otolaryng.*, **93**, 297.
Davis, P. K. B. and Jones, S. M. (1971), *Brit. J. plast. Surg.*, **24**, 405.
Farina, R. and Villano, J. B. (1971), *Plast. reconstr. Surg.*, **48**, 251.
Goldman, I. B. (1965), *Arch. Otolaryng.*, **83**, 151.
Heanley, C. (1973). Personal Communication.
Janeke, J. B. and Wright, W. K. (1971), *Arch. Otolaryng.*, **93**, 458.
Linn, L. and Goldman, J. B. (1949), *Psychosom. Med.*, **11**, 307.
Marquit, B. (1967), *Arch. Otolaryng.*, **85**, 78.
Millard, D. R. (1965), *Plast. reconstr. Surg.*, **36**, 48.
Millard, D. R. (1969), *Plast. reconstr. Surg.*, **44**, 545.
Neuner, O. (1971), *Brit. J. plast. Surg.*, **24**, 375.
Parkes, M. L. and Kamer, F. M. (1973), *Laryngoscope*, **83**, 157.
Rees, T. D. and Wood-Smith, D. (1973), *Cosmetic Facial Surgery.* Philadelphia: Saunders.
Rubin, F. F. (1967), *Arch. Otlaryng.*, **85**, 698.
Rubin, F. F. (1969), *Arch. Otolaryng.*, **89**, 602.
Safian, J. (1970), *Plast. reconstr. Surg.*, **45**, 217.
Sarnat, B. G. and Wexler, M. R. (1967), *Arch. Otolaryng.*, **86**, 463.
Skoog, T. (1966), *Arch. Otolaryng.*, **83**, 283.
Smith, T. W. (1973), *Arch. Otolaryng.*, **97**, 244.
Walter, C. D. (1969), *Arch. Otolaryng.*, **90**, 622.
Wexler, M. R. and Sarnat, B. G. (1961), *Arch. Otolaryng.*, **74**, 305.

67. RECONSTRUCTIVE SURGERY OF THE LARYNX AND LARYNGEAL PART OF PHARYNX:

Experimental Aspects
and
Their Clinical Application

JOSEPH H. OGURA
AND
GERSHON J. SPECTOR

INTRODUCTION

The past decade has seen rapid and far-ranging advances made in the field of reconstructive surgery of the larynx. The main objective has been the preservation or restoration of the airway, phonation and deglutition to a normal or near-normal state. With continued advances ever increasing improvement in voice quality and upper airway competency may be anticipated.

Advances in reconstructive management of laryngeal disorders have been achieved in three areas:

(1) Basic laboratory experiments.
(2) Surgical techniques.
(3) Instrumentation and prostheses.

EXPERIMENTAL ASPECTS OF LARYNGEAL RECONSTRUCTION

Basic laboratory experiments dealing with problems in laryngology have been aimed at two areas. The first is the elucidation of the normal embryology, anatomy and physiology of the larynx; this is described elsewhere in this book. The second is the experimental approach to certain key pathologic problems of the larynx. Some of the pertinent areas will be discussed in this section. Those studies which have been applied clinically will be discussed in the second section.

Neuromuscular Studies

Management of the paralyzed larynx has been a major problem facing the laryngologist. The present methods of clinical management of adductor and abductor vocal fold paralyses are discussed in the clinical portion of this chapter. Experiments in this area have dealt primarily with descriptions of lesions and of vocal fold (cord) position after selective neural sections, neural repair (neurorrhaphy), neural anastomosis to other nerves in the neck region and neuromuscular transplantation.

Galen, in the second century, described the anatomy including the musculature, and demonstrated the neural innervation of the larynx including the communication between the superior laryngeal and the recurrent laryngeal nerves (Galen's "anastomosis"). He also demonstrated that transection of the recurrent nerve resulted in dysphonia. Onodi (1902), and later Lemere (1932), demonstrated the specific neuromuscular innervation of the larynx, showing that the recurrent laryngeal nerve innervated the ipsilateral muscles and half of the transverse arytenoid (interarytenoid) muscle, and that the external laryngeal (external branch of the superior laryngeal) nerve supplied the ipsilateral cricothyroid muscle. Supraglottic sensory innervation was by means of the internal laryngeal (internal branch of the superior laryngeal) nerve. Later Rosenbach (1880), Semon (1881), Wagner (1890), Grossman (1906) and others postulated laws on vocal fold position following neural lesions. Today we support the Wagner–Grossman theory that states that, in the absence of cricoarytenoid joint fixation, an immobile vocal fold in the *paramedian position* is due to *unilateral recurrent nerve paralysis* and an immobile fold in the *intermediate position* has a *combined* recurrent and superior laryngeal paralysis. The paramedian position is assumed because of the adduction effect of the intact cricothyroid muscle. This finding was confirmed by many authors (Arnold, 1957; Dedo, 1970; Clerf, 1940; Evoy, 1960; Frazier and Erb, 1935; Faaborg-Anderson et al., 1960; Kirchner, 1966; Lemere, 1934; Murtagh and Campbell, 1948; Ogura, 1969; Onodi, 1902). The posterior cricoarytenoid is the dilator of the larynx (Arnold, 1961; Tschiassny, 1957). Loss of tension of the vocal fold or curling of the edges has been presumed to be due to superior laryngeal nerve paralysis. This is a debatable concept. Muller (1937), and later Husson (1950), postulated physiologic theories on phonation. Most of this information has been covered in some detail in previous chapters in this book.

Initial use of electromyography of the larynx by Weddell and his associates (1944) provided a possibility to study physiologically the neuromuscular mechanics of the larynx (Ogura et al., 1966; Dedo, 1970; Ueda et al., 1971; Koyama et al., 1969; Siribodhi et al., 1963; Gordon and McCabe, 1968; Takenouchi et al., 1968). Studies using such methods tend to support the hypothesis that partial reinnervation with misdirection of the regrowth of the recurrent laryngeal nerve fibers causes spasm of the vocal folds, thus resulting in little useful functional activity. This is primarily due to indiscriminate (misdirected) reinnervation of both abductors and adductors by the regenerating nerve. Thus all muscles are stimulated synchronously. There is no correlation of vocal fold motion with respiration (Siribodhi et al., 1963). In addition, electromyographic (EMG) studies demonstrated microcurrents in muscular tissue, but EMG cannot predict useful functional activity (Hiroto et al., 1968; Fex, 1970).

Evidence for recurrent nerve regeneration occurring in man has been presented, but its functional character has been questioned (Dedo, 1970; Murakami and Kirchner, 1971) both in total neural resection and in trauma (Blomstedt and Rydmark, 1960). Both Doyle and his colleagues (1967) and Gordon and McCabe (1968) have demonstrated that immediate accurate repair of sectioned recurrent

laryngeal nerve will generally result in recovery of function. Indeed, Blalock and Crowe (1926), Horsley (1909) and Ikeda (1934) have reported successful results following immediate repair. Experiments by Miehlke and his associates (1967), Boles (1966), Mounier-Kuhn (1968) and Lahey and Hoover (1938) have shown limited return of function. No return of function has been reported by Siribodhi and his associates (1963) and by Tomita (1967). Gutmann and Young (1944) have demonstrated end-plate degeneration after long-term denervation. Kirchner (1963) demonstrated progressive muscular atrophy after neural section. These may be factors which mitigate against normal recovery after delayed neurorrhaphy or neural "anastomosis". Although the laryngeal muscles can be reinnervated by repair of the recurrent laryngeal nerve after complete division, the vocal folds do not abduct and continue to act as an obstacle to the airway (Murakami and Kirchner, 1971; Kirchner et al., 1966).

Tashiro and his colleagues (1972) have demonstrated that accurate neurorrhaphy of the recurrent laryngeal nerve after a lapse of more than one year did not produce functional respiratory vocal fold motion. Such motion cannot be expected because of the misdirected reinnervation which is responsible for immobility of the reinnervated vocal fold. It thus appears that immediate neurorrhaphy of lacerated recurrent laryngeal nerves may be of value in surgical reconstruction as an initial attempt for functional reconstruction.

There have been many reports of direct anastomosis of the distal ends of the sectioned recurrent laryngeal nerve to other nerves (Serafini, 1969; Frazier and Erb, 1935; Colledge and Ballance, 1927; Lahey and Hoover, 1938; Miehlke et al., 1967). Direct anastomosis to the vagus nerve was reported by Doyle (1967), by Berendes and Miehlke (1968), by Ballance (1924), by Blalock and Crowe (1926), by Colledge (1925) and by McCall and Hoerr (1946). Anastomosis or implantation of the phrenic nerve has been reported by Barnes and Ballance (1927), by Fex (1970), by Colledge (1925) and by Ormerod (1941). The use of the accessory nerve was reported by Hoessly (1916) and by Ballance (1934). The upper root of the ansa cervicalis (N. descendens hypoglossi) was employed by Colledge and Ballance (1927), Ballance (1924), Frazier and Erb (1935) and by Navratil (1910). However, there was still poor functional restitution despite electromyographic evidence of reinnervation. The usual cause of failure has been misdirected reinnervation: i.e. abductor fibers reinnervating adductor muscles. Thus contraction of adductor muscles during inspiration causes obstruction of the airway [posterior cricoarytenoid muscle contraction during inspiration is nullified as an abductor force (Edwards, 1952)]. Murtagh and Campbell (1948; 1951) and Sunderland and Swaney (1952) have demonstrated the random distribution of nerve fibres in laryngeal nerve trunks which prohibits topognostic surgical repair regardless of the particular nerve selected for grafting or anastamosis (Hoover, 1932; Capps, 1958). Other attempts to circumvent this problem have been proposed. Murakami and Kirchner (1971) proposed the inactivation of adductor muscles by selective denervation within the larynx.

Kirchner (1966) has demonstrated that adductor muscles play only a slight role in respiratory function. Anatomic studies have demonstrated branching of the recurrent motor fibres after the nerve enters the larynx (Dedo, 1970). Amelioration of adduction in vocal fold paralysis has been attempted by Fischer (1952) by transection of the ipsilateral superior laryngeal nerve. Both Freedman (1956) and Tschiassny (1957) have transected the cricothyroid muscle. Tschiassny performed both cricothyrotomy and superior laryngeal denervation. The results have been unpredictable. These latter studies did not provide relief because of the valvular shape of the glottis. The vocal folds are sucked in during inspiration (Bernoulli effect). Fex (1970), describing the posterior cricoarytenoid muscle as respiratory, implanted the phrenic nerve (respiratory nerve) into the paralyzed homolateral muscle in cats. He described a respiratory motion of the vocal folds, abducting on inspiration and adducting on expiration. Similarly, the phrenic nerve has been implanted into the posterior cricoarytenoid muscle in dogs. Vocal fold function synchronous with inspiration was noted.

Muscle transplantation or replantation has been proposed as another method to activate the paralyzed arytenoid. It was considered by King (1939) in his original description of the treatment of adduction of the vocal folds due to bilateral recurrent laryngeal nerve paralysis. He used the cut end of the omohyoid muscle and attached it to the muscular process of the arytenoid cartilage. This proved to be of no real value. Evoy (1960; 1968) employed an external respiratory muscle, the sternothyroid, in sheep and transplanted it to the tendon of the posterior cricoarytenoid muscle. His results were equivocal.

English and Blevins (1969) have demonstrated that the intrinsic laryngeal muscles require almost perfect reinnervation in order to obtain acceptable function. They showed that the thyro-arytenoid, although a single muscle anatomically, comprises three separate entities functionally. Thus simple mass action would perhaps be acceptable for airway protection but would probably not provide a satisfactory voice. In addition, they have studied and mapped out the motor units of the intrinsic muscles of the larynx, and demonstrated a high motor neuron to muscle fibre ratio (the muscles of the middle ear were more richly innervated than those of the larynx). Tucker and Ogura (1971) used these principles to demonstrate a new method of reinnervation of the canine larynx. They used terminal neuromuscular islands and achieved excellent vocal fold function. They further demonstrated histologically that the recurrent laryngeal nerve-muscle pedicle is reinnervated rapidly and achieves good function as soon as the muscle is healed. The terminal cut fibres reinnervated the proper motor units.

Ohyama and his associates (1972) have demonstrated that reinnervated muscles needed greater intensity of indirect stimulation, were more susceptible to cold blockade, had increased sensitivity to suxamethonium chloride (succinylcholine), and had slower repolarization. Supramaximal stimulation of the RLN (recurrent laryngeal nerve) at low frequency failed to abduct the vocal folds in half of the cases and adducted the vocal folds at extremely high frequencies. These findings suggested that the reinnervated laryngeal muscles were supplied by a reduced number of motor fibres which were of smaller size.

Laryngopulmonary Mechanics

Partitioning the total airway system has shed light on the physiology of the larynx as part of the respiratory system. Studies by Wagner (1969), by Taylor (1953), by Ross (1957), by Rauwerda (1946) and by Thews (1967) have demonstrated that the pulmonary gas transport time (larynx to alveolus) involves the interaction of bulk flow and diffusion. They injected a bolus of carbon monoxide translaryngeally and measured photoelectrically the formation of carboxyhemoglobin in the capillaries on the surface of the lung. The rapidity of transit was 0·3 s.

Hyatt and Wilcox (1961; 1963) suggested that the larynx accounts for the greater part of upper airway resistance during mouth breathing. Ogura and his colleagues (1965) demonstrated a higher laryngeal resistance during mouth breathing than during nasal breathing. This was confirmed by Rattenborg (1961) using direct measurements. Ogura demonstrated that, during nasal breathing the larynx was the principal source of resistance in the upper airway. Ferris and his colleagues (1964), Hyatt and Wilcox (1963) and Schiratzki (1964) have all demonstrated that, during inspiration, the upper airway accounts for 55 per cent of the total pulmonary resistance and, during expiration, for 34 per cent. Heyden (1950) and Ogura (1960) indicated only minor changes in respiratory frequency and tidal volume in laryngectomized patients.

O'Neil (1959) reported that loss of vocal fold function secondary to paralysis resulted in decreased maximal breathing capacity and impaired mixing, thus resulting in measurable physiologic deficit of respiratory function. Ogura (1970) demonstrated, in addition, that the expiratory resistance increased with laryngeal obstruction. In experiments on dogs greater turbulence and increased pressure was noted subglottically during expiration. Rattenborg (1961), describing laryngeal respiration, indicated that the resistance of the larynx decreases when the resistance to expiration increased. The pressure drop across the larynx in anesthetized or decerebrate cats demonstrated a greater resistance during inspiration (Campbell et al., 1963). Ogura and his colleagues (1964) demonstrated that the respiratory resistance was greater during inspiration in the normal larynx but was reversed in the post-obstructive state. Hyatt and Wilcox (1963) demonstrated that upper airway resistance during mouth breathing is proportional to lung inflation. Ogura and his colleagues (1965) noted that, in the paralyzed larynx, the subglottic pressure changes in proportion to lung inflation. It would thus appear that the same mechanism governs the movement of the vocal folds during respiration, especially in the expiratory phase.

Ogura and Harvey (1971) reported that the total pulmonary resistance was increased in the presence of upper airway obstruction. They also demonstrated that laryngeal obstruction increases total pulmonary resistance. In the lower airway, the post-obstructional resistance was lower than in the pre-obstruction state. Thus laryngeal obstruction created by transecting both recurrent laryngeal nerves caused an increased mean pulmonary resistance, and increased expiratory and inspiratory resistance, which caused increased retention of pulmonary gases and decreased tidal volumes. Ogura (1971) demonstrated that, in laryngeal obstruction, the tidal volume did not change but both the pulmonary inspiratory and expiratory resistances were higher and that both of Rohrer's factors were elevated due to the narrowed airway. These changes were not noted in the lower airway resistance.

With the rise of total resistance due to laryngeal obstruction, higher values for P_{CO_2} (partial pressure of carbon dioxide) and lower values for P_{O_2} (partial pressure of oxygen) were noted. There were no changes in blood pH. Nadel and Widdicombe (1962) reported that the increased P_{CO_2} and decreased P_{O_2} in dogs with laryngeal obstruction increased the total pulmonary resistance. This was confirmed by Ogura (1971) who noted that CO_2 retention preceded the drop in P_{O_2}.

The study of afferent impulses transmitted as reflexes has also shed some knowledge on the larynx as a respiratory organ. Shimada and Ogura demonstrated that nasal obstruction caused increased pulmonary resistance, vocal fold adduction, increased laryngeal resistance with turbulent air flow, and increased pulmonary resistance with decreased lung compliance. In addition to the well known reflexes of the upper airway of sneezing and coughing, there is smooth muscle contraction of the trachea and bronchi following stimulation of the larynx or nose. Following laryngeal stimulation, Widdicombe (1954) demonstrated bronchospasm with eventual retention of CO_2. Sauerland and Mizuno (1968) and Lindquist and Martensson (1969) noted that afferent impulses transmitted through the hypoglossal nerve set up reflex discharges in the intrinsic laryngeal muscles. This reflex plays some part in swallowing and phonation. Teitelbaum and his associates (1936) elicited a pharyngeal reflex related to swallowing and mediated by the glossopharyngeal nerve. These reflexes may play a role in changing respiration from the nasal to the oral route. In apnea, aerodynamic conditions must be appreciably distorted to create these events. These possible changes of aerodynamics may also be related to the discrepancy of the resistance across the larynx due to different methods of respiration. In the inspiratory phase, the resistance of the laryngeal region is greater during nasal breathing than during mouth breathing. The lower airway resistance is greater during oral breathing than during nasal breathing. These airway resistances are variable and are phasic in nature. Hyatt and Wilcox demonstrated decreased upper airway resistance corresponding to increased lung volume and Widdicombe noted a direct relationship of tracheal volume to lung volume. It has been suggested that receptors for mechanical deformation may be present in the larynx. If that is true, they play an accessory role in respiration since intrinsic laryngeal muscle stimulation causes contraction of tracheal smooth muscle.

Nasal mucosal stimulation produces reflexes which affect the tracheobronchial tree. Dixon and Brodie (1903), Einthoven (1892), Ellis (1938), Kratschmer (1870),

Lasarus (1891), Rall and his colleagues (1945) and Sandmann (1890) have all noted increase in tracheobronchial tree tone following nasal mucosal stimulation. Sercer (1952) and Ogura (1958) have each demonstrated that nasal stimulation results in dilatation of the tracheobronchial tree. Sercer has described a biphasic response: weak stimulation produces constriction and strong stimulation dilatation of the human bronchial muscle. However Tomori and Widdicombe (1969) were unable to confirm this. These authors showed that nasal stimulation caused an increase in respiratory rate, in tidal volume, in intrapleural pressure and in tracheal diameter. Laryngeal stimulation produced constriction of the tracheobronchial muscle. Most other observers have confirmed these findings. If marked tracheal muscle contraction precedes laryngeal stimulation, dilatation may be produced. Widdicombe and Nadel (1963) and Nadel and Widdicombe (1962) postulate that this tonus helps to adjust dead space and airway resistance to optimum values where the mechanical work of breathing is minimal. Widdicombe reviewed the effects of mechanical and chemical stimulation of the larynx by inert dust, cigarette smoke, sulphur dioxide, ammonia, carbon dioxide and hypoxia. These all produced constriction of the tracheobronchial muscle. Bouhuys and van de Woestijne (1971) have demonstrated increased muscle tone and increased airway rigidity, particularly in forced expiration. Laryngeal stimulation results in initial suppression of respiratory activity and decrease in tracheal diameter. Widdicombe and Nadel suggest that laryngeal stimulation is a strong constrictor of the tracheobronchial tree. Thus the tracheobronchial tree gives opposite reactions to nasal and laryngeal stimulation. The tracheobronchial tree is maintained under constant tonus by vagal activity and laryngeal stimulation causing reflex contraction of the tree. This tonus itself depends greatly on the prestimulatory level of vagal tone. The nasal and laryngeal stimulation tend to cancel each other. Stimulation of the afferent laryngeal nerve causes bradycardia, hypotension, decreased respiratory activity, apnea, decreased respiratory rate and decreased tidal volume. It thus appears that the larynx can act as a fine honing device which regulates respiration and modifies the vagal tone of the tracheobronchial system.

One of the major problems in the area of partitioning and measuring the airway is the lack of uniformity in experimental models. This makes interpretation and extrapolation of data very difficult, for example, in determining upper airway resistance at different flow rates. We believe that the time is ripe for the standardization and definition of experimental parameters so that data from many experimenters may be pooled into a meaningful body of knowledge.

Phonation, voice production, neuromuscular activity of the larynx and laryngeal motion in relation to respiration and deglutition have been discussed in other chapters in this book.

Laryngeal Transplantation

Experiments in laryngeal transplantation have demonstrated the feasibility of this procedure from the surgical point of view. Inasmuch as the larynx is not an organ essential to life (in the sense that the heart or liver are) and that current conservative and reconstructive surgical procedures generally result in an adequate voice, it is most important that laryngeal transplantation must be both safe and functional.

Successful transplantation of the larynx requires:

(1) The establishment of an adequate blood supply.
(2) Proper reinnervation of at least one vocal fold after transplantation.
(3) Immunosuppression to prevent host rejection.
(4) Absolute safety of the surgical procedure.

Our initial efforts, performed on anesthetized dogs, were concerned with establishing the minimal blood flow requirements of the isolated larynx. The cranial thyroid artery averages 2·5 mm and the laryngeal artery 0·5 mm in diameter. The average blood flow volume through the larynx is 6·7 ml per minute. The volume passing through the laryngeal artery is 30–40 per cent and the cranial thyroid artery 50–60 per cent of the total. Any one of the four vessels provides sufficient blood supply for survival of the transplanted larynx. The minimal requirements for survival of an isolated canine larynx can be met by 40 per cent or more of the total blood flow. Adequate blood flow to the canine larynx was provided by retaining one or both cranial thyroid arteries (comparable to the lower branches of the superior thyroid arteries in man). These are kept intact as branches of the common carotid arteries which are in turn reanastomosed with those of the host. Using this method, the success rate for reimplanted larynges was 50 per cent (Cassisi et al., 1968). Venous drainage by the cranial laryngeal veins to the external maxillary vein was achieved. Nakayama's eyelet-rivet-clamp technique was the most reliable method of rejoining these vessels.

Carrel first described the circular suture method for vascular anastomosis in 1967. At present, there are more than 60 modifications of this technique. Progress in the field has led to the use of prosthetics and mechanical methods in small vessel anastomosis. Today there are three groups of techniques:

(1) Manual suturing.
(2) Prostheses used alone or combined with suture or tissue adhesives (Payr, 1900; Rohman et al., 1960).
(3) Mechanical anastomosis such as metal clips (Samuels, 1955), staples or rings.

In our experience, anastomotic techniques such as suture, various types of glue, and plastic eyelets were not as successful. If the diameter of the vessel which is to be anastomosed is small (2 mm ± 0·5 mm), thrombosis will occur (e.g. anastomosis of the cranial thyroid artery). Larger vessel anastomosis using the common carotid arteries (4·0 mm ± 0·5 mm diameter) is more successful.

Experiments with allotransplants* in the dog have substantiated our findings. Work and Boles (1965) have outlined the factors which are needed for laryngeal

* See Chapter 50 for terminology on transplants.

replantation in the dog. In one of their dogs the larynx could survive when isolated from its entire blood supply except the superior vascular pedicle. Boles (1966) isolated the larynx from all vessels except the cranial thyroid arteries which he left attached to the common carotids, then he divided and reanastomosed the carotids both proximal and distal to the cranial thyroid arteries. A major problem was thrombosis at the site of anastomosis. Ogura and his colleagues (1966) successfully performed both common carotid and venous anastomosis. Silver and his colleagues (1967) used a similar technique of anastomosis employing common carotid artery and external jugular vein anastomosis in dogs. The transplanted dog larynx was created with bilateral vascular pedicle flaps attached to the common carotid arteries. The attachments of both the cranial thyroid and the laryngeal artery to the larynx were not disturbed. Kluyskens and his associates (1969) sucessfully preserved the superior laryngeal vessels in the first human laryngeal transplantation. Newer methods such as microvascular anastomosis may be of value in the future in order to achieve anastomosis at a more distal level than the carotid artery. Takenouchi and his associates (1967) discussed the technical problems involved in microvascular anastomosis as well as the methods available and their application to laryngeal transplantation. Using immunosuppressive drugs and carotid cranio-thyroid anastomosis, Cassisi and his associates (1968) successfully transplanted the larynx in 13 out of 14 dogs.

Vineberg (1946) has described the use of the internal thoracic (mammary) artery implantation to establish collateral circulation in the ischemic heart muscle. Beck and Leighninger (1954), Sabiston and Blalock (1958), Brewer and Dana (1963) and others have substantiated these findings. More recently Goldsmith (1968) successfully used a revascularization technique in ischemic kidney disease. Schechter and Ogura (1969) demonstrated that carotid artery to perichondrium, and carotid artery to intrinsic laryngeal musculature is not a feasible procedure. However, carotid artery to cricothyroid muscle anastomosis demonstrated new vessel formation and definite revascularization. This method may have limited value in the future.

Physiologic studies on the replanted larynx by Yagi and his colleagues (1966) demonstrated the interrelationship of circulation and innervation. The blood flow volume through the larynx increased gradually with an increase in stimulation frequency of the laryngeal nerves until the stimulation frequency reached 15 Hz. At higher rates, there was a decrease in blood flow volume. Denervation caused an initial rise in blood flow volume (stimulating effect) and then a reduction of blood flow volume through the larynx. The laryngeal nerves are therefore necessary to maintain normal blood circulation of the larynx. This can also be seen by a delay in electromyographic variations in the laryngeal muscles following alterations in blood flow. Thus with complete vascular interruption the muscular action potentials disappear within 30 min. Therefore laryngeal reanastomosis must be done in a short period of time (30–45 min).

The importance of reinnervation of the larynx arises from the interdependence of two factors:

(1) Intrinsic motor control of the transplanted larynx is necessary to protect the airway and proper phonation.
(2) Normal or near normal sensation is needed for proper function during conscious or reflex activity such as deglutition.

Although reinnervation of the allotransplanted larynx ultimately depends on proper control of the rejection phenomena, another factor complicating the picture is the unreliability of reinnervation of the normal larynx. This is true when recurrent laryngeal nerves are sectioned and reanastomosed. Failure to achieve ideal results is attributed to a combination of factors:

(1) Mis-directed regeneration nerve fibres.
(2) Reduction in the number of functional motor units and nerve fibres.
(3) Trophic changes involving the muscle fibres.
(4) Retarded maturation of the neuromuscular junctions.
(5) Disturbances in nerve conductivity.

We have attempted to solve the problem in two ways (neuromuscular island grafts and acceleration of regenerating laryngeal nerves). The intrinsic laryngeal muscles require almost perfect reinnervation in order to achieve acceptable function. This is best achieved by means of neuromuscular island grafts. These methods cause denervation within the intrinsic muscles of the larynx at the level where the nerve is dispersed as individual neurofibrils. Thus regenerating fibres travel only a short distance and exhibit no further branching between the point of transection and the motor unit. A more extensive discussion on this topic is presented in the previous section. Weiss and Hoag (1946) have reported recent improvements in surgical technique.

Many workers have attempted to accelerate the rate of regeneration of nerve fibres (Hoffman, 1952; McCullough, 1959; Davanzo *et al.*, 1963; Harvey *et al.*, 1970). Davanzo and his colleagues have presented evidence that 1, 1, 3-tricyanoallylamine (Tricyanoaminopropene) accelerated peripheral nerve regeneration, and Harvey and his colleagues have studied its effect on the reinnervated canine larynx. Electromyographic recordings demonstrated an average recovery time, based on the appearance of the neuromuscular motor-unit complex (NMU) voltage, of 35 ± 5.2 days (40.0 ± 4.4 days for control group), appearance of normal NMU complex 49 ± 8.5 days (74 ± 7.5 days for control group) and functional restoration in 71 ± 7.8 days (103 ± 16.6 days in control group). Laryngologic examination at 10 months demonstrated better function in the experimental dogs than in the control animals. Experiments confirm that, besides the central effects of this drug, it also facilitates neuromuscular transmission. However, abductor disability was noted in spite of successful adduction function in 5 out of 9 animals.

Alternative technical approaches to the transplantation problem have been employed. Ogura (1958) devised a functioning sphincter or valve using the cricopharyngeal muscle about a collapsible first tracheal ring. Delahunty and his colleagues (1970) and Alonso and Chambers (1970) have described cricoid arch transplants which resorbed on long-term follow-up. Tracheal transplantation has been reported by Alonso and his colleagues (1971), Bailey and Calcaterra (1971) and Greenberg and his colleagues (1962). In all cases, the allografts were unsuccessful owing to extensive resorption, fibrosis and collapse of the transplanted segments. Delahunty and his colleagues (1969) and Cherry and his colleagues (1970) have reported vocal fold transplantation in dogs using the tendinous margin of the fold. They obtained good results over a 2-year interval without the use of immunosuppressive drugs.

Although transplanting a larynx is technically feasible, the suppression of the immune reaction and the rejection phenomenon require further study. The problems of typing and pairing the donor and the recipient by means of lymphocyte typing are unsolved. Russell and Monaco (1964) have summarized the biology of tissue transplantation. The use of antilymphocyte serum has been reviewed by Denman (1969), by Sell (1969) and by Starzl and his associates (1970). Cannulation of the thoracic duct for prolongation of transplant survival in animals and in man has been reported by many authors. Woodruff and Anderson (1963) reported the first use of ALS (antilymphocytic serum) as an immunosuppressive agent in skin rejection. This was combined with chronic cannulation of the thoracic duct for lymphocyte depletion to prolong renal transplant survival (Murray *et al.*, 1968). Mogi (1972) described the long-term results for thoracic duct esopharyngeal shunts for depletion of small lymphocytes Histocompatibility testing has been described by Brünings (1911), by Gibson (1967) and by Starzl and his associates (1970).

Mogi also described our method of preparing antilymphocytic serum and its purification. Anti-dog lymphocyte plasma was made by injecting suspensions of thymic lymphocytes into a horse. The first injection, with Freunds adjuvant, was given subcutaneously and the second intravenously 10 days later. One week later, blood was harvested, plasma separated in acid citrate dextrose and heated to remove complement. The purification of the crude gamma globulins (antibodies) was achieved by salting out with ammonium sulfate. G-200 Sephadex (cross-linked dextran) gel was used for filtration and separating it into 19S and 7S gamma globulins and DEAE cellulose column chromotography was used to further separate the 7S fraction. The IgG (immunoglobulin G) was eluted with phosphate buffer, concentrated and lyophilized. The IgG caused pronounced peripheral blood leukopenia and enhanced skin allograft survival. The immunosuppressive activity of ALS seemed to reside mainly in the IgG fraction.

Ideally, all donor-recipient pairs should be matched preoperatively in regard to histocompatibility of antigens. However, this is not always possible. The use of antiglobulin increases the sensitivity of cell typing techniques. The fluorescent antibody method further increases the sensitivity of the antiglobulin method. We are employing these methods at the present time to develop methods for tissue typing.

ALS activity is greatly prolonged if ALS administration is combined with thoracic duct cannulation or esophageo-duct fistula for peripheral lymphocyte depletion. This reduces a requirement for large quantities of ALS which is difficult to obtain. Suppression is further enhanced by pretreatment of the host with immunosuppressive medic-ation (procarbazine, azathioprine, prednisolone, cactin-omycin etc.)

The immune responses in vitamin deficient rats have been reported. Both pantothenic acid and pyridoxine deficiency prolonged skin graft survival. Harvey has recently demonstrated acceptance of allographic skin grafts between rats raised on diets deficient in certain B complex vitamins (pyridoxine and folic acid). A study is now under way to determine the efficacy of vitamin deficiency in transplantation experiments.

When Kluyskens and his colleagues (1969) transplanted the first human larynx, they were able to control to some extent the rejection reaction by immunosuppressive management. Unfortunately, the patient developed recurrent cancer and died. No further human trans-plantations have been attempted.

CLINICAL ADVANCES IN RECONSTRUCTIVE SURGERY

One of the major advances in the past decade was the clinical application of advanced surgical techniques and a cross-over from the experimental stages of laboratory methods to the practical stage of delivery of health services. This is especially true in the field of laryngology. In this section we would like to highlight some of the prominent clinical advances.

Postlaryngectomy Rehabilitation

Postlaryngectomy: there are three basic aims—to reconstruct the esophagus, to reconstruct the laryngeal part of the pharynx (hypopharynx), and, in certain instances, to construct a shunt by which air can be diverted from the permanent tracheostome to the oral cavity in order to produce intelligible speech, i.e. to construct a tracheoesophageal shunt.

Phonation

The concept of a tracheoesophageal shunt to improve speech in post-laryngectomy patients is old. In 1874, Billroth noted the restoration of a coarse bark in a dog after constructing a tracheopharyngeal communication. Gussenbauer (1874) designed a pharyngostome above a tracheostome, and then used a metal bivalved tube to create a continuous flow of air between the two. Czerny (1870) reported a series of experiments on dogs using tracheopharyngeal shunts to improve the bark. Scuri reported a spontaneous tracheoesopharyngeal fistula in a patient who consequently achieved an excellent voice. In 1959, Briani reported vocal rehabilitation after total laryngectomy. He created a pharyngstome just to the left and below the base of the tongue and connected it with the

tracheal tube by a valved prosthesis. Conley and his colleagues (1958) constructed a tracheoesophageal com-municatiion with a tube of split thickness skin (later vein graft). The voice was serviceable but a high incidence of stenosis occurred. Barton (1965) produced a tracheo-oral communication and used a silicone tube prosthesis implanted from the tracheotomy to the anterior floor of the mouth. It contained a valve to direct air into the mouth. In 1965, Asai presented a three-stage laryngoplasty procedure. In the first stage, a high pharyngostome is created and a second tracheostome made in the anterior tracheal wall below the cut edge of the trachea. Finally, the tracheostome and pharyngostome are connected by a skin-fashioned tube. Asai (1972) has since developed three types of laryngoplasty procedures, all modifications of the original scheme. Miller (1967) reported his success with this procedure, but subsequent events have pointed out some undesirable features. Montgomery and Gamble (1970) have described two types of modifications to this concept. One was the creation of an esophageal tube which is brought out through the anterior neck flap as a eso-phagostome and, later, covered by a skin-lined tube to provide communication with the tracheostome. Another type involved the creation of a valve pharyngostome. In both cases the tracheostome was lengthened and a silicone T-tube was used as a prosthesis. Both Putney and Bagley (1970) and Karlan (1968) have described a two-stage Asai procedure. Calcaterra and Jafek (1971) have described a tracheoesophageal shunt procedure. Kitamura and his associates (1970) found that the best shape for the tube cross-section was elliptical with a diameter of 5 mm. They noted that these shunting tubes have inherent vibratory characteristics which depend on the length, the diameter and the tension of the tube.

The concept of shunting air from the trachea to the oral cavity is sound but a satisfactory method of achieving this has not yet been found. Such shunts may stenose or they may be too large, thus permitting aspiration. Moreover, the voice is not uniformly good Furthermore, plugs of hair and debris may fill the lumen of these skin-lined tubes. The use of implanted foreign materials has also been of no practical value. Methods, such as those of Porres and Mersol (1968), Barton (1965), Briani (1952), De Vincentiis (1956), Czerny (1870) and Gussenbauer (1874), which use artificial material for shunting, do not seem to be acceptable as functional at the present time. Thus, although the concept is simple, implementation with uniformly good results has been unpredictable.

Another direction taken to resolve this problem is surgical reconstruction using a direct anastomotic technique (Hoffman-Sangez, 1951; Majer, 1959). Arslan (1972) and Serafini (1969) performed a series of experiments on dogs and on monkeys in which a total intraperichondrial subhyoid laryngectomy was performed and the upper trachea was anastomosed to the laryngeal part of the pharynx, the epiglottis and the hyoid bone. The method was used in 35 patients. The voice was good, but 70 per cent required tracheotomy tubes and many had prolonged or persistent difficulty with swallowing fluids, or displayed abnormal forms of swallowing. Our experience in 3

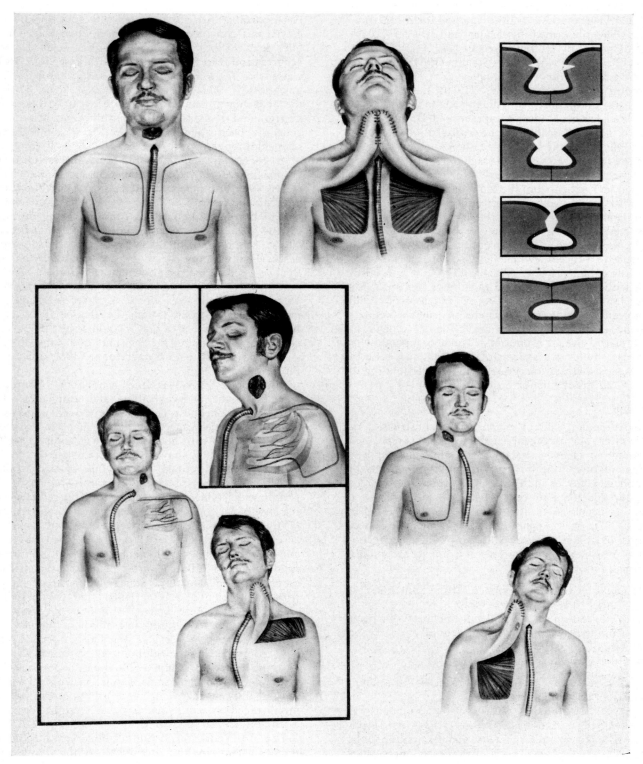

FIG. 1. Bilateral acromiopectoral flaps used to repair large midline pharyngeal fistula. Upper right insert—principle of the two stage technique. Lower left insert—medial based chest flap repair of lateral pharyngeal fistula. Lower right acromiopectoral flap repair of pharyngeal fistula.

patients demonstrated the need for later conversion to standard laryngectomies. Another method for reconstruction has been described by Majer and Rieder (1959) (cricohyoidpexy), by Hoffman-Sangez (1951), by Lapidot and his colleagues (1965) and by Serafini (1969) which are types of direct anastomosis techniques.

Kitamura and his colleagues (1970) described his technique for shunting air from the trachea to the laryngeal part of the pharynx. After a supracricoid laryngectomy using a vertical midline incision, he created a pseudoglottis which originated in the subglottic region and ended in the base of the tongue. In a second stage operation, a dermal tube is used to cover this trough-like region. This was performed in 9 patients but the long-term follow-up is not given. It may be a promising procedure.

In summary, two-thirds of laryngectomized patients can be expected to develop fair to good esophageal voice (Murphy *et al.*, 1964). The remaining third may need a reconstructive procedure. The use of internal (Czerny, 1877; Gussenbauer, 1874; Caselli, 1879; De Vincentiis and DeSantis, 1956) or external prostheses (Briani, 1952; Conley, 1953; Barton, 1965; Porres and Mersol, 1968) has not been satisfactory. Surgical reconstructive methods employing direct anastomosis are generally dangerous because of the risk of aspiration. Tracheoesophageal or pharyngeal shunts are successful in 40–60 per cent of cases. Stenosis, aspiration, poor voice or accumulation of debris or hair are the major problems.

Deglutition

In most patients direct esophageal reconstruction is possible after total laryngeal extirpation. However, when a tumour involves extralaryngeal areas, composite resections involving the laryngeal part of the pharynx or the esophagus may be indicated. The reconstruction of a large pharyngostome or cervical esophagus has been a problem to which much attention has been addressed in the past. The well-prepared surgeon anticipates these problems and plans the procedure so as to make reconstruction possible. There are several available techniques for reconstruction:

    (1) Creation of a neoesophagus from split thickness skin graft stented over a mold.
    (2) Mobilization of regional full thickness skin flaps from the cervical or pectoral region.
    (3) Use of the larynx.
    (4) Intestinal transplants.

In 1877, Czerny first recorded an unsuccessful attempt to reconstruct an esophagus.

The use of skin grafts to reconstruct the esophagus has been attempted in the past. Negus (1938) used split thickness skin over a plastic stent, and then sutured the pharyngeal and esophageal ends of the resection. Conley (1953) modified and popularized this concept. Split thickness skin grafts have been used over plastic, tantalum and stainless steel mesh stents (Edgerton, 1952; Figi, 1950; Klopp *et al.*, 1951). Harris and Tobin (1970) used an Edwards–Topp arterial graft as a stent. They achieved success in 4 out of 8 patients. Rob and Bateman (1949)

reported the use of fascia lata over a tantalum gauze tube. Nechiporuk (1961) experimented with split thickness skin grafts and concluded that this technique had much to offer in noncircumferential defects but delayed stenosis occurred following complete segmental resection. He also stated that the use of lyophilized aortic homografts was unsuccessful. This agrees with our experience. Owing to the frequency of fistula formation, stenosis and poor takes in irradiated tissue, the use of split thickness skin has now generally been abandoned in favour of circumferential segmental replacement.

In 1886, Mikulicz first reported successful cervical esophagus reconstruction using skin flaps. Von Hacker (1908) described a method of creating a skin tube made of cervical pedicle flaps. Evans (1933) reported the first success using this method. A concept Trotter introduced in 1913 was used by Wookey in 1942. In what became a classic technique, he modified the cervical pedicle flap and described a two-stage repair. He used a laterally-based full thickness cervical skin flap which was doubled over itself and sutured to the resected margins. The remaining anterior deformity was closed at a second stage. This procedure had two limitations, i.e. the length of the skin flap and the surface area that it could cover. These can be corrected by planning the incisions and flaps differently (Conley, 1965). Gaisford and Hanna (1962) used a lined thoracic pedicle flap.

Montgomery (1964) designed a polyvinyl chloride tube to connect the pharyngostome and esophagus. Using cervical full thickness flaps, he developed a two-staged procedure to reconstruct the esophagus. He reported 14 successful cases with no postoperative stenosis. Stell and his colleagues (1970) have used medially-based chest flaps. Ogura (1969) described a technique of using bilateral pedicle chest flaps (acromio-pectoral) to repair large pharyngeal fistulae. Using this method, large defects from the base of the tongue to the thoracic inlet can be repaired (Fig. 1). It is a two-stage technique and usually the acromio-pectoral flaps need not be delayed. Marchetta and his associates (1961) reported using full thickness rotational mucosal flaps from the pharynx to reconstruct the esophagus. This technique was not found to be successful with circumferential defects (Harris and Tobin, 1970).

Sisson (1969) described a method to reconstruct the deficit by using two sliding laterally-based cervical flaps. Others have used a cervical skin flap covering a muscle flap from the sternocleidomastoid to cover a pharyngostome defect. Bakamjian (1965) used a combination of pectoral and cervical skin flaps to reconstruct the pharynx. All full thickness skin flap reconstructions are inherently multi-staged procedures and, as such, require creation of a temporary pharyngostome.

Use of the anterior portion of the larynx and the upper trachea as anterior and lateral walls of the absent cervical esophagus segment was originally described by Asherson (1954) for postcricoid carcinoma. Both Som (1959) and Simpson (1960) report similar methods using this laryngo-tracheo-autograft technique. The posterior esophageal wall is covered by split thickness skin and the anterior and lateral walls are composed of the skeletonized larynx together with the upper tracheal rings. Sercer (1959) reported the use of the entire larynx to replace the cervical esophagus. These methods are one-stage techniques, not requiring a pharyngostome, but they are limited to those isolated cases of the postcricoid region when the lesion is in an appropriate resectable position. This operation is not appropriate for cancer of the upper one-third of the esophagus.

Technical advances in small blood vessel anastomosis and the use of the dissecting microscope have made revascularized intestinal autografts possible. Heibert and Cummings (1961) reported successful replacement of cervical esophagus, using revascularized free graft from the pyloric (gastric) antrum. Both Mustard (1960) and Iskeçeli (1962) have reported the use of free jejunal autografts. Nakayama and his associates (1964) modified this technique for free sigmoid colon grafts. In 1907, Roux performed the first successful jejunal replacement. Hyde performed experiments in dogs using revascularized colon as esophageal replacement. He achieved one successful result. Both Iskeçeli (1962) and Stoner and his associates (1972) have described the use of nonrevascularized jejunum and irradiated horse vein for anastomosis, but in all experimental dogs, strictures developed. Kaplan and Markowicz (1964) described the use of full thickness penile skin for replacement of the pharynx and upper esophagus but their good results were not confirmed. Both Bernatz and Hopkins (1963) and Harrison (1964) have reviewed the problems of cervical esophageal replacement.

The use of jejunal and colonic transplants has also been adopted for thoracic esophageal replacement. Hawk (1961) reported a technique, using reversed greater curvature gastric tube, which is attached to the cardia and anastomosed, through a submucosal tunnel, to the laryngeal part of the pharynx. Harrison (1964) reported another gastric anastomosis technique based upon a report by Beck and Carrell (1905). The use of the transposed stomach has also been reported by LeQuesne and Ranger (1966), by Stell and his colleagues (1970), by Leonard and Maran (1970) and by Ong and Lee (1960). Ogura and his associates (1962) reported on a method (von Hacker, 1908) of colon transplantation for total esophageal and pharyngeal reconstruction. Others who have written on this method are Mahoney and Sherman (1954), Petrov (1959), Robertson and Sarjeant (1950), Terracol and Sweet (1958), Burford and his colleagues (1953), Goligher and Robin (1954) and Harrison (1964).

Reconstructive Aspects of Laryngeal Trauma

In the past decade, surgery for laryngeal trauma has made great advances in two areas:

(1) The use and construction of endolaryngeal prostheses (discussed in the next section).
(2) The evolution of new and more comprehensive reconstructive techniques.

The treatment of chronic laryngeal stenosis has a long history. In 1870 Schroetter advocated laryngeal dilatation with hard rubber and tin bolts. The results were poor. O'Dwyer (1897) used intubation tubes. In 1890, Lefferts used metal dilators. Iglauer (1935) used an endoscopically placed rubber tube in the stenosed larynx with the lower end anchored to a tracheotomy tube. Schmiegelow (1929) advocated laryngo-fissure and scar excision, the use of a rubber stent, primary closure and tracheotomy. Arbuckle (1930) used the latter method but grafted the denuded endolarynx with a Thiersch graft, stented by sponge rubber. LeJeune and Owens (1935) used Arbuckle's method and plaster splints to prevent secondary stenosis. Negus (1938) also employed this technique. In 1936, Jackson advocated endoscopic scar excision and the use of graduated rubber core molds, laryngeal dilators. This was not an adequate procedure. In 1938, Looper advised hyoid bone grafts to the thyroid cartilage to widen the larynx in cases of marked laryngeal cartilage loss. Bennett (1960) reported a hyoid graft to cricoid cartilage. Both Erich (1945) and Figi (1947) used skin grafting and a postoperative endolaryngeal obturator to prevent stenosis. In 1950, McNaught introduced the tantalum keel for anterior web stenosis. In 1950, Woodward combined the thyrotomy approach for submucosal excision of scar with a Looper hyoid graft technique, and closed the incision over an acrylic mold. The submucosal scar excision eliminated the need for skin grafting. Holinger and his colleagues (1968), Poe and Seager (1948) and later Alonso and his colleagues (1971) advocated the endolaryngeal approach for anterior webs, using small metal splints with externally placed passing sutures. In 1962, Ogura and Roper described transhyoid pharyngotomy, resection of massive scar tissue and primary closure over a stent. This was essentially a supraglottic laryngectomy for external laryngeal trauma with primary anastomosis.

In the management of acute laryngeal injuries, the basic principle is early restoration of the injured parts to as nearly normal a position as possible and to splint them in a position of function. The best results have been obtained by early (6–8 days) management (Holinger et al., 1968; Shumrick, 1967; Fitz-Hugh and his colleagues, 1962; Ogura and his associates, 1969). The mucosal lacerations are repaired. If mucosa is missing, split thickness skin grafts are used. Cartilage fragments are realigned and sutured (32 gauge wire) in proper alignment. Generally, the arytenoid cartilage, if subluxated, is repositioned on the cricoid and preserved. Any laceration of the vocal folds is repaired and the vocal ligaments are realigned in proper position. In most cases stenting is required. In cases of acute soft tissue injuries without cartilage displacement (manifest as haemorrhage and ecchymosis of the aryepiglottic folds), both the vestibular (false cords) and vocal folds are observed and not treated surgically. Acute midline vertical thyroid fractures may be treated by insertion of a McNaught keel. If the base of the epiglottis is subluxated posteriorly, it may be resected and sutured forward (Ogura, 1971). Glottic fractures which involve depression and communications through the lamina (ala) of the thyroid cartilage, laceration of the vocal ligaments or associated cricoid fractures are repaired and realigned over a stent. Wire (32 gauge) is used to align the cartilage and 4–0 chromic gut to repair the mucosal laceration. In subglottic cricotracheal injuries the fragments are realigned and sutured with fine braided wire over a stent. In tracheal avulsion or separation, it is often necessary to elevate the retracted trachea from the superior mediastinum and anastomose it to the fractured larynx over a Portex stent (Chodosh, 1968). The recurrent laryngeal nerves, if lacerated, should be exposed and reanastomosed as soon as possible.

In minimal supraglottic injuries, the subluxated epiglottis may be sutured back to its normal position (Montgomery, 1966) or its base resected (Ogura, 1969). In most cases, anterior commissure involvement requires the use of a keel. However, most supraglottic injuries are extensive with depression of the thyroid notch and thyroid cartilage posteriorly, and are associated with a pharyngo-laryngeal fistula and sepsis. The stenosis involves both the vestibular folds and the aryepiglottic folds. Generally this requires anterior pharyngotomy and removal of the epiglottis, aryepiglottic folds and the vestibular folds. The mucosal lacerations are repaired with 4–0 chromic gut sutures, the arytenoids are replaced on the cricoid cartilage and the depressed thyroid cartilage fragments elevated into position and wired in place (Ogura, 1965). In all restorations preliminary tracheotomy is indicated (Fig. 2).

The treatment of chronic combined laryngeal and tracheal stenosis is more complicated and the results are not as predictable (Priest et al., 1967; Pennington, 1972; Chodosh, 1968; Middleton, 1966; Ogura et al., 1968; Curtin et al., 1966; Harris and Tobin, 1970; Shumrick, 1967; Holinger et al., 1968; Miles et al., 1971). Chronic supraglottic stenosis may be anterior, posterior or circumferential. The latter is usually associated with injury to the laryngeal part of the pharynx and the recognition of the glottic level may be extremely difficult since, in most instances, the vocal fold and the laryngeal ventricle have been fused by scar tissue. Usually there is superior and posterior displacement of the upper part of the thyroid cartilage. The anterior stenosis can be handled by the method of Montgomery by resection of the base of the epiglottis with V–Y closure of the endolaryngeal mucosa to the perichondrium. Posterior inlet stenosis can be resected submucosally in the interarytenoid space (window shade method described by Montgomery and Gamble, 1970). One arytenoid cartilage may be resected (Hoover, 1953; Knight, 1964; King, 1939; Scheer, 1953) or pinned (Montgomery, 1963). However, the majority of lesions are circumferential and involve the laryngeal part of the pharynx. These are best handled by a supraglottic resection with direct anastomosis (Ogura et al., 1966). If the vocal folds move, a midline thyrotomy is made and a McNaught keel inserted. If both vocal folds are paretic, a unilateral translaryngeal arytenoidectomy is performed (Hoover, 1953) and a stent is inserted (Woodman, 1955; Ogura, 1962). If the anteroposterior diameter of the glottis is fore-shortened, an excellent procedure is the use of the hyoid bone graft over the sternohyoid muscle. The endolaryngeal surface is lined with split thickness skin or mucosal graft [taken from the mouth or the undersurface of the epiglottis (Looper, 1938; Ogura, 1958)]. Stenoses involving both the laryngeal part of pharynx and the supraglottic region are repaired by a supraglottic laryn-

gectomy with end to end pharyngeal anastomosis (Ogura, 1961).

Glottic stenosis may be anterior, posterior or complete. Anterior stenosis is managed by midline thyrotomy and resection of the scar, followed by insertion of a McNaught keel. Posterior stenosis is approached through a midline incision and excised submucosally (Woodman, 1955). Arytenoidectomy is often necessary in fixation of the vocal folds. If mucosal flaps are inadequate, skin grafting is employed. In most cases stents are used. Total glottic stenosis require excision of the scar, submucosally if possible, and the use of a stent. Most often a Schmiegelow procedure with resection of scar and skin grafting is undertaken.

Chronic subglottic stenosis may be high or low. With high lesions, scar resection, skin grafting and stents are used. In low lesions, T-tubes (Montgomery and Gamble, 1970) or Portex tubes (Ogura, 1971) are employed. The scar can occasionally be excised and grafted over by split thickness skin. Ogura (1969) described a method of resection of cricoid cartilage with the first tracheal ring followed by a laryngotracheal end to end anastomosis. Similar methods are described by Conley (1965), by Shaw and his colleagues (1961) and by Rush (1961). Tracheal elongation techniques can increase the length of the resectable areas of stenoses (Grillo, 1965; Pressman and Simon, 1959).

Occasionally, unilateral vocal fold paralysis may follow laryngeal trauma, and is due to compression of the recurrent laryngeal nerve by the inferior laryngeal cornu. Decompression of the nerve by resection of a portion of the lamina of the thyroid cartilage and inferior cornu may improve chances for vocal fold movement (Ogura, 1970).

Cervical Trachea Reconstruction

Reconstruction of a stenosis or complete loss of a segment of the cervical trachea has always been a problem. Tracheal damage due to cuffed endotracheal tubes has been described by numerous observers (Aboulker et al., 1960; Flege, 1967; Foley et al., 1968; Gibson, 1967; Friedberg et al., 1965; Pearson et al., 1968; Grillo, 1966; Stiles, 1965; Watts, 1963; Yanagisawa and Kirchner, 1964). Looper (1938) and Pearson and his colleagues (1968) described the evolution of tracheal injuries secondary to ventilating assistance through a cuffed tube, and Florange and his colleagues (1965) and Cooper and his colleagues (1969) described the pathology. Tracheal injuries secondary to tracheostomy have been described by Bignon and Chretien (1962) and Stiles (1965). Injuries to the cervical trachea secondary to blunt trauma (Ogura and Dedo, 1965; Montgomery, 1964) or resection for malignancies (Sisson, 1969; Grillo, 1966) have been described by many authors.

Many methods for cervical trachea reconstruction have been employed. In 1881, Gluck and Zeller performed the first tracheal transection and reanastomosis, and in 1884 Kuester performed the first circumferential radical resection and anastomosis in a human. Thus far, there is no consistently satisfactory method for replacement of a

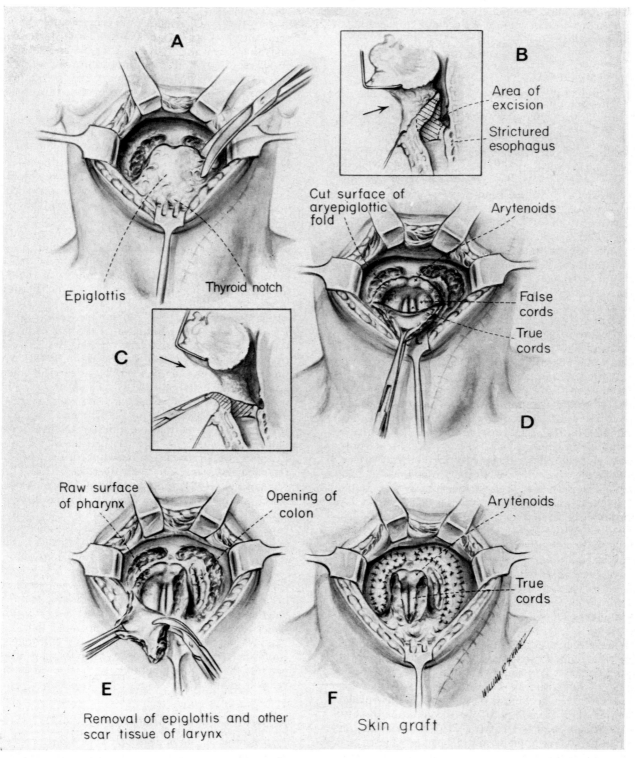

A

B

Area of excision

Strictured esophagus

Epiglottis   Thyroid notch

Cut surface of aryepiglottic fold

Arytenoids

C

False cords

True cords

D

Raw surface of pharynx

Opening of colon

Arytenoids

True cords

E

Removal of epiglottis and other scar tissue of larynx

F

Skin graft

WILLIAM P. X. MINK

FIG. 2. Chronic traumatic supraglottic stenosis. Repaired by means of a supraglottic resection and skin grafting. An important point is to identify the glottis prior to definitive resection and grafting, note D.

resected length of cervical trachea. Successful reconstruction should result in an adequately functioning larynx and tracheobronchial system without the use of a tracheotomy. It should provide:

(1) Lateral rigidity.
(2) Longitudinal elasticity.
(3) Adequate lumen.
(4) Air tight closure.
(5) Lining with ciliated columnar epithelium (Belsey, 1950).

Use of foreign materials has been adequately explored. Although some reports show a favourable trend (Miglets, 1971; Beall *et al.*, 1960), the results have not been consistently satisfactory. These rigid implants easily produce pressure necrosis with cervical motion, and eventually extrude (McCall and Hoerr, 1946; Montgomery, 1964; Miglets, 1968). Metallic mesh cylinders and plastic replacements have included stainless steel (Paulson, 1951), Nobilium (Harkins, 1952), Vitallium (Kay, 1951), tantalum, gelatin sponge (Bailey, 1966), polyethylene (Beall *et al.*, 1963; Miglets, 1968), polyethylene terephthalate, polyvinyl alcohol, Tygoflex (Moncrief and Salvatore, 1958) and Tylon. (Bailey used a variety of materials experimentally in dogs without success.) Animal experiments have demonstrated that tracheal allografts, lyophilized tracheal allografts and autografts do not survive (Greenberg *et al.*, 1962). However, autogenous bone and cartilage grafts have been successfully employed by Bryce and his colleagues (1963) and Montgomery (1964). Miglets (1968) attempted to create autogenous polyethylene tracheal grafts and noted a high incidence of stenosis. In some cases this could be ameliorated by large doses of steroids. Montgomery (1966) described a new method for cervical tracheal reconstruction. A trough, lined with split thickness skin graft, was used to form the posterior and lateral tracheal walls. A horizontal cervical pedicle flap fashioned on itself (trap door) and supported by strips of rib cartilage formed the anterior tracheal wall. A specially designed T-tube acrylic stent was used to maintain an airway. Alonso and his colleagues (1971) demonstrated the use of small tracheal allografts to reconstruct the anterior wall in dogs. In eight months these were resorbed and a flaccid fibrous membrane was formed. Transplantation of the total cervical trachea was unsuccessful (Greenberg, 1960).

There have been other reports of tracheal reconstruction utilizing autogenous cartilage, split thickness skin grafts and full thickness skin flaps (Fairchild, 1927; Serrano *et al.*, 1959; Edgerton, 1952). Grillo and his colleagues (1963) described a technique employing polypropylene rings buried in a skin flap to provide anterior-tracheal support. Bailey and Calcaterra (1971) reviewed the experience with development of tracheal prostheses and demonstrated experimentally that, at the present time, there is no suitable prosthesis for the reconstruction of extensive defects of the cervical trachea.

Another line of approach to this problem has been the development of a wide variety of tracheal lengthening procedures in order to maximize the length of trachea which can be resected and followed by direct end to end reanastomosis. Excessive tension on the line of anastomosis is the principal cause of failure (re-stricture or wound dehiscence). Cantrell and Folse (1961) demonstrated in dogs that a tension of less than 12 N (equivalent to 1200 gm) is required. Tension on the suture line of 22 N (2200 gm) results in re-stenosis. Primary end to end anstomosis is today recognized to be the best method of reconstruction of the trachea. Ogura and his colleagues (1962) demonstrated a method of cricoid resection with direct laryngotracheal anastomosis. Conley (1960) described a method for direct anastomosis of small subglottic defects. Dedo and Ogura (1965) described a method for sleeve resection of the tracheal stenotic segment, mobilization of the larynx by release from its hyoid and supraglottic attachment, and primary anastomosis. In all these methods only 2–4 cm of cervical trachea can be resected.

Grillo (1965), in a series of anatomical and animal experiment, has demonstrated that over half (5·7–6·4 cm) of the trachea may be resected and direct anastomosis performed. To achieve this amount of lengthening, mobilization of the right pulmonary hilum, division of the inferior pulmonary ligament (3·0 cm or 5·9 rings) intrapericardial dissection of pulmonary vessels (0·9 cm or 1·6 rings) and re-implantation of the left main bronchus into the trachea or bronchus intermedium (2·7 cm or 5·5 rings) was necessary (Rob and Bateman, 1949). Mobilization of the larynx or division of the cervical trachea can also increase length (2–3 cm). These observations have been supported by Michelson and his colleagues (1961) by Ferguson and his colleagues (1950) and by Kay (1951). Belsey (1950) stated that the limits of tracheal resection in man is 3–4 rings. On the basis of his elasticity studies, Ferguson stated that up to one-third of the trachea can be removed and reanastomosed with success. MacManus and McCormick (1954) emphasized tracheal mobilization in resections of lesions over 3 cm in length. Juvenelle and Citret (1951) proposed re-implantation of the main bronchi to facilitate resection. Barclay and his colleagues (1957) and Archer and his colleagues (1963) successfully performed extended resections and re-implantation of the left main stem bronchus, lengthening the trachea by 5–6 cm. Cantrell and Folse (1961) emphasized the loss of elasticity in aged individuals which mitigates against extensive lengthening manoeuvres. In patients more than 60 years old, circumferential resection of no more than two rings may be possible. Michelson and his colleagues (1961) confirmed these findings and stated that, in 50-year-old patients, half as much mobility was achieved as in 30–50-year-old patients.

Conservation Surgery of the Larynx

In a sense, laryngologists have always been conservationists in their attempts to save the respiratory and phonatory function of the larynx. In fact, the earliest procedures on the larynx were partial laryngeal resections. The first laryngofissure was performed for papillomata in 1833 by Brauers and in 1851 for cancer by Buck. Solis-Cohen (1907) developed subperichondral dissection and Gluck and Sorensen (1912) performed the first hemilaryngectomy. It was later revived by Som. Both Ogura (1958) and Som (1959) also demonstrated a partial supraglottic technique for epiglottic carcinoma. Trotter described lateral pharyngotomy in 1920. The anterior commissure resection for cancer was described by Jackson in 1922, window resection by Patterson in 1932 and wedge resection by Clerf in 1940. Bilateral thyrotomy was demonstrated by Kemler in 1947.

In the late 1940's a rebirth in conservation surgery occurred. Both Alonso and Ogura have demonstrated that, in selected cases, the glottis could be spared. The rationale was that the supraglottic larynx is derived separately from the glottis and subglottic larynx. The former is a derivative of the pharynx and the latter of the tracheobronchial complex. As a result these have two different and separate lymphatic systems. The supraglottis drains superiorly through the thyrohyoid membrane, while the glottic and subglottic region drains inferiorly through the esophagotracheal compartment into the lateral neck. Thus supraglottic resection is feasible without sacrificing the glottis. The pre-epiglottic space containing the superior network of lymphatics must be removed. Since most tumours are moderately well differentiated and slow in developing, they can be resected with narrow margins. Thus in 1947 Alonso introduced partial horizontal and partial vertical laryngectomy. This technique was a two-stage method, creating a pharyngostome initially and closing it several months later. In 1958 Ogura described supraglottic subtotal laryngectomy as a one-stage operation. In 1956 Leroux-Robert devised the frontolateral and frontoanterior laryngectomy and Norris in 1958 the extended frontolateral laryngectomy. In 1963, the Piquets described a modified partial vertical laryngectomy. Pressman (1954) and later Bailey (1966), described the laryngoplasty procedures.

Today, conservation surgery in selected cases of glottic, supraglottic, pyriform sinus, laryngeal part of pharynx and base of tongue lesions can be performed without compromising survival. The remaining postoperative laryngeal anatomy is adequate for normal physiological function. Approximately 60–70 per cent of all cancers seen in our centre can be treated in this fashion. Precise preoperative evaluation of the lesion, thorough knowledge of the surgical techniques, and understanding of rehabilitative physiology are necessary for consistent success. The methods described below may all be combined with *en bloc* radical neck dissection.

Resection of glottic lesions can be accomplished by a hemilaryngectomy, anterior commissure resection, or a frontolateral partial laryngectomy. These are subperichondral resections and are followed by immediate reconstruction. In the two latter cases a McNaught keel is needed. If the arytenoid is to be removed, the glottis is reconstructed by a variety of procedures, the most common of which is a pedicled muscular graft using thyrohyoid, or omohyoid muscles (Ogura *et al.*, 1962). On occasion, a Meurman (1952) procedure employing cartilage grafts may be indicated. This is applicable to those cases with glottic incompetence either after supraglottic or partial

laryngopharyngectomy or after extended hemilaryngectomy with total arytenoid removal (Fig. 3).

When the supraglottis needs to be resected for laryngeal stenosis or a tumour of the epiglottis, aryepiglottic folds or vestibular folds, a supraglottic subtotal laryngectomy is performed (Ogura, 1961). The procedure may be extended on one side to include the arytenoid cartilage. Thyroid cartilage invasion is a contraindication for this conservation surgery. At least one normal functional arytenoid and vocal fold must be present. The perichondrium of the thyroid cartilage is preserved, a portion of the thyroid cartilage and the supraglottic region (including the hyoid bone) is resected including an *en bloc* neck dissection. Primary hypopharyngeal perichondrial anastomosis is then performed, including a cricopharyngeal myotomy (Fig. 4) (Ogura and Powers, 1964). Midline glottic fixation is necessary if the arytenoid is totally resected. This must be anticipated and planned for prior to surgery. It can be achieved in a variety of ways. The vocal fold may be fixed in the midline to the cricoid cartilage. The involved vocal fold may be adducted in a variety of ways: muscle flaps (Ogura *et al.*, 1966) and cartilage (Meurman, 1952). An excellent method of reconstructing a resected vocal fold is achieved by the use of infractured thyroid cartilage lamina (pedicled on the internal perichondrium) forming a new fold (Ogura *et al.*, 1966). This cartilage is later covered by a piriform mucosal flap. The latter technique is most useful in the three-quarter laryngectomy, the most extensive conservation glottic procedure (Fig. 5).

For tumours involving the superior hypopharynx, base of tongue (posterior to vallate papillae), and vallecula, an extended supraglottic subtotal laryngectomy is performed. In these cases mucosal approximation may not be possible, but perichondrium to the anterior base of tongue closure is accomplished.

For lesions involving the piriform fossa, a partial laryngopharyngectomy is performed. This is not applicable to lesions involving the piriform apex, invading cartilage, extending beyond the laryngeal part of the pharynx, or involving the glottis or subglottic larynx. Lesions involving and extending beyond the paralaryngeal space are excluded from this procedure. An oblique cartilage incision is made and the piriform with the aryepiglottic fold and arytenoid is removed. Usually split thickness skin over a bipedicled scalene muscle flap is used to reconstruct the lateral pharyngeal wall (Ogura *et al.*, 1968). Primary closure anastomosis is performed at the time of resection. It is stressed that there is no mucosa to mucosa closure. For tumours of the hypopharynx a partial pharyngectomy can be performed through the same approach. Reconstruction is achieved with split thickness skin grafts over prevertebral muscle flaps. A Negus stent is employed to prevent stenosis and lateralization of the graft (Fig. 6).

The principles of conservation surgery demand that it be precision surgery. It is essential that the superior, inferior and lateral extent of the lesion be related to the glottis and that the glottis be visualized at all times. The initial indirect and direct laryngoscopy, as well as laryngograms, should be related to the maximal excision which is consistent with a functional repair. The basis for

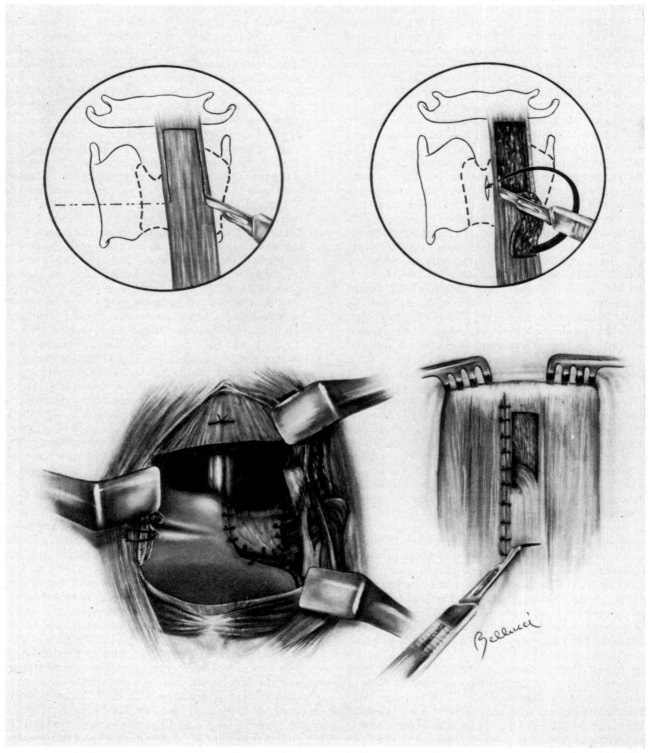

Fig. 3. Reconstruction following three-quarter frontolateral hemilaryngectomy with removal of the involved arytenoid. The repair employs an inferior based muscle flap from the overlying strap muscles to increase glottic bulk. The opposite vocal and vestibular folds are sutured to the perichondrium to reconstitute the new anterior commissure. The muscle flap may be lengthened or released (lower right corner).

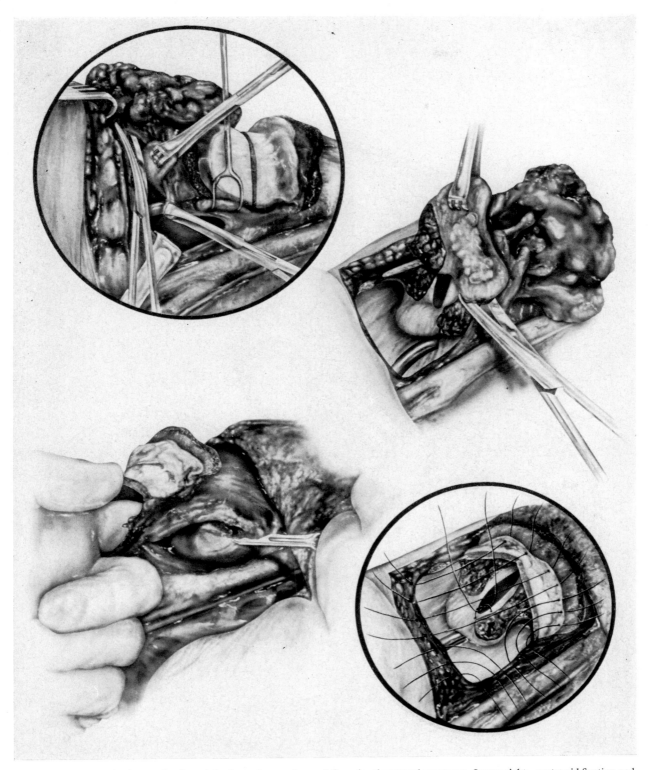

FIG. 4. Classic supraglottic resection for epiglottic carcinoma. Lower left—cricopharyngeal myotomy. Lower right—arytenoid fixation and perichondrial hypopharyngeal anastomosis.

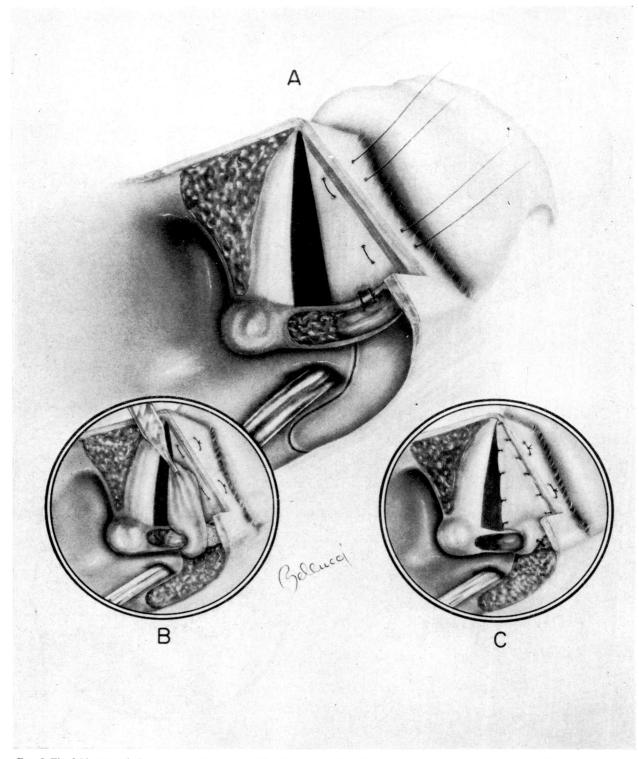

FIG. 5. The fold over technique to reconstitute the glottis. Thyroid cartilage based on the internal perichondrium is trimmed, infractured, and sutured in place (A). Piriform mucosa is used to cover the folded cartilage (B and C).

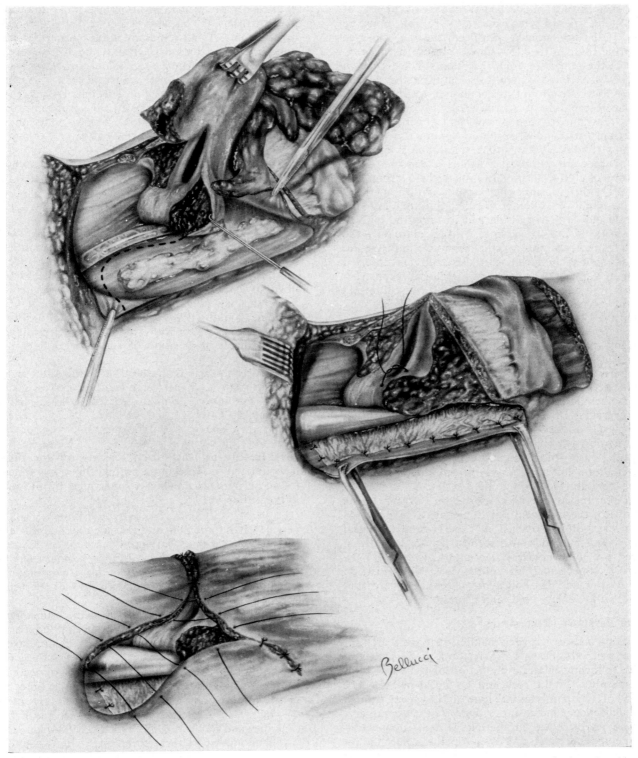

Fɪɢ. 6. Partial laryngopharyngectomy for a piriform fossa carcinoma. Top—resection of lesion. Middle—lining of prevertebral muscles with split thickness skin to reconstitute the hypopharynx. Bottom—closure with interrupted silk sutures.

rehabilitation depends upon adequate water tight glottic closure. This must be re-checked at the time of surgery. If the arytenoids are not removed, both vocal folds must be mobile. If the arytenoid is sacrificed, the fold must be fixed in the midline to allow glottic closure by approximation of the remaining fold. Fixation is achieved by a variety of ways, most generally by suturing the severed posterior fold margin (in the midline) to the cricoid cartilage. If the fold is sacrificed, a thyroid cartilage infolding procedure to form a new fold is instituted. Poor glottic reconstruction will result in continual aspiration and poor phonation. At this time, anesthesia is lightened be removal of all paralyzing agents to assure direct observation of glottic closure. In spite of these techniques, if delayed glottic insufficiency results, other methods should be employed. Politef (Teflon) injection into the fixed abducted cord will displace it towards the midline (Lewy, 1964). If, due to scarring, this procedure fails, the larynx is re-explored and a pedicled muscle flap (Ogura, 1970) or subperichondrial cartilage graft is inserted (Meurman, 1952). Other methods for glottic reconstruction have been advocated (Conley, 1960). Musculoplasty has been accomplished with bi-pedicled (Bailey and Calcaterra, 1971), uni-pedicled (Ogura, 1971) and transposed, muscle flaps. Free muscle grafts (Quinn, 1969) have been used. Coverage of the muscle with mucosal and skin flaps (Ogura et al., 1968 and Quinn, 1969) and perichondrium (Bailey and Kosoy, 1970) has been advised.

The incidence of complications in conservation surgery (excluding hemilaryngectomy in which they are extremely small) averages 18 per cent, with fistulae formation accounting for about 9 per cent, aspiration, 6·6 per cent, and airway obstruction, 0·8 per cent. With carcinoma, the success of conservation surgery with radiation is comparable to total laryngectomy with radiotherapy and is superior to total irradiation alone.

An important aspect of conservation surgery is the knowledge of the laryngeal function that it has provided and the vistas it has opened in experimental laryngeal surgery. New methods for reconstruction have been described by Quinn (1969), Bailey and Calcaterra (1971), Som (1970), Bocca and his colleagues (1967), Harrison (1964), Maran and his colleagues (1968), Leonard and Maran (1970), Conley (1965) and Ogura (1969).

Abductor Paralysis—Reconstruction

Increasing interest has been manifested in the search for the best method of achieving restoration of laryngeal function following bilateral abduction of the vocal folds due to paralysis of the recurrent laryngeal nerves. The majority of the paralyses are due to laryngeal trauma (whose incidence is increasing); thyroid or chest surgery; prolonged endotracheal intubation with assisted ventilation; neurogenic causes; or are idiopathic. Neel and his colleagues (1972), Huppler and his colleagues (1955) and Gorman and Woodward (1965) have classified the etiologic causes: approximately 76 per cent were secondary to thyroid surgery, 6 per cent were idiopathic, 6 per cent neurogenic, and 1 per cent traumatic.

The problem is essentially due to an inverse relationship between airway patency and good phonation. If the vocal folds are in the median position bilaterally, the voice may be good but the airway is poor; usually requiring a tracheotomy. If both folds are in the paramedian position, the patient can breath freely but the voice is weak and usually breathy. There are various gradations of these positions and functional consequences. The greatest problem is maintenance of an adequate airway, especially on exertion. The true reconstruction problem is to create an adequate airway and to maintain good phonation. This has been attained in various ways:

(1) Neural repair (neurorrhaphy) or anastomosis.
(2) Intralaryngeal techniques.
(3) Extralaryngeal techniques.
(4) Endoscopic methods.

In 1909, Horsley described complete return of vocal fold function following neurorrhaphy three months after gunshot trauma to the nerve. Lahey (1928) described similar results. Recent experiments in this field have been made by Doyle and his colleagues (1967), Miehlke and his colleagues (1967), Gordon and McCabe (1968) and Mounier-Kuhn (1968). Vocal fold functions were investigated by electrical stimulation, electromyograms and/or direct observation of active vocal fold measurements.

Reports on various anastomoses of the distal segment of the recurrent laryngeal nerve to other nerves in the neck region are fairly common (Serafini, 1969; Frazier and Erb, 1935; Colledge and Ballance, 1927; Doyle et al., 1967; Miehlke et al., 1967). Results are of dubious functional success.

There are at least seven reasons for the difficulties encountered in achieving a normal functional innervation of those muscles previously innervated by the recurrent laryngeal nerve:

(1) It is quite difficult to isolate and find the lacerated ends of a recurrent laryngeal nerve in scar tissue.

(2) Denervated muscle can be reinnervated by any motor nerve with no proclivity to its function or related to its behaviour (Weiss and Hoag, 1946; Bernstein and Guth, 1961).

(3) The recurrent laryngeal nerve innervates four different muscles and the posterior cricoarytenoid muscle is antagonistic to the others; i.e. it relaxes when the other three contract (Fex, 1970). For these reasons, the nerve axons following regeneration or nerve anastomosis will, at random, reinnervate muscle fibres belonging to abducting and adducting muscles (Hiroto et al., 1968). This clinical experience (Frazier and Erb, 1935; Lahey and Hoover, 1938; Ballance, 1934) has led to the abandonment of these techniques. It was noted that, after neurorrhaphy or anastomosis, spasticity of the vocal folds was present, presumably due to dual innervation of antagonistic muscles.

(4) Anastomosis over a long distance after nerve trauma, although technically not difficult to obtain, is associated with a high incidence of failure due to

formation of traumatic neuromas and improper nerve conduction.

(5) Longstanding vocal fold paralysis is associated with muscular degeneration, reduction of number of nerve fibres, and reduction in the number of motor end plates (Kirchner, 1963).

(6) Arthrodesis of the cricoarytenoid joint with arytenoid fixation is frequent in longstanding vocal fold paralysis (Montgomery, 1968).

(7) Synchronization of vocal fold motion to the respiratory cycle and deglutition is disturbed. Experimentally some of these problems and their solutions have been explored, and are described in the previous section.

Endoscopic techniques have focused on various areas of investigation:

(1) Lateral fold fixation.
(2) Cordectomy.
(3) Arytenoidectomy.
(4) Arytenoid pinning.

Most of these procedures have been abandoned because of poor results except for two methods which are still used successfully. In 1943, Thornell described intralaryngeal submucous arytenoidectomy. Both Montgomery and Gamble (1970) and Polisar (1959) have reviewed the literature and described the differential diagnoses of cricoarytenoid joint fixation. Montgomery described his cricoarytenoid joint pinning and lateral fixation procedure. A specially designed pin is used after endoscopic abduction of the arytenoid and vocal fold to fix them in a lateral position, and increase the airway.

Intralaryngeal methods to create a competent airway have been aimed at:

(1) Arytenoidectomy.
(2) Cordectomy.
(3) Lateral fixation of the vocal fold.

Most of these methods require a midline thyroidotomy incision. Jackson (1922) described the ventriculocordectomy procedure by which the vocal fold is resected. This procedure failed because the soft tissues readily formed a new fold with cicatricial stenosis of the lumen. Baker (1916) described arytenoidectomy through a laryngofissure technique in a 9-year-old boy: the result was excellent. Hoover (1953), realizing that scar tissue was the main cause of failure, developed submucous resection of the vocal cord and vocal process of arytenoid and its adjacent tissues through a laryngofissure. Lore (1936) and Stevenson (1937) employed the Hoover method of submucous resection of the vocal fold and went a step further by proposing the complete removal of the arytenoid. Moulonguet and his colleagues (1951) described and popularized the cordopexy procedure in France; Scheer (1953) and DeBord (1953) modified these techniques. They performed submucous resection of the arytenoid cartilage and fixed the vocal fold laterally by means of translaminar mattress sutures. There are many techniques described using the laryngofissure approach, but all have the common

factors of arytenoidectomy (usually submucous) and lateral fixation of the vocal fold. Generally, today, resection of the vocal fold has been abandoned as part of these procedures.

Extralaryngeal approaches have become more popular today. Essentially there are four types of procedures:

(1) Fixation of the arytenoid laterally.
(2) Partial or total arytenoidectomy and lateral fixation of the vocal fold and vocal process.
(3) Decompression of the laryngeal nerve.
(4) Sacrifice of other nerves and muscles.

King (1939) described a procedure whose basic principles were division of the capsule of the cricoarytenoid joint, mobilization of the arytenoid cartilage and vocal fold, and fixation to the thyroid cartilage in the abducted position. This was performed extralaryngeally by rotating the arytenoid cartilage 90°, transecting the omohyoid and inferior constrictor muscles and the inferior cricothyroid joint. A small hole was made in the thyroid lamina and the arytenoid fixed to it with a silk suture. In addition, the cut end of the omohyoid muscle was sutured to the muscular process of the arytenoid cartilage with the hope of thus obtaining some active movement of the vocal fold. Seed (1942) and Morrison (1945) described modifications of this procedure and have demonstrated that the use of the omohyoid muscle is not essential to rotation and lateralization of the disarticulated arytenoid cartilage. Galloway (1941) noted that the omohyoid did not move the arytenoid postoperatively.

Kelly (1941) described another approach to simplify the extralaryngeal procedure by creating a window in the thyroid lamina. This would, he said, release the tension on the vocal fold and allow it to "fall away" laterally, create scarring between the vocal fold and the thyroid lamina, and not disturb the anterior glottic relationships. Kelly (1943; 1944) finding that lateral fixation was not always adequate, began to use a suture placed through the thyroid cartilage window to lateralize the vocal fold after arytenoidectomy. Laryngoscopy was used to determine the amount of abduction achieved. Both McCall and Hoerr (1946) and Galloway (1941) modified the Kelly procedure by leaving the arytenoid cartilage after disarticulation for better lateral traction and by using the laryngoscope to determine the amount of lateral fixation achieved. McCall used endoscopic transillumination to identify the arytenoid cartilage. Wright (1943) sutured the posterior end of the transected vocal fold to the inner perichondrium of the thyroid cartilage. Orton (1943) described a method which would give better exposure for the extralaryngeal approach by removing the lateral half of the thyroid cartilage. After arytenoidectomy, he sutured the vocal ligament and thyroarytenoid muscle to the external perichondrium and to the anterior split sternothyroid and thyrohyoid muscles to achieve abduction of the vocal fold.

Woodman (1948) presented another method for extralaryngeal arytenoidectomy. The lateral border of the thyroid lamina is exposed and the larynx is rotated 90°. The cricothyroid joint is disarticulated and the arytenoid is completely dissected extralaryngeally so that the crico-arytenoid joint is disarticulated and the vocal process remains attached to the vocal fold. A suture placed through the vocal process is tied laterally to the inferior cornu of the thyroid lamina to achieve vocal fold abduction. The muscular process and body of the arytenoid are then removed. This method gave a more open and wide field approach for resection of the articular process of the arytenoid and is the most popular method employed at present.

The pathophysiology of unilateral idiopathic recurrent laryngeal nerve paralysis remains unexplained. Direct EMG measurements, which are necessary pre- and post-operatively, are not available. Usually recovery occurs within 4 months in 90 per cent of the cases. Ogura and Dedo (1965) described a method for decompression of the recurrent laryngeal nerve by disarticulation of the crico-thyroid joint and resection of the inferior thyroid cornu. The rationale was that the anterior branch of the recurrent laryngeal nerve entering the thyroid membrane was oedematous and was therefore compressed. Thus removal of this cartilaginous segment would improve the recovery rate. However, recovery in itself is not absolute proof that the surgery was the effective cause of the improvement. Fischer (1952) described improvement, both experimentally and clinically, of abductor paralysis by superior laryngeal nerve section. Freedman (1956) accomplished a similar result by cricothyroid muscle section.

Generally, we employ extralaryngeal methods or politef injection (if after 6 months) because they are better tolerated by the patients, have fewer complications, and are amenable to direct observation of the amount of abduction that is achieved or desired at the time of surgery.

REFERENCES

Aboulker, P., Lissac, J. and Saint-Paul, O. (1960), *Acta chir. belg.*, **59**, 553.

Alonso, J. M. (1947), *Trans. Amer. Acad. Ophthal. Otolaryng.*, **51**, 633.

Alonso, J. M. (1949), *Rev. Otorrinolaring. (Chile)*, **9**, 122.

Alonso, J. M. and Regules, J. E. A. (1957), *Arch. Otolaryng.*, **65**, 111–115.

Alonso, W. A. and Chambers, R. G. (1970), *Laryngoscope (St. Louis)*, **80**, 244.

Alonso, W. A., Bridger, G. P., Youngblood, J., Delahunty, J. E. and Bordley, J. E. (1971), *Laryngoscope (St. Louis)*, **81**, 1968.

Arbuckle, M. F. C. (1927), *Trans. Amer. laryng. rhinol. otol. Soc.*, **33**, 450.

Arbuckle, M. F. C. (1930), *Ann. Otol. (St. Louis)*, **39**, 134.

Archer, F. L., Harrison, R. W. and Moulder, P. V. (1963), *J. thorac. cardiovasc. Surg.*, **45**, 539.

Arnold, G. E. (1955), *Arch. Otolaryng.*, **62**, 1.

Arnold, G. E. (1957), *Arch. Otolaryng.*, **65**, 317.

Arnold, G. E. (1958), *Arch. Otolaryng.*, **68**, 284.

Arnold, G. E. (1959), *Arch. Otolaryng*, **70**, 444.

Arnold, G. E. (1961), *Laryngoscope (St. Louis)*, **71**, 687.

Arnold, G. E. (1962), *Arch. Otolaryng.*, **75**, 549.

Arnold, G. E. (1962), *Arch. Otolaryng.*, **76**, 358.

Arnold, G. E. (1963), *Ann. Otol. (St. Louis)*, **72**, 384.

Arslan, M. (1972), *Ann. Otol. (St. Louis)*, **81**, 479.

Asai, R. (1965), *Excerpta med. I.C.S.*, **92**, E25.

Asai, R. (1966), *J. Jap. broncho. Soc.*, **12**, 1.

Asai, R. (1972), *Arch. Otolaryng.*, **95**, 114.

Asherson, N. (1954), *J. Laryng.*, **68**, 550.

Baclesse, F. (1949), *Brit. J. Radiol.*, suppl. 3.

Baclesse, F. (1951), *Clin. Radiol*, **3**, 3.

Baerthold, W. and Budach-Gamaleja, A. K. (1969), *Z. Laryng. Rhinol.*, **48**, 178.

Bailey, B. J. (1966), *Trans. Amer. Acad. Ophthal. Otolaryng.*, **70**, 559.

Bailey, B. J. and Calcaterra, T. C. (1971), *Arch. Otolaryng.*, **93**, 232.

Bailey, B. J. and Kosoy, J. (1970), *Laryngoscope (St. Louis)*, **80**, 1553.

Bakamjian, V. Y. (1965), *Plast. reconstr. Surg.*, **36**, 173.

Bakamjian, V. Y. (1968), *N.Y. St. J. Med.*, **68**, 2771.

Bakamjian, V. Y. and Littlewood, M. (1964), *Brit. J. plast. Surg.*, **17**, 191.

Baker, C. H. (1916), *J. Mich. med. Soc.*, **15**, 485.

Ballance, C. (1924), *Brit. med. J.*, **2**, 349.

Ballance, C. (1934), *Proc. roy. Soc. Med.*, **27**, 1207.

Barclay, R. S., McSwan, N. and Welsh, T. M. (1957), *Thorax*, **12**, 177.

Barnes, E. B. and Ballance, C. (1927), *Brit. med. J.*, **2**, 58.

Barton, R. T. (1965), *Excerpta med. I.C.S.*, **92**, E26.

Beall, A. C., Jr., Harrington, O. B., Greenberg, S. D., Morris, G. C. and Usher, F. C. (1963), *Arch. Surg.*, **86**, 970.

Beall, A. C., Jr., Harrington, O. B., Greenberg, S. D., Usher, F. C. and Morris, G. C. (1960), *Surg. Forum.*, **11**, 40.

Beall, A. C., Jr., Harrington, O. B., Greenberg, S. D., Usher, F. C. and Morris, G. C. (1963), *J. Amer. med. Ass.*, **183**, 1082.

Beck, C. and Carrell, A. (1905), *Illinois med. J.*, **7**, 463.

Beck, C. S. and Leighninger, D. S. (1954), *J. Amer. med. Ass.*, **156**, 1226.

Belsey, R. (1950), *Brit. J. Surg.*, **38**, 200.

Bennett, T. (1960), *Laryngoscope (St. Louis)*, **70**, 973.

Berendes, J. and Miehlke, A. (1968), *Int. Surg.*, **49**, 319.

Bernatz, P. E. and Hopkins, D. M. (1963), *Surg. Clin. N. Amer.*, **43**, 1171.

Bernstein, J. J. and Guth, L. (1961), *Exp. Neurol.*, **4**, 262.

Bignon, J. and Chretien, J. (1962), *J. franç. Méd. Chir. thorac.*, **16**, 125.

Biller, H. F., Barnhill, F. R., Jr., Ogura, J. H. and Perez C. A. (1970), *Laryngoscope (St. Louis)*, **80**, 249.

Biller, H. F., Davis, W. H. and Ogura, J. H. (1971), *Laryngoscope (St. Louis)*, **81**, 1499.

Biller, H. F., Ogura, J. H. and Bauer, W. C. (1971), *Laryngoscope (St. Louis)*, **81**, 1323.

Biller, H. F., Ogura, J. H., Davis, W. H. and Powers, W. E. (1969), *Laryngoscope (St. Louis)*, **79**, 1387.

Biller, H. F., Ogura, J. H. and Pratt, L. L. (1971), *Arch. Otolaryng.*, **93**, 238.

Billroth, T. (1872), *Arch. klin. Chir.*, **13**, 65.

Billroth, T. (1874), *Verh. ostsch. Ges. Chir.*

Birck, H. G. and Manhart, H. E. (1963), *Arch. Otolaryng.*, **77**, 603.

Blalock, A. and Crowe, S. J. (1926), *Arch. Surg.*, **12**, 95.

Blomstedt, B. and Rydmark, K. E. (1960), *Acta Otolaryng.*, **52**, 150.

Bocca, E., Bozzi, E. and Cover, P. L. (1967), *Cancer of the Head and Neck* (J. J. Conley, Ed.). Washington, D.C.: Butterworth.

Boedts, D., Roels, H. and Kluyskens, P. (1967), *Arch. Otolaryng.*, **86**, 562.

Boles, R. (1966), *Laryngoscope (St. Louis)*, **76**, 1057.

Boles, R. and Fritzell, B. (1969), *Laryngoscope (St. Louis)*, **79**, 1405.

Bouhuys, A. and Van De Woestijne, K. P. (1971), *J. appl. Physiol.*, **30**, 670.

Bowden, R. E. M. (1955), *Proc. roy. Soc. Med.*, **48**, 437.

Brenman, A. K. (1961), *Trans. Amer. Acad. Ophthal. Otolaryng.*, **65**, 724.

Brewer, D. W. and Dana, S. T. (1963), *Ann. Oto-laryng. (Paris)*, **72**, 1060.

Briani, A. A. (1952), *Arch. ital. Otol.*, **63**, 469.

Briani, A. A. (1959), *L'Evolution Médicale*, **3**, 17.

Bruenings, W. (1911), *18. Verh. dtsch. laryng.*, pp. 93 (525), (151), (583).

Bryce, D. P., Ireland, D. P. and Rider, W. D. (1963), *Ann. Otol. (St. Louis)*, **72**, 416.

Bryce, D. P. and Lawson, V. G. (1967), *Ann. Otol. (St. Louis)*, **76**, 793.

Burford, T. H., Webb, W. R. and Ackerman, L. (1953), *Ann. Surg.*, **138**, 453.

Buschke, F. and Galante, M. (1959), *Radiology*, **73**, 845.

Calcaterra, T. C. and Jafek, B. W. (1971), *Arch. Otolaryng.*, **94**, 124.

Campbell, C. J., Murtagh, J. A. and Raber, C. F. (1963), *Ann. Otol. (St. Louis)*, **72**, 5.

Cantrell, J. R. and Folse, J. R. (1961), *J. thorac. cardiovasc. Surg.*, **42**, 589.

Capps, F. C. W. (1958), *J. Laryng.*, **72**, 1.

Cardwell, E. P. (1946), *Arch. Otolaryng.*, **44**, 560.

Caselli, A. (1879), *Atti Soc. med.- chir. Bologna.*

Cassisi, N. J., Harris, B. L., Kawasaki, M. and Ogura, J. H. (1968), *Surg. Forum*, **19**, 471.

Cherry, J., Davis, W., Rosenblatt, B. A. and Coleman, R. (1970), *Ann. Otol. (St. Louis)*, **79**, 1077.

Chodosh, P. L. (1968), *Arch. Otolaryng.*, **87**, 461.

Churchill-Davidson, I., Sanger, C. and Thomlinson, R. H. (1957), *Brit. J. Radiol.*, **30**, 406.

Clerf, L. H. (1931), *Ann. Otol. (St. Louis)*, **40**, 770.

Clerf, L. H. (1933), *Ann. Otol. (St. Louis)*, **42**, 1.

Clerf, L. H. (1940), *Arch. Otolaryng.*, **32**, 484.

Clerf, L. H. (1953), *J. Amer. med. Ass.*, **151**, 900.

Clerf, L. H. (1953), *Acta oto-laryng. (Stockh.)*, **43**, 108.

Colledge, L. (1925), *Brit. med. J.*, **1**, 547.

Colledge, L. and Ballance, C. (1927), *Brit. med. J.*, **1**, 553.

Conley, J. J. (1953), *Ann. Otol. (St. Louis)*, **62**, 477.

Conley, J. J. (1953), *Arch. Otolaryng.*, **58**, 645.

Conley, J. J. (1959), *Ann. Otol. (St. Louis)*, **68**, 990.

Conley, J. J. (1960), *Ann. Otol. (St. Louis)*, **69**, 1223.

Conley, J. J. (1961), *Arch. Otolaryng.*, **74**, 239.

Conley, J. J. (1965), *Arch. Otolaryng.*, **82**, 198.

Conley, J. J., Deamesti, F. and Pierce, M. K. (1958), *Ann. Otol. (St. Louis)*, **67**, 655.

Cooper, I. S. (1962), *J. Amer. med. Ass.*, **181**, 600.

Cooper, I. S. (1963), *New Engl. J. Med.*, **268**, 743.

Cooper, J. D. and Grillo, H. C. (1969), *Ann. Surg.*, **169**, 334.

Coutard, H. (1932), *Radiophys. radiother.*, **2**, 541.

Coutard, H. (1934), *Lancet*, **ii**, 1.

Coutard, H. (1937), *J. Radiol. Electrol.*, **21**, 402.

Coutard, H. and Baclesse, F. (1932), *Amer. J. Roentgenol.*, **28**, 293.

Curtin, J. W., Holinger, P. H. and Greeley, P. W. (1966), *J. Trauma*, **6**, 493.

Czerny, V. (1870), *Wien. med. Wachr.*, **20**, 557.

Czerny, V. (1877), *Centralbl. Chir.*, **4**, 433.

Davanzo, J. P., Matthews, R. J., Wingerson, F. and Barnes, M. B. (1963), *Arch. int. Pharmacodyn.*, **141**, 299.

DeBord, B. A., Jr. (1953), *Laryngoscope (St. Louis)*, **63**, 757.

Dedo, H. H. (1970), *Laryngoscope (St. Louis)*, **80**, 1455.

Dedo, H. H. and Ogura, J. H. (1965), *Laryngoscope (St. Louis)*, **75**, 201.

Dedo, H. H. and Sooy, F. A. (1968), *Ann. Otol. (St. Louis)*, **77**, 435.

Delahunty, J. E., Aloneo, W. A. and Bordley, J. E. (1970), *Laryngoscope (St. Louis)*, **80**, 137.

Delahunty, J. E., Cherry, J. and Brookhauser, P. (1969), *Laryngoscope (St. Louis)*, **79**, 2081.

Delsaux, V. (1909), *Brit. med. J.*, **2**, 1141.

Denman, A. M. (1969), *Clin. exp. Immunol.*, **5**, 217.

DeVincentiis, I. and DeSantis, M. (1956), *Ann. Oto-laryng. (Paris)*, **73**, 57.

Dixon, W. E. and Brodie, T. G. (1903), *J. Physiol. (Lond).*, **29**, 97.

Doyle, P. J., Brummett, R. E. and Everts, E. C. (1967), *Laryngoscope (St. Louis)*, **77**, 1245.

Duff, T. B. (1971), *J. Laryng.*, **85**, 947.

Edgerton, M. T. (1952), *Surgery*, **31**, 239.

Edgerton, M. T. and Zovickian, A. (1954), *Plast. reconstr. Surg.*, **13**, 167.

Edwards, T. M. (1952), *Ann. Otol. (St. Louis)*, **61**, 159.

Einthoven, W. (1892), *Pflügers Arch. ges. Physiol.*, **51**, 367.

Ellis, M. (1938), *Lancet*, **i**, 819.

Emery, E. W., Lucas, B. G. B. and Williams, K. G. (1960), *Lancet*, **i**, 248.

English, D. T. and Blevins, C. E. (1969), *Arch. Otolaryng.*, **89**, 778.

Erich, J. B. (1945), *Arch. Otolaryng.*, **41**, 343.

Erich, J. B. (1956), *Ann. Otol. (St. Louis)*, **65**, 799.

Evans, A. (1933), *Brit. J. Surg.*, **20**, 388.

Evoy, M. H. (1960), *Laryngoscope (St. Louis)*, **70**, 1268.

Evoy, M. H. (1968), *Arch. Otolaryng.*, **87**, 155.

Faaborg-Anderson, K. (1957), *Acta physiol. scand.*, **41**, 140.

Faaborg-Anderson, K. (1964), *Acta oto-laryng. (Stockh.)*, **57**, 50.

Faaborg-Anderson, K., Bress, F. B. and Brewer, D. W. (1960), *Acta oto-laryng. (Stockh.)*, **158**, 200.

Fabrikant, J. I. and Dickson, R. J. (1965), *Brit. J. Radiol.*, **38**, 28.

Fabrikant, J. I., Richards, G. J., Jr., Tucker, G. F. and Dickson, R. J. (1962), *Amer. J. Roentgenol.*, **87**, 822.

Fairchild, F. R. (1927), *Surg. Gynec. Obstet.*, **44**, 119.

Ferguson, D. J., Wild, J. J. and Wangensteen, O. H. (1950), *Surgery*, **28**, 597.

Ferris, B. G., Jr., Mead, J. and Opie, L. H. (1964), *J. appl. Physiol.*, **19**, 653.

Fex, S. (1970), *Acta oto-laryng. (Stockh.)*, **69**, 294.

Figi, F. A. (1940), *Ann. Otol. (St. Louis)*, **49**, 394.

Figi, F. A. (1947), *Sth. med. J. (Bgham, Ala.)*, **40**, 17.

Figi, F. A. (1950), *Ann. Otol. (St. Louis)*, **59**, 474.

Fischer, N. D. (1952), *Ann. Otol. (St. Louis)*, **61**, 352.

Fitz-Hugh, G. S., Wallenborn, W. M. and McGovern, F. (1962), *Ann. Otol. (St. Louis)*, **71**, 419.

Flege, J. B., Jr. (1967), *Ann. Surg.*, **166**, 153.

Fletcher, G. H. (1967), *Cancer of the Head and Neck*, Chap. 8 (W. S. MacComb and G. H. Fletcher, Eds.). Baltimore: William and Wilkins.

Florange, W., Muller, J. and Forster, E. (1965), *Curr. Res. Anesth.*, **22**, 693.

Foley, F. D., Moncrief, J. A. and Mason, A. D. (1968), *Ann. Surg.*, **167**, 251.

Frazier, C. H. (1924), *Ann. Surg.*, **79**, 161.

Frazier, C. H. (1924), *J. Amer. med. Ass.*, **83**, 1637.

Frazier, C. H. and Erb, W. H. (1935), *Ann. Surg.*, **101**, 1353.

Frazier, C. H. and Mosser, W. B. (1926), *Surg. Gynec. Obstet.*, **43**, 134.

Freedman, L. M. (1956), *Laryngoscope (St. Louis)*, **66**, 574.

Friedberg, S. A., Griffith, T. E. and Hass, G. M. (1965), *Ann. Otol. (St. Louis)*, **74**, 785.

Friedman, W. H. and Goldman, J. L. (1969), *Arch. Otolaryng.*, **89**, 766.

Gaisford, J. C. and Hanna, D. C. (1962), *Plast. reconstr. Surg.*, **29**, 561.

Galloway, T. C. (1941), *Arch. Otolaryng.*, **34**, 1197.

Gibson, P. (1967), *Thorax*, **22**, 1.

Gluck, T. and Sorrensen, J. (1912), *Jber. ärztl. Fortbild.*, **2**, 20.

Goff, W. F. (1960), *Trans. Pacif. Cst oto-ophthal. Soc.*, **41**, 77.

Goldman, L. (1967), *Biomedical Aspects of the Laser*. New York: Springer.

Goldman, L. (1967), *Cancer of the Head and Neck*, p. 401 (J. J. Conley, Ed.). Washington, D.C.: Butterworth.

Goldsmith, H. S. (1968), Presented AMA Convention, San Francisco.

Goligher, J. C. and Robin, I. G. (1954), *Brit. J. Surg.*, **42**, 283.

Gordon, J. H. and McCabe, B. F. (1968), *Laryngoscope (St. Louis)*, **78**, 236.

Gorman, J. B. and Woodward, F. D. (1965), *Sth. med. J. (Bgham, Ala.)*, **58**, 34.

Gray, L. H., Conger, A. D., Ebert, M., Hornsey, S. and Scott, O. C. A. (1953), *Brit. J. Radiol.*, **26**, 638.

Greenberg, S. D. (1960), *Arch. Otolaryng.*, **72**, 565.

Greenberg, S. D., Beall, A. C., Jr. and Wallance, S. A. (1962), *Exp. molec. Path.*, **1**, 141.

Grillo, H. C. (1964), *J. thorac. cardiovasc. Surg.*, **48**, 741.

Grillo, H. C. (1965), *Ann. Surg.*, **162**, 374.

Grillo, H. C. (1966), *J. Amer. med. Ass.*, **197**, 1085.

Grillo, H. C. (1966), *J. thorac. cardiovasc. Surg.*, **51**, 422.

Grillo, H. C. (1969), *Surg. Gynec. Obstet.*, **129**, 347.

Grillo, H. C. (1972), *Arch. Otolaryng.*, **96**, 31.

Grillo, H. C., Bendixen, H. H., Gephart, T., Dignan, E. F. and Miura, T. (1963), *Ann. Surg.*, **158**, 889.

Gross, C. W. and Crocker, T. R. (1970), *Laryngoscope (St. Louis)*, **80**, 532.

Grossmann, M. (1906), *Arch. Laryng. Rhin. (Berl.)*, **18**, 463.

Gussenbauer, C. (1874), *Arch. klin. Chir.*, **17**, 343.

Gussenbauer, C. (1874), *Verh. ostsch. Ges. Chir.*, 250.

Gutmann, E. and Young, J. Z. (1944), *J. Anat. (Lond.)*, **78**, 15.

Harkins, W. B. (1952), *Ann. Otol. (St. Louis)*, **61**, 663.

Harris, H. H. and Tobin, H. A. (1970), *Laryngoscope (St. Louis)*, **80**, 1376.

Harris, W., Kramer, R. and Silverstone, S. M. (1948), *Radiology*, **51**, 708.

Harrison, D. F. N. (1964), *Ann. Otol. (St. Louis)*, **73**, 1026.

Harrison, D. F. N. (1964), *Proc. roy. Soc. Med.*, **57**, 1104.

Harvey, J. E., Ohyama, M., Ueda, N., Moei, G. and Ogura, J. H. (1970), *Laryngoscope (St. Louis)*, **80**, 1646.

Harvey, J. E., Tucker, H. M., Sessions, R. and Ogura, J. H. (1971), *Laryngoscope (St. Louis)*, **81**, 1126.

Hawe, D. and Lothian, K. R. (1960), *Surg. Gynec. Obstet.*, **110**, 488.

Hawk, J. C., Jr. (1961), *Amer. J. Surg.*, **102**, 789.

Heibert, C. A. and Cummings, G. O., Jr. (1961), *Ann. Surg.*, **154**, 103.

Hendrickson, F. R. (1965), *Radiology*, **84**, 727.

Hendrickson, F. R. and Liebner, E. (1968), *Ann. Otol. (St. Louis)*, **77**, 222.

Heyden, R. (1950), *Acta oto-laryng. (Stockh.)*, suppl. 85.

Hiroto, I., Hirano, M. and Tomita, H. (1968), *Ann. Otol. (St. Louis)*, **77**, 296.

Hiroto, I., Hirano, M., Toyozumi, Y. and Shin, T. (1967), *Ann. Otol. (St. Louis)*, **76**, 861.

Hoessly, H. (1916), *Bruns' Beitr. klin. Chir.*, **99**, 186.

Hoffman, H. (1952), *Aust. J. exp. Biol.*, **30**, 541.

Hoffman-Sanguez, M. (1951), *Ann. Oto-laryng. (Paris)*, **68**, 736.

Holinger, P. H. and Johnston, K. C. (1958), *Ann. Otol. (St. Louis)*, **67**, 496.

Holinger, P. H. and Johnston, K. C. (1959), *Amer. J. Surg.*, **97**, 513.

Holinger, P. H. and Schild, J. A. (1972), *Ann. Otol. (St. Louis)*, **81**, 538.

Holinger, P. H., Schild, J. A. and Maurizi, D. G. (1968), *Laryngoscope (St. Louis)*, **78**, 944.

Holinger, P. H., Schild, J. A. and Maurizi, D. G. (1968), *Laryngoscope (St. Louis)*, **78**, 1462.

Hoover, W. B. (1932), *Arch. Otolaryng.*, **15**, 339.

Hoover, W. B. (1953), *Surg. Clin. N. Amer.*, **33**, 879.

Horsley, J. S. (1909), *Trans. Sth. surg. Ass.*, **22**, 161.

Huppler, E. G., Schmidt, H. W., Devine, D. and Gage, R. P. (1955), *Mayo Clin. Proc.*, **30**, 518.

Husson, R. (1950), *Thèse Fac. Sciences Paris*.

Husson, R. (1955), *Expos. ann. Oto-rhono-laryng.*, p. 187.

Hyatt, R. E. and Wilcox, R. E. (1961), *J. appl. Physiol.*, **16**, 326.

Hyatt, R. E. and Wilcox, R. E. (1963), *J. clin. Invest.*, **42**, 29.

Iglauer, S. (1918), *Ann. Otol. (St. Louis)*, **27**, 1233.

Iglauer, S. (1935), *Arch. Otolaryng.*, **22**, 597.

Ikeda, S. (1934), *Otol. Fukuoka*, **7**, 512.

Isambert, N. L., Thomson, S. C. and Colledge, L. (1930), *Cancer of the Larynx*. London: Routledge and Kegan Paul Limited.

Iskeçeli, O. K. (1962), *Surgery*, **51**, 496.

Jackson, C. (1922), *Arch. Surg.*, **4**, 257.

Jackson, C. (1936), *Trans. Amer. laryng. rhinol. otol. Soc.*, **42**, 12.

Jackson, C. and Jackson, C. L. (1939), *Cancer of the Larynx*, pp. 216–287. Philadelphia: W. B. Saunders Co.

Jackson, C. and Jackson, C. L. (1943), *Arch. Otolaryng.*, **38**, 413.

Jackson, C. L. (1939), *Surg. Clin. N. Amer.*, **19**, 1479.

Jackson, C. L. (1941), *Arch. Otolaryng.*, **33**, 520.

Jackson, T. L., O'Brien, E. J., Tuttle, W. and Meyer, J. (1950), *J. thorac. Surg.*, **20**, 598.

Jako, G. J. (1972), *Laryngoscope (St. Louis)*, **82**, 2204.

Jenkins, J. C. (1967), *J. Laryng.*, **81**, 385.

Juvenelle, A. and Citret, C. (1951), *J. Chir. (Paris)*, **67**, 666.

Kaplan, I. and Markowicz, H. (1964), *Brit. J. plast. Surg.*, **17**, 314.

Karlan, M. S. (1968), *Amer. J. Surg.*, **116**, 597.

Kay, E. B. (1951), *Ann. Otol. (St. Louis)*, **60**, 864.

Kelly, J. D. (1941), *Arch. Otolaryng.*, **33**, 293.

Kelly, J. D. (1943), *Ann. Otol. (St. Louis)*, **52**, 628.

Kelly, J. D. (1944), *Ann. Otol. (St. Louis)*, **53**, 461.

Kemler, J. I. (1947), *Laryngoscope (St. Louis)*, **57**, 704.

King, B. T. (1939), *J. Amer. med. Ass.*, **112**, 814.

King, B. T. (1939), *Trans. Amer. laryng. rhinol. otol. Soc.*, **61**, 264.

Kirchner, F. R., Toledo, P. S. and Svoboda, D. J. (1966), *Arch. Otolaryng.*, **83**, 350.

Kirchner, J. A. (1963), *Inst. Laryng. Otol. Rept.*, **14**, 27.

Kirchner, J. A. (1966), *Laryngoscope (St. Louis)*, **76**, 1753.

Kitamura, T., Kaneko, T., Togawa, K. and Unno, T. (1970), *Ann. Otol. (St. Louis)*, **79**, 1027.

Kitamura, T., Kaneko, T., Togawa, K., Unno, T., Kanda, T., Konno, A., Asano, H. and Miura, T. (1970), *Laryngoscope (St. Louis)*, **80**, 300.

Kleinsasser, O. (1961), *Z. Laryng. Rhinol.*, **40**, 276.

Kleinsasser, O. (1962), *Arch. Ohrenheilk.*, **180**, 724.

Kleinsasser, O. (1968), *Mikrolaryngoskopie und endolaryngeale Mikrochirurgie*. Stuttgart: Schattauer.

Klopp, C. T., Alford, C. and Pierpont, H. (1951), *Surgery*, **29**, 231.

Kluyskens, P., Boedts, D., Dhont, G., Van de Weghe, J. P., Vandenhove, P., Van Clooster, R., Bilo, F., Ringoir, B. and Daneels, R. (1969), *Acta oto-rhino-laryng. belg.*, **23**, 5.

Knight, J. S. (1964), *Laryngoscope (St. Louis)*, **74**, 564.

Knight, J. S. (1966), *Ann. Otol. (St. Louis)*, **75**, 392.

Koyama, J., Harvey, J. E. and Ogura, J. H. (1971), *Laryngoscope (St. Louis)*, **81**, 47.

Koyama, J., Harvey, J. E. and Ogura, J. H. (1972), *Laryngoscope (St. Louis)*, **82**, 210.

Koyama, J., Kawasaki, M. and Ogura, J. H. (1969), *Laryngoscope (St. Louis)*, **79**, 337.

Kratschmer, F. (1870), *S. B. Akad. Wiss, Wien*, **62**, 147.

Lahey, F. H. (1928), *Ann. Surg.*, **87**, 481.

Lahey, F. H. and Hoover, W. B. (1938), *Ann. Surg.*, **108**, 545.

Lapidot, A., Kouyoumgian, J. and Ramm, C. (1965), *Arch. Otolaryng.*, **82**, 38.

Lapidot, A., Sodagar, R., Ratanaprashtporn, S. and Silverman, R. (1968), *Arch. Otolaryng.*, **88**, 529.

Lasarus, J. (1891), *Arch. Anat. Physiol. (Physiol. Abt.)*, **19**, 1.

Lauerma, K. S. L., Harvey, J. E. and Ogura, J. H. (1972), *Laryngoscope (St. Louis)*, **82**, 447.

Lederman, M. (1961), *Brit. med. J.*, **1**, 1639.

LeJeune, F. and Owens, N. (1935), *Ann. Otol. (St. Louis)*, **44**, 354.

Lemariey, A. and Muler, H. (1960), *Ann. oto-laryng. (Paris)*, **77**, 288.

Lemere, F. (1932), *Amer. J. Anat.*, **51**, 417.

Lemere, F. (1932), *Anat. Rec.*, **54**, 389.

Lemere, F. (1934), *Ann. Otol. (St. Louis)*, **43**, 525.

Lenz, M. (1935), *Amer. J. Surg.*, **30**, 259.

Leonard, J. R. and Maran, A. G. D. (1970), *Laryngoscope (St. Louis)*, **80**, 849.

LeQuesne, L. P. and Ranger, D. (1966), *Brit. J. Surg.*, **53**, 105.

Leroux-Robert, J. (1956), *Ann. oto-laryng. (Paris)*, **65**, 137.

Leroux-Robert, J. and Ennuyer, A. (1956), *Ann. oto-laryng. (Paris)*, **73**, 521.

Lewy, R. B. (1954), *Laryngoscope (St. Louis)*, **64**, 693.

Lewy, R. B. (1963), *Laryngoscope (St. Louis)*, **73**, 547.

Lewy, R. B. (1964), *Acta oto-laryng. (Stockh.)*, **58**, 214.

Libersa, C., (1952), *J. franç. Oto-rhino-laryng.*, **1**, 480.

Lindquist, C. and Martensson, A. (1969), *Acta physiol. scand.*, **77**, 234.

Looper, E. A. (1938), *Arch. Otolaryng.*, **28**, 106.

Lore, J. M. (1936), *Ann. Otol. (St. Louis)*, **45**, 679.

Lynch, M. (1951), *Laryngoscope (St. Louis)*, **61**, 51.

MacCombe, W. S. and Fletcher, G. H. (1967), *Amer. J. Roentgenol.*, **77**, 397.

MacKenzie, M. (1960), "History of the Laryngoscope," in *Source Book of Medical History* (L. Clendening, Ed.). New York: Dover Publisher Inc.

MacManus, J. E. and McCormick, R. (1954), *Ann. Surg.*, **139**, 350.

McCabe, B. F. and Magielski, J. E. (1960), *Ann. Otol. (St. Louis)*, **69**, 1013.

McCall, J. W. and Hoerr, N. L. (1946), *Laryngoscope (St. Louis)*, **56**, 527.

McCoy, G. and Bordin, E. (1962), *Trans. Pacif. Cst. oto-ophthal. Soc.*, **43**, 35.

McCullough, A. W. (1959), *J. comp. Neurol.*, **113**, 471.

McGavran, M. H., Bauer, W. C. and Ogura, J. H. (1961), *Cancer, Philad.*, **14**, 55.

McNaught, R. C. (1950), *Laryngoscope (St. Louis)*, **60**, 264.

Mahoney, E. B. and Sherman, C. D., Jr. (1954), *Surgery*, **35**, 937.

Majer, E. H. and Rieder, W. (1959), *Ann. Oto-laryng. (Paris)*, **76**, 677.

Maran, A. G. D., Hast, M. H. and Leonard, J. R. (1968), *Laryngoscope (St. Louis)*, **78**, 1916.

Marchetta, F. C., Sako, K. and Creedon, P. J. (1961), *Amer. J. Surg.*, **102**, 854.

Marres, E. H. M. A., Wentges, R. T. H. R. and Brinkman, W. F. B. (1966), *Laryngoscope (St. Louis)*, **76**, 1979.

Meurman, O. H. (1950), *Acta oto-laryng. (Stockh.)*, **38**, 460.

Meurman, Y. (1952), *Arch. Otolaryng.*, **55**, 544.

Michelson, E. M., Solomon, R., Maun, L. and Ramirez, J. (1961), *J. thorac. cardiovasc. Surg.*, **41**, 748.

Middleton, P. (1966), *Ann. Otol. (St. Louis)*, **75**, 139.

Miehlke, A., Küsel, H. J., Dal Ri, H. and Schmidt, G. (1967), *Arch. Klin. exp. Ohr.-, Nas.- u. Kehlk.- Heilk.*, **188**, 668.

Miehlke, A., Schätzle, W. and Haubrich, J. (1967), *Arch. Ohrenheilk.*, **188**, 654.

Miglets, A. W. (1968), *Arch. Otolaryng.*, **87**, 494.

Miglets, A. W. (1971), *Arch. Otolaryng.*, **93**, 492.

Mikulicz, J. (1886), *Prag. med. Wschr.*, **9**, 93.

Miles, W. K., Olson, N. R. and Rodriguez, A. (1971), *Ann. Otol. (St. Louis)*, **80**, 710.

Miller, A. H. (1967), *Ann. Otol. (St. Louis)*, **76**, 829.

Mogi, G. (1972), *Laryngoscope (St. Louis)*, **82**, 252.

Mogi, G., Harvey, J. E. and Ogura, J. H. (1972), *Laryngoscope (St. Louis)*, **82**, 998.

Mogi, G., Harvey, J. E., Ohyama, M., Ueda, N. and Ogura, J. H. (1972), *Laryngoscope (St. Louis)*, **82**, 61.

Moncrief, W. H. and Salvatore, J. E. (1958), *Surg. Forum*, **9**, 350.

Montgomery, W. W. (1963), *Laryngoscope (St. Louis)*, **73**, 801.

Montgomery, W. W. (1964), *Ann. Otol. (St. Louis)*, **73**, 5.

Montgomery, W. W. (1966), *Ann. Otol. (St. Louis)*, **75**, 380.

Montgomery, W. W. (1968), *Ann. Otol. (St. Louis)*, **77**, 534.

Montgomery, W. W. and Gamble, J. E. (1970), *Arch. Otolaryng.*, **92**, 560.

Montgomery, W. W., Perone, P. M. and Schall, L. A. (1955), *Ann. Otol. (St. Louis)*, **64**, 1025.

Montgomery, W. W. and Toohill, R. J. (1968), *Ann. Oto-laryng. (Paris)*, **88**, 499.

Moore, I. (1929), *The Nose, Throat and Ear and Their Disease*, p. 713. Philadelphia: W. B. Saunders.

Morrison, L. F. (1945), *Ann. Otol. (St. Louis)*, **54**, 390.

Morrison, L. F. (1945), *Trans. Amer. laryng. rhinol. otol. Soc.*, 213–236.

Morrison, L. F. (1948), *Ann. Otol. (St. Louis)*, **57**, 945.

Moulonguet, A., Mayonx, R., Debain, J. J. and Bouche, J. (1951), *J. Soc. franç. oto-rhino-laryng.*, **58**, 39.

Mounier-Kuhn, P. (1968), *J. franç. oto-rhino-laryng.*, **17**, 297.

Muller, J. (1937), *Handbuch der Physiologie des Menchen Bd III*, p. 133. Abschnitt: 'Von der Sinne und Sprache.'

Muller, J. (1840), *Handbuch d. Physiol Coblenz*, pp. 184–222.

Murakami, Y. and Kirchner, J. A. (1971), *Arch. Otolaryng.*, **94**, 64.

Murphy, G. E., Bisno, A. L. and Ogura, J. H. (1964), *Laryngoscope (St. Louis)*, **74**, 1535.

Murray, J. E., Wilson, R. E., Tilney, N. L., Merrill, J. P., Cooper, W. C., Birtch, A. G., Carpenter, C. B., Hager, E. B., Guttman, R., Hampers, C. L., Dammin, G. J. and Harrison, J. H. (1968), *Trans. Amer. surg. Ass.*, **86**, 106.

Murtagh, J. A. and Campbell, C. J. (1948), *Ann. Otol. (St. Louis)*, **57**, 465.

Murtagh, J. A. and Campbell, C. J. (1951), *Laryngoscope (St. Louis)*, **61**, 581.

Mustard, R. A. (1960), *Surg. Gynec. Obstet.*, **111**, 577.

Nadel, J. A. and Widdicombe, J. G. (1962), *J. Physiol. (Lond.)*, **163**, 13.

Nadel, J. A. and Widdicombe, J. G. (1962), *J. appl. Physiol.*, **17**, 861.

Nakamura, F., Uyeda, Y. and Sonoda, Y. (1958), *Laryngoscope (St. Louis)*, **68**, 109.

Nakayama, K., Yamamoto, T., Makino, H., Odaka, M., Ohwada, M. and Takahashi, H. (1964), *Surgery*, **55**, 796.

Navratil, D. V. (1910), *Arch. Laryng. Rhin. (Berl.)*, **23**, 342.

Nechiporuk, V. M. (1961), *Khirurgiya (Mosk.)*, **37**, Pt. 6, 19.

Neel, H. B., Townsend, G. L. and Devine, K. D. (1972), *Ann. Otol. (St. Louis)*, **81**, 514.

Negus, V. E. (1938), *Ann. Otol. (St. Louis)*, **47**, 891.

Negus, V. E. (1947), *Proc. roy. Soc. Med.*, **40**, 849.

Negus, V. E. (1953), *Brit. J. plast. Surg.*, **6**, 99.

New, G. B. and Childrey, J. H. (1932), *Arch. Otolaryng.*, **16**, 143.

Nias, A. H. W. (1967), *Brit. J. Radiol.*, **40**, 166.

Nielsen, J. and Strandberg, O. (1924), *Acta radiol. (Stockh.)*, **23**, 189.

Norris, C. M. (1958), *Laryngoscope (St. Louis)*, **68**, 1240.

Norris, C. M. (1959), *Laryngoscope (St. Louis)*, **69**, 306.

O'Dwyer, J. (1897), *Trans. Amer. pediat. Soc.*, **9**, 180.

Ogura, J. H. (1958), *Laryngoscope (St. Louis)*, **68**, 983.

Ogura, J. H. (1960), *Arch. Otolaryng.*, **72**, 66.

Ogura, J. H., Powers, W. E., Holtz, S., McFauran, M. H., Ellis, B. and Voorhees, R. (1960), *Laryngoscope (St. Louis)*, **70**, 780.

Ogura, J. H. (1961), *Ann. Otol. (St. Louis)*, **70**, 451.

Ogura, J. H. (Ed.) (October, 1969), *Oto. Clin. N. Amer.*

Ogura, J. H. (1970), *Ann. Otol. (St. Louis)*, **79**, 1.

Ogura, J. H (1971), *Kopf und Hals Chirurgie*. Stuttgart: G. Thieme.

Ogura, J. H. (1972), *Trans. Amer. Acad. Ophthal. Otolaryng.*, **76**, 741.

Ogura, J. H. and Biller, H. F. (1969), *Arch. Klin. exp. Ohr.-, Nas.- u. Kehlk. Heilk.*, **194**, 339.

Ogura, J. H. and Biller, H. F. (1969), *Laryngoscope (St. Louis)*, **79**, 2181.

Ogura, J. H. and Biller, H. F. (1971), *Ann. Otol. (St. Louis)*, **80**, 492.

Ogura, J. H. and Biller, H. F. (1972), *J. Amer. med. Ass.*, **221**, 77.

Ogura, J. H., Biller, H. F., Calcaterra, T. C. and Davis, W. H. (1969), *Int. Surg.*, **52**, 29.

Ogura, J. H. and Dedo, H. H. (1965), *Laryngoscope (St. Louis)*, **75**, 588.

Ogura, J. H. and Dedo, H. H. (1965), *Laryngoscope (St. Louis)*, **75**, 865.

Ogura, J. H. and Harvey, J. E. (1971), *Acta oto-laryng.*, **71**, 123.

Ogura, J. H., Harvey, J. E., Mogi, G., Ueda, N., Ohyama, M. and Tucker, M. M. (1970), *Laryngoscope (St. Louis)*, **80**, 1231.

Ogura, J. H., Jurema, A. A. and Watson, R. K. (1960), *Laryngoscope (St. Louis)*, **70**, 1399.

Ogura, J. H., Kawasaki, M., Takenouchi, S. and Yagi, M. (1966), *Ann. Otol. (St. Louis)*, **75**, 295.

Ogura, J. H. and Mallen, R. (1966), *Excerpta med. I.C.S.*, **113**, 167.

Ogura, J. H. and Powers, W. E. (1964), *Laryngoscope (St. Louis)*, **74**, 1081.

Ogura, J. H., Powers, W. E., Holtz, S., McFauran, M. H., Ellis, B. and Voorhees, R. (1960), *Laryngoscope (St. Louis)*, **70**, 780.

Ogura, J. H. and Roper, C. C. (1962), *Laryngoscope (St. Louis)*, **72**, 468.

Ogura, J. H., Roper, C. L. and Burford, T. H. (1961), *Laryngoscope (St. Louis)*, **71**, 885.

Ogura, J. H., Saltzstein, S. L. and Spjut, H. J. (1961), *Laryngoscope (St. Louis)*, **71**, 258.

Ogura, J. H., Shumrich, D. A. and Lapidot, A. (1962), *Ann. Otol. (St. Louis)*, **71**, 532.

Ogura, J. H., Togawa, K., Dammkoehler, R., Nelson, S. R. and Kawasaki, M. (1966), *Arch. Otolaryng.*, **83**, 135.

Ogura, J. H., Unno, T. and Nelson, J. R. (1968), *Ann. Otol. (St. Louis)*, **77**, 367.

Ohnishi, T. and Ogura, J. H. (1969), *Laryngoscope (St. Louis)*, **79**, 1847.

Ohnishi, T., Ogura, J. H. and Nelson, J. R. (1972), *Laryngoscope (St. Louis)*, **82**, 712.

Ohyama, M., Ueda, N., Harvey, J. B., Mogi, G. and Ogura, J. H. (1972), *Laryngoscope (St. Louis)*, **82**, 237.

O'Neil, J. J. (1959), *Laryngoscope (St. Louis)*, **69**, 1494.

Ong, G. B. and Lee, T. C. (1960), *Brit. J. Surg.*, **48**, 193.

Onodi, A. (1902), *Die Anatomie und Physiologie der Kehlkopfnerven*. Berlin: O. Coblentz.

Opheim, O. (1955), *Acta oto-laryng. (Stockh.)*, **45**, 226.

Ormerod, F. C. (1941), *J. Laryng.*, **56**, 151.

Orton, H. B. (1943), *Laryngoscope (St. Louis)*, **53**, 709.

Orton, H. B. (1944), *Ann. Otol. (St. Louis)*, **53**, 303.

Palva, T. and Meurman, O. H. (1962), *Acta oto-laryng. (Stockh.)*, **54**, 376.

Park, R. (1886), *Ann. Surg.*, **3**, 28.

Patterson, N. (1932), *J. Laryng.*, **47**, 81.

Paulson, D. L. (1951), *Amer. Rev. Tuberc.*, **64**, 477.

Payr, E. (1900), *Arch. klin. Chir.*, **62**, 67.

Payr, E. (1916), *Dtsch. med. Wschr.*, **42**, 682.

Pearson, F. G., Goldberg, M. and Da Silva, A. J. (1968), *Arch. Surg.*, **97**, 380.

Pennington, C. L. (1964), *Laryngoscope (St. Louis)*, **74**, 317.

Pennington, C. L. (1972), *Ann. Otol. (St. Louis)*, **81**, 546.

Perez, C. A. and Olson, J. (1970), *Amer. J. Roentgenol.*, **108**, 396.

Petrov, B. A. (1959), *Surgery*, **40**, 890.

Piquet, J. C. and Piquet, J. J. (1963), *Laryngoscope (St. Louis)*, **73**, 1351.

Poe, D. L. and Seager, P. S. (1948), *Arch. Otolaryng.*, **47**, 46.

Polanyi, T. G., Bredemeier, H. C. and Davis, T. W., Jr. (1970), *Med. biol. Engng.*, **8**, 541.

Polisar, I. A. (1959), *Laryngoscope (St. Louis)*, **69**, 1129.

Porres, R. and Mersol, V. F. (1968), *Arch. Otolaryng.*, **88**, 413.

Powers, W. E., McGee, H. H., Jr. and Seaman, W. B. (1957), *Radiology*, **68**, 169.

Powers, W. E. and Ogura, J. H. (1965), *Arch. Otolaryng.*, **81**, 153.

Preibisch-Effenberger, R. (1966), *Arch. Klin. exp. Ohr.-, Nas.- u. Kehlk. Heilk.*, **186**, 146.

Preibisch-Effenberger, R. (1969), *Mschr. Ohrenheilk.*, **103**, 561.

Pressman, J. J. (1954), *Arch. Otolaryng.*, **59**, 395.

Pressman, J. J. and Simon, M. B. (1959), *Amer. J. Surg.*, **25**, 850.

Priest, R. E., Huff, J. S. and Banovetz, J. D. (1967), *Ann. Otol. (St. Louis)*, **76**, 786.

Proctor, D. F. and Edgerton, M. T. (1959), *Ann. Otol. (St. Louis)*, **68**, 187.

Putney, F. J. and Bagley, C. S. (1970), *Ann. Otol. (St. Louis)*, **79**, 1057.

Quinn, H. J. (1969), *Laryngoscope (St. Louis)*, **79**, 1980.

Rabbett, W. F. (1965), *Ann. Otol. (St. Louis)*, **74**, 1149.

Rall, J. E., Gilbert, N. C. and Trump, R. (1945), *J. Lab. clin. Med.*, **30**, 953.

Rattenborg, C. (1961), *Acta anaesth. scand.*, **5**, 129.

Rauwerda, P. E. (1946), Thesis, Groningen University, Groninger, Netherlands.

Rob, C. G. and Bateman, G. H. (1949), *Brit. J. Surg.*, **37**, 202.

Robertson, R. and Sarjeant, T. R. (1950), *J. thorac. Surg.*, **20**, 689.

Rohman, M., Goetz, R. H. and Dee, R. (1960), *Surg. Forum*, **11**, 236.

Rooney, D. R. and Powell, R. W. (1959), *J. Amer. med. Ass.*, **169**, 1.

Rosenbach, O. (1880), *Breslau arztl. Z.*, **2**, 14; **2**, 27.

Ross, B. B. (1957), *J. appl. Physiol.*, **10**, 1.

Rubin, H. J. (1960), *Arch. Otolaryng.*, **71**, 913.

Rubin, H. J. (1960), *Arch. Otolaryng.*, **72**, 207.

Rubin, H. J. (1965), *Arch. Otolaryng.*, **81**, 604.

Ruedi, L. (1945), *Pract. oto-rhino-laryng. (Basel)*, **7**, 186.

Rush, B. F. (1961), *Surg. Gynec. Obstet.*, **112**, 507.

Russell, P. S. and Monaco, A. P. (1964), *New Engl. J. Med.*, **271**, 502, 553, 610, 664, 718, 776.

Sabiston, D. C., Jr. and Blalock, A. (1958), *Surgery*, **44**, 406.

Salem, W. O. (1950), *Hospital, Rio de J.*, **38**, 143.

Salinger, S. (1942), *Ann. Otol. (St. Louis)* **51**, 273.

Samuels, P. B. (1955), *Arch. Surg.*, **70**, 29.

Sandmann, G. (1890), *Arch. anat. Physiol. (Physiol. Abt.)*, 252.

Sanfilippo, L. J., Lane, S. L., Sherman, P., Pauporte, J. and Steichen, F. M. (1969), *Amer. J. Surg.*, **118**, 701.

Sauerland E. K. and Mizuno N. (1968), *Brain Res.*, **10**, 256.

Scalco, A. N., Shipman, W. F. and Tabb, H. G. (1960), *Ann. Otol. (St. Louis)*, **69**, 1134.

Schechter, G. L. and Ogura, J. H. (1969), *Laryngoscope (St. Louis)*, **79**, 942.

Scheer, A. A. (1953), *Arch. Otolaryng.*, **57**, 173.

Schinz, H. R. and Zuppinger, A. (1937), *Siebzehn Jahre Strahlentherapie Der Krebse*, pp. 174–194. Leipzig: Thieme.

Schiratzki, H. (1964), *Acta Otolaryng.*, **58**, 535.

Schmiegelow, E. (1929), *Arch. Otolaryng.*, **9**, 473.

Schultz, M. D. (1967), *Cancer of the Head and Neck*, p. 577 (J. J. Conley, Ed.). Washington, D.C.

Seaman, W. B., Tapley, N. V., Sanger, C., Jacox, H. W. and Atkins, H. L. (1961), *Amer. J. Roentgenol.*, **85**, 816.

Seed, L. (1942), *Ann. Otol. (St. Louis)*, **51**, 66.

Seiffert, A. (1943), *Arch. Klin. exp. Ohr.-, Nas.- u. Kehlk. Heilk.*, **152**, 366.

Sell, S. (1969), *Ann. intern. Med.*, **71**, 177.

Semon, F. (1881), *Arch. Laryng. Rhin. (Berl.)*, **2**, 197.

Serafini, I. (1969), *Advanc. oto-rhino-laryng.*, **16**, 95.

Sercer, A. (1952), *Arch. Klin. exp. Ohr.-, Nas.- u. Kehlk. Heilk.*, **161**, 264.

Sercer, A. (1959), *J. Laryng.*, **73**, 589.

Serrano, A., Ortiz-Monasterio, G. and Andrade-Pradillo, J. (1959), *Plast. reconstr. Surg.*, **24**, 333.

Shaw, R. R., Paulson, D. L. and Kee, J. L., Jr. (1961), *J. thorac. cardiovasc. Surg.*, **42**, 281.

Shilovtseva, A. S. (1969), *Arch. Otolaryng.*, **89**, 552.

Shimada, T. and Ogura, J. H. To be published.

Shumrick, D. A. (1967), *Arch. Otolaryng.*, **86**, 691.

Silver, C. E., Liebert, P. S. and Som, M. L. (1967), *Arch. Otolaryng.*, **86**, 95.

Simpson, J. F. (1960), *J. Laryng.*, **74**, 300.

Singleton, G. T. and Adkins, W. Y. (1972), *Ann. Otol. (St. Louis)*, **81**, 784.

Siribodhi, C., Sundmaker, W., Atkins, J. P. and Bonner, F. J. (1963), *Laryngoscope (St. Louis)*, **73**, 148.

Sisson, G. A. (1969), *Oto. Clin. N. Amer.*, **2**, 617.

Sisson, G. A., Goldstein, J. C. and Becker, G. D. (1970), *Oto. Clin. N. Amer.*, **3**, 529.

Skolnick, E. M., Sobaroff, B. J., Tenta, L. T., Saberman, M. N. and Jones, H. C. (1968), *Trans. Amer. Acad. Ophthal. Otolaryng.*, **72**, 937.

Solis-Cohen, (1907), *J. Laryngoscope (St. Louis)*, **17**, 365.

Som, M. L. (1951), *Arch. Otolaryng.*, **54**, 524.

Som, M. L. (1956), *Arch. Otolaryng.*, **63**, 474.

Som, M. L. (1959), *Trans. Amer. Acad. Ophthal. Otolaryng.*, **63**, 28.

Som, M. L. *Oto. Clin. N. Amer.*, **2**, 631.

Som, M. L. (1970), *J. Laryng.*, **84**, 655.

Som, M. L. (1972), *J. Amer. med. Ass.*, **221**, 1256.

Staple, T. W. and Ogura, J. H. (1966), *Radiology*, **87**, 226.

Starzl, T. E., Penn, I., Brettschneider, L., Ono, K. and Kashiwagi, N. (1970), *Fed. Proc.*, **29**, 186.

Stell, P. M., Maisels, D. O. and Brown, G. A. (1970), *J. Laryng.*, **84**, 1113.

Stevenson, W. (1937), *Ann. Otol. (St. Louis)*, **46**, 531.

Stiles, P. J. (1965), *Thorax*, **20**, 517.

Stone, J. W. and Arnold, G. E. (1967), *Arch. Otolaryng.*, **86**, 550.

Stoner, J. C., Thomas, G. K. and Albo, D. C. (1972), *Arch. Otolaryng.*, **95**, 141.

Strome, M. (1969), *Laryngoscope (St. Louis)*, **79**, 272.

Strong, E. W., Henschke, U. K., Nickson, J. J., Frazell, E. L., Tollefsen, H. R. and Hilaris, B. S. (1966), *Cancer, Philad.*, **19**, 1509.

Strong, M. S. (1970), *Laryngoscope (St. Louis)*, **80**, 1540.

Strong, M. S. and Jako, G. J. (1972), *Ann. Otol. (St. Louis)*, **81**, 791.

Sunderland, S. and Swaney, W. E. (1952), *Anat. Rec.*, **114**, 411.

Tabb, H. G. and Kirk, R. L. (1962), *Laryngoscope (St. Louis)*, **72**, 1228.

Takenouchi, S., Koyama, T., Kawasaki, M. and Ogura, J. H. (1968), *Acta oto-laryng. (Stockh.)*, **65**, 33.

Takenouchi, S., Ogura, J. H., Kawasaki, M. and Yagi, M. (1967), *Laryngoscope (St. Louis)*, **77**, 1644.

Tardy, M. E. and Tenta, L. T. (1970), *Otol. Clin. N. Amer.*, **3**, 483.

Tashiro, T. (1972), *Laryngoscope (St. Louis)*, **82**, 225.

Taylor, G. (1953), *Proc. roy. Soc. Sec. A*, **219**, 186.

Teitelbaum, H. A., Ries, F. A. and Lisansky, E. (1936), *Amer. J. Physiol.*, **116**, 505.

Terracol, J. and Sweet, R. H. (1958), *Diseases of the Esophagus*. Philadelphia: W. B. Saunders.

Thews, G. (1967), *Physiological Basis of Circulation Transportation*, p. 327 (E. B. Reeve and A. C. Guyton, Eds.). Philadelphia: W. B. Saunders.

Tomita, H. (1967), *J. oto-rhino-laryng. Soc. Jap.*, **70**, 963.

Tomori, Z. and Widdicombe, J. G. (1969), *J. Physiol. (Lond.)*, **200**, 25.

Toomey, J. M. and Brown, B. S. (1967), *Laryngoscope (St. Louis)*, **77**, 110.

Trotter, W. (1920), *J. Laryng.*, **35**, 289.

Tschiassny, K. (1957), *Arch. Otolaryng.*, **65**, 133.

Tucker, G. (1935), *Arch. Otolaryng.*, **21**, 172.

Tucker, H. M., Harvey, J. and Ogura, J. H. (1970), *Arch. Otolaryng.*, **92**, 530.

Tucker, H. M. and Ogura, J. H. (1971), *Laryngoscope* (*St. Louis*), **81**, 1602.

Ueda, N., Ohyama, M., Harvey, J. E., Mogi, G. and Ogura, J. H. (1971), *Laryngoscope* (*St. Louis*), **81**, 1948.

Van den Brenk, H. (1963), *Dermal Application of Hyperbaric Oxygen*, p. 152. New York: Elsevier.

Vineberg, A. M. (1946), *Canad. med. Ass. J.*, **55**, 117.

Von Hacker (1908), *Verh. dtsch. Ges. Chir.*, **37**, 359.

Von Leden, H. and Rand, R. W. (1967), *Amer. J. Surg.*, **33**, 36.

Von Leden, H., Yanagihara, N. and Werner-Kukuk, E. (1967), *Arch. Otolaryng.*, **85**, 666.

Wagner, R. (1890), *Arch. Anat. Physiol.* (*Physiol. Abt.*), **120**, 437.

Wagner, W. W., Latham, L. P., Brinkman, P. D. and Filley, G. F. (1969), *Science*, **163**, 1210.

Waltner, J. G. (1958), *Arch. Otolaryng.*, **67**, 99.

Wang, C. C. and O'Donnell, A. R. (1955), *New. Engl. J. Med.*, **252**, 743.

Wang, C. C. and Schulz, M. D. (1963), *Radiology*, **80**, 963.

Watts, J. McK. (1963), *Brit. J. Surg.*, **50**, 954.

Weddell, G., Feinstein, B. and Pattle, R. E. (1944), *Brain*, **67**, 178.

Weiss, P. and Hoag, A. (1946), *J. Neurophysiol.*, **9**, 413.

Widdicombe, J. G. (1954), *J. Physiol.* (*Lond.*), **123**, 55.

Widdicombe, J. G. and Nadel, J. A. (1963), *J. appl. Physiol.*, **18**, 681.

Widdicombe, J. G. and Nadel, J. A. (1963), *J. appl. Physiol.*, **18**, 863.

Woodman, D. (1946), *Arch. Otolaryng.*, **43**, 63.

Woodman, D. (1948), *Ann. Otol.* (*St. Louis*), **57**, 695.

Woodman, D. (1949), *Arch. Otolaryng.*, **50**, 91.

Woodman, D. (1953), *Arch. Otolaryng.*, **58**, 150.

Woodman, D. (1953), *Laryngoscope* (*St. Louis*), **63**, 714.

Woodman, D. (1955), *Ann. Otol.* (*St. Louis*), **64**, 794.

Woodman, D. (1956), *Trans. Amer. Acad. Ophthal. Otolaryng.*, **60**, 130.

Woodman, D. and Pollack, D. (1950), *Laryngoscope* (*St. Louis*), **60**, 832.

Woodruff, M. F. A. and Anderson, N. A. (1963), *Nature* (*Lond.*), **200**, 702.

Woodward, F. D. (1950), *Ann. Otol.* (*St. Louis*), **59**, 488.

Wookey, H. (1942), *Surg. Gynec. Obstet.*, **75**, 499.

Wookey, H., Ash, C., Welsh, W. K. and Mustand, R. A. (1951), *Ann. Surg.*, **134**, 529.

Work, W. P. and Boles, R. (1965), *Arch. Otolaryng.*, **82**, 401.

Wright, E. S. (1943), *Ann. Otol.* (*St. Louis*), **52**, 346.

Yagi, M., Ogura, J. H., Kawasaki, M. and Takenonehi, S. (1966), *Ann. Otol.* (*St. Louis*), **75**, 849.

Yanagisawa, E. and Kirchner, J. A. (1964), *Arch. Otolaryng.*, **79**, 80.

68. TRACHEA: TRACHEAL STENOSIS

BRUCE W. PEARSON

INTRODUCTION TO THE ANATOMY AND PHYSIOLOGY OF THE TRACHEA

The word "stenosis" is derived from the Greek "stenos" meaning narrow, small, or close. Stenosis is a narrowing of the opening or cavity of any passage, tube or orifice. Incomplete stenosis is to be differentiated from total obliteration of a lumen or complete stenosis.

Knowledge of normal tracheal anatomy and physiology is fundamental to an understanding of what truly constitutes narrowing in the trachea. The tracheal lumen is a dynamic structure of D-shaped cross-section, 2 cm wide in the adult, larger in males than females. The transverse muscles in the posterior wall can slightly constrict the lumen. There are no antagonistic muscles, but the spring of the cartilaginous arches may be considered the dilators of the trachea. A balance between these tensions, and the intraluminal and extratracheal pressures accounts for the resting tracheal luminal size.

The lower half of the trachea lies within the thorax and is subject to variations in size according to intrathoracic pressures. On inspiration, the volume enlargement of the chest creates enough radial traction on the trachea to cause enlargement. On expiration, the positive intrathoracic pressure compresses the trachea slightly. The membranous posterior wall reflects these changes most dramatically. It stretches during inspiration to produce an almost circular tracheal lumen and protrudes forward slightly during expiration to give a more crescent shaped cross-section. The changes in calibre which occur during coughing offer impressive testimony to the wisdom of the "sprung-arch" construction, as opposed to a pile of rings. During a cough, after full inspiration, the glottis closes and pleural pressures reverse to as high as 20 kilopascals (150 mm of mercury). When the glottis opens, for just an instant pressure is released from the trachea. There is extreme momentary narrowing of the bronchi and trachea. This contributes to the high air speed (linear velocity approaching the speed of sound) and turbulence necessary to hurl tenacious mucous secretions up from the airway walls (to which they have been transported by the cilial activity and "tussive squeeze" of the lower respiratory tract).

To interpret tracheal stenoses and surgical resections as a percentage of total tracheal length, it is necessary to appreciate how short the normal trachea is. There is some discrepancy between cadaver and living subject measurements, attributable to the upright posture and less rigid tissues of the latter. The cadaver's carina lies at the level of the four-five thoracic interspace. In the living however, studied by bronchograms the carina lies opposite the seventh thoracic vertebra. Cadaver data (Pineau *et al.*, 1972) gives the average male tracheal length as 9·74 cm, and the female, 9·11 cm. The ranges are 7·2–11·8 and 7·2–11·2 cm respectively. Ten to 13 cm is a workable figure in patients. The number of rings varies between fourteen and twenty. The anomalous variations in these rings was described by Niculescu and his associates (1972). Partial, total or multiple fusions of adjacent rings are common.

Incomplete rings are occasional. The average trachea manifests seven departures from the simple ring structure with a variation of two to thirteen.

Blood Supply

The dependency of the trachea for its blood supply on the inferior thyroid arteries above and the bronchial arteries below was restudied by Miura and Grillo in 1966. They noted that extensive skeletonization of the trachea in an attempt to mobilize it following partial surgical resections could lead to ischemic necrosis. Our own studies show the mucosal lining to be supplied from one or two fine arteries travelling circumferentially in the soft tissue between each cartilaginous arch. This is not true for the posterior tracheal wall which has a more linearly disposed microcirculation. The segmental horizontal intercartilaginous arterioles are united externally by three to five vertical blood vessels which occur at different points on the circumference of the arch for each different level. Close dissection on the external surface of the trachea can therefore devitalize major sections of its anterior and lateral walls. Inside the trachea the intercartilaginous vessels are connected across each cartilage by many fine intercommunicating vertical arterioles. The area most readily susceptible to pressure necrosis, therefore, is the mucosa immediately overlying the midportion of any given tracheal ring.

Mucosal Lining

The trachea is dependent for its integrity on an intact mucosal lining. This is normally pseudostratified ciliated columnar epithelium. At 37°C (310 K), the cilia beat about a thousand times per minute and their co-ordinated activity moves the overlying mucous blanket along at about 1·5 cm/min (Toremalm, 1972). This admirable cleaning power is subject to certain variations according to the physical and chemical properties of the overlying secretions, gravity and desiccation.

The mucosa contains goblet cells, and tubulo-acinar glands which dip into the submucosa. Secretional products of these glands and goblet cells, along with normal mucosal transudation of fluid, total 10 ml/day. This can be considerably increased by pathological exudation, edema, or aspiration. Normal elimination of secretions depends on excretion (cilial transport and cough), evaporation and possibly, to some extent, resorption.

Taffel (1940) observed satisfactory re-epithelialization of 1 × 1 cm fascial repaired defects in dog tracheas at 3 weeks. The detailed sequences of tracheal re-epithelialization were described by Wilhelm in 1953. Using freshly curetted rat tracheas, he found migration of nonciliated flattened cells, derived from the marginal ciliated columnar cells, proceeded at the rate of 200 μm in 8 h and 2 mm in 48 h. The flat migrating cells were much wider than their parent cells, and hence the number required to bridge the defect was reduced. Occasional mitosis within the sheets of spreading cells added a minor contribution. Migration did not begin until gross infection had ceased. An intact basement membrane seemed helpful. Following coverage, the flattened cells increased in number, thickened and eventually differentiated to a full thickness layer of pseudostratified ciliated columnar epithelium.

Structural Support

As at sites elsewhere in the body, the regenerative capability of the tracheal supporting cartilages is nil. Defects heal with fibrous scars as originally described by Schüller in 1880. The work of Mori in 1932 and in 1936 and, subsequently, of Borrie (1957) has shown that subperichondrial excision of one ring produces little loss of tracheal support, of two rings collapses the lumen to half its normal cross-sectional area and the excision of three rings causes severe tracheal stenosis. It should be remembered that after most pathological tracheal injuries, devitalized cartilage remains. Exposed cartilage soon dies and must be removed by the demolition (macrophage) phase of the inflammatory response. Inflammation is therefore considerably prolonged, compared to other soft tissue wounds, even in the absence of infection. Collagen deposition is increased as a result and this may be part of the explanation of the trachea's propensity to cicatricial stenosis.

The Laryngeal Guardian

It has been mentioned that, an intact epithelial lining, adequate external mechanical support and a sufficiently competent blood supply are critical to the vitality of the trachea. The fourth and equally crucial factor is the integrity of the larynx above. By virtue of its sphincteric actions, it prevents the ingress of food, fluid and secretions during deglutition. It is essential to the performance of an effective cough. It will not be surprising that the assessment and treatment of tracheal stenosis depends to some extent on accurate knowledge of the larynx.

HISTORICAL FACTORS

Endotracheal Intubation

In 1540 Vesalius demonstrated the artificial ventilation of an animal through an endotracheal tube. The use of such tubes to ventilate humans was made known through the publications of MacEwen in 1880. It was generally admitted that endotracheal tubes could cause damage to the upper respiratory tract, but early interests centred largely on the larynx and most traumatic effects were ascribed to inept intubation. Little attention was given to the damage that might result to the trachea, after a tube was in place.

With the rapid advances in surgery and anesthesia which accompanied World War II, the endotracheal tube came into widespread use as an effective means of establishing and ensuring an airway. Its use in the management of coma was established by Rovenstine (1945) and Foregger (1946) was popularizing its extensive use for prolonged tracheo-bronchial toilet. Normal tracheas thus replaced diphtheritic ones as the most likely candidates for intubation.

In 1943, Lundy reported the autopsy finding of an acute inflammatory reaction to an endotracheal tube which had remained in place for 38 h. In the same year, Grimm and

Knight were able to link tracheal necrosis in a child to the pressure of an inflated endotracheal tube cuff. From that time forward a growing number of reports have documented the problems of acute injury and subsequent stenosis of the upper airway associated with the prolonged use of endotracheal tubes.

Endotracheal Tube Cuffs

Adriani and Phillips (1957) showed that the pressure exerted by an endotracheal tube cuff on the tracheal wall during positive pressure ventilation was equal to or greater than the peak airway pressures employed to ventilate the patient. By 1964, Bain and Spoerel had drawn attention to the causal relationship between rising ventilator pressures, progressively increased cuff pressures used to enforce a seal, and unforeseen tracheal damage from the cuff. Throughout the 1960's numerous studies clarified the relationships between tube materials, sizes, cuff pressures, duration of use, movement, infection, hypotension and other factors. Slowly, cheeringly, supportive ventilatory techniques and apparatus appropriate to the delicacy and sophistication of the trachea has ensued.

Tracheotomy

Among the earliest of references to tracheal stenosis following tracheotomy is the paper of Colles in 1886 in which 4 stenoses followed 57 recoveries after 103 tracheotomies for diphtheria. By 1911, Thost had related the degree of stenosis to the size of the tracheal cannula. Periodic reports of successful repairs of post-tracheotomy stenoses began to appear, starting with Howarth's (1923) staged trough and cover reconstruction of the lower larynx and upper cervical trachea. By 1940 Cummings was still able to state that high tracheotomy in diphtheria was the leading cause of the rather rare condition of tracheal stenosis and up to that time only one author (Jackson, 1937) provided textbook instructions for its management.

Tracheal stenosis following tracheotomy differed from that following cuffed tube intubation insofar as it often involved less than the total tracheal circumference. That reconstructive surgical techniques could deal with subtotal tracheal defects was first demonstrated in 1896, when König is said to have made up a defect in the trachea with a pedicle flap which gained its structural support from a rib graft. It was the laryngotracheal repairs of Fairchild (1927) and of Schmiegelow (1929), however, that appeared to guide subsequent surgeons in their attempts at subtotal tracheal repair. In 1940 Taffel demonstrated the dependability of the free fascial grafts introduced by Kirschner in 1909, in repairing window defects of the trachea. Variations of the König and Schmiegelow transcervical tracheoplasties were rediscovered, modified and applied by Gebauer, Paulson, Som, Consiglio, Aboulker, Meyer, Montgomery, Bryce and others often in an attempt to deal with post-tracheotomy stenoses, emanating from respiratory care units, in the 1950's and early 1960's. As hoped for advances in the employment of prosthetic materials for tracheal reconstruction failed to materialize,

the flap and graft techniques of these men reached states of development that continue to justify their selected employment today, as alternatives to segmental resection and end to end anastomosis.

Knowledge of the roles of the type of incision, tube size, placement, shape and flexibility, wound sepsis and the like grew a pace with the knowledge of endotracheal tube pathology, through the efforts of Florange, Pearson, Donnelly, Grillo, Goldberg, Bryant and others. Many of the stenoses associated with tracheostomy itself are becoming preventable, and it is possible that external trauma and violence will rival tracheotomy and intubation as the leading cause of stenosis.

Early Attempts to Treat Complete Circumferential Tracheal Stenosis

Experience with the healing powers of the trachea following mechanical injury dates back to the 1880's when Schüller incised pig trachea and found the cut edges united by fibrous tissue; the cartilage failed to regenerate. Gluck and Zeller performed tracheal transection and re-anastomosis in the dog in 1881, and, in 1884, Küster successfully treated a tracheal stricture in man by the resection and end to end anastomosis technique. Failure to re-exploit this method in the management of tracheal stenosis over the next 75 years is perhaps the most ironic feature of development of knowledge in this field.

Originally, as now, few surgeons had the opportunity of gaining more than a handful of experiences with tracheal stenosis. The high immediate mortality of crushing injuries to the larynx and trachea kept this a rare disease. This continued to be true, even as the motor car and high speed travel become prominent fixtures of modern life. The resuscitative techniques of the 1940's and 1950's, evolved in response to the needs of the war, poliomyelitis and the cardiovascular and thoracic surgeons, began salvaging these patients in significant numbers. More and more attention came to be paid to the possibility of repairing or replacing the damaged airway.

In 1948, Daniel cast the work of Schüller in doubt by stating that healing wounds following circumferential excisions of the canine trachea showed evidence of new cartilage in the granulation tissue. This in turn led to unfounded optimism in the ability of the trachea to regenerate. It was reasoned that earlier patients and animals may have succumbed to simple airway obstruction by granulation, before the injured trachea had been given a chance to regenerate. Efforts were therefore redirected toward stenting tracheal defects open during this period in the hope that regeneration would appear.

Other authors reasoned that just as the constant pressure of an aneurysm could cause bone to be resorbed, so the constant pressure of a core mold in the lumen of the trachea could cause resorption of stenotic scar tissue. In 1948, the futility of this approach was declared both by Clagett and his colleagues and by Longmire who described structural collapse after removal of stents they had placed to induce tube formations. Figi and co-workers at the Mayo Clinic were able to stop the ingress of granulation by skin grafting the luminal surface before supporting it with a stent, but the problem of subsequent rigid support remained for full circumferential defects. The first successful repair of a circumferential resection is the report of Belsey in 1946 in which fascia lata and a steel spring appeared to provide the right combination of a lined airtight repair and adequate structural support.

From this time forward, the idea of providing a lined tube with circumferential support as enunciated by Belsey seemed to guide most investigators. Simultaneously, the medical limelight fell on cardiovascular surgery and its success in arterial replacement with prosthetic vascular techniques. It was perhaps only natural that hope should arise that another flexible tube, the trachea, could be replaced with prosthetic materials. Perhaps porous varieties could even be incorporated and become lined with mucosa the way woven plastic arteries appeared to endothelialize their lumens.

Tracheal Prostheses

The long line of candidate materials for this job started with tantalum gauze in 1949 (Rob and Bateman). This was followed by stainless steel, Tygoflex (1958), polyethylene (Marlex) (1960), polyethylene terephthalate (Dacron) (1961), woven politef (Teflon) (1961), polyvinyl alcohol (formalinized) (1961), polyurethane, silicone rubber (1962), polyethylene implanted with omentum (1962), heavier polyethylene (1962), politef with polyethylene mesh (1963), politef mesh with polypropylene rings (1965), silicone rubber (1967 and 1968), and politef again in 1969. Despite the occasional success of individual prostheses, reliability was never established and failure was the general rule. The work of Craig (1953), of Ekeström and Carlens (1959) and of Borrie (1970), if closely studied, shows that such tubes occasionally work by virtue of their similarity to a stent. A granulating wound is simply held open, but the prosthesis which has been placed in a potentially infected connective tissue bed and remains mobile, bathed in secretions and unable to epithelialize, is treated like a foreign body which continues to induce a granulating mediastinitis so long as it is present and, on occasion, adds the threat of major vessel erosion and exsanguination from either the brachiocephalic (innominate) artery (Cummins and Waterman, 1957), or the common carotid (Keshishian et al., 1956) to an already unstable situation. Borrie's attempt to fashion a prosthesis that would extend intraluminally beyond the junction line with normal trachea in an attempt to hold back granulation at the anastomosis line somewhat extended his own success but, in general, prosthetic materials had failed to restore the lumen of circumferential tracheal defects; the greater the length of the defect, the less effective they had been.

Throughout this period a line of investigation into the biology of tracheal wound repair that led to current treatment methods may be traced. In 1958 Nelson confirmed Schüller's original observation that the trachea is incapable of regenerating. Greenberg in 1960 showed that tracheal segments simply removed and reimplanted as autografts failed to survive and was not surprised that tracheal allografts and lyophilized allografts also failed to

gain acceptance. Previous work on cartilage autografts, summarized by Peer in 1955, had shown that cartilage autografts themselves can survive if provided with coverage and an adequately vascularized bed. Correll and Beattie in 1956 further showed that tracheal epithelium was capable of regenerating so long as infection was absent. Taffel had previously described this phenomenon in his fascial autografts. The respiratory epithelium that resulted even regenerated cilia and mucosal glands but the muscularis and cartilage were never regenerated. It seemed then that, if infection were prevented, a vascular bed supplied and the job of support entrusted to living cartilage autografts, partial reconstructions larger than those of Taffel could be undertaken. The wire supported dermal grafts of Gebauer (1950) and Paulson (1951) gave way to the more ingenious all tissue reconstructions of Serrano in 1959 and Consiglio in 1969. The former author employed arch-shaped rib cartilage autografts on either side of a tracheal defect. These were then rotated medially to form a lined tracheal lumen and covered with a local rotation flap. The latter author provided experimental data and one clinical case of repair with auricular cartilage. Auricular cartilage with skin has been used as a composite graft by Farkas and his associates (1972) and nasal septum with its mucosa has been used as a composite graft by Krizek and Kirchner (1972).

Although such techniques could occasionally handle long stenoses the total management of circumferential tracheal stenosis continued to elude investigators until recent times. A review of sleeve resection and end to end anastomosis of circumferential tracheal stenotic defects as exemplified by the reports of Kay (1951) Flavell, (1959), Barclay and his associates (1957) and Miscall and his associates (1963) suggested that this was the management of choice, but only the latter two authors were successful with resections of greater than 3·5 cm in length and it was widely held that this method should not be attempted for defects beyond 2·5 cm. Cantrell and Folse (1961) established that recurrence of stenosis at such anastomoses was chiefly attributable to suture line tension. They found 16·7 newtons (1700 grams) of tension to be the upper limit of safety in dogs. In the same year Michelson and his associates showed that complete mobilization of the trachea could give 4–6 cm of release. This included division of the right pulmonary ligament (2·5 cm) and division and reimplantation of the left main bronchus (2·5 cm). Only half this much could be obtained in patients over 50 years of age. In 1964, Grillo and co-workers further established the value of intrathoracic release in permitting longer (4–5 cm) tracheal resections. In the same year, Ogura and Powers first mentioned gaining length proximal to an anastomosis by thyrohyoid release and laryngeal drop. This method was further defined and popularized by Dedo and Fishman (1969). Montgomery placed the site of release even higher (1973) to lessen the post-operative dysphagia. Mulliken and Grillo's cadaver studies (1968) and summary publications (1970) clarified the roles of neck flexion, tracheal mobilization (with preservation of the local vascular pedicles), hilar mobilization, and inferior pulmonary ligament division (without bronchial reimplantation) in securing new tracheal length at tensions which would not lead to dehiscence.

Future of Tracheal Reconstruction

The reliability of sleeve resection and end to end anastomosis with or without length gaining procedures remains imperfect to the present day. Two alternative lines of investigation deserve mention, although neither has passed beyond the stage of laboratory study as yet.

In 1902, Sacerdotti and Frattin observed bone formation in a kidney after ligation of the renal pedicle. In 1931 Huggins showed that transitional epithelium alone, without the presence of urine, was capable of inducing osseous metaplasia in certain connective tissue sites. This principle of metaplastic bone induction by transitional epithelium was applied to the problem of tracheal reconstruction by Rush and Clifton in 1956. They succeeded in inducing bony tube formation with out-turned bladder mucosa in dogs, but survival could not be maintained. Barker and Litton (1973) have re-explored this method, and appear to have better results.

Approaching the problem from a different direction, Schechter (1972) reported his experience with the concept of revascularized pedicled flaps. The first basic step has been to fashion the desired transplant with autogenous tissues on a muscular site in the dogs hind leg. When the fabrication has healed and incorporated a blood supply from the adjacent muscle the entire construction, including the underlying muscle and its nutrient vascular pedicle, is transplanted to the desired site of employment, and local vascular reanastomosis performed. Applying the concept to tracheal reconstruction, he has been unable to achieve success, but the ingenuity of the method may attract future investigators.

INCIDENCE OF TRACHEAL STENOSIS

The more patients that are resuscitated following major cervical or thoracic injury, heart and chest surgery, drug intoxication and coma, the higher will be the incidence of tracheal stenosis. The full impact of improved ventilatory techniques, for example, the use of the volume ventilator, the soft cuffed tubes, etc. has not yet been fully appreciated so that current figures on incidence may soon require revision.

Lindholm's (1969) report on the frequency of acute upper airway injuries following endotracheal intubation prolonged beyond 24 h is a classic review on this subject. As one might expect, the damage is directly related to where and with how much force the endotracheal tube contacts the airway. Primarily the medial surfaces of the arytenoids and posterior plate of the cricoid cartilage are affected when tubes are placed in the larynx, and the larger the tube proportional to the size of the glottis, the greater the damage.

Laryngeal stenosis is even more disabling than tracheal narrowing. In cases requiring ventilatory assistance beyond 48 h, most physicians try to spare the larynx by introducing the tube through a tracheotomy. This creates the highest risk population; patients sick enough to require

prolonged ventilatory assistance with a cuffed tube, necessarily introduced through a tracheotomy.

Definitive data on such patients was collected by Pearson and Andrews (1971). Four hundred and fifty eight severely ill admissions to a large hospital respiratory unit yielded 220 patients requiring tracheotomy and positive pressure ventilation through a conventional cuffed tube for prolonged ventilatory assistance. One hundred and twenty-one patients survived the first 3 weeks to be admitted to the study. Eighteen were lost to follow-up, but of the 103 studied prospectively, very careful data were collected. Clinical and radiological examinations were undertaken at extubation, at 3 weeks, and at 3 month intervals. Tomography and endoscopy were undertaken where indicated. Radiologically evident stomal stenosis was present in 100 per cent of these patients. Eighteen developed symptomatic stenosis, 12 at the stomal level and 6 at the cuff. Two of the stomal stenoses proved fatal. Anyone who had a circumferential defect at the first post-extubation examination went on to develop cuff-level stenosis. It is clear from these data that any figures on incidence must be interpreted in terms of the diligence of the investigators and the definition of stenosis.*

ETIOLOGY AND PATHOGENESIS

Tracheal stenosis may be classified according to its degree (partial, complete), its anatomical level (cervical, thoracic), or its pathophysiology (endotracheal mass, intramural constriction or malacia, extratracheal compression). An etiological classification will be followed in this chapter which allows inclusion of less common entities such as congenital narrowings of the trachea and specific inflammatory stenoses caused by microbiological agents or chemical and physical factors other than intubation or trauma (Table 1).

DEVELOPMENTAL TRACHEAL STENOSIS

A child may be born or present early in life with narrowing of the tracheal airway secondary to deficient development of the epithelial lining or the supporting structures in the tracheal wall itself (primary stenosis) or with cardiovascular, oesophageal or thyroid anomalies causing extraluminal compression or an intraluminal mass (secondary stenosis).

Embryology

The trachea and main bronchi form in the first 9 weeks of fetal life. From that time forward the pulmonary system enlarges and the lobular and eventually the alveolar systems elaborate. The tracheal endoderm is derived from a ventral outgrowth of the primitive foregut at $3\frac{1}{2}$ weeks. This gives rise to the tracheal epithelium and glands. The mesoderm surrounding this outgrowth differentiates to the cartilages, vessels and connective tissue.

---

*A satisfactory working definition of severe stenosis is "stenosis sufficient to produce symptoms and require surgical correction" (Bryce, 1972). This excludes the majority of anatomically present but physiologically insignificant stenoses and may allow comparisions of the work of various investigators.

TABLE 1

Tracheal Stenosis

I. *Developmental*
    A. Primary   (i) Atresia
                      (ii) Hypoplasia
                      (iii) Agenesis
    B. Secondary   (i) Vascular Arch Anomaly
                      (ii) Esophageal Anomaly
                      (iii) Ectopic Thyroid

II. *Inflammatory*
    A. Infectious   (i) Diphtheria
                      (ii) Scleroma
                      (iii) Tuberculosis
                      (iv) Syphilis
                      (v) Histoplasmosis
    B. Idiopathic   (i) Amyloidosis
                      (ii) Tracheopathia Osteoplastica
                      (iii) Histiocytosis "X"
                      (iv) Polychondritis
    C. Chemical
    D. Physical

III. *Traumatic*
    A. Exogenous   (i) Blunt Chest Injury
                      (ii) Blunt Neck Injury
                      (iii) Penetrating Neck Injury
    B. Endogenous   (i) Suprastomal
                      (ii) Stomal
                      (iii) Cuff
                      (iv) Tip

Arey (1958) calls attention to the fact that this development is not a progressive tubular downgrowth from the larynx but begins as a laryngotracheal trough running lengthwise on the floor of the foregut, caudal to the pharyngeal pouches. The pulmonary buds are lateral extensions that begin development as the tracheal lumen separates itself from the future esophagus. The lower portion of the larynx organizes around the cranial end of the trachea, but the major part of the larynx including the vocal cords arises from the pharyngeal floor and the laryngeal muscles and cartilages consequently originate from the branchial arch system.

Congenital Subglottic Stenosis

The region within the cricoid ring is a junctional zone in the separate embryologic evolutions of the laryngeal and tracheal primordia. Atresia occurring at this level ("congenital subglottic stenosis") is usually thicker than the occasional web seen in the trachea itself. The patient may escape detection at birth and later be discovered during the endoscopic evaluation of a child with repeated attacks of croup. Fearon (1966) indicated that occasional cases come to light when the child is undergoing anesthesia for unrelated surgery. The anesthetist is unable to pass an endotracheal tube which would normally meet no resistance in a child of that age and laryngoscopic examination reveals an annular subglottic stenosis within the cricoid

ring. Rare causes of stenosis in the same region mentioned by Leape (1973) are sclerotic resolution of a pre-existing subglottic hemangioma and posterior laryngotracheal redundancy following repair of a laryngotracheal cleft.

Although discussion of the treatment of this disorder is beyond the scope of this chapter, the alternatives debated in recent years include:

(1) Endoscopic dilatation with or without the addition of an indwelling subglottic upper tracheal silastic stent or T tube.

(2) Surgical division of the cricoid ring and wedging apart with a local thyroid cartilage graft.

(3) Bypass valved tracheostomy so that speech and respiration may continue while the larynx grows to adequate dimensions.

Congenital Tracheomalacia

Hypoplasia usually affects the entire length of the trachea when it occurs, causing stenosis or malacia. Congenital tracheomalacia implies an intrauterine insult at the fifth to sixth weeks of development since cartilage begins to appear from this time forward. There is a tendency to association with other major congenital abnormalities (especially of the heart and genitourinary tract). Although the severe cases have progressive respiratory difficulties at birth which lead to death in a few hours, the diagnosis being discovered only at autopsy, there are cases where the diagnosis of malacia or hypoplasia has been made during life and surgery has been undertaken.

One reported case presented at 3 months. The trachea would not pass a No. 12 French catheter. The patient died following surgery on her common bile duct atresia due to inability to maintain an airway, despite tracheotomy. At post-mortem, a generalized hypoplasia of the trachea (1·5 mm lumen) extended from 1 cm below the glottis to the carinal level.

Fonkalsrud and Sumida described a case in 1971 of severe congenital stenosis of the entire trachea with absence of the membranous portion. The patient suffered repeated episodes of lower respiratory tract infections since birth and was dyspneic by age $3\frac{1}{2}$. Acute respiratory obstruction at age $4\frac{1}{2}$ required emergency tracheal replacement. The oesophagus was transposed as a substitute and held open with a long tracheostomy cannula. The patient died 39 days post-operatively from asphyxiation by occlusion of the lower anastomosis with a mucous plug. The severity of narrowing of the trachea and the anomalous formations of the tracheal cartilages, which were complete rings rather than arches, was documented at autopsy.

Tracheal Agenesis

Total agenesis of the trachea is a rare anomaly incompatible with life, but autopsy specimens show that in such cases the larynx is normal with a lumen ending blindly just below the cricoid level (Hopkinson, 1972). Bronchi may arise directly from the midthoracic esophagus.

Vascular Compression of the Trachea

The embryonic ventral aortic root gives rise to the innominate arteries between branchial arches 4 and 6. Descent of the heart during the seventh and eighth weeks of gestation draws the origin of these vessels caudad. Degeneration of the dorsal retro-esophageal connections and right aortic arch breaks the vascular ring that surrounded the mediastinal viscera. The right innominate, left carotid and left subclavian ultimately arise in close proximity near the summit of the arch of a left-sided aorta. Anomalous expressions of this development lead to rearrangements compatible with life such as the double aortic arch or aberrant (retroesophageal) right subclavian artery (Congdon, 1922). The trachea develops in the presence of these contiguous embryonic events and for this reason the tracheal indentation associated with vascular rings may tend to persist, even after the pressure is released.

Of 68 infants who underwent operation for relief of tracheobroncho-esophageal obstruction secondary to anomalies of major vessels in the mediastinum, Nikaidoh et al. (1972) found 33 double aortic arches, 23 right aortic arches with a left ductus or ligamentum, 6 aberrant right subclavian arteries, 1 displaced innominate artery and 2 anomalous left pulmonary arteries. Gross (1954) reported the first successful surgical relief of tracheal obstruction secondary to double aortic arch and since that time vascular ring procedures have made up 1–2 per cent of cardiac operations performed in a pediatric hospital.

A good deal more controversial and according to some more common condition is the phenomenon of tracheal compression by the innominate artery in children without such a ring. Usually the origin of the innominate is directly over the trachea, about 1 cm above the carina. The diagnosis of innominate tracheal compression is said to be worth considering in children under the age of 3 who suffer recurrent attacks of croup. Bronchoscopy is reported to show a pulsatile transverse anterior indentation of the intra-thoracic tracheal wall involving 50 per cent of the lumen. Identification of the bar as the innominate is achieved by levering forward with the bronchoscope, and observing disappearance of the right temporal and radial pulses. Unfortunately, very similar observations can often be made in normal children.

The contrast esophagogram is the most helpful investigative procedure when the diagnosis of tracheo-esophageal obstruction secondary to vascular anomalies is suspected. Bilateral indentation of the esophagus almost always implies the presence of a vascular ring. Posterior compression implies an aberrant right subclavian artery. Both situations require confirmation by angiography, prior to surgical treatment. In the case of innominate artery compression, the tendency to outgrow the condition is such that more than 85 per cent of Mustard's series (1962) did not require operative suspension.

Esophageal Tracheal Compression

Minor degrees of tracheal stenosis have been described in association with congenital tracheo-esophageal fistula, but the supporting structures of the trachea have generally been adequate and the esophageal atresia, with or without aspiration, has proven to be the major problem.

A peculiar form of tracheal obstruction may arise from an excessive flaccidity of the tracheo-oesophageal party wall. The diagnosis may be suspected when an abnormal degree of tracheal collapse on expiration is seen by careful fluoroscopy. This condition is usually outgrown by the second year of life. Nevertheless, cases in which this phenomenon produced a nonproductive cough, dyspnea on exertion, and uncontrollable attacks of coughing progressing to syncope have been described. In addition to radiologic examination, Herzog et al. (1972) based their diagnoses on proof of respiratory obstruction with pulmonary function tests, and on bronchoscopic examination with direct intrabronchial measurement of pressures and flow resistances. They proposed reinforcing the tracheo-oesophageal party wall with rectus sheath fascia.

Giustra et al. (1973) have drawn attention to the occasional association between oesophageal achalasia and secondary tracheal compression by the sheer bulk of the distended oesophagus. Overspill and aspiration, with secondary bronchitis and pneumonia may hinder recognition of the tracheal compression factor.

Thyroid Tracheal Obstruction

Ectopic portions of an otherwise normal thyroid gland can project into the lumen of the trachea. They usually do so at the junction of the lateral and posterior cervicotracheal walls, suggesting they are rolled in as the tracheal groove separates from the oesophagus. Waggoner (1958) divides intralaryngotracheal thyroid masses into those that retain continuity with the gland, and those that become isolated intratracheal ectopic thyroid. Differentiation of ectopic thyroid from well differentiated locally metastatic or invasive thyroid carcinoma is not simple, for both conditions usually appear in adult life, and are associated with a defect in the tracheal wall. Associated anomalous courses of the recurrent laryngeal nerve can expose them to risk at surgery. The tissue is under the influence of TSH, and is therefore more likely to become clinically manifest in goiter, or after thyroidectomy (Dowling, 1962).

INFLAMMATORY TRACHEAL STENOSIS

Diphtheria

Diphtheria is an acute infectious disease produced by the exotoxin of corynebacterium diphtheriae. The organism is a gram positive non-sporulating nonmotile club-shaped pleomorphic metachromatic rod which only becomes toxogenic when infected itself with a bacteriophage. The toxin causes severe local necrotizing inflammation usually in the upper respiratory tract and exerts remote effects on the heart, peripheral nerves and adrenals. The organism is transmitted to man by droplets from active cases or carriers. At one time a common disease of childhood, it has been brought under control by active immunization of pre-school children with diphtheria toxoid (an immunogenic but non-pathogenic form of the toxin).

Debilitated adults who missed immunization in childhood are the more likely victims today.

The nose and pharynx are the usual sites of origin but about 10 per cent of cases spread to involve the larynx, trachea and bronchi. Although the organism remains localized, the powerful exotoxin is absorbed and causes necrosis and acute inflammation. A thick leathery bluish-white pseudo-membrane forms in patches and eventually becomes confluent over the entire site of involvement. Adherence to the underlying surface (which bleeds when the membrane is stripped) is a helpful diagnostic sign in the pharynx. In the trachea and bronchi, the membrane is more easily detached and may form a "cast" of the entire airway.

Patients may be asphyxiated by the laryngo-tracheal membrane itself, the bilateral vocal cord paralysis (neurotoxicity of the endotoxin) that may appear weeks after apparent recovery from the acute illness, or rarely, cicatricial tracheal stenosis.

It is difficult to be sure that tracheal stenosis of sufficient severity to produce permanent symptoms or warrant surgery was wholly attributable to the destructive effects of the intoxication alone. The intubation tubes in use for laryngeal diphtheria, devised by O'Dwyer in 1885, extended down into the trachea. High tracheotomy was thought to be the leading cause of post-diphtheritic tracheal stenosis by Cummings (1940). Suffice it to say, the combination of acute specific inflammation, blind peroral intubation and emergency tracheotomy provide ample opportunities for the loss of structural support and initiation of excessive fibrous repair.

Scleroma

Scleroma is a chronic infectious granulomatous disease of the nose and nasopharynx endemic in Latin America and central south-eastern Europe. Occasional cases are seen in the U.S.A. The onset resembles a cold and may begin in childhood. Tracheal lesions appear in 3 per cent of cases (Acuña, 1973), secondary to laryngeal involvement. When the trachea is involved its unyielding firmness may prevent intubation and necessitate emergency treatment with bronchoscopic dilatation or resection. Secondary pulmonary infection and atelectasis is frequently present.

Diagnosis is confirmed by a biopsy which reveals a chronic inflammatory infiltrate characterized by numerous plasma cells, lymphocytes and large foamy macrophages which contain the causative organism. The organism is a gram negative bacillus (Klebsiella rhinoscleromatis; von Frisch's bacillus) and the cells in which it is found are called Mikulicz cells. "Russell bodies" refer to degenerate plasma cells with acidophilic inclusion bodies also seen in this disease. Mikulicz cells and Russell bodies are not exclusive to scleroma, but also characterize the histopathology of leprosy and venereal granuloma. Since leprosy can involve the nose also, misdiagnosis is a possibility. Streptomycin and antituberculous regimens are usually applied but control of the disease is difficult. Dilatation and the use of an indwelling endotracheal stent have been reported to maintain the airway during medical management.

Tuberculosis

Tuberculosis is a chronic, infectious inflammatory disease caused by Mycobacterium tuberculosis and its predilection for the respiratory system and its ability to produce chronic cicatricial sequelae is well known. The host tissue's acute inflammatory response to introduction of the bacilli fails as the tubercle bacillus destroys polymorphs. Macrophages phagocytose but often fail to kill the bacilli. They may elongate (epitheloid cells) or fuse (Langhan's giant cells). Lymphocytes and fibroblasts surround the lesion. Central caseous necrosis occurs and the typical tuberculous follicle is formed. Another type of lesion, the exudative reaction characterizes tuberculosis involving epithelial surfaces. The lymphocytic component predominates, macrophage elements are scant, and a fibrin rich exudate is generated. Tuberculous tracheobronchitis which is always secondary to active pulmonary lesions does occur but the bronchi are much more severely affected than the trachea.

There is a difference in pathogenesis depending on previous exposure and age. Typically the childhood primary Ghon lung focus showers the mediastinal nodes with organisms. The resulting primary complex includes massive lymphadenopathy (sufficient to compress the trachea). It usually heals; if it spreads, the child dies of miliary tuberculosis.

In adults, pulmonary tuberculosis is combated at the primary (usually apical) site. Failure to control it results in cavitation. Intrabronchial dissemination of infectious debris carries the disease to the trachea and larynx, and the prognosis is diminished by this finding.

Reporting 1255 autopsies for tuberculosis in the pre-antibiotic era, Negus cites a 47·4 per cent incidence of laryngeal involvement and a 10·4 per cent incidence of tracheobronchial disease. Ulcerative and non-ulcerative tubercles are described as having a predilection for the posterior tracheal wall, the tips of the rings and the intercartilaginous areas. It should be noted that the treatment of tuberculosis is chemotherapy, but the treatment of cicatrix is surgery. The former is paramount: Tracheal involvement implies advanced and active disease. The latter is rarely required, as few survive disease active enough and longstanding enough to stricture the trachea severely.

Other Bacterial Inflammations

Other specific inflammatory diseases occasionally produce narrowing of the trachea. The author has witnessed one case in which a pyogenic mediastinal abscess in an infant produced severe tracheal compression. The child had developed a clinical syndrome mimicking asthma and heart failure (impeded airway and venous return). Bronchoscopic confirmation of the compression and its relief was obtained before and after transcervical drainage of the pus.

Syphilis

Negus claims treating a 17-year-old girl with syphilitic tracheal stenosis, presumably a sequel of secondary lues with mucositis and perichondritis. Jackson depicts a case of tracheal compression due to syphilitic aortitis with aneurysm formation.

Histoplasmosis

Histoplasma capsulatum is a highly infectious yeast like fungus which most frequently affects the reticuloendothelial system and may obstruct the trachea with mediastinal lymph node involvement (Greenwood and Holland, 1972). Dysphagia and superior vena caval syndrome may rarely occur due to the pressure of fibrosing mediastinitis. Histoplasma skin tests are usually positive, but the limitations of intradermal tests in an obvious endemic area must be recognized as only recent conversion would be significant. The acute phase of the infection is documented by demonstrating precipitating antibodies to histoplasmosis antigen by the micro-ouchterlony technique and by complement fixation titers. H and M bands appear in active cases. The H band may persist 12 months following recovery. Recommended management includes intravenous hydrocortisone and amphotericin B. The lympholytic effect of steroids results in some relief of the mediastinal compression and also alleviates the acute febrile side effects that accompany intravenous amphotericin B.

Amyloidosis

Amyloidosis of the respiratory tract was divided by House and Barrington (1950), into three categories:

(1) A solitary nodule affecting the larynx, trachea, bronchial tree or pulmonary parenchyma.
(2) Multiple amyloid deposits confined to the pulmonary parenchyma.
(3) Diffuse tracheobronchial amyloidosis.

The diffuse primary tracheobronchial variety may occur primarily (Attwood *et al.*, 1972) and mimic tuberculous tracheobronchitis. Patients develop wheezing, cough and mucopurulent sputum sometimes streaked with blood. The narrowing of the trachea may be moderate to severe, with increased rigidity of the tracheobronchial tree and pale nodules and distortion on bronchoscopy. A tracheobronchogram is frequently interpreted as malformation with stenosis. In the primary form, gingival and rectal biopsies are negative for amyloid but the tracheal biopsy specimen shows apple-green birefringence in polarized light following Congo red staining. Although the amyloid deposits are histologically relatively avascular, serious bleeding may accompany biopsy because of a failure of vessel retraction. Cartilaginous transformation, calcification and ossification may occur in tracheobronchial and pulmonary sites and give rise to confusion with tracheopathia osteoplastica. The multinodular form of this disease may be adequately treated by surgical removal with a satisfactory prognosis because it does not seem to be associated with amyloidosis in other sites. Secondary infection with *Proteus mirabilis*, *Pr. vulgaris* and *Klebsiella aerogenes* caused death in Attwood's case.

Tracheopathia Osteoplastica

Tracheopathia osteoplastica is an infrequent disorder marked by osseous and cartilaginous formation within the submucosa of the trachea and bronchi which may give little or no symptoms and is usually discovered at postmortem examination or endoscopy. As with amyloidosis, the etiology is completely unknown. Osseous metaplasia in connective tissue is usually a response to injury, hemorrhage, neoplasm or infection and Ashley (1970) felt longstanding inflammation was contributory in the 3 cases he gleaned from 700 autopsies. It does not appear to be a manifestation of ageing since 3 of 7 cases were under 50 and only 2 over 60. The slight male preponderance was ascribed by Ashley to the higher incidence of chronic respiratory infection in males.

Histiocytosis "X"

The problems of confusion between mycobacterial disease and histiocytosis "X" was reviewed by Lincoln and Gilbert (1972). Histiocytosis "X" includes the chronic granulomatous reticuloses known as Letterer-Siwe disease, Hand-Schüller-Christian disease and eosinophilic granuloma. Focal accumulations of large macrophages occur in various organs, but may cause chronic mediastinal lymphadenopathy with tracheal compression. Brickman's case (1973) was thought to be tuberculous (refractory to anti-tuberculous drugs) until lesions developed in the temporal and iliac bones that proved histiocytic on biopsy.

Polychondritis

Idiopathic polychondritis in a newborn has been cited as a cause of tracheal malacia and stenosis by Johner and Szanto (1970). The infant died of tracheal collapse and respiratory obstruction on the seventy-eighth day of life and 80 per cent of the tracheobronchial tree was affected by random confluent areas of tracheal cartilaginous inflammation or necrosis. A superimposed respiratory infection and previous bronchoscopy made interpretation difficult.

Chemical Stenosis

Tracheal stenosis following chemical injury has been reported by Leape *et al.* (1972). A 2-year-old girl ingested a paste oven cleaner (Easy-Off) then aspirated some of her vomitus. She required 12 h of endotracheal intubation for respiratory distress, but no cuff or pressure ventilation was employed. A very severe esophageal and tracheal stricture ensued, the latter escaping recognition until 3 months after the ingestion. An additional contributing factor may have been a mediastinal abscess secondary to perforation following esophageal dilatation. The tracheal stenosis was eventually corrected after sleeve resections with end to end anastomosis.

Radiation Stenosis

Radiation of tracheal neoplasms may result in fibrous tracheal stenosis. This has been reported for hemangioma and squamous cell carcinoma and may be suspected for adenoid cystic carcinoma. Endoscopic resection or cautery of laryngeal papillomata that spread into the trachea is associated with mild stenosis.

Mediastinal Masses

Several intrathoracic lesions deserve mention for their ability to compress the trachea, although a full discussion is beyond the scope of this chapter. Substernal thyroid enlargements may compress the trachea bilaterally ("scabbard" trachea). Mediastinal lymphomas may compress the trachea, but more often involve the bronchi. Thymomas, but not a large thymus, occasionally compress the trachea from in front. Pulmonary hilar metastases, usually from bronchogenic carcinoma, also appear.

TRAUMATIC TRACHEAL STENOSIS

The vast majority of tracheal stenoses seen today result from direct injury applied from without or within the trachea. The force of the closed injuries is received in an anteroposterior direction; penetrating neck wounds are AP oblique or lateral. The chin and sternum protect the trachea during cervical flexion. Extension raises it to an exposed position and reduces the relative protection afforded by its mobility.

Blunt Chest Trauma

Anterior blunt chest injuries (Shaw et al., 1961) may compress the trachea against the rigid posterior vertebral bodies and result in longitudinal tracheal tears, usually at the junction of the cartilaginous and membranous walls. Simultaneous rapid extension of the head decreases the mobility of the trachea and increases the sheer forces at points of relative fixation such as the carina. Associated tears of the bronchi and esophagus and ruptured lung, aorta and heart have been described. The pulmonary vessels are thought to escape injury because of their relative mobility and low pressure. If the glottis is closed at the time of chest compression the intraluminal air pressure may increase so rapidly as to produce a blow-out type of injury. Rupture separations within the thoracic cavity are followed by mediastinitis which may be aggravated by an esophageal tear or complicated by a tracheo-esophageal fistula. Massive stenosis is the likely sequel. The diagnosis of tracheal tear is suspected when a sharp blow to the sternum is followed by cough and subcutaneous emphysema. Hamman's sign (xiphisternal crunch) suggests the mediastinal air, and if no fractured ribs are demonstrated on X-ray, the diagnosis of a torn trachea or bronchus is almost certain. Dyspnea and cyanosis increase as hematoma and inflammatory swelling evolve. Hemoptysis and pneumothorax may or may not occur.

Tracheotomy to decompress the cough, chest tubes to aspirate pneumothoraces, and primary resuturing of tracheal ruptures will prevent most stenoses before they occur. If other injuries preclude primary (within the first 24 h) repair, it may be best to wait several months before undertaking any surgery. The inflamed trachea holds sutures poorly.

Blunt Cervical Injuries

Blunt injuries to the neck have been well described by Nahum and Siegel (1967). The patient, typically a female, in the seat beside the driver, is involved in an automobile accident. Her head strikes the windshield, extending her neck, and the cervical viscera receive a punishing blow from the dashboard. Cricotracheal avulsion, partial or complete with or without recurrent laryngeal nerve injury results. Occasionally one or two rings are left with the larynx. In complete separations, the trachea itself tends to retract into the mediastinum. Associated injuries of the cricoid arch and thyroid cartilage are usual. Occasionally the anterior wall of the esophagus is torn and a tracheo-esophageal fistula forms below the obliterated infracricoid airway.

A flat lower neck (if examination is undertaken before soft tissue swelling and subcutaneous emphysema obscure it) is superimposed on the clinical observations mentioned for blunt chest injury with tracheobronchial tears. One can be misled by the lack of dyspnea in complete crico-tracheal avulsion because the pretracheal fascia may form a sufficiently rigid tube for ventilation. At tracheotomy, the distal trachea is well retracted into the chest. Once again, appropriate treatment of the acute injury is the best prevention for future stenosis. Open reduction, with mucosal approximation, conservative debridement and support with a Montgomery T-tube silicone rubber stent are indicated. The duration of stenting varies with the degree of injury.

Penetrating Cervical Injuries

Penetrating wounds of the neck may injure the trachea and lead to severe stenosis, particularly when followed by suppuration. Gunshot wounds (Lemay, 1971) usually result in the loss of two tracheal rings. This makes them suitable for primary treatment by debridement and end to end closure. Stationary wires may produce injuries that lead to stenosis when they meet the oncoming neck of any unsuspecting minibike or snowmobile rider.

Tracheotomy might reasonably be considered a penetrating wound of the neck with potential for producing tracheal stenosis. It will be considered in detail with the endogenous traumatic causes of stenosis.

Endogenous traumatic tracheal stenoses are classified by level and according to the causative agent. Stomal stenoses outnumber the other three. Tube tip stenoses are least common.

Tracheotomy and Stomal Stenosis

In translating work on tracheotomy and cuff tube stenoses done in dogs, pigs, sheep, etc., to man it is helpful to appreciate that the dog trachea has a better longitudinal blood supply than that of man, is much more elastic and on the other hand, is much more susceptible to hemorrhagic tracheitis, excessive tracheal secretions and cannula blockage following tracheotomy. Most experimental animals are more difficult to intubate than man and following intubation there are technical difficulties in ensuring standardization of longitudinal and rotatory movements of the tubes. Finally, the type and duration of anesthetic gases used in experimental procedures can influence the outcome. Most desiccate the airway and impair mucociliary flow.

The typical tracheostomal stenosis is shaped like an isosceles triangle (Goldberg and Pearson, 1972). Cartilage has been excised from the anterior tracheal wall breaking the spring of the cartilages. More cartilage dies due to the pressure of the tube, lack of nutrition, exposure and infection and the extent of the loss is directly proportional to the size of the tube inserted. This process is aggravated by steroids. Granulation tissue appears in the presence of pyogenic infection and cartilage necrosis extends. Chronic inflammation due to a foreign body (the tube), pyogenic infection and the slow task of digesting necrotic cartilage results in considerable fibrosis which webs and unites what remains of the lateral walls and produces the wedge-shaped stenosis. Nelson (1958) showed in animals with various incisions but no cannula, no stenosis developed. Granulations and subsequent stenosis varied with the duration of intubation not with the type of incision. Murphy (1966) showed that when a cannula was used there was a higher incidence of stenosis with an H-type incision than a circumferential excision. Insertion of a tube buckles in any inadequately excised tissue at the upper margin of the stoma leading to anterior wall malacia with or without granuloma. The role of contamination and infection has been documented by Bryant (1972). Pearson (1968) had found his experimental dog tracheostomies universally contaminated by pathogens at 72 h. Bryant showed that aseptic techniques in the respiratory unit were inadequate to prevent tracheal contamination in patients with intubation or tracheotomy. The lower respiratory tree became contaminated quickly, 115 of 129 patients growing pathogens within 48 h of intubation. Treating simple colonization with antibiotics caused colonization with even worse pathogens. The differentiation between colonization, tracheobronchitis and pneumonia was a clinical one.

Stridor immediately or weeks after decannulation raises the possibility of stomal stenosis. The triangular or slit type stenosis at the second and third ring levels is visualized with a laryngoscope.

Prevention of Stomal Stenosis

The primary means of prevention is to anticipate the need for elective tracheotomy so emergency tracheotomy is avoided. Once the tracheotomy is accomplished, avoid unnecessary steroids; the ultimate fibrous tissue requirements are not reduced, but tolerance of infection may be (Greenberg, 1958). Local antisepsis (e.g. Betadine solution) is useful. Tracheotomy cultures should be interpreted with intelligence. Pathogens may represent colonization only, and the employment of antibiotic should depend on clinical appearances of the tracheotomy site, the sputum and the chest X-ray; otherwise, the pathogenicity of the offending organism once infection does occur is likely to be great.

Lindholm (1969) advocates inspection of the larynx before switching from an endotracheal tube to a tracheotomy. If the larynx was tolerating the tube well, tracheotomy could be avoided. He developed an endotracheal tube with much more physiologic curvatures than conventional tubes so that posterior leverage of the tube against the cricoid would be avoided. He also drew attention to the value of ultrasonic nebulization, fixation of the tube to a face bar and sedation.

Post-endotracheal Intubation Stenosis

Tracheal inflammations caused by endotracheal tubes were classified by Florange (1965) into four types which reflect the progression of events in post-intubation stenoses. Type 1: superficial irritation of mucosa by the cannula or cuff. Type 2: submucosa or perichondrial changes under the tube or cuff. Type 3: internal exposure of cartilage, intense purulent inflammation of intercartilaginous and extracartilaginous tissues with thrombosed paratracheal veins and lymphatics engorged with cellular debris. Type 4: circumferential mediastinitis around necrotic tracheal cartilage. These are circumferential stenoses and are positively correlated with the size of the tube compared to the size of the trachea and the use of steroid medications.

Lindholm's and Pearson's findings show conclusively that the size of the intubation tube relative to the airway is the most significant factor in endotracheal tube induced stenosis.

Intubation itself is responsible for some acute damage in just about every case. Hilding's studies of 1925 showed that a 10 g swab stroke cleaves respiratory epithelium off the interior of the trachea but leaves a basal layer and the basement membrane intact so that by a process of proliferation and differentiation from the basal cells the epithelial surface is regenerated in 10 days. Although Donnelly's series (1969) showed a positive correlation between the duration of intubation and the resulting airway damage, this factor has been shown to be less important than size discrepancies. No doubt age, general health, and the presence or absence of hypotension (Little, 1956) influence the outcome in individual cases.

Endotracheal Tube Cuff Stenosis

Tracheotomy cuff pressures have been studied by Hanson (1973), Knowlson (1970) and others and are crucial to an understanding of the circumferential stenoses caused by endotracheal tube cuffs. As one adds volume inflating the cuff, pressure rises slowly. Once the minimum occlusal volume is reached, the pressure curve rises steeply as the resistance of the tracheal wall is added to the elasticity of the cuff. Excellent data are available now to show that anything greater than the minimum occlusive pressure is dangerous (the arteriolar pressure in the tracheal mucosa itself is only 40 mm of mercury). The trachea is D-shaped not circular so that inflation to the point of seal necessarily causes pressure and distortion. Over-inflation of a cuff with acute tracheal rupture has been described by Couniot and Santy (1955) and König and Hackel (1958). Secretions pool above endotracheal tube cuffs. Cuff pressures are not equally distributed around the circumference of the cuff and vary with head position and levels of consciousness (Knowlson and Bassett, 1970).

Modern cuff materials themselves are usually not histo-toxic, but in 1972 Mantz drew attention to the hazards of residues following gas sterilization. Insufficient removal of the interaction products of ethylene oxide gas, poly-vinyl chloride tubing and water may allow alkalation or hydrolysis products to injure the tracheal mucosa.

Sackner et al. (1973) demonstrated that when mucosa occludes the eye of a suction catheter, the suction rises to full vacuum, the mucosa invaginates into the catheter, and a haemorrhagic lesion results. He designed a new suction catheter with a distal flange and four side holes to minimize the extent to which suctioning damages the trachea.

Post-intubation stenoses are often misdiagnosed as asthma. Shortness of breath on exertion is often neglected by ascribing it to the original chest disease that may have necessitated the ventilation. Grillo (1970) found the onset of symptoms to be 10–42 days after extubation. When frequent readjustments of the cuff are demanded, and the patient's distress is eventually solved by inserting a longer tube, subsequent cuff stenosis should be anticipated. At endoscopy, endotracheal tube stenoses are circumferential. They tend to be slightly higher than tracheotomy tube cuff stenoses. Tracheomalacia may occupy the distance between a tracheotomy stomal stenosis and a lower cuff stenosis.

Prevention of Endotracheal Tube and Cuff Stenosis

Efforts to make cuffs less traumatic began with pre-stretching the cuff or employing a soft cuff. It was soon learned that floppy cuffs may fold along their length. They may herniate over the end of the tube. They may allow the piston-like actions transmitted from the ventilator to move the tube itself at a point higher up in the trachea. They may be eccentric and allow the tube tip to irritate the tracheal wall.

Alternating double balloon cuffs were attempted to cut inflation time in half at a given site. However, if stenosis was induced, it was twice as long as usual.

The current atraumatic cuffed intubation tubes may not be completely free of ill-effects, but already their superiority is recognized. The Shiley* model (1971) exploits a very compliant cylindrical cuff; the Kamen-Wilkinson (1971) has a 4 cm diameter low pressure polyurethane foam filled cuff that is sucked flat for insertion, and the Lanz† tube employs a very compliant exterior pressure chamber that absorbs any pressure generated through over inflation.

CLINICAL EVALUATION OF POST-TRAUMATIC TRACHEAL STENOSIS

Shortness of breath on exertion of insidious onset is the usual mode of presentation. It is often unnoticed until the patient is ambulatory. To provide symptoms a stenosis must be greater than 50 per cent of the trachea. Two-way stridor is characteristic of tracheal stenosis but in Grillo's series (1970) did not appear until the lumen was reduced to

5 mm (from a normal of 2 cm in adults). This stenosis is likely to worsen signs of pre-existing chest disease because of the barrier it presents to raising secretions.

Adequate radiologic investigations are essential to reveal the degree of stenosis, its longitudinal extent and its precise localization with reference to the larynx and carina. Lateral soft tissue films are best taken with the head fully extended and the patient swallowing to raise the trachea as high as possible into the neck. Tomograms refine visualization without incurring any risks from the introduction of radiopaque materials. Fluoroscopy is quite useful in the demonstration of tracheomalacia, a factor which may coexist with fixed stenoses unsuspected.

Conventional tracheograms are helpful but not without risk. Iodine suspensions are not very radiopaque because of the low atomic number of iodine. Peanut oil, the usual suspending medium for contrast agents like Dionosil can be toxic in airways. If a large amount of a viscous contrast agent is used to obtain a tracheogram, small airway occlusion and pneumonitis may result. In 1968, Nadel introduced powdered tantalum as a high-resolution low-bulk contrast medium for bronchography. Stitik and Proctor (1973) have adequately demonstrated its suitability to the investigation of tracheal stenosis and malacia. Two milligrams are insufflated with a non-combustible gas (tantalum powder ignition is a hazard in the presence of oxygen insufflation) under topical anesthesia. The best X-rays are taken with no tracheotomy tube in place. If the patient cannot tolerate 5 min of extubation, they are sent to the X-ray Department with a temporary plastic non-radiopaque tracheotomy tube.

Pulmonary function studies can be very valuable preoperatively in determining whether or not a patient with co-existing severe lung disease can afford to lose his tracheotomy. They provide baseline values so that the success or failure of reconstructive procedures can be measured without necessitating endoscopy. The typical findings in tracheal stenosis are a normal distribution of ventilation but reduced FEV_1 (forced expiratory volume in 1 s). There is no improvement of airway resistance with the use of bronchodilators. However, one-third of the patients with chronic obstructive pulmonary disease are also unresponsive.

The use of flow volume loops to assess these patients has been well described by Miller and Hyatt (1969). In fixed tracheal obstruction the ratio of the peak expiratory flow rate and the peak inspiratory flow rate at mid-vital capacity is 1. In chronic obstructive pulmonary disease inspiratory flow is usually better than expiratory. Clear interpretation of findings depends on testing at significant transmural pressure gradients and these only occur during the forced ventilatory manoeuvres. Significant findings depend on tests involving forced ventilatory manoeuvres.

Endoscopy is usually reserved for assessment immediately prior to surgical correction, as it carries the danger of precipitating obstruction. Some times biopsy is useful to exclude tumours, amyloidosis, etc. Flexible fiberoptic bronchoscopy has decreased the morbidity of postoperative assessment by eliminating the need for extending the neck after a procedure which shortens the trachea.

---

* Shiley Laboratories, Inc. Santa Ana, Calif., U.S.A. 92705.
† Lanz Controlled Pressure Cuff Endotracheal or Tracheotomy Tube Extracorporeal Medical Specialties, Inc., King of Prussia, Pa., U.S.A. 19406.

TREATMENT

The general aim of treatment of tracheal stenosis is to provide a flexible, extensible, but non-collapsible airway which will undergo internal epithelialization (not necessarily respiratory) and will be impervious to the egress of air and organisms into the mediastinum. Reconstruction of the intrathoracic trachea must be a one stage procedure whereas cervical tracheal repairs allow the possibility of staging and leakage is not a lethal complication. Most authors feel that repairs should not be attempted in the presence of active infection but are better performed after scar maturity. The general health of the patient may exclude reconstruction and force one to fall back on the insertion of a tracheotomy tube through the stenosis to act as a permanent stent.

Careful consideration should be given to the larynx before undertaking repairs. Laryngeal reconstruction should precede or be concurrent with tracheal reconstruction. Laryngeal paralysis or incompetence must be carefully searched for preoperatively because complete tracheal obstruction can mask aspiration. Paralysis in abduction and inability to rehabilitate the larynx may be a contraindication to correcting stenosis if it simply unmasks a serious aspiration problem. Stenoses resulting from exogenous wounds are surrounded by scar and difficult to operate, but the typical patient has good pulmonary function. Stenoses from endogenous agents (e.g. a tracheotomy tube cuff) may present less of a technical challenge but often prove more difficult problems in management because of the patient's diminished pulmonary reserve. Careful consideration must be given to the choice of anesthesia and airway management before a procedure is initiated. The stenosis can usually be visualized with a laryngoscope under local anaesthesia. Geffin et al. (1969) found that if an airway was larger than 4 mm in diameter, anaesthesia could be maintained without hypercarbia. Airways under 4 mm may be gently dilated with progressive pediatric bronchoscopes, the final one being used for the administration of anaesthesia. If the stenosis is larger than 4 mm the patient is put to sleep with a tube that passes the glottis but stops short of the stenosis itself.

Granulations, where localized, are usually resected. Montgomery feels local steroid injection in the remaining base reduces recurrence. Zinc may be an important enzyme cofactor in healing wounds. Pullen (1970) felt oral zinc sulphate was helpful therapy in dealing with persisting granulations.

In Grillo's 1973 series of 84 post-intubation tracheal stenoses treated surgically, the avenue of exposure was transcervical in 50 patients. The cervical-mediastinal approach was used in 28 and only 5 transthoracic repairs were necessary. Most authors have abandoned endoscopic approaches and dilatation completely, although the occasional report still appears of individual endoscopic successes (e.g. McInnes, 1972). An unusual variation is the approach of Grahne and Poppious (1973) who reported 6 selected cases followed over 1 year where the trachea was approached through a vertically oriented transcervical route but the stenosis was resected intratracheally with long handled instruments and managed with a stent for 4 months.

It seems clear that lesions causing loss of cartilage with full thickness scarring cannot respond to dilatations or endotracheal resections no matter how long they are stented. An indwelling stent is also certain to aggravate pre-existing secretional retention difficulties. Reconstitution with local tissue after partial resection is probably worthwhile in cervical tracheal stenoses where the stenosis is incomplete and involves less than 50 per cent loss of mucosa. Free split thickness skin grafts or buccal mucosal grafts are thin and free of hair but require a healthy recipient bed and have greater potential for shrinkage than pedicled flaps. Details of transcervical tracheoplastic techniques are illustrated by Montgomery (1973).

Sleeve Resection

Resection and end to end anastomosis, the method of choice in most post-traumatic stenoses, can usually be performed through a cervical collar incision with or without upper sternal resection. The innominate artery and vein may be retracted downward. The division of the vein adds nothing since the trachea travels rapidly posteriorly. Removal of the manubrium and/or the head of the clavicle and the first rib allows working room particularly if an anastomosis will finally lie in the mediastinum. The recurrent laryngeal nerves may be avoided by sub-perichondrial dissection when near the cricoid cartilage. The trachea is divided near the lower end of the obstruction and reintubation is accomplished across the field while the surgeon follows the stenosis proximally to determine where the upper end of the resection should fall. Chromic gut sutures at least 2 mm from the cut edge through and through the full thickness tracheal wall give satisfactory purchase and swell slightly contributing to an airtight anastomosis. They eventually resorb avoiding the granulation problem that has been documented by numerous authors (Weerda et al., 1972; Attar et al., 1973) who employed non-absorbables.

Neck flexion is maintained by the use of a guardian stitch from chin to chest. Stenoses less than 3 cm in length are unlikely to require additional release procedures (other than cervical flexion). Extensive dissection from surrounding fascia adds very little mobility and may devascularize the trachea.

Stenoses Longer Than 3 cm

Length gaining procedures can be used to encompass defects up to 6·5 cm in length (Grillo, 1973). Laryngeal release gains about 2·5 cm. Thyrohyoid release was first described by Ogura and Powers in 1964 and detailed by Dedo and Fishman in 1969. The thyrohyoid membrane, thyrohyoid muscle and superior thyroid cornua are transected to gain the additional length. As well as reducing tension on the suture line this manoeuvre decreases the effect of swallowing on the healing anastomosis. It may occasionally be useful to aid transverse primary closure of a coexisting tracheo-oesophageal fistula (Pearson, 1974).

To decrease the morbidity to swallowing that may result from thyrohyoid release, Montgomery has employed even more proximal detachment of the larynx. The suprahyoid musculature and greater and lesser horns of the hyoid are freed and less trouble with deglutition is claimed.

When very short degrees (perhaps 1 cm) of additional length are desired but laryngeal release is not felt necessary, Som's principle of annular ligament incisions may be employed. Circumferential cuts would cause too much interference with the longitudinal interconnecting extra-cartilaginous blood vessels so that hemisections on one side proximal to the anastomosis and on the other side distal to it would be more appropriate. Worman and his colleagues (1966) described successful use of hemicircumferential incisions in the trachea every few rings including mucosa. The defects are made up with elliptical fascial patch grafts.

Intrathoracic mobilization (Grillo procedure) may be used during transthoracic procedures. The extra length is obtained by dividing the right inferior pulmonary ligament, mobilizing the hilum and in some cases sectioning the left main bronchus at its origin and reimplanting it further down on the right main bronchus.

REFERENCES

Aboulker, P. and Berge, Y. (1967), *Ann. Otolaryng. Chir. Cervicofac. (Paris)*, **84**, 764.

Acuña, R. T. (1973), *Ann. Otol.*, **82**, 765.

Adriani, J. and Phillips, M. (1957), *Anesthesiology*, **18**, 1.

Andersen, H. C. and Egknud, P. (1966), *Acta oto-laryng. (Stockh.)*, suppl., **224**, 29.

Andrews, M. J. and Pearson, F. G. (1973), *Brit. J. Surg.*, **60**, 208.

Arey, L. B. (1958), *Developmental Anatomy: A Textbook and Laboratory Manual of Embryology*, 6th edition, p. 260. Philadelphia: W. B. Saunders Company.

Aronstom, E. M., Nims, R. M. and Winn, D. F. (1961), *J. Surg. Res.*, **1**, 108.

Ashley, D. J. B. (1970), *J. Path.*, **102**, 186.

Atamanyuk, M. Y. and Melrose, D. G. (1965), *Brit. J. Surg.*, **52**, 95.

Attar, S., Hankins, J., Turney, S., Mason, G. R., Ramirez, R. and McLaughlin, J. (1973), *Ann. Thorac. Surg.*, **16**, 555.

Attwood, H. D., Price, C. G. and Riddell, R. J. (1972), *Thorax*, **27**, 620.

Bain, J. A. and Spoerel, W. E. (1964), *Can. Anaesth. Soc. J.*, **11**, 598.

Barclay, R. S., McSwan, N. and Welsh, T. M. (1957), *Thorax*, **12**, 177.

Barker, W. S. and Litton, W. B. (1973), *Arch. Otolaryng.*, **98**, 422.

Beall, A. C., Harrington, O. B., Greenberg, S. D., Morris, G. C. and Usher, F. C. (1963), *Arch. Surg.*, **86**, 970.

Belsey, R. (1946), *Thorax*, **1**, 39.

Belsey, R. (1950), *Brit. J. Surg.*, **38**, 200.

Beskin, C. A. (1957), *J. Thorac. Cardiovasc. Surg.*, **34**, 392.

Bone, R. C., Biller, H. F. and Irwin, T. M. (1972), *Ann. Otol.*, **81**, 424.

Borrie, J. (1957), *Proc. Univ. Otago med. Sch.*, **35**, 15.

Borrie, J. and Redshaw, N. R. (1970), *J. Thorac. Cardiovasc. Surg.*, **60**, 829.

Brickman, H. F., Nogrady, M. B. and Wiglesworth, F. W. (1973), *Amer. Rev. Resp. Dis.*, **108**, 1208.

Bryant, L. R., Trinkle, J. K., Mobin-Uddin, K., Baker, J. and Griffen, W. O. (1972), *Arch. Surg.*, **104**, 647.

Bryce, D. P. (1972), *J. Laryng.*, **86**, 547.

Bryce, D. P. and Lawson, V. G. (1967), *Ann. Otol.*, **76**, 793.

Cantrell, J. R. and Folse, J. R. (1961), *J. Thorac. Cardiovasc. Surg.*, **41**, 594.

Caputo, V. and Consiglio, V. (1961), *J. Thorac. Cardiovasc. Surg.*, **41**, 594.

Calgett, O. T., Grindlay, J. H. and Moersch, H. J. (1948), *Arch. Surg.*, **57**, 253.

Colles, C. J. (1886), *Ann. Surg.*, **3**, 499.

Colley, F. (1895), *Dtsch. Z. Chir.*, **40**, 150.

Congdon, E. D. (1922), *Contrib. Embryol.*, **14**, 47.

Consiglio, V. (1969), *Pan-minerva Med.*, **11**, 3.

Cooper, J. D. and Grillo, H. C. (1969), *Ann. Surg.*, **169**, 334.

Correll, N. O. and Beattie, E. J. (1956), *Surg. Gynec. Obstet.*, **103**, 209.

Couniot, J. and Santy, R. P. (1955), *Lyon chir.*, **50**, 104.

Craig, R. L., Holmes, G. W. and Shabart, E. J. (1953), *J. Thorac. Cardiovasc. Surg.*, **25**, 384.

Cross, D. E. (1973), *Resuscitation*, **2**, 77.

Cummings, G. O. (1940), *Ann. Otol.*, **49**, 801.

Cummins, C. F. A. and Waterman, D. H. (1957), *Dis. Chest*, **31**, 375.

Curtin, J. W., Holinger, P. H. and Greeley, P. W. (1966), *J. Trauma*, **6**, 493.

Daniel, R. A., Jr. (1948), *J. Thorac. Cardiovasc. Surg.*, **17**, 335.

Dedo, H. H. and Fishman, N. H. (1969), *Ann. Otol.*, **78**, 285.

Donnelly, W. H. (1969), *Arch. Path.*, **88**, 511.

Dowling, E. A., Johnson, I. M., Collier, F. C. D. and Dillard, R. A. (1962), *Ann. Surg.*, **156**, 258.

Dubost, C., Mathieu, J., Duranteau, A., Rollin, G. and Thomeret, G. (1957), *Mém. Acad. Chir.*, **83**, 717.

Ekeström, S. and Carlens, E. (1959), *Acta chir. scand.*, suppl., **245**, 71.

Erich, J. B. (1945), *Arch. Otolaryng.*, **41**, 343.

Fairchild, R. R. (1927), *Surg. Gynec. Obstet.*, **44**, 119.

Farkas, L. G., Farmer, A. W., McCain, W. G. and Wilson, W. D. (1972), *Plast. reconstr. Surg.*, **50**, 238.

Fearon, B. and Cotton, R. (1972), *Ann. Otol.*, **81**, 508.

Fearon, B., MacDonald, R. E., Smith, C. and Mitchell, D. (1966), *Ann. Otol.*, **75**, 975.

Flavell, G. (1959), *Proc. roy. Soc. Med.*, **52**, 143.

Florange, W., Muller, J. and Forster, E. (1965), *Anesth. Analg. Reanim.*, **22**, 693.

Fonkalsrud, E. W. and Plested, W. G. (1966), *J. Thorac. Cardiovasc. Surg.*, **52**, 666.

Fonkalsrud, E. W. and Sumida, S. (1971), *Arch. Surg.*, **102**, 139.

Foregger, R. (1946), *Anesthesiology*, **7**, 285.

Gebauer, P. W. (1951), *J. Thorac. Cardiovasc. Surg.*, **22**, 568.

Geffin, B. and Pontoppidan, H. (1969), *Anesthesiology*, **31**, 462.

Giustra, P. E., Killoran, P. J. and Wasgatt, W. N. (1973), *Amer. J. Gastro-Ent.*, **60**, 160.

Gluck, T. and Zeller, A., *cited by* Michelson, E., Solomon, R., Maun L. and Ramirez, J. (1961), *J. Thorac. Cardiovasc. Surg.*, **41**, 748.

Goldberg, M. and Pearson, F. G. (1972), *Thorax*, **27**, 678.

Grahne, B. and Poppius, H. (1973), *Acta oto-laryng.*, **75**, 64.

Greenberg, S. D. (1958), *Arch. Otolaryng.*, **67**, 577.

Greenberg, S. D. (1960), *Arch. Otolaryng.*, **72**, 565.

Greenwood, M. F. and Holland, P. (1972), *Chest*, **62**, 642.

Grillo, H. C. (July, 1970), *Current Probl. Surg.*

Grillo, H. C. (1972), *Arch. Otolaryng.*, **96**, 31.

Grillo, H. C. (1973), *Ann. Otol.*, **82**, 770.

Grillo, H. C., Dignan, E. F. and Miura, T. (1964), *J. Thorac. Cardiovasc. Surg.*, **48**, 741.

Grimm, J. E. and Knight, R. T. (1943), *Anesthesiology*, **4**, 6.

Gross, R. E. (1945), *New Engl. J. Med.*, **233**, 586.

Hanson, B., Hansson, P. and Nilsson, K. (1973), *Acta oto-laryng. (Stockh.)*, **75**, 391.

Herzog, H., Keller, R. and Allgower, M. (1972), *Thoraxchirurgie*, **20**, 239.

Hilding, A. C. (1971), *Ann. Otol.*, **80**, 565.

Hilding, A. C. and Hilding, J. A. (1952), *Ann. Otol.*, **71**, 455.

Holden, W. S. (1957), *Brit. J. Radiol.*, **30**, 530.

Hopkinson, J. M. (1972), *J. Path.*, **107**, 63.

Howarth, W. (1923), *J. Laryng.*, **38**, 375.

Huggins, C. B. (1931), *Arch. Surg.*, **22**, 377.

Kamen, J. M. and Wilkinson, C. J. (1971), *Anesthesiology*, **34**, 482.

Jackson, C. and Jackson, C. L. (1937), *The Larynx and Its Diseases*, p. 481. Philadelphia: W. B. Saunders Company.

Johner, C. H. and Szanto, P. A. (1970), *Ann. Otol.*, **79**, 1114.

Kay, E. B. (1951), *Ann. Otol.*, **60**, 864.

Keshishian, J. M., Blades, B. and Washington, W. C. (1956), *J. Thorac. Cardiovasc. Surg.*, **32**, 707.

Kirschner, M. (1909), *Beitr. Z. Klin. Chir.*, **65**, 472.

Knowlson, G. T. G. and Bassett, H. F. M. (1970), *Brit. J. Anaesth.*, **42**, 834.

König, F. (1897), *Verh. dtsch. Ges. Chir.*, **26**, 95.

König, G. and Hackl, H. (1958), *Arch. Ohr.-, Nas.-, u. Kehlk Heilk.*, **171**, 251.

Krizek, T. J. and Kirchner, J. A. (1972), *Plast. reconstr. Surg.*, **50**, 123.

Küster, E. (1884), *Verh. dtsch. Ges. Chir.*, **13**, 95.

Leape, L. L., Ashcroft, K. W. and Mann, C. M. (1972), *Surgery*, **72**, 357.

Lemay, S. R., Jr. (1971), *Arch. Otolaryng.*, **94**, 558.

Lincoln, E. M. and Gilbert, L. A. (1972), *Amer. Rev. Respir. Dis.*, **105**, 683.

Lindholm, C. E. (1969), *Acta anaesth. scand.*, suppl. 33.

Lindholm, C. E. (1973), *Acta Otolaryng.*, **75**, 389.

Little, D. M., Jr. (1956), *Controlled Hypotension in Anesthesia and Surgery*, p. 79. Springfield; Charles C. Thomas.

Longmire, W. P., Jr. (1948), *Ann. Otol.*, **57**, 875.

Lundy, J. S. (1942), *Clinical Anesthesia: a Manual of Clinical Anesthesiology*. Philadelphia: W. B. Saunders Company.

MacEwen, W. (1880), *Brit. med. J.*, **2**, 122.

Mantz, J. M., Tempe, J. D., Jaeger, A. and Vidal, S. (1972), *Sem. Hôp. Paris*, **48**, 3367.

McCall, J. W. and Whitaker, C. W. (1962), *Trans. Amer. laryng. Ass.*, **83**, 16.

McInnes, M. F. (1972), *Canad. med. Ass. J.*, **106**, 577.

Meyer, R. (1972), *Trans. Amer. Acad. Ophthal. Otolaryng.*, **76**, 758.

Michelson, E., Solomon, R., Maun, L. and Ramirez, J. (1961), *J. Thorac. Cardiovasc. Surg.*, **41**, 748.

Miller, R. D. and Hyatt, R. E. (1969), *Mayo Clin. Proc.*, **44**, 145.

Miscall, L., McKittrick, J. B., Giordano, R. P. and Nolan, R. B. (1963), *Arch. Surg.*, **87**, 726.

Miura, T. and Grillo, H. C. (1966), *Surg. Gynec. Obstet.*, **123**, 99.

Montgomery, W. W. (1964), *Ann. Otol.*, **73**, 5.

Montgomery, W. W. (1965), *Arch. Otolaryng.*, **82**, 320.

Montgomery, W. W. (1973), *Surgery of the Upper Respiratory System*, Vol. II. Philadelphia; Lea and Febiger.

Mori, N. (1936), *J. Okayama med. Soc.*, **48**, 1410.

Mulliken, J. B. and Grillo, H. C. (1968), *J. Thorac. Cardiovasc. Surg.*, **55**, 418.

Murphy, D. A., MacLean, L. E. and Dobell, A. R. C. (1966), *Ann. Thorac. Surg.*, **2**, 44.

Mustard, W. T., Trimble, A. W. and Trusler, G. A. (1962), *Canad. med. Ass. J.*, **87**, 1301.

Nadel, J. A., Wolfe, W. G. and Graf, P. D. (1968), *Invest. Radiol.*, **3**, 229.

Nahum, A. M. and Siegel, A. W. (1967), *Ann. Otol.*, **76**, 781.

Negus, V. E., *cited in* Thomson, S., Negus, V. E. and Bateman, G. H. (1955), *Diseases of the Nose and Throat: a Textbook for Students and Practitioners*, 6th edition, p. 885. London: Cassell and Company.

Nelson, T. G. (1958), *Tracheotomy: a Clinical and Experimental Study*. Baltimore: Williams and Wilkins Company.

Niculescu, V., Pineau, H. and Delmas, A. (1972), *Arch. Anat. Pathol. (Paris)*, **20**, 403.

Nikaidoh, H., Riker, W. L. and Idriss, F. S. (1972), *Arch. Surg.*, **105**, 327.

Ogura, J. H. and Powers, W. E. (1964), *Laryngoscope*, **74**, 1081.

Paulson, D. L. (1951), *Amer. Rev. Tuberc. Pulm. Dis.*, **64**, 477.

Pearson, B. W. and Harrison, D. F. N. (1974), *Laryngoscope*, **84**, In press.

Pearson, F. G. and Andrews, M. J. (1971), *Ann. Thorac. Surg.*, **12**, 359.

Pearson, F. G., Goldberg, M. and da Silva, A. J. (1968), *Ann. Otol.*, **77**, 867.

Peer, L. A. (1955), *Transplantation of Tissues*. Baltimore: Williams and Wilkins.

Pineau, H., Eralp, I. and Delmas, A. (1972), *Arch. Anat. Pathol. (Paris)*, **20**, 395.

Prowse, C. B. (1950), *Thorax*, **13**, 308.

Pullen, F. W. (1970), *Arch. Otolaryng.*, **92**, 340.

Rob, C. G. and Bateman, G. H. (1949–50), *Brit. J. Surg.*, **37**, 202.

Rovenstine, E. A. (1945), *Anesthesiology*, **6**, 1.

Rush, B. F. and Clifton, E. E. (1956), *Surgery*, **40**, 1105.

Sacerdotti, C. and Frattin, G. (1902), *Arch. Path. Anat. Physiol.*, **168**, 431.

Sackner, M. A., Landa, J. F., Greeneltch, N. and Robinson, M. J. (1973), *Chest*, **64**, 284.

Schechter, G. L. (1972), *Otolaryng. Clin. North Amer.*, **5**, 647.

Schmiegelow, E. (1929), *Arch. Otolaryng.*, **9**, 473.

Schüller, K. H. M. (1880), *Die Tracheotomie Laryngotomie Und Exstirpation Des Kehlkopfes*. Stuttgart: Von Ferdinand Enke.

Serrano, A., Ortiz-Monasterio, F. and Andrade-Pradillo, J. (1959), *Plast. reconstr. Surg.*, **24**, 333.

Shaw, R. R., Paulson, D. L. and Kee, J. L. (1961), *J. Thorac. Cardiovasc. Surg.*, **42**, 281.

Som, M. L. (1951), *J. Mt Sinai Hosp.*, **17**, 1117.

Stitik, F. P. and Proctor, D. F. (1973), *Ann. Otol.*, **82**, 838.

Taffel, M. (1940), *Surgery*, **8**, 56.

Thomson, S., Negus, V. E. and Bateman, G. H. (1955), *Diseases of the Nose and Throat: a Textbook for Students and Practitioners*, 6th edition, p. 740. London: Cassell and Company.

Thost, A. (1911), *Die Verengerungen der oberen Luftwege nach dem Luftrohrenschitt und deren Behrandlung* (Stenosis of the Upper Air Passages Following Tracheotomy and Their Treatment). Wiesbaden: J. F. Bergmann.

Toremalm, N. G. (1972), *Laryngoscope*, **82**, 108.

Trendelenburg, F. (1871), *Arch. klin. Chir.*, **12**, 112.

Waggoner, L. G. (1958), *Ann. Otol.*, **67**, 71.

Weerda, G. H., Gruntjens, L., Karnahl, T. and Streit, H. J. (1972), *Arch. Klin. exp. Ohr.-, Nas.-, u. Kehlk. Heilk.*, **203**, 115.

Wilhelm, D. L. (1953), *J. Path. Bact.*, **65**, 543.

Worman, L. W., Starr, C. and Narodick, B. G. (1966), *Amer. J. Surg.*, **111**, 819.

SECTION XV

FINALE

PAGE

69. ETHICAL AND LEGAL CONTROL OVER ACQUISITION AND APPLICATION OF
OTOLARYNGOLOGICAL KNOWLEDGE   935

69. ADMINISTRATIVE, ETHICAL AND LEGAL ASPECTS

D. HINCHCLIFFE and R. HINCHCLIFFE

INTRODUCTION

A quarter of a century ago, research workers would complain that it was difficult to conduct an experiment and write the report without a statistician looking over one's shoulder. Nowadays, the administrator, the ethical committee and the law have replaced the statistician as the *bête noire* of the research worker.

It might be argued that administration, ethics and law have no place in a book on the scientific foundations of a subject. However, Comte (1798–1857), the founder of modern sociology, regarded ethics as the highest (7th) in his hierarchy of sciences, with mathematics coming first, i.e. lowest, in the hierarchy. Comte ascribed to sociology the task of building up a science of human society based purely on the empirical approach of observation and experiment. Duguit (1859–1928) extended Comte's concepts to form the basis for a science of law and reiterated Comte's dictum that "the only right which any man can possess is the right always to do his duty" (Duguit's Principle of Social Solidarity—analogous to Malinowski's Doctrine of Reciprocity among pre-literate peoples). Ehrlich's (1912) scientific approach to law also relates it closely to the life of the particular society. Weber used the sociological approach to study the development of Buddhist, Chinese, English, German, Islamic and Roman systems of law. The study showed the influence on law of economic, political and social forces. Weber did not restrict his sociological analysis to law, but he also extended it to administration, with his concept of the "bureaucratic" (rational-legal) organization as technically the most efficient form or organization possible. Thus a discussion of the administrative, ethical and legal control of the acquisition and application of scientific knowledge in otolaryngology can be justified as a practical aspect of the relevance of sociological sciences.

In view of the dependence of administrative regulations, ethics and law on political systems, cultural bases and historical factors, this account must inevitably concern itself primarily with the country with which the authors are best acquainted, i.e. Britain. However, the use of Anglo-Saxon Law by all English speaking communities and the universal recognition of declarations of medical ethics should make this account of wider applicability.

It is convenient to discuss, first, law and ethics in regard to man and, then, similarly, in respect of other animals.

LAWS, REGULATIONS, CODES OF PRACTICE AND STANDARDS

A law is a rule governing (positively or negatively) external human action and enforced by a sovereign political authority. There are two sources of law, i.e. statute (code) law and case law. Statute law is enacted by legislation in Parliament. Examples of statutes are the Cruelty to Animals Act 1876, which regulates animal experimentation, the various Medical Acts, which govern both the level of competency and the professional conduct of medical practitioners, the Medicines Act 1968, which requires drug manufacturers to provide medical practitioners with standard information on their products, and the Misuse of Drugs Act 1971, which repealed the three preceding Dangerous Drugs Acts but re-enacted most of their provisions and introduced new and more extensive provisions for controlling the use of drugs.

British case law comprises two systems of law, common law and equity. Equity was a peculiar development in the Middle Ages which sought to counter the rigidity of the Common Law by proceeding on flexible principles of "good conscience". Common Law comprises the ancient unwritten law of the country. It developed tentatively and casually, based upon the decisions of judges in preceding cases.

There are also two systems of courts in Britain which deal with civil law and criminal law. At civil law, *the plaintiff sues the defendant for damages* (monetary compensation). At criminal law, *a prosecutor prosecutes the accused*, who, if found guilty, may be punished with a fine and/or imprisonment. Civil cases are reported as, for example, *Brown* v. *Jones* (spoken of as "Brown *and* Jones"), where "Brown" is the plaintiff and "Jones" is the defendant. Criminal cases are reported as, for example, *R.* v. *Brown* (spoken of as "Queen—or King if a King is ruling—*against* Brown"), where "Brown" is the accused. Some wrongs are actionable in both civil and criminal courts, e.g. assault and battery.

In Britain, there is now a considerable amount of what is termed "delegated legislation". A *Statutory Instrument* is the most important form of delegated legislation which also covers Regulations, Orders and Orders in Council. An example is Statutory Instrument 1966 No. 424 as amended by Statutory Instrument 1968 No. 1842. Under the London (Heathrow) Airport Noise Insulation Grants Scheme 1966 of the British Airports Authority, this instrument provides for financial assistance to residents in the neighbourhood of London Airport to enable them to provide sound insulation for their homes.

Examples of *Orders* are the Hexachlorophane Prohibition Order 1973 and the Town and Country Planning (Use Classes) Order 1963 (Statutory Instruments 1963 No. 708). The former governs the concentration of hexachlorophene in various preparations and the latter order defines a "light industrial building" as "an industrial building (not being a special industrial building) in which the processes carried on or the machinery installed are such as could be carried on or installed in any residential area without detriment to the amenity of that area by reason of noise, vibration. . . ."

Regulations are made under the authority of an Act of Parliament by a Secretary of State or a Minister for the purposes of prescribing the detailed methods by which local authorities shall carry out certain administrative functions. Examples are provided by the Electricity Special Regulations 1944 (made under the Factories Act) to guard against electrical hazards, the Prescribed Diseases Regulations 1959 (made under the National Insurance (Industrial Injuries) Act 1946) listing occupational disorders, and the Motor Vehicles (Construction and Use) Regulations 1969 (made under the Road Traffic Act 1930). Several Sections of the latter Regulations govern the generation of noise by motor vehicles.

Bye-Laws constitute another form of subordinate legislation. A bye-law was defined by Lord Russell (1898) in the case of *Kruse* v. *Johnson* as: "An ordinance affecting the public or some portion of the public, imposed by some authority clothed with statutory powers, ordering something to be done, or not to be done, and accompanied by some sanction or penalty for its non-observance. Further, it involves this consequence—that, if validly made, it has the force of law in the sphere of its limited operation." Bye-laws are made under the provisions of Section 249 of the Local Government Act 1933 for the good rule and government of a borough and are available to all local authorities. They are designed for the prevention of nuisances, including noise nuisances.

Outside the general body of law, there are a number of advisory and informative documents which have been produced for the purpose of administration. Government departments or other official bodies make their advice known to authorities by means of *circulars*. Circulars are expressed in terms of a Minister's or a body's beliefs, advice and requests, rather than instructions. As Milne and Chaplin (1969) point out, circulars are more mandatory than their form of wording suggests, although studies have shown that they are not always effective in bringing about the changes they recommend. In Continental Europe, where most countries follow the Romano-Germanic tradition of law, the internal regulations and instructions which various government administrative departments distribute to their officers are known as *circulaires*. Civil servants in these countries often know the law only from these *circulaires*; even if it were otherwise, they would prefer to observe these instructions rather than expose themselves to difficulties with their administrative superiors. Consequently, the adherents to the Sociological School of Law consider the *circulaires* to be sources of law *par excellence*. Examples of circulars in the U.K. are Circulars 5/68 (6.2.68) and 22/67 (18.4.67) issued from the Ministry of Housing and Local Government and the Welsh Office and dealing with the use of conditions in planning permissions and with industrial noise respectively.

Non-governmental advisory documents comprise Stand-

ards, Codes of Practice, Rules, Guides and Guidelines. *A Standard* is a specification for the attributes of a particular thing or the way of measuring some quantity. Standards adopt the best possible solutions to recurring problems consistent with achieving maximum economy and convenience in use and take into account all available scientific knowledge. This also provides a common medium of communication between contracting parties. Standards are prepared and issued not only by an international body (International Organization for Standardization) but also by a number of national bodies. The one in the U.K. is known as the British Standards Institution (B.S.I.). The B.S.I. dates from 1901 when an Engineering Standards Committee was set up by the Institution of Civil Engineers and a number of professional bodies. The present name was adopted in 1931, when it received a supplemental Royal Charter. Although financially assisted by the government, it is not under government control. In drawing up these voluntary standards and codes of good practice it fuses the interests of all concerned, i.e. manufacturing, consumer, distributive and professional. The use of Standards may be directed in Statutory Instruments. For example, Regulation 23 of the Motor Vehicles (Construction and Use) Regulations 1969 provides for the measurement of vehicular noise in accordance with B.S. 3425:1966.

Codes of Practice may be drawn up not only by the British Standards Institution but also by British government departments and by the Universities. A Code represents a standard of good practice and, therefore, like the Standard, takes the form of a recommendation. In certain bye-laws. particularly those Building Bye-laws based upon one of the models issued by the Ministry of Housing and Local Government and the Department of Health of Scotland, compliance with the provisions of certain British Standards or British Standard Codes of Practice is "deemed to satisfy" the requirements of certain of these bye-laws. An example of a British Standards Institution Code of Practice is the British Standard Code of Practice 3: Chapter III (1960): Sound Insulation and Noise Reduction. In 1972, the Department of Employment produced the "Code of Practice for reducing the exposure of employed persons to Noise". In 1964, the Department of Education and Science and the then Ministry of Health, published a Code of Practice for the Protection of Persons against Ionizing Radiations arising from Medical and Dental Use. At the moment, a Code of Practice for the Protection of Persons exposed to Laser Radiation is being prepared for British Universities.

Sometimes a set of recommendations designed to prevent possible harmful effects from biological, chemical and physical agents are set out in *booklets*. Thus, in 1960, H.M.S.O. published a booklet for the Post Office on "Safety Regulations relating to Intense Radio-Frequency Radiation".

LAW IN RESPECT OF MAN

Torts

The law of torts was a creation of the common law and it was evolved from the principle of providing a remedy for an unjustifiable injury done by one person to another. The law of torts governs the acquisition and the application of otolaryngological knowledge more strongly than any other branch of the law. The Common Law Procedure Act 1852 defined a tort as a wrong independent of contract. The various torts which will be discussed here are:

(1) Nuisance
(2) Negligence
(3) Trespass to Person (Assault and Battery)
(4) Deceit
(5) Defamation

Nuisance

A nuisance has been defined as "an inconvenience materially interfering with the ordinary comfort, physically, of human existence, not merely according to elegant or dainty modes of living, but according to plain and sober and simple notions among the English people". (*Walter* v. *Selfe*, 1851). A nuisance is thus an unlawful interference with a person's use or enjoyment of land, or of some right over or in connection with it.

It is no defence for the defendant to show that he has taken all reasonable steps and care to prevent the nuisance. This principle was upheld in a recent case where the plaintiff was granted both damages for loss caused by acid smuts from the defendants' depot and injunctions to restrain the making of noise at night and the emission of pungent smells at any time. This action was also of note because the plaintiff brought noise level measurements to Court in evidence.

Structure-borne sound (vibration) may also result in a successful action for nuisance. A particular case was in connection with pile driving operations which set up vibrations that damaged the plaintiff's building.

Noises other than those due to gunfire or machinery can also constitute a nuisance. In one case, it was held that noise resulting from moving milk churns when being loaded interfered with the personal comfort of the nearby residents and thereby constituted a common law nuisance. Noise from carts and shouts from their drivers during night-time, so that they made the plaintiff unable to sleep, also constituted a common law nuisance. Noisy animals can also constitute a common law nuisance, e.g. cockerels crowing. More recently, a plaintiff obtained an injunction with respect to the howling and barking of dogs kept in a police station compound. These noises had disturbed his sleep and made it difficult for him to work in his study even when he wore earplugs and had installed both double glazing and internal shutters in the bedroom.

Odours may also constitute a nuisance. In perhap the earliest recorded case of nuisance (*Aldred's Case*, 1610), the "foeted and insalubrious" stench from a "house for hogs" was held to have rendered the plaintiff's house practically uninhabitable.

Temporary nuisances, e.g. those due to noise from the demolition of a building, may not, if the operation is reasonably conducted and all proper reasonable steps taken to ensure that no undue inconvenience is caused to neighbours, form a basis for a successful action for nuisance at common law. Nevertheless, a teacher in New Zealand was successful in claiming damages in the New Zealand Supreme Court because nearby construction noise forced him to shout and this caused him to develop a tumour on the vocal folds.

At common law, prescriptive right is a defence in an action for nuisance. This arises after twenty years but the time begins only when the act in fact becomes a nuisance. Thus it was held that the defendant had no prescriptive right in a case where he had used noisy equipment for more than twenty years but the vibrations caused by it became a nuisance only when the plaintiff, a physician, put up a consulting room abutting the room with this equipment.

Negligence

Negligence is a failure to provide against reasonably foreseeable hazards. The concept of foreseeability is an essential element in all cases of nuisance and negligence (Privy Council in the Wagon Mound Case (*Overseas Tankship (U.K.) Limited* v. *Miller Steamship Co. Limited*, Wagon Mound (No. 2)—so called because it refers to the ship *S.S. Wagon Mound*. However, as Munkman (1962) points out, the concept of foreseeability has been shown up as vague, capricious and subjective when applied to anything much more complex than bows and arrows or horses and carts. Some learned judges are able to foresee very little; others, by taking a complex succession of events step by step, are able to foresee almost anything. Moreover, the same Court can reach opposite results on two cases based on the same happening. In the Wagon Mound case, different plaintiffs took action on the same occurrence. The lower court in one case held that a particular event was not reasonable foreseeable, whilst, in the second case, another lower court held that the same event might have been foreseeable.

In British courts, the concept of "foreseeability" is usually interpreted in the sense given to it by Lord Oaksey in the case of *Bolton* v. *Stone* (the plaintiff was injured by a cricket ball hit over a fence on to a road. It was held that the cricket club was not liable as the possibility of injury was so slight). The reasonable man does not take precautions against everything which he can foresee, but only against those things which he can foresee are reasonably likely to happen.

In an action for negligence, the plaintiff must prove that the defendant was under a duty of care to him, that there was a breach of such duty, and that, as a direct consequence, the plaintiff suffered damage. Thus, the essential requisites have been given as the "four Ds": "Duty of care, Dereliction of Duty, Damage, Directness".

In practice, there is usually no doubt about the existence of the duty of care and it is then assumed to exist. However, in the case of *Donoghue* v. *Stevenson* (1932), Lord Atkin formulated the general concept that "you must take reasonable care to avoid acts or omissions which you can reasonably foresee will be likely to injure your neighbour". He then defined "neighbours" as "persons so closely and directly affected by my act that I ought reasonably to have them in contemplation as being so affected when I am directing my mind to the acts or omissions which are called in question". Thus there will be a "duty" situation wherever the relationship of the parties is such that the likelihood that the plaintiff would be affected by the defendant's conduct ought reasonably to have been contemplated by the defendant. Although the Atkins formulations have not gone uncriticized, they have been accepted at English Common Law starting with the premises that all damage caused through failure to take reasonable care is actionable, as under French law.

The question of "dereliction of duty" relates to the "standard of care". A practitioner is not liable merely because some other doctor might have shown greater skill and knowledge. This principle applies to pathologists also. In a case relating to carcinoma, a pathologist was held not to be negligent even though the head of his department (another pathologist) had taken a different view of the case. In actions for negligence in respect of medical practice, the law is applied almost entirely on the expert evidence of medical witnesses—evidence from competent practitioners that, in the same circumstances, they would have done, or would not have done, what the defendant did.

It is normal for the plaintiff to establish that the defendant's negligence had caused him injury. However, the onus is on the defendant if the principle of "*res ipsa loquitur*" operates. For example, a patient went into hospital with two stiff fingers (due to Dupuytren's contracture) and came out with four. In reversing the decision of the trial court, Lord Denning held it to be a case of *res ipsa loquitur*. Two conditions are required before this doctrine will apply. First, the event which caused the damage must have rested within the control of the defendant. Secondly, the mere occurrence of the event itself implies that the defendant has been negligent.

In respect of the "*directness*" of the causation, actions for medical negligence may allow for a "chain of causation". Thus failure in the treatment of the infected finger of a pregnant woman was held to be the cause of a voice disorder. The chain of causation here was via a septicaemia and subsequent damage to the cranial nerves.

Defences available in an action for negligence are, apart from denying the alleged negligence, that:

(1) it was an inevitable accident (mishap);
(2) the negligence was that of someone else;
(3) the risk was assumed by the plaintiff ("*volenti non fit injuria*"); and
(4) there was contributory negligence by the plaintiff.

It is a defence to an action in tort that the defendant neither intended to injure the plaintiff nor could have avoided doing so by the use of a reasonable care. In respect of medical practice, Lord Denning has said that a doctor was not to be held negligent simply because something went wrong. He was liable only when he fell below the standard of care of a *reasonably competent* practitioner *in his field* so much that his conduct might be deserving of censure or be inexcusable. However, this holds only when the mishap cannot be avoided by any such precaution as a reasonable man may be expected to

take. Risks are inherent in most medical and surgical procedures but a practitioner must not take "an unwarranted and unnecessary risk". The "broken needle" cases best illustrate the law relating to medical mishaps. When the needle of a hypodermic syringe breaks off during a diagnostic or therapeutic procedure, the plaintiff must produce evidence of negligence as such. The evidence may be that the needle was not the appropriate one for the particular injection or that it was inserted wrongly.

Mistakes must be differentiated from mishaps. As a general rule in the law of torts, a mistake is no defence. However, the law appears to take a different view in respect of medical mistakes. The legal attitude appears to be different according to whether the error involves diagnosis or whether it concerns treatment. A mistake in diagnosis can be construed as an "error of judgement" but a mistake in treatment cannot.

A mistake in diagnosis is accepted as a risk inherent to the practice of medicine, but a mistake in treatment is not. Thus, in an action for damages brought by a widow in respect of the misdiagnosis of her late husband's chest pain, the judge ruled that the case was one of mistake and not of negligence because the doctor had examined the case carefully for an hour. However, failing to make a correct diagnosis must be differentiated from failure to adequately examine a patient. The latter may amount to negligence. Failure to use a stethoscope in a Casualty Department to diagnose fractured ribs in an intoxicated injured patient has been held to be negligent. Failure to request a radiological examination in possible bony disorders or injuries would probably be held to be negligent. But, surprisingly, failure to employ an endoscope which would have diagnosed a rare condition may not amount to negligence. If a doctor does not feel competent to diagnose a particular case, he may be held negligent for failing to refer the case to the appropriate specialist. Although, in cases concerning surgical treatment, the question of negligence hinges on what other competent practitioners would, or would not, have done, so often the principle of *res ipsa loquitur* (*vide supra*) is applied. This principle would hold where the wrong operation was performed or the wrong side was operated on. Lord Goddard held that the principle applied in "swab cases" also.

The institution of an experimental therapeutic procedure can be particularly hazardous—legally for the doctor as well as medically for the patient. The law governing the institution of new (experimental) treatment of patients was established over 200 years ago (*Slater* v. *Baker and Stapleton*, 1767). In this case, the plaintiff sued the then Head Surgeon (Mr. Baker) of St. Bartholomew's Hospital. Mr. Baker had re-fractured the plaintiff's healed leg so that it could go through the "operation of extension using a heavy steel invention with fearsome teeth". On appeal, the Chief Baron held that, "although the defendants in general may be as skilful in their respective professions as any two gentlemen in England, yet the Court cannot help saying that, in this particular case, they have acted ignorantly and unskilfully contrary to the known rules and usage of surgeons". The law applicable to actions for negligence in respect of new therapeutic procedures was systematized in a Scottish case (*Hunter* v. *Hanley*) by Lord President Clyde in 1955. Three facts must be established. Firstly, that there does exist a normal, usual practice. Secondly, that the defendant had not adopted that practice. Thirdly, that the course of management adopted was one that no professional man of ordinary skill would have taken if he had been acting with ordinary care.

A defence of *volenti non fit injuria* in medical cases of actions for negligence can only be made if *consent—informed consent*—has been freely given. Any medical or surgical procedure, including the simplest diagnostic examination which is conducted without the patient's consent (expressed or implied) is a trespass to person (*see later*). For minor diagnostic and therapeutic procedures, consent is usually implied. It is argued that, when a patient presents himself seeking treatment, he has clearly implied his consent to a physical examination and, at least, some minor therapeutic procedure. Sitting down in the examination chair or lying down on a couch may be taken as tacit consent. In other cases, written consent should be obtained. If an emergency operation is necessary to save a patient's life and consent cannot be obtained, the principle of "agency of necessity" is invoked.

In a recent claim for damages arising out of an unsuccesful stapedectomy, the plaintiff claimed that he had not carefully read the consent form and was under the impression that it signified authority only for a general anaesthetic and an examination. The plaintiff was employed as a claims manager by an insurance company where careful scrutiny of forms and their small print is all important. Not surprisingly, therefore, the Judge completely rejected the plaintiff's evidence. Failure to mention and explain to a patient the hazards of intra-nasal ethmoidectomy, especially following previous intra-nasal operations, would imply failure to obtain informed consent. Such a case which occurred recently and resulted in a medial rectus muscle damage was therefore settled out of Court.

In some experimental therapeutic procedures, actions for negligence have hinged not on whether or not an unusual course of action was adopted but on whether or not *informed consent* had been really given. In a recent case in the U.K., where a facial paralysis developed after an operation involving the insertion of an electronic device in the para-aural tissues to treat deafness, the Judge held that there was inadequate warning of all the risks involved. However, in *non-experimental* therapeutic procedures, the courts will admit to the necessity for "therapeutic misrepresentation". In an action for negligence arising from damage to the recurrent laryngeal nerve during a thyroidectomy, the trial judge said "on the evening before the operation, the surgeon told the plaintiff that there was no risk to her voice, when he knew that there was some sight risk, but he did that for her own good because it was of vital importance that she should not worry. He told a lie, but he did it because in the circumstances it was justifiable. The law does not condemn the doctor when he only does what a wise doctor so placed would do. . . . And none of the doctors called as witnesses have suggested that the surgeon was wrong".

Until 1945, *contributory negligence* was a complete defence to an action in tort. However, in that year, the Law Reform (Contributory Negligence) Act was enacted. Section 1 of that Act states that "where any person suffers damage as the result partly of his own fault and partly the fault of any other person, a claim in respect of that damage shall not be defeated by reason of the fault of the person suffering the samage, but the damages recoverable in respect thereof shall be reduced to such an extent as the court thinks just and equitable having regard to the claimant's share in the responsibility for the damage". In two decisions in 1971, 5 per cent and 20 per cent were deducted from damages awarded as the result of road accidents in which the plaintiff was not wearing a seat belt. Associated with the concept of contributory negligence is the doctrine of "hypothetical causation". About 15 years ago a steel erector was killed by a fall from a tower. Although on the day in question no safety belts were available, it was held, from the evidence given, that the deceased would not have worn one. The plaintiff's act of omission may therefore constitute a "*novus actus interveniens*".

The Common Law may have certain limitations imposed on it by Statute Law. In particular, the Limitation Act 1939 stated that actions founded on tort shall not be brought after the expiration of a certain duration (6 years) from the date on which the cause of action accrued. The Law Reform (Limitation of Actions) Act 1954 reduced this period to 3 years in connection with actions for damages for negligence, nuisance or breach of statutory duty where personal injury was concerned. The time commences on the date on which the cause of action accrues. Thus, until 1963, an injustice might have arisen in a case where an injury was inflicted in a way that could become discoverable only after a lapse of time. Such a manner is, of course, characteristic of many occupational disorders, noise-induced hearing loss *par excellence*. This injustice was removed by the Limitation Act 1963. This Act enables a plaintiff to bring a claim even though the 3 year limit is past, provided that he neither knew about the injury, nor ought to have known about it, and provided that he brings the claim within one year.

Trespass to Person

Trespass to the person is any direct, intentional interference with an individual without lawful justification. Trespass to person encompasses both *assault* (the threat or attempt to use force against another person) and *battery* (the actual application of force). Unlike the law of negligence, the plaintiff need not prove that the defendant was negligent or had a duty of care to him. He need only prove that the act was harmful to him. He must, however, establish an intention. Where the battery does not amount to a serious crime, a defence of *volenti* can be maintained, as in the law of negligence. Thus it is not a battery to make a medical examination of a patient who consents to it. But, a battery does take place if a person is exmained against his/her own will. However, Lord Justice Winn's Committee on Personal Injuries Litigation concluded

(Cmnd. 3691, 1968, para. 312) that it "entertained no doubt that every claimant for personal injuries must be bound to submit himself to medical examination of a reasonable character which is reasonably required, subject, of course, to proper safeguards and to the claimant's right to object to any particular doctor". Nevertheless, Mr. Justice Lawson has condemned the procedure whereby a person could be compelled to submit to a medical examination by indirectly staying proceedings as not being conducive to respect for the administration of justice (*Baugh* v. *Delta Walter Fittings*, 1971). Mr. Justice Lawson pointed out that a requirement to submit to a medical examination could be justified only where Parliament had specifically authorized it. Compulsory medical examinations are required by various statutes, e.g. of school children under the Education Act 1944. Even then, the examination can only be done after the requisite notice has been served on the parent.

Surgical operations which are technically successful may amount to a trespass if consent has not been obtained. Thus, during an operation on an ear, a surgeon in the U.S.A. found that the other ear was more extensively diseased. He therefore operated on both ears. Although he did so skilfully and successfully, the Court, on appeal, found for the plaintiff. Similarly in the U.S.A., an action was successful against a surgeon who had performed tonsillectomy on an 11-year-old child in the absence of consent from her parents.

The need to obtain informed consent freely given is particularly important in non-therapeutic human experiments. In these cases, there can be no question of employing the concept of "therapeutic misrepresentation" as can be done in non-experimental therapeutic procedures. In a Canadian case, the judge emphasized, on appeal, that the duty of experimenters towards their subjects was at least as great, if not greater, than the duty owed by the practitioner to his patients. In this case, a jury awarded $22 500 damages to a student who had to be resuscitated by open heart massage after his heart had stopped during an experiment with a new anaesthetic agent. The student had not been told that the drug was a new anaesthetic about which the experimenter (a Professor of Anaesthetics) had no previous knowledge.

Deceit

Also relevant to the question of informed consent is the tort of deceit. To establish liability here, it must be shown that

    (a) the defendant made a false statement of fact;
    (b) it was made fraudulently;
    (c) it was made with the intent that the plaintiff should act upon it;
    (d) that the plaintiff did in fact do so; and
    (e) that he thereby suffered damages.

Defamation

With the extremely wide publicity which can now be given to both the spoken and the written word, defamation, encompassing both slander and libel, has grown to be one of the largest sections of the law of tort. Lord Denning has drawn a distinction between libel and lawful criticism. Libel is personal and subjective—the lowering of the status of a man in the eyes of right-thinking people generally. Lawful criticism is impersonal and objective—criticisms of a thing, of a technique or of a system. However, in the same court, Lord Salmon considered that a man's name, practice or reputation could be so closely associated with a technique that a severe attack on the technique implied an attack on the plaintiff's reputation.

The main defences in an act for defamation are

    (a) justification or truth;
    (b) fair comment; and
    (c) privilege—either absolute or qualified.

Failure to prove the truth of every charge will not defeat a defence of justification. For a defence of fair comment to be upheld it must be shown that

    (i) the criticism is an expression of opinion, on
    (ii) a matter of public interest, and
    (iii) it must be fair and
    (iv) not actuated by malice.

In a case some years ago, it was held on appeal that, for the plaintiff to describe himself as "a specialist for the treatment of deafness, ear, nose and throat disorders" and the defendant a "quack of the rankest species" was fair comment. Any person who writes for publication or otherwise engages in public work, is said to invite comment or challenge public attention. Absolute privilege (complete immunity from an action for defamation) now applies only in a relatively few instances. Section 8 of the Defamation Act 1952 has withdrawn absolute privilege from the reports of many administrative and disciplinary tribunals. The occasions on which qualified privilege exists has been defined by Lord Atkinson in *Adams* v. *Ward* (1917). He said "A privileged occasion is, in reference to qualified privilege, an occasion where the person who makes a communication has an interest or a duty, legal, social or moral, to make it to the person to whom it is made, and the person to whom it is made has a corresponding interest or duty to receive it. This reciprocity is essential."

Contract

Breach of contract, like a tort, is a civil wrong. However, duties in respect of tortious liability are primarily fixed by law whereas duties in respect of contractual liability are primarily fixed by the parties themselves. Nevertheless, in practice, a claim for breach of contract may be essentially the same as a claim in tort. Indeed, as Lord Simons has pointed out, "It is trite law that a single act of negligence may give rise to a claim either in tort or for breach of contract". For example, where a dentist extracts a tooth so unskilfully that pieces of it remain in the upper jaw, he breaks his contractual obligation to treat his patient with proper care and attention and simultaneously commits the tort of negligence which arises from inflicting foreseeable harm.

Manslaughter

This is defined as the unlawful killing of another without malice express or implied. If a patient dies for want of either competent skill or sufficient attention this may be manslaughter. However, a single act of carelessness by a doctor, for example, by giving an overdose of a drug, as the result of which the patient dies is held not to be manslaughter.

The Law Relating to Transplants

So far as otolaryngology is concerned, cadavers are the most likely source for transplants. At Common Law, nobody has a right to his body after death. His directions as to its disposal can be ignored. Moreover his direction that his body should be used for transplant purposes will protect no one. However, the Common Law has been modified by the Corneal Grafting Act 1952 and the Human Tissue Act 1961. According to Section 1 of the last Act, if a person has expressed a request that his body should be used after his death for therapeutic purposes, the person lawfully in possession of the body after his death may authorize the removal from the body of any part for use in accordance with the request. An amendment to the 1961 Act has been suggested by Lord Kilbrandon to provide for any designated hospital to lawfully remove *any* organ required for medical or scientific purposes *unless* the hospital authorities have reason to believe that the deceased in his lifetime had forbidden this to be done. Lord Justice Davies also advocates legislation making it clear that an operation for transplant purposes will not *per se* give rise either to civil or to criminal liability, whilst still leaving unaffected the surgeon's duty of proper care in deciding whether the risk involved to the donor is so great as to render the operation inadvisable. Transplantation also involves wide ethical issues. As Daube says, the jurists certainly must adapt their rigid over-conceptualized thinking to novel conditions, and the doctors should perhaps acknowledge in increasing measure their accountability before a wider forum of society, ethics and law.

Copyright, Design and Patent Law

As well as laws protecting individuals who might be used to extend knowledge of otolaryngological science, or who might be subject to the application of such knowledge, there are also laws protecting the designs, inventions and writings of those who seek to extend this knowledge. Five particular statutes are so involved, i.e. the Copyright Acts of 1911 and 1956, the Design Copyright Act 1968, the Registered Design Act 1949, and the Patents and Design Act 1949.

Copyright is defined as the exclusive right to do, or to authorize other persons to do, certain acts in relation to original literary work. The latter also covers medical literature. Literary work consists of any work expressing in print or in writing, irrespective of the quality. As Mitchell (1974) points out, copyright exists in the way that ideas are expressed rather than in the ideas themselves. It is not necessary to use an author's actual words to infringe his copyright. A summary or paraphrase may be an infringement. The duration of copyright is:

(i) During the lifetime of the author, plus 50 years from the end of the calendar year in which he died.

(ii) In the case of joint authorship, 50 years after the death of the first to die, or during the lifetime of the author who died last, whichever is the longer.

After 25 years, provided appropriate notice of intention has been given to the author, a work may be reproduced on payment of royalties.

Copyright is vested in an employee where the work is done in his own time. Literary work relating to case reports which use X-ray films and other records relevant to a patient's case record, is the copyright of the employer.

Although copyright gives certain rights it is not a monopoly in that it can prevent the production of an identical work. There is such a thing as parallel evolution!

The Registered Design Act 1949 regulates *designs*, with the exclusion of artistic work protected by the Copyright Act 1956. In contrast to medical literary work, copyright in designs must be registered at the Patents Office and lasts for a period of 15 years only. It has been held that "substantial reproduction" constitutes an infringement of the Design Copyright Act and that "anything worth copying is *prima facie* worth protecting".

The term *patent* is defined as a privilege granted by letters patent from the Crown to the first inventor of any new manufactured contrivance that he alone be entitled to benefit, for a limited period (now 16 years), from his own invention. This thus constitutes an exception to the Statute of Monopolies 1623 by which the granting of monopolies is in general forbidden. It should be noted that the granting of a patent is not something in its own right, but an act of royal favour.

Applications for a patent for an invention may be made by a person claiming to be the true and first inventor, or by his representative, to the Comptroller of Patents, Designs and Trade Marks. The application must be accompanied by a complete, or provisional, specification. If provisional, the complete specification must be filed within 1 year. A patent is not invalidated by the publication or use of the invention but may be revoked on petition of an interested party by the court or by the Comptroller if found not to be new.

The Patents and Designs Act 1949 has special provisions relating to medical or surgical inventions. Following an application by an interested person, the Comptroller may order the grant of a licence to such a person to make, sell or use the invention for therapeutic, including surgical, purposes. Section 56 of the 1949 Act governs disputes between an employer and an employee concerning rights to an invention. An employee is not disqualified by a contract of service from taking out a patent in his own name notwithstanding that the invention was made in his employer's time and with his materials. The rights of the parties may, however, be influenced by the terms of service.

Section 46 of the 1949 Act empowers government departments to make, use and exercise any patented invention for the service of the Crown. The House of Lords has held that drugs used in hospitals of the NHS are used for the services of the Crown, even though for the benefit of patients. Consequently, the British government has been able to place contracts for the purchase of drugs to be acquired in countries where the patent law is not applicable at prices less than those requested by patentees.

ETHICAL CONSIDERATIONS—MAN

Despite the legal safeguards embodied in the law of negligence and the law of trespass to persons, considerable disquiet has been voiced regarding the conduct of clinical investigations. Following the receipt of a letter on this subject from certain of its members in 1966, the Royal College of Physicians of London appointed a Committee to consider how far supervision of clinical investigation was required, and, if it was required, how best it might be effected. The Committee considered the term "clinical investigation" to cover all forms of experiment on man. These were divided into two groups. First, those of direct diagnostic or therapeutic relevance to the individual patient concerned. Secondly, research carried on to advance knowledge which will benefit the community. In the first group, the doctor could perhaps be said to have failed in his duty to his patient if he had not performed such an experiment. In the second group, where the subject might be a patient or a normal individual, ethical problems might present in relation to this individual. The Committee recommended that the conduct of clinical investigations should be guided by a code of ethical practice. They recommended the Code of Ethics of the World Medical Association (Declaration of Helsinki). They pointed out that the Medical Research Council had also issued a statement on "Responsibility in Investigations on Human Subjects" (M.R.C. Annual Report, 1962-1963). This was reprinted, together with the Declaration of Helsinki, in the *British Medical Journal* in 1964. The Declaration of Helsinki is given in Appendix 4. The Committee also recommended that all hospitals where clinical investigations were carried out should have an informal advisory committee to ensure that the investigations were ethical and that the safety precautions were satisfactory. The report was endorsed by the then Ministry of Health and, by 1970, nearly all teaching hospitals had established active ethical committees. Ethical problems in research on man nevertheless persist. C.I.O.M.S. (Council for International Organizations of Medical Sciences) held a Round Table (VIII) Conference in 1973 specifically on "Protection of Human Rights in the Light of Scientific and Technological Progress in Biology and Medicine". The Conference drew up a list of ethical canons for medical-scientific investigations, to protect the welfare and human rights of participants (*see* Appendix 5). *Inter alia*, C.I.O.M.S. called for encouragement of investigations so designed to minimise ethical dilemmas. It was pointed out that this could be achieved through greater use of epidemiological methods.

At the time of writing (1974), it would seem that the establishment of ethical committees for every N.H.S.

hospital in the U.K. will be made mandatory by an Act of Parliament. The "Rights of Patients" Bill which is now before the House of Commons is designed to clarify the right of patients to privacy when receiving hospital treatment under the N.H.S., and in regard to medical experiments on human beings. The Bill would ensure that those who were particularly sensitive, nervous or unwilling had the right to refuse being subject to teaching if they could not face it.

The need to safeguard individual *privacy* is of current concern. The Younger Committee on Privacy was set up to consider this question and it gave its report in 1972. The Committee thought that the question of privacy should be played by ear. In medicine, it was not a matter for legislation, but for ethics. As the result of information which the M.R.C. submitted to the Younger Committee in 1971, the Council published a code of practice on "Responsibility in the use of Medical Information for Research". The Council accepts that medical information about identified patients can be made available for medical research without the patient's explicit consent. However, all medical information that can be related to an identified individual should be treated as confidential and should be communicated only to medical research workers who are engaged in investigations in the interests of the health of the community. There are grave fears that confidentiality will break down with the increasing use of computers. In an effort to safeguard privacy here, the British Medical Association's Planning Unit's Report No. 3 on "Computers and Medicine" stated that computer-based information systems which contained information concerning the health of identifiable individuals "must be isolated from all other information banks". The World Medical Association has also recommended that medical data banks should be available only to the medical profession and should be linked to other central data banks.

LAW IN RESPECT OF ANIMALS

In Liechtenstein, the law prohibits any form of animal experimentation. However, in the majority of other states in the world, animal experimentation is accepted at Common Law. Moreover, a large number of the states have legally defined controls over the use of animals in medical and scientific research. The law in Britain in this regard is probably more comprehensive than that in any other country.

United Kingdom

There are a number of statutes which regulate the use of animals in experimentation. The principal statute is the Cruelty to Animals Act 1876. The Act applies only to vertebrates (other than man). It requires that, in experimental animal procedures, pain shall be prevented by the use of anaesthetics and experimenters must possess a licence to conduct such experiments. If, however, the animal is being used to provide tissues for studies in comparative anatomy or pathology, no such licence is required, provided that the tissues are obtained after the animal has been killed following anaesthetization. Although the Act does not exclude research into surgical techniques, it prohibits experiments whose object is the acquisition of manual skill (this must therefore be performed on cadavers or patients!). If experiments other than simple inoculation or superficial venesection are required to be conducted without anaesthetics, then the experimenter must be in possession of certain certificates. It should be noted, however, that paralysing drugs are specifically prohibited from being used to immobilize a conscious animal. Certificate A permits the experimenter to conduct experiments without anaesthesia. Certificate B permits the experimenter to allow the animal to recover from the anaesthesia, i.e. as in chronic experiments. Neither Certificates A nor B, however, cover cats, dogs, asses, horses or mules. Certificates E and EE are required for unanaesthetized and recovery experiments respectively, to be done on cats and dogs. Certificate F is required for experiments on asses, horses and mules. Needless to say, Certificate F is granted only if it can be shown that the experiment cannot be done on any other animal, including cats and dogs. Certificates E and EE will be granted provided the experiment cannot be done on any animal other than these five. The Act provides for the control of vertebrate animal experimentation not only by granting licences and certificates but also by:

(1) Examination of the experimental procedure and its effects (immediate and remote).
(2) Inspection of the laboratories where the experiments are being conducted.
(3) Inspection of the rooms where the animals are being maintained.
(4) Requiring holders of licences to submit an annual report on the number and nature of experiments performed.

Licences and certificates are personal to the holder who may not delegate his authority under them, not even to another licence-holder. Despite these provisions, the Act has been continually criticized since its inception on the grounds that it is insufficiently stringent. Consequently, the British government set up a Departmental Committee under the chairmanship of Sir Sydney Littlewood to consider the existing control over experiments on living animals and to consider whether or not changes were desirable. The Littlewood Report (1965) made 83 recommendations for changes. Of these recommendations, about 50 items would have required new legislation. However, Lane-Potter (1970) and others consider that, under the present Act, experimental animals enjoy a real measure of protection against anything that could be construed as cruelty, while, at the same time, science is not prevented from pursuing a profitable course. Nevertheless, attempts are still being made to extend the legislation to restrict animal experimentation. The proposed Houghton amendment to the 1876 Act read:

"... it shall be a condition of every such licence that no experiment on a living animal shall be performed under the authority thereof if the purpose of the experiment can be achieved by alternative means not involving an experiment on a living animal".

Gowans (1974) has cogently argued against the establishment of such a provision. The replacement of all animal experiments by non-sentient systems is a completely unattainable ideal. Indeed, animal experiments will always be required to ascertain whether or not a given non-sentiment system is an appropriate substitute for the whole animal. It is therefore not surprising that the 1973 Cruel Experiments Bill was withdrawn from the House of Lords after criticism that it would be both impracticable and unenforcible.

A number of other statutes support the 1876 Act in controlling the acquisition and application of knowledge by means of animals. Thus the Therapeutic Substances Act 1956 controls the use of tests on animals for the establishment of the purity and potency of therapeutic substances when the tests cannot be carried out satisfactorily by chemical methods. The Dogs Act 1906 prohibits the giving or selling, for the purposes of vivisection, of any dog seized by the police. The Protection of Animals Act 1911 safeguards both captive and domestic animals from cruelty by either acts of commission or acts of omission. *Inter alia*, if an animal is to be killed, this must be done as speedily as possible.

In addition to these aspects of statute law which apply to experimental animals, there are particular aspects of case law which are relevant to experimental animals. There are special rules in tort governing the misdeeds of animals. The most important of these rules is the so-called "scienter" rule. The essence of this rule was summarized by Lord Devlin in 1957 (*Behrens* v. *Bertram Mills Circus Ltd.*). It is as follows:

"A person who keeps an animal without knowledge (*scienter retinuit*) of its tendency to do harm is strictly liable for damage it does if it escapes; he is under an absolute duty to confine or control it so that it shall not do injury to others. All animals *ferae naturae*, that is, all animals which are not by nature harmless, such as a rabbit, or have not been tamed by man and domesticated, such as a horse, *are conclusively presumed to have such a tendency*, so that the *scienter* need not in their case be proved. All animals in the second class, *mansuetae naturae*, are *conclusively presumed to be harmless* until they have manifested a savage or vicious propensity; proof of such a manifestation is proof of *scienter* and serves to transfer the animal, so to speak, out of its natural class into *ferae naturae*."

The decision as to whether a given animal is *ferae naturae* or *mansuetae naturae* is for the Court to decide. Previous legal categorizations of *ferae naturae* have been in respect of elephants and monkeys.

Other Countries

There is believed to be no legal control of animal experimentation in Canada, France, Greece, India, Luxembourg, Netherlands, New Zealand, Pakistan, Portugal, Yugoslavia and the U.S.S.R.

SI Derived Units with Special Names

Quantity	Name of Unit	Symbol	Expression in Terms of Other Units	Expression in Terms of SI Base and Supplementary Units
frequency	hertz	Hz		s^{-1}
force	newton	N		$m\ kg\ s^{-2}$
pressure, stress	pascal	Pa	$N\ m^{-2}$	$m^{-1}\ kg\ s^{-2}$
energy, work, quantity of heat	joule	J	$N\ m$	$m^2\ kg\ s^{-2}$
power, radiant flux	watt	W	$J\ s^{-1}$	$m^2\ kg\ s^{-3}$
quantity of electricity, electric charge	coulomb	C		$s\ A$
electric potential, potential difference, electromotive force	volt	V	$W\ A^{-1}$	$m^2\ kg\ s^{-3}\ A^{-1}$
capacitance	farad	F	$C\ V^{-1}$	$m^{-2}\ kg^{-1}\ s^4\ A^2$
electric resistance	ohm	Ω	$V\ A^{-1}$	$m^2\ kg\ s^{-3}\ A^{-2}$
conductance	siemens	S	$A\ V^{-1}$	$m^{-2}\ kg^{-1}\ s^3\ A^2$
magnetic flux	weber	Wb	$V\ s$	$m^2\ kg\ s^{-2}\ A^{-1}$
magnetic flux density	tesla	T	$Wb\ m^{-2}$	$kg\ s^{-2}\ A^{-1}$
inductance	henry	H	$Wb\ A^{-1}$	$m^2\ kg\ s^{-2}\ A^{-2}$
luminous flux	lumen	lm		$cd\ sr$
illuminance	lux	lx	$lm\ m^{-2}$	$m^{-2}\ cd\ sr$

Examples of Other SI Derived Units

Quantity	Symbol	Expression in Terms of SI Base and Supplementary Units	Quantity	Symbol	Expression in Terms of SI Base and Supplementary Units
area	m^2		heat flux density, irradiance	$W\ m^{-2}$	$kg\ s^{-3}$
volume	m^3		heat capacity, entropy	$J\ K^{-1}$	$m^2\ kg\ s^{-2}\ kgK^{-1}$
speed, velocity	$m\ s^{-1}$		specific heat capacity, specific entropy	$J\ kg^{-1}\ K^{-1}$	$m^2\ s^{-2}\ K^{-1}$
acceleration	$m\ s^{-2}$				
wavenumber	m^{-1}		specific energy	$J\ kg^{-1}$	$m^2\ s^{-2}$
density, mass density	$kg\ m^{-3}$		thermal conductivity	$W\ m^{-1}\ K^{-1}$	$m\ kg\ s^{-3}\ K^{-1}$
current density	$A\ m^{-2}$		energy density	$J\ m^{-3}$	$m^{-1}\ kg\ s^{-2}$
magnetic field strength	$A\ m^{-1}$		electric field strength	$V\ m^{-1}$	$m\ kg\ s^{-3}\ A^{-1}$
concentration (of amount of substance)	$mol\ m^{-3}$		electric charge density	$C\ m^{-3}$	$m^{-3}\ s\ A$
			electric flux density	$C\ m^{-2}$	$m^{-2}\ s\ A$
activity (radioactive)	s^{-1}		permittivity	$F\ m^{-1}$	$m^{-3}\ kg^{-1}\ s^4\ A^2$
specific volume	$m^3\ kg^{-1}$		permeability	$H\ m^{-1}$	$m\ kg\ s^{-2}\ A^{-2}$
luminance	$cd\ m^{-2}$		molar energy	$J\ mol^{-1}$	$m^2\ kg\ s^{-2}\ mol^{-1}$
angular velocity	$rad\ s^{-1}$		molar entropy, molar heat capacity	$J\ mol^{-1}\ K^{-1}$	$m^2\ kg\ s^{-2}\ K^{-1}\ mol^{-1}$
angular acceleration	$rad\ s^{-2}$				
dynamic viscosity	$Pa\ s$	$m^{-1}\ kg\ s^{-1}$	radiant intensity	$W\ sr^{-1}$	$m^2\ kg\ s^{-3}\ sr^{-1}$
moment of force	$N\ m$	$m^2\ kg\ s^{-2}$	radiance	$W\ m^{-2}\ sr^{-1}$	$kg\ s^{-3}\ sr^{-1}$
surface tension	$N\ m^{-1}$	$kg\ s^{-2}$			

Units in Use with the International System

Name	Symbol	Value in SI Units
minute	min	$1\ min = 60\ s$
hour	h	$1\ h = 60\ min = 3600\ s$
day	d	$1\ d = 24\ h = 86\ 400\ s$
degree	°	$1° = (\pi/180)\ rad$
minute	′	$1' = (1/60)° = (\pi/10\ 800)\ rad$
second	″	$1'' = (1/60)' = (\pi/648\ 000)\ rad$
litre	l	$1\ l = 1\ dm^3 = 10^{-3}\ m^3$
tonne	t	$1\ t = 10^3\ kg$

Units, in Use with the International System, whose Values are Obtained Experimentally

Name	Symbol	Approximate Value
electronvolt	eV	$1\ eV = 1·602\ 19 \times 10^{-19}\ J$
unified atomic mass unit	u	$1\ u = 1·660\ 53 \times 10^{-27}\ kg$
astronomical unit	AU*	$1\ AU = 149\ 600 \times 10^6\ m†$
parsec	pc	$1\ pc = 206\ 265\ AU$ $= 30\ 857 \times 10^{12}\ m$

* English abbreviation only, not international
† By definition

Further information about SI units, and international agreements relating to them, is given in *SI: The International System of Units*, the approved English translation of the publication *Le Système International d'Unités*. It is published by HMSO.

APPENDIX 3

CONVERSION TABLE FOR UNITS OF MEASUREMENT (CONVERSION OF UNITS IN OTHER SYSTEMS TO S.I. UNITS)

Non-S.I. Units	S.I. Units	Multiply by
inch	cm	2·54
foot	metre	0·3048
mile	kilometre	1·609
sq in	cm^2	6·4516
sq ft	m^2	9·29 $\times 10^{-2}$
cu ft	m^3	2·8317 $\times 10^{-2}$
ounce (avoirdupois)	gram	28·35
pound (avoirdupois)	kilogram	0·4536
dyne	newton	10^{-5}
kg weight	newton	9·80665
mm Hg	pascal	133·3
mm H$_2$O	pascal	9·8
atmosphere	pascal	101325
calorie	joule	4·1868

APPENDIX 4

DECLARATION OF HELSINKI

World Medical Association (1964)

I Basic Principles

1. Clinical research must conform to the moral and scientific principles that justify medical research and should be based on laboratory and animal experiments or other scientifically established facts.

2. Clinical research should be conducted only by scientifically qualified persons and under the supervision of a qualified medical man.

3. Clinical research cannot legitimately be carried out unless the importance of the objective is in proportion to the inherent risk to the subject.

4. Every clinical research project should be preceded by careful assessment of inherent risks in comparison to foreseeable benefits to the subject or to others.

5. Special caution should be exercised by the doctor performing clinical research in which the personality of the subject is liable to be altered by drugs or experimental procedure.

II Clinical Research Combined with Professional Care

1. In the treatment of the sick person, the doctor must be free to use a new therapeutic measure, if in his judgement it offers hope of saving life, re-establishing health, or alleviating suffering. If at all possible, consistent with patient psychology, the doctor should obtain the patient's freely given consent after the patient has been given a full explanation. In case of legal incapacity, consent should also be procured from the legal guardian; in case of physical incapacity the permission of the legal guardian replaces that of the patient.

2. The doctor can combine clinical research with professional care, the objective being the acquisition of new medical knowledge, only to the extent that clinical research is justified by its therapeutic value for the patient.

III Non-therapeutic Clinical Research

1. In the purely scientific application of clinical research carried out on a human being it is the duty of the doctor to remain the protector of the life and health of that person on whom clinical research is being carried out.

2. The nature, the purpose and the risk of clinical research must be explained to the subject by the doctor.

3a. Clinical research on a human being cannot be undertaken without his free consent after he has been informed; if he is legally incompetent the consent of the legal guardian should be procured.

3b. The subject of clinical research should be in such a mental, physical and legal state as to be able to exercise his power of choice.

3c. Consent should as a rule be obtained in writing. However, the responsibility for clinical research always remains with the research worker; it never falls on the subject even after the consent is obtained.

4a. The investigator must respect the right of each individual to safeguard his personal integrity, especially if the subject is in a dependent relationship to the investigator.

4b. At any time during the course of clinical research the subject or his guardian should be free to withdraw permission for research to be continued. The investigator or the investigating team should discontinue the research if in his or their judgement it may, if continued, be harmful to the individual.

APPENDIX 5

NATIONAL AND INTERNATIONAL CONSIDERATION OF ETHICAL CANONS FOR MEDICAL–SCIENTIFIC INVESTIGATIONS TO PROTECT THE WELFARE AND HUMAN RIGHTS OF CONCERNED PARTICIPANTS
(CIOMS, 1973)

The Conference, having considered that,

WHEREAS appropriate representatives of different nations, professions, disciplines and persuasions have all expressed deep concern for the development and implementation of suitable ethical as well as scientific standards for the protection of all concerned in medical and scientific investigations requiring the participation of human beings, and

WHEREAS these investigations now and in the future in such areas as assessment of the safety and effectiveness of drugs, devices, appliances, substances and also environmental exposures, medical, psychological, behavioural and educational methods, among others, may through known and speculative risks affect the physical and mental health, safety, well-being, status and condition of participants in these investigations,

URGES that health authorities, professional and similar bodies and other groups, including those representing the general public, and a wide range of interests and specialities, consider and act upon appropriate measures for protection of the human, personal and societal rights of parties involved in such investigation. With due regard to differences in philosophy, culture, goals, values and basic needs, as well as current problems, opportunities, resources and similar features, it is urged that, in the interest of a worldwide demonstration of social responsibility and recognition of fundamental human rights, the following subjects, among others, be given attention:

1. Promotion of reciprocally-acceptable medico-legal and ethical standards, similar to scientific requirements, based on existing codes, statutes or modifications as needed, including the preparation of mechanisms for periodic amendment as required;
2. Encouragement of professional and technical education of physicians, researchers and students in various disciplines concerning the ethical and psychological aspects of research on human beings;
3. Common education of professional and public representatives and in particular training for consideration and review of proposals for research investigation and demonstration;
4. Additional research on the value and effectiveness of ethical codifications and development of new approaches to the sharing of understanding among parties leading to appropriate consideration and consent, especially by the non-competent, minors and persons in situations which interfere with their ability to give free consent;
5. Consideration of risk and benefit deriving from proposals in terms of community as well as individual interests;
6. Protection of subjects harmed through participation by appropriate insurance and restorative measures;
7. Establishment of systems of publication and information for sharing determinations of ethical questions;
8. Encouragement of study designs to minimize ethical dilemmas through greater use of epidemiological methods and through other acceptable scientific means; and finally;
9. Formation of alliances for communication and education at various levels to ensure that the basic tenets be subject to constant surveillance and review.

REQUESTS the Council to bring the content of this resolution to the attention of appropriate governmental and non-governmental bodies concerned, as well as universities, research centres, medical societies, etc.

APPENDIX 6

SHORT MULTILINGUAL DICTIONARY

English	French*	German†
acute	aigu	akuter (akute, akutes)
adaptation, abnormal auditory	déterioration du seuil tonal; relapse	pathologische Hörermüdung; pathologische Höradaptation
address	adresse	Speicheradresse
allograft	homogreffe	allogenes Transplantat
array	série; suite; tableau	Feld
artery, brachiocephalic	tronc brachio-céphalique	Truncus brachiocephalicus
auricle	pavillon	Ohrmuschel
autograft	autogreffe	autologes Transplantat
base of stapes	platine	Fussplatte (des Steigbügels)
block	bloc	Speicherabschnitt
block, nasal	obstruction nasal	Nasenverlegung
canal, facial	acqueduc de Fallope	Facialiskanal
cells, hair	cellules ciliées	Haarzellen
chronic	chronique	chronischer (chronische, chronisches)
cochlea	cochlée	Schnecke
computer	ordinateur	Computer
concha	spiralé	Nasenmuschel
current, alternating	courant alternatif	Wechselstrom
current, direct	courant continu	Gleichstrom
data	données	Daten; Angaben
discharge, aural	écoulement de l'oreille	Ohrfluss; Ohrensekretion
discharge, nasal	écoulement nasal	Nasenabsonderung; Nasensekretion
discharge, postnasal	ecoulement rétronasal	Nasenrachensekretion
disk	disque	Magnetplatte
dizziness	étourdissement	Schwindel
drug	produit pharmaceutique; médicament	Arzneimittel
ear	oreille	Ohr
electrical	électrique	elektrisch
electro-oculography	électronystagmographie	elektro-okulographie (elektronystagmographie)
epistaxis	épistaxis; hémorragie nasale	Epistaxis; Nasenbluten
ethanol	éthanol	Äthanol
etacrinic acid	acide etacrinique	Etacrynsäure
examination	examen	Untersuchung
fetus	foetus	Fötus
file	fichier	Datei
flow chart	organigramme; diagramme de séquence	Flussrate
folds, vestibular	bandes ventriculaires	Taschenbänder; Taschenfalten
folds, vocal	cordes vocales	Stimmbänder; Stimmlippen
function, auditory	fonction auditive	Hörfunktion
function, vestibular	fonction vestibulaire	Vestibularfunktion
head	tête	Kopf
headache	mal de tête	Kopfschmerzen
hearing loss	perte d'audition	Hörverlust
hoarseness	enrouement	Heiserkeit
hyporeflexia	hyporéflexie	Hyporeflexie
injection	piqûre; injection	Spritze; Injection

SHORT MULTILINGUAL DICTIONARY

Italian‡	Spanish§	Serbo-Croat†
acuto	agudo	akutan (akutna, akutno)
anomalo addattamento uditivo (sposta- mento temporaneo della soglia)	adaptacion, auditiva patologica	abnormalna slušna adaptacija
indirizzo	direccion; dirigirse	adresa
omoinnesto	injerto homologo	alogeni transplantat
equipaggiamento-arrangiamento ordinamento	arreglo; orden; colocación	zona; oblast
arteria brachiocefalica	tronco braquio-cefalico	brahiocefalna arterija
padiglione uditivo	pabellon auditivo; oreja	ušna školjka
autoinnesto	auto-injerto	autologni transplantat
platina della staffa	platina del estribo	baza stapesa
blocco	bloqueo; obstruccion	blok
ostruziona nasale	obstruccion nasal	zapušenje nosa
canale del facciale	canal del facial	kanal ličnog živca
cellule ciliate	celulas ciliadas	dlakaste ćelije
cronico	cronico	hroničan
coclea	coclea	puž (u uhu), cochlea
calcolatore	computadora	računar; kompjuter
turbinato	cornete: concha	nosna školjka
corrente alternata	corriente alterna	naizmenična struja
corrente continua	corriente directa	jednosmerna struja
dati	datos	podaci
secrezione auricolare	escurrimiento auditivo	ušno curenje
secrezione nasale	escurrimiento nasal	nosno curenje
secrezione retronasale	escurrimiento retronasal	postnazalno curenje
disco	disco	kotur
vertigine	mareo	vrtoglavica
farmaco	medicamento; fármaco	lek
orecchio	oido	uho
elettrico	eléctrico	elektriçni
elettro-oculografia	electro-oculografía	elektro-okulografija; elektronistagmo- grafija
epistassi	epistaxis; hemorragia nasal	krvarenje iz nosa
etanolo	etanol	etil alkohol
acido etacrinico	acido etacrínico	etakrinska kiselina
esame	examen	pregled
feto	feto	fetus
schedario-scheda	fila; hilera	kartoteka
diagramma di flusso	diagrama de flujo	tekuća lista
false corde vocali	cuerda vocal falsa	vestibularni sloj
corde vocali vere	cuerda vocal verdadera	glasna žice
funzione uditiva	función auditiva	slušna funkcija
funzione vestibolare	función vestibular	vestibularna funkcija
capo	cabeza	glava
mal di capo	dolor de cabeza	glavobolja
diminuizione dell'udito (danno uditivo)	disminucion de la audicion	gubitak sluha
raucedine	ronquera	promuklost
iporeflessia	hiporeflexia	hyporeflexia
iniezione	inyeccion	injekcija

SHORT MULTILINGUAL DICTIONARY

English	French*	German†
insidious	insidieux	schleichend
language, high level	langage évolué	Hohe Programmsprache
language, machine code	langage machine	Maschinensprache
language, symbolic	langage symbolique	Symbolsprache
lightheadedness	éblouissement; étourdissement	Leichtsinn
membrane, tympanic	membrane tympanique	Trommellfell
neck	cou	Hals
nerve, vestibulocochlear	nerf cochléo-vestibulaire	Hör-und-Gleichgewichtsnerv
no	non	nein
noise	bruit	Lärm; Geräusch
nose	nez	Nase
nystagmus, slow phase of	phase lente du nystagmus	Nystagmus, langsame Phase
nystagmus, quick phase of	phase rapide du nystagmus	Nystagmus, schnelle Phase
otitis externa	otite externe	Gehörgangsentzündung
otitis media	otite moyenne	Mittelohrentzündung
otitis media, secretory	otite moyenne séromuqueuse	seromuköse Otitis media
otorrhoea	otorrhée	Otorrhoe
otosclerosis	otospongiose; otosclérose	Otosklerose
otoscopy	otoscopie	Otoskopie
pain	douleur	Schmerz
pharynx	pharynx	Pharynx
pharynx, nasal part of	naso-pharynx; cavum	Nasenrachenraum
prognosis	pronostic	Prognose
recess, epitympanic	attique	Epitympanon (Kuppelraum)
reflex	réflexe	Reflex
reliable	reproductible	reproduzierbar
sclerosis, multiple	sclérose en plaques	Multiple Sklerose
semicircular canal	canal semicirculaire	Bogengang
signs	signes	Zeichen
sinus, paranasal	sinus paranasale	Nasennebenhöhle
sneezing	éternuement	Niesen
speech	parole	Sprache
sudden	soudain	plötzlich
symptoms	symptomes	Symptome
tenderness	sensibilité	Schmerzen
test	épreuve; analyse	Prüfung; Test
throat	gorge	Hals
thyroid	thyroïde	Schilddrüse
tinnitus	bourdonnements; acouphènes	Ohrensausen
tube, auditory	trompe d'Eustache	Ohrtrompete
tube, tympanostomy	tube aérateur	Kunsstoffröhrchen zur Paukenbelüftung
tumour	tumeur	Geschwülst
unsteadiness	instabilité	Unsicherheit
valid	valide	gültig
vertigo	vertige	Schwindel
word	mot	Wort
xenograft	hétérogreffe	heterologes Transplantat
yes	oui	ja

* Prepared by S. D. G. Stephens and Y. Cazals.
† Prepared by A. Sokolovski.
‡ Prepared by Franca Merluzzi.
§ Prepared by J. A. Arroyo.

SHORT MULTILINGUAL DICTIONARY

Italian‡	Spanish§	Serbo-Croat†
insidioso	insidioso	podmukao
——	lenguaje "high level"	jezik, visoki nivo
linguaggio, codice di macchina	lenguaje a máquina	jezik, mašinski kod
linguaggio simbolico	lenguaje simbólico	jezik, simbolički
senso di testa vuota	sensacion de cabeza flotante; o vacia	slaboumnost
membrana timpanica	membrana timpanica	bubna opna
collo	cuello	vrat
nervo cocleo-vestibolare	nervio cocleo-vestibular; VIII par craneal	vestibulo-kohlearni živac
no	no	ne
rumore	ruido	buka
naso	nariz	nos
scossa lenta del nistagmo	fase lenta del nistagmus	nistagmus, spora faza
scossa rapida del nistagmo	fase rapida del nistagmus	nistagmus, brza faza
otite esterna	otitis externa	zapaljenje spoljnjeg uha
otite media	otitis media	zapaljenje srednjeg uha
otite media catarrale	otitis media secretoria	serozno zapalenje srednjeg uha
otorrea	otorrea	curenje iz uha; otorea
otosclerosi	otosclerosis; otoesclerosis	otoskleroza
otoscopia	otoscopia	otoskopija
dolore	doler	bol
faringe	faringe	ždrelo
nasofaringe; spazio retronasale	naso-faringe	nazofarinks;
prognosi	pronostico	prognoza
recesso epitipanico	receso epitimpanico	epitimpanični recesus
riflesso	reflejo	refleks
attendibile	responsible	pouzdan; reproducirni
sclerosi multipla	esclerosis multiple	multipla skleroza
canale semicircolare	canal semicircular	polukružni kanalić
segni	signos	znaci
seni paranasali	seno paranasal	paranazalni sinus
starnutire	estornudo	kijanje
linguaggio	habla	govor
improvviso	subito	iznenadni
sintomi	sintomas	simptomi
tenerezza	sensible; delicado	osetljivost; bol
esame	examen; analisis	proba; ispitivanje
gola	garganta	grlo; vrat
tiroide	tiroides	tireoidna šlezda
acufene	tinitus; acufeno	zujanje u ušima
tuba di Eustachio	trompa de Eutaguio	slušna truba
tubicino o valvola di drenaggio	tubo de ventilacion	cev za prozračivanje
tumore	tumor	tumor
incertezza nella deambulazione	inestabilidad	nestabilnost
valido	valido	važeći
vertigine	vertigo	vrtoglavica
parola	palabra	reč
eteroinnesto	injerto heterologo	heterologni transplantat
si	si	da

INDEX

Abacus, 32
Abductor paralysis, reconstruction, 912
Abductors, 541
Abnormal auditory adaptation, 354
ABO blood group system, 754
Absidia, 652
Absolute mortality, 137
Absolute pitch, 350
Absorbable gelatine sponge, 850, 856, 879
Absorbable gelatin sponge implant, 873
Absorption coefficient, 96
Acceptors, 54
Acetone, 508
Acetylcholine, 476
Acetylcholinesterase in taste bud, 476
Acetylsulfosalicylic acid, 480
Achalasia of the oesophago-gastric junction, 597
Acid mucopolysacharrides, 367
Acoustic analysis of speech, 490
Acoustic aspects of nasal function, 523–27
Acoustic automonitoring, 564
Acoustic cues, 608
Acoustic efficiency, 94
Acoustic feedback, 819
Acoustic filters, 158
Acoustic impedance, 281–90
Acoustic impedance
  bridge, 255
  definition, 282
  formula, 282
  history, 282
  internal ear, 243
  miscellaneous applications, 289
  principles, 281
  tympanometry and absolute measurement of, 286
Acoustic measurements, 779
Acoustic meatus
  external, 293, 296, 305
  internal, 228, 307, 429
Acoustic neuroma. *See* Vestibulocochlear schwannoma
Acoustic reflex, 268, 269
  as feedback system, 273
  linear analysis, 271
  models of, 273
Acoustic spectrography, 584
Acoustic stapedial reflex, 335
Acoustic structure of nasal consonants, 523
Acoustic test box, 809
Acoustic trauma, 276
Acousticolaryngeal reflexes, 564
Acoustics, 87–101
ACTH, 519, 454
ACTH gel, 450
Actinomycins, 728

Actinomycin D. *See* Dactinomycin
Actinomycosis, 658
Acute meningoencephalitis, 662
Adaptation, 349
Adductors, 541, 894
Adenocarcinomas, 676
Adenocystic carcinoma, 675
Adenoidectomy, 492, 749
Adenoids, 211, 492
Adenomas, 676
Adenovirus, 626
Adenyl cyclase, 476
Adhesives, 717, 765
Administrative aspects, 935
Ad-strial capillaries, 852
Afferent auditory pathway, 353
Afferent nerves, 221
Aflatoxins, 658
African histoplasmosis, 651
AGC. *See* Automatic gain control
Age-specific incidence rates, 136
Ageusia, 478
Aglycogeusia, 468
Air conditioning, 517
  and recycling, 503
Air sacs, 537, 539, 544, 545
Airway patency, 912
Airway resistance, 504, 896
Alar cartilages, 886, 887
Albumin, 752
Alcohol. *See* Ethanol
Alertness, 331
Alexander's law, 401
Alexandria, 10
Algorithm, 39
Alkylating agents, 726
Alleles, 121
Allergic bronchopulmonary aspergillosis, 659
Allergies, 659, 669
Allogenic adipose tissue, 879
Allogenic cartilage, 878
Allograft bone, 869
Allograft cartilage, 869, 871
Allograft reaction, 713
Allografts, 712, 713, 867–71, 874, 922
  composite, 875
Allotransplants, 898
Alloys, 714
Alpha particles, 707
Alphanumeric data, 33
Alport's syndrome, 125
ALS. *See* Antilymphocytic serum
Alternaria padwickii, 659
Alternate binaural loudness balance test, 354, 359, 794, 797
Alternating current, 57
Alveoli, 510
Amantadine, 636

Amblystoma punctatum, 177, 178, 181
Amenhotep II, 1
Aminoglycoside antibiotics, 849, 851
6-Amino-penicillanic acid, 703
Aminopterin, 725
Amitriptyline, 480
Ammonia, 508, 554
Amoebiasis, 662
Amoebic dysentery, 662
Ampere, 67
Amphotericin, 648
Amphotericin B, 649, 650, 703
Ampicillin, 703
Amplification factor, 73
Amplification, compression. *See* Linear dynamic compression
Amplifiers, 77
  chopper, 78, 278
  hearing aid, 817
  logarithmic, 815
  operational, 84
  sound, 830
Amplitude, 89
Ampullary crest, 376
Ampullary cristae, 369
Ampullary juxta-crista regions, 300
Amyloidosis of respiratory tract, 927
Anaesthesia, 18, 556
Analogue-to-digital convertor, 33
Analysis of variance, 26, 29
Analytical engine, 32
Angiogram, vertebral, 229
Angiography, 229
Angiostrongylosis, 663
Angular acceleration, 8
Animal parasites, 661
Animals
  comparative anatomy of the ear, 184–202
  ethical considerations, 944
  in experimentation, 942–44
  law in respect of, 942
Annulus tympanicus, 304, 336
Anode, 72
Anoxia, 293
  effect of, 291–92
Anoxic endolymphatic potential, 294
Anterior rhinoscopy, 490
Anterior sac, 214
Anterior saccule, 215
Anthracoids, 639
Antibacterial agents, 863
Antibiotics, 212
Antibiotics, 212, 703, 725, 728, 849–52, 856, 859, 861
  in infected tissue, 704
  in interstitial tissue fluid, 704
Antibodies, 633
  resistance to, 640

Antibody screen, 755
Anti-cholinergic agents, 863
Anti-convulsant drugs, 850, 863
Antidepressants, 863
Antidesma bunius, 480
Anti-heparinizing agents, 849, 855
Antihistaminics, 863
Antihypertensive agents, 863
Antilymphocytic serum, 713, 899
Antimetabolites, 725, 727, 732
Anti-protozoal agents, 849, 855
Antiseptics, 863
Antiviral drugs, 636
Apertures, 91
Aphasia, 610
    Language Modalities Test of, 617
Area ratio, of tympanic membrane, 238
Aristotle, 211
Arithmetical probability paper, 14
Arkansas, 25
Arterio-venous anastomoses, 515
Arthrokinetic reflex system, 552
Arthropods, 665
Articular mechanoreceptors, 564
Articulation, 603
Artificial ossicles, 869
Aryepiglottic folds, 530
Aryepiglottic musculature, 566
Arytenoidectomy, 913
Asbestos, 510
Ascaris lumbricoides, 663
Aspergilloma, 653
Aspergillosis, 653
Aspergillus flavus, 658
Aspergillus fumigatus, 659
Aspiration biopsy, 465
Assortive mating, 129
Asthma, 659
Athetosis, 550
Atomic number, 52, 706
Atoms, 52
ATP concentration in stria vascularis, 293
ATPase, 261, 292, 293, 295, 299, 300
    anion activated, 293
    myofibrillar, 265
    strial, 293
Atrophic rhinitis, 520
Atropine, 462
Atropinization, 519
Attack rate, 135
Attention, 331
Attenuation, 98
Attic see Epitympanic recess
Attributes, 9
Audio-dontics, 821
Audiogram,
    pure-tone, 339, 353, 828, 843
    self-recorded, 792
    stiffness tilt, 796
Audiologist, 344
Audiometers, 772–88
    calibration, 783, 786
    delayed auditory feedback, 778
    development of, 786
    masking, 784–86

Audiometers (*contd.*)
    masking zero reference level, 786
    paediatric, 777
    pure-tone, 772, 789
    Rudmose self-recording, 792
    self-recording automatic, 776
    signal monitoring, 775
    speech, 776
    surveys, 784
    types, 772
Audiometric thresholds, 45
Audiometric zero, 778
    standardization for air conduction, 780
    standardization for bone conduction, 782
Audiometry, 311, 788–800
    clinical, 790
    computer controlled automatic, 40
    conditions for, 800
    diagnostic, 797
    electric response, 804
    evoked response, 337
    in industry, 797
    masking procedure, 791
    monitoring, 169
    play, 802
    pure-tone, 353, 798, 802
    pure-tone threshold, 790
    recording, 798
    school screening, 798
    self-recording, 792
    speech, 786, 796
Auditory, 221
Auditory adaptation, 795
    abnormal, 354
Auditory analysis, law of, 312
Auditory centre, 264
Auditory control system, centifugal extra-reticular, 264
Auditory cortex, 264, 326, 347, 359
    single unit discharge patterns for, 327
    central, 352–61
    tests of, 355
Auditory evoked response, 338
Auditory fatigue, 795
Auditory function,
    electrophysiological investigation of, 334–43
    investigation of, 402
Auditory handicap, 141
Auditory localization in vertical planes, 358
Auditory nervous system, 312–34
Auditory network, 313
Auditory neurone, 7, 317
Auditory ossicles, 230
Auditory pathways, main ascending, 313
Auditory perception, 278, 279
Auditory processing, 250
Auditory prosthetic devices, 763
    see also Hearing aids
Auditory reaction times, 358
Auditory rehabilitation
    children, 839–46
    definition of, 839

Auditory response, 40
Auditory sensation, 344
Auditory system
    frequency analysis of, 312
    function, 312
    mechanics of, 237
    non-linearities in, 269
Auditory temporal integration, 346, 358
Auditory threshold, 310, 344
Auditory training, 831, 841
Auditory training units, 826
Auditory tubal block, 285
Auditory tubal function, 252–57
    anatomy, 252
    changes with age, 253
    changing ambient pressure, 256
    closing mechanism, 255
    draining function, 256
    gross structure, 252
    historical aspects, 252
    lymphatics, 253
    opening mechanism, 254
    opening time, 255
    physiology, 254
    testing draining function, 256
    testing ventilating function, 255
Auditory tubal irradiation, 29
Auditory tubes, 203, 492
    collapsed, 254
    comparative anatomy, 191
    function of, 283
    muscles, 253
Auerbach's plexus, 597
Aural myiasis, 665
Aural organogenesis, 214
Aural prostheses, 805
Auricle, 185, 238, 305, 350, 429
    hearing aid, 806
    tactile stimulation of, 287
Auriculectomy, 187
Autistic children, 614
Autogenous fascia, 868
Autografts, 712, 867, 868, 870, 922
    revascularized intestinal, 903
Auto-immune reaction, 467
Automatic gain control, 815, 826
Autonomic motor function, 439
Autonomic nervous system, 515
Averaged evoked potentials, 328
Averaged evoked responses, 858
A-weighting, 100
Azaserine, 728
Azathioprine, 671, 900

Babylonian civilization, 1
Bacillus, 638
Background noise, 100
Bacterial inflammations, 926
Bacterial multiplication, 638
Bacterial toxins, 641
Bacteriophages, 628, 629, 639
Baldwin's formulae, 582
Band-pass filter, 72
Bandwidth, 72
Bar chart, 10
Bárány chair, 379

Bárány box, 789
Barbecue experiments, 380
Barbiturates, 389
Barium titanate, 105
Barriers, 91
Basal ganglia, 385, 550
Base, 75
Base number, 1
Basidiobolus haptosporus, 652
Basilar membrane, 45, 246, 251, 308, 315, 320
  comparative anatomy, 196
  displacement, 51
  envelope of, 316
  resistance, 298–99
Bast's utriculoendolymphatic valve, 300
Bateriology, 638–45
Bats, 185, 187, 191, 196, 197, 199, 276
  larynx, 537–45
Bayes' theorem, 25
Beats, 91
Békésy audiogram 3, 20
Békésy audiometry, 345, 346, 349
Békésy patterns, 354
Bel, 6
Bell's palsy, 10, 148, 276, 279, 434, 446–52
Bence Jones protein, 680
Benign vocal nodule, 587
Benzene, 440
Benzylpenicillin. *See* Penicillin G
Beri-beri, 133
Bernoulli effect, 896
Bernoulli's phenomenon, 502
Beta particles, 707
Bilateral cortical lesions, 326
Binary digit, 34
Binary numbers, 34
Binary system, 1
Bing test, 791
Binomial distribution, 11
Biodegradation, 717
Biological clocks, 321
Biological growth, 8
Biological half-lives, 707
Biopsies, 223
Biopsy histopathology, 667
Bioreactive properties, 717
Bismuth subnitrate and iodoform paste, 445
Bit, 34
Bithermal caloric test procedures, 398
Blastomyces brasiliensis, 650
Blastomyces dermatitidis, 650
Blastomycosis, European. *See* Crypto-coccosis
Bleomycin, 698, 729
Blood,
  cadaver, 751
  use of, 751
Blood donors, 750
  screening, 759
  selection criteria, 751
Blood fractions, 751
Blood, grouping, 751, 753–57
  ABO system, 754

Blood loss, 18, 21
  adenoidectomy and tonsillectomy, 749
  major otolaryngological operations, 749–50
  microsurgery, 749
Blood pressure, 6
Blood transfusion, 749–61
  autologous, 750
  exchange, 756
  history, 749
  incompatible crossmatching, 760
  incompatibility, 757, 760
  incompatibility reactions, 760
  need for, 749
  request procedure, 757
  screening, 751
  selection of, 753
Blood vessels, 741
Blood volume, 749
Blowfllies, 665
Blowing, 490
Blunt chest trauma, 928
Blurring, 711
Bode plots, 72
Bodian protargol stain, 178
Body equilibrium, 361
Body plethysmograph, 581
Boilermakers' deafness, 151
Bondy operation, 212
Bone, 89, 741
Bone-conduction hearing level, 792
Bone-conduction tests, 790
Bone grafts, 885
Bone marrow, 741
Bone structure, 231
Bone vibrators, 782, 783
Boolean algebra, 1
Booster doses, 644
Bowley's coefficient of skewness, 15
Bowman's gland, 495, 496
Brachiocephalic artery, 922
Brain stem, 363
Brain stem ischaemia, 721
Brainstem lesions, 353, 358
Brain stem reticular system, 550
Brain tumour, 229, 708
Branchial arches, 425, 529
Branchial cyst, 530
Branchial ducts, 425
Branchial grooves, 425
Branchial pouches. *See* Pharyngeal pouches.
Breach of contract, 940
Bretylium tosylate, 863
Brickwork, 96
Broad band, 94
Brodmann's cortical Area 8, 384
Brodmann's cortical Area 17, 385
Bromide, tetrylammonium, 294
Bonchial carcinoma, 145
Bronchial catarrh, 659
Bronchiectasia, 466
Bronchioles, 510
Bronchoscope, 719, 720
Bronchoscopy, fiberoptic, 930

Bronchospasm, 555
Bronchus, carcinoma of, 25
Broomsliter-Creel test, 359
Brown tumour, 686
Brownian movement, 504
Buccal fat pad, 436
Buccopharyngeal membrane, 421
Bucrilate, 765, 876
Burkitt's lymphoma, 133
  epidemiology, 147
Burkitt's tumour, 137
Busulfan, 727
Butyl cyanoacrylate, 765
Bye-laws, 936

Cacogeusia, 478
Cactinomycin, 900
Calcium ions, 519
Calibration, 155
Callithrix jacchus, 199
Callitroga hominivorax, 665
Caloric test, 25, 381, 394
  bithermal, 398
  variations, 397
Calories, 115
Canal paresis, 394
Cancer,
  control by drug therapy, 725–26
  death rate from, 8
  epidemiology, 143, 145
  registries, 136
  stages, 4
  treatment kinetics, 7
Cancer cells, abnormal behaviour of, 730
Cancer-specific messenger RNA, 732
Candida albicans, 648
Candidiasis, 648
"Canal sickness" symptoms, 369
Canthariasis, 666
Capacitance, 59, 67
Capillary networks, 352
Capreomycin, 849
Capsid, 625
Capsomers, 625, 628
Carbenicillin, 703
Carbon dioxide, 554
Carbonic anhydrase, 293
Carcinogenesis, 8
Cardioderma cor, 185, 187
Cardiac syncope, 124
Carhart notch, 792
Carina, 504
Carollia perspicillata, 200
Carotid aneurysms, 233
Carotid canals, 226
Cartesian coordinates, 67
Cartilage, 741
  autografts, 922
  nasal, 513
Cascading, 72
Cassava, 133, 142, 147, 148, 208
Catecholamine depleting agents, 863
Catguts, 717
Catharanthus roseus, 729
Cathode, 72

Cathode follower, 81
Cathode-ray oscilloscope, 66
Cathode-ray tube, 33
Cavia porcellus, 200, 201, 259, 266
Cefaloridine, 703
Cell cycle time, 740
Cell reproductive cycle, 731
Cell survival curves, 736, 739
Cells of Böttcher, 199
Cells of Claudius, 199
Cells of Deiters, phalangeal, 204
Cellulosics, 718
Cements, 717, 765
Central auditory dysfunction, 352–61
    tests of, 355
Central masking, 348, 360
Central processor unit, 34
Centurio senex, 199
Cephalosporins, 703
Cercopithecus, 188
Cercospora apii, 657
Cerebellar nuclei, 385
Cerebellum, 363, 384, 550
Cerebral atrophy, 229
Cerebral cortex, 342, 385
    frontal regions of, 549
Cerebral cysticercosis, 664
Cerebral infarcts, 229
Cerebral palsy, 465
Cervical injuries
    blunt, 928
    penetrating, 928
Cervical posture tests, 390
Cervical sinus, 425
Cervical torsion nystagmus, 390
Cervical trachea, reconstruction of, 904
Cervicofacial actinomycosis, 658
Cercosporamycosis. *See* Verrucous
    mycosis
Chaetomium sps, 659
Characteristic curves, 72, 711
Characteristic frequency, 313
Characters, 9
Charge, 51, 67
Charge carriers, 74
Chemodectomas, 209
Chicleros, 662
Chiggers, 665
Childhood autism, 614
Children, auditory rehabilitation, 839–46
Chimaera, 199
Chinchilla, 192
Chip, 69
Chiroptera, larynx, 537–45
Chi-squared test, 14, 26
Chlorambucil, 480, 727
Chloramphenicol, 368
Chlordiazepoxide, 389
Chlorhexidine, 850
Chlormethine, 726
Chloroquine, 368, 849
Choanae, 513
Chocholle test, 359
Cholera, 133
Cholesteatoma, 8, 203, 211, 217, 233,
    234, 455, 457

Cholesterol granuloma, 673
Chomskian theories, 609
Chorda tympani, 436, 462
Chordal ridge, 216
Chordoma, 683
Chromosomal aberrations, 127
Chronic glossitis, 649
Chronic parotitis, 467
Chrysomyia bezziana, 665
Cigarette smoking, 144, 145, 507, 554
    costs, 722–23
Ciliary function, 518
Cinéfluorography, 489
Cinéfluoroscopy, 490
Circuits, integrated, 85
Circulaires, 936
Circulars, 936
Citellus, 652
Citric acid, 464
Cladosporium, 659
Cleft lip and palate, 427, 491
Clethrionomys, 190
Click pitch, 350
Clinical research, 949
Clinical trials, 721
Clipper, 73
Clonic facial spasm, 438
Closed-loop gain, 80
Clotrimazole, 647
Cloxacillin, 703
Cluster analysis, 25
Coccidioides immitis, 652
Coccidioidomycosis, 652
Coccus, 638
Cochlea, 221, 245, 281, 303, 342, 349,
    851, 854
    comparative anatomy, 195
    development, 206
    electrophysiology, 303–12
    peripheral bio-electric signals related
        to, 336
    preparations of, 219
    sensitivity for different frequencies,
        307
Cochlear aqueduct, 199
    abnormal patency, 125
Cochlear disorders, 797
Cochlear duct, electrical resistance of
    the individual walls of, 297
Cochlear duct enzymes, 292
Cochlear duct membrane, 292, 296
Cochlear endolymph, 290, 299
Cochlear function, 347
    loss of, 290
Cochlear hair cells, 247
Cochlear hydrodynamics, 316
Cochlear implant, 212, 342, 763, 822
Cochlear lesions, 346
Cochlear mechanics, 45
Cochlear membrane
    characteristics of, 296
    properties of, 297
Cochlear microphonic, 303, 305, 337,
    367
    from tympanic membrane, 304
Cochlear-microphonic potential, 334

Cochlear-microphonic response, 244,
    245
Cochlear nerve compound action poten-
    tial, 336
Cochlear nerve lesions, 354
Cochlear nonlinearities, 250
Cochlear nucleus, 221, 313, 319, 320,
    321, 550, 564, 612
Cochlear partition, 244
Cochlear potentials, 40
Cochlear receptor, 303
Cochlear reserve, 792
Cochleo-saccular degenerations, 232
Codes of Practice, 935, 936
Coefficient of association, 17
Coefficient of colligation, 17
Coefficient of curvilinear correlation, 24
Coefficient of determination, 20, 23
Coefficient of kurtosis, 14
Coefficient of variation, 14
Coendou prehensilis, 195
Coherence, 720
Coincidence, 89
Coincidence frequency, 95
Coincidence region, 95
Colestyramine, 480
Collagen, 682
Collector, 75
Coloboma, 125
Columella, 883
Comb filter, 350
Common carotid, 922
Common-mode rejection, 79
Communication, 599
    mathematical theory of, 609
Community physician, 134
Comparative incidence, 137
Comparing the means, 28
Competing message tests, 357
Compiler, 36
Complex number, 65
Complex stimuli, response to, 326
Composite allografts, 875
Compound benzoic acid ointment, 647
Compression amplification, 826
Compulsory medical examinations, 940
Computer-assisted diagnosis, 25
Computer languages, 35
Computer program, 34
Computers, 31–48, 585, 942
    general applications, 43
    on-line applications, 40
Concentrated erythrocytes, 750, 752
Concha of the auricle, 819
Conchae, 517
Conditional probability, 25
Conduction velocity, 442
Conductors, 53
Congenital aphasia, 610
Congenital malformations, 127
Congenital meatal atresia, 865
Congenital subglottic stenosis, 924
Congenital syphilis, 400
Congenital tracheomalacia, 924
Conjugation, 640, 641
Connecting materials, 717

Consonance, 326
Constant, 9
Contingency correlations, 17
Contraceptive pill, 863
Contract, breach of, 940
Contralateral routing of signals (CROS), 807, 828
Contrast, 711
Contrast media, 228, 711–12
Contrast radiography, 228, 711
Control system, 384
Control unit, 34
Controlled clinical trials, 26
Convergence, 385
Conversion table for units, 949
Coombs' test, 760
Copyright, 941
Copula of His. *See* Hypobranchial eminence
Cordopexy, 913
Cordylobia anthrophaga, 665
Cores, 34
Coriolis effect, 381
Coriolis forces, 369
Corneoretinal potential, 379
Corniculate cartilages, 531
Coronavirus, 626
Corpus trapezoideum, 321
Correlograms, 585
Corrosion, 717
Cortical projection systems, 549
Cortical responses, 337
Cortical stimulation, 822
Corticobulbar tract, 549
Corticosteroids, 519, 648, 671, 862, 863
Corvus corone, 199
Corynebacterium diphtheriae, 626
Cost-benefit analysis, 722
Coughing, 550
Coulomb, 67
Coupled ionic transport, 292
Coupler, 102
Coupling capacitor, 70
Cousins, 128
Covariance, 20
CPE. *See* Cytopathogenic effect
Cranio-facial hypoplasia, 480
Creaky voice, 601
Creatine phosphate concentrations in the stria vascularis, 293
Cretinism, 147
Crico-arytenoid joints, 552, 913
Crico-arytenoid muscles, 557
Cricoid cartilage, 531, 539
Cricopharyngeal sphincter, 594
Cricopharyngeus, 566
Cricopharyngeus muscle, 560
Cricothyroid joints, 552
Cricothyroid muscle, 548, 556
Cricotracheal avulsion, 928
Crista ampullaris, 375
Crista falciformis, 228, 430
Criterion, β, 345
Critical bands, 348
Critical bandwidth, 348
Critical flicker fusion frequency, 619

Critical period hypothesis, 840
Critical ratio, 348
Crocodile tear phenomenon, 441
Cross olivo-cochlear bundle, 313
Crossmatching, 753, 756–60
Cross-over trials, 26
Cross-resistance, 640
Crotalus cerastes, 190
Cruelty to Animals Act 1876, 942–44
Cryofibrinogen precipitate, 752
Cryosurgery, 114, 364, 721
Cryptococcosis, 650
Cryptococcus neoformans, 650
Ctenomys, 190
Cumulative frequency curve, 11
Cuneiform cartilages, 531
Cupula deflection, 378, 379, 380
Cupulograms, 380
Cupulolithiasis, 369
Curie, 707
Current, 51, 57, 67
    heating effect of, 57
Curve-fitting, 46
Cutaneous larval migrans, 663
Cutebria, 665
Cut-off frquency, 70
Cuticular plate, 248, 249
Cyanide, 133, 142, 294
Cyanoacrylate, 717
Cyanoacrylate, 717, 765
Cycle, 57
Cycle-histogram, 317, 321
Cyclophosphamide, 727, 731
Cymba conchae, 819
Cysteine, 480
Cytarabine, 637
Cytidine diphosphate, reduction of, 729
Cytopathogenic effect, 631
Cytotoxic drugs, 698, 699, 725–32, 748, 849, 856

D antigen, 755
Dactinomycin, 728, 748
Damping, 95
Damping factor, 312
Data, presentation of, 10
dc-shift, 328
    Keidel's, 343
Deafness, 151, 537, 565
    see also Hearing loss
Death rate from cancer, 8
Deceit, 940
Decibel, 1, 3, 6
Decisive, 26
Declaration of Helsinki, 942, 949
Decongestants, 862
Deep mycoses of the head and neck, 650
Defamation, 940
Degeneration, cochlear, 301
Deglutition, 591–97, 902
    nervous regulation of, 595
    oesophageal stage, 594
    oral stage, 591
    pharyngeal stage, 592
    see also Swallowing
Degrees of freedom, 27

Deiters' cells, 221, 248
Delayed auditory feed back, test, 778
Delayed paralysis, 456
Delayed speech feedback, 338
Demilunes of Gianuzzi, 460
Demultiplication, 323
Denes-Naunton test, 345
Dental auditory implants, 821
Dental lamina, 425
Dental radio receiver, 822
Deoxyribonucleic acid. *See* DNA
Deoxyuridilic acid, 728
Depigmentation, 125
Dermatobia hominis, 665
Dermatophagoides sps, 659
Dermatophytoses, 647
Design, 941
Design of experiments, 26
Desorption, 509
Detectability measure, 345
Detection theory, 344
Development factor, 711
Dexamethasone, 454, 456
Dextran, 753, 756
Diarthrognathus, 192
Diazepam, 342, 385
Dictionary, multilingual, 951–54
Dielectric constant, 60
Dielectrics, 53
Difference engine, 32
Difference limens, 345
Differentiator, 72
Diffraction, 92
Diffuse field, 93
Diffusion, 505
Diffusion potential, 291–92
Digit, 1
Digital computer, 32
Digital-to-analogue converter, 33
Dihydrostreptomycin, 365, 849
Dimethylsiloxane, 715
Dimetrodon, 192
Dimeticones, 715
Dimorphic fungi, 646
Dinitrophenol, 294
Diode, 72
Diphtheria, 925
Diphthongs, 605
Diploid organism, 121
Dipodomys, 190, 652
Direct currents, 57
Directional compensation, 362
Directional preponderance, 394
Directionality, 94
Discriminant analysis, 25
Dispersion, 13
Displacement activities, 615
Displacement transfer function, 242
Distortion, 348
Diuretics, 849, 855, 859
Divergence, 385
DNA, 122, 182, 726, 728, 729, 735, 748
DNA viruses, 133, 634
Dominance, 121
Donors, 53
Dopants, 53

Doppler shift, 187, 276
Dorsal nucleus of corpus trapezoideum, 321
Dorsal sail, 192
Dose-response curves, 7
Double-blind trial, 26
Down's syndrome, 127
Doxorubicin, 480
Droplet filtration, 508
Drug resistance, 640
Drugs, 703
  ototoxic, 207, 849–62
  rhinotoxic, 862–63
  see also Cytotoxic drugs
Ductus arteriosus, 530
Ductus reuniens, 300
Duration difference limen, 346
Duration discrimination, 346, 358
Duverney, Joseph, 211
Dysarthria, 549
Dysequilibrium, 368
Dysgeusia, 449, 478, 480
Dyskinetic diseases, 550
Dysostosis, mandibulo-facial, 125
Dysphonia, 549, 895
Dysplasia, 693

Ear
  abnormal histology, 230
  abnormal radiographic anatomy, 232
  acoustical properties of, 282
  anatomy, 213–19
  applied morphology, 211–35
    historical aspects, 211
  artificial, 110, 780
  as detector, 250
  capsule, 180
  comparative anatomy, 184–202
    methods of study, 185
    species studied, 185
  comparative morphology, 184
  decalcified bone sections, 184
  dissection, 213
  epidemiology, 137
  experimental pathology, 207
  external, 429
    comparative anatomy, 185–87
  histological examination of, 219
  hydrodynamics of, 312
  induction, 176
  internal, 231
    abnormalities, 878
    acoustic impedance of, 243
    comparative anatomy, 195–200
    histology of, 220
    hydrodynamics of, 317
    impedance, 242
    light microscopy, 219
    organogenesis, 175–83
    place/resonance theory (Helmholtz), 244
    protection, 243
    routes of access to, 850
  middle, 25, 183, 214

Ear (*contd.*)
  cavity, comparative anatomy, 189
  cavity, viruses isolated from, 635
  comparative anatomy, 187–95
  compliance, 285
  disease, 29
  dynamics of, 791
  examination of, 281
  function of, 281
  impedance change in relation to type of stimulus in various lesions, 288
  infection, 635
  model, 51
  mucosa, 202
  muscle contraction and its effects, 265–68
  muscle reflex, 276
  muscle reflex measurements, 287
  muscles, 243, 257, 266, 279, 286
    fibre arrangement, 263
  network, 241
  normal histology, 220
  organogenesis, 173–75
  pathology, 195
  pressure, 254, 285, 287
  pressure transformation, 241
  reflex, 267, 272, 274
  resonant loci of, 278
  transfer function, 242
  transformer mechanism, 238
  transformer ratio in Man, 240
  ultrastructure, 202–4
  neoplasms, 209
  occlusion effect, 791
  organogenesis, 173–84
  outer, 173, 183
    transformer mechanism, 238
  pathological aspects, 230–33
  reconstructive surgery, 865–81
  sensitivity of, 250
  surgical anatomy, 233–35
  techniques of structure examination and normal findings, 212–30
  time/frequency analysis, 250
  ultrastructure of, 202–11
Ear fluids, internal, 301
Ear function, 236
Early vertex potential, 342
Earmoulds, 819
  configuration, 820
  materials, 820
  vented, 820
Earmuffs, 160
Earphones, 778, 812
  calibration, 109, 110
  electrostatic, 105
  moving coil, 831
  noise excluding enclosure for, 781
Earplugs, 159, 160
Echinococcosis, 664
Echinococcus granulosus, 664
Echo reflectors, 187
Echoes, 350
Echolocation, FM pulses during, 276
Edetic acid, 750

EDTA. *See* Edetic acid
Educational sound amplification systems, 831
Effective half-lives, 707
Efferent nerves, 222
Efficacy, 25
Egyptian mythology, 1
Elastic limit, 715
Elasticity, 87, 715
Elastomers, 714
Electret, 108, 812
Electric current, 52
Electric field, 51
Electric response audiometry, *see* evoked response audiometry
Electrical instruments, 721
Electrical measurement, 66
Electrical potential, 67
Electrical potential changes in ototoxicity, 858
Electricity, 51–68
Electro-acoustic impedance bridge, 283, 284
Electro-acoustic instruments, 721
Electro-acoustic rehabilitation equipment, 830–38
  auditory trainers, 831
  induction loop system, audio-frequency, 834
  induction loop system, radio-frequency, 835
  radio-frequency free field system, 835
  self-contained individually worn unit, 836
  sound amplifying equipment, 831
  tactile vibrators, 838
  transposing equipment, 837
  types, 830, 831
  see also Hearing aids
Electroacoustic instrument, 772
Electroacoustics, 101
Electrocardiogram, 124
Electrocochleogram, 336
Electrocochleography, 306, 336
Electrode properties, 67
Electrodermal response, 335
Electroglottography, 51, 576
Electrogustometry, 439
Electrolaryngograph, 721
Electrolaryngology, 51
Electrolyte transfer, 300
Electro-mechanical impedance bridge, 283
Electromotive force, 52
Electromyography, 442, 456, 485, 489, 546, 586, 588
Electron microscopy, 202, 204, 222
Electronic averagers, 337
Electronics, 69–87
Electrons, 52, 706
  excited, 53
Electronvolt, 733
Electronystagmography *see* Electro-oculography
Electro-oculography, 45, 401
Electro-olfactogram, 8, 496

Electrophysiological investigation of auditory function, 334–43
Electrophysiological tests, 804
Elephas maximas, 196
EMI scanner, 229
Emitter, 75
Emotional disturbance, 614
Enamel organs, 425, 426
Enclosures, 91
Endocochlear potential, 291, 296
  change with age, 299
  dual nature of, 294, 297
Endolymph, 290, 366, 371, 374
  circulation, 297
  flow determination, 298
  function, 298
  pressure, 301, 310
Endolymphatic duct, 200
Endolymphatic hydrops, 301, 363, 703
Endolymphatic sac, 300
  endolymph, 301
  function of, 301
  obliteration of, 297
Endolymphatic surface, marginal cells at, 294
Endolymphatic system, 209
Endoscopes, 490, 718, 719, 720, 930
Endotoxins, 642
Endotracheal intubation, 920
Endotracheal tube, 920
Endotracheal tube cuff, 921
Endotracheal tube cuff stenosis, 929
  prevention of, 930
Energy producing enzymes, 293
Entamoeba histolytica, 662
Entomophthora coronata, 652
Entrapment syndromes, 445
Enzyme concentrations, 5
Enzyme inhibitors, 293, 727
Enzymes, energy producing, 293
Eosinophilic granular cell cyst, 690
Eosinophilic meningoencephalitis, 663
Eosinophilic myeloencephalitis, 664
Epibranchial placodes, 530
Epidemiology, 133–50
  ear, 137
  facial nerve, 148
  head and neck, 147
  history, 133
  methodology, 135
  methods for acquiring data, 136
  mouth, 144–45
  nose, 143–44
  oesophagus, 145
  prospective studies, 136
  retrospective studies, 135
  speech disorders, 148
  systematic, 137–48
  terminology, 135
  throat, 145
  uses, 133–50
Epidermis, 740
Epiglottic carcinoma, 909
Epiglottis, 427, 531, 540, 593
Episodic vertigo, 659
Epitympanic recess, 215, 217, 286, 456

Epitympanum, *see* Epitympanic Recess
Epstein-Barr virus, 133, 147, 634
  antibody, 144
Eptesicus fuscus, 651
Eptesicus rendalli, 194, 195
Equal-energy principle, 152
Equivalent Threshold Sound Pressure Level (ETSPL), 779
ERA. *See* Evoked response audiometry
Erosion, 717
Erythrocytes, 751
Etacrynic acid, 294, 295, 368 849, 855, 859
Ethacrynic acid *see* etacrynic acid
Ethanol, 389
Ethical aspects, 935
Ethical canons for medical-scientific investigations, 950
Ethical committees, 942
Ethical considerations, 942
  animals, 944
Ethmoidal arteries, 515
Ethmoidal veins, 515
Ethmoidectomy, 939
Ethosuximide, 850
Ethylene, 714
Ethyleneimines, 727
Euler formula, 716
Eustachian tube. *See* Auditory tube
Eustachias, Bartholomeus, 211
Evoked response audiometry, 19, 337
Exchange transfusion, 756
Excitation, 735
Excited state, 708
Excretory ducts, 460–61
Exotoxins, 641
Expansion of gases, 117
Expectancy wave, 328
Explantation, 712
Exponential function, 7
Exposure, 711
Expression, 599
Expressivity, 123
External acoustic meatus, 304, 350
  comparative anatomy, 187
  reconstruction, 865
External spiral sulcus, 293, 296, 305
External sulcus capillaries, 852
Extirpation experiments, 179
Extramedullary plasmacytoma, 680
Eye, 424
  lens of, 741
Eye movements, 386–400
  control systems, 383
  non-nystagmic induced, 389
  non-nystagmic spontaneous, 387
  spontaneous, 386

Face and neck operations, 22, 28
Facial muscles, 437
Facial nerve, 217
  course, 218
  epidemiology, 148
  functional tests, 289
  genu, 218
  sensory, 217

Facial nerve (*contd.*)
  canal, 211, 435
  canal, dehiscences in, 218
  dehiscence in, 219
  erosions, of, 233
Facial mask, 436
Facial muscles, 437
Facial neurorraphy, 718
Facial nerve, 429–59
  anatomical anomalies, 436
  arterial supply, 435
  conduction velocity, 438
  decompression, 451
  electrical excitability, 438
  electromyographic activity of, 437
  fibrous sheath of, 434
  functional tests for, 289
  injury effects, 440
  interconnections of, 434
  repair, 455
Facial nerve lesions, topognosis of, 442
Facial nerve nucleus, 437
Facial nerve surgery, 444
Facial nucleus, 217
Facial Palsy
  complicating head injury, 454
  complicating middle ear surgery, 455
  due to intratemporal trauma, 453
  due to intratemporal tumours, 458
  general management of, 443
  incidence and aetiology of, 446
Facial paralysis, 436, 663
  in otitis media, 457
  results of nerve grafting, 457
Facial primordia, 422
Facial prominence, 216
Facial sinus, 216
Facial structures, embryology of, 421–29
Factor analysis, 24
Factor IX, 753
Factorial, 12
Falling ball calibrator, 102
Fallopius, 211
Familial dysautonomia, 476, 480
Far field, 94
Farad, 67
Farmer's lung, 659
Fatality, 136
Fatigue, 349, 716
Favus, 647
Feedback, negative, 78
Felis concolor, 199
Fenestra cochleae, 336
Fenestra ovalis, 211
Fenestra vestibuli, 218, 219, 430
Fenestrae, comparative anatomy, 193
Fenestration operation, 212
Fentanyl, 401
Ferrous sulfate, 751
Fetuses, rabbit, 206
Fibres, 714, 715
Fibrillation potentials, 442
Fibrinogen, 752
Filial generation, 121
Film gamma, 711
Filtered clicks, 307

Fistula sign, 399
Fixation index, 393
Fixation system, 385
Flatworms, 664
Flesh fly, 665
Flexner-Wintersteiner rosettes, 683
Flies, 665
Flow charts, 402
Flow diagram, 37
Flucytosine, 650
Flukes, 664
Fluorouracil, 728
Flying buttresses, 190
Flying helmets, 163
Folded-histogram, 317
Foramen
    cecum, 427
    ovale, 226
    spinosum, 226
    stylomastoideus, 214, 226, 430
Forebrain prominence, 421, 423
Foreseeability, 937
Formaldehyde, 508, 856
Formants, 524, 605, 606
Fossa, piriform, 593
Fossa incudis, 217
Fossula fenestrae vestibuli, 218
Fourier components, 312
Framycetin, 849
Free zone, 710
Frenzel glasses, 386
Frequency, 57, 67, 89, 350
Frequency analyzers, 250
Frequency curve, 11
Frequency difference limens, 346
Frequency discrimination, 346
Frequency distribution, 11
Frequency domain, 314, 319
Frequency polygon, 11
Frequency response curves, 326
Frequency spectra, 99
Frequency spectrum, 94, 250
Frequency transposition, 842
Frequency tuning 315,
Frequentist philosophy, 30
Friedman's rank order test, 19
Frontal prominence, 421
Frozen sections, 667–68, 669
Frusemide. See Furosemide
Function, 6
Fungal infections, 646
Fungi, 645, 659, 698
Fungiform squamous papilloma, 676
Furosemide, 849, 859

Gadus callarius, 200
Gagging reflex, 490
Galactosaemia, 129
Galea, 196
Galen's anastomosis, 895
Gallamine triethiodide, 558
Gallium-67, 708
Galvanic test, 399
Gametes, abnormal, 127
Gamma-rays, 707, 734
Ganglionectomy, 455

Gas absorption, 508
Gas expansion, 117
Gastric muscular loop of Willis, 595
Gastrophilus intestinalis, 665
Gaucher's disease, 689
Gaussian distribution, 11, 13
Geiger-Müller counter, 710
Genetical counselling, 128
Genetics, 119, 121
Genicular ganglion, 218, 430
Geniculate body, single units of, 327
Geniculum, 218
Genome, 625
Genotype, 121, 122
Gentamicin, 367, 704, 849
Geotrichosis, 649
Geotrichum candidum, 649
Germanium, 75
Giant cell tumour, 685
Glioma, 682
Globus hystericus, 596
Glomus jugulare tumours, 233
Glottal area function, 604
Glottal stop, 602
Glottal wave, spectrum of, 605
Glottic fractures, 903
Glottic lesions, resection of, 907
Glottic slit, 533
Glottis, 582
    reconstruction, 910
Glottography, 576
Glucose concentration, 291
Glutamine antagonist, 728
Glycerol, 703
Glycocalyx, 296
Gnathostoma spinigerum, 663
Gnathostomiasis, 663
Goblet cells, 252
Goitre, 124, 147
Goitrogenic effect, 148
Gompertz function, 8, 46
Gompertzian tumour growth, 731
Gongylonema pulchrum, 664
Goodness of fit, 27
Gorilla gorilla, 188
Gossypium, 718
Graft preservation techniques, 875
Grafts, 885
Granular cell tumour, 692
Granulomas, 717
    non-healing, 670
Graph, 10
Gravity, 371
Gravity receptors, 374
Gravity sedimentation, 505
Greater petrosal nerve, 218
Greenbottle fly, see Phaenica sericata
Grid, 73
Griseofulvin, 647, 703
Groen and Hellema test, 357
Grommet see tympanostomy tube.
Ground state, 706
Grouping sera, 753
Guanethidine, 863
Guanyl cyclase, 476
Guarnieri body, 140

Guidelines, 936
Guinea-pig, see Cavia porcellus
Gypsum ceiling tiles, 96

Habenulae perforata, 221
Habituation, 331, 397
Haemagglutination, 629
Haemagglutination-inhibition tests, 633
Haemangioendothelioma, 678
Haemangiomas, 678, 690
Haemangiosarcoma, 678
Haemoglobin, 6, 750
Haemolytic disease of the fetus and the
    newborn, 756
Haemophilia, 123
Haemorrhage, effects of, 750
Haemotympanum, 454
Hair cells, 200, 201, 221, 222, 312, 318,
    366, 368, 374, 376, 851, 859
    inner, 204, 247
    outer, 294, 247
    stimulation, 247
    vestibular, 247, 248
Hair follicles, 740
Half-lives, 707
Hamman's sign, 928
Hanging rootogram, 14
Harmonic disorder, 250
Haploid, 121
Hardness, 715
Harmonic distortion, 813
Hay fever, 659, 722
Head, epidemiology, 147
Healing wounds, tensile strength of, 716
Hearing
    age effect, 795
    conditions for testing, 779
    cross, 790
    damaging effects of noise on, 797–98
    evaluation of hearing in infants and
        and young children, 798
    impairment of, 664, 830
    measurement of, 138, 788
    resonance theory of, 312
    threshold of, 135, 187, 250, 344
Hearing aids, 805–23
    acoustic coupler, 809
    AGC circuits, 815, 819, 826
    amplifiers 817
    binaural, 828
    body baffle effect, 812
    body-worn, 806, 813, 817, 825, 826
    bone-conduction, 809
    children, 843–44
    circuit design, 817
    CROS, 807, 828–29
    design and function of, 844
    developments, 806, 824, 843
    ear mould, 819
    educational, 809, 826
    efficiency of, 826
    electroacoustic characteristics of, 824
    electronic, 806
    environmental factors, 826
    evaluation of, 827, 845
    fitting of, 827, 843, 844

Hearing aids (*contd.*)
 frequency range, 825
 frequency response, 812, 816, 824
 gain, 816
 group, 832
 head-baffle effects, 812
 head worn, 807, 817
 history, 805
 implantable, 820–22
 in-the-ear, 809, 817, 826
 maximum acoustic output, 812, 813
 non-electric, 806
 non-wearable, 826
 output, 816, 825–26
 output limitations, 813
 performance, 816
 performance measurement, 809
 performance specification, 815
 post-aural, 826
 prescribing. *See* Hearing aids, selection of
 rated maximum sound pressure level, 813
 recoding devices, 819
 reverberation, 826–27
 saturation point, 812
 selection of, 824–30, 843, 844
 sensitivity of, 816
 spectacle type, 807, 808
 types, 806, 826
 uniformity of slope, 816
 unilateral hearing loss, 828
 Y-lead system, 813, 828
 see also Electroacoustic rehabilitation equipment
Hearing conservation, 151
Hearing disorders, 788
 X-linked, 125
Hearing impairment
 conductive component in, 287
 epidemiology, 140
 in child, 613
Hearing level, 20
Hearing loss, 123, 335
 and language disorder, 612
 assessment of, 796
 conductive, 141, 304, 791, 797
 congenital, 141, 756
 degree of, 817, 827–28
 nerve fibre, 797
 noise-induced, 167, 797–98
 non-organic, 288, 338, 339, 797
 occupational, 151, 797–98
 persistent, 152
 profound, 819
 sensorineural, 141, 287, 290, 302, 797
 strepomycin-induced, 342
 sudden, 142
 temporary, 152
Hearing mechanism, reconstruction, 865
Hearing protection, 158
 effects on communication, 167
 programme, 168
 provided in practice, 165

Hearing protectors, 159
 attenuation characteristics, 163
 cost, 166
 methods for the evaluation of, 164
 percentage of time worn, 165
 performance limitations and requirements, 162
 practical problems, 166
 special types of, 161
Hearing sensitivity of the very young, 288
Hearing tests, 788, 789
 conditions for, 800–4
 electrophysiological, 804
 free field, children, 800, 803
 objective, 804
Heat, 111–19
Heat transfer, 115
Heath's operation, 212
Helmholtz resonators, 545
Helper viruses, 626
Hemilaryngectomy, 907, 908
Hennebert's sign, 400
Henry, 67
Hensen's stripe, 205
Herpes simplex, 637
Herpes zoster, 637
Herpes zoster oticus, 452–53
Hertz, 67
Heterochromia, 124
Heterogeusia, 478
Heterograft. *See* Xenograft
Heteromyidae, 25
Heteroscedastic populations, 13
Heterozygotes, 129
Hexadecimal system, 1
Hexadimethrine bromide, 849, 855
Hiatus for the greater petrosal nerve, 218
Hiatus semilunaris, 514
High frequency losses, 316
High palate, 125
High-pass filter, 70
Hippocrates, 211
Hipposideros caffer, 197, 198, 199
Histamine, 5
Histidine, 480
Histiocytic lymphoma, 658, 671, 672, 673
Histiocytosis 'X', 927
Histocompatibility testing, 899
Histograms, 11, 13
Histopathology, 667–700
 larynx, 689–92
 ototoxicity, 851
 paranasal sinuses, 669
 techniques in, 667
 tonsils, 687–89
Histoplasma capsulatum, 651, 927
Histoplasmosis, 651, 927
HL-A *see* human leucocyte antigen system, 8
Hoarseness, 582–84
Hodgkin's disease, 648, 650, 688
 epidemiology, 147
Homeostasis
 endolymphatic, 294, 296, 299
 saccular, 300

Homer Wright rosettes, 683
Homograft. *See* Allograft
Homoscedastic populations, 13
Hooke's Law, 715
Horner's syndrome, 521
Horseradish peroxidase, 296, 301
House's bar, 217, 234
Human eye tracking system, 385
Human leucocyte antigen system, 713
Human rights, 942, 950
Huntington's chorea, 401
Hyaline mass, comparative anatomy, 197
Hyaluronic acid, 519
Hydrocephalus, 229
Hydrocortisone, 521, 713
Hydrocyanic acid, 207, 508
Hydroxycarbamide, 729
Hyoid arch, 425
Hyoid bone, 531, 565
Hyperactive children, 341
Hyperimmune animal sera, 636
Hyperkeratosis, 693
Hypernasality, 492
Hypertension, 135
Hypertrophic rhinitis, 520
Hyperventilation, 393
Hypobranchial eminence, 529, 531
Hypogeusia, 478, 480
Hypoglossolaryngeal reflex system, 556
Hyponasality, 492
Hypophysis, 425
Hyposmia, 480
Hypotensive procedures, 750
Hypothermic procedures, 750
Hypoxic cells, 738, 745
 chemical radiosensitizers of, 748

Iceterus gravis neonatorum
Idiopathic multiple haeomorrhagic sarcoma, 147
Idiopathic polychondritis, 927
Idoxuridine, 637
IgA, 643, 752
IgD, 644
IgE, 644, 752
IgG, 643, 899
IgM, 644
Illinois Test of Psycholinguistic Abilities, 614, 617
Imipramine, 863
Immunity, 642
Immunization, 644
 allotypic, 750
Immunobiology, 712
Immunoglobulins, 510, 636, 643, 752, 899, *also see* IgA, IgD, IgE, IgG and IgM
Immunosuppressant drugs, 713
Impaction of dust particles, 505
Impedance, 61, 64, 100
 input, 79
Impedance bridge, 281
Impedance matching, 237
Implantation. *See* Surgical implants

Impulse sounds, 46
Inborn error of metabolism, 129
Incidence, 135
Incudo-mallear disclocations, 233
Incudo-mallear joint, slippage in, 243
Incus
    allografts, 870, 871
    posterior ligament of, 217
    short process, 218
    transplant, 872
Indicant, 9
Indirect antiglobulin test, 760
Inductance, 59, 61, 67
Inductors, 61
Industrial dusts, 507
Inertia, 87
Inertial deposition, 505
Inertial reactance, 281
Infantile hemiplegia, 353
Infection with viruses, 628
Infectious mononucleosis, 133
Inferior colliculi, 322, 323
Influenza, 637
Influenza vaccine, 636
Inheritance, 121
    quantitative, 126
    recessive, 122
Innervation ratios, 264
Input, push-pull, 79
Input impedance, 79
Insects, 665
Insertion loss, 99
Instruments, 719
Insular-temporal region, bilateral lesions
    of, 327
Insulators, 53
Intelligence quotient (IQ), 355, 618
Intensity coding, 318
Intensity difference, 351
Intensity difference limen, 345
    tests, 354
Intensity functions, non-monotonic,
    320
Interarytenoid notch, 532
Interaural intensity differences, 322, 323
Interaural time differences, 323
Interdental cells of spiral limbus, 205
Interference, 91
Interference otoscope, 282
Interferon, 635
Integers, 3
Integrated circuits, 85
Integrator, 72
Intermaxillary segment, 425
Internal acoustic meatus, 228, 307,
    429
Inter-observer variation, 135
Interpreters, 36
Interquartile distance, 13
Interspike-interval histogram, 318, 323
Interstitial nuclei (of Cajal), 384
Interval-histogram, 317
Intonation indicator, 837
Intonation pattern, 601
Intonations, 599
Intra-observer variation, 135

Intratympanic muscles
    comparative anatomy, 194
    function, 275
Intubation granuloma, 690
Intubation tubes, 903
Inverse square law, 734
Inverted papilloma, 676
Iodine-131, 709
Iodine-132, 709
Ion, 53
Ion transporting enzymes, 292
Ionization, 735
Ionizing radiation, 733
    diagnostic, 706
    effect on cells, 735
    see also Radiation
Iridium-40, 739
Iron albuminate, 298
Iron dextran, 205
Irradiation in high pressure oxygen, 739
Islandotoxin, 659
Iso-intensity curves, 315, 326
Isoprene, 714
Iso-rate contours, 320
Iso-rate curves, 315, 321
Isotopes, 706
Isthmus, 252

Jaw
    malignancies, 133, 147
    upper, 425
Jenkins, 212
Jervell and Lange-Nielsen, 124
Joule-Thompson effect, 721
Joule, 114
J-receptor. See Juxtacapillary receptor
Jugular foramen, 233
Just noticeable difference, 345
Juxta-capillary receptors, 555

Kanamycin, 208, 290, 366, 849, 851, 852,
    856, 857, 860, 861
Kaposi's tumour see idiopathic multiple
    haemorrhagic sarcoma
Karyotype, 127
K-complex, 337
Keloidal blastomycosis, 651
Kelvin, 5
Keratoma see Cholesteatoma
Kernicterus, 124, 756
Kinocilia, polarization, 207
Kinocilium 248, 374
Kirchhoff's Laws, 55
Klebsiella rhinoscleromatis, 926
Koch's postulates, 638
Koerner's septum, 216
Kopfschüttelnystagmus, 390
Kurtosis, 14
Kveim test, 673

Labyrinth, 211, 221, 234, 371
Labyrinthine destruction, 364
Labyrinthine fluids,
    ototoxic antibiotic concentrations, 856
    physiology, 290

Labyrinthine surgery, 234
Lacrimal sac, 436
Lacrimation, 439, 440, 450
Lamina cribrosa, 515
Laminar flow, 770
Langenbeck's noise sudiometry, 348
Langhan's giant cells, 926
Language, 536, 609, 796
    acquisition of, 616, 840
    and behaviour, 616
    and memory, 615
    and personality and cortical arousal,
        619
    development of, 611, 845
Language disorder
    and environment, 617
    and hearing loss, 612
    and primary emotional disturbance,
        614
    definition of, 610
    in children, 609, 613
    motivational disturbance in, 613
    primary problem of, 615
    specific, classification of, 610
Language Modalities Test of Aphasia,
    617
Language performance, evaluating, 617
Language theory, 609
Laryngeal aditus, 530
Laryngeal afferent systems, 550
Laryngeal and tracheal stenosis, chronic
    combined, 904
Laryngeal arthrokinetic reflexogenic
    systems, 558
Laryngeal articular afferent systems,
    552
Laryngeal carcinoma, 145
Laryngeal chemoreceptor afferent
    systems, 554
Laryngeal cyst, 690
Laryngeal dilatation, 903
Laryngeal diphtheria, 926
Laryngeal function, tomographic studies
    of, 587
Laryngeal hyperkeratosis, 649
Laryngeal motoneurones, suprabulbar
    influences on, 549
Laryngeal notoneurone pools, 548
Laryngeal motor nerves, 547–49
Laryngeal motor systems, 546
Laryngeal motor units, 546
Laryngeal mucosal afferent systems, 550
Laryngeal mucosal reflexogenic in-
    fluences, 558
Laryngeal muscle activity
    lingual afferent systems influencing,
        556
    pulmonary afferent systems influenc-
        ing, 555
Laryngeal muscles
    disturbances of, 576
    electromyography of, 588
    extrinsic, 533, 541, 547, 548, 559, 560,
        565, 588
        myotatic reflexes in, 544
    intrinsic, 533, 546, 556, 560, 562

Laryngeal muscles (*contd.*)
  afferent discharges from myotatic mechanoreceptors in, 553
  myotatic mechanoreceptor systems, 552
  myotatic reflexes in, 553
Laryngeal myotatic afferent systems, 552
Laryngeal myotatic reflexogenic systems, 559
Laryngeal neoplasms, 584
Laryngeal nerves, 530
  extralaryngeal afferents in, 554
  neurorrhaphy of, 895
  recurrent, 550, 554, 912
  superior, 550, 551
  recurrent paralysis, 914
Laryngeal neurological systems, behavioural aspects of, 556
Laryngeal nodule, 689
Laryngeal stenosis
  and tracheal stenosis combined, 904
  chronic, 903
Laryngeal trauma, reconstructive aspects of, 903
Laryngeal tuberculosis, 651
Laryngeal vibrator, 721
Laryngectomy, 510
  intraperichondrial subhyoid, 900
  specimen, 668
Laryngofissure, 903, 906
Laryngograph, 602
Laryngopharyngectomy, partial, 907, 911
Laryngopulmonary mechanics, 896
Laryngostroboscopy, 575, 720
Laryngotracheal groove, 529, 530
Laryngotracheobronchial tree, 766
Laryngotracheo-oesophageal cleft, 532
Larynx, 593, 600, 653
  aerodynamic investigations, 577, 580
  allotransplanted, 899
  artificial. *See* Laryngeal vibrator
  carcinoma of, 668, 746
  Chiroptera, 537–45
  clinical advances in reconstructive surgery, 900
  comparative morphology, 536–45
  conservation surgery, 906
  developmental anatomy, 529–35
  electromyography of, 895
  embryology of, 530
  epithelium of, 532
  experimental aspects of reconstruction, 894
  functions in speech, 602
  histopathology, 689–92
  laboratory processing of specimen of, 668
  measurement of function, 574–91
  neurology, 546–74
  paralyzed, 894
  pathological conditions, 690
  primary aspergillosis of, 657
  reconstructive surgery, 894–919
  reinnervation of, 899
  replanted, 898
  squamous carcinoma of, 695

Larynx (*contd.*)
  transplantation, 897–900
  ultra-high speed cinematography, 577
  vibratory measurements on, 574
Lasers, 245, 364, 720
L-asparaginase, 730
Lassa fever, 142
Late vertex potentials, 342
Lateral nasal elevations, 421
Lateral semicircular canal, 217, 218
Lateral tympanic sinus, 216
Lateralization, 350 359
Latin Square design, 26
Law in respect of animals, 942
Law of auditory analysis, 312
Law of torts, 936
Law relating to transplants, 941
Laws, 935
Law's lateral oblique view, 223
Lead zirconate titanate, 105
Leakage current, 76
Legal aspects, 935
Legislation, public health, 134
Leishmania donovani, 651
Leishmaniasis, 661, 662
Lentiform process, 212
Lenz's law, 61
Leptokurtic, 14
Leuconostoc mesenteroides, 753
Leukaemia, 147
Leukapheresis, 753
Lidocaine, 307
Lidocaine, 363, 720
Linamarin, 142
Linear attenuation coefficient, 710
Linear dynamic compression, 815
Linear function, 6
Linguatula rhinaria, 666
Liomy pictus, 190
Lipidoses, 688
Litre, 5
Localization, 350, 359
Locus, 122
Logarithms, 6
Logistic function, 7
Longitudinal flow theory, 297
Lorentz equation, 54
Loudness, 347
  growth of, 347
  integration of, 348
  recruitment, 792–95
    objective test of, 287
Loudness Discomfort Level (LDL), 795
Loudness level, most comfortable, 349
Loudness reversal phenomenon, 354
Loudspeaker, 89
  electrostatic, 102
Low-pass filter, 70
Lung, carcinoma of, 25, 126, 137
Lung fluke, *see Paragonimus westermani*
Lung irritant receptors, 555
Lycopodium, 717
Lymph nodes
  cervical, block dissection, 668
  dissection of the cervical, 750
Lymphadenoma, epidemiology, 147

Lymphadenopathy, 147, 658
Lymphocytic lymphosarcoma, 671
Lympho-epitheliomas, 697
  Regaud type, 697
  Schminke type, 697
Lysosomal enzymes, 208

M. constrictor pharyngis superior, 484
M. levator veli palatini, 484
M. palatoglossus, 484
M. palatopharyngeus, 484
M. tensor veli palatini, 484
Macaca irus, 188
McNaught keel, 903
Macrophages, 300
Macrostomia, 125
Macula, 373
Macula sacculi, 375
Macula utriculi, 375
Macular epithelium, 178
Magendie-Hertwig phenomenon, 385
Magnetic field, 54, 834
Magnetic flux, 54, 67
Magnetic tape, digital, 34
Malacoplakia, 692
Malformation, Klippel-Feil, 128
Malignancy grading, 4
Malignant melanoma, 677, 678
Malignant neoplasm, 672
Malingering, 339, 797
  detecting, 335
Malleus, 211, 215, 316
Mandibular arch, 425
Mandibular fossa, 214
Mandibular joint, 214
Mandibular processes, 421, 425
Manioc utilissima, 208
Manslaughter, 941
Manubrium mallei, 238
Manubrium sterni, 585
Marikina geoffroyi, 197–98
Masking, 348
Masking level difference, 351, 359
Mass, 5
Mass law, 95
Mass number, 706
Mastication, 592
Mastoid, 211
Mastoid antrum, 217, 228, 233
Mastoid bowl, 866
Mastoid cavities, 456, 866
Mastoid emmisary vein, 214
Mastoid foramen, 214
Mastoid process, 188, 214, 216
Mastoidectomy, 211, 212, 850
  cortical (simple), 233
  modified radical, 233
  radical, 234
Mastoiditis, 231
  acute, 211
Materia otolaryngologica, general aspects, 703–25
Mathematical theory of communication, 609
Matzker test, 357
Maxillary bone, myxoma of, 681

Maxillary cysts, 427
Maxillary processes, 421, 423, 425, 513
Maximum likelihood solution, 24
Mean deviation, 13
Means, comparison of, 28
Measurement, 1–9
Meatal wall, 214
Mechanical force, 5
Mechanical impedance, 281
Mecrilate, 765
Medial geniculate body, 322, 324
Medial geniculate nucleus, 324
Medial nasal elevations, 421
Medial sac, 215
Medial saccule, 215
Median fronto-nasal process, 513
Mediastinal masses, 928
Medicines Act 1968, 935
Meiosis, 121
Mel scale, 348, 350
Membraneous labyrinth, 373
Memory, 615
Menadiol sodium phosphate, 756
Mendelian inheritance, 121
Ménière's disease, 25, 127, 143, 205, 208, 209, 223, 234, 290, 296, 297, 300, 301, 310, 363, 364, 365
    ultrasonic treatment of, 456
Meningiomas, 230
Meningitis, 124, 128
Mentoplasty, 886
Mercaptopurine, 713
Meriones crassus, 190
Merulius lacrymans, 659
Mesenchyme, 422
Mesons, 747
Mesotympanum, 286
Messenger RNA, cancer-specific, 732
Metabolic studies in ototoxicity, 858
Metals, 714
Metameter, 11
Metastable states, 706
Metastases, 708, 712
Methacholine, 480
Methacholine chloride, 463, 464
Methane sulphonates, 727
Methionine, 480
Method of least squares, 22
Methotrexate, 728, 748
Methyldopa, 863
Meticillin, 703
Metisazone, 636
Metronidazole, 748
Metropolitan Ear Institution, 211
Mexican free-tailed bat, *see Tadarida brasiliensis*
Mice, mutant strain, 178
Michaelis-Guttmann bodies, 692
Microdipodops pallidus, 190, 197–98
Microelectrics, 85
Microelectronics, 69–87
Microlaryngoscopy, 764
Microphones, 101
    calibration, 102
    directional, 108, 812
    electret, 812

Microphones (*contd.*)
    electrostatic capacitor, 102
    moving coil, 106
    piezo-electric, 105
    piezo-junction, 108
    probe-tube, 110
    sensitivity, 101
Micropolyspora faeni, 659
Microsaccades, 385
Microscopes, 719
Microvilli, 205, 206
Middle ear. *See* Ear, middle
Middle fossa dura, 214
Mid-line granuloma, *see* histiocytic lymphoma
Mikulicz cells, 926
Mistakes, 938
Misuse of Drugs Act 1971, 935
Mites, 665
Mitochondria, 295
Mitosis, 731, 740
Mixed tumours, 675
Modelling, 45
Modified Pearson coefficient, 15
Modified rhyme test (MRT), 797
Modiolus, 221
Mole, 5
Molluscous tumour, 211
Molossus ater, 191
Mongolism, 127
Mongoloid palpebral fissures, 125
Monosomy, 127
Mortality, 136
Mössbauer effect, 199, 245, 312, 316
Most comfortable loudness level (MCL), 794
Motion sickness experiments, 369
Moulds, 646
Mouth, 425, 591
    epidemiology, 144–45
    verrucous squamous carcinoma, 696
Moving coil meter, 66
Mucociliary system, 256
Mucoepidermoid tumour, 675
Mucor, 652
Mucormycoses, 652
Mucosa, 740
Mucosal folds, 217
Mucous blanket, 504, 509
Mufflers, 158
Multilingual dictionary, 951–54
Multiple sclerosis, 353, 354
Multi-terminally innervated fibres, 261
Muramidase, 510
Mus musculus, 196, 200
Muscle fibres
    focally innervated, 261
    histochemical classification of, 261
    intratympanic, 260
Muscle transplantation or replantation, 896
    facial, 437
    intratympanic, 194, 257–80
        function, 275
    salpingopharyngeus, 253
    stapedius, 218, 257, 272, 276–79

Mustela nivalis, 190, 193, 194
Mustine. *See* Chlormethine
Mutual conductance, 73
Myasthenia gravis, 596
Mycetismus, 646, 658
Mycogenous neoplasias, 646
Mycology, 645–61
Mycoses, 646
    classification of, 647
    superficial, 647
Mycosis fungoides, 658, 669
Mycotic disorders, 646
Mycotoxicoses, 646, 658
Mycotoxins, 658
Myiasis, 665
Myoblastoma, 692
Myogenic response, 42
Myotatic mechanoreceptor reflex system, 564
Myringoplasty, 866, 867
Myringotomy, 12
Myxine, 199
Myxoma, 681
Myxomatosis, 635
Myxoviruses, 626

NACE (Necrosis with Atypical Cellular Exudate), 671
Naegleria fowleri, 662
Naphazoline, 862
Nasal actinomycosis, 658
Nasal air flow, 503
Nasal bones, 514, 884
Nasal cancer, 143, 507
Nasal cartilages, 503, 514, 886
Nasal cavity, 502
    angiosarcoma of, 678
    effect of changes, 526
    embryonic rhabdomyosarcoma of, 680
    function of, 517
    haemangiopericytoma of, 679
    organizing haematoma of, 678
    plasmacytoma of, 681
Nasal concha, inferior, glioma of, 682
Nasal congestion, 862
Nasal consonants, acoustic structure of, 523
Nasal cryptococcosis, 650
Nasal cycle, 519
Nasal deformity, 891
Nasal deposition
    particulate matter, 503
    physics of, 504
Nasal filtration, 502–12
    experiments, 507
    in miners, 507
Nasal function, acoustic aspects of, 523–27
Nasal glands, 516
    neoplasms of salivary structure, 675
Nasal graft, 885
Nasal implants, 885
Nasal indicator, 837
Nasal irritants, 504

Nasal mucosa, 516
Nasal mucosal stimulation, 897
Nasal obstruction, 504, 674
Nasal papilloma, 653
Nasal placode. *See* Olfactory placode
Nasal polyposis, 669
Nasal polyps, 652
Nasal resonance, 523, 525
Nasal septum, 423, 424, 882
   neurofibroma of, 682
Nasal sinuses, ulcerating lesion, 672
Nasal stenosis, 522
Nasal stuffiness, 522, 863
Nasal tip, 886
   bifid, 890
   drooping, 890
   rhinoplasty, 884
   square, 890
Nasal turbinate. *See* Nasal concha
Nasality, 525
Nasalization of vowels, 524
Nasobronchial reflexes 504
Nasolacrimal duct, 514
Nasolacrimal reflex, 440
Nasolacrimal sulcus, 513
Nasopharyngeal angiofibroma, 687
Nasopharynoscopes, 719
Nasopharynx. *See* Pharynx, nasal part of
Nasopulmonary reflexes, 504
Natalus tumidirostris, 196
National Health Service, 942
National Insurance (Industrial Injuries) Act, 1946, 134
Near-field, 94
Neck, 425
   epidemiology, 147
   swelling in, 147
Neck lesions, experimental, 362
Neck operations, 22, 28
Negligence, 937
Negri bodies, 634
Nematodes, 662
Neomycin, 207, 366, 849, 850, 851
Neoplasias, mycogenous, 646
Neoplasms, 3
   head and neck region, 708
   morphology of, 4
   vocal folds, 586
Neoplastic reactions, 717
Neotoma, 188
Nephritis, 125
Nernst equation, 6, 291
Nerve excitability, 441
   thresholds, 449
Nerve fibres, regeneration of, 899
Nerve growth factor, 714
Nervus intermedius, 430
Nerve regeneration, recurrent, 895
Nervous system
   auditory, 312–34
   autonomic, 515
Network analysis, 237
Networks, 69
Neurapraxia, 440, 457
Neurocysticercosis, 664

Neuroepithelium of vestibular apparatus, 206
Neurofibromas, 682, 691
Neurofibromatosis, 341
Neurogenic tumour, 681
Neuroleptanaesthesia, 19
Neuromasts, 371
Neuron, 741
   single, temporal patterns of, 320
Neuronal information processing, 316
Neuronal periodicities, 321
Neuro-otology, 383, 419
   clinical practice of, 402
Neurorrhaphy, 894, 912
Neuroticism, 135
Neutrons, 52, 706
Newton's law of motion, 94
Nigerian Ataxic Neuropathy, 208
Nissl substance, 206
Nitrogen dioxide, 508, 509
Nitrogen mustard, 368, 726, 849–50, 856
Noise, 151, 208
   dosemeter, 154
   environmental factors, 142
   hazard assessment, 152
   impulse, 151, 155
   industrial, 151
   nuisance, 937
   steady-state, 151
   transient, 152
Noise communication, effects of, 167
Noise components in speech, 607
Noise control, 155
   and building design, 157
   by absorption, 157
   by barriers, 157
   by enclosure, 157
   summary, 158
Noise criterion curves, 100
Noise effect on communication, 167
Noise emission level, 4, 142
Noise exposure, 347
Noise level, measurement of equivalent continuous, 153
Noise pollution level, 4
Noise rating, 100
Noise reduction, 151
Noise transmission, 154
Non-acoustic stapedius response, 287
Non-healing granuloma, 670
Norm, measurement of, 134
Normal distribution, 13
North American blastomycosis, 650
Nose, 423, 494
   anatomy, 514
   baffles, 517
   congenital anomalies, 143
   embryology, 513
   epidemiology, 143–44
   heat and moisture exchanges, 518
   histopathology, 669
   innervation, 515
   saddle deformity of, 885
   specific infections, 143
   ulcerating lesion, 672

Nose (*contd.*)
   valves, 517
   vascularization, 515
Nose drops, rebound effect of, 522
Nose sound, 523
Nostrils, 513
Notch of Rivinus, 215
Notifiable diseases, 134
n-type material, 54
Nuclear isomers, 706
Nuclear otolaryngology, 706
Nuclear stability, odd-even rule of, 707
Nucleic acid, 625, 629
Nucleus, 706
Nucleus ambiguus, 548
Nuclides, 706
Nuisance, 937
Null hypothesis, 26
Number, 1, 3
Number systems, 947
Numerical taxonomy, 9, 25
Nystagmus, 361, 381, 383, 454
   investigation of, 400–2
   secondary phase of, 362
Nystagmusbereitschaft, 391
Nystatin, 648, 649, 703

Observer error, 135
Observer variation, 135
Occupational disorders, 136
Octal system, 3
Octodon, 190
Octodon degus, 193
Ocular kinetics, 383
Oculomotor decussation, 384
Oculomotor system, 361, 383
Odd-even rule of nuclear stability, 707
Odours, nuisance, 937
Oesophageal tracheal compression, 925
Oesophageal Voice, 902
Oesophagus, 594, 658
   carcinoma of, 145
   epidemiology, 145
   reconstruction, 902, 903
Oesophago-gastric junction, achalasia of, 597
Oesophagoscope, 720
Oesophago-tracheal fistula, 145
Oestrus ovis, 665
Ogive, 11
Ohm, 67
Ohm's Law, 54
Oil of Origanum, 219
Olfaction, 495–501, 537
Olfactory alloaesthesia, 499
Olfactory bulb, 497
Olfactory esthesioneuroblastoma, 682
Olfactory esthesioneurocytoma, 683
Olfactory neuroblastoma, 682
Olfactory organ, 495
Olfactory pigment, 496
Olfactory pits, 421, 423
Olfactory placodes, 421, 423
Olfactory spectrogram, 498
Onchocerciasis, 664
Open-loop gain, 80

Operator, 65
Optical density, 711
Optical instruments, 719
Optokinetic nystagmus, 383, 400
Optomotor nystogmus *see* Optokinetic nystagmus
Oral cancer, 145, 650
Oral candidiasis, 648
Oral cavity, 421
  anti-resonance produced by, 524
Oral manometer, 491
Orbicularis oculi, lacrimal part of the, 436
Orbital valency, 53
Order sequence effects, 26
Organizing haematoma, 678
Ornithorhynchus, 193
Orofacial structures, 420
Oronasal membrane, 423
Oropharyngeal membrane, 421
Oscillators, 79, 82
Oscilloscope, 155
Osmic acid, 222
Osmolality, 5
Osseous spiral lamina, 308
  canaliculi of, 221
Ossicles, 233, 286
  blood supply of, 217
  comparative anatomy, 192
Ossicular adhesives, 875
Ossicular chain, 266
Ossicular chain allograft, 871
Ossicular chain reconstruction, 869
Ossicular discontinuity, 242, 286
Ossicular lever, 239
Ossicular prostheses, 870
Ossifying fibroma, 684
Osteogenesis imperfecta, 126
Osteosarcoma, 684
Otic placode, 180
Otic vesicles, 177, 180
Otitis, 211, 635
Otitis externa, 647, 658
  epidemiology, 137
Otitis media, 127, 212, 457
  acute, 138
  epidemiology, 137
  secretory (seromucinous), 138
  suppurative, 231
Otoconia, 207, 373
Otocysts, 181, 183
Otogenic facial palsy, 457
Otolith organs, 373, 374
Otolithic end organs, 362
Otolithic membrane, 369, 373–74
Otomops martiensseni, 195
Otomycosis, 647
Oto-neuro-opthalmological syndrome, 133, 142
Otosclerosis, 126, 204, 211, 212, 233, 242 285, 304
  epidemiology, 140
Otoscopic examination, 281
Ototoxic drugs, 207, 849–62
Ototoxicity
  and renal status, 859
  electrical potential changes in, 858

Ototoxicity (*contd.*)
  histopathology of, 851
  mechanisms of, 859
  metabolic studies in, 858
  prevention of, 859
Ototoxic synergism, 850
Otus assio, 190
Ouabain, 293, 300
Overall SPL, 100
Overload phenomenon, 348
Oxacillin, 703
Oxidative metabolism, 293
  inhibitors of, 294
Oxygen, high pressure, 745
Oxygen effect, 738, 743
Oxyphenonium, 863
Ozaena, 521, 527

Packed cell volume, 750
Paget's disease, 230, 684, 685
Palatal dysfunction, 491
Palatal function, 484–93
  during food intake and swallowing, 485
  during respiration, 485
  during speech, 487, 490
Palatal papillae, 469
Palate, 426, 484
  topographic changes during growth, 484
Palatine processes, 426, 513
Palatoglossus muscles, 490
Palatopharyngeal partition, 485
Palatopharyngeus, 565
Palatopharyngeus muscles, 489
Panthera pardus, 199
Pan troglodytes, 188
Paper tape, 32
Papillae, 469
Papillary adenocarcinoma, 674
Papillary adenoma, 674
Papilloma
  fungiform squamous, 676
  inverted, 676
  transitional cell, 676
Papillomata, 906
Papillomatosis, 691
Paracoccidioides loboi, 651
Paracusis, 211
Paraformaldehyde, 659
Paragangliomas, 209, 692
Paragonimus westermani, 664
Parameters, 11
Parameters of central tendency, 13
Paramyxoviruses, 622, 626
Paranasal sinuses, 514, 652
  histopathology, 669
Paranystagmus, 387
Parasites associated with otolaryngological disorders, 661
Parasitology, 661–66
Parental generation, 121
Parkinson's disease, 550
Parotid gland, 460
Paroxysmal vertigo, 235
Pars magnocellularis, 324
Pars principalis, 324

Pascal, 155
Pascal's Triangle, 11
Passavant's ridge, 487
Passive resistance, 644
Patau's syndrome, 192
Patent law, 941
Pautrier's abscesses, 658
Pavlovian conditioning, 335
Pea, 121
Peak clipping, 813, 826
Peak-limiter, 73
Pearson's product-moment correlation coefficient, 19
Pearson's coefficient of skewness, 15
Pedestal experiments, 346
Pendred's syndrome, 124, 129, 709
Pendular chair, 394
Pendular eye tracking test, 389
Penetrance, 123
Penicillamine, 480
Penicillin, 658, 659, 703
Penicillin G, 703
Penicillinase, 640
Penicillium frequentans, 659
Penicillium glaucum, 659
Penicillium islandicum, 658
Pentastomids, 666
Pentobarbital, 342, 385
Perception, 344
Perilymph, 301, 365, 366
Perilymphatic perfusion, 296
Perilymphatic tracer material, 298
Period, 57
Period-histogram, 317, 319
Period phase locking, 322
Peri-saccular fibrosis, 301
Peristaltic wave, 592, 594, 595
Permanent threshold shift, 277, 795
Permeability, 54
Permeatal operation, 212
Permittivity, 60
Perognathus, 652
Perry-Robertson formula, 716
Persistent viruses, 634
Petromyzon, 199
Petrosquamosal lamina, 216
pH, 6
Phaenica sericata, 665
Phagocytosis of colloidal silver, 301
Phalangeal end plates, 248
Phantogeusia, 478
Pharyngeal recess, 502
Pharmacokinetics, 704
Pharyngeal dysphagia, 596
Pharyngeal fistula, repair, 901
Pharyngeal palsy, 593
Pharyngeal plexus, 548
Pharyngeal pouches, 425, 529
Pharyngotomy
  lateral, 907
  transhyoid, 903
Pharynx, 592
  cancer of nasal part of, 144, 658, 659
  cancer of oral part of, 746
  congenitally large, 492

Pharynx (contd.)
   epithelium of nasal part of, 697
   pathological processes, 687
   reconstructive surgery of laryngeal
      part of, 894–919
   rhabdomyosarcoma of nasal part of,
      680
   squamous carcinoma, 696
Phase difference, 57, 351
Phase-transfer function, 271
Phasors, 64
Phenobarbital, 850
Phenylalanine, 129
Phenylketonuria, 129
Phenylthiourea, 480
Phenytoin, 389, 850, 863
Pheromones, 499
Philtrum, 425
Phocaena phocaena, 200
Phon scale, 347
Phonation, 550, 554, 558, 561, 565, 574,
      580, 600, 602, 900, 912
   digital simulation, 589
Phonation quotient, 581
Phonatory disorders, 564
Phonatory reflex modulation, 563
Phonemes, 562, 603
Phonetically balanced word lists, 353
Phosphorous-32, 709
Phosphors, 710
Phosphorylate glucose, capacity to, 293
Photocathode, 710
Photoelasticity, 717
Photomultiplier tube, 710
Photons, 707
Phrenic nerve, 896
Physical half-life, 707
Physiotherapy, 443
Picornavirus, 626
Pictogram, 10
Pie chart, 10
Piezo-electricity, 105
Pigmentary anomalies, 125
Pinealoma, 354
Pinna. See Auricle
Pinocytosis, 298
Pions, 747
Piriform fossa, 907
   carcinoma, 911
Pistonphone, 102
Pitch, 90, 348, 350
Pitch discriminability, 312
Pituitary snuff, 863
Place Principle, 250
Placebo, 26
Plane waves, 93
Plasma, 756
   freeze-dried, 752
   platelet rich, 752
   protein fractions, 757
   substitutes, 753
Plasmacytoma, 671
Plasmapheresis, 751
Plasmids, 641
Plasmodium berghei, 147
Plastic sheeting, 876

Plastic surgery, 444
Plastics, 714, 815
   degradation of, 762
Platelet rich plasma, 752
Platelets, 752
Platyhelminthes, 664
Platykurtic, 14
Plecotus, 187
Pleomorphic adenoma, 675
Plethysmography, 721
pn junction, 74
Pneumatic test, 399
Pneumatization, 188
Pneumotachography, 578
Poikilorchis congolensis, 664
Points of inflection, 23
Poiseuille's equation, 770
Poisson distribution, 12
Poisson's ratio, 716
Polarization of sensory cells, 375
Poliomyelitis vaccine, 636
Poliovirus, 630
Politef, 764, 877, 878, 914, 922
Politef piston, 880
Pollutants, 502
Polly-beak deformity, 886
Polychondritis, 927
Polyethylene, 714, 877, 922
Polyethylene terephthalate, 715, 922
Polyethylene tubing, 212
Polyglycolic acid, 717
Polyhydroxylethylmethacrylate, 764
Polyisoprene, 714
Polymers, 714, 764
Polymyxins, 857, 858
Polynomial equation, 23
Polyphasic action potentials, 442
Polytomography, 227, 454, 710
Polyurethane, 922
Population, 13, 14
Porous layers, 96
Porus acousticus, 429
Positive secretion potential, 294
Positrons, 707
Post-auricular incision, 214
Post-auricular response, 336, 343
Post-endotracheal intubation stenosis,
      929
Posterior pharyngeal diverticulum, 597
Posterior sac, 216
Posterior tympanic sinus, 216
Post-herpetic neuralgia, 453
Postlaryngectomy, 900
   rehabilitation, 900
Post-stimulus time histograms, 315, 317
Post-strial capillaries, 852
Post-traumatic tracheal stenosis, clinical
   evaluation of, 930
Potential, 52
Potential difference, 52, 67
Povidone, 753
Powdered tantalum, 930
Power function, 8, 328
Power transfer function, 242
Predictability potential, 328
Prednisolone, 451, 900

Prednisone, 713
Premaxilla, 427
Premaxillary process, 513
Prephonatory tuning, 562
Presbyacusis, 167, 795
Prescribed diseases, 134
Pressure, 87
Pretectal nuclei, 384
Prevalence, 135
Primary medial palatal triangle, 425
Primates, 369
Primitive pharynx, 421
Principle of correspondence, 1
Principle of position, 1
Privacy, 942
Probability, 9, 28
Procaine, 294
Procarbazine, 900
Processus trochleariformis, 430
Product-moment correlation coefficient,
      17
Proechimys, 190
Profound childhood deafness, 124
Prolabium, 425
Promethazine, 342
Prominence of the lateral semicircular
   canal, 218
Promontory, 303
Promontory versus external ear elec-
   trode, 305
Proof stress, 716
Proportional morbidity, 136
Proportional mortality, 137
Prostheses, 719
   auditory, 763
      see also Hearing Aids
   aural, 805
Protection of Human Rights, 942
Protein fraction, 752
Protons, 52, 706
Protozoa, 661
Protympanum, 252
Provocation nystagmus, 390
Provokationsnystagmus, 390
Prussak's space, 216
Pseudodysautonomia, 480
Pseudohypoparathyroidism, 480
Pseudomycoses, 646, 658
Pseudonystagmus, 387
Pseudostratified ciliated epithelium, 517
Psittacosis-lymphogranuloma venereum
   group of organisms, 625
PST histograms, see Post-stimulus time
   histograms
Psychoacoustics, 344–52
Psychogalvanic skin response. See
   Electrodermal response
Psychophysical law, 7
Pteronotus parnelli, 187, 267
Pteropus giganteus, 193
p-type material, 54
Public Health Act 1936, 134
Public health legislation, 134
Pulmonary afferent systems, 558
   influencing laryngeal muscle activity,
      555

Pulmonary function studies, 581, 930
Pulmonary mechanoreceptors, stretch-sensitive, 555
Punched card, 33
Pyramidal ridge, 216
Purkinje cells, 385
Push-pull input, 79
Pythagoras theorem, 64, 68

Quantum, 707
Quartz, 105
Quinine, 849, 855

Rabbit fetuses, 206
Rad, 735
Radial flow theory, 297
Radiation, 699
    distribution in tissues, 734
    dose unit, 735
    dose rate, 739
    dose-time fractionation relationships, 737
    effects on normal tissues, 740
    effects on solid tumour, 742
    fractionation, 738
    ionizing, diagnostic, 706
    multidose fractionation, 739
    repair of injury, 737
    stenosis, 927
    tolerance, 741
Radioactive labelled elements, 297
Radiography, 212, 223, 226, 710
    abnormal anatomy of the ear, 232
    body section, 227
    contrast, 228, 711
    views, 223
Radiological instruments, 720
Radiology, 586
Radionuclide activity, measurement of, 710
Radionuclides, 706
Radiosensitivity, 735, 748
Radiosialography, 708
Radiotelemetry, 401
Radiotherapy, 658, 733–49
    and cytotoxic drugs, 748
    and surgery, 744
    clinical, 742
    external beam, 739
    fast neutron, 747
    fractionated, 743
    future developments in, 745
    high pressure oxygen, 745
    interstitial, 839
    palliative, 744
    post-operative, 745
    pre-operative, 744
    prophylactic, 744
    radical, 742, 744
    supervoltage, 735
    therapeutic ratio of, 742
    total dose in, 737
Radium needle implant, 739
Radium sources, 739
Ramsay Hunt syndrome, 434

Rana pipens, 177
Rana sylvatica, 180
Range, 13
Rat, 469, 477
Rate-intensity functions, 319
Rathke's pouch, 421, 425
Rational number, 3
Reactance, 61
Rebound effect of nose drops, 522
Rebound nystagmus, 850
Reconstructive surgery, 864
Record linkage, 136
Records, 941
Recovery potentials, 442
Recruitment of loudness, 792–95
Rectifier, 73
Recurrent laryngeal nerve, 530
Reference coupler, 781
Reference Equivalent Threshold Sound Pressure Level (RETSPL), 780
Reflex responses, 335
Reflexes, middle ear, muscle measurements, 287
Refraction, 719
Regeneration, 440, 714
Registration, 136
Regression equation, 21
Regulations, 935, 936
Reichert-Gaupp theory, 192
Reichert's cartilage, 217
Re-innervation, defects of, 441
Relative humidity, 118
Relative likelihood model, 25
Reliability, 17
Remote masking, 348
Renal insufficiency, 861
Renal status and ototoxicity, 859
Renshaw cell system, 549
Repair, 714
Reserpine, 863
Resistance, 67, 642
Resonance, 64, 92
Resonance curves, 245
Resonance frequency, 64
Respiration, 554, 600
Respiratory activity, 556
Respiratory function tests, 581
Respiratory syncytial virus, 635
Response decline, 394–97
Response pattern of single unit, 323
Reticular lamina, 291
Retinitis pigmentosa, 124
Retrocochlear lesion, 797
Rets (rad equivalent therapy) 738
Revascularized pedicled flaps, 923
Reverberant field, 93
Reynold's criterion, 770
Rhabdomyosarcomas, 209, 458, 679
Rhesus system, 755
Rhinitis, 499
Rhinitis atrophicans, 527
Rhinitis caseosa-pseudo-cholesteatoma, 674
Rhinocerebral mucormycosis, 652
Rhinocerebral phycomycosis, 652
Rhinoentomophthoromycosis, 652–54

Rhinolophus ferrumequinum, 187, 196
Rhinomanometry, 520
Rhinophycomycosis. See Rhinoentomo-phthoromycosis
Rhinoplasty, 882–94
    age in, 890
    complications, 887
    post-operative problems, 888
    results of, 893
    selection and preparation of patients, 891
    surgical techniques, 882
Rhinoscleroma, 651
Rhinosporidiosis, 652, 655, 656
Rhinosporidium seeberi, 652
Rhinotoxic drugs, 862–63
Rhinovirus, 510
Rhizopus, 652
Rhythm indicator, 837
Rhythm perception, 359
Ribonuclease, 713
Ribonucleic acid. See RNA
Ringertz tumour, 676
Rinne response, 13, 18
RNA, 181, 182, 625, 728, 729
RNA polymerase, 728
RNA tumour viruses, 634
RNA viruses, 133, 634
Rochelle salt, 105
Roentgen, 711
Rotatory tests, 393
Rousettus aegyptiacus, 260
Rouvière's diagram, 668–69
Rubber stent, 903
Rubbers, 714
Rubella, 124, 128
Rubella virus, 636
Rudolph's sign, 481
Rules, 936
Russell bodies, 926

'S' indicator, 837
Saccade, 383
Saccadic eye movement, 384
Saccadic system, 383
Saccular dc potential, 300
Saccular macula, 362
Saccular membranes, 300
Saccule, 300
Saccus endolymphaticus, 363
Saddle deformity of nose, 885
Saguinus, 188
Saimiri sciureus, 188, 199
Salicylates, 367, 849, 855
Salivary apparatus, 460–67
Salivary flow, 440
Salivary glands, 460, 461, 741
    diagnosis of disorders of, 465
    examination of, 463
    radiographic examination of, 464
    scanning, 708
    secretory rate of, 464
    tumours, 145, 709
Salivary secretion under normal and pathological conditions, 463
Salivary tissue, 540

Salpingopharyngeus muscle, 253
Salt, 7
Sampling distribution, 28
Sarcoidosis, 673
Sarcoptes scabei, 665
Scabbard trachea, 928
Scala media, 300
Scala media perfusion, 296
Scala tympani, 301
Scala vestibuli, perfusion of, 294
Scales, 1, 3
Scanning electronmicroscopy, 223
Scarlet fever, 145
Scattergraph, 10
Schirmer's test, 440
Schuster bridge, 282
Schwann cells, 206, 682
Schwannoma, 682
Schwannoma of VIIIth nerve, *see* vestibulocochlear nerve schwannoma
Scintillation counter, 710
Scleroma, 926
Screening, 134
Screw worm fly, *see Chrysomia bezziana*
Seasonal variation, 138
Secobarbital, 342
Secretion, 519
Secretory otitis media, 12, 457, 718
Sedation, 331
Segregation, 121
Semicircular canals, 211, 299, 376, 386
Semicircular ducts, 376
Semiconductor diode, 75
Semiconductors, 53
Semon's Law, 547
Sense organs, 221, 371
    vestibular, 221
Sensitivity, 17
Sensitivity test, 135
Sensorineural acuity level (SAL), 791
Sensory cells, 178
    polarization of, 375
Sensory hairs, 249
Septal haematoma, 884
Septoplasty, 883
Septum, 882
Sequential trials, 29
Serological test, 633
Seromucinous glands, 252, 674
Sex distribution, 11
Shear modulus, 716
Shear waves, properties of, 249
Sheet implants, 875
Short increment sensitivity index (SISI), 354 778, 794
Short-term memory, 326
Shunts, 66
SI units, 4–6, 947–49
Sialectasis, 466
Sialography, 464
Sialometry, 464
Sickle-cell anaemia, 122
Sigmodon, 188
Sigmodon hispida, 189, 258

Sigmoid sinus, 214
Sigmoid sinus thrombosis, 522
Signal analysis, 250
Signal detectability, theory of, 345
Signal extraction methods, 342
Signal monitoring, audiometers, 775
Silica, 510
    particles, 508
Silicon, 75
Silicone rubber, 714, 764, 876, 885, 922
Silicosis, 507
Similarity coefficient, 25
Simple harmonic motion, 89
Simultaneous midplane lateralization, 359
Sinodural angle of Citelli, 214
Sinoscopy, 719
Sinusitis, epidemiology, 143
Sinusoid, 138
Sjögren's syndrome, 466
Skew deviation, 385
Skewness, 14, 15
Small biopsy, 667
Smell
    abnormalities of, 499
    disorders, 708
    tests of, 498
    theories of, 497
Smoothing, 73
Snell's Law, 719
Snoring, 490
Snuff, 143, 863
Social Medicine, 134
Soddy-Fajans radioactive displacement law, 708
Sodium carboxymethylcellulose, 718
Sodium cyanide, 208
Sodium pertechnetate, 708
Sodium potassium tartrate, 105
Soft palate, 484, 490
Solid angle, 214
Sonagram, 524
Sonagraphy, 582
Sone scale, 348
Sono-ocular test, 400
Sound, 87
Sound, 87, 237
    absorption, 96
    compactness of, 348
    speed of, 88
South American blastomycosis, 650
Sound amplifiers, 830, 831
Sound-conducting mechanism, 872
Sound insulation, 95
Sound lateralization, 323
Sound level, A-weighted, 96
Sound level meter, 154
Sound power level, 98
Sound pressure, 96
    tympanic membrane, 238
Sound pressure level, 96, 97, 779, 796, 809, 813
Sound reduction index, 98
Sound reflection, 281
Sound sources, 94
    localization of, 323

Sound spectrography, 582
Sound transmission, 94, 281, 870
Speaking tubes, 806
Spearman's rank order or rank-difference, correlation coefficient, 18
Specific heat, 114
Specific resistance, 643
Specificity test, 135
Spectrum, 99
    frequency, 151
    vocal, 583
Spectrum level, 99
Speculae, 718
Speech, 250, 275, 523, 599
    acoustic analysis of, 490
    acquisition of, 840
    compressed, 842
    conversational, 153
    low sensation level, 256
    masked, 356
    noise components in, 607
    palatal function, 487, 490
    perception of, 355
    periodically interrupted, 357
    source function, 604
    synthetic, 842
    system function, 604
    time compressed, 356
Speech audiogram, 11, 23
Speech discrimination, 310, 353, 356
Speech disorders, epidemiology, 148
Speech hearing level, 20
Speech intelligibility, 245
Speech material, tests using, 355
Speech mechanism as acoustic system, 604
Speech Reception Threshold (SRT), 796
Speech tests, 796
    binaural, 357
    low-redundancy, 355
    monaural, 356
Spheno-ethmoidal recess, 514
Spheno-palatine artery, 515
Spheno-palatine foramen, 515
Spindle cell carcinoma, 696
Spiral canal, 221
Spiral ganglion, 221, 313
Spiral ligament, 199, 296
Spiral limbus, interdental cells of, 205
Spiral nerve endings, 553
Spiral organ, 204, 221, 245, 247, 293, 303, 308, 313, 337
Spiral vessel, 301
Spirillum, 638
Spirochaete, 638
Splendore-Hoeppli phenomenon, 652
Spondaic word lists, 353
Sporangium, 655
Sporotrichosis, 657
Sporothrix schenckii, 657
Squamotympanic suture, 214
Squamous carcinoma
    differentiation of, 694
    growth patterns of, 694
    histogenesis of, 693

Squamous carcinoma (*contd.*)
  histological effects of treatment on, 698
  nasal part of pharynx, 693
  non-surgical therapy of, 699
  upper respiratory tract, 692–700
  with infiltrating and pushing margins, 694
Squamous differentiation after treatment by irradiation and cytotoxic drugs, 699
Squamous papillomas, 691
Squint, 385
Squirrel monkey platform runway test, 361
Squirrel monkey rail test, 361
Stachybotryotoxicosis, 658
Stachybotrys alternans, 658
Stack, 211
Stackburn disease, 659
Staggered spondaic tests, 357
Stainless steels, 714, 922
Stammering, 563
Standard deviation, 13, 14
Standard error, 28
Standing wave, 93
Standards, 935, 936
Stapedectomy, 18, 212, 234, 850, 873, 877, 880, 939
Stapedial acoustic reflex, 264
Stapedial artery, comparative anatomy, 191
Stapedial tenotomy, 26
Stapedius, 263
Stapedius muscle, 218, 257, 272, 276–79,
Stapedius reflex, 437
Stapes, ankylosis of, 211
Stapes fixation, 792
Stapes mobilization, 212
Stapes piston implant, 874
Stapes prostheses, 880
Stapes replacement studies, 870
Statistically significant, 25
Statistics, 9–31
Statoconia, 207
Statutory Instrument, 935
Steady-state events, 250
Steel-Richardson-Olszewski syndrome, 401
Steels, 714
Stent, 718
Stenvers' views, 454
Stereocilia, 374
Sternocleidomastoid muscle, 530
Sternohyoid, 548
Sternothyroid muscles, 548, 650, 565
Steroid therapy, 450
Stiffness reactance, 281
Stiffness tilt audiogram, 796
Stimulus click, 307
Stimulus response curve, 321
Stimulus response theory, 609
Stomach, transposed, 903
Stomal stenosis, prevention of, 929
Stomodeum, 421
Stop consonants, 607

Strabismus, 385
Strain, 715
Strenght-duration measurements, 442
Streptococcus pyogenes, 145
Streptomyces antibiotics, 850, 859
Streptomyces verticillus, 698, 729
Streptomycin, 207, 232, 365, 704, 849, 851, 852, 859
Streptomycin-induced hearing loss, 342
Stress-strain curve, 715
Stria vascularis, 199, 291, 292, 294, 296, 299, 853, 858
Strial capillaries, 296
Strial function, 296
Strial intercellular spaces, 295
Strial marginal cell, 296
Striate (visuosensory) cortex, 385
Striola, 207
Stroboscopes, 720
Stroboscopic examination, 575
Stroboscopic laminagraph, 587
Stromal cells, atypical, 670
Strontium-90, 29
Struts, 716
Student's *t*, 28
Stycar tests, 778
Styloid ridge, 216
Stylomastoid foramen, 214, 226, 430
Stylopharyngeus, 565
Subcutaneous phycomycosis, 652
Subepithelial cells of Langhans, 554
Suberosis, 659
Subglottic mucosa, 551
Subglottic pressure, 579
Subglottic space, 518
Subglottic stenosis, 904
  congenital, 924
Submandibular gland, 460, 674
  extirpation, 467
Submandibular salivation, 450
Submaxillary gland, 460
Submucous resection, 882
Substernal thyroid enlargements, 928
Succinylcholine. *See* Suxamethonium
Sudomotor reflex, 335
Sulcus terminalis, 428
Sulphonamides, 212
Sulphur dioxide, 508
Sulphur granules, 658
Summating potential, 303
Superior sac, 216
Supplementary motor area, 549
Suprabulbar palsy, 549
Supraglottic mucosa, 550
Supraglottis resection, 907, 909
Supraglottic stenosis, chronic traumatic, 905
Suprahyoid muscles, 566
Supramastoid crest, 214
Supranuclear ophthalmoplegias, 401
Suprapyramidal recess, 216
Supra-strial capillaries, 852
Surface specimen technique, 222
Surgery and radiotherapy, 744
Surgical implants, 712, 762–66, 865, 866
  carcinogenicity, 762

Surgical implants (*contd.*)
  cochlear, 212, 763
  general aspects, 762
  ideal material, 762
  metal, 763
  plastics, 762
  sterilization, 762
Surgical morcellizer, 883
Surinam, 655
Sutures, 717
Suxamethonium chloride, 896
Swallowing, 486, 554, 558, 560, 561
  action of, 592
  closure of larynx during, 593
  normal mechanism of, 592
  see also Deglutition
SWAMI test, 357
Swinging speech tests, 357
Sydenham's chorea, 550
Symbols, 5
Synchronstroboscope, 575
Syndromes, 133
Synotia dorsalis, 178
Syphilis, 926
Système International, 947

Tactile vibrators, 838
Tadarida, 276
Tadarida brasiliensis, 267
Tadarida thersites, 191
Taenia solium, 664
Talbot's law, 575
Talpa, 190
Tangier disease, 688
Tantalum gauze, 922
Tape recorders, 155
Tapeworms, 664
Taphozous, 191
Tastant-receptor interactions, 475
Taste, 439, 468–83
  abnormalities in man, 479
  central brain terminals which subserve, 477
  integrative mechanisms, 477
  laboratory techniques, 481
  measurement techniques and nomenclature, 477
  neural depolarization and transmission, 477
  neural transmission of the generator potential, 476
  pathological processes affecting, 478–82
  stimulus-receptor binding mechanisms, 475
  thresholds for, 144
  transduction of binding energy to form generator potential, 476
Taste acuity, 478
Taste blindness, 468
Taste buds, 469
  cells, 471
  characteristics, 471
  function of, 471
  receptor characteristics, 475

Taste detection threshold, 477
Taste disorders, 708
Taste recognition threshold, 477
Taste stimulus characteristics, 468
Taste support systems, 469
Taste testing, 439
Tatera, 187
Tatera indica, 197
Taxonometry, 25
Technetium-99m, 440, 708
Tectal nuclei, 550
Tectorial membrane, 204, 245–47, 299
Teeth, 425
epidemiology, 145
Telecanthus, 125
Teleprinter, 32
Teletype, 32
Temperature, 112
units, 5
Temporal bone, 214
dissection of, 213
fractures of, 233, 454
fracture of petrous part of, 231
holder, 213
Temporal coding, 316
Temporal fascia, 214
Temporal integration function, 358
Temporal line, 214
Temporal lobe lesions, 353, 354, 357, 358, 359, 353
Temporal order perception, 358
Temporal patterns of single neurons, 320
Temporalis fascia grafts, 867–69
Temporary immunological inertia, 712
Temporary threshold shift, 46, 349, 795
Tensile creep modulus, 717
Tensile force, 715
Tensile strain, 715
Tensile stress, 715
Tensor tympani muscle, 211, 253, 258, 263, 268, 272, 276, 278, 279
Tensor tympani response, 287
Tensor veli palatini muscle, 253
Tent-pole deformity, 890
Test, 2×2 probability, 28
Tests of significance, 25
Tetracosactide, 722
Tetracyclines, 703, 857
labelling techniques, 871
Tetrahydrofolic acid, 728
Tetrodotoxin, 294
Tetrylammonium bromide, 294
Thai adults, 15
Thalamic nuclei, 325
Therapeutic doses, 5
Therapeutic misrepresentation, 940
Therapeutic procedures, economics and efficiency of, 722
Therapeutic trials, 26, 722
Thermal capacity, 115
Thermal conductivity, 115
Thermal instruments, 720
Thermal radiation, 116
Thermionic emission, 72
Thermocouple, 113

Thermodynamics, second law of, 503
Thermoelectric psychrometer, 518
Thermography, 116
Thermometers, 112
Thévenin, theorem of, 82
Thiazinanium, 863
Thiotepa, 727
Thiouracil, 148
Thonzylamine, 27
Threshold of overload, 351
Threshold differences in man and animals, 269
Throat, 528
epidemiology, 145
Thrush, 648
Thymidylic acid, 728
Thyroarytenoid muscle, 530, 557
Thyro-epiglottic joints, 552
Thyrohyoid, 548
Thyrohyoid joints, 552
Thyrohyoid muscle, 560, 565
Thyrohyoid release, 931
Thyroid cartilages, 538, 565
Thyroid disorders, 709
Thyroid function, 25, 709
Thyroid gland, epidemiology, 147
Thyroid hormones in bloodstream, 709
Thyroid tracheal obstruction, 925
Thyroidectomy, 939
Thyropharyngeus muscle, 560, 565
Ticks, 665
Time base, 67
Time constant, 70
Time difference, 351
Time domain averaging, 40, 47
Time locking, 322, 323
Time series, 10
Time varying events, 250
Tinnitus, 142, 232, 402, 664, 849
Tissue cages, 704
Tissue-culture experiments, 868
Tissue reactions, 717
Tissue-typing, 713
TNM classification, 3
Tobramycin, 368, 849
Tomography, 212, 226, 710
computerized, 229
hypocycloidal, 228, 233
Tonal density, 348
Tonal volume, 348
Tone pitch, threshold, 350
Tones, 94
Tongue, 427, 469, 591
cancer of, 145
Tonotopic organization, 325
Tonsillectomy, 749, 940
Tonsillitis, 127, 635
Tonsils
enlarged, 687
histopathology, 687–
Topical aural preparation, 850, 856
Torsion, 716
Torsion swing, 380, 4
Torts, law of, 936
Torulosis. *See Crypto*

Toxic effects, 722
Toxicology, 848
Toxocara canis, 663
Toxocara cati, 663
Toxoplasmosis, 662
Trabeculae, 190
Trabeculation, 217
Tracers, 134, 708
Trachea, 504
anatomy, 919
blood supply, 920
cervical, reconstruction of, 904
embryology, 923
intrathoracic mobilization, 932
mucosal lining, 920
physiology, 919
reconstruction, 906
sleeve resection and end-to-end anastomosis, 931
vascular compression, 925
Tracheal agenesis, 924
Tracheal allografts, 922
Tracheal prostheses, 922
Tracheal reconstruction, future of, 923
Tracheal stenosis, 919–33
chemical, 927
developmental, 923
early attempts to treat complete circumferential, 921
etiology, 923
incidence of, 923
inflammatory, 925
pathogenesis, 923
traumatic, 928
Tracheal stenotic defects, anastomosis of circumferential, 922
Tracheal wound repair, biology of, 922
Tracheobronchial tree, 897
Tracheoesophageal shunt, 900
Tracheograms, 930
Tracheomalacia, congenital, 924
Tracheopathia osteoplastica, 927
Tracheostomal stenosis, 928, 929
Tracheostomy, 556, 558, 766,
dead space, 766
effects of making, 766
purposes of, 767
Tracheostomy tubes, 556, 718, 766–72
Alder Hey, 769
design, 767
Durham's, 767
Durham's, 767, 770
Edinburgh, 767
Fuller's, 767
lobster-tail, 768
Morrant Baker, 768
Negus, 768–69
plastic, 770–71
shape and bore, 770
ler, 770
oretical ideal design, 770
Wilson, 769
Tracheotomy, 921, 926
Trait, 122
Transcendental number, 3

Transducers, 101
  electrodynamic, 105
  magnetic, moving iron, 107
  piezo-electric, 105
  ribbon, 107
Transduction 639, 641
Transfer characteristic, 73
Transfer function, 71
Transformation, 630, 640
Transformation constant, 707
Transformer, 61
  impedance-matching, 237
Transhyoid pharyngotomy, 903
Transients, 312
Transistor, 75, 77
Transitional cell carcinoma, 697
Transitional cell papilloma, 676
Transmembrane potential, 6
Transmission coefficient, 98
Transmission loss, 98
Transplant ossicle, 872
Transplants, 177, 712
  law relation to, 941
Transposing equipment, 837
Transtympanic electrode, 336
Transudation, 518
Transverse crest, 228
Trautmann's triangle, 214
Travelling-wave concept (Békésy), 244
Travelling-wave patterns, 245, 247
Travelling-wave properties, 248
Travelling-wave theory, 308
Treacher Collins syndrome, 125
Trespass to person, 939
Trichloroacetic acid, 8
Trichosurus, 193
Trigeminal nerve, 214,
Triode, 73
Triphenylphosphate, 506
Triple-S triangle, 218
Trisomy, 127
Tritiated thymidine, 731
Tritium, 365, 708
Trochleariform process, 234
Trophocytes, 653, 655
Tuberculoid granulomas, 673
Tuberculosis, 510, 926
Tullio phenomenon, 400
Tumour blush, 230
Tumour grading, Broder's method of, 694
Tumour growth
  Gompertzian, 731
  kinetic law of, 7
Tumour kinetics, 730
Tumour size, 743
Tumours inside internal acoustic meatus, 310
Tuning curves, 245, 314–16, 322, 326
  double-peaked, 322
Tuning fork tests, 788
Tunnel of Corti, 221
Turbulence, 502
Turbulent flow, 70
Turner's syndrome, 127
Two-tone-inhibition, 318, 319

Tympanic bone, 214
Tympanic cavity, 211, 214
Tympanic membrane, 211, 214, 238, 250, 251, 281, 285, 307, 336
  chalk patches in, 231
  cochlear microphonic from, 304
  comparative anatomy, 187
  displacement profiles of, 239
  perforation, 8, 138, 286
  replacement, 866
Tympanic mucosa, 230
Tympanic muscle contractions, 276
Tympanic sinus, 216, 218
Tympanogram, 285
Tympanomastoid suture, 214
Tympanometry, 285
Tympano-ossicular allografts, 874
Tympano-ossicular auditory implants, 820
Tympano-ossicular mechanism, 286
Tympanoplasty, 3, 26, 233, 234, 718, 850, 870
  experimental, 873
  silicone rubber insert, 872
Tympanosclerosis, 217, 231
Tympanostomy tube, 11, 718

Ultimate tensile strength, 716
Ultimobranchial body, 529
Ultra-high speed cinematography, 577
Ultrasonic irradiation, 364
Ultrasonic treatment of Ménière's disease, 456
Ultrasound, 364
Unilateral vocal paralysis, 587
Units, 4, 947–49
  conversion table, 949
Unsharpness, 711
Upper respiratory tract, squamous carcinoma, 692–700
Urethane, 729
Usher's syndrome, 124
Utricle, 373
Utricular dc potential, 300
Utricular endolymph, 299
Utricular nerve section, 362

V-51R ear protectors, 159
Vaccination, 644
Vaccinia gangrenosa, 637
Vacuum tubes, 72
Validity, 17
Valsalva manoeuvre, 393, 593
Valve, 72
Vancomycin, 849
Vapour, saturated, 117
Variable, 9
Variance, 13, 1
Variate, 9
Varicella-zoster infection, 453
Vascular stria, 205
Vasculitis,
Vasoconstriction, 862

Vasomotor conditions, 721
Vasomotor rhinitis, 516, 520
Vectornystagmography, 401
Vectors, 64, 67
Vein grafts, 868
Velolingual closure, 485
Velopharyngeal closure, 487
Velopharyngeal competence, 491
Velopharyngeal muscles, 485
Velopharyngeal port, 487
Ventilating tube. See Tympanostomy tube
Ventilograph, 581
Verbotonal procedure, 842
Vergence, 385
Verrucous mycosis, 657
Verrucous squamous carcinoma, 695
Vertebral artery function, 721
Vertebro-basilar insufficiency, 359
Vertex potential, 330, 337, 342
Vertiginous disorder, 25
Vertigo, 142, 302, 364, 454, 650, 663, 664
Vestibular apparatus, neuroepithelium of, 296
Vestibular disorders, 45
Vestibular end organs, 362
Vestibular endolymph, electrochemical constitution, 299
Vestibular folds, 560, 566
Vestibular function, 383, 402
Vestibular ganglion, 8
Vestibular labryinth, 199, 299
Vestibular membrane, 205, 246, 293, 297
  cells of, 296
  rupture of, 296
Vestibular nerve cells, 221
Vestibular neurones, 207
Vestibular nystagmus, induced, 390
Vestibular otoxicity, 364
Vestibular physiology, 371–82
Vestibular sense organs, 221
Vestibular system, 852
  experimental pathophysiology, 361–71
Vestibular trauma experiments, 369
Vestibulocochlear nerve, 221, 303, 341
  tuning curves of single fibres, 314
Vestibulocochlear nerve compound action potential, 303, 306, 307
Vestibulocochlear nerve tumours, 209, 217, 233, 438,
Vestibulocochlear schwannomas, 230, 393
Vestibulo-oculomotor investigation, 383
Vibration
  isolation, 158
  nuisance, 937
Vigilance, 331
Vinblastine, 480, 730
Vinca alkaloids, 729
Vincristine, 480, 730
Viomycin, 366, 849
Virion, 625
Virology, 625–37
Virus diseases
  diagnosis of, 631

Virus diseases (*contd.*)
   pathogenesis of, 634
   prevention of, 636
   treatment of, 636
Virus infection, resistance to, 635
Virus vaccine, 636
Viruses
   classification of, 626
   definition, 625
   growing in laboratory, 630
   identification of, 629
   infection with, 628
   isolated from middle ear cavity, 635
   persistent, 634
   structure of, 628
Visco-elastic material, 717
Visual devices, 837
Visual display units, 33
Visual area, subjective magnitude of, 23
Vital capacity, 581
Vocal folds, 530, 540, 600, 693, 720
   abductor, 894
   carcinoma of, 587, 694
   functions, 912
   mathematical model of, 588–89
   motion, 913
   movements of, 574
   myo-elastic properties of, 561
   paralyzed, 764
   spindle cell carcinoma, 696
   tumour on, 937
   vibration, 601, 602
   vibratory pattern of, 574
Vocal fry, 601

Vocal function, 581
Vocal ligament, 531
Vocal nodule, 586
Vocal processes, 531, 537
Vocal tract, 45, 603
   acoustical resonating system, 604
   synthesizer, 589
Vocal velocity index, 581
Vocalis muscle, 588
Voice, 599
   acoustical evaluation of, 582
   frequencies, 601
   quality, 582
Voice print, 583
Volt, 67
von Recklinghausen's disease, 682, 692
von Tröltsch, 211
Vowels, 582
   nasalization of, 524
V-potential. *See* Vertex-potential

Waardenburg's syndrome, 124
Wagner-Grossman theory, 895
Wall absorbers, 97
Waldeyer's ring, 688
Wallerian degeneration, 440
Warble flies, 665
Washed erythrocytes, 752
Waveforms, 250
   of mechanical vibration, 308
Wavelength, 90
Wax, epidemiology, 137
Weber, 67

Weber test, 18, 790
Weber-Fechner Law, 7, 345
Wechsler Intelligence Scale for Children, 618
Wegener's granuloma, 670
Weightlessness, 371
Wever and Bray phenomenon, 334
Whistling, 490
Wildervanck's syndrome, 128
Wohlfahrtia magnifica, 665
Word lists, 796

X chromosome, 123
Xenografts, 712, 713, 865, 866, 869, 870
Xenon-133, 708
Xerostomia, 464, 465
X-ray films, 711, 941
X-rays, 733, 737
   attenuation of, 7, 710
   exposure to, 711
   radiodiagnostic properties, 710

Y chromosome, 123
Yeasts, 646
Yield point, 716
Young's modulus, 716

Zinc metabolism, 481
Zonograms, 227, 233
Zonography, 227–28, 710
Zonulae occludentes, 294, 299
Zwislocki's acoustic impedance bridge, 283